Fundamentals of Nursing

CONCEPTS, PROCESS, AND PRACTICE

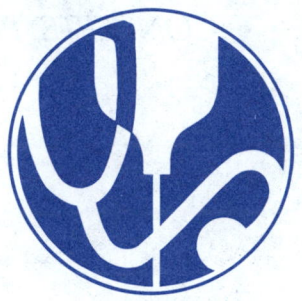

Fundamentals of Nursing

CONCEPTS, PROCESS, AND PRACTICE

PATRICIA A. POTTER, RN, MSN

Clinical Director of Surgical Nursing,
Nursing Service, Barnes Hospital,
St. Louis, Missouri

ANNE G. PERRY, RN, MSN, ANP

Associate Professor,
St. Louis University School of Nursing,
St. Louis, Missouri

with 767 illustrations including 16 in color

The C. V. Mosby Company

ST. LOUIS • TORONTO • PRINCETON   1985

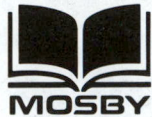

MOSBY

A TRADITION OF PUBLISHING EXCELLENCE

Editor: Alison Miller
Assistant editor: Bess Arends
Developmental editor: Thomas Lochhaas
Design: Suzanne Oberholtzer
Production: Jeanne Genz, Judith Bamert, Mary Stueck

Printed in the United States of America

The C.V. Mosby Company
11830 Westline Industrial Drive, St. Louis, Missouri 63146

Library of Congress Cataloging in Publication Data

Potter, Patricia Ann.
  Fundamentals of nursing.

  Includes bibliographies and index.
  1. Nursing.   2. Nursing—Examinations, questions, etc.
3. Nursing—Study and teaching—Audio-visual aids.
4. Nurse and patient.   I. Perry, Anne Griffin.
II. Title.   [DNLM: 1. Nurse-Patient Relations.
2. Nursing Care.   3. Nursing Process.   WY 100 P868f]
RT42.P68   1985   610.73   84-25479
ISBN 0-8016-3828-3

C/VH/VH   9 8 7 6 5 4 3 2 1   01/D/032

Contributors

Bobbie Bloch, *RN, MSN*

School of Nursing
University of Michigan
Ann Arbor, Michigan

Lois Bodinski, *RN, MEd*

Professor and Department Chairman
Community College of Rhode Island
Lincoln, Rhode Island

Debra C. Broadwell, *RN, MN, ET, PhD*

Associate Professor
Emory University
Nell Woodruff School of Nursing
Atlanta, Georgia

Nancy Dickenson-Hazard, *RN, PNP, MSN*

Executive Director
National Board of Pediatric Nurse Practitioners
    and Associates
Rockville, Maryland

Gordon L. Dickman, *MA*

Sex Counselor and Educator
Co-Director, Seattle Sexual Health Center
Seattle, Washington

Catherine Fogertey Doerrer, *RN, MSN*

Director, Surgical Nursing
Barnes Hospital
St. Louis, Missouri

Mary Ann English, *RN, MSN*

Associate Professor
Department of Nursing
Pennsylvania State University
New Kensington, Pennsylvania

Virginia M. Fitzsimmons, *RN, CEdD*

ANA Certified Gerontological Nurse
Assistant Professor, College of Nursing
Keane College of New Jersey
Union, New Jersey

Cheryl Hall Harris, *RN, BSN*

Lecturer in Medicine
University of Missouri at Kansas City Medical Center
Kansas City, Missouri

Gail Kieckhefer, *RN, MSN*

Doctoral Candidate
Children's Orthopedic Hospital
University of Washington
Seattle, Washington

Sr. Kathleen Krekeler, RN, PhD

Associate Professor
St. Louis University
School of Nursing
St. Louis, Missouri

Carolyn A. Livingston, RN, AA, SECT, PhD

Certified Sex Therapist
Seattle Sexual Health Center
Seattle, Washington

Sharon Merritt, EdD, RN

Associate Professor
Graduate Program in Nursing
Southern Illinois University—Edwardsville
Edwardsville, Illinois

Modesta S. Orque, RN, EdD

Director of Public Health Nursing
Public Health Department
Fresno County
Fresno, California

Consultant Board

To Grace Louis Potter

a loving mother whose belief in the value of hard work and commitment to purpose has been a gift of priceless value

To William Noble Potter

a caring father who gives his love unselfishly

To Florence Bowmaster Griffin

for her love and her belief that learning continues throughout one's life and the knowledge acquired should be shared with others

To Mike, Rebecca, and Chip Perry

for their love, good humor, support, and encouragement

Preface

As society changes, so too do the art and science of professional nursing practice. In response to new consumer needs and demands, health care services are increasingly moving into the home and into community and alternative care settings. As a consequence of this, and of changes within the profession, the nurse's roles and responsibilities are expanding to meet new challenges and expectations. More than ever before, the nurse today must be able to apply a broad knowledge base in providing proficient and skillful care to individual clients, families, and communities. The development of nursing theories, the growing body of nursing research, and the continued expansion of knowledge in the physical, social, and behavioral sciences have combined by provide nurses with the fundamental tools to promote, maintain, and restore a client's well-being. Knowledge alone, however, is insufficient. If nurses are to provide quality care, they must also be sensitive to clients' needs as unique individuals and committed to achieving standards of excellence in nursing practice. This awareness leads to a nursing perspective that is truly holistic.

Fundamentals of Nursing: Concepts, Process, and Practice is a basic textbook designed for beginning students in professional nursing programs. Comprehensive in scope and complete in its coverage, this text will not only introduce students to the basic concepts, process, skills, and techniques of nursing practice, but also provide them with a firm foundation for more advanced areas of nursing study. Empha-sizing cognitive, interpersonal, and psychomotor skills, the text presents the theoretical and practical knowledge needed to make sound clinical judgments and carry out fundamental nursing activities.

APPROACH

All units and chapters of the text have been designed to meet the specific needs of the learner. Learning objectives at the beginning of each chapter help students focus on the relevant issues in subject matter. A glossary of the terms that will be introduced in each chapter is presented next to familiarize students with the terms and basic concepts they will encounter in the detailed text discussion. Special attention has been paid to the reading level and clear presentation of material. In all chapters the subject is approached in a logical, building-block fashion. Realistic clinical examples are offered throughout to illustrate clearly the application of theoretical concepts in clinical practice. To help students recognize and understand key issues and principles, tables, boxed material, and step-by-step procedural guides present information graphically, logically, and succinctly. Over 700 illustrations and photographs highlight the major concepts and procedures to supplement discussion with accurate and meaningful visual aids. Each chapter closes with a brief summary followed by a list of key concepts that emphasize the most important nursing principles presented in the chapter. The references and suggested readings for each chapter can be used as guides for students who desire to explore further the information in the nursing and applied sciences literature.

Although the emphasis of the text is on the clinical aspects of nursing care, we fully recognize that technical expertise alone will not prepare today's nurses to deliver care creatively and effectively. Fundamental concepts such as the health-illness continuum, basic human needs, self-awareness, the nurse-client relationship, and client teaching are therefore discussed in depth in individual chapters and referred to throughout the text. This approach helps students begin to incorporate nursing theory in clinical practice situations. For example, an entire unit is devoted to the principles of growth and development and the appropriate health care concerns of each developmental stage, but other chapters discuss developmental health care needs of clients throughout the life span along with appropriate nursing interventions.

The five-step nursing process serves as a framework in chapters discussing the physiological, psychosocial, and special needs of clients. Students learn to assess a broad range of factors related to the nature and extent of clients' health status and to cluster assessment data in order to identify actual or potential health problems. Nursing diagnoses, both those approved at the National Conferences for the Classification of Nursing Diagnoses and some new diagnoses not yet approved, are explored in these chapters. The value of nursing diagnoses for planning the direction and scope of nursing care is considered. Within the planning phase students learn to establish goals of care, to set priorities for different aspects of care, and to integrate nursing activities within a care plan. In the implementation step nursing interventions are discussed along with scientific rationales and practical considerations for making nursing therapies more effective. Current nursing research findings help broaden the student's understanding of independent nursing functions. The ongoing evaluation of nursing care is discussed in terms of specific outcome criteria reflecting the long- and short-term goals of care.

The approach used throughout the text reflects the major premise that students must understand and master the performance of basic clinical skills. Skills and procedures are discussed in depth in the relevant chapters and presented in tabular form. The step-by-step, two-column format for each procedure provides the appropriate nursing action and the rationale for the action. The procedures incorporate current scientific principles and research results to help students understand the reason for specific nursing interventions. Text discussions elaborate on the objectives and purposes of the procedures and relate the nursing

actions to meaningful client assessments. In addition, the procedures include opportunities for heightened nurse-client interactions and integrate client teaching activities with the performance of skills.

ORGANIZATION

The text is comprised of 11 units organized to enhance teaching strategies. Unit 1 introduces the student to the profession of nursing by presenting a historical overview of nursing practice. Current nursing theories are then discussed to help the student understand the health care consumer, the range of health care needs, and different approaches to health care. The health-illness continuum, basic human needs, homeostasis, and stress and adaptation are considered as a foundation for clinical application of theory.

Unit 2 discusses the use of the nursing process as a whole and considers each component in detail. The unit introduces the skills needed to assess the client's health status through the nursing history and physical assessment, to cluster and analyze data in order to formulate nursing diagnoses, to organize and write the nursing care plan, to select and implement appropriate nursing interventions, and to evaluate the care plan on an ongoing basis. The unit concludes with a chapter on recording and reporting techniques and the methods for accurate and complete documentation and communication of nursing care.

The nurse learns to apply certain basic concepts of professional nursing practice in all encounters with clients. Unit 3 offers a comprehensive review of values, ethics, legal issues, and principles of communication and teaching. In the chapter dealing with values, students learn the importance of clarifying their personal and professional values, as well as assisting clients in defining and understanding their values related to health care beliefs and practices. Because of new ethical issues related to technology and a greater societal emphasis on clients' rights, the nurse must be aware of the importance of ethical decision making in health care. The chapter on ethics discusses the significance of an ethical code for nursing and provides guidelines for the resolution of ethical dilemmas in health care. The chapter discussing communication provides a solid introduction to communication principles, particularly as used in therapeutic nurse-client relationships. Client teaching is increasingly important in nursing, and the chapter on teaching and learning focuses on factors that promote or hinder learning and draws parallels between the teaching-learning process and the nursing process for establishing effective teaching plans for clients. The legal issues chapter helps students become acquainted with clients' legal rights and the increasingly complex legal issues that confront nurses in practice.

Unit 4 explores the psychosocial needs of individuals both in the community and in institutional settings. The student learns how a client's self-concept, sexuality, spiritual health, culture, and family background influence the client's health beliefs and practices. The chapters in this unit explain how to assess needs in these areas and incorporate interventions in the nursing care plan.

Because the student nurse cares for clients of all ages, and because normal developmental tasks influence how the nurse promotes health and prevents illness, the student can gain from a developmental perspective in all areas of practice. In Unit 5, individual chapters are devoted to the neonate, infant, and toddler, the school-age child and adolescent, the young and middle adult, and the older adult. In addition to describing theoretical views of growth and development for each stage, the unit explores the primary and developmental health care needs of all age groups.

Unit 6 provides information about fundamental skills essential for all areas of nursing practice. The unit progresses from the simple skills of vital sign measurement to the more complicated techniques of physical assessment, medication administration, and medical and surgical asepsis. Throughout this unit numerous illustrations and photographs and step-by-step descriptions clearly show how each skill should be performed. Each chapter also describes ways to implement skills with minimum stress to clients and to combine client teaching with skills performance.

A client's need for comfort and security is one of the most important needs, and one that the client is often unable to meet because of health problems. In Unit 7 the student learns the importance of maintaining a safe environment for clients and assisting them with hygiene, sleep, relief from pain, and other comfort measures. These chapters also emphasize ways in which nurses can help clients meet their own comfort and security needs.

Unit 8 details nursing care for clients with basic physiological needs in the areas of nutrition, urinary and bowel elimination, oxygenation, fluid and electrolyte balance, and acid-base balance. Each chapter discusses both normal physiology and alterations that result in or from client's health problems. The emphasis on the physiological nature of health alterations, as well as a comprehensive look at assessment criteria in each area, helps prepare the student to develop individualized therapies in a clinical setting.

Units 9 and 10 focus on the care of clients with special needs—those who have sensory alterations, are experiencing grief or impending death, or are encountering surgery. Because the student nurse often works with such clients in early clinical experiences, a conceptual foundation and a familiarity with nursing interventions are important. Each chapter provides the student with a broad understanding of the nature of clients' problems and gives specific guidelines for innovative nursing therapies.

Unit 11, unique in this fundamentals text, introduces the student to the principles of nursing leadership and management and the process of nursing research. The leadership and management chapter discusses theories of effective leadership and the student's participation in the health care team. The student also gains valuable knowledge on ways to assume a leadership role in client care. The nursing research chapter is an introduction to the process of research and helps the student learn to pose basic research questions, locate current nursing research findings and apply them in nursing practice, and participate in data collection.

In organizing the text, every attempt was made to ensure a logical progression of concepts and skills and a meaningful grouping of related subjects. Only rarely, however, is a textbook read in sequence. Recognizing that instructors may assign chapters in different sequences, we make exensive use of cross-references throughout the text and include a thorough index. We hope this approach will provide easy access to information of particular interest.

TEACHING AND LEARNING PACKAGE

To help students and instructors use the text to its fullest potential, four ancillary materials have been developed: an instructor's resource manual, a student study guide, a computerized and printed testbank, and a set of overhead transparencies. The *Instructor's Resource Manual* comprises 50 chapters, each coordinated to one chapter in the text. The chapters include learning objectives, a list of key terms introduced in the chapter, lecture notes and suggestions for classroom- and clinically based activities. In addition, performance checklists for the basic skills presented throughout the text are included at the end of the manual in a format that allows convenient duplication for class use. Instructors or students may use these checklists as guides to evaluate skills performance in laboratory or clinical settings.

A Modular Study Guide to Fundamentals of Nursing, by Lorraine Watson, RN, MEd, and the authors, has been developed to furnish a meaningful self-instructional tool focusing on the essential concepts, principles, and skills presented in the text. More than just the usual workbook approach, each module parallels a text chapter and includes learning objectives, requisite reading, learning activities, self-checks, and posttests. The modules provide students with an opportunity for self-paced learning.

Questbank is a testbank of over 500 multiple-choice questions directly related to the learning objectives and content presented in the text. *Questbank* is available both in printed form and on floppy disks along with a computerized test creation system for the IBM-PC and the Apple II, Apple II Plus, and Apple IIe.

The overhead transparency set includes nearly 100 illustrations and photographs from this new text, selected for their value as instructional tools. Many of the transparencies are in two colors.

Throughout the text the clinical examples depict both men and women who practice nursing in a variety of health care settings. The construction of the English language, however, sometimes makes it awkward to avoid using feminine and masculine pronouns. In the interest of clarity and to avoid using cumbersome terms such as "he/she" and "his/her," we have used the feminine pronoun to refer to the nurse and the masculine pronoun to refer to the client.

We acknowledge the differences in opinion related to use of the terms "client" and "patient." We have chosen to use the term "client" because it suggests a more active, participatory role for the person who has entered the health care delivery system. In its broadest sense "client" refers to the client-family unit and the client–significant other unit as well as the individual.

Writing this book has been challenging and exciting for us, as has been the process of working with a team of expert reviewers and editors to produce a text of the highest quality. Of the many goals we set for ourselves during the development of the book, the first and foremost was to prepare a comprehensive resource to meet the varied needs of both students and instructors. At the same time, however, we have attempted to remain responsive to the needs of the profession, and for this reason we welcome the comments and suggestions of readers. As practicing clinicians and instructors, we have during the writing of the book felt particularly close to our own clients, students, and colleagues, as if communicating directly with them rather than writing on a page. In this spirit we hope that the reader too may participate in this larger communication we believe is essential for nursing education.

Patricia A. Potter
Anne G. Perry

Acknowledgments

The creation of this textbook has been a true labor of love. We wish to extend our thanks and gratitude for the many contributions made by the following individuals:

Our friend and developmental editor Bess Arends, for her limitless energy, commitment, and love for this project. She is a special person who always has the ability to instill confidence and support when it is most needed. Without her this textbook would have remained a dream.

Alison Miller, our editor and friend, who created the idea for this text and continually nurtured and shaped our efforts so we would strive for excellence. Her experience in developing textbooks has been invaluable.

Our developmental editor Tom Lochhaas, a talented man who has taught us many lessons as authors. The long hours Tom contributed to this project have resulted in a textbook we believe is unique.

Robert Bishop, a highly creative individual whose photographs are visually realistic. Through Bob's patience and a determination to achieve visual perfection his photographs make each chapter very special.

Our illustrator Vicki Friedman, for her meticulous line and full-color drawings. The images she creates on paper seem to come alive.

The professional nursing staff of Barnes Hospital. Their commitment to excellence in nursing care has instilled many ideas for this text. A special thanks to members of the administrative staff for their support and belief in this project.

St. Louis University School of Nursing for providing an environment in which faculty and students can achieve their highest potential. Thanks to faculty members and students who lent their time and expertise for many of the photographic sessions.

Karen Walch, our typist, who spent long hours from her family preparing the manuscript. Her good humor and hard work helped us to meet all last-minute deadlines.

Vicki Boyer, an excellent typist whose secretarial expertise and speed helped to keep this project on schedule.

Our family and friends for their patience, understanding, and support during times that were often difficult at best. They provided an emotional strength that made all our efforts worthwhile.

Our nursing advisory panel, whose knowledge, recommendations, and support helped develop this text to meet the needs of beginning nursing students.

The book editing and production staff at The C.V. Mosby Company, whose talents and commitment to quality resulted in a visually appealing and much more readable textbook.

We also wish to acknowledge a friendship that has weathered many difficult decisions, crises, and revisions and will continue to be the basis for future creative efforts.

Contents

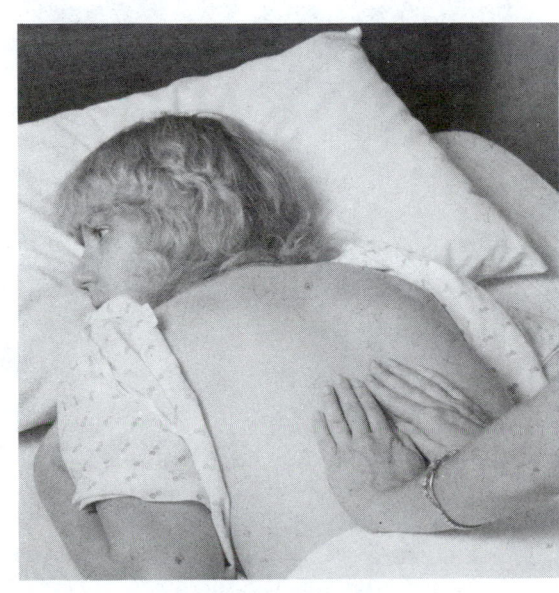

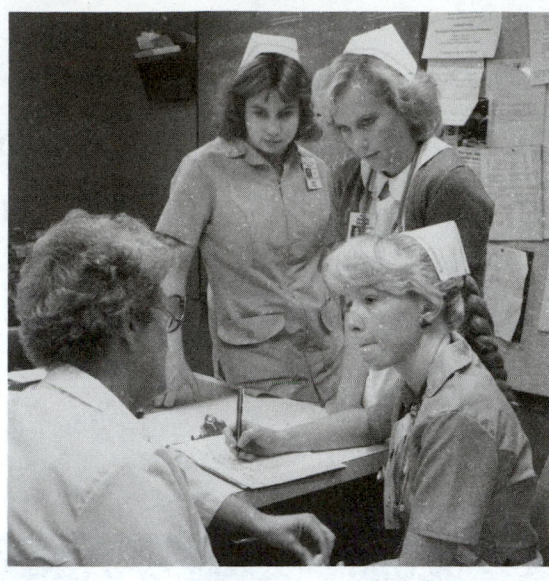

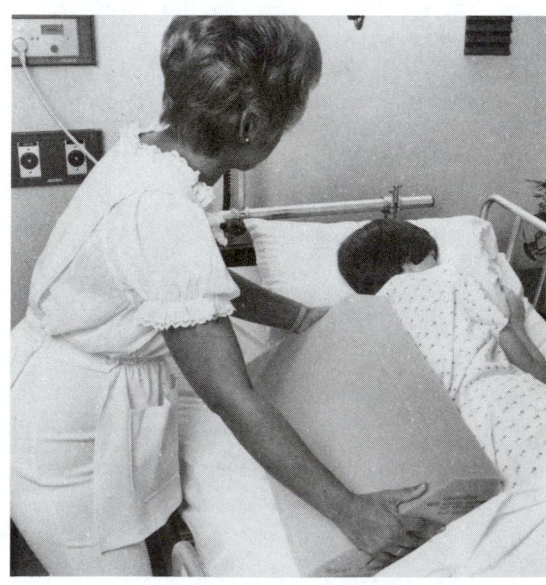

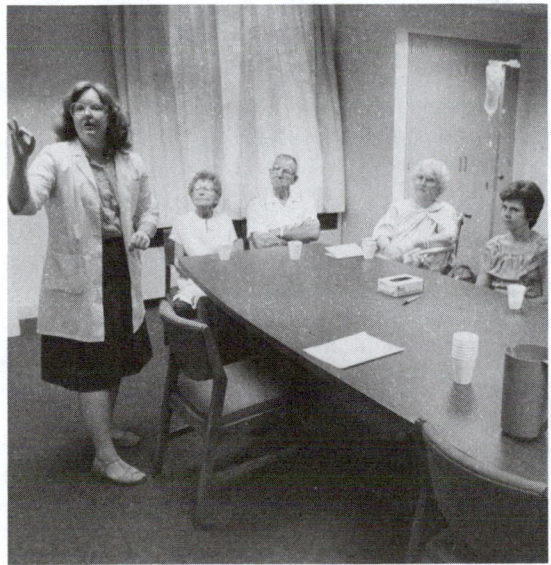

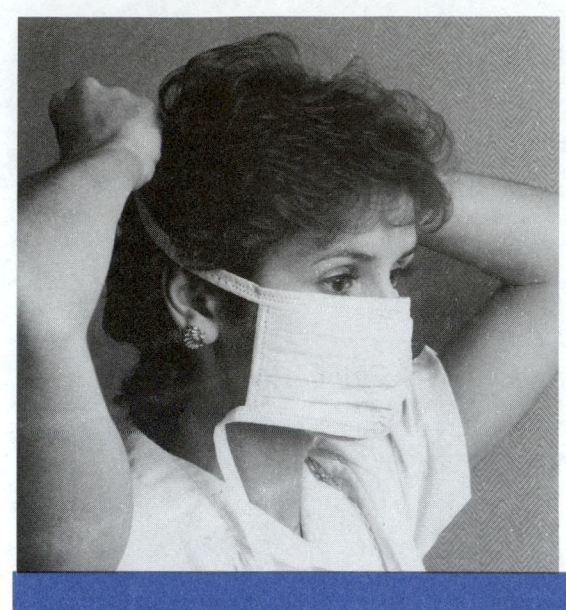

Detailed Contents

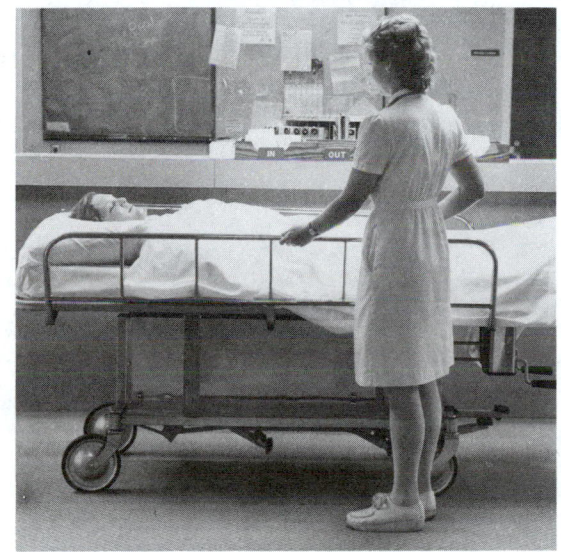

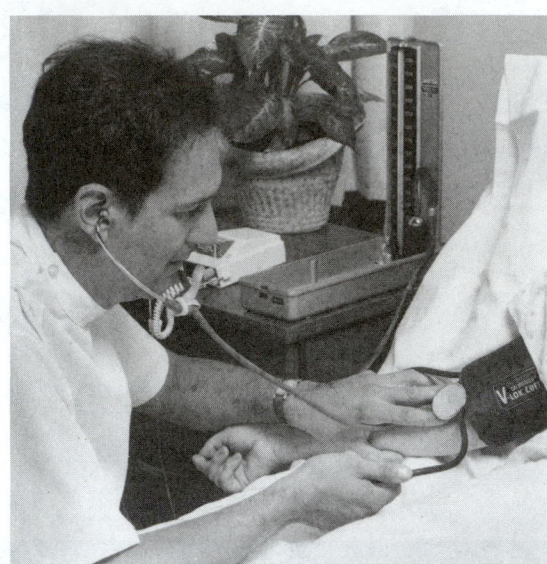

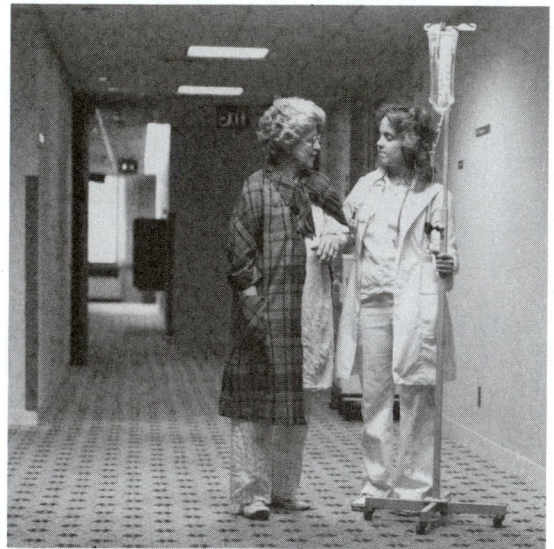

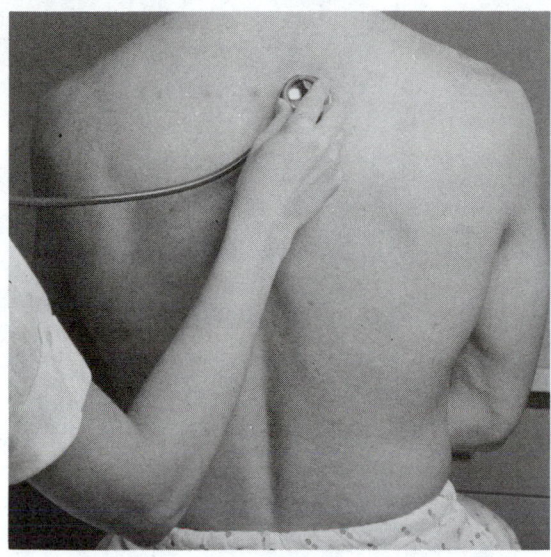

UNIT 2

The Nursing Process

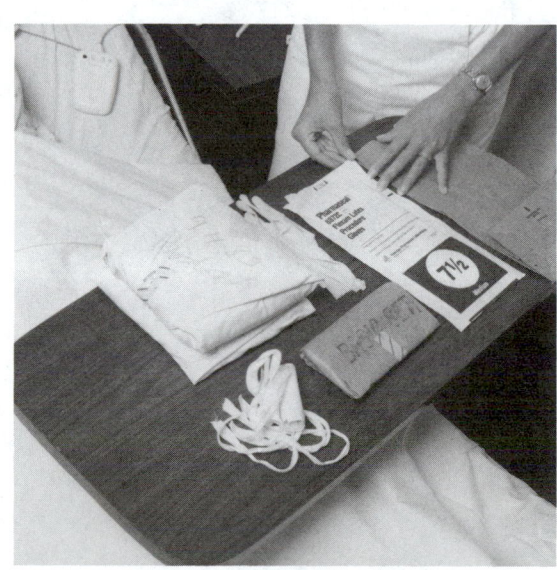

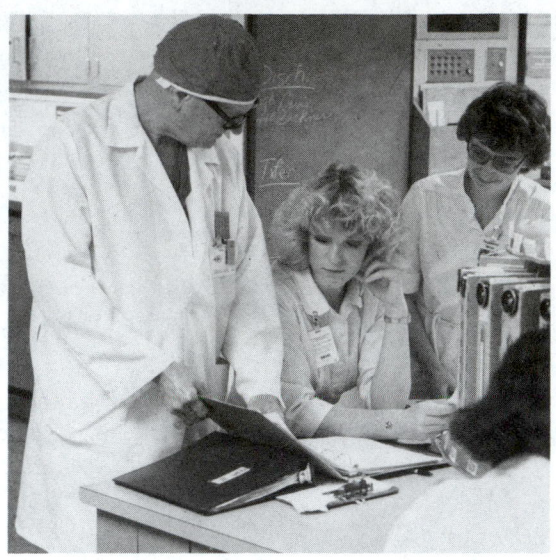

UNIT 3

Concepts for Professional Nursing Practice

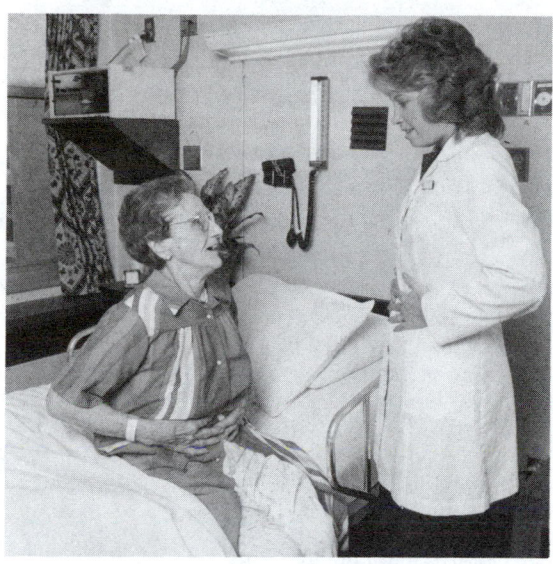

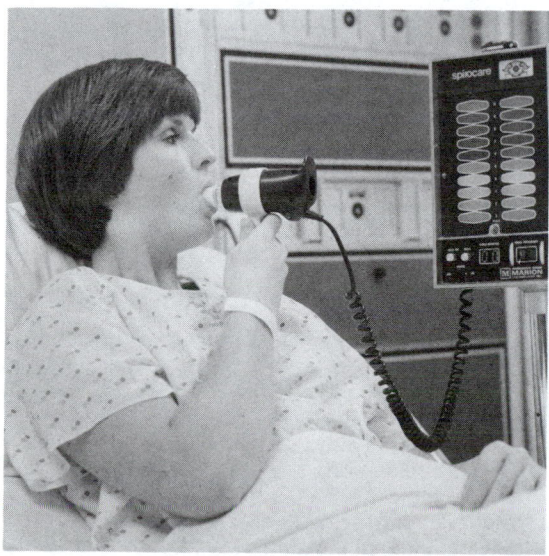

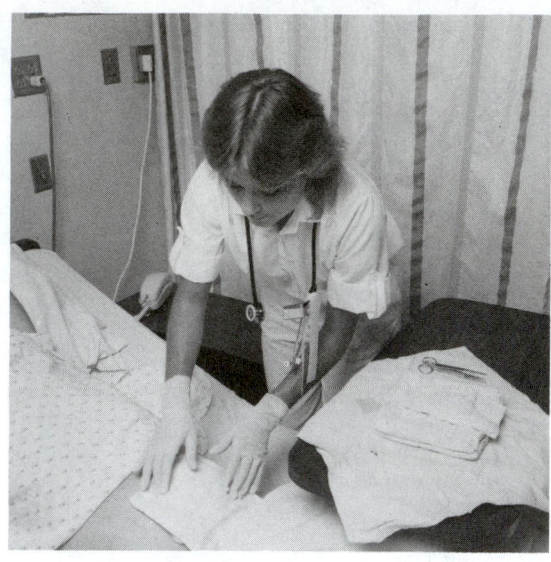

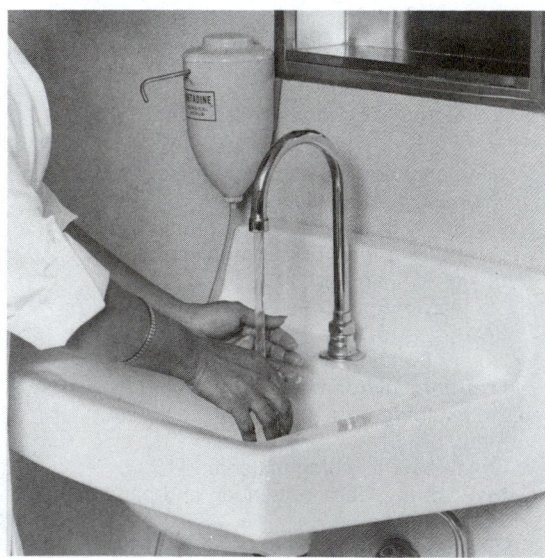

UNIT 4

Caring for Clients with Psychosocial Needs

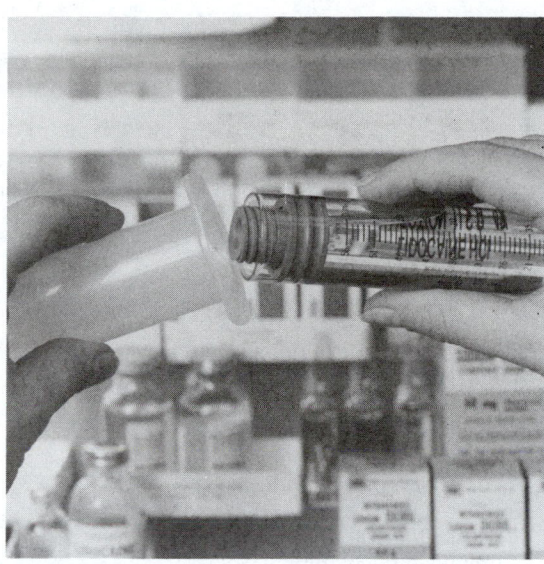

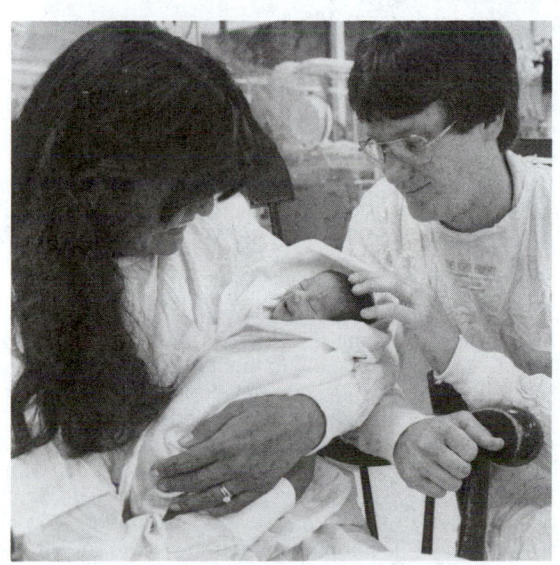

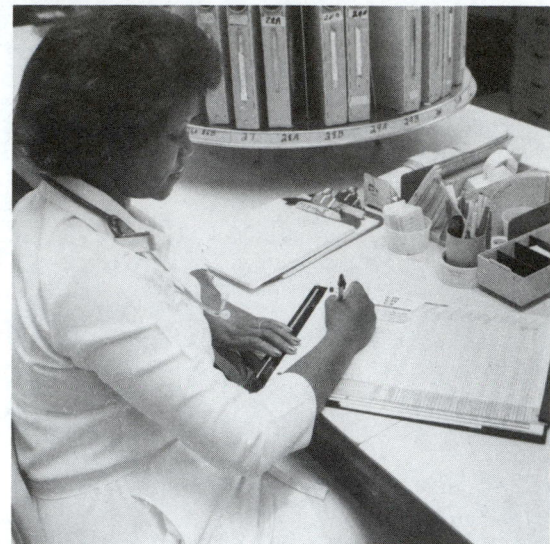

UNIT 5

Growth and Development

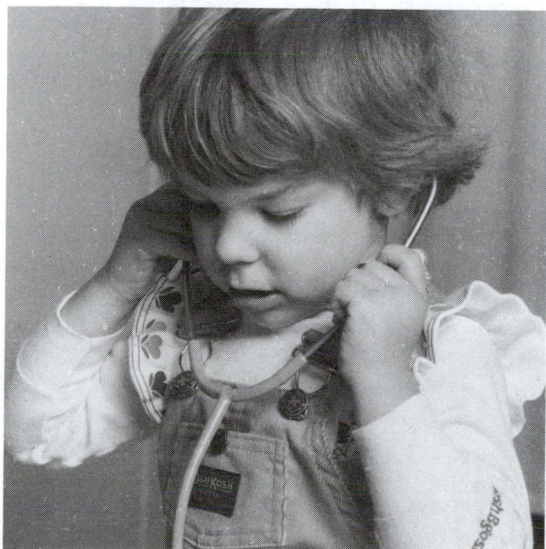

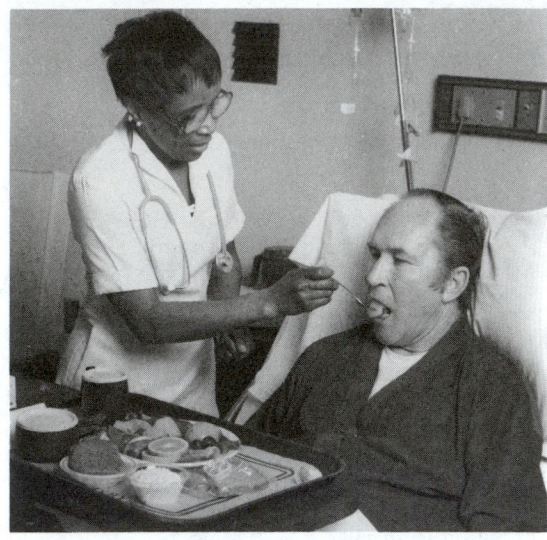

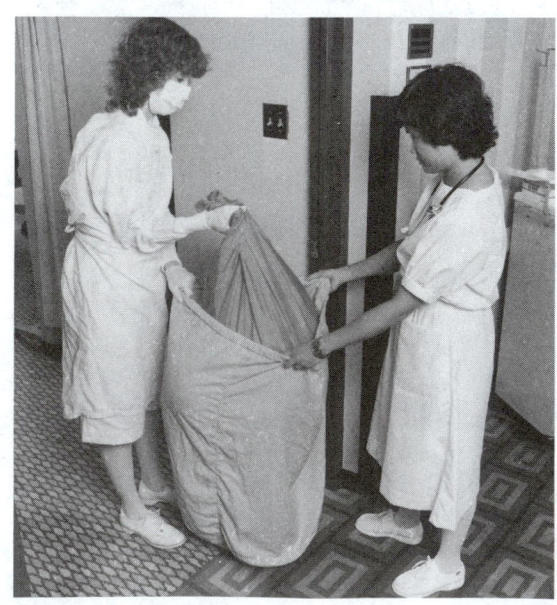

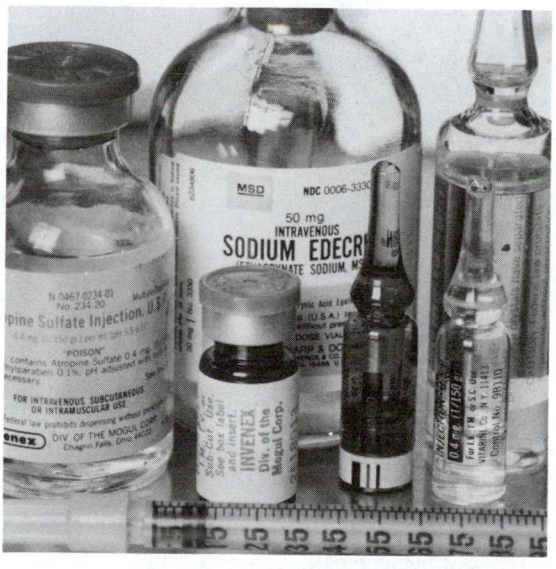

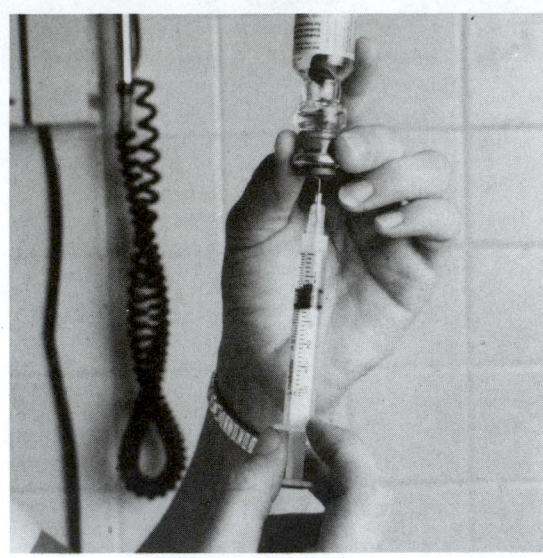

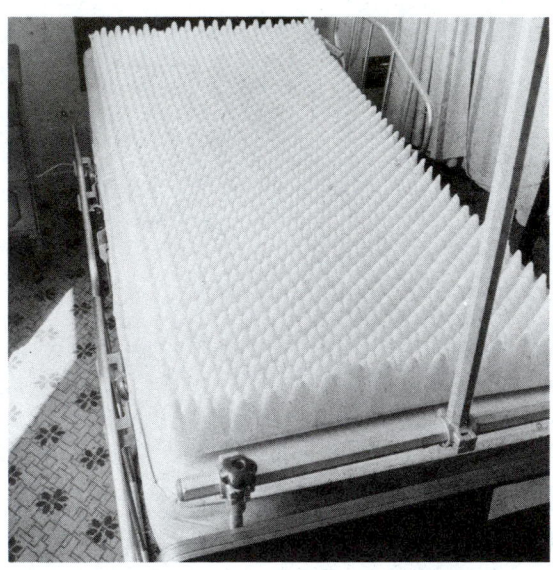

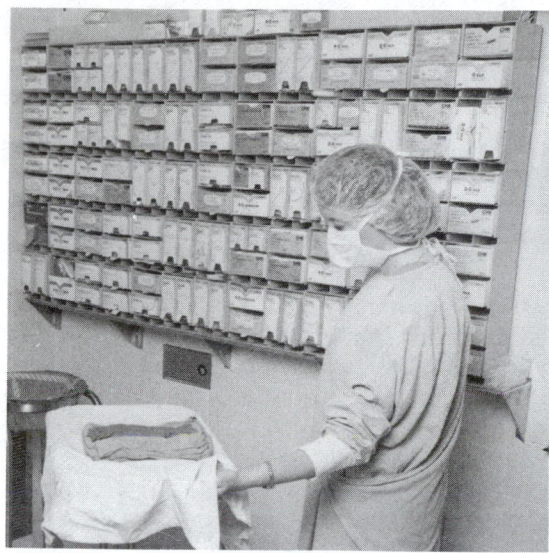

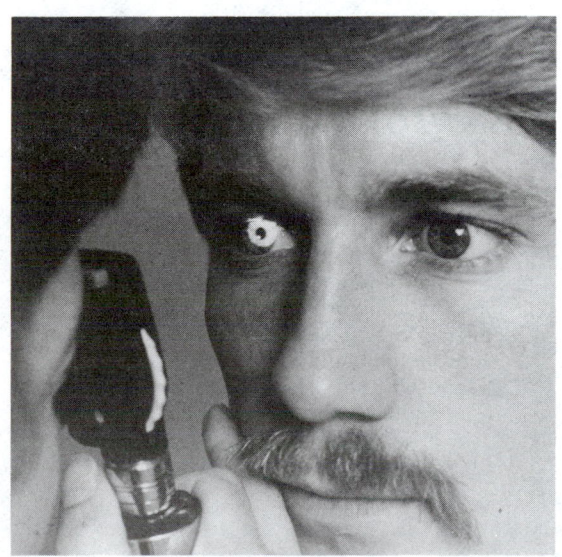

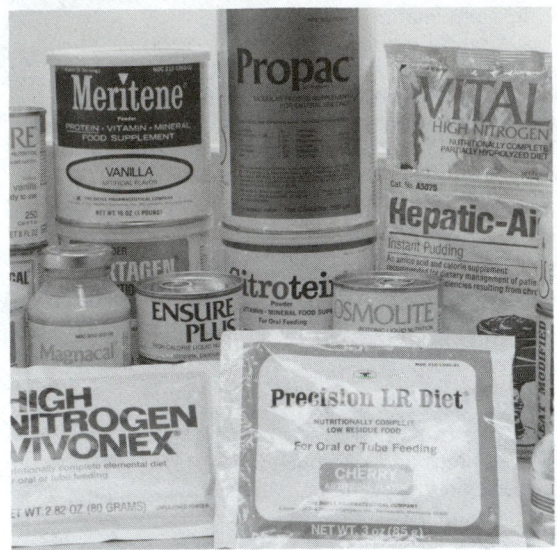

UNIT 8

Caring for Clients with Physiological Needs

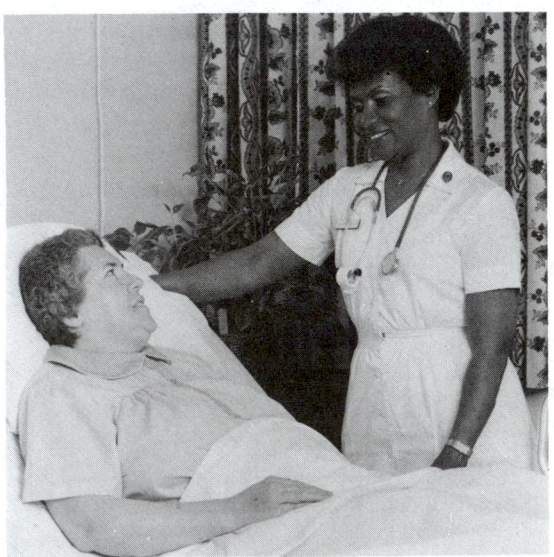

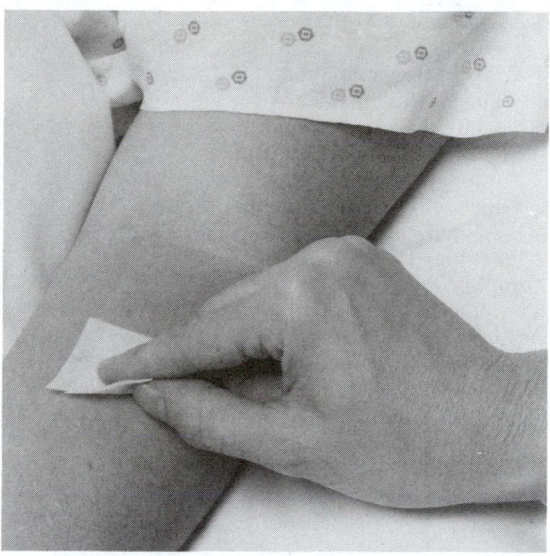

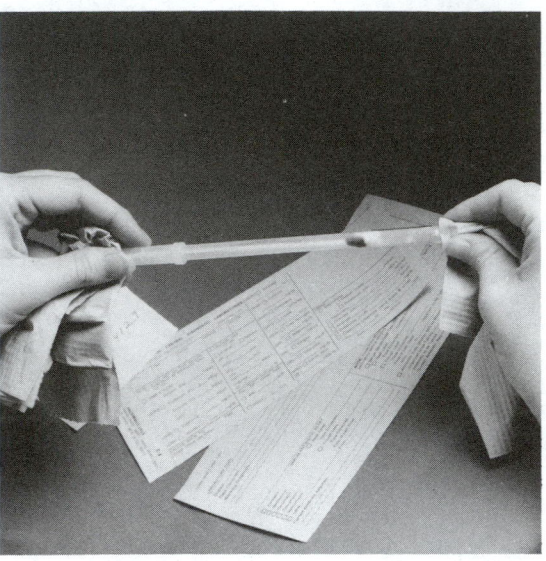

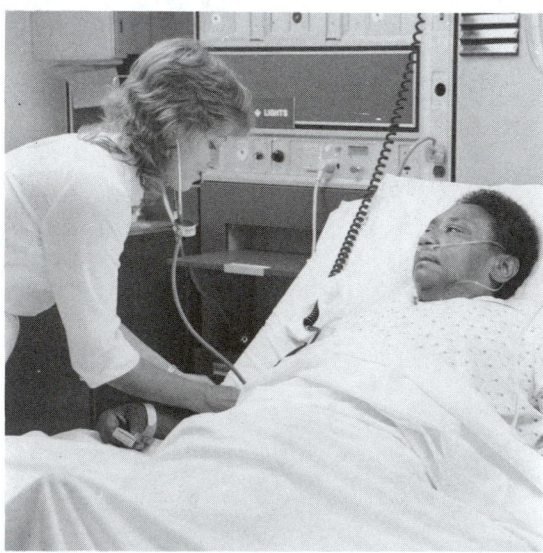

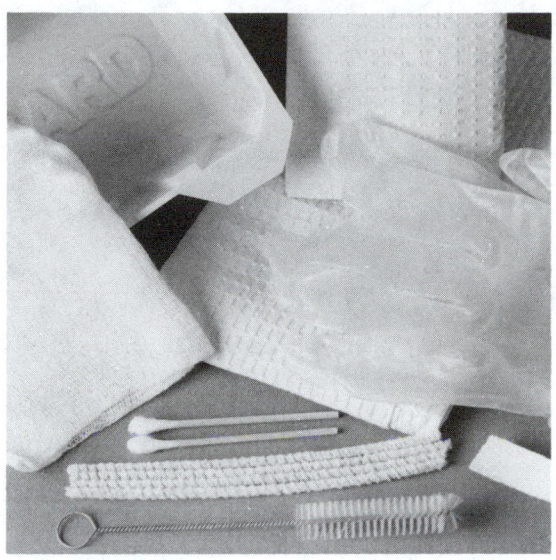

UNIT 9

Caring for Clients with Special Needs

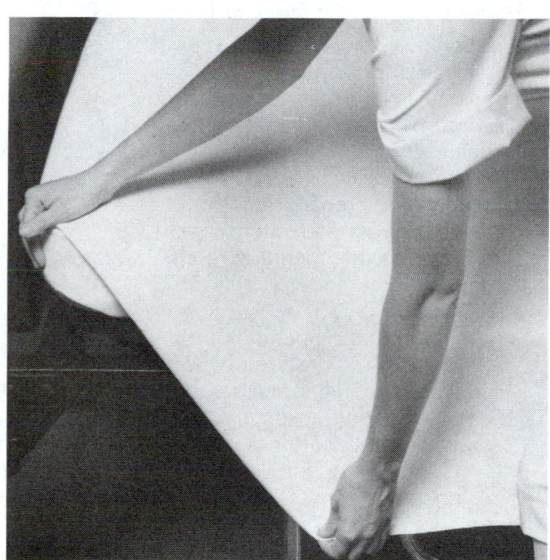

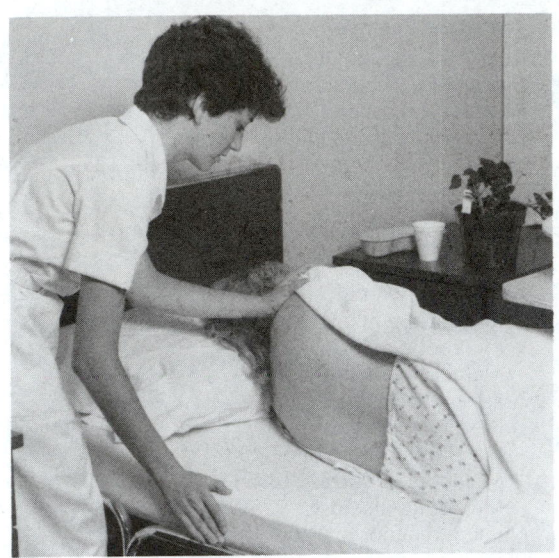

UNIT 10
Caring for the Perioperative Client

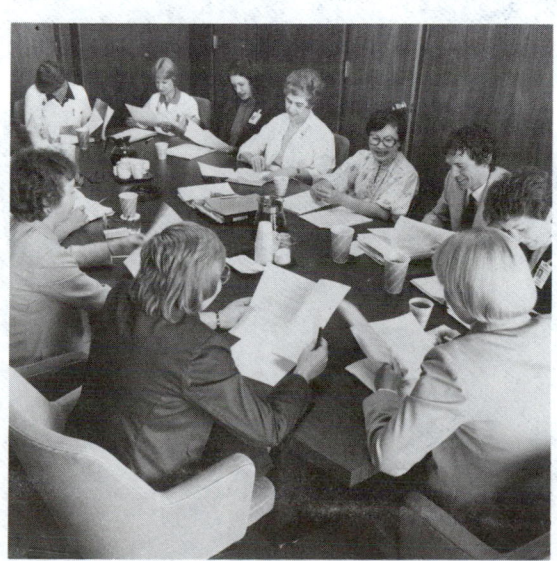

1

The five chapters in Unit 1 introduce many of the fundamental aspects of nursing by examining the profession itself, basic concepts of health and illness, and the world of health care services. Because nursing is a dynamic, growing profession and the roles of nurses have expanded to address the needs of the whole person in both illness and health, these chapters focus on the larger context of nursing as it is practiced today.

Nurses practice in a variety of settings and assume many different roles as they provide care. The first chapter explores these roles, prominent philosophies of nursing and the meaning of nursing as a profession, and current trends in nursing. The succeeding chapters consider basic human needs, stress adaptation, and the relationship of health and illness, with emphasis on health promotion and illness prevention for the family and community as well as the individual client. The complexities of the present health care system and the client's rights within it are also discussed.

The Nurse,
the Consumer, and
Health Care Practices

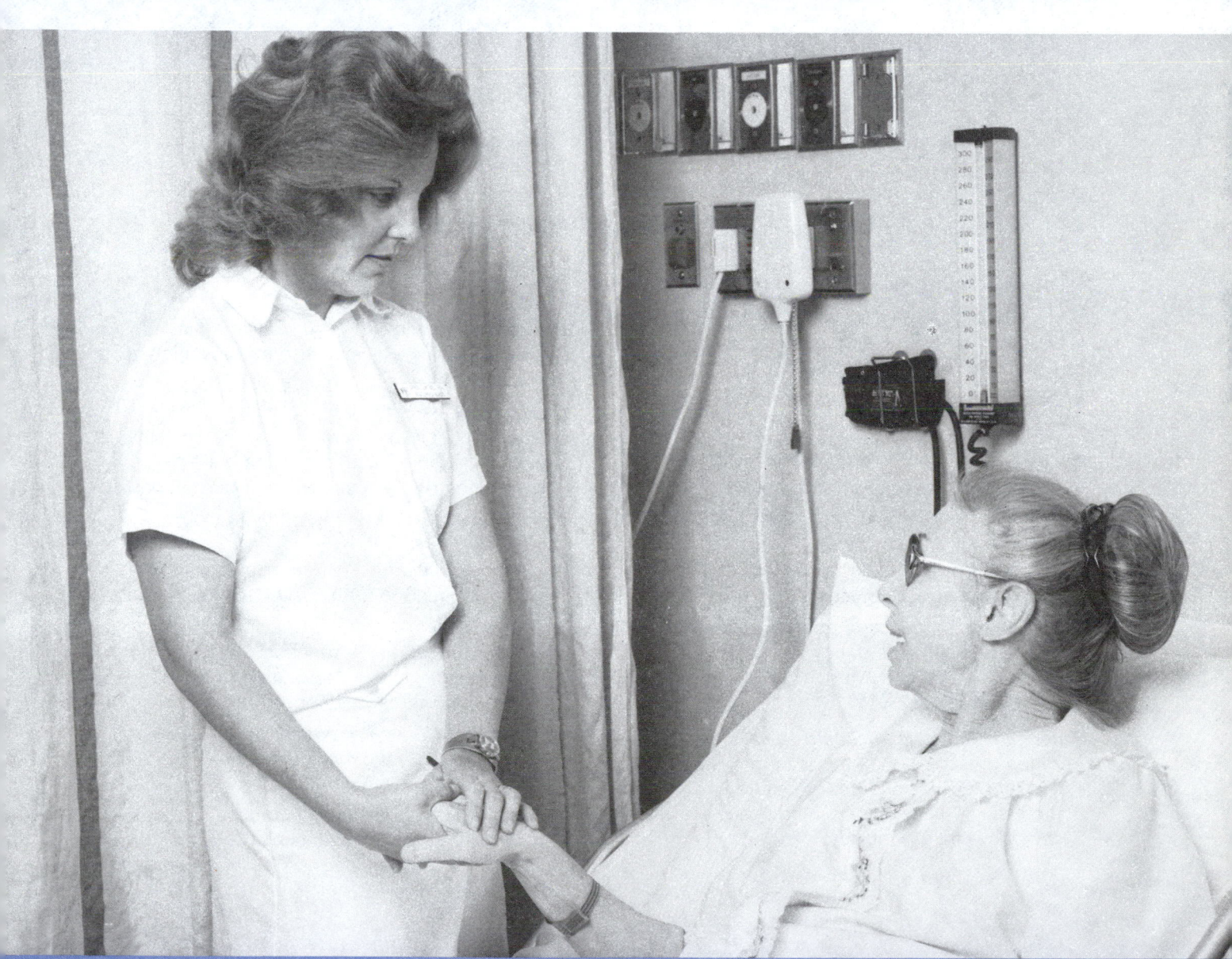

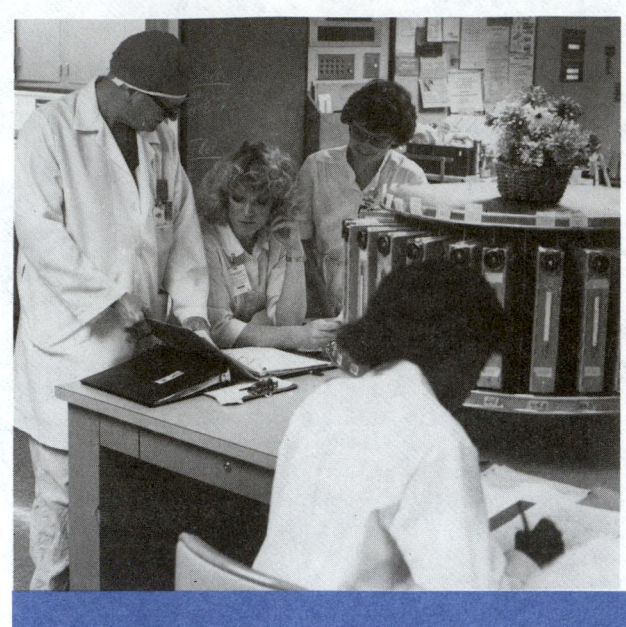

OBJECTIVES

Mastery of content in this chapter will enable the student to:

- Define the terms in the glossary.
- Discuss the historical development of professional nursing.
- Discuss the modern definitions and philosophies of nursing.
- Describe the different educational programs for becoming a registered nurse.
- Describe the different practice settings and roles for nurses.
- Describe at least three career roles for nurses.
- List the five characteristics of a profession and discuss how nursing demonstrates these characteristics.
- Discuss the influence of social and economic changes on nursing practice.
- Discuss the influence of nursing on political issues and health care policy.

GLOSSARY

American Nurses' Association (ANA) Organization of professional nurses in the United States that focuses on standards of health care, nurses' professional development, and economic and general welfare of nurses.

Canadian Nurses' Association (CNA) Organization of professional nurses in Canada similar to the ANA.

certified nurse-midwife Nurse who is educated in midwifery and possesses certification in accordance with criteria of the American College of Midwives.

clinical nurse specialist Nurse with a master's degree in nursing and expertise in a specific area of practice.

Congress for Nursing Practice Unit of the ANA whose activities concern the scope of nursing practice, legal aspects of nursing practice, public recognition of the significance of nursing practice in health care, and implications of health care trends for nursing practice.

continuing education Formal educational programs designed to further the knowledge, skills, and professional attitudes of practicing nurses.

in-service education Instruction or training provided by an agency or institution to nurses practicing within the agency or institution.

International Council of Nurses (ICN) International organization for professional nurses of which the ANA and CNA are part.

licensed practical or vocational nurse Person trained in basic nursing techniques and direct client care who practices under the supervision of a registered nurse.

1 The Profession of Nursing

National League for Nursing (NLN)   Organization of nurses and lay people concerned with improving nursing education, nursing service, and the delivery of health care in the United States. The NLN is the official accrediting agency for nursing schools.

nurse administrator   Nurse whose management position within an agency focuses on the delivery of nursing services.

nurse anesthetist   Nurse with advanced training and accreditation in the speciality of nurse anesthesia; manages the anesthetic care of clients in certain surgical situations.

nurse educator   Nurse with a background in clinical nursing who works in a school of nursing as a faculty member, in a staff development department of a health care agency, or in an inpatient education department.

nurse practitioner   Nurse with advanced training or education who provides primary care for nonemergency clients, usually in an outpatient or community setting.

nurse researcher   Nurse with graduate nursing education who investigates problems related to nursing practice.

nursing   Profession concerned with the diagnosis and treatment of human responses to actual and potential health problems.

nursing theory   Organized framework of concepts and purposes designed to guide the practice of nursing.

occupational therapist   Health care professional certified to develop and use adaptive devices that help the chronically ill or handicapped carry out activities of daily living.

pharmacist   Licensed professional who formulates and dispenses medications.

physical therapist   Health care professional licensed to assist in the management of physically disabled or handicapped clients through techniques such as special exercise, application of heat and cold, and sonar wave methods.

physician   Health care professional who has the degree of Doctor of Medicine (MD) or Doctor of Osteopathy (DO) and is licensed to provide medical, surgical, and other treatment.

physician assistant   Health care professional trained in aspects of the practice of medicine to provide support to physicians.

professional organization   Association of professionals created to deal with issues of concern to the profession as a whole.

registered nurse   Health care professional who has completed a course of study at an accredited school of nursing and has passed an examination administered by a state board of nursing or the Canadian Nurses' Association Testing Service.

respiratory therapist   Health care professional licensed to deliver treatment to improve ventilatory function or oxygenation.

social worker   Professional trained to counsel clients and their families.

Modern nursing involves many different kinds of activities, concepts, and skills related to the health sciences, social sciences, and other areas. Nursing as a profession is unique in that it addresses in a humanistic and holistic manner the responses of individual clients and their families to actual and potential health problems. The nurse in practice has many roles, such as care giver, decision maker, client advocate, and teacher, and often acts in several roles at the same time. Because of this complex interrelationship of roles, practicing nurses need a philosophy of nursing to guide their delivery of care. Over the years nurses have developed many such philosophies and definitions of nursing. The definition by the International Council of Nurses (1973) is a concise statement with which most nursing theorists would agree:

> The unique function of the nurse is to assist the individual, sick or well, in the performance of those activities contributing to his health, its recovery, or to a peaceful death that he would perform unaided if he had the necessary strength, will, or knowledge.

The profession of nursing is complex and multifaceted in other ways as well. Nurses practice in many different settings, which emphasize different aspects of nursing care and different nursing roles. In addition, there are a variety of educational programs by which one becomes a registered nurse and a variety of career opportunities open to nurses as they gain experience and continue their education. This chapter presents an overview of educational and career opportunities for nurses in the United States and Canada to give beginning nursing students an understanding of the profession as a whole and specific career paths.

The profession of nursing continues to evolve as society in general and health care in specific continue to change. Nursing responds and adapts to such changes and meets new challenges as they arise. Nursing is also influencing political decisions related to health care and decisions of health care policy, as the profession responds to new issues and trends in health care.

Historical Perspective

Nursing is an essential part of society, out of which it has grown and with which it evolves. Nursing can be said to have always been directed to serving the health care needs of society. Nursing originated with the desire to keep people healthy, as well as to provide comfort, care, and assurance to the sick. Although these general goals of nursing have remained relatively stable over the centuries, the practice of nursing has been influenced by characteristics of society that have changed with time, and thus nursing has gradually evolved into a modern profession from its roots in ancient cultures. A general understanding of this historical development can help the nursing student better comprehend the profession as it is today.

In ancient cultures nurses generally had a subservient role. Many ancient societies did not value human life in the same way we do today, and the caretakers of human life were less respected. Nurses delivered custodial care and depended for direction on physicians or priests (Kelly, 1981). Under the direct supervision of a physician the nurse tended to the hygiene of clients in the home. Nurses did not participate in any activities to promote health, nor did they teach families how to care for their ill.

Under the influence of Christianity, however, nurses gained increased respect and the practice of nursing expanded. In the first century of the Christian Church the Order of the Deaconesses, a group somewhat like today's public health or visiting nurses, was formed. Their goals included meeting the following basic needs of the society (Dolan, 1978):

1. To feed the hungry
2. To give water to the thirsty
3. To clothe the naked
4. To visit the imprisoned
5. To shelter the homeless
6. To care for the sick
7. To bury the dead

The Benedictine order marked the entrance of men into nursing; they created infirmaries and placed the care of the sick above all other duties (Dolan, 1978). By the fifth century infirmaries for persons with leprosy were established in Ireland.

Although with the influence of religion nursing became increasingly humanistic, there was still no formal education or training for nurses. Nurses were often employed as servants, caring for infants and children to free the mistress of the household for social duties. In early institutions for the physically and mentally ill, uneducated nurses gave care as best they could, generally under the orders of a physician.

In the Middle Ages the Crusades were a stimulus for expanded nursing and health care. Military nursing orders were formed for men, and hospitals were established. After the Crusades, with the decline of feudalism, large cities began to develop. The growth of cities led to certain health problems (see boxed material) and an increased need for health care. Some of these health problems still exist in urban areas today, although the mortality associated with them has greatly declined. During the Middle Ages secular groups were formed to meet specific health needs, such as the Hospital Brothers of St. Anthony to care for those with the disease called St. Anthony's fire, the Misericordia in Italy to provide transportation services for the ill (Fig. 1-1), and the Alexian Brothers (a group still active today) to care for victims of bubonic plague. The practice of midwifery also flourished in the Middle Ages.

In the fifteenth to seventeenth centuries the lack of hygiene and sanitation and the increasing poverty in urban centers resulted in serious problems in health care. Societal factors, such as laws punishing the poor and the Window Tax, which led to decreased ventilation as landlords bricked in windows to avoid the tax, created conditions and health needs to which nursing responded. The early visiting nurse association called the Order of the Visitation of Mary brought nurses into the homes of the poor and ill. The Sisters of Charity, established in the sixteenth century by Louise de Gras, an associate of St. Vincent

> ## Health Problems Associated with the Growth of Cities
>
> - Overcrowding and related stresses
> - Poor ventilation
> - Poor heating and cooling
> - Poor sanitation, garbage collection, and plumbing
> - Poor water supply
> - Inadequate methods of preserving foods
> - Ignorance of elementary hygiene

de Paul, was perhaps the first nursing order with a systematic educational program. Soon after the French colonies were established in Canada, the Augustinian Sisters arrived to staff hospitals and provide nursing care for the Indians. In the English colonies in America midwifery was common, and nurses along with clergymen and their wives cared for the ill.

In the eighteenth century the growth of cities brought an increase in the number of hospitals and a greater role for nurses. The smallpox epidemics in the French colonies and the Revolutionary War in the English colonies increased the need for nursing services. Nursing skills and knowledge were generally passed on by experienced nurses; there was still little formal education for nurses.

In the nineteenth century Florence Nightingale brought about major reforms in nursing when caring for the wounded and ill in the Crimean War. Nightingale's reforms included providing cleanliness and comfort in hospitals, meeting the basic needs of the ill, and educating the ill and their families about health and health promotion. In addition, she estab-

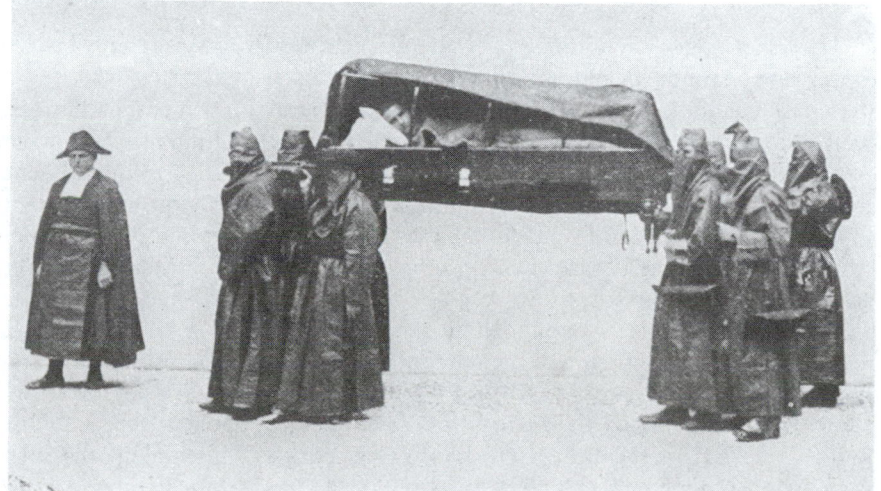

Fig. 1-1 The Brothers of Misericordia taking a patient to the hospital in Florence.

Courtesy Dolan Collection.

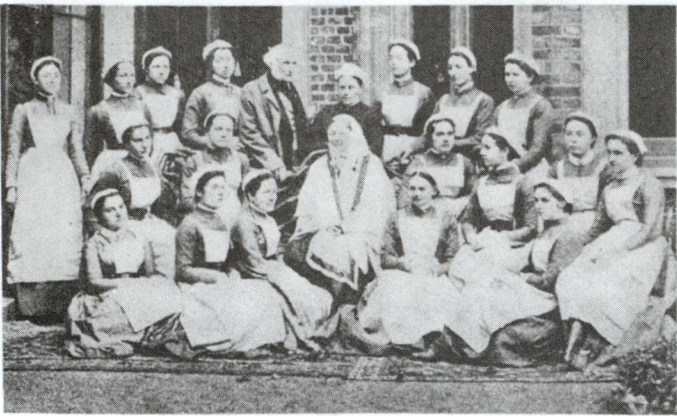

Fig. 1-2 Florence Nightingale *(center)* and students at St. Thomas' Hospital, London, 1887.
Courtesy Dolan Collection.

lished formal nursing educational programs and founded the Nightingale Training School at St. Thomas' Hospital in London (Fig. 1-2). Her educational reforms began the evolution of nurse training (see boxed material). Nightingale did not limit nursing activities to clients within a hospital but expanded professional nursing practice to the home (Woodham, 1951). Her philosophy of nursing practice reflected the changing needs of society. She saw the role of nursing as having "charge of somebody's health" based on the knowledge of "how to put the body in such a state to be free of disease or to recover from disease" (Nightingale, 1860).

The Civil War (1861-1865) stimulated the growth of nursing in the United States. Clara Barton (who was to found the American Red Cross in 1882) tended soldiers on the battlefields, cleansing their wounds, meeting their basic needs, and comforting them in death. While Barton was not the only nurse on the Civil War battlefields, she is one of the best remembered.

After the Civil War nursing schools in the United States and Canada began to follow the Nightingale plan. Such schools provided classroom instruction as well as clinical practice. In 1884 the Canadian Nurses' Association (CNA) was established through the efforts of Mary Agnes Snively, and in 1886 Isabel Hampton Robb helped found the Nurses Associated Alumni of the United States, which later became the American Nurses' Association (ANA).

Nursing in hospitals expanded in the late nineteenth century, but nursing in the community did not increase significantly until in 1893 Lillian Wald and Mary Brewster opened the Henry Street Settlement, which focused on the health needs of New York's poor living in tenements. Nurses working in this settlement had greater responsibility for their clients than nurses working in hospitals at the time, because they frequently encountered situations that required action independent of a physician's orders. In addition to the treatment of illness, the poor needed nursing therapies aimed at restoring nutrition, providing shelter, and maintaining hygiene.

Early in the twentieth century there were advances in hospital care, public health, and nursing education. Mary Adelaide Nutting, a member of the first graduating class at Johns Hopkins Hospital, was instrumental in the affiliation of nursing education with universities; she became the first professor of nursing in a university in 1907. In 1923 the Rockefeller Foundation funded a survey of nursing education, which has become known as the Goldmark Report. The report concluded that nursing education needed financial support and suggested that such support be given to university schools of nursing. As a result of the Goldmark Report, the Rockefeller Foundation funded the expansion of nursing programs at Yale University, Vanderbilt University, and the University of Toronto. Frances Payne Bolton provided financial support for the nursing school at Western Reserve University.

As nursing education developed, nursing practice also expanded. In 1901 the Army Nurse Corps was established, followed in 1908 by the Navy Nurse Corps. Nursing specialization was occurring. In the 1920s graduate nurse-midwifery programs were initiated, and beginning in the 1950s specialty nursing organizations were formed, such as the Association of Operating Room Nurses (1953-1954), Association of Critical Care Nurses (1969-1972), and Oncology Nursing Society (1975). (See Appendix A for a comprehensive list of professional organizations.)

In 1965 the National Commission on Nursing and Nursing Education took up issues including the supply of and demand for nurses, clarification of nursing roles and functions, education of nurses, and career opportunities available to nurses. Their report, often called the Lysaught report after Jerome P. Lysaught, the director of the study, called for clarification of nursing roles and responsibilities in relation to those of other health care professionals. It also advocated greater financial support for nurses and more career opportunities to attract nurses and retain them in the profession (Lysaught, 1970).

Over the past three decades the growth of nursing as a health care profession and science has led to the development of philosophies of nursing and theoretical models on which nursing practice can be based. The following section describes several important nursing theories and demonstrates how far nursing has come from Florence Nightingale's day.

Modern Definitions and Philosophies of Nursing

As nursing has continued to evolve, expanding its roles, concepts, and emphases, theorists have defined nursing in a variety of ways. Nursing definitions not only reflect changes in the practice of nursing but also help bring about changes by identifying the domain of nursing practice and guiding research, practice, and education. Nursing definitions or philosophies are

useful in the following ways:
1. Formulating legislation governing nursing practice
2. Formulating regulations interpreting nurse practice acts so that nurses and others better understand the laws
3. Developing curriculum plans for nursing education
4. Establishing criteria for measuring the quality of nursing care
5. Preparing job descriptions used by employers of nurses
6. Guiding the development of nursing care delivery systems

These aspects of nursing practice are discussed separately in later sections in this chapter. In addition, a nursing definition can help the nursing student understand how the different roles and actions of nurses fit together in the unified profession of nursing. The following sections describe, in chronological order, the general focus of several important theories of the philosophy of nursing. Table 1-1 presents a summary of these nursing theories for comparison.

Peplau's Theory

Hildegard Peplau's theory (1952) focuses on interpersonal relationships that people formulate as they pass through various developmental stages. Nursing's overall purpose is to educate the client and family and help the client reach mature personality development. Therefore the nurse strives to develop a nurse-client relationship in which the nurse serves as a resource person, counselor, and surrogate.

When the client seeks help, the nurse first discusses the nature of the problem with the client and explains the services available. As the nurse-client relationship develops, the nurse helps the client identify the problem and potential solutions. The client gains from this relationship by using available services to meet needs. When the original needs have been resolved, new needs may emerge.

Abdellah's Theory

The nursing theory developed by Faye Abdellah and her colleagues (1960) emphasizes delivering nursing care for the whole person to meet the physical, emotional, intellectual, social, and spiritual needs of clients and their families. In this approach the nurse needs knowledge and skills in interpersonal relations, psychology, growth and development, communication, and sociology, as well as the basic sciences and specific nursing skills. The nurse is seen as a problem solver and decision maker. The nurse formulates an

TABLE 1-1

Summary of Nursing Theories

Theorist	Goal of Nursing	Framework for Practice
Hildegard Peplau (1952)	To develop an interpersonal interaction between the client and the nurse	Interpersonal theoretical model emphasizing the relationship between the client and nurse
Faye Abdellah (1960)	To deliver nursing care for the whole individual	Problem solving based on Abdellah's 21 nursing problems
Virginia Henderson (1964)	To help the client gain independence as rapidly as possible	Henderson's 14 basic needs
Joyce Travelbee (1966)	To help the client and family cope with and find meaning in the experience of illness	Interpersonal theory emphasizing nurse-client relationship
Dorothy Johnson (1968)	To reduce stress so the client can recover as quickly as possible	Adaptation model based on seven behavioral subsystems
Martha Rogers (1970)	To help the client achieve a maximal level of wellness	"Unitary man" evolving along a life process
Imogene King (1971)	To use communication to help the client reestablish a positive adaptation to his environment	Nursing process defined as a dynamic interpersonal state between the nurse and the client
Dorothea Orem (1971)	To care for the client and help the client attain self-care	Self-care deficit theory
Myra Levine (1973)	To use conservation activities aimed at optimal use of client's resources	Adaptation model of human as an integrated whole based on "four conservation principles of nursing"
Sister Callista Roy (1976)	To identify the types of demands placed on a client and the client's adaptation to the demands	Adaptation model based on four adaptive modes: physiological, psychological, sociological, and independence

individualized view of the client's needs, which may occur in four areas:

1. Comfort, hygiene, and safety
2. Physiological balance
3. Psychological and social factors
4. Sociological and community factors

In these four areas Abdellah and colleagues identified the following specific needs clients may have, which are often referred to as "Abdellah's 21 nursing problems":

1. To maintain good hygiene and physical comfort
2. To achieve optimal activity, exercise, rest, and sleep
3. To prevent accident, injury, or other trauma and prevent the spread of infection
4. To maintain good body mechanics and prevent and correct deformities
5. To facilitate the supply of oxygen to all body cells
6. To facilitate the maintenance of nutrition to all body cells
7. To facilitate the maintenance of elimination
8. To facilitate the maintenance of fluid and electrolyte balance
9. To recognize the physiological responses of the body to disease conditions—pathological, physiological, and compensatory

10. To facilitate the maintenance of regulatory mechanisms and functions
11. To facilitate the maintenance of sensory function
12. To identify and accept positive and negative expressions, feelings, and reactions
13. To identify and accept the interrelatedness of emotions and organic illness
14. To facilitate the maintenance of effective verbal and nonverbal communication
15. To facilitate the development of productive interpersonal relationships
16. To facilitate progress toward achievement of personal spiritual goals
17. To create and/or maintain a therapeutic environment
18. To facilitate awareness of self as an individual with varying physical, emotional, and developmental needs
19. To accept the optimum possible goals in light of limitations—physical and emotional
20. To use community resources as an aid in resolving problems arising from illness
21. To understand the role of social problems as influencing factors in the cause of illness

Henderson's Theory

Virginia Henderson's nursing theory (1964) involves basic needs of the whole person. Henderson (1964a) defines nursing as

assisting the individual sick or well in the performance of those activities contributing to health or its recovery that he would perform unaided if he had the necessary strength, will, or knowledge. And to do this in such a way as to help him gain independence as rapidly as possible.

The following needs, often called "Henderson's 14 basic needs," provide a framework for nursing care (Henderson, 1964b):
1. Breathe normally
2. Eat and drink adequately
3. Eliminate by all avenues of elimination
4. Move and maintain a desirable position
5. Sleep and rest
6. Select suitable clothing; dress and undress
7. Maintain body temperature within normal range
8. Keep the body clean and well groomed
9. Avoid dangers in the environment
10. Communicate with others
11. Worship according to faith
12. Work at something that provides a sense of accomplishment
13. Play or participate in various forms of recreation
14. Learn, discover, or satisfy the curiosity that leads to normal development and health

Travelbee's Theory

Joyce Travelbee (1966), like Peplau, emphasizes nursing as an interpersonal process involving the nurse and client. Travelbee defines nursing as

an interpersonal process whereby the . . . nurse practitioner assists an individual or family to prevent, or cope with, the experience of illness and suffering, and, if necessary, assists the individual or family to find meaning in these experiences.

Because the client's whole self may be involved in coping with the experience of illness, this definition also addresses the individual in all dimensions.

Johnson's Theory

Dorothy Johnson's theory of nursing (1968) focuses on how the client adapts to his illness and how actual or potential stress can affect the client's ability to adapt. For Johnson the goal of nursing is to reduce stress so that the client can move more easily through the recovery process. Johnson's theory focuses on basic needs in terms of seven categories of behavior:
1. Security-seeking behavior
2. Nurturance-seeking behavior
3. Mastery of oneself and one's environment according to internalized standards of excellence
4. Taking in nourishment in socially and culturally acceptable ways
5. Ridding the body of waste in socially and culturally acceptable ways
6. Sexual and role identity behavior
7. Self-protective behavior

According to Johnson, the nurse assesses the client's needs in these categories of behavior, called behavioral subsystems. Under normal conditions the client is able to function fairly effectively in his environment. When stress disrupts normal adaptation, however, the client's behavior becomes erratic and less purposeful. The nurse identifies the client's inability to adapt and provides nursing care to resolve problems in meeting the client's needs.

Rogers' Theory

In her theory, Martha Rogers (1970) considers the client as a whole person, whom she calls the "unitary man." The unitary man is continually evolving and changing, and thus the nurse is concerned with the client's evolutionary patterns and helps him achieve maximal wellness. Rogers describes nursing this way:

Nursing is concerned with people—all people—well and sick, rich and poor, young and old. The arenas of nursing's services extend into all areas where there are people; at home, at school, at work, at play, in hospitals, nursing homes, and clinics—on this planet and now moving into outer space.

Rogers views nursing primarily as a science and is committed to nursing research. Nursing therefore incorporates knowledge of the basic sciences and physiology as well as nursing knowledge.

The science of nursing aims to provide a body of abstract knowledge growing out of scientific research and logical analysis and capable of being translated into nursing practice. Nursing's body of scientific knowledge is a new product specific to nursing . . . . Nursing is a humanistic science.

King's Theory

Imogene King's theory (1971) also focuses on the interpersonal relationship between client and the nurse. In the King theory the nurse-client relationship is the vehicle for the nursing process, which is defined as a dynamic interpersonal process in which the nurse and the client are affected by each other's behavior as well as by the health care system. The nurse's goal is to use communication to assist the client in reestablishing or maintaining a positive adaptation to his environment.

Orem's Theory

Dorothea Orem (1971) developed a definition of nursing that emphasizes the self-care needs of the client. Orem describes her philosophy of nursing in this way:

Nursing has as a special concern man's needs for self-care action and the provision and management of it on a continuous basis in order to sustain life and health, recover from disease or injury, and cope with their effects. Self-care is a requirement of every person—man, woman, and child. When self-care is not maintained, illness, disease, or death will occur. Nurses sometimes manage and maintain required self-care continually for persons who are totally incapacitated. In other instances, nurses help persons to maintain required self-care by performing some but not all care measures, by supervising others who assist patients, and by instructing and guiding individuals as they gradually move toward self-care.

The goal of Orem's self-care deficit theory of nursing is helping the client care for himself. According to Orem, nursing care is necessary when the client is unable to fulfill his biological, psychological, developmental, or social needs. The nurse determines why a client is unable to meet his self-care needs, what must be done to enable the client to meet these needs, and how much the client is able to do for himself.

Levine's Theory

Myra Levine's nursing theory (1973) views the client as an integrated being who interacts with and adapts to his environment, with conservation of energy as a primary concern. In this theory health is viewed in terms of the conservation of energy in four areas, which Levine calls the "four conservation principles of nursing":
1. Conservation of client energy
2. Conservation of structural integrity
3. Conservation of personal integrity
4. Conservation of social integrity

With this approach, nursing care involves conservation activities aimed at optimal use of the client's resources.

Roy's Theory

Sister Callista Roy's adaptation theory (1976) views the client as an adaptive system. Roy believes that the need for nursing care arises when the client cannot adapt to internal and external environmental demands. All individuals must adapt to four demands:
1. Meeting basic physiological needs
2. Developing a positive self-concept
3. Performing social roles
4. Achieving a balance between dependence and independence

The nurse determines what demands are causing problems for a client and assesses how well the client is adapting to these demands. Nursing care then helps the client adapt.

American Nurses' Association Definition

In 1955 the ANA published the following official definition of nursing practice*:

The practice of professional nursing means the performance for compensation of any act in the observation, care, and counsel of the ill, injured, or infirm or in the maintenance of health or prevention of illness of others, or in the supervision and teaching of other personnel, or the administration of medications and treatments as prescribed by licensed physician or dentist, requiring substantial specialized judgment and skill and based on knowledge and application of the principles of biological, physical, and social sciences. The foregoing shall not be deemed to include acts

---

*From American Nurses' Association: Am. J. Nurs. 55:1474, 1955.

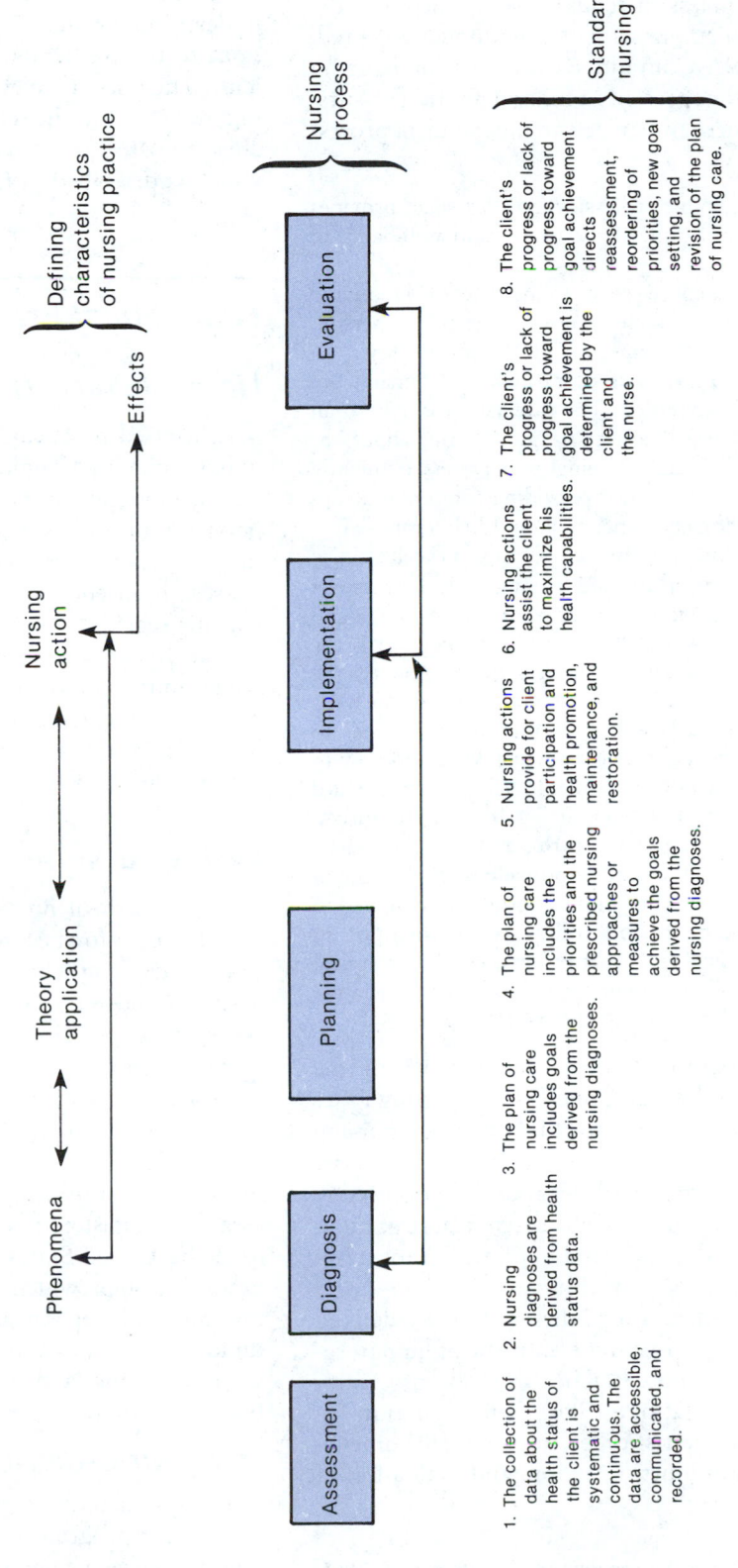

Fig. 1-3 Defining characteristics of nursing practice: relationship to the nursing process and the standards of nursing practice.

Modified from American Nurses' Association: A social policy statement, Kansas City, 1980, The Association.

of diagnosis or prescription of therapeutic or corrective measures.

This early definition by the ANA is significant in its attempt to define nursing practice in a fairly specific manner. Nonetheless, it tends to stress nursing's dependent role, an emphasis that is no longer accepted. In 1965 the ANA Committee on Education issued a position paper that presents a fuller definition of nursing and emphasizes nursing as an independent profession*:

Nursing is a helping profession and, as such, provides services which contribute to the health and well-being of people.

Nursing is a vital consequence to the individual receiving services; it fills needs which cannot be met by the person, by the family, or by other persons in the community.

The essential components of professional nursing are care, cure, and coordination. The care aspect is more than "to take care of", it is "caring for" and "caring about" as well. It is dealing with human beings under stress, frequently over long periods of time. It is providing comfort and support in times of anxiety, loneliness, and helplessness. It is listening, evaluating, and intervening appropriately.

The promotion of health and healing is the cure aspect of professional nursing. It is assisting patients to understand their health problems and helping them to cope. It is the administration of medications and treatments. And it is the use of clinical nursing judgment in determining, on the basis of patients' reactions, whether the plan for care needs to be maintained or changed. It is knowing when and how to use existing and potential resources to help patients toward recovery and adjustment by mobilizing their own resources.

Professional nursing practice is this and more. It is sharing responsibility for the health and welfare of all those in the community, and participating in programs designed to prevent illness and maintain health. It is coordinating and synchronizing medical and other professional and technical services as these affect patients. It is supervising, teaching, and directing all those who give nursing care.

In 1979 the Committee of Chairpersons of the ANA determined that the Congress for Nursing Practice should define the nature and scope of nursing practice. The Congress for Nursing Practice is the part of the ANA concerned with legal aspects of nursing practice, public recognition of the significance of nursing practice to health care, and implications for nursing practice of trends in health care.

In 1980 the Congress for Nursing Practice defined nursing as the diagnosis and treatment of human responses to actual or potential health problems (American Nurses' Association, 1980). This definition involves four characteristics of nursing: phenomena, theory application, nursing action, and evaluation of

the effects of action (Fig. 1-3). *Phenomena* are the human responses to actual or potential health problems. The nurse identifies the client's responses by assessing the client's health status and obtaining data about the client. The nurse uses nursing *theory* to understand the client's responses. The nurse takes *actions* to resolve actual or potential health care problems. The nurse then evaluates the *effects* of the nursing actions on the client's responses. These four characteristics are related to the nursing process, which is described in Unit 2.

Educational Preparation

Licensed Practical Nurse Education

A licensed practical or vocational nurse is trained in basic nursing techniques and direct client care. The licensed practical nurse (LPN) practices under the supervision of a registered nurse in a hospital or community health practice setting. Licensed practical nurses, licensed vocational nurses (LVNs), and in Canada registered nurse's assistants (RNAs) generally receive 1 year of education and training in a hospital, community college, or other agency. The licensed practical nurse is licensed by the state board of nursing after completing the educational program and passing the licensure examination.

Registered Nurse Education

The growth of nursing stimulated various educational routes for becoming a registered nurse (RN). Initially training schools were usually associated with a specific hospital. The primary purpose of such a school was to train nurses who would work within that institution after completing the training program.

As nursing increasingly defined its own body of knowledge, formalized educational processes developed to ensure a consistent level of nursing education in various institutions. Such consistency was also necessary for registered nurse licensure.

In the United States there are three types of programs through which an individual can become a registered nurse: the associate degree program, the diploma program, and the baccalaureate degree program. In Canada there are diploma programs and baccalaureate degree programs.

ASSOCIATE DEGREE EDUCATION

The associate degree program in the United States is a 2-year program usually offered by a college or junior college. The major focus of this program is on

---

*From American Nurses' Association: Am. J. Nurs. **65**:106, 1965.

theoretical and practical courses related to the practice of nursing. Graduates of the associate degree program take the state board examination for registered nurse licensure.

DIPLOMA EDUCATION

The diploma program in the United States is a 2- or 3-year program that is usually associated with a hospital. Some diploma programs are affiliated with a college or university, which grants college credit for nonnursing courses. Graduates of a diploma program receive a diploma from the hospital and take the state board examination for registered nurse licensure. In Canada diploma programs are offered in community colleges or hospitals and are 2-year programs (or 3 years in some hospital-based programs) comparable to associate degree programs in the United States.

BACCALAUREATE EDUCATION

The baccalaureate degree program is within a college or university and usually encompasses 4 years of study. The baccalaureate program focuses on theoretical and practical courses but also includes courses in the social sciences, basic sciences, and humanities to support nursing theory. In Canada either a Bachelor of Science in Nursing (BScN) or a Bachelor in Nursing (BN) is the equivalent to the Bachelor of Science in Nursing (BSN) in the United States.

ACCREDITATION AND LICENSURE

Associate degree, diploma, and baccalaureate degree programs must meet certain standards to remain accredited. These criteria are established by the state board of nursing and the National League for Nursing (NLN). The boxed material below and on pp. 14 to 17 describes the competencies expected of graduates from the three programs for basic nursing education in the United States.

Registered nurse licensure for practice in most states and provinces requires that the nurse complete a prescribed course of study in an accredited program. In the United States registered nurse candidates must pass the National Council Licensure Examination for Registered Nurses (NCLEX-RN), which is administered by each state's board of nursing. In Canada the Canadian Nurses' Association Testing Service (CNATS) administers the test to qualified candidates in each province. Whether a nurse in the United States or Canada can practice in a state or province other than her own depends on the reciprocal agreement between the two states or provinces involved. In some instances reciprocity is considered on an individualized basis.

Graduate Nursing Education

As expressed by the ANA (1969), the purpose of a graduate program in nursing is to prepare nurse

Text continued on p. 18.

Assumptions Basic to the Scope of Practice of the Associate Degree Nurse on Entry into Practice

The practice for graduates of associate degree nursing programs:

- Is directed toward clients who need information or support to maintain health
- Is directed toward clients who are in need of medical diagnostic evaluation and/or are experiencing acute or chronic illness
- Is directed toward clients' responses to common, well-defined health problems
- Includes the formulation of a nursing diagnosis
- Consists of nursing interventions selected from established nursing protocols where probable outcomes are predictable
- Is concerned with individual clients and is given with consideration of the person's relationship within a family, group, and community

- Includes the safe performance of nursing skills that require cognitive, psychomotor, and affective capabilities
- May be in any structured care setting but primarily occurs within acute- and extended-care facilities
- Is guided directly or indirectly by a more experienced registered nurse
- Includes the direction of peers or other workers in nursing in selected aspects of care within the scope of practice of associate degree nursing
- Involves an understanding of the roles and responsibilities of self and other workers within the employment setting

Continued.

From National League for Nursing: Competencies of the associate degree nurse on entry into practice, Pub. No. 23-1731, New York, 1978, The League.

Assumptions Basic to the Scope of Practice of the Associate Degree Nurse on Entry into Practice, cont'd

ROLES OF PRACTICE

Five interrelated roles have been defined for graduates of the associate degree nursing program based upon the above assumptions underlying the scope of practice. These roles are: provider of care, client teacher, communicator, manager of client care, and member within the profession of nursing. In each of these roles, decisions and practice are determined on the basis of knowledge and skills, the nursing process, and established protocols of the setting.

Role as a Provider of Care

As a provider of nursing care, the associate degree nursing graduate uses the nursing process to formulate and maintain individualized nursing care plans by:

Assessing

- Collects and contributes to a data base (physiological, emotional, sociological, cultural, psychological, and spiritual needs) from available resources (e.g., client, family, medical records, and other health team members)
- Identifies and documents changes in health status which interfere with the client's ability to meet basic needs (e.g., oxygen, nutrition, elimination, activity, safety, rest and sleep, and psychosocial well-being)
- Establishes a nursing diagnosis based on client needs

Planning

- Develops individualized nursing care plans based upon the nursing diagnosis and plans intervention that follows established nursing protocols
- Identifies needs and establishes priorities for care with recognition of client's level of development and needs, and with consideration of client's relationship within a family, group, and community
- Participates with clients, families, significant others, and members of the nursing team to establish long- and short-range client goals
- Identifies criteria for evaluation of individualized nursing care plans

Implementing

- Carries out individualized plans of care according to priority of needs and established nursing protocols

- Participates in the prescribed medical regime by preparing, assisting, and providing follow-up care to clients undergoing diagnostic and/or therapeutic procedures
- Uses nursing knowledge and skills and protocols to assure an environment conducive to optimum restoration and maintenance of the client's normal abilities to meet basic needs
  - Maintains and promotes respiratory function (e.g., oxygen therapy, positioning, etc.)
  - Maintains and promotes nutritional status (e.g., dietary regimes, supplemental therapy, intravenous infusions, etc.)
  - Maintains and promotes elimination (e.g., bowel and bladder regimes, forcing fluids, enemas, etc.)
  - Maintains and promotes a balance of activity, rest, and sleep (e.g., planned activities of daily living, environmental adjustment, exercises, sensory stimuli, assistive devices, etc.)
  - Maintains an environment which supports physiological functioning, comfort, and relief of pain
  - Maintains and promotes all aspects of hygiene
  - Maintains and promotes physical safety (e.g., implementation of medical and surgical aseptic techniques, etc.)
  - Maintains and promotes psychological safety through consideration of each individual's worth and dignity and applies nursing measures which assist in reducing common developmental and situational stress
  - Measures basic physiological functioning and reports significant findings (e.g., vital signs, fluid intake and output)
  - Administers prescribed medications safely
- Intervenes in situations where:
  - Basic life support systems are threatened (e.g., cardiopulmonary resuscitation, obstructive airway maneuver)
  - Untoward physiological or psychological reactions are probable
  - Changes in normal behavior patterns have occurred
- Participates in established institutional emergency plans

Evaluating

- Uses established criteria for evaluation of individualized nursing care
- Participates with clients, families, significant others, and members of the nursing team in the evaluation of established long- and short-range client goals
- Identifies alternate methods of meeting client's needs, modifies plans of care as necessary, and documents changes

Role as a Communicator

As a communicator, the associate degree nursing graduate:

- Assesses verbal and non-verbal communication of clients, families, and significant others based upon knowledge and techniques of interpersonal communication
- Uses lines of authority and communication within the work setting
- Uses communication skills as a method of data collection, nursing intervention, and evaluation of care
- Communicates and records assessments, nursing care plans, interventions, and evaluations accurately and promptly
- Establishes and maintains effective communication with clients, families, significant others, and health team members
- Communicates client's needs through the appropriate use of referrals
- Evaluates effectiveness of one's own communication with clients, colleagues, and others

Role as a Client Teacher

As a teacher of clients who need information or support to maintain health, the associate degree nursing graduate:

- Assesses situations in which clients need information or support to maintain health
- Develops short-range teaching plans based upon long- and short-range goals for individual clients

- Implements teaching plans that are specific to the client's level of development and knowledge
- Supports and reinforces the teaching plans of other health professionals
- Evaluates the effectiveness of client's learning

Role as a Manager of Client Care

As a manager of nursing care for a group of clients with common, well-defined health problems in structured settings, the associate degree nursing graduate:

- Assesses and sets nursing care priorities
- With guidance, provides client care utilizing resources and other nursing personnel commensurate with their educational preparation and experience
- Seeks guidance to assist other nursing personnel to develop skills in giving nursing care

Role as a Member within the Profession of Nursing

As a member within the profession of nursing, the associate degree nursing graduate:

- Is accountable for his or her nursing practice
- Practices within the profession's ethical and legal framework
- Assumes responsibility for self-development and uses resources for continued learning
- Consults with a more experienced registered nurse when client's problems are not within the scope of practice
- Participates within a structured role in research (e.g., data collection)
- Works within the policies of the employee or employing institution
- Recognizes policies and nursing protocols that may impede client care and works within the organizational framework to initiate change

Role and Competencies* of Graduates of Diploma Programs in Nursing

The graduate of the diploma program in nursing is eligible to seek licensure as a registered nurse and to function as a beginning practitioner in acute, intermediate, long-term, and ambulatory health care facilities. In order to fulfill such roles, graduates should demonstrate the following competencies:*

ASSESSMENT

- Establishes a data base through a nursing history including a psychosocial and physical assessment
- Utilizes knowledge of the etiology, pathophysiology, usual course, and prognosis for the prevalent illnesses and health problems
- Establishes priorities when providing nursing care for one or more patients
- Recognizes the significance of nonverbal communication

PLANNING

- Formulates a written plan of nursing care based on the assessment of patient needs
- Includes in the nursing care plan the effects of the family or significant others, life experiences, and social-cultural background
- Involves the patient, family, and significant others in the development of the nursing plan of care
- Incorporates the learning needs of the patient and family into an individualized plan of care
- Applies principles of organization and management in utilizing the knowledge and skills of other nursing personnel

IMPLEMENTATION

- Meets the health needs of individuals and families
- Utilizes concepts, scientific facts and principles when providing nursing care
- Performs technical nursing procedures
- Initiates appropriate intervention when environmental and safety hazards exist
- Initiates preventive, habilitative, and rehabilitative nursing measures according to the needs demonstrated by patients and families
- Performs independent nursing measures and/or seeks assistance from other members of the health team in response to the changing needs of patients.
- Collaborates with physicians and members of other disciplines to provide health care
- Documents nursing interventions and patient responses
- Utilizes effective verbal and written communication
- Communicates pertinent information related to the patient through established channels
- Assists the physician in implementing the medical plan of care
- Applies knowledge of individual and group behavior in establishing interpersonal relationships
- Teaches individuals and groups to achieve and maintain an optimum level of wellness
- Utilizes the services of community agencies for continuity of patient care
- Protects the rights of patients and families

EVALUATION

- Evaluates the effectiveness of nursing care and takes appropriate action
- Initiates and cooperates in efforts to improve nursing practice

PROFESSIONALISM

- Recognizes the legal limits of nursing practice
- Demonstrates ethical behavior in the performance of nursing
- Practices nursing in a nondiscriminatory and nonjudgmental manner
- Respects the rights of others to have their own value systems
- Accepts responsibility and accountability for professional practice
- Pursues independent study and continuing education
- Demonstrates flexibility in functioning in a changing society
- Adjusts with minimal difficulty to the role of employee

*Competency, as used in this document, is the ability to apply in practice situations the essential principles and techniques of nursing and to apply those concepts, skills, and attitudes required of all nurses to fulfill their role, regardless of their specific position or responsibility.

From National League for Nursing: Role and competencies of graduates of diploma programs in nursing, Pub. No. 16-1735, New York, 1978, The League.

Characteristics of Baccalaureate Education in Nursing

The baccalaureate program in nursing, which is offered by a senior college or university, provides students with an opportunity to acquire: (1) knowledge of the theory and practice of nursing; (2) competency in selecting, synthesizing, and applying relevant information from various disciplines; (3) ability to assess client needs and provide nursing intervention; (4) ability to provide care for groups of clients and ability to work with and through others; (5) ability to evaluate current practices and try new approaches; (6) competency in collaborating with members of other health disciplines and with consumers; (7) an understanding of the research process and of its contribution to nursing practice; (8) knowledge of the broad function the nursing profession is expected to perform in society; (9) a foundation for graduate study in nursing.

Nurses are prepared as generalists at the baccalaureate level. They provide within the health care system a comprehensive service that assesses, promotes, and maintains the health of individuals and groups. These nurses are prepared to: (1) be accountable for their own nursing practice; (2) accept responsibility for the provision of nursing care through others; (3) accept the advocacy role in relation to clients and, (4) develop methods of working collaboratively with other health professionals. They practice in a variety of health care settings—hospital, home, and community—and emphasize comprehensive health care, including prevention, health promotion, and rehabilitation services, health counseling and education, and care in acute and long-term illness.

Baccalaureate nursing programs are organized according to conceptual schema consistent with the stated philosophy and objectives of the parent institution and the unit in nursing. These programs provide the general and professional education essential for understanding and respecting people, various cultures, and environments; for acquiring and utilizing nursing theory upon which nursing practice is based; and for promoting self-understanding, personal fulfillment, and motivation for continued learning. The structure of the baccalaureate degree program in nursing follows the same pattern as that of baccalaureate education in general. It is characterized by a liberal education base at the lower division level on which is built the upper division major. In baccalaureate nursing education, the lower division consists of foundational courses drawn primarily from the scientific and humanistic disciplines inherent in liberal learning. The major in nursing is built upon this lower division general education base and is concentrated at the upper division level. Upper division studies also include courses that complement the nursing component or increase the depth of general education. Consistent with the foregoing characteristics and directly related to criteria as outlined in the Criteria for the Appraisal of Baccalaureate and Higher Degree Programs in Nursing, the graduate of the baccalaureate program in nursing is able to:

1. Utilize nursing theory as the basis for making nursing practice decisions
2. Use nursing practice as a means of gathering data for refining and extending that practice
3. Synthesize theoretical and empirical knowledge from the physical and behavioral sciences and humanities with nursing theory and practice
4. Assess health status and health potential, plan, implement, and evaluate nursing care with clients—individuals, families, and communities
5. Improve service to the client by continually evaluating the effectiveness of nursing intervention and revising accordingly
6. Accept individual responsibility and accountability for nursing actions
7. Evaluate research for applicability of its findings to nursing theory and practice
8. Utilize leadership skills through the involvement of others in meeting health needs and nursing goals
9. Collaborate with citizens and colleagues on the interdisciplinary health team to promote the health and welfare of people
10. Participate in identifying and effecting needed change to improve delivery within specific health care systems
11. Participate in identifying community and societal health needs and in designing nursing roles to meet these needs

These characteristics are developed by the professional nurse membership of the Council of Baccalaureate and Higher Degree Programs and are an expression of professional accountability to the consumer—student and/or client.

From National League for Nursing: Characteristics of baccalaureate education in nursing, New York, 1978, The League.

clinicians capable of improving nursing care through the advancement of nursing theory and sciences. Those completing a graduate program can receive the degree of Master of Arts in Nursing (MA), Master in Nursing (MN), or Master of Science in Nursing (MSN). The National League for Nursing has described the characteristics of and standards for accredited master's degree nursing programs (see box).

A master's degree in nursing can be valuable for nurses seeking expanded roles such as that of nurse educator or clinical nurse specialist. These roles are described in a later section of this chapter.

As nursing theory has developed, many nurses have desired the advanced knowledge and research skills required for a doctoral degree to further develop and test nursing theories. Nurses first earned doctoral degrees in the related fields of education, psychology, physiology, and sociology, because until the 1960s there were no doctoral programs in nursing. The doctoral degree further prepares the nurse for education, administration, research, and clinical practice.

Continuing Education

Changes are occurring continually in the sciences, in technology, and in nursing procedures. Continuing education programs have been developed to help nurses remain current in skills, knowledge, and theory related to nursing practice.

Continuing education involves formal, organized, educational programs offered by educational and health care institutions. As expressed by the ANA (1975), the goals of continuing education in nursing are (1) to improve and maintain nursing practice, (2) to promote and exercise leadership in effecting change in health care delivery systems, and (3) to fulfill professional learning needs. Other goals include helping nurses become specialized in a particular area of practice and teaching nurses new skills and techniques.

In general, continuing education programs are short term and are designed for all professional nurses. The ANA or the state board of nursing is the accrediting agency for continuing education programs. The ANA awards continuing education units on completion of specific courses. Some states require nurses to take continuing education courses for license renewal (Table 1-2).

In-Service Education

In-service education programs are instruction or training that is provided by a health care agency or institution in which nurses are employed. An in-service program is held in the institution and is de-

---

Characteristics of Graduate Education in Nursing Leading to the Master's Degree

The master's program in nursing is offered by an educational institution of higher learning and is built upon a baccalaureate curriculum that has included an upper division major in nursing. It provides students with an opportunity to: (1) acquire advanced knowledge from the sciences and the humanities to support advanced nursing practice and role development; (2) expand knowledge of nursing theory as a basis for advanced nursing practice; (3) develop expertise in a specialized area of clinical nursing practice; (4) acquire the knowledge and skills related to a specific functional role in nursing; (5) acquire initial competence in conducting research; (6) plan and/or initiate change in the health care system, and in the practice and delivery of health care; (7) further develop and implement leadership strategies for the betterment of health care; (8) actively engage in collaborative relationships with others for the purpose of improving health care; and (9) acquire a foundation for doctoral study.

Modified from National League for Nursing: Characteristics of graduate education in nursing leading to the master's degree, New York, 1978, The League.

---

signed to increase the knowledge, skills, and competencies of nurses and other health care professionals employed by the institution. For example, a hospital might offer an in-service program to inform nurses about primary nursing before it is implemented at the hospital.

All nurses have access to continuing education and in-service programs organized and conducted by a university, private hospital, private continuing education service, or the employing institution or agency. Such programs assist the practicing nurse in acquiring new knowledge and skills necessary for today's highly technical and fast-changing health care delivery system.

Career Mobility and Clinical Ladder

Education continues to be important after the nurse begins to practice as a registered nurse. In addition to continuing and in-service education designed to give practicing nurses new knowledge and skills, educational programs are designed to help nurses advance in their careers. Career advancement is often linked to the ongoing debate concerning the three

TABLE 1-2

Mandatory Continuing Education

State	CE contact hours required
For registered nurses	
California	30 hours every 2-year relicensure period (all 30 may be in home study)
Colorado	20 hours every 2-year relicensure period (5 may be in home study)
Florida	24 hours every 2-year relicensure period (all 24 may be in home study)
Iowa	45 hours every 3-year relicensure period (15 may be in home study)
Kansas	30 hours every 2-year relicensure period: '82-'84 (6 may be in home study in '82-'84)
Kentucky	15 hours every 1-year relicensure period (home study permitted only for licensees living or working outside of United States)
Massachusetts	10 hours every 2-year relicensure period: '82-'84 15 hours every 2-year period: '84-'86 (all 10, 15 may be in home study)
Minnesota	30 hours every 2-year relicensure period (all 30 may be in home study)
Nebraska	75 hours every 5 years *or* 20 hours + 200 hours of practice every 5 years (licenses must be renewed every year; no provision for home study)
Nevada	30 hours every 2-year relicensure period (10 may be in home study)
New Mexico	30 hours every 2-year relicensure period (all 30 may be in home study)
For nurse practitioners	
Alaska	30 hours every 2-year relicensure period (home study provision is pending)
Idaho	60 hours every 2-year relicensure period (30 may be in home study)
Mississippi	40 hours every 2-year relicensure period (no home study permitted)
New Hampshire	20 hours every 2-year relicensure period (no home study permitted)
Oregon	100 hours every 2-year relicensure period + 25 hours pharmacological CE if NP prescribes (50 may be in home study)

types of educational programs for registered nurses. The ANA Committee on Education in a 1965 position paper differentiated between what it called the "professional nurse" with a baccalaureate degree and the "technical nurse" with an associate degree or diploma. This debate involves complex issues and need not be described here. Different institutions and health care agencies approach the issues of educational preparation in different ways, however, and the nurse in a particular practice setting may require further education for career advancement. If more career opportunities in a given setting are open to a baccalaureate graduate, for example, an associate degree or diploma nurse may at some point choose to pursue a baccalaureate degree. There are various kinds of specialized educational programs designed specifically to help nurses meet educational requirements for career advancement.

In the past, career mobility for nurses was some-what limited. However, with expanding roles in nursing practice, this situation has changed. The clinical ladder approach to advancement (Fig. 1-4) has been discussed in many nursing journals and put into practice in various settings (Anderson and Denyes, 1975; Colavecchio, Tescher, and Scalzi, 1975; Zimmer, 1972). The clinical ladder unifies clinical practice and nursing administration, fosters collaboration between nursing education and nursing service, and is a professional advancement system. This approach recognizes that nursing is practiced at several levels of skill and competence and that clinical nurses should be rewarded according to their level of expertise. (Knox, 1980). This kind of advancement program encourages and motivates nurses who remain in the health care setting. In addition, it induces both new and experienced nurses to increase their expertise by upgrading their skills, knowledge, and educational preparation. Finally, it gives nurses the opportunity for

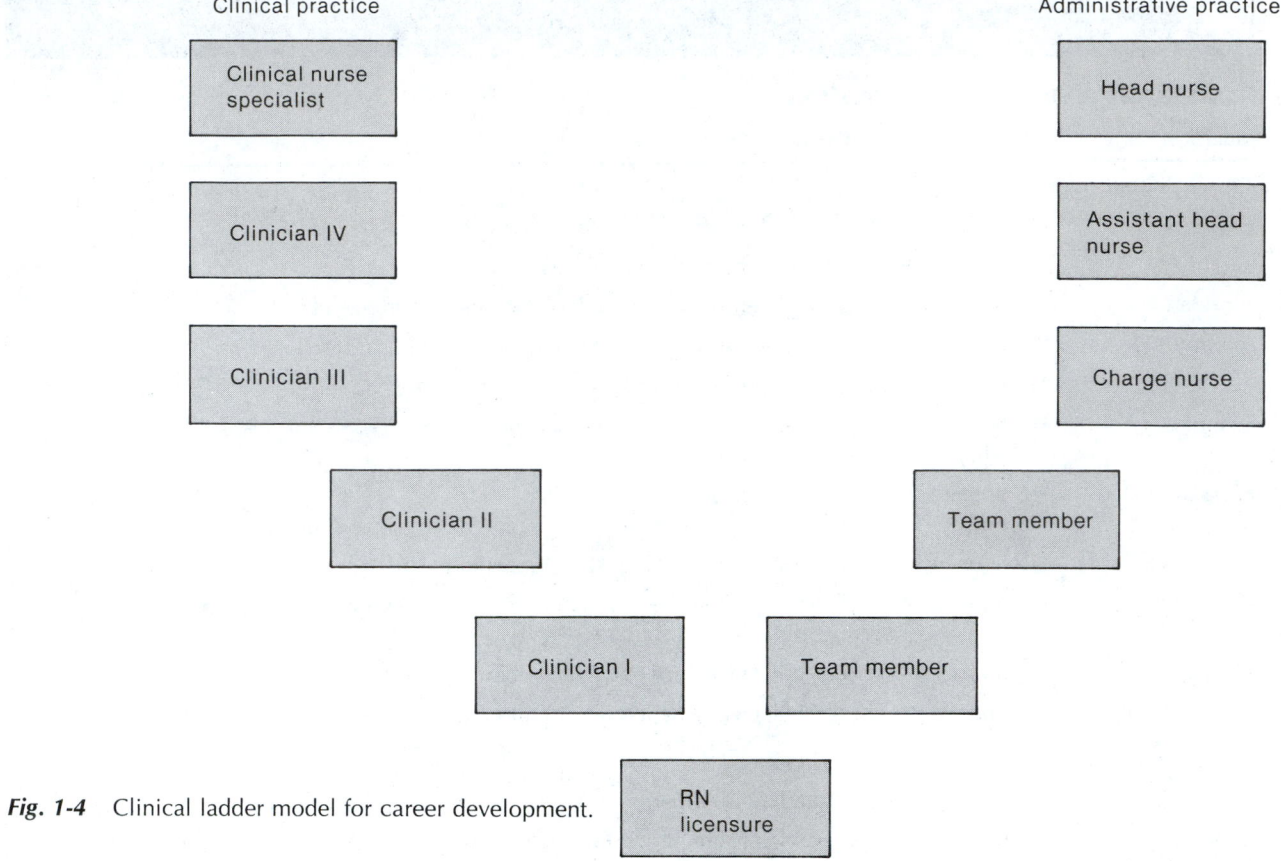

Clinical practice

Administrative practice

Fig. 1-4 Clinical ladder model for career development.

advancement through clinical practice, whereas previously most nurses in hospitals could advance only in administration.

Nursing Practice

Nurses practice in a variety of settings, in many roles within those settings, and with other care givers in the allied health professions. The practice of nursing is guided only in part by administrators in hospitals and other health care agencies and institutions. State and provincial nurse practice acts establish specific legal regulations for nursing practice, and professional organizations establish standards of nursing practice as criteria for nursing care.

Standards of Nursing Practice

As nursing has become more independent as a profession, it has increasingly set its own standards for practice. Such standards are important both as guidelines for providing care and as criteria for evaluating care. When standards are clearly defined, clients can be assured they are receiving high-quality care, nurses know exactly what is necessary to give nursing care, and administrators can determine that care meets acceptable standards. Moreover, standards of practice are important if a legal dispute arises over whether adequate care was provided in a particular case (see Chapter 17). Both the ANA and the CNA have published standards of nursing practice (Tables 1-3 and 1-4).

Nurse Practice Acts

In all states in the United States and all provinces in Canada, nurse practice acts regulate the licensure and practice of nursing. Each state or province defines for itself the scope of nursing practice, but most states and provinces have similar practice acts. The definition of nursing practice published by the ANA in 1955 (see p. 10) is in some ways representative of the scope of nursing practice as defined in most states and provinces. In the last decade, however, many states have revised their nurse practice acts to reflect nursing's growing autonomy and the expanded roles of nurses in practice. The 1955 ANA prohibition against diagnosis and treatment, for example, has been removed from nurse practice acts in many states or

TABLE 1-3

American Nurses' Association Standards of Nursing Practice

Standard	Rationale
1. The collection of data about the health status of the client/patient is systematic and continuous. The data are accessible, communicated, and recorded.	Comprehensive care requires complete and ongoing collection of data about the client/patient to determine the nursing care and needs of the client/patient. All health status data about the client/patient must be available for all members of the health care team.
2. Nursing diagnoses are derived from health status data.	The health status of the client/patient is the basis for determining the nursing care needs. The data are analyzed and compared to norms when possible.
3. The plan of nursing care includes goals derived from the nursing diagnoses.	The determination of the results to be achieved is an essential part of planning care.
4. The plan of nursing care includes priorities and the prescribed nursing approaches or measures to achieve the goals derived from the nursing diagnoses.	Nursing actions are planned to promote, maintain, and restore the client/patient's well-being.
5. Nursing actions provide for client/patient participation in health promotion, maintenance, and restoration.	The client/patient and family are continually involved in nursing care.
6. The nursing actions assist the client/patient to maximize his health capabilities.	Nursing actions are designed to promote, maintain, and restore health.
7. The client/patient's progress or lack of progress toward goal achievements is determined by the client/patient and the nurse.	The quality of nursing care depends upon comprehensive and intelligent determination of nursing's impact upon the health status of the client/patient. The client/patient is an essential part of this determination.
8. The client/patient's progress or lack of progress toward goal achievement directs reassessment, reordering of priorities, new goal setting, and revision of the plan of nursing care.	The nursing process remains the same, but the input of new information may dictate new or revised approaches.

From American Nurses' Association: Standards of nursing practice, Kansas City, Mo., 1973, The Association.

rephrased to differentiate between nursing diagnosis and treatment and medical diagnosis and treatment. Nurse practice acts are discussed in more detail in Chapter 17.

Practice Settings

As nursing's role in the health care system has expanded, the settings in which nurses practice have also increased. Table 1-5 gives statistics on the numbers of nurses in various practice settings. The most common practice settings for nurses are described in the following sections.

HOSPITALS AND OTHER INSTITUTIONS

More nurses are employed in hospitals than in any other type of practice setting. A 1980 survey indicated that 65.6% of all employed nurses practice in hos-

pitals (Department of Health and Human Services, 1982). In hospitals, nursing services operate 24 hours a day. Hospitals use various staffing patterns to meet the need for nursing care. Some hospitals have three 8-hour shifts, whereas other hospitals use three 10-hour shifts that overlap during the early morning and late afternoon.

The roles and responsibilities of nurses employed in hospitals vary because hospitals themselves vary widely in size and bureaucratic structure. Hospitals usually have many policies and regulations governing nursing activities, as well as other health care activities, and responsibilities tend to be clearly divided among nurses and other health care professionals.

Clients in hospitals generally require 24-hour nursing care. Hospital settings include those providing acute, long-term, and rehabilitational care. The nurse in an acute care setting usually cares for clients with

TABLE 1-4

Summary of Canadian Nurses' Association Standards for Nursing Practice

Standard	Elements
I. Nursing practice requires that a conceptual model for nursing be the basis for the independent part of that practice.	1. Nurses are required to have a clear idea or conception of the distinct goal of nursing. 2. Nurses are required to have a clear idea or conception of the client. 3. Nurses are required to have a clear idea or conception of their role in response to the health needs of society. 4. Nurses are required to have a clear idea or conception of the source of client difficulty. 5. Nurses are required to have a clear idea or conception of the focus and modes of nursing intervention. 6. Nurses are required to have a clear idea or conception of the expected consequences of nursing activities.
II. Nursing practice requires the effective use of the nursing process as the method for carrying out the independent, interdependent, and dependent functions of nursing practice.	1. Nurses are required to collect data in accordance with their conception of the client and consistent with their interdependent and dependent functions. 2. Nurses are required to analyze data collected in accordance with their conception of the goal of nursing, their role, and the source of client difficulty, and consistent with their interdependent and dependent functions. 3. Nurses are required to plan their nursing actions based upon the identified actual and potential client problems, in accordance with their conception of the focus and modes of intervention and consistent with their interdependent and dependent functions. 4. Nurses are required to perform nursing actions that implement the plan. 5. Nurses are required to evaluate all steps of the nursing process in accordance with their conceptual model for nursing and consistent with their interdependent and dependent functions.
III. Nursing practice requires that the helping relationship be the nature of the client-nurse interaction.	1. Nurses are required to increase the likelihood that the client will perceive the health service experience as understandable, manageable, and meaningful at the outset. 2. Nurses are required to set mutually agreed upon expectations as a means of increasing the likelihood that the client will perceive the health service experience as understandable, manageable, and meaningful. 3. Nurses are required to ensure a successful termination of the helping relationship.
IV. Nursing practice requires nurses to fulfill professional responsibilities in their independent, interdependent, and dependent functions.	1. Nurses are required to respect statutes and policies relevant to the profession and the practice setting. 2. Nurses are required to comply with the Code of Ethics of their profession. 3. Nurses are required to function as members of a health team.

Modified from Canadian Nurses' Association: A definition of nursing practice standards for nursing practice, Ottawa, 1980, The Association.

TABLE 1-5

Employment Setting of Primary Position of Registered Nurses Employed in Nursing

Employment Setting	United States*	Canada†
Hospital	835,646	118,494
Nursing homes or extended care facilities	101,209	9,608
Public/community health	83,436	14,838
Physicians' or dentists' offices	71,972	4,260
Student health services	44,906	—
Nursing education	47,501	4,650
Other	81,916	5,451
Not known	7,249	3,769
TOTAL	1,272,851	161,070

*Data from Department of Health and Human Services: The registered nurse population: an overview, DHHS Pub. No. HRS-POD-83-1, Washington D.C., 1980, U.S. Government Printing Office.
†Data from Health Division Statistics Canada, Health Manpower Statistics Section, Revised Registered Nurse Data Series, 1981.

severe illnesses and more complex problems. Clients in an acute care setting are usually more dependent and more seriously ill than in the past because periods of hospitalization are now shorter (Department of Health and Human Services, 1982). As a result, nursing practice in acute care settings has become more specialized and complex. The skills and knowledge a nurse needs to practice in an acute care setting depend on the clinical area.

The rapid rise in the number of the elderly, clients with chronic illnesses, and clients with functional impairments has resulted in the growth of long-term care facilities. Most long-term care is provided in institutions such as chronic disease hospitals, psychiatric hospitals, and nursing homes. Nursing homes are the most common agencies providing in-house long-term care.

Rehabilitation institutions generally employ many types of health professionals. The goal of such institutions is to teach the client how to achieve a maximal level of function and his family how to help him reach that level.

In both chronic care and rehabilitation institutions, as in hospitals, nurses generally have multiple roles and responsibilities. The extent of specialization and nurses' independence from other health care professionals varies from institution to institution.

COMMUNITY SETTINGS

Since 1974 the number of nurses employed in community-based practice settings has increased substantially. The escalating costs of institutional care have underscored the need for community-based nursing services aimed at health promotion and disease pre-

vention. Approximately 2% of the North American population is in acute, long-term, or other institutional settings at any given time. The remaining population receives health care in the community, at home, at school, and at work.

Nursing in community-based settings is concerned primarily with health promotion, health maintenance, health education and management, and coordination and continuity of care within the community. Community-based nurses try to determine the health needs of individuals, families, and communities and help their clients cope with threats to their health and with problems of illness. Whereas institutional health care focuses on the individual and his family, community-based nursing is directed toward the health of the community and the interaction of individuals within that community. A community can be a particular location, as in an urban or rural area, or a group of people related by occupation, school, or some other common interest or characteristic. Thus, community-based nurses are employed in a variety of practice settings: community health centers, schools, occupational health, home health care, and private practice.

COMMUNITY HEALTH CENTERS. A community health center offers comprehensive programs for health maintenance, health promotion, health education and management, and coordination of care within the community. Community health centers provide ambulatory care as well as care within the home. Persons seeking health care at a community health center usually live near the center.

Nurses employed in community health centers often work more independently than nurses working in institutional settings. Community health centers also employ other health professionals, but generally nurses provide most of the care. In some settings physicians are called in only when specific needs arise. Examples of community health centers are planned parenthood clinics, family care centers, and mental health centers.

SCHOOLS. Community-based health services are common in schools and on college campuses. Nursing services include health education in such areas as disease prevention, health promotion, and sex education. In addition, nurses working in schools may provide care for students with nonemergency acute illnesses such as upper respiratory tract infections, influenza, and viruses. School nurses also make referrals for students and their families when additional, more specialized health care is needed.

OCCUPATIONAL HEALTH. Health services are provided by many companies in large office buildings and factories. Nursing care in such settings involves five areas. First, the nurse may develop programs aimed at increasing health and safety in the workplace by reducing occupational accidents, the risk of occupational disease, or the transmission of a contagious disease among the work force. The nurse may provide programs for health promotion, disease prevention, and health education to employees. The nurse also treats nonemergency acute illnesses and provides first aid. In emergency situations, such as heart attacks or trauma, the nurse gives emergency care and arranges transportation to a hospital. The nurse in an occupational setting also refers employees to additional health resources.

HOME HEALTH CARE AGENCIES. Often a client needs specific nursing care that can be given efficiently in the home. A home health care agency provides this care. Such agencies include visiting nurse associations, public health nursing agencies, and private home care agencies.

OTHER SETTINGS

The settings described previously are the most common areas in which nurses are employed, but there are a number of other practice settings, in which nurses' roles and responsibilities vary widely. A nurse employed in a physician's office, for example, may have little independent responsibility, but a nurse in sole practice or joint practice with other nurses or other health care professionals may provide nursing care with much independence. Nurses are also employed in educational and research positions.

Roles and Functions of the Nurse

Contemporary nursing requires that the nurse possess knowledge and skills in a variety of areas. In the past the principal role of nurses was to provide care and comfort as they carried out specific nursing functions, but changes in nursing have expanded the roles of nurses to include an increased emphasis on health promotion and illness prevention, as well as a concern for the client as a whole. The contemporary nurse functions in the interrelated roles of care giver, decision maker, client advocate, manager, rehabilitator, comforter, communicator, and teacher.

CARE GIVER

As care giver, the nurse helps the client regain health through the healing process. Healing is more than just curing a specific disease, although treatment skills that promote physical healing are important to the nurse in this role. The nurse addresses the holistic health care needs of the client, including measures to restore the client's emotional and social well-being. The nurse as care giver helps clients and their families set goals and meet those goals with a minimal cost of time and energy.

DECISION MAKER

To provide effective care, nurses use decision-making skills throughout the nursing process. Before undertaking any nursing action, whether it is assessing the client's condition, giving care, or evaluating the results of care, the nurse plans the action by deciding the best approach for the individual client. In some situations the nurse makes such decisions alone or with the client and family, and in other cases she works with other nurses or health care professionals in planning nursing care.

PROTECTOR AND CLIENT ADVOCATE

As protector the nurse helps maintain a safe environment for the client and takes steps to prevent injury and to protect the client from possible adverse effects of diagnostic or treatment measures. Confirming that a client does not have an allergy to a medication to be administered in a hospital and providing immunization against disease in a community-based practice are examples of the nurse's protective role. In the role of client advocate, the nurse protects the client's human and legal rights and assists him in asserting those rights if the need arises. The nurse may also defend clients' rights in a general way by speaking out against policies or actions that might endanger clients' well-being or conflict with their rights.

MANAGER

In various situations in which nursing care is provided, the nurse acts as manager and coordinator. Management of a client's care may include delegating some responsibility to and supervising other health care workers. Nurses must also manage their own time and the resources of the practice setting when providing care to several clients concurrently. The nurse coordinates the activities of others in the health care team, such as nutritionists and physical therapists, in managing the client's total care.

REHABILITATOR

Rehabilitation is the process by which a person returns to maximal functioning after an illness, accident, or other disabling event. Many such clients experience alterations that change their lives, and the nurse as rehabilitator helps them adapt as fully as possible. Rehabilitative activities range from teaching a client how to walk with crutches to helping a client cope with severe exacerbations of chronic illness.

COMFORTER

The role of comforter, caring for the client as a person, is a traditional and historical one in nursing and has continued to be important as nurses have assumed new roles. Because nursing care must be directed to the whole person rather than simply the body, comfort and emotional support are often important in giving the client strength to recover. While carrying out nursing activities, the nurse can provide comfort by demonstrating care for the client as an individual human being with unique feelings and needs. As comforter, the nurse should help the client reach therapeutic goals rather than encouraging him to become emotionally or physically dependent on the nurse.

COMMUNICATOR

The role of communicator is central to all other nursing roles. Without clear communication it is impossible to give care effectively, make decisions with the client and family, protect the client from threats to his well-being, coordinate and manage client care, assist the client in rehabilitation, offer comfort, or teach the client. Nursing involves almost constant communication with clients and families, other nurses and health care professionals, resource persons, and the community. The quality of communication is a critical factor in meeting the health needs of individuals, families, and communities.

TEACHER

Teaching involves many kinds of activities beyond what is often considered the traditional classroom teacher's role. As teacher, the nurse explains to clients concepts and facts concerning health, demonstrates procedures such as self-care activities, determines that the client fully understands, reinforces learning or client behavior, evaluates the client's progress in learning, and so on. All of these, in addition to the direct presentation of information, can be considered teaching. Some kinds of teaching are unplanned and informal, as when a nurse responds to a client's question about a health issue in casual conversation. Other teaching activities may be planned and more formal, as when the nurse teaches a diabetic client how to administer his own injections. Teaching is involved in the full range of nursing activities directed toward helping the client achieve a high level of health. To help the client learn, the nurse uses teaching methods that match his capabilities and needs and incorporates other resources, such as the family, in teaching plans.

Career Roles

The preceding roles and functions of the nurse are true of most nurses in most practice settings. *Career roles,* on the other hand, are specific employment positions. Table 1-6 gives a statistical breakdown of nursing positions classified by job title. This table shows that most registered nurses are general duty or staff nurses practicing in institutional or community settings, as described previously. With increasing educational opportunities for nurses and the growth of nursing as a profession, along with a greater concern for job enrichment, nursing now involves expanded roles offering different kinds of career opportunities. These include the nurse as educator, clinical nurse specialist, nurse practitioner, certified nurse-midwife, anesthetist, administrator, and researcher. Many physicians and other health care professionals, in addition to nurses themselves, support these expanded nursing roles (White, 1977).

NURSE EDUCATOR

Nurse educators work primarily in three areas: schools of nursing, staff development departments of health care agencies, and client education departments. Nursing educators generally have a background in clinical nursing, which provides them with practical skills as well as theoretical knowledge. A faculty member in a school of nursing prepares students to perform as nurses. Nursing faculty members are responsible for teaching current nursing practice as well as necessary skills in laboratory or clinical settings.

Nurse educators in staff development departments of health care institutions provide educational programs for nurses within their institution. Such pro-

---

TABLE 1-6

Position Titles of Registered Nurses Employed in Primary Nursing Jobs

Position Title or Type of Position	United States*	Canada†
Administrator	61,414	11,640
Clinical nursing specialist	19,070	1,971
General duty/staff nurse	824,841	104,986
Head nurse	90,202	16,503
Instructor	60,322	4,164
Other	202,513	7,904
Not known	6,547	13,897
TOTAL	1,272,851	161,065

*Data from Department of Health and Human Services: The registered nurse population: an overview, DHHS Pub. No. HRS-POD-83-1, Washington D.C., 1982, U.S. Government Printing Office.
†Data from Health Division Statistics Canada, Health Manpower Statistics Section, Revised Registered Nurse Data Series, 1981.

---

grams include orientation of new personnel, critical care nursing courses, and instruction about new equipment or procedures.

The primary focus of the nurse educator in an agency's department of client education is to teach the ill or disabled client and his family how to provide care in the home. In most health care agencies, however, the budget does not permit a separate client education department. Therefore staff nurses usually incorporate education into a client's plan of care.

Nurse educators are usually required to have graduate nursing education. In addition, they generally have a specific clinical specialty and advanced clinical experience.

CLINICAL NURSE SPECIALIST

The clinical nurse specialist has a master's degree in nursing and expertise in a specialized area of practice. Clinical nurse specialists work in critical care, acute care, long-term care, and community health care agencies. In addition, a clinical nurse specialist may specialize in the management of a disease such as cancer, diabetes, or cardiovascular or pulmonary disease or in a specific field such as pediatrics or gerontology. The clinical nurse specialist functions as a clinician, educator, manager, consultant, and researcher within the area of practice to plan, or improve the quality of, nursing care for the client and his family.

NURSE PRACTITIONER

The nurse practitioner provides health care to clients, usually in an outpatient or community setting

(Roy and Obloy, 1978). A nurse practitioner may work with clients in a specific group or with clients of all ages. There are four practitioner categories: adult nurse practitioner, family nurse practitioner, pediatric nurse practitioner, and obstetrics-gynecology nurse practitioner. A nurse practitioner should have the knowledge and skills necessary to detect and manage both acute self-limited and chronic stable conditions. The nurse practitioner's educational preparation includes either a practitioner program or a master's degree in nursing.

An *adult nurse practitioner* (ANP) provides primary, ambulatory care to adults with a nonemergency acute or chronic illness. ANPs are usually employed in ambulatory care centers or outpatient clinics and work in collaboration with a primary physician.

A *family nurse practitioner* (FNP) provides primary, ambulatory care for families, usually in collaboration with a family care physician. The FNP meets the family's general health care needs, manages some illnesses by providing direct care, and guides or counsels the family as needed.

A *pediatric nurse practitioner* (PNP) provides health care to infants and children.

An *obstetrics-gynecology nurse practitioner* provides primary ambulatory care to women seeking obstetrical or gynecological health care. If she is also a certified nurse-midwife, she may independently deliver infants.

CERTIFIED NURSE-MIDWIFE

A certified nurse-midwife (CNM) is educated in both nursing and midwifery and is certified by the

American College of Nurse-Midwives. The practice of nurse-midwifery involves providing independent care for women during normal pregnancy, labor, and delivery and for the newborn. It may include some gynecological services such as routine Pap smears, family planning, and treatment for minor vaginal infections. Nurse-midwives practice in conjunction with a health care agency that provides medical consultation, collaborative management, and referral.

NURSE ANESTHETIST

A nurse anesthetist is a registered nurse who has received advanced training in an accredited program in anesthesiology. Nurse anesthetists provide surgical anesthesia under the guidance and supervision of an anesthesiologist, who is a physician with advanced knowledge of surgical anesthesia. Nurse anesthetists frequently administer anesthetics to clients undergoing minor surgery.

NURSE ADMINISTRATOR

A nurse administrator manages client care and the delivery of specific nursing services within a health care agency. She may hold a middle management position, such as head nurse or supervisor, or an upper-level management position, such as assistant or associate director or director of nursing services. Middle management positions usually require at least a baccalaureate degree in nursing, and upper-level positions generally require a master's degree in nursing.

NURSE RESEARCHER

The nurse researcher investigates nursing problems to improve nursing care and to further define and expand the scope of nursing practice. The nurse researcher may be employed in an academic setting or in an independent professional or community service agency. The minimum educational requirement is a graduate degree in nursing.

Health Care Team

In most practice settings the nurse works with other health care professionals to provide total care for clients. The health care team is comprised of four general types of professionals: nurses, physicians, allied health professionals such as technicians, and other specialists such as social workers and chaplains. The involvement of many different persons in the client's health care, however, holds the risk of fragmenting care. Because nurses have the greatest opportunity to interact with all the other professionals in the health care team, they often have the role of coordinating and integrating various services within the plan of care. The following sections briefly describe the professionals with whom the nurse most commonly collaborates in practice settings.

PHYSICIAN

A physician is a professional who has earned a degree of Doctor of Medicine (MD) or Doctor of Osteopathy (DO). The physician has completed a required curriculum, has had a specific period of postgraduate training, and has passed a licensing examination. A physician is licensed for the medical diagnosis and treatment of clients.

Most physicians specialize in diseases that involve one body system (for example, a cardiologist specializes in heart diseases) or in one specific disease, (for example, an oncologist specializes in cancer). Physicians may also specialize in surgery or in treating a certain age group.

Nurses work with physicians in various capacities. One nurse may work in a setting in which most of the nursing care depends on the physician's orders. An intensive care nurse may follow written guidelines that permit more independent nursing actions. A clinical nurse specialist or nurse practitioner may function in a collaborative capacity with a physician; for example, in preparing a client with newly diagnosed diabetes for discharge, the nurse and physician work together to teach the client and family about home care.

PHYSICIAN ASSISTANT

A physician assistant (PA) is trained in certain aspects of the practice of medicine to provide support to physicians. PAs practice in the United States but not in Canada. A PA must work under the direction and supervision of a physician. PAs practice in hospitals, clinics, or private physicians' offices.

Nurses usually work with PAs in the same way they work with physicians. In some rural areas the PA is always present in the hospital or clinic and may assume some of the tasks of the physician.

ALLIED HEALTH PROFESSIONALS

THERAPIST. A *physical therapist* (PT) is licensed to assist in the examination, testing, and treatment of physically disabled or handicapped people through the use of special exercises, the application of heat and cold, the use of sonar waves, and other techniques. PTs usually receive their training in a 4-year college course leading to a bachelor of science degree in physical therapy. They practice in hospitals, clinics, rehabilitation centers, and community-based agencies.

An *occupational therapist* (OT) is licensed or certified to develop and use adaptive devices that help the chronically ill or handicapped carry out activities of daily living. OTs usually receive their education and training in a 4-year college program. Like PTs, OTs work in a variety of settings.

A *respiratory therapist* (RT) is licensed to deliver treatment that is designed to improve clients' ventilatory function or oxygenation. Educational and training programs for RTs vary from 6-month training programs to educational programs in 4-year colleges. RTs are usually employed in institutional health care settings.

Nurses work with PTs, OTs, and RTs in a collaborative capacity. The care initiated by a PT, OT, or RT is frequently continued and evaluated by a nurse. Nurses and therapists together consider the client's progress and develop goals and discharge plans that include the client and the family. In addition, nurses refer clients to therapists for further care. For example, a nurse caring for a person with severe pulmonary disease may refer the client to a PT to learn exercises for strengthening the upper arm muscles, to an OT to learn energy-saving techniques for activities of daily living, and to an RT for techniques to promote airway clearance.

PHARMACIST. A pharmacist is a licensed professional who formulates and dispenses medications. The pharmacist may practice only within a pharmacy or may be involved in client care conferences or in the development of medication administration systems (see Chapter 32). The pharmacist's education ranges from a bachelor of science degree to a doctorate in pharmacology. Pharmacists practice in institutional and outpatient settings.

The pharmacist is a valuable resource for nurses. For example, the nurse can request information about new drugs from the pharmacist. The nurse must know the action, desired effect, correct dosage, and side effects of all drugs that are administered. If this information is not available in standard reference books such as textbooks or hospital formularies, the nurse should consult the pharmacist.

Pharmacists also provide information about which drugs are compatible and can be mixed or administered together. In addition, the pharmacist can tell the nurse which over-the-counter drugs may interact adversely with prescribed drugs so that the nurse can incorporate this information into the discharge teaching plan for the client.

SOCIAL WORKER. A social worker is trained to counsel clients and their families. Counseling services provided by a social worker may include providing emotional support for a client and family during a severe or terminal illness, arranging placement in an extended care facility, and locating financial resources for clients. The social worker generally has a baccalaureate or master's degree in social work. Social workers are employed in every type of agency in the health care system.

Nurses frequently refer clients to social workers. The social worker and the nurse work together to identify resources for meeting the client's present and future health care needs.

CHAPLAIN. Chaplains offer spiritual support and guidance to clients and their families. A chaplain may be employed by an agency or institution or be provided by a church within the community. A client may request to see a chaplain, or the nurse may initiate a referral.

Nursing as a Profession

Professionalism

Nursing is not simply a collection of specific skills, and the nurse is not simply a person trained to perform specific tasks. Nursing has evolved into a profession. As is implied by the number and complexity of roles the nurse assumes in the practice of nursing, the contemporary nurse is a professional.

There is no one factor that absolutely differentiates a job from a profession, but the difference is important in terms of how nurses practice. When we say a person acts "professionally," for example, we imply that the person is conscientious in actions, knowledgeable in the subject, and responsible to self and others. What does it mean, then, for an occupation to be a profession? How should professionalism guide the behavior of the members of the profession and shape the attitudes and activities of the profession as a whole?

Etzioni (1961) describes professions in terms of five primary characteristics:

1. A profession requires an extended education of its members in addition to a basic liberal foundation.
2. A profession has a theoretical body of knowledge leading to defined skills, abilities, and norms.
3. A profession provides a specific service.
4. Members of a profession have autonomy in decision making and practice.
5. The profession as a whole has a code of ethics for practice.

Nursing clearly shares, to some extent, each of these characteristics of a profession. Nursing is still evolving as a profession, however, and faces controversial issues as nurses strive for greater professionalism.

EDUCATION

An earlier section describes the three types of educational preparation for registered nurses. As a profession, nursing requires that its members possess a significant education, and the issue of standardization of education is a major controversy in nursing today. Most nurses agree, however, that nursing education is of great importance to practice and that nursing education must respond to the changes in health care created by scientific and technological advances. The ANA's 1965 position paper on nursing

---

Eight Premises for ANA's First Position Paper on Education for Nursing

- Nursing is a helping profession and, as such, provides services which contribute to the health and well-being of people.
- Nursing is of vital consequence to the individual receiving services; it fills needs which cannot be met by the person, by the family, or by other persons in the community.
- The demand for services of nurses will continue to increase.
- The professional practitioner is responsible for the nature and quality of all nursing care patients receive.
- The services of professional practitioners of nursing will continue to be supplemented and complemented by the services of nurse practitioners who will be licensed.
- Education for those in the health professions must increase in depth and breadth as scientific knowledge expands.
- In addition to those licensed as nurses, the health care of the public, in the amount and to the extent needed and demanded, requires the services of large numbers of health occupation workers to function as assistants to nurses. These workers are presently designated: nurses' aids, orderlies, assistants, attendants, etc.
- The professional association must concern itself with the nature of nursing practice, the means for improving nursing practice, the education necessary for such practice, and the standards for membership in the professional association.

From American Nurses' Association: Am. J. Nurs. **65**:106, 1965.

---

education emphasizes the role of education in the profession (see boxed material).

THEORY

As nursing has emerged as a profession, nursing knowledge has been developed through nursing theories. Theoretical models serve as a framework for both nursing curricula and clinical practice. Nursing theories also lead to research that increases the scientific basis of nursing practice.

A theory is a way of understanding a reality, and in this general sense all practicing nurses use the theories they have learned. Several of the approaches described previously in the section on definitions and philosophies are parts of fully developed nursing theories.

SERVICE

Nursing, like other professions, provides a specific service. Nursing has always been a service profession, although in the past the service was usually viewed as a charitable one. Today, nursing is a vital and indispensable component of the health care delivery system.

AUTONOMY

Autonomy means that one is reasonably independent and self-governing in decision making and practice. It has been difficult for nurses to attain the degree of autonomy enjoyed by some other professionals. In the past, physicians, hospital administrators, and others in the health care delivery system have found nursing autonomy difficult to understand and support. Through clinical competence and greater educational preparation, however, nurses are increasingly taking on independent roles in nurse-run clinics, collaborative practice, and advanced nursing careers.

With increased autonomy come greater responsibility and accountability. Accountability means that the nurse is held responsible, professionally and legally, for the type and quality of nursing care provided to clients. The nurse is accountable for keeping abreast of the technical skills and knowledge needed to perform nursing care. The nursing profession itself regulates accountability through nursing audits and standards of practice.

CODE OF ETHICS

Nursing has the final characteristic of a profession, a code of ethics. The code of ethics defines the principles by which nurses function. In addition, nurses incorporate their own values and ethics into their practice. Chapter 14 gives several examples of specific nurses' codes of ethics.

Professional Organizations

A professional organization is created to deal with issues of concern to those practicing in the profession. In North America the major professional nursing organizations are the American Nurses' Association (ANA), the Canadian Nurses' Association (CNA), and the National League for Nursing (NLN). The CNA and the ANA were formed in the late nineteenth century to improve standards of health and the availability of health care, to foster high standards for nursing, and to promote the professional development and general and economic welfare of nurses. The ANA and CNA are part of the International Council of Nurses (ICN). The objectives of the ICN parallel those of the CNA and ANA in that the ICN promotes national associations of nurses, improves standards of nursing practice, seeks a higher status for nurses, and provides an international power base for nurses.

The NLN is concerned with the improvement of nursing education, nursing service, and health care delivery in the United States. In Canada the Canadian Association of University Schools of Nursing and the Canadian Association of Practical and Nursing Assistants perform similar functions.

Nursing students also take part in organizations such as the National Student Nurses' Association (NSNA) in the United States and the Canadian Student Nurses' Association (CSNA) in Canada. These organizations consider issues of importance to nursing students and often cooperate in activities and programs with professional organizations such as the ANA, CNA, and NLN.

Some professional organizations are special interest groups that focus on specific areas of nursing such as critical care, nursing administration, nursing research, or nurse-midwifery. The goal of such organizations is to improve the standards of practice, expand nursing roles, and foster the welfare of nurses within the specialty areas. Some representative specialty organizations are discussed in the following paragraphs. Appendix A gives a comprehensive list of specialty nursing organizations in the United States and Canada.

The Association of Operating Room Nurses (AORN) is the national organization of operating room nurses in the United States. The National Conference of Operating Room Nurses is the equivalent Canadian organization. Both organizations are concerned with continuing education for operating room nurses, higher standards for operating room care, and increased research activities.

The Nurses' Association of the American College of Obstetricians and Gynecologists (NAACOG) includes Canadian and American nurses. The NAACOG promotes standards of practice in obstetrical and gynecological nursing, encourages professional growth for its members, and is an accrediting body for advanced programs in obstetrical and gynecological nursing.

The National Association of Pediatric Nurse Associates/Practitioners (NAPNAP) is the national organization of nurses prepared by training or experience to give primary care to children. NAPNAP works in conjunction with the American Academy of Pediatrics.

The American Association of Critical Care Nurses (AACN) is the national organization of nurses who work in critical care areas. The AACN is concerned with nursing education, practice, and research as they involve critical care nursing.

Society's Influence on Nursing

Throughout its history nursing has responded to changes in other areas of society. The contemporary nursing profession continues to respond to the needs and influences of society as a whole. Some of the societal changes to which nursing is currently responding are technological advances, demographic changes, the consumer movement, the increased emphasis on health promotion, the women's movement, and the human rights movement.

TECHNOLOGICAL ADVANCES

In recent years scientific and technological advances have affected almost every aspect of life. Health care has changed in many ways, including the use of new equipment, new diagnostic tests and treatment measures, and new drugs. Nursing had adapted and will continue to respond to such changes with continuing education and in-service programs and other educational approaches. Nursing is also uniquely concerned with the *human* side of technological advances. Society as a whole seems to accept technological advances in health care, but individual clients often experience problems related to technology. For example, dialysis machines have been used for many years to treat clients with kidney problems, but that does not lessen the emotional conflict a client may experience on learning he needs to undergo dialysis. As health care technology becomes increasingly complex and sophisticated, nurses have the growing role of helping clients adjust to the use of technology in their care.

DEMOGRAPHIC CHANGES

Demographic changes are changes in the population as a whole. Changes that in recent decades have influenced health care include the population shift from rural areas to urban centers, the increasing life span, the higher incidence of chronic, long-term illness, and increases in the incidence of certain diseases such as alcoholism and lung cancer. Nursing as a profession responds to such changes by exploring new methods for providing care, by changing educational emphases, by establishing practice standards in new areas, and so on. The individual nurse also responds to demographic changes in the population served by her practice setting to better meet the changing health care needs of clients.

CONSUMER MOVEMENT

Consumers in recent years have become increasingly knowledgeable and concerned about all kinds of products and services. The consumer movement is a heightened awareness of the value and costs of products and services; in short, consumers want their money's worth. Health care in general has been influenced by the consumer movement in ways as diverse as new kinds of health care agencies such as health maintenance organizations, new forms of health insurance, and concern about the rising costs of health care. Also, consumers are more knowledgeable about health and illness and are becoming more vocal in their desire for high-quality care. Because nurses generally interact more with clients than do other health care professionals, they often must answer consumer questions about the quality and costs of health care. Health care consumers are also more aware of their rights as clients, and the nurse supports these rights in the role of client advocate, as discussed previously.

HEALTH PROMOTION

Related to the consumer movement is a greater emphasis in society on health promotion and illness prevention, rather than waiting until illness occurs and then treating it. Exercise and nutrition are subjects that interest an increasing number of people. Nursing has responded to this greater concern for health promotion in a number of ways, ranging from programs in the community to specific health promotion and teaching activities for clients in hospitals and other health care settings. As discussed previously, health promotion actions are a part of many of the roles of nurses, including those of care giver, client advocate, rehabilitator, communicator, and teacher.

WOMEN'S MOVEMENT

The women's movement has brought about many changes in society as women have increasingly sought economic, political, occupational, and educational equality. Nursing is responding in two ways. First, since most nurses are women, nurses are increasingly asserting their equal rights as human beings, as employees, and as health care professionals. The women's movement has encouraged nurses to seek greater autonomy and responsibility in providing care. Second, the women's movement has caused women clients to seek more responsibility for and control over their bodies, their health, and their lives in general. As women become more aware of their own needs and unique qualities, they seek health care that can help them meet those needs.

HUMAN RIGHTS MOVEMENT

Like the women's movement, the human rights movement is changing the way society views the rights of *all* its members, including minorities, clients with terminal illness, pregnant women, and the elderly. Many groups have special health care needs, and nursing has responded by respecting all clients as individuals with a right to good care and with basic human rights. Nurses advocate the rights of all clients, but they have also recognized the special needs of some groups and thus have created bills of rights for dying clients, hospitalized clients, pregnant clients, and other groups as a way of ensuring that quality care is provided without sacrificing the client's rights.

Trends in Nursing

This chapter has emphasized that nursing is not a static, unchanging profession but is continually growing and evolving as society changes, as health care emphases and methods change, as the life-styles of clients change—and as nurses themselves change. To speak of nursing at all is to speak of nursing as it is at a given time, and in this sense this chapter is about trends in nursing.

The current philosophies and definitions of nursing demonstrate the holistic trend in nursing—to address the whole person in all dimensions, in health and illness, as an individual but also in interaction with the family and community. Nursing continues to draw on the social sciences and other fields as the focus of nursing care expands.

One trend in nursing education is the growing number of students who are receiving their basic nursing education in community colleges and universities. Professional nursing organizations continue to stress the importance of education for nurses seeking new and expanded roles.

Nursing practice trends include a growing variety of settings in which nurses practice and greater independence in many settings. Nurses continue to gain autonomy and respect as members of the health care team. Nursing roles continue to expand along with the broadening focus of nursing care. The clinical ladder and new career roles also represent current trends in nursing practice.

Trends in nursing as a profession include the growing emphasis on those aspects of nursing that characterize it as a profession: education, theory, service, autonomy, and ethical codes. The activities of nursing's professional organizations reflect all the trends in nursing education and practice. Finally, all the influences of society on nursing described in the preceding sections also reflect trends in contemporary nursing.

Two other trends remain to be discussed: the increasing political influence of nursing and nursing's influence on health care policy and practice.

Political Influence of Professional Nursing

Historically, nurses' involvement in politics has been limited. Although individual nurses such as Florence Nightingale and Margaret Sanger have influenced decision making in such areas as sanitation, nutrition, and birth control, nurses have accomplished less as a group. The recent women's movement, however, has inspired nurses to address health care issues. In addition, as more college-educated people enter the profession, they bring to nursing the activism and involvement of the university campuses (Deloughery and Gebbie, 1975).

Nurses' involvement in politics is receiving greater emphasis in nursing curricula, in the professional organizations, and in various health care settings (Stanhope and Belcher, 1982). Professional nursing organizations have employed lobbyists to urge state legislatures and the U.S. Congress to improve the quality of health care. Kalisch and Kalisch (1982) note that the ANA

works for the improvement of health standards and the availability of health care services for all people; fosters high standards of nursing, stimulates and promotes the professional development of nurses, and advances their economic and general welfare. The purposes are unrestricted by considerations of nationality, race, creed, lifestyle, color, sex, or age.

The ANA employs registered nurses as lobbyists at the federal level, and state nursing organizations also hire lobbyists and legislative specialists to work on state nursing issues and assist with federal efforts as needed. Finally, lobbyists who work on behalf of nursing are employed in Washington by professional interest groups such as the American Federation of Teachers, National League for Nursing, American College of Nurse Midwives, American Public Health Association, and American Association of Colleges of Nursing. The overall political purposes of these groups are to remove financial barriers to health care, to increase the quality of nursing care available, to increase economic rewards to nurses, and to expand professional nursing roles (Aiken, 1982).

In addition, individual nurses work to effect change in the health care system. According to Mullane (1975), if nurses become serious students of social needs, activists in influencing policy to meet those needs, and generous contributors of time and money to nursing and their organizations and to candidates working for universal good health care, then the future is bright indeed.

Nursing's Influence on Health Care Policy and Practice

Nurses are still on the outer edge of the health care power system, perhaps partly because the public has assumed that nurses, most of whom are women and thus traditionally viewed as followers, do not need representation on advisory committees or boards. In addition, many nurses seem to be content with "over-the-fence" methods, offering assistance individually on specific issues but avoiding political involvement (Deloughery and Gebbie, 1975).

Political activism and commitment are a part of professionalism, however, and politics are an important aspect of the delivery of health care. Therefore nurses should not view politics as "dirty business" but as a reality that includes the arts of influence, compromise, and social interaction. Nurses have been involved in a different sort of politics in schools of nursing and in health care settings when seeking additional resources, more self-direction, and accountability with authority, and the skills gained in such experiences can be transferred to the politics of health care policymaking.

So long as nurses avoid involvement in health care policy and practice, misinformed outsiders can attempt to impose their will on nursing and nursing practice. Nonnursing groups, often led by other health care providers, have made attempts to impose institutional licensure, mandatory continuing education, curtailment of advanced nursing practice, and other constraints on a profession that should have its own voice in decisions made in these and numerous other areas affecting the quality of nursing care. Although nurses have often successfully prevented infringement on the profession's self-governance, the future of nursing requires that nurses individually and collectively seek a greater influence on health care policies that affect nursing practice.

✓ Nursing is an essential part of society, out of which it has grown and with which it evolves.

✓ Nursing has responded to the health needs of society, which were influenced by economic, social, and cultural variables of a specific era.

✓ Formalized education programs for professional nursing were established in the nineteenth century by Florence Nightingale.

✓ The growth of nursing and nursing education in the United States was stimulated by the Civil War.

✓ The Canadian Nurses' Association and the American Nurses' Association were established in the late nineteenth century.

✓ The opening of the Henry Street Settlement by Lillian Wald and Mary Brewster marked the expansion of nursing into the community setting.

✓ Nursing education became affiliated with universities early in the twentieth century.

✓ Expansion of nursing into the military occurred in the early twentieth century, and the development of specialty nursing organizations began in the 1950s and has continued to the present.

✓ The Lysaught Report (1970) emphasized the need for clarification of nursing roles and responsibilities, greater financial support for nurses, and more career opportunities.

✓ Nursing definitions reflect changes in the practice of nursing and help bring about changes by identifying the domain of nursing practice and guiding research, practice, and education.

✓ Peplau's nursing theory focuses on interpersonal relationships that people establish as they pass through various developmental stages.

✓ Abdellah's theory emphasizes the delivery of nursing care for the whole person as an individual.

✓ Henderson's theory involves 14 basic needs of the whole person through which the nurse assists "the individual, sick or well, in the performance of those activities contributing to his health [or] its recovery . . . that he would perform unaided if he had the necessary strength, will, or knowledge."

✓ Travelbee emphasizes nursing as an interpersonal process involving the nurse-client relationship and the client's ability to cope with the experience of illness.

✓ Johnson's theory focuses on the client's ability to adapt to his illness and the impact of actual or potential stressors on his adaptation. The client's adaptation is based on basic needs in terms of seven categories of behavior.

✓ Rogers' theory approaches the client as a whole person ("unitary man") who is continually evolving and changing.

✓ King's theory focuses on the relationship between the client and the nurse. This relationship is the vehicle for the nursing process in which the nurse uses communication to help the client adapt to his illness.

✓ Orem's theory emphasizes the self-care needs of the client, in which the goals of nursing care are to help the client care for himself.

✓ Levine's theory views the client as an integrated whole interacting with and adapting to his environment with the conservation of energy as a primary concern.

KEY CONCEPTS, *cont'd*

✓ Roy's theory views the client as an adaptive system, in which the need for nursing care developed when the client was unable to adapt to internal and external environmental demands.

✓ Educational preparation of the registered nurse can be through one of three programs in the United States or one of two programs in Canada.

✓ A license for a registered nurse in each state or province is granted after a candidate has completed a prescribed course of study in an accredited program and passed a licensing examination.

✓ Graduate nursing programs prepare nurse clinicians to improve nursing care through the advancement of nursing theory and sciences.

✓ Continuing education programs help the nurse remain current in skills, knowledge, and theory related to nursing practice.

✓ Continuing education programs can be accredited by the American Nurses' Association or the state board of nursing.

✓ In-service education is instruction or training provided by a health care agency or institution in which the nurse is employed.

✓ The clinical ladder is a mechanism for career mobility that incorporates opportunities for advancement in nursing through either an administrative or a clinical track.

✓ Nursing standards provide the guidelines for implementing and evaluating nursing care.

✓ Rapid rise in the elderly population, chronic illnesses, and functional impairments has resulted in an increased number of long-term care facilities.

✓ Community-based agencies focus primarily on health promotion, health maintenance, health education and management, and coordination and continuity of care within the community.

✓ The multiple roles and functions of the nurse include care giver, decision maker, client advocate, manager, rehabilitator, comforter, communicator, and teacher.

✓ Specific employment positions include educator, clinical nurse specialist, nurse practitioner, certified nurse-midwife, nurse anesthetist, administrator, and researcher.

✓ The health care team is multidisciplinary and may include a physician, physician assistant, physical therapist, occupational therapist, respiratory therapist, pharmacist, social worker, and chaplain.

✓ Nursing is a profession in which there are established educational preparation for the nurse, nursing theory, a service provided, autonomy, and a code of ethics.

✓ Professional nursing organizations deal with issues of concern to various specialist groups within the nursing profession.

✓ Changes in society, such as increased technology, new demographic patterns, consumerism, health promotion, and the women's and human rights movements, have led to changes in nursing.

✓ Nurses are becoming more politically sophisticated and as a result are able to increase nursing's influence on health care policy and practice.

REFERENCES

Abdellah, F.G., et al.: Patient-centered approaches to nursing, New York, 1960, Macmillan, Inc.

Aiken, L.H.: The impact of federal health policy on nursing. In Aiken, L.H., editor: Nursing in the 80's: crises, opportunities, challenges, Philadelphia, 1982, J.B. Lippincott Co.

Anderson, M.I., and Denyes, M.J.: A ladder for clinical advancement in nursing practice, J. Nurs. Adm. 5(2):16, 1975.

American Nurses' Association: Statement on graduate education in nursing, New York, 1969, The Association.

American Nurses' Association: Standards for continuing education in nursing, Kansas City, Mo., 1975, The Association.

American Nurses' Association: Nursing and social policy statement, Kansas City, Mo., 1980, The Association.

American Nurses' Association Committee on Education: A position paper, New York, 1965, The Association.

Colavecchio, R., Tescher B., and Scalzi, C.: A clinical ladder for nursing practice, J. Nurs. Adm. 4(5):54, 1974.

Deloughery, G.L., and Gebbie, K.M.: Political dynamics: impact on nurses and nursing, St. Louis, 1975, The C.V. Mosby Co.

Department of Health and Human Services: The registered nurse population: an overview, DHHS Pub. No. HRS-P-00-83-1, 1982, Washington, D.C., U.S. Government Printing Office.

Dolan, J.A.: Nursing in society: a historical perspective, Philadelphia, 1978, W.B. Saunders Co.

Etzioni, A.: The semiprofessions and their organization, New York, 1961, The Free Press.

Henderson, V.: The nature of nursing, Am. J. Nurs. 64:62, 1964a.

Henderson, V.: The nature of nursing, New York, 1964b, Macmillan, Inc.

International Council of Nurses: Code for nurses, Geneva, 1973, The Council.

Johnson, D.: Theory in nursing: borrowed and unique, Nurs. Res. 11:206, 1968.

Kalisch, B.J., and Kalisch, P.A.: Politics of nursing, Philadelphia, 1982, J.B. Lippincott Co.

Kelly, L.Y.: Dimensions of professional nursing, New York, 1981, Macmillan, Inc.

King, I.M.: Toward a theory for nursing, New York, 1971, John Wiley & Sons, Inc.

Knox, S.L.: A clinical advancement program, J. Nurs. 10(7):29, 1980.

Levine, M.C.: An introduction to clinical nursing, ed. 2, Philadelphia, 1973, F.A. Davis Co.

Lysaught, J.P.: An abstract for action, New York, 1970, McGraw-Hill Book Co.

Mullane, M.K.: Nursing care and the political arena, Nurs. Outlook 23:699, 1975.

Nightingale, F.: Notes on nursing: what it is and what it is not, London, 1860, Harrison & Sons.

Orem, D.E.: Nursing: concepts of practice, New York, 1971, McGraw-Hill Book Co.

Peplau, H.E.: Interpersonal relations in nursing, New York, 1952, G.P. Putnam & Sons.

Rogers, M.E.: An introduction to the theoretical basis of nursing, Philadelphia, 1970, F.A. Davis Co.

Roy, C.: An introduction to nursing: an adaptation model, Englewood Cliffs, N.J., 1976, Prentice-Hall, Inc.

Roy, C., and Obloy, S.M.: The practitioner movement—toward a science of nursing, Am. J. Nurs. 79:1698, 1978.

Stanhope, M., and Belcher, A.E.: Political imperatives for nursing practice. In Lancaster, J., and Lancaster, W., editors: Concepts for advanced nursing practice, St. Louis, 1982, The C.V. Mosby Co.

Travelbee, J.: Interpersonal agents of nursing, Philadelphia, 1966, F.A. Davis Co.

White, S.: The expanded role for nurses, Nursing 77 7:90, 1977.

Woodham, S.C.: Florence Nightingale, New York, 1951, McGraw-Hill Book Co.

Zimmer, M.J.: Rationale for a ladder for clinical advancement, J. Nurs. Adm. 5:18, 1975.

ADDITIONAL READINGS

Chinn, P.L., and Jacobs, M.K.: Theory and nursing: a systematic approach, St. Louis, 1983, The C.V. Mosby Co.

Donaldson, S.K., and Crowley, D.M.: The discipline of nursing, Nurs. Outlook 26:113, 1978.

Etzioni, A.: A comparative analysis of complex organizations, New York, 1961, The Free Press.

Leininger, M.: Conference on the nature of science and nursing: introductory comments, Nurs. Res. 17:484, 1968.

Stevens, B.J.: Nursing theory: analysis, application, evaluation, Boston, 1979, Little, Brown & Co.

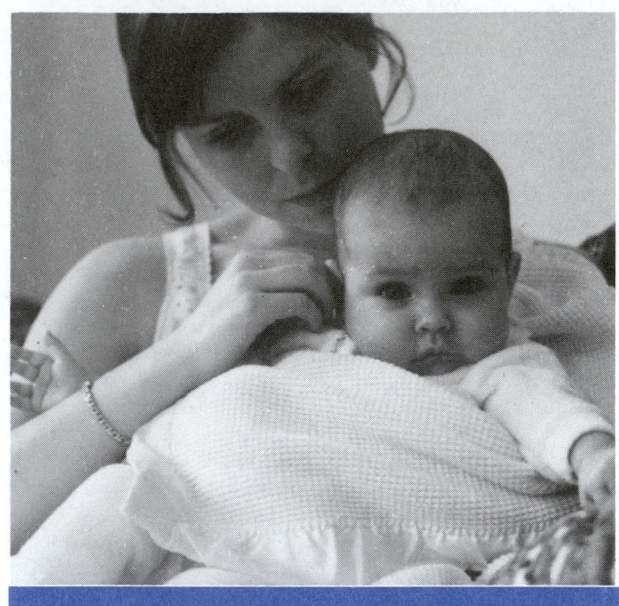

OBJECTIVES

Mastery of content in this chapter will enable the student to:

- Define the terms in the glossary.
- Discuss health definitions and concepts.
- Discuss the health belief model, the health-illness continuum model, the agent-host-environment model, and the high-level wellness model.
- Describe health promotion and illness prevention activities.
- List and discuss the three levels of preventive care.
- List and explain four kinds of risk factors.
- Describe the variables that influence a person's health beliefs and practices.
- Describe the variables that influence illness behavior.
- State and discuss the stages of illness behavior.
- Describe the impact of illness on the client and family.
- Discuss the nurse's role for clients in health and illness.

GLOSSARY

active strategies of health promotion Activities that depend on the client being motivated to adopt a specific health program.

acute illness Illness characterized by symptoms that are of relatively short duration, are usually severe, and affect the functioning of the client in all dimensions.

agent Element of the agent-host-environment model of health and illness; any biological, chemical, physical or mechanical, or psychosocial factor whose presence or absence can lead to disease or illness.

anxiety Feeling of apprehension, uneasiness, agitation, uncertainty, and fear resulting from the anticipation of something perceived as negative.

body image Person's subjective concept of his physical appearance.

chronic illness Illness that persists over a long period of time and affects physical, emotional, intellectual, social, and spiritual functioning.

denial Mechanism by which emotional conflict and anxiety are avoided through refusal to acknowledge facts that are consciously or unconsciously intolerable.

external environment Set of factors outside and distinct from a person that may influence his health, including the physical environment, social relationships, economic variables, and so on.

2 | *Health and Illness*

health   Dynamic state in which an individual adapts to his internal and external environments so that there is a state of physical, emotional, intellectual, social, and spiritual well-being.

health behavior   Activities through which a person maintains, attains, or regains good health and prevents illness.

health belief model   Conceptual framework that describes a person's health behavior as an expression of his health beliefs.

health promotion   Health education programs or activities directed toward maintaining or enhancing the health and well-being of clients.

health-illness continuum   Scale by means of which a person's level of health can be described, ranging from high-level wellness to severe illness. The scale takes into account the presence of risk factors.

host   Element of the agent-host-environment model of health and illness. A host is a person or group who, because of risk factors, may be susceptible to disease or illness.

illness   Abnormal process in which any aspect of a person's functioning is diminished or impaired as compared with his previous condition.

illness behavior   Ways in which persons monitor their bodies, define and interpret their symptoms, take remedial actions, and use the health care system.

illness prevention   Health education programs or activities directed toward protecting clients from threats or potential threats to health or well-being and toward minimizing risk factors.

internal environment   Set of factors inside a person that may influence his health, including genetic factors, physiological processes, psychological variables, and intellectual and spiritual dimensions.

passive strategies of health promotion   Activities that involve the client as the recipient of actions by health care professionals.

primary nursing   System of nursing care in which the care of a client is managed for the entire day by one nurse, who directs and coordinates other nurses and other personnel and schedules all tests, procedures, and daily activities for the client. When on duty, the primary nurse cares for the client personally.

risk factor   Any internal or external variable that makes a person or group more vulnerable to illness or an unhealthy event.

sick role   Pattern of behavior in which a client admits the symptoms of a physical or mental disorder in order to be cared for, sympathized with, and protected from the demands and stresses of life.

social interaction   Participation in activities involving two or more persons.

related to health care. Nurses therefore need to be aware of variables that influence a client's health beliefs and practices, in order to provide nursing care individualized for the client.

People also have different attitudes toward illness and react in different ways to illness. Medical sociologists describe the reaction to illness as illness behavior. The nurse needs to understand both how clients react to illness and how illness affects clients and their families. Illness can have an enormous impact on a client and his family, and the nurse who recognizes this impact and the factors involved can take steps to minimize the effects of illness and assist the client and family in maintaining normal levels of functioning.

The nurse also identifies actual and potential risk factors that predispose a person or a group to illness. Nursing actions involving health promotion and illness prevention activities assist the client not only in regaining optimal health but also in maintaining and enhancing a high level of health.

The nurse assesses the whole person, including his physical, intellectual, emotional, and spiritual dimensions and his interactions with his family and his community. Nursing care involves understanding the client's psychosocial, cultural, and economic backgrounds as well as his physical being, so that he can be assisted in health maintenance and promotion, illness prevention, and adaptation to changes that illness produces in every dimension of his functioning.

In the past, most individuals and societies have viewed health as the opposite of disease or the absence of disease. This attitude toward health still remains popular with many health professionals. It assumes that people are normally healthy and that people with disease are unhealthy and in an abnormal state. Perhaps the major reason for this simple, either-or attitude toward health is that such a definition can be easily applied: a person is simply considered either healthy or ill, with no range in between. There are two problems with this attitude: it ignores states of health between disease and full health, and it emphasizes the physiological dimension of a person, considering only the body as being either ill or healthy and overlooking the complex interrelationships among a person's physiological, emotional, intellectual, sociocultural, and developmental dimensions.

Today's health and medical care services are shaped largely by how health professionals define health and illness (Balog, 1982). Health professionals therefore *must* define health and illness; these definitions serve as a basis for determinations about the types and quality of health care services that should be provided. Not all health care professionals, however, agree about how these concepts should be defined.

The definition of health adhered to by health care workers also may not always correspond with a client's concept of health, which is unique to each person. An individual's life-style, cultural background, and economic and psychosocial status influence what he believes about health and his practices

Definition of Health

Health is not merely the absence of illness. Defining health is difficult, because every person has his own concept of health. Health is not an acquired piece of scientific knowledge, nor is it a thing, a part of the body, or a function of the body, like hearing, seeing, or breathing. Health is a state of being that each person defines in relation to his own values.

Health care professionals are still struggling to develop a definition of health that is acceptable to all health care workers and to consumers. The World Health Organization (WHO) defines health as a "state of complete physical, mental and social well-being, not merely the absence of disease or infirmity" (1974). Yet this definition of health has not been totally accepted. Those opposed to it believe that for underdeveloped countries and for persons of low economic status, the WHO definition of health is unrealistic because many people, according to this definition, would not be considered healthy (Fuchs, 1974). In addition, with the WHO definition it is difficult to determine scientifically who is or is not healthy or to determine the point at which a person becomes ill rather than healthy (Breslow, 1972).

Thus it is difficult for health care professionals to agree on a clear, workable definition of health. A related issue is the unique attitude of each client toward health. A person's attitude toward health involves much more than the absence of illness or disability. For example, an adult with hypertension does have a documented disease process, but if his condition is being controlled with medication, he may consider himself healthy and experience no change in his functioning. A blind person does not have normal vision, but if he has fully adapted to his visual disability he is able to live much as he wants and therefore views himself as a healthy adult. A client's concept of health is thus very important to the nurse in helping him reach his health goals, which may not be the same for all clients.

Nurses also have an attitude toward health. Nurses plan care for a client in order to help him meet his health care needs and achieve maximal independence. Nurses plan care based on a definition of health and accepted standards of health care. Health in its broadest sense is a dynamic state in which the individual adapts to changes in his internal and external environments so that he maintains a state of well-being in all dimensions. The internal environment comprises many factors that may influence a person's health, including genetic variables, physiological processes, psychological variables, intellectual and spiritual dimensions, and physical disease processes. The external environment comprises factors outside the person that may influence health, including the physical environment, social relationships, economic variables, and so on. Because both environments may be continually changing, the person must adapt in order to maintain a state of well-being.

"Health" and "illness" therefore must be defined in terms of the individual client. Health can include conditions the client or nurse may previously have considered illness; a condition such as a temporary disability may be illness for one client, whereas if the same disability is permanent for another client, who has adjusted to his condition, the second client can be considered healthy. Health is also closely related to an individual's life-style, and some illnesses can be considered manifestations of a person's life-style. A client who neglects personal hygiene and makes little attempt to stay warm and dry in winter, for example, may have frequent respiratory infections. In such a case, treating the infection may have no effect on the pattern of the person's behavior, and he may even not consider such an infection an illness at all if it seems to him a "normal" or usual aspect of his life. A rigid attitude toward health and illness by a health professional may have little meaning for such a person's future health, since the whole person is not being considered.

Therefore, because the attitudes of client and nurse toward health may not coincide exactly, the nurse works with the client and his family throughout the nursing process to establish mutually the goals of care and to plan individualized nursing care.

Models of Health and Illness

A model is a theoretical way of understanding a complex phenomenon. Because health and illness are complex concepts involving attitudes that may differ between the client and the nurse, and because a client's beliefs about health and his behaviors related to health are both influenced by other variables, it is helpful to use models of health to understand the relationship between health and illness and the relationship between clients' attitudes toward health and their health practices.

A person's health beliefs are his ideas, convictions, and attitudes about health and illness. Health beliefs may be based on factual information or misinformation, common sense or common myths, reality or false expectations. Thus a person's health beliefs can support activities that maintain or promote health, or they may negatively affect a person's health. Health behaviors usually result from a person's health beliefs, and therefore they can either positively or negatively affect the person's health. Positive health behaviors are activities related to maintaining, attaining, or regaining good health and preventing illness. Common positive health behaviors include adequate exercise, adequate diet and nutrition, immunizations, and proper sleep patterns. Negative health behaviors include practices actually or potentially detrimental to health, such as smoking, drug or alcohol abuse, poor diet, and refusal to take necessary medications.

To understand the health behaviors and beliefs of clients so that effective health care can be provided, nurses have developed health models. Models allow a nurse to understand and predict a client's health behavior, including the use of health services and compliance with recommended therapies. If a nurse understands a client's health behavior, the nurse can better help the client to regain and maintain a high level of wellness. The nurse assesses the client's risk factors, illness patterns, life-style, use of health services, and physiological and behavioral functioning. The nurse then plans care accordingly, as in the following:

Mr. Price is a 68-year-old asthmatic, whose asthmatic attacks are controlled with medication. Mr. Price takes his medication every day but usually forgets to renew his prescription. Forty-eight hours after he has been without his medication he enters an emergency room in an asthmatic attack. This sequence has occurred five times during the past 12 months. A nurse notes this past behavior and designs a nursing care plan with the goal of maintaining a consistent level of wellness. The nursing care plan includes (1) a request to the physician to order a 3-month supply of medication and (2) a notice to be sent to Mr. Price 2 weeks before the end of his supply to remind him to renew his prescription.

A client's health beliefs depend on many factors, including his perception of his level of health, modifying factors such as demographics, his personality, and his perception of benefits resulting from positive health behaviors. Health models usually consider these components. Four health models are described in this chapter: the health-illness continuum, the high-level wellness model, the agent-host-environment model, and the health belief model. The first three models describe the relationship between health and illness, and the fourth model is designed to explain and predict a client's health behaviors. Two other health models—basic human needs and stress adaptation—are discussed in Chapters 4 and 5.

Health-Illness Continuum

According to the health-illness continuum model, health is as a dynamic state that is continually changing as a person adapts to changes in the internal and external environments to maintain a state of physical, emotional, intellectual, social, and spiritual well-being. Illness is an abnormal process in which the functioning of a person is diminished or impaired in one or more dimensions as compared with the person's previous condition. Because both health and illness are relative qualities, existing in varying degrees or levels, it is more accurate to consider health

and illness in terms of a scale or continuum rather than as either-or, absolute states (Fig. 2-1).

A nurse can locate a client's level of health at any point on the health-illness continuum. High-level wellness and severe illness are the opposite ends of the continuum, with a full range of states in between. As Fig. 2-1 suggests, a client's risk factors (variables in any of the person's dimensions that make illness more likely) are important in identifying the client's level of health. Risk factors include variables related to genetic and physiological factors, age, life-style, and the environment (see later section in this chapter). As a person progresses through the developmental stages of life, certain risk factors are more common than others. An adolescent, for example, is more likely than an adult to experience stresses related to body image and self-concept, and an older adult is more likely than a child to develop cardiac illness. In addition, within any one developmental stage, a person may experience various health-illness states, as the following shows:

Before reaching her teens, Dorothy Helms, now age 19, a college sophomore, had good health most of her life. The only illnesses she had were minor viruses and colds. Before reaching her teens, therefore, she maintained high-level wellness. At 13, however, she began to smoke; and for the next 3 years she smoked two packs of cigarettes a day. About 2 years ago she developed a bad respiratory infection with a productive cough, which remained for 3 months. Then she began to get a cold about every 3 months, which was always accompanied by a productive cough. Although she was encouraged to quit smoking, her attempts to quit were unsuccessful, primarily as a result of peer pressure. Her friends would tell her that it was OK to smoke, that it was a popular thing to do, and they continued to offer her cigarettes. Smoking is a risk factor for respiratory illness, and by taking up smoking Dorothy moved along the continuum from health toward illness. Finally, Dorothy developed severe bronchitis, which was the single factor that motivated her to stop smoking. Dorothy has not smoked for the last 13 months, during which time she has had only one respiratory tract infection. She has now moved back toward the health end of the continuum.

Fig. 2-1 The health-illness continuum, ranging from high-level wellness to severe illness, provides a method of identifying a client's level of health at a given time. The most important point to remember in regard to this continuum is that a person's level of health is a reflection of his level of functioning in all dimensions.

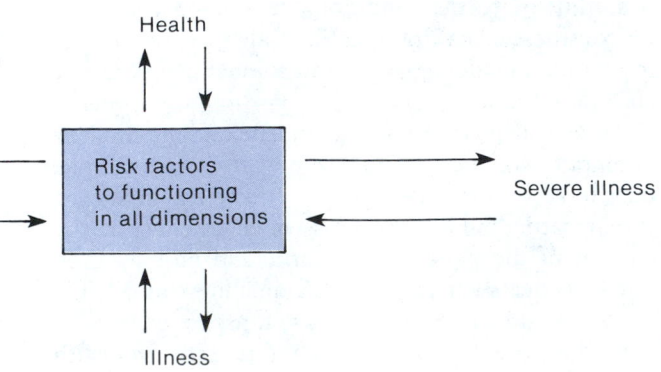

This hypothetical case illustrates how a person at the health end of the health-illness continuum can add a risk factor and move to a different point on the continuum. After a period of exposure to a risk factor the person may develop an illness. Dorothy's later development of severe bronchitis could easily be traced to the continuous smoking. Although Dorothy knew she should stop smoking, she also experienced increased social and peer pressure to continue to smoke. It was the severe bronchitis that motivated Dorothy to completely stop smoking. The final result was a return to a higher level of health.

How the client himself views his present level of health depends on his attitude toward health, his values, his beliefs, and his perception of his physical, emotional, intellectual, social, and spiritual well-being. The nurse's role in this respect is to help the client identify his position on the health-illness continuum in order to plan nursing care to assist him in reaching an optimal level of health.

The drawback of the health-illness continuum is that it is not always easy to describe a client's level of health in terms of one point between the two extremes. For example, is a man who has his broken leg in a cast but who has adapted to his limited mobility more or less healthy than the same man a year later who is experiencing severe depression following the death of his spouse but who is physiologically healthy? The model is effective, nonetheless, when it is used for comparing a client's present level of health with previous levels and for setting goals for nursing care to attain a future level of health.

High-Level Wellness Model

Dunn (1961, 1977) developed a model in which optimal health, or high-level wellness, is described as a state in which all aspects of a person's functioning are balanced, purposeful, and directed toward attaining his full potential. This approach is holistic and focuses on integrated well-being in all dimensions as the basis of health. Dunn differentiated between good health, which is simply a state of not being ill, and high-level wellness, which involves an upward and forward movement to achieve full potential.

Health care directed toward helping a client achieve high-level wellness emphasizes health promotion and illness prevention activities rather than focusing only on treatment for illness. High-level wellness is a dynamic process rather than a passive, static state. Using this model when providing care for a client with a permanent physical disability, for example, a nurse would plan care not only to help the client reach maximal physical functioning within limitations imposed by the disability, but also to help him adapt emotionally, intellectually, socially, and perhaps even spiritually to the disability in order to continue developing his human and individual potential.

The high-level wellness model is applicable also to family and community health. Families and communities both have many functions, and high-level wellness, as with the individual, involves successful functioning in an integrated manner. Families, for example, have the following functions: child rearing, providing security and emotional support for family members, and assisting family members in solving problems. Family health care, then, includes an emphasis on how the family works together in these areas, with the goal being the attainment of the fullest potential for both the individual family members and the family as a whole.

Agent-Host-Environment Model

The agent-host-environment model of health and illness originated in the community health work of Leavell and associates (1965) and has since been expanded as a model for describing the causation of illness in other health areas. According to this approach, the level of health or illness of an individual or group depends on the dynamic relationship among three variables: (1) the agent, any factor, internal or external, that by its presence or absence can lead to disease or illness; (2) the host, the individual person or group, who may or may not be susceptible to a particular illness or disease; and (3) the environment, including physical, social, economic, and other factors that may make it more likely that the person or group will experience disease or illness. This model emphasizes that both health and illness depend on the

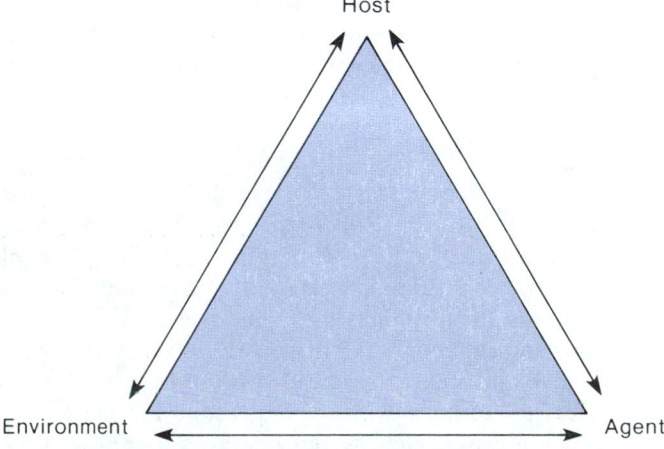

Fig. 2-2 Interaction of agent, host, and environment as causes of disease and illness. The double arrows indicate that each factor can be affected by the other two factors.

dynamic interaction of all three variables (Fig. 2-2). For example, a person does not contract a respiratory infection simply because a microorganism has entered his respiratory system. The microorganism alone does not *cause* the illness, which depends on host and environmental factors as well. It has been shown that the presence of an infectious organism may affect one individual in one environment but not affect another in a different environment.

Within each of the three areas, several factors influence a person's state of health or illness.

AGENT

Agents can be classified as biological, chemical, physical, mechanical, or psychosocial. Biological agents are living organisms, including parasites, bacteria, and viruses. Chemical agents are any liquids, gases, or solids that may adversely affect health, including drugs, poisons, toxic gases, and some food additives. Physical and mechanical agents include heat and cold and forces that can injure body tissues, such as the forces produced by an automobile accident. Psychosocial agents include emotional stress, problems related to social interaction, and psychological forces. The presence of any of these agents does not mean that a person necessarily will become ill, but an agent must be present (or absent, as in nutritional deficiencies) if a particular illness is to occur.

HOST

Host factors are those physical or psychosocial situations or conditions that put an individual or group at risk for becoming ill. Such factors may be related to the host's family history, age, or life-style. A person who smokes cigarettes, for example, is at greater than normal risk for cardiac disease, as is a person with a family history of cardiac disease. The presence of host factors does not mean that a person will become ill, but illness is more likely in such cases. A later section in this chapter discusses risk factors in more detail.

ENVIRONMENT

Environmental factors may make illness more or less likely for a person or group. The environment consists of all factors outside the host. The physical environment includes climate, living conditions, and elements such as light and sound levels. The social environment consists of many factors involving a person or group's interaction with others, including stresses, conflicts with others, economic hardships, and life crises such as the death of a spouse. Like agents and host factors, environmental factors do not cause illness in themselves, but they can increase or decrease susceptibility to disease.

The three sets of factors are continually interacting, in both health and illness. No one can be totally free of all agents of illness; for example, we are frequently exposed to microorganisms in food and water, to toxic fumes such as automobile emissions, and to psychosocial stresses. But in health the defense mechanisms of the body and mind allow us to resist or minimize the threats of such agents, depending on host and environmental factors. Health, then, can be considered a state in which these three areas are interacting positively and maintaining a dynamic state of adaptation to changes in any of the areas. Illness occurs when the interaction of two or more factors in these areas leads to a failure of the person to adapt.

The agent-host-environment model has been expanded into a general theory of the multiple causation of disease. Until recent decades, it was commonly believed that single causes of diseases could be identified. Infectious diseases in particular were thought to have single causes: the bacterium or virus that is the agent was considered solely responsible. It is now recognized that most diseases have multiple causes, as the agent-host-environment model demonstrates. Lung cancer, for example, is related to cigarette smoking, a host factor. A family history of cancer, another host factor, also increases a person's susceptibility. Environmental factors, such as peer pressure, may intensify a person's smoking habits and may produce emotional stresses, which some research suggests may also increase susceptibility. The agent of cancer is not yet fully understood, but clearly biological or chemical agents are involved. Because all these factors can in a sense be considered "causes" of the disease of lung cancer, health care directed toward the prevention of the disease must focus on all of them. The theory of the multiple causation of disease is important to nurses because nursing emphasizes holistic care of the client, which is based on knowledge of environmental, psychosocial, and life-style factors, among others.

Health Belief Model

Rosenstock's (1974) health belief model (Fig. 2-3) provides a way of understanding and predicting how clients behave in relation to their health and how they will comply with health care therapies. The model considers the individual's perception of his susceptibility to an illness, his perception of the seriousness of the illness, psychosocial and demographic modifying factors, and the likelihood that he will take recommended actions. The first component in this model involves how the individual perceives his susceptibility to a specific illness, as shown in the following:

■ ■ ■ ■ ■

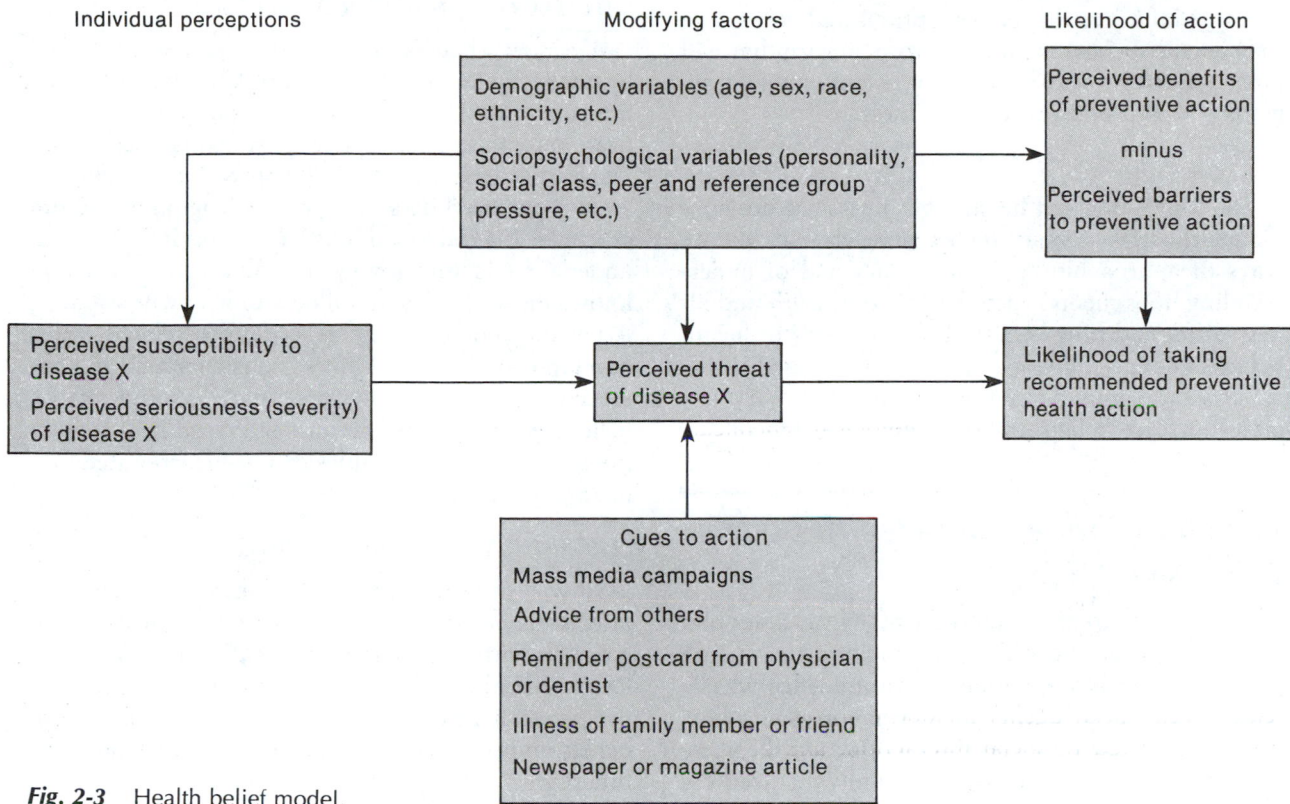

Individual perceptions   Modifying factors   Likelihood of action

Fig. 2-3   Health belief model.
From Becker, M.H., and Maiman, L.A.: *Med. Care* **13**:12, 1975.

Neither Mrs. Duke nor Mrs. Wales, who are friends of similar age and socioeconomic status, had chickenpox as a child. Mrs. Duke has recently been in contact with two neighborhood children who developed chickenpox, and her own son now has chickenpox. Mrs. Wales, on the other hand, has not been in contact with the illness, and in a recent telephone conversation teased Mrs. Duke about Mrs. Duke's possibly contracting this childhood disease.

Thus Mrs. Duke believes that she is susceptible to this illness, whereas Mrs. Wales does not believe herself to be susceptible.

The second component is the individual's perception of the seriousness of the illness. In the hypothetical situation just described, Mrs. Duke probably would consider the illness a short-term annoyance rather than a serious threat. This perception is influenced by modifying factors, the third component, which include psychosocial variables. Because Mrs. Duke is teased by family and friends about the chance of getting chickenpox, she shares in their lighthearted attitude toward the threat of this illness. The opposite is true in the following:

Mr. Best, age 43, a business executive, has a family history of coronary disease. His father died of a heart attack at age 50, and his older brother had a serious heart attack at age 45. His sister frequently advises him to slow down in his fast-paced work life.

Mr. Best, because of the modifying factors of his family history, age, and life-style, perceives a high susceptibility to coronary disease. Because of his family's experience, he also perceives the disease as a serious threat.

The fourth component—the likelihood that a person will take preventive action—involves the person's perception of the benefits of taking action. Mrs. Duke believes she will either get chickenpox or not get it, and she continues her daily activities as usual. Even if she comes down with the illness, she is unlikely to take action, since she does not perceive the disease as a serious threat, unless her symptoms change her perception of how serious the disease may become. Mr. Best, on the other hand, understands that smoking, being overweight, and stress all increase the risks of cardiac disease, and thus he perceives strong benefits in changing his life-style in ways that decrease his risks. If he enters the health care system, such as for an annual physical examination, and with a nurse plans a program for weight reduction and other changes, all the components that influence his behavior make it likely that he will comply with these recommended changes.

The health belief model addresses the relationship between what a person believes and how he acts. Nurses using this approach can better understand factors that influence clients' perceptions and beliefs and thus clients' behavior, in order to plan care that will most effectively assist clients in maintaining or regaining health and preventing illness.

■ ■ ■ ■ ■

The four models of health and illness are not conflicting theories among which a nurse chooses but are ways of approaching complex issues and of understanding how clients' attitudes toward health and illness differ and thus lead to different kinds of health behaviors. The following section continues this discussion by examining in more detail the primary variables of these beliefs and practices.

Variables Influencing Health Beliefs and Practices

Nurses need to understand the many variables that influence clients' health beliefs and practices. Both internal and external variables can influence what a client thinks and how he acts. Understanding how these variables affect a specific client allows the nurse to plan and deliver nursing care individualized for that client.

Internal Variables

Internal variables include a person's developmental stage, his intellectual background, his perception of his own functioning, and emotional and spiritual factors.

DEVELOPMENTAL STAGE

A person's thought and behavior patterns change as he progresses through the stages of life, and thus a nurse must consider a client's level of growth and development when planning care based on the client's health beliefs and practices. A young child, for example, is generally not able to conceptualize the potential seriousness of illnesses and thus needs to be motivated according to his developmental level to act in ways beneficial to a treatment plan or to develop habits for illness prevention. The emotional development of an adolescent may influence his beliefs about health-related matters, such as the use of contraception, and the nurse thus uses different techniques of health teaching than would be used for a young adult. Knowledge of the stages of growth and development helps the nurse predict the client's behavior in response to illness or the threat of illness, and the planning of nursing care is then adapted to these expectations as well as to the individual client's abilities to participate in his own care.

INTELLECTUAL BACKGROUND

A person's beliefs about health are shaped in part by intellectual variables, including knowledge (or misinformation) about body functions and illnesses, educational background, and past experiences from which the person learned. These variables influence what a person thinks; in addition, cognitive abilities shape *how* a person thinks, including his ability to understand factors involved in illness and to apply knowledge of health and illness to his own practices. A person's cognitive abilities are also related to his developmental stage. A nurse considers a client's intellectual background in order to understand why he believes what he does about health and health practices, so that these variables can be incorporated into nursing care.

PERCEPTION OF FUNCTIONING

How a person perceives his physical functioning affects his health beliefs and practices. For example, a person with a chronic heart condition perceives his level of health differently from someone who has never had a heart problem. As a result, the health beliefs and practices of these two persons tend to be different.

In addition, a person who has successfully recovered from a severe acute illness may change his health beliefs and practices as a result of the illness.

Although Mr. Hare had been overweight for the last 10 years, he continued to eat a high-fat, high-cholesterol diet with almost no fresh fruits or vegetables, and he did not exercise. Mr. Hare's physician had encouraged him to exercise or lose weight, but he did not do so because he had always perceived himself as being in good health and he believed that his weight, dietary habits, and exercise patterns did not affect his level of health. But then Mr. Hare had a severe myocardial infarction that required immediate coronary bypass surgery. Mr. Hare was fortunate and recovered fully from his cardiac illness without any chronic disability. After the acute illness Mr. Hare changed his health practices: he began to exercise regularly, and he soon lost 30 pounds.

When nurses assess a client's level of health, they gather subjective data about how the client perceives his physical functioning, as well as objective data about his actual functioning. Such information about the client's health beliefs and practices allows nurses to plan and implement nursing care more successfully.

EMOTIONAL AND SPIRITUAL FACTORS

Emotional and spiritual factors also influence a client's health beliefs and practices. A person who experiences a stress response with each change in his life tends to respond stressfully to any sign of illness (see Chapter 5).

Judy Kay has always overreacted to problems that arise during the course of her daily activities. If a problem occurs at work, Judy immediately becomes worried that she will be fired from her job. Anytime she becomes ill, she immediately thinks that she has a severe illness and goes to her doctor to request diagnostic tests.

A person who generally is very calm may have very little emotional response during illness or after being informed of a life-threatening diagnosis. A person who is unable to cope emotionally with the threat of illness may deny the presence of symptoms and thus not take actions to prevent illness because he believes the symptoms are a normal response. A man who finds he is short of breath and coughs frequently may blame this condition on cold weather if he cannot emotionally accept the possibility of a respiratory illness. Because much media attention has been given to cancer, for example, many people have strong emotional reactions against even thinking about the risk of this disease, and thus they deny symptoms and refuse to take preventive action when otherwise they might seek health care.

If a person's religious beliefs include the belief that physical health is necessary for spiritual health, his practices will reflect that belief. On the other hand, if the person's religious beliefs require that the person abstain from certain kinds of medical treatment, he may avoid health care in general. In some cases a client may believe that illness is a punishment he deserves or must accept and thus does not act to regain or maintain his health. Thus, as with emotional variables, a nurse must understand a client's spiritual values to involve the client effectively in nursing care.

External Variables

External variables that influence a person's health beliefs and practices include family practices, socioeconomic factors, and cultural variables.

FAMILY PRACTICES

How a client's family has used health care services generally affects the client's health practices. If a client's parents treated every childhood virus and illness as a potentially severe disease and immediately sought health care, the person as he grows into adulthood also generally views each cold as a severe illness and seeks treatment. This is one reason why some people stay home from school or work each time they have colds, while others attempt to carry on as usual. In addition, if a client's family practiced preventive health care, the client as an adult is also more likely to practice prevention. For example, usually people whose parents had them immunized against childhood diseases also immunize their own children.

SOCIOECONOMIC FACTORS

Social and psychosocial factors can increase a person's risk for illness as well as influence how the person defines and reacts to illness. Psychosocial variables can include the stability of the person's marital or intimate relationship, various life-style habits, and his occupational environment.

A person's social network has also been shown to be related to his health behavior (Steele, 1982; Parsons, 1958). An individual's neighbors, peers, and co-workers are usually aware of his level of health, and if the person is unexpectedly absent from work or a planned activity, or if he shows that he is experiencing a symptom of illness, a member of his social network may assist him in obtaining medical attention. A client's social interaction involves family, neighborhood or community, peer group, church, and occupation. People generally seek approval and support from their social groups, and this desire for approval and support affects their health beliefs and practices. For example, if it is socially acceptable in a particular peer group for teenage girls to smoke, the young women in that group may not view the practice of smoking as being potentially harmful to their health.

Social variables partly determine how the health care delivery system provides medical care. Because the health care system is organized in certain ways, it determines how clients can obtain the care they seek. The system provides care for clients with health problems society considers "legitimate" and "acceptable." In addition, the system defines the treatment method, the economic cost to the client, and potential reimbursement to the health care agency or the client. The health care system is a complex structure on which clients are dependent for care. Chapter 3 describes this system in detail.

Economic factors, like social factors, can affect a client's level of health by increasing the client's risk for disease, by influencing how or at what point the client enters the health care system, or by limiting the client's compliance with a prescribed treatment plan.

Epidemiological studies have documented that persons at low economic levels have a greater risk for pulmonary disease, cancer, and diabetes mellitus than do persons at higher levels (Goldsmith, 1975; Davidson, 1971). In addition, a large proportion of people at low economic levels live in urban areas and therefore have a greater risk for disease because of their environment.

Economic factors also influence how a client enters the health care system. A worker who has health insurance benefits is more likely to seek care and treatment for a chronic cough than is an individual who is out of work and no longer has insurance to cover the cost of treatment and hospitalization.

Finally, a person's compliance with treatment designed to maintain or improve his level of health is affected by his economic status. A person with high utility bills, a large family, and low income tends to give higher priority to food and shelter than to costly drugs or treatment or to expensive foods for special diets.

CULTURAL BACKGROUND

Cultural background influences an individual's beliefs, values, and customs. It influences how he enters the health care system as well as his health practices. For example, a study of the illness referral practices of Spanish-speaking cultural groups showed that most individuals in such a group generally did not use health care services but believed in self-medication (Allinger, 1977). When a person perceived himself to be ill, he sought treatment within his social network rather than from the health care system.

Sociocultural differences between clients and nurses can affect the nurse-client relationship and therefore the quality of nursing care delivered. If nurses are not aware of their own cultural patterns of behavior, language, and action, they may not be able to recognize and understand a client's behavior and beliefs and may have difficulty interacting with the client. For example, a client from a culture that strongly values and expects close, warm, and supportive family relationships may experience cultural conflict with a nurse who does not value or has not experienced close kinship ties (Leininger, 1977).

Cultural factors must be identified and incorporated into a client's plan of care in order to avoid conflict between the goals and methods of care and the client's cultural background (see Chapter 21).

Health Promotion and Illness Prevention

Nurses have increasingly emphasized health promotion and illness prevention activities as important forms of health care, since they assist clients in maintaining good health and improving their levels of health instead of merely providing care after illness occurs. Health promotion and illness prevention are closely related concepts and in practice overlap to some extent. Health promotion activities seek to help a client maintain his present level of health or enhance it in the future. Illness prevention activities are directed toward protecting a client from actual or potential threats to his health. Both types of activities are oriented to the future. The difference between them involves motivations and goals. Health promotion activities are intended to motivate a person

to act positively to reach the goal of a higher level of health and well-being. Illness prevention activities are designed to motivate a person to avoid a negative condition rather than to take a positive action, with the goal of maintaining, rather than attempting to improve, a level of health.

Health promotion activities can be either passive or active. With passive strategies, an individual gains from the activities of others without acting himself. The fluoridation of municipal drinking water and the fortification of homogenized milk with vitamin D are two examples of passive health promotion strategies. Fluoride is added to drinking water to promote healthy teeth and reduce the risk of tooth decay. The addition of vitamin D to milk promotes better nutrition for all consumers and decreases the incidence of rickets in persons who live in environments with limited sunshine.

With active strategies of health promotion, an individual becomes motivated to adopt a specific health program. Weight reduction and smoking cessation programs require clients to be actively involved in measures to improve their present and future levels of wellness while at the same time decreasing the risk of disease.

Health promotion and illness prevention activities have become an important focus of health care for three reasons. First, although scientific and medical advances since the 1940s have resulted in cures for infectious diseases, there are still no cures for many chronic diseases. Thus there is greater motivation for preventing the occurrence of these diseases. Second, the rapid escalation of health care costs has motivated consumers to seek ways of decreasing the incidence and minimizing the results of illness or disability. Third, society as a whole has become increasingly conscious of health and the value of maintaining or increasing the level of health rather than allowing problems to arise and then treating them.

Many programs for health promotion and illness prevention have been developed. The goal of a total health program is to improve a client's level of well-being in all dimensions, not just his physical health. Total programs are based on the belief that many different factors can affect a person's level of health (Fig. 2-4). Health can be influenced by an individual's practices, such as poor eating habits, little or no exercise, and other habits. Health can also be affected by physical stressors, a poor living environment, exposure to air pollutants, and an unsafe environment. Psychological stressors can influence an individual's level of health, as can hereditary factors. The following seven habits have been shown to promote total health, help prevent illness, and improve life expectancy (Belloc and Breslow, 1972):

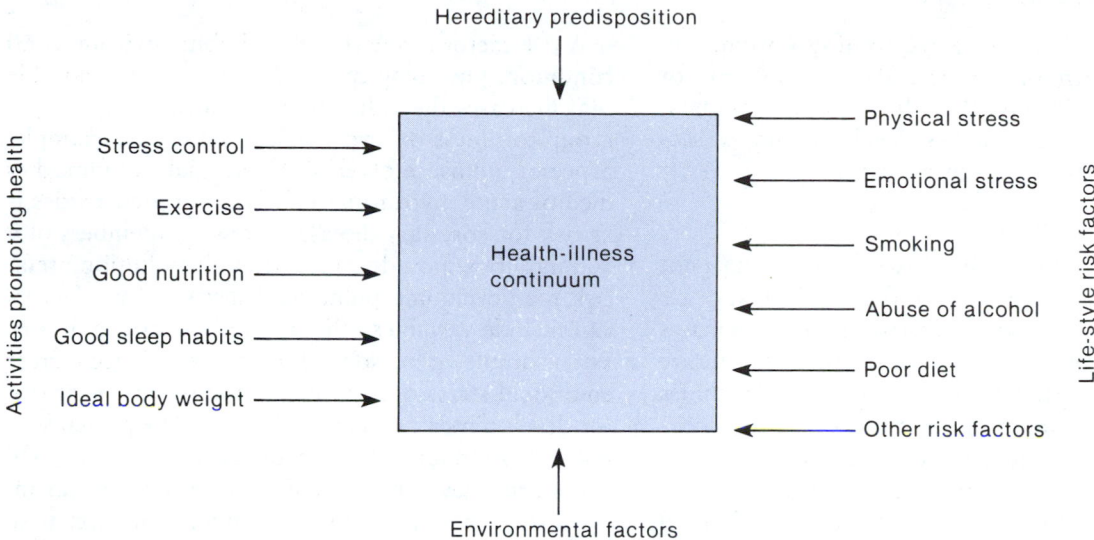

Fig. 2-4 Multifactorial health-illness dynamics.
From Milsum, J.H.: Family Community Health **3:**1, 1981.

1. Three meals a day with no snacking
2. Breakfast every day
3. Moderate exercise two or three times a week
4. Seven to 8 hours uninterrupted sleep a day
5. No smoking
6. Ideal body weight for sex, age, height, and body build
7. Alcohol only in moderation

Total health promotion programs are directed toward changing a person's total life-style so that he develops habits that can improve his level of health. Another type of program is aimed at a specific health care problem. For example, the American Lung Association has developed client-centered smoking cessation clinics that include group support (Fig. 2-5). An exercise program encourages participants to schedule exercise in their weekly calendars. A stress reduction program teaches participants how to cope with stressors in their personal lives.

Some health promotion and illness prevention programs are operated by health care agencies, and thus nurses may be actively involved. Most health promotion centers are independent of health care agencies, however, although nurses may still be involved as consultants or by giving referrals. Many corporations have developed health promotion activities for their employees. Likewise, colleges and community centers offer health promotion and illness prevention programs. The goal of these activities is to improve the client's level of health through preventive health services, environmental protection, and health education.

Health promotion and illness prevention activities are new to the consumer as well as the health care provider. Whether an activity is an active or passive strategy, the overall goal is to maintain or improve the level of the client's physical, emotional, intellectual, social, and spiritual well-being. Although activities are often organized in specific programs, nurses in all areas of practice often have opportunities to assist clients in adopting activities to promote their health and decrease the risks of illness.

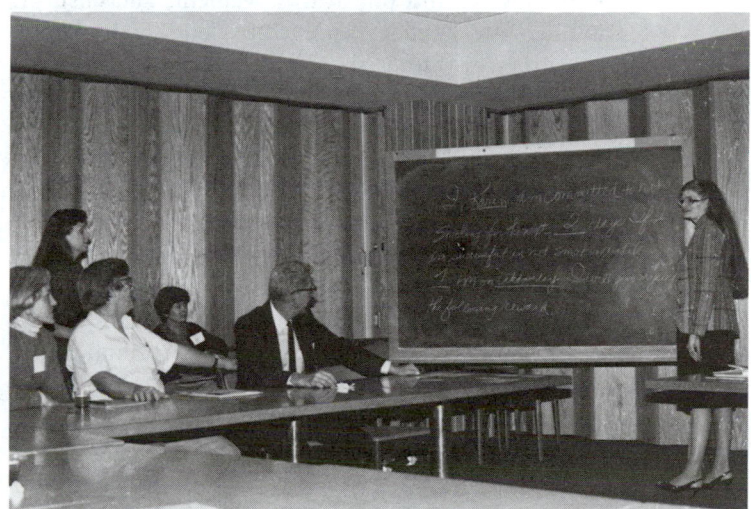

Fig. 2-5 Total health promotion programs are directed toward changing a person's total life-style so that the person develops habits to improve his level of health. The American Lung Asssociation has developed client-centered smoking cessation clinics that include group support.

Courtesy American Lung Association of Eastern Missouri.

Levels of Preventive Care

Nursing care that is oriented to health promotion and illness prevention can be understood in terms of health care activities on three levels. Leavell and associates (1965) described these levels as primary, secondary, and tertiary preventive care.

PRIMARY LEVEL

Primary preventive care focuses on individuals not currently experiencing health problems. Primary care activities are thus oriented to assisting clients in maintaining and improving health and preventing future illness. Primary preventive care by nurses includes health education programs in areas as diverse as dental hygiene, nutrition, and sexuality and reproduction. Also included are nursing activities such as providing immunization against common childhood diseases. Primary preventive care may be provided to a general population or may focus on particular groups identified as being at risk for developing health problems.

SECONDARY LEVEL

Secondary preventive care focuses on individuals who are experiencing health problems or illnesses and who are at risk for developing complications or worsening conditions. Much nursing care delivered in hospitals and other institutions is at the secondary level, designed to prevent complications. Examples include preventing wound infection, administering intravenous fluids, helping with personal hygiene, assisting with exercise and physical movement, and ensuring an adequate oxygen supply for clients with respiratory illnesses. Other secondary-level nursing actions may include educating clients about self-care and providing emotional support to help clients adapt to illness and continue to comply with therapy.

TERTIARY LEVEL

Tertiary preventive care focuses on individuals with short- or long-term disabilities or reduced functioning resulting from illness. The goal of care at this level is to help clients adapt as fully as possible to limitations caused by illness or overcome problems related to limited functioning; such care is often termed "rehabilitation." This level of care is called preventive care because it involves preventing further disability or reduced functioning. A nurse who provides tertiary care to a recently blinded client, for example, not only assists the client in adapting to the disability through activities such as teaching him how to perform the tasks of personal hygiene, but also directs his attention to the goal of preventing future problems such as accidents in the home, potential problems with child rearing, or emotional difficulties related to a changed self-concept.

Risk Factors

A risk factor is any situation, habit, environmental condition, physiological condition, or other variable that increases the vulnerability of an individual or a group to illness or an unhealthy state. For example, a person whose mother and maternal grandmother died of acute myocardial infarction in their forties is at risk for coronary disease. Likewise, members of a community exposed to industrial air pollution are at risk for developing pulmonary disease. Risk factors can include variables other than physical conditions. For example, a person who has experienced great emotional stress over a long period of time is at risk for developing many kinds of illness. The presence of risk factors does not mean that a disease state will necessarily develop, but risk factors increase an individual's vulnerability to a particular disease. Risk factors can occur in different aspects of a person's internal or external environment, because, as discussed previously, factors in either of these environments can influence a person's health. Nurses and other health care professionals are concerned with risk factors for several reasons. As discussed earlier, in the section on the health-illness continuum, risk factors play a major role in how a nurse identifies a client's present health status. Risk factors can also influence a person's health beliefs and practices, if the person is aware of the presence of the risk factor; the health belief model includes, for example, the component of the client's perception of his susceptibility to illness. Identifying risk factors is also important for health promotion and illness prevention activities, which are often based on reducing or eliminating the risk factors. For example, cigarette smoking is a risk factor for respiratory illness, and smoking cessation clinics offer illness prevention programs to eliminate the risk. For clients with high blood pressure, a risk factor for cardiac disease and other illnesses, medication therapy to lower the blood pressure is directed toward lessening the risk of developing these illnesses.

Risk factors can be placed in four categories: genetic and physiological factors, age, physical environment, and life-style. These factors are often interrelated.

GENETIC AND PHYSIOLOGICAL FACTORS

A physiological risk factor involves the physical functioning of the body. Certain physical conditions, such as pregnancy or being overweight, place increased stress on a person's physiological systems, such as the circulatory system, increasing the person's susceptibility to illness in these areas. Heredity, or an individual's genetic predisposition to specific illness, is a major physical risk factor. For example, a person with a family history of diabetes mellitus is at risk for developing the disease later in life. Other documented genetic risk factors include family histories of cancer, coronary disease, and renal disease.

AGE

Age is often a factor that increases an individual's susceptibility to illness. For example, the risk of cardiovascular disease increases with age for both sexes. The risks of birth defects and complications of pregnancy increase after a certain age, usually considered to be about 35. Many kinds of cancer pose a greater risk for persons over age 45 than for younger persons. Age risk factors are often closely associated with other risk factors, such as family history and personal habits. For example, a man at age 60 who has smoked for 40 years is at greater risk for developing lung cancer than a man at age 30 who has smoked for 10 years.

ENVIRONMENT

The physical environment in which a person works or lives can increase the likelihood that certain illnesses will occur. Studies have shown, for example, that some kinds of cancer and other diseases are more likely to develop in industrial workers exposed to certain chemicals. Black lung disease, for instance, once afflicted many coal miners inadequately protected from coal dust. The workplace may include other kinds of risk factors as well, such as high noise levels or increased emotional stress.

TABLE 2-1

Social Readjustment Rating Scale

Rank	Life Event	Mean Value	Rank	Life Event	Mean Value
1	Death of spouse	100	23	Son or daughter leaving home	29
2	Divorce	73	24	Trouble with in-laws	29
3	Marital separation	65	25	Outstanding personal achievement	28
4	Jail term	63	26	Wife begins or stops work	26
5	Death of close family member	63	27	Begin or end school	26
6	Personal injury or illness	53	28	Change in living conditions	25
7	Marriage	50	29	Revision of personal habits	24
8	Fired at work	47	30	Trouble with boss	23
9	Marital reconciliation	45	31	Change in work hours or conditions	20
10	Retirement	45	32	Change in residence	20
11	Change in health of family member	44	33	Change in schools	20
12	Pregnancy	40	34	Change in recreation	19
13	Sex difficulties	39	35	Change in church activities	19
14	Gain of new family member	39	36	Change in social activities	18
15	Business readjustment	39	37	Mortgage or loan less than $10,000	17
16	Change in financial state	38	38	Change in sleeping habits	16
17	Death of close friend	37	39	Change in number of family get-togethers	15
18	Change to different line of work	36	40	Change in eating habits	15
19	Change in number of arguments with spouse	35	41	Vacation	13
20	Mortgage over $10,000	31	42	Christmas	12
21	Foreclosure of mortgage or loan	30	43	Minor violations of the law	11
22	Change in responsibilities at work	29			

Reprinted with permission from J. Psychosom. Res. **11**:213. Holmes, T.H., and Rahe, R.H.: Social readjustment rating scale. Copyright 1967, Pergamon Press Ltd.

TABLE 2-2

Hospital Stress Rating Scale

Rank	Event	Mean
1	Possibility of loss of function of senses (e.g., eyesight, hearing)	116.8
2	Admission for life-threatening illness	107.1
3	Possibility of loss of an organ	92.1
4	Anticipated bad experience with medications	80.3
5	Inadequate insurance to cover hospitalization	78.5
6	Possibility of disfigurement	75.8
7	Anticipated future loss of income as a result of illness	75.5
8	Admission for surgery	73.7
9	Inadequate explanation of diagnosis	71.8
10	Undiagnosed ailment at time of admission	71.1
11	Inadequate finances for family during hospital stay	71.0
12	Being away from home	60.4
13	Inadequate explanation of treatment	58.0
14	Presence of severely ill roommate	57.8
15	Isolation for contagious condition	57.5
16	Anticipated improvement in functioning	56.8
17	Unconcerned attitude of hospital staff	56.4
18	Spouse at home	55.7
19	Anticipated pain or discomfort as a result of treatment	54.6
20	Dependent children at home	53.9
21	Hospitalization at considerable distance from home	53.2
22	Hospitalization as the result of an accident	50.7
23	Anticipated relief of pain or discomfort	50.2
24	Emergency admission	50.0
25	Experience of esthetically unpleasant surroundings	47.7
26	Admission for diagnostic tests only	46.2
27	Not having visitors	44.5
28	Prior hospitalization experience	43.3
29	Anticipated improved appearance	43.0
30	Change in amount of physical activity	41.6
31	Holiday or special family occasion during hospitalization	41.3
32	Change in amount of independent behavior	41.0
33	Major change in eating habits	40.1
34	Cared for by unfamiliar physician	39.6
35	Major change in sleeping habits	38.8
36	Being away from job	38.0
37	Language problem in communication with staff	36.2
38	Presence of unfamiliar machines or mechanical devices	35.1
39	Isolation from friends	34.5
40	Acquaintance with someone else with the same medical problem	34.3
41	Change in amount of personal privacy	33.6
42	Change in amount of interaction with other people	32.2
43	Extensive medical knowledge	30.7
44	Change in awareness of world or local events	27.2
45	Being away from school	26.3

Air and water pollution increases the risk of illness. High crime rates or overcrowding can lead to stresses that make individuals more susceptible to disease.

In the home the physical environment may include conditions that pose risks to an individual or to a whole family. Unclean, poorly heated or cooled, or overcrowded dwellings increase the likelihood that infections and other diseases will be contracted and spread. Within the family, conflicts or other problems may create stresses that put individual members, or the family as a whole, at increased risk of illness.

LIFE-STYLE

Many of a person's activities, habits, and practices can involve risk factors, as do the stresses of life crises and frequent life-style changes.

As discussed earlier, a person's health practices and behaviors can have either a positive or a negative effect on health. Practices with potential negative effects, therefore, are risk factors. Such practices include overeating or poor nutrition, insufficient rest and sleep, and poor personal hygiene. Other habits that put a person at risk for illness include smoking, alcohol or drug abuse, and activities that involve a threat of accidents. Some habits are risk factors for specific diseases. For example, excessive sunbathing increases the risk of skin cancer, and being overweight increases the risk of cardiovascular disease.

Any emotional stress can be a risk factor if the stress is severe or prolonged or the person is unable to cope adequately with it. In such a case, emotional stress may increase the chance that the individual will develop an illness. Emotional stresses may occur with such events as divorce, pregnancy, and arguments with others. Any area of life that leads to long-term emotional stresses can be a risk factor. Job-related stresses, for example, may overtax a person's cognitive skills and decision-making ability, leading to what is sometimes called "mental overload" or "burnout." Often there is a close relationship between mental health risk factors and emotional stresses.

Holmes and Rahe (1967) have developed a social readjustment rating scale (Table 2-1), which correlates life-style changes with the risk of illness. Research has shown that when a person has a change in life-style, there is a greater risk that illness will occur. Chapter 5 describes many kinds of illness that have been shown to be related to stress.

The adjustment that clients must make in hospitals and other health care settings can also involve a risk for further illness. Volicer (1974) has developed a hospital stress rating scale (Table 2-2), which closely parallels the Holmes and Rahe scale. The objective of the scale is to predict the risk of a long hospital stay, complications, and pain, all of which may be linked to further disability or prolonged illness. The hospital stress rating scale assigns a numerical value to actual or potential stresses experienced during hospitalization. The higher the client's total score, the greater the risk that complications will develop, that pain medications will be necessary, and that the hospital stay will be prolonged. A high score on the scale does not necessarily mean that a client will experience complications or a long hospital stay. However, the scale predicts general risks and therefore helps a nurse identify the risks for a particular client in order to develop nursing interventions to reduce hospital stress and the incidence of complications (Volicer, 1974).

Illness and Illness Behavior

Illness is not merely the presence of a disease process. Illness is an abnormal state in which a person's physical, emotional, intellectual, social, or spiritual functioning is diminished or impaired compared with that person's previous experience. Cancer is a disease process, but one client with leukemia who is respond-

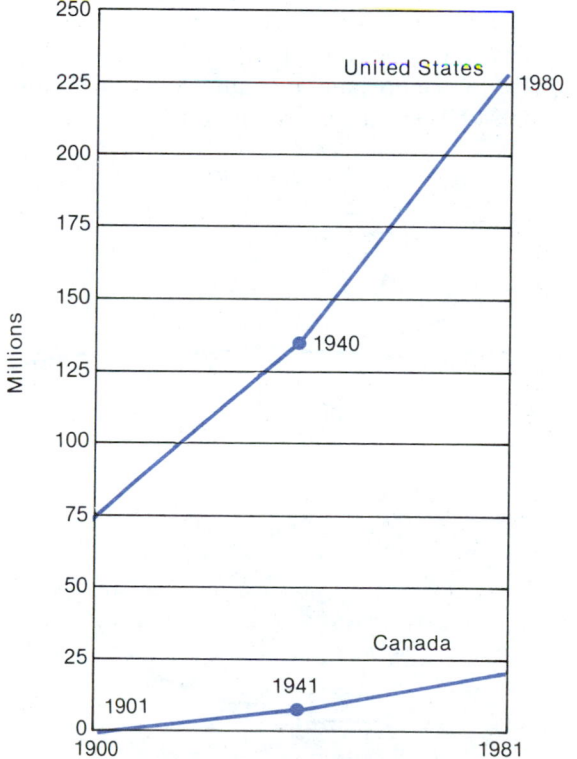

Fig. 2-6 Increases in population in the United States (1900-1980) and Canada (1901-1981).

Data from Department of Commerce, Bureau of the Census: Population profile of the United States, 1980, series P, No. 363, Washington D.C., 1981, U.S. Government Printing Office; Statistics Canada, Census of Canada, Ottawa, 1981, Minister of Supplies and Services, p. 6.

ing to treatment may not perceive himself as ill and may continue to function as usual, whereas another client with breast cancer who is preparing for surgery may perceive herself as ill and be affected in dimensions other than the physical.

Illness therefore is not synonymous with disease, although nurses must of course be familiar with different kinds of diseases and their treatments. Fig. 2-6 displays increases in population in the United States and Canada; Table 2-3 and Figs. 2-7 to 2-9 list leading causes of death and indicate the utilization of health care services in each country. Such statistics show only the potential physical effects of disease. Nurses are concerned more with illness, which includes disease but which also involves effects on an individual's functioning and well-being in all dimensions.

People who are ill generally act in a way that medical sociologists call "illness behavior." Illness behavior involves how persons monitor their bodies, define and interpret their symptoms, take remedial actions, and use the health care system (Mechanic, 1982). If an individual perceives himself to be ill, illness behavior can serve as a coping mechanism. For example, illness behavior may serve as a means of obtaining reassurance. If a person has been off work for a week because of illness, one result may be that he is reassured that his employer missed his contribution and that others care about him. The health team can also be a source of support and reassurance for the client. Such support is particularly important for a client

with a chronic disease. A person with severe cardiac impairment who is unable to care for himself looks to the health team for support. The client may need reassurance that his inability to care for himself is due to the physical disease and not to his own lack of motivation or desire. In addition, illness behavior can result in the client being released from a role, social expectation, or responsibility. For a housewife, for example, the "flu" may be a temporary release from child care and household responsibilities.

TABLE 2-3

Major Causes of Death in Canada and the United States, All Ages, 1977

Cause of Death	Canada*	United States†
Diseases of the circulatory system	81,474	Heart: 3426 Stroke: 740
Cancers	36,419	1332
Accidents, suicides, and violence	16,001	450

*Data from Causes of deaths in perspective in Canada. In Statistics Canada, catalogue No. 84-203, Ottawa, 1980, Minister of Supplies and Services, p. 68.
†Data from National Center for Health Statistics, Division of Vital Statistics, Washington, D.C., 1977.

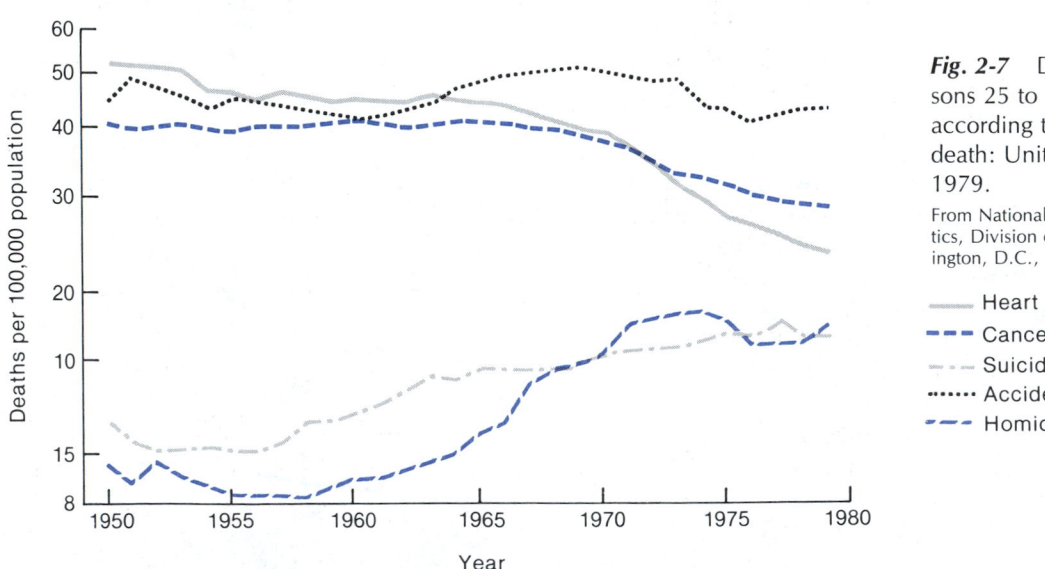

Fig. 2-7 Death rates for persons 25 to 44 years of age, according to leading causes of death: United States, 1950 to 1979.

From National Center for Health Statistics, Division of Vital Statistics, Washington, D.C., 1977.

—— Heart disease
- - - Cancer
—·— Suicide
······ Accidents
– – Homicide

Note: Causes of death are assigned according to the International List of Causes of Death. Because of the decennial revisions and changes in rules for cause-of-death selection, there may be some lack of comparability from one revision to the next. The beginning dates of the revisions are 1949, 1958, 1968, and 1979.

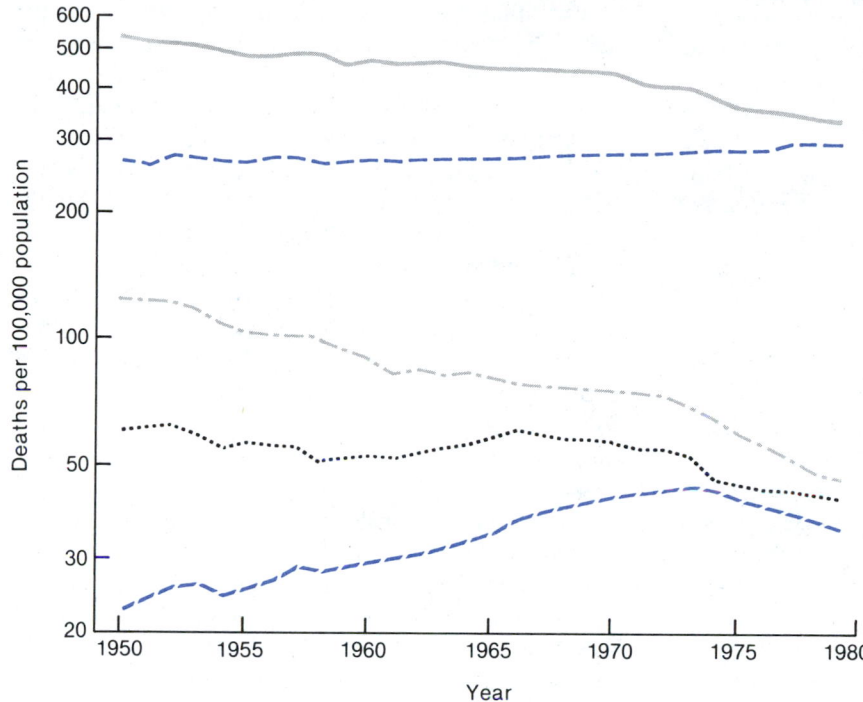

Fig. 2-8 Death rates for persons 45 to 64 years of age, according to leading causes of death: United States, 1950 to 1979.

From National Center for Health Statistics, Division of Vital Statistics, Washington, D.C., 1977.

——— Heart disease
– – – Cancer
–·–·– Stroke
·········· Accidents
– – – Cirrhosis of liver

Note: Causes of death are assigned according to the International List of Causes of Death. Because of the decennial revisions and changes in rules for cause-of-death selection, there may be some lack of comparability from one revision to the next. The beginning dates of the revisions are 1949, 1958, 1968, and 1979.

Fig. 2-9 Age-adjusted death rates for person 65 years of age and over, according to leading causes of death: United States, 1950 to 1979.

From National Center for Health Statistics, Division of Vital Statistics, Washington, D.C., 1977.

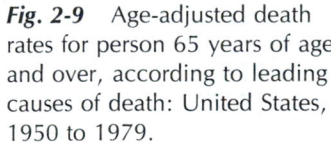

——— Heart disease
– – – Cancer
–·–·– Stroke
·········· Influenza and pneumonia
– – – Diabetes mellitus

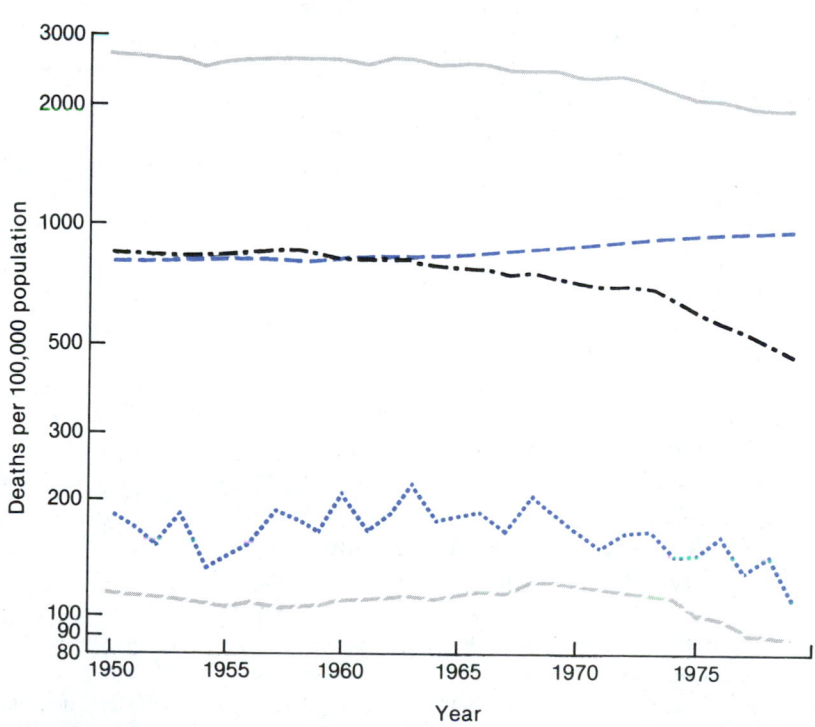

Note: Causes of death are assigned according to the International List of Causes of Death. Because of the decennial revisions and changes in rules for cause-of-death selection, there may be some lack of comparability from one revision to the next. The beginning dates of the revisions are 1949, 1958, 1968, and 1979.

Variables Influencing Illness Behavior

Just as health behavior is affected by internal and external variables, so also is a client's illness behavior. The nurse needs to understand the influences of these variables in order to understand the client's behavior and plan individualized nursing care. These variables tend to be complex in their origins and effects. Not all of the variables can be discussed here, but later chapters continue this discussion in relevant sections.

INTERNAL VARIABLES

Two important internal variables that influence how a person behaves when he is ill are his perception of his symptoms and the nature of the illness itself.

If a client believes that the symptoms of his illness are disrupting his normal routine, he is more likely to seek health care assistance than he would be if he did not perceive the symptoms to be disruptive. A client with persistent, severe headaches, for example, is likely to seek health care sooner than a client with a mild toothache. If a client perceives his symptoms as serious or perhaps life threatening, he is also more likely to seek assistance. A person awakened in the middle of the night with crushing chest pain generally views this as a symptom of a potentially serious and life-threatening illness and will probably be motivated to seek assistance. However, such a perception can also have the opposite effect. A person may fear that he has a serious illness, react by denying this possibility, and thus not seek medical assistance.

A client's illness behavior can also be affected by the nature of the illness. Acute illnesses involve symptoms of relatively short duration that are usually severe and that may affect the client's functioning in any dimension. Acutely ill clients are generally passive; they do not expect, and are not expected, to participate in the health care decisions made for their immediate treatment. A person with an acute respiratory tract infection, for example, is more interested in obtaining antibiotic treatment as soon as possible than in actively participating with the health care team.

Chronic illnesses are those that persist over a long period of time; they, too, can affect the functioning of a client in any dimension. Several variables influence the illness behavior of a client with a chronic illness. He may fluctuate between a state of maximal functioning and serious exacerbations that may be life threatening. A diabetic client, for example, may remain stable when his disease process is under control, but if he alters his food intake or his activity level he can run the risk of diabetic ketoacidosis.

If a chronic illness cannot be cured and the symptoms are only partially relieved by therapy, the client is generally not highly motivated to comply with the therapy plan (Aiken, 1976). An adolescent with diabetes may resent the fact that he cannot be cured and that he must remain on a diet different from that of his friends, and because of this resentment and frustration he may not follow his diabetic diet properly. In addition, in the present health care system, health care professionals are sometimes not highly motivated to remain involved in a client's care (Aiken, 1976), and the client's own motivation may lessen correspondingly. The present system is geared to short, intensive client interactions; continuity is often lacking in the provision of health care, and health care services and community support systems vital for management of chronic illness do not always maintain adequate communication with one another (Aiken, 1976).

Clients with acute illness, then, are more likely to seek health care and to comply readily with therapy. Chronically ill clients, because of the factors discussed previously, may become less actively involved in their care, may experience greater frustration, and may comply less readily with care. Because nurses generally spend more time with chronically ill clients than other health care professionals do, they are in the unique position of being able to assist the chronically ill in overcoming problems related to illness behavior.

EXTERNAL VARIABLES

External variables that can influence a client's illness behavior include the visibility of symptoms, the person's social group, the person's cultural background, economic variables, and the accessibility of the health care system.

The visibility of the symptoms of an illness can affect a client's body image and thus his illness behavior. For example, a person who has a draining sore on the lip may seek assistance sooner than a person with a sore throat of the same duration, because more people may comment on the sore, the sore changes the person's appearance, and the drainage requires continual care by the client.

A client's social group can influence his illness behavior. The social group may assist the client in recognizing the threat of an illness, or the group may support his denial of a potential illness. Assume, for example, that two 35-year-old women in two different social groups have identified a breast mass while performing self-breast examination. Both women discuss the finding with their friends. The first woman's friends might encourage her to seek medical attention to determine if a biopsy is necessary, while the second woman's friends might tell her that the lump represents only fibrocystic disease and that she does not need to go to a doctor. In a third situation, the social group might forbid the discussion of such subjects altogether, with the result that a woman would neither seek medical attention nor feel reassured that there is no risk. These examples illustrate the influence that friends may have on a client; the client's interaction with family members, peers, and others in his social group may have similar results.

A person's reactions to both his illness and the therapy for that illness are influenced by his cultural beliefs, values, and experiences. Therefore a nurse needs to understand a client's cultural background in order to develop individualized nursing therapy. For example, two studies of how cultural groups respond to pain (Leininger, 1977; Zborowski, 1952) demonstrated several cultural variations. Older New Englanders, for instance, were found to be stoical in their response to pain; they tended to suffer in silence and not seek pain relief. Members of the Irish cultural group tended to deny their pain. Members of the Italian and Jewish cultural groups sought relief of pain, but Italians were more concerned about the implications of pain for their future levels of wellness and functioning. With an understanding of how cultural factors influence a client's illness behavior, a nurse can more effectively assess the client's level of health and provide care.

Economic variables also influence how a client reacts to an illness. Because of economic constraints an individual may delay treatment, and in many cases a client continues to work, rear children, or go to school despite an illness. People of higher economic status tend to practice preventive health care more frequently than people of lower economic status, perhaps because middle- and upper-class persons have more resources to devote to preventive health care. Frequently the resources of lower-class and lower-middle-class persons are devoted to the basic needs of food and shelter.

Closely related to the influence of economic factors is the effect of the client's accessibility to the health care system. The health care system is a socioeconomic system that a client must enter, interact in, and exit. To many clients entry into the system itself is complex or confusing. As a result some clients may seek nonemergency medical care via an emergency room, simply because they do not know how to obtain health services otherwise. The physical proximity of a client to a hospital, clinic, or health care agency often influences how soon he enters the system after deciding to seek care. In addition, some clients are reluctant to seek care from a large, complex medical center but would more readily visit a community agency if one were available. Clients frequently feel that a large medical center is impersonal, that care is provided in a mechanized, assembly-line approach, and that health care personnel in such a center are always looking for the worst. Some clients, however, may seek care only from a large medical center because they believe diagnosis and treatment procedures are more current.

The present health care system is better equipped to treat acute illnesses than chronic or moderate illnesses, and as a result the system is more accessible to clients with acute illness (Aiken, 1976). For example, consider three people who are new in a community, and do not have personal physicians. Over the weekend the first suffers an acute myocardial infarction, is taken to the local emergency room, and is subsequently admitted for treatment. On the same weekend, the second person develops a severe, productive cough with green sputum. Because she has no other access to medical care, she also visits the local emergency room after attempting by telephone to arrange an appointment with a personal physician. Af-

---

Ten Determinants of Illness Behavior

- The visibility and recognizability of the illness's symptoms
- The extent to which the person perceives the symptoms as serious (the person's estimate of the present and future risks)
- The person's information, knowledge, and cultural assumptions and understanding related to the perceived symptoms
- The extent to which symptoms disrupt family, work, and social activities
- The frequency of the appearance of the symptoms and their persistence
- The extent to which others who are exposed to the person tolerate the symptoms
- The extent to which basic needs are denied because of the illness
- The extent to which meeting other needs competes with illness responses
- The extent to which the person gives other possible interpretations to the symptoms
- The availability and physical proximity of treatment resources and the psychological and monetary costs of taking action (including costs in time and effort, as well as such costs as stigma, social distance, and feelings of humiliation)

Modified from Mechanic, D.: The epidemiology of illness behavior and its relationship to physical and psychological distress. In Mechanic, D.: Symptoms, illness behavior, and help seeking, New York, 1982, Prodist.

ter a lengthy wait she obtains an antibiotic but receives no follow-up treatment or evaluation. The third person has an infected laceration of the foot. Frustrated by the thought of a long wait in the emergency room, or afraid that he may be denied treatment because he does not have health insurance, he decides not to visit the emergency room, which leads to his illness becoming worse. In each case the person's condition is affected by the person's accessibility to the health care system.

■ ■ ■ ■ ■

All these internal and external factors can interact in various ways to influence how a person behaves when ill and how and when he seeks health care. Mechanic (1982) has summarized the influences on illness behavior to produce a list of 10 primary determinants (see boxed material on p. 55). A nurse who knows the variables affecting illness behavior can better understand a client's illness behavior. As a result nursing care can be planned and delivered in a way that involves the client's resources so that he is restored to a maximal level of health.

Stages of Illness Behavior

Although the behavior of individuals when they become ill is influenced in different ways by internal and external variables, people generally pass through five stages of illness behavior (Fig. 2-10). This be-

havior pattern involves how a person seeks, finds, and completes health care. Suchman (1965) identified these stages as follows:
1. Symptom experience
2. Assumption of the sick role
3. Medical care contact
4. Dependent client role
5. Recovery and rehabilitation

Nurses encounter clients in various stages of illness behavior. Knowledge of these stages enables a nurse to assess a client's behavior, determine his stage of illness behavior, and develop nursing interventions to enable him to achieve optimal physical, emotional, intellectual, social, and spiritual functioning throughout the illness experience.

STAGE 1: SYMPTOM EXPERIENCE

During this initial stage a person is aware that "something is wrong." He usually recognizes a physical sensation or a limitation in his functioning, but does not suspect a specific diagnosis.

The person's perception of a symptom includes three components. First, he becomes aware of a physical change such as pain, a rash, or a lump. Second, he evaluates this change and decides that it is a symptom of an illness. Last, if the person decides that an illness may be present, there is an emotional response. Assume, for example, that a 38-year-old woman feels a lump in her left breast during her monthly self-examination. She knows because she recently completed her menstrual period that the lump is not related to hormonal changes. She decides that the pres-

Fig. 2-10 Stages of illness behavior.
From Suchman, E.A.: J. Health Hum. Behav. **6:**114, 1965.

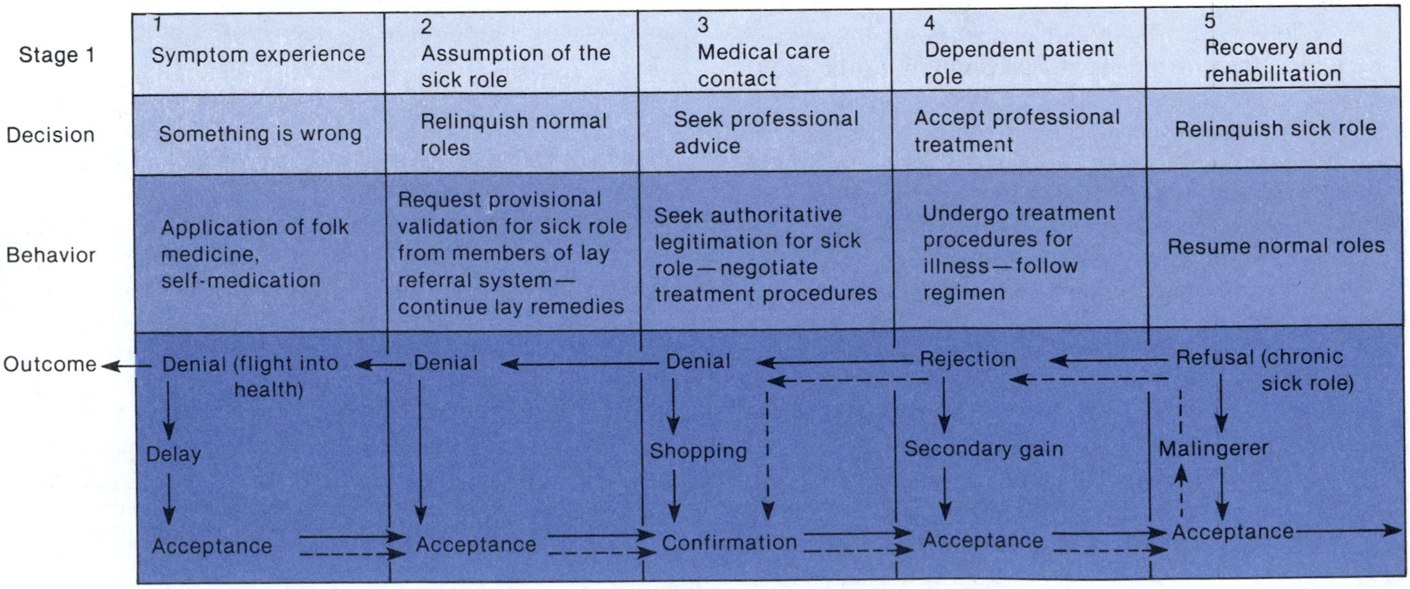

	1	2	3	4	5
Stage 1	Symptom experience	Assumption of the sick role	Medical care contact	Dependent patient role	Recovery and rehabilitation
Decision	Something is wrong	Relinquish normal roles	Seek professional advice	Accept professional treatment	Relinquish sick role
Behavior	Application of folk medicine, self-medication	Request provisional validation for sick role from members of lay referral system—continue lay remedies	Seek authoritative legitimation for sick role—negotiate treatment procedures	Undergo treatment procedures for illness—follow regimen	Resume normal roles
Outcome ←	Denial (flight into health) ← Delay Acceptance	Denial ← Acceptance	Denial ← Shopping Confirmation	Rejection ← Secondary gain Acceptance	Refusal (chronic sick role) Malingerer Acceptance →

the lump means "something is wrong" and that it may be the symptom of an illness. Because she knows that the lump may indicate the presence of cancer, she may become anxious and fearful about this potential diagnosis.

Once a person acknowledges the presence of a symptom or symptoms he may behave in various ways. If he regards the symptoms as mild or not life threatening, as in the case of a cold, he may attempt various self-medication strategies rather than seek health care. Most commonly he treats himself with over-the-counter drugs and home remedies.

If the person regards the symptoms as severe or life threatening, he may either seek immediate care or deny the symptoms' presence or implications. If he denies the symptoms or their meaning for his future level of wellness, he delays seeking advice or treatment. Before progressing to the next stage of illness behavior, the person must first acknowledge the presence of a health problem.

STAGE 2: ASSUMPTION OF THE SICK ROLE

If the symptoms persist and become severe, the person assumes the sick role, the second stage. At this point the illness becomes a social phenomenon, and the sick person seeks confirmation from his family and social group that he is indeed ill and that he should be excused from normal duties and role expectations (Coe, 1978). The social group validates the person's illness. In addition, the social group may support the person's continued self-medication.

The assumption of the sick role results in emotional changes as well as physical changes. Emotional changes may be simple or complex, depending on the severity of the illness, the degree of disability, and the anticipated length of the illness.

In the case of an illness that requires intervention from health professionals, the person may deny that such intervention is necessary and thus delay contact with the health care system.

Once the person accepts the persistent nature of the symptoms or the potential threat to his present and future levels of wellness, he seeks contact with the health care system and becomes a client, the third stage of illness behavior.

STAGE 3: MEDICAL CARE CONTACT

If the symptoms persist despite home remedies, become severe, or require emergency care, the person is motivated to seek professional health services. In stage 3 the client seeks expert validation of his illness as well as treatment. In addition, he seeks an explanation of the symptoms, the cause of the symptoms, the course of the illness, and the implications of the illness for his future health.

The severity of the illness influences how long the person waits before making contact with health professionals. Life-threatening illnesses or trauma result in immediate contact, whereas a person with a persistent skin rash may delay contact for several weeks or months. In addition, the psychosocial and cultural variables that affect illness behavior may influence how long the person delays.

The client's illness can be validated at any point on the health-illness continuum. A health professional may determine that the client does not have an illness or that an illness is in fact present and may be life threatening. The client then accepts or denies this diagnosis, depending on several factors. First, the variables that affect illness behavior in general also influence how the client reacts to his illness. If he accepts the diagnosis, he usually follows through with the prescribed treatment plan. If he denies the diagnosis, he may begin "shopping" within the health care system. In such a case the client consults various health care providers until he finds one who makes the diagnosis he desires or until he changes his mind and accepts the initial diagnosis. A client who considers himself ill even if health professionals regard him as healthy may explore nontraditional health settings to obtain the desired diagnosis of illness. Conversely, a client who is initially diagnosed as ill, particularly with a life-threatening illness, may seek a different expert to tell him that his health or life is not threatened. Clients with diagnosed cancer may seek opinions from several physicians in an attempt to avoid facing the diagnosis.

STAGE 4: DEPENDENT CLIENT ROLE

Once the client accepts the fact of his illness and seeks treatment, he enters the fourth stage of illness behavior. In this stage the client depends on health professionals for the relief of his symptoms. In the dependent role the client accepts care, sympathy, and protection from the demands and stresses of life. A client can adopt the dependent role in a health care institution, at home, or in a community setting.

In the dependent role, it is socially permissible for the client to be relieved of his normal obligations and tasks. The more ill the client, the more he is exempted from responsibilities. Nonetheless, being ill is socially undesirable, and therefore the client is expected to get well as soon as possible.

Once the client enters the dependent stage of illness, he must also adjust to the disruption of his daily schedule. This disruption affects the client's role in his occupation, in his family, and in his community and may lead to stress in his emotional, intellectual, social, and spiritual dimensions.

STAGE 5: RECOVERY AND REHABILITATION

The final stage of illness behavior—recovery and rehabilitation—can arrive abruptly, such as with the subsiding of a fever, or long-term care may be required, as in the case of a fractured leg, before the client is able to resume his optimal level of functioning. In the case of chronic illness, the final stage may involve adjustment to a prolonged reduction in the level of health and functioning.

■ ■ ■ ■ ■

Not all clients go through each of these five stages, nor do all clients move through them at the same rate or in the same manner. A person who has been in good health but suddenly has a myocardial infarction and is taken to an emergency room, for example, is put immediately into the dependent client role, even though he has not progressed emotionally through the earlier stages. Nonetheless, this pattern of illness behavior occurs in many cases, and an understanding of these stages helps a nurse identify a client's changing illness behavior to provide effective nursing care.

Impact of Illness on Client and Family

Illness is never an isolated event; the client and his family must deal with the changes resulting from the illness and its treatment. Each client responds uniquely to illness, and therefore nursing interventions must be individualized. The client and his family commonly experience behavioral and emotional changes, changes in roles, changes in body image, changes in self-concept, and changes in family dynamics.

Behavioral and Emotional Impact

Different people react differently to illness or the threat of an illness. Individual behavioral and emotional reactions depend on the nature of the illness, the client's attitude toward the illness, the reaction of others to the illness, and the variables of illness behavior described previously.

Short-term, non-life-threatening illnesses evoke few behavioral changes in the functioning of the client or the family. A husband and father who has a cold, for example, may lack the energy and patience to spend time in family activities, and he may be short tempered and prefer not to interact with his family. This is a behavioral change, but the change is subtle and does not last long. Some may even consider such a change to be a normal response to illness.

Severe illnesses, particularly those that are life threatening, can lead to more extensive emotional and behavioral changes, such as anxiety, shock, denial, anger, and withdrawal. These behaviors are common responses of the client and family to the stress of illness. The nurse develops interventions to assist the client and family in coping with this stress because usually the stressor itself cannot be changed (see Chapter 5).

ANXIETY

Anxiety is a feeling of apprehension, uneasiness, agitation, uncertainty, and fear that occurs when a person anticipates some threat. The symptoms of an illness do not necessarily create as much anxiety for clients and their families as their anticipation of how the illness may affect the clients' future health. For some, the anxiety is a fear of a possible diagnosis, particularly a diagnosis of cancer. Other clients may become more anxious over impending surgery and anticipated pain. The anxiety response varies from client to client, from family to family, and from stage to stage in illness behavior, but the nurse who is attuned to the signs of anxiety develops appropriate nursing interventions (see Chapter 5).

SHOCK

When a client or his family is informed of the presence of a severe or life-threatening illness, a shock response may occur. The shock response is a powerful emotional state. Some people describe themselves as "numb" or "immobilized." People hearing that they have cancer or a severely debilitating disease, such as parkinsonism, may react with shock. They hear what has been said to them but fail to respond, or they respond in a totally inappropriate manner. For example, on hearing that he has cancer, a client may ask how the physician's family is. For some clients the state of emotional shock may be an adaptive mechanism allowing them time to absorb what they have been told (see Chapter 46).

DENIAL

Denial is a mechanism by which the client or family avoids emotional conflict and anxiety by refusing to acknowledge facts that are intolerable. A family that learns a loved one has cancer may deny the diagnosis and attempt to carry on as though nothing were wrong. Denial, however, can be an effective way for a client or family to cope wth an illness. The nurse must determine when a client or family's denial is no longer productive and may be a hindrance to therapy (see Chapter 5).

ANGER

The client or family may experience anger because of the illness. The anger of family members might be directed toward the client because his illness has disrupted their routine, their plans, and in some cases their economic support. The family members' anger might also be directed toward themselves. Assume, for example, that a 50-year-old man has a heart attack while cleaning the garage and that throughout his hospitalization and the recovery phase his teenage son is very angry and makes no attempt to hide his anger. After much discussion the nurse could very well discover that the son has been angry at himself for not cleaning the garage, because he thinks that if he had cleaned the garage his father would not have had the heart attack. In addition, the client or family could become angry with the health care team for making the diagnosis.

Anger, like other emotions, may take irrational forms. A client might be angry at the disease process itself, as if it had singled him out. Anger also may have effects on a client's social or spiritual dimensions; for example, a client may become unsociable or blame the Supreme Being for his illness (see Chapter 20). Regardless of the kind of anger, the nurse helps the client and family work through this emotion and cope with the associated stresses.

WITHDRAWAL

Illness, particularly long-term or severe illness, may cause a client to withdraw. Regardless of whether he is in a hospital or in his own home, he may avoid interacting with people, remain in his room, or resort to solitary activities such as continuously watching television. Withdrawal is a symptom of depression and may be an effect of the illness or the diagnosis. Family members may also withdraw from contact with the ill person as a result of anger or depression, in which case the nurse needs to plan care activities that promote the continuation of family functioning and family support for the client.

Impact on Family Roles

People have various roles in life, such as wage earner, decision maker, professional, and parent. When an illness occurs, the roles of both client and family may change. Such a change may be subtle and short term or drastic and long term. Clients and families generally adjust more easily to subtle, short-term changes. In most cases the client knows that the role change is only temporary. Assume, for example, that the mother of two preschool children acquires a viral infection and that her illness continues for a week, during which time she relinquishes her roles of house-wife and child care provider. Initially she may welcome giving up these roles to be able to care for herself. As she gets better, however, she begins to look forward to resuming her role.

With short-term role changes a client does not go through prolonged adjustment phases. Long-term changes, however, require an adjustment process similar to the grief process (see Chapter 47). Often the client and family members require specific counseling and guidance to assist them in coping with the role changes. The following illustrates how such changes can occur.

Mr. Lampe is a married 40-year-old construction worker with three sons. The family is very active in outdoor activities and goes hiking and camping every 2 weeks during the summer and fall. Mr. Lampe is injured while hiking, and his injury necessitates the amputation of one leg. Because of the injury Mr. Lampe has to change jobs, with the result that he receives a lower salary. The family activities change from active outdoor ones to passive indoor ones. Mrs. Lampe becomes angry because the reduction in income makes it difficult for the family to maintain its previous standard of living. The three sons become angry because their dad no longer takes them camping and hiking. Mr. Lampe becomes angry because he feels that his wife and children should be grateful that he is alive and should not worry about material things. The anger in the family gradually increases to the point that Mr. Lampe becomes unable to function at his highest level. The visiting nurse notices these changes in the family and observes the family members' angry outbursts. She refers the family for counseling sessions with a family therapist to help the family members cope with the anger resulting from the changes in Mr. Lampe's roles.

In some cases the family takes over all the roles of the client, including those of wage earner and decision maker, because family members mistakenly believe that this is the only way to help the client. When illness causes role changes for a person, the family often tries to relieve the ill person of all responsibilities and decisions. Families tend to assume that the ill person needs to be free of decisions and responsibilities in order to recover. Although a person who is ill does need to recover physically from his illness, this does not mean that he must relinquish all his roles in his family. If the family attempts to relieve him of all responsibility, he may feel isolated from the family and withdraw from it. Because changes in a client's role affect his family, nurses must incorporate the family into the plan of care.

Impact on Body Image

A person's body image is his subjective concept of his physical appearance. Some illnesses result in changes in the client's physical appearance, which can affect the client and his family. Different clients and families react differently to changes in body image.

Mrs. Lacey and Mrs. Avery are both 53-year-old housewives, and each has two children. Eight months ago, each woman had a modified mastectomy for breast cancer. Mrs. Lacey does not perceive any change in her relationship with her husband or children. She has also resumed an active social life. Mrs. Avery has not gone out socially or entertained guests in her home since the surgery. In addition, she says that her husband will not look at her scar or resume sexual activity.

The reactions of a client and his family to a change in body image depend on (1) the type of change (for example, loss of a limb, loss of a special sense, or loss of an organ); (2) the adaptive capacity of the client and family; (3) the rate at which the change takes place; and (4) supportive services available to the client and family (see Chapter 18).

When a change in body image occurs, the client generally adjusts in four phases: shock, withdrawal, acknowledgment, and rehabilitation. Initially the client may be shocked by the change or impending change in his body image. He may depersonalize the change and talk about it as though it were happening to someone else. As the client and his family are increasingly forced to recognize the reality of the change, they become anxious and may withdraw, refusing to discuss the change. At this point it is not therapeutic to force the client to face reality. Withdrawal is an adaptive coping mechanism and can assist the client in making the adjustment. As the client and family acknowledge the change, they move through a period of grieving. At the end of the acknowledgment phase they accept the loss. During rehabilitation the client is ready to learn how to adapt to the body image change through use of a prosthesis, changes in life-style, and changes in goals.

Because a change in body image can be traumatic and frightening for the client and the family, the nurse develops a care plan to assist the client in adjusting to the change. Chapters 18 and 46 discuss nursing principles and interventions for clients undergoing the grief process and changes in body image.

Impact on Self-Concept

A person's self-concept is his mental image of himself, including how he views his strengths and weaknesses in all aspects of his personality. A person's self-concept depends in part on his body image and roles but also includes other aspects of his psychological and spiritual self. The impact of illness on the self-concepts of the client and the members of his family may be more complex and less readily observed than changes in roles.

Mr. Martin's self-concept had always involved strong self-confidence, a feeling of certainty that he could cope with anything that happened to him. He contracted a severe respiratory infection that required hospitalization for a week. Although he fully recovered his former level of health, he felt more vulnerable than he had felt previously, and although he maintained all the same roles in his family and occupation, he was no longer as self-confident. His self-concept had changed in a subtle way.

A person's self-concept is important in his relationships with other family members. For example, a client whose self-concept changes because of illness may no longer meet the expectations of family members, leading to family tensions or conflicts.

Mr. Martin's young daughter had always asked her father's advice and depended on his strength when she had school problems. Now that he was less self-confident, he hesitated to offer his advice, and she perceived this hesitation as emotional withdrawal from her. Thus the change in self-concept had led to emotional conflict within the family.

In the course of providing care, a nurse is able to observe such changes in the client's self-concept—or in the self-concepts of family members—and to develop the care plan to help the client and family adjust to this impact of illness.

Impact on Family Dynamics

Because of the various effects of illness on the client and his family, family dynamics is often changed. Family dynamics is the process by which the family as a whole functions, makes decisions, gives support to individual members, and copes with everyday changes and challenges. If a parent in a family becomes ill, often family activities and decision making come to a halt as the other family members wait for the illness to pass or delay acting because they are reluctant to assume the ill person's roles or responsibilities. Particularly in cases of prolonged illness, the family often has to shift to a new pattern of functioning, a change that can lead to emotional stresses. Young children, for example, may experience a strong sense of loss if either parent is hospitalized or unable to provide affection and a sense of security as usual; such emotional difficulty may persist even when the other parent or other family members are successful in assuming the roles and responsibilities of the hospitalized parent. If a parent of an adult becomes ill and cannot carry out usual activities, often the adult child assumes many of the parent's responsibilities and in essence becomes a parent to his own parent; such a reversal of the usual situation can lead to emotional stresses, conflicting responsibilities for the adult child, or even direct conflict over who is to make what decisions.

Chapter 22 discusses in more detail family dynamics and the impact of illness on family functioning. Illness can disrupt a family's patterns of living, just as it can disrupt the functioning of the client himself in all dimensions; a nurse must view the whole family as a client and plan care to meet the same goal that must be met for the ill person—to regain the maximal level of functioning and well-being.

Summary

Health is not merely the absence of illness or disability; it is a dynamic state, in which an individual adapts to his internal and external environments to maintain a condition of physiological, emotional, intellectual, sociocultural, and developmental well-being.

To provide effective nursing care and assist clients in regaining and maintaining high levels of wellness, nurses must understand each individual client's concept of health and his health beliefs and practices. This understanding is important in all steps of the nursing process: assessment, nursing diagnosis, planning, implementation, and evaluation (see Unit 2). Successful nursing care requires that nurses work with clients and their families, and the success of this relationship depends on nurses' awareness of the unique feelings, beliefs, and practices of clients and family members.

At present most nurses practice in hospitals, and most clients who enter the health care system to receive care perceive themselves as ill. Nurses who practice within home health care or community agencies also care for many clients, whose health beliefs and practices also vary.

Health professionals are increasingly emphasizing health promotion and illness prevention activities, which are designed to help clients reduce the risks of illness and maintain maximal levels of health. Consumers of health care are also giving a higher priority to health promotion activities.

When a person becomes ill, he progresses through stages of illness behavior. Illness behavior is influenced by psychosocial and cultural factors, the accessibility of the health care system, and the nature of the illness itself. If the illness is serious enough that the person enters the health care system and receives nursing care, a nurse should be able to identify the factors influencing his behavior and the impact of the illness on both the client and his family. In this way the nurse establishes a nursing care plan that helps the client achieve a high level of wellness in all dimensions. Nursing care is thus directed toward preventing illness and promoting health, helping the client adjust to an illness and its impact, and helping him regain maximal functioning.

KEY CONCEPTS

✓ Health is a dynamic state in which the individual adapts to changes in the internal and external environment and thus maintains a state of well-being in all dimensions.

✓ An illness may be a disease but also includes reduced functioning in any of the human dimensions.

✓ A person's state of health or illness should be considered in relation to individual values, personality, and life-style rather than measured by any absolute standard.

✓ According to the health-illness continuum model, health and illness are in a dynamic, relative relationship; this model allows a nurse to compare a client's state of health with past states.

✓ The high-level wellness model describes health as balanced, integrated, and purposeful functioning directed toward attaining one's full potential.

✓ The agent-host-environment model describes disease or illness as being the result of the dynamic interaction of factors related to the agent, the host, and the environment, no one factor of which is alone the cause of disease or illness.

KEY CONCEPTS

✓ The health belief model considers various factors that influence a person's health beliefs; this model helps nurses understand and predict the behaviors of clients in seeking or complying with health care.

✓ A person's health beliefs and practices are influenced by internal variables, including developmental stage, intellectual background, perception of functioning, and emotional and spiritual factors, and by external variables, including family practices, socioeconomic factors, and cultural factors.

✓ To individualize care for a client and ensure his maximal participation in that care, the nurse considers the client's health beliefs and practices when planning care.

✓ Health promotion activities seek to maintain or enhance a person's health.

✓ Illness prevention activities seek to protect a person against risk factors and thus maintain his level of health.

✓ Nursing incorporates health promotion and illness prevention activities rather than simply treating illness once it occurs.

✓ Primary preventive care helps healthy people maintain and increase their levels of health.

✓ Secondary preventive care seeks to help already ill persons avoid complications or further health problems.

✓ Tertiary preventive care helps clients adapt to or overcome disability or reduced functioning caused by illness.

✓ Risk factors threaten a person's health, influence health practices, and are important considerations in illness prevention activities.

✓ Risk factors are commonly associated with genetic or physiological variables, age, environment, and life-style.

✓ A person's illness behavior, like his health practices, is influenced by a number of variables and must be considered by the nurse when planning care.

✓ Although no two individuals behave in exactly the same way when they are ill, most people pass through five stages of illness behavior: symptom experience, assumption of the sick role, medical care contact, the dependent role, and recovery and rehabilitation.

✓ Illness can have a number of effects on both the client and the family, including behavioral and emotional changes and changes in roles, body image, self-concept, and family dynamics.

✓ A nurse must consider all the effects of an illness on a client and his family in order to plan and implement holistic nursing care that assists both client and family in attaining a state of maximal functioning and well-being.

REFERENCES

Aiken, L.H.: Chronic illness and responsive ambulatory care. In Mechanic, D.: The growth of bureaucratic medicine, New York, 1976, John Wiley & Sons, Inc.

Allinger, R.L.: Study of illness referral in a Spanish speaking community, Nurs. Res. 26:53, 1977.

Balog, J.E.: The concepts of health and disease: a relativistic perspective, Health Values: Achieving High Level Wellness 6:7, 1982.

Belloc, N.B., and Breslow, L.: Relationship of physical health status and health practices, Prev. Med. 1:409, 1972.

Breslow, L.: A quantitative approach to the World Health Organization definition of health: physical, mental and social well-being, Int. J. Epidemiol. 1:347, 1972.

Coe, R.: Sociology of medicine, ed. 2, New York, 1978, McGraw-Hill Book Co.

Davidson, J.K.: Diabetes in socioeconomically deprived neighborhoods. In Diabetes mellitus: diagnosis and treatment, New York, 1971, American Diabetes Association.

Dunn, H.: High level wellness, Arlington, Va., 1961, R.W. Beatty, Ltd.

Dunn, H.: What high level wellness means, Health Values: Achieving High Level Wellness 1:9, 1977.

Fuchs, V.R.: Who shall live? health, economics, and social choice, New York, 1974, Basic Books, Inc.

Goldsmith, J.R.: Health effects of air pollution, Basics R. D. 4(2):4, 1975.

Holmes, T.H., and Rahe, R.H.: Social readjustment rating scale, J. Psychosom. Res. 11:213, 1967.

Leavell, H.R., et al.: Preventive medicine for the doctor in his community, ed. 3, New York, 1965, McGraw-Hill Book Co.

Leininger, M.: Cultural diversities of health and nursing care, Nursing Clin. North Am. 12(1):5, 1977.

Mechanic, D.: Medical sociology, ed. 2, New York, 1978, The Free Press.

Mechanic, D.: The epidemiology of illness behavior and its relationship to physical and psychological distress. In Mechanic, D.: Symptoms, illness behavior, and help seeking, New York, 1982, Prodist.

Parsons, T.: Definitions of health and illness in light of American values and social structures. In Joco, E.G., editor: Patients, physicians, and illness, New York, 1958, The Free Press.

Rosenstock, I.: Historical origin of the health belief model, Health Educ. Monogr. 2:334, 1974.

Steele, R.L.: Social networks as a means of health maintenance, Health Values: Achieving High Level Wellness 6(6):6, 1982.

Suchman, E.A.: Stages of illness and medical care, J. Health Human Behav. 6:114, 1965.

Volicer, B.J.: Perceived stress levels of events associated with the experience of hospitalization: development and testing of a measurement tool, Nurs. Res. 22:491, 1973.

World Health Organization: Chronicle of WHO, Geneva, 1974, The Organization, Interim Commission.

Zborowski, M.: Cultural components in response to pain, J. Soc. Issues 8:16, 1952.

ADDITIONAL READINGS

Andreoli, K.G.: Future directions: organizational settings for practice. In Lancaster, J., and Lancaster, W., editors: Concepts for advanced nursing practice, St. Louis, 1982, The C.V. Mosby Co.

Brown, B.J.: Reorganizing hospital-based nursing practice: an analysis of patient outcomes, provider satisfaction and costs. In Aiken, L.H., editor: Health policy and nursing practice, New York, 1981, McGraw-Hill Book Co.

Jonas, S.: Hospitals adopt new role, Hospitals 53:84, 1979.

Milsum, J.H.: Health, risk factor reduction and life-style changes, Fam. Comm. Health 3:1, 1980.

Newman, M.: Theory development in nursing, Philadelphia, 1979, F.A. Davis Co.

Parsons, T.: The social system, New York, 1951, The Free Press.

Steinfels, P.: The concept of health: an introduction, The Hastings Center Studies 1(3):3, 1973.

Suchman, E.A.: Health attitudes and behavior, Arch. Environ. Health 20:105, 1970.

Volicer, B.J.: Patient's perception of stressful events associated with hospitalization, Nurs. Res. 23:235, 1974.

Volicer, B.J., and Bahannon, M.W.: A hospital stress rating scale, Nurs. Res. 24:354, 1975.

Wolinsky, F.D.: The sociology of health: principles, professions and issues, Boston, 1980, Little, Brown & Co.

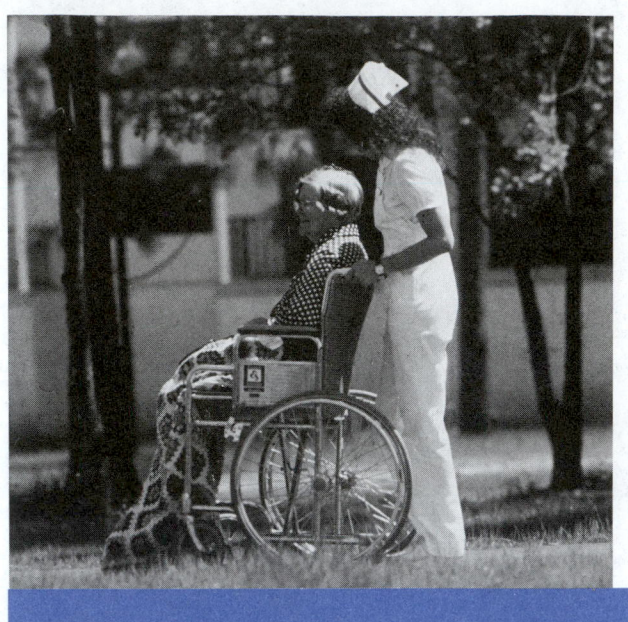

OBJECTIVES

Mastery of content in this chapter will enable the student to:

- Define the terms in the glossary.
- Describe society's influence on the health care delivery system.
- Discuss the client's entry into the system.
- Discuss how a client can use the system.
- Describe the seven types of health care agencies.
- Discuss the client's right to health care and describe client rights within the health care delivery system.
- State various methods for financing health care.
- Describe the problems of the present system.

GLOSSARY

Alcoholics Anonymous   International, nonprofit organization of recovered alcoholics whose purpose is to help alcoholics stop drinking and maintain sobriety through group support, shared experiences, and a faith in a power greater than themselves.

crisis intervention centers   Agencies providing emergency psychiatric and counseling assistance to clients experiencing extreme stress or conflict, often involving attempted suicide, drug or alcohol abuse, or other crisis behaviors.

day-care centers   Agencies that provide health care during the day.

diagnostic related groups   Groups of patients classified for measuring a hospital's delivery of care; classification is based on the following variables: primary and secondary diagnosis, primary and secondary procedures, age, and length of stay.

drug rehabilitation centers   Agencies providing long-term care for a gradual return to the community of a person with chemical or drug dependency.

extended care facility   Institution providing medical, nursing, or custodial care for clients over a prolonged period.

governmental agencies   Clinics, hospitals, and health services that are supported by local, state or provincial, or national taxes.

3 | Health Care Delivery System

health care industry   Total complex of preventive, remedial, and therapeutic services provided by hospitals and other institutions, governmental and voluntary agencies, health care professionals, pharmaceutical and medical equipment manufacturers, and governmental and private insurance agencies.

health maintenance organization   Group health care agency that provides basic and supplemental health maintenance and treatment services to voluntary enrollees who prepay a fixed periodic fee that is set without regard to the amount or kind of services received.

home health agency   Organization providing health care in the home.

hospice   System of family-centered care designed to help terminally ill persons be comfortable and maintain a satisfactory life-style throughout the terminal phase of their illness.

informed consent   Process of obtaining permission from a client to perform a specific test or procedure, after describing all risks, side effects, and benefits.

Medicaid   Joint federal and state health insurance program for a population of low-income persons, families with dependent children, and aged, blind, or disabled clients.

Medicare   U.S. federal health program that provides both medical and hospital insurance for people who are over 65 years of age or disabled or both.

nursing care strategy   Detailed nursing care plans that include direct and indirect care for the client.

outpatient setting   Physician's office, clinic, or other ambulatory care facility for treatment of nonhospitalized clients.

preferred provider organization   Group of physicians or hospital that provides companies with comprehensive health services at a discount.

prospective payment   Procedure by which the federal government sets rates for hospitals in advance for treatment of specific illnesses; this replaces the previous policy of reimbursing each hospital based on actual cost.

psychiatric hospital   Institution providing inpatient and outpatient counseling services to clients with behavioral or emotional illnesses.

rehabilitation   Restoration of an individual to normal or near-normal function following a physical or mental illness, injury, or chemical addiction.

rehabilitation center   Facility that provides therapy and training to restore a client to his optimal level of functioning and independence.

voluntary agencies   Not-for-profit health care agencies established within a community to meet specific needs.

ing is such an important part of the health care system, and because the delivery of nursing services is intertwined with other components of the health care delivery system, the nurse needs to understand the system in order to most effectively deliver quality care within it. The health care delivery system has changed in recent decades, and a complex array of agencies now provides specialized care in different areas. This complexity may at times threaten the client's rights or complicate the client's entry into the system. The present system also involves problems such as a fragmentation of care because of increased specialization. In these areas the nurse is in a unique position among health care professionals; she not only provides clients with care within the health care delivery system but also assists clients in coping with the system itself.

*I*n the last decade the emphasis in health care has shifted from diagnosis and treatment to health promotion and disease prevention. This change has resulted in part from the increased participation of the client in his health care and in part from the need to hold down costs in the delivery and use of health services.

As a result of consumer demand and federal involvement in the form of grants, loans, and legislation, the health care delivery system has been expanding for several decades in terms of its services, size, and complexity. We now have a health care delivery system that has developed in response to some of society's needs and influences and that is continually growing as biomedical technology and knowledge increase. Now more than ever, health care services are provided in a great number of settings, across all age groups, and for the chronically ill as well as the acutely ill.

Although some changes in the health care delivery system have been in response to health care consumers, the system today is complex and, for some clients, confusing or difficult to enter. Health care costs continue to rise at a rapid and somewhat frightening rate. The financing of health services has become expensive both for persons with private health insurance and for government agencies that provide assistance to meet health care costs.

Nursing is a major component of the health care delivery system, and nurses comprise the largest single employment group within the system. Nursing services are necessary for virtually every client seeking care of any type, including health promotion, diagnosis and treatment, and rehabilitation. Because nurs-

Changes in Health Care Delivery

The health care delivery system provides services related to health promotion, illness prevention, diagnosis and treatment of diseases, and rehabilitation. Such services are provided by many kinds of agencies in different settings, including outpatient settings such as hospital clinics and physicians' offices, community settings such as day-care centers and home health care, and institutional settings such as hospitals or nursing homes. The health care system has evolved over a long period of time, but within the last two or three decades change has accelerated. The present system is the result of changes associated with the health care industry, new knowledge and technology, societal and consumer influences, and economic and political factors.

Health Care Industry

The health care industry is the business side of the health care delivery system. It involves a complex of preventive, remedial, and therapeutic services provided by hospitals and other institutions, governmental and voluntary agencies, health care professionals, pharmaceutical and medical equipment manufacturers, and governmental and private insurance agencies. In the 1960s and 1970s the health care industry exploded in size and complexity, the number of hospital beds increased, the types of services increased, new diagnostic testing services were developed, and health professionals increasingly specialized. The health care industry became so complex that the consumer was confused in all aspects of his involvement with the system. Money was needed to train technicians and buy the equipment developed as a result of scientific advances. The system increasingly became a business, and business objectives sometimes seemed to threaten service goals. Therefore there was a risk that the system would lose touch with the needs of the consumer. Planners of health care services still need to remain aware of consumer needs rather than requiring the consumer to fit into the services of the system (Brown, 1979).

Societal and Consumer Influences

By the late 1970s and early 1980s society was gaining an increased influence on health care and the delivery of health care. Slowly this influence has resulted in changes within the system and has counteracted to some extent the changes in the health care industry. The system has become increasingly sensitive to the needs of the consumer and the community. The health care delivery system is still complex, but it is responding to changing health care beliefs and practices, new knowledge and technology, and economic and political influences.

Chapter 2 discusses health care beliefs and practices and the variables that affect client's beliefs and practices. As consumers have become more knowledgeable about health in general, they have gained a greater awareness of the impact of life-style on health. As a result consumers of health care have expressed a greater need for knowledge and services related to illness prevention and health promotion. Consumers still need the diagnosis and treatment of illness, but no longer is this exclusively or even primarily the focus of health care.

In addition, clients with chronic disease or disability increasingly seek information about self-care and wish to remain as independent as possible. Thus clients have demanded more health maintenance services, which allow those with chronic disease to achieve their highest level of wellness and functioning. This consumer influence has resulted in more research into health maintenance and thus more services available to these clients.

The health care beliefs and practices of society in general are as complex as those of an individual client, depending on continually evolving values, ethics, concepts of health, and other factors. In general, however, consumers' desire for health promotion, health maintenance, and new cures and treatments has led to changes in the health care delivery system. Many institutions and community-based agencies provide a wide range of health promotion and health maintenance programs to clients on a regular basis. Voluntary agencies have arisen to meet specific needs in health maintenance and promotion, and consumers have become more active in fund raising to support research in these areas.

Influence of New Knowledge and Technology

The different health care professions and the health care system as a whole are experiencing a knowledge explosion. Scientific knowledge continues to grow rapidly. Research has led to new treatments and cures for life-threatening diseases such as cancer, cardiovascular diseases, and diabetes mellitus. Clients have the opportunity to receive the most advanced treatment for specific illnesses. A disadvantage of the knowledge explosion, however, is that it is becoming increasingly difficult for health care professionals to remain well informed about all advances in their fields.

Because of advances in technology, biomedical equipment has changed rapidly, and new and increasingly sophisticated machines are continually coming into use. Such equipment is usually designed to provide the nurse, physician, or therapist with information used to diagnose a client's disorder or to determine the response to a treatment. It assists nurses working in operating rooms, labor rooms, and critical care areas, for example, in the assessment and constant monitoring of clients. Such equipment can provide lifesaving information about clients, but there is also a risk that the nurse or other health care professional may give more attention to the machine than to the person. In addition, the frequent changes in equipment and the acquisition of new equipment further increase the cost of health care services.

Another problem associated with advanced technology is whether new developments can be fully utilized. Equipment is becoming more specialized and more costly; a very expensive and sophisticated piece of equipment such as a gallium scanner may be needed for relatively few clients. Should every hospital in a community have a sophisticated scanner? Will the scanner be used effectively or remain underused even though it added significantly to the hospital's operating costs? The health care delivery system must investigate the best uses for new knowledge and technology. The ultimate factors in the use of new technology may be the economic resources available and the wants and needs of society as a whole.

Economic Influences

Ultimately someone must pay for all health care services delivered. Clients with private resources or insurance policies are generally able to seek health promotion and health maintenance services, but too often those with lower economic status have to defer seeking health services until they become very ill because their income goes to meet other needs. As the total economy of a community or a country declines, its overall use of health care services also declines.

Inflation and the economic recession in the late 1970s and early 1980s have resulted in changes in the use of health care services. As more people began to defer seeking diagnosis and treatment for illness, use of the health care delivery system decreased. In some communities the health care delivery system has been forced to respond to declining use of services by decreasing the amount and type of services offered to clients.

A specific result of general economic decline is increased unemployment, which also influences the health care delivery system. As unemployment increases, potential consumers of health care services lose their employment-based health insurance, and often they then delay seeking care for minor or even major health care problems. Government insurance programs assist these consumers in meeting their health care needs, but eligibility for such programs and benefits vary considerably from state to state and province to province.

Political Influence

The health care delivery system is also influenced by political decisions and factors. Through health care legislation, government at all levels affects how health care is provided. A federal administration that makes health care a high priority, for example, can benefit the provision of health care by introducing legislation that increases funding for health education and research.

Although politics influences the health care delivery system, it is the client who must adjust to changes caused by health care legislation. The poor frequently must delay seeking care because of economic restraints resulting from government policies.

Present Health Care Delivery System

With the passage of the Medicare and Medicaid amendments to the Social Security Act in 1965, the U.S. government established a national and state health insurance program for certain segments of the population. The Medicare program provides medical and hospital insurance for a population of 27 million persons who are either over 65 years of age or disabled. The Medicaid program provides a joint federal and state health insurance program for a population of 21 million low-income persons in specific groups: families with dependent children, the aged, the blind,

the disabled, and those who cannot afford medical care (The Social Security Act, 1976). In Canada, similar but more inclusive medical services are provided by provincial medical care plans.

In 1972 another amendment to the Social Security Act provided for professional standards review organizations (PSROs) to monitor medical care given to Medicaid, Medicare, and Maternal and Child Health Program recipients. The PSRO program was designed to improve quality of care and to guarantee appropriate use of health care services. Initially, PSROs concentrated on reviewing inpatient care in hospitals, but PSROs and similar programs are used now to evaluate and to ensure the quality of all types of care.

The National Health Planning and Resources Development Act of 1974 (PL 93-641) introduced a comprehensive system of health planning. This law brought together into one system the previously existing but fragmented federal programs involved in health planning and resource development in the United States: the Hill-Burton program for health facility construction, Regional Medical Programs for categorical health delivery programs, and the Comprehensive Health Planning Act of 1966. This law created a network of 205 health systems agencies (HSAs) throughout the nation. These HSAs were designated by governors of each state and approved by the Secretary of Health, Education and Welfare (now Health and Human Services).

In addition, this act specified that nurses have voting membership in the HSAs and provided for a statewide health coordinating council to advise state health planning and development agencies about state health planning issues. The law created a national council on health planning and development to make recommendations regarding national health policy to the Secretary of Health and Human Services, but the focus of planning remained at the HSA level. HSAs are charged with the improvement of the health of area residents by increasing the accessibility, continuity, and quality of health care services, restraining cost increases, and preventing unnecessary duplication of services. To date, reports indicate that HSAs have been successful in these aims.

Finally, the Rural Health Clinics Act of 1978 exemplifies the U.S. government's willingness to allow nurse practitioners to deliver primary health care. This act provides for the development of rural health clinics in areas that are medically underserved, for the use of nurse practitioners as clinic staff, and for direct reimbursement to the clinics for services provided by nurse practitioners to Medicare and Medicaid recipients. This law demonstrates the trend toward involving nurses in primary health care delivery.

Types of Health Care Services

The health care system offers four broad types of services to clients: health promotion, illness prevention, diagnosis and treatment, and rehabilitation.

HEALTH PROMOTION

Health promotion services have developed rapidly within the health care delivery system. Health promotion activities, including specific health education programs, are designed to help clients reduce the risk of illness, maintain maximal function, and promote habits related to good health. Health promotion activities take place in many settings. Hospitals, for example, offer programs such as prenatal nutrition classes, in which pregnant women are taught the essentials of good nutrition during pregnancy, after childbirth, and for the infant; classes thus promote the general health of both the woman and the infant. Within the community are many kinds of health promotion activities. For example, exercise classes such as aerobic dance encourage participants to exercise the body and cardiovascular system, thereby promoting a healthy, active life-style.

Nurses can promote good health by conducting educational programs and participating in health promotion activities. For example, nurses can both teach and participate in classes on stress management. When working individually with clients, nurses engage in health promotion through teaching activities and by setting an example.

ILLNESS PREVENTION

Illness prevention is a second type of service provided by the health care delivery system. The nurse helps prevent illness by assisting the client and family in reducing risk factors to avoid the need for primary, secondary, or tertiary health care. Prevention activities usually directly involve the client and include such things as periodic physical examinations and identification of familial risk factors for illnesses, such as cardiovascular disease. Once a risk factor is identified, the client, with the assistance of nurses, can engage in positive health practices to prevent illness, such as giving up smoking. Community and family mental health programs have been created to prevent mental health problems.

Illness prevention activities also include environmental programs to reduce the threat of illness or disability. For example, controlling the breeding of mosquitoes with insecticides during hot, humid weather can reduce the risk of an encephalitis outbreak.

Occupational safety measures and educational programs also are illness prevention activities. In the painting and construction industry, for example, the use of respirators by employees exposed to dust and paint fumes reduces the risk of lung disease.

Public education programs and legislation are also involved in illness and injury prevention. Laws requiring the use of an approved infant or toddler restraint seat in automobiles, for example, are directed toward preventing severe injury or death if a child is involved in an automobile accident.

Preventive health education and health practices are generally very effective in reducing the risk of disease and disability, and prevention activities help to improve the level of health of both the client and the community. Furthermore, it is becoming increasingly evident that preventive measures reduce the overall costs of health care.

DIAGNOSIS AND TREATMENT

The diagnosis and treatment of illness have traditionally been the most commonly used services of the health care delivery system. In the past, most people tended to seek health care only when they felt ill.

Advances in scientific knowledge and space-age technology and computers have resulted in more sophisticated diagnostic procedures and a greater chance for early diagnosis. Many new diagnostic tests are noninvasive and painless. Although the advanced technology has improved the diagnostic and treatment capacity of the health care delivery system, it has also increased the complexity of the system; in some instances the machinery itself poses a threat and increases the client's anxiety.

Nurses' activities in the community can be directed toward early diagnosis. For example, nurses teach female clients about breast self-examination (Chapter 30), enabling them to discover a breast mass at an early stage and thus to seek early treatment. In other community settings, such as schools, special programs have been organized to detect certain illnesses in early stages.

Nurses are also involved in early diagnosis when they take the client's history in the assessment phase of the nursing process (Chapter 7).

While interviewing 35-year-old Mrs. Brunner, the nurse notices that Mrs. Brunner has had all of her teeth extracted. When she asks Mrs. Brunner about her teeth, Mrs. Brunner replies, "I never knew how to take care of my teeth, so they had to be pulled." When the nurse inquires about the oral hygiene of Mrs. Brunner's two children, ages 8 and 10, she notes that they have never been to a dentist. After performing an oral examination of the children, the nurse identifies early signs of dental decay and makes appointments for the children at a dental clinic.

Although the nurse does not assume the role of medical diagnostician, she is responsible for client education during the diagnostic process. When the client understands the procedure, anxiety about it and about equipment used is reduced. The client is better informed and can participate more fully and efficiently in the diagnostic tests.

Treatment methods have also expanded as a result of advances in technology and knowledge. Clients are receiving newer, more innovative health care treatments based on the most recent research. The treatment of illnesses has also expanded outside hospitals and other institutions. Even when treatment is initiated within an institution, nurses teach the client and family how to complete the treatment plan at home and in outpatient settings.

REHABILITATION

Rehabilitation is the restoration of a person to normal or near-normal function after a physical or mental illness, injury, or chemical addiction. Rehabilitation was once available primarily for clients with illnesses or injury to the nervous system, but the health care delivery system has increasingly expanded its rehabilitative services. Today cardiovascular rehabilitation programs help clients and their families adjust to changes in life-style that become necessary after a heart attack. Pulmonary rehabilitation programs aim to increase the exercise tolerance of clients with chronic pulmonary diseases. In addition, specific rehabilitation programs have been designed for clients with physical impairments such as stroke, spinal cord trauma, or orthopedic injuries; clients with chemically induced impairments such as alcohol or drug dependencies; and clients with mental illnesses such as depression.

Rehabilitation services begin the moment a client with a chronic illness or injury enters the health care system. Initially rehabilitation may focus on the prevention of complications related to the illness or injury. As the client's physical condition stabilizes, rehabilitation is directed toward maximizing the client's functioning and increasing his level of independence.

Effective rehabilitation involves the client, the family, and the whole health care team, which may include a physician, social worker, physical and occupational therapists, speech therapist, dietitian, or psychiatrist. The rehabilitation team is individually designed for each client. For example, a client recovering from a chemical dependency may not need a speech therapist but may rely heavily on the services of a psychiatrist or counselor, whereas a person recovering from a stroke needs speech, physical, and occupational therapists more than a dietitian. Each member of the health care team supplies expertise for the rehabilitation of clients. The specific roles and functions of the members of the health care team are outlined in Chapter 1.

Rehabilitation programs take place in various health care settings, including specific rehabilitation institutions. Frequently clients needing long-term rehabilitation have severe disabilities that affect their ability to carry out the activities of daily living. Rehabilitation services are also provided by outpatient settings in which the client receives treatment at specified times during the week but remains at home the rest of the time.

Many rehabilitation services are provided in the home or community, particularly when rehabilitation strategies are to be applied to the client's home environment so that he can achieve a maximal level of function and independence. Nurses and other members of the health care team visit the client's home and help the client and family learn to adapt to the illness or injury.

Rehabilitation can be a long process. Clients and their families involved in rehabilitation rely on the members of the health care team for their expertise as well as emotional support. Both the client and the family generally require assistance in adjusting to a chronic disability from illness or injury.

Types of Agencies

As a result of the expansion of the health care system and increasing specialization, the variety and numbers of health care agencies have also increased. Services once delivered primarily by hospitals are now provided in many other types of settings. The range of health care agencies includes outpatient, community-based, voluntary, institutional, hospice, governmental, and health maintenance agencies.

OUTPATIENT AGENCIES

Clients who do not require hospitalization can receive treatment in a physician's office, a clinic, or other ambulatory care facility. Most clients receive health care through these outpatient services. Outpatient services are generally directed toward the diagnosis and treatment of both acute and chronic illnesses.

Physicians' offices provide primary care for a large segment of the population. During 1980 in the United States, approximately 44% of the population received some form of primary care in physicians' offices (Department of Health and Human Services, 1982) (Table 3-1). Physicians in office practice tend to focus on the diagnosis and treatment of specific illnesses rather than on health promotion and other health services. Some physicians' offices have complete laboratory facilities for analyzing blood specimens and urine samples and obtaining electrocardiograms and radiographs. Nurses employed in physicians' offices can

TABLE 3-1

Office Visits (Per Person) to Physician According to Physician Specialty and Selected Client Characteristics, United States, 1980

Selected Characteristics	All Specialties*	General and Family Practice	Internal Medicine	Obstetrics and Gynecology	Pediatrics	General Surgery
AGE						
Under 15 years	2.21	0.54	0.03	0.01	1.20	0.05
15-44 years	2.36	0.81	0.20	0.48	0.40	0.12
45-64 years	2.99	1.08	0.58	0.12	0.00	0.20
65 years and over	4.22	1.56	0.95	0.06	0.00	0.22
SEX						
Male	2.25	0.73	0.28	0.00	0.39	0.12
Female	2.98	0.98	0.33	0.44	0.34	0.13
RACE						
White	2.73	0.89	0.31	0.23	0.39	0.13
All other	2.03	0.70	0.24	0.23	0.25	0.08

From Division of Health Care Statistics, National Center for Health Statistics: Data from the National Ambulatory Medical Care Survey, Pub. No. PHS 83-1232, U.S. Department of Health and Human Services, Washington, D.C., 1982, U.S. Government Printing Office.
*Includes other specialties not shown separately.

assume a variety of roles. Some nurses have the traditional role of registering clients, taking vital signs, preparing the client for examination or laboratory studies, and providing basic information. Other nurses working with physicians have the expanded role of nurse practitioner with responsibility for the primary care of clients in stable health states.

Clinics traditionally involve two kinds of settings: (1) a department in a hospital where clients not requiring hospitalization receive medical care and (2) a group practice of physicians such as the Leahy Clinic in Boston or the Mayo Clinic in Rochester, Minnesota. The roles of nurses in a clinic closely parallel the roles of nurses in a physician's office; a nurse can be employed in a traditional role or in the expanded role of nurse practitioner.

Ambulatory care centers, like clinics, provide health services on an outpatient basis. Nurses providing primary care in an ambulatory setting work in a more expanded role as a nurse practitioner or clinical nurse specialist. Such nurses have a specific caseload of clients and provide follow-up care for these clients at each of their visits to the care center.

COMMUNITY-BASED AGENCIES

Community-based health care agencies are facilities that focus on providing health care to clients within their neighborhoods. Examples of community-based agencies are day-care centers, home health agencies, crisis intervention centers, drug rehabilitation centers, and specialized agencies such as Alcoholics Anonymous. Within community-based agencies nurses may have a variety of roles.

Day-care centers provide health care to specific client populations during the day. Day-care centers may be associated with a hospital or other institution or may function independently. Frequently the clients of such centers do not require hospitalization but need continuous health care services while their family or support persons are working. Such clients include elderly clients who need daily physical rehabilitation, clients with emotional illnesses who need daily counseling, and clients with chemical dependence problems who are involved in a rehabilitation program. Some day-care health centers provide minor surgical services such as excision of skin lesions and tubal ligation. Day-care centers reduce the cost of health care and allow the client to retain more independence by living at home.

Nurses who work in day-care centers provide continuity between the care delivered in the home and the care delivered in the center. For instance, nurses can ensure that the client continues to take his medication, can administer specific treatments, and can assist the client through counseling sessions.

Home health agencies are organizations that provide health care in the home. Community health nursing is one such type of service. Community health nurses employed by various agencies deliver continuing and comprehensive care that can be preventive, curative, and rehabilitative. Home health agencies, like community health agencies in general, provide care based on the belief that care directed to the individual, the family, and the group contributes to the health of the population as a whole.

Crisis intervention centers provide emergency psychiatric care and counseling to clients experiencing extreme stress or conflict, often involving suicide attempts or drug or alcohol abuse. These centers, which are usually self-contained units within a hospital or community health center, provide services 24 hours a day. The services may be delivered directly on the premises, or counseling may be provided over the telephone. The primary objectives of crisis intervention centers are to help the person cope with the immediate problem and to offer guidance and support for long-term therapy (see Chapter 5).

Nurses working in crisis centers must be skilled in communication and counseling techniques. Many nurses working in these settings have a master's degree in psychiatric or mental health nursing. Usually the primary role of the nurse is to quickly identify clients in crisis and to take actions to assist the person in coping with the immediate problem. Later the nurse may refer the client to other resources for long-term support.

Drug rehabilitation centers provide long-term care and a gradual return to the community of a client with chemical drug dependency. Such rehabilitation centers may operate in association with a hospital or other institution or may function independently. Clients in drug rehabilitation programs desire to be free of drug dependence and to function within the community. Nurses employed in drug rehabilitation centers must be knowledgeable about chemical dependencies and community resources, as well as counseling and communication techniques.

Alcoholics Anonymous is an international nonprofit organization of recovered alcoholics whose purpose is to help alcoholics stop drinking and remain sober through group support, shared experiences, and a faith in a higher power. Meetings are held in central community locations such as a church, a school, or a hospital. Alcoholics Anonymous has developed a group called Al-Anon to assist families in helping an alcoholic family member and another group called Alateen to help teenagers cope with alcoholism in their families. Nurses may become involved with Alcoholics Anonymous by referring clients to the agency or by providing care in other settings to which a client has been referred by the agency.

VOLUNTARY AGENCIES

Voluntary agencies are not-for-profit health care agencies established nationally or within a community to meet a specific need. Examples are the American Lung Association and the American Cancer Society and, in Canada, the Canadian Lung Association and the Canadian Heart Foundation. Most such voluntary agencies do not provide treatment but have programs focused on the prevention and detection of specific illnesses. In addition, some voluntary agencies provide financial support for training of physicians and nurses, as well as for biomedical research directed toward the prevention, detection, or treatment of certain diseases.

Voluntary agencies depend heavily on professional and lay volunteers to carry out many of the activities of the agency. Financial support is generally derived from fund-raising activities, federal grants, and donations from individuals who support the agency. Many health professionals donate time and resources to agencies within their specialty. Cardiologists and nurses working with cardiac patients, for example, may participate regularly in the activities and programs of the American Heart Association.

INSTITUTIONAL SETTINGS

Institutional settings include hospitals, nursing homes, extended care facilities, and some rehabilitation centers that offer health care services to inpatients (clients admitted to a stay within the institution for the purpose of diagnosis, treatment, or rehabilitation).

Hospitals traditionally have been the major agency of the health care system. Hospitals vary in size from small rural hospitals of perhaps only 20 beds to large urban medical centers with hundreds of beds. Throughout Canada and the United States there are public and private hospitals. A public hospital is financed and operated by a government agency at either the local or the national level. Many of the clients in public hospitals cannot afford to pay for care. Private hospitals are owned and operated by groups such as churches, corporations, businesses, and charitable organizations. Clients of private hospitals generally have some type of insurance or medical assistance to pay for hospital care.

Hospitals generally provide inpatient, outpatient, and support group services to answer the needs of the community. Because of the variety of services, nurses working in hospitals have a variety of roles, including opportunities for specialization.

The length of hospital stay for clients varies from

hospital to hospital. Some hospitals are strictly acute care settings where clients stay from a few days to perhaps a month. Other hospitals focus on long-term rehabilitation and admit clients for much longer periods of time.

The expansion of health care services has resulted in the growth of hospitals. Many hospitals have increased their bed capacity and have expanded their range of services to include such activities as research and teaching.

An *extended care facility* is an institution that provides long-term medical, nursing, or custodial care for clients with a chronic illness or a disability. Extended care facilities include intermediate care facilities, skilled nursing facilities, convalescent homes, nursing homes, and some residential institutions.

Extended care facilities offer the client various levels of skilled nursing care. One client may require only minimal nursing care, such as ensuring that medications are taken each day, and the presence of health care professionals in case other problems develop. Another client may need some assistance with the activities of daily living, such as dressing himself. Still another client may need considerable assistance with bathing, dressing, and feeding himself.

Extended care facilities provide round-the-clock nursing coverage. Nurses employed in such a setting have expertise in the nursing skills required for the clients to whom the facility provides care.

A *rehabilitation center* is a residential institution that provides therapy and training to restore a client to his optimal level of functioning and independence. Rehabilitation centers actively involve the client and his family in providing health care. The goal of rehabilitation is gradually to decrease the client's dependence on the care provided so that little by little he assumes responsibility for his own care.

Rehabilitation centers employ persons from nursing, medicine, and the allied health fields. Many rehabilitation centers focus on physical rehabilitation programs to teach the client and family how to achieve maximal physical function after a stroke, spinal cord injury, or physical impairment. Drug rehabilitation centers help the client become free from drug dependence and return to the community. Mental health rehabilitation centers assist the mentally ill to cope with their problems and return to independent functioning.

Nurses employed in rehabilitation centers are committed to long-term continuity of nursing services. They must be knowledgeable in their specialized area of rehabilitation. In physical rehabilitation, for example, nurses must have knowledge and expertise about normal physical function and adaptive devices designed to assist clients in functioning at their maximal level. In drug and mental health rehabilitation, nurses have knowledge and expertise in counseling techniques and other specialized skills.

Rehabilitation centers teach clients how to live independently. Frequently, part of a rehabilitation program is the controlled return of the client to his home, often beginning with weekend and other brief visits.

Psychiatric hospitals or mental health hospitals provide inpatient and outpatient counseling services to clients with behavioral or emotional illnesses. Treatment in psychiatric hospitals is directed toward helping the client control his behavior or restore his behavior to his preillness state. Psychiatric hospitals may be operated within large medical centers or hospitals or may be independent, government-supported or private hospitals.

Nurses who work in psychiatric hospitals use communication skills as a basis for nursing care (see Chapter 15). Nursing care may involve participating with the client in group, occupational, or recreational therapies. As in other settings, the psychiatric nurse involves the client's family or significant others in the plan of nursing care. Effective nursing care depends on the nurse's use of communication and other skills to develop a nurse-client relationship as a basis for care.

HOSPICES

The trend of health care consumers to seek care outside of institutions has led to the development of hospices to meet the needs of the terminally ill. A hospice is a system of family-centered care designed to make the terminally ill person comfortable and to ensure a satisfactory life-style through the terminal phase of the illness. Hospice care is not solely for cancer patients as is widely assumed. Hospice care can benefit any client in the terminal phases of a disease, such as a cardiomyopathy, multiple sclerosis, emphysema, or renal disease.

The hospice concept originated in England with the work of Dame Cicely Saunders. Dame Saunders founded St. Christopher's Hospice to meet the total physical, social, and environmental needs of dying people and their families. Dying clients were actively involved in their care and were not isolated from their families and friends.

Clients who enter a hospice have reached the terminal phase of their illness, and the client, family, and physician have agreed that no further treatment could reverse the disease process. The client and family must accept the fact that the hospice will not use emergency measures, such as cardiopulmonary resuscitation, to prolong life. Instead, the hospice provides pain control and comfort measures for the terminally ill to maintain the quality of life. Hospices do not have rigid visiting policies or other prescribed limits, and the environment for the clients and the health care workers is very relaxed.

Hospices are operated in a variety of settings. Independent hospices provide only hospice care and are not affiliated with a specific hospital or medical center. Other hospices operate within a hospital setting, and many hospitals are now developing hospice units in a separate area of the institution. Many home care agencies also offer hospice services and involve neighborhood and community resources in providing care and emotional support for the terminally ill client and his family.

Nurses who work in hospices are employed in both institutional and community settings. A hospice nurse is committed to the philosophy and objectives of a hospice. The nurse provides care and support for the client and family during the terminal phase and continues to give the family emotional support throughout the grieving period. Hospice nurses generally function independently, are dedicated to the supportive rather than the curative function of the hospice, and are skilled in communication techniques.

GOVERNMENTAL AGENCIES

Governmental agencies are clinics, hospitals, and other health services that are supported by local, state or provincial, or national taxes. Local governmental agencies include city hospitals and public health clinics. Agencies at the state or provincial level include state psychiatric hospitals and hospitals for clients with pulmonary disease. National agencies include primary research institutions, such as the National Institutes of Health (NIH), and agencies that administer health and welfare programs for a country, such as the Canadian Department of Health and Welfare.

The types of local and state or provincial agencies and the allocation of resources for these agencies vary from one city, state, or province to another. Usually agency funds originate in the tax base and are controlled by elected or appointed officials in the city, state, or province.

Health departments at the city or county level are generally concerned with specific health needs of the community and may receive additional support from the state or provincial health organization. Federal agencies provide specific kinds of health services on a national level. Of the many health-related national agencies in the United States and Canada, three representative agencies are described in the following paragraphs: the Veterans Administration hospitals, the Public Health Service, and the Canadian health care system.

The *Veterans Administration (VA) hospitals* were established after World War II to provide care for injured veterans. VA hospitals have since expanded eligibility for care to include all veterans with service- and non-service-related illnesses or disabilities.

VA hospitals are generally near major medical centers with teaching and training functions and a medical school. Many of the medical staff in a VA hospital are supplied by the medical school.

Nursing services in VA hospitals are provided around the clock. Nursing services and nursing roles in the VA hospitals are similar to those in nongovernmental hospitals.

The *Public Health Service* (PHS) is a federal health agency and a branch of the Department of Health and Human Services. The PHS is being restructured, but its responsibilities currently include assistance to communities in planning and developing health services, and financing and providing adequate personnel to carry out these services.

The PHS provides health care services according to the needs of the area. For example, in rural poverty areas most of the available health care services may be supplied by the PHS. In an urban area, however, the PHS may offer only the service of tuberculosis control.

The PHS also provides grants to support research and training in the health field. This research includes projects both for the early detection of an illness and for its treatment. Training grants from the PHS support educational programs and seminars for physicians, nurses, and other members of the health care team.

The *Canadian health care system* comprises provincial medical care plans that cover medical care for all residents of Canada. All clients receive the same type of care within the same institutions.

Most general and specialized hospital costs are financed by provincial hospital insurance plans. Each province organizes and administers its own plan for its residents, but these plans have many common features and each plan must meet certain federal standards (Soderstrom, 1981). In all provincial plans, insured services must be available to all residents. Members of the military and the Royal Canadian Mounted Police and inmates of federal prisons are excluded because their insurance is financed through other federal agencies.

These insurance plans are financed jointly by the federal and provincial governments. Usually the financing from the provinces comes out of the province's general revenues; only a few provinces levy special taxes for this purpose.

In structure the Canadian health system closely parallels that of the United States. There are public and private hospitals, clinics, community health centers, and other agencies like those in the United States.

HEALTH MAINTENANCE ORGANIZATIONS

A health maintenance organization (HMO) is a group health care agency that provides basic and supplemental health maintenance and treatment services to voluntary enrollees who prepay a fixed periodic fee. This fee is set without regard to the amount or kind of services the client receives. Key features of the HMO are the following (Luft, 1981):

1. The HMO assumes a contractual responsibility to provide or ensure the delivery of a stated range of health services, including ambulatory care and inpatient hospital services.
2. The HMO serves only enrollees in the plan.
3. Enrollment is voluntary.
4. The client pays a fixed annual or monthly payment that is independent of the client's use of services.
5. The HMO assumes at least part of the financial risk or gain in the provision of services.

In 1973 the U.S. Congress passed the Health Maintenance Organization Act in an effort to control the accessibility, quality, and cost of health care. This act helped private agencies develop new models of health care delivery and provided some financial support. There are now HMOs across the United States. The Kaiser-Permanente Medical Care Program, the largest group, serves clients in California, Oregon, Hawaii, Ohio, and Colorado. Other examples are the Group Health Association, Inc., based in Washington, D.C., and the Medical Care Group of Washington University, serving the greater St. Louis metropolitan area.

The focus of health care in HMOs is health maintenance, and these agencies employ many health care professionals. HMOs differ from hospitals and other agencies primarily in their mode of financing and thus their organizational structure. A person with private health insurance can generally seek health services from any hospital or other agency, which is reimbursed for most or all of the services by the insurance company. In an HMO the client must use the agency's facilities, but the client has the advantage that such services are prepaid. Thus HMOs are motivated to hold down the costs of care and are generally less expensive for the client.

Nurses employed in HMOs generally function in the same roles as in hospitals and other agencies providing comprehensive services.

The Client and the Health Care Delivery System

While in good health a person may have little or no interaction with the health care delivery system. However, if the person becomes ill, feels illness threat-

ening, or is motivated for other reasons to seek health care, he must enter the health care delivery system. Some clients enter the system easily by walking into a clinic or hospital emergency room or by making an appointment with a physician in private practice. Other clients experience difficulties in entering the system because of confusion or unfamiliarity with the various agencies or because of low economic status.

Clients who enter the system have different rights. Society generally believes that all people have a right to health care. Once a person enters the health care delivery system, he becomes a client and thus has certain rights *within* the system. Finally, people as health care consumers have a general right to determine *what kind* of health care should be available for present and future needs. Each of these clients' rights affects how health care is delivered, but practices ensured by these rights are also influenced by society's attitudes and the delivery system itself.

Client Rights

RIGHT TO HEALTH CARE

Society has generally come to believe that all people have a right to health care, regardless of cultural, economic, or other factors. In the 1960s this belief led to the development of the federal Medicare and Medicaid programs, directed toward providing health care for those otherwise unable to afford care. These two programs continue to seek to meet the health care needs of the elderly and the poor, the groups generally least able to afford health care on their own.

Through the 1970s and into the early 1980s, these federal programs reimbursed health care providers after the care was provided, and thus the health care delivery system was not encouraged to hold down costs. As health care costs rose dramatically, changes were gradually made in Medicare and Medicaid programs, and in some situations clients had to pay an increased portion of the cost of their care. Some people objected that these increased costs to the individual threatened the right of all people to health care, while others asserted that the system of payments after the fact allowed health costs to rise at an unnecessarily fast rate, thus threatening the right to care.

To control rising costs, Medicare and Medicaid were changed in 1983 so that payments for services would become prospective, meaning that rates for reimbursement to health care agencies are standardized under federal policy for all clients receiving health care in these programs. These rates are determined on the basis of 467 diagnostic related groups (DRGs).

It may take some time before the full impact of this change is known. If, as planned, health care costs are kept from rising unreasonably, the client may gain and the right to health care will be protected. On the other hand, since a hospital or other agency is reimbursed only a set amount regardless of the actual costs of providing care for a particular client, the agency in some cases may be reluctant to accept clients whose long-term care is anticipated to exceed the standard amount or may be less likely to provide certain kinds of expensive treatments, thus posing a threat to the client's right to health care.

Specific financial changes in Medicare and Medicaid are discussed in the later section on financing health care.

RIGHTS WITHIN THE SYSTEM

In 1973 the American Hospital Association developed a Patient's Bill of Rights (see Chapter 17), which lists 12 specific rights of hospitalized clients. The bill offers some guidance and protection to clients by stating the responsibilities of the hospital and staff toward them and their families; however, it is not a legally binding document. The Patient's Bill of Rights supports consumer activities for clients in the health care system. The client has the right to information pertaining to diagnosis and treatment, fees for services, and continuity of care. The client has the right to refuse diagnostic or treatment procedures. Above all, the Patient's Bill of Rights reaffirms the client's right to both information and privacy while receiving health care.

One of the client's specific legal rights is informed consent. Informed consent is the obtaining of permission from the client to perform certain kinds of actions. Informed consent must be obtained before beginning any invasive procedure, administering an experimental drug, or placing a client in a research study. Informed consent must meet six criteria:

1. The consent document must be written in language that the client or guardian can understand.
2. The consent document must delineate all possible risks and the actions of the physician or researcher to minimize the risks.
3. The consent document must list the benefit of the procedure to the client; if there is no known benefit at present, the consent document must state that fact.
4. Any alternatives to the procedure must be specified even if the only alternative is nonparticipation.
5. The document must state that participation is voluntary and that clients can refuse to participate or withdraw from participation without having further health care withheld.
6. Clients who give informed consent must be ra-

tional and competent or represented by a competent guardian, and they must be told how they can reach the physician or researcher who is performing the procedure.

Clients' rights and informed consent affect how the health care system delivers care. Most agencies now have committees to evaluate clients' suggestions and complaints about the delivery of health care; in many institutions this committee is called a patient care committee. A second committee, an institutional review board, ensures that elements of informed consent are consistent with federal guidelines. Although the need to protect clients' rights sometimes results in increased paperwork and extra work, this protection is necessary to ensure that all clients maintain their rights within the health care delivery system.

As clients become better informed about their rights within the health care system, they take a more active consumer role. As a result, the health care industry is increasingly listening to consumers and developing services to fit client needs.

Entry of the Client into the System

Clients can enter the health care system by various routes. The three most common forms of entry are (1) entry by referral from a health team member, (2) entry when the client has a specific health need, and (3) entry related to financial resources.

A client may enter the system by referral from a health team member in the case of an acute, potentially life-threatening problem, such as the presence of an angina-like chest pain, or in the case of a less threatening problem such as a rash of unknown cause. The nurse is frequently the professional who is in a position to refer clients to the system. Such referrals may be given to neighbors who seek advice, children and their families at a school where the nurse practices or does volunteer work, and families of clients to whom the nurse has previously provided care.

Clients also enter the system on their own because of a specific need. For example, a college student may seek health care for treatment of a complaint such as a sore throat or gastrointestinal upset and so may enter the health care system at the primary care level through the student health center. A different student may be involved in a severe automobile accident and enter the health care system through a hospital emergency room.

Finally, the entry of clients into the health care system may be influenced by their financial situation. An employed person with insurance may readily enter a hospital for elective surgical or diagnostic procedures, because he has the financial resources to seek and pay for primary health care. On the other hand, an unemployed person with limited resources may seek care only if an illness becomes acute and then go to a hospital emergency room. Frequently the only type of care some clients can obtain is that which is supported by local, state or provincial, or federal programs.

Regardless of their manner of entry into the system, all clients encounter nurses and nursing services. The first impression the client has of nursing services may stay with him and become a significant and lasting impression of nursing. Nurses therefore have the opportunity to increase clients' awareness of nursing services and the types of quality nursing care they can and should expect.

Financing Health Care Services

The rapid rise in health care costs has been the subject of discussion by governmental officials, the media, health care professionals, and consumers. It has become increasingly difficult for people to meet these costs with their own resources, and therefore government agencies and private companies have developed a variety of prepaid health care programs, insurance programs, and social services to subsidize the cost of health care.

Private and Group Health Plans

Private health insurance can be obtained by the individual alone or through a group plan offered by employers. Health insurance programs pay for some, most, or all of the expenses of health care for the client, as specified by the policy. Such payments are called third-party reimbursements because the costs of health care services are met, not by the health care agency or the client, but by the third party, the insurer. Ultimately, of course, consumers bear the costs through the insurance premiums.

Group health plans are another method of financing health care services. Health maintenance organizations (HMOs), as discussed earlier in this chapter, deliver care based on a prepaid fee set in advance. HMOs provide all types of health care services and often emphasize health promotion and illness prevention more than other agencies.

A second type of group health plan is a preferred provider organization (PPO). A PPO is a group of physicians or a hospital that agrees to provide comprehensive health services at a discount to companies under contract. Such plans are also called industry-based health plans. The PPO benefits both the client and the hospital. The client receives care at a reduced rate, and the hospital gains because it can provide services at lower cost when its services are used by more clients.

Governmental Support

The U.S. government's commitment to financing medical care for the elderly and poor has been reduced by federal budget cuts. Changes in federal health policy have led to reductions in Medicare and Medicaid payments.

Before 1983 the federal government, through Medicare and Medicaid, reimbursed hospitals for services already provided. However, in March 1983, the U.S. Congress approved a Medicare prospective pricing plan for most inpatient services as part of the Social Security Amendments of 1983, thus initiating the prospective reimbursement as the basis for payments for hospital services. The amount of reimbursement is based on diagnostic related groups (DRGs), the type of hospital, and the geographical region. The new prospective Medicare system is gradually being phased in over a 4-year period. DRGs are categories of clients designed for measuring the quality and extent of a hospital's health services. They were developed at Yale University's Center for Health Studies based on the following variables: primary and secondary diagnoses, primary and secondary procedures, the client's age, and the length of stay. The 467 DRGs were formulated through research into usual procedures and treatments for different illnesses.

The prospective pricing plan using DRGs for Medicare reimbursement will be phased in as follows (American Hospital Association, 1983):
1. During year 1 Medicare will pay 75% of the hospital-specific cost per case and 25% of the regional average price for the client's DRG.
2. During year 2 Medicare will pay 50% of the hospital-specific cost per case, 37.5% of the regional average price for the client's DRG, and 12.5% of the national average price for the client's DRG.
3. During year 3 Medicare will pay 25% of the hospital-specific cost per case, 37.5% of the regional average price for the client's DRG, and 37.5% of the national average price for the client's DRG.
4. In year 4 Medicare payments will be based on the urban or rural national average price for each DRG, adjusted for differences in area wages.

Prospective pricing affects all hospitals except children's, psychiatric, rehabilitation, and long-term hospitals. Separate psychiatric and rehabilitation units of general hospitals are also exempt.

In theory the objective of the prospective payment system is to provide incentives for hospitals to lower costs. For example, the DRG fee for gallbladder removal requiring an 8-day hospital stay might be set at $2500. This figure has been set on the basis of what all the services for such a client should total. In hospital X, however, these services have typically been billed at $3000. Because Medicare reimburses the hospital only $2500, regardless of actual costs, the hospital has the incentive to investigate other methods of providing quality care. The hospital is also motivated not to keep the client hospitalized longer than necessary, since the reimbursement is the same regardless of length of stay. In theory, then, prospective payments should help contain costs. On the other hand, some people are concerned that this policy might in certain cases reduce the quality of care. The hospital might, in the example here, be tempted to discharge the client before 8 days even though, by its past standards, the client would have remained in the hospital another day or two. While DRGs provide incentives for hospitals to lower costs, it is also necessary to protect clients from premature discharge. Protection of the clients is ensured by audits of client records by federal auditors. If these audits identify a hospital's trend of premature discharging, resulting in clients' readmission to the hospital within 7 days or less, the hospital is at risk for curtailment of reimbursement funds.

At present prospective payments are intended only for federally supported health insurance programs, implemented near the end of 1983. At the time of writing, the prospective payment system applies only for the hospital stay, not for physician services. However, the Health Care Financing Administration has been ordered by Congress to study the feasibility of applying DRGs to physician services and to report its findings by 1985 (Hunt, 1983).

One can only speculate on the benefits or harm of the prospective payment system. If it proves beneficial, a similar system may be adopted by private and group insurers.

Problems with the Present System

Although the health care delivery system is increasingly responsive to the needs of the community it serves, such as by offering more services for health promotion and health maintenance, it still has a number of problems. These include the high costs of care, fragmentation of care, inability to meet the special needs of the chronically ill and elderly, and uneven distribution of services. These problems are not particularly new in the health care delivery system but in many cases have been aggravated by modern conditions.

Because nurses comprise the largest segment of health professionals and because they are able to provide 24-hour-a-day care for their clients, they have an opportunity to work toward solutions to the problems of the health care system.

High Costs of Care

Over the last decade the costs of overall health care in the United States and Canada have tripled, and the total spent on health care services is expected to top $1 trillion by 1993 (Soderstrom, 1983). The following are some of the causes of the increasingly high costs of care:

1. Increased population and demand for services
2. Greater number of people with chronic illnesses
3. Growing cost of new technology and equipment
4. Inflation
5. Increased specialization of care

To gain some control over skyrocketing health costs, companies are increasingly turning to health maintenance organizations and preferred provider organizations for their health care services. The U.S. government is introducing the system of prospective payments for Medicare recipients, also to hold down costs.

Nursing must also address the need for cost containment. If the prospective hospitalization payment system proves to be an effective method of reducing costs, nursing should also determine the costs of nursing service based on DRGs. One method for determining price rates for nursing services based on DRGs is to use nursing care strategies—detailed nursing care plans that include direct and indirect client care and that should allow for variances in both the independent and interdependent functions of nurses. According to Curtin (1983), nursing care strategies should reflect the nursing time needed to deliver care to clients, thus quantifying nursing care. To establish nursing care strategies, the nurse must correctly assess the client's needs and develop an individualized and accurate nursing care plan (see Unit 2).

Fragmentation of Care

Advanced scientific knowledge and technology have resulted in increasing specialization of health care. Many physicians and nurses specialize in certain areas, such as cardiac disease, kidney disease, and cancer. One result of such specialization is that clients often require care from many different health care providers. Although specialization allows each professional on the health care team to provide clients with highly advanced care, the delivery of the total care for the client is often fragmented among many different providers.

The number of primary physicians and primary care givers has gradually declined, and many families find themselves in the position of having a different physician for each family member or each illness. As a result care is not provided for the family as a unit or for the whole person. The care giver is not able to assess family or personal dynamics and its impact on the person's level of health. In 1 day in a hospital, for example, a patient might interact with a radiologist, a physical therapist, a laboratory technician, and several orderlies or other aides, in addition to nurses. In such cases the client may see each member of the health care team only briefly. It is easy to understand how the client could feel that no one provider is responsible for his total care and that his condition may not be fully understood if specialists "cannot see the forest for the trees." Such an emotional climate is obviously not advantageous for regaining a high level of health.

With so many specialists involved in the care of clients, there is also a potential for the client to become lost to health care follow-up simply because it is too difficult for the client to cope with specialization. Furthermore, as the client goes from one specialist to another the cost of care increases, there is a potential for the client to be overmedicated or undermedicated, and the client's quality of life is changed because of the time involved in obtaining health care.

Nurses employed in community health, outpatient, psychiatric, and institutional settings have the opportunity to reduce the fragmentation of care. Primary care nursing reduces fragmentation, for example, because in this system one nurse manages the total care of the client. The primary nurse coordinates care given by other nurses, physicians, and other personnel and schedules all tests, procedures, and daily activities for the client. In addition, the primary nurse personally cares for the client when on duty. The primary nurse can thus continually monitor and assess the client's condition, relate information to the client, and maintain continuity between specialists who may make recommendations for the client's care. Also, the nurse can give support to the client and help him cope with what otherwise might be a confusing situation.

Special Needs of the Chronically Ill and Elderly

The health care delivery system, and particularly the hospital, has been developed primarily to meet the needs of the acutely ill. The needs of the chronically ill are frequently not met, or met only partially, in this system. The chronically ill commonly receive care in health care settings such as outpatient clinics, where there is little continuity of care. In such cases clients and their families receive very little support to help them adapt to changes in life-style that result from chronic illness.

Chronic illnesses affect the elderly more frequently than young or middle-aged adults, and because people are living longer in North America, the population of clients with chronic diseases is growing. Thus there is an increasing need for the health care system to address the special care requirements of the elderly. These include adaptation to changing roles, changes in family structure, and changes in cognitive and functional abilities, as well as physical and other needs related to disease processes.

The nursing profession is giving increased attention to the special needs of geriatric and chronically ill clients. The rapidly growing specialty of gerontological nursing prepares nurses to design nursing strategies aimed at helping elderly clients maintain their functioning and independence. Geriatrics involves the collaboration of all the health care disciplines. Nurses are able to coordinate the health care team in the care of the individual client and in many cases direct this care.

Nursing is also increasing its knowledge and expertise in caring for the chronically ill in all age groups. Nurses coordinate efforts to provide care designed to return the chronically ill client to his home and to achieve and maintain the highest possible level of functioning.

Uneven Distribution of Services

The numbers of health care workers in North America have increased, but for several reasons low-income and rural areas still lack adequate health care professionals and services. First, low-income communities often do not have the fiscal resources necessary to establish or maintain major health care services. Second, rural and low-income regions frequently lack the kinds of social and cultural activities that can attract health care professionals into the area to practice. Third, increased specialization by health care professionals has led to fewer family and general practitioners being available to meet the need in some rural areas, and such areas often do not need or cannot support the services of specialists. Finally, some rural areas have seasonal population fluctuations that result in varying needs for health care services.

Nursing is able to meet some of these special health care needs in low-income and rural areas. Nurse practitioners who specialize in family, pediatric, adult, and obstetrical-gynecological services can provide needed services. Many community health agencies have expanded their nursing staff in rural areas to provide better care. School health nurses can provide health education and referral to members of the community.

■ ■ ■ ■ ■

Nursing alone certainly cannot solve all the problems of the present health care delivery system, and nurses should not expect to solve all of these problems. However, nursing can influence the system by:

1. Implementing cost containment measures
2. Providing primary care to coordinate the client's care and decrease fragmentation
3. Designing nursing strategies to meet special needs of the elderly and chronically ill
4. Providing low-income and rural regions with more nursing services

Summary

The health care industry is the most rapidly growing and changing industry in North America. As a result of its rapid expansion, patterns of use by clients have changed and new emphases are emerging. Consumers of health care have increasingly demanded health promotion and maintenance services, and the health care delivery system is changing to meet these needs.

The costs of health care are growing as rapidly as the health care system itself. This trend has led to the development of new and different kinds of outpatient and community-based health agencies, as consumers increasingly desire to receive health care outside the traditional hospital setting.

Today's health care delivery system is certainly much better than in the past, but it is not without problems. The financing of health care puts an increasing burden on private and governmental resources. Technological advances have resulted in high-quality specialized care, but specialization has led to fragmentation of care. Finally, health care services are still unevenly distributed.

KEY CONCEPTS

✓ Health care services are provided in a great number of settings, across all age groups, and for the chronically as well as the acutely ill.

✓ The explosion of the health care industry has resulted in specialization of health care professionals.

✓ Consumers are requesting more information, especially on services related to illness prevention and health promotion.

✓ Chronically ill and disabled clients are seeking knowledge and skills to maximize their levels of wellness and independence.

✓ Increased technology and new biomedical equipment increase the risk of health care professionals giving greater attention to the machine than to the client.

✓ A nation's economy directly affects the fiscal resources of the health care delivery system.

✓ Legislation, such as the Social Security Act and its amendments, National Health Planning and Resources Development Act, and Rural Health Clinics Acts, affects the types of services available to health care clients.

✓ Health promotion activities are designed to help clients reduce the risk of illness, maintain maximal function, and promote life-style habits related to good health.

✓ Illness prevention activities are directed toward helping the client and family reduce risk factors to avoid the need for primary, secondary, or tertiary health care.

✓ Diagnosis and treatment activities are usually disease specific, with the goal of curing the client.

✓ Rehabilitation is the restoration of an individual to normal or near-normal function following a physical or mental illness, injury, or chemical dependency.

✓ Community-based agencies focus on providing health care to clients within their neighborhoods.

✓ Crisis intervention centers provide emergency psychiatric treatment and counseling to clients experiencing extreme stress or conflict.

✓ Drug rehabilitation centers provide long-term care of the client with chemical drug dependency and assist in the gradual return of the client to the community.

✓ Voluntary agencies are not-for-profit health care agencies established nationally or within a community to meet a specific need.

✓ Extended care is the provision of medical, nursing, or custodial care for clients who need long-term care because of chronic illness or disability.

✓ Rehabilitation centers use a multidisciplinary health care team to gradually restore the client to the maximal level of physical, emotional, or mental wellness.

✓ Psychiatric mental health agencies provide inpatient and outpatient counseling services to clients with behavioral or emotional illnesses.

✓ A hospice provides family-centered care to help clients maintain a satisfactory level of comfort and life-style through the terminal phase of illness.

✓ Governmental agencies can be local, regional, or national and are supported by revenues obtained through taxes.

✓ Prepaid health care can be obtained through health maintenance organizations or preferred provider organizations.

✓ Clients may enter the system through referral and specific health need.

✓ Financing of health care services is primarily through private and group health plans or governmental support.

✓ The high cost of health care is the result of increased population and demand for services, increased number of people with chronic illness, cost of technology, inflation, and specialization.

✓ Nursing is able to reduce health care costs by implementing cost containment measures, implementing primary care, meeting special needs of the elderly and chronically ill, and expanding nursing activities into low-income and rural regions.

REFERENCES

American Hospital Association: AHA Medicare payment: special report 3, Chicago, 1983, The Association.

Brown, R.E.: Consumerism in health care delivery: the harbinger of opportunity. In Cooper, P.D., editor: Health care marketing, Germantown, Md., 1979, Aspen Systems.

Curtin, L.: Determining costs of nursing services per DRG, Nurs. Management 14(4):16, 1983.

Department of Health and Human Services: Health United States, Pub. No. (PHS) 83-1232, Washington, D.C., 1982, U.S. Government Printing Office.

Hunt, K.: DRG: what it is, how it works, and why it will hurt, Med. Econ., September 5, 1983, p. 262.

Luft, H.S.: Health maintenance organizations: dimensions of performance, New York, 1981, John Wiley & Sons, Inc.

Soderstrom, L.: The Canadian health system, London, 1981, Croom Helm, Ltd.

Soderstrom, L.: Soaring hospital costs, the brewing revolt, U.S. News and World Report, August 22, 1983.

ADDITIONAL READINGS

Flomann, M.P., and Shaffer, F.A.: DRG's as one of nine approaches to case mix in transition, Nurs. Health Care 4(8):438, 1983.

Fox, R.T.: DRGs: a management control tool in hospitals and multi-institutional systems, Hosp. Prog. 62:52, 1981.

Inglehart, J.K.: Federal health policies and the poor, N. Engl. J. Med. 307:836, 1982.

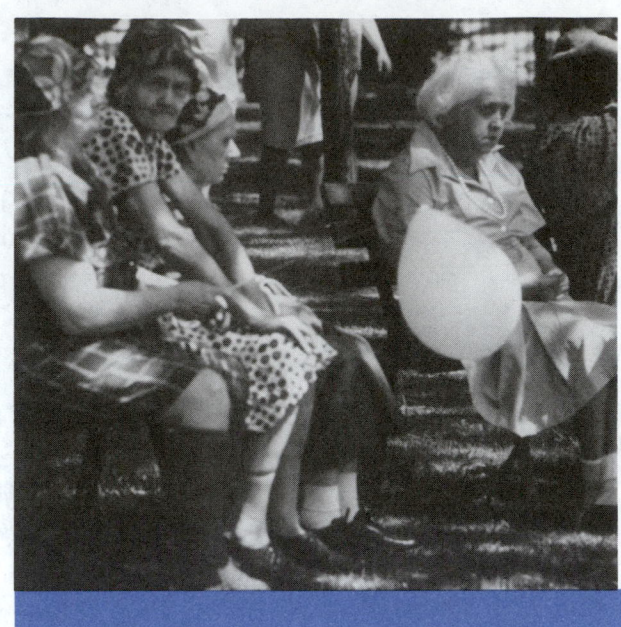

OBJECTIVES

Mastery of content in this chapter will enable the student to:

- Define the terms in the glossary.
- Discuss each component of Maslow's hierarchy of needs.
- Identify conditions that are an actual or potential threat to fulfillment of a client's needs.
- Describe the basic nursing implications concerning unmet needs.
- Describe relationships among the different levels of needs.
- State factors that influence the individual client's need priorities.
- Identify resources for information about meeting specific needs.

GLOSSARY

aerobic metabolism Production of energy and body fuels by the tissues in the presence of oxygen.

anaerobic metabolism Production of energy and body fuels by the tissues without oxygen.

basic human needs Needs for things, such as food, water, safety, and love, that people require to survive and be healthy.

carbon dioxide Respiratory gas formed in the body as an end product of tissue metabolism.

cyanosis Bluish discoloration of the skin and mucous membranes caused by a decreased level of oxygen in the blood.

dehydration Excessive loss of water from the body tissues, accompanied by a disturbance of body electrolytes.

edema Excessive accumulation of fluid in certain spaces in the body.

frostbite Traumatic effect of extreme cold on the skin and subcutaneous tissues, first manifest by distinct pallor.

hierarchy of basic human needs Categorization of human needs from the most basic to those at a higher level.

physiological needs Needs necessary for human survival, including those for oxygen, fluid, nutrition, temperature, elimination, and shelter.

safety and security needs Needs for freedom from threats to one's physical and psychological well-being.

self-actualization State of being in which one is fully achieving one's potential and is able to cope realistically with problems.

self-esteem Feeling of self-worth characterized by feelings of achievement, adequacy, self-confidence, and usefulness.

4 | Basic Human Needs

Basic human needs are needs for those things such as food, water, safety, and love that are necessary for human survival and health. Although each person has other, unique needs, these basic human needs are shared by all people, and the extent to which a person's health needs are met is a major factor in determining his level of health and position on the health-illness continuum (see Chapter 2). Nurses are therefore concerned that the basic human needs of clients seeking health care are being met.

Abraham Maslow's hierarchy of needs is a theory nurses can use to understand the relationships among basic human needs when providing nursing care. Maslow assigned priorities to basic needs. According to his theory, certain human needs are more basic than others; that is, some needs must be met before the individual directs his attention to meeting others. For example, a starving person is more likely to seek food than to engage in activities that increase his self-esteem. The hierarchy of human needs arranges the basic needs in five levels according to priority (Fig. 4-1). On the most basic, or first, level are physiological needs such as air, water, and food. On the second level are safety and security needs, including the need for both physical and psychological security. On the third level are needs for love and a sense of belonging, including needs for friendship, social relationships, and sexual love. On the fourth level is the need for self-esteem, the feeling of self-confidence, usefulness, achievement, and self-worth. The final level is the need for what Maslow calls self-actualization, the state in which one is fully achieving one's potential and is able to solve problems and cope realistically with life's situations.

At any one time an individual's basic human needs may be unmet, partially met, or wholly fulfilled. According to this theory, a person whose needs are all met is healthy, and a person with one or more unmet needs is at risk for illness or may be unhealthy in one or more of the human dimensions—physically, emotionally, intellectually, socially, or spiritually.

The hierarchy of needs is a theoretical model; that is, the priorities given human needs are *generally* true of people but not necessarily true of all individuals. A man who attempts to meet his self-esteem needs by working 18 hours at a time, for example, may ignore physiological needs for adequate sleep and nutrition because for him the need for self-esteem takes priority. Eventually, however, this man may be forced to give more attention to his physiological needs if he can no longer function as usual because he has been weakened by inadequate nutrition and rest. Thus the hierarchy of needs can still be applied to individuals who seem to have different priorities. In providing care to those with unmet needs, the nurse should always take into account the individual's own priorities, as well as other factors, such as his environment and social interactions, that influence how well he can meet his needs.

Clients entering the health care system generally have unmet needs or may be unable to continue meeting their needs. A person brought to an emergency room with a cardiac arrest has an unmet need for air, the most basic physiological need. An elderly client in a declining neighborhood may believe that his

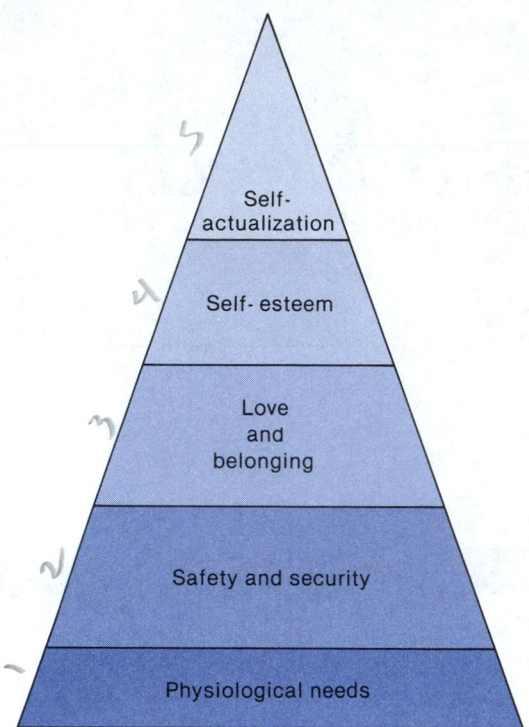

Fig. 4-1 Maslow's hierarchy of needs.

physical safety is threatened and while hospitalized may have an unmet need for psychological security if he fears that his home will be burglarized in his absence. A widowed homemaker whose children have recently married and moved away may feel that she does not belong or is not loved by others. Nurses in all practice settings encounter clients whose needs are actually or potentially unmet, and nursing care includes helping clients, and often the family, meet these needs.

The hierarchy of needs is a useful way for nurses to evaluate and understand the needs of all clients. Although one need may take priority and the nurse often must first be concerned with the highest-priority need (such as restoring an adequate airway before helping the client adjust to an emotional conflict), often the nurse simultaneously addresses needs on different levels, such as assisting a client in meeting the need for social belonging while also helping him achieve adequate nutrition. The nurse first assesses the client's needs and then considers how nursing care can best help him meet those needs.

Physiological Needs

Physiological needs have the highest priority in Maslow's hierarchy. An individual who has several unmet needs generally seeks first to fulfill his phys-

iological needs (Maslow, 1970). For example, a person who lacks food, safety, and love usually searches for food before seeking safety or love.

Physiological needs are needs for things necessary or important for survival. Humans have eight such basic needs: oxygen, fluid, nutrition, temperature, elimination, shelter, rest, and sex.

An infant requires someone to meet his needs for food, shelter, fluids, adequate temperature, and elimination. As the individual grows and progresses developmentally, he is increasingly able to satisfy his physiological needs. A 2-year-old who wants a drink of water usually knows where the water is and how to get it. Although the child's efforts may not be very efficient, if his motivation is great enough and no one else will meet the need, he will get his water. Healthy adults are usually able to meet physiological needs without assistance.

The very young, the very old, the poor, the ill, and the handicapped frequently depend on others for assistance in meeting their basic physiological needs. The nurse often has the role of helping the client meet physiological needs.

Oxygen

Oxygen is the most essential physiological need. The body depends on oxygen for moment-to-moment survival. Certain tissues, such as skeletal muscles, can survive for a time without oxygen through anaerobic metabolism, a process by which these tissues provide their own energy in the absence of oxygen. In long-distance running, for example, the runner's skeletal muscles undergo anaerobic metabolism so that the available oxygen can be used by the more vital organs—the heart, brain, and lungs.

Tissues that carry out only aerobic metabolism, the process of providing energy in the presence of oxygen, depend totally on oxygen for survival. The brain, for example, cannot function without oxygen for longer than 4 to 5 minutes.

For the various body tissues to receive necessary oxygen, oxygen must be adequately delivered from the environment to the lungs, the bloodstream, and finally the tissues. At any point in the life span, clients are at risk for not meeting their oxygen needs. The need can be acute, as with a cardiac arrest, or chronic, as in a long-term smoker with emphysema.

ASSESSMENT

Nurses continually evaluate clients' oxygenation to determine if this need is being met. The assessment of the client's need for oxygen is basically the same in chronic and acute situations. The client may be confused or lethargic because the level of oxygen in his blood and tissues is decreased. When oxygen needs are unmet, the client is unable to lie flat because of his air hunger; he is forced to remain upright so that gravity can assist in expanding his lungs with each breath. The client breathes more quickly to deliver more oxygen to the lungs, and his respirations are usually shallow. Frequently this effort fatigues the client rather than meeting his need for oxygenation. (Other signs of inadequate oxygenation include nasal flaring and sternal, substernal, and suprasternal retractions, so that the client appears to be tugging for air.)

Clients with a progressive long-term decrease in tissue oxygen show cyanosis, the bluish discoloration of the skin and mucous membranes caused by decreased oxygen in the blood. Because cyanosis is a late sign of poor oxygenation, the nurse should be aware of the earlier, more subtle indicators described previously (see also Chapters 41 and 43).

NURSING IMPLICATIONS

Because many organs such as the brain and heart cannot survive without oxygen, oxygen has the highest priority of all physiological needs. The nurse must be able to identify a client's need for oxygen and to assist the client in meeting this need. The problem can be corrected in some instances by controlling anxiety. People when anxious have a tendency to hyperventilate. This decreases the intake of oxygen and increases the expiration of carbon dioxide, causing the person to become more anxious and confused and feel a tingling of the hands and feet, numbness around the lips, and dizziness. In such a case the nurse can first help the client control the imbalance of respiratory gases by having him breathe into a paper bag, which will cause him to rebreathe his carbon dioxide and slow his respiratory rate. Once the client has adequate oxygen, the nurse may use reassurance, teaching, and counseling techniques to help him control his anxiety.

In other instances the nurse uses specific techniques to help the client meet oxygen needs. For example, a 50-year-old man has a 30-year smoking history and a medical diagnosis of chronic obstructive pulmonary disease. He has chronic breathlessness and requires 1 liter per minute of oxygen every night administered through nasal cannulae. Because of the client's frequent breathlessness, the nurse first helps plan daily care activities so that he has adequate opportunity to meet his needs for hygiene, nutrition, and rest. The nurse also teaches the client how to rest in a position that increases his respiratory volume and thus his level of oxygen.

Nursing measures to meet the oxygen needs of clients range from emergency cardiopulmonary re-suscitation in the case of cardiac arrest to supportive measures such as administering oxygen to clients with pulmonary disease while they exercise. Chapter 41 discusses in detail the measures necessary for meeting oxygen needs of the client.

Fluids

The human body requires a balance between the intake and output of fluids. Fluids are taken in by mouth or parenterally by administration into a vein or other area, and fluids leave the body from the intestines, lungs, and skin and as urine from the kidney. Clients of any age can have unmet fluid needs, but the very young and the very old have the greatest risk. Severely ill, traumatized, or handicapped clients are also more likely to have unmet fluid needs.

Two conditions indicate unmet fluid needs: dehydration and edema. Dehydration is the excessive loss of water from the body tissues and is accompanied by a disturbance of body electrolytes. Dehydration may result from excessive and prolonged fever, vomiting, diarrhea, trauma, or any condition that causes a rapid fluid loss. Edema is the abnormal accumulation of fluid in interstitial spaces of tissues, the pericardial sac, the intrapleural space, the peritoneal cavity, or joint capsules. Edema is also accompanied by a disturbance of body electrolytes and may occur in a nutritional, cardiovascular, renal, malignant, traumatic, or other disorder that results in a rapid accumulation of fluids.

ASSESSMENT

The nurse examines clients for an actual or potential fluid imbalance. A number of signs and symptoms can reveal dehydration: poor skin turgor, flushed dry skin, decreased tearing or salivation, coated tongue, decreased urine output, confusion, and irritability. Skin turgor is the normal elasticity of the skin, which becomes lax with dehydration; when grasped and raised between two fingers, the skin only slowly returns to its former position.

The dehydrated client's skin is dry because the body transfers the fluid that is present to the circulation and the more vital organs. The skin may be flushed because of an elevated body temperature that can accompany dehydration. The tongue is coated and dry. A person may cry but not have any tears. Oliguria, a diminished ability of the kidneys to form and excrete urine, is frequently caused by dehydration.

Because of the fluid and associated electrolyte imbalances, the mental status is altered, and the client may be irritable and confused. In cases of severe dehydration the client may even be comatose.

The presence of excessive body fluids is most commonly manifest as edema. Edema may be caused by decreased serum protein, severe burns, altered functioning of the cardiovascular, renal, or hepatic system, or drugs. Edema is first observed in lower body regions; when the person is standing, the edema is seen in his feet and legs. A client with edema may complain that his shoes are too tight, particularly in the evening. To determine whether edema is present, the nurse applies light fingertip pressure to the suspected region and watches to see if the fingertip leaves an imprint on the skin. The client with edema may also have a daily weight gain, shortness of breath, or an increased heart rate. The skin of a client with excessive body fluids is smooth and shiny and very susceptible to breakdown.

NURSING IMPLICATIONS

The overall nursing goal for clients with unmet fluid needs is to restore body fluid and electrolyte balances to normal. The nurse uses simple or complex measures to meet this goal. For example, if the client has diarrhea without vomiting, an appropriate nursing intervention is to increase the client's oral intake of fluids. If the fluid loss is greater, as with a client who has a severe burn, nursing interventions are more complex and include intravenous administration of fluids.

If the client has excessive fluids, nursing actions are directed toward restricting the client's fluid intake and facilitating elimination of the excess fluids from the body.

Chapters 42 and 43 describe in more detail the knowledge and techniques the nurse needs for restoring fluid, electrolyte, and acid-base balances.

Nutrition

The human body has an essential need for nutrients, although the body can survive without food longer than without oxygen and fluids. Like other physiological needs, nutritional needs may be unmet in a person of any age.

The metabolic processes of the body control the digestion and storage of nutrients and the elimination of waste products. The digestion and storage of nutrients are essential in meeting the body's nutritional demands.

After food is eaten, digestive processes break down the nutrients into usable compounds such as glucose, amino acids, and fatty acids, which meet the immediate nutritional needs of the body. Glucose is a body sugar that satisfies the body's immediate energy requirements. Nutrients not needed immediately are stored as glycogen, protein, or fat.

When a person skips a meal, eats insufficiently or sporadically, or fasts, the body uses its stored reserves to meet nutritional needs. Glycogen, stored in the liver and muscles, is used first because it is readily available and can be quickly converted to glucose. If the person still has not eaten when the glycogen is depleted, his body begins to use protein and fat stores to meet nutritional needs.

The body also needs vitamins and minerals to function with full efficiency. For example, deficiencies in vitamin C impair wound healing. Deficiencies in calcium and vitamin D retard bone growth and bone metabolism.

ASSESSMENT

To determine whether a client is meeting his nutritional needs, the nurse considers many factors in addition to body weight. Clients with appropriate body weight may still have particular nutritional deficits. Nutritional assessment should include measurement of body muscle mass, laboratory data, and food intake patterns (see Chapter 38).

Signs and symptoms indicating that a client is not meeting his nutritional needs include a failure to grow or gain weight, unplanned weight loss, fatigue, pallor, and recurring sores in the mouth and gums.

NURSING IMPLICATIONS

Clients require adequate nutrition to carry out activities of daily living, promote wound healing, and maintain a high level of wellness. In some cases the nurse takes a direct role in meeting the client's nutritional needs. For example, when caring for an infant with the syndrome known as the failure to thrive, the nurse and the health care team assume total responsibility for ensuring that the child has adequate nutrition.

Sometimes a nurse assists a client in meeting nutritional needs through a teaching role. An adult with recently diagnosed insulin-dependent diabetes mellitus, for example, needs to be taught to balance his nutritional needs, insulin intake, and exercise habits.

To help clients meet their nutritional needs, the nurse must understand the digestive and metabolic processes of the body. The nurse may use various nutritional supplements and techniques to correct nutritional deficits. Chapter 38 discusses in detail nursing measures related to the nutritional needs of clients.

Temperature

The body can function normally within only a narrow temperature range, between 35° C (97° F) and 41° C (106° F) (Mountcastle, 1983). Body temperatures outside this range can result in impairment, permanent effects such as brain damage, or death.

The body can temporarily regulate its temperature by certain mechanisms. For example, a person shivers when he moves from a warm environment to an environment at 55° F. Shivering is an adaptive response that can temporarily increase body temperature. Chapter 30 discusses other adaptive responses.

Nurses care for clients with conditions related to both heat and cold exposures. When the body is unable to regulate its temperature, severe illness or death may result. Rapid change in temperature or exposure to temperature extremes is most critical for the very young, the very old, and the chronically ill.

ASSESSMENT

The body has a physiological response to extreme environmental temperatures. Prolonged exposure to cold decreases the body's rate of metabolism and use of oxygen. If body temperature is lowered beyond the point at which the body can adapt, the vital signs decrease, consciousness decreases, the person is more difficult to arouse, the skin is pale and cold, and urinary output decreases. A localized exposure to cold, as occurs when hands are bare in the winter, leads to the injury known as frostbite. Frostbite is a traumatic effect of extreme cold on the skin and subcutaneous tissues and is first manifested as distinct pallor. Blood circulation in the area is impaired, leading to decreased oxygen in the tissues and tissue death.

Prolonged exposure to heat increases the body's metabolic activity and increases tissue oxygen demand. Extreme or prolonged heat exposure can also have specific physiological effects. Local exposure to heat can result in first-, second-, or third-degree burns. Overexposure to the sun can lead to sunstroke, which is characterized by high fever, convulsions, and coma. Elderly persons living in poorly ventilated homes without air conditioning are at risk for heatstroke during prolonged hot weather. Symptoms are an elevated body temperature, dehydration, and fluid and electrolyte imbalances. If untreated the person becomes disoriented and confused, enters a coma, and dies.

NURSING IMPLICATIONS

Nursing care for clients exposed to extreme heat or cold is directed toward restoring normal body temperature and temperature regulation. In addition, the nurse helps clients avoid exposure to heat or cold and thus meet the body's temperature needs.

To treat frostbite, the nurse gently warms the affected area. The nurse should not rub the area in an attempt to increase circulation, since this can further damage the skin and underlying tissues.

A client with sunstroke needs emergency treatment to reduce his body temperature. Nursing measures include a tepid sponge bath (Chapter 35).

Nursing care related to heat and cold exposure is directed primarily to prevention. The nurse assesses the client's environment and life-style to determine whether there is a risk for extreme temperature exposures, and if there is, helps the client and family minimize the risk.

Elimination

The elimination of waste materials from ingested food is one of the metabolic processes of the body. Waste products are eliminated by the lungs, skin, kidneys, and intestines.

The lungs primarily eliminate carbon dioxide (CO_2). CO_2 is a gas formed in the body during tissue metabolism. Most of the CO_2 formed by tissue metabolism is carried to the lungs by the venous system and excreted by the lungs through expiration. If a client has difficulty eliminating CO_2, as with acid-base imbalances that originate in the respiratory system, nursing measures are needed to prevent severe impairment or death (see Chapter 43). The water eliminated by the lungs with every expiratory cycle amounts to about 200 ml a day. The nurse considers this amount in calculating the fluid needs of a dehydrated client.

The skin eliminates water and sodium, most noticeably in the form of sweat. Sweat also assists in temperature regulation because the evaporation of sweat lowers the body temperature and helps maintain a normal range in body temperature in a hot environment. Sweat cannot always be seen, but the skin excretes water continuously, approximately 200 ml a day. A client with fever or prolonged exposure to hot humid weather has an increased water loss from the skin. The nurse considers water loss from the skin when caring for a client with actual or potential dehydration.

The kidneys are the body's primary means of excreting excess body fluids, electrolytes, hydrogen ions, and acids. Urinary elimination normally depends on fluid intake and circulatory blood volume; if either is decreased, urinary output decreases. Urinary output is also changed in persons with kidney disease, which affects both the quantity of urine and the content of waste products within the urine. Severe kidney disease can be life threatening.

The intestines eliminate solid waste products and some fluid from the body. The elimination of solid waste by bowel evacuation usually becomes a pattern at about 30 to 36 months of age. Each person has a different pattern for bowel evacuation.

ASSESSMENT

A client whose urinary elimination needs are unmet may be incontinent. Incontinence can occur because the person is unable to perceive the urge to void, as when waking from general anesthesia or after a stroke or spinal cord injury. Urinary incontinence may also occur if an immobilized person is unable to reach a bedpan or urinal or obtain assistance.

Unmet urinary elimination needs also result in fluid and electrolyte imbalances. A fluid volume loss such as that occurring with dehydration or shock may lead to an imbalance in waste products eliminated by the kidney. Electrolyte imbalance may result from an acute or chronic kidney disorder.

A client's unmet needs for bowel elimination may lead to changes in elimination patterns or diet patterns. Changes in bowel elimination patterns include incontinence, constipation, and diarrhea. Altering the dietary intake of fluids and foods can also change elimination patterns and elimination needs.

NURSING IMPLICATIONS

Nursing care assists the client in meeting elimination needs. The nursing intervention may be simple, such as providing privacy or changing the diet, or complex, such as inserting a catheter or administering a soapsuds enema. In helping clients meet urinary and bowel elimination needs, a nurse uses knowledge of anatomy and physiology along with specific skills and techniques. Chapters 39 and 40 describe in detail the knowledge and skills needed to meet the elimination needs of clients.

Shelter

All humans need shelter. Although most people have some kind of shelter, sometimes it is substandard and does not offer full protection from the elements, such as heat, cold, wind, and rain. Disasters such as floods, fire, and tornadoes can render a family or an entire community homeless. Disaster agencies such as the Red Cross are excellent resources in helping clients obtain shelter.

ASSESSMENT

Often the nurse can identify environmental risk factors in a client's home that could lead to the client's shelter needs not being met. Such risk factors include exposure to temperature extremes, as in a poorly insulated, drafty home or a poorly ventilated home without air conditioning. Other risk factors may involve the physical safety of the home and its environment. A home with a leaky roof is inadequate shelter, as is an unprotected home in a high-crime neighborhood.

Clients at risk for unmet shelter needs include those with limited financial, social, and family resources. Frequently such clients are elderly or handicapped or have limited job skills. Often they feel trapped in their environment because they are unaware of resources that can help them relocate.

In assessing whether a client is meeting his shelter needs, the nurse seeks to identify conditions that put the client at risk for illness or injury. Environments that are dirty and may attract insects or rodents increase the risk for infections and other illness. If a home is poorly lighted or cluttered, the client has an increased risk of accidental injury. Other kinds of environmental conditions may produce stress or affect the client's health in other dimensions by leading to frustration or feelings of hopelessness.

NURSING IMPLICATIONS

In many situations it is unrealistic for a nurse to seek new shelter for a client and family, but the nurse can refer the client to community agencies that can help him improve his present shelter. Community agencies can establish standards for rental housing and help a client pay utility bills or repair his home. Such agencies can also help the client identify available alternatives for shelter.

The nurse can directly help the client make changes within the home to make it a healthier environment. Her role in health promotion and illness prevention often involves teaching clients about the relationship between home environment and health.

Rest

Every person has a basic physiological need for rest on a regular basis. The amount of sleep an individual needs varies, depending on the person's quality of sleep, health status, activity patterns, life-style, and age. An infant, for example, requires a great deal of sleep, frequently as much as 16 to 20 hours a day. The infant's sleeping cycle is irregular, however, and sleep is frequently interrupted by the need for food or elimination. As the child grows, the sleep-wake cycle becomes more regular.

A person's need for rest and sleep changes throughout life. A young adult generally needs less rest than a middle-aged or elderly adult. A client with a chronic disease requires more rest than a healthy person of the same age. Pregnancy and lactation increase the need for rest, as do health status changes such as recovery from surgery.

Physical and emotional stress may also increase a client's need for rest. Rest and sleep often provide temporary relief from stress, and thus rest can be therapeutic in helping a person cope with stress. But rest can also provide an escape from stress such that a client may depend on it as a nonproductive method for resolving stress.

A person's need for rest and sleep may be unmet because of life-style, temporary activities that prevent him from getting sufficient sleep, sleep pattern disturbances such as insomnia, pain caused by illness or injury, and other factors.

ASSESSMENT

When a person goes without rest or sleep for a time or regularly gets insufficient sleep, his appearance and behavior begin to change. He may have circles under his eyes, appear pale, and be disheveled. He may have less energy, seem less motivated, be more irritable or withdrawn, stare into space, have difficulty concentrating, be restless, and fall asleep during the day.

NURSING IMPLICATIONS

Whenever possible, the nurse should plan nursing care to fit the client's usual sleep-wake cycle. If the client usually retires to bed at 10 PM, for example, the care plan should not include activities that routinely disturb him after that time. If the client has certain habits before retiring, such as walking, bathing, reading, or drinking warm milk or a glass of wine, this activity should be incorporated into the plan of care.

Frequently a client's pattern of rest is changed by an illness or pain. The nurse uses specific methods to promote comfort and relieve pain so that the client's need for rest can be anticipated and met (see Chapters 36 and 37). If the client is unable to meet his needs for sleep and rest because of other factors, such as life-style or chronic stress, the nurse directs care toward resolving the underlying cause while also helping the client meet these needs.

Sex

Sex is considered by Maslow (1970) to be a basic physiological need that generally takes priority over higher-level needs. Sexual needs and the manner in which they are expressed and met are influenced by age, sociocultural background, ethics, values, self-esteem, and level of wellness.

The health professions as a whole are giving increasing attention to human sexuality as a component of health. As nurses too become more knowledgeable about clients' sexual needs, nursing care takes into account factors related to clients' sexuality. Sexuality involves much more than simply physical sexual activity; it may be associated with needs in other dimensions, including emotional, social, and spiritual needs. Sexuality in all dimensions can be affected by illness, and chronic conditions and hospitalization can prevent an individual from meeting sexual needs.

ASSESSMENT

A client who is unable to meet sexual needs may behave in a way indicating that these needs are unmet. Some clients seek other outlets, which may not meet their sexual needs or may lead to other conflicts, such as excessive sexual language, excessive masturbation, or exposing sexual organs. Other clients engage in behavior such as flirting with a member of the health care team or sublimate the sexual need through physical exercise, overeating, or overwork. A client unable to meet sexual needs may feel emotionally frustrated or show signs of stress.

Changes in hormonal levels throughout life, particularly during puberty, menopause, and pregnancy, can influence a client's ability to meet sexual needs. Illnesses and altered functioning of the sexual organs can change how a client perceives and expresses himself sexually.

Changes in the body's appearance such as with paralysis or after mastectomy or colostomy can affect how a person feels about his or her sexuality and ability to fulfill sexual needs. A change in physical appearance must be accepted by the client as well as the client's sexual partner, and their pattern of sexual behavior, including activities other than those involving the sexual organs, may require readjustment.

Clients experiencing depression, grief, or life-style changes are at risk for having unmet sexual needs. In some cases the meeting of sexual needs is only temporarily interrupted. In other situations, especially with clients experiencing severe depression, sexual needs are unmet for a longer period of time and may resolve only with professional counseling.

NURSING IMPLICATIONS

Nursing care designed to help a client meet needs related to sexuality must be individualized according to the client's age, maturity, developmental level, values, habits, level of health, sexual partner, and sexual practices. To help a client meet sexual needs, the nurse must be comfortable in discussing sexuality in general.

Not all nurses feel competent to discuss sexuality with their clients, but it is important that a nurse recognize when a client is unable to meet sexual needs so that other resources, such as another nurse, a physician, or a social worker, can help the client in this area. Chapter 19 discusses sexuality in more detail.

Safety and Security Needs

Next in priority after physiological needs are needs for physical and psychological safety and security.

Physical Safety

An infant enters the world totally dependent on others for his physical safety. As the infant grows and develops, he gradually achieves greater independence in meeting his needs. Adults are generally able to provide for and maintain their own physical safety, but the ill, handicapped, and elderly may not be able to meet their physical safety needs unassisted.

Maintaining physical safety involves reducing or eliminating threats to a person's body or life. The threat may be an illness, an accident, a danger, or environmental exposure. When ill, a client may be unable to protect himself from threats such as infection, and the client therefore depends on professionals in the health care system to protect him from such threats.

Occasionally the meeting of physical safety needs takes precedence over a physiological need. For example, a nurse may need to protect a disoriented client from falling out of bed before providing care to meet his nutritional needs.

ASSESSMENT

When assessing the physical safety needs of a client, the nurse considers both actual and potential threats. Clients with limited movement or total immobilization of an extremity are at risk for developing joint contractures, skin breakdown, and muscle atrophy. Clients taking medication are at risk for side effects related to the medication. Clients with indwelling intravenous lines or Foley catheters are at risk for secondary infections.

Clients with acute or chronic illnesses, disability, or handicaps may require assistance in meeting their safety needs. The nurse assesses the total environment, whether it is the client's home or a hospital setting, to identify potential or actual threats to the client's physical safety.

Health problems in other dimensions may also present a safety risk to a client. A client under emotional stress, for example, may behave in a manner that would potentially threaten his safety. A client who is socially isolated may be unaware of environmental factors that could threaten his physical safety.

NURSING IMPLICATIONS

The early identification of potential threats to a client's physical safety is perhaps the most beneficial means of maintaining the client's safety. For example, nurses teach parents about potential risk to their children throughout the developmental stages (see Chapters 25 and 34).

The nurse teaches clients receiving medication or therapy in either the hospital or the home about the side effects, interaction effects, and potential hazards of treatments, as well as the specific desired effects of the drug or treatment. The nurse individualizes education techniques for all clients and their families to best assist clients in meeting their needs. Chapter 16 details the teaching-learning process by which the nurse incorporates the client's learning needs into the plan of care.

Psychological Safety

To be safe and secure psychologically, a person must understand what to expect from others, including family members and health care professionals, as well as what to expect from procedures, from new experiences, and from encounters within his environment. Everyone feels some threat to psychological safety when encountering new and unfamiliar experiences. A student entering college may feel insecure if he is not sure what to expect, a person starting a new job may feel threatened by having to interact with unfamiliar people, and a client about to undergo a diagnostic test may be psychologically threatened by the technology involved or unfamiliar physical sensations. In such cases people generally do not directly state that they feel their psychological safety is threatened, but their conversation may indirectly reveal their feelings. The student may say, "I feel kind of strange about starting college." The new worker might tell his boss repeatedly, "Please let me know if there is anything wrong with my work." The client might say to the nurse, "The diagnostic tests are going to be OK, don't you think so?"

Frequently an explanation of the procedure or experience by the nurse is enough to counteract the psychological threat. In some cases, however, the nurse must take more active steps with clients and their families to meet their psychological safety needs.

ASSESSMENT

Assessment of the client's psychological safety needs is often difficult because the nurse may have to interpret the client's language and behaviors. Because a perceived threat causes stress, the client may act in various ways to adapt to the stress (see Chapter 5). The client's behavior may change radically. For example, an outgoing, active person may become withdrawn, or a previously cooperative client may suddenly refuse to participate in his care. Most clients want to be active and cooperative, and a drastic change in a client's behavior is a clue that he may be feeling some threat to his psychological safety.

NURSING IMPLICATIONS

The nurse can use teaching methods with the client and family to reduce a threat to psychological safety, particularly when the potential threat includes a change in role, a change in body image (see Chapter 18), or an invasive diagnostic or surgical procedure. Because people often fear or have unrealistic expectations about the unknown, telling clients and their families what to expect greatly reduces their anxiety and increases their participation in health care.

Healthy adults are generally able to meet physical and physiological safety needs without help from health care professionals. But a person who is ill or is handicapped by illness or injury is more susceptible to threats to his physical and emotional well-being, and therefore the nurse intervenes to help the client protect himself from actual or potential harm.

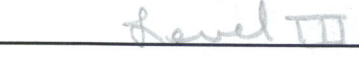

Love and Belonging Needs

The next priority after physiological and safety needs is the need for love and belonging. People generally need to feel that they are loved by members of their family and that they are accepted by their peers and members of the community. This need generally arises after physiological and safety needs are already met, because only when the individual feels safe and secure does he have time and energy to seek love and belonging and to share that love with others (Rogers, 1961).

Even a person who is generally able to meet his needs for love and a sense of belonging is often unable to fulfill these needs when illness or injury interrupts his life. When a client enters the health care system, it becomes even more difficult for him to meet these needs. The client is forced to adapt to aspects of the health care delivery system such as organization, routines, environmental limitations, and visiting hours, and as a result he has little time or energy left to meet the needs for love and belonging with his family or significant others.

ASSESSMENT

A client of any age in any health care setting may have difficulty meeting love and belonging needs. The ways in which these unmet needs are manifested depend on the client. The client's behavior may be similar to the adaptive behaviors of a person responding to stress (see Chapter 5).

Discussion with the family and significant others is important as the nurse compares the client's present needs for love and belonging with how he normally meets these needs. The nurse may identify changes in the family or in the client's relationship with a significant other that can provide insight about his needs for love and belonging.

Physical and behavioral changes may indicate that a client is unable to meet love and belonging needs. The client's appearance and hygiene habits may change; a normally neat and well-groomed person may seem sloppy and uncaring about his appearance. The client may complain of physical ailments such as headaches or gastrointestinal problems when separated from family and significant others. Sleep and eating habits may also change.

A person's conversation often demonstrates that his needs for love and belonging are not being met. A hospitalized client may speak often of family or friends expected to visit, or a client who becomes anxious because family or friends have not yet visited him may attempt to cope with his unmet needs by insisting it does not matter. A child separated from parents because of illness or injury may seem to adopt the nurse as surrogate parent. A client may attempt to interact with the nurse as with a close friend or may even become possessive about the amount of time spent with the nurse. All these are manifestations of the normal human need for love and affection.

If a person's need persists for a long period without being met, his behavior may change in more noticeable ways. A usually mild-tempered person may become easily irritated. An outgoing person may withdraw from interaction with co-workers and friends. The person's work habits may change, leading to increased absenteeism or overcommitment to his job.

NURSING IMPLICATIONS

The nursing care plan for all clients should include means by which the client can meet his needs for love and belonging. For example, if the client is a young child hospitalized for some time, the nursing care plan should include specific opportunities for the child and family to interact. In some cases it may be important for the mother or father to remain overnight with the child.

A client suddenly isolated from his family and others by illness or injury cannot meet his needs for love and belonging in his usual ways. If opportunities for social interaction are limited, the client may come to feel that he does not belong and thus may begin to withdraw. The nurse can take specific actions to help the client maintain social contacts so that he can meet love and belonging needs. A hospitalized client isolated because of a wound infection may benefit from short social visits by members of the health care team. Resources in the community may help; for example, an elderly client can be helped to meet his need for contact with others through a Meals on Wheels program or a senior citizens' center.

Finally, the nurse works with the client and family to adapt the nursing care plan in any way that might help the client meet his needs for love and belonging.

The more actively involved the client is in developing his plan of care, and the more control he has over his environment while receiving care, the easier it will be for him to meet all his needs independently and with the assistance of family members, significant others, and the nurse.

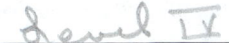

Esteem and Self-Esteem Needs

All people need a stable sense of self-esteem, as well as the feeling that they are held in regard by others. The need for self-esteem is linked to the desire for strength, achievement, adequacy, mastery and competence, confidence when facing the world, and independence and freedom. People also need recognition or appreciation from others. When both of these needs are met, a person feels self-confident and useful. If a person's needs for self-esteem and esteem of others are unfulfilled, he may feel helpless and inferior (Maslow, 1970).

ASSESSMENT

A change in a person's roles in life may threaten his esteem or self-esteem. The change may be planned and anticipated, such as retirement, or sudden, as with an injury or being unexpectedly laid off from work. Along with the change in role comes a change in the person's independence and relationship with others; frequently people who were formerly independent become more dependent, and strains are put on relationships with others. A person may become more dependent on family members, social agencies, or health care professionals and may begin to question his usefulness and importance—he may lose self-esteem. If he is no longer functioning in a former role, such as that of worker, he may feel he has lost the esteem of others as well.

Changes in a person's body image, such as those caused by illness or injury, may also influence self-esteem. Body image changes include both obvious changes such as the amputation of a leg and unobservable changes such as a hysterectomy. Normal developmental changes such as those of puberty or menopause can change a person's image.

It is not the magnitude of a change in body image or role that affects a person's self-esteem, but rather how the person perceives himself after the change. A person's sense of self-esteem and the esteem of others therefore depends on his values and beliefs, his support from others, and his self-concept.

There are many indications that a client has unmet needs for self-esteem or the esteem of others. A client who feels helpless or inferior may defer all decisions to the nurse rather than expressing his own wishes.

The client may "put himself down" or seem unusually lethargic or apathetic about anything involving himself, including his appearance. His general attitude may be summed up as a feeling of hopelessness. In some cases a client with low self-esteem may avoid or ignore opportunities for actions that could increase his self-esteem because he is certain he would fail. The loss of self-esteem can thus become a self-fulfilling prophecy.

A client who feels he lacks the esteem of other people may test others by making statements that call for their approval or praise. Conversely, he may act in a way that prevents such approval if he has little self-esteem and is sure that he will fail.

NURSING IMPLICATIONS

Helping the client meet his need for self-esteem begins with the first contact between the client and nurse. The nurse from the beginning must convey respect for the client as an individual. Even though the client and nurse may have different beliefs and values, the nurse needs to accept, not judge, the client's values (see Chapter 13).

If the client's self-concept is changed by illness or injury, nursing care involves improving his self-concept and body image. Specific nursing actions depend on the cause of the client's altered self-concept, his support system, his personality, and the resources available to him (see Chapter 18). If the client's level of self-esteem is so low that he fails to care for himself, the nurse may have to help him meet other needs, such as those for nutrition and safety, while taking steps to increase his self-esteem.

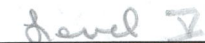

Need for Self-Actualization

Self-actualization is the highest-level need in Maslow's hierarchy of human needs. When a person has met all the lower-level needs, it is by self-actualization that he achieves his fullest potential (Maslow, 1970).

The self-actualized person is autonomous, easily motivated, and not self-centered. He is generally able to solve his own problems and accepts and assists others. Self-actualization is not the same as being well-adjusted or successful because a person can have these qualities and still not have met all other needs. A self-actualized person is mature in all dimensions. Although he may have failings and doubts, he is generally able to deal with them realistically.

How well a person meets his need for self-actualization depends on his present needs, environment, and stressors. To be self-actualized, the client needs to achieve a balance among his needs, stressors, and ability to adapt to the changes and demands of his body and environment.

ASSESSMENT

Illness or injury can threaten or disturb a client's self-actualization. A client's loss of self-actualization occurs when he can no longer achieve his fullest potential because of the limitations imposed by the illness or injury. This loss may result in behavioral changes. The client may feel frustrated because his illness prevents him from making decisions, being creative, and solving his problems independently. Instead, because of the illness, he is forced to be more self-centered, more dependent on others, and motivated more by external factors.

NURSING IMPLICATIONS

The major focus for nursing care is to restore the client as much as possible to his self-actualized state. Nursing care is planned to encourage the client to make his own decisions whenever possible, particularly in regard to his health care. Thus the nurse seeks the active involvement of the client in the planning and delivery of nursing care (see Chapter 9).

Because the self-actualized person tends to be creative and highly individual in many ways, nursing care should include the opportunity for the client to fulfill his creative needs. He should be encouraged to continue with specific projects, and if he is hospitalized, time should be set aside for such projects. Frequently hospital routines leave the client with little free time for relaxing activities.

The client's need for privacy must be respected and met. When in good health the self-actualized person generally has a strong need for periods of privacy, and illness, especially in a hospital setting, can greatly reduce a person's privacy. Nurses can help meet this need by planning and coordinating health care so that the client's privacy will not be interrupted during specific times throughout the day.

Finally, although the self-actualized person may seen unconventional in some respects, the nurse should avoid judging his behavior or imposing undue restrictions on activities that may be necessary to his self-actualization.

Application of Basic Needs Theory

Although Maslow's theory of human needs can provide a basis for the nursing care of clients of all ages in all health settings, when the nurse applies this theory in practice the focus is on the needs of the individual client rather than rigid adherence to Maslow's hierarchy. Maslow's hierarchy is a generaliza-

tion about the need priorities of most people—not all people. In all cases an emergency physiological need takes precedence over a higher-level need, but with one client the need for self-esteem may be a higher priority than a long-term nutritional need, whereas for another client these priorities may be reversed. To provide the most effective care, the nurse needs to understand the relationships among different needs for the individual client and the factors that determine priorities for the individual client. Furthermore, although the hierarchy of needs suggests that one need should be met before another, nursing care often addresses more than one need simultaneously.

Relationships among Needs

In some nursing situations it is unrealistic to expect a client's basic needs to occur in the fixed hierarchical order. For example, a client enters the health care system because he has a chronic respiratory infection. While providing care, the nurse learns that he has not eaten adequately, slept well, or maintained any social relationships since his wife died 6 weeks before. In this case the client has several unmet needs, including the physiological needs for nutrition and rest and lower-priority needs for love and a sense of belonging. For the client these separate needs are closely related. Nursing care in this situation would not simply be directed to helping the client meet the higher-priority needs for nutrition and rest, because these needs in part occurred because the client was not meeting his lower-priority needs. Nursing care for this client focuses also on assisting him through the grief process (see Chapter 46) so that, once he has resolved his feelings of grief and loneliness, he is able to return to his former eating and sleeping habits and thus meet these physiological needs.

An opposite relationship among similar needs may be true of a different client. For example, a woman is receiving treatment for severe arthritis and often feels pain or discomfort when engaging in certain activities. Because of this, she has changed her habits and no longer visits family members and friends as she once did. The nurse realizes that the woman also now has unmet needs for love and belonging. As with the client in the preceding example, these two sets of needs are clearly related and the nurse provides care directed to meeting both. In this situation, however, the priority is to provide relief from pain, which will then allow the woman to return to former activities that meet the lower-priority needs.

For different individuals, needs on different levels may be related in different ways. One person may give the sexual need higher priority than the need for love, whereas for another person the sexual need is deferred until the need for love is met, so that the sexual relationship follows love. Similarly, a person with an unmet need for self-esteem may be unable to seek fulfillment of his need for love if his level of self-esteem is so low that he feels inferior and fears rejection. In these and many other ways, needs on different levels may be closely related for an individual client, and the nurse in assessing the client's needs and planning care must be careful not to assume that a lower-level need always takes priority. As with all other aspects of providing care, the nurse individualizes the nursing care plan for the client as a person with unique needs and desires.

Simultaneous Meeting of Needs

In many nursing situations the nurse provides care for clients with several different needs, because illness often disrupts the client's ability to meet the needs on different levels. After identifying the client's specific needs, the nurse generally has to set priorities for providing care to help the client meet these needs. However, setting priorities does not mean that the nurse provides care for only one need at a time. The nurse does not, for example, simply begin with the need lowest in the hierarchy and move up to another need only after the first has been met. In emergency situations, of course, physiological needs take precedence, but even then the nurse is aware of the client's other needs. Even in an emergency case, such as stopping profuse blood flow from an injury, the nurse considers the client's higher-level needs and treats the client's body and person with respect.

A young man who is hospitalized with paraplegia resulting from a severed spinal cord, for example, certainly needs assistance in meeting his physiological needs. But this client may also have low self-esteem related to his condition. The nurse is faced with the challenge of simultaneously meeting his physiological needs and his need for self-esteem because, if the client does not feel good about himself, he may not eat properly or participate in his physical care. The nurse should not offer the client false hopes about future recovery, but while planning care to meet his physiological needs, she can include measures that will help gradually restore his self-esteem.

Factors That Influence Need Priorities

Although the nurse ideally can direct nursing care toward the simultaneous meeting of several needs, in practice one need often takes precedence over another and priorities must be determined so that care can be more focused and effective. Life-threatening situations always take first priority, and unmet physiological needs that pose a potential threat to life certainly have a high priority. In other situations, however, the nurse has to consider various factors that influence which needs take priority over others for the individual client.

First, a person's personality and mood affect how he perceives and is able to meet any particular need. A depressed person may react negatively to a suggestion for an activity that could increase his self-esteem, although at another time and in another mood the person might respond with enthusiasm. Thus, when providing care to help a client meet several needs, the nurse can adjust the care plan to correspond most effectively to the client's personality and mood.

Second, some needs must be deferred until the client is in better health. A client recovering from an acute gastrointestinal infection should not be encouraged to resume physical activities related to his need for self-esteem until his needs for physical safety and security have been met by achieving full health. Similarly, a diabetic whose condition is unstable may have to defer other needs until he has satisfied nutritional needs related to his insulin therapy.

Third, the client's perception of his needs varies among cultural groups (see Chapter 21). One group may encourage a woman to become independent and self-actualized through working, whereas another culture may discourage the woman from meeting this need. In addition, the client's perception of some needs, such as sexual needs, varies between the sexes and among age groups. The nurse considers the client's perception of his needs when planning care and does not impose her own perceptions about the client's need priorities.

Fourth, the client's family structure can influence how he seeks to satisfy his needs (see Chapter 22). A mother may, for example, place the needs of an infant before her own needs, such as by interrupting a meal or sleep to feed the child. The nurse considers family patterns and habits when planning care to help a client meet needs.

Last, and perhaps most important, when setting need priorities the nurse considers the fact that, since the person's physiological functioning is closely related to his body systems, his environment, and his values, ethics, and culture, his basic needs are also interrelated. One need does not occur independent of other needs. For example, if a person's nutritional need is unmet for a long time, he begins to show signs of malnutrition, his body deteriorates, he becomes weak, and he is unable to recognize or meet the lower-priority needs of safety, love, and self-esteem. Needs are interrelated in unique ways for each person, and the nurse considers such relationships in planning care. The nurse involves the client and family in this planning so that the care plan reflects the need priorities of the client rather than simply following the hierarchical priorities described by the human needs theory.

Summary

Healthy adults are usually able to meet most of their basic needs. But as an adult ages or if he becomes ill or handicapped, the risk of not being able to meet basic needs increases.

Maslow's theory of human needs postulates a hierarchical relationship among different levels of human needs. A client entering the health care system may have one or more unmet needs at different levels, and nursing care addresses all the client's needs. In general the essential, life-sustaining needs take priority over others. The client's different needs may be interrelated in ways unique to him, and the nurse considers the client's own priorities when planning

care to help him meet his needs. Nursing care may be directed toward meeting several needs simultaneously. The nursing care plan is based on the nurse's assessment of the extent to which the client is meeting, and is able to meet, all his needs.

Nursing involves providing care for the whole person. The nurse applies knowledge about the body systems and also about the client's family, social system, emotions, values, ethics, and goals of health care. In this way the theory of human needs corresponds to nursing's holistic perspective by addressing the client's needs in his physical, emotional, intellectual, social, and spiritual dimensions. Basic needs theory is appropriate and applicable in community health, psychiatric, outpatient, and institutional settings, including critical care units and rehabilitation centers. This theory can provide a basis for nursing care for clients of all ages at all developmental stages, from the neonate to the geriatric client. Human needs theory is therefore a set of concepts important for the nurse's understanding of health and illness and the client's position on the health-illness continuum.

KEY CONCEPTS

✓ Basic human needs are the needs for things such as food, water, safety, and love that people require to survive and be healthy.

✓ Some human needs are more necessary to survival than others and must be met first.

✓ Maslow's hierarchy of needs is a theoretical representation of the levels of basic needs.

✓ The very young, the very old, the chronically ill, and the handicapped are generally less able than others to meet their needs without assistance.

✓ The highest priority is given to physiological needs: for oxygen, fluid, nutrition, temperature, elimination, shelter, rest, and sexuality.

✓ Oxygen is the most essential physiological need. A chronic or acute oxygen need can be identified by confusion, lethargy, rapid shallow respirations, an inability to lie flat, nasal flaring, retractions, a decreased level of consciousness, and cyanosis.

✓ Fluid needs require a balance between the intake and output of fluids. Dehydration or edema indicates unmet fluid needs.

✓ Dehydration may result in flushed, dry skin, poor skin turgor, coated tongue, dry mucous membranes, decreased saliva, decreased tears, and oliguria.

✓ Edema may result in the swelling of a dependent body part, weight gain, shortness of breath, increased heart rate, and smooth and shiny skin.

KEY CONCEPTS

✓ Nutritional needs require an adequate intake of foods to allow the body to carry on metabolic processes. Unmet nutritional needs may be indicated by weight loss or failure to grow or gain weight, fatigue, pallor, and recurring sores in the mouth and gums.

✓ The body is able to function within only a very small temperature range, 35° C (97° F) to 41° C (106° F). Unmet temperature needs may result from exposure to either cold or heat.

✓ Prolonged exposure to cold decreases the body's rate of metabolism and oxygen requirements and may be indicated by lowered vital signs, decreased level of consciousness, cold and pale skin, decreased urinary output, and localized frostbite.

✓ Prolonged exposure to heat increases the body's metabolic activity and tissue oxygen demands and may be indicated by high fever, increased pulse, convulsions, and coma.

✓ Elimination needs involve the body's removal of excess fluids and wastes. The body meets these needs by elimination through the skin, lungs, kidneys, and intestines.

✓ The need for shelter is a physiological need. Unmet needs can be identified through assessment of a client's environment.

✓ Sleep and rest needs vary depending on the individual's quality of sleep, age, health status, activity patterns, and life-style. Unmet needs may result in a decreased level of energy, disheveled appearance, irritability, decreased concentration, and restlessness.

✓ People have different needs related to sexuality at different times in life, and the manifestation of unmet sexual needs can take many forms.

✓ Safety and security needs include both physical and psychological safety.

✓ Clients in the health care system may be unable to meet their needs for love and belonging because of changes in relationships with others and the separation often imposed by illness.

✓ People need stable self-esteem as well as the esteem of others. Illness, role changes, or changes in body image may threaten a person's ability to meet these needs.

✓ The self-actualized person is autonomous, easily motivated, and not self-centered. The need for self-actualization can be threatened by changes that occur with illness or injury.

✓ To apply basic needs theory in practice, the nurse considers the relationships among the client's specific needs, sets priorities for meeting needs by considering the client's own priorities, and when possible assists the client in meeting needs on different levels simultaneously.

REFERENCES

Maslow, A.H.: Motivation and personality, ed. 2, New York, 1970, Harper & Row, Publishers, Inc.

Mountcastle, V.R.: Medical physiology, St. Louis, 1980, The C.V. Mosby Co.

Rogers, C.: On becoming a person, Boston, 1961, Houghton Mifflin Co.

ADDITIONAL READINGS

Maslow, A.H.: Toward a psychology of being, ed. 2, New York, 1968, Van Nostrand Reinhold Co.

Maslow, A.H.: Toward a humanistic biology, Am. Psychol. 24:724, 1969.

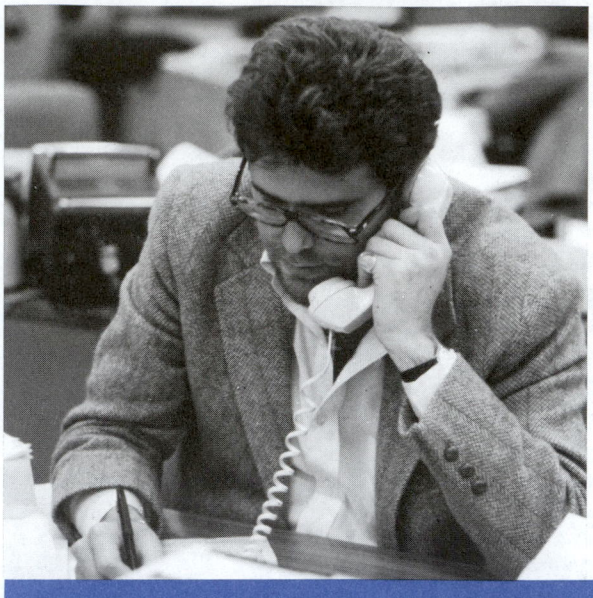

OBJECTIVES

Mastery of content in this chapter will enable the student to:

- Define the terms in the glossary.
- Describe three mechanisms of homeostasis.
- Discuss the limitations of homeostatic control.
- Discuss four models of stress as they relate to nursing practice.
- Describe how adaptation occurs in each of the five dimensions.
- Describe two forms of local physiological adaptation.
- Describe the three phases of the general adaptation syndrome.
- List and discuss task-oriented behaviors that are responses to stress.
- List and discuss the most common ego-defense mechanisms that are responses to stress.
- Discuss the effects of prolonged stress on each of the five dimensions of a person's functioning.
- Describe stress management techniques that nurses can help clients to use.
- Discuss techniques of crisis intervention.
- Describe stress management techniques that can benefit nurses themselves

GLOSSARY

adaptation   Process by which changes occur in any of a person's dimensions in response to stress.

attack behavior   Psychological response to stress in which a person uses either constructive or destructive mechanisms in an attempt to remove or overcome the stressor.

compensation   Adaptive ego-defense mechanism in which a person avoids feelings of inferiority or inadequacy in one area through achievement in another area.

compromise   Changing one's usual behavior, substituting goals, or delaying satisfaction of needs in one area to reduce stress in another.

conversion   Adaptive ego-defense mechanism in which emotional conflicts are transformed into physiological symptoms.

coping mechanism   Any effort directed toward stress management, including task-oriented and ego-defense mechanisms.

crisis   Stressful encounter with a change or obstacle to life goals that is perceived as insurmountable.

crisis intervention   Use of therapeutic techniques directed toward helping a client resolve a particular and immediate problem.

denial   Defense mechanism by which a person avoids emotional conflicts and anxiety by refusing to acknowledge thoughts, feelings, desires, impulses, and other factors that would cause intolerable pain.

displacement   Unconcious method of avoiding emotional conflict and anxiety by transferring emotions, ideas, or wishes from a stressful object or situation to a substitute that is less anxiety producing.

ego-defense mechanism   Unconscious behavior that protects a person from an emotional stress.

external stressor   Stressor originating outside a person.

5 | Homeostasis and Adaptation to Stress

"flight-or-fight" syndrome Set of physiological responses to a stressor that prepares a person to attempt to overcome or avoid stress.

general adaptation syndrome Generalized defense response of the body to stress, consisting of three stages: alarm, resistance, and exhaustion.

homeostasis State of relative constancy in the internal environment of the body, maintained naturally by physiological adaptive mechanisms.

identification Adaptive mechanism by which a person consciously or unconsciously attributes to himself the qualities and characteristics of another person as a means of avoiding or coping with stress.

internal stressor Stress-causing stimulus that arises within a person.

job stress Condition in which some factor or combination of factors at work disrupts the worker's psychological or physiological balance.

local adaptation syndrome Localized response of tissue, an organ, or a system that occurs as a direct reaction to stress.

medulla oblongata Portion of the brain that controls vital functions necessary for homeostasis and survival.

mild stress situation Type of stress situation that is encountered by most people on a daily or weekly basis.

moderate stress situation Stress situation that lasts from several hours to a number of days.

pituitary gland Small gland attached to the hypothalamus that supplies numerous hormones for the control of vital functions and the maintenance of homeostasis.

regression Ego-defense mechanism by which a person assumes the behaviors associated with an earlier developmental period to reduce or avoid present stress.

reticular formation Small cluster of neurons in the brainstem and spinal cord that continuously monitors and controls vital functions to maintain homeostasis.

severe stress situation Chronic stress situation, which may last from several weeks to years.

situational crisis Crisis occurring suddenly in response to a specific external event or conflict.

stress Physiological or psychological tension that threatens homeostasis or a person's psychological equilibrium.

stress behaviors Changes from a person's normal behaviors in response to a stressor.

stressor Any event, situation, or other stimulus encountered in a person's external or internal environment that necessitates change or adaptation by the person.

task-oriented behavior Actions involving a person's cognitive abilities in an attempt to solve problems, resolve conflicts, and gratify the person's needs in order to reduce or avoid stress.

withdrawal behavior Physical or psychological removal of oneself from a stressor.

describes what occurs in the human body during a stress response. Selye also introduced the concept of stressors, those internal or external stimuli that cause stress (Selye, 1976).

Selye's research into stress and stressors has been important for the health care professions and is the primary focus of this chapter. The GAS model is readily applicable to all areas of nursing practice. As a nurse cares for clients experiencing various kinds of stress, she helps clients use their own adaptive resources—through various techniques, including crisis intervention–to return to their highest levels of wellness.

Homeostasis

Homeostasis is the body's tendency to maintain itself in a state of relative constancy. Homeostasis is a dynamic form of equilibrium in the body's internal environment, because that environment is constantly changing and the body's adaptive mechanisms are continually functioning to adjust to these changes and thus to maintain equilibrium.

The concept of homeostasis can be understood in relation to the basic human physiological needs (see Chapter 4). A healthy person is maintaining homeostasis if he is meeting his physiological needs, even though these needs may be changing with time. For example, by means of the respiratory system the body takes in oxygen and eliminates carbon dioxide. If the need for oxygen increases, as during strenuous exercise, the body responds by increasing the respiratory rate in order to take in more oxygen. If the need is satisfied, even though the process of breathing is changed, the person maintains homeostasis. Homeostasis therefore is not the same as stasis, a state of absolute nonchange, but is a condition of *relative* constancy, in which the various body systems continually adapt to changes. Homeostasis, then, is a state of health.

Homeostasis is maintained by physiological mechanisms that control various body functions and monitor body organs. For the most part these mechanisms are controlled by the nervous system and do not involve conscious behavior. As an analogy, consider the process of driving an automobile at a constant speed along a straight road; environmental factors such as winds, bumps in the road, and hills require continual small adjustments of the steering wheel and the accelerator, and an experienced driver is seldom consciously aware that he is making these adjustments to keep the car going straight. Similarly, the body makes adjustments in heart rate, respiratory rate,

Every person experiences various forms of stress throughout his life span. The presence of stress can provide the stimulus for change and growth, and in this respect some stress can be positive. However, too much stress can result in poor judgment, physical illness, and inability to cope with the stressor.

The term "stress" is derived from the Latin word *stringere,* which means "to draw tight" (Skeat, 1958). Although the concept of stress can be traced through the history of civilization, it became important in the sciences of physiology and health only in the mid-1800s.

Claude Bernard, in 1867, was one of the first physiologists to recognize the potential consequences of stress for an organism. He proposed that changes in the internal and external environments disrupted the functioning of an organism. In addition, he noted that it is essential for an organism to adapt to a stressor in order to survive. Although Bernard studied primarily the physiological response to stress, he also noted specific psychological adaptations that an organism makes in order to cope with stress and survive.

In 1920 Walter Cannon introduced the term "homeostasis" to describe how an organism successfully responds to stress. Cannon studied specific mechanisms that organisms use to adapt to stress and in turn to maintain a balance, homeostasis, within the internal environment.

Perhaps the most important contemporary researcher in stress is Hans Selye. Selye developed a biochemical model of stress known as the "general adaptation syndrome" (GAS). The GAS model clearly

blood pressure, temperature, fluid and electrolyte balances, hormone secretions, level of consciousness, and so on—all directed toward maintaining homeostasis.

Mechanisms

When a person becomes aware of an unmet physiological need, such as a need for food or warmth, he can take deliberate actions to meet the need. For the most part, however, homeostasis involves adjustments the body makes automatically to maintain equilibrium. These homeostatic mechanisms are self-regulatory, in the sense that they are automatic in a healthy person. In a person with an illness or injury, however, the mechanisms may not be able to maintain homeostasis. In a case of severe emphysema, for example, the increased respiratory rate initiated by physiological mechanisms may be insufficient to meet the person's oxygen needs. Homeostatic mechanisms function also through a process of negative feedback, the process by which the controlling mechanism senses an abnormal state, such as a lowered body temperature, and makes an adaptive response to return the state to normal, such as initiating shivering to generate heat. In this way homeostatic mechanisms compensate for abnormal conditions.

Three of the major homeostatic mechanisms are controlled by the medulla oblongata, the reticular formation, and the pituitary gland. These three mechanisms serve as examples of the different ways in which the body maintains homeostasis.

MEDULLA OBLONGATA

The medulla oblongata controls vital functions—such as heart rate, blood pressure, and respiration—that are necessary to survival. Impulses traveling to and from the medulla oblongata can either increase or decrease these vital functions. For example, the regulation of the heart beat is the result of sympathetic or parasympathetic nervous system impulses traveling from the medulla oblongata to the heart. The heart rate increases in accordance with impulses from the sympathetic fibers and decreases in accordance with discharges from the parasympathetic branches. These impulses are generated by the medulla oblongata in response to needs related to vital functions.

RETICULAR FORMATION

The reticular formation, a small cluster of neurons in the brainstem and spinal cord, controls vital functions as well but also continuously monitors the physiological status of the body through connections with sensory and motor tracts. For example, certain cells within the reticular formation can cause a sleeping person to regain consciousness or can increase a person's level of consciousness when a need arises.

PITUITARY GLAND

The pituitary gland, a small gland attached to the hypothalamus, supplies numerous hormones that control vital functions. The pituitary gland produces hormones that are necessary for adaptation to stresses, as well as growth hormone; in addition, the pituitary gland regulates the secretion of thyroid hormones, gonadal hormones, and parathyroid hormone. Hormone secretion, like other homeostatic mechanisms, is normally regulated by a feedback mechanism, which continuously monitors hormone levels in the blood. When hormone levels drop, the pituitary gland receives a message to increase hormone secretion. When hormone levels rise, the pituitary gland decreases hormone production. One of the pituitary hormones, for example, controls the production of thyroxine in the thyroid gland, which in turn controls rates of metabolism. Thus this homeostatic mechanism helps the body meet energy and other needs.

Limitations of Homeostatic Control

Homeostatic control mechanisms work together through complex relationships in the nervous system, hormone levels, and other body systems to maintain relative constancy within the body. In a healthy person these mechanisms are effective in maintaining homeostasis so that physiological needs are met. However, homeostatic mechanisms can provide only a short-term form of control over the body's equilibrium; these mechanisms cannot adapt to long-term changes in hormone secretion or vital functions. Thus illness, injury, or prolonged stress can decrease the adaptive capacity of homeostatic functions. Decreased functioning can take either of two forms: continued but inadequate homeostatic control or breakdown of the feedback mechanism that allows control; in either situation the result is illness or death.

In severe stress situations, for example, the pituitary gland continues to supply the body with necessary hormones to cope with stress. However, these hormones may be insufficient in quantity to provide the physiological energy necessary for the person to cope with the stressor, in which case the person's condition deteriorates and functioning declines. This physiological response to stress is described in detail later in this chapter in the section on the psychophysiological response to stress.

The feedback mechanism of homeostatic control

may break down because of an abnormality within an organ. For example, people with pituitary tumors have decreased hormone production, which in turn can lead to abnormalities in sex and endocrine organs. The feedback system breaks down because the hormones in the system are absent or at minimal levels.

For clients with homeostatic limitations, the health care professional directs therapeutic interventions toward restoring physiological balance. Often such interventions are successful, as with hormone replacement therapy or blood transfusion following massive hemorrhage. If interventions are ineffective, the body may no longer be able to function properly, resulting in illness or death.

Concepts of Stress and Adaptation

Stress and Stressors

We are all familiar with the general concept of stress, since the word itself has come into common usage in a variety of contexts. We speak of the stress of everyday living, job stress, the stress of rearing children, the stress of divorce, and so on. Everyone experiences some form of stress from time to time, and normally the healthy person is able to adapt to long-term stress or cope with short-term stress until it passes. Stress can place heavy demands on a person, however, in any or all of the human dimensions, and if the person is unable to adapt to or cope with the stress, illness can result.

Stress is any physiological or psychological tension that threatens a person's total equilibrium. In the physical dimension, stress can threaten a person's homeostasis. In the emotional dimension, stress can lead to negative or counterproductive feelings or threaten emotional well-being. In the intellectual dimension, stress can threaten the way a person normally perceives various aspects of reality, solves problems, or thinks in general. In the social dimension, stress can threaten a person's relationships with others, the support he receives from others, and his sense of belonging. In the spiritual dimension, stress can threaten a person's general outlook on life and attitude toward a Supreme Being. In essence, stress can affect how an individual satisfies all his basic human needs, as described in the preceding chapter. Stress is an important concept in nursing because stress affects the whole person.

Any factor that causes a person to experience stress is called a stressor. A stressor is any thing, event, situation, or person, encountered by an individual in his internal or external environment, that requires the individual to respond or adapt in order to avoid or minimize stress (Ivancevich and Matteson, 1980). A disease process is a stressor, but so is an event such as a test a student faces, or a person such as an unpleasant job supervisor, or an emotion such as a major disappointment. Stressors can generally be classified as internal or external. Internal stressors originate inside a person, such as a fever, a condition such as pregnancy or menopause, or an emotion such as guilt. External stressors originate outside a person, such as a marked change in environmental temperature, a change in family or social role, a life crisis such as the death of a spouse, or an event such as peer rejection. Both internal and external stressors can produce stress that adversely affects a person in one or more dimensions.

Models of Stress

The origins and effects of stress can be understood in terms of various medical and behavioral theoretical models. A stress model is used to predict what constitutes stressors for an individual and how the person will respond and to understand how various stressors and the individual interact. For the nurse, the overall purpose of any stress model is to help a client avoid unhealthy, nonproductive responses to stressors. This chapter focuses primarily on the psychophysiological response to stress described by Selye. The four alternative stress models described in the following sections are useful in gaining an understanding of stress and the human responses to stress in all dimensions.

PSYCHOSOMATIC MODEL

The psychosomatic model is based on the premise that stressors in one dimension can have pathological effects in other dimensions. Frequently, for example, stressors that arise in the emotional dimension are manifested in physiological ways. A college freshman may enter a university fearful of "failing." Even though he studies hard, completes assignments satisfactorily, and meets deadlines, he is continuously preoccupied with a fear of failure. At midsemester he experiences stomach pains, headaches, and inability to sleep. His symptoms can be traced directly to his fear of failing. Thus the physical symptoms are the result of a psychosomatic response to stress. Once the student is able to control his emotional response to the stressor of college, his fear of failure is controlled, and the physical symptoms subside.

In the psychosomatic model of stress, as in other models, what is important is for a person to control his response to a stressor. Many kinds of stressors cannot be altogether avoided, but a person's response to a stressor can be controlled. In the example just given, the student cannot eliminate the stressor, college, except by leaving school, but there is much he can do to control his response to this stressor.

ADAPTATION MODEL

The adaptation model of stress proposes that four factors determine whether a situation is stressful (Mechanic, 1962). The first factor is the ability of a person to cope with stress. This ability usually depends on the person's previous experience with similar stressors, his support system, and his overall perception of the stressor. For example, a nursing student who is preparing for a state licensure examination may adapt well to this stressor if she has scored satisfactorily on previous standardized tests, if her friends have helped her prepare for the test, and if she does not *view* the upcoming examination as a stressor.

The second factor in the adaptation model comprises the practices and norms of the person's peer group. If the peer group considers it normal to talk about the stress of the upcoming test, the student may respond to this stress by complaining or worrying aloud. This stress response may then help the student adapt to the stress, or the student may respond in this way simply because she is trying to conform to the expected peer group behavior, rather than actually being concerned about the examination.

The third factor in the adaptation model is the means the social environment provides an individual to adapt to a stressor. For example, a college freshman who suspects that he has a sexually transmitted disease may confide this fear to an upperclassman, who may then refer him to a student health service, where a diagnosis could be made and treatment initiated if necessary. In this example the resources of both the older student and the student health service offer the freshman the means to reduce the severity of the stressor, the possibility that he has a sexually transmitted disease.

The last factor in the adaptation model is the nature of the process that determines where and how an individual can use resources in the social environment to deal with stress. In the example just given, the student needs only a valid student identification card to use the prepaid health benefits, and the health service is open 7 days a week from 9 AM to 9 PM. Both of these factors make the resource easily accessible to help the student cope with the stress. However, if the process for using the health service were complex, if the service offered health care only on a limited basis, or if the student had to pay a significant fee to use the service, it is possible that the solution to the problem could increase the original stress resulting from the problem itself.

The adaptation model of stress is based on the understanding that when people feel unprepared to cope with a stressful situation they are uncomfortable and experience anxiety and often increased stress. This concept is essential for members of the health professions. With this understanding nurses can anticipate stresses their clients are likely to experience, in connection with such events as labor, diagnostic tests, discharge from the hospital to home, and illness itself. With appropriate interventions nurses can help clients and their families to reduce the effects of stress in all human dimensions.

SOCIAL ENVIRONMENT MODEL

The social environment model of stress is concerned with the effects of a person's work role on his health (French and Kahn, 1962). The model focuses on six

Fig. 5-1   Social environment stress model.

From Ivancevich, J.M., and Matteson, M.T.: Stress and work: a managerial perspective, Glenview, Ill. Copyright © 1980 by Scott, Foresman and Company. Reprinted by permission.

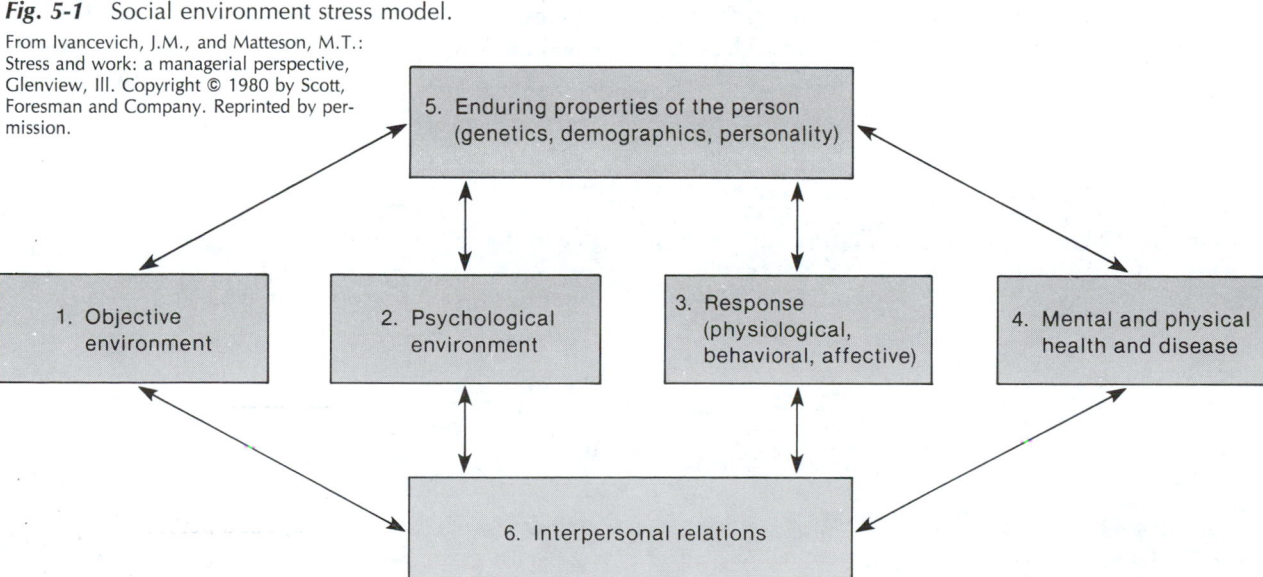

variables that determine how a person's work role interacts with his health (Fig. 5-1). The model explains how a person's personality, external and internal environments, individual responses to stressors, and interpersonal relationships influence how he responds to the stresses of work and ultimately affect his physical and mental health.

When assessing clients' levels of wellness, nurses should identify both actual and potential stressors in clients' work environments. Although nurses may not be able to remove stressors, they can plan nursing interventions directed toward helping clients change their responses to stress.

Nurses themselves can experience stress resulting from their work environments. Stressors in nursing environments include complex technical equipment, such as in specialized care units; difficult schedules, such as rotating shifts; increased demands to perform nonnursing functions, such as ordering supplies; and the responsibility of providing care to many clients. To adapt to stressors in their work environments, nurses should identify both actual and potential stressors, determine which stressors can be changed, devise courses of action to change them, and learn to control their personal responses to unavoidable work-related stressors.

PROCESS MODEL

The process model of stress is concerned with how a person chooses among alternative responses to stress with the overall goal of changing the stress situation and thus reducing the stress (McGrath, 1976). The process model describes a stress situation as a four-stage, closed-cycle set of processes. As shown in Fig. 5-2, the four stages are linked by four processes: cognitive appraisal, decision, performance, and outcome. In the first stage, the person encounters the stress situation. The individual's thought processes, previous experiences with similar stressors,

and coping mechanisms all affect what and how he thinks of the situation; the person thus perceives the situation as a stressor, or he does not. If he perceives stress, the second stage, he then decides how to respond to the stressor, the third stage. The person then acts in some way, the fourth stage, and finally assesses the situation again to determine whether it has changed and whether stress is reduced. If the level of stress remains high, the person moves through the process again and attempts new responses to the stress.

The process model of stress is useful in understanding stress situations within organizations, and it is helpful for nurses who are caring for clients with disabilities or chronic illnesses. Such clients must continually evaluate their levels of health and modify their daily activities in order to maintain optimal levels of wellness. The nurse can use the process model of stress to teach clients with chronic diseases and their families how to adapt to changes in functioning and life-style. Application of the process model in nursing situations requires active participation by clients' families and therefore is not effective in all cases. The individual needs of each client will determine which model of stress can be used effectively for stress management.

COMPARISON OF MODELS

Each of the four models of stress emphasizes a different aspect of stress. The psychosomatic model focuses on how emotional stress in one dimension usually has measurable physiological consequences in another dimension, such as when emotional stress results in a physical illness. The adaptation model emphasizes factors that influence how an individual adjusts to a stressor. If a person is able to change in response to the stressor, the stress response is minimized and the stressor does not lead to negative results. The social environment model focuses on the

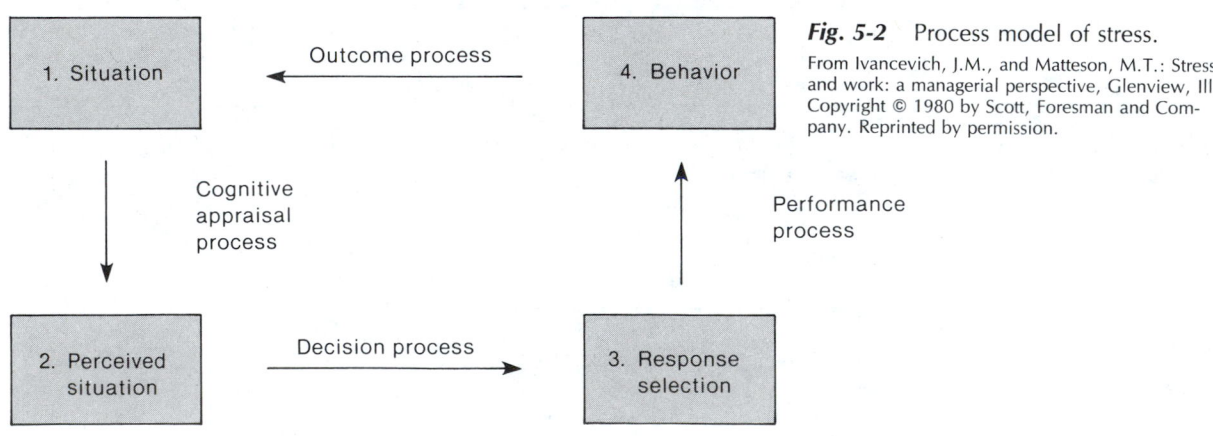

Fig. 5-2 Process model of stress.

From Ivancevich, J.M., and Matteson, M.T.: Stress and work: a managerial perspective, Glenview, Ill. Copyright © 1980 by Scott, Foresman and Company. Reprinted by permission.

relationship between a person's work role and his health. Last, the process model emphasizes a person's ability to solve a stress problem by changing the stress situation.

These theoretical models view stress in different ways, but all are concerned with *how* stress affects individuals. Because of their differences in emphasis, these models can be applied in different practice settings, according to which is most appropriate for the particular situation of the client and his ability to adapt to stress. Thus, as with other aspects of nursing care, the nurse's care plan is individualized for each client.

Despite differences in emphasis, all four models agree on the primary principle of stress management: since stressors themselves cannot always be controlled or minimized, a person experiencing stress must learn to change his response to the stressor. This concept is discussed in more detail later in this chapter, in the section on stress management.

Factors Influencing the Response to Stressors

A person's response to any stressor depends both on the characteristics of the person himself and on the nature of the stressor. Personal variables, such as personality and past experience with similar stressors, were discussed earlier. The nature of the stressor involves four factors, each influencing how a person responds:

1. Intensity of the stressor
2. Scope of the stressor
3. Duration of the stressor
4. Number and nature of other stressors present

A person may perceive the intensity or magnitude of a stressor as minimal, severe, or somewhere in between. For example, a parking ticket may be a low-intensity stressor, but an arrest for driving while intoxicated may be a high-intensity stressor. Obviously, the greater the magnitude of the stressor, the greater the stress response.

Likewise, the scope of a stressor can be described as limited, medium, or extensive (Sundeen et al., 1981). A laceration in the arm that requires sutures, for example, has a limited scope because, as long as the trauma is limited to the arm, the total body is not involved. If the potential for serious infection were present, however, the scope would be greater, and if the person used the arm in his work, the injury could have an even more extensive scope. Pregnancy is a stressor of extensive scope because it involves physiological, emotional, and social changes (Sundeen et al., 1981). The greater the scope of a stressor, the greater the stress response.

A stressor may be of short, medium, or extended duration. A person with a broken arm, for example, experiences short-term stress, whereas paralysis following a cerebrovascular accident is a long-term stress. The greater the duration, the greater the stress response.

The presence of several stressors at the same time means that a person needs more energy to adapt to any one of them than would ordinarily be required. For example, consider two women in their mid-thirties who are both in the middle of divorce proceedings.

Susan Clay has no children, has been married for 5 years, is successful in her career, and anticipates a smooth divorce. Mary Green has also been married for 5 years, but she has one child, she is just beginning her career, and she is having difficulty reaching a property settlement with her husband. Both women are experiencing the stress of divorce, but Mary Green must adapt to additional stressors: single parenting, a new career, and the conflict of property settlement. Six months later Susan Clay's divorce has been granted, but Mary Green's is still being negotiated. Susan is healthy and fulfilling her career goals. Mary, however, is experiencing unwanted physiological and psychological responses to the intense stress; she has been ill with minor viruses and feels that she is barely able to get through a working day, let alone establish or achieve any career or parenting goals.

Thus, the presence of a number of stressors at the same time reduces a person's adaptive capability.

Concepts of Adaptation

Thus far we have been discussing various aspects of stressors and stress. Adaptation is the process by which the body or the whole person changes in response to stress. Since many kinds of stressors cannot be avoided, the focus in health care is often on how a person, family, or community adapts to stress.

Adaptation to stress has many forms, just as stress has many forms. Homeostatic mechanisms, as described earlier, make possible a continuous physiological adaptation to the constant changes and stresses in the body's internal environment. A similar process of adaptation, however, may occur in all of a person's dimensions, as well as in those of a family, group, or community.

An adaptive response occurs when a stimulus from the internal or external environment causes a departure from the balanced state of the organism. Adaptation thus is an attempt to maintain optimal functioning. Included in adaptation are reflexes, automatic body mechanisms for protection, coping mechanisms, and instincts (Coelho, Hamburg, and Adams, 1974). A stressor that stimulates adaptation may be short term, such as a fever, a sudden change in environmental temperature, or a temporary change in one's job, or long term, such as paralysis of a limb, the addition of a new family member, or relocation to a new community. To function optimally, a person must be able to respond to such stressors and adapt to the required demands or changes. Adaptation is therefore not a simple or passive process, because it requires an active response from the whole person.

Like an individual, a family, a group, or a community may need to adapt to a stressor. Family adaptation is the process by which a family maintains a balance so that it can fulfill its purposes and tasks, deal with stress, and promote the growth of individual family members. For a family to adapt successfully, there must be (1) good communication skills, (2) mutual respect for all family members, (3) adequate resources available for adaptation, and (4) previous experience with stressors.

Many kinds of stressors affect a family, and the impact of any stressor is unique to each family. Examples of stressors encountered by families include a chronic or life-threatening illness of a family member, the loss of a job, divorce, return of the mother to work, the addition of a new family member, or relocation to a new community.

A family's adaptive behaviors generally require attitudes of cooperation, support, patience, and sharing. These attitudes encourage affection among family members and a strong sense of cohesion, which is important for the family's effective adaptation to stressors.

The adaptive response of a group is similar to that of a family. Most people belong to a group of some kind, whether it be an informal peer group, a formal professional organization, or anything in between. Groups vary according to purpose, size, and complexity. When a group encounters a stressor, the group as a whole must adapt, usually by some type of change in tasks or purpose. Such change is necessary to maintain an equilibrium within the group.

Common stressors encountered by groups include changes in organizational structure, the addition of new members, the departure of old members, changes in purpose or goals, and changes in location. Because each group reflects the personalities of its members, stressors have different effects on different groups.

A community is a network of social systems, political units, institutions, associations, organizations, agencies, and groups. A community has physical or geographical boundaries and includes various resources and facilities designed to help community members meet their needs. Some stressors encountered by communities include changes in financial re-

sources, new legislation, natural disasters, and political changes.

A person seeking nursing care is usually part of a family, one or more groups, and some type of community. Therefore a client's stressors may include stressors acting on these units, as well as his own individual stressors.

Dimensions of Adaptation

Any kind of stress can have effects in any of the human dimensions—physical, emotional, intellectual, social, and spiritual. Adaptive resources exist in each of these dimensions; therefore, when evaluating how a client is adapting to the stress of illness or any other type of stress, a nurse must consider the total person. Responses in dimensions other than the physical often influence how a person adapts to the stress of physical illness.

PHYSICAL-DEVELOPMENTAL DIMENSION

As noted in Chapter 4, a person must meet basic physiological needs in order to survive. Physiological adaptation is the process by which the body responds to a stressor in order to maintain functioning compatible with survival.

Physiological adaptive responses are stimulated by demands either in the internal environment, such as fever or inflammation, or in the external environment, such as changes in altitude or ambient temperature. A physiological response to stress may be limited to a particular body area, or it may involve the entire body. The sections on the local and general adaptation syndromes, later in this chapter, will discuss physiological adaptive responses in more detail.

Unit 5 describes the developmental stages of the human life span—neonate, infant, toddler, preschooler, school-age child, adolescent, young adult, middle-aged adult, and older adult. Each developmental stage poses particular tasks and thus involves particular potential stressors. A young adult, for example, may have to adapt to such stressors as establishing a career and rearing children. At the same time, each developmental stage is characterized by certain potential adaptive resources by means of which an individual can respond to stress. An older adult, for example, because of his greater past experience with certain kinds of stressors, may be better able to adapt to some stresses than a young adult. The chapters in Unit 5 discuss such developmental differences in detail.

EMOTIONAL DIMENSION

Adaptation in the emotional dimension involves the use of normal psychological coping mechanisms to resolve stress. Because every client has a different personality, every client copes with stress in a slightly different way, although certain basic forms of psychological adaptation are common. Adaptive behavior is most successful when it leads to a sense of discovery and creativity. A person may not always be happy and content in adapting to stress, but the goal of adaptation is to live constructively. Psychological adaptive behaviors are of two types: task-oriented behaviors and ego-defense mechanisms; the former are deliberate problem-solving methods, and the latter are unconscious protective processes. A later section in this chapter describes both in more detail.

INTELLECTUAL DIMENSION

A person's intellectual dimension includes not only his intellectual development and education, but also his perceptions of other people and the world in general, his problem-solving ability, and his communication patterns. Intellectual adaptive responses to stress include activities involving gathering information, solving problems, and communicating with others in order to adjust to a stressor. For example, a person with diagnosed diabetes mellitus may adjust to the stress of this diagnosis by learning more about the disease and its treatment.

Intellectual adaptation can be strongly influenced by a person's emotions. If a person is unable to adapt emotionally to the changes necessitated by an illness, for example, he may be less able to adapt intellectually by learning more about the illness. Similarly, helping a client to adapt emotionally can lead to more effective intellectual adaptation. Nurses are often in a unique position to assist clients in intellectual adaptation to stress.

SOCIAL DIMENSION

Everyone has social relationships with others, including spouse, family members, co-workers, and peers. This social network can be important in helping a person adapt to stresses of all kinds. The social group may provide psychological support and can help direct a person to resources available for coping with stress. For example, friends often can help a person adjust to the stress of a change such as the death of a loved one by encouraging the person to express his feelings. In addition, organized social groups, such as Alcoholics Anonymous, can help people adapt to specific stresses in the social dimension.

A client's social dimension is often closely interrelated with his other dimensions. A client who is unable to cope emotionally with stress may, for example, withdraw from contact with people who could potentially assist him in adapting to the stress.

SPIRITUAL DIMENSION

A person's spiritual dimension can include beliefs about a Supreme Being, a feeling of oneness with nature and the world as a whole, and a positive sense of life's meaning and purpose. These beliefs or attitudes can be a powerful resource for adapting to stress of any kind. Chapter 20 discusses ways in which nurses can help clients meet their spiritual needs and use their spiritual strength to cope with the effects of illness and other stressors.

Psychophysiological Response to Stress

The discussion of concepts of adaptation emphasized that the total person is involved in responding and adapting to stresses. Most research into stress responses, however, has focused on the psychological, or emotional, response and the physiological response, even though these dimensions overlap and interact with the other dimensions of a person's functioning.

When stress occurs, a person uses both emotional and physical energy to respond and adapt. The amount of energy required, as well as the effectiveness of the attempt to adapt, depends on the intensity, scope, and duration of the stressor and on the number of other stressors present. This adaptive response can be understood in terms of its physiological and psychological components.

Physiological Component

The two forms of physiological response to stress are the local adaptation syndrome (LAS) and the general adaptation syndrome (GAS). The LAS is a response of body tissue, an organ, or a part of the body to the stress of trauma, illness, or other physiological change. The GAS is a defense response of the whole body to stress.

LOCAL ADAPTATION SYNDROME

The human body produces many kinds of localized responses to stress. These include blood clotting, wound healing (see Chapter 48), accommodation of the eye to light (see Chapter 30), and response to pressure (see Chapter 31). Two localized responses, the reflex pain response and the inflammatory response, are described here as examples of the local adaptation syndrome. Nurses encounter these two responses in many health care settings.

All forms of the LAS share four characteristics. First, the response is localized; it does not involve entire body systems. Second, it is an adaptive response, meaning that a stressor is necessary to stimulate the response. Third, it is a short-term response; it does not persist indefinitely. Fourth, it is a restorative response, meaning that the LAS assists in restoring homeostasis to the body region or body part.

REFLEX PAIN RESPONSE. The reflex pain response is a localized response of the central nervous system to the stimulus of pain (see Chapter 37). Pain may be caused by extreme temperature, excessive pressure, or tissue damage. The reflex pain response is an adaptive response and serves to protect the tissue from further damage. The response involves five physiological components: (1) a sensory receptor, (2) a sensory nerve to the spinal cord, (3) a connector neuron within the spinal cord, (4) a motor nerve from the spinal cord, and (5) an effector muscle. For example, if a person accidentally places his hand on a hot radiator, he immediately jerks the hand away. Because this is a reflex response, the person does not need to think or consciously act to move his hand.

The reflex pain response serves to protect body tissue from further damage from whatever stimulus is causing the pain. Like other forms of the local adaptation syndrome, this response is directed toward restoring the normal state.

INFLAMMATORY RESPONSE. The inflammatory response is stimulated by trauma or infection. The purposes of the inflammatory response are to localize the inflammation, thus preventing the spread of the infection, and to promote wound healing. The inflammatory response may produce localized pain, swelling, heat, redness, and changes in functioning.

The inflammatory response is a process that occurs in three phases. The first phase involves changes in cells and the circulatory system. Initially vasoconstriction, or narrowing of blood vessels, occurs at the site of injury to control bleeding. Then histamine is released at the site of injury, which results in increased blood flow to the area and an increase in the number of white blood cells, or leukocytes, in the region to combat infection. As a result of this increased blood flow the site of injury appears red and becomes warm to the touch. Almost simultaneous with the release of histamine is the release of kinins, which increase capillary permeability to permit the flow of proteins, fluid, and leukocytes to the site of injury. This increased flow may lead to some swelling. At this point the localized blood flow decreases, keeping leukocytes in the area of injury to fight infection.

The second phase of the inflammatory response is characterized by the release of exudate from the wound. Exudate is a combination of fluid, cells, and other substances produced in the area of injury. The type and amount of exudate vary from injury to injury and from person to person. Exudate is usually released at the site of injury, which may be a cut, laceration, or surgical incision. With all such injuries the nurse continually assesses the wound to monitor healing as well as to identify any early signs of infection.

The last phase of the inflammatory response is the repair of tissue. Injured tissues are repaired by either regeneration or scar formation. Regeneration is the replacement of damaged cells by identical or similar cells. The cells of the skin are easily regenerated; for example, after sunburn new cells are produced to replace those that die and peel off. Tissues of the gastrointestinal and respiratory tracts, as well as skin, bone, and lymph nodes, usually regenerate easily. Musculature tissue, such as heart tissues; nervous system tissues, such as brain tissues; and highly elastic tissue, such as in the intestine, do not regenerate; in these tissues healing is accomplished by the formation of scar tissue, which replaces the original tissue but is not functional.

The inflammatory response alerts the nurse that the body is adapting to a local injury. During the adaptation the inflammatory response serves to protect the body from infection and to promote wound healing through the regeneration of new cells or the development of scar tissue.

GENERAL ADAPTATION SYNDROME

The general adaptation syndrome is a physiological response of the whole body to stress. The GAS involves several body systems, primarily the autonomic nervous system and the endocrine system; some textbooks, in fact, refer to the GAS as the "neuroendocrine response."

The GAS consists of three stages—the alarm reaction, the resistance stage, and the exhaustion stage (Fig. 5-3). The alarm reaction involves a number of physiological changes that prepare a person to adapt to a stressor. In the resistance stage the body stabilizes to allow the person to make an adaptive response. If this response fails to alleviate the stress, the person enters the exhaustion stage when he no longer has sufficient energy to attempt adaptation. Although everyone generally goes through the first two stages and possibly the third stage, the duration and effectiveness of each stage vary from individual to individual, depending on both the person and the nature of the stressor. A long-term critical illness, for example, is more likely to lead to exhaustion than a short-term, minor infection. A client with a high level of wellness is often more able to adapt to stress, including psychological stress, than a client who is not as healthy. The number and nature of other stressors also affect the duration and effectiveness of each stage.

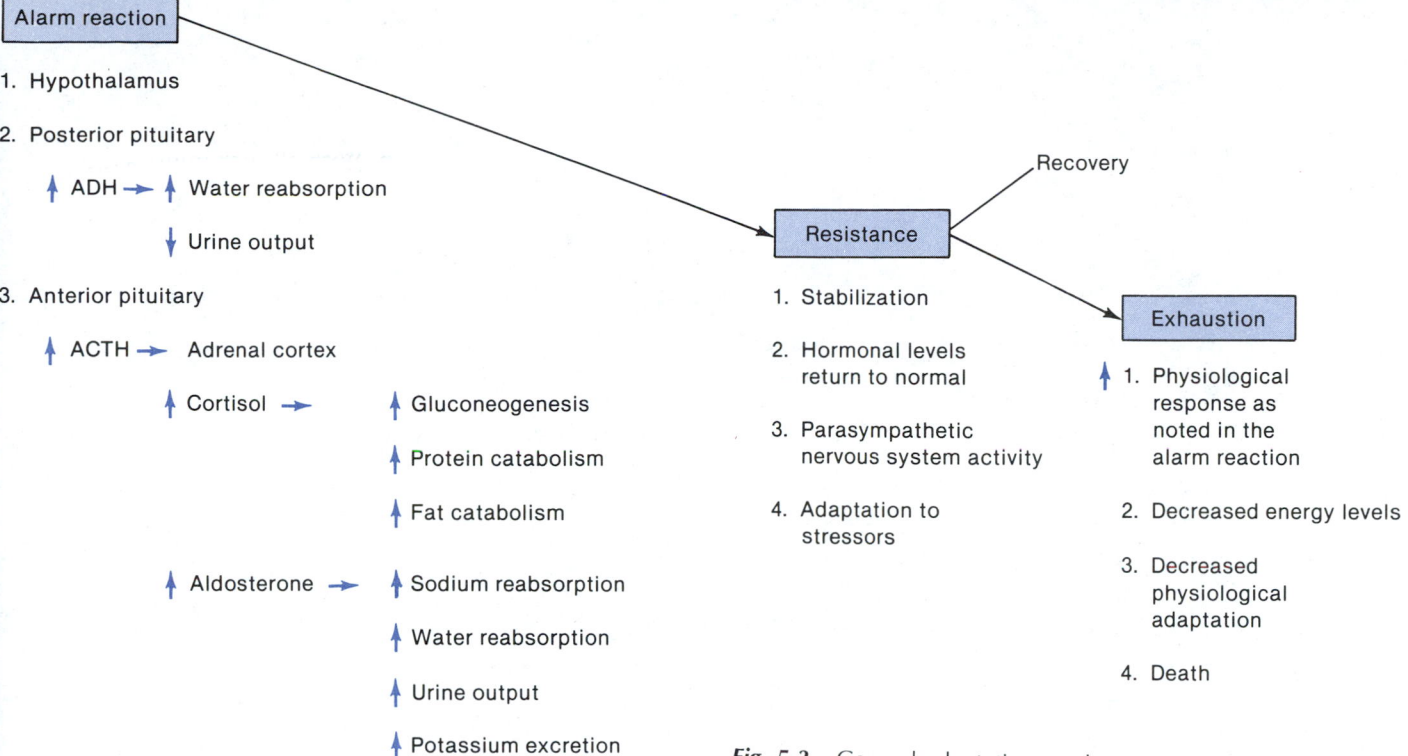

Alarm reaction

1. Hypothalamus

2. Posterior pituitary

    ↑ ADH → ↑ Water reabsorption

        ↓ Urine output

3. Anterior pituitary

    ↑ ACTH → Adrenal cortex

        ↑ Cortisol → ↑ Gluconeogenesis

                ↑ Protein catabolism

                ↑ Fat catabolism

        ↑ Aldosterone → ↑ Sodium reabsorption

                ↑ Water reabsorption

                ↑ Urine output

                ↑ Potassium excretion

4. Sympathetic nervous system and adrenal medulla

    ↑ Epinephrine → ↑ Heart rate

                ↑ O₂ intake

                ↑ Blood sugar

                ↑ Mental acuity

    ↑ Norepinephrine → ↑ Blood flow to skeletal muscle

                ↑ Arterial blood pressure

5. "Flight-or-fight"

Recovery

Resistance

1. Stabilization

2. Hormonal levels return to normal

3. Parasympathetic nervous system activity

4. Adaptation to stressors

Exhaustion

↑ 1. Physiological response as noted in the alarm reaction

2. Decreased energy levels

3. Decreased physiological adaptation

4. Death

Fig. 5-3 General adaptation syndrome.

ALARM REACTION. The alarm reaction is characterized by the mobilization of the various defense mechanisms of the body or mind to cope with the stressor. Hormone levels rise to increase blood volume and thereby prepare the person to act. Other hormones are released to increase blood sugar levels to make energy available for adaptation to the stressor. Increased levels of still other hormones—epinephrine and norepinephrine—result in increased heart rate, increased blood flow to muscles, increased oxygen intake, and greater mental alertness.

This extensive hormonal activity prepares the person for the "flight-or-fight" response, in which cardiac output is increased, oxygen intake is increased, respiratory rate is speeded up, the pupils of the eyes are dilated to produce a greater visual field, the heart rate is increased for more muscular and other energy, and other changes occur to prepare the person to act (Fig. 5-4). With increased mental energy and alertness that result, the person is prepared to choose either to flee or to fight the stressor.

During the alarm reaction the person is faced with a specific stressor. The physiological response is extensive, involving major systems of the body, and may last from a minute to many hours. If the stressor is extreme or remains for a long time, there may be a threat to the person's life. If the stressor is still present after the initial alarm reaction, the person progresses to the second phase of the general adaptation syndrome, resistance.

RESISTANCE STAGE. In the resistance stage the body stabilizes and hormone levels, heart rate, blood pressure, and cardiac output all return to normal. In this stage the person is attempting to adapt to the stressor. If the stress can be resolved, the body then repairs any damage that may have occurred. However, if the stressor remains present, as in continued blood loss, debilitating disease, or long-term severe mental illness, and the person is unable to adapt, he enters the third phase of the general adaptation syndrome, exhaustion.

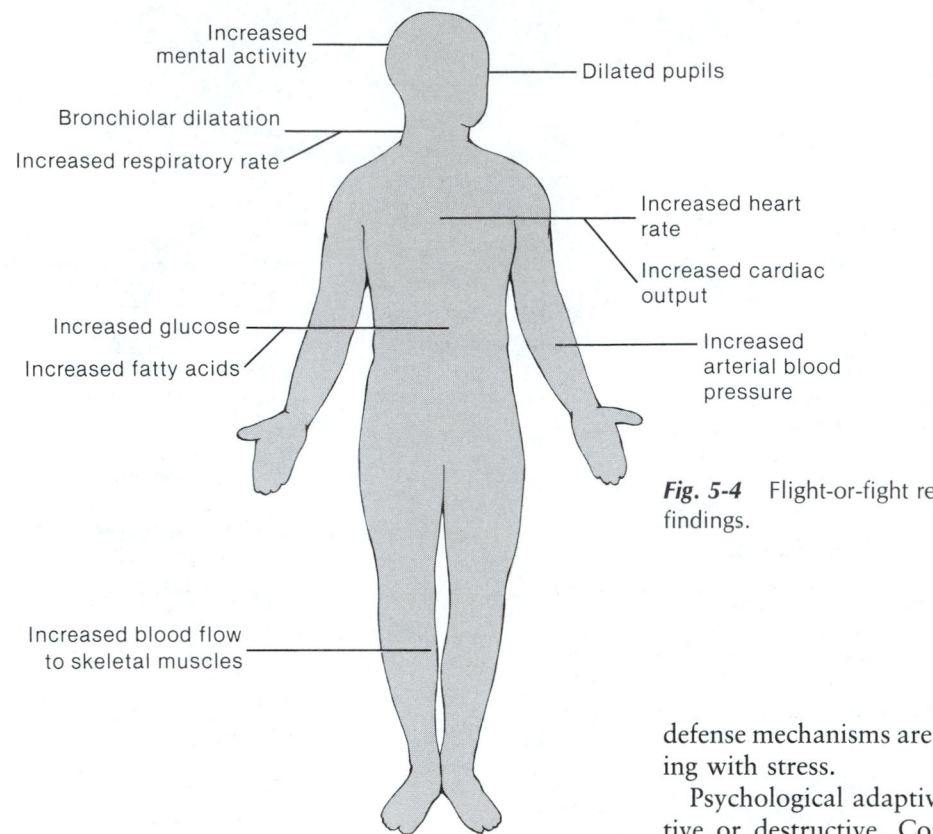

Increased
mental activity

Dilated pupils

Bronchiolar dilatation

Increased respiratory rate

Increased heart
rate

Increased cardiac
output

Increased glucose

Increased fatty acids

Increased
arterial blood
pressure

Increased blood flow
to skeletal muscles

Fig. 5-4 Flight-or-fight response—physical assessment findings.

EXHAUSTION STAGE. The exhaustion stage occurs when the body can no longer resist the stress, when the energy necessary to maintain adaptation is depleted. The physiological response is intensified, but the person's energy level is compromised and adaptation to the stressor diminishes. The body is unable to defend itself against the impact of the stressor, physiological regulation diminishes, and, if the stress continues, death may result.

Psychological Component

Exposure to a stressor results in psychological as well as physiological adaptive responses. Healthy individuals as they encounter life stressors develop psychological adaptative behaviors to cope with the stressors. These behaviors are acquired through learning and experience, as a person learns what behaviors are both acceptable and successful in dealing with the stressors. Psychological adaptive behaviors, also referred to as coping mechanisms, are thus efforts directed at stress management. Such mechanisms can be task oriented, involving the use of direct problem-solving techniques to cope with the threats themselves, or they can be ego-defense mechanisms, whose purpose is to regulate one's emotional distress and thus protect oneself from anxiety and stress. Ego-

defense mechanisms are thus indirect methods of coping with stress.

Psychological adaptive behaviors can be constructive or destructive. Constructive behaviors help an individual accept the challenge to resolve the conflict that is causing stress. Even anxiety can be a constructive behavior, when it signals that a threat is present so that a person can take measures to reduce the severity of the threat.

Destructive behaviors are those that do not help a person cope with a stressor. Destructive behaviors affect an individual's reality orientation, his problem-solving abilities, his personality, and, in severe circumstances, his ability to function. Anxiety can be destructive, for example, if a person is so overcome that he is unable to act to remove the stressor. Another example is abuse of alcohol or drugs, which may seem an adaptive behavior to an individual, when in reality it may increase rather than decrease the stress.

A healthy individual in normal circumstances is able to cope with everyday and moderate stresses by means of task-oriented behavior and ego-defense mechanisms. Illness, however, can diminish a person's capacity to cope with even relatively mild stress, and severe or prolonged stress can overcome the effectiveness of the adaptive behaviors of even a very healthy individual.

TASK-ORIENTED BEHAVIORS

Task-oriented behaviors involve a person's cognitive abilities in an attempt to reduce stress, solve problems, resolve conflicts, and gratify his needs (Stuart and Sundeen, 1983). The goal of task-oriented behaviors is to enable a person to cope realistically with the demands of a stressor. Three general types of task-oriented behavior are attack behavior, withdrawal behavior, and compromise.

ATTACK BEHAVIOR. Attack behavior, which can be either constructive or destructive, is action taken to remove or overcome a stressor or to satisfy a need. The following example of a stress situation illustrates the use of constructive attack behavior.

Cathy Johnson, a second-year nursing student, is assigned to care for Mrs. Paul, a 28-year-old mother of two young children who has a diagnosis of cancer. Cathy has successfully developed a plan of care to meet Mrs. Paul's physical needs. However, although Cathy knows that Mrs. Paul needs help in adjusting to her illness, the changes in her role and body image, and the threat to independent functioning, Cathy feels that she is unable to meet many of Mrs. Paul's emotional needs. Cathy therefore requests the help of her nursing instructor in planning further care, and the instructor works with Cathy in the planning process. In addition, Cathy's instructor helps her gain confidence in providing emotional support to patients with cancer.

In this case, Cathy has used a constructive method of coping with the stress of being unsure of how to provide emotional support. She might have used a destructive method, however, such as denying that Mrs. Paul had unmet emotional needs. This denial might have temporarily seemed to have reduced Cathy's stress, but the problem would have remained and the client's needs would not have been met.

WITHDRAWAL BEHAVIOR. Withdrawal behavior, another type of task-oriented reaction, can be physical or psychological. A person simply removes himself physically or emotionally from the stressor. A person who has been unable to resolve a long-term conflict with his employer, for example, may simply quit his job and thereby withdraw from the stressor. Physical withdrawal can be either a positive or a negative method of adapting to a stressor, depending on the total impact on the person. In the example just mentioned, it would be positive if it led to a new, less stressful job; it would be negative if it led to prolonged unemployment, increased stress within the family, and so on. A task-oriented behavior is generally positive if it is carefully considered and is realistic.

Psychological withdrawal, although not as obvious a reaction as physical withdrawal, is another means of dealing with a stressor. In the preceding example, the man might have chosen to remain in his present job but to alleviate the stress by interacting less with his employer, thus avoiding conflicts. Psychological withdrawal also can be positive or negative. If the employee's withdrawal were extreme, he might be passed over for promotions and thereby could experience more stress. But if the behavior were realistic and he withdrew only enough to avoid conflict, this could be an effective means of reducing the stress.

COMPROMISE BEHAVIOR. Compromise, a third type of task-oriented behavior, involves changing one's usual method of operating, substituting goals, or omitting the satisfaction of needs in order to meet other needs or avoid stress (Stuart and Sundeen, 1983). In most circumstances compromise is constructive, and it can be extremely useful when attack behavior or withdrawal behavior is not appropriate or has failed. However, if an individual is continually forced to compromise to deal with a stressor, compromise can have negative results such as increased anxiety or loss of self-esteem.

EGO-DEFENSE MECHANISMS

Ego-defense mechanisms, first described by Sigmund Freud, are unconscious behaviors that offer psychological protection from a stressful event. These mechanisms are used by everyone at one time or another, and they help protect a person against feelings of worthlessness and anxiety. Occasionally a defense mechanism can become distorted and no longer able to assist a person in adapting to a stressor.

There are many kinds of ego-defense mechanisms. The mechanisms described in this section are the ones that are commonly observed in a variety of people in a variety of health care settings. These mechanisms are frequently activated by short-term stressors and usually do not result in psychiatric disorders. This section is meant to serve as an orientation to these mechanisms, not as a guide to psychiatric nursing.

COMPENSATION. The mechanism of compensation allows a person to avoid unpleasant or painful emotions that result from a feeling of inferiority or inadequacy in some situations. The person makes up for a deficiency in one aspect of his self-image by strongly emphasizing a feature that he regards as an asset (Stuart and Sundeen, 1983). For example, a person who is having difficulty in a personal relationship may compensate for a feeling of inadequacy in this area by becoming increasingly involved in job activities, which produce a greater sense of satisfaction. Compensation usually occurs as a means of adapting to short-term, situational stressors.

CONVERSION. Conversion is an unconscious defense mechanism by which emotional conflicts that might ordinarily result in anxiety (especially extreme anxiety) are repressed and transformed into symptoms that have no organic basis, such as loss of sensation in an extremity, pain, or blindness. A conversion reaction, the only pathological defense mechanism included in this section, often follows a traumatic event. A nurse in an emergency room, critical care unit, hospital, or community health center may be the first health professional to recognize such a reaction.

Mrs. Brown is driving her car when she strikes and kills a 9-year-old child who runs into traffic from between parked vehicles. Mrs. Brown sustains a mild concussion in the accident and is unconscious for 30 minutes. After treatment in an emergency room and subsequent admission to the hospital, Mrs. Brown is informed of the child's death. After hearing about the child's death, Mrs. Brown complains of a headache and goes to sleep for an hour. When she awakes, she becomes hysterical and says she is blind. In addition, she has no memory of the accident or her subsequent admission to the hospital. Several diagnostic tests are performed to determine if the blindness has resulted from her concussion. The results of the tests are negative. No organic cause for her blindness is found, and it is determined that the condition is the result of a conversion reaction. Appropriate psychiatric treatment is then initiated.

A stressor that initiates a conversion reaction tends to be an extreme stressor—one with which a person cannot cope in any other way. Conversion reactions are rare and require the therapeutic and communication skills of specially trained professionals.

DENIAL. Denial is a defense mechanism by which a person avoids emotional conflicts and anxiety by refusing to consciously acknowledge thoughts, feelings, desires, impulses, or external factors that would cause intolerable emotional pain. Denial is a common defense mechanism and is used by everyone at one time or another. Denial can be a means of adapting to a short-term stressor; for example, a person might refuse to admit to himself that he is having difficulty performing a job task in an area in which he feels especially competent. Denial can also be activated by a major, long-term stressor, such as the discovery that one has cancer. Initially a client in such a situation might refuse to acknowledge the presence of the illness or the need for its treatment.

Denial can be protective because it can give a person the opportunity to begin to adjust to a stressor. When a person has been told that he is dying from an illness, he usually experiences a period of denial, and his loved ones often undergo a similar period. The denial phase of the dying and grieving processes is discussed in Chapter 46.

DISPLACEMENT. Displacement is an unconscious method of avoiding emotional conflict and anxiety by transferring emotions, ideas, or wishes from a stressful object or situation to a substitute that is less anxiety producing. Throughout the life span, most people experience this mechanism. A young child who has been spanked may release his anxiety by then spanking or striking a toy or doll. A teenager who has not been selected for a role in the school play may pick a fight with a brother or sister. An adult may follow a tense, frustrating day at the office with physical activity in the local gym.

Displacement can be an effective means of releasing frustration, stress, and anxiety. In some cases, however, displacement can be destructive; child or spouse abuse, for example, can be the result of an attempt to displace stress through physical or emotional violence to others.

IDENTIFICATION. Identification is a process in which a person patterns his personality on that of another person and assumes the other person's qualities, characteristics, and actions. A certain amount of identification normally occurs throughout life and in the learning process. Children and adolescents learn by example. As a child grows he learns from his parents to some extent and acquires their values, ethics, and interests. In addition, children identify with teachers, athletes, celebrities, and peers.

Identification can permit an individual to avoid or escape stress by basing his self-concept on the attitudes and behaviors of someone else. A teenager who feels inadequate in social interaction, for example, may overcome this feeling by identifying strongly with a popular musical star, or a student athlete may identify with a well-known professional athlete. Identification can be positive if it motivates a person in positive ways, but it can be negative if a person becomes unrealistic in coping with his own situation or if he adopts negative behaviors, such as drug use, of the person with whom he identifies.

REGRESSION. Regression is an unconscious mechanism by which a person copes with a stressor through actions and behaviors associated with an earlier developmental period. Persons in any age group can react to stressors by regressive behavior.

Regression is commonly seen, for example, in an older child who is confronted with a new infant sibling in the home. The older child may feel that he is receiving less attention or love from his parents, and to cope with this anxiety he may use regressive behavior such as speaking in baby talk or throwing temper tantrums. Regression generally occurs because a person is unconsciously motivated to try to reduce stress by methods that formerly were successful. The behavior is temporary and usually corrects itself—in this example, as soon as the older child no longer feels threatened by the new sibling.

Ill adults may also experience regression. Assume, for example, that a woman who manages a family, a home, and a career develops a long-term illness; after a time the family and members of the health team may notice that this independent person is beginning to assume a passive role and to avoid responsibility for decisions concerning her family or her health care. In this case the woman would be avoiding the stress of assuming responsibility while she is ill by regressing to the passive behavior of childhood, when her parents made the important decisions. This regressive behavior may be temporary; as she begins to feel well, she may resume her preillness independent roles.

Regression can be initiated by many stressors, such as the loss of a family member, loss of a job, job role anxiety, and relocation in a new community.

■ ■ ■ ■ ■

Like physiological adaptive responses, psychological adaptive responses can be effective in dealing with a stressor on a short-term basis. But as a person is continually exposed to a stressor or as the stressor becomes more severe, psychological adaptive mechanisms become less effective for stress management. Nonetheless, the person may use the same coping mechanisms even after they are no longer helpful in resolving the stress, because the coping behaviors may still permit the person to consciously ignore the stressor. In such cases, specific counseling techniques are used to help the person cope with the continuing stress and return to normal functioning.

Mind-Body Interaction

Health care professionals are becoming increasingly aware of the relationship between psychological stress and the onset, course, and outcome of medical illness. The link between psychological stress and disease is frequently called the mind-body interaction. Scientific research has increasingly shown that stress can affect illness and disease patterns (Pelletier, 1977). At the turn of the century, infectious diseases were the leading causes of death, but since then antibiotics, improved living conditions, increased knowledge of nutrition, and better sanitation methods have lowered the death rate from infection. Now the leading causes of death are diseases that are highly correlated with life-style stressors.

Mild stress situations do not usually produce long-lasting physiological damage, but moderate and severe stress situations can place a person at risk for medical illness. Mild stress situations are stressors that everyone encounters on a daily or weekly basis,

such as oversleeping, traffic jams, a flat tire, or criticism from a superior. Such situations usually last from a few minutes to a few hours. Such short-term, isolated stress situations are not likely to increase the risk of illness, unless a person experiences them on a continuous basis (Ivancevich and Matteson, 1980).

Moderate stress situations last longer, from several hours to a number of days. For example, an unresolved disagreement with a co-worker or family member, work overload, new job expectations, and the prolonged absence of a family member are moderate stress situations. These situations can be significant because they increase the risk of a physical illness in a person with a predisposition to that illness. The relationship between illness and moderate stress situations has been documented in cases of myocardial infarction in men who are predisposed to coronary disease (Ivancevich and Matteson, 1980).

Severe stress situations are chronic situations, which may last several weeks to several years, such as continual marital disagreements, prolonged financial difficulties, and long-term physical illness (Ivancevich and Matteson, 1980). The more intense and the longer the stress situation, the higher the risk for a negative health outcome.

Stress is manifested by the psychophysiological responses described earlier. A person's specific response to stress, however, is unique, because of the interaction of various factors in the person's different dimensions (Sutterly, 1979). How illness develops in cases of diseases related to stress can be understood in terms of the health-illness continuum (Fig. 5-5). As a person's stress increases, he engages increasingly in stress behaviors. Stress behaviors are changes from the person's normal behaviors that are made in an attempt to adapt to the stressor. Such changes may be consciously or unconsciously motivated. The following are some common stress behaviors:

1. Changes in eating patterns or appetite
2. Increase in the use of substances such as tobacco, alcohol, and drugs
3. Changes in activity patterns
4. Changes in sleep patterns
5. Inappropriate behavior, such as crying or laughing at unusual times, or a rapid speech pattern
6. Increase in the number of physical complaints
7. Increase in the frequency of illness

Understanding the mind-body interaction is crucial for predicting whether a person is at risk for developing a stress-related illness. Health professionals are becoming increasingly aware of the relationship between stress and illness, and a nurse is frequently in a position to consider the possible effects of a client of a stressful life-style or stressful events and to assess how well a client is able to adapt to a stressor.

Stage 1	Stage 2	Stage 3	Stage 4	Stage 5	Stage 6	Stage 7
Short stress situation (no risk)	Moderate stress situation (at risk)	Severe stress situation	Early clinical signs	Symptoms	Disease or disability	Death

Health.. Illness.. Death

Predictive and preventive medicine.............. .... Medical care...................................

Fig. 5-5 Stages of illness development in stress-related diseases.

Results of Prolonged Stress

The presence of stress is a fact of life. Everyone encounters stress because no one is isolated from stressors. How a person responds to stress can affect his overall level of health. Although short exposures to stress can be productive and can promote change, longer exposures can affect a person's health.

When stress is prolonged, a person's ability to adapt to it is diminished in each of the five dimensions. If the person is unable to adapt in one or more dimensions, he is at increased risk of having an accident or developing an illness. The point at which stress is sufficiently prolonged or intense to present this risk depends on the individual and on factors described earlier. The intensity, scope, and duration of the stressor and the number and nature of other stressors present all affect the person's capacity to adapt to stress. In addition, the person's general level of wellness influences his ability to cope with stress. When a person is ill, his ability to cope with prolonged stress is diminished because the illness is consuming energy that is necessary to adapt to the stress. Finally, a person's past experience in coping with stress helps determine how he is able to deal with current stress. People frequently have learned to cope with stress through past experiences with stressors.

Physical Results

Although the causes of specific diseases are multifaceted, three characteristics in general determine whether illness is likely to develop in a given person: the individual's susceptibility to the disease, the presence of the disease-producing agent, and the environment (Ivancevich and Matteson, 1980). The individual's susceptibility is linked to factors such as heredity, personality, life-style, health status, health beliefs, and health practices. Susceptibility is a more important factor in cases of diseases related to chronic stress than in cases of infectious disease.

The disease-producing agent is a major cause in many illnesses. With infectious diseases, variations in strength and other characteristics of bacteria and viruses help account for varying intensities of infectious diseases in different people. In cases of illnesses related to chronic stress, the intensity of a stressor and its duration are crucial variables in the onset, course, and recovery stages of the illnesses.

Several illnesses have been shown to be closely associated with high levels of stress. These illnesses include cardiovascular illness, gastrointestinal illness, and cancer.

A strong correlation has been shown between coronary artery disease and stress. Stress is linked to coronary artery disease because the primary pathological change in coronary artery disease is atherosclerosis. Atherosclerosis is characterized by the accumulation of yellowish plaques of cholesterol and cellular debris in the inner layers of the wall of large and medium-sized arteries. Blood flow through the affected vessels is decreased, and greater pressure is therefore required to propel the blood through the vessels. When a person with atherosclerosis experiences stress, his heart rate and blood pressure rise as a normal response. As the heart rate increases, the heart has a greater demand for oxygen, but because of the atherosclerosis, the blood flow to the heart is restricted. Thus the heart is unable to meet the need for more oxygen and the person is at risk for myocardial infarction. Other cardiovascular conditions that are associated with stress include angina pectoris, hypertension, and cerebrovascular accidents.

Gastrointestinal disorders associated with stress can occur in both the upper and lower gastrointestinal systems. It has been hypothesized that gastrointestinal disease is linked to stress because stress increases the secretion of adrenocorticotropic hormone (ACTH) and cortisol. Both of these hormones can cause gastric irritation and in some cases bleeding. If a person is in a high-stress state, the circulatory levels of ACTH and cortisol are elevated, thereby increasing the person's susceptibility to stress-induced gastrointestinal diseases such as duodenal ulcer, colitis, and irritable bowel syndrome.

The interaction between stress and cancer has not been as clearly defined; however, there is increasing evidence that stress is associated with cancer. Current studies are showing that such factors as smoking, poor nutrition, and depression increase a person's risk for cancer. Certainly the link between smoking and lung cancer has been well documented, and smoking is associated with stress. Smokers who encounter a stressor have a tendency to increase the number of cigarettes they smoke. The greater the stressor, the greater the number of cigarettes smoked and the greater the risk for lung cancer.

Recent studies of nutritional patterns have shown that high-fat, high-calorie, low-bulk diets are associated with colon cancer. Nutritional patterns are linked to stress; for some people stress behavior includes a change in eating habits, which frequently results in an increase in the consumption of high-calorie "junk" foods.

Finally, there is some evidence of a link between prolonged depression and the development of leukemia and lymphomas. At present, surveys have identified a potential association but have not documented the pathophysiological basis of a relationship between depression and leukemia or lymphoma.

The physiological impact of prolonged stress is becoming increasingly evident. Because nursing involves care of the client in all dimensions, nurses have an opportunity to use preventive measures to reduce the physiological impact of stress by helping clients change their responses to stressors. As health care consumers become increasingly knowledgeable about the causes of chronic illness, they will begin to expect nursing care to involve more health maintenance and health promotion.

Developmental Results

A person in any developmental stage can experience prolonged stress, and such stress can result in effects related to his particular stage. In any developmental stage a person normally faces certain characteristic tasks and engages in certain characteristic behaviors, and prolonged stress can interrupt or impede his passage through the stage. In extreme forms, prolonged stress can lead to a maturational crisis, which itself can generate stress.

An infant or young child generally encounters stressors within the home environment. For example, an infant must learn trust through his relationship with his parents; however, if parental figures are absent or fail to provide the infant with the security he needs to develop a sense of trust, this void can become a stressor for the infant. If the infant does not develop a sense of trust in this stage, in later life he may experience chronic distrust, resulting in withdrawal and limited interpersonal relationships. This situation can then lead to increased stress in other areas.

As the infant progresses into childhood, he normally develops a sense of autonomy. Gradually the child is given independence by his parents, and he attempts to meet some of his needs by himself and to exert some control over his parents. If parents or the environment prevent the child from developing autonomy, he may experience stress and may become overly dependent on others to meet his needs. In later life he may experience stresses related to feelings of inadequacy or low self-esteem.

A preschool child normally develops through exploring his surroundings, exploring differences between males and females, and developing a conscience based on being taught right from wrong. The child is ashamed when he is caught being "bad" and wants to be told when he is being "good." Prolonged stress, such as discomfort or decreased parental attention, can result in decreased initiative in the exploration of new skills, rigidity and guilt in interpersonal relationships, and a confused psychosexual role (Aguilera and Messick, 1982). These problems also can persist into later life.

A school-age child normally develops a sense of adequacy. He begins to realize that he can accumulate knowledge and master skills to accomplish his goals, and his self-esteem develops through friendships and sharing with peers. A common major stress in this developmental stage is a threat or potential threat to the support he receives from his family. Prolonged fear of being separated from his family, as may occur with illness, can result in feelings of inadequacy and inferiority.

An adolescent normally develops a strong sense of identity and at the same time has a need to be accepted by his peer group. Physical development includes changes in secondary sexual characteristics. There are many stressors in this age group, including conflicts involving sexual drive and expected standards of behavior. Prolonged conflict may result in indecision and confusion, rebelliousness, depression, or anxiety, which if not resolved can remain troublesome in later years.

A young adult is in transition from youthful experiences to adult responsibilities. The young adult must prepare for a career, for living on his own, and perhaps for forming a family. He may experience conflict between responsibilities to his work and his new family and his desire to maintain an active social life. Stressors in this developmental stage include conflicts between expectations and desires, such as the conflict between the expectation to marry and the desire to maintain open social relationships. Effects of being unable to cope with such stresses can include indecision and confusion in establishing goals, anxiety about relationships with others, and inability to form long-range commitments in the area of work or family.

Middle-aged adults are usually involved in family building, creating stable careers, and perhaps caring for their own elderly parents. Middle-aged adults are generally able to control their desires, and in some cases substitute the needs of spouses, children, or parents for their own needs. Stress can result, however, if they feel that too many responsibilities have been placed on them. Prolonged conflict can lead to making poor decisions, avoiding decisions, or becoming totally dependent on others.

An older adult is commonly faced with the task of adapting to changes in his family as children grow and leave the home, and perhaps to the death of a spouse. The older adult must also adjust to changes in physical appearance and physiological functioning. In addition, he experiences the stress of decreasing social interactions, as friends die or become unable to maintain contact. Prolonged fear and stress can make an older adult overly dependent, which may cause further stress on family or social relationships.

Older adults are more likely to have lower levels of wellness, and thus are at greater risk for developing stress-related illnesses.

Emotional Results

Prolonged stress results not only in physical illness but also in mental illness. Emotional changes are a direct and sometimes obvious result of prolonged stress. Frequently a nurse can observe the emotional impact of stress through changes in behavior.

When they are experiencing intense or prolonged stress, people tend to increase their use of substances such as alcohol, drugs, caffeine, and tobacco. Alcoholics account for about 6% of the U.S. population, and it is estimated that another 10% are problem drinkers; some 6 billion doses of prescription tranquilizers and 9 billion doses of amphetamines and barbiturates are consumed annually. This is strong evidence that in modern society many people are experiencing high levels of tension, anxiety, and stress (Ivancevich and Matteson, 1980).

Stress has many effects on a person's emotional well-being (see boxed material). Because everyone's personality involves a complex relationship between many factors, an individual's reaction to prolonged stress depends on his support systems, his prior experience with stressors, his coping mechanisms, and his overall stress response. A change in behavior should alert a nurse, family members, or friends that the person is experiencing stress to which he is no longer able to adapt, and that help is needed. Ideally, coping problems should be anticipated and preventive measures taken, but often it is difficult to anticipate a person's unique psychological reaction to stress.

Effects of Stress on Emotional Well-Being

- Anxiety
- Depression
- Burnout
- Increased use of chemical substances
- Changes in eating habits
- Changes in sleep and activity patterns
- Mental exhaustion
- Feelings of inadequacy
- Loss of self-esteem
- Increased irritability
- Loss of motivation

Intellectual Results

Prolonged stress can reduce a person's ability to acquire new knowledge and skills and can result in less effective communication and problem solving. Many stressors can affect a person intellectually, depending on the person's adaptive capacities.

Carol Messer and Janet King both recently were told that they have insulin-dependent diabetes mellitus and that they will have to learn to give themselves insulin injections. Both Carol and Janet cried when told of the diagnosis, and both expressed a "fear of needles." When the girls took diabetes education classes, however, Janet progressed through the program rapidly, and as her knowledge level increased her fear of needles and fear of diabetes decreased. Carol, however, was unable to learn to give herself injections because she was unable to remember how to administer the insulin. The prolonged stress of the illness and the injections resulted in her being unable to adapt; she was unable to acquire the knowledge and skills she needed to cope independently with her diabetes.

Social Results

Each person has a unique sociocultural role and set of social expectations and norms. Prolonged stress often results in changes in a person's "normal" roles, expectations, and practices. Changes in behavior in the social dimension can involve a person's family interaction, job performance, social activity, and community interaction. For example, a stressor such as a work conflict or a life crisis can cause a person to become withdrawn from family members in ways that sometimes then increase the stress, since social support systems are a means of coping with stress.

Spiritual Results

People use their spiritual resources to adapt to stress in many ways, but stress can also threaten a person in the spiritual dimension. Severe stress may result in a person becoming angry at the Supreme Being, or the person may view the stressor as punishment for a wrong action. Stressors such as acute illness or the death of a loved one may threaten a person's sense of the meaning of life and can lead to spiritual depression. In providing care to a client who is affected spiritually by stress, a nurse should not judge the appropriateness of religious feelings or practices but should assist the client in using his own spiritual resources to adapt to the stress.

■ ■ ■ ■ ■

Prolonged stress can affect a person in one or more dimensions. Stress not only can contribute to physical illness but can also lead to changes in a person's emotional behavior, social role, intellectual processes, and spiritual beliefs and practices. Nurses are in a unique position to help clients cope with stress, since nurses are able to spend a great deal of time with clients and their families or friends. Nurses also provide care for clients in various settings, the two most common of which are hospital and the home, and thus nurses are often able to observe how clients react to stress. The nurse notes a client's risks for developing a stress-related illness and provides care that includes stress management techniques. The following section focuses on the management of stress—not only for clients and their families but also for nurses themselves.

Management of Stress

Society's increased concern with health promotion and health maintenance has provided the nursing profession with an increased responsibility for the health care of clients. In addition to helping clients develop behaviors for better health, nurses also need to develop behaviors that promote their own high-level wellness (Claus and Bailey, 1980). Such behaviors for both the client and the nurse include techniques of stress management.

Stress Management for Clients

In normal circumstances a person adapts to stress effectively with his own coping methods. When stress is more severe or more prolonged than usual, however, a person may need a nurse's help in coping with the stress. To assist clients in this regard, nurses can use a number of stress management techniques, which are described in the following section. Most of these methods are long-term strategies for coping with stress. If there is an immediate need for reduction of stress, crisis intervention techniques may be required.

Long-term coping strategies can help a client relieve the stresses of everyday life or the prolonged stress of an illness or a major stressful event. Long-term coping strategies are applicable to clients with various levels of health and can also be used by their families.

Before a nurse uses any method of stress management, however, she assesses the client to understand how much stress is present and whether the client is adequately coping. There are various behavioral, physical, and emotional signs of potential or actual stress (see boxed material on p. 118). The number and types of these indicators present when a person is experiencing stress vary from client to client.

In general, stress management techniques involve the use of health-enhancing habits that can reduce the

Indicators of Stress in Clients

BEHAVIORAL INDICATORS

- Decreased productivity and quality-of-job performance
- Tendency to make mistakes—poor judgment
- Forgetfulness and blocking
- Diminished attention to detail
- Preoccupation—daydreaming or "spacing out"
- Inability to concentrate on tasks
- Reduced creativity
- Increased use of alcohol and/or drugs
- Increased smoking
- Increased absenteeism and illness
- Lethargy
- Loss of interest
- Accident proneness

PHYSICAL INDICATORS

- Elevated blood pressure
- Increased muscle tension (neck, shoulders, back)
- Elevated pulse and/or increased respiration
- "Sweaty" palms
- Cold hands and feet
- Slumped posture
- Tension headache
- Upset stomach
- Higher pitched voice
- Change in appetite
- Urinary frequency
- Restlessness—difficulty in falling asleep or frequent awakening

EMOTIONAL INDICATORS

- Emotional outbursts and crying
- Irritability
- Depression
- Withdrawal
- Hostile and assaultive behavior
- Tendency to blame others
- Anxiousness
- Feeling of worthlessness
- Suspiciousness

From Claus, K.E., and Bailey, J.T.: Living with stress and promoting well-being: a handbook for nurses, St. Louis, 1980, The C.V. Mosby Co.

---

impact of stress on a person's physical and mental health. These are often common-sense approaches that provide a sound basis for effective, low-stress living. General prerequisites for stress management include regular exercise, good nutrition and diet, adequate rest, a successful support system, and effective time management.

REGULAR EXERCISE

It has been clearly shown that a regular exercise program improves muscle tone and posture, controls weight, reduces tension, and promotes relaxation. In addition, exercise reduces the risk of cardiovascular disease and improves cardiopulmonary functioning.

Clients who have a history of a chronic illness, who are at risk for developing an illness, or who are over the age of 35 should begin a physical exercise program only after discussing the plan with a physician. In general, for a fitness program to have positive physical effects, a person should exercise at least three times a week for 30 to 40 minutes.

Anyone who follows an exercise program should use warm-up exercises prior to vigorous exercise such as jogging, aerobic dancing, or tennis. Warm-up exercises stimulate blood flow to the muscles and increase flexibility. The goal of warm-up exercises is to reduce the risk of damage to the musculoskeletal system during the exercise. Similarly, after vigorous exercise it is recommended that a person do a series of cool-down exercises rather than stop abruptly. For example, after jogging or aerobic dancing a person should walk around at a moderate pace, gradually slowing down and stopping. Cool-down exercises allow the cardiovascular, pulmonary, musculoskeletal, and metabolic systems to gradually return to their resting functional states.

Physical exercise programs have been shown to be effective in decreasing the severity of such stress-related conditions as hypertension, overweight, tension headaches, fatigue, mental exhaustion, irritability, and depression. Adults, particularly, need routine exercise plans; because adults frequently are occupied with rearing children, developing careers, and establishing homes, their life-styles are often sedentary.

NUTRITION AND DIET

Nutrition and exercise are closely related, because a person's diet provides his body with fuel for activity and because increased exercise improves circulation and the delivery of nutrients to body tissues.

Everyone is encouraged to maintain his weight according to standard ranges for sex, age, and body build. In addition to avoiding overeating or undereating, one should be aware of the nutritional quality of the foods one eats. Too much caffeine, salt, or sugar can upset the body's metabolic functioning, as can deficiencies in vitamins, minerals, and nutrients.

Poor dietary habits can exacerbate a stress response and make a person irritable, hyperactive, and anxious, thus impairing his ability to meet his personal, family, and job responsibilities. The nursing measures for helping clients meet their nutritional needs are detailed in Chapter 38. In general, dietary goals should be based on the following three objectives endorsed by the U.S. Senate Committee on Nutrition and Human Needs:

1. Reduce the consumption of salt, refined sugar, fat, and cholesterol.
2. Increase the consumption of fruit, vegetables, and whole grains.
3. Limit meat consumption, substituting poultry and fish.

REST

An established, habitual pattern of sufficient rest and sleep is also important to stress management. A person experiencing stress may need to be encouraged to allow enough time for rest and sleep. Rest and sleep not only refresh the body but also help a person to become mentally relaxed so that he is able to use problem-solving methods to deal with stressors and resolve conflicts. A client may need specific help in learning to relax in order to fall asleep.

SUPPORT SYSTEMS

The saying "No man is an island" is of particular importance for stress management. A support system of family, friends, and colleagues who will listen and offer advice and emotional support is very beneficial to a person who is experiencing stress. Support systems can reduce stress reactions and promote physical and mental well-being. Thus a person experiencing stress should be encouraged to expand his social and personal contacts.

Nurses can use various methods to help clients build their support systems. Nurses can use therapeutic communication skills to encourage clients to express their feelings and begin to identify causes of stress in their lives. When stress is the result of confusion or wrong information, a nurse can use teaching techniques to help relieve client's stress. If a client's stress results from disparities between expectations and realities, a nurse can use methods to help the client gain a stronger self-concept or body image. All these methods generally help clients indirectly to build stronger support systems. If a client's stress is the result of social isolation, nursing strategies are aimed directly at helping the person develop a new social network.

> ### Advanced Techniques of Stress Management
>
> - Biofeedback
> - Progressive muscular relaxation
> - Autogenic training
> - Transcendental meditation
> - Relaxation therapy
> - Stressor-directed interventions

TIME MANAGEMENT

A person who uses time efficiently generally experiences less stress related to social, family, and job activities. For some clients, time management techniques may include developing a list of tasks to be performed in order of priority. This technique can be very beneficial for a client who is unable to get anything done because there seems too much to do.

Another time management measure is learning to say "no" to potential disruptions in one's work and to some tasks requested of one. Time management may also include scheduling appointments realistically so that one is not always rushing from task to task, meeting to meeting, or errand to errand.

Controlling the demands of others is essential for effective time management. Few people are always able to meet all the requests made by others. It is important for a client, or a nurse, to learn to recognize which requests can be realistically met, which requests are impossible to meet, and which requests are negotiable.

■ ■ ■ ■ ■

The stress management techniques briefly described above are common-sense strategies to help clients deal with life stressors. There are other, more sophisticated techniques for stress reduction (see boxed material), which require advanced education and training and should not be implemented by inexperienced nurses.

CRISIS INTERVENTION

Crisis intervention is a therapeutic technique for helping a client resolve a particular, immediate stress problem. Crisis intervention does not involve an in-depth analysis of a client's situation but addresses the immediate, urgent need for stress reduction. The goal is to restore the person as quickly as possible to the precrisis level of functioning in all dimensions.

A crisis occurs when a person encounters a problem or stress situation that he is unable to cope with in

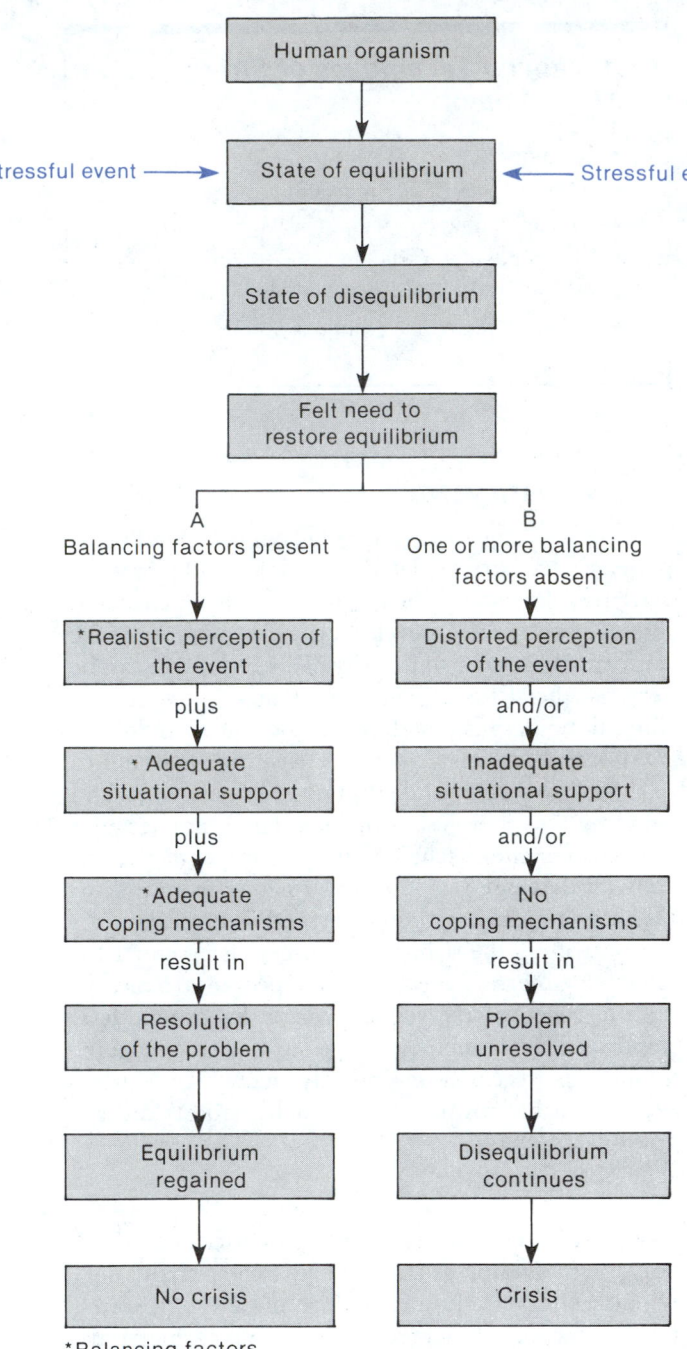

*Balancing factors

Fig. 5-6 Crisis intervention model.

From Aguilera, D.C., and Messick, J.M.: Crisis intervention: theory and methodology, ed. 4, St. Louis, 1982, The C.V. Mosby Co.

are transient, and the episode itself is brief. Situational crises include giving birth, major role changes, acute physical illness, physical assault or rape, family changes such as remarriage or the death of a family member, and unexpected unemployment.

Developmental crises occur when a person is unable to complete the developmental tasks of a psychosocial stage and is therefore unable to continue developing. A developmental crisis can occur at any point in life, if circumstances prevent a person from meeting the challenge of his particular stage. A child in need of developing a sense of trust may experience a crisis, for example, if his parents are emotionally cold or physically abuse him. A young adult may experience a developmental crisis if on graduation from high school or college he is unable to find a job and thus cannot plan for the future. An older adult may experience a situational crisis when a friend of the same age dies; a developmental crisis may also result, since the death may evoke the need for the person to continue his own personal development in spite of his age. A developmental crisis may thus originate in a situational crisis.

When a nurse assesses a client and determines that he is experiencing a crisis, the nurse plans and implements specific measures directed toward helping him resolve the crisis. Aguilera and Messick (1982) have developed an approach to crisis intervention that can be used for both types of crises (Fig. 5-6). This approach enables the nurse to understand how a stressful event has lead to a state of disequilibrium, or crisis. Resolution of the crisis depends on the person's perceiving the stressful event realistically, having adequate support, and using adequate coping mechanisms. If the client is lacking in one or more of these three areas, the nurse and the client plan specific methods to restore the client to equilibrium. If the crisis has arisen because the client's perception of the event is distorted, then the nurse uses techniques to help the client perceive the stressful event realistically. If the crisis has arisen because of a lack of situational support or coping mechanisms, then the nurse initiates measures to assist the client in these areas by maximizing the client's available coping mechanisms and developing additional supports. The nurse then evaluates the extent to which the client is able to resolve the crisis with these means.

any of his usual ways. His behavior tends to be disorganized, and he may make only abortive attempts at resolving the problem (Aguilera and Messick, 1982).

Both clients and nurses are at risk for experiencing two types of crises, situational and developmental. A situational crisis arises suddenly in response to an external event or conflict involving a specific circumstance. Symptoms associated with situational crises

This approach to crisis intervention is based on effective communication between the nurse and the client. The nurse listens to the client's concerns and helps him to develop new methods of coping with stressors. Crisis intervention techniques also involve teaching clients about resources and methods that can be effective in solving problems, so that the clients will be able to use them with subsequent stressors.

Stress Management for Nurses

Rapid changes in society, health care technology, and health care knowledge, as well as changes in the nursing profession, can all place stress on nurses. Job stress is "the condition in which some factor or combination of factors at work interact with the worker to disrupt his psychological or physiological balance" (Margolis and Kroes, 1974).

Most nurses experience stress within their work environments. Stressors can be related to rotation of shifts, severity of clients' illnesses, number of clients per nurse, interactions with other nurses and other health care workers, and institutional policies. A nurse's reaction to a job-related stressor depends on the nurse's individual personality, health status, previous experience with stress, and coping mechanisms.

Job stress is frequently associated with a condition called "burnout," which is characterized by emotional, physical, and spiritual exhaustion. In the work setting an individual experiencing burnout may withdraw from others, exhibit negative feelings toward others, have increased absences from work, and perform work tasks less effectively than he used to (Claus and Bailey, 1980).

Nurses are at risk for job stress as a result of three factors. First, new graduates generally have high expectations, which may not be accomplished in the work setting, leading to feelings of frustration. Second, nurses usually work in close interaction with others, specifically, clients and other health care professionals; such continuous interaction can lead to conflicts and other stresses. Finally, the work setting itself increases the risk for job stresses. Most nurses work in institutional settings that are frequently unable to meet all the individual needs of either clients or nurses.

Nurses can reduce these stresses by using all the stress management techniques that they use on behalf of clients. Those common-sense techniques improve the nurses' physical and mental well-being, enabling them to cope more successfully with stressors. In addition, nurses should identify specific stressors in their work environments and if possible eliminate or minimize them. Finally, nurses can use a problem-solving

---

Problem-Solving Process for Reducing Stress in the Work Environment

1. Define overall needs, purposes, and goals.
2. Define the problem.
3. Analyze capabilities, constraints, and interest groups.
4. Specify an approach to problem solving.
5. State behavioral objectives.
6. Generate alternative solutions.
7. Analyze alternatives.
8. Choose the best alternative.
9. Implement and control the action chosen.
10. Evaluate the effectiveness of the action.

Modified from Bailey, J.T., and Claus, K.E.: Decision making in nursing: tools for change, St. Louis, 1975, The C.V. Mosby Co.

---

process directed toward stress reduction and conflict resolution (see boxed material).

Summary

Stress is present to some degree in everyone's life. Each person reacts to stress differently, according to his perception of the stressor, his personality, his prior experience with stress, and his use of coping mechanisms. Various models of stress—and Selye's general adaptation syndrome, the most commonly used model—help the nurse understand the causes of stress and responses to stress.

Stress can be positive if it results in necessary changes in a person's life-style and work environment. However, prolonged stress can affect a person's level of health, resulting in physical or mental illness. Stress management techniques are directed toward changing how a person reacts to a stressor. Many of the techniques presented in this chapter are common-sense approaches to coping with stress and developing healthy personal habits.

A nurse, like anyone else, is exposed to stressors, but the practice of nursing exposes a person to additional stressors. Management of job stress requires an ability to solve problems and thus avoid job burnout.

Stress is a fact of life, but it need not control one's life. How a person responds to stress can be controlled and changed. Through the use of health promotion and health maintenance strategies, nurses can help clients to manage stress successfully.

KEY CONCEPTS

✓ Homeostasis is a state of relative constancy in the internal environment.

✓ Key homeostatic mechanisms are controlled by the medulla oblongata, the reticular formation, and the pituitary gland.

✓ Homeostatic mechanisms regulate vital functions, level of consciousness, fluid and electrolyte balance, and hormone secretion.

✓ Prolonged stress decreases the adaptive capacity of homeostatic mechanisms.

✓ Stress is a physiological or psychological tension that can affect a person in any or all of the human dimensions.

✓ Stressors are events, situations, or other stimuli that an individual may encounter in the internal or external environment.

✓ Stressors necessitate change or adaptation so that a state of equilibrium can be maintained.

✓ The various models of stress agree that when a person cannot cope with stress, it is usually the person's response to stress that requires changing, rather than the stressors.

✓ A person's response to stress is influenced by the intensity, duration, and scope of the stressor and by the number of stressors present at one time.

✓ Adaptation is the process through which a person changes in response to stress.

✓ A person adapts to stress by using resources in all his dimensions—physical and developmental, emotional, intellectual, social, and spiritual.

✓ Physiological adaptation is the body's attempt to maintain optimal functioning.

✓ The two forms of physiological response to stress are the local adaptation syndrome and the general adaptation syndrome.

✓ The local adaptation syndrome involves several specific responses to stress, including the reflex pain response and the inflammatory response.

✓ The general adaptation syndrome is a multisystem physiological response to stress.

✓ The three stages of the GAS are the alarm reaction, the resistance stage, and the exhaustion stage.

✓ The alarm reaction involves physiological changes that prepare the person for "flight or fight" behavior.

✓ The resistance stage provides the body with an opportunity to stabilize and return to normal, to continue adapting to the stressor.

✓ The exhaustion stage occurs if the body no longer has energy to continue attempting to adapt.

✓ Psychological responses to stress include task-oriented behaviors and ego-defense mechanisms.

✓ Task-oriented behaviors include attack behavior, withdrawal, and compromise.

✓ Ego-defense mechanisms are unconscious behaviors that offer a person psychological protection from stressful feelings or events.

✓ Stress has been shown to have an impact on the onset, course, and outcome of illness.

KEY CONCEPTS, cont'd

✓ Prolonged stress decreases a person's ability to adapt to the stress and affects the person in all five dimensions.

✓ People generally learn to use both short- and long-term strategies to cope with stress.

✓ Stress management techniques include health-enhancing habits, crisis intervention, and methods of reducing job stress.

✓ Crises are either situational and developmental in origin; both types can be resolved with crisis intervention techniques.

REFERENCES

Aguilera, D.C., and Messick, J.M.: Crisis intervention: theory and methodology, ed. 4, St. Louis, 1982, The C.V. Mosby Co.

Claus, K.E., and Bailey, J.T.: Living with stress and promoting well-being: a handbook for nurses, St. Louis, 1980, The C.V. Mosby Co.

Coelho, G., Hamburg, D., and Adams, J., editors: Coping and adaptation, New York, 1974, Basic Books, Inc., Publishers.

French, J.R.P., and Kahn, R.L.: A programmatic approach to studying the industrial environment and mental health, J. Soc. Issues 18:1, 1962.

Ivancevich, J.M., and Matteson, M.T.: Stress and work: a managerial perspective, Glenview, Ill., 1980, Scott, Foresman & Co.

Margolis, B., and Kroes, W.: Occupational stress and strain. In McLean, A., editor: Occupational stress, Springfield, Ill., 1974, Charles C Thomas, Publisher.

McGrath, J.E.: Stress and behavior in organizations. In Dannette, M.D., editor: Handbook of industrial and organizational psychology, Chicago, 1976, Rand McNally & Co..

Mechanic, D.: Students under stress, Glencoe, Ill., 1962, The Free Press.

Pelletier, K.: Mind as health, mind as slayer, New York, 1977, Dell Publishing Co., Inc.

Selye, H.: The stress of life, ed. 2, New York, 1976, McGraw-Hill Book Co.

Skeat, W.W.: A concise etymological dictionary of the English language, Oxford, 1958, Oxford University Press.

Stuart, G.W., and Sundeen, S.J.: Principles and practice of psychiatric nursing, ed. 2, St. Louis, 1983, The C.V. Mosby Co.

Sundeen, S.J., et al.: Nurse-client interaction: implementing the nursing process, ed. 2, St. Louis, 1981, The C.V. Mosby Co.

Sutterly, D.C.: Stress and health: a survey of self-regulation modalities, Top. Clin. Nurs. 1:1, 1979.

ADDITIONAL READINGS

Hurst, M.W., Jenkins, C.D., and Rose, R.M.: The relation of psychological stress to onset of medical illness. In Garfield, C.A., editor: Stress and survival: the emotional realities of life-threatening illness, St. Louis, 1979, The C.V. Mosby Co.

Gherman, E.M.: Stress and the bottom line, New York, 1981, American Medical Association Communication.

Randell, B., Tedrow, M.P., and Van Landingham, J.: Adaptation nursing: the Roy conceptual model applied, St. Louis, 1982, The C.V. Mosby Co.

Selye, H.: The general adaptation syndrome and the diseases of adaptation, Clin. Endocrinol. 6:117, 1946.

2

The five chapters in Unit 3 focus on concepts of professional nursing practice that are important in all health care areas. These concepts involve five aspects of the nurse-client relationship: values, ethics, communication, teaching and learning, and legal issues.

Values clarification helps the nurse and client understand their values and the effects of values on attitudes and health practices in order to work together to meet the client's health care goals more effectively. Because nurses are both responsible and accountable for their actions, they need to understand the profession's code of ethics and ethical issues that may arise in client care. Similarly, because nurses continually communicate with clients and other professionals, nurses use principles of communication to provide care most successfully. Client teaching is also an essential aspect of nursing, requiring the nurse to individualize methods for each client and apply basic teaching principles throughout the nursing process. Finally, because of the legal complexities of the health care system, nurses must be aware of the potential legal implications of their actions.

The Nursing Process

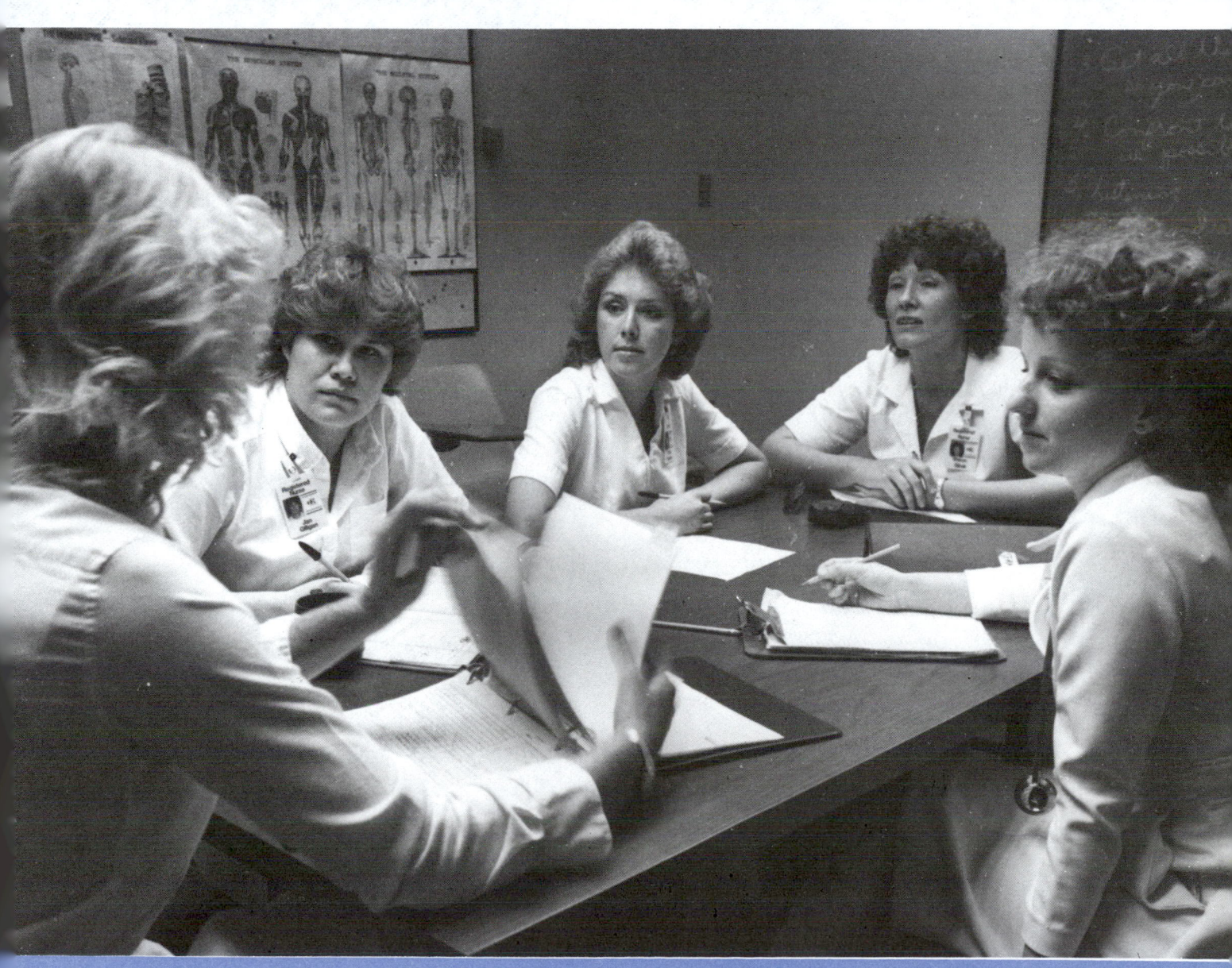

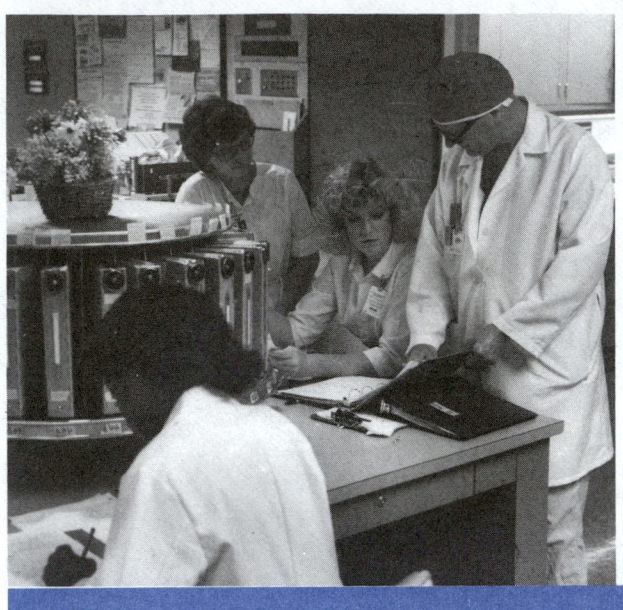

OBJECTIVES

Mastery of content in this chapter will enable the student to:

- Define the terms in the glossary.
- Describe the five components of the nursing process.
- Discuss the historical development of the nursing process.
- Describe systems theory, the problem-solving method, and the scientific method.
- Compare and contrast systems theory, the problem-solving method, and the scientific method with the nursing process.

GLOSSARY

analysis Interpretation and synthesis of collected data resulting in the identification of the client's health care problems, the selection of client goals and nursing care prescriptions, and the validation of the effect of nursing care.

assessment Gathering, verifying, and communicating data about a client so that a data base is established.

closed system System that does not interact with its environment.

data base Information obtained about a client's past or present level of health; information for the data base is derived during the assessment phase.

evaluation Determination of the extent to which the established client goals have been achieved.

feedback Process in which the output of a given system is returned to the system.

general systems theory Framework for dealing with complex problems and the changing relationships inherent within and among them.

goal Desired result of nursing actions, set realistically by the nurse and client as part of the planning stage of the nursing process.

health care need Condition or problem that results when a client is unable to meet his physiological, psychological, sociocultural, developmental, and spiritual needs within the context of daily living.

6 | Overview of the Nursing Process

hypothesis Unproven theory or proposition tentatively accepted to explain certain facts or to provide a basis for further investigation using the scientific method.

implementation Initiation and completion of the nursing actions necessary to help the client achieve health care goals.

input Information or material that enters a system.

intervention Action performed to prevent harm from occurring to a client or to improve the mental, emotional, physical, or social function of a client.

nursing care plan Written document based on the data obtained during assessment, the nursing diagnosis, and priorities and goals developed during the planning component.

nursing diagnosis Statement of the client's potential or actual health problem that the nurse is licensed and competent to treat.

nursing process Systematic method for organizing and delivering nursing care.

open system System that interacts with its environment.

outcome Condition of a client at the end of therapy, including the degree of wellness and the need for continuing care, medication, support, counseling, or education.

output End product of a system.

planning Designing of nursing strategies to achieve the goals for an individual client, based on the nursing diagnosis.

priority setting Process of setting an order of importance for meeting a client's health care needs.

problem Question proposed for solution or consideration.

problem solving Specific method or system used to obtain the solution to a problem.

process Specific method of achieving a goal, generally involving a number of steps or components.

scientific method Systematic procedure for gathering data, testing hypotheses, and solving problems.

system Unit made up of separate parts or elements; the parts rely on each other, are interrelated, have a common purpose, and together form a collective whole.

The nursing process provides the organizational structure and framework for nursing care, yet is creative and flexible enough to be used in various nursing settings. The nursing process has the three characteristics listed above. The purposes are to identify the client's health care needs, to establish a nursing care plan to meet those needs, and to complete the nursing interventions designed to meet the needs. A health care need is a problem that results when a client is unable to meet physiological, psychological, sociocultural, developmental, and spiritual needs within the context of daily living. For example, a client who cannot maintain proper nutrition because of poor teeth would have inadequate nutrition as a health care need. After identifying the client's health care needs, the nurse develops a nursing care plan, a written document based on the data obtained during assessment of the client, on the nursing diagnosis, and on the priorities and goals developed during the planning component.

The components of the nursing process—assessment, nursing diagnosis, planning, implementation, and evaluation—provide the organizational structure for achieving the purpose of the process (Fig. 6-1). Throughout the process the nurse collects and analyzes data to identify actual or potential health care needs. The nurse then develops and implements an individualized nursing care plan. The nurse evaluates the client's response to the plan, determining whether the health care needs have changed or remain the same. If they have changed, the nurse may modify the original plan of care.

Evaluation and modification bring creativity to the nursing process. In addition, the evaluation and modification of the existing care plan provide for the continual growth of the nursing process. With this pro-

The nursing process is a method for organizing and delivering nursing care. To understand the functions, components, and interactions of the nursing process, it is helpful to have working knowledge of the nature of a process. A process is a series of steps or components leading to achievement of a goal. The three general characteristics of a process are purpose, organization, and creativity (Bevis, 1978). The first characteristic, purpose, is the goal or specific aim of the process. The second characteristic, organization, is the series of steps or components needed to achieve the goal. The third characteristic, creativity, concerns the continual development of the process itself. Thus a process is a continuous progression from one point to another to achieve a specific goal.

TABLE 6-1

Evolution of the Five-Step Nursing Process Model

Hall (1955)	Johnson (1959)	Orlando (1961)	Wiedenbach (1963)	Knowles (1966)	WICHE (1967)
"Nursing is a process"	1. Assessment	1. Behavior of the client	1. Identify	1. Discover	1. Perception and communication
				2. Delve	
	2. Decision	2. Reaction to the nurse		3. Decide	2. Interpretation
	3. Action	3. Nursing action	2. Act	4. Do	3. Intervention
			3. Evaluate	5. Discriminate	4. Discrimination

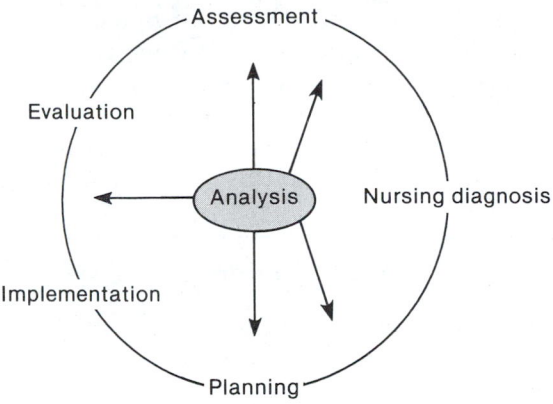

Fig. 6-1 Five-step nursing process model.

cess the nurse is able to meet the client's health care needs as they arise or change. The creativity of the nursing process is also demonstrated by its application in a wide variety of health care settings. For example, the nursing process is readily applicable for the neonate or the geriatric client, in critical care units or general medical-surgical units, and in inpatient or community-based settings.

Each step of the nursing process requires the nurse to analyze information about the client. Analysis is the interpretation and synthesis of the data resulting in the identification of the client's health care problems, the selection of the client goals and nursing care prescriptions, and the validation of the effect of the nursing care. The nurse analyzes assessment data to develop nursing diagnoses. The nursing diagnoses are analyzed to establish priorities, set goals, and select nursing interventions during the planning step. As the nurse implements the nursing care plan, she analyzes the client's response to nursing therapies, determines

their effectiveness, and incorporates new assessment data into the nursing process. Thus the new assessment data are analyzed and the care plan is modified as necessary.

Subsequent chapters in this unit discuss each of the five components of the nursing process in depth and elaborate on the purposes and objectives of each. The cognitive, affective, and psychomotor skills needed to use each component correctly are discussed. To facilitate application of the nursing process, these chapters fully describe the history, physical examination, and nursing care plan and discuss how to carry out each step of the process.

Historical Perspective

The nursing process has traditionally been defined as a systematic method for assessing the client's health status, diagnosing his health care needs, formulating a plan of care, initiating the plan, and evaluating the effectiveness of the plan. The use of the nursing process in providing individualized care requires the nurse to rely on scientific knowledge to make clinical nursing judgments and set priorities.

The term "nursing process" was first introduced by Lydia Hall in 1955. Although this term has been used in education and practice for 30 years, the definition of the process has evolved and been modified (Table 6-1). Hall described four types of relationships between nursing and the client: nursing at the client, to the client, for the client, and with the client (Hall, 1955).

During the late 1950s and early 1960s, Dorothy Johnson (1959), Ida Orlando (1961), and Ernestine Wiedenbach (1963) each introduced a three-step

Catholic University (1967) (Yura and Walsh [1983])	Little and Carnevali (1969)	Freeman (1970)	Gebbie and Lavin (1970)
1. Assessment	1. Health assessment and designation of the problem	1. Establishment of working relationship	1. Assessment
		2. Assessment	2. Nursing diagnosis
2. Planning	2. Goals	3. Development and negotiation of action goals	3. Planning
3. Intervention	3. Nursing action	4. Implementation of step-by-step actions	4. Intervention
4. Evaluation	4. Evaluation	5. Validation of action taken	5. Evaluation

nursing process model into nursing education and practice. In each of these models the nurse must first identify or assess client needs. However, these authors then diverge so that steps two and three of their nursing process models differ. Only Wiedenbach includes an evaluation component within her nursing process model.

In 1967, Lois Knowles presented a process model that she called the "five D's": discover, delve, decide, do, and discriminate. During the first two phases (discover and delve) the nurse collects data on the health status of the client. Next the nurse selects a plan of action (decide) and carries out the plan (do). During the last phase of the model (discriminate) the nurse establishes the health care priorities and assesses the client's reaction to the nursing actions (Knowles, 1967).

In 1967 the Western Interstate Commission of Higher Education (WICHE) and the Catholic University of America studied the nursing process. WICHE defined the nursing process as "the interrelationship between a patient and a nurse in a given setting; it incorporates the behaviors of patient and nurse and the resulting interaction." They listed the steps in the process as perception, communication, interpretation, intervention, and evaluation. The faculty at the Catholic University of America divided the nursing process into four phases: assessment, planning, intervention, and evaluation (Yura and Walsh, 1983).

In 1969 Dolores Little and Doris Carnevali used a four-step process in the development of written nursing care plans. In this model they combined health assessment and designation of the problem into the first step.

The nursing process is a model for delivering nursing care in a variety of settings. In 1981 Ruth Freeman and Janet Heinrich introduced a six-step nursing process to community health nursing. The first step of the process is the establishment of a working relationship. Second is the assessment of the situation as it relates to health and nursing care, as well as to the balance between health conditions and the reinforcing or counteracting forces that mediate them. The third and fourth steps are the development and negotiation of action goals with the client and the collaboration between nurse and client to decide possible courses of action. The fifth step is the implementation phase in which the step-by-step course of action is taken. The sixth and final step is validation of the effectiveness of the action taken. In this model the decisions and actions of multiple health care professionals are continually coordinated.

In 1973 Kristine Gebbie and Mary Ann Lavin at St. Louis University School of Nursing initiated national conferences on the classification of nursing diagnoses. In addition, at that time nursing educators and practicing nurses began to use the five-step nursing process model on a regular basis. Since 1973, conferences on the classification of nursing diagnoses have been held every 2 years.

Five-Step Nursing Process Model

The five-step nursing process model has the nursing diagnosis as a separate component. Like all nursing process models, the five-step process is continuous and changes as the client's needs change. The five components in the model require continual analysis of the client's status and incorporation of new data into the plan of care (Table 6-2).

Assessment

Assessment is the gathering, verification, and communication of data about a client to establish a data base. The data selected focus on the client's health status and actual or potential nursing care problems. The nurse gathers and verifies data in various ways, such as by obtaining a nursing health history, conducting a physical examination, and evaluating laboratory and diagnostic test results. The nurse can obtain data by observing the client and his family and asking them questions, checking past medical records, or consulting another health care professional. The nurse may also gather data during routine care. Once the assessment is completed, the nurse synthesizes and analyzes the collected data.

Nursing Diagnosis

The nursing diagnosis is a statement of the client's potential or actual health problems that the nurse is licensed and competent to treat. To develop a nursing diagnosis, the nurse uses a process that includes three major elements: analysis and interpretation of data gathered during assessment, identification of client problems, and formulation of a nursing diagnostic statement.

Nursing diagnoses are developed for an individual client, a family, or a community, taking into account the physical, developmental, intellectual, emotional, social, and spiritual dimensions of the client, family, or community.

Planning

Planning is designing nursing strategies to achieve the goals of care. During the planning phase the nurse and client determine the goals, establish priorities,

TABLE 6-2

Summary of Nursing Process

Component	Purpose	Steps
Assessment	To gather, verify, and communicate data about client so data base is established	1. Collecting nursing health history 2. Performing physical examination 3. Collecting laboratory data

Nursing diagnosis	To identify health care needs of client; to formulate nursing diagnoses	1. Interpreting data
		   a. Data validation
		   b. Data clustering
		2. Formulating nursing diagnoses

Planning	To identify client's goals; to determine priorities of care; to design nursing strategies to achieve goals of care; to determine outcome criteria	1. Identifying client goals 2. Selecting nursing actions 3. Delegating actions 4. Consulting 5. Writing nursing care plan
Implementation	To complete nursing actions necessary for accomplishing plan	1. Reassessing client 2. Reviewing and modifying existing care plan 3. Performing nursing actions
Evaluation	To determine extent to which goals of care have been achieved	1. Establishing evaluation criteria 2. Comparing client response to criteria 3. Analyzing reasons for results and conclusions 4. Modifying care plan

develop the nursing care plan, and project expected outcomes of the nursing interventions. The care plan involves the client and his family, anticipates the client's needs, provides for his comfort and maintenance of optimal functioning, and sets forth nursing measures. In addition, the nurse functions within the health care team to ensure that care is coordinated and that appropriate health resources are made available to the client.

Implementation

Implementation is putting the plan of care into action. Once the nursing care plan has been developed according to the client's needs and priorities, the nurse carries out specific nursing interventions to meet the needs of the client. The interventions can be of three general types: dependent, independent, or interdependent. A dependent intervention is based on the instruction or written orders of another professional, such as a medication order. An independent intervention involves aspects of professional nursing prac-

tice that are encompassed by licensure and do not require supervision from others, such as turning an immobilized client every 2 hours. Interdependent interventions are performed by the nurse in collaboration with another health care professional, in which the nurse uses judgment within the framework of a standard protocol. Implementation can take various forms. For example, the nurse may actually perform the care, the client or family member may be counseled and taught how to perform the activity, or the nurse may delegate the nursing care to another member of the health care team.

Evaluation

In evaluation, the final step of the nursing process, the nurse determines the extent to which the client's goals have been achieved. In addition, evaluation provides the nurse with information concerning the client's response to the intervention, allowing her to determine if the health care need is still present or if new needs have developed.

Theoretical Approaches

The focus of the nursing process is problem identification and resolution. Systems theory, problem solving, and the scientific method are theoretical approaches used to identify and resolve problems in nursing as well as other professions. These approaches are well defined, and most professional nurses are already familiar with them. The beginning student should learn to use systems theory, problem solving, and the scientific method to identify problems and solutions and should apply these theoretical approaches to the nursing process model.

Systems Theory

A system is made up of separate parts or elements. The parts rely on one another, are interrelated, have a common purpose, and together form a whole (Bailey and Claus, 1975). A system has a specific purpose or goal and uses a process to achieve that goal. The system's content is the product and information obtained from the system. For example, a farm is a system. A farm is composed of people, machinery to run the farm, the land itself, and so on. Each part or component of the farm is essential to the running of the farm. Also, each of these parts must interact with other components of the system. The purpose of the farm is to grow and sell crops. The process is the work of the people and the machinery. The content is the crops produced and the information obtained during the process, such as crop control, harvesting methods, and care of the livestock. When the farming system functions properly, sufficient crops are produced, harvested, and sold to maintain the system.

A system consists of several components: input, output, and feedback. Input is the information or materials that enter the system. On a farm the input includes the seeds to grow the crops, fertilizers, water, and so on. The output is the end product of a system. On a farm the output consists of the crops and profits. In addition to input and output, a system maintains a feedback mechanism. Feedback is the process through which the output of a given system is returned to that system (Fig. 6-2). On the farm seeds from the crop and profits are returned to the system

for the following year's crops, enabling the farm to maintain itself.

In addition to having input, output, and feedback, a system can be either open or closed. An open system interacts with its environment. There is an exchange of information between the system and the environment. Factors that change the environment also can have an impact on the system. In the farming example, if a change in the environment occurs, such as unusually heavy spring rains, the product (harvest) of the farm is affected. The heavy rains delay the planting and hinder the growth of the vegetables, and the end product is a poor harvest.

A closed system is one that does not interact with environment. An example of a closed system is a chemical reaction occurring under specific conditions.

Finally, a system continually builds up and breaks down as the elements within the system change and affect the input, output, or feedback of the system. Again using the farm as an example, the crops are planted in the spring and there is a buildup or growth of fruits and vegetables, but there is very little output from the farming system at this point. However, once the fruit and vegetables ripen, they are harvested and sold, thus increasing the output of the system. As the output of the farm increases, the system breaks down because the fruits and vegetables are no longer within the system, and the system begins to recycle as preparation for a new planting season begins.

Systems theory can be a framework for dealing with complex health problems and their changing relationships (Yura and Walsh, 1983). This theory can be used to examine the components of a system, by investigating input information, the process, and the output, and thereby to determine if the system is indeed fulfilling its purpose. When systems theory is applied to the farm, each component of the farm, such as the input and the output, is examined. The information obtained is measured against the purpose of the farming system, which is to grow and sell crops and maintain itself.

The nursing process demonstrates the three characteristics of a system: purpose, process, and content. The purpose is providing systematic, individualized, and appropriate nursing care to the client. The process is the five components: assessment, nursing di-

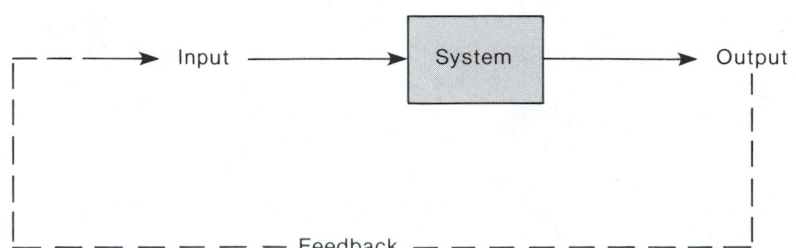

Fig. 6-2 Feedback control of a system.

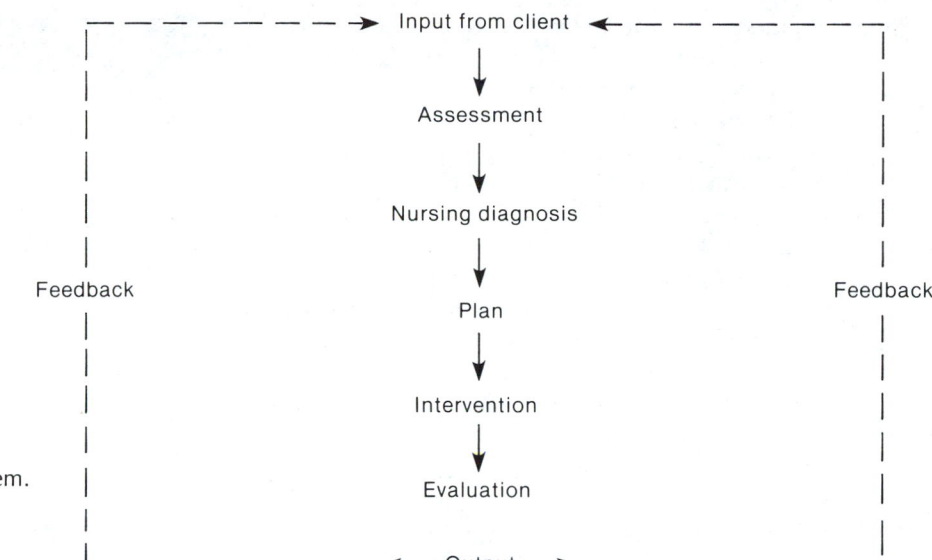

Fig. 6-3   Nursing process as a system.

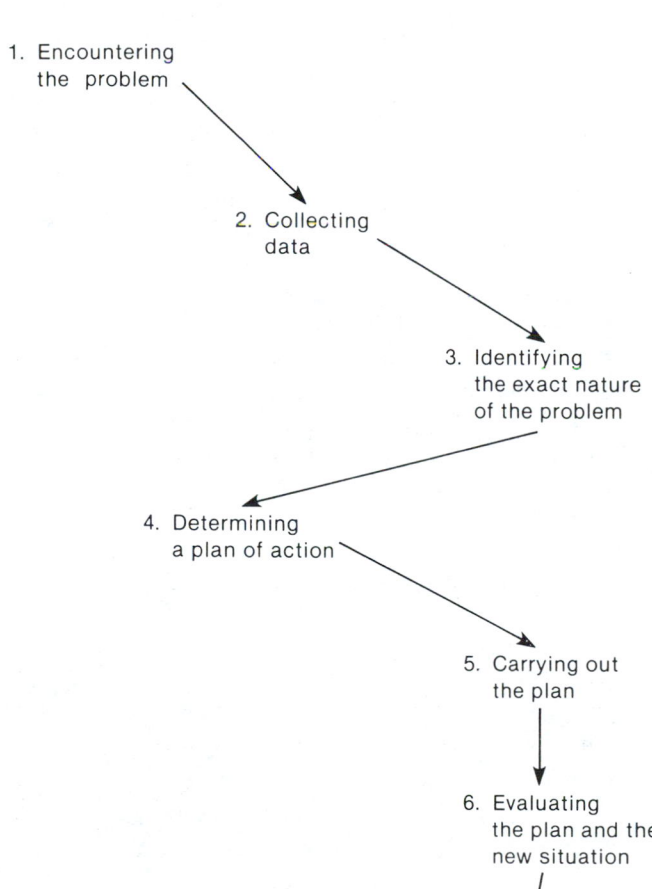

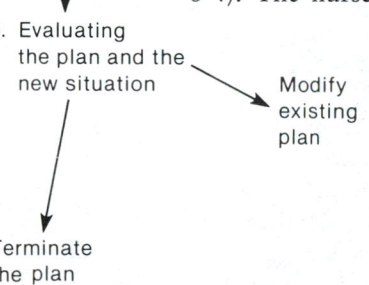

Fig. 6-4   Problem-solving method.

agnosis, planning, implementation, and evaluation. The content is the information obtained and used from each component. The nursing process is an open system because it interacts with its environment, continually changing as the client's nursing needs change. The input to the system comes from the client through assessment and from the nurse through interventions. The output, the evaluation component, is returned as feedback to the nursing process system, and reassessment occurs on the basis of the client's health care needs (Fig. 6-3).

Problem-Solving Method

Problem solving is the foundation for the nursing process. A problem is a question that is proposed for solution or consideration. In nursing a problem arises when clients are unable to meet their health care needs. Problem solving is a specific method for obtaining a solution. In nursing practice, problem solving is used to assist clients in meeting their health needs.

The problem-solving method used in clinical nursing practice is a six-step model that enables the nurse to make judgments and be accountable for them (Fig. 6-4). The nurse may encounter many problems in clinical practice. The problems may be client oriented, personnel oriented, or equipment oriented. The nurse should first be able to recognize that a problem exists and then move quickly to the second step.

In the second step the nurse collects data about the problem. For example, the nurse might obtain information on the frequency and duration of a client's symptoms, on personnel workload, or on a piece of equipment. Whatever the problem, the nurse must collect data on what is occurring, when it is occurring, and what is the deviation from the normal. In addition, the nurse needs to know the duration of the problem, what may cause it, and what makes it worse or better. As this data collection takes place, the nurse is able to draw some conclusions about the nature of the problem.

Identifying the exact nature of the problem is the crucial third step in the problem-solving method. Data must be grouped into similar categories and interpreted. Categorization and interpretation involve understanding relationships among the facts gathered and drawing a conclusion (Johnson, Davis, and Beletch, 1970). If the problem requires nursing action, a plan is developed.

The more specific the problem statement, the easier it will be to carry out the fourth step, developing a plan of action. The plan depends on the cause and urgency of the problem and the availability of resources, such as health care personnel and equipment. The nurse tailors the plan to the client's needs, the setting, and the limits of time and resources. In determining the plan of action, the nurse consults the client and family so that their needs and priorities are being considered.

Having decided on a plan of action, the nurse implements the plan in step five. After each step of the plan has been carried out, the evaluation process, step six, is begun.

The evaluation provides additional data about the problem and the new situation. Evaluation includes comparison of observable results such as a subsidence of symptoms, improvement in personnel morale, or proper functioning of equipment. Positive evaluations can lead the nurse to conclude that the plan was effective and thus can be terminated. Negative evaluations indicate that the problem was not solved and that the plan must be modified. In addition, the evaluation process can identify factors that resulted in the success or failure of the plan.

The nursing process shares several characteristics with the problem-solving method (Table 6-3). During the assessment component of the nursing process the nurse gathers and verifies data about actual or potential health care problems. With problem solving the nurse first identifies the problem and then collects

TABLE 6-3

Comparison of Steps in Problem Solving and the Nursing Process

Problem Solving	Nursing Process
Encountering the problem Collecting data	Assessment
Identifying the exact nature of the problem	Nursing diagnosis
Determining a plan of action	Planning
Carrying out the plan	Implementation
Evaluating the plan in the new situation	Evaluation

data about it. In both the nursing process and the problem-solving method, information from multiple sources, such as the patient, the family, other members of the health care team, and the medical record, is used to complete the data base.

After the collection of data, the nursing process includes an analysis component in which the interpretation and synthesis of data lead to the formulation of a nursing diagnosis. In the problem-solving method data are categorized and interpreted to define the exact nature of the problem. Both of these approaches result in the identification of nursing care problems that are individualized to the client.

The planning component of these two approaches is also similar. In both methods the plan involves designing strategies to meet the health care need. These strategies are individualized to the client's needs and resources, as well as to the resources of the health care agency.

The components of carrying out the plan (implementation) and evaluation are similar in both methods. After the specific actions devised in the plan are implemented, the nurse evaluates the extent to which the health problem has been alleviated. In both approaches the evaluation component provides the nurse with additional information concerning the client's response to the nursing action.

Scientific Method

The scientific method is a systematic procedure for solving problems that includes seven sequential steps (Fox, 1975) (Fig. 6-5). In some ways the nursing process is similar to the scientific method. Step one in the scientific method is the recognition of the problem. As with the problem-solving method, the prob-

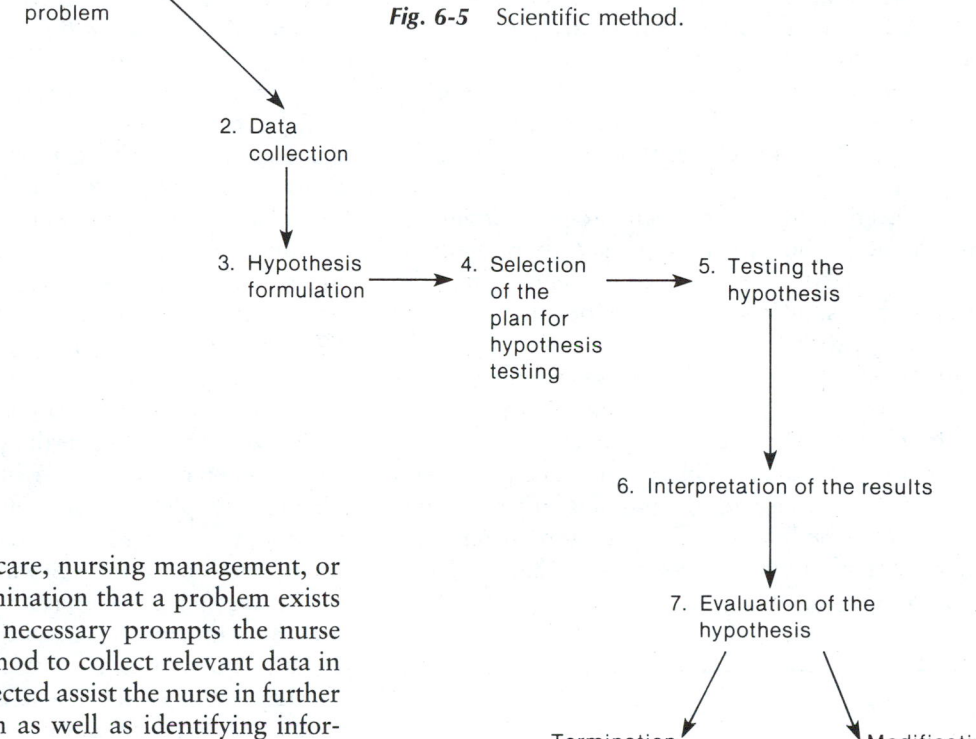

Fig. 6-5 Scientific method.

lem can exist in client care, nursing management, or technology. The determination that a problem exists and that a solution is necessary prompts the nurse using the scientific method to collect relevant data in step two. The data collected assist the nurse in further identifying the problem as well as identifying information that may later result in the success or failure of the plan.

The third step of the scientific method differs somewhat from the nursing process and the problem-solving method. Once the problem has been identified and data have been collected, the nurse formulates a hypothesis. A hypothesis is an unproven theory or proposition tentatively accepted to explain certain facts or to provide a basis for further investigation. In the clinical nursing setting the hypothesis serves several functions: (1) it determines the specific problem to be tested, (2) it provides an organizational framework for nursing care, and (3) it details objective criteria on which the evaluation is based. In terms of the first of these functions, the hypothesis is somewhat similar to the nursing diagnosis step in the nursing process.

Once the hypothesis is formulated, the nurse proceeds to step four, selection of the plan for testing the hypothesis. The nurse initially develops several plans and from these selects the one that seems to have the greatest probability of success. The nurse then tests the hypothesis by implementing the plan in step five.

In step six the results of the hypothesis testing are interpreted.

Frequently, these results are placed in categories. The nurse looks for significant trends, either positive or negative, in these results. In step seven the nurse evaluates the results to see if they support the hypothesis being tested. At this point the nurse deter-

mines if the hypothesis should be accepted or rejected. If the hypothesis is accepted and the results are evaluated as positive, the plan is terminated; if, on the other hand, the hypothesis is rejected, the plan is modified.

As it does with the problem-solving method, the nursing process shares some characteristics with the scientific method (Table 6-4). In the nursing process

TABLE 6-4

Comparison of Steps in the Scientific Method and the Nursing Process

Scientific Method	Nursing Process
Recognition of the problem Data collection	Assessment
Formulation of the hypothesis	Nursing diagnosis
Selection of the plan for testing the hypothesis	Planning
Testing of the hypothesis	Implementation
Interpretation of the results Evaluation of the hypothesis	Evaluation

the collection of data occurs in the first component, assessment. The scientific method requires that a problem be identified before relevant data are collected. The formulation of the hypothesis in the scientific method and the nursing diagnosis in the nursing process require the interpretation and synthesis of the collected data to specify a problem to be resolved.

The selection of a plan is similar in the scientific method and in the nursing process. In both methods a plan is selected to resolve the problem. Testing the hypothesis is similar to the implementation step of the nursing process.

Finally, in both methods the effectiveness of the plan is evaluated. The scientific method evaluates the validity of the hypothesis and the plan, and the nursing process evaluates the validity of the diagnosis and the client's response to the nursing interventions. With both methods the evaluation determines whether the plan was successful and what modifications are needed.

Summary

The five steps of the nursing process are assessment, nursing diagnosis, planning, implementation, and evaluation. The five-step nursing process model has the characteristics of a process: purpose, organization, and creativity. The nursing process identifies and meets the client's health care needs, the components comprise the organizational structure of the process, and the adaptability of the process to varying clinical settings, clients, and health care needs demonstrates the creativity of the process.

Since its introduction in 1955, the nursing process has evolved into the current five-step process. The five-step nursing process model fulfills specific objectives that are essential to nursing practice. It includes creating an individualized health data base, which includes all relevant data on the client's level of wellness. Actual or potential health problems are identified, and priorities of nursing action are established. Organized and individualized nursing care is planned, and innovative nursing care is implemented in accordance with established health problems and priorities. The five-step model of assessment, nursing diagnosis, planning, implementation, and evaluation provides for creative nursing actions, as well as being a method for communication of relevant client data.

The five-step model has advanced the professional growth of nursing. Through the nursing care plan the focus of nursing care is established because specific nursing responsibility has been defined. Nursing autonomy and accountability are enhanced through the identification of health care problems within the domain of nursing practice. By establishing a plan of care, nurses have become more accountable not only for their actions, but also for the client's response to the nursing interventions.

KEY CONCEPTS

✓ The nursing process is a method for organizing and delivering nursing care.

✓ The purpose of the nursing process is to identify the client's health care needs, establish a nursing care plan, and complete nursing interventions designed to meet the needs.

✓ The nursing process has evolved from a three-component to a five-component process.

✓ The organization of the nursing process is based on its five components: assessment, nursing diagnosis, planning, implementation, and evaluation.

✓ The role of creativity in the nursing process is in the continual evaluation and modification of the nursing care plan.

✓ The nursing process can be used in all health care settings and with all age groups.

✓ Nursing assessment is the gathering, verifying, and communicating of data about a client.

KEY CONCEPTS, cont'd

✓ Nursing diagnoses state the actual or potential problems in the client's health status.

✓ In planning, nursing strategies are developed to achieve the client's goal.

✓ Implementation puts the plan of nursing care into action.

✓ Evaluation determines the extent to which the client's health care goals have been achieved.

✓ The nursing process is an open system, continually changing as the client's nursing needs change.

✓ The nursing process closely parallels the problem-solving and scientific methods.

REFERENCES

Bailey, J.T., and Claus, K.E.: Decision making in nursing: tools for change, St. Louis, 1975, The C.V. Mosby Co.

Bevis, E.M.: Curriculum building in nursing: a process, St. Louis, 1978, The C.V. Mosby Co.

Fox, D.J.: Fundamentals of research in nursing, ed. 3, New York, 1975, Appleton-Century-Crofts.

Freeman, R.B., and Heinrich, J.: Community health nursing practice, ed. 2, Philadelphia, 1981, W.B. Saunders Co.

Gebbie, K., and Lavin, M.A.: Classification of nursing diagnosis, Am. J. Nurs. 75:250, 1974.

Hall, L.E.: Quality of nursing care, address given at the Department of Baccalaureate and Higher Degree Programs of the New Jersey League for Nursing, Public Health News, New Jersey State Department of Health, June 1955.

Johnson, D.: A philosophy of nursing, Nurs. Outlook 7:198, 1959.

Johnson, M.M., Davis, M.L.C., and Beletch, M.J.: Problem-solving in nursing practice, Dubuque, Ia., 1970, Wm. C. Brown Co.

Knowles, L.: Decision making in nursing: a necessity for doing, ANA Clinical Sessions, 1966, New York, 1967, Appleton-Century-Crofts.

Little, D.E., and Carnevali, D.L.: Nursing care planning, Philadelphia, 1969, J.B. Lippincott Co.

Orlando, I.: The dynamic nurse-patient relations, New York, 1961, Putnam.

Western Interstate Commission of Higher Education: Defining clinical content, Graduate Nursing Programs, Medical and Surgical Nursing, 1967.

Wiedenbach, E.: The helping art of nursing, Am. J. Nurs. 63:64, 1963.

Yura, H., and Walsh, M.: The nursing process: assessing, planning, implementing and evaluation, ed. 4, New York, 1983, Appleton-Century-Crofts.

ADDITIONAL READINGS

Carlson, J.H., Craft, C.A., and McGuire, A.D.: Nursing diagnosis, Philadelphia, 1982, W.B. Saunders Co.

Carnevali, D.L.: Nursing care planning, diagnosis and management, ed. 3, Philadelphia, 1983, J.B. Lippincott Co.

Carrieri, V.K., and Sitzman, J.: Components of the nursing process, Nurs. Clin. North Am. 6:115, 1971.

Marriner, A.: The nursing process: a scientific approach to nursing, ed. 3, St. Louis, 1983, The C.V. Mosby Co.

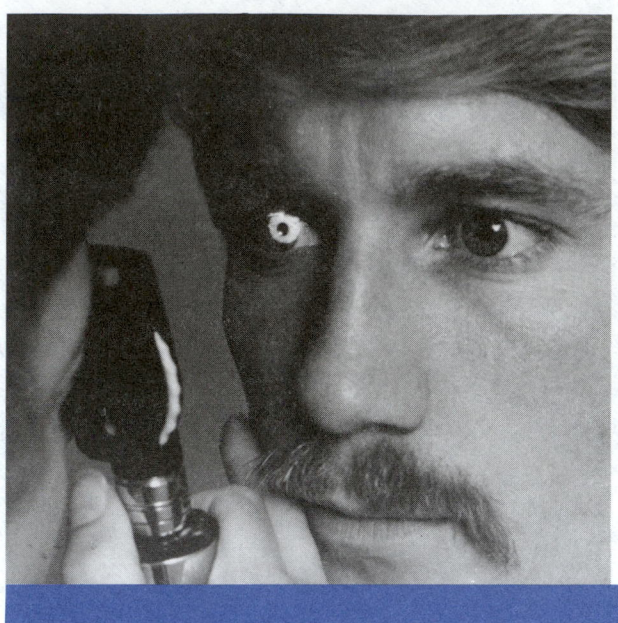

OBJECTIVES

Mastery of content in this chapter will enable the student to:

- Define the terms in the glossary.
- Describe the three components of the nursing assessment.
- Discuss the purposes of nursing assessment.
- Differentiate between objective and subjective data.
- State the sources of data for a nursing assessment.
- Describe interviewing techniques.
- State the purpose of a nursing history.
- State the purpose of a physical examination.
- Demonstrate the skills of physical examination.
- Conduct and record a nursing assessment.

GLOSSARY

auscultation   Method of listening for sounds within the body to evaluate the status of the cardiovascular, respiratory, or gastrointestinal system.

data source   Origin of information relevant to the client's level of wellness and health patterns.

direct-question interview   Type of inquiry that requires one- or two-word answers.

inspection   Assessment process during which the nurse observes the client.

interview   Type of communication with a client initiated for a specific purpose and focused on a specific content area.

norm   Measure of a phenomenon generally accepted as the ideal standard performance against which other measures of the phenomenon may be measured.

nurse-client relationship   Association between the nurse and the client that has as a mutual concern the well-being of the client.

nursing health history   Data collected about a client's present level of wellness, changes in life patterns, sociocultural role, and mental and emotional reactions to illness.

objective data   Data observed or measured by the data collector.

observation   Report of what is seen or noticed by the nurse about the client.

open-ended question interview   Inquiry aimed at obtaining a full client response and discussion between the client and the nurse.

palpation   Use of the hands and the sense of touch to gather data.

percussion   Tapping of various body organs and structures to produce vibration and sound.

physical examination   Scrutinization of all body parts through the use of inspection, palpation, percussion, and auscultation.

problem-seeking interview   Type of inquiry that focuses on gathering data to identify problems the client needs to resolve.

problem-solving interview   Type of inquiry that focuses on specific problems that have been identified by the client or nurse.

standard   Measure or guide that serves as a basis for comparison for evaluating similar phenomena or substances.

subjective data   Client's or significant other's perceptions, ideas, and sensations about a health problem.

7 | Assessment

The nursing assessment is the process of gathering, verifying, and communicating data about a client. The purpose of the assessment is to establish a data base about the client's level of wellness, health practices, past illnesses and related experiences, and health care goals. The information contained in the data base is the basis for an individualized plan of nursing care that is developed throughout the nursing process.

The collection of data involves the nursing health history, the physical examination, and the results of laboratory and diagnostic tests. The data gathered during the health history are obtained when the nurse interviews the client. To collect data from an interview, the nurse initiates the nurse-client relationship, uses various interview techniques, and progresses through three phases of an interview: orientation, working, and termination. The skills of inspection, palpation, percussion, and auscultation permit the nurse to collect data from the physical examination. Laboratory and diagnostic tests validate the findings of the history and examination and can lead to identification of other problems not previously noted.

Data Collection

Data collection during the assessment is an important aspect of the nursing process. Data should be descriptive, concise, and complete and should not include interpretative statements. Descriptive data originate in the client's perception of any symptom, the nurse's observations, or reports from other members of the health team. For example, a client may describe his pain as a "sharp, throbbing pain in the abdomen." The nurse's observation may be, "The client lies on his side holding his abdomen. Facial grimacing present throughout the assessment." The nurse records only what is observed and does not interpret the client's behavior such as by writing, "The client is in extreme pain." Concise data briefly describe the information obtained. The information is summarized in a short format using correct medical terms, for example, "Patient describes a constant sharp throbbing pain in the upper right quadrant of his abdomen. Pain began 48 hours before hospitalization, 2 hours following a high-fat meal. Pain was not relieved by antacids." A complete data collection results when the nurse has obtained all the information relevant to the actual or potential health problem. To confirm that complete data have been collected, the nurse might ask herself, "Do I have the information to answer the questions: when, where, and what are the duration and influencing factors?" For example, a nurse in an outpatient clinic might write the following on the assessment form of a client who is seeking treatment for recurrent headaches:

Mrs. Cooper is seeking treatment for recurrent headaches. She describes the headaches as occurring every morning after she arises from her bed. The pain is localized over the left front maxillary sinus and is described by Mrs. Cooper as "pulsating." She states, "The pain pulsates with my heartbeat." The headaches last anywhere from 1 hour to "all day." In the past the pain has been relieved with 10 grains of aspirin, but client states that during the past 10 days the aspirin has not been effective. Mrs. Cooper notices an increase in the intensity of the headache during cold, damp weather.

The collection of inaccurate, incomplete, or inappropriate data leads to incorrect identification of the client's health care needs. Inaccurate data result if the nurse fails to collect information that is relevant to a specific area or if the nurse is disorganized or unskilled in assessment techniques. Data are incomplete if the nurse neglects to obtain all information about a specific area, jumps to conclusions about a potential problem, or makes assumptions without validation. Inappropriate data are those not related to the area being assessed.

Types of Data

During the assessment the nurse obtains two types of data: objective and subjective. Objective data are observations or measurements by the data collector. Identifying the presence of a total body rash is an example of observed objective data. The measurement of objective data is based on an accepted standard, such as a thermometer or unit of measure. An elevated body temperature and measurement of a child's head circumference are examples of measured objective data.

Subjective data are the client's perceptions about his health problem. Only the client can provide this kind of necessary information. For example, the presence of pain is a subjective finding. Only the client perceiving the pain can provide information about the frequency, duration, location, and intensity of the pain. Subjective data usually include feelings of anxiety, physical discomfort, or mental stress. While only the patient can provide subjective data relevant to such feelings, the nurse must be aware that these problems can result in physiological changes, which are identified through objective data collection.

Ms. Johnson is taking care of Mr. Woods 1 day after an appendectomy. Ms. Johnson asks Mr. Woods about any pain or discomfort. He replies, "I have an occasional twinge in my right side, but I'm fine." Ms. Johnson observes that he is diaphoretic, he has tachycardia, and his blood pressure is elevated.

Mr. Woods' description of his pain is subjective, but the physiological changes of elevated blood pressure, tachycardia, and diaphoresis are the basis for objective data.

Sources of Data

A data source can be the client, the family or significant others, health team members, the health record, other records, and pertinent nursing and medical literature. Each source of data provides information regarding the client's level of wellness, risk factors, health practices, health goals, and patterns of illness, as well as additional information relevant to the client's health needs. The physical examination and diagnostic and laboratory tests are also sources of data and are described later in the chapter.

Client

In most situations the client is the best source of information. The client who is not disoriented and answers questions appropriately can provide the most accurate information regarding his health care needs, life-style patterns, and present and past illnesses. If a client is critically ill, disoriented, confused, mentally handicapped, or quite young, additional sources of data are necessary to complete an adequate nursing history.

Family or Significant Others

The family or significant others can be interviewed as primary sources of information about infants, children, the critically ill, and disoriented or unconscious clients. In cases of severe illness or emergency situations, the family or significant others may be the only available source of data about the client's health-illness patterns, current medications, allergies, onset of illness, and other information needed by nurses and physicians.

In addition to serving as a primary source of information, the family or significant others can supply additional relevant data about the client's health status. The family may also be able to indicate how the client reacts to changes in level of wellness and functioning. Finally, the family or significant others can make pertinent observations about the client's needs that can affect the delivery of care.

Health Team Member

Because assessment is an ongoing process, the nurse talks with other health team members, such as other nurses, physicians, physical therapists, clergy, social workers, and community health workers, to obtain additional information as to how the client interacts within the health care environment, how he reacts to information about diagnostic tests, and how he responds to visitors. Every member of the health team who interacts with a client is a potential source of information, and the health care team can identify and communicate data as well as verify information from other sources. The health team is comprised of physicians, nurses, allied health professionals, and nonprofessional employees employed in a health care setting (Chapter 3).

Medical Records

The present and past medical records of the client can verify information given by the client about past health patterns or provide new information for the nurse. By reviewing medical records the nurse can identify past patterns of illness and past methods of coping that the client may use again.

Other Records

In addition to the client's medical record, other records such as educational, military, and employment records may contain pertinent health care information. If the client received services at a community health center or day-care clinic, the nurse should obtain data from these records. To consult other records for health information the nurse must first obtain written permission from the client or guardian to see the record. Any information obtained is treated as confidential and as part of the client's legal medical record. The legal issues pertaining to the confidentiality of medical and personal records are detailed in Chapter 17.

Literature Review

Reviewing nursing and medical literature on the client's illness helps to complete the data base. The review increases the nurse's knowledge about the symptoms, treatment, and prognosis of specific illness. The knowledgeable nurse is able to obtain pertinent information for the assessment and for planning the client's care.

Methods of Data Collection

The nurse uses various methods of data collection to establish the data base: the interview, the nursing health history, the physical examination, and results of laboratory and diagnostic tests. Each method provides the nurse with the opportunity to collect complete information about a client's past and present level of wellness. Each method has specific purposes and requires certain cognitive, affective, or psychomotor skills.

Interview

The interview is a pattern of communication initiated for a specific purpose and focused on a specific content area. In nursing, the major purposes of the interview are to obtain a nursing health history, identify the client's health needs and risk factors, and determine specific changes in the client's level of wellness and pattern of living. The interviewer elicits information on the client's health state, life-style, support systems, patterns of illness, patterns of adaptation, strengths and limitations, and resources.

In conducting the interview the nurse uses specific communication skills to focus attention on the client's level of wellness and attends to the business of helping the client better understand the changes that are occurring or will occur in his pattern of living. The communication skills introduced in this chapter are broadly described within the context of conducting the interview. Chapter 15 discusses the total communication process and details the various communication techniques necessary for nursing practice.

The nursing interview achieves several objectives. First, the nurse-client relationship is initiated. A nurse-client relationship is the association between the nurse and the client that has a mutual concern, the client's well-being. The nurse-client relationship encourages the sharing of information, ideas, and emotions. This exchange of information between the client and nurse assists in obtaining an accurate and complete data base.

Second, the interview obtains information from the client concerning his physical, developmental, emotional, intellectual, social, and spiritual dimensions. Physical and developmental information reflects both normal functioning and the pathological changes induced by illness, trauma, or developmental stage as they affect the client's pattern of living. Emotional information includes the behavioral responses of the client to changes in health and pattern of living. Relevant emotional information includes the client's mood, perceptions, body image, self-concept, and attitudes about sexuality. Intellectual information includes intellectual performance, problem-solving ability, educational level, communication patterns, and attention span. Social information involves environmental, cultural, ethnic, or social patterns that can affect the client's present or future level of wellness. The nurse also collects information about the client's values, beliefs, and religious practices, which are part of the spiritual dimension.

Third, the interview provides the nurse with the opportunity to observe the client. The nurse is able to observe any interaction between the client and his family, as well as between the client and the health care environment, and the client's use of eye contact, nonverbal communication, and other body language. As the nurse observes the client's behavior, appearance, and interaction with the environment, she is able to determine whether the data obtained by observation are consistent with the data obtained by verbal communication. For example, if the client says he is not concerned about an upcoming diagnostic test but appears anxious and irritable, the data are conflicting. The observation provides additional data for the health history.

Fourth, the interview is a mechanism by which the client can obtain information. If a good nurse-client relationship has been established, the client will feel comfortable enough to ask the nurse questions about the health care environment, treatments, diagnostic testing, and available resources. The client needs such information to participate in establishing goals and planning care.

Finally, the interview is a first step toward establishing a therapeutic relationship between the nurse and the client so that necessary health interventions such as education or counseling of the client and family can occur.

To interview a client successfully and to achieve the purpose and objectives of the interview, the nurse needs skills in initiating the nurse-client relationship, using the various types of interviews, and moving from one phase of the interview to the next (Chapter 15).

INITIATING THE NURSE-CLIENT RELATIONSHIP

The role of interviewer is new in nursing. Perhaps the most difficult client interview for a nurse to conduct is her first interview. Likewise, for some clients being interviewed by a nurse is a new experience. Therefore, it is important that the nurse establish an effective nurse-client relationship before proceeding to the nursing health history.

The first step in initiating the relationship is for the nurse to introduce herself as the interviewer, stating her name, position, and the purpose of the interview.

Good afternoon, Mr. Carney. I am Miss West, the student nurse who will be taking care of you tomorrow. I would like to interview you for about 30 to 40 minutes to talk about your health and any questions you may have concerning your care. The reason for the interview is so that I can plan your nursing care. Do you have any questions at this time? May I take the time to talk with you now?

In this example the nurse introduced herself as the interviewer, gave an estimate of the time needed for the interview, and told Mr. Carney the reason for conducting the interview. Indicating the interview length is important because it clarifies for the client in advance how long the process will take and thus helps ensure his cooperation. Clients, even those in a hospital, should not be considered captive audiences, and the nurse should take steps to ensure that a client's time is not used inappropriately. Stating the length of the interview demonstrates to clients that their time will not be abused. In the example the nurse also gave Mr. Carney an opportunity to ask questions. It is important to determine if the client has any pressing questions before beginning the interview. By answering these questions the nurse immediately meets some of the client's needs, and the client may feel more comfortable about completely answering the nurse's questions. If the client is unsure how his hospital bed operates, for instance, he may be thinking about the bed instead of the interviewer's questions and therefore may not provide complete information for the data base. Finally, the nurse asked if it was all right to conduct the interview at that time, which demonstrated respect for the client by giving him a choice rather than seeming to demand his compliance.

The next step in initiating the nurse-client relationship is to communicate trust and confidentiality to the client. Illnesses that cause people to seek help are often accompanied by anxiety, helplessness, disruption of family relationships, and changes in self-image. Frequently clients are asked to provide very personal information about themselves and their families. Generally people share such information only with close friends, and there is a certain amount of trust that this information will not be shared with others. The nurse assures the client that the interview is confidential before asking him to share personal information concerning his past or present level of wellness or his family.

Finally, the nurse-client relationship is enhanced by the professionalism and competence conveyed by the nurse. The nurse's attitude of professionalism encourages a supportive therapeutic relationship with the client, so that the nurse and client can communicate freely, thereby allowing the nurse to identify health care needs and objectives. The nurse is involved with the client and family or significant others and becomes an advocate for the client. The nurse as a client advocate frequently intercedes for the client and encourages others to put the client's needs high on their list of priorities. The nurse demonstrates competence throughout the interview process and in the performance of nursing care.

TYPES OF INTERVIEW TECHNIQUES

The client's personality and health care needs and the health care setting all affect the interview process. An emergency situation may require one type of interview technique, while a chronic illness requires another technique. The interview in an emergency room usually centers on the present illness or trauma, precipitating factors, medications the client is taking, and allergies. In contrast, an interview with a client undergoing extensive rehabilitation may focus on past and present illnesses and coping strategies, family and community resources, the client's goals for rehabilitation, and the client's present limitations.

The nurse is able to use various types of interview techniques to elicit necessary information from the client or other data source. Four types of interview techniques are used in obtaining information from the client: problem seeking, problem solving, direct questioning, and open-ended questioning.

PROBLEM-SEEKING TECHNIQUE. The problem-seeking technique focuses on gathering data to identify problems that the client needs to resolve (Yarnall and Atwood, 1974). For example, the nurse may ask the client if there are changes in his digestion such as lack of appetite, nausea, vomiting, or diarrhea. If the client says that some of these symptoms are present, the nurse may proceed with problem-solving questions.

PROBLEM-SOLVING TECHNIQUE. The problem-solving interview technique focuses on gathering in-depth data on specific problems that have been identified by the client or nurse (Yarnall and Atwood, 1974). If, for example, the client says he has experienced nausea, the interviewer gathers information about the onset of the nausea, aggravating factors, associated symptoms, and relief measures the client has tried. Thus the nurse gathers data as to how the client solves some of his health problems, as well as data that will be used later in designing the nursing care plan.

DIRECT-QUESTION TECHNIQUE. The direct-question technique is a structured format that requires one- or two-word answers and is frequently used to clarify previous information or provide additional information (Enelow and Swisher, 1979). With the direct interview technique the questions do not encourage the client to volunteer more information than is directly requested. This type of questioning is useful in obtaining biographical data from the client, as well as specific information about health problems, such as symptoms, precipitating factors, and relief measures.

OPEN-ENDED QUESTION TECHNIQUE. The open-ended question is aimed at obtaining a response of more than one or two words. The open-ended technique leads to a discussion between the client and the nurse in which the client assumes the active role of describing his health status. The open-ended interview method strengthens the nurse-client relationship

because it demonstrates that the nurse wants to invest time in hearing the client's thoughts. Examples of open-ended questions are: What are your health care needs? How have you been feeling? What can you tell me about your problem?

PHASES OF THE INTERVIEW

The interview is carried out in three phases: orientation, working, and termination. Before interviewing the client, the nurse should prepare by reading the past medical record, obtaining information about the client's present illness, reviewing literature on the client's health problem, and creating an environment conducive to an interview. An interview with a hospitalized client should be scheduled for a time when interruptions by other health professionals or families will be minimal and the client will not be receiving visitors. An environment in which the client is comfortable and relaxed is also conducive to a good interview. For some clients their hospital room is appropriate, while other clients may wish to be interviewed in the solarium or lounge. Clients interviewed at home may prefer that the interview take place in a bedroom away from other family members. Finally, the nurse should select a place for the interview that is private enough to allow the client to be comfortable when providing the nurse with personal information.

ORIENTATION PHASE. Before beginning the interview the nurse reviews the purposes for the interview, the types of data to be obtained, and the methods most appropriate for conducting this interview. The review encourages the nurse to consider why the interview is being done, what specific data she needs from the client, and which interview techniques she will use to obtain those data. The interview helps establish the nurse-client relationship; therefore, as the nurse conducts the interview, she should be aware that the client is at this time forming an impression about nursing that may persist.

The nurse opens the interview by orienting the client to the purposes of the interview. The nurse also tells the client what types of questions she will ask and what the client's role in the interview process will be. Then the nurse spends 5 to 10 minutes becoming acquainted with the client.

Mr. Coffey is preparing an admission history on Mr. Rose, a 21-year-old hospitalized for the first time for removal of 18 plantar warts on the sole of his right foot.
Mr. Coffey: Good afternoon, Mr. Rose. I'm Bill Coffey and I'm your primary nurse for your hospital stay.
Mr. Rose: Hi, Bill. Please call me Jim. What is a primary nurse?
Mr. Coffey: Jim, "primary nurse" means that I'm totally

responsible for all your nursing care while you are hospitalized. Although other nurses will sometimes take care of you when I'm off, I'm the nurse who plans your care.

Mr. Rose: I guess that's a lot like being a coach. You may not play the game, but you're responsible for winning or losing.

Mr. Coffey: I suppose that's one way of looking at it. Sometime this afternoon I'd like to ask you some questions about your health; we call this a health interview. The interview is done so I can best plan your care, and any information you give me is confidential. The total interview process should take about 20 to 30 minutes. When could I interview you?

Mr. Rose: Could we do it now? My girl friend is coming to visit later this afternoon. We coach a Little League team in the evenings, so she'll have to be at the game tonight.

Mr. Coffey: That's fine. Since you're in a private room, is it OK if we stay here? (Mr. Rose nods yes.) Good, let me close the door. Before we start, do you have any questions about anything in your room?

Mr. Rose: Yes. Why is there an outlet for oxygen on the wall above my bed? Does that mean that I'm really sick— did they put me in a special room?

Mr. Coffey: No, that's not it. Every bed in this hospital has an oxygen outlet located on the wall above the head of the bed. The reason is that this hospital has a central oxygen delivery system, and when a patient needs oxygen we are able to supply it quickly, easily, and more safely.

Mr. Rose: OK. I wasn't worried actually, I was basically just curious. That was the only piece of equipment I couldn't explain.

Mr. Coffey: (pause) Jim, you mentioned that you and your girl friend are coaches for a Little League team. What's that like?

In this example Mr. Coffey introduced his role to the client. He reviewed the interview process, the objectives and confidentiality of the process, and the length of the process. The nurse and client agreed mutually on an interview time. Before beginning the interview, Mr. Coffey asked his client if he had any questions. Mr. Coffey's answer about the oxygen allowed the client to clarify his concern so that he would not be distracted during the interview. Mr. Coffey used the client's experience with coaching as a means of becoming acquainted before proceeding to the health interview. He chose coaching because the client had made two references to his coaching experience. Mr. Coffey asked an open-ended question about coaching to encourage Mr. Rose to talk.

WORKING PHASE. As the interview progresses, the nurse poses questions to the client that will form a data base from which the nursing care plan will be developed. The four techniques of interviewing are implemented as needed. In addition, the nurse uses 10 strategies to facilitate communication and ensure that both nurse and client clearly understand what the other is saying:

1. Silence
2. Attentive listening
3. Conveying acceptance
4. Planning related questions
5. Paraphrasing
6. Clarifying
7. Focusing
8. Stating observations
9. Offering information
10. Summarizing

Silence during the interview is helpful for making observations about the client, such as noting if he is in pain, anxious, or angry. Silence also provides the client with time to organize his thoughts and present complete information in response to the interviewer's questions.

Attentive listening means that the nurse is interested in the client's needs, concerns, and problems. The nurse acquires the skill of attentive listening through practical experience. Listening is essential in an interview; important data can be lost or ignored if the nurse is a poor listener. Listening can be facilitated through maintaining eye contact with the client, remaining relaxed, and using appropriate touch techniques.

Throughout the interview the nurse remains nonjudgmental about a client's life-style, values, and ethics. Acceptance by the nurse communicates a willingness to listen to the client's beliefs and values without conveying disapproval or disagreement.

The interviewer plans questions that are related to a specific topic or system and that use language understood by both nurse and client. The use of common language means that the nurse uses words and word patterns in the client's normal sociocultural context. The choice of language depends on the client's educational level, ethnic background, developmental level, and experiences. The interviewer uses medical terms only with caution. If a term is necessary to obtain data, the nurse clearly defines it for the client. For example, if a client refers to a tumor as a "lump," the nurse also refers to the tumor as a lump, asking questions such as, "When did you first notice the lump?" and "How does the lump affect your living patterns?" If the client does not understand the words and phrases in the question, inaccurate or incomplete data are likely to be obtained. The effective interviewer asks only one question at a time and plans the questions to follow a logical sequence. For example, if one purpose of the interview is to obtain information about a client's past illnesses, the interviewer should complete questioning on that topic before moving to another broad area.

Paraphrasing is the interviewer's formulation of what the client has said in words that are more specific. Paraphrasing provides an opportunity for the interviewer to validate information from the client, but the interviewer should be careful to avoid changing the client's meaning. For example, if a client said that the area of swelling was the size of a quarter and red, it would be appropriate for the nurse to draw a circle the size of a quarter to demonstrate an understanding of the information and confirm the size. However, it would be wrong for the nurse to say the swelling was as hard as a rock because this statement does not paraphrase the original statement but changes its meaning.

The nurse's techniques of clarifying also facilitates the correct communication of information. The nurse can clarify data by asking the client to restate the information or by providing an example. A client who is trying to describe back pain, for instance, may find it helpful if the interviewer asks whether the pain was throbbing or burning.

The technique of focusing helps to eliminate vagueness in communication, limits the area of discussion for the client, and helps the nurse direct attention to the pertinent aspects of a client's message. For example, if a client describes weakness in his left hand, the nurse follows this with questions that center on the problem: "Is the weakness always present? Does it occur at the same time every day? Does it occur following exercise? Is there any pain, numbing, or tingling associated with the weakness?"

The nurse states observations to provide the client

Do's and Don'ts in Interviewing

- DO be assured of a quiet private setting without distractions and interruptions.
- DO use the most reliable source of information—if not the patient, the closest family member.
- DO use prior knowledge of diagnoses (if known) to plan information you want to focus upon—to obtain facts you need.
- DO explain before starting that the purpose of so many questions is to provide better nursing care by knowing more about the patient and family.
- DO write brief notations during your interview. Record dates, times, durations of hospitalizations and onsets of illness, etc. accurately.
  DON'T rely on memory.
  DON'T try to write finished sentences.
- DO be calm, unhurried, and sympathetic. Show genuine interest and concern. (Sensitivity encourages the patient to express his feelings.)
  DON'T show annoyance or exasperation when the patient hits a memory block. If you react with understanding, he may recall the information later, in a related question.
- DO use eye contact—appropriately. Observe facial expressions and "body language" while doing so.
  DON'T stare at the patient or your outline.
- DO use neutral, open-ended questions to elicit the verbalization of feelings and additional information. Use leading questions sparingly and judiciously—only to focus in on hazy comments.
  DO use the patient's pertinent words to add to clarification. "By 'knife-like' pain, you mean sudden and intense?"
- DO use the terminology the patient understands. If not sure of his understanding, ask what it means to him; or ask him to describe what the word means to him. "Explain the 'nauseated feeling' you have."
- DO ask about the patient's complaints first, to have him feel purpose and expediency in your interviewing.
  DON'T start with delicate, personal questions too soon.
- DO allow the patient to finish his sentence, even if he's rambling. Then direct questioning.
  DON'T continually jump between unrelated topics.
  DON'T repeat questions unnecessarily. If a repeat question is necessary, reword the question for better comprehension.
- DO accept what the patient says. A simple nod, um-hm, or glance will encourage him to go on.
- DO call the patient by name. Express friendliness, pleasure, and concern.
  DON'T lose professional perspective or mannerisms.
- DO speak clearly, slowly and distinctly.
- DO listen.

with feedback as to how the message is received. For example, if the client becomes teary eyed and is unable to continue speaking when describing a past hospitalization, the nurse says, "You appear very upset about the events of your last hospitalization." This feedback may encourage the client to provide more information that may be relevant to nursing care.

The interviewer can also convey information, such as health education, to the client while conducting the interview. This process is pertinent throughout the nurse-client interaction.

The nurse's summary condenses the data into an organized review. The summary has two purposes. First, it is another means of validating data because the client has the opportunity to confirm that the data are correct. Second, it indicates an end to a particular part of the interview or the interview itself. The summary method is useful for clients who have difficulty staying with one topic or clients who try to control the interview.

The success or failure of the interview depends on how the interviewer conducts the process. The boxed material on p. 145 gives some specific tips about what to do and not to do during an interview.

TERMINATION PHASE. As in the other phases of the interview, termination requires skill on the part of the interviewer. Ideally the client should be given a clue that the interview is coming to an end. For example, the nurse may say, "There are just two more questions," or "We'll be finished in 5 to 6 minutes." With this method the client can maintain directed attention without being distracted by wondering how much longer the interview will last. Also, he has an opportunity to raise any final questions before the interview ends.

The nurse should be as organized during this phase as in opening the interview. The interview is terminated in a friendly manner with the nurse indicating specifically when there will be additional contact. For example, an appropriate way to end an interview would be, "Thank you for answering these questions. They will be helpful in planning your nursing care. Another nurse will be caring for you this evening, but I'll be back on duty tomorrow morning. Do you have any other questions? Is there anything I can do for you now?"

The nurse's interviewing skills and techniques are essential in the development of a data base. The skillful interviewer is able to adapt interview strategies to various clients and health care environments. Pertinent health data are obtained from the client when the nurse is prepared for the interview and is able to carry out each of the three phases of an interview: orientation, working, and termination.

Nursing Health History

The nursing health history is the data collected about the client's level of wellness, changes in life patterns, sociocultural role, and mental and emotional reactions to illness. The nursing history is obtained during the interview and is the first step in carrying out the nursing assessment. The objectives of the nursing health history are to identify the client's patterns of health and illness, the presence of risk factors for physical and behavioral health problems, any deviations from normal, and the client's available resources for adaptation (Perry, 1982).

Patterns of health and illness are identified by collecting data concerning the physical, developmental, intellectual, emotional, social, and spiritual dimensions of the client (Fig. 7-1). Incorporating data from all these dimensions into the nursing health history ultimately enables the nurse to develop a holistic plan of care. Directing attention to all dimensions assists the nurse in determining the presence of risk factors in the environment, in the client's family history, or in the client's support system.

Many formats for the nursing health history have been given in the literature (Figs. 7-2 and 7-3). The format of the nursing health history contains the following basic components:

1. Biographical information
2. Client's reason for seeking health care and present illness
3. Client's expectations of health care providers
4. Past health status
5. Family history
6. Environmental history
7. Psychosocial history
8. Present health status and review of symptoms

Biographical information is factual data about the client. The sample nursing health history developed for this text (see Fig. 7-3) includes the type of biographical information obtained in the nursing health history.

The nurse asks the client his reason for seeking health care because the information contained on the client's admission form may differ greatly from the client's subjective reason for seeking health care.

Mr. Jones is being admitted to the hospital. His admission slip indicates that he is scheduled for a series of gastrointestinal diagnostic tests to evaluate his chronic diarrhea. During the nursing health history the nurse asks Mr. Jones his reason for seeking health care. "To find out why I have this pain in my stomach," the client replies. The information can make the nurse aware of any discomfort that Mr. Jones has that may or may not be related to his chronic diarrhea.

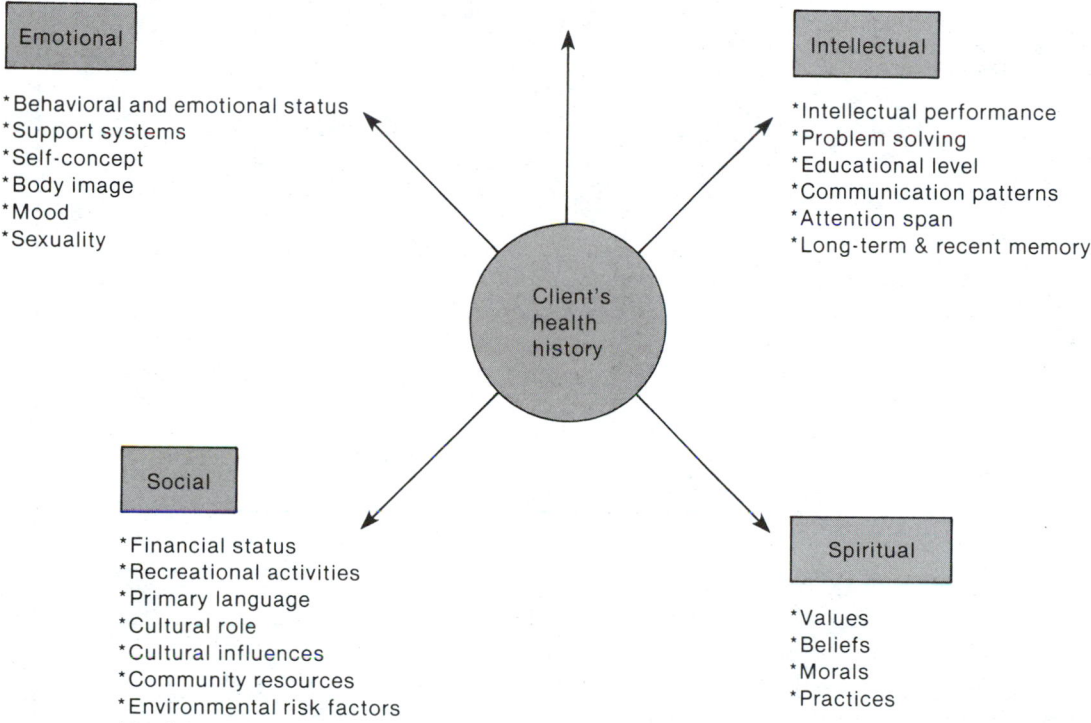

Physical & developmental
* Past health problems & therapies
* Present health therapies
* Risk factors
* Activity and coordination
* Review of symptoms
* Developmental stage
* Effect of health status on developmental stage
* Members of household, marital problems
* Growth & maturation
* Occupation

Emotional
* Behavioral and emotional status
* Support systems
* Self-concept
* Body image
* Mood
* Sexuality

Intellectual
* Intellectual performance
* Problem solving
* Educational level
* Communication patterns
* Attention span
* Long-term & recent memory

Client's health history

Social
* Financial status
* Recreational activities
* Primary language
* Cultural role
* Cultural influences
* Community resources
* Environmental risk factors
* Social relationships

Spiritual
* Values
* Beliefs
* Morals
* Practices

Fig. 7-1 Dimensions for gathering data for a health history.

The statement made by the client is not a diagnostic statement but is the client's perception of his reasons for seeking health care. When recorded, the statement is enclosed in quotation marks to indicate that it is the client's own words.

If an illness is present, the nurse gathers essential and relevant data about the onset of the symptoms. Did the symptoms begin suddenly or gradually? What is the duration of the symptoms? Are the symptoms always present or do they come and go? In the section of the history on present illness the nurse should record specific information about the symptoms, such as location, intensity, and quality of a symptom. The nurse needs to know if any action precipitates the symptoms, makes them worse, or provides relief.

While the nurse is discovering why the client is seeking health care, it is appropriate to learn the client's expectations of the health care providers. Does the client expect to be "cured," "free of pain," or "able to care for myself?" This information assists in establishing the goals of nursing care as well as determining whether the client's expectations of himself and the health care providers are realistic. In addition, the client's expectations provide the nurse with information on the client's perceptions regarding any patterns of illness or changes in life-style.

The information collected about the client's past history provides data on the client's health care experiences. The nurse determines if the client has ever been hospitalized or undergone surgery. Also essential in planning nursing care are descriptions of any allergies, including if the allergic reaction is caused by

90017

C-2

Barnes Hospital
NURSING ADMISSION NOTES AND CARE PLAN

PRIMARY NURSE _____

Adm. Date	Age

Diagnosis and other pertinent medical information:

_____

_____

ADDRESSOGRAPH PLATE

_____

_____

Condition

Allergies (Drugs, food, other)

Identifying Characteristics

Smoker   Non-smoker

Prosthesis/Supportive Devices:

Dentures (circle): Upper Lower Partial	Glasses	Contact Lenses R L	Hearing Aid

Important Phone No.'s

	Doctor	Religion
Service:	Resident:	Intern:

NURSING ADMISSION DATA   INFORMANT_____

Date_____Time_____   Accompanied by_____

Via ☐ Ambulatory   ☐ Wheelchair   ☐ Stretcher

Temp._____Pulse_____Respirations_____BP_____Ht._____Wt._____

Reason for this hospitalization_____

Previous hospitalizations/other illnesses_____

Meds/Procedures/Equipment at home (list)_____

Time of last medication_____With patient_____Taken home_____

PHYSICAL STATUS

Appearance_____

Skin condition_____

Motor Ability_____

Sensory defects (hearing, vision, other)_____

Emotional Status_____

Speech/Language problems_____

Fig. 7-2 Nursing admission notes and care plan.
Courtesy Barnes Hospital, St. Louis.

Date _____

Biographical information

Name _____ Date of birth _____ Sex _____

Address _____

Family member or significant other name _____

_____ Address _____

Marital status   S   M   D   W   Religious preference _____

_____ Religious practices _____

Occupation (present) _____

Length of occupation _____

_____

_____

Source of health care _____

Insurance _____

Client's reason for seeking health care _____

_____

Present illness

Onset _____ , Sudden or gradual _____

Duration _____

Symptoms _____

Precipitating factors _____

Relief measures _____

Expectations of health care providers _____

Past history

Illnesses: Childhood _____

Injuries & hospitalizations _____

Operations _____

Major illnesses _____

Allergies: Type _____

Reaction _____

Treatment _____

Immunizations: _____

Habits: ETHANOL _____ SMOKING _____ CAFFEINE _____ DRUGS _____

Duration of each _____

Medications: Prescribed _____

Self-medicated _____

Sleep patterns _____

Exercise patterns _____

Nutritional patterns _____

Work patterns _____

Fig. 7-3   Nursing health history.

Family history

Health of parents, siblings, spouse, children _____

Risk factor analysis: cancer, heart disease, diabetes mellitus, kidney disease,
                       hypertension, mental disorders

Environmental history

           Cleanliness _____

           Hazards _____

           Pollutants _____

Psychosocial/cultural history

    Primary language _____

    Cultural group _____ Community resources _____

    Mood _____ Attention span _____

Developmental stage _____

_____

_____

Review of systems (ROS) _____

Head, eyes, ears, nose, and throat (HEENT)

    Head: Headaches_____ Dizziness_____

    Vision: Last eye exam_____

              Glasses_____ Contacts_____ (Hard_____ Soft_____ Long wearing_____)

              Blurring_____

              Diplopia_____ Pain_____ Inflammation _____

              Surgery_____

    Hearing: Impaired _____ Type of hearing aid_____

                       Date of new batteries_____

              Pain _____ Drainage_____ Tinnitus_____

    Nose: Allergic rhinitis _____ Type allergen_____

                       Relief measures_____

              Frequency of colds per year _____

              History of polyps_____

              Sinuses _____

              Nose bleeds _____

    Throat & mouth: Last dental exam _____

                     Dentures_____

                     Speech disorders_____

                     Swallowing problem _____

    Respiratory: Cough _____ Sputum _____

                  Dyspnea_____ Dyspnea on exertion_____

                  Activity tolerance _____

                  Last chest x-ray_____

                  Pain _____ Hemoptysis_____

Fig. 7-3, cont'd Nursing health history.

Circulatory: Pain _____ Palpitations _____

                   Edema _____ Numbness _____ Tingling _____

                   Changes in color _____ Changes in hair _____

                   Distribution on extremities _____

                   Syncope _____ Dizziness _____

                   PND _____

Nutritional: Appetite _____ Type of diet _____

                   Nausea _____ Vomiting _____

Elimination (bowel):

         Routine pattern _____ Use of laxatives _____

         Colostomy _____ Ileostomy _____

         Constipation _____ Diarrhea _____

         Melena _____

         (Urine) incontinence _____ Infections _____

         Hematuria _____ Catheter _____

Reproductive:

         Pregnancies _____ Children _____

         Last Pap test _____ Results _____ LMP _____

         Excessive bleeding _____ Vaginal discharge _____

         Self breast exam

         Prostate problems

Neurological:

         Confusion _____ Convulsions _____

         Paralysis _____ Paresthesia _____ Weakness _____

         Incoordination _____ Headaches _____

Musculoskeletal:

         Pain _____ Stiffness _____

         Exercise patterns _____

         Adaptive responses _____

Skin: Rashes _____ Lesions _____ Color _____

       Texture _____ Turgor _____

Fig. 7-3, cont'd Nursing health history.

food, drugs, or pollutants. If an allergy is present, the specific allergic reaction and specific treatment are noted on the assessment form.

While collecting information on the client's history, the nurse identifies the client's habits and life-style patterns. Use of alcohol, tobacco, caffeine, or drugs can place the client at risk for diseases involving the liver, lungs, heart, nervous system, or thought processes. Noting the type of habit as well as the frequency and duration of use provides essential data.

Assessing patterns of sleep, exercise, and nutrition is important in planning nursing care. Whenever possible the nursing care plan should be correlated with the client's life-style patterns. Frequently individual variations in sleep, exercise, and nutritional patterns can be accommodated. If a client is used to jogging a half mile daily, can this activity be part of a care plan? If in a hospital setting it is unrealistic for the client to jog, a substitute exercise could be arranged through the physical therapy department.

The purpose of the family history is to obtain data about the client's immediate and blood relatives. The overall objectives are to determine whether the client is at risk for illnesses of a genetic, familial, or environmental nature and to identify areas of health promotion and illness prevention. The family history also provides information about the family structure, interaction, and function that may be useful in planning care. For example, a cohesive, supportive family can be a resource in helping a client adjust to an illness or disability and should be incorporated into the plan of care. On the other hand, if the client's family is nonsupportive, it may be preferable not to involve them in his care, particularly if the family history reveals that the client is experiencing stress related to familial relationships.

The environmental and psychosocial histories provide data about the client's home environment and any support systems that the client or family may need to use in the future. The environmental history, for example, identifies exposure to pollutants that can affect the client's health, high crime that prevents the client from walking around his community, and resources that can assist the client in the return to the community.

The psychosocial history includes information as to how the client and family cope with stressors. Questions about resolved stressors indicate to the nurse the types of stressors encountered by the client and the resources available to the client to deal with any impending stressors (see Chapter 5).

The review of the systems (ROS) is a systematic method for collecting data on all body systems. During the ROS the nurse asks the client about the normal functioning of each system, as well as any changes in functioning noted by the client. Changes in function noted by the client are usually subjective data because they are described as perceived by the client.

As the nurse proceeds through the nursing health history, the data obtained are recorded in a clear, concise manner using appropriate terminology (see Chapter 12). A clear, concise record is necessary because other health care professionals may use the nursing health history in delivering health care. The sample in Fig. 7-4 shows the correct way to record information on a nursing health history.

Physical Examination

The physical examination is the taking of vital signs and other measurements and the scrutinization of all body parts using the techniques of inspection, palpation, percussion, and auscultation. The examiner looks for abnormalities that may yield information concerning past, present, and future health problems. The physical examination is conducted after the nursing health history, so that data gathered during the nursing health history can be verified. In addition, new data are obtained during the examination.

Throughout the examination data are measured against a standard, which is an established rule or basis of comparison in measuring or judging capacity, quantity, content, and value of objects in the same category. The term "norm" is frequently used synonymously with "standard" in the literature. Selected standards are reliable and relevant for the category being compared. For example, there are established standards for ideal height and weight. The standards are used to determine if an individual is taller or shorter than the standard or is overweight or underweight. Likewise there are standards for the components of body fluids; for example, an individual may have too many or too few red blood cells. The nurse conducting the physical examination uses the skills of inspection, palpation, percussion, and auscultation to verify information and collect further data, which are compared with the standards to determine whether the findings are normal or abnormal. Chapter 29 discusses these skills in more detail; they are presented here as an overview of the physical examination.

The techniques of inspection, palpation, percussion, and auscultation are basic to the physical examination. Before conducting the physical examination, the nurse prepares the client, the environment, and the necessary equipment. The nurse informs the client about the process of the physical examination, specifically its purposes, the nurse's role, the client's role, and the approximate duration.

Date *April 10, 19--*

Biographical information

Name *William Brown*   Date of birth *06/20/19*   Sex *M*

Address *4511 Front Street*

Family member or significant other name *Hannah — 40 years*

                        Address *same*

Marital status   S Ⓜ D W   Religious preference *Methodist*

                          Religious practices *Attends church weekly*

Occupation (present) *carpenter*

Length of occupation *32 years*   *client has owned his own remodeling firm for the past 20 years*

Source of health care *private doctor, Dr. Kelly*

Insurance *Blue Cross - Blue Shield*

Client's reason for seeking health care *"To find out why I've had diarrhea for 3 weeks"*

Present illness

Onset *3 weeks ago*, Sudden or gradual *sudden*

Duration *continued to present*

Symptoms *watery diarrhea, no cramping or GI pain noted*

Precipitating factors *occurs following a meal, diarrhea is sudden*

Relief measures *some relief noted when client eats small meals*

Expectations of health care providers *"to stop diarrhea" and "to tell me I don't have stomach cancer"*

Past history

Illnesses: Childhood *measles, mumps, and chickenpox*

              Injuries & hospitalizations *(1) age 12 - tonsillectomy, (2) age 46 - broken leg*

              Operations *see above*

              Major illnesses *none*

Allergies: Type *roses, no drugs or food allergies stated*

              Reaction *sneezing, runny nose*

              Treatment *Allerest tablets*

Immunizations: *current*

Habits: ETHANOL *6-pack/day*   SMOKING *2 packs/day for 20 years*   DRUGS *none*

              Duration of each

Medications: Prescribed *none*

              Self-medicated *Allerest*

Sleep patterns *usually retires at 11 pm and rises at 6 AM*

Exercise patterns *plays tennis or racquetball 3 times a week*

Nutritional patterns *large breakfast-lunch, salad for evening meal*

Work patterns *works 50-60 hours a week*

Fig. 7-4   Nursing health history.

Family history

Health of parents, siblings, spouse, children _____

Risk factor analysis: cancer, heart disease, diabetes mellitus, kidney disease,
        hypertension, mental disorders

mother died at 58 from stomach cancer; father died at 75 from heart attack; brother died at 42 from stomach cancer; 2 sisters, 50 and 48, alive and well; 1 son, 35, alive and well

Environmental history

      Cleanliness *lives in rehabilitated city home* _____

      Hazards *some street crime* _____

      Pollutants *auto fumes* _____

Psychosocial/cultural history

    Primary language *English* _____

    Cultural group *neighbors* _____ Community resources *his church* _____

    Mood *sociable, talkative, asked if symptoms were cancer related.*

Developmental stage *an adult male who appears to assume the responsibilities of an adult role.*

Review of systems (ROS) _____

Head, eyes, ears, nose, and throat (HEENT)

    Head: Headaches *occasional* _____ Dizziness *no* _____

    Vision: Last eye exam *2 months ago* _____

               Glasses *yes, bifocals* Contacts _____ (Hard_____ Soft_____ Long wearing_____)

               Blurring *no* _____

               Diplopia *no* _____ Pain *no* _____ Inflammation *yes, during allergy season*

               Surgery *no* _____

    Hearing: Impaired *no* _____ Type of hearing aid_____

               Date of new batteries_____

               Pain *no* _____ Drainage *no* _____ Tinnitus *occasionally*

    Nose: Allergic rhinitis *yes* _____ Type allergen *roses*

                                  Relief measures *Allerest tablets*

               Frequency of colds per year *1* _____

               History of polyps *no* _____

               Sinuses *no problems* _____

               Nose bleeds *none* _____

    Throat & mouth: Last dental exam *6 months ago* _____

               Dentures *no* _____

               Speech disorders_____

               Swallowing problem *no* _____

    Respiratory: Cough *yes* _____ Sputum *yes on rising in the morning*

               Dyspnea *no* _____ Dyspnea on exertion *no*

               Activity tolerance *plays racquetball 3 times per week*

               Last chest x-ray *this hospitalization*

               Pain *no* _____ Hemoptysis *no*

Fig. 7-4, cont'd Nursing health history.

Circulatory: Pain _no_   Palpitations _no_

                Edema _no_   Numbness _no_   Tingling _no_

                Changes in color _no_   Changes in hair _no_

                Distribution on extremities _no_

                Syncope _no_   Dizziness _no_

                PND _no_

Nutritional: Appetite _good until 3 weeks ago_

                Nausea _____ Vomiting _____

Elimination (bowel):

        Routine pattern _every other day_ Use of laxatives _none_

        Colostomy _____ Ileostomy _____

        Constipation _____ Diarrhea _began 3 weeks ago_

        Melena _____

        (Urine) incontinence _no_   Infections _once — 10 years ago_

        Hematuria _no_   Catheter _no_

Reproductive:

        Pregnancies _N/A_   Children _____

        Last Pap test _____ Results _____ LMP _____

        Excessive bleeding _____ Vaginal discharge _____

        Self breast exam

        Prostate problems

Neurological:

        Confusion _no_   Convulsions _no_

        Paralysis _no_   Paresthesia _no_   Weakness _no_

        Incoordination _no_   Headaches _relieved with ASA 10 gr_

Musculoskeletal:

        Pain _no_   Stiffness _no_

        Exercise patterns _racquetball 3 times a week_

        Adaptive responses _no_

Skin: Rashes _no_   Lesions _no_   Color _white_

        Texture _smooth_   Turgor _good_

Fig. 7-4, cont'd Nursing health history.

INSPECTION. Inspection is the process of the nurse observing the client. The nurse inspects the client's body and observes his mood, including all responses and nonverbal behavior. The inspection begins with the nurse's first contact with the client. The nurse continues to inspect the client while taking the nursing history.

PALPATION. With palpation the examiner uses her hands and sense of touch to gather data. Palpation is used to detect tenderness, temperature, texture, vibration, pulsations, masses, and other changes in structural integrity. Each body part is palpated, usually following a systematic assessment pattern.

PERCUSSION. Percussion is the tapping of various body organs and structures to produce vibration and sound. The sounds indicate the density of the underlying tissue. For example, percussion over a hollow organ such as the stomach produces a high-pitched, drumlike sound called tympany, whereas percussion over a dense organ such as the liver produces a low-pitched, thudlike sound called dullness. The technique of percussion requires that the examiner place the palmar surface of one hand against the client's body while tapping with the other.

AUSCULTATION. Auscultation is the process of listening to sounds produced by the body. Three systems produce sounds for the examiner to auscultate: the cardiovascular system, the respiratory system, and the gastrointestinal system. For auscultation of these systems the nurse uses a stethoscope, an instrument that amplifies sounds produced by internal organs.

ORDER OF EXAMINATION

The physical examination is carried out in a systematic manner that is similar to the review of systems (see Chapter 29). This component of the assessment usually begins with data on the client's height, weight, and vital signs.

Next the examiner writes a general statement about her perceptions of the client and the client's level of health. This statement, usually labeled the general survey, includes information about the client's mental status, body development, nutritional status, sex and race, chronological versus apparent age, appearance, and speech.

Last is a head-to-toe examination of the body systems. The examiner records objective data obtained during the examination, using clear, concise, and appropriate language in describing each system examined.

LABORATORY DATA

The final source of assessment data is the results of laboratory tests. Laboratory data provide verification of alterations identified in the nursing health history and physical examination. The data are baseline information concerning the client's response to illness and information about the effects of later treatment measures.

Laboratory data are compared with the established norms for a particular test, client age group, and sex. The nurse identifies variations from the normal and interprets the findings according to the client's disease process and treatments. In addition, laboratory data can be used to evaluate the success or failure of nursing measures.

Laboratory tests are selected according to the client's symptoms or disease. However, there are common laboratory tests that may be used for a large number of clients (see the boxed material at left). Specific laboratory tests and the nursing responsibilities associated with them are detailed in Unit 8.

The laboratory data are one more source of information that the nurse uses in completing a data base. In addition to verifying abnormal findings noted in the history and examination, laboratory data can

---

Common Laboratory and Diagnostic Tests

BLOOD

- Complete blood count (CBC)
- Electrolytes—SMA_6, SMA_{12}
- Arterial blood gases (ABGs)
- Fasting blood sugar (FBS)
- Glucose tolerance test (GTT)

URINE

- Urine analysis (UA)
- Urine culture and sensitivity

RADIOLOGICAL EXAMINATIONS

- Chest roentgenogram (CXR)
- Upper gastrointestinal (UGI)
- Lower gastrointestinal (LGI)
- Scans: body, head, chest, bone

STOOL

- Guaiac
- Ova and parasites

SPUTUM

- Culture and sensitivity
- Acid-fast bacilli (AFB)
- Cytology

identify actual or potential health care problems not previously noted by the client or the examiner.

Summary

The nursing assessment is the gathering and verifying of data about a client to establish a data base. The nursing health history, physical examination, and collection of laboratory data are all components of the nursing assessment. To complete the assessment phase, the nurse implements proper interview techniques, is systematic, and correctly inspects, palpates, percusses, and auscultates the client's body systems.

The professionalism, competency, and organization of the nurse promote an environment in which the client is able to share appropriate, pertinent data about previous levels of wellness, health practices, past illness, and health care goals. The data gathered about the client enable the nurse to draw conclusions about the client's needs and to plan individualized nursing care.

KEY CONCEPTS

✓ Assessment is the gathering, verification, and communication of data about a client by means of the interview, nursing health history, physical examination, and laboratory and diagnostic tests.

✓ Written data statements should be descriptive, concise, and complete and should not include interpretative statements.

✓ Collection of inaccurate, incomplete, or inappropriate data may result in incorrect identification of the client's health care needs.

✓ Objective data are observations or measurements by the data collector.

✓ Subjective data are the client's perceptions.

✓ The client is the principal source of data.

✓ Families or significant others can be a primary source of information about the client's health status.

✓ Every member of the health care team who interacts with the client is a potential source of information.

✓ Other data sources include the health record, other records, and pertinent literature.

✓ Review of the pertinent literature increases the nurse's knowledge about the symptoms, treatment, and prognosis of specific illnesses.

✓ The interview is the mechanism for obtaining the nursing health history.

✓ The interviewer identifies the client's needs and risk factors, as well as specific changes in the client's level of wellness and pattern of living.

✓ The use of effective communication skills enables the nurse to initiate the nurse-client relationship and complete the interview.

✓ The interview is comprised of three phases: orientation, working, and termination.

✓ During the interview process information is obtained about the dimensions of the client: physical, developmental, intellectual, emotional, social, and spiritual.

KEY CONCEPTS, cont'd

✓ The interview allows the nurse to observe the client and any interaction between the client and his family.

✓ The interview is a mechanism by which information about the client can be obtained.

✓ The four primary interview techniques are the problem solving, problem seeking, direct question, and open-ended question.

✓ The physical examination requires the skills of inspection, palpation, percussion, and auscultation.

✓ Laboratory and diagnostic tests add to the data base and verify data gathered through the nursing health history and physical examination.

REFERENCES

Enelow, A.J., and Swisher, S.N.: Interviewing and patient care, ed. 2, New York, 1979, Oxford University Press.

Perry, A.G.: Analysis of the components of the nursing process. In Carlson, J.H., Craft, C.A., and McGuire, A.D., editors: Nursing diagnosis, Philadelphia, 1982, W.B. Saunders Co.

Yarnall, S., and Atwood, J.: Problem-oriented practice for nurses and physicians, Nurs. Clin. North Am. 9:215, 1974.

ADDITIONAL READINGS

Alexander, M.M., and Brown, M.S.: The why and how of examination, Nursing 73 3:25, 1973.

Alexander, M.M., and Brown, M.S.: The why and how of examination. II. History taking, Nursing 73 3:35, 1973.

Bermost, L.S.: Interviewing: a key to therapeutic communication in nursing practice, Nurs. Clin. North Am. 1:205, 1966.

Eggland, E.T.: How to take a meaningful nursing history, Nursing 77 7:22, 1977.

Kesler, A.R.: Pitfalls to avoid in interviewing outpatients, Nursing 77 7:70, 1977.

McCain, R.F.: Nursing by assessment—not intuition, Am. J. Nurs. 65:82, 1965.

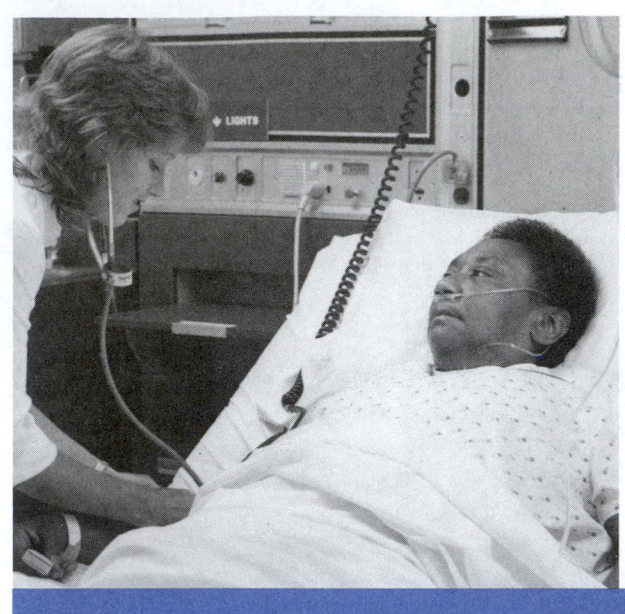

OBJECTIVES

Mastery of content in this chapter will enable the student to:

- Define the terms in the glossary.
- Differentiate between a nursing diagnosis and a medical diagnosis.
- List and discuss the four steps of the nursing diagnostic process.
- Demonstrate the nursing diagnostic process.
- Explain what makes a nursing diagnosis incorrect.
- Discuss the advantages of nursing diagnoses for the client.
- Discuss the advantages of nursing diagnoses for the profession of nursing.
- Discuss the limitations of nursing diagnoses.
- Formulate nursing diagnoses, nursing goals, priorities, and projected outcomes from a nursing assessment.

GLOSSARY

actual health care problem Health problem currently being perceived or experienced by the client.

clinical reasoning Cognitive skills by which the nurse gathers relevant data about the client, analyzes the client's response to the health care problem, organizes the data, and formulates the nursing diagnosis.

data clustering Grouping of related information from the nursing health history, physical examination, and laboratory results as part of the process of determining the nursing diagnosis.

data validation Process of determining if information gathered during assessment is complete and accurate.

diagnosis Identification of a health problem by analyzing the assessment data about a client's health status.

diagnostic process Process of determining a client's health status and evaluating the factors influencing that status.

discharge planning Set of decisions and activities involved in providing continuity and coordination of nursing care when a client is discharged from a health care agency.

error of commission Mistake resulting from over-diagnosis or diagnosing a nonexistent health problem.

error of omission Mistake resulting from failure of the nurse to diagnose a health problem.

medical diagnosis Identification of a specific disease or pathological process.

peer review Appraisal, by professional co-workers of equal status, of the way a nurse conducts practice, education, or research.

potential health care problem Health problem for which the client is at risk.

quality assurance Evaluation of nursing services provided and the results achieved as compared with accepted standards.

8 | Nursing Diagnosis

After completing the nursing assessment the nurse proceeds to the second component of the nursing process, the nursing diagnosis. A nursing diagnosis is a statement of the potential or actual problem in the client's health status that the nurse is licensed and competent to treat. The overall purpose of the nursing diagnosis is to interpret assessment data and thus identify health problems involving the client, the family, and significant others.

The statement of a nursing diagnosis is the culmination of a diagnostic process. During this process the nurse analyzes assessment data to determine the client's health problems. The problems are then stated as a nursing diagnosis.

Nursing Diagnostic Process

The diagnostic process includes three major elements: analysis and interpretation of data, identification of client problems, and formulation of nursing diagnoses (Fig. 8-1). Analysis and interpretation of data require data validation and data clustering. Data validation is the process of determining whether the data gathered during assessment are complete and accurate. It is important for the nurse to validate data early in the diagnostic process, since the formulation of correct, appropriate nursing diagnoses depends on accurate data collection. The nurse uses data clustering to group related data from the nursing health history, physical examination, and laboratory findings. The statement of the client's needs then describes the general health care problem, after which the nurse

formulates a statement of the client's present or potential health problems. The specific problem is written as a nursing diagnosis.

Analysis and Interpretation of Data

As the nurse examines assessment data, information about the client's health status is validated. Validation involves determining the relationship between data and health needs and confirming their accuracy. Data obtained during assessment are valid if they are related to the area being examined. For example, data collected about a client's eating habits, nausea, vomiting, diarrhea, weight, height, muscle mass, adipose tissue, serum albumin, and hemoglobin are valid for assessment of nutritional status. However, these data would not be valid for assessment of the client's ability to complete activities of daily living.

The nurse continually revises the data base to include changes in the client's physical and emotional status, as well as the results of laboratory and diagnostic tests. These data must also be validated as accurate. Various sources are used to validate data, including the client, family, health care team members, and the medical record. The nurse validates data through several methods. First, the nurse can verify data obtained from another source of information. For example, if a family member of a client who is an outpatient says that the client is unable to leave his home because he is easily fatigued, the nurse can validate this information by asking the client about his activity patterns and his fatigue. Second, the nurse validates data obtained during the nursing history by the physical examination. For example, if a client says

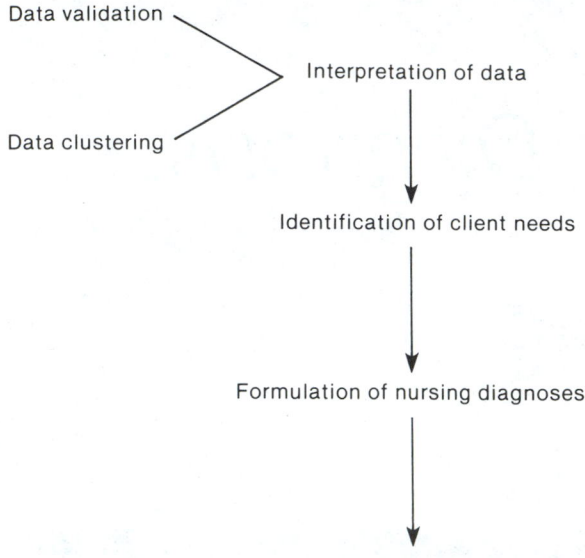

Data validation
Data clustering

Interpretation of data

Identification of client needs

Formulation of nursing diagnoses

Fig. 8-1 Nursing diagnostic process.

that she has a lump in her left breast, the nurse can verify the presence of the lump by physical examination. Third, the nurse can validate physical examination findings by reexamining the client later or requesting a colleague to verify the data by physical examination. For example, a client with pulmonary disease may have a slight inspiratory wheeze auscultated during the physical examination. The nurse can reevaluate the lung later to determine if the wheeze is still present, or she may request a more experienced colleague to auscultate the lung. Last, the nurse validates data obtained with the history or physical examination by the results of laboratory or diagnostic tests. For example, during the history the client says he feels fatigued continuously, and during physical examination the nurse notes that the client's pulse is 108 and his blood pressure is 110/60. The nurse knows that fatigue, a rapid pulse, and a lowered blood pressure are signs of anemia. She checks the laboratory results regarding the client's hemoglobin level, which is 9.6 g. While validating existing data the nurse also verifies that findings in the physical examination are based on fact rather than intuition.

The clustering of data is the process the nurse uses to group related data. These data are usually signs and symptoms indicating a general problem. The nurse clusters data as they relate to the client's mental or emotional status, to individual body systems, to risk factors, to family data, or to community factors. For example, as the nurse analyzes Mr. Brown's assessment, she notes the following related data: a smoking history for 20 years, rales noted on auscultation of the lung fields, and emphysematous changes noted on chest roentgenogram. These data are from

the history, physical examination, and laboratory studies, respectively. As the nurse analyzes the total assessment, she begins to cluster common data. In the example here, the clustered data were related to the respiratory system.

The clustering of data identifies related changes in the client's needs and ultimately leads to the formulation of a nursing diagnosis. Mr. Brown's smoking history, rales, and x-ray changes are all related to a general problem with the respiratory system. Data clustering may also identify missing data that must be collected.

During the assessment the nurse gathers a large amount of data that at first may appear irrelevant and unrelated. However, as data are clustered, a pattern begins to emerge. The nurse begins clustering once the information is obtained in the nursing assessment and continues throughout the analysis process.

Identification of Client Need

Before formulating the nursing diagnosis the nurse identifies the client's general health care need. It may be helpful for the beginning nurse to think of the identification of client needs as the general health care problem and the formulation of the nursing diagnosis as the specific health care problem. Thus in the second and third steps of the diagnostic process the nurse, in describing health care problems, is moving from general to specific. After the general health care problem has been identified, the assessment data are refined to support a nursing diagnosis.

To identify the client's need, the nurse first determines what the client's health problems are and whether they are actual or potential problems. An actual health care problem is one that is currently being perceived or experienced by the client, such as a sleep pattern disturbance caused by a noisy environment. A potential health care problem is one for which the client is at risk, such as an overweight smoker being at risk for ineffective airway clearance related to incisional pain.

When identifying the client's needs, the nurse considers all aspects of the assessment. Often the client and family are important in helping the nurse identify needs. The nurse can actively solicit the family's involvement in conversation. Throughout the nursing process the nurse should remain receptive to the family's response to the identification of needs and the nursing diagnosis, as well as to the care provided.

The problem identification step brings the nurse closer to the formulation of a nursing diagnosis. The step prepares the nurse to make general analyses of the clustered data, thus initiating the development of a nursing diagnosis.

TABLE 8-1

Comparison of Care Plans for Health Care Problems with Different Causes

Nursing Diagnosis	Interventions
CLIENT A	
Ineffective airway clearance related to obesity	1. Place in high Fowler's position. 2. Cough and deep breathe every 2 hours while awake: 8-10-12-2-4-6-8-10. 3. Start weight reduction diet (1200 calories) to decrease obesity.
Self-care deficit in feeding related to bilateral arm casts	1. Encourage family to visit during meals. 2. Be certain staff or family members are available to feed client. 3. Provide high-calorie milkshakes with straw at 3 PM and 8 PM.
Social isolation related to wound infection	1. Plan staffing patterns to include visits to client's room four times a day. 2. Relax visiting hours for client's family. 3. Cleanse wound with antibiotic solution every 4 hours, maintaining strict surgical asepsis.
CLIENT B	
Ineffective airway clearance related to poor coughing	1. Teach deep breathing and coughing. 2. Have client demonstrate deep breathing and coughing.
Self-care deficit in feeding related to inability to grasp feeding utensils	1. Provide large-handled eating utensils. 2. Offer finger foods cut in large pieces for between-meal snacks: 10-2-8.
Social isolation related to recent move into neighborhood	1. Provide client with phone numbers and location of local senior citizens' center. 2. Draw client a map of neighborhood stores, restaurants, libraries.

Formulation of Nursing Diagnoses

The formulation of the nursing diagnosis follows from the analysis of clustered assessment data. The nursing diagnosis is a statement of an actual or potential health problem that a nurse is licensed and competent to treat. The diagnostic statement should include the problem and its cause. The problem is the current or the potential client need that can be resolved by nursing interventions. The cause may be a direct or a contributing factor in the development of the health problem. Inclusion of the cause helps individualize the nursing diagnosis and subsequent plan of care. Examples of diagnostic statements that include the problem and cause are ineffective airway clearance related to obesity, self-care deficit in feeding related to bilateral arm casts, or social isolation related to wound infection. A client may have one of

these problems but a different cause. Such a client would require a different plan of care (Table 8-1). Examples of diagnostic statements for a client who has one of the problems mentioned previously but a different cause are ineffective airway clearance related to poor coughing, self-care deficit in feeding related to inability to grasp eating utensils, or social isolation related to inability to adjust to a recent move into a new neighborhood.

As the client's needs change, the nursing diagnosis is modified. For example, a client's pertinent assessment data included decreased dietary fiber and limited fluid intake, no bowel movement for 5 days, presence of bowel sounds, distention of lower abdomen, hard fecal material extracted in digital rectal examination, and guaiac-negative stool specimen. The nursing diagnosis was constipation related to limited fiber in

Summary of Relevant Data for Mr. Brown

PHYSICAL AND DEVELOPMENTAL

- Diarrhea for 3 weeks
- Productive cough upon rising each morning
- Occasional rales in lung bases
- 15-pound weight loss 2 weeks before hospitalization
- Hemoglobin 12 g
- Slight change of emphysema shown on chest roentgenogram
- Distended abdomen
- Squamous cell cancer
- Smoked for 20 years, 2 packs a day (40 pack-years)
- Family history of stomach cancer
- Family history of heart attack
- Married 40 years
- Self-employed for 20 years
- One adult son, 35 years old
- Two sisters, 50 and 48 with no major health problems

INTELLECTUAL

- Talkative
- Frequently asks nurses if he has cancer
- Good attention span

EMOTIONAL

- Anxious
- Withdrawn after biopsy report of squamous cell cancer

SOCIAL

- Plays tennis three times a week
- Active in his neighborhood

SPIRITUAL

- Methodist
- Attends church weekly
- Reads Bible daily

diet and fluid intake. After appropriate nursing interventions, the client's constipation was resolved and the nursing diagnosis was modified to read, "Potential for constipation related to diet and fluid intake." Once the health problem has been resolved, the nursing diagnosis for that problem is no longer relevant. In addition, as the client's physiological and emotional status changes, the health problem may remain relevant but the cause may change. Therefore the

nursing diagnosis must be restated. New nursing diagnoses are developed as the client's needs and status change.

The modification of nursing diagnoses is ongoing. As the client's level of nursing care and level of wellness change, these changes are reflected in the statement of nursing diagnoses. Outdated nursing diagnoses do not accurately reflect the client's current needs and result in a lower quality of nursing care.

Chapter 7 includes a sample nursing assessment to demonstrate how to collect and record data (see Fig. 7-4). At left is a summary of the pertinent data that may lead to the identification of an actual or potential health care problem. Table 8-2 demonstrates data clustering, identification of client need, and formulation of nursing diagnoses in the analysis process for some of the nursing diagnoses for Mr. Brown. Relevant data are clustered; an understanding of the client's needs and the specific nursing diagnoses are based on these clusters.

Nursing Diagnosis

Nursing Diagnosis and Medical Diagnosis

Up until recent years the term "diagnosis" was almost exclusive to the medical profession. A medical diagnosis is the identification of a disease condition based on a specific evaluation of physical signs, symptoms, history, laboratory tests, and procedures. During the last two decades the term "nursing diagnosis" has appeared more frequently in the literature. A nursing diagnosis identifies any of the client's health care needs. It can reflect the client's present level of health or present response to a disease or pathological process. A medical diagnosis identifies a client's need that physicians are better prepared to handle. Both medical and nursing diagnoses are derived from the physiological, psychological, sociocultural, developmental, and spiritual dimensions of the client (Fig. 8-2). In some institutions physicians and nurses use the same data base in formulating diagnoses.

The goals and objectives of a nursing diagnosis differ from those of a medical diagnosis. The goal of a nursing diagnosis is to identify actual and potential health problems of the client; the goals of a medical diagnosis are to identify and cure the disease or the pathological process. The objective of a nursing diagnosis is to develop a plan of care so that the client and family are able to adapt to changes resulting from health problems; the objectives of the medical diagnosis are to prescribe treatment and cure the client. Thus the focus of a medical diagnosis is curative, whereas the nursing diagnosis focuses on helping the

TABLE 8-2

Development of Mr. Brown's Nursing Diagnoses

Clustering Data	Identification of Client Need	Nursing Diagnosis Formulation
Diarrhea for 3 weeks Distended abdomen Family history of stomach cancer	Alteration in elimination patterns ⟶	Alteration in bowel elimination related to diarrhea of unknown cause
Weight loss: 15 pounds total Diarrhea Surgery scheduled for 11/29/85 Anemia, hemoglobin level 12 g	Excessive weight loss ⟶	Potential alteration in nutrition: less than body requirements related to chronic diarrhea for 3 weeks
40 pack-year history of smoking Slight change of emphysema shown on chest roentgenogram Rales auscultated in lung fields Scheduled for abdominal surgery	At risk for postoperative respiratory complications ⟶	Potential ineffective airway clearance postoperatively related to abdominal incision
Temporary colostomy Abdominal incision	Change in body image ⟶	Potential disturbance in self-concept related to change in body image
Verbalize fear of stomach cancer Became withdrawn following biopsy report	Changes in interpersonal interactions ⟶	Potential ineffective coping related to fear of medical diagnosis

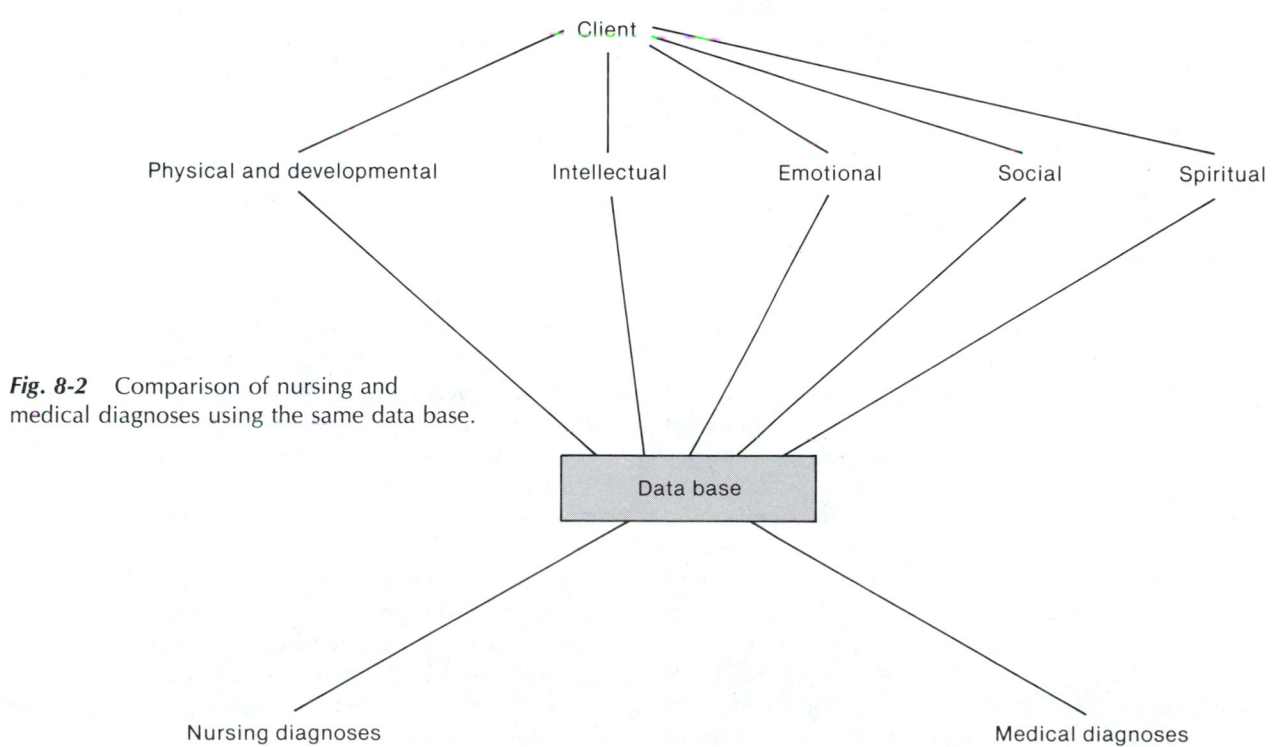

Fig. 8-2 Comparison of nursing and medical diagnoses using the same data base.

client reach his maximal level of wellness. A medical diagnosis of appendicitis, for example, requires the physician to remove the infected appendix. After the appendectomy the client may have a nursing diagnosis of impaired mobility related to surgical incision. The nursing care of the client would be directed toward gradually increasing his mobility to his preoperative level.

Advantages of Nursing Diagnoses

The nursing diagnosis is advantageous for both nurses and clients. It facilitates communication among nurses about a client's level of wellness and discharge planning. The health care delivery system today is highly advanced and uses highly technical equipment that has required increases in the numbers of health care professions and professionals. As more people become responsible for the health care of a single client, it is essential that these professionals be able to communicate with one another. Nursing diagnoses facilitate communication in several ways. First, the initial list of nursing diagnoses is an easily obtainable reference to the client's current health care needs. Second, the diagnostic process and the subsequent development of the list of nursing diagnoses encourage the nurse to develop organizational skills. As the nurse communicates with other professionals, the use of the nursing diagnoses encourages organized communication that is relevant to the client's goals and priorities. Third, nursing diagnoses are used for charting in the nurse's notes, writing referrals, and providing effective transition of care from one unit to another, from one clinic to another, or from the hospital to the community setting. Discharge planning is the set of decisions and activities involved in giving continuity and coordination to nursing care (McKeehan, 1979). Discharge planning is necessary when a client is discharged from one hospital to another or from the hospital to the community. In discharge planning, nursing diagnoses are the mechanism for communicating and delineating the nursing care the client still requires.

Nursing diagnoses can also serve as a focus for quality assurance and peer review. Quality assurance is the evaluation of nursing services provided and the results achieved as compared with accepted standards. In nursing, peer review is an appraisal by professional co-workers of equal status of the way a nurse conducts practice, education, or research. Both quality assurance and peer review use accepted standards as measures against which performance is weighed. The nursing diagnosis is a method of identifying the focus of nursing activity. In focusing on the nursing diagnosis, the reviewer can determine whether the nursing care was correct and delivered according to standards of practice.

All these benefits of the nursing diagnosis for the profession are, of course, also important for the client and the family. Better communication among health care professionals helps eliminate potential problems in giving care and maintains a focus on meeting the client's health care goals. Similarly, the ultimate reason for quality assurance and peer review is to ensure that high-quality care is given clients and their families. Furthermore, the client benefits from the individualization of nursing care that results from appropriate goal setting, correct selection of priorities, selection of appropriate intervention, and establishment of outcome criteria.

Limitations of Nursing Diagnoses

The primary limitation of the nursing diagnosis is an incomplete taxonomy. The 51 nursing diagnoses at right, developed by the Task Force of the National Group for the Classification of Nursing Diagnoses, are obviously only the beginning of a total classification system. Through the formulation and use of other nursing diagnoses, the taxonomy will grow and thus expand the focus of professional nursing.

Sources of Error

The diagnostic process is not without potential for errors. An error is the failure to identify a client need correctly or the identification of a need that is important to the nurse and not the client. Errors in the diagnostic process result in the development of an incomplete or inappropriate nursing care plan.

Gordon (1982) groups errors into two categories: errors of omission and errors of commission. An error of omission occurs when the nurse has failed to identify a health care problem, which can occur when incomplete data are collected from the client, when data are clustered incorrectly in the analysis process, or when data are interpreted improperly. Errors of commission occur from overdiagnosis, or diagnosing nonexistent health care problems.

Although errors of omission and commission occur during any step of the diagnostic process, such errors often have their origins in the nursing assessment. When collecting data the interviewer can fail to use the problem-solving interview technique. As Chapter 7 explains, in the problem-solving technique the interviewer asks specific questions focused on a particular problem. For example, when a client says he has abdominal pain, the nurse uses the problem-solving technique to determine the location, intensity, dura-

Approved Nursing Diagnoses

- Activity intolerance
- Activity intolerance, potential
- Airway clearance, ineffective
- Anxiety
- Bowel elimination, alteration in: constipation
- Bowel elimination, alteration in: diarrhea
- Bowel elimination, alteration in: incontinence
- Breathing pattern, ineffective
- Cardiac output, alteration in: decreased
- Comfort, alteration in: pain
- Communication, impaired: verbal
- Coping, family: potential for growth
- Coping, ineffective family: compromised
- Coping, ineffective family: disabling
- Coping, ineffective individual
- Diversional activity, deficit
- Family process, alteration in (formerly Family dynamics)
- Fear
- Fluid volume, alteration in: excess
- Fluid volume deficit, actual
- Fluid volume deficit, potential
- Gas exchange, impaired
- Grieving, anticipatory
- Grieving, dysfunctional
- Health maintenance, alteration in
- Home maintenance management, impaired
- Injury, potential for: (poisoning, potential for; suffocation, potential for; trauma, potential for)
- Knowledge deficit (specify)
- Mobility, impaired physical
- Noncompliance (specify)
- Nutrition, alteration in: less than body requirements
- Nutrition, alteration in: more than body requirements
- Nutrition, alteration in: potential for more than body requirements
- Oral mucous membrane, alteration in
- Parenting, alteration in: actual
- Parenting, alteration in: potential
- Powerlessness
- Rape trauma syndrome
- Self-care deficit: feeding, bathing/hygiene, dressing/grooming, toileting
- Self-concept, disturbance in: body image, self-esteem, role performance, personal identity
- Sensory-perceptual alteration: visual, auditory, kinesthetic, gustatory, tactile, olfactory
- Sexual dysfunction
- Skin integrity, impairment of: actual
- Skin integrity, impairment of: potential
- Sleep pattern disturbance
- Social isolation
- Spiritual distress (distress of the human spirit)
- Thought processes, alteration in
- Tissue perfusion, alteration in: cerebral, cardiopulmonary, renal, gastrointestinal, peripheral
- Urinary elimination, alteration in patterns
- Violence, potential for: self-directed or directed at others

From Kim, M.J., McFarland, G.K., and McLane, A.M., editors: Classification of nursing diagnoses: proceedings of the fifth National Conference, St. Louis, 1984, The C.V. Mosby Co.

tion, precipitating causes, and relief factors of the pain. Even without this method it may be possible to identify a problem, but important information and potential solutions remain undetected because incomplete, inaccurate, or irrelevant data have been collected.

Failure of the nurse to identify correctly the client's response to health problems during assessment can result in incorrect data collection, leading to an incorrect or inaccurate nursing diagnosis. While analyzing the client's response to actual or potential health care problems, the nurse relies on the client's verbal and nonverbal communication patterns. The alert nurse changes interview techniques to obtain the most complete, accurate, and relevant data base.

Errors in data clustering can lead to errors of commission because the data are clustered prematurely, incorrectly, or not at all (Gordon, 1982). Premature closure of clustering occurs when the nurse jumps to the nursing diagnosis before all the similar data have been grouped. For example, a nurse is assessing a client who has a cast on his right arm. Data concerning the immobilized arm are clustered, but the nurse does not include relevant information on the client's perception of his ability to carry out activities of daily living. Because the similar data are not all together, the nurse develops an incorrect nursing diagnosis. Incorrect clustering of the data occurs when the nurse tries to make the nursing diagnosis fit the signs and symptoms obtained in data collection. For example, a nurse has assessed a client with a medical diagnosis of an acute myocardial infarction. From her knowledge base the nurse is aware that chest pain occurs with a myocardial infarction, and she includes "pain due to myocardial ischemia" as a nursing diagnosis. However, she did not validate the presence of pain with the client. The nursing diagnosis should be arrived at from the data, not the other way around. The absence of a nursing diagnosis can affect the quality of care, just as an incorrect nursing diagnosis can.

Another type of error can occur in the manner in which the nursing diagnosis is stated. While the nursing diagnosis should be stated in the format designated by a particular school or agency, some common guidelines will reduce errors in the diagnostic statement itself. First, the statement should be worded in appropriate, concise, and precise language. Appropriate language involves using correct terminology that reflects the *nursing* needs of the client. The diagnostic statement should be concise so that the nursing need can be easily communicated intraprofessionally and interprofessionally. Finally, the diagnos-

tic statement should be precise, identifying unique nursing needs. The nursing diagnosis should be stated in the problem-cause format. A diagnostic statement such as "unhappy and worried about health" can lead to errors; the language needs to be more precise and appropriate, such as "potential ineffective coping related to fear of medical diagnosis of cancer."

There are three other potential sources of error in writing the diagnostic statement: (1) nursing diagnoses that are stated as medical diagnoses, (2) use of medical terminology to describe the cause, and (3) stating the nursing diagnosis as an intervention. These are errors because they shift the focus of the statement from nursing to medicine or they shift the focus from the cause to the intervention. Table 8-3 states the correct nursing diagnoses formulated from Mr. Brown's assessment data and compares them with the three errors of medical diagnosis, medical terminology, and nursing intervention.

As the nurse gains expertise with the diagnostic process, the likelihood of errors is reduced, and the nurse is able to develop the nursing diagnoses based on the actual or potential nursing needs of the client.

TABLE 8-3

Examples of Errors in Formulating the Nursing Diagnostic Statement

Correct Nursing Diagnostic Statement	Nursing Diagnosis Stated as a Medical Diagnosis	Nursing Diagnosis in Medical Terminology	Nursing Diagnosis Stated as a Nursing Intervention
Alteration in bowel elimination related to diarrhea of unknown cause	Diarrhea	Alteration in bowel elimination related to lesion in descending colon	Offer bedpan frequently because of alteration in elimination.
Potential alteration in nutrition: less than body requirements related to chronic diarrhea for 3 weeks	Potential malnutrition	Potential alteration in nutrition: less than body requirements owing to malnutrition	Client needs high-protein diet owing to potential alteration in nutrition.
Potential ineffective airway clearance postoperatively related to abdominal incision	Potential pneumonia	Potential ineffective airway clearance owing to emphysema	Cough frequently because of ineffective airway clearance.
Potential disturbance in self-concept related to change in body image	Avoidance reaction to colostomy	Potential disturbance in self-concept owing to colostomy	Client needs to be encouraged to interact with others.
Potential ineffective coping related to fear of medical diagnosis	Fear of cancer	Potential ineffective coping owing to squamous cell cancer	Client needs to verbalize fear.

KEY CONCEPTS

✓ The statement of nursing diagnoses is the result of the diagnostic process.

✓ The diagnostic process includes analysis and interpretation of data, identification of client problems, and formulation of nursing diagnoses.

✓ The interpretation of data requires the nurse to validate and cluster data.

✓ Nursing diagnoses are written for the physical, developmental, intellectual, emotional, social, and spiritual dimensions of the client.

✓ Nursing diagnoses are necessary to develop a plan of care that will help the client and family adapt to changes resulting from an illness or change in life-style.

✓ Nursing diagnoses improve communication between nurses and other health professionals.

✓ Nursing diagnoses can serve as a focus for quality assurance and peer review.

✓ Nursing diagnostic errors can occur by either omission or commission.

✓ Errors of omission occur when the nurse has failed to identify a health problem.

✓ Causes of errors of omission are incomplete data collection, incorrect data clustering, or improper interpretation of data.

✓ Errors of commission occur when the nurse overdiagnoses or diagnoses nonexistent health problems.

✓ Causes of errors of commission are incomplete data collection and incorrect data clustering.

✓ Diagnostic statement errors include using inappropriate or imprecise language, stating a nursing diagnosis as a medical diagnosis, using medical terminology to describe the cause, and stating the nursing diagnosis as an intervention.

Summary

The analysis of data obtained during the nursing assessment results in the formulation of nursing diagnoses. Nursing diagnoses are developed through a process in which data are validated and clustered, the client's needs are identified, and the specific nursing diagnoses are formulated. The stated nursing diagnoses reflect the client's individual needs and response to a disease or pathological process.

Formulation of the nursing diagnosis is a cognitive activity that focuses on the client's health care needs and expectations. The formulation of nursing diagnoses enables the nurse and client together to determine client goals, priorities, and projected outcomes of nursing care in the planning component.

REFERENCES

Gordon, M.: Nursing diagnosis: process and application, New York, 1982, McGraw-Hill Book Co.

McKeehan, K.M.: Nursing diagnosis in a discharge planning program, Nurs. Clin. North Am. 14:517, 1979.

ADDITIONAL READINGS

Aspinall, M.J.: Nursing diagnosis—the weak link, Nurs. Outlook 24:433, 1976.

Aspinall, M.J.: Use of a decision tree to improve diagnostic accuracy, Nurs. Res. 28:182, 1979.

Campbell, C.: Nursing diagnosis and intervention in nursing practice, New York, 1978, John Wiley & Sons, Inc.

Gebbie, K.M., and Lavin, M.A.: Classifying nursing diagnoses, Am. J. Nurs. 74:250, 1974.

Gleit, C.J., and Tatro, S.: Nursing diagnoses for healthy individuals, Nurs. Health Care 8:456, 1981.

Gordon, M.: Classification of nursing diagnoses, J. N.Y. Nurses Assoc. 9:5, 1978.

Gordon, M.: The concept of nursing diagnoses, Nurs. Clin. North Am. 14:487, 1979.

Kim, M.J., McFarland, G.K., and McLane, A.M., editors: Classification of nursing diagnoses: proceedings of the fifth National Conference, St. Louis, 1984, The C.V. Mosby Co.

Kim, M.J., and others: Pocket guide for nursing diagnoses, St. Louis, 1984, The C.V. Mosby Co.

Price, B.R.: Nursing diagnoses: making a concept come alive, Am. J. Nurs. 80:668, 1980.

Shoemaker, J.: How nursing diagnoses helps focus your care, RN 8:56, 1979.

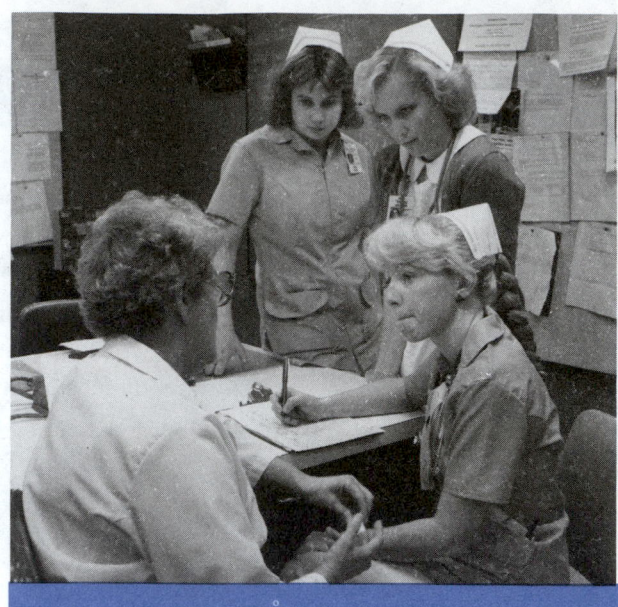

OBJECTIVES

Mastery of content in this chapter will enable the student to:

- Define the terms in the glossary.
- List the purposes of the nursing care plan.
- Discuss differences between institutional and student care plans.
- Describe the differences between care plans used in a hospital and a community health setting.
- Identify incorrect nursing interventions developed during the planning component.
- Develop a nursing care plan from a nursing assessment.
- List the six steps involved in obtaining a consultant.
- Discuss the consultant process.

GLOSSARY

anticipatory guidance Psychological and physical preparation of a client to help relieve fear and anxiety of an event or outcome that is expected to be stressful.

consultation Process in which the help of a specialist is sought to identify ways to handle problems in client management or the planning and implementation of programs.

Kardex Trade name for a card-filing system that allows quick reference to the particular need of the client for certain aspects of nursing care.

nursing goal Specific aim planned by the nurse to assist the client in achieving his maximal level of wellness.

projected outcome Expected condition of a client at the end of therapy or of a disease process, including the degree of wellness and the need for continuing care, medications, support, counseling, or education.

scientific rationale Reason, based on supporting literature, why a specific nursing action was chosen.

9 | *Planning*

The nursing assessment and the formulation of nursing diagnoses initiate the individualization, coordination, and continuity of nursing care that is planned during the third component of the nursing process. Planning is a category of nursing behaviors in which the goals of care are set for an individual client and a strategy is designed to achieve goals. During planning the client's goals are determined, priorities are established, outcomes of nursing care are projected, and a nursing care plan is written. The planning of nursing care includes consulting other health professionals, modifying care, and recording information relevant to client management.

Determining Goals of Care

Nursing care that is planned and organized around specific nursing diagnoses is individualized to the client's health care needs, goals, and priorities. The nursing diagnoses are based on the client's response to change in his level of wellness or life-style patterns. Because each person responds in his own way to a given situation, the health problems of each individual and therefore the goals of care differ.

Individualized nursing diagnoses facilitate the development of the nursing goal. A nursing goal is a specific aim planned by the nurse to assist the client in achieving his maximal level of wellness. A goal for a postpartum, lactating mother may be, "Prevent skin irritation and breakdown around the nipple," while a goal for a man with a myocardial infarction may

be, "Return client to total self-care." Setting goals is an activity that includes the family and significant others as well as the client. Ultimately the goal is the intended outcome of the nursing intervention. The setting of goals follows from the second step of the nursing process, the identification of client needs and the nursing diagnosis.

Goals include prevention and rehabilitation as well as meeting emergency needs of the client. Two types of goals are developed for the client: short-term and long-term. A short-term goal is one that can be achieved quickly, such as during a clinic visit, the present hospitalization, or a home visit. A short-term goal for a client with a myocardial infarction, for example, might be "self-care for all hygiene needs." A long-term goal is one that is to be achieved in the future. A long-term goal for a client with a myocardial infarction might be to "stop smoking within 6 months." Long-term goals often focus on prevention, rehabilitation, and health education. Failure to set long-term goals may prevent the client from achieving his maximal level of wellness.

Goal setting establishes the framework for the nursing care plan. Table 9-1 shows the short-term and long-term goals for Mr. Brown, whose assessment and nursing diagnoses were presented in the preceding chapters. The goals are individualized to meet his needs. Through the goals for Mr. Brown the nurse is able to provide continuity of care during the hospitalization and convalescent phases. In addition, goal setting promotes appropriate use of time and resources.

TABLE 9-1

Goal Setting for Mr. Brown

Nursing Diagnoses	Client Goals	
	Short-Term Goals	Long-Term Goals
Alteration in bowel elimination related to diarrhea of unknown cause	Maintain privacy for Mr. Brown's elimination needs.	Presurgery bowel elimination patterns will return in 1 month.
Potential alteration in nutrition: less than body requirements related to diarrhea for 3 weeks	Maintain present weight.	Return Mr. Brown's weight to preillness level.
Potential ineffective airway clearance postoperatively related to abdominal incision	Mr. Brown's lungs remain clear postoperatively.	Mr. Brown stops smoking 1 month after surgery.
Potential disturbance in self-concept related to change in body image	Mr. Brown views the incision and colostomy by fifth postoperative day.	Mr. Brown cares for colostomy independently 2 weeks after surgery.
Potential ineffective coping related to fear of medical diagnosis	Mr. Brown asks pertinent questions about cancer.	Mr. Brown will attend the "I can cope" classes at the Cancer Society.

Establishing Priorities

After specific nursing diagnoses have been formulated and the goals set, the nurse establishes priorities for each of the diagnoses during the planning component. Establishing priorities ranks the nursing diagnoses and goals in order of importance. The nurse begins the nursing care plan with the nursing diagnoses having the highest priorities.

Maslow's hierarchy of needs can be useful in designating priorities. Basic physiological needs are given priority over safety needs; the needs for love, esteem, and self-actualization follow. The nurse may encounter situations in which there are no emergency physical needs but in which high priority must be given to psychological, sociocultural, developmental, or spiritual needs of the client. Chapter 4 discusses in detail Maslow's hierarchy of needs and its implications for nursing practice.

Priorities are classified as high, intermediate, or low. High-priority nursing diagnoses reflect the emergency or immediate needs of the client. High priorities occur in the psychological as well as the physiological dimensions, and the nurse should avoid classifying only physiological nursing diagnoses as high priority. Intermediate-priority nursing diagnoses reflect non-emergency, non-life-threatening needs of the client. Low-priority nursing diagnoses reflect client goals that are not directly related to his specific illness or prognosis. As with long-term goals, high-, intermediate-, and low-priority nursing diagnoses involve all dimensions of the client. The use of priorities does not necessarily mean that the low-priority diagnoses are ignored until high-priority goals are met—the nurse may simultaneously give care to meet several different goals. But a high-priority goal, such as the need to establish a clear airway, obviously requires attention before a lower-priority goal, such as meeting the client's social needs.

Whenever possible, the client should be involved in priority setting. In some situations the client and the nurse will assign different priority rankings to the nursing diagnoses. If the nurse and the client place a different value on health care needs and treatments, these differences in priorities can be resolved through open communication between the client and the nurse. However, when the client's physiological and emotional needs are at stake, the nurse may need to assume primary responsibility for setting the priorities.

When the nurse assigns priorities to nursing diagnoses, the needs of the client, the resources of the health care system, and the limitations of time are variables that are considered. The priorities established for Mr. Brown reflect some of his needs and the resources and limitations of the health care system (Table 9-2).

TABLE 9-2

Priority Setting for Mr. Brown

Nursing Diagnosis	Rationale
HIGH PRIORITY	
Potential ineffective coping related to fear of medical diagnosis of cancer	Dealing with ineffective coping early will help Mr. Brown prepare for surgery and his postoperative and restorative care.
Potential ineffective airway clearance postoperatively related to abdominal incision	Because of the risk of postoperative complications, the nurse will institute preventive client education early in nursing care.
Potential disturbance in self-concept related to change in body image	Early intervention will help Mr. Brown begin to accept his change in body image and increase his independence in self-care.
INTERMEDIATE PRIORITY	
Alteration in bowel elimination related to diarrhea of unknown cause	Neither of these nursing diagnoses affects the client's immediate physiological or emotional status. Also, the future surgery will assist the nurse in resolving the diagnoses.
Potential alteration in nutrition: less than body requirements related to chronic diarrhea for 3 weeks	
LOW PRIORITY	
Potential for chronic respiratory infections related to history of smoking for 20 years	This nursing diagnosis reflects the long-term needs of the client.

Projecting Outcomes

In addition to facilitating goal and priority setting, nursing diagnoses enhance the development of projected outcomes. The projected outcome is the change in the client's condition that the care plan is designed to bring about, including the degree of wellness and the need for continuing care, medications, support, counseling, or education.

Projecting the outcomes will assist the nurse later in evaluating the extent to which the problem has been resolved. Outcomes are projected before nursing actions are implemented and are measurable behaviors related to goals (Gordon, 1982). The projected outcomes serve as a basis for the criteria the nurse uses to evaluate the effectiveness of the nursing care plan. Achievement of the outcomes implies that the client has reached the desired level of health. The specific nature of the outcome criteria provides the basis for the evaluation component of the nursing process.

The projected outcomes for Mr. Brown are based on the nursing diagnoses, the nursing goals, and the established priorities (Table 9-3). The outcomes presented are measurable and predict the end point of the nursing care for a particular nursing diagnosis. Projected outcomes should be realistic and attainable within the time periods specified.

Nursing Care Plan

The final product of the planning component is the nursing care plan. The nursing care plan is based on the data obtained during assessment and the nursing diagnosis, priorities, and goals developed during analysis. Generally nursing care plans involve the four areas of the nursing care problem, the goals, the specific actions by the nurse, and the projected evaluation of the client's responses to the nursing actions. Specific care plans may in some settings include the additional area of assessment, and in some settings they may not include evaluation. The written nursing care plan describes the actions to be taken in the last two

TABLE 9-3

Projected Outcomes for Mr. Brown

Nursing Diagnosis	Client Goals		Projected Outcomes
	Short-Term Goals	Long-Term Goals	
Potential ineffective coping related to fear of medical diagnosis of cancer	Mr. Brown asks pertinent questions about cancer.	Mr. Brown will attend "I can cope" classes at the Cancer Society.	Mr. Brown asks pertinent questions related to his nursing care. Mr. Brown follows preoperative teaching plan.
Potential ineffective airway clearance postoperatively related to abdominal incision	Mr. Brown's lungs remain clear postoperatively.	Mr. Brown stops smoking 1 month after surgery.	Lungs are clear to auscultation. No consolidation or infiltration noted on postoperative chest roentgenograms.
Potential for chronic respiratory infections related to history of smoking for 20 years			
Alteration in bowel elimination related to diarrhea of unknown cause	Maintain privacy for Mr. Brown's elimination needs.	Presurgery bowel elimination pattern will return in 1 month.	Bowel patterns return to preillness elimination patterns.
Potential alteration in nutrition: less than body requirements related to chronic diarrhea for 3 weeks	Maintain present weight.	Return Mr. Brown's weight to preillness level.	Weight returns to preillness status.
Potential disturbance in self-concept related to change in body image	Mr. Brown views the incision and colostomy by the fifth postoperative day.	Mr. Brown cares for colostomy independently 2 weeks after surgery.	Mr. Brown independently cares for colostomy. Mr. Brown returns to prehospitalization activities 2 months after surgery.

components of the nursing process, implementation and evaluation.

Purpose of the Nursing Care Plan

The nursing care plan is a written guideline for client care so that the specifics of nursing care can be quickly grasped. Written nursing care plans document the individual health care needs of the client determined by assessment and the nursing diagnosis, priorities, and goals formulated during planning; coordinate nursing care; promote continuity of care; and list outcome criteria that will be used in the evaluation of nursing care (Little and Carnevali, 1983). In addition, the written care plan communicates to other nurses and other health professionals pertinent assessment data, a list of problems, and therapies. A written care plan decreases the risk of incomplete, incorrect, or inaccurate care.

The nursing care plan is organized in such a way that any professional nurse can quickly identify the nursing actions to be delivered to each client. Often in hospitals and outpatient and community-based settings the client receives care from more than one nurse, more than one physician, various allied health professionals, and many health technicians. The written nursing care plan makes possible the coordination of nursing care, subspecialty consultations, and scheduling of diagnostic tests.

The care plan can also identify and coordinate the resources that are used to deliver nursing care. The listing of specific equipment and supplies necessary for nursing actions is an economically efficient mechanism for selecting equipment. If all the equipment and supplies needed are included in the nursing care plan, the nurse will not have to leave the client to locate necessary supplies.

The nursing care plan enhances the continuity of

nursing care through listing the specific nursing actions necessary to achieve the goals of care. The nursing activities listed can be carried out throughout the day and from day to day. A correctly formulated nursing care plan facilitates the continuity of care from one nurse to another. As a result all nurses caring for a client have the opportunity to deliver the same quality of care.

The written nursing care plan organizes the information exchanged by nurses in the change-of-shift report. Nurses focus their report on the nursing care and treatments delineated in the nursing care plan. At the end of a scheduled shift, the nurse discusses the care plan with the next care giver. Thus all nurses are able to discuss current and pertinent information about the client's plan of care.

The written care plan can also be adapted to the discharge needs of the client. Incorporating the goals of the care plan into the client's discharge is particularly important for a client who will be undergoing long-term rehabilitation in the community setting. The adaptation of the care plan enhances the continuity of nursing care between the nurses in the hospital and the nurses in the community.

In developing an individualized care plan the nurse involves the family during the planning phase. The family is a resource the nurse can use to help the client meet health goals. In addition, meeting some of the family's needs can improve the client's level of wellness.

The last item documented on the nursing care plan is the projected outcome criteria used in the evaluation of care. Proper listing of the outcome criteria provides the nurse with objective statements that help determine whether the goals of care have been achieved.

The development of the nursing care plan is the end point of the planning phase. The complete nursing care plan is the blueprint for nursing action, providing direction for implementation of the plan and a framework for evaluation of the client's response to nursing actions.

Types of Nursing Care Plans

The structure of the nursing care plan varies from one health care setting to another. The nursing care plan used in a hospital is different from one used in a community health setting. First, the nursing care plan developed for the client who has returned to his home is usually based solely on long-term health needs. Second, because the client is receiving nursing care in his home, the client and the family or significant others are more involved and assume more responsibility for compliance. While the structure varies, the overall purpose remains the same. The beginning student will be exposed to two types of nursing care plans: institutional (staff) care plans and student care plans.

INSTITUTIONAL (STAFF) CARE PLANS

Staff care plans are concise documents that become part of the client's medical record. Most hospitals use the Kardex nursing care plan. Kardex is a trade name for a card-filing system that allows quick reference to the particular needs of the client for certain aspects of nursing care. Each card is folded once. Information concerning medications, activity levels, level of self-care, diet, treatments, and procedures is usually included on the outside of the card (Fig. 9-1). The nursing care plan is commonly placed on the inside (Fig. 9-2). Each institution has its own format for the Kardex, but the basic information contained on the Kardex is universal. The nursing care plan section of the Kardex also has institutional variations. One institution might use a three-column nursing care plan, which includes the problem, the goal, and the nursing action (Fig. 9-3). Another institution may incorporate a four-column nursing care plan on the Kardex, which includes the problem, the goal, the nursing action, and the evaluation (Fig. 9-4). As the five-step nursing process has gained popularity, the nursing care plan on the Kardex in many hospitals has been revised to include the components of the nursing process: assessment, nursing diagnosis, planning, implementation, and evaluation (Fig. 9-5).

STUDENT CARE PLANS

The nursing student learns to write and use a nursing care plan as part of her training. The student care plan is essential for learning the problem-solving technique, the nursing process, skills of written and verbal communication, and organizational skills needed for nursing care. Most important, by using the nursing care plan, students can apply the knowledge gained from nursing and medical literature and the classroom in a practice situation.

The student care plan is more elaborate than the care plans in hospital or community health agencies because its purpose is to teach the process of planning care. To learn the care-planning process, the student must progress in a step-by-step manner, beginning with assessment and ending with evaluation. Student care plans vary from one educational program to another and between beginning and more advanced students. Some educational institutions model the student care plan on the care plan used in the affiliated health agency. The only modification may be that the

Text continued on p. 181.

Medical Diagnosis and other pertinent medical information:

Condition

Allergies (Drugs, food, other)

Adm. Date	Age	Religion	Mode of Travel	
Service	Doctor	Resident	Intern	

Stamp Addressograph Plate Here

FREQUENTLY ORDERED ITEMS

	Date	Specimens/Daily Lab	Date	Treatments
Temp.				
Pulse & Resp.				
BP				
I & O				
Weights				
Spot Checks				
Chest P.T.				
Incentive Spirometer				
P.T.				

ACTIVITIES | **NUTRITION**

			Date	Diagnostic Procedures
Ad lib	Diet			
Ambulate				
Chair				
BRP				
Bedrest				
Bath	Feedings			
Self	Assist c̄ meals			
Tub	**FLUID BALANCE**			
Shower	Force			
Bed	D E N			
Assist.	Restrict			
	D E N			

Orderlies Needed

Family:

NURSING CARE PLAN

140962 Rev. 2/83

Date	Nursing Diagnosis	Expected Outcomes	Nursing Plan/Orders

Discharge Planning: Destination: Transportation: Probable Date:

Referral Agencies: Appointment:

Supplies:

Patient Name

Fig. 9-1   Nursing Kardex.

Medical Diagnosis and other pertinent medical information:

10/23 LBP c̄ RLE Sciatica
10/26 Laminectomy L4-L5 c̄ Bone graft

Condition: _Satis_   PMH:

Allergies (Drugs, food, other): PCN, ASA, Codeine   DM

| Adm. Date 10/23 | Age 64 | Religion Cath | Mode of Travel |
| Service Ortho | Doctor Ford | Resident Kowalski | Intern |

Stamp Addressograph Plate Here

1083 13160 23-4
Deaney, Phil

FREQUENTLY ORDERED ITEMS

Temp.	
Pulse & Resp.	q 4°
BP	

Specimens/Daily Lab	Date	
10/23	Adm. blood work	
10/23	UA c̄ Micro	
10/24	BS	

Treatments	Date	
10/24	BR and logroll q 2°	

Diagnostic Procedures	Date	
10/23	Myelogram CT scan	
10/24	Spinal diff	
10/24	CXR	
10/24	EKG	

ACTIVITIES
- Ad lib
- Ambulate
- Chair
- BRP
- Bedrest

NUTRITION
- Diet
- Feedings
- Bath
- Self
- Tub
- Assist c̄ meals
- Shower

FLUID BALANCE
- Bed
- Force   D   E   N
- Assist.
- Restrict   D   E   N

Orderlies Needed

Family:

I & O
Weights
Spot Checks
Chest P.T.
Incentive Spirometer
P.T.

NURSING CARE PLAN

14096Z Rev. 2/83

Date	Nursing Diagnosis	Expected Outcomes	Nursing Plan/Orders
10/24	Alterd comfort, pain	1. Pt. requests for pain med. decreased	1. Encourage patient to splint abdominal incision when turning
		2. Pt. respiratory expansion 1.	2. Instruct patient in relaxation exercises
			3. Splint incision when coughing & deep breathing

Discharge Planning: Destination:

Transportation:

Probable Date:

Referral Agencies:

Supplies:

Appointment:

Patient Name

Fig. 9-2 Nursing care plan on nursing Kardex.

Problem	Goal	Nursing action
Potential alteration in nutrition: less than body requirements related to sensation of fullness c̄ meals	Maintain present weight of 185 lbs	1. Weigh daily 2. Small frequent high caloric feedings 8-10-12-2-4-6

Fig. 9-3 Three-column nursing care plan.

Problem	Goal	Nursing action	Evaluation
Potential alteration in nutrition: less than body requirements related to sensation of fullness c̄ meals	Maintain weight of 185 lbs	1. Weigh daily 2. Small frequent high caloric feedings 8-10-12-2-4-6	1. Weight remains 185 lbs 2. Consumes all food delivered on meal tray

Fig. 9-4 Four-column nursing care plan.

instructor requires the beginning student to include the scientific rationale for the nursing actions selected (Table 9-4). A scientific rationale is the reason, based on supporting literature, why a specific nursing action was chosen.

Format of the Nursing Care Plan

As an initial step in planning, the nurse assigns a priority to each nursing diagnosis. The nursing diagnosis with the highest priority is the beginning point for the nursing care plan and is followed by other nursing diagnoses in order of assigned priority.

When using the five-column plan, in the assessment column the nurse includes all data relevant to the corresponding nursing diagnosis. Next the nurse includes the previously developed goals in the planning column. At this point the nurse begins to translate the short- and long-term goals into action plans that anticipate the needs of the client, to coordinate nursing care, and to select the appropriate nursing measures.

The nurse writes the action plan in the implementation column of the nursing care plan. Each nursing action is written to include the information necessary to implement nursing care. It may be helpful to the beginning nurse to ask if the stated interventions answer the following questions: *What* is the intervention? *When* should each intervention be implemented? *How* should the intervention be performed? *Who* should be involved in each aspect of intervention? In addition, the nurse should understand the reason for a specific intervention. Nonspecific nursing interventions result in incomplete or inaccurate nursing care, lack of continuity among care givers, and poor use of resources.

Common omissions in writing nursing interventions include what is to be done, the frequency, the quantity, the method, or who is to carry out the intervention. Such errors can occur if the nurse is unfamiliar with the planning process. Table 9-5 illustrates these types of errors by showing incorrect and correct statements of nursing interventions.

The final column in the nursing care plan contains the projected outcome criteria previously identified. Listing the criteria on the nursing care plan gives a written indication of when the goal of care has been achieved, thus indicating when a particular nursing diagnosis is no longer relevant to the plan of care.

Assessment	Analysis Nursing diagnosis	Plan	Intervention	Evaluation
Weight loss: 15 lbs in 10 days. Eats only portion of meal due to full feeling immediately after beginning a meal	Potential alteration in nutrition: less than body requirements related to sensation of fullness c̄ meals	Maintain present weight 185 lbs	1. Weigh daily 2. Small frequent high calorie feedings 8-10-12-2-4-6	Weight remains 185 lbs. Consumes all food delivered on meal tray

Fig. 9-5 Five-column nursing care plan.

TABLE 9-4

Scientific Rationale for the Student Care Plan

Assessment	Analysis (Nursing Diagnosis)	Plan	Implementation	Scientific Rationale	Evaluation
Fever: greater than 102° R for 72 hours Incontinent of urine	Potential impairment of skin integrity	1. To reduce pressure on bony prominences	1. Primary nurse will turn client every 2 hours in the following sequence: 8 AM—supine 10 AM—left side 12 noon—prone 2 PM—right side Repeat, begin with supine position.	Critical time for skin tissue breakdown is between 1 and 2 hours of constant pressure.*	No skin breakdown noted. Skin remains dry.
Secretions draining from abdominal fistula		2. To avoid skin breakdown and the formation of decubitus ulcers	2a. Primary nurse or nursing assistant will massage bony prominences for 5 minutes after turning client.	Massage to bony prominences after relieving pressure increases circulation and nutrition to the affected areas.†	No skin breakdown noted. Skin remains dry.
Decreased skin turgor Comatose No skin breakdown noted			2b. All nursing personnel will keep client's skin dry at all times.	Moisture increases maceration of the skin and promotes bacterial growth.‡	

*Data from Berecek, K.H.: Etiology of decubitus ulcers, Nurs. Clin. North Am. **10**(1):160, 1975.
†Data from Gruis, M.L., and Innes, B.: Assessment essential to prevent sores, Am. J. Nurs. **76**: 1764, 1976.
‡Data from Kavchack-Keys, M.A.: Four proven steps for preventing decubitus ulcers, Nursing 77 **7**:60, 1977.

Sample Nursing Care Plan

A nursing care plan developed for Mr. Brown is shown in part in Table 9-6. The nursing care plan for Mr. Brown is individualized to his needs. In addition, the care plan is developed from the nursing diagnoses, priorities, and goals established during analysis. To illustrate the development of a nursing care plan, two of Mr. Brown's nursing diagnoses are shown.

Mr. Brown has frequently voiced concern over a medical diagnosis of cancer. The astute nurse recognizes his concern and plans nursing care and activity so that he receives prompt, correct information about the results of his laboratory and diagnostic tests.

Anticipating the needs of the client, referred to as anticipatory guidance, is the psychological and physical preparation of a client to help relieve fear and anxiety about an event or outcome that is expected to be stressful. Anticipating the physical, developmental, intellectual, emotional, social, and spiritual needs of the client can increase the client's participation in and cooperation with nursing care, help control the client's stress response, and provide an efficient and economical use of health care resources.

Preoperative teaching, shown on the nursing care plan, is an example of anticipatory guidance because it is designed to familiarize Mr. Brown with the surgical procedure and postoperative care in order to reduce his emotional stress. This preoperative teaching also anticipates a physiological need. Because of Mr. Brown's smoking history, his age, and an abdominal incision, he is at risk for postoperative respiratory complications. The preoperative teaching prepares him for the postoperative care and what is

TABLE 9-5

Frequent Errors in Writing Nursing Interventions

Type of Error	Incorrectly Stated Nursing Intervention	Correctly Stated Nursing Intervention
Failure to indicate what is to be done	Primary nurse will turn client every 2 hours.	Primary nurse will turn client every 2 hours, using the following schedule: 8 AM—supine 10 AM—left side 12 noon—prone 2 PM—right side Repeat sequence at 4 PM and 2 AM
Failure to indicate frequency	Primary nurse will observe client cough and deep breathe.	Primary nurse will observe client cough and deep breathe at 10 AM–2 PM–6 PM–10 PM.
Failure to indicate quantity	Primary nurse will provide hydrogen peroxide (H_2O_2) mouthwash to client every 2 hours while awake: 8-10-12-2-4-6-8-10.	Primary nurse will provide 50 ml of H_2O_2 mouthwash to client every 2 hours while awake: 8-10-12-2-4-6-8-10.
Failure to indicate method	Primary nurse will change client's dressing once a shift: 6 AM–2 PM–10 PM.	Primary nurse will replace client's dressing with Neosporin ointment to wound and two dry 4 × 4's secured with hypoallergenic tape once a shift: 2 PM–10 PM–6 AM.
Failure to indicate who will carry out the action	Irrigate nasogastric (NG) tube every 2 hours round the clock with 30 ml of normal saline (NS).	Primary nurse will irrigate NG tube every 2 hours round the clock with 30 ml NS.

expected of him, which increases the effectiveness of the postoperative nursing measures.

The nursing interventions designed for Mr. Brown include both present and future nursing actions so that the nursing care plan will reflect the continuing needs of the client. As Mr. Brown progresses through the postoperative course, the nursing interventions are revised according to changes in his needs.

Including the outcome criteria (evaluation column) in the nursing care plan provides all nurses caring for Mr. Brown with a measurable end point for termination of nursing care for a particular diagnosis.

Consultation with Other Health Care Professionals

Planning nursing care involves consultation with other members of the health care team. Consultation may occur at any step in the nursing process but is needed most often in the planning and intervention steps, because at these points the nurse is more likely to identify a problem requiring additional knowledge, skills, or resources. Consultation is a process in which the help of a specialist is sought to identify ways to handle problems in client management or the planning and implementation of programs. Consultation is based on the problem-solving approach, and the consultant is the stimulus for change.

In clinical nursing, consultation is used to solve problems in the delivery of nursing care or use of resources. Nurse consultants are most frequently approached for advice about difficult clinical problems. Nurses are consulted for their clinical expertise, patient education skills, or staff education skills.

Nurses also obtain consultations from other members of the health care team, such as physical therapists, nutritionists, and social workers. Again the consultant focuses on problems in nursing.

When to Consult

The need for consultation in nursing occurs when the nurse has identified a problem that cannot be

TABLE 9-6

Mr. Brown's Nursing Care Plan

Assessment	Analysis (Nursing Diagnosis)	Plan	Implementation	Evaluation (Projected Outcome)
Verbalizes fear of cancer	Potential ineffective coping related to fear of medical diagnosis	1. Client receives information about diagnostic tests promptly	1. Each morning provide Mr. Brown with the current information on his diagnostic tests or have physician talk to Mr. Brown.	1. Mr. Brown asks pertinent questions related to nursing care and diagnosis.
Became withdrawn following biopsy report		2. Preoperative teaching a. Turn, cough, and deep breathing	2a. Demonstrate to Mr. Brown turn, cough, and deep breathing techniques on 11/22, 10 AM–2 PM–8 PM.	2a. Mr. Brown correctly demonstrates procedure two times a shift on 11/23, 11/24, 11/25.
		b. Surgical procedure	2b. Discuss the surgical procedure with patient and wife, including (a) location of incision, (b) location of colostomy.	2b. Mr. Brown points out location of incision and colostomy.
		3. Enrolls in "I can cope" classes	3a. On fourth postoperative day (POD) discuss "I can cope" classes with Mr. Brown and wife.	3a. By 1 month after discharge, Mr. Brown and wife have inquired about "I can cope" classes.
40 pack-year history of smoking	Potential ineffective airway clearance postoperatively related to abdominal incision	1. Preoperative teaching: turn, cough, and deep breathing	1. Demonstrate turn, cough, and deep breathing.	1. Mr. Brown correctly demonstrates procedure.
Chest roentgenogram shows slight change of emphysema		2. Maintain a patent airway postoperatively	2. Turn, cough, and deep breathe every 2 hours around the clock on first and second POD.	2a. Lung fields clear on auscultation. 2b. Patient remains afebrile. 2c. Chest roentgenogram does not show infiltrate or consolidation.
Rales auscultated in lung fields				
Scheduled for abdominal surgery		3. Mr. Brown is given information on smoking cessation	3. On sixth POD provide Mr. Brown with smoking cessation literature and support groups.	3. Mr. Brown stops smoking 1 month postoperatively.

solved using the nurse's present knowledge, skills, and resources. The consultation process increases the nurse's knowledge about the identified problem and helps the nurse learn the necessary skills and resources needed to resolve the problem. After the consultation process the nurse may be able to resolve similar problems that arise in the future. For example, a nurse who encounters a patient with a recent colostomy might request a consultation from an enterostomal therapist to determine what materials are needed to clean the colostomy site and the specific techniques to use during the procedure.

Consultation is also used when the exact problem remains unclear. A consultant objectively entering a situation is able to more clearly assess and identify the exact nature of the problem, whether it be client oriented, personnel oriented, or equipment oriented. Often a nurse with consistent exposure to a problem area is less able to clearly identify and solve the problem because she is "unable to see the forest for the trees." A consultant who enters the environment unbiased can objectively identify the problem and outline a method for resolving it.

How to Consult

Once the nurse decides to consult, she initiates the consultation process. The first step in obtaining a consultant is to identify the general problem area if possible. Identification of the general problem will give the consultant a starting point for identifying the specific problem.

Second, the consultation should be directed to the appropriate professional, who may be another nurse or another member of the health care team. Consultations requested of the wrong individual delay problem solving and alter the quality of care being delivered to the client. For example, Mr. Brown had a nursing diagnosis of ineffective coping related to fear of medical diagnosis. Once the diagnosis of colon cancer was made, Mr. Brown's coping became increasingly ineffective until he became totally withdrawn and did not respond to the nursing interventions developed by the nursing staff. At this point there was a problem of ineffective coping, and the staff nurses were unable to develop a solution. The decision for a nursing consultation was made. The request for a consultation was directed to the oncology clinical nurse specialist because of the specialist's theoretical knowledge and clinical competence in cancer nursing, which would be used to develop nursing strategies to resolve Mr. Brown's ineffective coping.

Third, the nurse provides the consultant with pertinent information and resources that concern the problem area. The pertinent information includes a brief summary of the problem, methods used so far to resolve the problem, and outcome of those methods. Additional resources can include the patient's medical record, nurses and other members of the health team, and the client's family.

Fourth, it is important that the nurse not bias the consultant. The consultant is in the clinical setting to identify and resolve a nursing problem, and biasing the consultant can hinder problem resolution. Bias can be avoided by not overloading the consultant with subjective and emotional conclusions about the client and the problem. For example, saying that a client is acting "childish" or is "not really having a problem" can bias a consultant who is trying to identify and resolve a particular nursing problem.

Fifth, the nurse requesting consultation should be available to discuss the consultant's findings and recommendations. When a consultant is requested, the nurse provides a private, comfortable atmosphere in which the consultant and the client can meet. However, this does not mean that the nurse becomes totally absent from the environment. A common mistake is turning the whole problem over to the consultant. The consultant is not there to take away the problem, but rather to teach the nurse how to resolve the problem. Thus the nurse requesting assistance should request the consultation for a day when she is scheduled to work and at a time when distractions are minimal. Thus the consultant is available to the nurse, and the nurse is also available to the consultant.

Finally, the nurse incorporates the consultant's recommendations into the nursing care plan. The consultant's role is to analyze the problem and advise the nurse on the best possible solution. The nurse then integrates these suggestions into the nursing care plan. The success of the consultant's advice depends on the nurse's implementation of the problem-solving technique suggested by the consultant in the care of the client.

The use of consultants is a valuable adjunct to nursing care. In clinical nursing practice even a competent and experienced nurse encounters problems that are beyond her knowledge or experience. The professional and competent nurse recognizes her limitations, seeks appropriate consultation, and learns from the consultant's findings and recommendations.

Summary

The planning component of the nursing process results in the development of the nursing care plan, which details the selected nursing interventions and the appropriate evaluation criteria for each client. The nursing student learns the process of planning care in both the educational and the clinical settings. Although the format of the nursing care plan varies from one educational institution to another and from one health care setting to another, the student nurse will encounter both the student care plan and the institutional care plan throughout the educational process.

Planning nursing care involves a cognitive and a written process. The student learns how to solve a client's health care problems by selecting appropriate nursing interventions. In addition, the student learns how to communicate the client's health care needs through the written nursing care plan. The individual nursing care plans developed for clients are the result of the nurse's knowledge and expertise, as well as knowledge and expertise gained through use of consultants.

Adequate planning of nursing care results in the individualization, coordination, and continuity of nursing care. Planning establishes the framework of nursing care to be delivered during the fourth component of the nursing process, implementation.

KEY CONCEPTS

✓ During the planning component client goals are determined, priorities are established, projected outcomes of nursing care are developed, and a nursing care plan is written.

✓ Nuring care is planned and organized around specific nursing diagnoses, resulting in an individualized nursing care plan.

✓ The goal is the intended outcome of the nursing intervention.

✓ Goals include prevention and rehabilitation, as well as crisis or emergency needs of the client.

✓ Goal setting establishes a framework for the nursing care plan.

✓ Establishing priorities ranks the nursing diagnoses and goals in order of importance.

✓ The nurse begins the nursing care plan with the nursing diagnoses having the highest priority.

✓ Projected outcomes serve as a basis for the criteria that the nurse uses to evaluate the effectiveness of the nursing care plan.

✓ In general, nursing care plans include the nursing care problem, the goals, the specific actions by the nurse, and the projected client response to the nursing action.

✓ The nursing care plan is a written guideline for client care so that specific nursing care can be quickly grasped.

✓ The nursing care plan increases communication between nurses and facilitates the continuity of care from one nurse to another and from one health care setting to another.

✓ The development of an individualized care plan requires involvement of the family or significant others during the planning phase.

✓ Staff care plans may become part of a client's medical record.

KEY CONCEPTS, cont'd

✓ The nursing care plan is a method for teaching students how to transfer knowledge gained from nursing and medical literature and the classroom into practical experience.

✓ A scientific rationale is the reason, based on supporting literature, why a specific nursing action was chosen.

✓ Poorly written nursing care plans result in incomplete or inaccurate nursing care, lack of continuity among care givers, and poor use of resources.

✓ Correct nursing interventions include what is to be done, the frequency, the quantity, the method, and who is to carry out the intervention.

✓ Planning nursing care often involves consultation with other members of the health care team.

✓ The need for consultation in nursing occurs when the nurse identifies a problem that cannot be solved using the nurse's present knowledge, skills, and resources.

REFERENCES

Gordon, M.: Nursing diagnosis: process and application, New York, 1982, McGraw-Hill Book Co.

Little, D.E., and Carnevali, D.C.: Nursing care planning, ed. 3, Philadelphia, 1983, J.B. Lippincott Co.

ADDITIONAL READINGS

Caplan, G.: The theory and practice of mental health consultation, New York, 1970, Basic Books, Inc.

Hendrix, M.J., and LaGodna, G.E.: Consultation: a political process aimed at change. In Lancaster, J., and Lancaster, W., editors: Concepts for advanced nursing practice, St. Louis, 1982, The C.V. Mosby Co.

Mayers, M.G.: A systematic approach to the nursing care plan, ed. 2, New York, 1978, Appleton-Century-Crofts.

Yura, H., and Walsh, M.B.: The nursing process: assessing, planning, implementing, evaluating, ed. 3, New York, 1978, Appleton-Century-Crofts.

OBJECTIVES

Mastery of content in this chapter will enable the student to:

- Define the terms in the glossary.
- Discuss the differences between dependent, independent, and interdependent interventions.
- List and discuss the five steps of the implementation process.
- Describe the five different implementation methods.
- Select appropriate implementation methods for an assigned client.

GLOSSARY

activities of daily living   Activities usually performed in the course of a normal day in the client's life, such as eating, dressing, bathing, brushing the teeth, or grooming.

adherence   Process in which a client follows the prescriptions and recommendations of a regimen of care.

adverse reaction   Harmful or unintended effect of a medication, diagnostic test, or therapeutic intervention.

counseling   Implementation method that helps the client recognize and manage stress and that facilitates interpersonal relationships between the client and the family, significant others, or the health care team.

dependent intervention   Action based on the instruction or written orders of another professional.

independent intervention   Action pertaining to certain aspects of professional nursing practice that are encompassed by applicable licensure and law and require no supervision or direction from others.

interdependent intervention   Actions carried out by the nurse in collaboration with another health care professional.

lifesaving measure   Independent, dependent, or interdependent nursing intervention that is implemented when a client's physiological or psychological status is threatened.

nurse practice act   Statute enacted by the legislature of any of the states or by the appropriate officers of the districts or possessions.

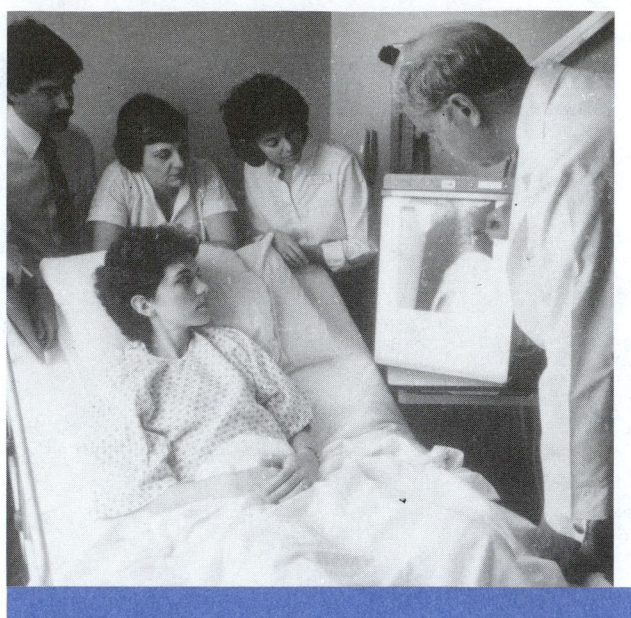

nursing intervention   Any act by a nurse that implements the nursing care plan or any specific objective of the plan.

preventive nursing action   Interventions directed toward preventing illness and promoting health to avoid the need for primary, secondary, or tertiary health care.

protocol   Written plan specifying the procedures to be followed during an assessment or in providing treatment for a client.

standing order   Written document containing rules, policies, procedures, regulations, and orders for the conduct of client care in various stipulated clinical settings.

teaching   Implementation method used to present correct principles, procedures, and techniques of health care; to inform the client about his health status; and to refer the client and family to appropriate health or social resources in the community.

teaching-learning process   Interaction between the teacher and learner in which specific learning objectives are achieved.

technique   Method followed in performing a specific procedure such as administering medications, changing a patient's dressing, or inserting a Foley catheter.

10 | *Implementation*

In theory the implementation of the nursing care plan follows the planning component of the nursing process. However, in practice settings implementation may begin directly after nursing assessment. Immediate implementation is necessary when the nurse identifies emergency needs of the client, such as a threat to the client's physiological status (for example, a cardiac arrest), psychological status (for example, a sudden death of a loved one), or socioeconomic status (for example, sudden loss of a home in a fire).

Implementation is a category of nursing behavior in which the actions necessary for accomplishing the health care plan are initiated and completed. Implementing includes the nurse's performing or assisting in the performance of the client's activities of daily living, counseling and teaching the client or client's family, giving care to achieve therapeutic goals and to facilitate the achievement of the client's health goals, supervising and evaluating the work of staff members, and recording and exchanging information relevant to the client's continued health care.

The purpose of implementation is to carry out the nursing care plan developed in the previous component of the nursing process. A nursing intervention is any act by a nurse that implements the nursing care plan or any specific objective of the plan. The client may require intervention in the form of support, medication, treatment for the current condition, or treatment to prevent future health problems.

Like other components of the nursing process, implementation is continuous and interacts with the other components. During implementation the nurse reassesses the client, modifies the plan of care, and rewrites projected outcomes as necessary. To complete the implementation component effectively, the nurse is knowledgeable about types of interventions, the implementation process, and specific implementation methods.

Types of Nursing Interventions

There are three general types of nursing interventions: dependent, independent, and interdependent.

Dependent Interventions

A dependent nursing intervention is based on the instruction or written orders of another professional. Commonly, dependent nursing interventions are delineated by a physician's order. Examples of dependent nursing interventions include following physician's orders as to type, dosage, and frequency of a medication; completing an invasive procedure, such as inserting a Foley catheter; and requesting specific diagnostic and laboratory tests. Each dependent nursing intervention involves specific nursing responsibilities.

When administering medications, the nurse is responsible for knowing the classification of the drug, its physiological action, the normal dosage, the side effects, and nursing interventions related to the drug's actions or side effects.

Ms. Kline is caring for a preoperative client, Mrs. Wells, who has the following medication order: "Atropine sulfate 0.4 mg IM at 8:00 AM today." The nursing interventions

189

associated with the administration of the medication depend on the order written by the physician. Ms. Kline recalls that atropine is an anticholinergic drug and that the desired preoperative effect is to control salivation, bronchial secretions, and rhinorrhea during surgical anesthesia. She consults a resource to determine that 0.4 mg is a normal preoperative dose. Ms. Kline prepares Mrs. Wells for the injection and tells Mrs. Wells to expect an increase in thirst caused by medication. After administration of the drug she observes the client for any side effects such as flushing, tachycardia, restlessness, or disorientation, and she records in the client's medical record that the drug has been administered.

This example illustrates the nursing responsibilities associated with carrying out a dependent intervention of a medication order. Chapter 32 discusses in detail the medication procedure and the associated nursing skills and responsibilities.

With an invasive procedure the nurse is responsible for knowing when a specific procedure is necessary, the clinical skills necessary to complete the procedure, the expected outcome of the procedure, possible side effects of the procedure, adequate preparation of the client, and proper communication of the results of the procedure.

Ms. Myer is caring for Mr. Smith, who underwent abdominal surgery 3 days before. Ms. Myer reviews the physician's orders and notes the following order: "Insert nasogastric (NG) tube if abdomen becomes distended and bowel sounds are absent. Attach NG tube to low Gomco suction and irrigate tube every 2 hours with 30 ml normal saline (NS)." Six hours later Ms. Myer assesses Mr. Smith and observes that he is complaining of nausea, his abdomen is distended, and bowel sounds are absent. A review of Mr. Smith's record indicates that he has had 800 ml of clear liquids during the previous 12 hours. Through the assessment process Ms. Myer has determined that Mr. Smith needs to have a nasogastric tube inserted. She then implements the skills to complete the procedure: gathering proper equipment, explaining the procedure to the client, positioning the client, and inserting the tube. The desired outcome of the procedure is a return of gastric contents from the nasogastric tube into the Gomco suction receptacle. Following the procedure Ms. Myer reassesses Mr. Smith and observes that his nausea and bowel sounds remain absent.

This example demonstrates the nurse's responsibility in completing a dependent intervention of an invasive procedure. Chapter 38 details the procedure of inserting a nasogastric tube, as well as other nursing procedures associated with nutrition.

When a specific diagnostic or laboratory test is ordered by a physician, the nurse is responsible for scheduling the test, preparing the client, and knowing the normal findings and the nursing implications associated with the test.

The evening nurse, Mr. Fellows, following physician's orders, has scheduled a client for a barium enema the next morning. His immediate responsibilities are to explain the procedure to the client, administer cleansing enemas the night before, ensure that the client is not served breakfast in the morning, and record pertinent information in the medical record.

In the morning a second nurse, Ms. Green, RN, is responsible for answering any of the client's questions, making sure that breakfast has not been served, administering the third enema, sending the client to the radiology department for the procedure, and assessing the client after the procedure. Ms. Green records the following information in the medical record:

7:30 AM	500 ml normal saline enema, clear return with no evidence of solid fecal material
8:00 AM	breakfast held until after barium enema
9:15 AM	to special procedures in radiology via wheelchair
10:15 AM	return from barium enema, breakfast served
1:00 PM	ii Ducolax tablets PO to client. Client instructed to notify nurse when he has a bowel movement or to notify the nurse if he does not have a bowel movement within 36 hours.

The preceding example illustrates the nurse's responsibility in preparing a client for a diagnostic test. Chapter 40 discusses in detail the barium enema and other diagnostic tests related to bowel elimination.

While it is not within the legal practice of nursing for the nurse to prescribe and order medications, invasive procedures, and diagnostic tests, it is within the practice of nursing to complete such orders. Administering medications, implementing an invasive procedure, and preparing a client for diagnostic tests are dependent nursing interventions. The student nurse becomes familiar with dependent nursing interventions throughout the educational process. As the student continues to practice, the awareness of a professional nurse's responsibility in dependent interventions grows.

When encountering an order for a dependent intervention, the nurse does not automatically implement the order. She stops to determine whether the requested order is appropriate for the client. Every nurse encounters an inappropriate or incorrect order at some time. The nurse with a strong knowledge base will recognize the error and seek clarification of the order. Being able to recognize incorrect orders is of particular importance when administering medications or implementing procedures. An error can occur in writing the order or transcribing the order to the Kardex or medication card. Clarifying an order is competent nursing practice, and it protects the client as well as the health care delivery system. The nurse who carries out an incorrect or inappropriate order is as much in error as the person who wrote or transcribed the original order. A nurse who carries out an inappropriate order is liable for any complications resulting from the error. Chapter 17 explains such legal issues affecting nursing practice.

Independent Interventions

Independent interventions involve certain aspects of professional nursing practice that are encompassed by applicable licensure and law and require no supervision or direction from others. Examples of independent interventions include assisting the client with activities of daily living, giving skin care to prevent the formation of a decubitus ulcer, offering health education, counseling clients and their families, and supervising and evaluating the care of others.

Independent nursing interventions do not require a physician's order or an order from another professional. Physicians frequently include in their written orders the specifics of independent nursing interventions. However, according to the nurse practice acts in a majority of states, nursing actions pertaining to activities of daily living, health education, health promotion, and counseling are in the domain of nursing practice. These acts delineate the legal scope of the practice of nursing within the geographical boundaries of the jurisdiction (see Chapter 17).

In Chapter 9 a sample nursing care plan was developed for Mr. Brown (see Table 9-6). All the nursing interventions in this care plan are independent nursing interventions. For each independent intervention the nurse is responsible for assessing the need for the intervention, obtaining the necessary knowledge and skills to carry out the intervention, and evaluating the client's response to the intervention.

Interdependent Interventions

Interdependent interventions are carried out by the nurse in collaboration with another health care professional. One type of interdependent intervention is following activities listed in a protocol. A protocol is a written plan specifying the procedures to be followed during an assessment or in providing treatment for a client. For example, nurses providing primary care for a caseload of clients in an outpatient setting follow a protocol. In such a setting the nurse assesses the client and identifies abnormalities. The established protocol delineates the conditions the nurse is permitted to treat and the types of treatment the nurse is permitted to administer.

Ms. Roth provides primary care for a caseload of 20 clients with chronic obstructive pulmonary disease (COPD) in an outpatient setting. One of her protocols is the treatment of an exacerbation of bronchitis. During the physical assessment the client describes or has the following symptoms:

1. Cough, fever less than 101° F
2. Change in sputum color to yellow or green
3. "Coldlike" symptoms
4. Rales on auscultation
5. Infiltration noted on chest roentgenogram

The following treatment prescribed by a physician is instituted by the nurse:

1. Rest
2. Increased fluids
3. Use of a humidifier
4. Increased chest physiotherapy
5. Aspirin X gr 4 hours for fever
6. Ampicillin 500 mg q.i.d. for 10 days by mouth; if allergic to penicillin, tetracycline 250 mg q.i.d. for 10 days by mouth

Another example of an interdependent interaction is a standing order. A standing order is a written document containing rules, policies, procedures, regulations, and orders for the conduct of client care in various stipulated clinical settings. Standing orders are commonly found in critical care settings, in which the nurse continually assesses the client's emergency needs and intervenes appropriately. An example of such a standing order is one that specifies a certain drug for an irregular heart rhythm. When the critical care nurse assesses the client and identifies the irregular rhythm, she gives the appropriate medication without first notifying the physician. Standing orders are also common in the community health setting, in which the nurse encounters situations that do not permit her to contact a physician immediately. Thus standing orders and protocols give the nurse the legal protection to intervene appropriately in the client's best interest. The nursing interventions are interdependent because the implementation of the nursing action is specified by the written physician's orders delineated in the protocol. The written orders name the condition and prescribe the action to be taken by the nurse.

■ ■ ■ ■ ■

The nursing interventions implemented during the fourth component of the nursing process can include dependent, independent, and interdependent interventions. The nurse who implements any intervention has the responsibility to obtain correct theoretical knowledge and to develop the clinical competency necessary to carry out the intervention. The nursing responsibility is equally great for all types of interventions.

Implementation Process

The implementation component of the nursing process has five steps: reassessing the client, reviewing and modifying the existing nursing care plan, identifying areas of assistance, implementing nursing strategies, and communicating nursing strategies.

Reassessing the Client

As has been described previously, assessment is a continuous process. Each time a nurse interacts with a client she is gathering data that reflect the client's physical, developmental, intellectual, emotional, social and spiritual needs. In the nursing process the student nurse begins to reassess the client's needs each time the client and student interact. Whenever new data are assessed and a new client need is identified, the nurse modifies the nursing care.

During the initial phase of implementation the nurse reassesses the client. This is a partial assessment and may focus on one dimension of the client or on one body system. The purpose of the reassessment is to gather data that can affect the implementation or outcome of nursing care.

A nursing care plan has been developed for Mrs. Coyle (Table 10-1). The nursing diagnosis, "Impaired urinary elimination related to perineal swelling following vaginal delivery of 8-pound, 15-ounce baby girl," provided the focus for the plan. Before inserting the straight catheter, the nurse conducts reassessment to determine that Mrs. Coyle has not voided spontaneously, for if she has, the catheterization procedure would no longer be appropriate.

The reassessment phase of the implementation component thus provides a mechanism for the nurse to determine that the proposed nursing action is appropriate for the client's level of wellness.

Reviewing and Modifying the Existing Nursing Care Plan

Although the nursing care plan was developed according to the health care needs identified during assessment and the nursing diagnoses then established, changes in the client's status can necessitate modification of the planned nursing care. Before beginning the care of a client, the nurse reviews the plan of care and compares the established plan with the client's current needs. The review is done to validate the stated nursing diagnoses and to determine if the nursing interventions are the most appropriate for the clinical situation. If the nurse discovers that the client's status has changed and the nursing diagnosis and the related nursing interventions are no longer appropriate, the nursing care plan needs to be modified.

Modification of the existing nursing care plan includes several steps. First, the data in the assessment column are revised to reflect the client's current status. New data entered in the nursing care plan should be dated to inform other members of the health team when the client's status changed. Whenever possible, new data should be recorded in a different color to alert other care givers to changes in a client's status.

Second, the nursing diagnoses are revised. Nursing diagnoses that are no longer relevant are deleted, and new nursing diagnoses are added. Because the client's status and health care needs have changed, the priorities, goals, and projected outcome criteria need revision. These revisions are also dated and noted in a different color on the nursing care plan.

TABLE 10-1

Nursing Care Plan for Mrs. Coyle

Assessment	Nursing Diagnosis	Plan	Implementation	Evaluation
1. Has not voided in 10 hours 2. Fluid intake for last 8 hours 2400 ml 3. Patient status: she "feels the urge to void" 4. Bladder palpable to 2 cm below umbilicus	Impaired urinary elimination related to perineal swelling following vaginal delivery of 8-pound, 15-ounce, baby girl	Promote excretion of urine	The primary nurse to 1. Insert straight catheter, using sterile technique, if patient has not voided in 8 hours and bladder is palpable	1. 1000 ml of clear yellow urine returned via straight catheter 2. Bladder not palpable 3. Patient no longer has sensation to void

Third, the specific implementation methods are revised to correspond to the new nursing diagnoses. This revision of the expanded proposed methods for implementing nursing care reflects the client's present health status. The new implementation methods indicate the client's greater independence from or dependence on nursing. In addition, the revised implementation can include the client's specific needs for health care resources.

Finally, the evaluation section of the nursing care plan is changed to correspond to the other modifications in the plan. Changes in the evaluation criteria further project the desired level of wellness for the client and indicate when the need has been resolved and the nursing diagnosis is no longer relevant.

In Chapter 9 a preoperative nursing care plan was developed for Mr. Brown. As he progressed through the postoperative period, his nursing needs changed. New data were noted in blue ink and dated. The nurse made modifications in the nursing care plan for one nursing diagnosis: potential ineffective airway clearance postoperatively related to abdominal incision (Table 10-2).

On the second postoperative day the nurse assessed Mr. Brown and noted decreased chest wall movements, basilar rales, and elevated temperature (101° F). Mr. Brown had a standing order for a chest roentgenogram, which was taken immediately and revealed a right lower lobe atelectasis. The nursing diagnosis was revised to read "Ineffective airway clearance related to abdominal incision." The plan of "maintaining a patent airway" was still appropriate. Specific

TABLE 10-2

Modified Nursing Care Plan for Mr. Brown

Assessment	Analysis	Plan	Implementation	Evaluation
Has smoked two packs/day for 20 years; chest roentgenogram shows slight change of emphysema; rales auscultated in lung field; scheduled for abdominal surgery	Potential ineffective airway clearance postoperatively related to abdominal incision	Maintain a patent airway	1. Mr. Brown demonstrate turn, cough, and deep breath.	1. Mr. Brown correctly demonstrates procedure.
12/2	12/2		12/2	
Decreased chest wall movements; rales in bases, does not clear with coughing	Ineffective airway clearance postoperatively related to abdominal incision	Mr. Brown is given information on smoking cessation	1. Nurse administers chest physiotherapy to all lobes of the lung: 8-12-4-8-12-4. 2. Mr. Brown coughs and deep breathes every 2 hours around the clock.	1. Lung fields are clear on auscultation. 2. Patient becomes afebrile. 3. Chest roentgenogram demonstrates atelectasis resolving.
Chest roentgenogram shows right lower lobe atelectasis; 101° R			3. Nurse to suction nasotracheally every 2 hours if patient is unable to cough productively.	
			1. On sixth postoperative day the nurse provides Mr. Brown with smoking cessation literature and support groups.	1. Mr. Brown stops smoking 1 month postoperatively.

nursing interventions were developed to assist in achieving a patent airway. Finally, the projected evaluation criteria were rewritten to reflect the desired level of wellness and to indicate when the need had been resolved.

The astute nurse is sensitive to the changes in the client's status and readily incorporates the changes into the nursing care plan. The health status of clients is dynamic and continuously changing. Therefore the plan of care established for a client needs to be flexible to incorporate the necessary changes. An out-of-date or incorrect nursing care plan compromises the quality of nursing care being delivered to a client, whereas review and modification of the existing nursing care plan enable the nurse to provide nursing care that meets the client's current needs.

Identifying Areas of Assistance

Most nursing situations require the nurse to seek assistance of some type. The assistance can fall in three categories: additional personnel, additional knowledge, and additional nursing skills. Before implementing nursing care, the nurse evaluates the plan to determine the need for assistance and the type of assistance required.

Situations requiring additional personnel vary. For example, a nurse assigned to care for an overweight, immobilized client may need additional personnel to help turn, transfer, and position the client because of the physical work involved. Advanced education or years of nursing experience will not enable this nurse to care independently for such a client. The nurse also needs to determine when the personnel are needed. If the client is to be turned and repositioned every 2 hours, additional personnel will be needed every 2 hours. The nurse then must determine how many persons are needed and must discuss the need for assistance with potential resources. Finally, the nurse needs to take time to plan the nursing care so that the additional personnel do not become overburdened.

Additional personnel are also required when a client's health status declines or when the number of clients in a unit increases. In both situations the required level of nursing care is too much for one nurse to deliver safely.

Mr. Douglas is assigned to care for two postoperative patients, Mr. West and Mrs. Jade. Two hours into the shift Mr. West begins to hemorrhage and goes into shock. Mr. Douglas spends the next hour stabilizing Mr. West's condition. At this point he reviews the care plan for Mrs. Jade and the new care plan for Mr. West. The nurse's assessment of the situation is that for next 2 hours he will need to spend all of his time with Mr. West. He approaches his supervisor with this assessment and requests additional help for the next 2 hours.

Some nursing situations require additional knowledge and skills as well as additional personnel. A nurse needs additional knowledge when administering a new medication or implementing a new procedure. Such information can be obtained from a hospital's formulary or procedure book. If the nurse still is uncertain about the new medication or procedure, other members of the health care team can be consulted.

Because of the continual growth of the health care professions and the related technology, a nurse may find herself in a situation in which she lacks the skills needed to carry out a procedure. When this occurs the nurse should obtain as much information as possible about the procedure from the current literature and the agency's procedure book. Next she collects all the equipment necessary for the procedure. Finally, she seeks out another nurse who has completed the procedure correctly and safely and asks for assistance. The assistance can come from another staff nurse, a supervisor, an educator, or a nurse specialist.

Ms. Jacobs, a student nurse, is caring for Mrs. Sutter, who is receiving intravenous (IV) antibiotics. During the morning the IV catheter infiltrates into the subcutaneous tissues. Ms. Jacobs discontinues the nonfunctioning IV catheter and notifies the physician. The physician asks her to insert a new catheter. She has never inserted an IV catheter. First she looks up the procedure in her nursing textbook and hospital procedure book. She learns that it is a sterile procedure and that the purpose is to insert the catheter into a vein so that fluids and drugs can be given intravenously. Ms. Jacobs also learns the equipment that is needed:

1. Sterile intravenous catheter
2. Sterile intravenous tubing
3. Sterile intravenous solution, as ordered
4. Bacteriostatic ointment
5. 4 × 4 dressings
6. Nonallergenic tape
7. Alcohol swabs

She collects the equipment and seeks out her nursing instructor. She tells her instructor what she has learned about the procedure. The instructor first answers all her questions and confirms correct knowledge and principles. Next her instructor reviews the function and purpose of all the equipment and each step of the procedure. Finally, Ms. Jacobs and her instructor return to Mrs. Sutter's room, and Ms. Jacobs inserts the IV catheter. After the procedure is completed, the instructor reviews the total procedure with her, identifying strengths and offering suggestions for completing the procedure again.

Requesting assistance occurs frequently in all types of nursing practice. Asking for assistance is a learning process that continues throughout the nurse's educational experiences and into the nurse's professional development.

Implementing Nursing Strategies

The nurse implements nursing strategies to achieve the goals of care. The nurse can select various methods to achieve the goals of nursing care:

1. Assisting in the performance of the activities of daily living
2. Counseling and education
3. Giving care to achieve the therapeutic goals for the client
4. Giving care to facilitate attainment of therapeutic goals by the client
5. Supervising and evaluating the work of other staff members

The nurse is responsible for knowing when one of these methods is preferred over another and for having the necessary theoretical knowledge and psychomotor skills to implement each method. A later section introduces the general theoretical information for each method and refers to subsequent chapters, which detail the necessary theoretical and psychomotor skills.

Communicating Nursing Strategies

Nursing strategies are communicated in writing or verbally. When written, nursing strategies are incorporated into the nursing care plan and the client's medical record. The nursing care plan usually reflects the proposed nursing strategies. After the strategies are implemented, pertinent information is written in the client's record. Usually the information incorporated in the record includes a brief description of the nursing assessment, the specific procedure, and the client's response to nursing care.

A brief description of pertinent assessment findings in the client's medical record validates the need for a specific nursing intervention. Writing the time and the details of the intervention document that the procedure was completed. A summary of the client's response to the procedure evaluates the effectiveness of the procedure.

Ms. Nettle, a student nurse, determines that her 2-day postoperative client is diaphoretic and has a pulse of 100 and a blood pressure of 130/90. She asks her client if he is comfortable and notes his complaint of incisional pain. After administering 75 mg of meperidine hydrochloride IM as ordered for pain, she includes the following information in the client's medical record:

10:00 AM   Client diaphoretic, pulse 100, BP 130/90, incisional dressing dry
10:15 AM   75 mg meperidine hydrochloride IM

10:45 AM   Client skin dry, pulse 76, BP 110/80, client relaxing with book, states pain relief

Nursing strategies are also communicated verbally from one nurse to another or to other health professionals. Nurses commonly communicate verbally when changing shifts, transferring a client to another unit, or discharging a client to another health agency. Whether the nursing strategy is communicated verbally or in writing, the language should be clear, concise, and to the point. Chapter 15 discusses communication skills necessary in nursing practice, and Chapter 12 describes skills needed to record pertinent information in the client's medical record.

Implementation Methods

The nurse carries out the nursing care plan by using several implementation methods. For example, the client with a nursing diagnosis of "impaired mobility related to bilateral arm casts" may require assistance in performing activities of daily living. The client who is coping inadequately because of fear of a medical diagnosis requires counseling as a method of nursing action. The client with a diagnosed knowledge deficit needs interventions through health education. The client who is totally immobilized or is disoriented requires nursing interventions that provide total client care. Yet another method of implementation of the nursing care plan involves the supervision and evaluation of other members of the health care team.

For each nursing diagnosis the nurse is able to identify the need for one specific implementation method rather than another. Each method of implementation includes specific theoretical knowledge and clinical skills.

Assisting with Activities of Daily Living

The activities of daily living (ADLs) are those activities usually performed in the course of a normal day in the client's life, such as eating, dressing, bathing, brushing the teeth, or grooming. Conditions that result in the need for assistance with ADLs can be acute, chronic, temporary, permanent, or rehabilitative. An acute disease is characterized by symptoms that are usually severe and that are present for a relatively short period of time. An episode of acute disease results in (1) recovery to a state of health and activity comparable to the client's state before the disease, (2) passage into a chronic phase of the disease, or (3) death. For example, the postoperative client is unable to complete ADLs independently because of the acute health problem, surgery. As the client progresses through the postoperative period, he gradually depends less on nurses for completing ADLs.

A chronic disease persists for a longer period than an acute disease. Although the symptoms of chronic disease are usually less severe than those of the acute phase of the same disease, chronic disease may result in complete or partial disability. A client with partial paralysis following a cerebrovascular accident has a chronic impairment that requires long-term assistance with ADLs.

The client's need for assistance with ADLs may be temporary, permanent, or rehabilitative. In the case of temporary assistance with ADLs there is a specific time period during which the client needs assistance. A client with impaired mobility because of bilateral arm casts has a temporary need for assistance. After removal of the casts the client will gradually assume responsibility for ADLs. A client who has a total self-care deficit related to an injury high in the cervical spinal cord has a permanent need for assistance. Because of the client's spinal cord injury it is unrealistic to plan a rehabilitation program with the goal that the client will be able independently to complete all ADLs. This client may have a rehabilitative need for assistance with ADLs; that is, through rehabilitation the client will learn new ways to perform certain ADLs, thus becoming more independent and decreasing his self-care deficit.

Through the nursing assessment the nurse collects data that verify the need for assistance with ADLs. As the nurse analyzes the data, she formulates nursing diagnoses related to such assistance.

For example, if the nurse is meeting the client's nutritional needs, she must be able to draw from the knowledge base of nutrition. In addition, the nurse needs specific psychomotor skills to feed the client adequately and safely. If the client requires bathing and grooming, the nurse uses skills related to proper hygiene measures. The essential knowledge and skills that the nurse uses in carrying out ADLs for clients are detailed in Chapters 35 and 38.

Counseling and Teaching

Counseling is an implementation method that helps the client recognize and manage stress and that facilitates interpersonal relationships between the client and the family, significant others, or the health care team. Nurses provide counseling to help the client accept the actual or impending changes that result from stress. Counseling is emotional, intellectual, and psychological support (Duff and Hollingshead, 1968). Clients and their families in need of nursing counseling are those who have "normal" adjustment difficulties to change and are upset or frustrated at the beginning of counseling, but who are not psychologically disabled (McGowan and Schmidt, 1962). Clients who are psychologically disabled require counseling by nurses specializing in psychiatric nursing, social workers, psychiatrists, or psychologists.

Clients and their families or significant others needing counseling support include clients who must adjust their life-style patterns, such as stopping smoking, reducing weight, or decreasing their activity levels. Clients coping with chronic or disabling diseases require counseling to help them accept changes in life-style or body image as the disease progresses. During life-threatening illnesses, clients and particularly their families or significant others need counseling support to cope with the possibility of death.

The activity of counseling is closely aligned to teaching. Both teaching and counseling involve using communication skills to result in a change in the client. However, with counseling the change results in the development of new attitudes and feelings, whereas in teaching the focus of change is an intellectual growth or the acquiring of new knowledge or psychomotor skills (Redman, 1984).

Teaching is an implementation method used to present correct principles, procedures, and techniques of health care to the client, to inform the client about his health status, and to refer the client and family to appropriate health or social resources in the community. As a nursing responsibility, teaching is implemented in all health care settings. The nurse is responsible for assessing the learning needs of the client and is accountable for the quality of education that is delivered.

The teaching-learning process is an interaction between the teacher and learner in which specific learning objectives are achieved (Redman, 1984). The teaching-learning process provides the organizational structure and framework for client education. The teaching-learning process is much like the basic nursing process but has four components: assessment, planning, implementation, and evaluation.

During assessment the nurse determines the client's learning needs and readiness to learn. In planning, the nurse and the client establish the learning goals. Implementation is the initiation of the teaching strategies designed to achieve the learning goal. Finally, evaluation measures the learning that has occurred. The purpose of the teaching-learning process is to develop and implement a teaching plan that is individualized for the client's needs, level of knowledge, and learning resources.

Both counseling and teaching require theoretical knowledge and practical experience. The nurse who is beginning clinical practice needs to have a background in communication skills (see Chapter 15) to implement counseling or teaching. The use of the teaching method also requires the nurse to have an in-depth knowledge of the teaching-learning process (see Chapter 16).

Giving Care to Achieve the Therapeutic Goals for the Client

To achieve the therapeutic goals for the client, the nurse initiates interventions to compensate for adverse reactions, uses precautionary and preventive measures in providing care, applies correct techniques in administering care and preparing the client for special procedures, and initiates lifesaving measures in emergency situations. The following sections briefly discuss the nursing interventions in these areas. The specific knowledge and skills needed to carry out these nursing procedures are detailed in subsequent chapters to which the student is referred.

COMPENSATION FOR ADVERSE REACTIONS

An adverse reaction is a harmful or unintended effect of a medication, diagnostic test, or therapeutic intervention. Adverse reactions can follow independent, dependent, or interdependent nursing interventions. Nursing actions that compensate for adverse reactions are those that either reduce or counteract the adverse reaction. As the nurse intervenes to compensate for an adverse reaction, she uses her knowledge about the potential undesired effects. For example, when administering a medication, the nurse understands the known and potential side effects of the drug. Following administration of the medication the nurse assesses the client for any side effects. The nurse should be aware of drugs that can counteract the side effects of a medication administered. For example, a client may have an unknown hypersensitivity to penicillin. Hives develop after three doses of penicillin have been administered. The nurse records the reaction, stops administration of the drug, and administers an antipruritic to relieve the itching from the hives and an antihistamine to reduce the allergic response to penicillin.

In caring for a client who is undergoing or has undergone a particular diagnostic test, the nurse uses her understanding of the test and its potential adverse effects. For example, a client has not had a bowel movement in the 24 hours since he had a barium enema. Since a bowel impaction is a potential side effect of a barium enema, the nurse administers increased fluids, gives a stool-softening medication, and instructs the patient to let the nursing personnel know if he has a bowel movement or becomes uncomfortable.

Therapeutic interventions may also have potential harmful side effects.

Ms. Rice, the nurse, assesses that Mr. Allen has a small area of skin breakdown. Ms. Rice develops interventions designed to prevent further skin breakdown and to promote wound healing for Mr. Allen. She plans a heat lamp treatment to the skin for 20 minutes twice a day, selects the wattage for the bulb of the lamp, places the lamp 24 inches from the client's skin, and plans to check the client after 10 minutes. When reassessing the client's skin, Ms. Rice finds that there are no adverse effects of the treatment and resumes the treatment for another 10 minutes. After the second 10 minutes of treatment the nurse notices that the skin is reddened and the area of breakdown has increased. To counteract the increased skin breakdown, the nurse discontinues the treatment and institutes another skin care measure to reduce skin breakdown and promote wound healing.

Although adverse effects are not common, they do occur. The nurse learns the potential side effects, is able to recognize the presence of an adverse reaction, and is able to intervene accordingly. The medication process includes specific steps designed to reduce the chance of error when administering medications (see Chapter 32). Likewise, diagnostic procedures related to bowel elimination have specific nursing implications for reducing the occurrence of an adverse reaction (see Chapter 40). The application of heat as a nursing technique has specific procedures to limit the development of any side effects (see Chapter 48).

PREVENTIVE MEASURES

Preventive nursing actions are directed toward preventing illness and promoting health to avoid the need for primary, secondary, or tertiary health care. Prevention includes such nursing actions as assessment and promotion of the client's health potential application of prescribed measures such as immunizations, health teaching, early diagnosis and treatment, and development of rehabilitation potential.

In the case of a client who has a hypersensitivity to penicillin, the nurse can implement several preventive measures. First, the nurse indicates in the client's medical record that he is allergic to penicillin. Second, the nurse informs the client and his family of the need for a Medic Alert bracelet and teaches them actions that they should take if the client is given penicillin again.

Preventive nursing actions are one type of intervention used to meet the therapeutic goals for the client. Through preventive actions the nurse is able to help the client attain the highest level of wellness.

CORRECT TECHNIQUES IN ADMINISTERING CARE AND PREPARING A CLIENT FOR PROCEDURES

The administration of nursing care requires the nurse to be experienced in various techniques. A technique is the method followed in performing a specific procedure such as administering medications, changing a client's dressing, or inserting a Foley catheter. Client care, particularly in the hospital setting, involves many techniques. Every procedure that the nurse does for the client is carried out by a specific method.

To carry out a procedure, the nurse must be knowledgeable about the procedure itself, when it is needed, how to do it, and the expected outcome. In a hospital the nurse is required to complete many procedures each day. Some of these procedures might be new to the nurse. Before entering into a new procedure the nurse assesses her competencies and determines the need for assistance, new knowledge, or new skills.

LIFESAVING MEASURES

A lifesaving measure is an independent, dependent, or interdependent nursing intervention implemented when a client's physiological or psychological state is threatened. The purpose of the lifesaving measure is to restore physiological or psychological equilibrium. Such measures include administering emergency medications, instituting cardiopulmonary resuscitation (CPR), restraining a confused or violent client, and obtaining immediate counseling from a crisis center for a severely anxious client.

The initiation of lifesaving measures is an essential component of nursing practice. As with any procedure the nurse must be knowledgeable about the lifesaving procedure itself, when it is necessary, how to do it, and the expected outcome. If an inexperienced nurse happens on a situation requiring emergency measures, the proper nursing action is to get an experienced professional.

Giving Care to Facilitate the Client's Attainment of Health Goals

The nurse facilitates the attainment of health goals by providing an environment conducive to attaining the client's health care goals, adjusting care in accordance with the client's expressed or implied needs, stimulating and motivating the client, thereby enabling him to achieve self-care and independence, and encouraging the client to accept care or adhere to the treatment regimen. In each of the nursing interventions the nurse and the client work together to meet the goals that they developed during the analysis component. In some of the interventions the nurse assumes a more active role, and in others she assumes a more passive role.

Nurses have the capacity to create a health care environment conducive to achieving the client's goals. Ideally the nurse develops an environment that provides the client with adequate privacy for his basic needs and that allows him to feel safe and free to interact with the health care team. An early step in creating an appropriate environment is to orient the client and his family to the health care agency. If it is a hospital, the client needs to be acquainted with his room, the health care team, and other clients. A client in a clinic should be made acquainted with clinic policies and procedures, location of restrooms and cafeterias, and the health care team. When the client is receiving care in his home, the nurse should take time to acquaint the client and family with the purposes of and expectations about the home visit.

Whether the client is in the hospital, an outpatient clinic, or a community setting, the nurse takes measures to provide for the client's privacy. Obviously clients need privacy to carry out activities of hygiene, grooming, and elimination. In addition, they need privacy to talk with their families, friends, or members of the health care team. In an environment of privacy the client feels free to share concerns, ask questions about diagnosis and treatment, and resolve personal problems. The perceptive nurse recognizes the client's need for privacy and creates an appropriate environment.

Nursing care and other therapeutic measures are designed to meet the client's needs. As a further aid in the attainment of health care goals, the nursing care plan includes some flexibility so that the client is not placed into a fixed routine. Obviously the degree of flexibility depends on the nature of the need, the severity of the client's disability or illness, and the client's dependence on nursing care. However, even the smallest degree of flexibility, giving the client an opportunity to have some choice about the type or timing of nursing care, is valuable.

Mrs. Duncan has severe osteoarthritis and is in the hospital for reevaluation of the limitations of the disease. The nursing care plan designed for Mrs. Duncan includes physical therapy every morning at 10:00. The care plan also notes that Mrs. Duncan is able to carry out hygiene, grooming, and elimination activities independently. Ms. Flemming, a student nurse, is assigned to care for Mrs. Duncan on the second day of hospitalization. Ms. Flemming observes Mrs. Duncan during her bed bath and notes that Mrs. Duncan is indeed able to care for herself, but because of her arthritis she is very slow in completing her bath and grooming. Mrs. Duncan is unable to get to physical therapy until 10:30. Ms. Flemming asks the nurse who wrote the original care plan why the 10:00 AM physical therapy time was chosen. The nurse replies that there was no specific reason and says that the time can be changed. Mrs. Duncan and Ms. Flemming talk about the care plan. Mrs. Duncan definitely wants to be able to give herself her morning care, but she also feels that the physical therapy is necessary for increasing her mobility. The care plan is modified to have the physical therapy at 2:00 PM, a time when Mrs. Duncan will not be having visitors.

The flexibility in implementing the care plan for Mrs. Duncan achieved two purposes. First, the physical therapy was continued, thereby increasing Mrs. Duncan's mobility. Second, Mrs. Duncan was able to meet her need for independence by having enough time to complete her morning care.

Clients with severe and chronic diseases need to be encouraged to increase their level of self-care and independence, a difficult task that is often disheartening for both the client and the nurse. To avoid discouraging the client, it is best to attempt to achieve this nursing goal gradually. The nursing care plan is implemented so that the client successfully achieves one level of independence before attempting the next level.

Mr. Porter is a 50-year-old executive, husband, and father of three teenagers. He is recovering from a severe myocardial infarction and cardiac arrest. For the past 10 days all of Mr. Porter's hygiene and grooming needs have been met by the nursing staff. One day Mr. Porter expresses doubts of ever getting his energy back and being able to care for himself. That evening Mr. Martin, a student nurse, assesses Mr. Porter and develops a nursing care plan. One of the goals is complete self-care by Mr. Porter within 1 week. With the help of his instructor, Mr. Martin implements the following nursing care plan, which is designed to achieve the overall goal of independence in various phases:

Day 1   Wash face and comb hair
Day 2   Wash face, shave, and comb hair
Day 3   Feed himself breakfast, wash face, shave, and comb hair
Day 4   Feed himself meals, wash face, shave, and comb hair
Day 5   Perform grooming activities and feed himself
Day 6   Perform grooming activities and feed himself
Day 7   Shower

Each day included achievable tasks for Mr. Porter. Placing the tasks in sequential order served three purposes: (1) each task was developed with the knowledge that Mr. Porter could indeed successfully complete the activity, (2) a sequence of successes motivated Mr. Porter to continue with the plan, and (3) the sequence was designed to increase gradually Mr. Porter's activity tolerance.

Clients with chronic diseases are frequently on a regimen that requires strict adherence to the treatment modalities. Client adherence means that the client and family must invest time in carrying out the required home treatments. For example, a client with chronic obstructive pulmonary disease must spend several hours a day performing various respiratory therapies designed to keep the airway open and the client at an acceptable level of wellness.

Some treatment plans include the need for the client and the family to adjust to functional changes as a result of the medications. For example, a hypertensive client treated with methyldopa (Aldomet) occasionally feels increasingly fatigued during the early stages of treatment, or a client with cancer who is undergoing chemotherapy has changes in energy level and body image as a result of the medication.

Finally, adherence to treatment plans can require an increased financial investment by the client and family. For example, a cardiac client may find that his two-story house is no longer suitable, and he and his family must invest in a new house. A client with a pulmonary disease may discover that the weather decreases his level of wellness and that he and his family must move to a more suitable climate.

Investments of time, money, and personal resources for a long period of time can discourage the client and his family. The discouraged client may neglect the treatment regimen. Once the client begins to reduce his adherence to treatment, his level of wellness declines.

Nurses are able to intervene and assist clients in their adherence to a treatment plan. First, adequate discharge planning and education of the client and family help promote a smooth transition from one health care setting to another or to the home and help to increase the client's level of knowledge about his treatment plan. Second, counseling the client and family helps them adapt to change resulting from the disease process or treatment. Third, continuity of care provides the client with a supportive professional who is familiar with the client's pattern of living, pattern of wellness, and treatment. Finally, reinforcing the client's successes with his treatment plan encourages the client to adhere to the regimen.

Supervising and Evaluating the Work of Other Staff Members

Frequently the nurse who develops the nursing care plan does not perform all the nursing interventions. Some of these interventions may be delegated to another member of the health care team. Noninvasive interventions such as skin care, range of joint motion exercises, ambulating, grooming, and performing hygiene measures are assigned to another staff nurse, a nursing assistant, or a licensed practical nurse. The nurse assigning tasks is responsible for ensuring that each task is assigned to an individual who is skilled in that task. The nurse is also responsible for ensuring that the delegated task was completed according to the standard of care.

Summary

In the fourth component of the nursing process, implementation, the nurse initiates and carries out the objectives of the nursing care plan. During implementation the nurse completes dependent, independent, and interdependent nursing interventions.

As with the other components of the nursing process, implementation itself is a process. It is comprised of five sequential steps: reassessing the client, reviewing and modifying the existing nursing care plan, identifying areas of assistance, implementing nursing strategies, and communicating nursing strategies. During reassessment the nurse focuses on one part of the total nursing assessment to determine the presence of changes that can affect the nursing interventions. The nurse gathers and analyzes data from the reas-

sessment and reviews or modifies the nursing care plan as needed. The review and modification of the nursing care plan reflect the client's current health care needs and the appropriate nursing actions. Before implementing nursing strategies the nurse identifies areas of assistance requiring additional personnel, additional knowledge, and additional nursing skills. Following the implementation of nursing strategies the nurse communicates either in writing or orally the specific nursing intervention and the client's responses.

Nursing strategies are selected from five methods: assisting with activities of daily living, counseling and teaching, giving care to achieve the therapeutic goals for the client, giving care to facilitate the attainment of health care goals by the client, and supervising and evaluating the work of other staff members. Each implementation method requires the nurse to use theoretical knowledge and clinical skills.

Knowledge of the implementation process and the selection of appropriate nursing strategies enable the nurse to provide individualized and competent care to a client. Through implementation, strategies are designed to accomplish the goals delineated in the nursing care plan.

KEY CONCEPTS

- ✓ The purpose of implementation is to carry out the nursing care plan developed in the planning component.
- ✓ There are three types of interventions: dependent, independent, and interdependent.
- ✓ Dependent nursing interventions are based on the instruction or written orders of another professional.
- ✓ Independent nursing interventions involve certain aspects of professional nursing practice that are defined by applicable licensure and law and require no supervision or direction from others.
- ✓ Interdependent nursing interventions are carried out in collaboration with another health care professional.
- ✓ Implementation requires the nurse to reassess the client, review and modify the existing nursing care plan, identify areas in which assistance is needed, implement nursing strategies, and communicate nursing strategies.
- ✓ The nursing care plan is modified as a client's level of wellness and health care needs change.
- ✓ The implementation of nursing care may require more knowledge, additional nursing skills, and the assistance of more personnel.

✓ Following implementation the nurse writes in the client's record a brief description of the nursing assessment, the specific procedure, and the client's response to nursing care.

✓ Implementation methods fall into five categories: assisting with activities of daily living, counseling and teaching, giving care to achieve the therapeutic goals, giving care to facilitate the client's attainment of health goals, and supervising other personnel.

✓ Activities of daily living are the activities usually performed in the course of a normal day.

✓ Counseling helps the client recognize and manage stress and facilitates interpersonal relationships between the client and his family, significant others, or the health care team.

✓ Teaching is used to present correct principles, procedures, and techniques of health care to the client, to inform the client about his health status, and to refer the client and family to appropriate resources.

✓ Nursing actions to achieve therapeutic goals include compensation for adverse reactions, preventive measures, correct techniques for administering care and preparing the client for procedures, and lifesaving measures.

✓ Nursing actions to facilitate the client's attainment of health goals include providing a conducive environment, adjusting care to fit the client's needs, and stimulating and motivating the client.

✓ Delegating care to other personnel involves ensuring that the individuals assigned are skilled in the tasks and evaluating that each task was completed according to the standard of care.

✓ To complete any nursing procedure the nurse must be knowledgeable about the procedure, when it is needed, how to do it, and the expected outcome.

REFERENCES

Duff, R.S., and Hollingshead, A.B.: Sickness and society, New York, 1968; Harper & Row Publishers, Inc.

McGowan, J.F., and Schmidt, J.F.: Counseling: readings in theory and practice, New York, 1962, Holt, Rinehart & Winston, Inc..

Redman, B.K.: The process of patient teaching in nursing, ed. 5, St. Louis, 1984, The C.V. Mosby Co.

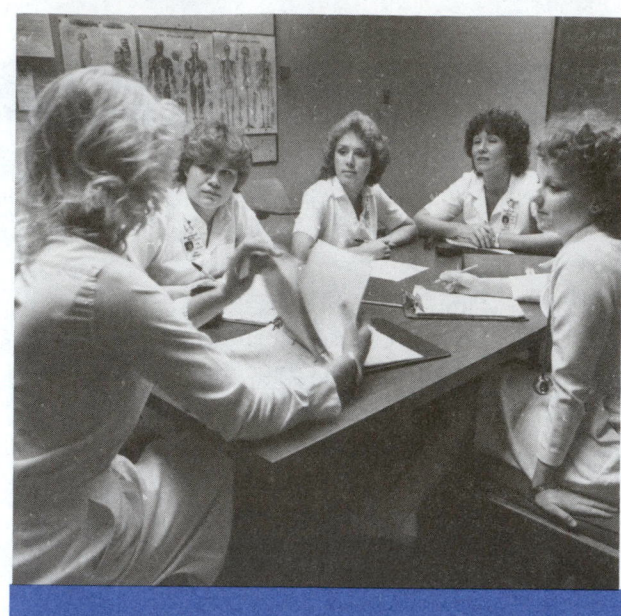

OBJECTIVES

Mastery of content in this chapter will enable the student to:

- Define the terms in the glossary.
- State and discuss the four steps of the evaluation process.
- Describe the interaction between the components of the nursing process.
- Evaluate the nursing actions selected for an assigned client.

GLOSSARY

concurrent nursing audit Evaluation of nursing care while the client is receiving the care.

nursing audit Thorough investigation designed to identify, examine, or verify the performance of certain specified aspects of nursing care using established professional standards.

nursing research A detailed process in which a systematic study of a problem in the field of nursing is performed.

The evaluation component of the nursing process measures the client's response to nursing actions, the client's progress toward achieving the health care goal, the quality of nursing care provided in an institution or agency, and the level of nursing care for an individual client. Evaluation is a category of nursing behavior in which a determination is made and recorded regarding the extent to which the goals of care have been met.

The nursing care is evaluated through a continuous process determining:

1. The client's response to nursing actions as measured against the projected outcomes established during the planning component
2. The client's progress toward achieving short- and long-term goals
3. The presence of new health care needs
4. The need to modify the existing nursing care plan

Evaluation includes comparison of observed results, such as subsidence of symptoms, improving energy level, and proper use of equipment by the client, with the outcome criteria. Positive evaluations can lead the nurse to conclude that the plan was effective in meeting nursing goals. Negative evaluations indicate that the problem was not solved and that modifications in the plan are necessary. In addition, the evaluation process can identify specific factors resulting in the success or failure of the plan.

The evaluation component of the nursing process is oriented toward the client who is receiving nursing care, as well as toward the institution that is providing the care. Individual evaluation focuses on the client's response to nursing therapies, the progress of the

11 | *Evaluation*

client toward achieving the goals of nursing care, and the development of new health care needs. Institutional evaluation uses legal criteria and professional standards to judge the quality of care being delivered to clients.

Evaluation Process

The evaluation of nursing care is a process that includes four steps:
1. Establishment of evaluation criteria
2. Comparison of client response to the criteria
3. Analysis of variables affecting outcomes and conclusions
4. Modifications in the nursing care plan

Establishment of Evaluation Criteria

First, the evaluation criteria for the effectiveness of the nursing actions are based on the projected outcomes developed during the planning component. Projected outcomes are stated in behavioral terms to describe the desired effect of nursing actions. Inclusion of projected outcomes in the nursing care plan gives the nurse an objective determinant as to when and how the nursing goal has been achieved.

Second, scientific principles, supported by nursing research findings, increase the theoretical base from which the projected outcomes are derived. Nursing research is a detailed process in which a systematic study of a problem in the field of nursing is performed (see Chapter 50). The problem may be identified in various areas of clinical practice, and the scientific

method is implemented to solve the problem. Nursing research is essential for the continued development of the scientific aspects of professional nursing.

Third, the evaluation process determines the quality of nursing care in relation to accepted standards of care. A standard is an established basis of comparison in measuring or judging capacity, quantity, content, and value of objects in the same category. The American Nurses' Association (ANA) has developed eight standards of nursing practice used to promote high-quality care (Table 11-1). The ANA standards encourage the nurse to assess the total client, to analyze his health care needs, to develop goals and nursing actions, and to evaluate the client's response to the nursing actions (Barba, Bennett, and Shaw, 1978). Furthermore, the ANA standards are based on the nursing process (Table 11-1). The evaluation of the quality of nursing care is also based on the correct use of the components of the nursing process.

Last, each hospital uses evaluation to establish its own system for nursing audits. These audits resulted from the 1972 and 1973 revisions of the standards of the Joint Commission on Accreditation of Hospitals. Basically the revisions required medical and nursing audits in hospitals that were seeking accreditation (Barba, Bennett, and Shaw, 1978).

A nursing audit is a thorough investigation designed to identify, examine, or verify the performance of certain specified aspects of nursing care using established professional standards. At present only a concurrent nursing audit—an evaluation of nursing care while the client is receiving the care—is required of health care agencies. The concurrent nursing audit frequently occurs while the client is in the hospital.

TABLE 11-1

Correlation of the American Nurses' Association Standards of Practice and the Components of the Nursing Process

Standard	Nursing Process
1. The collection of data about the health status of the client is systematic and continuous. The data are accessible, communicated, and recorded.	Assessment
2. Nursing diagnoses are derived from health status data.	Analysis
3. The plan of nursing care includes goals derived from the nursing diagnoses.	Planning
4. The plan of nursing care includes priorities and prescribed nursing approaches or measures to achieve the goals derived from the nursing diagnoses.	
5. Nursing actions provide for client participation in health promotion, maintenance, and restoration.	Implementation
6. Nursing actions assist the client to maximize his health capabilities.	
7. The client's progress or lack of progress toward goal achievement is determined by the client and the nurse.	Evaluation
8. The client's progress or lack of progress toward goal achievement directs reassessment, recording of priorities, new goal setting, and revision of the plan of care.	

The purpose of the audit is to evaluate the overall nursing care that the client receives. Frequently the person who performs the audit is a nurse who works in a different nursing unit from the one in which the audit is taking place. To ensure consistency in audits from one nurse to another, each agency develops its own audit form. The audit form is a checklist including specific criteria for each category of care (Fig. 11-1). Although different in structure and style, audit forms are consistent in evaluating all levels of nursing care activities as included within the nursing process and the ANA standards of nursing practice.

The establishment and use of evaluation criteria provide a standard for determining the client's response to a specific nursing action, as well as the quality of nursing care being delivered. The criteria are a mechanism for improving the delivery of health care to clients.

Comparison of Client Response to the Criteria

After establishing the evaluation criteria, the next step in the evaluation process is comparing the client response to a nursing action with the criteria. After the nursing action is completed, the client is reassessed and new data are obtained. The new data are compared with the projected outcomes to determine what changes have occurred and if the changes were the predicted ones. In the care plan developed for Mr. Brown's nursing diagnosis of "potential ineffective airway clearance postoperatively, related to abdominal incision," the projected outcomes for the second nursing action included: "lung fields clear on auscultation," "patient remains afebrile," and "chest roentgenogram does not show infiltrate or consolidation" (Table 11-2). The nursing actions were carried out as written for the first 36 hours postoperatively. During that period Mr. Brown's response to the nursing actions was as predicted. However, after 36 hours Mr. Brown developed right middle lobe rales that did not clear with auscultation and a fever of 102° F as measured by a rectal thermometer. These responses were not predicted and indicate that the plan of care was not successful.

As in the case of Mr. Brown, the comparison of new client data derived from the nursing action with the projected outcomes determines the degree of success of the plan of care. The comparison may lead the nurse to conclude that the care plan must be modified and reimplemented.

Analysis of Variables Affecting Outcomes and Conclusions

The data and comparisons obtained during the second step of the evaluation process enable the nurse to determine the degree to which the plan was effec-

Quality Monitoring Incident

SECTION A

Information to be Obtained from Recorded Patient Information

1.302	ARE RESPIRATORY RATE AND QUALITY RECORDED?	No	1
		Yes	2
	Applies to patients with respiratory conditions, conditions in which respiratory involvement is anticipated, or when otherwise necessary, e.g., stroke patient, patient on respirator, hyperglycemic patient, etc.	Not Applicable	3
	Quality refers to descriptions, such as shallow, labored Cheyne-Stokes, retracting, etc. Must be recorded within past 48 hours. Both rate and quality necessary for yes answer.		
1.408	IS THE PLAN FOR TURNING AND POSITIONING THE PATIENT STATED IN WRITING, E.G., IN THE NURSING CARE PLAN, KARDEX, ETC.?	No	1
		Yes	2
	If not stated in writing to see if applicable, may ask nurse: "IS MR. ABLE TO TURN AND POSITION HIMSELF?"	Not Applicable	3
	Code NA only if patient does not need to be turned or positioned. Accept only written plan.		
2.603	IF ATTENTION TO THE PATIENT'S ORAL FLUID INTAKE IS INDICATED, E.G., ENCOURAGE, FORCE OR RESTRICT FLUIDS, ARE THE FOLLOWING STATED?		
	A. TIME FLUIDS ARE TO BE GIVEN.	No	1
		Yes	2
		Not Applicable	3
	B. KINDS OF FLUIDS TO BE GIVEN	No	1
		Yes	2
		Not Applicable	3
	C. AMOUNT OF FLUIDS TO BE GIVEN.	No	1
		Yes	2
		Not Applicable	3

4001, 01

Courtesy Barnes Hospital, St. Louis.

Fig. 11-1 Nursing audit form.

tive. In addition, the nurse is able to draw conclusions about possible factors that led to the success or failure of the plan of care.

The new data collected on Mr. Brown indicate that the plan (Table 11-2) was not effective for "maintaining a patent airway postoperatively." After the nurse concludes that the plan was ineffective, she must reassess, reanalyze client data, and evaluate the nursing plan to determine why the plan was ineffective.

To determine why the plan failed, the nurse first reassesses the client for new data. During the reassessment of Mr. Brown, the nurse notes that Mr. Brown is well hydrated, has symmetrical chest wall movements, has rales in the right middle lobe, has a rectal temperature of 102° F, does not splint the abdominal incision, has requested an analgesic only five

times since surgery, and has clear chest roentgenograms. During reanalysis the significant new assessment findings of not splinting the abdominal incision and frequent need for analgesia lead the nurse to revise the nursing diagnosis to read "ineffective airway clearance related to abdominal incisional pain."

Perhaps one reason for the failure of the initial plan for Mr. Brown was that an incorrect nursing diagnosis was initially developed. The first nursing diagnosis of "potential ineffective airway clearance postoperatively related to abdominal incision" did not include incisional pain as a probable cause. Therefore the plan and subsequent implementation did not provide any nursing actions for the control of incisional pain.

TABLE 11-2

Nursing Care Plan for Mr. Brown

Assessment	Nursing Diagnosis	Plan	Implementation	Evaluation
40 pack-year history of smoking	Potential ineffective airway clearance postoperatively related to abdominal incision	1. Preoperative teaching: turn, cough, and deep breathe.	1. Demonstrate turn, cough, and deep breathing.	1. Mr. Brown correctly demonstrates procedures.
Chest roentgenogram shows flattened diaphragms and hyperinflated lungs		2. Maintain a patent airway postoperatively.	2. Turn, cough, and deep breathe every 2 hours around the clock on first and second postoperative days.	2a. Lung fields clear on auscultation. 2b. Patient remains afebrile. 2c. Chest roentgenogram does not show infiltrate on auscultation.
Rales auscultated in lung fields Scheduled for abdominal surgery		3. Give Mr. Brown information on smoking cigarettes.	3. On sixth postoperative day provide Mr. Brown with smoking cessation literature and support groups.	3. Mr. Brown stops smoking 1 month postoperatively.

A second factor in the failure of the plan can be found in the implementation. Nursing actions should be safe, effective, and efficient and should provide comfort. The nursing action of turn, cough, and deep breathe every 2 hours is a safe intervention. Nursing research has documented that this is an effective, efficient, and comfortable method for controlling pulmonary secretions postoperatively. However, because the initial nursing diagnosis for Mr. Brown was incorrect, he was uncomfortable during the procedure and was unable to cough as productively as he might have if the nursing actions implemented had included measures for minimizing his abdominal incisional pain.

Therefore the plan for Mr. Brown was ineffective because of an inaccurate nursing diagnosis and subsequent nursing strategies. With these conclusions the nurse knows why the plan failed and what modifications are necessary.

Modifications in the Nursing Care Plan

Modifications in the plan of nursing care are based on the conclusions developed during the third step of the evaluation process. Two conclusions were made for Mr. Brown. First, the nursing diagnosis should have read "potential ineffective airway clearance related to abdominal incisional pain." Second, the nursing actions developed for the implementation component should have included nursing strategies to control his incisional pain. Once these conclusions were reached, the nursing care plan for Mr. Brown was modified (Table 11-3).

The modifications alone are not enough. The nurse must implement the new plan of care and reevaluate the client's response to the nursing actions. Therefore the evaluation of nursing care is a continuous process. Reevaluation showed that Mr. Brown was afebrile, coughing productively, and properly splinting his incision, and that his lung fields were clear on auscultation.

TABLE 11-3

Modification of Nursing Care Plan for Mr. Brown

Assessment	Nursing Diagnosis	Plan	Implementation	Evaluation
40 pack-year history of smoking	Ineffective airway clearance related to incisional pain	2. Minimize incision pain while maintaining a patent airway	2a. Administer analgesics every 4 hours during first 48 hours.	2a. Pain controlled by analgesics and splinting of incision
Chest roentgenogram shows no evidence of consolidation			2b. Splint abdominal incision with two pillows during coughing.	2b. Lung fields clear on auscultation
Rales present in right middle lobe			2c. Turn, cough, and deep breathe every 2 hours around the clock for 48 hours.	2c. Afebrile 2d. Chest x-ray clear
Rectal temperature of 102° F				
Does not splint abdominal incision				
Used analgesics only five times since surgery				

Summary

The evaluation process determines the effectiveness of the nursing care plan, it is continuous, and it interacts with the other components of the nursing process. During evaluation the nurse compares the client's response to nursing actions with the projected outcomes, which serve as evaluation criteria. As the nurse assesses the client's response, she concludes whether the plan was a success or failure and why the plan succeeded or failed.

If the plan was successful and the goals of nursing were achieved, the nurse can terminate the plan. A successful plan can be individualized for use with other clients who have similar health care needs and goals.

If the plan failed, the nurse uses problem solving to determine why. Was the initial client assessment incomplete or inaccurate? Did the nurse incorrectly analyze the client's health care needs? Were the planned short- and long-term goals inappropriate for the health care need or unrealistic for the client? Perhaps the nursing strategies developed for implementation were incorrect, unsafe, or inefficient, or perhaps the evaluation of the client response was inaccurate. Whatever the cause for failure of the nursing plan, the nurse must determine why it failed before the problem can be resolved.

If a plan has failed to meet the client's health care needs and the goals of nursing care, the client's needs must be reassessed and rediagnosed and the plan must be modified, reimplemented, and reevaluated, thus enhancing the continuous nature of the nursing process.

KEY CONCEPTS

✓ Evaluation determines the extent to which the goals of care have been met.

✓ The nurse evaluates the client's response to nursing actions as measured against projected outcomes established during the planning component.

✓ The nurse evaluates the client's progress toward achieving his goals.

✓ The evaluation may uncover new health care needs.

✓ The nursing care plan is modified based on the data obtained during evaluation.

✓ Projected outcomes are stated in behavioral terms to describe the desired effect of nursing actions.

✓ Projected outcomes provide an objective determinant as to when and how the nursing goals have been achieved.

✓ Evaluation of client response determines the degree of success of the nursing care plan.

✓ Assessment data gathered during evaluation determine the need to revise and modify the plan of care.

✓ The evaluation process enables the nurse to determine why the nursing plan was successful or unsuccessful.

REFERENCES

Barba, M., Bennett, B., and Shaw, W.J.: The evaluation of patient care through use of ANA's standards of nursing practice, Superv. Nurse 9:42, 1978.

Standards of nursing practice, Am. Nurse 6:11, 1974.

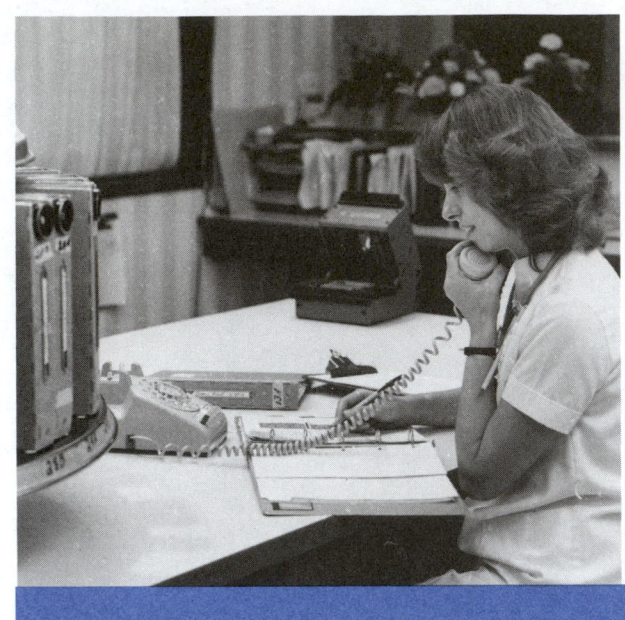

OBJECTIVES

Mastery of content in this chapter will enable the student to:

- Define the terms in the glossary.
- Discuss the role of records and reports in health team communication.
- Describe each characteristic of a good report or record.
- Identify ways to maintain confidentiality of records and reports.
- Describe the purpose of a change-of-shift report.
- Identify six purposes of a health care record.
- Compare and contrast advantages of source-oriented and problem-oriented records.
- Write a narrative SOAP note.
- Discuss legal guidelines for recording.

GLOSSARY

audit Methodical examination or review of written records with the intent to verify or deny the accuracy of information based on established standards.

chart *n.*, Informal term for the client's record; *v.*, to enter data into a client's record.

documentation Act of authenticating events or activities by keeping written records.

inpatient Client who receives treatment within a hospital.

litigation Practice of taking legal action.

oral report Verbal exchange of information.

outpatient Client who has not been admitted to a hospital but receives treatment in a clinic or facility associated with the hospital.

precipitating factor Element that causes or contributes to the occurrence of a symptom.

problem-oriented record (POR) Method of recording data about the health status of a client that fosters a collaborative problem-solving approach by all members of the health care team.

record Written form of communication that permanently documents information relevant to health care management.

relieving factor Element that alleviates a symptom.

SOAP Acronym for *s*ubjective, *o*bjective, *a*ssessment, and *p*lan, the four parts of the written account of a client's health problem in a problem-oriented record.

symptom Subjective indication of a disease or a change in condition as perceived by a client; some symptoms, such as numbness of a body part, may be objectively confirmed.

12 | Recording and Reporting

The client's care plan becomes more useful when it is communicated to all members of the health care team. Usually several persons in a hospital are involved in the care of a client. Records and reports allow each team member to become aware of other members' actions and decisions in delivering care. In an outpatient setting a client may visit several clinics (such as psychiatric, internal medicine, and surgical) many times over the course of a year. A method for communicating the client's changing health care needs is required so that each department is aware of the client's current health status. A community health nurse caring for a client in his home may be taken off the case or decide to change jobs. Unless the nurse has documented the client's care thoroughly, the next nurse assigned to the client will be unable to determine immediately the client's health history and provide continuity in his care. All health team members rely on reports and records to administer care that is directed toward the same goals.

Reports and records contain specific information related to a client's health care. A report involves a verbal or written exchange of information. When nurses complete a shift or tour of duty, they give a verbal report to the nurses on the succeeding shift. A client's overall condition and response to therapy are reported to keep the nurse assigned to the client well informed. Support services such as the laboratory and the radiology department issue written reports describing the results of diagnostic tests. These reports are incorporated into the client's permanent medical record.

A client's record is a written communication that permanently documents information relevant to his health care management. An example is the clinic record or chart. After each clinic visit, information about why the client sought medical care, diagnostic tests, the physician's diagnosis, and choice of therapy is recorded. When the client returns to the clinic, this record is available to the physician and nurse. It becomes a continuing account of the client's health care needs.

Information about the client's health care is also communicated through discussions among members of the health care team. Discussions may be informal, such as one nurse describing to another how a client responded to a medication, or formal, such as a conference of physicians and nurses to discuss a client's treatment plan.

Characteristics of Good Reporting and Recording

All members of the health care team depend on the reported and recorded information. If a vital piece of information has not been recorded or is illegibly written or poorly organized, the client's welfare may be threatened, as in the following two situations:

Mr. Ryan has been teaching his client, Mr. Adams, about the benefits of a low-salt diet. The nurse fails to document in the record the steps of his teaching plan. A new nurse, Ms. Warren, is assigned to Mr. Adams. Because the information regarding the client's teaching needs was not communicated, she must reassess the client's level of knowledge.

Ms. Jackoway has had a busy day in her medical unit.

All of her clients seem to be making requests at the same time. She forgets to record the administration of a medication to her client, Miss Sloan. After the change of shift Mr. Kaiser prepares to administer Miss Sloan's medications. He notes that the record does not show that an earlier dose of medication was administered. Ms. Jackoway is not available to verify the error, and the client cannot remember what medications she received.

The nurse is responsible for ensuring that all information pertinent to the client's nursing care is successfully communicated. Five characteristics of reporting and recording help ensure that communicated information is of high quality: accuracy, conciseness, thoroughness, currentness, and organization.

Accuracy

Information must be correct. The nurse does not report or record what she thinks might have happened or what another nurse has described, but only objective data concerning her own observations or measurements she has made. An example of an objective description is "abdominal wound, approximately 4 cm long, without inflammation or drainage." If subjective data are communicated, they should be acknowledged as such, for example, "Client stated she felt dizzy while standing."

It is important to differentiate between observations of the client's behavior and interpretations of those observations, as shown in the following two descriptions: "Mrs. Wilson walked with a staggering gait to the bathroom." "As Mrs. Wilson walked to the bathroom, she acted as though she was drunk." The latter statement is a subjective interpretation. Mrs. Wilson's staggering gait could have been associated with any of a number of different illnesses. Because interpretation of the client's behavior can be misleading, information should be factual and specific and should avoid assumptions.

Use of precise measurements also helps ensure accuracy. Reporting the actual amount of fluid a client drinks or drainage collected from a wound helps prevent misinterpretation of data. The nurse provides descriptions such as "intake 360 ml at 6:00 PM" (rather than "drank an adequate amount at dinner") or "10 ml bloody drainage from wound" (rather than "drainage from wound was minimal"). Most institutions use the metric system of measurement (see Chapter 32). The nurse should avoid using a system, such as household measures, that differs from the institution's standards.

It is important to use correct spelling and accepted abbreviations when recording information. Terms can easily be confused, for example, hyperemia or hypernatremia, apnea or eupnea, and dram or gram.

A simple spelling mistake might result in a serious treatment error. Medications such as digitoxin or digoxin, Keflex or Keflin, and Nitrospan or Nitrostat must be spelled carefully to allow for clear differentiation. Most major health care institutions provide a list of standard abbreviations and symbols. Although a nurse might be tempted to complete recording in a hurry by using her own abbreviations, inappropriate abbreviations or ambiguous phrases can easily lead to misinterpretation. Any abbreviations or symbols used should have the same meaning to everyone who reads them.

Any descriptive entry in the client's record ends with the health team member's signature. The nurse's signature includes the first initial, complete surname, and status, such as registered nurse, for example, "S. Miller, RN." Nicknames are not to be used. The signature makes the nurse accountable for information she has recorded and facilitates referral to her as a source of information regarding the client.

Conciseness

Concise communication makes information easy to understand. Health team members are more likely to take the time to read brief, well-written notes than lengthy, irrelevant ones. A long, drawn-out report wastes time and is usually boring. In both reporting and recording the nurse provides only essential information, avoiding unnecessary words and irrelevant detail. A report should resemble a telegraph message in which only key words are communicated.

CONCISE ENTRY	LENGTHY ENTRY
Ⓛ toes are warm, color pink, nail beds show good capillary return, dorsalis pedis pulse strong 4 +, no inflammation or pain present.	The client's left toes appear to be warm with color pink. There is no inflammation. There is good capillary return present. Dorsalis pedis pulse in left foot is strong. The client denies pain.

Thoroughness

A good report or record is thorough as well as concise. With experience the nurse learns what criteria to use when describing certain nursing activities (Table 12-1). When a client is in pain, the nurse reports the location, severity, type, duration, radiation, and frequency of the pain, any factors that precipitate, aggravate, or relieve it, and any associated symptoms. Incorporating relevant descriptive data into a record or report ensures that information is complete. For example:

TABLE 12-1

Examples of Criteria for Reporting and Recording

Topic	What to Report or Record
Symptom (such as pain, nausea, headache, dizziness)	Description of episode Location of symptom Severity Onset Precipitating factor(s) Frequency Duration Aggravating factor(s) Relieving factor(s) Associated symptom(s)
Nursing care measures (such as enema, bath, dressing change)	Time administered Equipment used if appropriate Client's response (positive* or negative†) Nurse's observations
Client behavior (such as anxiety, confusion, hostility)	Time of occurrence Behaviors exhibited Precipitating factor(s) Nurse's response or action taken Client's response to nurse's action
Medication administration (such as analgesic)	Time administered Any required preliminary observations (such as pulse, blood pressure) Client's response (positive‡ or negative§) Nursing measures taken if negative response occurs

*For example, client denied pain during dressing change.
†For example, client experienced severe abdominal cramping during enema.
‡For example, client reports pain was reduced by analgesic.
§For example, rash noted on abdomen.

7:15 PM Client states he is experiencing a sharp, throbbing, localized pain in the fingers of his Ⓡ hand. Pain began approximately 5 minutes ago. Client denies previous episode. Pain is increased during movement and slightly relieved with elevation of hand on pillow. Radial pulse is strong; fingers are swollen and inflamed.

Currentness

Information that is recorded or reported must be current. It is easy to omit pertinent information if communication is delayed. After a client leaves the clinic office, the nurse charts a note immediately rather than waiting until the next day. In a hospital, immediate charting of such routine activities as administering a bath, changing a bed, or delivering a meal tray is not crucial. However, certain activities must be communicated at the time they occur: administration of medications; preparation of clients for diagnostic tests or surgery; admission, transfer, or discharge of a client; changes in status of a client;

TABLE 2-2

Comparison of Military and Civilian Times

Military Time	Civilian Time
0100	1:00 AM
0200	2:00 AM
0215	2:15 AM
1200	12:00 Noon
1300	1:00 PM
1420	2:20 PM
1800	6:00 PM
2400	12:00 PM
0001	12:01 AM

and treatment initiated for sudden changes in a client's condition. Many institutions use military time, a 24-hour system that avoids the misinterpretation of AM and PM times that can occur with the 12-hour system. A four-digit number indicates the hours and minutes (Table 12-2).

Decisions about the client's care are based on currently reported information. The nurse charts or reports pertinent information before leaving for lunch or a coffee break. Unnecessary delays in communication may prevent the client from receiving timely attention and care.

Organization

An organized report or recorded note is easy to understand. Information is communicated in a logical order by topics. The following example compares a well-organized note with a disorganized note:

ORGANIZED NOTE	DISORGANIZED NOTE
Client reports sharp pain in left lower quadrant of abdomen, aggravated by turning. Positioning on left side offers minimal relief. Abdomen is tender to touch, rigid, dull to percussion. Bowel sounds are absent. Dr. Phillips notified. He ordered MS 10 mg IM for pain and a CT scan of abdomen.	Client experiencing sharp pain in lower quadrant of abdomen. MD notified. Abdomen tender to touch, rigid with bowel sounds absent. Percussion note is dull. MS 10 mg IM ordered for pain. Positioning on left side offers minimal relief of pain. CT scan ordered of the abdomen.

The organized note above describes three primary topics: the client's pain, the nurse's assessment, and the physician's orders. Information in the organized note flows logically in order of the occurrence of events. The disorganized note is fragmented and does not clearly show what happened first. The nurse should describe all assessment data before proceeding to a description of treatment strategies. An organized report or record addresses each topic thoroughly before a new topic is introduced.

Confidentiality

A confidential communication is information given by one person to another under circumstances of trust and confidence with the understanding that such information must not be disclosed. The law protects information about a client that is gathered by examination, observation, conversation, or treatment. Information communicated in the client's record and through the nurse's report is to be kept secret. Nurses must keep confidential any information noted in the record and avoid repeating what is heard about clients from other staff members, mentioning a client's diagnosis to others, and discussing a client with other clients. The nurse is legally and ethically obligated to keep information pertaining to a client's illness and treatment confidential. A legal suit can be brought against any nurse who discloses information about a client without his consent. Only staff members who are directly involved in the client's care have legitimate access to the client's record. Nurses and other health care professionals may have reason to use records for purposes of data gathering, research, or continuing education; these are not breaches of confidentiality as long as the records are used as specified.

Written documentation of a client's health care is accessible to many personnel. It is important that confidentiality be maintained. Nurses are responsible for protecting records from unauthorized readers such as visitors. The nurse should know the location of the client's record at all times. If it is misplaced, every effort is made to find it. The client's health care record is stored by the health care agency once the client's treatment ends.

Reporting

The two most common forms of reporting that nurses use are the change-of-shift report and telephone reporting. The change-of-shift report is a formal exchange of information between nurses involved in clients' care. This report is in addition to the nurses' written report. Telephone reporting occurs between any members of the health care team at any time of day.

Change-of-Shift Report

At the end of each shift the nurse gives a report about her assigned clients to a nurse working in the succeeding shift. The major purpose of the report is to provide continuity of care from one shift to the next. If a dressing is changed a certain way during the day shift, it should be changed the same way on the evening shift unless a physician's order changes the procedure. If the day nurse was unable to complete a discussion with the client concerning his disease process, the evening nurse can resume the discussion without wasting time giving repetitive information. A complete report is important for establishing the nurse's accountability in the eyes of the client. When the client sees different nurses performing the same procedure in different ways, he may become anxious and wonder if all the nurses are providing good nursing care.

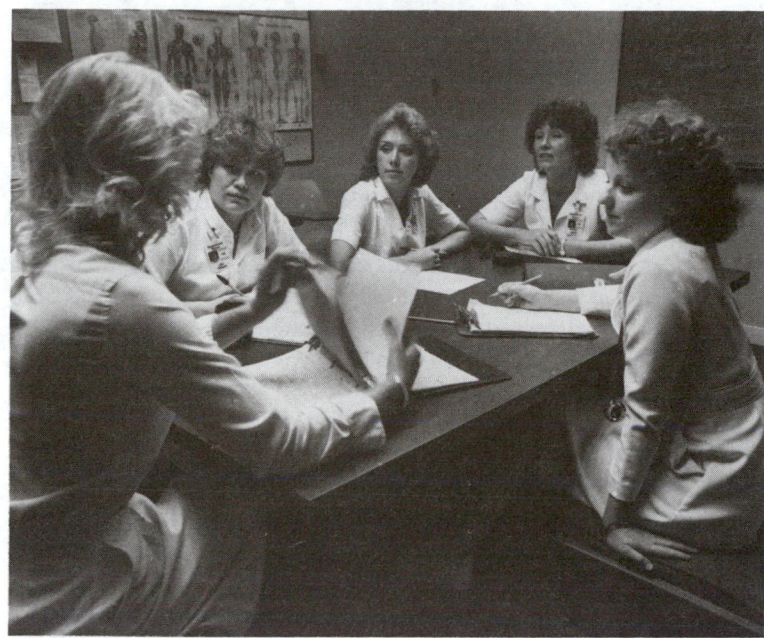

Fig. 12-1 Members of the nursing team meet at the change of shift for a report on each client's progress and specific health care needs.

Change-of-shift reports are given orally in person or by audio tape recordings. Reports given in person permit nurses to obtain immediate feedback. Consider the following information given in a taped report:

Mrs. Roberts' blood pressure was 160/100 at 10:00 PM. Apresoline 20 mg was given at 10:15 PM for the elevated blood pressure. The client also had a poor appetite.

Did the medication lower Mrs. Roberts' blood pressure? If the nurse who gave the taped report has left for the day, the nurse listening to this report will have to look through the client's record to see if the blood pressure value is available. An in-person report allows nurses to ask those on the preceding shift questions and to clarify explanations.

The change-of-shift report may be conducted in a conference room or during the nurses' "walking rounds" (Fig. 12-1). During walking rounds the nurses visit all clients to review their condition as report is given. Making rounds has several advantages: the client meets the staff who will care for him, he is informed of activities to expect during the shift, and the nurse observes and meets the client as report is given. Any information that might alarm the client is reported out of the client's hearing. The nurse giving the report ensures the client's privacy by speaking in a low voice to prevent others from overhearing the information.

Time is at a premium during a report. Report should be given quickly and efficiently without idle chatter or gossip. The sequencing of specific types of information helps to keep a report organized. In a hospital, report is usually given in order of the clients' room numbers. The nurse begins with basic information pertaining to the reason for the client's hospitalization, followed by a detailed description of the client's progress during the shift. A clinic nurse may choose to give report in order of the clients' appointments, detailing the reason for each client's visit. Whatever method is used, an organized sequence allows each nurse to anticipate the flow and direction the report is taking.

The report on each client typically includes the following information:

1. Client's name, age, and sex
2. Physician's name
3. Medical diagnosis
4. Nursing diagnosis or problems
5. General description of client's physiological and psychological condition
6. Tests, procedures, or surgery scheduled
7. New therapies ordered, such as medications or intravenous fluids
8. Dietary restrictions
9. Significant medications and their effects
10. Client's response to nursing care measures and therapies
11. Teaching plan
12. Significant information concerning family members

It is especially important to report any recent changes in the client's condition. The nurse also relays priority situations to the next shift.

Mrs. Rose began having problems about an hour ago. After returning from a chest x-ray, she began to have shortness of breath. Chest excursion was decreased with lung sounds clear in all lobes. Mrs. Rose denied chest pain. Vital signs were respirations 32, pulse 98, and blood pressure 132/90. I called Dr. Boles and he ordered oxygen 40% at 5 liters.

The nurse has reported a significant change in the client's health status: shortness of breath. The next nurse assigned to Mrs. Rose's care is thus informed of the need to monitor closely the client's breathing pattern and respiratory status. The information communicated during report serves as a baseline for determination of a client's condition, level of progress, and need for nursing care. A good report tells the next nurse who enters a client's room what to expect and what actions to take for the client's welfare.

When giving a report the nurse discusses the client or his family in a professional and dignified manner. It is often necessary to describe the interactions between client, nurse, and family members in behavioral terms. The nurse avoids using such labels as "uncooperative," "difficult," or "bad" when describing client behaviors. Any derogatory statements overheard by the client could lead to a lawsuit against the nurse (see Chapter 17). A good report is objective and nonjudgmental. Value-laden terms are not conducive for establishing working relationships between staff members and the client. Staff members may unintentionally form a prejudicial opinion about the client before even meeting him. The content of the report should be pertinent to the client's health care. The following is a good report:

Mrs. Jean Wilson is a 67-year-old client of Dr. Tucker and has the diagnosis of left foot stasis ulcer. Vital signs were blood pressure 132/70, pulse 80, respirations 18, and temperature 37.5° C. Mrs. Wilson says her foot has not been as painful today as it was yesterday. The wet-to-dry dressing was changed at 11:45 AM. The ulcer is on the left heel, about 2 cm in diameter and 1 cm deep, which is unchanged from yesterday. The ulcer is erythematous with no drainage. The night shift reported a minimal amount of pink drainage. The skin around the ulcer remains slightly inflamed and tender. I gave Mrs. Wilson Tylenol 600 mg at 2:00 PM. I was just in her room and she said the medication relieved her pain. This is the first time the Tylenol has helped. Mrs. Wilson told me she is worried about the possible need for surgery. The doctors are considering performing a skin graft. If you get a chance, talk with her. She enjoys company. Her family has not yet visited this afternoon.

The report on Mrs. Wilson is relevant; the nurse receiving it can use all of the information shared. The description of the ulcer's appearance, Mrs. Wilson's response to pain medication, and the reported vital signs can be used as a basis for assessing change. The nurse will know what to expect and look for when caring for Mrs. Wilson. If the evening nurse's observations come in conflict with reported information, the new findings will reveal either an improvement or a worsening of Mrs. Wilson's condition. The report also indicates a possible nursing care problem: Mrs. Wilson's concern about surgery. Mrs. Wilson may need an explanation of any impending surgical procedures. The nurse on the evening shift will be able to assess this problem further and perhaps include family members who have come to visit Mrs. Wilson.

Telephone Report

Health care workers frequently communicate with one another by telephone (Fig. 12-2). For instance, a nurse may inform a physician of changes in a client's condition, relay information to the nursing division to which a client is being transferred, or receive the results of laboratory tests by telephone. Because there may be no permanent documentation of what is communicated by telephone, reports are carefully made. Information must be clear and concise. If there is any doubt as to what is being said over the telephone, the recipient repeats the message back to the sender.

Nurse: This is Ms. Ryan from 4 West. Do you have the results of Mrs. Gladys Oney's blood glucose level?
Laboratory technician: Yes, Mrs. Gladys Oney's blood glucose is 118.
Nurse: 118?
Laboratory technician: Yes, that's correct.

Any information concerning the client's care that is communicated by telephone must be verified. Re-

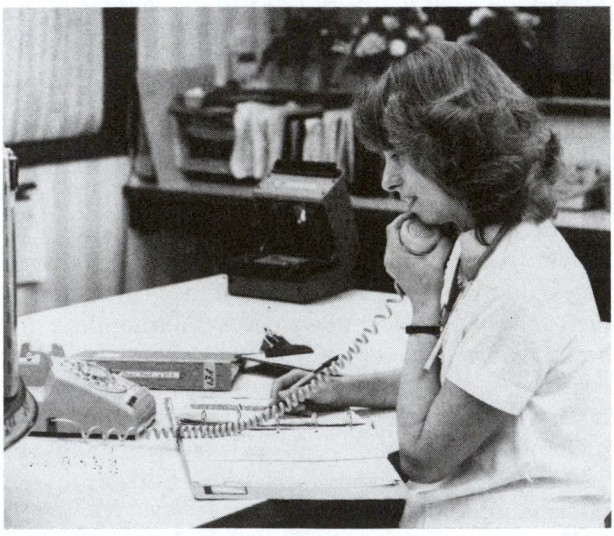

Fig. 12-2 When receiving a telephone report, the nurse must verify the accuracy of all pertinent information.

peating messages clearly and precisely allows for verification. If a physician gives an order over the telephone, the nurse repeats it for accuracy, charts the order in the client's permanent record, and signs it. A physician must later verify the telephone order by signing it within a set time period.

It is always helpful to be courteous when communicating with other health team members (see boxed material). Basic telephone techniques require minimal effort. Courtesy conveys a sense of professionalism and promotes cooperation among health team members.

Recording

Various types of records are used to communicate information about the client's health status and care. Records are kept current while the client uses a health agency's facilities. Although each agency uses a different record format, all records contain basically the same type of information:

1. Demographic data
2. Consent forms
3. Admission nursing histories
4. Client's medical history
5. Reports of physical examinations
6. Reports of diagnostic studies
7. Client's medical diagnosis
8. Therapeutic orders
9. Progress notes
10. Nursing care plans
11. Record of care and treatment
12. Discharge summary

Purposes of Records

Records serve numerous purposes, including communication, education, assessment, research, auditing, and legal documentation.

COMMUNICATION

The client's record is the vehicle by which health team members communicate their contributions to the client's care. Those in each health care discipline (nursing, medicine, social work, physical therapy, and others) document the type of care they administer. Good record keeping improves communication among all of those caring for the client, providing a common focus on the client's problems.

EDUCATION

A client's record offers a wealth of information: diagnoses, related symptoms, successful and unsuccessful therapies, diagnostic findings, and behaviors.

Students of nursing, medicine, dietetics, social work, and other health-related disciplines use these records as a valuable educational resource. An effective way of learning the nature of a given illness and the client's response is to read a client's medical record. Although no two clients have identical records, patterns of information can be identified in records of clients who have similar medical problems. With this information, students learn the patterns to look for in various diseases. As a result, they become better able to anticipate the type of care required for a specific client.

ASSESSMENT

The nurse or other health care worker is unable to plan appropriate interventions for the client unless sufficient data are gathered and interpreted to reveal relevant problems and resources. The client's record is an invaluable source of data. The nurse analyzes physiological and psychological indicators of the client's status before making nursing diagnoses. The

---

Telephone Techniques

INCOMING CALLS

- Cue yourself to smile before picking up the phone.
- Identify the nursing division and yourself.
- Be natural; use your real voice, tone, and volume.
- Treat each call as important.
- Give the caller your full attention.
- Listen carefully.
- Use words of courtesy and politeness.
- Take notes as pertinent information is communicated.
- If there are any questions, ask them after the caller has finished speaking.
- End the call graciously.
- Let the caller hang up first.

OUTGOING CALLS

- Place your call.
- When the other person answers, identify yourself.
- Use the person's name. State *why* you are calling.
- If the report is lengthy, have notes in front of you.
- Ask the other person if he has any questions.
- End the call graciously.

physician reviews results of laboratory tests and x-ray examinations before planning surgery. The dietitian assesses the client's medical history and food preferences before planning diet therapy. Anyone directly involved in the client's care uses the record as a primary source of assessment data.

Information from the record supplements the nurse's own observations and assessment. The client's medical history, for example, can be found in the medical record. Thus it is unnecessary for the nurse to collect information that is already available unless she doubts the authenticity of information in the record.

The nurse continuously observes the client's physiological and psychological responses. These observations are not isolated happenings. Each observation is part of a larger puzzle, which when solved reveals the client's health status. The record contains data to explain and confirm observations or refute interpretations. After inspection of a client's wound, for example, the nurse may conclude that it is healing poorly. What clues to understanding the problem might be found in the record? What has the client's appetite been like? Have nurses on previous shifts also described the wound's poor appearance? Are there any laboratory results indicating onset of infection? Has the physician observed the wound in the last 24 hours? Any observations or interpretations made by the nurse are compared with data from the client's record. The record helps to explain the reasons for and implications of any findings the nurse gathers.

RESEARCH

Client records serve as a source of data for research. Statistical data related to the frequency of disorders, complications, use of specific medical and nursing treatments, deaths, and recovery from illness can be gathered from client records. The effects of experimental drugs and treatments are also available in client records.

Records contain data describing characteristics of the client population using a health agency. Patterns of age, sex, occupation, place of residence, and health alterations can easily be determined. An epidemiological study looks at the occurrence, distribution, and causes of health and disease. Epidemiological research helps in planning preventive health care for large client populations.

AUDITING

A regular review of information available in client records provides a basis for the evaluation of health care administered. The Joint Commission on Accreditation of Hospitals (JCAH) requires that hospitals establish quality assurance programs to conduct on-going objective assessments of important aspects of client care and the correction of identified problems. The JCAH has set standards for information to be found in reviewing recorded nursing histories, care plans, goals of nursing intervention, and client responses to care. For example, a client's care plan must show that the plan is individualized and incorporates client teaching and family participation. Nurses conduct audits regularly throughout the year to determine the degree to which quality assurance standards are met. Deficiencies identified during audits are shared with all members of the nursing staff so corrections can be made. Quality assurance programs keep nurses informed in order to maintain excellence in nursing care.

Medical records are also audited to establish a client's health care bill. Private insurance carriers and auditors from the federal government review records to determine the reimbursement due a client or a health care agency. Unless a nurse carefully records medications administered, a private insurer may judge that the client did not receive the therapy and thus withhold reimbursement. The economic survival of many health care agencies depends on thorough documentation by nurses.

LEGAL DOCUMENTATION

The client's record becomes a legal document if it is used as evidence in a court of law. In a nursing malpractice suit (see Chapter 17) the jury decides whether the nurse adequately met expected standards of care. Proper charting documents the level of care provided. Accurately reported facts are the best defense against litigation.

In many states clients can obtain copies of medical records. The clients' access to records serves as a reminder to health care professionals to write records legibly and incorporate the characteristics of good recording. A client has a legal right not only to adequate health care but also to accurate and truthful records.

Guidelines for Recording

There are some useful guidelines for recording that may protect the nurse and the employing institution against a lawsuit. *If an error is made while recording, the nurse should not erase it or scratch it out.* The nurse draws a single line through the error, writes the word "error," and signs her name or initials. Then the nurse records the note correctly.

error P.S.
Administered ~~75 mg~~ 50 mg Demerol IM in right gluteus medius for abdominal pain.

Erasures or alterations of recorded data create suspicion that a deliberate attempt to conceal information was made. It is important to correct errors promptly. Under no circumstances should erroneous records be removed from the overall record and new pages submitted.

Only facts should be recorded. This maintains accuracy of a record and communicates exactly what occurred in an incident. For example, a nurse should not record that a client fell out of a chair if she did not see the client fall. If she heard the client cry out, walked to the room, and found the client on the floor, she records exactly what happened and what she observed.

While walking down the hall, nurse heard client call for help. Client found lying on floor with right knee bent under leg. Client was alert and able to answer questions. He stated he tripped over shoe. No bruises or lacerations noted. Client able to extend and flex knee in full ROM. Vital signs before fall: BP 136/68, pulse 82, resp. 16; after fall: BP 140/58, pulse 88, resp. 20. Client denies pain in knee. Physician notified.

It is important that the information recorded be true and complete. A nurse who accedes to a physician's demands that she omit information from the record may find herself in trouble. A deliberate omission of the facts could ultimately lead to loss of license or even a jail sentence.

Entries into the record should be legible. A jury may equate sloppy charting with sloppy nursing. An illegible entry can easily be misinterpreted and become the basis for a lawsuit.

The nurse should not rely on recall when charting. Many nurses have the habit of delaying charting until the end of their assigned shift. The dangers of such a practice are obvious. During a busy day it is easy to forget important details that should be documented in the client's record. A change in the client's condition, implementation of new procedures or treatments, or an incident involving the client should be charted immediately.

If the nurse questions an order, she should chart it. On occasion the nurse questions the accuracy of a physician's order. For example, the dosage of a medication may seem too high. After the nurse questions the order, the physician may decide to reaffirm it. If the order is carried out and the client is harmed, the nurse can be held responsible if the record does not show she questioned the order.

Nurses can never be too cautious in the practice of recording. Taking a few extra minutes to write a clear, concise description of the client's care can save hours spent in a court of law.

Documentation Standards

The professional nurse is responsible for documenting elements of the nursing process. The JCAH requires that the "nursing process shall be documented for each hospitalized patient from admission through discharge" (Joint Commission on Accreditation of Hospitals, 1982). Standards for documentation ensure the nurse's professional accountability in delivering care.

The JCAH recommends that the client's record show evidence that an assessment of his health care needs has been conducted. Any identified problems or nursing diagnoses are then used to develop a client-centered plan of care. The record should show that goals are realistic, measurable, and consistent with the client's prescribed medical therapy. The nursing care instituted for a client should reflect current standards of nursing practice. For example, if a nurse documents client education, the record should include a description of what was taught, the client's response, and the client's ability to demonstrate learning.

It is important that the record include the nursing measures taken to restore, maintain, or promote the client's well-being. Relevant physiological, psychosocial, and environmental measures are documented. The record must show that the client was thoroughly prepared for his eventual discharge. The standards set by the JCAH merely support those that have long been proposed by the nursing profession. The nurse must assume responsibility for and document the care she provides. Documentation of the client's care should provide a yardstick for measuring the quality of care provided by all health care professionals.

Types of Records

Two types of record-keeping systems are used by various health agencies: traditional source records and problem-oriented records. The primary difference between these types is the manner in which information is organized. In the source record, information is grouped according to the source, or the health care department contributing the information. For example, the record is divided into the physician's record, nurse's notes, laboratory reports, radiology reports, and miscellaneous flow sheets. In contrast, the problem-oriented record groups information from all health departments into sections according to the client's specific problems. With the problem-oriented system all information relating to each of the client's problems can be found in a single section.

TABLE 12-3

Organization of Traditional Source Record

Section	Contents
Admission fact sheet	Specific demographic data about the client: name, identification number, sex, age, marital status, occupation, employer, health insurance, nearest relative
Physician's order sheet	Record of the physician's orders; each order entered with date, time, and physician's signature; orders prescribe specific therapies for the client
Graphic/flow sheet	Record of repeated observations and measurements such as vital signs and weight
Medical data base	All observations and interpretations of the client's condition made by physicians; includes physical examination, history, and progress notes
Nursing notes	Narrative record of the nursing process: assessment, nursing diagnosis, planning, implementation, and evaluation of care provided
Medication records	Accurate documentation of all medications administered to the client; the date, time, and signature of the nurse are recorded
Health care disciplines	Entries made into the record by all health-related disciplines: physical therapy, dietary department, radiology, social work, and laboratories
Discharge summary	Summary of client's condition, progress, prognosis, rehabilitation, and teaching needs at time of dismissal from hospital or agency

---

SOURCE RECORDS

Most health care institutions have traditionally used the source record, in which the nurse, physician, radiologist, laboratory technician, and social worker each have a separate section to record data (Table 12-3). The advantage of a source record is that care givers in each discipline can easily locate the proper section of the record in which to make their entries.

A disadvantage of source records is the fragmentation of data. Information is well organized but not according to the client's problems. Details about a particular problem may be distributed throughout the record. For example, in the case of a wound infection, the nurse describes the appearance of the wound in the nurse's notes. The physician notes in a separate section the progress of the wound's healing and the proposed course of therapy. The results of tests measuring growth of bacteria from the wound can be found in the laboratory test section. Thus data relevant to a single problem are dispersed, and considerable time may be needed to locate all the information about the problem.

The source record may contain detailed information pertaining to the client's problems. However, this method of data organization does not show how information from the various health care disciplines is related or how care was coordinated to meet all of the client's needs.

In the source record the nurse charts a narrative description of nursing care delivered. In a hospital an entry is made in the client's record for each shift of duty (Fig. 12-3). If a client is seen in a clinic or at home, the nurse documents the care provided at each visit. The nurse's description summarizes pertinent observations relating to the client's condition, nursing care performed, medical therapy administered, and evaluation of the client's response to nursing and medical therapy.

NURSING KARDEX. Nursing information needed for the daily care of a client is readily accessible in the Kardex (Fig. 12-4). The Kardex is a flip-over card that is usually kept in a portable index file at the nurse's station. Nurses refer to the Kardex frequently throughout the day and during the change-of-shift report. The Kardex contains pertinent information concerning the client's ongoing plan of care. The updated information in the Kardex eliminates the need for the nurse to refer continually to the client's chart for information. Information commonly found in the Kardex includes:

1. Basic demographic data
2. Primary medical diagnosis
3. Current physician's orders to be carried out by the nurse
4. Nursing care plan
5. Nursing orders
6. Scheduled tests and procedures

C - 6

BARNES HOSPITAL
NURSING RECORD NOTES

63-8 NEW 7/75

STAMP ADDRESSOGRAPH PLATE HERE

DATE	TIME	
3/10/84	1500	Client states "I was able to take a little nap this afternoon." Currently resting in bed. Cast to Ⓛ leg dry and intact. Ⓛ toes are warm, color pink, blanching with normal capillary return. Able to wiggle toes with ease. Client denies pain, numbness or tingling. Able to discriminate sharp pin prick sensation when tested. Discussed plans for discharge; able to explain principles of cast care — will practice stair climbing with crutches this evening. Transfers from bed to chair s̄ assistance.
		(S. Anderson, R.N.)

Fig. 12-3 Nursing notes are made daily into the client's record for the change-of-shift report.
Courtesy Barnes Hospital, St. Louis.

Medical Diagnosis and other pertinent medical information: COPD, pneumonia

Condition *Fair*

Allergies (Drugs, food, other) *Tetracycline, shellfish*

Adm. Date 11/2/84	Age 63	Religion *Catholic*	Mode of Travel *Ambulated*
Service *Medicine*	Doctor *Snow*	Resident *Phillips*	Intern *Meadows*

FREQUENTLY ORDERED ITEMS

		Date	Specimens/Daily Lab	Date	Treatments
Temp.		11/2	CBC, UA	11/2	O₂ 2L per nasal mask c̄
Pulse & Resp.	every 4°	11/3	ABG's daily		humidity
BP				11/3	Postural drainage c̄
					percussion q 4°
I & O	q shift				
Weights	daily				
Spot Checks					
Chest P.T.	8-12-4-8				
Incentive Spirometer					
P.T.			Diagnostic Procedures		
		Date			
		11/3	Pulmonary function		
		11/3	Chest X-ray		

ACTIVITIES

NUTRITION

Ad lib	Diet *Soft*
Ambulate	
Chair	
BRP	✓
Bedrest	
Bath	Feedings
Self	Assist c̄ meals
Tub	**FLUID BALANCE**
Shower	Force ✓
Bed	D 1500 cc E 1000cc 500N
Assist.	Restrict
	D E N

Orderlies Needed

Family: *Wife* (862-1999)

Stamp Addressograph Plate Here

140962 Rev. 2/83

NURSING CARE PLAN

Date	Nursing Diagnosis	Expected Outcomes	Nursing Plan/Orders
11/3	Reduced airway clearance related to COPD	1. Increased tidal volume 2. Productive cough 3. Respiratory rate within normal range 4. Lung clearon auscultation	1. Patient will learn diaphragmatic breathing and controlled coughing 2. Administer low-flow oxygen and humidity 3. Position for postural drainage for RLL congestion

Discharge Planning: Destination: Home Transportation: Probable Date: 11/20

Referral Agencies: VNA Appointment:

Supplies: O₂ per nasal prongs

Patient Name Gregory Phillip

Courtesy Barnes Hospital, St. Louis.

Fig. 12-4 The Kardex provides nurses with a means to communicate the client's nursing care plan. Written entries ensure continuity of care between all nursing personnel.

7. Safety precautions to be used in the client's care
8. Diet orders
9. Factors related to activities of daily living

Kardex entries should be written in ink, with frequent revisions made as new orders are written and the client's needs change. In many institutions the Kardex becomes a permanent part of the client's record. For the nurse unfamiliar with a particular client, the Kardex is a handy resource outlining the client's basic care.

In traditional record-keeping systems, the Kardex is the central source for recording the nursing care plan (see Chapter 10). The Kardex care plan can be a valuable resource. Often the simplest entries prove to be the most useful for delivering nursing care. When making up a Kardex care plan the nurse should not standardize nursing care measures but should always ask herself, "What is unique about the client? What information will be useful to the nursing staff?"

For example, for a client who has a urinary tract infection and is required to drink large amounts of fluids, a Kardex entry of "increase fluid intake" is relevant but not particularly individualized. If, however, the nurse's assessment has revealed that the client prefers iced tea and orange juice, a Kardex entry of "offer orange juice and iced tea, 1000 ml per shift" addresses the client's preferences and tailors the care plan to the client's needs.

The care plan should not be a reflection of routine nursing responsibilities. For example, nurses who work in orthopedic nursing divisions know the routine observations to make during the client's recovery: condition of a cast, character of circulation to the affected extremity, and level of pain. A Kardex care plan alerting the nurse to make such observations would simply be a waste of space.

A well-written care plan designed by one nurse makes the job of another nurse easier and more efficient. When all nurses who have worked with the client collaborate to write a plan of care, greater continuity of care is achieved. Each member of the nursing team will know what the client needs, what measures are best suited to meet those needs, and the best method to carry out each measure. The boxed material summarizes a few basic guidelines for Kardex care plans.

The Kardex care plan has some disadvantages. Access is usually limited to nursing members of the health care team. Also, the Kardex does not offer space for writing an extensive plan for the client with multiple problems.

FLOWSHEETS. A flowsheet is used when certain routine observations or specific measurements of a prob-

---

Tips on Writing Kardex Care Plans

WHEN TO WRITE A CARE PLAN

- During a report as nurses discuss client's problems and needs
- On rounds after client's problems are identified and reviewed
- After discussions with other health team members responsible for client's care
- After interactions with the client and family members

WHAT TO INCLUDE

- Pertinent nursing assessment data
- Nursing diagnosis
- Nursing orders
  - Observations to make and frequency required
  - Nursing measures aimed at restoring, maintaining, or promoting health
  - Specific methods used to implement nursing measures
  - Appropriate inclusion of family participation
  - Discharge planning
- Expected outcomes of nursing care

---

lem are made repeatedly. It is unnecessary to chart a narrative note each time a medication is administered, a bath is given, or vital signs are checked. The flowsheet is a quicker and more efficient way to record information. Fig. 12-5 is an example of a vital sign flowsheet. Each nursing unit may develop a flowsheet suited to the specific activities of the area. For example, a neurological flowsheet includes measurements of the client's level of consciousness, reflexes, and pupillary reactions. An orthopedic flowsheet might include measurements for checking traction and casts and observation of circulation to the extremities. Most general nursing divisions use flowsheets for vital signs and routine nursing care activities.

PROBLEM-ORIENTED RECORDS

The problem-oriented approach to recording client care places emphasis on the client and his problems. Developed by Dr. Lawrence Weed in the 1960s, the problem-oriented records (POR) system fosters collaboration among all health care team members. Each member of the team contributes to a single list of identified client problems. With the POR system the client's problems are easy to recognize and locate. The nurse, physician, dietitian, social worker, and

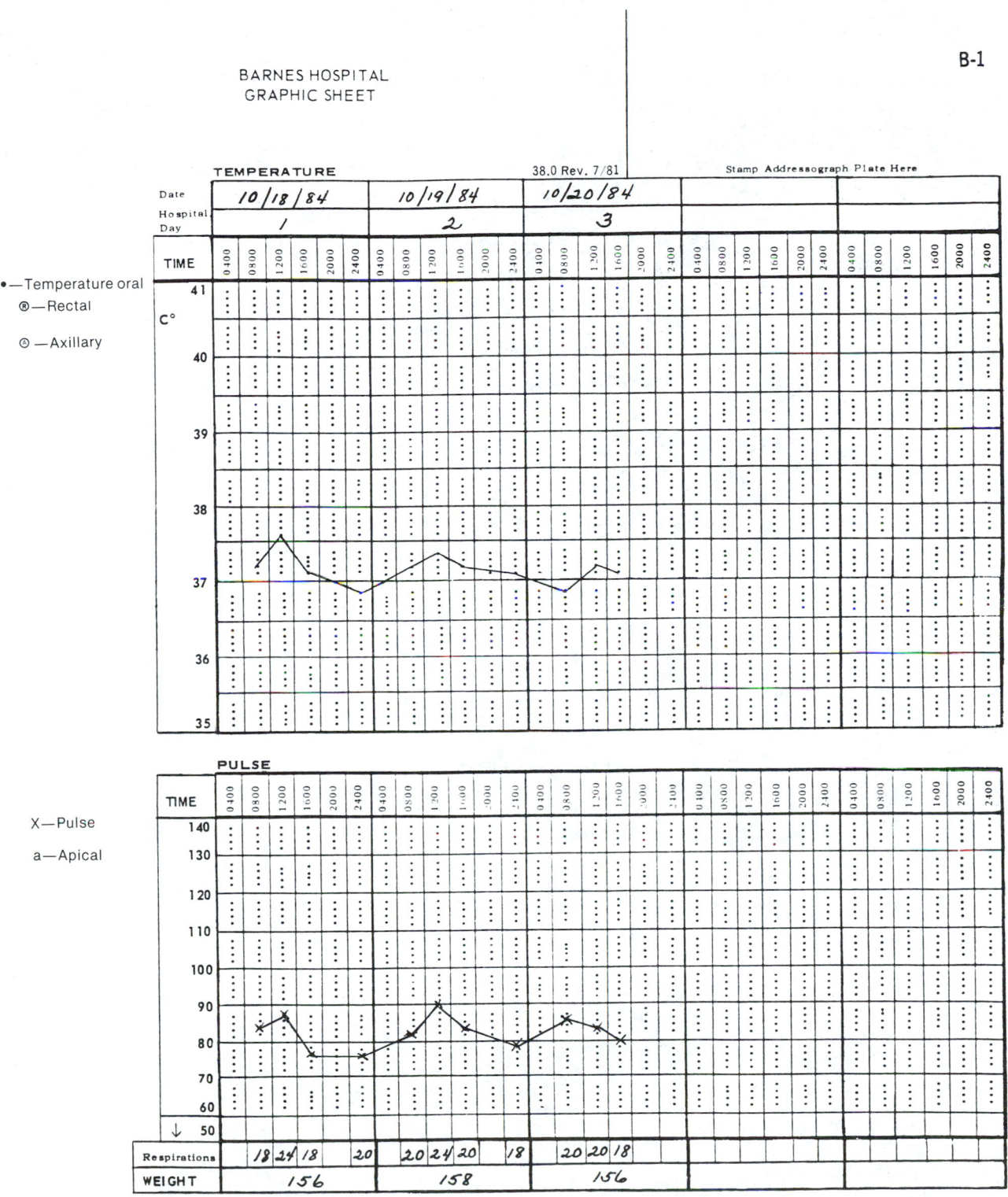

Fig. 12-5 Flowsheet is used whenever certain routine data or specific measurements of a problem are repeatedly recorded.

Problem number	Date	Problem	Date	Inactive or resolved
1	9/28/	Diabetes mellitus	10/28/	Controlled
	10/1/	Hyperglycemia and diabetic coma related to diabetes mellitus	10/28/	Controlled
2	9/28/	Inadequate knowledge related to diet	10/28/	Resolved
3	9/30/	Isolation — lives alone		
4	10/1/	Alteration in elimination, constipation	10/3/	Resolved
5	10/2/	Renal failure		
6	1/20/	Gangrene of ℞ large toe manifested as pain and sensitivity to cold		

Fig. 12-6 Problem record.

others enter notes in one common section. For example, a client's problem may be inadequate nutrition related to a bowel resection. Within a single record section the surgeon who removed a portion of the client's intestine describes the client's progress, the nurse notes the client's appetite, and the dietitian suggests a diet suitable to the client's digestive capabilities. The client benefits from the POR approach because team members in each discipline contribute to the creation of the most effective plan of care.

The POR has four major sections: data base, problem list, initial plan, and progress notes.

DATA BASE. The data base consists of all available assessment information pertaining to the client: the physician's physical examination and the medical history, the nurse's admission history and assessment, laboratory reports, and diagnostic test results. The data base serves as the foundation for planning the client's health care. As data are collected and interpreted, client problems are identified.

The data base should remain active and current. Revisions are made as new data become available. There should be only one data base in the client's active record, which accompanies the client through successive hospitalizations or clinic visits. An active data base ensures continuity of care between inpatient and outpatient facilities.

PROBLEM LIST. Once data are analyzed, problems are identified and a problem list is made (Fig. 12-6). The problems are listed in chronological order according to the date each was identified (not in order of acuteness or priority). A problem may be a well-defined and documented medical diagnosis such as diabetes or heart failure. Signs, symptoms, or syndromes may be stated as problems when insufficient data have been recorded to establish a specific diagnosis. Examples of signs or symptoms that reflect problems are pain, confusion, and diarrhea. Problems should encompass the client's physiological, psychosocial, cultural, spiritual, and environmental needs. Nursing diagnoses, such as a client's knowledge deficit concerning the disease process or fear of loss of a body part, also may be added to the problem list.

One difficulty encountered in developing a problem list is failure to make each problem concise and representative of all data. If a diagnosis can be reasonably established, the diagnostic term is used rather than a less specific term. For example, the problem of alteration in comfort is frequently manifested by a verbal expression of pain, restlessness, grimacing, and withdrawal from social contact. Manifestations of pain should not be listed as separate problems, even

though the nurse can plan activities to deal with a specific manifestation. If a separate plan of care is instituted to meet each manifestation of pain, nursing care becomes fragmented. Integration of data to form comprehensive descriptions of problems or diagnoses will result in more goal-directed care.

The essence of the POR is the structuring of health care information around the client's problems. A list of problems is filed in the front of the client's record to serve as an organizer or table of contents. New problems are added as they are identified. Once a problem has been resolved, the date of resolution is recorded and a line is drawn through the problem and its number on the problem sheet. The number for a resolved problem is not used again. This system keeps the problem list simple yet meaningful. Once a problem list is developed, succeeding record entries are coded by the problem number.

INITIAL PLAN. An initial plan is developed for each problem identified. The plan includes a diagnostic workup, proposed therapy, and client education. The physician indicates what diagnostic studies or forms of therapy should be initiated first. Setting priorities prevents duplication of efforts and delay in dealing with the client's immediate needs. Identifying the client's educational needs addresses the long-term implications of an illness. The plan notes the types of information or skills required by the client to adapt to the effects of illness.

PROGRESS NOTES. During the course of the client's health care management, notes are entered into the record describing the client's progress. Narrative notes and discharge summaries provide an overview of the client's progress from admission to discharge. All members of the health care team contribute to the progress notes.

NARRATIVE NOTES. The SOAP format is used to write narrative notes (Fig. 12-7). SOAP is an acronym for *s*ubjective data, *o*bjective data, *a*ssessment, and *p*lan. Each note is titled and numbered according to the problem it addresses. The numbering system makes it easier to find notes that relate to the same problem. All health team members learn from each other because descriptions of each problem are located in a single section.

The subjective data section includes information from the client, such as the client's description of pain or the acknowledgment of fear. Including subjective input from the client aids in his participation in the plan of care. Whether the narrative notes include subjective data depends on the acuteness of the client's illness or the nature of the problem.

BARNES HOSPITAL
NURSING RECORD NOTES

63-8 NEW 7/75

STAMP ADDRESSOGRAPH PLATE HERE

DATE	TIME	
9/23/	3:00 PM	#3 Isolation — lives alone
		S "I just don't have any friends or family close by to help take care of me. I'm afraid I may make a mistake when I give myself a shot."
		O Client is learning to administer self insulin injections. Has no resources at home to supervise injections. Client has the psychomotor skills needed to perform injections correctly. Has been able to correctly administer injection for the last 2 days.
		A Client fearful of returning home without available resource to supervise injections.
		P Call visiting nurse association to refer client.
		Continue practice sessions with injections and offer encouragement appropriately.
		Assist client in planning for acquisition of necessary syringes and supplies.

Courtesy Barnes Hospital, St. Louis.

Fig. 12-7 The SOAP format is used to write narrative notes that convey the client's problems to the health care team.

BARNES HOSPITAL
Patient Discharge Summary

C-16

Date: _3/8/84_ Time: _0900_
Discharge Diagnosis: _Right sided weakness related to CVA_

Stamp Addressograph Plate Here

562 New 8/80

Patient Aware of Diagnosis yes ☒ no ☐ Comment: _Discussed_

METHOD OF DISCHARGE

M.D. ☒ Name: _Tyson_
AMA with release signed ☐
AMA without release signed ☐
Elopement ☐
Deceased ☐   Release signed ☐

MEANS OF DISCHARGE

Ambulatory ☐   Wheelchair ☐   Stretcher ☐

DISCHARGED TO

Home ☒
Nursing Home ☐
  Name _____
  Address _____
  Forms completed:
    Summarization of today's care ☐
    Chart xeroxed ☐
    Nursing Home Forms ☐
Other ☐ Specify _____

DISCHARGE ACCOMPANIMENT

Left unaccompanied ☐
Left with other ☒
  Name _____
  Relationship _Wife_

FOLLOW UP

Clinic ☐ Date _4/8/84_
Name of clinic _Neurology_
Private Physician ☐ Date _____
Name of Physician _____
Patient and/or significant other verbalize understanding of above
  yes ☒   no ☐

REFERRAL MADE TO

VNA ☐   Call made ☐   Forms completed ☐
Social Service ☐
  Name of Social Worker _____
Other ☐ Specify _____

DISCHARGE CONSIDERATIONS

Valuables from cashier ☐   PTA meds returned ☐
Sent to Patient Accounts ☐   Discharge meds given ☒

NURSING ASSESSMENT

T _37.2_ P(rate/quality) _84 regular_ R(rate/quality) _18 deep_ B/P _132/78_
Afebrile for 24 hrs. (↓38) Y ☒ N ☐ Dr. _____ notified if T ↑ 38.

EMOTIONAL STATUS COMMENT	SENSORY/MOTOR IMPAIRMENT COMMENT
Accepting limitation in physical strength and dexterity. Able to discuss realistic goals for self.	_Weakness R arm and leg — Has attended physical therapy daily. Occupational therapy has taught client to dress and bathe self with deficits. Uses cane with little hesitation._

CONDITION OF SKIN   COMMENT

Normal — without signs of excessive drying, pressure or breakdown.

ADL STATUS	DEPEND.	PARTIAL ASST.	INDEPEND.
Eating		X	
Personal hygiene			X
Dressing			X
Ambulation		X	
Elimination			X

If not independent - specify and describe
Must open containers on meal tray. Is using cane with greater confidence.

Courtesy Barnes Hospital, St. Louis.

Fig. 12-8 A discharge summary describes the status of the client's remaining problems, future therapies, and need for additional resources before and after his return home.

Objective data are information that can be measured. Physical examinations, laboratory data, observations, and results of x-ray examinations are sources of objective information.

Once subjective and objective data are collected, the health team member writes an assessment of the information into the SOAP note. The assessment is an interpretation of the client's condition or level of progress. The conclusions made in the assessment are more than a restatement of the original problem. The assessment determines whether the problem has been resolved or if further care is required.

The final portion of the SOAP note is the plan. Plans may include specific orders designed to manage the client's problem, collection of additional data about the problem, individual or family education, and goals of care. The plan in each SOAP note is compared with the plan in previous notes. A decision is made to revise, modify, or continue previously proposed interventions. Most institutions require that a complete SOAP note be written every 24 hours or when the status of the client's problem changes.

Plans written by the physician and nurse are complementary. The physician directs attention to diagnostic studies and therapies. The nurse's plan for the same problem focuses on how the client's response to illness and therapy is to be observed and modified. With each health care discipline addressing the client's problems, health care becomes better integrated.

DISCHARGE SUMMARY. Before a client's discharge from a hospital or agency, the nurse and physician write a discharge summary that describes the status of the client's remaining problems, future proposed therapy, and need for additional resources before and after he returns home. For example, the physician's summary notes whether the client requires further treatment in the form of medications or physical and occupational therapy. The nurse assesses the client's ability to perform activities of daily living and documents instructions given to prepare the client to adjust to any remaining impairments in function. Fig. 12-8 is a sample nurse's discharge summary.

A discharge summary is frequently used by a referral agency such as a home health care agency or a nursing home. A detailed description of the client's health status at discharge enables the referral agency to anticipate the client's continuing needs. Continuity of health care between the inpatient agency (hospital) and the outpatient agency (community center) is therefore ensured.

Computerized Information Systems

The age of computers is here. The use of computerized information systems has wide benefits for health care delivery. Automated technology provides both improved integration of informational resources

Fig. 12-9 The nursing staff uses computer terminals to communicate with other health care departments, order services, review information pertinent to the client's care, and document nursing care provided.

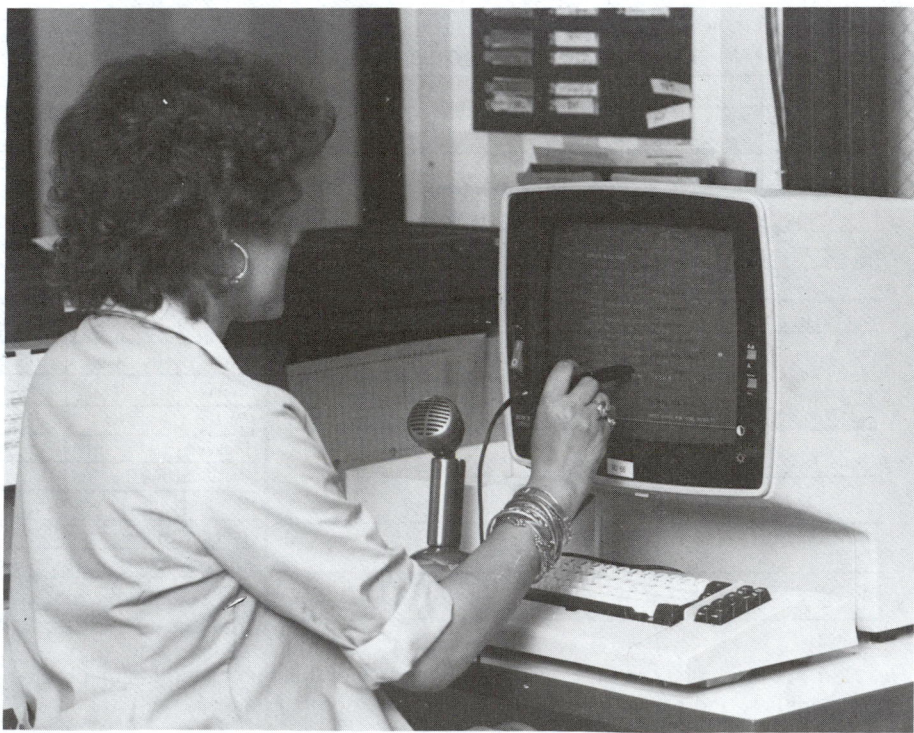

Potential Uses for Computerized Information Systems

- Communication of medical orders
- Recording of medications, flowsheet data, and nursing procedures
- Listing of client care plans
- Recording and analysis of quality assurance information
- Recording of client classification information
- Mechanism for charging supplies
- Centralization of a library of standard nursing care plans, policies and procedures, and educational information
- Hospital formulary

and improved accessibility to information by all health care personnel.

In many hospitals client records have been programmed for computerization (Fig. 12-9). Physician's orders, nursing care plans, flowsheets, and multiple interdepartmental communications are entered via a computer terminal. The quality of client care is enhanced when nurses are relieved of clerical duties, charting errors are reduced, and client information is immediately available (see boxed material). Nurses are freed for professional nursing care.

In the future it is likely that manual recording of information will become obsolete. Any information relating to the client's health care will be at the nurse's fingertips through a computer terminal. It is essential for nurses to become familiar with the potential that computerization has for nursing. Nurses must become instrumental in writing and implementing computer programs for their profession's use.

Summary

The health care of any client involves collaboration by many individuals. Communication is a key element in uniting the contributions of various health care professionals for the client's benefit. Recording and reporting are methods of communicating information related to a client's health care management. In any setting the success of a client's plan of care depends on intelligent reporting and precise record documentation.

To achieve high quality in communication, the nurse incorporates five characteristics in all records and reports: accuracy, conciseness, thoroughness, currentness, and organization.

Any information about a client must remain confidential. The nurse is legally and ethically obligated to use information about the client only in the delivery of nursing care. It is legally acceptable to use the client's record for purposes of research and education if confidentiality is maintained.

The two most common forms of reporting nurses use are change-of-shift reports and telephone reports. When a nurse on one shift transfers the care of a client to a nurse on the succeeding shift, she provides information that prepares the next nurse to assume the client's care. Telephone reports are made between members of all health care disciplines. Any information reported by telephone is carefully verified to ensure its completeness and accuracy.

Health care records are resources for communication, education, client's assessment, auditing, and legal documentation. Good record keeping establishes a level of communication that assists the health team in sharing a common perspective of the client's problems. Students of health care disciplines use records as valuable learning tools when managing a client's care. The record serves as a supplement to the nurse's own health assessment. The client's record also facilitates the nursing audit. Health care records are used to determine nurses' success at meeting established standards of care. Finally, the written record is representative of the level of health care provided for a client and is a legal documentation of that care.

Good charting practices follow basic guidelines. Information entered into the record must be factual. Errors are not erased or removed from the record. Notes are written legibly to avoid misinterpretation. Chart entries are made at the time treatments and procedures are performed or when pertinent observations are made.

Two methods are used for health care record keeping: traditional source recording and the problem-oriented method. The traditional source record organizes information according to the health care discipline contributing the information. With the record divided into specific sections, data from each discipline are easy to locate, but it is more difficult to acquire a multidisciplinary orientation. The problem-oriented record organizes data according to the client's specific problems. The record is composed of four sections: data base, problem list, plan, and progress notes. Information is organized so that all disciplines can collectively contribute to the client's care. The data base contains current assessment information collected by all health team members. As the client's problems are identified, a central problem list is developed. Problems or diagnoses are numbered and listed in order of occurrence. The initial plan proposes measures for the diagnosis and management of the client's problems. Each plan is numbered to correspond with its appropriate problem. The progress notes, written in the SOAP format, describe the daily progress made by the client. Each note includes subjective and objective findings and assesses the meaning of the data identified. Each SOAP note proposes a plan to revise, modify, or continue existing therapy. The advantage of the problem-oriented method is that emphasis is placed on the client and his problems, resulting in more organized and better-coordinated health care.

It is important for nurses to become aware of technological advances in record keeping. Computerized health information systems improve the integration of informational resources and their accessibility to health care personnel. They make it possible for nurses to devote more time to nursing care and less time to clerical duties.

KEY CONCEPTS

✓ A client's health care record is a written documentation of the care he receives.

✓ Accurate record keeping requires an objective interpretation of data with precise measurements, correct spelling, and proper use of abbreviations.

✓ When a nurse places her signature on an entry in a client's record, she assumes accountability for the contents of that entry.

✓ A concise record or report eliminates nonessential information that can be misleading or confusing.

✓ Any change in a client's condition warrants immediate recording and reporting.

✓ An organized record presents information logically in order of the occurrence of events.

✓ All information pertaining to a client's health care management that is gathered by examination, observation, conversation, or treatment is confidential.

✓ The major purpose of the nurses' change-of-shift report is to maintain continuity of care between shifts.

✓ Any verbal report is delivered in a professional manner emphasizing objectivity and a nonjudgmental viewpoint.

✓ When information pertinent to a client's care is communicated by telephone, the information must be verified.

✓ The client's record serves as a resource to explain and confirm observations or refute interpretations of data.

✓ Because the client's record may become a legal document, only factual information is to be recorded.

✓ Errors made while recording should never be erased or made illegible.

✓ The traditional source record and the problem-oriented medical record contain basically the same information but differ in the way information is organized.

✓ The nursing Kardex provides a concise overview of the client's plan of care in a readily accessible form.

REFERENCE

Joint Commission on Accreditation of Hospitals: Accreditation manual for hospitals, Chicago, 1982, The Commission.

ADDITIONAL READINGS

Atwood, J., et al.: The POR: a system for communication, Nurs. Clin. North Am. **9:**229, 1974.

Bergerson, S.R.: Charting with a jury in mind, Nurs. Life **2:**30, 1982.

Bernzweig, E.P.: The nurse's liability for malpractice, ed. 3, New York, 1981, McGraw-Hill Book Co.

Bower, F.L.: The process of planning nursing care, ed. 3, St. Louis, 1982, The C.V. Mosby Co.

Creighton, H.: Law every nurse should know, ed. 4, Philadelphia, 1981, W.B. Saunders Co.

Niland, M.B., and Bentz, P.M.: A problem-oriented approach to planning nursing care, Nurs. Clin. North Am. **9:**235, 1974.

Vasey, E.K.: Writing your patient's care plan efficiently, Nursing 79 **9:**67, 1979.

Vaughan-Wrobel, B.D., and Henderson, B.S.: The problem-oriented system in nursing, ed. 2, St. Louis, 1982, The C.V. Mosby Co.

Yarnall, S.R., and Atwood, J.: Problem-oriented practice for nurses and physicians, Nurs. Clin. North Am. **9:**215, 1974.

3

The five chapters in Unit 3 focus on concepts of professional nursing practice that are important in all health care areas. These concepts involve five aspects of the nurse-client relationship: values, ethics, communication, teaching and learning, and legal issues.

Values clarification helps the nurse and client understand their values and the effects of values on attitudes and health practices in order to work together to meet the client's health care goals more effectively. Because nurses are both responsible and accountable for their actions, they need to understand the profession's code of ethics and ethical issues that may arise in client care. Similarly, because nurses continually communicate with clients and other professionals, nurses use principles of communication to provide care most successfully. Client teaching is also an essential aspect of nursing, requiring the nurse to individualize methods for each client and apply basic teaching principles throughout the nursing process. Finally, because of the legal complexities of the health care system, nurses must be aware of the potential legal implications of their actions.

Concepts for Professional Nursing Practice

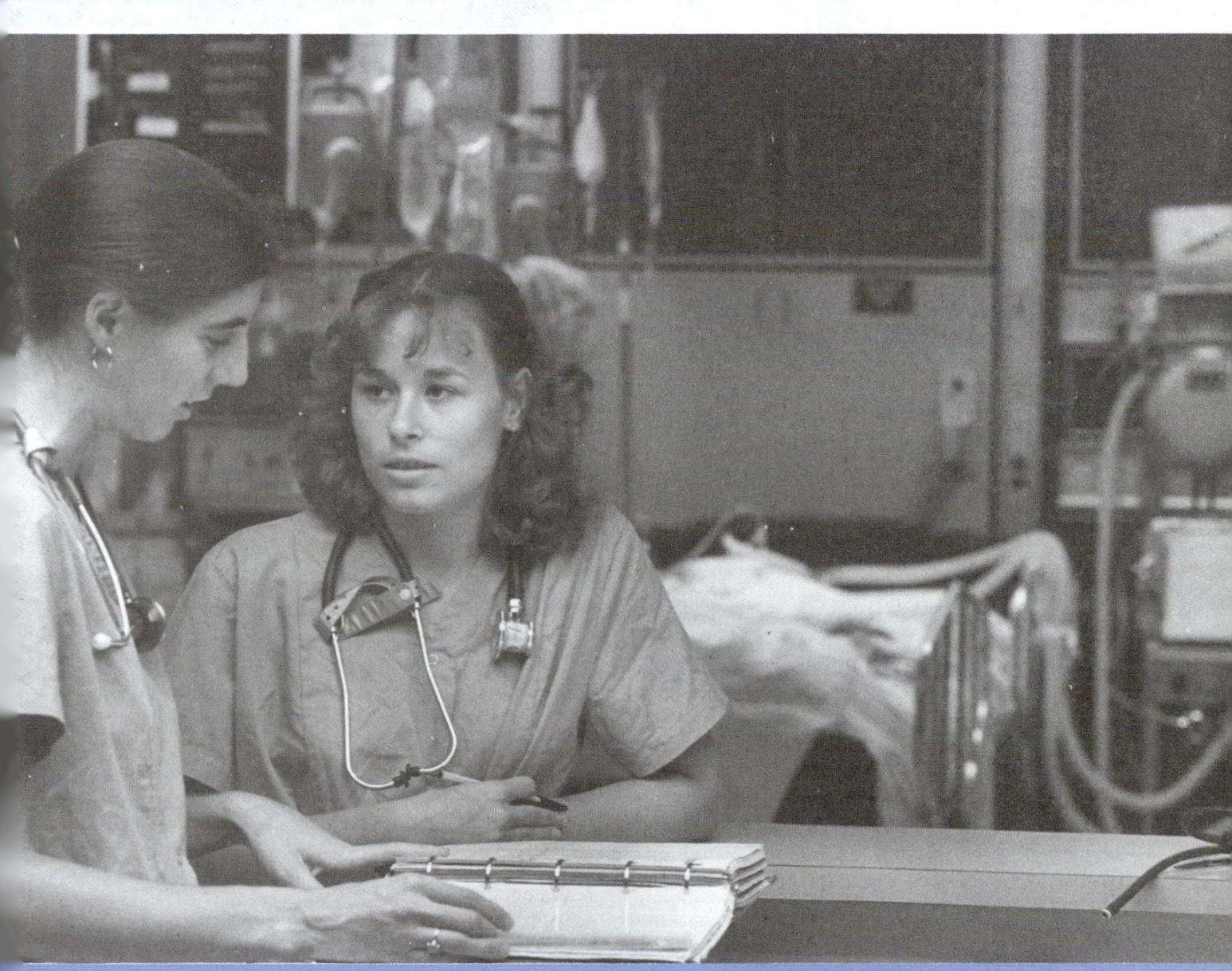

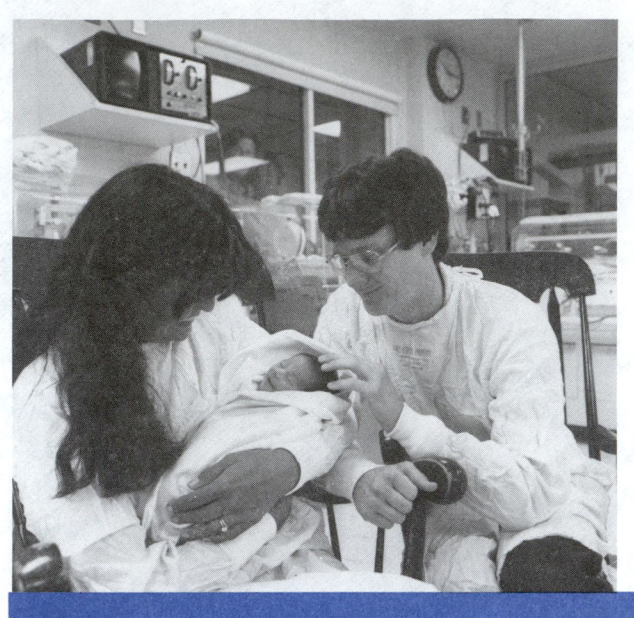

OBJECTIVES

Mastery of content in this chapter will enable the student to:

- Define the terms in the glossary.
- Describe how values influence behavior and attitudes.
- Differentiate between terminal and instrumental values.
- Discuss the ways in which values are learned.
- Contrast and compare modes of value transmission.
- Compare how values are formed at different stages of development.
- Discuss the influence of ethnicity on value formation.
- Describe the process of values clarification.
- Discuss the advantages of values clarification in nursing.
- Use a values clarification strategy to examine personal values.
- Discuss the techniques used to help patients clarify values.
- Analyze personal values as a student of nursing.

GLOSSARY

autonomy Ability or tendency to function independently.

industry Diligence in the pursuit of a goal.

initiative Energy displayed in starting an action.

instrumental value Principle concerning a desirable mode of conduct.

laissez-faire Philosophy characterized by an individual freedom of choice and action.

moralize Explain or interpret behavior on the basis of rigid principles of right or wrong.

modeling Technique in which a person learns a desired response by observing it performed.

terminal value Principle concerning a desired end state or goal.

value Personal belief about the worth of a given idea or behavior.

values clarification Technique for clarifying values, developed by Louis Raths; process designed to give an individual the opportunity to find meaning and significance in personal values.

values clarification strategy Exercise used to clarify one's values.

13 | Values in Nursing

Facing decisions with a clear perspective and purpose is no simple task. Every day brings situations that require thought, decision making, and action. Frequently the person deciding is confused over the multiplicity of options involved in a decision. How is a decision made? Who will be affected by the decision? What influences a person's thoughts when deciding? What are the implications of the decision? A decision is based in part on the person's conscious or unconscious values. A value is a personal belief about the worth of a given idea or behavior. To value a particular behavior or idea is to find it preferable to others. The values an individual holds reflect his personal needs, the culture and society in which he lives, and the significant others to whom he relates. Values vary from person to person, developing and changing as a person grows and matures. A person with clearly defined and well-reasoned values feels less frustration and conflict as he faces daily decisions.

The nurse practices under a personal and a professional set of values when entering a relationship with a client. Each client possesses a value system unique to his own needs and preferences. The nurse should not allow her values to conflict with those of clients. Objectivity enhances the nurse's ability to act in a disciplined and knowledgeable way when assisting clients with health-related problems. The nurse who accepts what she is and what she can do strives for a self-awareness that allows her to understand her attitudes and feelings and control her own behavior in professional relationships with clients.

In the health care setting, the values of the nurse, client, and society interact. The client may find himself dependent on the nurse in a role inconsistent with the independent role he values. Society expects the client to conform to the behaviors of the sick role (see Chapter 2). The nurse attempts to disregard any personal values about the client's behavior and assists him in adapting to his reduced level of function.

A client threatened by a serious illness may need to resolve his conflicting attitudes over whether illness is simply a part of living or a threat to his overall well-being. Ignoring an illness can have a serious outcome. On the other hand, a person who elects to view illness as a part of living may need the nurse's assistance to differentiate between an illness that requires health care intervention and one that does not.

Once the nurse becomes aware of the values that motivate her personal and professional behavior, she finds it easier to assist clients in identifying values that influence their own attitudes and behaviors. The threats posed by illness cause an individual to reassess his health-related values. The frequency and intensity with which a person practices health-promoting behaviors depend on the value he places on reducing the threat of illness and promoting health. The nurse helps the client clarify personal values, reorder value priorities, minimize conflict, and achieve consistency among values and behaviors related to illness prevention and health promotion. The nurse's competence rests on her ability to help clients understand themselves and the impact of certain behaviors on their well-being.

Nature and Function of Values

The values a person chooses are a part of his identity. These values are necessary for the person's satisfaction, security, and comfort as an individual. Rokeach (1973) has made the following observations about values:

1. The total number of values a person possesses is relatively small.
2. Values are organized into value systems.
3. The origin of human values can be traced to culture, society, institutions, and personality.
4. The consequences of human values will be manifested in all phenomena social scientists might consider worth studying and understanding.

The values a person consciously acknowledges as important are relatively few. The values we deem most significant in influencing our lives are even fewer. It is easy to identify a large number of values: courage, creativity, intellect, independence, imagination, spirituality, love, responsibility, and devotion. However, only a few values have a consistent and predictable impact on a person's behavior. No two individuals give equal importance to the same values. The values that hold the greatest importance in shaping a person's thoughts and actions are a part of his unique identity.

People hold values in a continuum of relative importance. Values related to one another form a value system. Examples of value systems are those related to religion, health, freedom, and self-respect. A person's value system provides meaning and practical guidance to his life. For example, a person may value health as essential for satisfaction in life. Eating a balanced diet, exercising, and seeking early medical attention during illness are valued behaviors that become a routine part of that person's life. It is important that the behaviors a person assumes as a result of his values are realistic. A young man with severe heart disease cannot set unrealistic expectations for the maintenance of his physical strength and endurance. A realistic value system allows the person to be flexible and to attain greater satisfaction from the attitudes, behaviors, and feelings that are influenced by his values.

Two types of values are terminal and instrumental values (Rokeach, 1973). A terminal value concerns desired end states or goals. World peace, happiness, career success, and a fulfilling life are terminal values. An instrumental value involves desirable modes of conduct, such as honesty, benevolence, and maintaining one's health. A person's instrumental values change as he encounters new experiences in life. Terminal values are the individual's ultimate goals, which

are achieved through behaviors that are motivated by instrumental values. For example, a person whose terminal value is a high quality of life will reach this goal by practicing good health habits.

Values serve numerous functions in shaping a person's life. His perceptions of other individuals are influenced by his values. When meeting someone for the first time, how does the person act? What aspect of his personality does he choose to show? What behaviors does he look for in another individual? Values direct people's responses toward one another. The nurse who grasps the outstretched hand of a dying client values the subtleties of interpersonal communication and the importance of compassion. The nurse also perceives the dying client's value of being able to maintain courage during a time of suffering. Values reflect a person's identity. His values guide how he presents himself to others and form a basis for his evaluation of himself and others.

Values serve as the basis for a person's positions on personal, professional, social, political, or philosophical issues. In health care, values are pivotal in determining how to attain high-quality care for all clients. For example, if a nurse values humanistic, individualized, and coordinated efforts at providing nursing care, it is likely that the care she provides will be of high quality. Nurses make decisions about the care of their clients on the basis of their personal and professional values. The values nurses hold serve to establish standards of excellence for the profession.

A nursing skill is not a value. However, the nurse practices good nursing skills based on the values of health and respect for the client's individuality and independence. For example, the nurse practicing in a neighborhood health clinic may work with many adolescents who contract sexually transmitted diseases. The nurse teaches them ways of avoiding such a disease and preventing its spread because she values health and the ability of young adults to produce normal children.

Values motivate behavior. Values are expressed through feelings, actions, and the knowledge a person pursues. The nurse who values compassion and caring will interact with clients in a manner that displays sensitivity and a genuine interest in the client's welfare. During a conversation or while performing care, the nurse is aware of the behaviors that exhibit her value of compassion. She strives to learn new communication techniques that enable her to express compassion more effectively. Values provide goals toward which people direct their behavior. As motivators, values provide the reasons to act. For example, the value of life motivates nurses to find ways to meet each client's basic needs.

Values give meaning to life, fulfilling the need for

self-esteem and promoting self-actualization (the understanding and achievement of a person's potential in life). Values involve a search for meaning and a desire for self-understanding. What makes a person happy? How does he become satisfied with a choice or a decision? What ideas does he share with others or defend? As a person forms and tests values, he retains those that provide the most reliable and satisfying solutions to problems.

Formation of Values

Values are learned through observation and experience. An individual observes not only behavior but also the setting in which it occurs and the response it evokes. He repeats and values behavior that he observes as being successful or productive. For example, a beginning nursing student closely observes her clinical instructor's actions at the client's bedside. The student watches the client's reactions as the instructor demonstrates her nursing skill. If the client remains relaxed and accepting as the instructor administers care, the student learns to value being a competent nurse. The instructor's competence as a professional nurse becomes incorporated into the student's value system.

Values are also acquired through experience. After repeatedly experiencing the same situations, a person is wise to look back on his successes and failures. What behaviors led to desirable effects? How did other people respond to those behaviors? The nature of the response a person receives after acting a certain way determines whether he acquires the behavior permanently. The nursing student who receives an instructor's praise after performing a task well will probably continue to set high standards of achievement. Repeated reinforcement results in the student becoming a skilled clinician.

Brill (1973) has summarized the manner in which attitudes and behaviors are learned or acquired:

1. A particular circumstance demands a reaction from an individual.
2. The individual responds on a trial-and-error basis or on the basis of principle.
3. The individual selects an effective response.
4. The individual comes to believe that this is the "right" response because it works for him.
5. The individual believes that people who respond differently in the same situation are "wrong."

People learn or acquire values by observing and interacting with others. Each person holds values that he believes to be important for a satisfying life. People often transmit their values to others in an effort to influence the attitudes and behaviors of those with whom they live.

Modes of Value Transmission

Values are initially learned in childhood. This is not a deliberate process whereby an individual consciously chooses the values he wishes to have throughout life. Values become a part of the individual during his socialization in the family, school, church, and other social groups. As a child observes parents, family, and friends, he internalizes behaviors that become a part of his value system (Fig. 13-1). The child may not know why he behaves in a certain way in a given situation, but often his response becomes invested

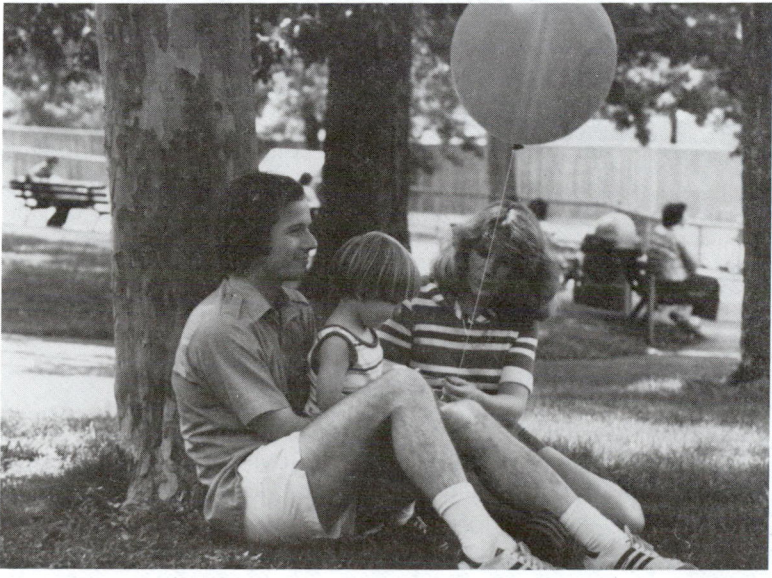

Fig. 13-1 A child's relationship with his parents can influence the values he forms as an adult.
Courtesy Tom Morton.

with an almost ritualistic and emotional significance. For example, a child observes his father saying prayers in church and offering a prayer of thanks at the dinner table. If feelings of happiness are conveyed by family members during these times, the child may begin to value religious activities. Saying a simple bedtime prayer may become the child's way of incorporating his father's religious values.

The people who influence a child are generally unaware of the way they transmit their values. For example, if a parent consistently demonstrates honesty in his dealings with others, his child will likely see the value of telling the truth. The child becomes honest without his father's insistence or threat. However, the process of imposing values can be deliberate, as when a parent says to a child who has lied, "You should be ashamed of yourself. Good boys don't lie."

There are four traditional modes of value transmission: modeling, moralizing, laissez-faire, and responsible choice. As discussed in a later section, these four modes are variably effective at different developmental stages.

MODELING

Parents commonly wish their children to be like them or to acquire values similar to their own. By setting a model or example, they show their children the preferred way to behave. Early in their development most children wish to model or be like their parents. Through modeling a child behaves in a way that epitomizes his perception of an ideal set of values.

Modeling may not always lead to socially acceptable behavior. A parent who consistently uses physical force during an argument presents a model that may lead the child to use aggressive behavior. Modeling can become ineffective in promoting any single value as a child becomes exposed to more and more models. Parents, movie and rock stars, and peers all model different value systems. Unless a parent deliberately points out which values are most desirable, the child is free to follow any model. Most people acquire values from a variety of role models.

MORALIZING

Each person has standards for right and wrong behavior. In traditional institutions such as churches, the teaching of values sometimes becomes an opportunity for moral indoctrination. Moralizing can become a rigid and authoritarian approach to value transmission. A moralizing parent may be unwilling to consider alternative values for his child and may insist that his way is the only way. If a child fails to conform to his parents' set of values, the parent may inflict guilt or even fear upon the child. Moralizing is effective only when all persons who influence a child agree about what constitutes "desirable" values. However, since in most cases a child is influenced by a number of groups and each group usually affirms a different set of desirable values, he is again left to make a choice. Young people reared by moralizing adults often have difficulty making responsible choices because they have had no experience in selecting for themselves the values that are truly beneficial.

LAISSEZ-FAIRE

"Doing your own thing," or behaving without restrictions or limitations from others, is a popular attitude. Many parents want their children to be free to explore a variety of life experiences. The laissez-faire philosophy assumes that no one value system is right for everyone and that the child should form his own values without his parents' rigid guidance. The child is permitted to be inquisitive and learn from his experiences. Parents generally refrain from disciplining the child for fear of interfering with the development of his value system. A drawback of the laissez-faire approach is that no one assumes responsibility for the child's behavior. He may experience conflict and confusion when adults in his life offer little support or guidance. The child tests many behaviors yet he gains no consistent rewards. He becomes unsure of which behaviors will offer predictable beneficial results.

RESPONSIBLE CHOICE

Values should be more than a list of do's and don'ts dictated by others. The imposition of values does not guarantee that a child will be able to make independent decisions later in life. As the child becomes capable of selecting his own values, parents, other family members, and teachers need to provide a healthy balance of freedom and restriction. A parent's attempt to increase control of an adolescent may only lead to the youth's rebellion and rejection of the parent's values. Restrictions and guidance should be tempered to give the child an opportunity to explore new behaviors and experience their consequences. A child who is able to discuss freely his behavior and its effects will learn to understand his own values. As the child succeeds in choosing behaviors that lead to personal satisfaction and earn parental support, he gains a greater awareness of his personal values.

Influence of Development

The formation, modification, and reinforcement of values take place throughout life. A person's cognitive and emotional development influences the way he acquires and learns values and his response to the different modes of value transmission.

INFANT

The newborn seeks emotional and physical security from his parents. Although an infant possesses no real ability to reason, he senses the emotions and behaviors of people around him. The manner in which parents react to and discipline their children is often a function of their values. For example, a parent who values being in control or having a "perfect" child may reward a baby who does not cry with a smile or a hug. If the child becomes irritable, such a parent may become angry, shout at the child, and frighten him. When the parents' values regarding methods of discipline conflict with the child's needs for security, the child may ultimately express fear, anger, or mistrust. The infant gains emotional security through prompt, predictable, and consistent responses to his needs (see Chapter 24).

TODDLER

The toddler learns through imitating others and gaining the approval of others when he engages in acceptable behavior. The child's experiments and exploration of his environment lead to an understanding of the world around him. As he strives for a sense of autonomy (self-direction), he begins to form an identity, shaped by the values of the people with whom he associates.

Parents who do not overly criticize or restrict the child's behavior help him attain a healthy independence. As the child is helped to achieve new physical skills, such as walking up stairs, he learns to value his parents' direction and becomes more assertive.

The parents must balance the child's need for independence against the necessity for protecting him. A toddler is too young to judge what behaviors are safe. When parents fail to provide sufficient supervision, the child can easily injure himself. A child needs a safe environment in which to explore. However, every new encounter is a valuable learning experience, and restrictions imposed by parents who value a highly protective environment inhibit the child's testing of normal behaviors.

PRESCHOOL CHILD

The preschool child is at the stage of cognitive development when concept formation begins. Concepts are objects, events, and experiences that have acquired meaningful labels: dogs bark, trees have leaves, a mother holds and comforts. The preschooler begins to think concretely but not yet abstractly; that is, the child can name what he sees or hears, but hearing the name does not conjure up a mental image of the object. The words "right" and "wrong" do not elicit thoughts of an array of acceptable or unacceptable behavior. What is right or wrong can only be associated with single acts. If the child is repeatedly told not to put toys in his mouth, he learns that this act is wrong, but he does not yet have an abstract awareness of all "wrong" behaviors.

The preschool child strives for a sense of initiative, or the ability to set goals independently and act on them. Play becomes the vehicle for the child to demonstrate initiative. The preschooler uses his imagination to act out his fantasies in play. Parents who value a child's need for creative and imaginative play are less likely to instill guilt in the child when he fails.

Consistent, fair, and kind limits for behavior let the child know that his parents care about him. The preschool stage of development is a suitable time for parents to begin directing the child toward behaviors they value. The child learns kindness when the parent encourages him to share toys and accept playmates. When the child initiates a behavior that reflects a desirable personality characteristic, the parents reinforce it so that the behavior becomes valued.

The nurse is particularly challenged by preschool children who are chronically ill. The parents and siblings of a chronically ill child frequently envelop him, preventing him from asserting initiative. The nurse demonstrates ways in which the preschooler can be independent within his physical limitations.

SCHOOL-AGED CHILD

The school-aged child is influenced by people holding diverse values, such as school personnel and peers in his neighborhood, school, and church. As the school-ager becomes socialized with other children, he becomes less self-centered and more aware of the group (Fig. 13-2). The child is involved in a competitive environment, motivated by peer pressure and a desire to satisfy the adults in his life. It is important for the child to acquire a sense of industry and to feel that he contributes to his peer group and family. As the school-ager matures, he generally comes to value self-motivation and productiveness rather than being manipulated by his peer group.

Parents and teachers promote a sense of industry by providing the school-aged child with constructive guidance. Planning specific school activities, setting aside times for study, and allowing a variety of activities with the child's peer group give the school-ager opportunities to compare his behaviors with those of his peers and to see the products of his efforts. In teaching values, parents who offer alternatives of behavior help the child learn to solve problems and make responsible decisions. For example, when a school-aged child asks his father for money to buy a radio, the father might refuse to give the child money or might challenge the child to think of ways to earn the money. As the child seeks opportunities to per-

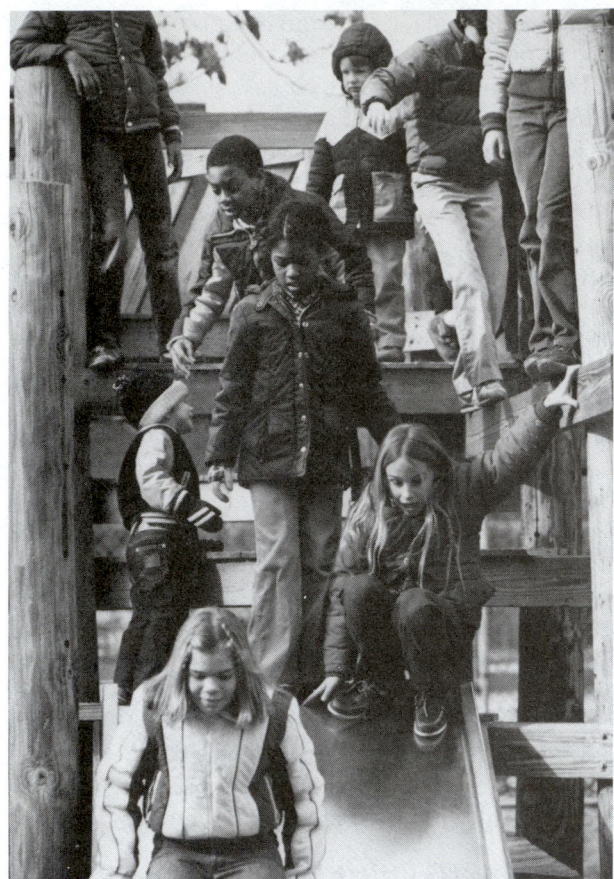

Fig. 13-2 The school-aged child learns the values of children his own age through socialized play.
Courtesy Richard Benkof.

form chores around the home, he gains the experience of working toward a meaningful goal. Once he earns the money for the radio, he will value the product of his efforts and realize the benefits of hard work and commitment.

ADOLESCENT

Adolescence is a critical developmental period during which the youth gains greater freedom and responsibility. It is also a time of rapid learning, with the adolescent being exposed to a multitude of new ideas and values. The adolescent undergoes dramatic physical changes that may affect his ability to develop a stable self-concept. The parents of an adolescent must be patient, supportive, and understanding of their child's need for independence. If the adolescent feels free to be himself and is also able to rely on his parents for support, he will value the family's relationship.

The adolescent's primary concern is to develop an identity that conveys his uniqueness. He experiments with a number of roles, often aimlessly, until he begins to acquire behaviors that are distinctively his own. Most adolescents are unable to identify the specific values or attitudes that comprise their identity. However, as the adolescent matures, he gradually develops a workable philosophy of life, a personally meaningful set of values, and worthy ideals. The adolescent often adopts the values of his parents, but they are no longer the only source of direction and support.

ADULT

The mature adult ideally is able to test values and freely determine which ones are acceptable. At each level of adulthood (young, middle aged, and elderly) the adult has certain experiences that lead to confrontations over the most desirable values.

Marrying, rearing children, and choosing a career often require the young adult to redefine his values.

The middle-aged adult begins to redefine his self-concept to suit the needs of later life. Middle-aged adults whose values have been reinforced through time have a growing sense of security. However, the onset of aging may pose a threat to adults who value youth and vitality. During middle age an insecure adult may sacrifice previously held values in an effort to regain lost years. For example, a married man might flirt with younger women to prove his virility. In contrast, the well-adjusted adult values each year of his life for the pleasures gained and the opportunities afforded. As old age approaches, an individual suffers less emotional turmoil if he is satisfied with his life and his values.

During late adulthood an individual faces significant changes in life including retirement from work, the physical alterations of aging, and the loss of close friends. It is important for the older adult to remain active and independent so that life continues to be enriching. Maintaining social relationships beyond the immediate family helps the older adult fulfill many of the values he holds significant, such as friendship, love, and an active way of life. The older adult may see many of his values threatened as he becomes inactive and less able to maintain meaningful interpersonal relationships. It is therefore essential for the adult to remain open to new ideas and values so that the opportunity for growth exists despite advancing age.

■ ■ ■ ■ ■

Developmental needs significantly influence the manner in which values are formed and expressed. The nurse who is familiar with a client's developmental level and corresponding needs is better able to help the client identify values, understand the impact illness has on values, and realistically modify values as needs arise.

Sociocultural Influences

Values are formed in social settings where the educational, socioeconomic, spiritual, and cultural backgrounds of people vary. Leininger (1975) describes culture as "a way of life belonging to a designated group of people." Each culture has many subcultures with different value systems. In the United States, for example, many people in the Midwest hold traditional and conservative values about issues such as abortion, but on the West Coast people tend to hold more liberal values about these issues. It is difficult to establish norms for any subculture, since no absolute agreement about what values are acceptable exists within a particular culture. The nurse is expected to respect the values of clients even when her cultural background is different from theirs.

Traditional values regarding health maintenance differ significantly among people of different subcultures. For example, clients in some cultural groups seek health care for the slightest problem, whereas those in other groups seek care only when their condition is serious. Clients from lower socioeconomic levels tend to value health promotion behaviors less than clients from higher socioeconomic levels. Individuals who belong to a lower socioeconomic subculture are often less motivated to seek health care early and thus may have a lower level of overall health.

A person's sociocultural background and ethnic heritage influence the ways he maintains his health. For example, a Puerto Rican may rely on a *curandera* or folk healer who uses herbs or special lotions to cure an ailment. A middle-class American typically tries home remedies and, if these fail, visits a licensed physician for treatment. The Chinese use acupuncture, the insertion of thin needles into body sites to produce analgesia, alter a system function, or treat effects of disease. There are a few black Americans who believe that the practice of voodoo will magically drive away evil spirits perceived to cause illness.

Consider the role your own background played in the development of your beliefs, practices, and values. What influence did your grandparents or other family members have on your socialization into the family's way of life? What standards or expectations did your parents set to shape your daily habits? Many children, for example, learn that brushing their teeth immediately on awakening and after meals is important for good hygiene and health. A parent might brush his own teeth with the child present to convey the importance of good dental care. If this child becomes hospitalized, he needs the nurse's support and assistance so that his tooth brushing practices can continue.

People of every ethnic group have unique customs and habits that become a permanent part of their lives. A person may continue to hold many of the tenets of his culture even after he leaves his cultural group. People find security in the values they choose to accept from their cultural upbringing. These values permeate their consciousness and later influence the way they respond to others, the decisions they make, and the directions they follow in their lives.

Changing Values

As individuals mature and experience new situations, their values change. It would be unusual if any one value remained the primary motivating factor throughout a person's life. Value changes may involve a reordering of values or the replacement of old values with new ones. As a result of changing values, the person modifies his attitudes and behavior. The willingness to change shows a healthy attitude toward life and the ability to adapt to new experiences.

Personal and Professional Values in Nursing

The person entering the profession of nursing has a set of personal values that guide actions. These values are the result of personal choice or habit. An adolescent just out of high school probably does not possess a value system similar to that of a professional nurse. However, the adolescent who chooses nursing as a career has found some aspect of nursing to be in agreement with personal values. For example, a young woman may choose nursing because she values respect and sees nurses as members of a helping profession that commands respect from others. A student who values drama or excitement may see the life-and-death situations nurses face as a reason for this career choice. A young adult entering nursing will find that she is unable at first to identify herself with all the attributes of a professional nurse. As she becomes socialized into the nursing profession, she soon finds her personal and professional values interacting.

Two primary values that Hall (1973) identifies are self-value and equal worth. Self-value is one's belief that one is of worth to significant others. Self-value is related to trust, the expression of emotions, and the ability to become involved with other people. The value of equal worth is a belief that other people are equal in worth to oneself. Hall suggests that the two primary values must exist together. Having a positive feeling for others requires that a person first value self. These two primary values are guiding forces in a nurse's personal and professional life. A nurse has difficulty helping and caring for others when she does not feel good about herself.

There are other values, such as accountability and competence, that the nurse acquires as she becomes socialized into the profession. When the nurse's personal and professional values are similar, she assumes a professional role with little difficulty. When her personal and professional values are inconsistent, she will likely feel frustrated and dissatisfied.

Values Clarification

For an individual to change his values in a manner that suits his needs and preferences, he must be aware of what he values. In addition, the individual must realize the implications his values have for his own behavior. Yet a person does not suddenly become aware of his values, and many people are unable to define their values clearly and meaningfully. To achieve the necessary awareness of one's personal values, a cognitive process of values clarification is invaluable.

Values clarification, or valuing, is a process of self-discovery that helps a person gain a clearer insight into his values. It is not a set of rules that interferes with conscientious decision making. The process of values clarification does not imply that a specific set of values should be accepted by all persons. It is also

---

The Seven Steps in Values Clarification

Choosing one's beliefs and behaviors
1. Choosing from alternatives
2. Choosing freely
3. Considering all consequences

Prizing one's beliefs and behaviors
4. Prizing and cherishing the choice
5. Publicly affirming the choice

Acting on one's beliefs
6. Making the choice part of one's behavior
7. Acting with a pattern of consistency and repetition

Modified from Raths, L.E., Harmin, M., and Simon, S.B.: Values and teaching, ed. 2, Columbus, Ohio, 1966, Charles E. Merrill Publishing Co.

---

not a method of indoctrination to religious, moral, or cultural standards. As a person clarifies his values, he learns what choices to make when alternatives are presented and how to determine whether choices are rationally made. The result of valuing is greater self-awareness and personal insight.

The nurse can use values clarification to clarify her own values and thus avoid conflict between her personal and professional behaviors. The process is also a useful intervention in helping clients understand their values and how they influence health-related behaviors.

Louis Raths (Raths, Harmin, and Simon, 1979) pioneered values clarification as an approach to an individual's appraisal of his values. Valuing involves three steps: choosing, prizing, and acting (see boxed material). By using the values clarification process the person is able to rank his values in a hierarchical order that provides a guide for personal conduct, life-style, and interpersonal interactions.

The person must choose his values freely. A nurse does not direct a client to adopt a predetermined set of values. The freedom to select among alternatives allows a person to cherish his final choice. However, the individual must understand what alternatives exist. For example, an older woman may experience the sudden loss of her husband. As she shares her concerns with a community health nurse, it is clear that she has several choices. She can continue to live alone and grieve for her husband, become active in a senior citizens' group, or begin to socialize with a male companion. The nurse helps the woman examine her choices without passing judgment or offering advice. A clear understanding of all alternatives and their consequences will ensure that the woman's final choice is the right one for her.

Prizing is showing private and public satisfaction with the value chosen. A person holds a value in esteem, feeling good about his choice. When a nurse stays late at work to be sure she has completed charting accurately, she prizes doing a thorough and competent job. When a nurse helps a client use values clarification, the client reaches a point in the process when he is able to affirm his values in the presence of significant others. When a terminally ill client chooses to die without emergency resuscitation, he prizes his decision by being able to share it with family members. By announcing his values a person reaffirms their importance or relevance.

Acting on a chosen value solidifies its acceptance. Acting requires a translation of values into behavior. A young man permanently disabled by a serious injury to his leg chooses to retain his independence by living alone. He acts further on his choice by entering a rehabilitation program to learn to use an artificial leg. Whatever value a person acts on must be consistently followed in similar experiences or circumstances. The young man who consciously values his independence continues to act independently in his work and social life.

Nurses' Values Clarification

When a nurse uses values clarification for her own benefit, she undergoes personal growth and gains professional satisfaction. During encounters with clients, peers, physicians, and other health care professionals, the nurse's values are challenged and tested. How does the nurse demonstrate a willingness to be accountable for her actions as a professional? How do the nurse's attitudes about a client influence the care she provides? When another nurse performs some action unsafely, what should be done? What are the nurse's beliefs about the quality of life? The nurse has difficulty assuming the role of a professional when her personal values are poorly conceived and unclear. Values clarification helps the nurse explore her values and decide whether to act on her beliefs. The nurse is able to establish more effective relationships with clients once her own values are clearly defined. A clear perspective of personal values permits the nurse to give greater attention to clients' needs. Values clarification facilitates decision making and problem solving for the nurse in her professional endeavors.

The process of values clarification can be used on an ongoing basis between nurses and other health care workers who face similar value conflicts daily. In working relationships, nurses develop confidence in colleagues on whose responses and decisions they can rely. The nurse who is aware of her own values acts quickly and decisively. Such a nurse can help her colleagues clarify their values in dealing with clients and performing health care. What type of client frustrates the nurse? What makes the nurse feel more satisfied about her job? When frustration with a fellow staff member arises, what is the cause? Sharing values about clients, their families, and colleagues with peers assists nurses in recognizing their commonly held values. This sharing helps nurses understand the behavior of colleagues. Communication lines become more open when dealing with a controversial issue. The quality of working relationships is enhanced as nurses gain insight into themselves and their co-workers.

Clients' Values Clarification

Valuing is also a useful tool in helping clients and their families adapt to the stress of illness and other health-related problems. The nurse helps the client sort out his emotions to clarify their meaning and significance. Values clarification is a consciousness-raising activity through which clients gain an awareness of personal priorities, identify ambiguities in values, and resolve major conflicts between values and behavior. The nurse's goal is to help the client establish health-protecting or -promoting behaviors. Communication with a client becomes more effective, since the nurse is able to focus her attention on what the

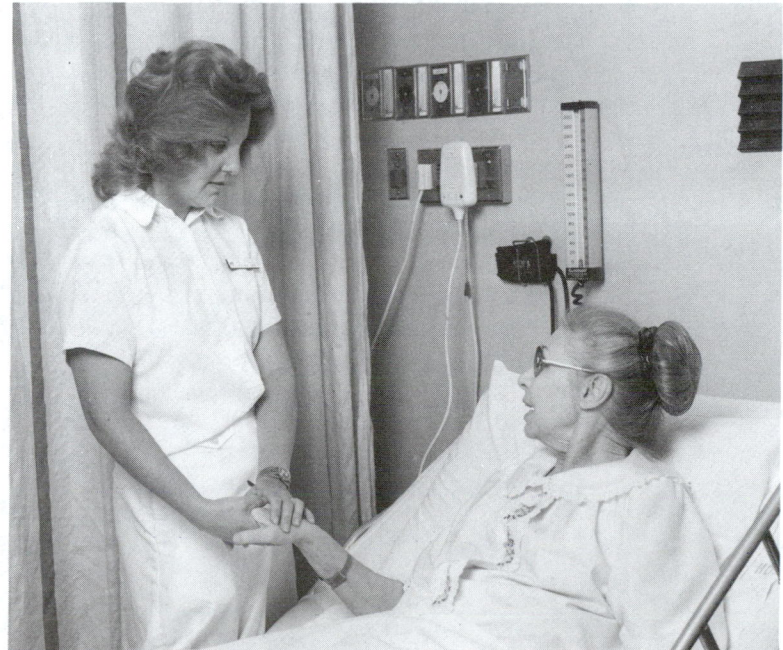

Fig. 13-3 Through values clarification the nurse helps the client become more aware of personal values and their influence on the client's behavior.

client is expressing and why. The client becomes more willing to express his problems and true feelings, and thus the nurse is able to establish an individualized plan of care (Fig. 13-3).

A nurse has the responsibility of educating the client about health-promoting behaviors. Frequently a client is taught facts and concepts about his condition but his health behavior remains unchanged. The nurse who learns what the client values and wants to know is able to devise a successful teaching program. Giving the client meaningful and practical information increases the likelihood that he will assume behaviors that promote his well-being.

Strategies for Values Clarification

A system of strategies can be used to make valuing more insightful, practical, and meaningful for the person whose values are unclear. These strategies are actually exercises to help an individual clarify his values using the three steps of valuing. The nurse can use the strategies with clients or to clarify her own values. For example, the strategy of completing unfinished sentences (see box below) can help the nurse determine and explore her own attitudes, beliefs, interests, and goals, which are indicators of her professional values. The finished sentences can be shared with a group to give the nurse an opportunity to affirm her choices.

The strategy of rank ordering (see box at right) requires the selection of priorities among different values. The nurse in practice can develop a similar exercise to help clients order their values in specific situations. This strategy demonstrates that many issues require more consideration of values than is usually given in decision making.

Sentence Completion

Complete the following sentences. Use them to examine your feelings and values.

I feel I succeed as a nurse when . . .

A patient has a right to . . .

I wish the director of nursing would . . .

Physicians and nurses work together best when . . .

I fail as a nurse if I cannot . . .

The most difficult patient is one who . . .

Modified from Simon, S.B., et al.: Values clarification: a handbook of practical strategies for teachers and students, New York, 1978, Hart Publishing Co.

The health value scale (see box on p. 247) is another device for setting value priorities. It consists of 10 values that a client ranks in order of importance. The client is encouraged to rank items in a way that accurately reflects his value hierarchy. If health is ranked in one of the top four positions, the client places a high value on health. The value placed on health is moderate if ranked 5, 6, or 7 and low if ranked 8, 9, or 10. Information obtained from this exercise can

---

Rank Ordering

The following questions require you to make value judgments. Rank the choices to the questions below according to your value preferences. Write the number "1" to the left for the most important value. Continue in the same manner until all four values are ranked. Share your feelings with a colleague and examine the available alternatives.

If you had the time, money, and skill to solve problems of nurses on your division, you would

___ Increase nurses' salaries

___ Enhance staff education

___ Increase the number of nurses to staff the division

___ Give staff more positive feedback

In developing a professional relationship with a physician, the nurse should

___ Respond promptly to all requests

___ Demonstrate knowledge of the patients assigned to the physician

___ Look attractive and be neatly dressed

___ Share ideas about the clients' needs

When assigned to a client's care, it is most important to

___ Make him as physically comfortable as possible

___ Let him know you are interested in his ideas and feelings

___ Be competent and skilled in the performance of all procedures

___ Allow the client to make decisions about his care

What would you prefer to have happen to you if you had a serious health problem?

___ Not be told

___ Be told immediately by the physician

___ Learn by accident

___ Keep it secret from your family

Modified from Uustal, D.B.: Am. J. Nurs. **78:**2058, 1978.

help the nurse in planning health care teaching methods.

Behaviors Reflecting the Need for Values Clarification

Sometimes it is difficult for the nurse to determine when a client might benefit from values clarification. Not all clients share such socially preferable values as the desire to maintain one's health, a willingness to work hard, or the importance of having a successful career. For example, a client may be unconcerned about his health and may ignore his physician's orders. Any attempts at changing his values would be rejected. Yet in some cases a client's behaviors suggest to the nurse that his values are unclear. Such behaviors could ultimately interfere with the nurse's efforts at promoting good health care. The nurse's role in each of the following situations should be to determine if the client is unhappy with or unsure of his value system or is experiencing a conflict of values that could be detrimental to his health. In such cases, values clarification might be appropriate for the client.

Apathy. Mr. Smith has reentered the hospital numerous times for the same health problem. His wife reports that he will not consistently follow his diet restrictions. During a discussion with the nurse, Mr. Smith cannot remember when he should take his medications. He does not seem to care about health promotion activities. When asked if he understands his physician's orders, Mr. Smith replies, "Oh, I suppose so. I just have trouble remembering sometimes. It's hard to always do the right thing."

Flightiness. Mrs. Jones is visited at home by a public health nurse, who is giving advice on the care of Mrs. Jones' newborn infant. Mrs. Jones tells the nurse, "I'm so glad you are here; I have questions about the baby." Before the nurse is able to answer questions about breast feeding, Mrs. Jones changes the subject and discusses her new kitchen curtains. Even Mrs. Jones' actions seem poorly directed. She places the infant in bed but returns in a moment and picks the child up again.

Uncertainty. Ms. Nelson has been suffering a gradual loss of vision. Her physician has proposed a new type of experimental surgery. Ms. Nelson has not been able to decide whether to follow the physician's recommendations. She has asked her family and friends for their opinions. She asks each nurse who cares for her whether surgery is the right choice.

Inconsistency. Mr. Wall has had serious heart disease for 3 years. He rarely follows the exercise plan prescribed by his physician. In a conversation with a nurse, Mr. Wall remarks that people should become more concerned about maintaining their health.

Drifting. Mr. Rush has had back pain for 3 years. His first physician recommended surgery to correct his problem. Since that time Mr. Rush has also visited a chiropractor and an osteopath. He believes in physical fitness and wants to find a cure for his pain. However, he tries each remedy for only a short time.

Overconforming. Mrs. Wade has gone to a physician for advice on weight reduction. The physician has ordered a diet of 1500 calories per day and a program of regular exercise. Mrs. Wade has bought four diet books to help her count calories and a scale to weigh foods. She keeps a chart on the refrigerator door to record each day's meals. Once Mrs. Wade eats the limit of 1500 calories, she refuses to eat for the remainder of the day, even if it means missing dinner. Each day she runs a mile at 7:15 AM and 5:45 PM.

Role Playing. Mrs. James might be called the "perfect" patient. She always has a smile for the nurses, never talks about her predicament, and rarely complains about pain. This is despite the fact that Mrs. James, age 24 and mother of three children, is dying of cancer.

Values Clarification as a Tool in Client Care

Merely encouraging a client to express his feelings may provide inadequate information if the real problem is a conflict in values. For example, a middle-aged man has a diagnosed terminal disease. His values of health, economic security, and family unity are threatened. When encouraged to discuss his feelings,

---

Health Value Scale

Below you will find 10 values listed in alphabetical order. Arrange the values in order of their importance as guiding principles in your life. Study the list carefully and choose the one value that is most important to you. Write the number "1" in the space to the left of that value. Write the number "2" for the value that ranks second in importance. Continue in the same manner for the remaining values until you have included all ranks from 1 to 10. Each value will have a different rank.

___ A comfortable life (a prosperous life)

___ An exciting life (a stimulating, active life)

___ A sense of accomplishment (lasting contribution)

___ Freedom (independence, free choice)

___ Happiness (contentedness)

___ Health (physical and mental well-being)

___ Inner harmony (freedom from inner conflict)

___ Pleasure (an enjoyable, leisurely life)

___ Self-respect (self-esteem)

___ Social recognition (respect, admiration)

Modified from Uustal, D.B.: Am. J. Nurs. **78:**2058, 1978.

he may be unable to describe clearly how he feels. The nurse who is familiar with values clarification can help the client define values, clarify goals, and seek solutions.

Providing a means for clarifying values is not an attempt at psychoanalysis. The nurse's role is to shape her responses to the client's questions or statements in a manner that stimulates the client's introspection. The nurse's clarifying verbal response is generated from her awareness that the valuing process will motivate the client to examine his thoughts and actions. Such responses can help the client choose a value freely, consider alternatives, prize the choice, affirm the choice with others, act on the choice, and incorporate into his life the behaviors that reflect the value selected.

When the nurse makes a clarifying response, it should be: (1) brief, (2) selective, (3) nonjudgmental, (4) thought provoking, and (5) spontaneous. A good clarifying exchange between nurse and client lasts only a short time. The nurse's response is designed to make the client think about his values after the exchange is over. Clarifying responses are used only when values conflict is the issue. For example, when the nurse sets out to explain a medical procedure, an attempt at values clarification is unwarranted. A nurse makes a clarifying response only for situations in which no right or wrong answer exists. Situations lacking answers are those involving beliefs, aspirations, feelings, and attitudes.

The nurse's response does not judge the client's values. A client will be unable to find comfort in his values if the nurse moralizes or advises on choices. The nurse's response must evoke the client's creative thinking. For example, a client might be undecided whether to seek another physician's opinion about his medical problem. It would be simple (although unethical) for the nurse to advise the client as to which physician is the most skillful in a given area. Likewise, the nurse could easily explain the hazards of proposed surgery. However, it is the client who must live with his choice; the focus must be on the client and what he views as the possible outcomes of any decision.

A nurse's spontaneity can help a client think creatively. The nurse often has little warning when the client seeks solutions to his values dilemma. With experience, a nurse can learn to make clarifying responses without advanced planning. Although the response is consciously and deliberately designed to stimulate thought, it should not appear contrived.

Values clarification can occur in any setting. The client's bedside, a clinic office, or the client's home is a suitable place for the client to express his feelings. Valuing is often more successful when the nurse has the opportunity for repeated contact with the client.

It is difficult for the nurse to help the client meaningfully achieve each step of the valuing process when she spends little time with him.

Ultimately the client gains a perception of how valuing provides personal satisfaction. Values clarification promotes effective reasoning and decision making. The client becomes more aware of how his values influence his actions, and this awareness is an essential component of problem solving.

CASE STUDY

Mrs. James is a 73-year-old woman who fractured her ankle in a fall at home. Mrs. James' daughter is concerned about her mother's welfare and wants Mrs. James to live with her family. The daughter has voiced concern to the nurse that Mrs. James is incapable of caring for herself. Mrs. James' rehabilitation has progressed well. One day Mrs. James asks the nurse, Ms. Fryer, "What should I do? I know my daughter worries about me, but I don't want to be cared for like a child."

Ms. Fryer realizes that Mrs. James is experiencing a conflict in her values for her independence, her love for her daughter, and her health. The nurse thinks the values clarification process would help Mrs. James make her choice. Ms. Fryer begins by helping Mrs. James choose from the alternatives available.

Choosing from Alternatives. The nurse's response depends partly on Mrs. James' age, education, and level of maturity. Mrs. James is an alert woman, knowledgeable about her needs and capable of making decisions for herself. She has demonstrated motivation in her rehabilitation.

Examining All Consequences. Mrs. James loves her daughter and knows that the offer to join the daughter's family is genuine. Mrs. James says that she has many friends in her apartment building and that moving to her daughter's home would make it very difficult for her to socialize with her friends. Mrs. James' present apartment is on the second floor, which requires her to climb two flights of stairs. A downstairs apartment will soon be vacant.

The nurse says, "Perhaps it would be helpful to weigh the advantages and disadvantages of joining your daughter against moving into the downstairs apartment." In making this suggestion the nurse carefully avoids letting her own values influence Mrs. James' thinking, even though she has a close relationship with her own daughter and has been very happy when they shared her house on extended visits.

Choosing Freely. The next day, Ms. Fryer enters Mrs. James' room during breakfast. The nurse's goal is to determine if Mrs. James was able to make a decision of her own. Mrs. James says, "I've decided to move into the downstairs apartment." Ms. Fryer asks, "Was this a difficult choice to make?"

Prizing the Choice. Mrs. James acknowledges that she does not want to hurt her daughter's feelings; however, she knows her decision was the best one. "I still have many friends and they have encouraged me to stay in the apartment. I still feel spry and able to take care of myself." The nurse recognizes that it is important for Mrs. James to be satisfied with her choice.

Affirming the Choice. It is important that Mrs. James be able to speak out in support of her decision. She may need assistance from the nurse in thinking of ways to affirm the choice. An appropriate response by Ms. Fryer is, "What will be the best way to share your decision with your daughter?" Mrs. James replies, "My daughter and son-in-law are coming by to visit this evening. I've decided to let them know tonight."

Acting on the Choice. Mrs. James has made the decision to retain her independence. She is able to share her choice and the rationale for it with her daughter. The nurse using values clarification recognizes Mrs. James' need to act on her decision. She asks, "What can you do to begin planning for your move?"

Mrs. James calls the apartment manager to arrange for her new home. She is going to stay with her daughter for a week after discharge from the hospital. Meanwhile, she will have the opportunity to select new paint and wallpaper for the apartment. Mrs. James' value of independence remains alive in the measures she has taken to accomplish her move.

Acting with a Pattern. A month after discharge, Mrs. James returns to her physician's office for a checkup. She stops by the nursing division to say hello to Ms. Fryer. Ms. Fryer is interested in learning if Mrs. James has continued to retain her independence. A value must be kept alive. For independence to be meaningful to Mrs. James, it must become integrated into her life-style. Ms. Fryer asks, "Was your choice to remain in the apartment the right one?" Mrs. James responds, "For now, yes. I am feeling much better and there are many friends to help me. My daughter visits every week. You know, though, I do have to be cautious in the way I walk around. I know someday I may have to live with my daughter."

As Mrs. James becomes more physically dependent, a conflict will arise between the independence she prizes and her ability to act on that value. The value of the genuine love and concern expressed by Mrs. James' daughter may become a higher priority than the value of independence. Mrs. James' maturity will be reflected in her eventual ability to modify her values. As she becomes more physically dependent, she must adapt her values accordingly. Mrs. James will still be alert and capable of making decisions. The daughter's ability to provide a safe environment for her mother without compromising Mrs. James' ability to make her own decisions should prove to be mutually satisfying.

As in the preceding case study, it takes time for the nurse to develop values clarification as a tool for a client's care. The nurse cannot attempt to help clients explore their values unless she has insight into her own. Values clarification can be a valuable means of helping clients sort out their true feelings and beliefs and gain a better awareness of their goals in life.

Summary

A person's unique set of values about ideas and behaviors influences his decisions and actions and in part determines his identity. Although values may be acquired and held unconsciously, a person's conscious awareness of his values helps him reach decisions and avoid conflicts. A client who is conscious of his values related to health and health behaviors is able to participate more fully in his health care, and a nurse who is conscious of her own values is better able to help clients clarify their values and make decisions.

People form values through observation and experience, noting the responses evoked by their own and others' behaviors. Values are acquired from parents, family, and significant others in a continuous process that begins in infancy. Values are transmitted through one or more modes: modeling, moralizing, laissez-faire, and responsible choice. The differing cognitive and emotional capabilities of the individual as he progresses through developmental stages influence how he acquires values.

Nurses have both personal and professional values. The personal values of a student nurse may already be similar to the professional values of a nurse in practice, such as respect for clients as individuals and the value of health. With socialization into the nursing profession these two sets of values may converge into one. The process of values clarification can be valuable in increasing the nurse's awareness of the impact of personal values on professional behavior and in avoiding conflicts within the nurse's value system or between the nurse's and the client's values.

Values clarification is the use of various strategies to explore the meaning of one's values and behaviors. The valuing process involves choosing, prizing, and acting on one's beliefs. Values clarification can be an important intervention for clients whose behavior suggests that their values may be ambiguous or nondirected. When values are clearly detailed and positively affirmed, the client is more capable of making objective decisions about health care.

KEY CONCEPTS

✓ When a nurse can clearly differentiate her personal values from her professional values, she is better able to help clients understand their values.

✓ A person's perceptions of others are shaped by his values.

✓ Values provide a standard for acceptable behavior.

✓ A person acquires values after observing behaviors that prove successful or productive for others.

✓ A child acquires values from his parents, other family members, school, church, and other social institutions.

✓ Setting a model for another person shows that individual the proper values to acquire.

✓ A moralizing person shows little tolerance for behaviors that do not fall within his own value system.

✓ A laissez-faire approach allows a child to experiment and explore different behaviors but provides little direction for right or wrong behavior.

✓ Restrictions that parents set for a child should be balanced with opportunities for the child to explore behaviors and their consequences.

✓ Value formation begins in the early developmental stages and continues through the life span.

✓ A person's sociocultural background influences his values toward health and health care.

✓ Values clarification is not an indoctrination method but a process that promotes an individual's understanding of what his values are.

✓ A person must be able to choose his values freely from available alternatives and understand the consequences of his choice.

✓ The process of valuing ultimately allows a person to act consistently on his chosen values.

✓ Values clarification helps a nurse explore personal values and feelings and decide whether to act on her beliefs.

✓ The nurse who learns about what a client values is better prepared to help the client assume health-protecting or -promoting behaviors.

✓ Values clarification strategies are useful tools to help clients understand their own values.

✓ Nurses who use values clarification with clients offer clarifying responses that stimulate the clients' introspection about their values and behavior.

✓ Values clarification promotes effective reasoning and decision making.

REFERENCES

Brill, N.I.: Working with people, the helping process, Philadelphia, 1973, J.B. Lippincott Co.

Hall, B.P.: Value clarification as learning process, New York, 1973, Paulist Press.

Leininger, M.: Transcultural nursing: concepts, theories, and practices, New York, 1978, John Wiley & Sons, Inc.

Raths, L.E., Harmin, M., and Simon, S.B.: Values and teaching, ed. 2, Columbus, Ohio, 1979, Charles E. Merrill Publishing Co.

Rokeach, M.: The nature of human values, New York, 1973, The Free Press.

ADDITIONAL READINGS

Coletta, S.S.: Values clarification in nursing: why? Am. J. Nurs. 78:2057, 1978.

Ford, J.G., Trygstad-Durland, L.N., and Nelms, B.C.: Applied decision making for nurses, St. Louis, 1979, The C.V. Mosby Co.

Howe, L.W., and Howe, M.M.: The values clarification approach. In Howe, L.W., and Howe, M.M., editors: Personalizing education, values clarification and beyond, New York, 1975, Hart Publishing Co.

McNally, J.M.: Values: part I, Superv. Nurse 11:27, 1980.

Murray, R.B., and Zentner, J.P.: Nursing assessment and health promotion through the life span, ed. 2, Englewood Cliffs, N.J., 1979, Prentice-Hall, Inc.

Simon, S.B., et al.: Values clarification: a handbook of practical strategies for teachers and students, New York, 1978, Hart Publishing Co.

Spector, R.E.: Cultural diversity in health and illness, New York, 1979, Appleton-Century-Crofts.

Steele, S.M., and Harmon, V.: Values clarification in nursing, ed. 2, New York, 1983, Appleton-Century-Crofts.

Uustal, D.B.: Values clarification in nursing: application to practice, Am. J. Nurs. 78:2058, 1978.

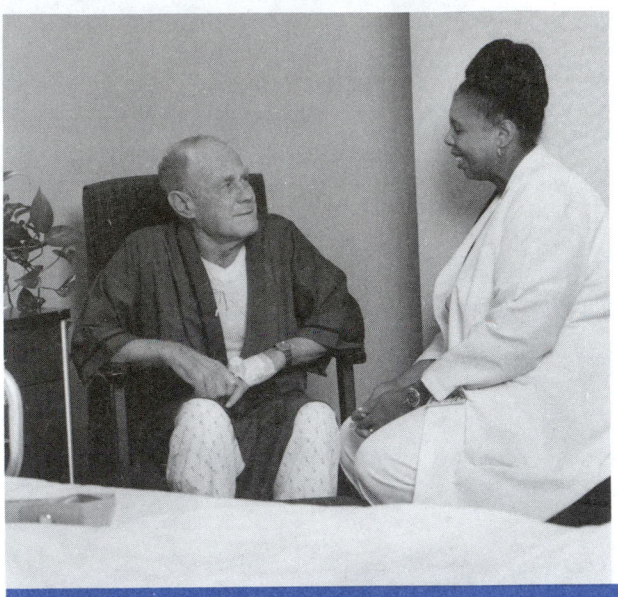

OBJECTIVES

Mastery of content in this chapter will enable the student to:

- Define the terms in the glossary.
- Describe the role of ethics in nursing practice.
- Differentiate ethical issues from moral and legal issues.
- Explain the influence of historical changes in health care on nursing ethics.
- Describe the influence of personal and professional values on ethical decisions.
- Contrast and compare responsibility and accountability.
- Explain the relationship between accountability and ethics.
- Identify the purposes of a professional code of ethics.
- Discuss the nature of ethical conflicts confronted by nurses.
- Discuss the process used to resolve ethical problems.

GLOSSARY

abortion Spontaneous or induced termination of pregnancy before the fetus has developed enough to be expected to live if born.

accountability State of being answerable for one's actions: the professional nurse answers to herself, the client, the profession, the employing institution, and society for the effectiveness of nursing care performed.

advocacy Process whereby a nurse objectively provides a client with the information he needs to make decisions and supports the client in whatever decisions he makes.

code of ethics Formal statement that delineates a profession's guidelines for ethical behavior; a code of ethics sets standards or expectations for the professional to achieve.

confidentiality Privacy; a nurse must maintain the confidentiality of information related to a client's health care.

contraception Prevention of pregnancy by means of a medication, device, or method that blocks or alters one or more of the processes of reproduction in such a way that sexual union can occur without impregnation.

ethics Principles or standards that govern proper conduct.

euthanasia Deliberately bringing about the death of a person who has an incurable disease or condition, either actively, by administering a lethal drug, or passively, by withholding treatment and allowing the person to die.

legal right Claim that is due according to legal guarantees.

living will Instrument by which a dying person makes his wishes known to those who are caring for him; a living will has no legal validity in most states.

morality Principles on which definitions of absolute right and wrong in behavior are based.

profession Vocation requiring specialized knowledge and intensive academic preparation.

psychosurgery Surgical interruption of certain nerve pathways in the brain; performed in selected cases of agitation, unremitting anxiety, and other forms of abnormal behavior.

psychotherapy Treatment of mental and emotional disorders by any of a large number of psychological techniques rather than by physical means.

sterilization Rendering a person unable to produce children; accomplished by surgical, chemical, or other means.

transplantation Transfer of an organ or tissue from one person to another or from one part of the body to another in order to replace a diseased structure or to restore function.

14 | *Ethics in Nursing*

The uniqueness of the nursing profession lies in the complexity and diversity of the roles and responsibilities assumed by its members. During the last decade, technological advances in health care have expanded the scope of duties nurses perform. Because today's professional nurse is a member of a multidisciplinary health care team, the nurse cannot make decisions and judgments in isolation from other health team members. Moreover, the client as a consumer has become more aware of his right to high-quality health care. The nurse acts as a liaison between the client and other health professionals to ensure that the client's rights are honored. Finally, nurses are better educated, are more independent, and possess more responsibility than ever before. The professional nurse therefore is able to strive toward the goal of providing a more thorough and comprehensive service to a wider range of clients.

The nurse's relationship with clients is unique. It is usually the nurse who spends the most time with clients—giving baths, offering comfort in times of pain, providing support when fears and anxieties are expressed. During times of crisis, the nurse is often more available than the physician, the social worker, or family members. The nurse's role is multifaceted, regardless of whether she is involved with the routines of health care or with dramatic life-and-death events. The nurse is ever present and thus frequently must assume the role of client advocate when ethical dilemmas develop.

Health care is administered within a pluralistic society, where many faiths and belief systems exist. With such a cultural and moral diversity it is often difficult to define common health care values. Who decides what is best for a client? What should clients know about their health? What is a nurse's responsibility when a client's right to good care is threatened? Value conflicts frequently cause nurses to be unsure of the nature of their relationships with clients, physicians, and other health care professionals. It therefore is mandatory that nurses know clearly what they value and why; otherwise they will be unable to make, and help clients make, responsible ethical decisions.

Definition of Ethics

Ethics comprises the principles or standards that govern proper conduct. The term originates from the Greek word *ethos,* meaning "custom." Put more simply, ethics speaks to what is right or wrong, to duties and obligations. Ethics addresses how human beings relate to each other in a philosophy of fairness. Characteristic of all professions, ethics serves to protect the rights of human beings.

Nurses are confronted with various types of ethical dilemmas in situations that may seem ordinary or routine. What should a nurse do in the following situations?

The nurse, Ms. Fryer, enters room 52B to give the client his medication. After taking the capsule, the client says, "I haven't seen this blue and red capsule before; what's it for?" Ms. Fryer tells the client that she is unsure but will find out. Later, when checking the client's chart, Ms. Fryer realizes that the client had no order for the blue and red capsule. He had received the wrong medication. Should Ms. Fryer fill out an incident report, which may damage the reputation of a colleague, even though the client had no ill effects from the medication?

The head nurse is walking by a client's room and overhears a conversation between the client and one of her nurses, Ms. Shelley. The client says, "Oh, please, my back is killing me. I need something for the pain." Ms. Shelley responds, "Now, now, just relax. The pain is only psychological." The head nurse is concerned, having discussed with Ms. Shelley only the week before the importance of not judging a client's behavior. Should the head nurse counsel Ms. Shelley about her judgmental behavior or ignore the incident?

The community health clinic where Mr. Green is employed operates along with other clinics under a city contract. Mr. Green has been a community health nurse for 12 years. He has gained personal and professional benefits from his community health experiences. His clients welcome his visits and encourage him to return to their homes. One day a fellow nurse asks Mr. Green if he will join other health care professionals in a strike against the city for higher wages. Should Mr. Green join the strike effort or continue to visit the clients who need his services?

Each of these three situations represents a typical ethical dilemma in which conflicts arise over philosophies, values, and professional duties. A dilemma is a situation that necessitates a choice between what appear to be equally desirable or undesirable alternatives. For example, a student faces a dilemma when he has to choose an academic major between two areas of study. His dilemma may be a difficult one, but it is not an ethical dilemma. In an ethical dilemma there is a conflict in values and a person is unsure of what constitutes proper conduct. In any ethical dilemma there is no absolute right or wrong; the person instead faces a difficult choice between conflicting values. Mr. Green, for example, must choose between loyalty to his clients and loyalty to his colleagues, neither choice being necessarily more "right" or ethical than the other.

Nurses face ethical dilemmas every day. The process of making an ethical decision can be a complicated one; choices cannot be made blindly or haphazardly. Nurses must make conscious efforts to resolve ethical problems intelligently and in ways that do not compromise their values.

A client receiving health care expects a nurse to be knowledgeable, skillful, and supportive of his rights as a consumer. A nurse's actions are guided by personal and professional beliefs and values, a philosophy of life and of nursing, and cultural and emotional variables. The multiplicity of factors that shape a nurse's ethical standards makes it difficult for the nurse to perceive ethical dilemmas clearly. Some basic questions can help to clarify a nurse's ethical perspective. What should be the philosophy of nursing? What constitutes good nursing practice? What qualities should nurses possess? How should personal values influence professional decision making? Nurses study ethics in order to prepare themselves to behave ethically when they are confronted with dilemmas and to function in ways that are consistent with what they believe.

Ethical, moral, and legal values are not necessarily related. A moral belief is the conviction that something is absolutely right or wrong in all situations. A person is generally unwilling to compromise or change his opinions on issues of a moral nature. To one person, for example, abortion may be an absolute moral wrong—in other words, there are no acceptable reasons for any woman to attempt to terminate her pregnancy prematurely. If this person holds morally consistent views, he may also believe that capital punishment is a moral wrong. Not all persons hold the same moral views, and what is a moral issue for some can be an ethical dilemma for others. In regard to the example of abortion, another person may be willing to accept abortion under certain situations. The values of the woman undergoing the abortion or the expected nature of the future life of the unborn child may make a difference in regard to whether abortion is acceptable. A moral issue becomes an ethical one when the choice is no longer clearly between right and wrong.

A difference also exists between ethical and legal issues. Frequently the two are inextricably related, as in the case of a family's willingness to halt life-support measures for a terminally ill child. The parents have the legal right to stop all efforts to keep their child alive when physicians agree that therapy is no longer beneficial. However, they must struggle with the ethical issue of whether it is right to end the life of a human being so young. Both ethics and the law refer to rules of conduct based on underlying principles of what is right or wrong. A legal right can be defined as a just claim or something that is due according to legal guarantees and moral principles, or as a moral, ethical, or legal principle considered as an underlying cause of truth, justice, or morality (Fromer, 1981). There are obvious legal and ethical overtones that accompany a definition of a right. The legal view implies that if there are rights, legal obligations also exist. For example, a physician is obligated to honor a client's request to stop therapy when an illness is determined to be terminal.

In contrast, an ethical right involves no legal guarantees, as in the example of the right to health care. If it is assumed that health care is a right, it must be assumed that ethical obligations are involved. But if health care is a right, who is obligated to provide it? The right to health care is not legally enforceable because it is not a legal right. Health professionals do, however, feel obliged to provide health care to those seeking it; they are motivated to provide health care as though it were a legal right.

The law attempts to resolve only major wrongs against an individual or society, while ethics deals with all the wrongs in humans' interactions with one another. Thus, ethical issues are not always translatable into law.

The profession of nursing is practiced within certain legal constraints (see Chapter 17) that ensure safe and effective care. However, there are also ethical considerations involved in the nurse's daily performance of care. Ethics provides standards that govern the nurse's decisions and actions. In today's society the nurse's role has become more complex, and thus ethical dilemmas have become more complex. Nursing ethics must keep pace with the diversity in nursing practice in order to remain relevant to that practice.

Historical Perspective

As nursing has changed, so too have its ethical standards. At the turn of the century a nurse did not have to resolve the issues facing the professional nurse of today. The nurse's role focused primarily on tending to a client's basic needs. Purity, honesty, dedication, obedience, and loyalty were standards against which a nurse's performance was measured. The nurse functioned in a dependent role under the watchful eye of the physician. Nursing ethics were relatively simple when all a nurse had to do was follow rules and the physician's orders.

The nurse of today has assumed more independence and responsibility. Nurses are educated to practice self-sufficiency and assertiveness as they participate actively in health care decisions. The nurse has become an equal to the physician with respect to involvement in the client's total health care plan. In some settings nurses are able to practice in roles independent of physicians' influence, such as nurse practitioners or clinical specialists. As nurses have expanded their realm of responsibility, the scope of ethical decision making has enlarged.

The system of ethics in nursing originates in the Judeo-Christian heritage. The sanctity of human life is assumed, and it is the duty of society to give care and compassion to the sick. Nursing's Judeo-Christian ethical orientation has not changed. However, advances in medicine and technology have brought about rapid social changes that have given rise to ethical dilemmas. Genetic engineering, whole-organ transplantation, and mechanical life-support systems, for example, have raised serious questions for ethically minded people. The nurse is faced with difficult ethical decisions as complex technology threatens to treat human beings as mere collections of body parts. The sanctity of human life is often forgotten when the maintenance of machines and equipment seemingly takes precedence over nurturing and compassion. The prolongation of life sometimes seems to have become more important than the quality of life.

As the profession of nursing continues to expand its roles and corresponding responsibilities, nurses must be informed about the ethical issues of the day. Standards for professional competence not only encourage the nurse to be informed but also establish guidelines for maintaining a nurse's ethical accountability.

Personal Values

Values are a person's beliefs about the worth of given ideas or behavior (see Chapter 13). Formed as a result of a person's experiences and cultural background, values provide a way to view the world. Some of a person's values may be shared by some or many other people, but a person's complete set of values is unique. One person may view the death of an individual as a natural part of life, as something to be understood and not feared. Another person may believe that every effort should be taken to preserve life, even if it means the endurance of considerable suffering. A person's set of values is one means by which he is known by others and by which he identifies himself. Becoming aware of her own personal values helps a nurse to understand their impact on her professional development and nursing actions.

Professional values are a reflection of personal values. The ability of a nurse to protect a client's right to privacy or accept responsibility for maintaining nursing skills depends on the nurse's personal view of the importance of confidentiality and professional development. When a person enters the nursing profession, she does not suddenly develop values, nor does she abruptly change them to meet life circumstances. With time, she adapts existing personal values to professional experiences and expectations. Experiences in nursing broaden the horizons of her thinking as she encounters new situations. It is of course beneficial for a beginning nurse to recognize and understand any differences between her personal values and her professional values. Most nursing students begin their professional socialization after they already have a clear sense of their personal values; however, because their health care experiences are limited, there is considerable room for growth in applying values to new experiences. As a nurse's personal values complement and reinforce professional values, it becomes easier for her to practice nursing as an ethically responsible individual. Only then can a nurse assist clients in the clarification of their values.

When an ethical dilemma arises, ideally the nurse analyzes it and then acts with foresight and reasoning. Too often, however, ethical questions are clouded by the emotions that accompany her personal values and attitudes and the specific situations that evoke the dilemmas. A nurse who devoutly values the creation of life will encounter an ethical dilemma if she is asked to assist with an abortion. She knows that, from an ethical standpoint, a woman having an abortion deserves the same care and respect as any other client. However, the value the nurse places on life makes the ethical commitment to avoid a value judgment extremely difficult.

Thus, a nurse's personal values shape the manner in which she assumes her professional responsibilities. When personal and professional values exist in harmony, a nurse is best able to resolve ethical dilemmas calmly and reasonably.

Professional Ethics

What makes nurses professionals? What responsibilities are involved in the role of a professional? Fromer (1981) lists the following characteristics of a professional:

1. The profession is worked at full time and is the professional's principal source of income.
2. The professional sees his work as a commitment to a calling. It is more than just a job.
3. Professionals are organized with their peers for professional reasons—that is, for reasons that transcend money and other tangible benefits.
4. The professional possesses useful knowledge and skills based on an education of exceptional duration and difficulty.
5. Professionals exhibit a service orientation that goes beyond financial motivation.
6. The professional proceeds in his work by his own judgment.

As a professional, the nurse makes a commitment to clients and the nursing profession to provide the best possible quality of health care. A nurse's education prepares her with the necessary knowledge and skills to help fulfill her professional commitment. Clinical experiences promote the nurse's socialization into the profession, as she learns the standards and norms set by colleagues within nursing and other health care disciplines. The process of becoming a

professional is complete only when the values of the profession are integrated into the values of the person.

Codes of Ethics

The nursing profession has codes of ethics that affirm professional regard for high ideals of conduct. A profession's ethical code is a collective statement about the group's expectations, a standard of behav-

---

American Nurses' Association Code of Ethics

1. The nurse provides services with respect for human dignity and the uniqueness of the client unrestricted by considerations of social or economic status, personal attributes, or the nature of health problems.
2. The nurse safeguards the client's right to privacy by judiciously protecting information of a confidential nature.
3. The nurse acts to safeguard the client and the public when health care and safety are affected by the incompetent, unethical, or illegal practice of any person.
4. The nurse assumes responsibility and accountability for individual nursing judgments and actions.
5. The nurse maintains competence in nursing.
6. The nurse exercises informed judgment and uses individual competence and qualifications as criteria in seeking consultation, accepting responsibilities, and delegating nursing activities to others.
7. The nurse participates in activities that contribute to the ongoing development of the profession's body of knowledge.
8. The nurse participates in the profession's efforts to implement and improve standards of nursing.
9. The nurse participates in the profession's efforts to establish and maintain conditions of employment conducive to high quality nursing care.
10. The nurse participates in the profession's effort to protect the public from misinformation and misrepresentation and to maintain the integrity of nursing.
11. The nurse collaborates with members of the health professions and other citizens in promoting community and national efforts to meet the health needs of the public.

From American Nurses' Association: Code for nurses, Kansas City, Mo., 1976, The Association.

ior. An ethical code for nurses serves as a reminder of the special responsibilities assumed by those who care for the sick. Nurses deal with people who, because of illness or injury, are often vulnerable and dependent on the professional's knowledge and skill. The nursing profession must formulate and adhere to high ideals of conduct to assure the public and society that individual nurses will not exploit their positions.

A code is a set of ethical principles that are generally accepted by all members of a profession, even though different professional organizations may describe the principles differently. Ethical codes provide standards of conduct and thus allow a profession to discipline its members. These standards indicate some of the factors that nurses must take into consideration in deciding on proper conduct. Ethical codes also provide a common foundation for professional nursing curricula. As a nurse makes the transition from ethical theory to ethical practice, she realizes that she alone is responsible for following ethical standards in her

behavior and in the care she delivers to her clients.

It is difficult to codify all of the principles to which one must adhere in order to resolve dilemmas in a field as ethically complex as nursing. Nurses face ethical dilemmas that are not always clearly governed by ethical codes. A useful code of ethics must be brief, yet detailed enough to offer clear guidance and attain widespread acceptance. The American Nurses' Association (ANA) and the International Council of Nurses (ICN) have established widely accepted codes that the professional nurse should attempt to follow (see boxed material). Although these codes differ somewhat in specific emphasis, they reflect the same underlying principles.

Accountability and Responsibility

Each nurse assumes responsibility for carrying out specific nursing activities for the care of a client. "Responsibility" also refers to the scope of functions and

---

International Council of Nurses Code for Nurses

The fundamental responsibility of the nurse is fourfold: to promote health, to prevent illness, to restore health, and to alleviate suffering.

The need for nursing is universal. Inherent in nursing is respect for life, dignity, and rights of man. It is unrestricted by considerations of nationality, race, creed, color, age, sex, politics or social status.

Nurses render health services to the individual, the family and the community and coordinate their services with those of related groups.

Nurses and People

The nurse's primary responsibility is to those people who require nursing care.

The nurse, in providing care, promotes an environment in which the values, customs and spiritual beliefs of the individual are respected.

The nurse holds in confidence, personal information and uses judgment in sharing this information.

Nurses and Practice

The nurse carries personal responsibility for nursing practice and for maintaining competence by continual learning. The nurse maintains the highest standards of nursing care possible within the reality of a specific situation.

The nurse uses judgment in relation to individual competence when accepting and delegating responsibilities.

The nurse when acting in a professional capacity should at all times maintain standards of personal conduct which reflect credit upon the profession.

Nurses and Society

The nurse shares with other citizens the responsibility for initiating and supporting action to meet the health and social needs of the public.

Nurses and Co-Workers

The nurse sustains a cooperative relationship with co-workers in nursing and other fields. The nurse takes appropriate action to safeguard the individual when his care is endangered by a co-worker or any other person.

Nurses and the Profession

The nurse plays the major role in determining and implementing desirable standards of nursing practice and nursing education.

The nurse is active in developing a core of professional knowledge.

The nurse, acting through the professional organization, participates in establishing and maintaining equitable social and economic working conditions in nursing.

From International Council of Nurses: ICN code for nurses: ethical concepts applied to nursing, Geneva, 1973, Imprimeries Populaires.

duties associated with the nurse's role. As nurses assume more functions, these functions become part of the nurse's responsibility. In the case of administering a medication, a nurse has responsibilities to assess the client's need for the medication, to ensure that the medication is given safely and correctly, and to evaluate the client's response to the medication. By being responsible for her actions, the nurse is reliable and worthy of trust from colleagues and clients. A responsible nurse is competent in knowledge and skills. It is also imperative that the nurse possess an ethical responsibility to her client. A nurse delivers care to a client who is at least partially dependent on the nurse's choice of actions and who has placed his trust in the nurse's abilities. The responsibility of a nurse entails a willingness to perform appropriately within the ethical guidelines of the profession.

Whenever a nurse performs nursing care for a client, she must be able to answer for her actions; in other words, the nursing profession is characterized by accountability. If during the administration of a medication a nurse gives the wrong dose, she is accountable to the client who received it, the physician who ordered it, and the nursing administrators who set standards of expected performance. A responsible nurse reports the error and initiates care to prevent any further injury to the client. Accountability calls for an evaluation of a nurse's effectiveness in performing her responsibilities.

A nurse is accountable to herself, to the client, to the profession, to the employing institution, and to society. A nurse assumes accountability to herself through a willingness to report to appropriate authorities any conduct on her part that endangers clients. The nurse's highest priority is the safety and well-being of clients. Whenever a nurse makes an incorrect judgment or acts in a manner that is harmful, or potentially harmful, to a client, she is accountable for her behavior. No one else is accountable for a nurse's own actions, even when she acts on another's orders. For example, if a physician orders the wrong dosage of a medication and the nurse administers it without questioning the order, the nurse can be held accountable for the medication's effects.

Being accountable to the client means that the nurse provides the client with information about his care. When caring for a client, a nurse is responsible for informing him about nursing procedures and providing information that helps him make decisions about his care. The nurse is accountable for being sure that the information given to him is accurate. A client can easily be misled or confused if a nurse, either consciously or unknowingly, gives him inaccurate information. A nurse must either have correct information or know where to get it.

The nurse maintains accountability to the profession and therefore to society by maintaining high ethical standards in her own practice and by encouraging other professionals to do the same. If a nurse observes conduct of another nurse or a physician that endangers a client, she must assume responsibility for reporting the incident. If she does not do so, she can be held accountable for failure to report her colleague's unethical behavior. For example, if a nurse observes another nurse change a sterile dressing using unsterile technique or perform a procedure that is contraindicated by a client's condition, the first nurse is obligated to report the incident to the appropriate authorities.

The nurse is also accountable to the institution that employs her. Nursing administrators and physicians are usually the persons to whom a nurse is answerable. Institutions develop policies and procedures to provide consistent guidelines for performing health care activities. Policies and procedures prevent confusion and error as nurses deliver care. If a nurse performs a procedure in a manner that is inconsistent with the institutional policy, she is accountable for the results of her actions.

The nurse's primary ethical concern is helping each client receive high-quality health care. In performing her professional functions, a nurse has the potential not only to help clients but also to inflict some discomfort or stress. When helping a client regain use of a badly fractured arm, a nurse may unavoidably cause pain as she assists the client in performing active exercises. If a nurse is to facilitate a client's acceptance of a terminal illness, it may become necessary to discuss emotionally stressful concerns. It often is difficult to discriminate beneficial actions from unnecessarily stressful ones. A nurse can be most responsible to a client if she weighs carefully the benefits and disadvantages of her actions. By being responsible the nurse ultimately becomes more accountable. A nurse's accountability rests on choosing the best possible alternative for meeting a client's needs.

Conflicts frequently arise over issues of responsibility and accountability. For example, a nurse's professional values may conflict with the policy of an institution. Should the nurse be obligated to behave in a way the institution expects? Often a nurse feels caught in the middle between nursing administrators and physicians and is unsure to whom she should be accountable. Policies and procedures provide uniformity in basic standards of nursing care, thus maintaining the quality of care within an institution. If a nurse disagrees with the expectations of an institution, it is possible to work within the system to change them, perhaps by refining and modifying outdated policies and procedures. Participation with the institution gives nurses more accountability.

Society at large has the goal of providing health care to everyone. As a member of the health care delivery system, the nurse functions within the rules of that system. Bureaucratic barriers are often imposed by the system, which can create conflicts involving a nurse's ethical values. For example, a client who is affluent, powerful, and educated generally is aware of his health care rights, or has little difficulty learning what they are. In contrast, a client who is poor, weak, and uneducated may be unaware of his rights and may have great difficulty learning what they are. Thus, nurses may experience conflict when attempting to protect the rights of the disadvantaged and vulnerable. Unless nurses support the rights of all clients, however, they are not complying with society's demands.

Professional accountability serves four basic purposes:

1. To evaluate new professional practices and reassess existing ones
2. To maintain standards of health care
3. To facilitate personal reflection, ethical thought, and personal growth on the part of health professionals
4. To provide a basis for ethical decision making

Without accountability a nurse's behavior may be unpredictable, preventing her from attaining professional competence.

Can an individual nurse's performance be measured? A recent trend in health care is the establishment of standards of care. The Joint Commission on Accreditation of Hospitals has recommended certain standards for the delivery of nursing care. Standards of nursing care provide a basic structure against which to measure whether competent nursing care is being delivered. Performance can then be measured objectively, as well as critically. Tucker and associates (1984) have provided an example of a set of standards to follow in providing general physical comfort to a client (see Table 14-1). These standards do not eliminate the need for an individual plan of care. However, nurses who incorporate these standards into a client's plan of care meet their ethical responsibility for delivering competent care in regard to physical comfort. Accountability is ensured because the quality of care achieved can be measured.

It is essential for nurses to be accountable for nursing care and not to let members of other disciplines assume that responsibility. Therefore nurses must be actively involved in the ethical decisions that are made. Accountability is achieved when a nurse assumes responsibility for professional competence and uses a systematic process to resolve ethical dilemmas.

TABLE 14-1

Standards for Physical Comfort on Which Accountability May Be Based

Observations	Ongoing Care
Condition of bed and linen	Change bed daily and as necessary. Keep linen neat, dry, wrinkle free, and clean.
Comfortable position	Change client's position as necessary.
Warmth and dryness	Provide adequate blankets for warmth; keep bedclothes dry.
Freedom from pain	Provide comfort measures to relieve discomfort and pain: Give soothing backrubs Change position Offer warm drinks Administer analgesics as ordered
Correct body alignment	Maintain body alignment: Prevent contractures and foot-drop with exercises and footboard Support dependent parts with pillows

Modified from Tucker, S.M., et al.: Patient care standards, ed. 3, St. Louis, 1984, The C.V. Mosby Co.

Client Advocacy

Ethical standards govern the behavior of professionals and institutions toward clients. In contrast, laws govern the licensing of professionals and prescribe the boundaries of legal practice. It is usually true that if a nurse practices ethically she will also be practicing legally. Of the two, ethics and the law, only the law is readily enforceable.

As Kohnke (1982) has pointed out, the concept of advocacy bridges the gap between ethics and the law. In nursing, advocacy consists of informing a client and then supporting him in whatever decision he makes. Properly informing a client meets a nurse's legal responsibilities, and supporting a client meets the ethical requirement of honoring a person's right to self-determination.

Advocacy is more than simply giving a client information and hoping he will use it in decision making. It is a complex process that first requires the nurse to gain an understanding of her own attitudes, values, and beliefs. Then she learns to approach a client with an open mind, recognizing that he may have different values and beliefs. Advocacy is not the same as values clarification (see Chapter 13); however, in order to be an advocate, a nurse may need to clarify what her own or the client's values are.

The two primary functions of advocacy are to inform and to support. To inform a client properly, a nurse must have accurate information or know where to get it. A nurse should not feel like a failure if she admits to not knowing something, as long as she attempts to find a resource for the correct information. A nurse advocate must also *want* the client to have the information. Frequently, nurses are fearful that if a client knows too much, his knowledge may cause him to question or even refuse the care he needs. However, a client must agree to knowing the information; he has the right *not* to know. In addition, a nurse advocate presents information in a way that is meaningful to the client. This may involve providing basic explanations or timing discussions so that the client is receptive to the nurse's descriptions. Finally, a nurse advocate recognizes that many persons, such as family members, physicians, and health care administrators, do not want clients to have information. This situation makes advocacy very difficult. The role of advocate becomes a careful balancing act between telling a client what he needs to know and not threatening the client's relationship with his physician or his family.

The supportive aspect of advocacy requires a nurse to support a client without falling into a defensive or rescuing position. The responsibility for decision making rests with the client and not the advocate. The nurse advocate refrains from giving advice, passing judgment, or offering approval. This is not an easy task. The nurse is well aware of the risks that are inevitable if a client makes a wrong decision about his health care. For example, a client may refuse a treatment or refuse to participate in his care. Either decision could seriously impede his recovery and rehabilitation. A nurse gives a client the knowledge he needs, thereby placing him in a position to make his own decision. If the decision is a wrong one, the nurse teaches the client how to accept it and how to make a better one in the future.

The beginning nursing student will frequently encounter clients who are asking for help in decision making: "Should I take my bath now, before I go to x-ray?" "Do you think I need this medication?" "Is it OK if I try to feed myself?" Such simple questions may be very significant to a client who is ill. However, they provide excellent opportunities for the nurse to help the client learn to make decisions for himself. When bigger decisions arise, the client will be more capable of making them. In helping clients to make seemingly small decisions, a nurse gains practice in the advocate's role.

Consider the following hypothetical situation:

Mr. Tate comes to the clinic 2 weeks after being discharged from the hospital following removal of a cataract. He tells a nurse, "My doctor said I shouldn't bend over or lift heavy weights for 6 weeks. Do you think it's OK to pick up my 1-year-old little boy if I'm careful?"

The nurse could simply tell Mr. Tate to avoid picking up anything weighing more than 10 pounds. However, to help Mr. Tate make his own decision, the nurse first explains why the lifting restriction is made and the effects lifting would have on his eye. The nurse clarifies with Mr. Tate how heavy his son actually is. The nurse and the client also discuss whether there is anyone at home during the day to watch the infant, since Mrs. Tate works.

At the end of the discussion the nurse says, "Well, Mr. Tate, I really can't tell you what to do. We've talked about the pros and cons of restrictions related to your surgery. What do you think is best?"

Mr. Tate still has a choice. He can decide to avoid lifting his son until 4 more weeks have passed, or he can risk injuring his eye by ignoring the physician's and nurse's warnings. What if Mr. Tate chooses to ignore the restrictions? The nurse might feel guilty for not insisting that the client make the safer decision. However, even then the nurse would have no assurance that the client would follow the restrictions at home. Using an advocate's approach places the responsibility for decision making with the client. The nurse fulfills her ethical responsibility by providing the client with a means to choose his own course of action.

There is one key point to remember when a nurse pursues an advocacy role. Not all clients require an advocate. There are clients who are quite capable of making their own decisions without a nurse's support. However, it is always appropriate for a nurse to share pertinent and meaningful information with a client.

Ethical Problems in Nursing

Diverse ethical issues are involved in health care today. Issues may arise in any of the five areas in which the nurse is accountable: self, profession, client and family, employing institution, and society. In addition, in any area or specialty of nursing practice, a nurse will be confronted with ethical issues unique to that practice. The following outline is not all inclusive:

Community health nursing
    Abortion
    Artificial insemination by a donor

Contraception
Genetic counseling
Right to health care
Nursing of children
Allowing severely ill or deformed neonates to die
Child abuse
Child experimentation
Mental health nursing
Behavior control
Involuntary hospitalization
Psychotherapy
Suicide
Medical-surgical nursing
Definition of death
Living will
Prolonging life artificially versus euthanasia
Transplantation
Nurse-physician-client relationships
Confidentiality
Informed consent
Role conflicts
Issues between nurses
Interdependent roles
Common licensure

Each of the following sections attempts to illustrate the nature of the ethical dilemmas in one area of nursing practice. For each area of practice only one example of an ethical dilemma is discussed.

Community Health Nursing

In community clinics, as well as in physicians' offices and hospital settings, the nurse will encounter couples raising questions about contraception. The nurse has an obligation to provide clients with information about the types of contraception, their benefits, and their disadvantages. If a man and a woman disagree about whether to have children, serious ethical questions arise. The nurse's role is to understand the attitudes and values each partner has regarding contraception. A values clarification approach will help each partner understand the other's views (see Chapter 13). The nurse cannot choose for her clients the actions to follow. However, she can provide information to allow each partner to make his or her own free choice so that ultimately the partners can agree on a course of action.

Nursing of Children

The question of whether a person should be allowed to die is one of the most difficult faced by health care professionals and society. The issue is even more value laden when it involves children; it is difficult to understand why a young child must lose his life without having had the opportunity to experience living. If a child suffers from a terminal illness or a serious brain injury, parents and family members may have to decide between preserving life artificially and allowing the child to die with dignity. Advocates of "death with dignity" believe that a person should not be forced to endure pain, suffering, or humiliation, and that he has the right to choose relief in dying. Those who support the "right to life," however, believe that hope should never be discarded; they argue that no individual has the right to determine when life is over, that only God can decide such a matter.

The physician, bound by the Hippocratic Oath, is committed to preserving life. The nurse has the responsibility to support any measures ordered by the physician, as well as to maintain the dignity of the dying person.

The parents and other family members experience the emotions of fear, guilt, and anger when the question of death is raised. The infant or child facing death cannot make a choice. The responsibility rests entirely with the parents. If the child is an only child, if the illness occurred suddenly rather than gradually, or if the parents have never been faced with the death of a family member before, a decision will be extremely difficult. Often the parents will seek the nurse's advice as to what choice is best. The nurse, influenced by her own emotions and philosophy of life, must help the parents clarify their own values. As a client advocate, the nurse helps the parents to understand their child's predicament and supports them in the difficult decision they face (Fig. 14-1).

Mental Health Nursing

What is acceptable behavior? Usually it is defined by the people who observe the behavior. Conflict can arise between groups of people who define acceptable behavior in different ways. For example, a person who starts a fistfight is seen by some as one who is willing to defend his opinions and beliefs at all costs; others see him as a troublemaker and a threat to society. The setting in which a person behaves also determines whether behavior is acceptable. For example, a public display of emotion is viewed one way in the U.S. House of Representatives and a different way in a neighborhood restaurant. Society evaluates the behavior of its members on the basis of whether that behavior is disruptive to its well-being. A severely mentally ill person who murders, rapes, or steals is removed from society until he is able to return as a contributing member. The disruption that persons suffering from milder forms of mental illness cause to society may not be as overt. If a person's behavior becomes sufficiently out of tune with society's expec-

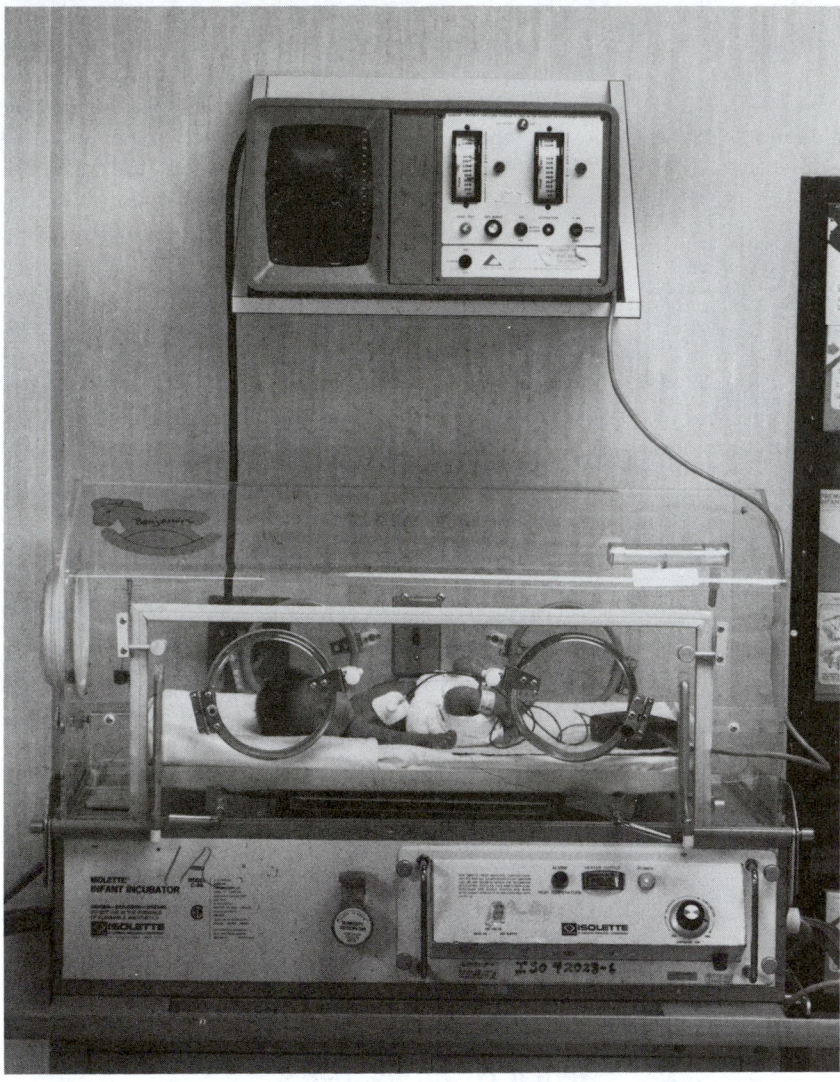

Fig. 14-1 Whether a child should be allowed to die peacefully, without aggressive medical care, is a difficult ethical issue for a nurse to face.

tations, then society decides that he needs to conform to more acceptable behavioral standards.

Mental illness and deviant behavior have traditionally not been accepted by society. The judgment that a person is mentally ill is based on social, ethical, and behavioral standards. At one time a person suffering mental illness was believed to be possessed by evil spirits. Today many types of mental illness are classified as biological disorders rather than behavioral disturbances. As society changes, so too do ideas about acceptable behavior.

Controlling a person's behavior can be considered an infringement of liberty. Confinement in a mental institution is an extreme example of depriving a person of his freedom. However, mental health care professionals have a variety of less extreme methods to control behavior in the interest of the person's own health and welfare and the welfare of society. Tran-

quilizers, electric shock, psychosurgery (removal of a portion of brain tissue that controls behavior), and psychotherapy are examples. Various ethical questions arise: Who decides whether any given behavior is normal or desirable? Who is expert enough to identify normal behavior? If a person has difficulty adjusting to his role in society, whose goals should influence behavior therapy—the client's, the family's, the therapist's, or society's? Should a person's behavior be changed if he does not wish it to be? Society and mental health professionals generally agree that behavior that is destructive to an individual or to others, as well as behavior that prevents an individual from being able to function independently, is abnormal and undesirable. However, the issue is far from clear cut, because judgment is still required as to what behavior fits these criteria. A nurse is able to observe a client's behavior over a longer period of time than a physician or a therapist. In addition, the nurse develops a relationship with family members, whose lives are affected by the client's behavior. The nurse will often find herself in a position to identify accurately the rationale for the client's behavior. The perspective of the nurse can help determine to what extent behavior should be modified or controlled.

Medical-Surgical Nursing

Transplantations of organs or tissues from one human being to another have been performed since the seventeenth century, when the first successful blood transfusion was accomplished. Since that time, organ transplantations have come to include hearts, kidneys, corneas, bone marrow, and lungs. However, the availability of organs from living donors and cadavers is limited, making transplantation an expensive procedure.

The overall success rate of transplants has increased with scientific advancements, and with that increase has come an array of ethical concerns. Members of some religious groups consider it wrong to mutilate a person's body. An opposing view suggests that parts of the body exist for the good of the whole and that a nonfunctioning part may be removed if preservation of the whole body is achieved.

It may seem surprising that there are strong views against organ transplantation. However, consider the ethical situation that exists in the case of a 14-year-old boy who has suffered brain death as a result of injuries sustained in an automobile accident. Mechanical life support is the only thing keeping the boy's body alive. Meanwhile, a 58-year-old man suffering from renal failure lies in a hospital bed waiting for a kidney donor. Should attempts to preserve the young boy's life be halted in order to use the boy's kidneys? Should the family feel obligated to donate the boy's kidneys?

The issue of organ transplantation can be extremely emotional. Guilt and coercion are commonly involved in a person's decision to give up a kidney or bone marrow to a family member. At a time when the relatives of a dead person are experiencing considerable grief, they are asked to make a calm, rational decision about donating an organ to a needy recipient. The recipient of a transplanted organ experiences the anxiety of wondering whether the new organ will function in his body.

A nurse may be confronted with questions from clients and families as to whether organ transplantation is the right choice. Many recipients have suffered from chronic diseases. A nurse who has cared for a chronically ill client may be particularly in favor of transplantation if it means relief of the client's

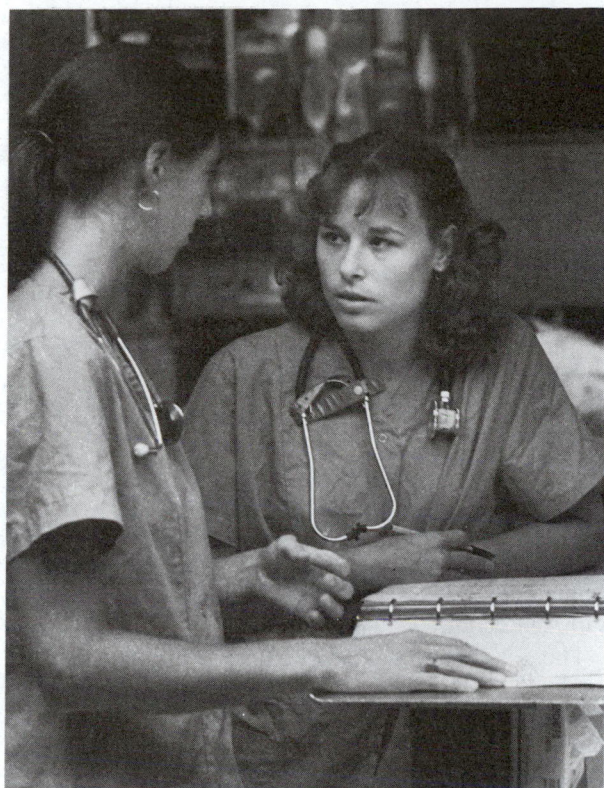

Fig. 14-2 With advances in medical technology, the care of critically ill clients poses numerous ethical dilemmas for nurses who work in intensive care settings.

suffering. Yet there is significant risk involved in organ transplantation, as with other types of major surgery, with no guarantee that the health of the recipient will improve. These issues must be raised before a client or his family makes the decision to have a transplant (Fig. 14-2).

Nurse-Physician-Client Relationships

One of the more common problems the nurse faces is role conflict. Not only are nurses responsible for the clients in their care, they are also accountable to families, health care administrators, and physicians. These differing roles give rise to ethical problems unique to nurses.

Smith and Davis (1980) have summarized factors within institutional settings that influence a nurse's ability to make ethical decisions:

1. Nurses, as employees, work under policies established by others.
2. Conflicts arise between the professional model of nursing education and the bureaucratic model of health care institutions.
3. Nurses are often given responsibility and accountability but not authority.

4. Nurses experience role conflicts with other health care professionals.
5. Nurses experience conflicts between meeting a client's needs and following institutional procedures.
6. Nurses generally have either limited or no input into decisions that they are responsible for implementing.

Several of these factors may operate simultaneously. Assume, for example, that a nurse is caring for a client whose wife has died during his hospitalization. The client asks frequent questions regarding why his wife has not visited. The client's physician has left orders not to tell the client of his wife's death for fear that an emotional setback would worsen his condition. The nurse's duty to the client's needs conflicts with her duty to follow the physician's orders. The nurse's role of providing psychological support has been made more difficult, since she cannot share the truth with the client.

The nurse often faces a dilemma when she attempts to clarify her role among health care professionals. Clients need compassionate and skilled nursing care. Health care administrators need good consumer relations and a realistic budget. Physicians expect nurses to follow the proposed plans of treatment. If a tight budget results in understaffing, the number of nurses may be inadequate to provide compassionate care. A physician may write an order that a nurse knows to be inappropriate to the situation, yet she faces great pressure to carry out the order. Again, the same questions arise: To whom is the nurse most accountable? How can the nurse resolve an ethical dilemma so that she retains her professionalism in delivering quality care?

Issues between Nurses

In most areas of nursing practice nurses work together. Because of the interdependent relationships between nurses, one nurse's practice affects and is affected by the practice of others. Failure of a nurse to maintain ethical standards in practice can have serious negative effects on her colleagues if they are unwilling to hold her accountable. For example, if a nurse arriving on a hospital's evening shift finds the narcotic count inaccurate, she should question each of the day shift personnel to see if they can account for the missing medication. If the nurse chooses not to pursue the matter, a subsequent investigation could cast doubt on her own professional integrity.

Several factors add to the complexity of ethical issues between nurses. All registered nurses hold the same license, but educational preparation may vary considerably. There is disagreement within the profession as to the preferred way to reach professional nursing status. Thus, situations can arise in which nurses with differing educational backgrounds question each other's ability to make sound judgments and decisions. In addition, levels of experience vary widely. A nurse who is experienced in her area of practice and who has kept informed about current developments in nursing is likely to be more clinically qualified than a recent graduate, even a graduate of a prestigious school. Nurses place differing degrees of importance on theoretical models of nursing as well as on activities involved in the nursing process. It is not uncommon to find two nurses correctly performing the same procedure in two entirely different ways.

Nurses practice in various settings and under various staffing arrangements. Settings within hospitals include intensive care units, nurseries, rehabilitation units, pediatric units, operating rooms, medical and surgical inpatient units, and in-service education departments. Settings outside of hospitals include extended care facilities, clinics, schools, industries, offices, and clients' homes. Each setting presents a nurse with different types of ethical dilemmas.

Staff assignment practices vary in terms of the level of responsibility nurses assume in managing the care of clients. For example, a nurse's role in team nursing is quite different from that in primary nursing. As a team leader, a registered nurse supervises the care of a large group of clients. The team members—fellow registered nurses, licensed practical nurses, and nurse assistants—deliver the actual client care. The team leader plans and coordinates the care of all clients being cared for by her team and serves as a resource person for team members. In contrast, a primary nurse provides direct, total care for a small group of clients. In addition, the primary nurse coordinates the activities of client, physician, family members, and other health care workers.

Because of the various roles and responsibilities nurses assume, a variety of ethical dilemmas arise between nurses. Consider the following ethical problems:

A client, Mrs. Gregory, tells her nurse, Mr. Owens, that the nurse assigned to her care the previous evening was rude and slow in responding to her calls. Mrs. Gregory asks Mr. Owens not to mention the incident for fear that the other nurse would become angry. Should Mr. Owens report the incident?

Ms. Matthews is responsible for interviewing all applicants for registered nurse positions in a hospital. During an interview with Ms. Douglas, a staff nurse with 2 years' experience in another hospital, Ms. Matthews learns that Ms. Douglas once had a drug problem. The young nurse is honest about her problem, stating that she had gone through a rehabilitation program and now wants another chance. Should Ms. Matthews recommend Ms. Douglas for a job?

During an emergency procedure, Mr. Hawkins, head nurse of a surgical intensive care unit, observes a staff nurse using the wrong technique for inserting an intravenous catheter. However, unless the catheter is inserted immediately, the client may not be saved. Should Mr. Hawkins say something now to the nurse about her improper technique?

In each of these situations the nurse faced with the ethical dilemma has difficult questions to answer. In the first case, Mr. Owens learns that a colleague has been accused of being rude, which would be contrary to her obligation to remain courteous, pleasant, and supportive of clients' needs. Mr. Owens knows that if the client, Mrs. Gregory, continues to be assigned to the rude nurse, there may be additional problems. The client may also begin to assume that all nurses caring for her are unpleasant. Mr. Owens recognizes that the nurse accused of being rude should be allowed to tell her side of the story. He decides to talk with the nurse in question, inform her of the client's concerns, and learn how the nurse interprets her encounter with the client.

Ms. Matthews has a difficult decision as to whether to offer Ms. Douglas a job. A nurse who has a history of drug abuse might be tempted to steal medication that is available in the work setting. However, the young nurse has been honest, and perhaps she has broken her habit. Ms. Matthews decides to check the nurse's work references and obtains her permission to speak to her therapist at the rehabilitation center.

In the situation involving Mr. Hawkins, the timing of the event creates the real problem. If he took the staff nurse aside to correct her for poor technique, there might not be enough staff nurses to attend to the client's emergency needs. Mr. Hawkins decides to discuss the event with the nurse once the emergency is over. He reasons that directing the nurse to change her technique will prevent similar occurrences in the future.

Throughout one's experience as a nurse there will always be situations involving other nurses that raise ethical questions. A nurse cannot be ethically responsible if she ignores the unethical conduct of colleagues. Careful judgment and a methodical decision-making process help a nurse to make sound ethical decisions.

Process for Resolving Ethical Problems

For the beginning nursing student, solving an ethical dilemma may seem impossible, but making a careful analysis of the variables involved in the dilemma

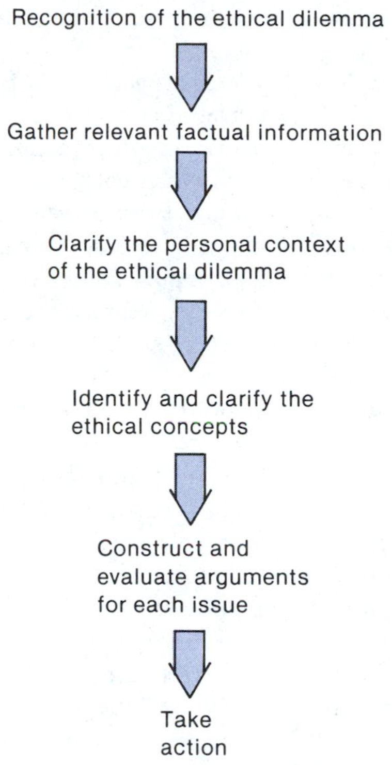

Recognition of the ethical dilemma

Gather relevant factual information

Clarify the personal context of the ethical dilemma

Identify and clarify the ethical concepts

Construct and evaluate arguments for each issue

Take action

Fig. 14-3 Process for resolution of ethical dilemmas.

will help her plan an intelligent course of action (Fig. 14-3). First, the nurse obtains relevant factual information related to the ethical issue. It is unwise to make an ethical decision on the basis of another person's opinions or emotions. The nurse gathers as much objective information as possible that is pertinent to the issue as well as to the individuals involved.

The nurse also clarifies the personal context of the ethical dilemma. What emotions, attitudes, or values influence the nurse's own perception of the dilemma? To clarify the real ethical issues in any given situation, a nurse needs to be aware of her own responses. Using standards clarified within a code of ethics helps the nurse view dilemmas more objectively.

The complexity of ethical decision making requires the nurse to make a conceptual analysis of any dilemma. What are the real issues? Who is involved? What are the implications? Are a client's rights being jeopardized? Is this an issue of a nurse's professional integrity? A nurse's analysis will help to clarify such concepts as "health," "disease," "death with dignity," "benefit," and "wrong." Unless the nurse and the individuals involved in an ethical dilemma clarify the concepts involved, ethical debates become frustrating and fruitless. Conceptual analysis prepares the nurse to take a defensible, intelligent position on one issue without being committed, possibly less defensibly, to a similar position on a completely different issue.

Once the nurse has a clear perception of the ethical dilemma, she constructs and evaluates arguments for and against each position involved and attempts to determine the extent to which each reason provides a solution to the dilemma. Ethical issues are not always clear cut. Weighing both sides of the dilemma helps the nurse to determine whether reasons for a position are valid and sound. A code of ethics is useful in evaluating the basis of any ethical position and in determining priorities.

The nurse acts on her ethical decision after carefully weighing all alternative courses of action. She responds in a systematic, principled manner rather than behaving capriciously or arbitrarily. Once she acts the nurse must be prepared to respond to objections or arguments from others. Regardless of how careful she is in resolving the dilemma, there will be individuals who reject her solution or opinion.

The following illustrates the ethical decision-making process:

Mr. Williams, 42 years old, has exploratory surgery for the removal of a substernal tumor. His surgeon, Dr. Allen, is reputed to be one of the best. On Mr. Williams' return to the surgical nursing unit, the nurse, Ms. Case, assesses his ventilatory movements, noting that he is having some difficulty breathing. The nurse takes the necessary measures to keep Mr. Williams' airways clear and helps him assume a comfortable breathing position. She calls the intern on duty to check the client's status. When the intern arrives, he asks the nurse to come to the conference room and proceeds to tell her that Dr. Allen accidentally severed the client's phrenic nerve. The intern says, "You should continue to keep a close eye on Mr. Williams. He is going to have some breathing difficulties." After the intern leaves, the nurse is upset but says nothing. She continues to monitor Mr. Williams closely and goes home at the end of her shift. The next day, Ms. Case goes to her head nurse to report: "I learned from the intern yesterday that Mr. Williams' phrenic nerve was accidentally cut during surgery. I think something should be done."

The head nurse faces a very delicate problem. Before forming an opinion, she takes the necessary steps to gather as much information as possible. First, she talks with Ms. Case to learn exactly what events occurred after Mr. Williams returned to the nursing unit. She discovers that the nurse's physical assessment findings could be indicative of phrenic nerve paralysis; however, she also knows that the client was still under the effects of anesthesia, which can depress normal ventilatory movement. The head nurse also goes to the client's medical record to determine what actually occurred during surgery. The surgeon's notes make no mention of phrenic nerve damage; in fact, the record suggests that the surgery was uncomplicated. However, a chest x-ray film, taken the evening after surgery, confirms the presence of diaphragmatic paralysis, a complication of phrenic nerve damage. The client's medical history contains no evidence of previous respiratory problems. Finally, the head nurse talks with the intern who reported the incident. He confirms his story but says, "I'll get shot if you report this. You know, Dr. Allen's done this before, but there have never been any problems as a result of his mistakes."

The head nurse considers her own feelings about the dilemma. First, she is angry that a physician has failed to acknowledge his mistake. She knows full well that if one of her nurses made a similarly dangerous error the nurse would be held accountable. It is also extremely dangerous to the client's welfare if all personnel are not aware of Mr. Williams' physical condition. Therefore the head nurse is concerned that the client's physical needs will not be managed properly. The head nurse values integrity on the part of all health care personnel and feels that Dr. Allen has compromised himself by not informing the client or the nursing personnel of the accident. The client, Mr. Williams, has been an extremely pleasant person to care for and has not complained about the measures taken by the nurses to maintain his respiratory function. Furthermore, Mr. Williams is very pleased with Dr. Allen and believes he is an excellent surgeon. However, the head nurse believes that Mr. Williams should be made aware of the incident.

What are the ethical problems that this situation poses for the head nurse? First, the client has the right to know whether there have been any complications from the surgery, and whether additional complications are possible in the future. Should the client suffer serious complications resulting from the phrenic nerve damage, Dr. Allen could be held legally responsible. Second, the professional integrity of Dr. Allen is in question. The nurses would not be aware of the client's situation had the intern not informed them of Mr. Williams' problem. The absence, in the record, of any admission of error suggests that Dr. Allen attempted to cover up his mistake. Third, there is the issue of the head nurse's responsibility. A staff nurse has reported a serious problem. Should the head nurse refuse to take action, what would this mean in terms of her own accountability and her reputation with her staff?

The head nurse methodically considers all the pros and cons that support or argue against possible courses of action. If Mr. Williams recovers successfully from his surgery, would he be better off not knowing what happened? He would continue to be well satisfied with his care and with Dr. Allen. The other side of this argument is that Mr. Williams needs to be aware of his health risks. Future surgery or illness could easily be complicated by the damaged phrenic nerve. The issue of Dr. Allen's integrity also must be looked at from different viewpoints. Can the head nurse assume that the intern's story is accurate? He could easily be misinformed or confused; after all, he did not perform the surgery, even though he assisted in the operating room. The staff nurse's physical assessment and findings from the chest film raise serious concern that the phrenic nerve was damaged. Perhaps Dr. Allen had reasons for not reporting the accident, thinking that Mr. Williams, a generally healthy individual, would have no difficulty. Finally, the head nurse's responsibility is the clearest of the three ethical problems. Regardless of the arguments involving the other issues, the head nurse knows she must report the information she has. It will not be the head nurse's responsibility to judge whether Dr. Allen made a mistake.

The head nurse decides to take the issue to the chief of surgery. He is in the position of being responsible for allowing Dr. Allen to practice on the staff. The head nurse prepares herself for the meeting by reviewing the client's chart and the notes that she has taken regarding the comments of the nurse and the intern. She anticipates that the chief of surgery might vigorously defend Dr. Allen's reputation. However, she knows the problem must be addressed for the client's welfare.

She brings the chart and her notes to the meeting. She does not take an accusing stand but instead shares the information in an objective, nonjudgmental fashion. She does express her concern for Mr. Williams' welfare and for the nursing staff who share responsibility for his care.

The chief of surgery is appreciative of the head nurse's professional approach to the problem. He investigates the situation more thoroughly, which ultimately leads to a reprimand for Dr. Allen. The members of the nursing staff gain satisfaction in knowing that the issues have been addressed and that Mr. Williams has been totally informed.

No two ethical dilemmas are the same. Without a systematic approach to ethical decision making, a nurse cannot resolve ethical issues in a consistent and objective manner.

Summary

Ethics consists of the principles that govern proper conduct. The professional nurse must assume roles that include diverse responsibilities wherein complex ethical dilemmas can develop. The nurse has a unique relationship with clients and other health care professionals, which puts her in the forefront of making ethical decisions.

Ethical issues are frequently confused with legal and moral issues. An unethical act is not necessarily illegal, nor is an illegal act necessarily unethical. Both ethics and the law refer to rules of conduct based on underlying principles of what is right or wrong. A legal right provides a person guaranteed protection from interference by others. An ethical right involves no legal guarantees but is validated by moral principles. A person's moral principles are his absolute beliefs about what is right or wrong. From an ethical standpoint, there may not be clear guidelines as to what is right or wrong.

The state of the art of nursing has changed significantly over the years. Because of rapid social and technological advancement, the role of the nurse has become more diverse and the nurse has become more independent. The ethical principles governing nursing practice have changed to become compatible with a growing profession.

Values are personal beliefs about the worth of given ideas or actions. Each person's values result from his life experiences. A nurse's professional values are a reflection of her personal values. The experiences that a nurse has in her professional life broaden her perspective on the values she holds. When personal values complement professional values, a nurse is best equipped to practice as an ethically responsible person. As a professional, a nurse practices under an ethical code designed to protect the rights of all human beings.

A responsible practitioner of nursing exhibits competence and skill in performing required nursing actions. The nurse is morally responsible to the client, who depends on her expertise. The principle of accountability necessitates an evaluation of the nurse's effectiveness in performing the responsibilities of nursing care. As a professional practitioner, the nurse must be answerable for acts performed in that role. The nurse is accountable to herself, the client, her profession, the employing institution, and society. Being accountable, the nurse is able to maintain high ethical standards of behavior.

Nurses face a variety of ethical problems in connection with their professional experiences. There are ethical issues that are unique to each health care setting and each area of nursing practice. A nurse must be familiar with the issues involved in her daily practice.

In order to resolve an ethical problem, a nurse uses a systematic process to understand the nature of the problem and to plan a responsible course of action. She first gathers any objective information relevant to the problem and reviews the personal context of the ethical dilemma. She uses the ethical codes of professional nursing as points of reference in order to further analyze the dilemma objectively. She then clarifies the ethical concepts that are involved, so that she can determine a clear course of action. Evaluating the arguments that support or challenge each possible course of action helps her to make a decision critically. No ethical dilemma is easily resolved. A nurse must be willing to dedicate the time and to make the personal commitment necessary to arrive at logical, fair, and humane ethical decisions.

KEY CONCEPTS

✓ Technological advances in health care have created many different types of ethical dilemmas.

✓ The nurse's role has become multifaceted, a situation that has increased the number and diversity of the ethical dilemmas that a nurse encounters in practice.

✓ A moral belief is the conviction that something is absolutely right or wrong.

✓ An ethical dilemma results from conflicts in values, causing uncertainty in decision making.

✓ A person's legal rights are ensured by legal guarantees.

✓ Personal values can make the ethical commitment to avoid value judgments difficult for the nurse.

✓ A code of ethics is a set of shared ethical principles that are accepted by the members of a profession.

✓ A professional nursing code of ethics protects the vulnerable and dependent members of society.

✓ "Responsibility" refers to the scope of functions and duties a nurse is required to perform.

✓ A nurse is accountable when she demonstrates a willingness to assume responsibility for her nursing care.

✓ Whenever a nurse is witness to an act that may potentially endanger a client, she is obligated to report that act.

✓ Established standards of care represent minimal expectations in regard to health care.

✓ Client advocacy requires a nurse to present a client with accurate, meaningful information without jeopardizing the client's relationship with physician or family.

✓ There are ethical issues unique to each area of nursing practice.

✓ The supportive role of advocacy protects a client's right to self-determination.

✓ A methodical approach to the resolution of ethical dilemmas requires the nurse to clarify personal values.

✓ Taking a stance in an ethical dilemma is easier when both sides of the dilemma are evaluated.

REFERENCES

Fromer, M.J.: Ethical issues in health care, St. Louis, 1981, The C.V. Mosby Co.

Kohnke, M.F.: Advocacy: risk and reality, St. Louis, 1982, The C.V. Mosby Co.

Smith, S.J., and Davis, A.J.: Ethical dilemmas: conflicts among rights, duties and obligations, Am. J. Nurs. 80:1463, 1980.

Tucker, S.M., et al.: Patient care standards, ed. 3, St. Louis, 1984, The C.V. Mosby Co.

ADDITIONAL READINGS

Ackerman, T.: Perspectives: resolving an ethical dilemma, Nursing 80 10(5):39, 1980.

Aroskar, M.A.: Anatomy of an ethical dilemma: the theory, Am. J. Nurs. 80:658, 1980.

Aroskar, M.A.: Anatomy of an ethical dilemma: the practice, Am. J. Nurs. 80:661, 1980.

Benjamin, M., and Curtis, J.: Ethics in nursing, New York, 1981, Oxford University Press, Inc.

Davis, A.J., and Krueger, J.C.: Patients, nurses, ethics, New York, 1980, American Journal of Nursing Co.

Mahon, K.A., et al.: Moral development and clinical decision making (symposium on bioethical issues in nursing), Nurs. Clin. North Am. 14:3, 1979.

Rust, L.: The ethical implications of artificial and transplant organ surgery for today's critical care nurse, Focus, vol. 22, January-February, 1980.

Shelly, J.A.: Dilemma: a nurse's guide for making ethical decisions, Downers Grove, Ill., 1980, Inter-Varsity Press.

Stanley, T.: Ethics as a component of the curriculum, Nurs. Health Care 1(2):63, 1980.

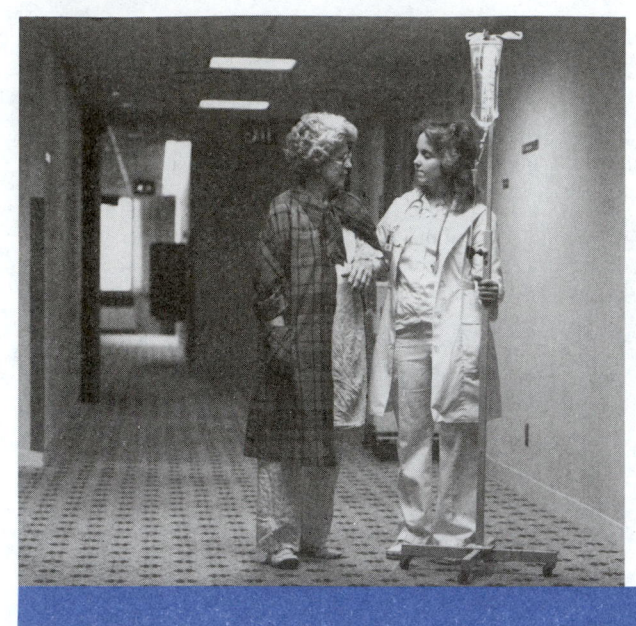

OBJECTIVES

Mastery of content in this chapter will enable the student to:

- Define the terms in the glossary.
- List factors that influence the communication process.
- Describe the nature of communication.
- Explain the purposes of communication.
- Describe each element of the communication process.
- Describe characteristics of verbal and nonverbal communication.
- Explain the role communication plays in the nursing process.
- List and discuss the phases of a therapeutic helping relationship.
- Describe the role communication plays in the performance of nursing care measures.
- Discuss effective communication techniques.
- Describe factors or conditions that create barriers to effective communication.

GLOSSARY

auditory Related to, or experienced through, hearing.

change agent Nursing role in which nurses use communication skills, education, and other resources to help a client adjust to changes caused by illness or disability.

communication Ongoing, dynamic series of events that involves the transmission of meaning from sender to receiver.

interpersonal communication Exchange of information between two persons or among persons in a small group.

intonation Rise and fall in pitch of the voice in speech.

intrapersonal communication Communication that occurs within an individual; for example, a person "talks with himself" silently or forms an idea in his own mind.

message Information sent or expressed by sender in the communication process.

paraphrasing Restating a passage or phrase to give the same meaning in another form.

perception Person's mental image or concept of elements in his environment, including information gained through the senses.

public communication Interaction between one person and a large group of people.

receiver Person to whom message is sent during the communication process.

referent Factor that motivates a person to communicate with another individual.

sender Person who initiates interpersonal communication by conveying a message.

tactile Relating to the sense of touch.

territoriality Persistent attachment of a person to a specific area or space.

therapeutic Of or pertaining to a treatment or beneficial acts.

visual Of or pertaining to the sense of sight.

15 Communication Skills in Nursing

All persons have the basic need to relate to others in a meaningful way. Communication allows a person to establish, maintain, and improve contacts with others. When two persons converse, more is exchanged than a mere assortment of words or series of gestures. Human communication is a complex process that involves behaviors and relationships and allows individuals to associate with others and the world around them.

An important component of nursing practice is the ability to communicate. A nurse uses a wide range of communication techniques with a client. Listening to a client's fears, describing the measures of care, and holding an outstretched hand are examples of ways the nurse interacts with the client through communication. Communication is the process that enables the nurse to establish a working relationship with a client and eventually help him meet his health care needs.

The failure to communicate leads to serious problems for both the nurse and the client. If a nurse ignores the nonverbal messages of a client in distress, ultimately the client could lose his life. Failure to convey important information to colleagues on the health care team can cause dangerous delays in the client's treatment. Avoiding interactions through communication at a time when the client seeks the nurse's support can threaten the nurse's professional credibility. Communication is a basic element in the nurse's delivery of total health care.

Through communication the nurse creates ways to effect change. A client must decide that he will maintain or acquire healthy behaviors. The nurse's success in helping the client achieve his desired level of health may rest on her ability to communicate effectively. The nurse deliberately speaks and acts in ways to initiate change that promotes the client's well-being.

Communication is also the foundation on which relationships are developed between the nurse and other members of the health care team. Because nurses collaborate with others in giving care, a nurse's competence may depend on her ability to express ideas and insights clearly to fellow professionals.

The process of communication is not something a nurse simply memorizes and puts into practice. Communication is complex and requires an intelligent application of principles. Having mastered the techniques of effective communication, the nurse will be able to establish meaningful relationships with clients and colleagues.

Definition of Communication

A nursing instructor lecturing on child abuse, a group of students posing questions to one another for an upcoming test, and a nurse listening to an anguished husband whose wife has died are all examples of communication. Human communication is an ongoing, dynamic series of events in which meaning is generated and transmitted. The instructor's descriptions, a student's question, and the nurse's empathetic gestures create responses in those who observe, listen, and interact. Meaning is not simply transferred from one person to another; it is mutually negotiated between the persons communicating. Not all the students who listen to a lecture on child abuse will acquire the same meaning initially. Many variables have significant impact on the meaning conveyed. The instructor's style of speech, the student's values regarding child rearing, and the amount of classroom noise around the student influence the student's interpretation and understanding of the instructor's words. For the instructor to communicate her intended message successfully, there must be a mutual search for meaning. The instructor fields questions, clarifies terms, and uses graphic slides to convey specific messages. For communication to be effective, the meaning acquired by the person listening must be similar or identical to the message intended by the speaker.

Factors That Influence Communication

Each person is unique and makes different associations and interpretations of messages communicated. A frown may convey unhappiness to one person and pain to another. A person's perceptions, values, emotions, cultural background, and levels of knowledge influence the way he sends and receives messages. The role an individual plays in any communication exchange and the setting in which it occurs also affect the communication process.

Perceptions

No two individuals perceive a situation in the same way. For example, a nurse enters a hospitalized client's room and says, "I've noticed you have been very quiet since your doctor spoke with you. Would you like to talk about it?" A client who at that moment is looking for emotional support might perceive the nurse's words as conveying concern and understanding. In contrast, a client who is angered by the situation of being hospitalized might perceive the nurse as intruding on his thoughts. Each person senses, interprets, and understands his surroundings differently. Perception is a person's personal view of the events occurring around him.

Our perceptions are closely linked to past experiences. We make decisions about another person's personality as a result of previous experiences in observing people's behaviors. It is difficult to change perceptions that have been shaped from years of similar experiences. If you perceive a person as selfish, rude, and egotistical, it may take a great deal of communication to change your initial impressions about him.

Perception begins with sensory input. The senses receive information that is organized and interpreted in the brain as perceptions. The sights we see, the sounds we hear, and the sensations we feel are combined to form our images of the world. Yet perceptions can be misleading. Shadows cast by light, the interference of environmental noise, and the dulled sensations caused by certain drugs can interfere with the accuracy and clarity of perceptions.

Perceptions are also formed as a result of an individual's goals or expectations for a particular observation or experience. A student who begins a conference with his instructor may perceive the situation as threatening if he feels unprepared. The instructor, in contrast, sees the conference as an opportunity to get to know the student better. The instructor's and student's perceptions may conflict unless both individuals together clarify the purpose of the conference. Differences in perceptions are often obstacles to effective communication. Before two persons can successfully communicate, each must understand his own perceptions and the influence he has on the perceptions of others.

Values

Values are our personal beliefs (see Chapter 13). The way we relate to life's events is influenced by the convictions we hold about certain ideas or behaviors. Our values reflect what we consider valuable and important in life and thus have significant influence on the way we communicate our thoughts and ideas.

No two individuals possess the same values. Diverse experiences throughout our lives shape the values we hold. Whenever we engage in communication, our values influence the way we express ideas and the way we interpret the ideas and behaviors of others. When communicating with a client and his family, the professional nurse cannot afford to let her values conflict with theirs. Judging a client's values will have detrimental effects on the nurse-client relationship. For example, a nurse in a community health clinic may highly value the maintenance of physical well-being. When a teenager comes to the clinic with a history of drug abuse, the nurse will likely find fault with his behaviors. The teenager is seeking help and support but may quickly feel rejected if the nurse allows her values about drug abuse to affect the way she communicates with him.

It is important that nurses come to grips with their personal and professional values. To facilitate values clarification with clients, the nurse must communicate in a nonjudgmental and supportive fashion. The nurse remains aware of her personal values as well as those of the client in order to interact with him therapeutically.

Emotions

Emotions are a person's subjective feelings about the events occurring around him. Emotions strongly influence how a person uses his capacities and how he relates to others. It may be difficult for others to understand or accept the emotions a person reveals.

To help a client, a nurse must become emotionally involved. In caring for a dying client, the nurse must feel his grief and suffering in order to help him gain comfort. However, the nurse must remain aware of what she is feeling and experiencing. She cannot allow her emotions to blind her to what is occurring in a relationship with the client. If the nurse permits her emotions solely to direct her nursing care, the client's needs will remain unmet. If she becomes too involved with the client's suffering, she may withdraw needed therapies. The nurse must assume responsibility for her emotions and act professionally in the client's care.

One should not underestimate the power of emotion in communication. For example, a young nurse has had an argument with her husband before coming to work. Her husband is just out of law school and establishing his practice. The nurse's income is needed for the family's survival. Her husband has proposed that they begin having children. The nurse knows that she and her husband would have difficulty rearing a family now, particularly since she would soon have to take a leave from work. The nurse goes to work angered by her husband's lack of understanding. The first client she sees is a 24-year-old mother of three who is divorced and living on welfare. The nurse cannot allow herself to transfer her anger at her husband to the client's situation. This would prevent her from understanding this client as an individual. If the nurse is to communicate effectively with the client, she must be aware of her emotions.

It is important for the nurse to have a healthy emotional life both professionally and personally. The nurse can benefit from clarifying the nature of her relationships with family, friends, and colleagues. A social support system provides avenues for the nurse to ventilate potentially damaging emotions. Nurses need support persons to share the emotional frustrations of their work. The client is not the appropriate person with whom to ventilate emotions. A competent professional nurse is knowledgeable about her emotional well-being and takes measures to prevent personal feelings from affecting or threatening her relationships with clients.

Sociocultural Background

A person's sociocultural background influences his ways of communicating. It is common, for example, for Arabs to wail with grief after a family member's death; crying is considered natural. A middle-class American man often refrains from crying openly after the loss of a loved one. His grief is internalized so that he may appear strong to other family members. Our culture forms our generalizations and preconceptions about the world. The influence of culture may be subtle, but it sets limits for the way we act and communicate.

Our language, our gestures, and the attitudes we communicate reflect our cultural origins. A nurse learns to acknowledge and accept a client's cultural norms. If a client speaks with an unfamiliar accent, the nurse courteously attempts to understand his words. If a client's cultural upbringing causes him to question the importance of health-promoting activities, the nurse explores his attitudes and introduces ideas he might be willing to consider. A person's culture creates the frame of reference for the events in his life. When the nurse is able to communicate with a client and share his frame of reference, the client becomes more receptive to the nurse's efforts to form a helping relationship.

Knowledge

Communication can be difficult when those communicating have different levels of knowledge. A message will not be clear if the words or phrases are not part of the listener's vocabulary. "The incision is well approximated without drainage" means the same as "The incision is clean and healing fine," but the latter would be understood by a greater number of people.

Nurses communicate with clients and professionals who have different levels of knowledge. A social worker may find it difficult to understand the nurse's explanation of a disease process. A nurse may be perplexed by a physician's explanation of cell development. A client may not understand the nurse's technical explanation of a drug's action. An individual's level of knowledge may be so far above that of the people he is addressing that they lose the message entirely and do not seek clarification or explanation of his words. The speaker who fails to use language his listeners can understand will lose their attention and interest. The most effective communication uses language common to those interacting.

Knowledge is a product of development as well as education. A nurse may encounter and communicate with clients of different age levels. The toddler is able to use only two- or three-word sentences and cannot use words in the past tense. A school-age child has a rapidly growing vocabulary and can exchange thoughts and ideas with others. The nurse learns to communicate at the client's level of language development.

Roles and Relationships

We communicate with others in a style appropriate to the roles and relationships we assume with those individuals. A student talks with a friend in a different way than he talks with his instructor, physician, or minister. The words, facial expressions, tone of voice, and gestures used to convey an idea depend on the person receiving the communication.

A nurse may feel comfortable communicating in a relaxed manner with colleagues, joking about the events of the day and sharing amusing stories. However, communicating with a client entering a clinic for the first time requires the nurse to assume a different role. Anticipating that the client may be apprehensive, the nurse avoids jokes or humor until she can determine how the client relates to her. The client is probably looking for support rather than funny stories. Later, when the relationship between the nurse and client is stronger, casual conversation may be appropriate.

The better we know an individual, the more liberty we can take in expressing ideas. We feel more comfortable in expressing ideas to individuals with whom we have developed positive, satisfying relationships. As a nurse-client relationship develops, both the nurse and the client gain confidence in relating ideas and feelings. Communication is more effective when the participants remain aware of the role each assumes in their relationship.

Environmental Setting

People tend to communicate better in a comfortable environment. A warm room, free of noise and distractions, is the optimal setting for communication. Noise or lack of privacy or space may create confusion, tension, or discomfort for the persons interacting. For example, a client fearful of the implications of the diagnosis of cancer would hesitate to discuss his illness in a busy, crowded waiting room. Environmental distractions can distort the messages sent between two people.

The nurse has some control when selecting the setting for communicating with clients. A quiet office or lounge is ideal. When the client is visited at home, a bedroom or den may be best suited for conversation. It is important that the nurse's efforts to convey information are not blocked by environmental distractions.

Levels of Communication

Communication occurs at three levels: intrapersonal, interpersonal, and public. Intrapersonal communication is that which occurs within an individual. When a nurse walks into the client's room and thinks, "He looks very uncomfortable. I'd better turn him onto his side," she is communicating intrapersonally. Communication occurs constantly within our consciousness. Intrapersonal communication helps us remain alert to the events around us. By considering our thoughts internally, we can better express ourselves to others.

Interpersonal communication is communication that occurs between two people or in small groups. A significant part of our lives involves activities with others. Interpersonal communication is essential in meeting people's social needs as they join together to share ideas, solve problems, make decisions, and take action.

In nursing there are many situations that challenge the nurse's interpersonal communication skills. Each encounter with a client, such as collecting a blood specimen or taking the client's medical history, requires an exchange of information. Meetings with staff members, physicians, social workers, and therapists test the nurse's communication skills with people who may have different opinions and experiences. Being a member of a nursing committee challenges the nurse's ability to express ideas clearly and decisively. Interpersonal communication is at the heart of nursing practice. A nurse can assist a client only by communicating at a meaningful interpersonal level.

Public communication is interaction with large groups of people. Giving a lecture to a roomful of students and speaking to a consumer group on health education are examples of public communication. Special platform skills are necessary to be proficient in public speaking.

Communication is both an art and a science. It takes more than just knowledge to be an effective communicator; practice and an awareness of the communication process are needed. Just as a craftsman becomes skilled in using the tools of his craft to produce a work of art, the professional nurse masters communication skills to help clients give a purposeful direction to their lives.

Elements of the Communication Process

There is no one best way to analyze the communication process. However, to understand communication, one should examine the components of the process. A model can simply and graphically demonstrate the most complex of processes, but it can also make a process look simpler than it actually is. A model of communication provides the nursing student with a framework for observing, understanding, and predicting what occurs as two people communicate.

The model in Fig. 15-1 depicts interpersonal communication as a simple process involving two people. The sender transmits a message to the receiver, who responds by giving feedback. The model fails to show all the levels of involvement that normally occur between two people communicating. When a mother scolds her child for misbehaving, the child does more than passively listen to his mother's words. He may frown, cry, or think to himself that his mother no longer loves him, and the mother may sense or perceive this reaction and change her communication. As two people communicate, they mutually interact in the sharing of information.

The basic elements of communication are shown in Fig. 15-2. Communication occurs on a social level with the participants engaged in intrapersonal and interpersonal interactions. The process is dynamic, with the meaning of messages mutually negotiated by the participants. As a person communicates, he may or may not be consciously aware of each element of communication. During casual conversation the participants do not bother to analyze the meaning of every gesture or word expressed. For example, a person may become quite animated, using his hands to express an idea, without consciously thinking, "I'll wave my hand to stress this point." The nurse, how-

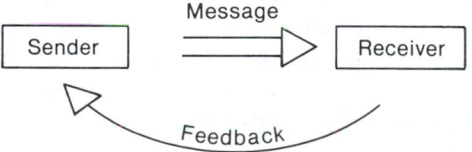

Fig. 15-1 Communication as a simple two-way process. The sender transmits a message to the receiver, who then provides feedback.

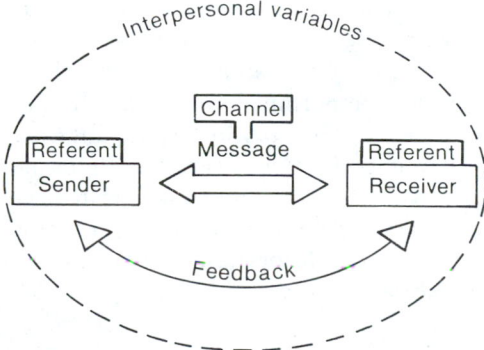

Fig. 15-2 Communication as an active process between sender and receiver.

ever, does learn to be conscious of each element of the communication process. In this way she can control interactions effectively with clients and remain aware of how communication affects them. Each of the elements described in the following paragraphs can be considered from the perspectives of both natural, uninhibited communication and consciously manipulated communication.

The referent is the factor that motivates an individual to communicate with another person. It may be an object, experience, emotion, idea, or act. If the individual consciously considers the referent during an intrapersonal interaction, he can carefully develop and organize the message he ultimately sends.

The sender is the person who initiates the interpersonal communication. The role of sender may switch back and forth between participants at any time when information is transmitted.

The message is the information that is eventually sent or expressed by the sender. The most effective message is clear, organized, and expressed in a manner familiar to the person receiving it. The message may be comprised of both verbal and nonverbal information, that is, spoken words, tone of voice, or facial expressions.

The message is sent along a channel of communication. Channels are means of conveying messages such as through the visual, auditory, and tactile senses. The sender's facial expression visually conveys a message to the person with whom he communicates. The spoken word travels via auditory channels. Placing a hand on an individual while communicating uses the channel of touch. Generally, the more channels the nurse uses to send a message, the better the client will understand it. For example, when a nurse attempts to relieve a client's pain, she verbalizes her concern, her expression reflects compassion, and her gentle movements lessen the pain.

The receiver is the person to whom the message is sent. For communication to be effective the receiver must perceive or become aware of the sender's message. The message generated by the sender then acts as one of the receiver's referents. It prompts the receiver to respond to the sender's message. The nurse learns to engage in intrapersonal communication while analyzing and interpreting what the client has to say.

The process of communication is ongoing. The receiver returns a message in the form of feedback to the sender. Feedback helps to reveal whether the meaning of the sender's message was received. The mere intent to communicate is insufficient to ensure that a message is accurately received. The receiver's own verbal and nonverbal response sends feedback to the sender to reveal the receiver's understanding of the message. The nurse must be open to feedback from a client to be sure he understands her explanations.

The roles of sender and receiver are dynamic. The person who is first the sender assumes the role of receiver when a message is transmitted back to him. Because of the reciprocal relationship involved in communication, the model tends to oversimplify a very complex process.

Both the sender and receiver are influenced by an array of intrapersonal variables as described previously. The individual's perceptions, values, cultural background, knowledge, and roles and the setting of the interaction all come into play to influence the content of a message and the manner in which it is shared. Interpersonal communication is made more complex by the fact that each person is influenced differently by these intrapersonal variables. Intrapersonal variables make each interpersonal communication a unique experience.

Each element of the communication process is crucial; information and meaning can be gained or lost if any element is altered. By understanding each element and the factors influencing it, a nurse can communicate with others more effectively. The nurse can control elements of the process to enhance communication. For example:

The nurse working with a hearing-impaired client uses visual and tactile channels to communicate a message more clearly.

If a nurse's values conflict with those of a client, she attempts to clarify her perceptions of the client's beliefs so mutual understanding is gained.

After a nurse explains the method for crutch walking, she seeks feedback by asking the client to demonstrate the technique.

Modes of Communication

Messages are conveyed in two primary modes: verbal and nonverbal. The two modes are closely bound together during interpersonal interaction. As we speak, we express ourselves through movements, tone of voice, facial expressions, and general appearance. These modes can convey the same or very different messages. The nurse learning the skills of communication masters the techniques of each mode.

Verbal Communication

Verbal communication involves the use of the spoken or written word. Language is a code that conveys specific meaning. The addition of a single word can change the entire meaning of a phrase or sentence. Language is effective only when both the sender and the receiver understand a message clearly.

A nurse encounters clients of various cultures who speak languages different from her own. Some clients speak the same language as the nurse but use subcultural variations of certain words. For example, the word "pig" may mean a farm animal to one person and a law enforcement officer to another. Often a nurse works with clients who speak the same language as she but interpret her messages differently from the way she intended. To make a message clear and relevant, the nurse employs techniques of effective verbal communication.

DENOTATIVE AND CONNOTATIVE MEANING

A single word can take on several meanings. A denotative meaning is one shared by individuals who use a common language. For example, the word "baseball" has the same meaning for all individuals who speak English, and the word "code" denotes cardiac arrest to professional nurses. A connotative meaning refers to the meaning a word assumes apart from what it explicitly describes. Using the word "serious" to describe a client's condition may suggest to his family that he is close to death, but the nurses caring for the client may not consider him to be near death unless the word "critical" is used. Connotations are shades or interpretations of a word's meaning rather than different definitions.

Since words can take on a variety of connotative meanings that may elicit powerful or negative emotions, the nurse should not be casual in her selection of words. The nurse should consider the manner in which a client may interpret her words and should clarify the client's meaning when she is unfamiliar with the connotations his words may have.

VOCABULARY

Communication is unsuccessful if the receiver is unable to translate the sender's words and phrases. In nursing and medicine there is a vast vocabulary of technical terms that most lay people do not understand. If the nurse uses many technical terms, the client may become confused and unable to follow instructions or learn important information. Rather than telling the client, "Sit up while your lungs are auscultated," it might be better to say, "Sit up for me while I listen to your lungs." The former statement might make the client feel anxious about why he needs to sit up. A simple, straightforward statement communicates the message more effectively.

PACING

Verbal communication is more successful when expressed at an appropriate speed or pace. Talking rapidly, using awkward pauses, or speaking very slowly and deliberately can convey an unintended message. Consider the nurse who uses awkward pauses during an explanation to a client.

Client: Do you know if the doctor found anything wrong?
Nurse: No (pause), but I'm sure if he did (longer pause) he would have come to explain things to you. (then very rapidly) Now let's get back to where we were.

The long pauses and the rapid shift to another subject give the client the impression that the nurse is hiding the truth.

The speed with which a message is verbalized, in addition to the presence, absence, and length of pauses, can determine the degree to which communication satisfies the listener. The nurse should not talk so quickly that enunciation is unclear. Pauses should be used to accentuate or stress a particular point. Pauses also give the listener time to digest and comprehend the meaning of the speaker's words.

One achieves proper pacing by thinking through what to say before speaking. Looking for any nonverbal cues from the listener that might suggest confusion or misunderstanding is also useful. Asking a listener if the pace of a message is too fast or too slow helps in determining if the pace is effective.

INTONATION

The tone of the speaker's voice can have a dramatic impact on the meaning of a message. Depending on intonation, the simple phrase "How are you?" can express enthusiasm, concern, indifference, and even annoyance. A person's emotions can directly influence his tone of voice. Often this effect is an unconscious one, and the words send one message while the tone of voice conveys an opposite one. The nurse must be aware of her emotions when interacting with clients. The intention of conveying sincere interest in a client's welfare can be blocked if the nurse's tone of voice imparts a totally different mood or meaning.

CLARITY AND BREVITY

Effective communication is simple, short, and to the point. Fewer words spoken result in less confusion. Because of the intrapersonal variables involved, human communication is imprecise in many ways. Ambiguous phrases such as "you know" or "well, that's how it goes" add little to the clarity of a message.

Clarity is achieved through speaking slowly and enunciating clearly. Using examples can make an explanation easier to understand. For instance, instructing an arthritic client on self-care measures at home is more meaningful when the nurse provides specific examples of how the client can help himself.

Brevity is best achieved by using words that express an idea simply. The word "use" is more quickly understood than "utilize." A client will respond better to an explanation of how "sitting up straight makes it easier to breathe" than how "sitting in an erect posture facilitates the chest's expansion." Clients are easily overwhelmed by long, drawn-out discussions. Explanations should be kept precise and brief.

TIMING AND RELEVANCE

Timing is critical to a person's reception of a message. If the boss is in a bad mood, the time is wrong to ask for a raise. If a client is crying in pain, the time is wrong to explain the risks of surgery. Even though a message is clearly and concisely stated, poor timing can prevent it from being accurately received. Therefore the nurse must be sensitive to the appropriate time for discussions with clients. Often the best time for interaction is when a client expresses an interest in communicating. By asking a simple question such as, "Would you like to talk about your surgery?" the nurse can avoid wasting time and energy if the client does not feel like talking.

A person is more likely to communicate when a message holds importance for him. For example, when a client is facing open-heart surgery the next day, a discussion of the risks of cigarette smoking has less relevance than a review of preoperative procedures. An explanation of the side effects of birth control pills is relevant to the young woman who has received her first prescription for the medication. Verbal communication is more likely to have impact when messages pertain to an individual's interests and needs.

Nonverbal Communication

Often actions speak louder than words. Nonverbal communication is the transmission of messages without the use of words. We continually communicate nonverbally in every face-to-face encounter. A nod of the head, a wink of the eye, or the grasp of a hand imparts meaning that is often more significant than the words we utter. Nonverbal messages help us judge the reliability of verbal messages. Ekman (1965) described the ways in which nonverbal communication and verbal communication are interrelated. Nonverbal cues add meaning to what is being said in verbal communication (Table 15-1).

A nurse needs to be aware of both the verbal and the nonverbal messages she sends to clients. Her perception and interpretation of a client's nonverbal cues require that she sense the client's basic intentions while communicating. For example, a client who says he feels fine but grimaces with each movement and

TABLE 15-1

Relationships between Verbal and Nonverbal Communication

Relationship	Example
Repeating—verbal and nonverbal cues saying the same thing but in different ways	When a mother describes how tall her son is, she also holds her hands at a distance above the floor equal to the child's height.
Contradicting—verbal and nonverbal cues conveying different messages	The nurse tells the client that obtaining a blood specimen "won't hurt a bit," but her sarcastic grin delivers a different message.
Complementing—nonverbal messages adding to verbal messages	A client says she is afraid to be admitted to the hospital, and her anxious expression and trembling hands leave little doubt of her fear.
Accenting—nonverbal cues emphasizing what is stated verbally	A wave of the hand while saying hello accentuates the word spoken.
Relating and regulating—nonverbal cues indicating when to begin or stop talking	A client who continually opens and closes her mouth briefly as her physician is talking is seeking an opportunity to speak.
Substituting—a nonverbal cue being used instead of words	The nurse nods vigorously to show approval of the client's decision.

cradles his side is communicating two different messages. Nonverbal messages are usually more subtle than verbal messages. Becoming an astute observer of nonverbal behavior requires time and practice. The nurse who watches the client's movements, expressions, and gestures while listening to the client's words can more accurately interpret what the client is actually communicating.

Because the nurse is on display during interactions with clients and their families, it is important that her nonverbal communication match what she says verbally. Any conflict arising from a mismatch between the nurse's verbal and nonverbal communication can threaten the nurse-client relationship. For example, a nurse who instructs a new mother on the importance of bathing an infant regularly will be less convincing if her appearance is unkempt. A nurse who verbally assures the client that he will feel better but simultaneously reveals an expression of doubt will not relieve the client's anxieties. The client's acceptance of the nurse as a professional may depend on the manner in which she presents a professional and caring image.

There are numerous nonverbal communication channels. Each channel serves to add significant meaning to any words that are expressed.

APPEARANCE

A person's appearance is one of the first things noticed during an interpersonal encounter. Physical characteristics, the manner of dress and grooming, and the presence of jewelry and other adornment provide clues to the person's physical well-being, personality, social status, occupation, religion, culture, and self-concept. We have instant impressions when seeing a nurse's uniform, a gold band on the third finger of the left hand, a policeman's badge, or a fashionable hairstyle.

Physical characteristics, such as the condition of the hair, color of the skin, weight, energy level, and presence of a physical deformity, also communicate information about a person's level of health. There are no established standards for physical characteristics that demonstrate good health. Each individual displays various combinations of physical characteristics. The nurse remains alert for changes in a person's physical appearance, since they can be significant signs of disease.

Physical appearance often leads to lasting impressions about the personality and self-concept of an individual. Unfortunately, stereotyped views regarding the characteristics of the "perfect body" influence the image that body features communicate. According to Knapp (1978), Americans initially respond more favorably to people perceived as physically attractive than to those seen as unattractive. The nurse should assess the importance of physical appearance to a given client, particularly when illness or surgery threatens the loss of a body part or its function. For example, a young woman facing surgery for the removal of a breast may be fearful of losing her husband's love and acceptance.

An individual's clothing and adornment are an important part of physical appearance. Clothes fulfill a variety of functions: decoration, protection (psychological and physical), sexual attraction, self-assertion, group identity, and role display (Knapp, 1978). A person's clothes are a reliable indicator about that person and his personality. Picture the following two men:

Mr. Hill is 6 feet tall and weighs 190 pounds. His dark brown hair is well styled, cut short at the neck with sideburns just below the top of his ear. Mr. Hill wears a dark, three-piece suit with a coordinated tie and shirt. His shoes are clean and polished. He wears no jewelry except a simple gold wedding band.

Mr. Thompson is 5 feet, 8 inches tall and weighs 240 pounds. His black hair looks greasy and reeks of hair lotion. A print sportshirt barely stretches over Mr. Thompson's protuberant abdomen. His brown loafers are scuffed, and his denim slacks are frayed at the knees.

Both men's descriptions communicate images of and expectations about their personalities, social status, and self-concept. The images may be false, but they are communicated before there is opportunity for verbal communication to occur.

The nurse's interest in clients' clothes can become a method of intervention. To stimulate a positive sense of worth in hospitalized clients, it is helpful to allow them to dress in their own clothes. Hospital gowns are drab and ill fitting. Being able to dress in his own clothes can give a client a sense of physical recovery and mental alertness.

The nurse's physical appearance influences the client's perception of the care he receives. Each client has a preconceived image of what a nurse should look like. The traditional white nurse's uniform and nurse's cap are secular adaptations of the religious habit and thus are symbols of purity. To many clients the white uniform symbolizes cleanliness. In many hospitals, however, nurses are allowed to wear colorful uniforms and rarely wear caps. Although the uniform is not a reflection of the nurse's abilities, it may become more difficult to establish a sense of trust and reliability if the nurse fails to meet the image conceived by the client. The nurse committed to establishing an effective relationship with a client must consider the style and fit of her uniform, length and style of hair, care of fingernails, and use of jewelry. A professional nurse wears a comfortable, clean-looking uniform and minimal jewelry so she can perform her duties in an unencumbered manner.

POSTURE AND GAIT

Leaning forward or back, standing with arms on hips or at one's sides, standing straight or stoop shouldered, and walking with knees high or heels shuffling are variations of posture or gait. The way people stand and move is a visible form of self-expression. Posture and gait reflect one's emotions, self-concept, and physical wellness.

An erect posture and a quick, purposeful gait communicate a sense of well-being and assuredness. A slumped posture and slow, shuffling gait may indicate depression or discomfort. A bent-over posture may be a protective response to physical disease and injury.

Nurses can collect useful information by observing clients' posture and gait. Specific illnesses cause identifiable gaits such as the shuffling gait in Parkinson's disease. Gait may be altered by numerous factors such as pain, the effects of drugs, fractures, and emotional depression. Gait and posture cannot be the sole basis for a diagnostic analysis, but they do provide important clues regarding the client's well-being.

FACIAL EXPRESSION

The face is rich in communication potential. As the most expressive part of the body, it supplies overt and subtle cues that assist in the interpretation of messages. Studies have shown that the face reveals six primary emotions: surprise, fear, anger, disgust, happiness, and sadness (Knapp, 1978). Hundreds of facial movements can be made to express a person's emotions. Facial expressions often become the basis for important interpersonal judgments.

Because of the diversity in facial expressions, the meaning of a facial expression may be difficult to judge. The face may reveal genuine emotions, an expression may contradict true emotions, or facial expressions may be suppressed. Frequently people are unaware of the messages their expressions communicate. Providing clear feedback helps to lessen any confusion created by conflicting messages and expressions. The receiver's expression can tell the sender whether a message was effectively communicated. If the sender communicates a message designed to make the receiver happy, the receiver's smile will confirm the sender's success. When facial expressions fail to reveal clear messages, verbal feedback should be sought to be sure of the speaker's intent.

Nurses are frequently under the scrutiny of clients. Consider the impact a nurse's facial expression might have on a client who asks the following questions: "Am I going to die?" "Is my doctor competent?" "Do you know what my tests showed?" The slightest change of expressions of the eyes, lips, or face can reveal the nurse's true feelings. It is difficult to control all facial expressions. However, the nurse learns to be aware of what her expressions can reveal to a client. For example, when caring for a debilitated or deformed client, the nurse should avoid expressions of disgust. When a client is embarrassed because he has vomited or urinated on himself, the nurse does not show expressions of anger or frustration. In general, however, communication is less effective when one remains expressionless. A nurse learns to convey a feeling of concern and compassion to clients through her facial expressions.

Eye contact is an important part of facial expressions conveyed by eye movements: wide eyes are associated with frankness, terror, and naiveté; downward glances reflect modesty; raised upper eyelids reveal displeasure; and a constant stare is frequently associated with hatred and coldness.

When two people confront each other, eye contact often prefaces a message. Initiating eye contact with another person demonstrates a willingness to communicate. Averting the eyes is a signal that the person does not wish to interact. Persons who seek to maintain eye contact during a conversation are perceived as believable and sincere. Greater mutual eye contact can be seen between friends.

Maintaining eye contact allows one to become an astute observer of another individual. It has been suggested that the level at which eye contact occurs significantly influences communication. The nurse should avoid looking down at a client during a discussion; she appears less dominant and threatening if she sits across from the client at the same eye level.

HAND GESTURES

A salute, a wave of the hand, and a thumb pointed up in the air are hand gestures. In gesturing, the hands are visual italics, emphasizing, punctuating, and clarifying the spoken word. Gestures alone may reveal specific meanings, or they may create messages in conjunction with other communication cues. A baseball umpire's outstretched hands clearly convey that the runner is safe. A finger pointed toward a person may communicate several meanings, but when the pointed finger is accompanied by a frown and an ominous tone of voice, the gesture becomes a sign of accusation or threat.

A nurse learns to view gestures as a part of the client's total pattern of communication. A hand held lightly over the abdomen does not convey the same message that a grimace, bent posture, and hand on the abdomen do when expressing pain. Gestures are combined with expressions and other nonverbal cues to create specific messages.

TOUCH

Touch is a very personal form of communication. Persons engaged in communication must be in close proximity when touch is used. Because touch is more spontaneous than verbal communication, it generally seems more authentic. Various messages are conveyed through touch, such as affection, emotional support, encouragement, tenderness, pain, and seeking attention (Fig. 15-3). Touch is an important part of the nurse-client relationship, but it must be used with discrimination.

Strong social norms govern the use of touch. In Russia men commonly kiss and embrace each other during a friendly greeting. In the United States greetings between men are accompanied by a handshake. Who, when, why, and where people touch are determined by unwritten sociocultural guidelines. Many persons mistakenly perceive touch as having only sexual implications. Although touch involves physical closeness with an individual, it is not just a sexual expression.

Nurses rely on touch when carrying out various interventions. Nurses touch clients while performing physical assessments, giving baths, providing backrubs, and assisting with dressing. The nurse who is unaccustomed to touching or being touched may feel uncomfortable when performing interventions.

The person who assumes the sick role must permit

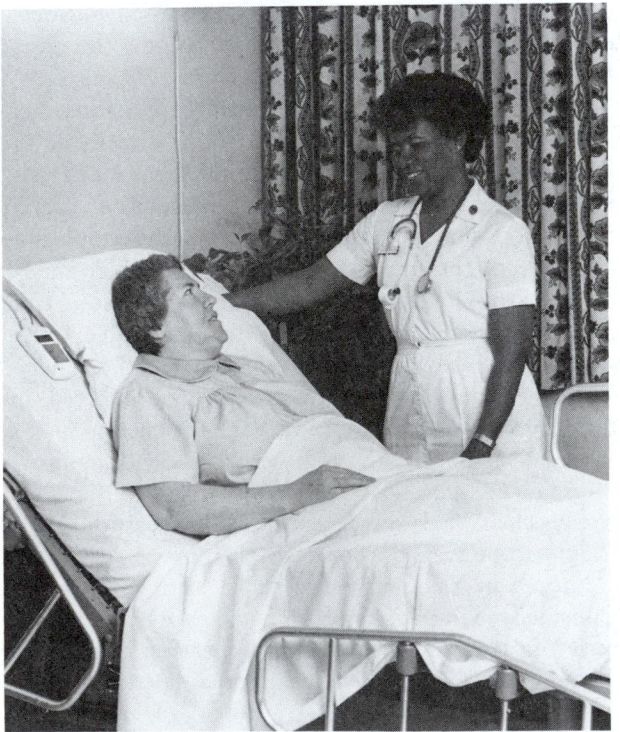

Fig. 15-3 Nurse and client communicating.

closer physical contact than is normally tolerated. Illness places a person in a dependent role that calls for the nurse to initiate and maintain closer interpersonal contact. It is important to remain sensitive to the client's disposition toward touching. If the client shies away from the nurse's efforts to touch him or refuses to hold the nurse's hand during an episode of pain, probably he is uncomfortable with being touched. The nurse must not alienate a client who rejects touch. When touch is necessary during a nursing procedure, the nurse explains its purpose carefully to the client.

Touch can be a useful therapeutic tool. Holding the hand of a grieving client can often convey understanding better than words or other gestures. Since the meanings of touch are varied and its use may evoke significant emotions, nurses must be sure to use touch purposefully during interactions. Although touch can be helpful to a client, its use must always be clearly understood and accepted.

SPACE AND TERRITORIALITY

Territoriality is the drive to gain, maintain, and defend one's exclusive right to an area of space (Pluckhan, 1978). During social interaction, people consciously maintain a distance between themselves. Personal space is invisible and mobile—it goes with a person. Territory can be separated and made visible to others, such as a fenced-in yard, a towel on the beach, or the bed in a hospital room. Whenever personal space becomes threatened by intrusion, a defensive response occurs, preventing effective communication.

Nurses frequently work with clients in situations where space and territory are important factors. As in the case of touch, the distance separating nurse from client must be judged by the nature of the situation. Physically restraining a client in danger of injuring himself, giving mouth-to-mouth resuscitation, holding a crying infant, and facilitating the excretory functions of an incontinent client require that an intimate distance be maintained between nurse and client. Hein (1973) describes intimate distance as 18 inches or less. The client receiving care is sensitive about how the nurse uses distance. The nurse must convey a sense of confidence as well as gentleness when close physical contact with a client is required.

As the distance between them becomes greater, both the client and the nurse feel more at ease. Greater flexibility is afforded when intimate contact is not required. Sitting with a client, observing intravenous fluids, and supervising the client's dressing change in the home are examples of nursing measures in which *personal distance* (18 inches to 4 feet) provides the closeness needed in interpersonal relationships. In-

creasing the physical distance makes it easier for the client and nurse to communicate because the nurse's actions and appearance become less imposing.

Social distance (4 to 12 feet) is needed when dealing with groups of people. Making rounds with physicians, waving hello to clients in a hospital lounge, and addressing a class of expectant mothers about childbirth are all examples of group interactions. The nurse is able to convey her presence to the client without close physical contact. Communication is less threatening than with intimate or personal space because an intimate sharing of thoughts and feelings is generally not required.

Communication and the Nursing Process

Communication is an important part of every step of the nursing process. A nurse cannot conduct the process without knowing a client and his nursing needs. Communication skills are necessary if the nursing process is ultimately to be successful (Table 15-2).

Assessment

Assessment, the initial stage of the nursing process, calls for the collection of information from a variety of sources. The nurse must be skilled in interviewing clients and observing their behavior to ensure that the information collected is objective and accurate. The nurse uses physical assessment skills (which employ the communication channels) to gather information reflecting the client's physical well-being (see Chapters 7 and 29). Medical records, medical and nursing literature, and diagnostic test results are forms of written communication the nurse uses to complete an assessment.

Nursing Diagnosis

During the nursing diagnosis the nurse uses communication skills to involve the client, family members, and health care professionals in identifying health care needs and determining priorities of nursing care. It is important for the nurse to communicate clearly to colleagues the nursing diagnoses identified for the client.

Planning

In developing a plan of care the nurse interacts with clients to determine their preferences for the methods of delivering nursing care. For example, before a

TABLE 15-2

Communication in the Nursing Process

Steps of Nursing Process	Modes of Communication
Assessment	Interviewing and history taking
	Physical examination (use of visual, auditory, tactile channels)
	Observing nonverbal behavior
	Reviewing medical records, literature, diagnostic tests
Nursing diagnosis	Written analysis of assessment findings
	Discussing health care needs and priorities with client and family
Planning	Written care plans
	Health team planning sessions
	Discussions with client and family to determine methods of implementation
Implementation	Discussion with other health professionals
	Health teaching
	Providing therapeutic support
	Contacting other health resources
	Recording clients' progress in care plan and nurse's notes
Evaluation	Acquiring verbal and nonverbal feedback
	Writing results of expected outcomes
	Updating written plan of care
	Explaining revisions to clients

nurse implements diet teaching, she must incorporate the client's food preferences in the diet. The nurse communicates with clients on an ongoing basis to familiarize them with health care options.

A written nursing care plan communicates to all health care personnel the measures of care to be delivered. Often members of the health care team conduct planning sessions to discuss a client's progress and treatment plan.

Implementation

During the implementation phase of the nursing process, the nurse engages in a wide range of activities that require communication skills. These activities generally fall into two categories: those that attend to a client's physical needs and those that meet psychosocial needs. Teaching health care measures, providing emotional support, explaining a procedure, and demonstrating dexterity with physical skills all involve interpersonal communication. Effective use of communication enhances the success of any intervention.

The nurse is also responsible for concisely documenting the care clients receive. In community clinics, home care agencies, hospitals, and other settings, written records are used to communicate clients' progress and needs. Better continuity of care is achieved when records are precise and accurate.

Evaluation

Nurses communicate with clients to evaluate the outcomes of nursing care. After presenting a class on the techniques of breast feeding, for example, the nurse requests feedback from the mothers to determine their comprehension of the information. While applying an elastic bandage to a client's leg, the nurse observes the client's nonverbal reactions to determine if the procedure is painless. Without communication the nurse is unable to determine whether implementation of care was successful.

The evaluation process may reveal the need to revise the plan of care. The nurse updates the written care plan and communicates any change in therapy to the appropriate personnel. The nurse also discusses with the client the rationale for proposed therapeutic changes.

■ ■ ■ ■ ■

During all steps of the nursing process the nurse is the center of a communication network. She is constantly gathering, assimilating, and transmitting information. The nursing process provides a reliable framework for delivering comprehensive care, but the process is useless unless the nurse masters therapeutic communication.

Therapeutic Communication

Beginning nursing students are frequently told to "get to know your client" as they attempt to enter into interpersonal relationships with clients. This is not an easy task, and frequently it becomes the one barrier to an effective relationship. A nurse cannot "get to know" a client without being able to appreciate his uniqueness. Without knowing the unique needs of a client, the nurse is unable to help him cope with the stress of health alterations. Through therapeutic communication the nurse can encounter, perceive, react to, and respect the client's uniqueness. The nurse who is an effective communicator will be accepted by the client as someone who shares a genuine concern for his welfare.

Therapeutic communication is not a casual pastime but a planned, deliberate, professional act. However, preoccupation with the various techniques of communication can cause the nurse to forget the client as a person. When the nurse first uses therapeutic communication techniques, the communication process may seem artificial and contrived. It is more helpful to perceive each client interaction as an opportunity to achieve a positive human relationship that results in the attainment of nursing care goals. The nurse should not place more emphasis on the mechanics of interpersonal communication than on the establishment of a meaningful and productive relationship with a client.

Social Interaction

The first attempt at communicating with a client usually results in a brief social interaction. The messages conveyed are superficial in that neither the nurse nor the client discusses deeply personal matters of concern. Any interpersonal exchange tends to be based on intuitive, unthinking, and automatic responses. A superficial interaction makes the participants feel safe, since the discussion holds no hidden intent for personal disclosures.

A nurse often uses superficial social interaction at the beginning of a conversation with a client. For example, the nurse might greet a client by saying, "Good morning, Mrs. Sears, it's nice to see you today," or "Hi, Mr. Simpson, how do you like the great weather we're having?" The nurse's purpose is to initiate friendly contact, which lays the foundation for a closer relationship of trust.

The skillful nurse does not allow social interaction to dominate a conversation, but she does maintain a congenial and warm style of communicating to elicit the client's trust. The nurse's ultimate goal is to help the client feel comfortable in sharing his true attitudes and feelings. The nurse cannot adequately assess the nature of a client's problems until he is willing to share relevant information about himself.

Developing a Helping Relationship

The nurse-client relationship is more than a mutual partnership. Travelbee (1971) calls it a human-to-human relationship. The facades of "nurse" and "client" disappear as each person tries to understand the humanity of the other. The nurse uses skills of interpersonal communication to develop a relationship with the client that allows her to understand the client as a total person. The relationship is therapeutic, promoting a psychological climate that facilitates positive change and growth in the client. The relationship also focuses on the goal of meeting the client's needs. Although the nurse may gain considerable satisfaction from the relationship, the client should be the primary recipient of any benefits.

The creation of a therapeutic environment rests on the nurse's ability to provide physical and psychosocial comfort for the client. Basic to the nurse's role is the assurance that the client's physiological needs are satisfied. For example, the nurse positions the client so he can breathe normally, acquire nutrients necessary for the repair of injured tissues, and sleep comfortably without interruption. The nurse's actions are not delivered without concern for the client's preferences. The nurse and client become actively involved in mutually determining how the client's needs are to be met.

Mrs. Greer is a 63-year-old widow who is hospitalized for cancer of the lung. She makes frequent requests for pain medication before a dose is due. When a nurse delivers the medication, Mrs. Greer criticizes her for being late. Nothing the nurses do seems to satisfy Mrs. Greer.

Ms. Edwards has cared for Mrs. Greer for the past 2 days. She could easily be tired of Mrs. Greer but chooses to be assigned to her for another day. Ms. Edwards enters her client's room and begins to straighten out the bed linen. Ms. Edwards asks, "Are you comfortable in that position, Mrs. Greer? Would you like a pain shot now?" Mrs. Greer accepts the offer of the pain shot and begins to relax in Ms. Edwards' presence. The nurse helps Mrs. Greer assume a more comfortable position on her side.

Once the client's pain has diminished, Ms. Edwards sits by her bed and says, "I know you've been experiencing much discomfort. Over the past few days we have not always been able to help you feel better. Can you help me to know the best way to make you feel comfortable?"

The nurse's efforts at improving Mrs. Greer's comfort make the client more amenable to a discussion of her problems. The nurse soon learns of Mrs. Greer's great fear of death. The client has made frequent requests of the nurses to avoid feeling lonely. By discussing the nature of Mrs. Greer's fears, the nurse and client are able to find ways to minimize Mrs. Greer's loneliness. The nurse's endeavor to show a real concern for Mrs. Greer leads to helpful solutions to the client's problems.

A helping relationship between nurse and client does not just "happen." It is built with care as the nurse logically employs therapeutic communication techniques.

Carl Rogers (1961), an eminent behavioral psychologist, extensively studied the therapeutic relationship. He theorized that is is not what one does but *how* one does it in the relationship that promotes the therapeutic conditions necessary for change. Rogers has identified three basic factors critical to forming a helping relationship:

1. The helper must be genuine and knowledgeable about himself.
2. The helper must show empathy.
3. The person being helped must feel free to explore himself in the relationship.

GENUINENESS

To help a client, the nurse must be aware of her values, feelings, and attitudes toward the client. What the nurse thinks and feels about a person with whom she is interacting is invariably communicated to that person, either verbally or nonverbally. The nurse who is able to show genuineness has an awareness of her attitudes toward clients but learns to communicate them in an appropriate fashion. The nurse does not deny any negative personal feelings she may have toward a client. However, she masters the ability to express her feelings in a way that does not blame or condemn the client.

It is not always easy to be genuine. To become confident about one's own feelings and values requires considerable self-development. However, once a nurse is able to say what she wants in the client's presence in a nonthreatening manner, her capacity for achieving helping relationships will be increased.

Ms. Bowman has seen Mrs. Thomas during her visits to the community health clinic for 3 years. Recent tests have confirmed that Mrs. Thomas has leukemia. Ms. Bowman senses that Mrs. Thomas is looking for an opportunity to talk about her condition but is finding it hard to do so. Ms. Bowman could say, "Now don't you worry, Mrs. Thomas. Everything is going to be all right." This would be an unhelpful response, and Mrs. Thomas would probably not feel encouraged to discuss her concerns. Instead, Ms. Bowman gives a more genuine response that acknowledges her true feelings: "Mrs. Thomas, we've talked together many times before. I have the feeling you'd like to be able to talk about your condition. I want you to know I'm interested in how you feel." Ms. Bowman's comments leave little doubt of her genuine concern for Mrs. Thomas. The client feels comfortable in communicating because she knows Ms. Bowman will be understanding and supportive.

EMPATHY

Empathy is the nurse's understanding and acceptance of the client's feelings and her ability to sense the client's private world as if it were the nurse's own. Empathy is a fair, sensitive, and objective look at what another person experiences. In contrast, sympathy is the inclination to think or feel as the client does. Sympathy is a subjective look at another person's world that prevents a clear perspective of all sides of the issues confronting that person.

Empathy tends to depend on similarities of experiences between the persons communicating. A nurse can empathize more easily with the client in pain if she too has experienced pain. When a client dies, the nurse who has lost a family member herself will be more accepting of the family's grief. Since it is difficult to empathize unless one has a similar experience or situation with which to relate, nurses cannot be empathetic in all situations. Nevertheless, empathy is a key to communicating concern and support for a client.

The empathetic nurse strives to understand exactly what the client is feeling or experiencing. Empathy is expressed in many ways—being available when needed, putting into words what the nurse thinks the client is feeling, and showing an awareness of what the client is going through. Empathy allows the nurse to participate momentarily in the client's emotions. A nurse who empathizes with another person avoids impulsive judgments about that person and is more likely to be sensitive and genuine.

Ms. Vincent has been caring for Mr. Pierce since his admission to the hospital 2 days ago. Mr. Pierce is scheduled to have open-heart surgery tomorrow. Ms. Vincent enters the client's room, makes eye contact with him, and sits in the chair beside his bed. The following conversation occurs:

Ms. Vincent: Hello, Mr. Pierce. You look as though you're rather deep in thought.
Mr. Pierce: Oh, I suppose I do. It's just that I can't help but think about what tomorrow will bring.
Ms. Vincent: Would you like to talk about your surgery? I imagine you have a lot of questions.
Mr. Pierce: Yes, I would like to know more.

The nurse could easily have avoided Mr. Pierce's true concerns and even attempted to change the subject. An unhelpful remark would be, "Don't worry about tomorrow, Mr. Pierce. Would you like me to get you something to read?" Such a comment would ignore Mr. Pierce's fears about the impending surgery and prevent the development of a meaningful relationship between the nurse and the client. The skillful nurse moves the conversation forward to learn more about the client and his concerns.

WARMTH

The helping relationship is structured to allow the client to explore his feelings and values freely. By conveying warmth, the nurse encourages the client to express and act out his feelings without fear of reprisal or scorn. A warm, permissive, nonthreatening atmosphere demonstrates the nurse's acceptance of the client. The client will likely share more pertinent information about himself, which allows the nurse greater opportunity to understand his needs.

Mrs. Stiles is a 42-year-old woman whose left leg has been amputated above the knee as a result of an injury suffered in an automobile accident. She is lying still in bed, her eyes reddened from a recent episode of crying. Ms. Wells, the nurse, comes in and sits beside the bed. She says, "You obviously are feeling really low this morning. Would it help to talk?"

Ms. Wells would fail to show warmth or concern if, as she entered Mrs. Stiles' room, she ignored the woman's expressions of sadness. A statement such as, "Come on now, Mrs. Stiles, let's get you up in a chair and I'll make your bed for you," would totally disregard the client's feelings. Ms. Wells' approach tells the client that the nurse acknowledges and accepts her sorrow.

Warmth can also be communicated nonverbally. A calm, reassuring tone of voice, a facial expression displaying concern, and the gentle grasp of the client's hand all reveal the nurse's compassion. When communicating warmth and understanding, the nurse should be sure the client understands that what he says or does is accepted.

Phases of a Helping Relationship

The helping relationship is established and maintained by the professional nurse. The relationship is reciprocal; nurse and client establish a relatedness to each other as they progress through the phases that eventually lead to therapeutic rapport. A helping relationship progresses over time as the nurse and client interact while the nurse carries out the nursing process, but the helping relationship is not the same as the nursing process. The nursing process is a series of steps the nurse takes to manage a client's health problems. A helping relationship is a bond between nurse and client that allows the nurse to be more effective in carrying out the nursing process. The nurse is responsible for directing the client through the phases of a helping relationship to ensure that the client's needs are met.

Chapter 8 discusses the interview as a method for obtaining a nursing health history and identifying changes in the client's level of wellness and living patterns. Although the three phases of an interview and of a helping relationship are the same, the communication patterns are different. The interview can serve to initiate a nurse-client relationship, since it may be the first encounter between the nurse and client. However, the interview is not the mechanism for maintaining a long-term therapeutic relationship. A helping relationship goes beyond the scope of an interview. It establishes a rapport between the nurse and client that is the basis for an ongoing resolution of the client's health problems.

ORIENTATION

The orientation phase begins when the nurse and the client first meet. This phase sets the tone for the remainder of the nurse-client relationship. The relationship in the orientation phase is superficial and is often marked by uncertainty and exploration on the part of both nurse and client.

As in the interview process, the nurse plans the orientation phase by gathering information about the client. The medical record and nursing history provide information the nurse can use to initiate and direct the discussion. For example, the client's past hospitalizations may be a useful topic for conversation, during which the nurse and client can get to know each other. During any initial encounter both participants closely observe each other. The nurse and client make inferences and form judgments about each other's behaviors. For this reason the nurse will be more effective if she conveys the genuineness, empathy, and warmth that characterize therapeutic communication.

The nurse and client meet and identify each other by name. It is wise to address the client formally using his last name at first, for example, "Good morning, Mr. Spencer. My name is Ms. Tucker. I am a student nurse assigned to take care of you today." After a while a client may ask the nurse to call him by his first name. This is appropriate as long as it is mutually agreeable.

Failure of the nurse to identify herself can create uncertainty, since the client often encounters many personnel from various agencies or departments when seeking health care.

At the beginning of the relationship, neither individual is able to perceive the other's uniqueness. The nurse perceives a person who has come to the health care agency or institution with a health-related problem. The client perceives the nurse as one of many health care professionals whose job is to help resolve his problem. The nurse's task is to get to know the client better as a person and to allow the client to get to know the nurse. Engaging in a social interaction initially helps the nurse and client to become relaxed in conversing.

Nurse: It certainly is a lovely day, Mrs. Spier.
Client: Yes, isn't it. If I were home and feeling better, I'd be planting my garden.
Nurse: You're a gardener? What types of plants do you enjoy growing?

Client: Oh, a little of everything. I like some tomatoes, lettuce, radishes, and maybe some squash.

The nurse directs the conversation so that she and the client feel at ease. It serves no purpose to rush into a therapeutically oriented discussion if the client feels uncomfortable in the nurse's presence. If a social interaction is directed properly, the nurse and client come to know each other better and a meaningful relationship begins to develop.

TESTING. The client often tests the nurse during the orientation phase of a relationship because of the client's difficulty in acknowledging the need for help, his fear of expressing true feelings, and his anxiety over facing the need to change. The nurse who is aware of the client's doubts and concerns attempts to display confidence and competence.

Mr. Miles is a 52-year-old businessman who has been hospitalized for treatment of a bleeding stomach ulcer. He has an independent personality and is accustomed to making decisions for himself. Ms. Rains, the nurse, enters the client's room.

Ms. Rains: Good morning, Mr. Miles. My name is Ms. Rains and I will be caring for you today.

Mr. Miles: You will, huh? Tell me, how long have you been a nurse?

Ms. Rains: About 2 years. I have worked in this hospital since graduating from nursing school.

Mr. Miles: Well, you won't have to worry about me. I can take care of myself.

Ms. Rains: I can imagine it's frustrating to be very independent one minute and then suddenly become ill and feel as though everyone is telling you what to do.

Mr. Miles: You can say that again. I'm just not used to needing help.

Ms. Rains: Mr. Miles, I'm not here to take away your independence. There are a number of things I need to do for you, but there are also many things I want you to be able to do for yourself. Let me explain some of the procedures I will be doing.

Mr. Miles: OK, I appreciate that.

In this situation the nurse recognized Mr. Miles' attempt to test her competence. It was also clear that the client was fearful of losing his independence. A nurse who has had minimal experience in developing relationships with clients may feel the need to remain superficial and nondirective. The client will sense the nurse's superficiality during testing and avoid any meaningful discussion. In Mr. Miles' care the nurse acknowledged the client's concerns and acted to eliminate his fears.

The nurse should not become defensive during testing but should be open and convey a genuine interest in the client's concerns. The client may use silence to avoid communicating. Even in this situation the nurse can show her desire to help by explaining her actions and performing care smoothly.

BUILDING TRUST. Trust is being able to rely on someone without doubt or question. Confidence, dependability, confidentiality, and credibility result when a trusting relationship develops. It is not easy for a client to perceive the need for help or to ask for it. Often a client trusts the nurse but is incapable of requesting assistance. Trust provides the needed foundation for effective communication as individuals become more open in expressing feelings and thoughts.

Trusting another person involves a certain amount of risk. As the client begins to share his feelings and attitudes with the nurse, he becomes vulnerable. When a client shares gut-level feelings with another person, he may fear being ridiculed or rejected. The client must become comfortable in revealing his true self. The nurse who is insecure in developing relationships with clients may choose superficial methods to build trust: sharing secrets, telling private jokes, encouraging the client to establish the relationship on a first name basis, or spending extra time with the client as though he has priority over other clients. Some clients accept such behaviors, but others may resent being treated differently from other clients. Instead of enjoying the nurse's extra attention, they become distrustful. There is no room for game playing or facades in developing a helping relationship.

Genuine caring is a powerful method for acquiring the client's trust. The nurse shows a sensitivity and understanding of the client's needs. Expressing concern for the client's welfare is one way to establish trust. By showing concern the nurse encourages the client's growth and progress.

Client: I've been home now for 4 days and I just don't know what to do.

Nurse: You're obviously upset. Tell me what the problem is. I'd like to help.

Client: The doctor put me on that new diet. It seemed easy in the hospital but I'm afraid I'm not eating right.

Nurse: You've improved so much since before your hospitalization. Let's sit down together and see what kind of foods you should eat. Then we'll look at the type of foods you like that are allowed in your new diet.

The client begins to trust the nurse who shows a willingness to help, not out of duty but out of a desire to meet his needs.

Client: You shouldn't have to go to so much trouble for me.

Nurse: You're not causing me trouble at all. An important part of my job is to help you stay healthy. If I can help you understand your diet better, I'll feel I did my job.

Client: Well, if I can learn to fix and eat the right foods, my doctor says I may stay out of the hospital longer this time.

Nurse: Your doctor is right. Now let's go over what you know so far.

Another element that facilitates the establishment of trust is recognizing the client's individuality. The client realizes that the nurse respects him as a unique person.

Client: The doctor said I should eat more vegetables and fruits. I really don't like many vegetables.

Nurse: Well, let's make a list of what you do like. You know there are different ways to prepare the same kinds of foods. If you're able to eat the things you like, you'll be able to follow the diet more easily.

Client: That sounds good. Before I left the hospital, I didn't think I would have much choice in what I ate.

Nurse: Sure you do. I'll show you that you can have a lot of variety in your diet and even enjoy it. It's important that the diet be planned for you and not someone else.

Trust develops on a foundation of caring. The nurse's time, patience, and conscientiousness show her concern for the client's welfare.

IDENTIFICATION OF PROBLEMS AND GOALS. At the initial encounter with the client, the nurse begins assessing his health status. Through observations and interaction the nurse begins to make diagnostic conclusions concerning the client's health problems. The problems may be simple, such as moving without discomfort, choosing foods that will be easily tolerated, or getting out of bed safely. The relationship with the client is strengthened if the nurse discovers what problems are important to him. The client may not be able to recognize his problems. During the orientation phase the nurse uses communication techniques to direct the client toward an awareness of problems, focus on the nature of the problems, and explore potential solutions. As problems are identified, the nurse and client mutually set goals. When the client is able to participate in goal setting and see the desired benefits, nursing interventions are more effective.

Identification of problems uses the techniques of attentive listening, open-ended questioning, paraphrasing, and clarifying. These techniques are discussed later in this chapter. Initially the nurse avoids identifying a large number of actual or potential problems. Bombarding the client with too many questions can result in his emotional and physical fatigue. Also, it makes the client less trusting and more suspicious of the nurse's intentions. Limiting problem identification facilitates the client's understanding of what his role and the nurse's role will be. Goals are more easily attainable when problems are clearly defined and understood.

Mr. Sachs is a 58-year-old man who has suffered a partial paralysis of his right side. Mr. Sachs needs to regain function in his right hand to retain his job as a telephone repairman. He is also fearful of damage to his self-image. He feels deformed and unable to live normally again.

Mr. Sachs: So much has happened to me. I know I may never again be able to do the things I once enjoyed.

Nurse: I know it's a difficult time for you now, but there are many things we can do to help you regain normal function.

Mr. Sachs: But there are so many things wrong with me.

Nurse: Let's take one at a time. What is most important to you?

Mr. Sachs: If only I could use my hand.

Nurse: Your doctor has ordered some exercises to increase the strength in your hand. I'll show you how to do each one. Are you willing to try them?

Mr. Sachs: You bet I am. If only I could use my hand again to work.

Nurse: Let's start with some simple goals. First we'll help you gain strength in your fingers so you can grasp eating utensils, a comb, or a razor. After that we'll try some more strenuous exercises.

Mr. Sachs: OK, that sounds reasonable. Show me what I need to do.

CLARIFICATION OF ROLES. Once a helping relationship is initiated, the roles of nurse and client must be clarified. Clarification of roles occurs through a sharing of information: what the nurse has assessed as the client's immediate needs, how the client perceives those needs, when various nursing care measures are to be instituted, and how the client can participate in his care. The helping relationship requires participation from both parties, but the nurse assumes the leadership role. Leadership does not mean control in the manipulative sense as in saying, "We *will* do your exercises now." Instead the nurse takes the initiative in determining the client's point of view by asking, "When would you prefer to start your exercises?" The client assumes a role as receiver of care, but he also assumes an ongoing role as collaborator and participant in his care.

CONTRACT FORMATION. Once goals and roles are clearly defined, the nurse establishes a contract with the client. Generally this involves a brief verbal interchange. Elements of the contract include location, frequency, and length of contacts with the client and duration of the relationship. The nurse should not present the contract in an overly formal way, since a client may perceive the nurse's businesslike style as cold or impersonal. The nurse outlines a contractual agreement in a way that clarifies both the client's and the nurse's expectations. The nurse thus informs the client of what he and the nurse must do to facilitate his progress toward health.

Nurse: Mr. Sachs, I'll be seeing you each morning for the next 4 days. After we practice your exercises together, I'd like you to do them on your own. Practice the exercises as often as you can without feeling pain or fatigue. On Friday I'll introduce you to the nurse who will work with you next week. I'll be sure she knows the types of exercises you're doing.

It is important to let the client know at what point the relationship will be terminated. If the relationship is successful, the nurse and client frequently share close bonds of respect and concern. The closer the nurse and client become in working together, the more difficult it is to end the relationship. If the client can anticipate how long the relationship will last, termination will be less stressful. This is particularly important for the student nurse, who often is able to spend considerable time with one or two clients. The client becomes accustomed to the student's constant attention. Unless the student prepares the client early for the end of their relationship, the client is likely to become angry or disappointed when termination occurs.

WORKING

During the working phase of a helping relationship, the nurse strives to meet the goals set during the orientation phase. The nurse and client work together to improve the client's health. The relationship broadens and becomes more flexible as the nurse and client become more willing to share feelings and discuss problems hampering the client's attainment of goals.

INTEGRATING COMMUNICATION WITH NURSING ACTIONS. Nursing actions can generally be divided into three groups: physiological, psychological, and socioeconomic. Bradley and Edinberg (1982) categorize the three groups by their level of visibility. Physiological actions that attend to a client's physical needs, such as nutrition, elimination, and comfort, have high visibility. Feeding a client, administering an enema, and applying a warm compress are tasks that require manual skill and are easily observed and measured. Most physiological actions are nonverbal and routinely performed. Traditionally emphasis has been placed on a nurse's ability to perform physiological actions. The high visibility of such actions allows the client to recognize the nurse as an adept practitioner.

In contrast, psychological and socioeconomic nursing actions have low visibility. Psychological actions such as listening attentively and providing reassurance attend to a client's emotional needs. Socioeconomic actions such as referring a client to a community health agency and providing health care education assist the client in adapting to a given environment. Low-visibility tasks are not readily observed or measured by others. Both psychological and socioeconomic actions require cognitive and affective skills that are not routine and have traditionally led to less reward for the nurse clinician (Fig. 15-4).

Communication is important in performing both high- and low-visibility tasks. Giving emotional support, educating the client's family, and similar psychosocial measures obviously require effective communication, but so do basic nursing care procedures. Consider the following two examples of nurses performing the physiological action of administering a pain medication:

The nurse, Ms. Thomas, silently enters Mr. Richards' room. She tells the client, "It's time for your pain shot."

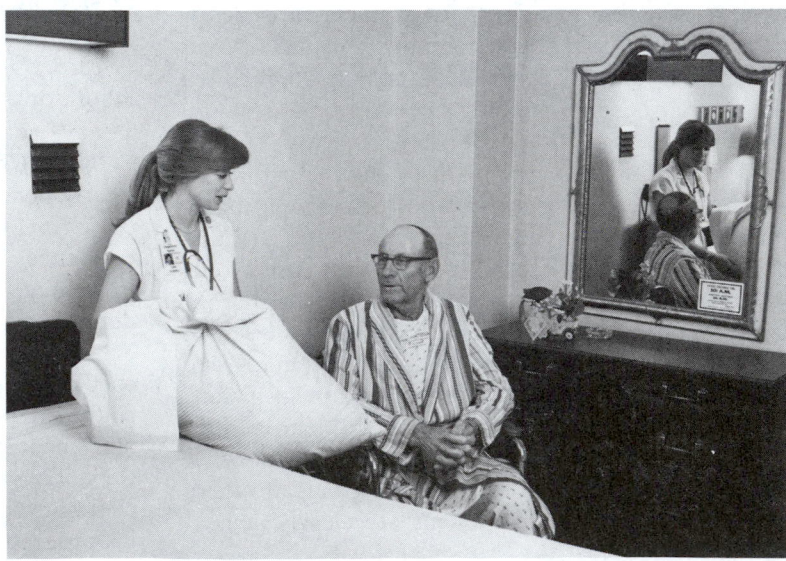

Fig. 15-4 The nurse integrates therapeutic communication skills into the delivery of basic nursing care.

The client is mildly startled and grimaces as he turns to see the nurse. As Mr. Richards starts to ask the nurse a question, she quickly reaches for his arm and prepares to inject the needle.

The nurse, Mr. Ives, enters Mr. Richards' room and says "I have that pain medication you requested. Are you still feeling uncomfortable?" The client turns and replies, "Yes, my back feels like a knife went through it. Will the pain ever go away?" Mr. Ives lays the syringe on the table, sits down next to the client, and says, "It's normal to have pain the first few days after surgery. Let me give you that shot and then I can show you how to move more carefully in bed to avoid worsening the pain."

Most clients would welcome Mr. Ives for their nurse but would like to bar the door when Ms. Thomas appeared. A few words of concern and reassurance (low-visibility communication skills) make receiving an injection more acceptable and encourage the client to express his feelings.

Communication facilitates all nursing care measures. Integrating high- and low-visibility tasks allows the nurse to accomplish several goals simultaneously. In the preceding situation, nurse Ives quickly and efficiently assessed the client's pain, provided a reassuring explanation, and demonstrated an alternative way of relieving pain. Therapeutic communication during high-visibility tasks increases the client's acceptance and understanding of procedures, lessens anxiety, and improves the client's willingness to cooperate.

ESTABLISHING A CLIMATE FOR CHANGE. During the working phase the nurse develops a positive climate for change as she helps the client explore and understand his thoughts, feelings, and actions. Rogers (1961) describes the nurse-client relationship as one "in which at least one of the parties has the intent of promoting the growth, development, maturity, improved functioning, and improved coping with life of the other."

Communication is the means by which the nurse helps clients adjust to the changes imposed by illness. For example, a young woman confined to a wheelchair as a result of multiple sclerosis may see little hope for a fulfilling or prolonged life. In most cases clients seek the opportunity to return as productive members of society following an illness. However, multiple sclerosis creates an imposing barrier to any goals the woman may have in maintaining a "normal" life-style. The nurse caring for the woman establishes a relationship that allows her to identify the client's values about life. Together the client and nurse seek out ways in which the client can adjust to her limitations and still achieve a satisfying level of existence.

In a helping relationship the client is supported in making decisions and taking actions within his abilities. Change becomes less of a threat as the nurse helps a client express his feelings about change, accepts his temporary setbacks, and encourages even the slightest progress toward the attainment of healthier behaviors.

TERMINATION

During the orientation phase the nurse tells the client when to expect the conclusion of their relationship. When termination occurs, the client should not be surprised. The nurse and client have remained aware of the goals of the relationship, and the client should be prepared to function effectively without the nurse's support. Termination can nonetheless be a difficult and painful experience. Frequently the client and nurse attempt to avoid the reality that termination is at hand. The primary objective at the end of any helping relationship is termination in a mutually planned and satisfying manner.

EVALUATING GOAL ACHIEVEMENT. Vital to termination of the relationship is the evaluation of the goals agreed on by the nurse and client. The nurse encourages the client to assess the appropriateness and outcome of the goals established.

Ms. Garner has worked with the client, Mr. Adams, during his 4-week stay in the hospital. Mr. Adams had surgery for the repair of a fractured leg. Together Ms. Garner and Mr. Adams set goals for the client's physical rehabilitation and eventual return home.

Ms. Garner: Well, Mr. Adams, your doctor has discharged you for tomorrow morning. How do you feel about going home?

Mr. Adams: Oh, I'll be glad to get out of here. My leg feels pretty good.

Ms. Garner: Do you feel comfortable walking with the crutches?

Mr. Adams: Yes, I do. As you suggested, I practiced climbing stairs quite a bit in physical therapy. As you know, I have five stairs to climb up to my front door. I can climb now without losing my balance.

Ms. Garner: You've also worked hard on learning to transfer from the bed and chair to a standing position with the crutches.

Mr. Adams: It's a lot easier now. All the practice you suggested helped. Since you've explained all of the right ways to hold the crutches, they feel like a natural part of me. I do hope I can get rid of them soon.

Ms. Garner: Well, it sounds like you're ready to leave. Continue your leg exercises as you've done them here and soon you won't need those crutches.

Mr. Adams: Thanks again for your help. I didn't think I'd ever be able to walk with these things, but now the crutches are no problem.

Both the nurse and the client experience a sense of satisfaction in meeting goals, particularly if the goals were mutually set. If goals are left unaccomplished, the reasons are examined and plans are made for attainment in the future. In the preceding situation, Mr. Adams had not achieved the ability to walk without his crutches. The nurse encouraged him to continue his exercise regimen so he would become strong enough to walk independently.

SEPARATION. Depending on the nature of the relationship between nurse and client, the client may have feelings of anxiety or ambivalence as termination nears. Ideally the client freely expresses his feelings regarding termination of the relationship. The nurse plans time to allow the client to share his concerns or fears.

If the client remains in the health care setting and the nurse is the one leaving, the client may feel abandoned. The nurse makes sure the client's care is uninterrupted by her departure. She introduces the client to the new nurse who will be providing his care. Orienting a fellow nurse to the client's plan of care provides continuity in the methods for managing the client's problems. The nurse shares with her colleague any information that might foster the development of a helping relationship between the colleague and the client. For example, information about a client's use of eye contact, acceptance of touch, and tendency to ask questions will help the new nurse communicate more effectively with the client.

TABLE 15-3

Techniques for Communicating with Children of Various Developmental Levels

Developmental Level	Child's Language and Thought Processes	Communication Techniques
Infant	Child communicates primarily nonverbally (coos, smiles, cries). Child seeks comfort.	Avoid loud harsh sounds and sudden movements. Gentle close physical contact helps a child become quiet. Keep mother in view while holding and interacting with child.
Toddler or preschooler	Child communicates verbally and nonverbally. Child is egocentric with all activities focused on *self*. Speech and thought processes are concrete.	Focus discussion on child's personal needs and concerns. Tell child specifically what he can do and how he will feel. Allow child to explore his environment (handle a stethoscope, play with tongue blade). Use simple, short sentences, familiar words, and concrete explanations. Avoid ambiguous phrases the child cannot interpret, such as "the shot will just feel like a bee-sting" or "take this medicine for your tummy ache."
School-age child	Speech is primarily verbal. Child seeks explanations of world around him and is interested in functional aspects of objects and events. Child is concerned about body integrity.	Give simple explanations. Demonstrate how equipment works; allow child to manipulate equipment (hold percussion hammer, wear stethoscope). Allow child to express any fears or concerns.
Adolescent	Adolescent thinks more abstractly, fluctuates between childish and adult thinking and behavior, and likes talking with adults outside of family.	Avoid imposing values or judgments. Allow the adolescent time to talk. Be attentive; avoid interrupting or showing gestures of disapproval. Avoid embarassing questions or the impulse to give advice. Adolescents frequently use a language of their own; clarify terms.

Communicating with Children

Communication with a child requires special considerations so that the nurse can develop a working relationship with both the child and his family. The nurse receives much of her information about a child from his parents. Because contact between parent and child is usually close, the information communicated by parents can be assumed to be reliable, although naturally some parents may exaggerate in some respects. If the client is a young child, it is helpful to offer him toys or materials to play with so the parent can give full attention to the nurse during a conversation. The nurse gives periodic attention to infants and younger children as they play to make them participants in the discussion. An older child can be actively involved in the communication process.

To communicate effectively with children, the nurse must understand the influence of development on language and thought processes. Both factors affect the way a child communicates and the manner in which the nurse can successfully engage a child in an interaction. Table 15-3 summarizes the developmental levels and corresponding language and thought processes for each developmental group.

Children, particularly young ones, are more responsive to nonverbal messages than to verbal messages. A child is very observant and notices any gestures or moves a person makes. Sudden movements or threatening gestures can frighten a child. The nurse walking into an examination room with a broad grin and animated hand movements will likely inhibit the formation of a relationship with a child. The nurse should remain calm and gentle in her movements. It helps to let the child make the first move in interpersonal contacts. A quiet, friendly, confident tone of voice is best when interacting with a child, even when he is having a temper tantrum.

Children dislike being stared at. Adults looking down on them make them feel vulnerable. While communicating with a young child, the nurse should meet him at eye level. The child feels helpless in most situations involving health care personnel. Sitting in a low chair, kneeling, or squatting places the nurse in a less threatening position during an interaction with a child.

Whenever it is necessary to give explanations or directions, the nurse uses simple, direct language. The child will be more likely to understand explanations involving the fewest words possible. The nurse must be honest with children. Deceiving a child into thinking a painful procedure is painless will only make him angry. A child should always be told what to expect. To minimize the child's fear and anxiety, explanations about a procedure should be given immediately before it begins.

Drawing and play are two very effective ways of communicating with young children. Drawing provides an opportunity for the child to communicate nonverbally (by making the drawing) and verbally (by explaining the picture). A child's drawing usually reveals something about himself and his experiences, and analysis of such drawings is a technique used by psychologists. The nurse can use a child's drawing as a basis for initiating a conversation with the child.

Play is the universal language of children. During play a child's defenses are lowered and the nurse is able to get to know the child more intimately (Fig. 15-5). Therapeutic play distracts the child from the anxieties and discomfort associated with illness. Play is particularly useful when the nurse needs to be close

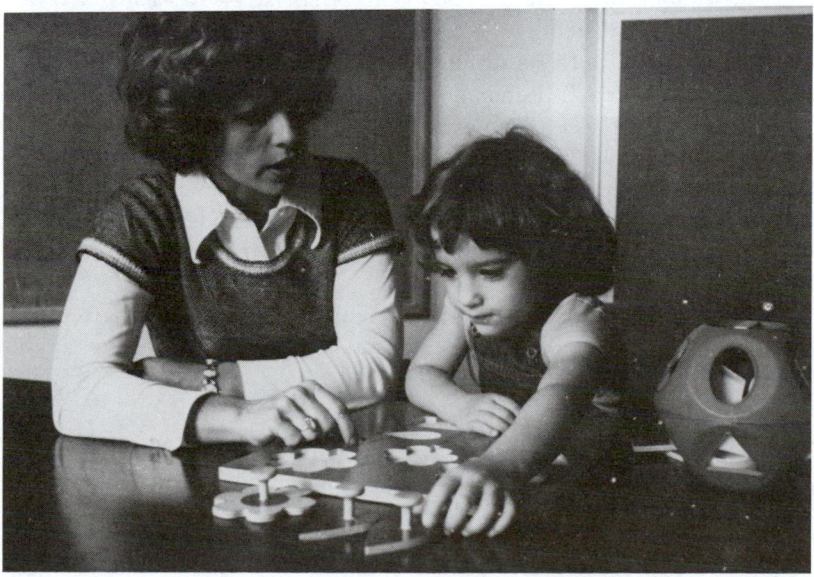

Fig. 15-5 The nurse is able to initiate communication more effectively with children during play activities.
Courtesy Tom Morton, St. Louis.

to the child to conduct a physical assessment but does not want to frighten him.

Skills That Promote Effective Communication

The nurse employs various communication skills while establishing a therapeutic relationship. There is no special formula that the nurse can use to form a relationship with a client. Each person communicates in his own way, and each client the nurse encounters requires a different consideration of communication techniques.

Ideally the nurse remains flexible in the techniques she chooses to foster effective communication. With experience and practice a nurse learns which techniques work best in given situations. For example, silence may prove useful in encouraging one client to express his feelings, whereas asking related questions may be the only method that prompts another client to converse.

The following techniques will prove useful if the nurse simultaneously applies knowledge of each phase of a helping relationship.

Maintaining Silence

Silence provides opportunity for the nurse and client to organize their thoughts. The use of silence can be very effective but is difficult, since pauses in conversation that last several seconds or minutes can make both the client and the nurse uneasy.

The use of silence requires skill and timing. Silence allows the client an opportunity to communicate intrapersonally and to process information. It gives the client time to search for the words or feelings he wants to express. Silence is particularly useful when the client is confronted with a difficult decision that he is not sure how to share with the nurse.

Silence also affords the nurse an opportunity to observe clients unobtrusively. The nurse pays particular attention to any nonverbal messages conveyed, as by a worried expression or loss of eye contact. Remaining silent demonstrates the nurse's willingness to wait patiently for a response. Often the nurse has many questions to raise with clients. Some clients, especially the elderly, are unable to reply quickly. Any impatience expressed by the nurse frustrates the client's efforts at communicating. Silence shows the client that the nurse is interested and will accept any response he can express.

Many nurses feel uncomfortable in using silence. Once a conversation reaches a pivotal point conducive to silence, the nurse may become ill at ease and break the silence. As a result the client's opportunity to gather his thoughts is lost. A premature interruption of silence can prevent important issues from surfacing during a discussion.

Observe your own behavior when silence prevails. Do you feel an urge to interrupt the silence? Are you uncomfortable around people who do not talk very much? Learning to use silence effectively requires a continuous evaluation of the effects silence has on you and your client.

Listening Attentively

Nurses spend much of their day listening to clients and colleagues. Unfortunately, information may go in one ear and out the other unless the nurse is attentive to what is being said. Attentive listening involves an attempt to understand the entire message a person is communicating, verbally and nonverbally.

By being attentive the nurse conveys the impression to the client that he has the nurse's total attention. The nurse shows interest by facing the person who is speaking, maintaining eye contact, assuming a relaxed open posture, avoiding distracting movements, nodding in acknowledgment, and leaning toward the speaker.

The nurse must appear natural while listening to clients. The use of nonverbal cues, such as leaning toward the speaker, should not become overbearing or threaten the client's intimate space. Listening skillfully while carrying out a nursing procedure is both beneficial and an efficient use of time. For example, much can be learned as well as conveyed by the attentive nurse who listens while giving the client a bath. In such a case it is the client who is the center of attention and not the bath procedure.

Walker (1969) offers six steps to more effective listening:

1. Be selective in what you listen to.
2. Remember words are only symbols—we impose our meanings on other's words.
3. Concentrate on the speaker's central theme rather than on isolated statements.
4. Judge content rather than style or delivery.
5. Listen openly—do not focus on emotionally charged words.
6. The average person listens four times faster than he can speak—take time to summarize what you have heard.

Conveying Acceptance

To show acceptance means that one is nonjudgmental of another person. This is a difficult behavior at times. Because nurses meet clients of diverse backgrounds and interests, often a client's values and ideas are in direct conflict with those of the nurse. Acceptance is not synonymous with agreement. Acceptance is a willingness to hear the person's message without conveying doubt or disagreement.

Certainly a nurse does not accept all aspects of a client's behavior, nor does she accept a client's illness. The nurse works to bring about purposeful change that improves a client's level of health. Acceptance is the tolerance and approval toward others that foster a relationship between nurse and client.

To convey acceptance the nurse remains aware of her nonverbal expressions. She should avoid facial expressions and gestures that suggest she disagrees or disapproves of a client's statements, such as frowning, rolling her eyes upward, or shaking her head in disbelief. The following show a client that the nurse accepts what he has to say:

1. Listening without interrupting
2. Providing verbal feedback that demonstrates understanding of what the client says
3. Being sure nonverbal cues match verbal communication
4. Avoiding arguing, expressing doubts, or attempting to change the client's mind

Asking Related Questions

Questioning is a direct method of communicating with a client. Usually the nurse's aim is to elicit specific information from the client. Questions used during a conversation set the tone of the verbal interaction and control its direction. Questions are most effective when they are related to the topic or subject being discussed.

During an assessment of the client's health status, questions follow a logical sequence.

Nurse: Mr. James, can you tell me where you are having pain?
Client: Well, it seems to be in my back.
Nurse: What part of your back?
Client: Here, in the lower part.
Nurse: How would you describe the pain?
Client: It feels like a knife went through me.

The nurse's line of questioning helps the client tell a story. Each question focuses on a specific aspect of the story. The nurse is careful not to move on to another subject until the current topic is adequately explored. The nurse selects a question on the basis of the client's previous response so that information discussed flows logically.

If the nurse wants the client to elaborate on the subject being discussed, open-ended questions are most effective. Such a question cannot be answered with a simple "yes" or "no." Frequently a client has much to communicate, and an open-ended question gives him the freedom to respond in any way he chooses. The open-ended question demonstrates the nurse's interest in what the client has to say. Examples of open-ended questions are: "What were you doing when you first noticed the pain?" "What seems to be the problem?" "How have you felt since your doctor talked with you today?" Asking the client open-ended questions allows the nurse to assess a number of factors. How the client responds verbally and nonverbally to a question can reveal his genuine emotions. The nurse may be able to judge the level of the client's vocabulary and understanding of his health by his response. Often the nurse seeks the details of physical signs and symptoms, and the open-ended question elicits more accurate and detailed descriptions. Since the open-ended question prompts a lengthy response, the nurse can assess gaps or discrepancies in the information shared.

There is a wealth of information to be shared by client and nurse. Questions allow the nurse to explore subjects that reveal information pertinent to the client's care.

Paraphrasing

Paraphrasing is restating the client's message in the nurse's own words. Usually a paraphrased statement uses fewer words than the original statement. Through paraphrasing the nurse sends feedback that lets the client know if his message was understood and prompts further communication.

Client: I've had it. My doctor won't tell me what is going on. He doesn't seem to care what I think.
Nurse: You're saying that you're angry with your doctor?
Client: Yes, he obviously doesn't know what it's like to be sick.

Practice is required to paraphrase accurately. If the meaning of a message is misconstrued or distorted through paraphrasing, communication may become ineffective. For example, a client may say, "I've been overweight all my life and never had any problems. I can't understand why I need to be on a diet." Paraphrasing this statement by saying, "You mean you don't care if you're overweight or not?" is incorrect. "It seems that you're not convinced you need a diet, since you've remained healthy," is a proper way of paraphrasing the statement.

Clarifying

Despite efforts at paraphrasing, the nurse may not understand the client's message. When a misunderstanding occurs, the nurse momentarily stops the progress of the discussion to clarify the client's meaning. Without clarification valuable information can be lost. Information critical to the client's care plan can be incomplete unless confusing or conflicting data are clarified. The nurse can either attempt to repeat the client's message or admit confusion and ask the client to restate the message. For example, a client has come to the clinic for a checkup:

Client: I knew I might have a problem. It seems to be in my family. The last time I was here, though, it wasn't bad so I didn't mention it.

Nurse: I'm sorry, Mr. Brewer, can you tell me what type of problem you're having?

It is also important for the nurse to clarify messages given to clients. Examples can be used to clarify a vague, abstract idea. When using examples, the nurse employs ideas or situations to which the client can easily relate. In the following dialog a nurse is explaining activity restrictions to a client who has had eye surgery:

Nurse: Now, Mr. Lee, once you go home you are not supposed to place stress on your eye.

Client: I'm not sure I know what you mean.

Nurse: Well, you're not allowed to stoop or bend over with your head down. For example, if you want to pick up your slippers off the floor or pick up a basket of laundry, don't bend over. Instead, bend your knees and keep your head up.

Client: I have a dog at home. I guess I can't bend over to pick him up?

Nurse: That's right. Bend your knees to lower yourself down if you want to pet your dog.

The more specific a clarifying message, the more likely it will be understood. Clients who are easily confused by the complex terms and jargon of medicine appreciate a simple, down-to-earth explanation that uses familiar examples.

Focusing

As the client discusses various topics related to his health, frequently the messages become vague or ill defined. A client may say to the nurse, "Well, I've just been feeling funny lately. It doesn't really bother me that much. It's just this feeling I'm having in my head." The client's description tells the nurse very little except that he does not feel well. If the nurse does not help the client focus specifically on his physical complaint, the client will likely continue his vague descriptions.

Focusing helps to limit the area of discussion to which the client can respond. The nurse might respond to the client by saying, "You said you've been

feeling funny lately. Tell me when this feeling first started," or "Describe the feeling in your head." As in clarifying, the nurse seeks meaning in the client's message. In the case of focusing, however, the nurse understands the client's message but realizes it is nonspecific or vague.

Once a client becomes involved in describing his problems, opinions, or concerns, it is important to encourage his verbalization. The nurse should not use focusing if it requires interrupting the client while he is discussing an important issue. If the conversation begins to drag on without new information or the client begins to repeat himself, focusing is a useful communication technique.

Stating Observations

When communicating, a person is often unaware of how his messages are received. Feedback from others tells him if he communicated the intended message. One way the nurse can provide feedback is by sharing with the client her observations of his behavior as he communicates. The nurse describes the impressions created by the client's nonverbal cues.

Miss Tucker is sitting in the waiting room of her physician's office. She is slumped in the chair, her body movements are slow, and she yawns while speaking with the nurse. The nurse says, "Miss Tucker, you appear to be quite tired."

If the client's verbal message conflicts with his nonverbal cues, the nurse's observation may help the client convey a truer and clearer message. Stating observations often leads the client to communicate more clearly without the need for extensive questioning, focusing, or clarifying by the nurse.

The nurse does not state observations that might embarrass or anger the client. The nurse in the preceding example would not say, "Miss Tucker, you look a mess." Even if such an observation is made with humor, the client can easily become resentful.

Offering Information

When two people communicate, the process is rarely one sided. In an interaction with a client the nurse frequently offers information that gives the client additional data or insight about the topic of discussion. The client in the following dialog is scheduled to have surgery the next day for a simple hernia repair.

Client: My doctor has told me I'm first on the schedule for surgery tomorrow.

Nurse: Yes, we'll be awakening you about 6:00 AM.

Client: My family would like to be here then.

Nurse: That's no problem. They are free to come at 6:00 and we'll show them where to wait for you once you've left for the operating room.

Frequently, providing the client with additional information encourages him to respond further based on the nurse's input. Offering information on an ongoing, timely basis not only facilitates communication but also promotes health teaching.

It is not helpful to withhold information from the client, particularly when he seeks it. If the nurse avoids sharing information or imparts only partial information, the client may lose trust in the nurse. The nurse cannot share information that the physician chooses to withhold from the client. However, there is a wide range of information the nurse can share (see Chapter 16). The nurse must avoid giving advice to a client when giving information. Information can facilitate a client's decision making, but the nurse should not make the decision for him.

Summarizing

Summarization is a concise review of the main ideas that have been discussed. A summary sets the tone for any further interactions between the nurse and client. Beginning a new interaction by summarizing a previous interaction helps the client recall the topics discussed and shows the client how the nurse has analyzed their communication.

Ms. Spier has been working for several days to help Mrs. Ramos learn about diabetes. Ms. Spier enters the client's room and says, "Good morning, Mrs. Ramos. I've come to talk with you more about your diabetes. If you recall, yesterday we discussed the purpose of insulin, its side effects, and how to give an injection."

Summarizing helps the nurse review key aspects of an interaction. Further communication can then focus on the relevant issues. The client will be able to sense whether the nurse understood his part of the message. With a summary the client is able to review information and make additions or corrections.

The client often adds critical information at the time of summarization, including information the nurse has perhaps forgotten but the client views as essential or relevant. During a summary the nurse should not add new material that might cloud previously discussed issues or facts.

Factors That Inhibit Communication

Just as there are ways to promote effective communication, there are also techniques or styles that cause interactions to be nontherapeutic. The nurse

tends to block effective communication when she has feelings of uncertainty or anxiety during an interaction. The nurse may be unsure of her ability to communicate or may feel threatened by the topic of discussion, such as whether the client will live or die. Many of the techniques that normally promote effective communication can be detrimental if used improperly. Failure to listen or clarify statements can be a costly mistake that jeopardizes the nurse-client relationship.

Giving an Opinion

When a client asks questions, the nurse may be tempted to give her opinion. However, a goal of a helping relationship is to promote the client's independence and ability to make decisions. Offering opinions transfers decision making from client to nurse. The client is no longer self-directed. When a client asks for an opinion, it is usually an attempt to validate an idea or feeling. The nurse's opinion inhibits the client's spontaneity, stalls his problem solving, and creates doubt.

Nurse: Mr. Jones, you look like you're deep in thought.
Client: Oh, no, not really. I was just thinking about whether my daughter is coming to see me.
Nurse: Well, if you ask me, she should have been here before now. It would mean so much to you.

Often the client simply needs an opportunity to express his feelings. Giving an opinion prevents the client from developing solutions to his own problems.

There may be times when clients require suggestions. For example, when a client is selecting foods from a special diet, he may require the nurse's help in choosing the right types of food. Suggestions are best presented to clients in the form of options, since the final decision rests with the client.

Client: What do you think is the best type of exercise for me to try?
Nurse: Well, Miss Raines, you've said you enjoy biking and swimming. Either one is an excellent way to exercise.

Offering False Reassurance

A nurse can easily become overinvolved with the emotions of sick clients. The client reaches out for acknowledgment that he is a person, possessing worth and dignity. The nurse may be tempted to remove all the client's fears and anxieties by telling him he is all right. Although this might make the nurse feel better, it could do the client more harm than good. In an effort to reassure the client, the nurse might promise something that will not occur ("You'll be fine") or say something that is untrue ("There's nothing to worry about").

Bradley and Edinberg (1982) have identified six conditions about which a client can safely be reassured:

1. That there is hope
2. That the nurse is listening
3. That care is available
4. That certain undesirable changes can be expected
5. That the client will be treated like a person
6. That the client's problem is understood

The following example shows how the nurse conveys a willingness to listen to and understand a client's concerns without falsely reassuring the client that the illness is a minor one.

Mrs. Stevens is a 58-year-old woman with terminal cancer. Her nurse, Ms. Fry, is sitting by her side.
Mrs. Stevens: I sometimes think this isn't happening to me. It seems so unfair . . . . Oh, I'm sorry. You don't want to hear my problems.
Ms. Fry: No, please, Mrs. Stevens, I do want to hear how you feel.

Being Defensive

When a person becomes defensive, the mood is easily conveyed through his words and nonverbal behavior. Frequently clients criticize a nurse, some other member of the health care team, or even the institution. The tendency may be for the nurse to defend herself or the person being criticized. If the nurse becomes angry or argumentative and refuses to listen to the client's concern, her relationship with the client is jeopardized. The nurse's defensiveness may imply that the client has no right to express an opinion.

Mr. Locke has been a regular visitor to the health clinic for several years. The last time he visited the clinic Mr. Locke had symptoms that resulted in his hospitalization. He now is returning to the clinic for a checkup 1 week after his discharge from the hospital.
Mr. Locke: Well, I hope I don't have to see Dr. Warren today.
Nurse: I don't understand, Mr. Locke, is something wrong? Dr. Warren has been your doctor here for some time.
Mr. Locke: I don't care. He was the one who put me in the hospital and that was a waste of time.
Nurse: That's silly. Dr. Warren is an excellent physician.
Mr. Locke: You think so, huh? He hasn't put you in the hospital for no reason.
Nurse: You were very ill, Mr. Locke. I know Dr. Warren made the right decision.

The nurse has threatened her relationship with Mr. Locke. Mr. Locke will probably not trust the nurse to keep his concerns confidential. She is ignoring the client's feelings and will probably not take any action to remedy his problem. After this conversation the nurse will have difficulty developing a rapport that will prompt the client to discuss additional problems.

When a client expresses criticism, the nurse should listen to what he has to say. Listening does not imply agreement. The nurse avoids becoming defensive in order to learn the real reasons behind the client's criticism. There are two sides to any story, and the nurse attempts to learn why the client has become angry or dissatisfied.

Mr. Locke: Well, I hope I don't have to see Dr. Warren today.
Nurse: You seem upset, would you like to talk about it?
Mr. Locke: I just don't think he should have put me in the hospital.
Nurse: You believe hospitalization was unnecessary?
Mr. Locke: Yes, they really didn't do much of anything. They took a few tests and did some x-rays.
Nurse: Mr. Locke, did your doctors tell you what the tests showed?
Mr. Locke: No, not really. That's why I'm so angry.

The nurse's patience with the situation led to an identification of the client's real concern, not knowing the results of his diagnostic tests. By avoiding defensiveness the nurse defused Mr. Locke's anger so he could describe his true concerns.

Problems at home or with colleagues can make the nurse more likely to feel defensive when criticized. When that occurs, it is wise for the nurse to avoid potentially volatile interactions. Talking with a supervisor or fellow staff member may help the nurse work out any anger or frustration.

Showing Approval or Disapproval

Expressing excessive approval can be as harmful to a nurse-client relationship as stating disapproval. Offering excessive praise implies that the behavior being praised is the only acceptable one. Often the client shares a decision with the nurse, not in an effort to seek approval but to provide a means to discuss his feelings.

Client: I've decided that when I leave the hospital I'll stay with my son. He doesn't want me to go home and be alone.
Nurse: Oh, I'm so glad to hear that. I think you definitely made the right decision. It's best for you to be with your son.

This nurse's comment will likely end any further discussion of the topic. The client may see the nurse's response as an affirmation of the son's view that the client should not live alone. Perhaps the client would be better off with his son. On the other hand, the client may have had a strong desire to remain independent, and now that desire has been repressed. The nurse's excessive approval did not allow the client to think or act freely and inhibited his potential for decision making.

Disapproval implies that the client must meet the nurse's expectations or standards.

Client: Oh, I feel good. I was able to get up in the chair once today.
Nurse: Only once? You're going to have to get up more often than that!

It would have been better for the nurse to say, "You're making fine progress. Your doctor would like you to try to be up at least three times today. Do you think you'd like to sit up just before going to bed?"

A disapproving statement causes the client to feel rejected. The client may avoid further interaction with the nurse, thus potentially slowing his recovery.

Asking Why

Whenever one disagrees with or fails to understand another person's statement or actions, the temptation is to ask why he believes or has acted in such a way. A client frequently interprets a "why" question as an accusation. The client may also think the nurse knows why and is simply testing him. Regardless of what the client perceives the nurse's motivation to be, "why" questions can cause resentment, insecurity, and mistrust.

If the nurse wants additional information, there are more effective ways of phrasing questions than beginning them with "why." For example, rather than asking, "Why didn't you do your exercises?" the nurse could say, "You didn't do your exercises. Is something wrong?" Rather than asking, "Why are you so anxious?" the nurse could say, "You appear upset. Would you like to talk about it?"

Changing the Subject Inappropriately

A nurse might inadvertently stop a client from discussing a subject of importance to him by changing the subject. Abruptly interrupting the flow of a conversation is rude and shows a lack of empathy.

Nurse: Good morning, Mr. Jones. How are you feeling?
Mr. Jones: (facial expression shows discomfort) Oh, not so good. My incision is rather sore.
Nurse: Well, let's get you up in a chair. We need to discuss your exercises.

The nurse's comment shows an unwillingness to discuss Mr. Jones' discomfort. The opportunity for a therapeutic assessment of the nature of Mr. Jones' discomfort is lost. In this example changing the subject was nontherapeutic, since the nurse ignored a potentially serious problem.

Changing the subject stalls the progress of a therapeutic communication. The client's thoughts and spontaneity are interrupted, his ideas become tangled, and as a result, the information he provides may be inadequate. It is particularly important to avoid changing the subject during an assessment. If the client has the opportunity to complete his message, the information shared will be more thorough and useful in meeting his needs.

Forming Communication Barriers

It is easy to inadvertently use a phrase or exhibit a behavior that blocks a client's communication. Interpersonal communication is a delicate process and anything can go wrong at any point. Nevertheless, the nurse should not hesitate to communicate freely for fear she might say something wrong to a client. Mistakes can be corrected. If a nurse blocks a client's communication, she can acknowledge her mistake and make an effort to restore communication by saying, "I've made a mistake in offering my advice. You have a difficult decision to make. The decision must be yours, but I want to understand your feelings and concerns."

■ ■ ■ ■ ■

A nurse is ineffective without good communication skills. Gaining such skills and learning to avoid factors that might inhibit communication take practice, an awareness of one's own behavior, and a willingness to evaluate personal performance.

Communication and Change

As a person develops the values, knowledge, attitudes, and feelings that shape his identity, change can be a threat. Change requires the person to trade his sense of security for something that is unknown and unpredictable. The risks can be significant. In our fast-paced society, change is ever present in our lives.

The client faces considerable change as a result of alterations in health. Hospitalization requires an immediate and often unplanned change in the client's life-style. Depending on the nature or type of illness, there may be permanent changes in the client's physical or emotional health. Long-term illness often interrupts the client's ability to maintain a job, thus threatening his economic security. The changes related to illness have an impact on family members as well as on the client. Often they must assume new roles as a result of a loved one's illness.

The nurse frequently has the important role of change agent. Clients and families require assistance in understanding and accepting the changes imposed by illness. The medium for change is communication.

For change to occur, an individual must communicate intrapersonally as well as interpersonally. He must first consider what effects a change will have. He reviews the implications of change for his existing beliefs, attitudes, and philosophies. For example, the client who loses the function of an arm considers the value of that body part for his body image, economic survival, and familial acceptance. Will he be looked at as a freak? Can he ever work again? How will his family accept the change? Before the client can successfully discuss the implications of change with others, he must address them himself.

Most interpersonal communication is centered on change. For example, the nurse and client influence each other to accept new ideas and share feelings. Through interpersonal communication, the client becomes aware of the perceptions of others and may learn to question previously held values and beliefs. His new way of viewing the world challenges his previous resistance to change.

Nurses facilitate change in a variety of ways. Education of clients and families serves to alter their perceptions of illness, clarify their misconceptions, and provide information for clients to use in maintaining health. Referring a client to resource persons such as social workers and physical therapists can help him accept a new life-style. The nurse is a catalyst for change, using communication skills to assist the client in acquiring self-understanding, seeking solutions to problems, and making relevant decisions.

Without communication skills the nurse holds little authority in the eyes of the client and has little chance to create change. A skillful communicator conveys confidence and ability. The client is more likely to consider the value of change if the nurse uses an innovative and individualized approach in discussing it.

Mr. Green is a 33-year-old business executive who has lost the function of his right arm as the result of an injury suffered in an automobile accident. Mr. Green's appearance is very important to him. The nurse realizes it will take time for Mr. Green to adjust to the physical and psychological changes created by his injury. When she enters Mr. Green's room, he sits slumped in bed and stares out the window rather than looking at her.

Nurse: Hi, Mr. Green. Do you mind if I spend some time with you?

Mr. Green: Sure, if you really want to.

Nurse: I do. Tell me how you're feeling.

Mr. Green: I'm thinking about my job and my family. With my arm the way it is, I know things will be different.

Nurse: Your wife was here this morning. Were you able to discuss this with her?

Mr. Green: She's a sweetheart. I just don't want to worry her.

Nurse: The two of you seem close. Have you talked about your injury together?

Mr. Green: Not really. Every time she starts to talk to me about it, I change the subject. I know we need to talk.

Nurse: She's concerned about you. I know because she always asks me how you've been feeling.

Mr. Green: Well, I don't want her to worry more. I'll try to tell her how I feel.

The nurse could simply have tried to convince the client that everything will be all right, but this approach would give little consideration to his feelings and values about his appearance. Instead, she used an individualized approach suited to Mr. Green's needs. Mr. Green shared the fact that he cares about his wife and is hesitant to let her know about his concerns. To initiate change, the nurse will attempt to involve Mrs. Green in her husband's plan of care. The nurse will interact with Mr. Green further in an attempt to bring client and wife together to communicate. Once Mr. and Mrs. Green are able to share their feelings, they will find it easier to accept Mr. Green's disability.

Communication is an effective force in creating change. The nurse's role as change agent encompasses many of the responsibilities of a professional nurse, such as introducing new therapies, providing new information, or assisting with the clarification of values. When she successfully fills that role, the rewards are limitless.

Summary

Communication is one of the most important skills for a nurse to master. Through communication a nurse establishes a relationship with a client to help him acquire healthy behaviors. A nurse's competence depends on her ability to convey meaningful messages in a timely and intelligent manner as the client's needs dictate and on her ability to understand the client's communications.

Communication is affected by many variables, including one's perceptions, values, emotions, sociocultural background, knowledge, roles and relationships, and environment. Communication between nurse and client is a complex process that includes both verbal and nonverbal communication. The nurse communicates more effectively when she is conscious of all the factors influencing the sending and receiving of messages and when she is receptive to the client's feedback.

Communication skills are essential throughout the nursing process. Therapeutic communication with the client involves planned, deliberate interactions that foster a helping relationship. The nurse conveys genuineness, warmth, and empathetic understanding in all phases of the relationship: orientation, working, and termination. Throughout the relationship the nurse uses the specific skills that promote effective communication and avoids words and actions that inhibit communication. Effective communication is necessary for the nurse's role in helping the client adapt to the changes resulting from health alterations.

KEY CONCEPTS

✓ Effective communication is the process that allows nurses to establish working relationships with clients.

✓ Successful communication requires the message intended by the speaker to be similar or identical to the meaning acquired by the receiver.

✓ The nurse does not ventilate her personal emotions with a client.

✓ The way a person perceives a message depends on his past experiences, sensory function, and personal expectations.

✓ Sources of environmental distraction create serious barriers to communication.

✓ Words that have different connotative meanings can be easily misinterpreted by the person receiving the message.

✓ The nurse must often translate technical terms into simple words to enhance a client's understanding of a message.

✓ Effective verbal communication requires appropriate voice intonation, clear and concise phrasing of words, and a proper pacing of statements.

✓ When the sender's verbal and nonverbal communications complement each other, a receiver is unlikely to misinterpret a message.

✓ Establishing eye contact with an individual signals an intent to communicate.

✓ A nurse must avoid using facial expressions that imply judgment of what a client says.

✓ Whenever a person senses that he has communicated unsuccessfully, he should seek feedback from the receiver.

✓ Touch can be an effective method of communication but should be used with discrimination.

✓ Social interaction is useful in initiating communication but should not be the principal means of maintaining a nurse-client relationship.

KEY CONCEPTS, cont'd

✓ The orientation phase of a helping relationship does not evolve from the nurse's use of complicated communication techniques but rather from her effort to facilitate the client's communication.

✓ Establishment of trust between the nurse and client allows the client to more openly express his thoughts and feelings.

✓ A contract between nurse and client clarifies their expectations of each other and tells the client when the relationship will be terminated.

✓ Communication aids the nurse in performing nursing care measures effectively and efficiently.

✓ Communication is a means for the nurse to help clients adjust to changes imposed by illness.

✓ During the termination of a nurse-client relationship the nurse and client evaluate goals achieved and discuss feelings about ending the relationship.

✓ Methods that facilitate communication with children include sitting at eye level with a child, using simple direct language, and incorporating play into a discussion.

✓ A nurse does not use all of the skills that promote effective communication for every client.

✓ Many skills that normally promote communication can be detrimental to nurse-client relationships if used improperly.

✓ Ineffective communication skills tend to inhibit the client's willingness to express ideas or concerns openly.

REFERENCES

Bradley, J.C., and Edinberg, M.A.: Communication in the nursing context, New York, 1982, Appleton-Century-Crofts.

Ekman, P.: Communication through nonverbal behavior: a source of information about an interpersonal relationship. In Tomkins, S.S., and Izard, C.E., editors: Affect, cognition, and personality, New York, 1965, Springer Publishing Co.

Hein, E.C.: Communication in nursing practice, Boston, 1973, Little, Brown & Co.

Kemp, C.G.: Perspectives on the group process, Boston, 1964, Houghton-Mifflin Co.

Knapp, M.: Nonverbal communication in human interaction, New York, 1972, Holt, Rinehart & Winston.

Pluckhan, M.L.: Human communication: the matrix of nursing, New York, 1978, McGraw-Hill Book Co.

Rogers, C.R.: On becoming a person: a therapist's view of psychotherapy, Boston, 1961, Houghton-Mifflin Co.

Travelbee, J.: Interpersonal aspects of nursing, ed. 2, Philadelphia, 1971, F.A. Davis Co.

Walker, R.: Effective listening, Am. J. Med. Technol. 35:8, 1969.

ADDITIONAL READINGS

Berlo, D.K.: The process of communication: an introduction to theory and practice, New York, 1960, Holt, Rinehart & Winston.

Murray, R.B., and Zentner, J.P.: Nursing concepts for health promotion, ed. 2, Englewood Cliffs, N.J., 1979, Prentice-Hall, Inc.

Purtilo, R.: Health professionals—patient interaction, ed. 2, Philadelphia, 1978, W.B. Saunders Co.

Whaley, L.F., and Wong, D.L.: Nursing care of infants and children, ed. 2, St. Louis, 1983, The C.V. Mosby Co.

Wilson, H.S., and Kneisl, C.R.: Psychiatric nursing, Menlo Park, Calif., 1979, Addison-Wesley Publishing Co.

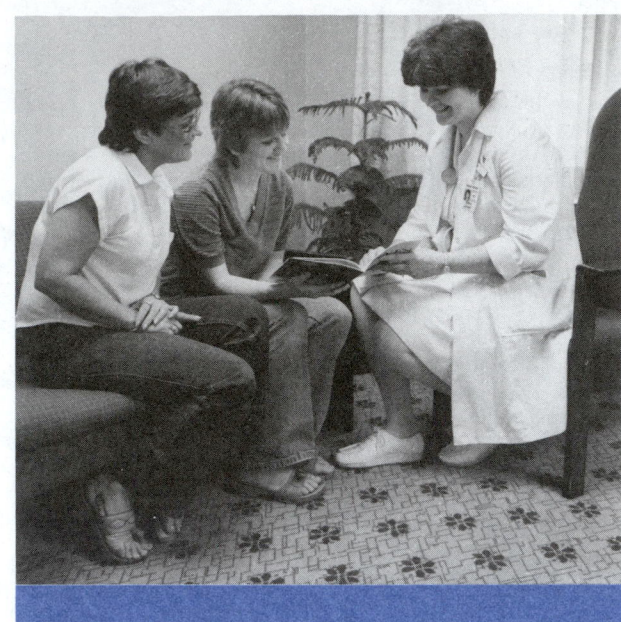

OBJECTIVES

Mastery of content in this chapter will enable the student to:

- Define the terms in the glossary.
- Describe the similarities and differences between teaching and learning.
- Identify the purposes of client teaching.
- Compare the communication process with the teaching process.
- Describe the domains of learning.
- Differentiate factors that determine the readiness to learn from those that determine the ability to learn.
- Identify principles of effective teaching.
- Use client teaching in the nursing process.

GLOSSARY

affective learning Acquisition of behaviors involved in expressing feelings in attitudes, appreciations, and values.

cognitive learning Acquisition of intellectual skills that encompass behaviors such as thinking, understanding, and evaluating.

compliance Person's fulfillment of prescribed course of treatment.

learning Acquisition of new knowledge and skills as a result of reinforcement, practice, and experience.

learning objectives Written statement that describes the behavior a teacher expects from an individual following a learning activity.

motivation Internal impulse that causes a person to take action.

psychomotor learning Acquisition of ability to perform motor skills.

reinforcement Provision of a contingent response to a learner's behavior that increases the probability of the behavior recurring.

teaching Interaction between a teacher and a learner in which the goal is to promote learning.

16 The Teaching-Learning Process

It is impossible to separate teaching from learning. Teaching is an interactive process that promotes learning. It consists of a conscious and deliberate set of actions that helps individuals either gain knowledge they previously lacked or perform new skills. Teaching is most effective when it is responsive to a learner's needs. The teacher is responsible for identifying these needs by fielding questions, inquiring into the learner's interests, sensing feelings of frustration, or acknowledging looks of bewilderment. The process of teaching thus relies on principles of interpersonal communication to send messages of significance to the learner and to receive the learner's feedback.

Telling a person to do something, describing an idea, or even giving advice are isolated acts; they are not examples of teaching. However, if a teacher applies the principles of learning when interacting with a student, these same acts can become teaching. The interdependent relationship between teaching and learning can be illustrated by the experience of a student sitting in a huge lecture hall, listening to the droning words of the lecturer. The student pays less attention to the lecturer's words than to thinking about his plans for after class. Despite the lecturer's intent, the student is probably learning absolutely nothing. The key to the teaching-learning process is knowing what a person wants to learn and in what way that person will learn best. If the lecturer discusses a topic of interest to the student and presents it in a less formal fashion, the chances are that the student will learn a great deal.

To learn is to acquire new knowledge or skills through reinforced practice and experience. Nursing students learn to describe and perform the steps of the nursing process, to implement the process of ethical decision making, to give a backrub, and to administer a medication. Each newly acquired behavior or skill reflects the teacher's efficacy in promoting learning. Nursing students also learn to use a variety of teaching techniques on their own, which inevitably will help their clients to learn.

Alterations in health create changes in a person's life-style. For example, a person may need to take a medication for the rest of his life, undergo an operation that causes a permanent disability, or simply postpone a day's activities to keep a physician's appointment. Such changes compel clients to seek out new ways to improve or maintain their health status. The person requiring health care is the central figure in the teaching-learning process. No one can force a client to learn—not the nurse, physician, or therapist. The client must become willing and able to learn before a nurse can begin to implement any teaching strategy.

A nurse is usually eager to teach a client as much as possible about his health. The opportunities, which occur during almost any encounter with a client, are limitless. The nurse should not, however, forget the individuality of the client. It is essential to recognize teaching as a collaborative effort between nurse and client, since a client will use the information a nurse gives him only if he chooses to. Thus the reward of teaching comes in finding creative ways to apply teaching strategies that ultimately help the client gain the information and skills he seeks.

With health maintenance and illness prevention as current focuses in health care, client education is a skill vital to the nurse's professional success. The Patient's Bill of Rights of the American Hospital Association (see Chapter 17) clearly recognizes that clients have the right to specific types of information. It is the nurse's responsibility to be aware of what information clients require. Although the physician is ultimately responsible for providing information pertinent to a client's diagnosis, treatment, and prognosis, the nurse is readily available to clarify information and help clients understand the physician's explanations. The nurse is the primary provider of information pertaining to all nursing care measures delivered.

Teaching and nursing are united philosophically. By helping clients learn, the nurse improves their ability to function independently. Regardless of the practice setting, the nurse works with clients to enhance their understanding of health and illness and to improve their compliance with medical and nursing therapies.

Purpose of Client Teaching

The nature of health care today calls for comprehensive nursing practice. The emphasis is more on maintaining a person's health than on simply treating disease. Clients are now more knowledgeable about health and seek to become actively involved in their own health maintenance. As a result of shorter hospital stays, the nurse must act early to prepare hospitalized clients for their convalescent period at home. A long-term illness or disability requires the client and family to gain a better understanding of illness and its implications.

Comprehensive client education includes three important purposes, each involving a separate phase of health care: maintenance of health and illness prevention, restoration of health, and coping with impaired functioning.

Maintenance of Health and Illness Prevention

During the last 10 years an increased number of people have sought to learn how to preserve their health. Hundreds of books about diet and exercise are available in bookstores. Television contributes time for self-help groups to appeal to the public about issues such as alcoholism and drug abuse. We have become a very health-conscious society.

The nurse is a convenient resource for any health-minded client who wants to learn how to improve his physical and psychological well-being. In the school, home, clinic, or workplace the nurse provides clients with information and skills that will allow them to assume healthier behaviors (see the boxed material). For example, in childbearing classes nurses teach expectant parents what to anticipate and do during pregnancy. The expectant parents learn about the stages of fetal (unborn child) development and factors that can alter normal growth. The physical and psychological changes the woman undergoes during pregnancy also are a part of the class content. After learning about normal childbearing the mother is more likely to eat healthy foods, engage in physical exercise, and avoid drugs or other substances that might harm the development of the fetus. Promoting healthy behavior through education increases a

---

Topics for Health Teaching

Health promotion/illness prevention
    First aid
    Avoidance of risk factors: smoking, alcohol
    Growth and development
    Hygiene
    Immunizations
    Normal childbearing
    Nutrition
    Exercise
    Safety (in home and hospital)
Restoration of health
    Client's disease or condition
        Anatomy and physiology of body system affected
        Cause of disease
        Origin of symptoms
        Expected effects on other body systems
        Prognosis
    Rationale for treatment
        Medications
        Tests and therapies
        Nursing measures
        Surgical intervention
    Expected duration of care
    Hospital/clinic environment
    Hospital/clinic staff
    Methods for client participation in care
Coping with impaired functions
    Home care
        Medications
        Diet
        Activity
        Self-help devices
    Rehabilitation of remaining function
        Physical therapy
        Occupational therapy
    Prevention of complications
        Knowledge of risk factors
        Implications of noncompliance with therapy

client's self-esteem by making it possible for him to assume more responsibility for his own health. With greater knowledge a person can maintain better health habits. When clients become more health conscious, they are more likely to seek early diagnosis of health problems.

Restoration of Health

When a client is injured or becomes ill, he needs information or skills that will allow him to regain an improved level of health.

Ms. Thorne, a 26-year-old student, fractured her leg in a skiing accident. It is the first time she has ever been hospitalized. The nurse senses Ms. Thorne's anxiety and explains to her who the nursing and medical personnel are so that their faces become familiar. Ms. Thorne's leg is in a cast that she will likely wear for 6 to 8 weeks. To ensure her eventual recovery, the nurse sets aside time to explain the principles of cast care. The nurse allows Ms. Thorne to ask questions about her injury and the cast so she can learn to manage her cast properly at home.

Once a client recovers from the initial stress of illness or injury and accepts the associated limitations, he often seeks information related to his condition. However, clients who find it difficult to adapt to illness may become passive and uninterested in learning. The nurse learns to identify clients' receptivity to acquiring new knowledge and institutes methods to motivate their interest in learning.

The family is often a vital part of a client's return to health. It is frequently as important for the family as for the client to know what to expect during an illness. If the nurse excludes the family from a client's teaching plan, conflicts may arise for the nurse. For example, if the family does not understand a client's need to regain independent function, their efforts may cause the client to become unnecessarily dependent and thus retard his progress. To restore a client's health, both the client and his family learn ways to reestablish his preillness level of functioning.

Coping with Impaired Functioning

Not all clients fully recover from illness or injury. Many must learn to cope with permanent health alterations. New knowledge and skills are often necessary for clients to continue normal activities of daily living. For example, the client whose ability to speak is lost following surgery of the larynx learns new ways of communicating with others, and the client with severe heart disease learns to avoid physical activities that place him at risk for further heart damage.

In the case of serious disability the client's role within the family may change, necessitating understanding and acceptance by family members. The family's ability to provide support comes as a result of education. Education begins as soon as the client's needs are identified and the family displays a willingness to help. The nurse teaches family members how to assist clients with health care management, for example, giving medications and baths and applying dressings. Families of clients with other kinds of alterations, such as alcoholism, mental retardation, or drug dependence, learn to adapt to the emotional effects of these illnesses.

A nurse learns to recognize what types of information to teach clients at different levels of wellness. She considers their needs in relation to their ability to meet them. Learning occurs when information is practical and useful to the learner. Comparing the client's desired level of health with his actual state enables the nurse to plan a meaningful and productive teaching program.

Teaching as a Form of Communication

The teaching process closely parallels the communication process. In fact, teaching is a form of interpersonal communication. A teacher applies each element of the communication process while imparting information to students (see Chapter 15). As in the case of a sender and receiver communicating, the teacher and student become actively involved in a process that ultimately increases the student's knowledge and skills.

Communication and teaching help the nurse establish a meaningful relationship with the client. In a therapeutic nurse-client relationship, change results from the trust and understanding formed between the nurse and client. In a teacher-learner relationship, learning also evolves from trust and understanding. The nurse builds trust by teaching information the client perceives as important and is able to understand. Teaching takes time, and the nurse must be committed to helping a client learn at his own speed. A client will sense the nurse's commitment and become more receptive to teaching endeavors.

The steps of the teaching process can be compared to those of the communication process (Table 16-1). In teaching, the referent represents the need to provide the client with information. The client may request information, or the nurse may perceive that the client needs new information or skills because of changes in his health. Once the nurse perceives the need to teach a client, she identifies specific learning objectives. A learning objective describes what the learner will be able to do after successful instruction.

TABLE 16-1

Comparison of Terms Used in Teaching and Communication

	Communication	Teaching
Referent	An idea that initiates the reason for communication	Perceived need to provide the person with information; teacher establishes relevant learning objectives
Sender	Person who conveys the message to another	Teacher who performs activities aimed at assisting the other person to learn
Intrapersonal variables (sender)	Knowledge, values, emotions, and sociocultural influences that affect the sender's thoughts	Teacher's philosophy of education, which stems from learning theory; knowledge of teaching content; experiences in teaching; the teacher's own emotions and values
Message	That which is expressed or transmitted by the sender	Content or information to be taught
Channels	Methods used to transmit a message: visual, auditory, touch	Methods used to present content: visual, auditory, touch, taste, smell
Receiver	Person to whom the message is transmitted	The learner
Intrapersonal variables (receiver)	Knowledge, values, emotions, and sociocultural influences that affect the receiver's thoughts	Willingness and capability to learn: physical and emotional health, education, development
Feedback	Information revealing that the true meaning of a message was received	Determination of whether learning objectives were achieved

The client, Mr. Lewis, has a newly diagnosed diabetic condition, and he will require daily insulin injections as part of his therapy. Mr. Lewis is mentally alert and physically capable of caring for himself. The nurse recognizes his need to learn to self-administer injections. The learning objective is that the client will self-administer correct insulin injections using the proper technique.

The nurse in the role of teacher is the sender, whose aim is to convey a message to the client. The nurse promotes learning by communicating in language recognizable to the learner.

A simple vocabulary is chosen for Mr. Lewis, who is unfamiliar with technical terms. Describing the method for using a "clean" technique lessens any confusion that might arise over the use of a more technical term such as "asepsis."

Numerous intrapersonal variables influence the nurse's style and approach toward teaching. The nurse's attitudes toward the client, her values about the type of information being taught, her own emo-

tional state, and her knowledge of adult learning theory influence the way she sends messages. Past experiences with teaching help the nurse choose the most effective way to present information to a client.

The nurse working with Mr. Lewis knows that an optimal learning environment is one that allows the client to assume some responsibility for learning. In the past the nurse has had good results in giving clients the opportunity to help themselves. The nurse will inform Mr. Lewis of the implications of improper insulin administration; she will stress the importance of his use of good injection techniques. The nurse will also be sure to provide Mr. Lewis with all the skills he needs to safely assume responsibility for his own care.

As is the case with communication, the message or content to be taught is delivered clearly and precisely. The nurse organizes information to be taught in a logical sequence so the client will more easily understand the skills or ideas. Each lesson presents content in a meaningful progression from simple to more complex skills or ideas.

Before instructing Mr. Lewis about insulin injections, the nurse identifies the order of content presentation:
1. The purpose and action of insulin
2. A description of an injection
3. A discussion of principles of sterility
4. Explanation of parts of a syringe
5. Demonstration of how to fill a syringe
6. Demonstration of an injection

The nurse may use a variety of channels to present teaching content. All the senses—visual, auditory, touch, smell, and taste—serve as channels for presenting information. The auditory channel is the simplest method for imparting information, as in a lecture or discussion. But the learning process becomes more active and stimulating when several sensory channels are used to present information.

While discussing the purpose of insulin injections, the nurse relies on Mr. Lewis' hearing. The nurse also uses a chart to let him see how an injection is administered correctly. She then allows Mr. Lewis to feel a syringe and manipulate its parts.

The receiver in the teaching-learning process is the learner. As with communication, a number of intrapersonal variables affect the client's willingness and ability to learn. The client is ready to learn once he expresses a desire to learn. He is more likely to receive the nurse's message when he perceives and understands the content being taught. The client's attitudes, anxiety, and values are a few of the factors influencing his ability to perceive a message. Whether he is capable of learning depends on his emotional and physical health, education, stage of development, and previous knowledge; these factors are discussed in a later section.

Mr. Lewis returns to his hospital room after a day of diagnostic testing. Fatigue is likely to impair his receptivity to teaching because he has little energy available to devote to the learning process. Thus the nurse postpones a discussion about injections until Mr. Lewis has rested.

An effective teacher provides a mechanism for evaluating whether a teaching plan was successful and if learning occurred. A familiar form of feedback following instruction is a written examination. Whatever form of feedback the nurse chooses, it must reflect the success of the teacher's learning objectives—that is, the learner displays or relates what he has learned.

The nurse sets an objective for Mr. Lewis: "The client will successfully administer an insulin injection to himself." To obtain the needed feedback indicating success, Mr.

Lewis must give himself an injection correctly without the nurse's assistance.

Comparing teaching and communication helps the nursing student recognize the basic elements of teaching. The effective teacher presents information in a creative and meaningful fashion at a time when the learner is most receptive to information.

Domains of Learning

Learning involves a number of domains. It prepares a person to perform functions of which he once was incapable. New knowledge provides a person with the ability to solve problems. Learning to clarify personal values helps a person choose the right course of action when confronted with an ethical dilemma. Gaining an improved level of physical coordination prepares a person to perform complex motor activities.

Learning behaviors can be classified in three principal domains: cognitive learning, affective learning, and psychomotor learning. The nurse often works with clients who need to learn behaviors in each domain. The characteristics of learning within each domain affect the eventual selection of teaching methods and the method of evaluating learning.

Cognitive behaviors encompass all intellectual behaviors such as the acquisition of knowledge, comprehension (ability to understand), application (using abstract ideas in concrete situations), analysis (relating ideas in an organized manner), synthesis (assembling parts into a whole), and evaluation (judging the worth of a body of information).

The following shows how a learner acquires cognitive behaviors:

Mrs. Spencer is a 45-year-old woman who has undergone the surgical removal of her left breast because of cancer. Her nurse, Ms. Lyles, provides Mrs. Spencer with the information she needs to learn to live with this permanent alteration. As a result of the nurse's efforts, Mrs. Spencer knows the purpose of her surgery *(knowledge)*. Mrs. Spencer further understands how her initial physical limitations will affect her ability to perform household chores *(comprehension)*. The nurse warns Mrs. Spencer that, because of the surgery, the risk of acquiring an infection in her left arm is now greater. Mrs. Spencer assures the nurse that once she returns home to resume her favorite activity of gardening she will protect herself from injury by wearing gloves *(application)*. Mrs. Spencer also learns the warning signs of recurrent cancer. Ms. Lyles asks her to describe when she thinks the signs are more likely to be detected and how she will use this knowledge during her routine activities at home *(analysis and synthesis)*. Before Ms. Lyles completes her instruction, she helps Mrs. Spencer explore whether she has gained sufficient information to care for herself. Mrs. Spencer considers the values of the information with respect to coping with the limitations created by surgery *(evaluation)*.

Affective learning behaviors deal with the expression of feelings related to attitudes, opinions, or values. (Chapter 13 describes an example of affective learning through values clarification.) A person acquires the skills necessary to become aware of his personal values, to acknowledge the significance they hold for him, and to show an acceptance of those values. The nurse uses therapeutic communication skills to teach clients ways to develop affective behaviors.

The nurse recognizes that Mrs. Spencer's loss of a breast can seriously impair her body image. Ms. Lyles uses the skills of attentive listening, focusing, and clarifying in directing Mrs. Spencer to discuss her feelings about cancer and the loss of her breast. The client learns that her concerns and fears are normal following such a traumatic experience. However, she also learns ways to express her feelings constructively and to gain a better feeling about herself.

Psychomotor behaviors involve the acquisition of skills that require the integration of mental and muscular activity such as the ability to walk, use an eating utensil, or climb a series of stairs. The nurse directs clients in psychomotor activities that maintain existing skills, restore lost skills, or develop new skills. For example, the nurse teaches an immobilized client exercises designed to maintain muscle strength and tone. The exercises will allow the client to retain function of his arms and legs despite activity restriction. The client with a partially paralyzed arm requires assistance in restoring lost function. A series of graded exercises will help the client regain the use of his arm. The nurse also teaches the client alternative ways to dress or bathe until function returns. Often clients experience alterations that require learning totally new psychomotor skills. For example, a client with a fractured leg needs to learn the proper method of crutch walking.

Teaching the client a specific behavior often involves incorporating behaviors from all three learning domains. Consider the client being taught the proper method of giving an injection. He must first understand why he requires injections and then must know the proper location for administering the injection and the importance of using sterile technique *(cognitive)*. The techniques of locating an acceptable area on the skin and introducing the needle use the senses of touch and vision *(psychomotor)*. The client must be willing to accept the fact he needs injections and must overcome any fear or distaste for injections *(affective)*.

An understanding of each learning domain prepares the nurse to select the proper teaching techniques. However, the nurse needs to know more than the type of learning that occurs. Teaching is unsuccessful without an application of basic learning principles.

Basic Learning Principles

To teach effectively and efficiently the nurse must first understand how people learn. The nurse forms teaching strategies to promote the manner in which a client learns best.

The ability to learn depends on three conditions: the readiness to learn, the ability to learn, and the learning environment. A person's emotional readiness to learn is a reflection of his internal will or desire to learn. Readiness means that a person is willing to take the necessary action to become involved in learning. Previous knowledge, attitudes, and sociocultural influences combine to form a person's experiential readiness.

The ability to learn depends on the learner's physical and cognitive attributes. Age, physical wellness, and intellectual thought processes determine whether a person is capable of learning. If a person's learning ability is impaired, a teacher postpones teaching activities or modifies strategies to better meet the learner's needs.

The environment has a significant impact on a person's ability to learn. One of the teacher's major tasks is to manipulate conditions within the environment to facilitate learning. The teacher who ignores the influence of the learning environment will miss numerous opportunities for stimulating a student's learning.

Readiness to Learn
ATTENTIONAL SET

Our minds generally function with some sort of mental picture. While a teacher explains how to give support to a dying client, we might envision ourselves grasping the fragile hand of a person as he struggles to take his last breath. Before we can learn anything, we must give attention to, or concentrate on, the information to be learned. An attentional set is an internal state of the learner that enables him to focus on and comprehend stimuli. A number of factors can influence a learner's ability to attend: physical discomfort, anxiety, and environmental distractions.

Any physical condition that impairs a person's ability to concentrate interferes with learning. Severe pain, excessive fatigue, hunger, thirst, and even the urge to urinate or defecate create barriers to learning. Therefore the nurse determines the client's level of comfort and energy before beginning a teaching plan and asks the client if he feels comfortable enough to discuss a particular topic. Nonverbal cues such as grimacing, maintaining a bent posture, or holding a body part securely also reveal that a client is not ready to learn.

Anxiety is one factor that may either increase or decrease the ability of a person to attend. Anxiety is a feeling of uneasiness or uncertainty resulting from the anticipation of some threat or danger. Anytime a person faces change or the need to act differently from usual, anxiety normally results. Learning requires a change in behavior and thus produces a certain degree of anxiety in a learner. A mild level of anxiety may motivate a person to learn. If a student did not become anxious about an upcoming examination, it is unlikely he would study. However, a high level of anxiety prevents learning from taking place. Severe anxiety incapacitates a person, making him unable to attend to anything other than measures aimed at the immediate relief of the anxiety. When manifestations of severe anxiety such as altered memory, inability to understand, nausea, and headaches occur, the nurse avoids inducing more anxiety by placing unrealistic expectations on the client to learn.

MOTIVATION

Motivation is an internal impulse that causes a person to take action. A motivator may be an idea, an emotion, or a physical need. If a person does not want to learn, there is little probablility that learning will occur. Motivation exists when one sees value or benefit from participating in learning.

There are three types of motives that stimulate a person to learn: social, task mastery, and physical. Social motives are a person's need for affiliation, social approval, or self-esteem. For example, often a student works hard to learn in order to elicit praise from a teacher. Task mastery motives are based on needs such as achievement and competence. A nursing student will repeatedly work in a laboratory to learn the proper technique for giving an injection because she is motivated to master the task or skill. Once a person gains success in a chosen task, there is usually even greater motivation to achieve further accomplishments. A good teacher learns how to cultivate and promote a student's motivational drives to enhance the learning process.

Often the motives of a health care client are of a physical nature. A client who has an acute debilitating illness seeks to meet the physiological needs of comfort, rest, and nourishment. Since these basic needs take temporary precedence over needs for affiliation or self-esteem, the nurse directs teaching strategies accordingly.

Mr. Truman is hospitalized for the removal of a ruptured appendix. He has considerable pain associated with the condition. His nurse knows that although Mr. Truman may benefit from learning about the implications of his surgery, the relief of pain is the client's first priority. The nurse teaches Mr. Truman relaxation exercises and comfortable methods for positioning in bed. The client's motivation to learn arises from the hope that each method will bring relief of his discomfort.

Not all persons are interested in maintaining their health. A person with lung disease may continue to smoke. A woman whose obesity worsens her heart condition may refuse to follow her diet. All the therapies in the world will have little effect unless a person is motivated to comply by the belief that his health is important. The trend in health care is to treat clients in their own homes after they recover from the acute phase of illness. Treatment in the home can be successful only if the client complies with the recommendations of his physician and the health care team. The obese woman will not reduce her weight unless she becomes motivated by the benefits to be gained from weight loss. Compliance is the client's fulfillment of the prescribed course of therapy and the nurse's ultimate goal in any health teaching plan.

A person's *health beliefs* can be powerful motivators, and they are influenced by a number of variables (see Chapter 2). Four health beliefs are critical to a client taking a health action (Rosenstock, 1960):

1. The person believes himself susceptible to the disease in question.
2. The person believes the disease would have serious effects on his life if he contracted it.
3. The person believes that he can take certain actions to reduce the likelihood of contracting the disease or lessen its severity.
4. The person believes the threat of taking these actions is not as great as the threat of the disease itself.

The nurse's knowledge of a client's health beliefs helps her determine what factors will motivate the client to learn. However, there is no standard method for motivating learning in a person with a given health belief. Health teaching often involves a changing of attitudes and values that are not altered by the simple teaching of facts. Therefore the nurse gives attention to ideas or beliefs that motivate a person to learn, and she applies the motivating factor to her teaching plan.

Mr. James is a 42-year-old businessman with high blood pressure. The nurse recognizes that Mr. James needs to learn a great deal about his condition, the type of treatment, and the implications of his illness for his busy life-style. Mr. James is a highly motivated man who works hard for success. He admits that he has always felt himself invincible to any physical malady. Now he tells the nurse that he knows he cannot continue his hectic work pace unless he regains his health.

The nurse's teaching plan will integrate two principal motivators that Mr. James has acknowledged: the desire to succeed and the concern that high blood pressure will seriously affect his work life. The nurse will use Mr. James' motivation for success as the means to help him acquire better health habits. Mr. James will learn how high blood pressure impairs physical function and the ways in which he can avoid factors in his work environment that can aggravate blood pressure problems.

PSYCHOSOCIAL ADAPTATION TO ILLNESS

A loss of health, whether temporary or permanent, is difficult for a person to accept. The process of grieving allows the person time to adapt psychologically to the emotional and physical implications of illness. The stages of grieving (see Chapter 46) encompass a series of responses clients experience during illness. People experience the stages at different rates and in different sequences; some people fail to complete all the stages. The implication for learning is that a person's readiness to learn is significantly related to his stage of grieving (Table 16-2). Learning will not occur when a client is unwilling or unable to accept the reality of his illness. The nurse identifies the client's stage of grieving on the basis of typically displayed behaviors. When the client enters the stage of acceptance, which is compatible with learning, the nurse begins to introduce the teaching plan. Continuous assessment of the client's behaviors determines what stages of grieving the client moves into and out of. Teaching continues as long as the client remains in a stage conducive to learning.

TABLE 16-2

Relationship between Psychosocial Adaptation to Illness and Learning

Stage of Adaptation	Clients' Behaviors	Learning Implications	Rationale
Denial	Client avoids discussion of illness ("There's nothing wrong with me"), withdraws from others, and disregards physical restrictions.	Provide support, empathy, and careful explanations of all procedures while they are being done. Let the client know you are available for discussion when he is ready. Explain to the family what is happening to the client. Teach in the present tense, e.g., explain current therapy.	Any attempt to convince or tell the client he is ill will result in further anger or withdrawal (client is not prepared to deal with his problem). Provide only information he pursues or absolutely requires.
Anger	Client blames and complains and often directs anger toward the nurse.	Do not argue with the client. Listen to his concerns, and teach in the present tense. Reassure the family of the client's normality.	Client needs opportunity to express feelings and anger; he is still not prepared to face the future.
Bargaining	Client offers to live a better life in exchange for promise of better health ("If God lets me live, I promise to be more careful").	Continue to introduce only reality. Teaching remains in present tense.	Client is still unwilling to accept his limitations.
Resolution	Client begins to express emotions openly, realizes illness has created changes, and begins to ask questions.	Encourage expression of feelings. Begin to share information needed for the future, and set aside formal times for discussion.	Client begins to perceive the need for assistance and is ready to accept responsibility for learning.
Acceptance	Client recognizes the reality of his condition, actively pursues information, and strives for independence.	Focus teaching on future skills and knowledge required. Continue to teach about present occurrences. Involve family in teaching information for discharge.	Client is more easily motivated to learn. Acceptance of his illness reflects a willingness to deal with implications.

Readiness to learn is critical to the success of any teaching endeavor. Active participation by the learner implies an eagerness to acquire new learning behaviors. Successful teaching is possible when the learner acknowledges the teacher's message as meaningful and when he is emotionally and experientially ready to participate in learning. Further assurance that learning will occur depends on the learner's cognitive and physical abilities.

Ability to Learn

DEVELOPMENTAL CAPABILITY

A person's cognitive development influences his ability to learn. A nurse can be a competent teacher, but if she disregards her client's intellectual abilities, teaching will be unsuccessful. Sometimes a nurse is happily sharing teaching booklets and brochures with a client when she suddenly discovers that the client cannot read. A client who is unable to perform simple mathematical calculations will have difficulty learning to measure medication doses or dietary supple-

ments. Learning is an evolving process, as is developmental growth. The nurse must know the client's level of knowledge and intellectual skills before beginning a teaching plan. Table 16-3 shows the types of learning problems clients may have when their intellectual skills are not fully developed.

There is a requisite level of maturation and cognitive development before an individual becomes capable of learning new information. The nurse makes an error if she assumes the client has a certain level of knowledge. Thus she should assess the client's level of knowledge before starting any teaching plan. Learning occurs more readily when new information complements existing knowledge.

AGE GROUP. A person's age often reflects his developmental capability for learning and the type of learning behavior he can acquire. The following examples illustrate these principles.

Infant. An infant relies totally on the adults in his world for basic needs. He learns to trust adults when they convey love and compassion. If an infant suffers pain or discomfort, the nurse can teach him to trust

---

TABLE 16-3

Cognitive Skills and Learning Implications

Intellectual Skill	Examples of Potential Learning Problems
Math calculation	Computing drug dosages; measuring liquid or solid food allotments; reading a thermometer or syringe calibrations
Reading	Reading directions and instructions in teaching booklets and on medication labels
Problem solving	Learning how to regulate insulin dosages on the basis of signs and symptoms
Comprehension and application	Understanding physical restrictions imposed by illness; following directions in performing self-care in accordance with limitations

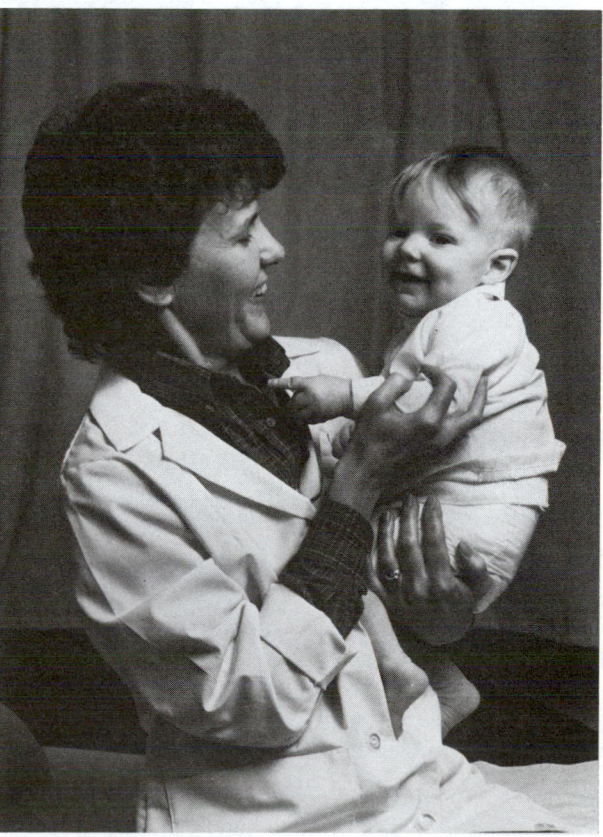

Fig. 16-1 The nurse's firm but gentle touch conveys love and trust to the infant.

her by holding him firmly, smiling, speaking softly, and gently moving his injured part (Fig. 16-1).

Toddler. During the toddler stage a child learns to understand words and to begin expressing his feelings verbally. The child also learns by associating words with objects. Play is an important technique for promoting a toddler's learning. Through play a toddler develops physically and learns to interact with the world around him.

If a toddler comes to a clinic for treatment of a laceration, the nurse wants the child to learn how the physician will repair his injury. The nurse may use a doll that has a cut on its arm to show the toddler how stitches and bandages are applied. The nurse also has picture books that describe the story of a young child in the clinic. Using simple words such as "cut" instead of "laceration," or "patch" instead of "bandage," promotes communication with the child (Fig. 16-2).

Preschooler. The preschooler's language becomes more complex and precise as his vocabulary expands rapidly. During play the child expresses his feelings more through words than actions. The preschooler learns by asking questions and imitating adults.

If a parent wants to teach the preschooler good health habits such as brushing teeth or washing hands, he uses simple explanations and demonstrations. Showing the child how to brush his teeth properly will increase the likelihood of the child learning the behavior. Preschoolers also find pleasure in being with other children. Most preschools or nurseries encourage the children to learn together through pictures, short stories, and demonstrations of how to follow hygiene practices.

School-Age Child. The school-age child learns by interacting with adults outside his immediate family. This child is less likely to feel threatened by nurses or health care workers than are younger children. The child matures physically, gaining improved muscle strength and coordination. Play becomes more formal and imaginative.

A school-age child is capable of learning a great deal about his health. He is also able to assume more responsibility for his health. A young school-age child who contracts juvenile diabetes, for example, can learn how to administer self-injections, perform urine tests, and understand the nature and complications of his disease. The child may need extensive practice to learn intricate psychomotor skills such as filling or injecting a syringe, but eventually he will be able to handle a syringe properly. Pamphlets describing health care measures can be comprehended by the school-age child. It is especially important to give this child, who is typically very inquisitive and asks numerous questions about his health, an opportunity to discuss any health problems.

Adolescent. The adolescent characteristically struggles between childlike feelings of dependence and the independent drives of an adult. He wants to be in control, but if illness occurs, he fears loss of self-concept and body image. A nurse helps the adolescent learn about his feelings and need for self-expression. Teaching must be a cooperative, shared activity because the adolescent becomes threatened easily by anyone who forces authority on him.

Since adolescents assume greater responsibility for their own actions, the nurse can be successful in teaching health-promotion activities to this age group. Safety and sex education, health care maintenance, and the dangers of drug abuse are just some of the topics a nurse can explore with adolescents.

If an adolescent becomes seriously ill, it is important to teach him all the information he needs to cope with his illness. The adolescent is capable of solving abstract problems and hypothesizing relationships.

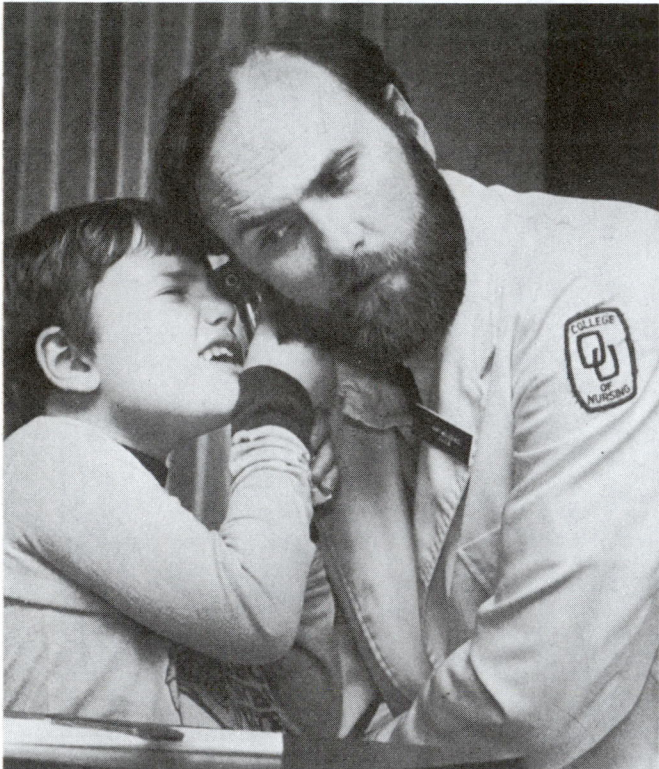

Fig. 16-2 The toddler learns not to be afraid of medical equipment by being allowed to handle it. The nurse shows the child how to use the equipment correctly.

From Davis, A.J.: Listening and responding, St. Louis, 1983, The C.V. Mosby Co.

Older Adult. The principles in this chapter apply to the learning habits of most adults. However, there are some special considerations in teaching older adults. Many older adults have undergone sensory alterations, especially visual and hearing impairments. When necessary the nurse must teach older clients by using methods that enhance a sensorially impaired individual's communication (see Chapter 44).

It is a common misconception that an older person cannot learn or is slow in learning. An older client takes considerable pride in helping himself and does not wish to lose his independence. For this reason the nurse will find most older clients to be very interested and active in teaching sessions.

If the older adult client suffers from memory loss, the nurse must exercise patience and keep each teaching session short. It may be necessary to repeat information frequently. It is especially important to teach the client at a time when he is most alert and rested.

PHYSICAL CAPABILITY

A person's ability to learn often depends on his level of physical development and overall physical health. To learn various psychomotor skills, a client must possess the necessary level of strength, coordination, and sensory acuity. For example, it will be useless to attempt to teach a client how to transfer from a bed to a wheelchair unless he has sufficient upper body strength. An elderly client cannot learn to apply an elastic bandage if his eyesight is poor and his fingers cannot grasp the bandage tightly. Therefore the nurse should not overestimate the client's physical development. The following physical attributes are required to learn psychomotor skills:

1. Size (height and weight match the task to perform or the equipment to use; for example, crutch walking)
2. Strength (ability of client to follow any strenuous exercise program)
3. Coordination (dexterity needed for complicated motor skills, such as using utensils or changing a bandage)
4. Sensory acuity (visual, auditory, touch, taste, and smell: sensory modalities needed to receive and respond to messages taught)

The nurse assesses a client's physical capabilities before beginning instruction.

Mrs. Lyon is a 68-year-old woman who received a prescription from her physician for a new heart medication that works by slowing the heart's rate. It is important that Mrs. Lyon learn how to check her pulse to be sure her heart does not beat too slowly. The nurse's assessment reveals that Mrs. Lyon is unable to feel an arterial pulse because

her fingers are stiff and callused. No one who lives with Mrs. Lyon can check her pulse for her. However, Mrs. Lyon's hearing is still good. The nurse chooses an alternative: teaching Mrs. Lyon how to listen to her heartbeat with a stethoscope.

In larger hospitals, clinics, or community health agencies the services of physical therapists can be highly valuable in assessing a client's physical capabilities.

Any condition that depletes a person's energy will also impair his ability to learn. If a client spends the entire morning undergoing a rigorous schedule of x-ray studies and tests, it is unlikely that he will be capable of the effort needed for any learning discussion. When a client's illness becomes aggravated by complications such as a high fever or respiratory difficulty, teaching should be postponed. After working with a client the nurse can sense his energy level by his willingness to communicate, the amount of activity he initiates, and his responsiveness toward questions. The nurse need not become discouraged if she has to halt teaching activities temporarily so a client can rest; instead she will achieve greater teaching success when the client is an active participant in learning.

Learning Environment

Factors in the physical environment where teaching takes place make learning either a pleasant or a difficult experience. The nurse chooses a setting that helps the client focus attention on the learning task. The following factors are important when choosing the setting:

1. Number of persons being taught
2. Need for privacy
3. Room temperature
4. Room lighting
5. Noise
6. Room ventilation
7. Room furniture

The ideal environment for promoting learning is a room that is well lit and has good ventilation, appropriate furniture, and a comfortable temperature (Fig. 16-3). A darkened room will interfere with the client's ability to watch the nurse's actions, especially when she is demonstrating a skill or using visual aids such as posters or pamphlets. A room that is too cold or too hot or that is humid and stuffy will make the client too uncomfortable to attend to the nurse's activities. Comfortable furniture helps to eliminate distractions such as the need to change position or shift body weight.

It is also important to choose a quiet setting. In a hospital the nurses' station is a site of constant activity, with telephones ringing and several conversations

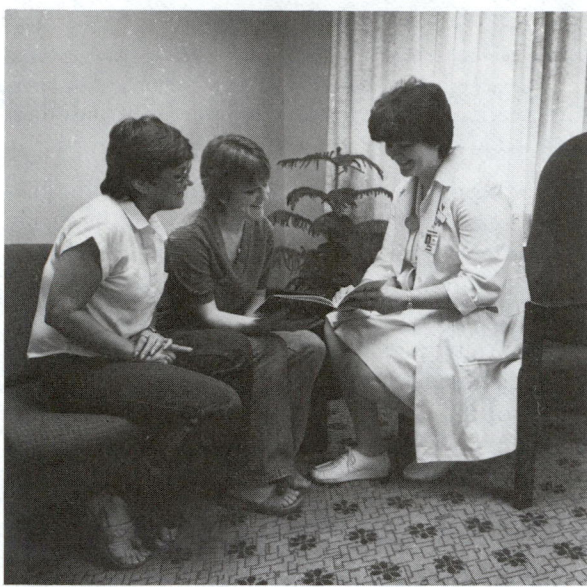

Fig. 16-3 Choosing a comfortable, pleasant environment enhances the learning experience. This nurse is using a teaching booklet to explain health care principles to the client and a family member.

occurring simultaneously. In a client's home the sounds of the television in the living room prevent a person from listening attentively. These sounds, instead of the teacher, become the focus of attention.

When a nurse is working with an individual client, the best setting is a quiet one that offers privacy—a location where frequent interruptions are unlikely to occur. The nurse can provide for a client's privacy even in a busy hospital by closing the cubicle curtains, using a conference room near the nurses' station, or taking the client in a wheelchair to a quiet spot near the nursing division. In a client's home a bedroom might separate the client from household activities. If the client desires, family members might share in any discussions. However, often a client is reluctant to discuss the nature of his illness when other persons, even close family members, are in the room.

Teaching a group of clients requires a room that allows all persons to be seated comfortably and within hearing distance of the teacher. The size of the room should not overwhelm the group, tempting participants to sit outside the group along the room's perimeter. Arranging the group to allow participants to observe one another further enhances learning. More effective communication occurs as learners observe others' verbal and nonverbal interactions.

■ ■ ■ ■ ■

Principles of learning encompass many variables, any combination of which can either enhance or deter

the learning process. A client may be ready to learn, but if the setting is not conducive to active participation, efforts at teaching may fail. A client may possess all the necessary intellectual skills to learn, but if he is highly anxious, a helpful explanation will go unnoticed. A nurse may plan to use a conference room to teach a class, but if an elderly client cannot remain attentive during the late evening hours when the room is available, teaching efforts will be wasted. Many elements must fall into place for learning to be successful.

Basic Teaching Principles

Teaching, or instruction, is the process of leading someone to learn. Just as there are basic principles that promote learning, there are also principles that enhance a teacher's effectiveness. The realm of teaching deals with (1) the teacher's behavior, (2) the reason why teachers behave the way they do, and (3) the effects of their behavior on students. There is no single right way to teach. Each learning situation has different implications for the best way to teach. The principles of teaching are basically techniques that incorporate the principles of learning.

Timing

When is the right time to teach? When a client first enters a clinic or hospital? When a client learns he has a serious illness? When the time arrives for discharge from the hospital? Actually, each of these may be an appropriate time for instruction. Once a client enters the health care system, the nurse's role as teacher begins. The client will continue to have learning needs and opportunities as long as he remains in the health care system. However, teaching must be timed to coincide with the client's readiness to learn.

The nurse should plan teaching activities for a time when the client is most attentive and receptive. She should determine the time of day when the client is most alert. Most people know if they are more receptive to teaching sessions in the morning hours, late in the afternoon, or in the evening. The client's activities should be organized to provide time for rest as well as time for teaching-learning interactions. The client who receives medications that cause drowsiness or impair concentration should be taught before the medications are administered.

The length of teaching sessions also influences learning ability. Prolonged sessions cause clients to lose concentration and attentiveness. Frequent sessions lasting 20 to 30 minutes are more easily tolerated and retain the client's interest in the material being taught. The nurse can assess a client's loss of concentration by observing for signs of poor eye contact, slumped posture, preoccupation with other activities in the room, or extraneous movements such as finger tapping and frequent change of position. Once the client's loss of concentration is noted, the session should be brought to a close. However, teaching sessions should not be too brief. The client needs time during each session to comprehend the information and to give feedback regarding his understanding.

Teaching sessions should be held frequently enough to document the client's learning. The frequency of sessions depends on the learner's abilities and the complexity of the material. Describing what it means to have a fractured arm takes less time than explaining the steps in filling a syringe. Intervals between teaching sessions should not be so long that the client might forget information.

Organizing Teaching Material

A good teacher gives careful consideration to the order in which to present information. Usually an outline of content helps to organize information into a logical sequence. Material should progress from simple to complex ideas because a person must learn simple facts and concepts before learning how to make associations or complex interpretations of ideas.

Ms. Willis is a client with diabetes who is to learn how to determine a 1200-calorie diet. The final task is a complex one. Ms. Willis will ultimately need to know how to calculate the number of calories from measurements of protein, fat, and carbohydrate food sources. She will also use mathematical skills to make accurate determinations.

The nurse knows that success in teaching Ms. Willis depends on starting instruction with simple concepts. First, the client needs to learn what calories, proteins, and carbohydrates are. Teaching content will cover identification of food items that fit into each food group. It will also be helpful for the nurse to give Ms. Willis simple mathematical calculation problems. Ultimately, Ms. Willis will be able to take knowledge of simple concepts and synthesize the information to calculate a proper diet.

It is also helpful to begin instruction with essential content. There is usually a certain amount of information that is critical for a client to learn. For example, following the surgical removal of a cancerous lung tumor, the client's predisposition to cancer recurrence makes learning about the warning signs of cancer crucial. Once the nurse discusses essential information with a client, she may choose to end a teaching session with informative but less critical content.

Maintaining Learner Attention and Participation

What was the most interesting class you ever attended? Was it a long lecture given by a soft-spoken professor, or was it a discussion with slides and group participation? Chances are that the latter class was more interesting and provided a more enriching learning experience.

Client involvement in the learning process is important. We learn better when more than one of the body's senses are stimulated. The field of audiovisual education has mushroomed, and the use of instructional aids such as filmstrips, audiotape cassettes, and motion pictures conforms to the principle of increasing a learner's attention and level of participation to promote learning. Role playing, an activity that allows an individual to acquire knowledge by acting out a set learning experience, is also a helpful teaching strategy. By actively experiencing a learning event, the person will likely retain the knowledge gained.

A lecturer who uses slides, demonstrations, and printed materials creates more interest in a discussion topic than a lecturer who merely reads notes. A variety of instructional resources that complement one another is helpful in the presentation of a learning topic. For example, a film will graphically show how to perform a breast self-examination. A teaching pamphlet will highlight the key points to remember in doing the examination correctly. A demonstration of a self-examination will help a learner acquire the necessary psychomotor skills.

A teacher's actions can also increase learner attention and interest. When conducting a discussion with a client, the teacher should stay active by changing tone and intensity of voice, making eye contact, and using gestures that accentuate key points of discussion. A teacher who speaks in a monotone is a sound cure for insomnia. An effective teacher often uses as much energy as the learner, talking and moving among the group rather than remaining stationary behind a lectern or table. A client remains interested in a teacher who is actively enthusiastic about the subject under discussion.

Building on Existing Knowledge

A client learns best on the basis of preexisting cognitive abilities and knowledge. Thus a teacher will be more effective by presenting information that builds on a learner's existing knowledge. The key to this principle is assessing the learner's level of knowledge by asking him to explain what he knows about a given topic or directing questions that will reveal his level of knowledge.

Mr. Casey is scheduled to have a diagnostic test to determine whether renal calculi (kidney stones) are present. His nurse wants to explain the test's purpose and the method in which it is conducted.

Nurse: Mr. Casey, have you ever had this test before?

Mr. Casey: No, this is the first time.

Nurse: Can you tell me what you know about kidney stones?

Mr. Casey: Well, my doctor has said that they're actual stones that form from calcium or some such thing. They collect inside the kidney and can't always pass into the urine.

Nurse: That's basically correct. Here, let me draw you a diagram and then explain how the test works.

By assessing the client's knowledge, the nurse is able to determine where to start with the teaching plan. The client senses that the nurse will adjust her explanations to his specific needs. A client will quickly lose interest if the nurse begins with information he already possesses. In addition, the nurse who is aware of her client's level of knowledge can determine how complex explanations need to be. If the client uses simple terminology, she uses the same level of language in her explanations.

Reinforcement

The principle of reinforcement applies to the process of learning; however, it is often the teacher who must be the source of reinforcement. A reinforcer is a stimulus that increases the probability of a response. When a learner receives reinforcement before or after a desired learning behavior, he will likely repeat the behavior. Feedback is a common form of reinforcement. A student's learning efficiency increases when he learns about the results of his performance.

Reinforcers are either positive or negative. A positive reinforcement, such as a smile, praise, or approval, is one that produces the desired responses. A reinforcement is negative if its removal from a situation following a response produces the desired behavior. Threatening, complaining, and criticizing are examples of negative reinforcers. People usually respond better to positive reinforcement. The effects of negative reinforcement are less predictable and often undesirable.

There are three types of reinforcers: social, material, and activity. When a nurse works with a client, most reinforcers are social—a smile, a compliment, a word of encouragement, or physical contact. A nurse uses verbal and nonverbal communication when acknowledging that a client has learned a skill well.

Examples of material reinforcers are food, toys, and music. This type of reinforcer works best with young children. For example, a child will be more likely to try to use a toothbrush correctly if he knows that afterward he will receive a new toy.

Activity reinforcers rely on the principle that a person is motivated to engage in an activity if he is promised that, after its completion, he will have the privilege of engaging in more desirable activity. For example, a hospitalized client may be more willing to perform difficult, even painful, exercises if given the opportunity to go to the cafeteria afterward.

Choosing an appropriate reinforcer involves careful thought and attention to a person's preferences. Observing a client's behavior often helps reveal the best type of reinforcer to use. Reinforcers should never be used as a threat, and it should be recognized that reinforcement is not effective all the time with every client. Younger children tend to respond more to social reinforcers such as a kiss or a hug than do older children or adults. An adult with whom the nurse has a good relationship is more effectively reinforced than an adult with whom the nurse has a poor relationship. Thus effort required in building a trusting relationship with a client yields results when the nurse attempts to provide meaningful positive reinforcers for learning behaviors.

Matching Teaching Methods with Learners' Needs

The efficacy of a teaching method depends in part on the client's learning need. Clients with psychomotor deficits learn best through demonstrations and supervised practice. The client masters skills by manipulating equipment and practicing manual skills. Discussions, question-and-answer sessions, and formal lectures are effective methods for promoting cognitive learning. Clients with intellectual deficits are given the opportunity to explore new ideas, recognize new relationships, and apply knowledge to their unique needs. A highly effective method for stimulating affective learning is the group discussion. Clients learn to share ideas and values with one another, realizing there are alternative ways to view the world. Whatever the method, it should complement the client's needs.

Teaching Process in Nursing

Teaching can become habitual for an experienced nurse. After working in a particular specialty area such as a family planning clinic, a grade school, or an intensive care unit, the nurse becomes familiar with the knowledge and skills clients need to care for themselves and understand their health problems. A nurse working in an orthopedic nursing unit will be much more comfortable teaching a client how to use crutches than will a nurse who works in a gynecologist's office. Achieving spontaneity in teaching does not eliminate the need for a methodical approach toward teaching, however. Spontaneity has the benefit of making both nurse and client more at ease during the teaching process, but regardless of a nurse's familiarity with certain educational topics, each learner is different. Thus an individualized approach toward the teaching process ensures that the nurse will meet a client's learning needs.

The nursing process provides a useful framework for individualizing the teaching process. The two processes are not the same. The nursing process requires an assessment of all sources of data to determine a client's total health care needs. The teaching process focuses primarily on the client's learning needs in addition to his willingness and capability to learn. Table 16-4 compares the teaching and nursing processes. As is the case with any important function the nurse performs, teaching cannot be undertaken haphazardly.

Assessment

Success in teaching a client requires the nurse to assess all factors that influence the content to be taught, the client's ability to learn, and the resources for instruction. The client's learning needs determine the choice of teaching content. The nurse assesses the client's cognitive, affective, or psychomotor knowledge and skill deficits. When the nurse assesses for learning deficits, two primary sources of information are the client's medical and nursing histories. The type of illness, its course, the diagnostic and therapeutic plan of choice, the client's physical and emotional response to therapy, and the client's familiarity with his condition are just a few of the factors that influence learning. Nursing literature often supplements the nurse's identification of the type and amount of information a client needs to know. The nurse is responsible and accountable for identifying what a client needs to know and the extent to which he knows and understands the information.

There are important questions to consider when reviewing a client's history. How long has the client known about his condition? What does the client need to know to understand his condition and all of its implications? What aspects of therapy should the

TABLE 16-4		

Comparison of the Nursing Process and the Teaching Process

Basic Steps	Nursing Activities	Teaching Activities
Assessment	Identify the client's physical, psychological, social, cultural, developmental, and spiritual needs. Sources of data are the client, family, diagnostic tests, medical record, nursing history, and literature.	Identify the client's learning needs, willingness to learn, ability to learn, and teaching resources. Sources of data are the client, family, learning environment, medical record, nursing history, and literature.
Diagnosis	Identify appropriate nursing diagnoses.	Identify client's learning needs on the basis of the three domains of learning.
Planning	Develop an individualized plan of care. Set diagnosis priorities on the basis of client's immediate needs. Nurse and client collaborate on plan of care.	Establish learning objectives, stated in behavioral terms. Identify priorities regarding client's learning needs. Nurse and client collaborate on teaching plan. Identify type of teaching method to use.
Implementation	Perform nursing care therapies. Include client as an active participant in care. Involve family in client's care as appropriate.	Implement teaching methods. Actively involve client in learning activities. Include family participation as appropriate.
Evaluation	Identify success in meeting desired outcomes of nursing care.	Determine outcomes of teaching learning process. Measure client's ability to achieve learning objectives.

client understand to participate in his health care? In what way can the client be prepared to know what to expect in his care? Has the client had similar experiences in the past that will influence what he needs to learn? What information does the family require to help support the client's needs?

After assessing the type of knowledge or skills the client lacks, the nurse assesses his readiness and ability to learn. What is his ability to attend to the teaching process? What motivates him to learn? Does he have the cognitive and physical capabilities to learn? The nurse observes the client's behavior, asks directive questions, and applies simple tests of his capabilities (for example, asking the client to read a pamphlet or magazine to assess reading level and comprehension, or having the client sit upright to determine his potential for learning to transfer from the bed to a chair). The nurse can assess the client's attention span, memory, and ability to concentrate by noting his reactions to questions during the nursing history. If the client seems uninterested in a discussion topic (such as medical or family history) or is unable to recall significant events (for example, date of last hospitalization), learning may be difficult for him. A short attention span may be attributable to poor physical health, anxiety, fatigue, or inability to understand questions and concepts.

If the decision is made to include family members in the client's teaching plan, the nurse assesses their perception of the client's illness and its implications. Any confusion on their part may slow the nurse's progress in helping the client understand his health status. Unless the family's perceptions match those of the client, their expectations will conflict with the nurse's teaching plan. The nurse should ask the client if he wants his family to be involved and if he agrees to having his family receive explanations about his condition. Any information pertaining to the client's health care is confidential unless the client chooses to share it (see Chapter 14).

Involvement of the family in a client's teaching plan is particularly important during discharge planning. In such a situation an assessment of the home environment and available resources helps the nurse prepare the client for the return home. The resources available may be personal (assisting the client with procedures such as the administration of medications, bathing, and cooking), material (providing financial aid or equipment such as handrails on stairs), or architectural (moving the client's bedroom to the first floor). The nurse involves the client and family early in the assessment process in order to anticipate all the client's needs. A teaching plan is nonproductive if a client learns something he can never fully use as a result of constraints by family members. For example,

teaching a client how to meet hygiene needs independently with impaired arm function is useless if family members insist on performing the actions for the client. Often the nurse has the serious disadvantage of never meeting the client's family. In that situation it is important to learn the client's perceptions of the nature of his family's support.

An assessment of the learning environment can be done quickly. The nurse considers what environmental conditions would be most conducive to learning and whether or not they are available. When a demonstration is the likely teaching method, the nurse should assess the room's lighting. For slides or a movie, does the room contain a screen or can one be set up? The nurse may wish to explore several rooms in a client's home or in the hospital and clinic before deciding on the best location for a teaching session. In a large hospital or clinic the availability of conference rooms is often limited. Thus, when scheduling a room, the nurse should be sure it is available for the necessary period of time to avoid interruption midway into the class.

A final assessment involves an inventory of available teaching resources. What types of printed brochures or pamphlets are available? Do the brochures present subject matter clearly and logically? Are there slides or movies to complement the printed teaching materials? The nurse should also be sure that the teaching materials she chooses are available when they are needed.

The assessment phase brings into focus the scope of what a teaching plan must entail. A thorough assessment helps the nurse choose the best teaching methods and ensures a more creative approach toward client education.

Diagnosis

After assessing information related to the client's ability and need to learn, the nurse interprets the data to form definite diagnoses that reflect the client's specific learning needs. Unless the nurse analyzes information related to the teaching-learning process and establishes diagnoses, her teaching efforts will not be adequately goal directed or individualized. If a client appears to have several learning needs, analysis allows for setting priorities.

The range of learning needs amenable to health teaching falls within the scope of nursing diagnoses. Each diagnostic statement describes the specific type of learning need and its cause. Classifying diagnoses by the three learning domains helps the nurse focus specifically on what and how to teach. For example, a cognitive knowledge deficit requires teaching methods different from those required for a psychomotor skill deficit. Typical diagnostic statements are: "Cognitive knowledge deficit related to poor understanding of activity restrictions" or "Psychomotor skill deficit related to weakness in right hand."

Each diagnosis aids the nurse in developing a plan to fit each of the client's major learning needs. Without diagnoses a nurse's teaching plan is poorly organized, and important information may be omitted.

Planning

During development of a teaching plan the nurse determines the desirable outcomes of the plan and elicits the client's involvement in selecting learning experiences. A teacher must know what she wants a student to accomplish following any teaching session. This is the purpose of learning objectives. Objectives describe what the client is to learn, providing both nurse and client with guidelines during any teaching session.

Objectives are either short term or long term. Short-term objectives relate to the client's immediate learning needs, such as acquiring an understanding of the nature of gallbladder disease in order to understand an upcoming test. Long-term objectives relate to the client's needs once short-term objectives have been met—for example, learning to plan a proper diet within the restrictions posed by gallbladder disease.

When writing objectives, the nurse should make them specific. Specific objectives provide structure to a teaching plan, indicating what behavior the learner should master, under what conditions, and under what acceptable standards. Knowledge of learning objectives makes the teacher and learner more comfortable in knowing what to expect from the teaching-learning process, and specific objectives clarify these expectations.

Each learning objective involves three aspects: statement of a behavior and content, identification of the conditions for learning, and identification of criteria for achieving the behavior.

Each objective points to a *behavior,* reflecting the learner's ability to do something at the end of a learning experience. A behavioral objective contains an active verb describing what the learner will do once the objective is successfully met, such as *to identify, to diagram, to walk.* These behaviors are measurable and observable. The nurse observes for behavioral changes in the client as a result of the teaching plan. Active verbs leave little doubt as to what to expect from a learner. More ambiguous verbs such as *to know* or *to assimilate* do not lend themselves to simple measurement.

If content is missing, the objective cannot guide teaching and learning. A behavioral objective also indicates the content to be learned, for example: "to describe the *purpose for daily insulin injections*" or "to perform the *three-point crutch walking gait.*" The objectives describe precise behaviors and content. This precision sets the standard for eventual feedback that reflects a client's learning and forms the basis for eventual evaluation of the teaching plan.

An objective is more precise when it also describes the *conditions* under which the behavior occurs. Will the behavior occur in a classroom, in the client's home, or during an interaction with the nurse? The conditions should be realistic and designed for the learner's needs. It is also helpful to consider the conditions under which the client or family will typically perform the learning behavior. Examples of objectives that include conditions for learning are: "to transfer from the bed to a wheelchair *in the client's bedroom*" or "to discuss *in class* the problems of sibling rivalry."

The criteria for acceptable performance set a standard by which the achievement of an objective is measured. A teacher sets criteria on the basis of a desired level of accuracy, success, or satisfaction. For example, a nursing student must *accurately answer 75% of a test's questions* to pass. A client undergoing rehabilitation for a fractured leg will walk on crutches *to the end of the hall within 3 days.*

Criteria are more acceptable when established jointly by the teacher and learner. However, the nurse serves as a resource in setting the minimal criteria for success. For example, the nurse knows the ideal distance a client should be able to walk on crutches before going home or the degree of success needed in administering an injection safely and correctly. Mutually agreed on criteria help to define the expected behaviors and the quality of performance. The client uses the criteria as a form of self-evaluation, which is a powerful motivator of behavior.

After formulating objectives the nurse and client work together to establish a teaching plan. Teaching priorities are set to reflect the priorities of the nursing diagnoses. For example, if a client with a permanent leg injury has a knowledge deficit regarding the nature of his injury and its associated implications, he will likely need to have the deficit filled before he is able to learn new ways of coping with his disability.

During planning the nurse chooses appropriate teaching methods and encourages the client to offer any suggestions regarding the learning experiences. If the nurse plans to demonstrate a skill, perhaps the client will choose to have a family member present. The nurse and client also collaborate to choose the best time for conducting a teaching session. For example, if a community health nurse plans to teach her client the proper method for bathing an infant, it will be best to teach at a time that is convenient to the mother and when the infant is less likely to be asleep.

In a hospital, extended care facility, or clinic setting, nurses develop written teaching plans for use by colleagues. The written plan may be extensive, or it may be set in outline format. If more than one nurse is to be involved with a client's teaching, the written plan should be specific to facilitate continuity among nurses. Any modifications in the plan should be communicated to the client and health care team before a teaching session. A step-by-step description of teaching content is useful if several teaching sessions are necessary. It is easier to implement a teaching plan when the nurse knows at what point the last teaching session ended.

Since few people are excellent teachers at first, nurses should try to learn from their mistakes rather than be frustrated by them. It is helpful, with each successive teaching plan, to include ideas acquired from past experiences.

Implementation

Implementation of a teaching plan involves the application of all teaching and learning principles, from knowing the client and his learning needs to personal teaching ability. Implementation involves anticipating each interaction with a client as an opportunity for maximal learning experiences; watching for behaviors during a teaching session that suggest the client is losing interest or the ability to attend; and using a diversified approach to create an active student-teacher exchange of ideas.

There are numerous ways to teach information or skills. Many nurses find that they can teach more effectively while delivering nursing care. An informal, unstructured style relies on the positive therapeutic relationship between nurse and client, which fosters a spontaneity in the teaching-learning process. This is not to suggest that teaching should occur without a formal plan. When the nurse follows a teaching plan in an informal way, the client feels less pressure to perform, and learning becomes more of a shared activity with the nurse. A nurse generally feels comfortable when delivering routine measures of care. Therefore this is a good time to engage a client in the teaching-learning process.

When a nurse is responsible for teaching groups of clients or families, a more formal teaching method is appropriate. Group discussions provide the opportunity for the open sharing of ideas and attitudes among participants (Fig. 16-4). Clients and families learn from each other as they review common experiences. A productive group discussion helps participants solve problems and arrive at solutions to-

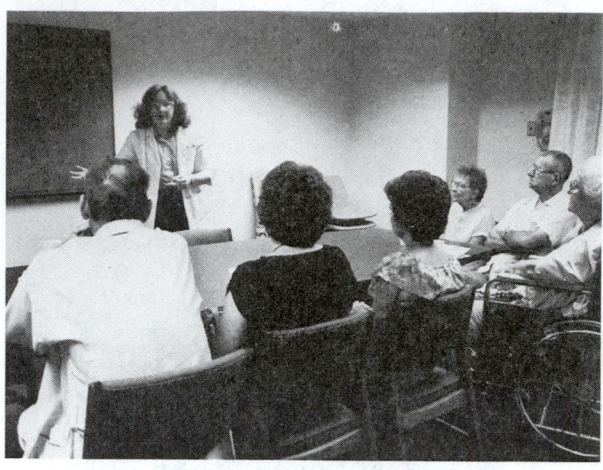

Fig. 16-4 Group teaching encourages active participation of all learners.

ward improving each member's health. To be an effective group leader, the nurse must be able to guide the participation of all group members. Acknowledging a group member's look of interest, asking questions, and summarizing key issues are methods that foster group involvement. However, not all clients will benefit from group discussions, and a client's physical or emotional level of wellness may prohibit active group participation.

A more specialized teaching method is preparatory explanation. Frequently clients face unfamiliar tests or procedures that create significant anxiety. Providing information about typical procedures assists the client in forming a realistic image of what to anticipate. When the actual experience coincides with the client's expectations, the client is more apt to attend to the nurse's future explanations. A nurse gains authority and respect when her preparatory explanations prove useful.

There are three guidelines for giving preparatory explanations:

1. Physical sensations during the procedure are described but not evaluated. For example, Mr. Reynolds is to have blood drawn as a routine admission test. The nurse explains that he will feel a sticking sensation as the needle punctures the skin. The nurse does *not* say, "It won't hurt very much."

2. The cause of the sensation is described, preventing misinterpretation of the experience. For example, the nurse tells Mr. Reynolds that often a needle insertion burns because the alcohol used to clean the skin frequently enters the puncture site.

3. Clients are prepared only for aspects of the experience that have commonly been noticed by

other clients. For example, the nurse explains that while blood is being drawn, often the tight tourniquet causes the hand to tingle and feel numb.

The client finds comfort in knowing what to expect. When the nurse's descriptions accurately portray the actual experience, the client is able to cope more effectively with the stress of procedures and therapies. The known is less threatening than the unknown.

Demonstrations are useful methods for teaching psychomotor skills. An effective demonstration requires advanced planning:

1. Review the rationale and steps of the procedure.
2. Assemble and organize equipment.
3. Perform each step in sequence while analyzing the knowledge and skills involved.
4. Determine at what step explanations are to be given, considering the client's learning needs.
5. Judge the proper speed and timing of the demonstration.

The nurse demonstrates a procedure or skill in the same order in which the client will perform it. In addition, she encourages the client to ask questions so that each step is clearly understood. To enable the client to easily observe each step of the procedure, she avoids rushing. The nurse gives the client an opportunity to practice the procedure under her supervision after the client has practiced handling any equipment involved in the procedure. Ultimately the client demonstrates the procedure independently to ensure his acquisition of the skill. The independent demonstration should occur under the same conditions the client will experience at home. For example, if a client is learning to walk with crutches, the nurse simulates the home environment. If short, narrow steps lead to the client's bedroom, the client should learn to climb similar stairs in the hospital.

Evaluation

Client education is not complete until the nurse evaluates the outcomes of the teaching-learning process. Did the client learn what was intended? The nurse evaluates the client's success at meeting each learning objective by observing the client's performance of each expected behavior under the desired conditions. Success depends on the client's ability to meet the established performance criteria.

If the evaluation process continues to indicate a knowledge or skill deficit, the nurse repeats or modifies the teaching plan. Alternative teaching methods often help to clarify information or skills the client was unable to comprehend or perform originally.

Evaluation may reveal the presence of new learning needs or the existence of new factors that may inter-fere with the client's ability to learn. The nurse reassesses those factors to update the teaching plan and make it relevant to the client's needs. As with the nursing process, the teaching process is continuous and ever changing.

CASE STUDY

Mrs. Clemmons is a 58-year-old woman seen in the clinic for treatment of arthritis. She repeatedly returns to the clinic as a result of her poor compliance with therapy. The nurse, Ms. Bingham, decides that Mrs. Clemmons might benefit from a teaching program directed toward improving her ability to cope with her disease.

ASSESSMENT	RELEVANT DATA
The nurse's assessment reveals that Mrs. Clemmons weighs 158 pounds (71 kg) and is 5 feet, 1 inch (153 cm) tall. Her arthritis affects primarily the joints of her hands and knees.	Obesity adds stress to affected joints
She has difficulty picking up small objects such as a pen, a dime, or a safety pin. Her grasp is also quite weak. Because of the involvement in her knees, Mrs. Clemmons has difficulty rising from a sitting to a standing position.	Psychomotor deficits
In discussing Mrs. Clemmons' condition, the nurse learns that her client knows only that arthritis is a "disease of the joints." However, the client does not understand how obesity can increase stress on her joints. She also does not know that there are measures that can help her perform more activities of daily living without added discomfort. Mrs. Clemmons is unaware of how her various medications act to relieve the symptoms of arthritis.	Knowledge deficits
Ms. Bingham is concerned that if Mrs. Clemmons has history of poor compliance she may not benefit from a teaching plan. However, she learns that Mrs. Clemmons has an interest in learning more since she asks the nurse several questions. The client is unfamiliar with many of the terms Ms. Bingham uses to describe arthritis. Mrs. Clemmons is married to a	Readiness to learn
	Cognitive capability

ASSESSMENT	RELEVANT DATA
carpenter. She tells the nurse that her husband becomes distressed over her inability to feel better: "It's hard for him to understand why I can't do more. He doesn't know how arthritis can cripple you." When asked if Mr. Clemmons would be interested in attending a teaching session, Mrs. Clemmons says, "Yes, I know he will come if I ask.	Family support
The nurse reserves a conference room for the first teaching session. She also arranges to use a film titled *Arthritis, a Crippling Disease*. Ms. Bingham locates pamplets on self-care devices and arthritic medications.	Teaching resources

DIAGNOSES

The nurse's assessment reveals a number of diagnoses:

Psychomotor deficits related to impairment in joint mobility and muscle strength

Knowledge deficit related to poor understanding of arthritis

Knowledge deficit related to poor understanding of measures to minimize arthritic symptoms and complications

PLANNING

On the basis of the diagnoses, Ms. Bingham sets specific learning objectives. After proper instruction Mrs. Clemmons will be able to:

Perform fine motor skills with activities of daily living in the home within 1 month

Stand from a sitting position without assistance

Describe the nature of how arthritis affects the joints of the body

Develop a low-calorie meal plan for a week

Describe the actions and side effects of arthritic medications

The nurse does not plan to cover all topics in one teaching session. Mrs. Clemmons expresses interest in first learning about arthritis and beginning to use some of the motor skills Ms. Bingham has proposed. The nurse and client decide that the best time to have the teaching session is on a Tuesday evening when Mr. Clemmons can come to the clinic with his wife. Ms. Bingham prepares a teaching plan for the first session (Table 16-5). She will also prepare teaching plans for later sessions to meet the other learning objectives.

IMPLEMENTATION

Ms. Bingham begins the session by getting to know Mr. Clemmons and observing how he and Mrs. Clemmons interact. She recognizes that Mr. Clemmons is interested in helping his wife if he can. Both the client and her husband are attentive and responsive to Ms. Bingham's questions.

The nurse shows the film to give Mr. and Mrs. Clemmons a thorough introduction to arthritis. After the film the nurse and her clients discuss aspects of the film relevant to Mrs. Clemmons' condition, and the nurse answers the couple's questions. Then they discuss how arthritis has affected Mrs. Clemmons' ability to perform activities of daily living. The nurse asks questions designed to help Mr. Clemmons gain an understanding of the long-term impact of his wife's disease. Throughout the discussion, Ms. Bingham uses simple terms to explain key concepts. Whenever the Clemmonses show confusion regarding the nature of arthritis, Ms. Bingham clarifies information with illustrations on the blackboard.

Ms. Bingham uses the remaining class time to demon-

TABLE 16-5

Teaching Plan for Mr. and Mrs. Clemmons

Diagnoses	Content	Methods	Objectives
Knowledge deficit related to poor understanding of arthritis	Normal function and structure of joints; the pathological process of arthritis	Film: *Arthritis, a Crippling Disease;* pamphlet on arthritis; informal discussion; question-and-answer session; blackboard for illustrations	To describe the nature of how arthritis affects the joints of the body
Psychomotor deficits related to impairment in joint mobility and muscle strength	Exercises designed to maintain joint mobility and muscle strength; types of self-help devices designed to minimize stress on joints	Demonstration of exercises; client participation in exercises; discussion	To perform fine motor skills with activities of daily living in the home within 1 month; to stand from a sitting position without assistance.

strate some simple exercises to maintain Mrs. Clemmons' joint mobility and muscle strength. This is a type of teaching strategy that gets Mr. and Mrs. Clemmons actively involved. The nurse shows Mrs. Clemmons how to do the exercises and then assists Mr. Clemmons in learning how to direct his wife appropriately.

The nurse also discusses types of self-help devices with the Clemmonses. Mr. Clemmons' carpentry skill can be put to use to build several of the devices. One device is wooden blocks or platforms to elevate chairs and the bed so that Mrs. Clemmons will not have to raise herself up so far from a sitting position.

EVALUATION

The nurse asks the Clemmonses to explain briefly the nature of arthritis. After viewing the film they are able to give a simple but complete description of how joints are injured. The nurse knows that it is easy to forget information unless it is reinforced. She gives the Clemmonses a pamphlet to review before the next class and asks them to write down any questions they might have.

It is too early to evaluate Mrs. Clemmons' joint mobility or muscle strength. The client is given an exercise plan to follow for a week. Ms. Bingham asks Mr. Clemmons to come to the next class with ideas on types of self-help devices he might be able to construct for his wife. Thus the nurse has begun a constructive teaching plan that will enable Mrs. Clemmons and her husband to cope more effectively with her disease. As the teaching process continues, Ms. Bingham will work with Mr. and Mrs. Clemmons to reach all the objectives based on the diagnoses.

Summary

During any interaction with a client the nurse has the opportunity to teach him something about his health. Whether the goal is to maintain good health habits, regain impaired function, or develop new skills for coping with permanent disability, the nurse teaches clients to function more independently. Client education focuses on the client's unique needs and his capacity for learning. The most effective teaching plan is one in which the nurse and client work together to define the type of information and skills the client needs to learn.

A nurse cannot teach effectively without understanding the basic learning domains: cognitive, affective, and psychomotor. Each involves the acquisition of different types of behaviors. The characteristics of each domain affect the selection of the teaching methods and the manner in which learning is evaluated. Learning depends on a person's readiness and ability to learn. Psychological and physical factors influence whether a person can master new skills, acquire new knowledge, or devote sufficient energy to the learning process.

A good teacher uses basic teaching principles to promote a student's participation in learning. Teaching sessions convene when the learner is most receptive to the teacher's efforts. A teacher organizes teaching material in a format that progresses from simple to more complex ideas. The teacher's actions and use of instructional resources help to stimulate a student's interest in learning.

The nursing process provides a useful framework for organizing the teaching process. As a teacher, the nurse assesses all factors that reflect the client's learning needs, his ability to learn, and the teaching resources available. Diagnoses focus on specific types of learning needs. The teaching plan involves the nurse and client in a collaborative effort, setting realistic learning objectives. During implementation the nurse uses a variety of teaching methods to engage the client actively in learning. To determine whether a client has gained the necessary knowledge or skills, the nurse evaluates the success of the plan on the basis of expected learning outcomes.

KEY CONCEPTS

✓ Teaching is most effective when it is responsive to learners' needs.

✓ An effective teacher uses the principles of learning when interacting with students.

✓ With the primary emphasis in health care on the maintenance of a person's health, client education is a primary responsibility of the nurse.

✓ Educating family members is often a vital part of a client's return to health.

✓ Teaching is a form of interpersonal communication with teacher and student actively involved in a process that increases the student's knowledge and skills.

✓ Teaching a client a specific behavior can involve incorporation of behaviors from all three learning domains.

✓ The client's ability to attend to the learning process depends on his physical comfort and anxiety level and the presence of environmental distraction.

✓ Because it is unlikely that a person will learn unless he wants to, the nurse applies principles of motivation when teaching.

✓ A person's health beliefs influence his willingness to gain knowledge and skills necessary to maintain his health.

✓ A person's readiness to learn is significantly related to his status within the grieving process.

✓ Clients of different age groups require different teaching strategies as a result of their developmental capabilities.

✓ The ideal environment for promoting learning is a room that is well lit and free of distractions and that has good ventilation, appropriate furniture, and a comfortable temperature.

✓ An effective teacher plans teaching activities when the client is most receptive and alert.

✓ Presentation of teaching content should progress from simple to more complex ideas.

✓ The use of instructional resources involves the principles of promoting active learner participation.

✓ A combination of teaching methods improves the learner's attentiveness and involvement.

✓ A teacher is more effective when presenting information that builds on a learner's existing knowledge.

✓ When a learner receives reinforcement for a desired learning behavior, he will likely repeat the behavior.

✓ Teaching methodologies should match the client's type of learning need.

✓ An informal teaching style fosters spontaneity between teacher and learner.

✓ Learning objectives describe in behavioral terms what a person is to learn.

REFERENCE

Rosenstock, I.M.: What research in motivation suggests for public health, Am. J. Public Health **50:**295, 1960.

ADDITIONAL READINGS

Bille, D.A.: Educational strategies for teaching the elderly patient, Nurs. Health Care **5:**256, 1980.

Bille, D.A.: Practical approaches to patient teaching, Boston, 1981, Little, Brown & Co.

Huckabay, L.M.D.: Conditions of learning and instruction in nursing, St. Louis, 1980, The C.V. Mosby Co.

Joyce, B., and Weil, M.: Models of teaching, ed. 2, Englewood Cliffs, N.J., 1980, Prentice-Hall, Inc.

Marlow, D.R.: Textbook of pediatric nursing, ed. 5, Philadelphia, 1977, W.B. Saunders Co.

McHugh, N.G., Christman, N.J., and Johnson, J.E.: Preparatory information: what helps and why, Am. J. Nurs. **82:**780, 1982.

Pohl, M.L.: The teaching function of the nursing practitioner, ed. 2, Dubuque, Iowa, 1973, William C. Brown Group.

Redman, B.K.: The process of patient teaching in nursing, ed. 4, St. Louis, 1980, The C.V. Mosby Co.

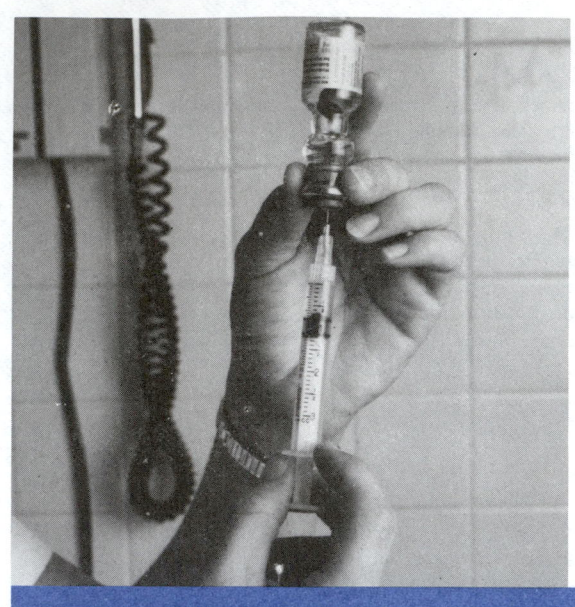

OBJECTIVES

Mastery of the content of this chapter will allow the student to:

- Explain legal concepts that nurses encounter.
- Give examples of legal issues that arise in nursing practice.
- Describe legal responsibilities and obligations of nurses.
- Discuss the legal implications of negligence.
- List various sources for standards of care for nurses.
- Define legal aspects of nurse-client, nurse-physician, and nurse-employer relationships.

GLOSSARY

assault Unlawful threatening or inflicting of harm on another.

battery Touching of another's body without consent.

crime Act that violates a law and that may include criminal intent.

libel Written false statement about a person that may injure his reputation.

malpractice Injurious or unprofessional actions that harm another.

negligence Careless act of omission or commission that results in injury to another.

slander Utterance of a false statement about another that harms his reputation.

tort Act that causes injury for which the injured party can bring civil action.

witness Person who is present and can testify that he has observed something (such as the signing of a will or consent form).

17 Legal Issues in Nursing

ontemporary law is a composite of all the rules and regulations by which our society governs itself. Without law, society could not deal with disputes and problems in an orderly fashion. The laws of any society are flexible and ever changing through either legislative process or judicial decisions.

The general public is better informed than in the past about health and illness. Through reports in newspapers and magazines and on television, more information is available to consumers of health services. Many clients are knowledgeable about their rights, and nurses are challenged to become advocates for their clients. In 1972 the American Hospital Association developed and adopted a Patient's Bill of Rights. In 1974 the Dying Person's Bill of Rights was completed, and in 1975 The Pregnant Patient's Bill of Rights was written. Although these documents are not considered legally binding, many hospitals use them to provide guidelines for the care they administer.

Many nurses view the law with apprehension because they fear being named in a malpractice lawsuit. With the increased emphasis on clients' rights, a nurse in practice today must understand her legal obligations and responsibilities to clients. Nurses who give competent care based on their education will seldom need to worry about being involved in a malpractice lawsuit.

The law serves many valuable functions when it is applied to nursing practice. It differentiates nursing practice from the practice of other health care professions. The law also describes and protects the rights of clients and nurses. For these reasons nurses should understand basic legal concepts as they relate to nursing practice.

General Legal Concepts

There are two basic sources for contemporary law. Statutory law is created by elected legislative bodies such as state or provincial legislatures, the U.S. Congress, or the Parliament of Canada. Common law is created by judicial decisions made in various courts as individual cases are decided. From these two sources two categories of law are defined: civil law and criminal law.

Civil law essentially is concerned with the protection of a person's rights. Although violations of civil law might cause harm to an individual or his property, there is usually no grave threat to society as a whole. For example, defamatory statements made about a person might lead to problems for him but do not threaten society in general. Civil law is also considered the portion of law that does not pertain to crimes.

Criminal law is concerned with acts that threaten society and its order but may involve only an individual. Willful assault and battery is an example of criminal activity in which nurses have sometimes been involved. Misuse of controlled substances is another example of criminal conduct for a nurse. A nurse who functions within professional standards of practice would have little chance of being named in a case involving misuse of controlled substances (Fenner, 1980).

From a legal standpoint a nurse who performs nursing care assumes three roles: provider of service, employee of an institution (or occasionally independent contractor for service), and private citizen. She performs these roles as she takes care of her clients and works with physicians and for her employing institution. If a nurse does not adhere to standards of care as she performs these roles, she may face legal consequences.

Legal Limits of Nursing

Standards of Care

One of the functions of law, as applied to nursing practice, is to define the standards of care the nurse must provide. All U.S. state legislatures and Canadian provincial parliaments have passed *nursing practice acts* that define the scope of nursing practice in that state or province. These acts, which vary among states and provinces, set educational requirements for nurses, distinguish between nursing practice and medical practice, and generally define the ways in which a nurse should practice. All nurses are responsible for knowing the provisions of the act for the state or province in which they work.

Professional organizations are another source for standards of care. The American Nurses' Association (ANA) has developed standards for nursing service in policy statements and similar resolutions. These standards are very general and include such recommendations as the obligation of nursing service departments to provide continuing education programs for nurses.

Finally, the written policies and procedures of the employing institution detail how the nurse is to perform her duties. These policies are usually quite specific and are set down in procedure manuals found in most nursing units. For example, a procedure policy that outlines the steps a nurse should take when she changes a client's dressing or administers medication gives specific information about how the nurse is to perform these tasks. These policies provide another definition of standards of care.

The standards of care, defined by all the sources mentioned, are very important. If a nurse is a defendant in a malpractice lawsuit, these standards may be used to determine if she has acted as any reasonably prudent nurse with the same level of education and experience would. In other words, standards of care serve as guidelines for determining whether a nurse performed her duties in an appropriate manner. If a nurse is named as a defendant in a malpractice lawsuit and it is proved that she did not follow the accepted standards of care as outlined by the nursing practice act of her state or province, the policies of her em-

ploying institution, or both, her legal liability is clear.

A 1966 case, *Darling v. Charleston Community Memorial Hospital,* involved an 18-year-old man with a fractured leg. When the cast was applied to his leg, the physician placed insufficient padding under the plaster. The man's toes became swollen and discolored, and he had decreased sensation in them. He complained to the nursing staff many times but the cast was left on. During the next 4 days gangrene developed, and the man's leg had to be amputated. The physician in the emergency room was liable for incorrectly applying the cast. The nursing staff was also liable because they had not adhered to the standards of care appropriate to this client's symptoms (Rocereto and Maleski, 1982).

Another issue in this case was inadequate nurse staffing in the emergency room. Since the Joint Commission for the Accreditation of Hospitals (JCAH) standard for the number of staff was not met, the institution was also liable in this lawsuit.

Standards of care basically concern a nurse's accountability for nursing care. A general duty nurse is legally responsible for meeting the same standards as other general duty nurses in a similar setting. However, specialized nurses such as nurse anesthetists, intensive care nurses, certified nurse-midwives, or operating room nurses are held to standards of care and skill exercised by those in the same specialty as defined by national standards. Every nurse should know the standards of care she is expected to meet.

In summary, standards of care are guidelines by which a nurse should practice. If a nurse does not perform her nursing duties within accepted standards of care, she may place herself in jeopardy of legal action.

Licensure

All registered nurses or licensed practical nurses are licensed by the board of nursing of the state or province in which they practice. The requirements for licensure vary among states in the United States and provinces in Canada, but in most nurse licensing acts there are requirements for education and the nurse must pass an examination. Currently all states use the National Council Licensure Examinations (NCLEX) for registered nurse and licensed practical nurse examinations. Nurse licensing statutes usually require that the nurse be 21 years of age, be a citizen, and exhibit good moral character (Cazalas, 1978).

A nurse's license can be suspended or revoked by the board of nursing if her conduct violates provisions contained in the licensing statute. For example, if a nurse performs an illegal act such as selling controlled substances, she is jeopardizing her licensed status. Before a nurse's license is revoked, she must be notified of the charges against her and permitted to attend a hearing in which she has an opportunity to present evidence on her behalf. These hearings are not court proceedings but are usually conducted by the state or provincial board of nursing. Some states and provinces do provide for judicial review of such cases if the nurse has exhausted all other forms of appeal (Cazalas, 1978).

Student Nurses

If a client suffers harm as a direct result of a nursing student's action, the liability for the incorrect action is generally shared by the student, the instructor, and the hospital or health care facility. A student nurse should never be assigned to a task for which she is unprepared and should be carefully supervised by her instructor as she learns new procedures. Although the student nurse is not considered an employee of the hospital, the institution does have a responsibility to monitor the acts of nursing students. A student nurse is expected to perform as a professional nurse would at that point in her experience. Usually the faculty member is responsible for instructing and observing students, but in some situations a staff nurse may share these responsibilities. Every nursing school should provide clear definitions of responsibility (Cazalas, 1978).

Sometimes student nurses are employed as nursing assistants or nurse's aides when they are not attending classes. If a student nurse is employed in this capacity, she should not perform tasks that do not appear in a job description for a nurse's aide or assistant. For example, even if a student has learned to administer intramuscular medications in class, she may not perform this task as a nurse's aide.

Legal Liability in Nursing

Crimes

A crime is an offense against society that violates a law. Criminal acts are prosecuted in the criminal justice system. A felony is a crime of a serious nature that usually carries a penalty of imprisonment or death. A misdemeanor is a crime of a less serious nature than a felony, and the penalty is usually a fine or imprisonment for less than a year. In nursing there are few crimes a nurse would commit if she practiced within accepted standards of care. For the purpose of this chapter, flagrant criminal activity such as murder and illegally dispensing controlled substances will not be discussed; laws pertaining to such offenses apply to nurses as to all individuals.

Torts

A tort is a civil wrong committed against a person or property. Torts may be subtle and difficult to define, but for this discussion two categories will be described: unintentional torts such as negligence and intentional torts such as a willful act that violates another's rights (for example, assault and battery). If a nurse performs an act that could be considered a tort, the case is tried in a civil (not a criminal) court with the intent to assess compensation for the client (plaintiff) who brought suit. The purpose of the judgment is not to punish the nurse, as it would be in a criminal proceeding.

NEGLIGENCE

If a nurse gives care that does not meet appropriate standards, she may be held liable for negligence. Negligence may involve carelessness such as not checking a client's armband and consequently administering the wrong medication. However, carelessness is not always the cause. If a nurse attempts a procedure for which she has not been trained and does it carefully but still harms the patient, a claim of negligence could be made (Hemelt and Mackert, 1982).

There are several common negligent acts in which nurses have been involved. Errors in sponge counts in surgical cases are among the most common of these. Such an error may result in a sponge being left inside the client by mistake. If an infection or other problem develops because of the sponge, a claim of negligence and liability for the physician, nurse, or both would be justified.

Another common negligent act is causing a burn. If a nurse applies a heating device that is too hot and the client sustains a burn, the nurse is legally liable for negligence. There have also been cases in which electronic equipment malfunctioned and the client sustained an electrical burn from a monitor probe. The nurse should never use equipment that she knows is malfunctioning, and she must make sure electrical equipment is grounded to prevent the chance of shock.

Many possible negligent acts may occur when administering medications. Incorrect dosages, mixups that result in the wrong medication being given to a client, medication administered incorrectly, and inaccurate computations of concentration are among the most common errors. Nurses must use extreme care whenever they are involved in the administration of medications because the possibility for error is so great.

A claim of negligence could also be made when infection can be traced to a nurse's actions or her failure to use aseptic technique when required. Therefore nurses must be concerned with the cleanliness of the client's environment, as well as with accepted standards of care regarding prevention of cross-contamination.

Nurses are responsible for performing all procedures correctly and for exercising professional judgment as they carry out the orders of physicians. Any nurse who does not meet accepted standards of care as she discharges her duties or who performs her duties in a careless fashion runs a risk of being found negligent in her nursing care.

INVASION OF PRIVACY

Another tort that might be brought against a nurse or other care giver by a client is a claim of invasion of privacy. A client is entitled to confidential health care. All aspects of a client's care should be free from unwanted publicity or exposure to public scrutiny.

One form of invasion of privacy is the release of information to an unauthorized person. In an Alabama case in 1973, *Horne v. Patton,* a physician revealed medical information about a client's condition to the client's employer. The client lost his job. A lawsuit found the physician liable for releasing information to the employer, who did not have a legitimate interest in the client's health history (Hemelt and Mackert, 1982).

Gossiping about a client's activities is another form of invasion of privacy and could lead to a charge of slander. If a client has a venereal disease, for example, the nurse should not discuss that information except as it directly relates to the care and treatment of the client. The nurse is required in some areas to report certain communicable diseases and is immune from prosecution when she does make a report.

Another example of invasion of privacy is a nurse's unwanted intrusion in private family matters. A nurse has no right to intrude in matters that are not directly related to her client's well-being. For example, if a client is terminally ill and does not want his family informed, the nurse could try to persuade the client that it would be in his best interest and beneficial to his family if he informed them, but the nurse should not tell the family without the client's permission.

An individual's right to privacy may conflict with the public's right to information. For example, a threat or benefit to public health may override the individual's right to privacy. Disclosures of private information were made about individuals who had toxic shock syndrome and in the Tylenol poisoning cases. Sometimes the client is a public figure whose physical condition is considered newsworthy. There are also cases in which information is given out about a scientific discovery or a major medical breakthrough, as with the first heart transplant cases or the first artificial heart recipient. If an event falls into any

of these categories, information should be channeled through the public relations department of the institution to ensure invasion of privacy does not occur; the nurse should not attempt to decide the legality of disclosing information herself.

DEFAMATION OF CHARACTER

Defamation of character is another type of tort in which a nurse could be involved. Any communication about a person that injures his reputation and is disseminated by another person is considered libel (written) or slander (oral). For example, if a nurse tells a client that his physician is incompetent, the nurse could be held liable for slander. If she writes such a comment, she could be sued for libel. The important issue in a claim of defamation of character is whether harm is done to the reputation of the plaintiff (Cazalas, 1978).

ASSAULT AND BATTERY

Although assault and battery might be considered criminal in the context of this chapter, only the civil aspects will be discussed. If a nurse is accused of assault and battery, the client could bring a civil lawsuit against her in order to recover damages. Such a case would be tried in a civil (not a criminal) court.

Assault is an act intended to provoke fear in a victim. The victim believes harm will come to him as a result of the threat. Assault may be subtle; for example, a nurse might attempt to coerce a client into taking a medication he does not wish to take. A more blatant example might involve a nurse handling an uncooperative client in the emergency room. If the exasperated nurse yells, "If you don't take off those filthy clothes, I'm going to rip them off you!" and moves toward the client, a claim of assault could be made.

Battery is willful, angry, or negligent touching of another's body, anything he is wearing or holding, or anything that is attached to him, without his consent (Creighton, 1981). There have been instances of abuse of confined clients by personnel in mental institutions. In a less drastic case, if a nurse attaches fetal electrodes during labor without the consent of the mother, a claim of battery could be made. The important issue is the client's informed consent. In some situations consent is implied. For example, if a nurse says, "I have your injection for you, Mr. Jones," and he holds out his arm, he is giving implied consent to the injection.

Whether the procedure that constitutes battery (without consent) ultimately helps the client is unimportant. In a classic case in 1905, *Mohr v. Williams,* the client gave written consent for surgery on his right ear. Once the client was anesthetized, the physician discovered that the left ear was more seriously affected, and he operated on the left ear. The client sued because surgery was performed on the "wrong" ear (Cazalas, 1978).

PROCEDURE IN A MALPRACTICE LAWSUIT

In a malpractice lawsuit against a nurse the following criteria must be established: (1) the nurse (defendant) owed a duty to her client (the plaintiff), (2) she did not carry out that duty, (3) the client (plaintiff) was injured, and (4) the client's injury was a result of the nurse's failure to carry out her duty. The best way for a nurse to avoid being named in a lawsuit is to follow standards of care as described earlier, give competent health care, and develop empathetic rapport with her client. A client who believes that the nurse did all she could is unlikely to initiate a lawsuit.

MALPRACTICE INSURANCE

All nurses should have their own malpractice insurance, even if the employing institution has malpractice coverage for nursing employees. Some institutional coverage provides only the cost of legal counsel in the event a nurse is named in a lawsuit, and in such cases the nurse is responsible for payment of any judgments awarded against her. If the employing institution does not cover a nurse's legal expenses, it may be very costly for her to prove her innocence.

Legal Concepts and the Nurse-Client Relationship

In nursing practice the nurse deals with many people: the client and his family, physicians, other nurses, other health care professionals, and the employing institution. In the nurse-client interaction several legal issues may arise. The Patient's Bill of Rights, adopted by the American Hospital Association, is an unofficial statement of guidelines related to nurse-client interaction (see box). Informed consent and legal issues involving death and dying are discussed in the following sections.

Informed Consent

A signed consent form is required for any potentially hazardous procedure such as surgery, for some treatment programs such as chemotherapy, and for

---

The Patient's Bill of Rights

1. The patient has the right to considerate and respectful care.
2. The patient has the right to obtain from his physician complete current information concerning his diagnosis, treatment and prognosis in terms the patient can be reasonably expected to understand.
3. The patient has the right to receive from his physician information necessary to give informed consent prior to the start of any procedure and/or treatment. . . . Where medically significant alternatives for care or treatment exist, or when the patient requests information concerning medical alternatives, the patient has the right to such information [and] to know the name of the person responsible for the procedures and/or treatment.
4. The patient has the right to refuse treatment to the extent permitted by law, and to be informed of the medical consequences of his action.
5. The patient has the right to every consideration of his privacy concerning his own medical care program.
6. The patient has the right to expect that all communications and records pertaining to his care should be treated as confidential.
7. The patient has the right to expect that within its capacity a hospital must make reasonable response to the request of a patient for services.
8. The patient has the right to obtain information as to any relationship of his hospital to other health care and educational institutions insofar as his care is concerned [and] any professional relationships among individuals, by name, who are treating him.
9. The patient has the right to be advised if the hospital proposes to engage in or perform human experimentation affecting his care or treatment [and] has the right to refuse to participate.
10. The patient has the right to expect reasonable continuity of care.
11. The patient has the right to examine and receive an explanation of his bill regardless of source of payment.
12. The patient has the right to know what hospital rules and regulations apply to his conduct as a patient.

From American Hospital Association: Nurs. Outlook **24**:29, 1976.

THE CHILDREN'S MERCY HOSPITAL
Kansas City, Missouri
Hospitalization Record
To Be Filled Out By A Physician

CHART COPY

Code	Diagnosis (es) at Discharge (Most Important, Admission Related First)	Condition

Operations		Dates

Primary Attending Physician's Signature

Resident Physician's Signature

A

PATIENT'S COMPLETE NAME	ADM SOURCE	ADMISSION DATE & TIME	ROOM BED	ACC CODE	CITY OR COUNTY OF PATIENT'S BIRTH	ADMISSION NO.

ATTENDING PHYSICIAN	CODE	DATE OF BIRTH	AGE	SEX	RACE	REV CODE	DISMISSAL DATE & TIME	TOTAL DAYS	MEDICAL RECORD NO.

PATIE REET ADDRESS	PATIENT	CITY	STATE	ZIP	COUNTY	CODE	CLERK

DIAGNOSIS	REFERRING PHYSICIAN	REFERRING PHYSICIAN'S ADDRESS

PARENT OR GUARDIAN	PARENT OR GUARDIAN ADDRESS	CITY	STATE	ZIP	HOME PHONE

EMPLO ER	EMPLOYER ADDRESS	EMPLOYER	CITY	STATE	ZIP	EMPLOYER PHONE

PARENT/GUARDIAN RELATION	PARENT/GUARDIAN OCCUPATION	DISMISS TO:	PHONE	MOTHER'S MAIDEN NAME

NAME OF LOCAL CONTACT	RELATIONSHIP	ADDRESS	CITY	STATE	ZIP	PHONE

GUARANTOR NAME	GUARANTOR ADDRESS	GUARANTOR CITY	STATE	ZIP	GUARANTOR PHONE

GUARANTOR EMPLOYER	GUARANTOR EMPLOYER ADDRESS	GUARANTOR EMPLOYER CITY	STATE	ZIP	GUARANTOR WORK PHONE

GUARANTOR RELATIONSHIP TO PATIENT	GUARANTOR OCCUPATION	GUARANTOR SOC. SEC. NO.	GR MO. INC. — # HOME

INSURANCE CARRIER #1	CODE	INSURANCE CARRIER #2	CODE	FATHER'S NAME

POLICY NUMBER/GROUP/ADC #	POLICY NUMBER/GROUP #	ADDRESS

NAME OF INSURED	GROUP	NAME OF INSURED	GROUP	CITY	STATE	ZIP	PHONE

Fig. 17-1   Sample consent form for admission to the hospital.

THE CHILDREN'S MERCY HOSPITAL
Kansas City, Missouri

TERMS AND CONDITIONS OF ADMISSION

NECESSARY MEDICAL TREATMENT:

Recognizing the need for hospital care for the child whose name appears herein, consent is hereby given to The Children's Mercy Hospital for hospital services rendered under the general and specific instructions of the attending physician and treatment to be necessary for the safety, welfare and health of the child.

PROFESSIONAL CARE:

The patient is under the professional care of an attending physician who arranges for services for the care and treatment of the patient. The attending physician is usually selected by the patient's parent or guardian, but may when not designated or under emergency circumstances be otherwise selected.

RELEASE OF INFORMATION:

The Hospital is authorized to furnish information from the patient's medical record to any insurer, compensation carrier or welfare agency who may be providing financial assistance for hospital care.

PHOTOGRAPHS:

Photographs of the patient may be taken under the supervision of The Children's Mercy Hospital by members of the Staff or other persons for teaching, medical research purposes or for publicity as deemed proper by the Hospital and the taking of pictures, unless specifically denied in writing, shall not be deemed an invasion of privacy.

PERSONAL VALUABLES:

The Hospital shall not be liable for loss or damage to any personal property of the patient brought into The Children's Mercy Hospital.

PAYMENT FOR HOSPITAL CARE:

I/We do hereby assume financial responsibility for and agree to make payment in full to The Children's Mercy Hospital for all charges for services or medical supplies furnished the above patient. Payment is to be made within 30 days as bills are presented with settlement in full, or arrangements for same to be made in the Financial Counseling Department before departure of the patient.

I/We do certify that the financial information given is true, accurate and complete to the best of my/our knowledge, and further authorize The Children's Mercy Hospital to investigate any and all financial information given on this admission under their normal investigative procedures.

I/We do hereby assign and authorize payment directly to the above named Hospital and physician(s) of all hospitalization or insurance benefits and physician fee benefits and guarantee to pay any balance, with the understanding that the account is not settled or closed until after the insurance benefits are received by the Hospital and if there is a remaining balance I/we agree to pay the same. I/We are aware of the above contents.

I/We hereby certify that I/we have read all parts of this Admission Form and agree and accept all terms and conditions hereon and state that all representations made by me are true.

I am aware of the above contents.

A photocopy of this agreement shall be considered as valid and effective as the original.

B

SIGNED	ADDRESS	PHONE

RELATION TO PATIENT	DATE

Patient approved for admission to The Children's Mercy Hospital under the terms hereon

WITNESS	DATE

SECOND WITNESS (TELEPHONE CONSENTS)	DATE

Courtesy The Children's Mercy Hospital, Kansas City, Mo.

THE CHILDREN'S MERCY HOSPITAL

Consent for Operation, Anesthesia, or Special Procedures

Hospital # _____

Patient's name _____

I consent for Dr. _____ or physicians whom he may designate
to perform the following procedures: _____
_____
_____
_____

(Describe the procedure in terms meaningful to the person signing.)

I consent to extensions or modifications of this procedure or to additional
procedures that may be required to diagnose or treat the condition described
below.

_____
_____
_____

(Describe the condition for which the patient is to receive the treatment that
requires this consent.)

I consent to anesthetic procedures in connection with these procedures.

I consent to disposal by The Children's Mercy Hospital of any tissue or parts
removed.

I consent to the taking of photographs for medical purposes.

I have discussed the procedures to which I am consenting with a physician, and
I understand that there is a chance of complications or permanent harm.

_____

| _____ | _____ |
| signature | witness |

address _____   address _____

| _____ | DATE ___/___/___ TIME _____ a.m. |
| relationship | p.m. |

MR-(10/75)

Fig. 17-2 Sample consent form for operations, anesthesia, or special procedures.
Courtesy The Children's Mercy Hospital, Kansas City, Mo.

experimentation involving clients. For a consent to be valid: (1) the person giving consent must be mentally and physically competent and be legally an adult; (2) the consent must be given voluntarily—no coercive measures may be used to obtain it; (3) the person giving consent must thoroughly understand the procedure and its risks and benefits, as well as alternative procedures; and (4) the person giving consent has a right to have all questions answered to his satisfaction. If a client is deaf or has some other impediment to communication (such as speaking a foreign language), he should have an interpreter available to explain the terms of consent. Fig. 17-1 is an example of a consent form for admission to the hospital.

Since the nurse is not the person who will perform the surgery or direct the medical procedure, she should not be the person who obtains the client's consent. However, in many institutions the nurse is the person who assumes the responsibility for confirming that the client has given consent. If a nurse takes a consent form for the client to sign, she should ask if he understands the procedure for which he is giving consent. If he answers that he does not understand, the nurse is obligated to notify the physician and to make certain that the client is informed before he signs the consent document. The court says that a client's right to self-determination gives him the right to clear information with which to make a decision for informed consent (Hemelt and Mackert, 1982). Fig. 17-2 is a sample consent form for operations, anesthesia, or special procedures.

If a client refuses surgery or other medical treatment, he must be informed about any deleterious consequences of his refusal. If he persists in refusing the treatment, his rejection should be written, signed, and witnessed.

Parents are usually the legal guardians of pediatric clients, and therefore they are the persons who must sign consent forms for treatment. Occasionally a parent or guardian refuses treatment for a child. For example, in a recent Texas case a child whose parents were Jehovah's Witnesses refused a lifesaving blood transfusion for the child. The child was made a ward of the court, and the blood transfusion was administered. The court ruled that although parents are adults and may choose to become martyrs, they cannot make a martyr of their child (Creighton, 1981). The practice of making a child a ward of the court, administering necessary treatment, and then returning legal guardianship to the parents is relatively common in such cases. If a nurse is involved in a similar case, she should inform her nursing supervisor, who will enlist the aid of the appropriate hospital administrator to handle the problem.

In some instances obtaining informed consent is difficult. If the client is unconscious, for example, consent must be obtained from a person who is legally authorized to give consent on the client's behalf (Cazalas, 1978). If a person has been declared legally incompetent in a judicial proceeding, consent must be obtained from the person's legal guardian. In emergency situations, if it is impossible to obtain consent from either the client or an authorized person, the procedure required to benefit the client (or perhaps save his life) may be undertaken without liability for failure to obtain consent (Cazalas, 1978).

Death and Dying

Many legal issues surround the events of death, including a basic definition of the actual point at which a person is considered dead. Current literature generally agrees that death occurs when there is an absence of brain function, irrespective of the function of other body organs. One reason for the development of this definition has been to facilitate heart and other organ transplantation. This definition is also useful when there is a question of whether to continue life support. Nurses must be aware of legal definitions of death because they must document all events that occur during the time the client is in their care.

There are ethical (see Chapter 14), as well as legal, questions raised by the issue of euthanasia. Active euthanasia—intentionally administering a lethal dose of morphine to a client, for example—is defined as murder. The less well-defined area of passive euthanasia, such as removing ventilatory support or withholding a blood transfusion from a terminally ill client with irreversible brain damage, raises legal questions that have not been resolved. There are heated arguments between those who believe in a person's right to die and those who believe in the sanctity of life no matter what the quality of that life (Hemelt and Mackert, 1982). The Dying Person's Bill of Rights is a set of guidelines used in many settings in the care of dying clients (see box on p. 336).

HANDLING OF BODIES

Nurses have the legal obligation to treat a deceased person's remains with dignity. Wrongful handling could cause emotional harm to the survivors. In one case, for example, survivors sued when a mislabeling of bodies led to an Orthodox Jew's body being prepared for a Roman Catholic funeral and a Roman Catholic's body being prepared for a Jewish burial.

AUTOPSY AND ORGAN DONATION

Consent for an autopsy must be given by either the decedent (before his death) or a close family member. Laws in many states and provinces give an order of

The Dying Person's Bill of Rights

I have the right to be treated as a living human being until I die.

I have the right to maintain a sense of hopefulness, however changing its focus may be.

I have the right to be cared for by those who can maintain a sense of hopefulness, however changing this might be.

I have the right to express my feelings and emotions about my approaching death in my own way.

I have the right to participate in decisions concerning my care.

I have the right to expect continuing medical and nursing attention even though "cure" goals must be changed to "comfort" goals.

I have the right not to die alone.

I have the right to be free from pain.

I have the right to have my questions answered honestly.

I have the right not to be deceived.

I have the right to have help from and for my family in accepting my death.

I have the right to die in peace and dignity.

I have the right to retain my individuality and not be judged for my decisions which may be contrary to beliefs of others.

I have the right to discuss and enlarge my religious and/or spiritual experiences, whatever these may mean to others.

I have the right to expect that the sanctity of the human body will be respected after death.

I have the right to be cared for by caring, sensitive, knowledgeable people who will attempt to understand my needs and will be able to gain some satisfaction in helping me face my death.

From Rothman, D.A., and Rothman, N.L.: The professional nurse and the law, Boston, 1977, Little, Brown & Co.

priority for family members who may give consent for autopsy. For an adult male, for example, his wife, then his children, then any other family member may be asked to give consent for autopsy.

Autopsies may resolve both legal and medical questions. They are required in certain circumstances such as death resulting from suspected child abuse or other criminal activity. Sometimes an autopsy consent stipulates specific exclusions (such as no studies involving the brain). As with any consent, the physician should not use coercion to obtain consent for autopsy.

If a person is legally competent to give consent and is over 18 years of age, he is free to donate his body or organs for medical use. Consent forms are available for this purpose. A nurse may serve as a witness when a person wishes to give consent for the donation of organs or his body.

WILLS

A will legally declares a person's intentions when he dies. It usually contains provisions for how he wishes his property to be divided, the guardianship of his children, and how his estate should be administered. A nurse should be knowledgeable about wills because she may sometimes be asked to be a witness. A witness must watch the person sign the will, know that it was voluntarily signed, and, to the best of his judgment, know that the person was of sound mind and memory at the time of signing.

Most wills are written, and the number of witnesses required varies from one to three, depending on the state or province in which the person making the will resides. If a client informs a nurse that he wishes to make an oral will, the nurse should write down his statements and send a written memorandum to the hospital administrator. A client might declare several wills during a prolonged illness, and the nurse should follow the same procedure each time (Cazalas, 1978).

∎ ∎ ∎ ∎ ∎

There are many possible legal questions involved in nurse-client interactions. If a nurse finds herself confounded by some particularly difficult legal question, help is always available. In the hospital setting she could begin her search for answers in the hierarchy of nursing administration. Hospitals generally have the benefit of legal counsel, and someone should be able to address the particular problem encountered.

Legal Concepts and Nursing Practice

In addition to encountering legal problems in their care of clients, nurses may share liability for errors made by physicians and other health care personnel or for inadequate care provided by their employing institution. Legal aspects of nursing practice involved in nurse-physician and nurse-institution interactions include issues concerning physician orders, staffing, and other areas as discussed in the following sections.

Physician Orders

The physician is responsible for directing the medical treatment for a client. The nurse is obligated to follow the physician's order unless she believes the order is in error or would be detrimental to the client.

Therefore the nurse must assess all orders, and if she determines that one is erroneous or harmful, she should seek further clarification from the physician. If the physician confirms the order, and the nurse still believes it is inappropriate, she should inform her supervising nurse. A written memorandum to the supervisor detailing the events in chronological order and the reasons for refusing to carry out the order should protect the nurse from disciplinary action (Hemelt and Mackert, 1982). The supervising nurse should help resolve the questionable order. A nurse who carries out an inaccurate order may be legally responsible for any harm suffered by the client.

The physician should write all orders, and the nurse should transcribe them carefully. Verbal orders are not recommended because they leave possibilities for error. If a verbal order is necessary, such as during an emergency, it should be written and signed by the physician as soon as possible.

A difficult area regarding physician orders involves an order of "no code" or "do not resuscitate" for a terminally ill client. Many physicians are reluctant to write such an order because they fear legal repercussions for "abandoning" their clients. Cushing (1981) suggests that if a physician has documented in his progress notes that the client's condition is deteriorating and that he has decided not to administer cardiopulmonary resuscitation, he is perfectly justified in writing a "no code" order. The physician should discuss the order in advance with the client if he is mentally competent unless the physician decides that such a discussion would be detrimental to the client's condition. In that case the physician should discuss the order with the client's family. A "no code" order should be written, not given verbally. The physician should review the order periodically in case the client's condition necessitates a change.

According to guidelines adopted by the American Heart Association, cardiopulmonary resuscitation is not intended for use when a client has an irreversible illness in which death is expected (Cushing, 1981). Partial code or "slow code" verbal instructions have occasionally been suggested as a way for a physician to avoid writing a "no code" order. "Slow code" may be defined differently by various institutions but usually means performing resuscitative procedures more slowly than recommended by the American Heart Association. If a nurse assists in a "slow code," however, this may be interpreted as not performing resuscitative procedures as a competent person would and therefore be the basis for a lawsuit.

Short Staffing

The JCAH has established guidelines to determine the number of nurses required to give care to specific numbers of clients (staffing ratios). Legal problems may arise if there are not enough nurses to provide competent care. If a nurse is assigned to take care of more clients than is reasonable, she should attempt to reject the assignment by informing the nursing supervisor that it is inappropriate. If the nurse is required to accept the assignment, she should make a written protest to the nursing administrators. Although the nurse's protest would not relieve her of responsibility if one of her clients suffered because of inattention, it would show that the nurse was attempting to act in good faith. The nurse should not walk out when staffing is inadequate, since a charge of abandonment could be made (Horsley, 1981).

Controlled Substances

Another legal issue that might arise for nurses involves the use of controlled substances. In 1970 the Comprehensive Drug Abuse Prevention and Control Act was passed in the United States. It controls substances such as narcotics, depressants, stimulants, and hallucinogens. The act regulates the hospital distribution system, rehabilitation programs for drug abuse, and research into the medical treatment of addiction. Canadian law similarly regulates controlled substances. Nurses may administer controlled substances only under the direction of a licensed physician.

Controlled substances should be kept securely locked up and only authorized personnel should have access to them. There are criminal penalties for misuse of controlled substances. There have been cases in which a physician illegally prescribed and dispensed controlled substances, and if a nurse employed by such a physician failed to report these activities, she would be legally accountable for aiding and abetting them (Cazalas, 1978).

"Floating"

Nurses are sometimes required to "float" from the area in which they normally practice nursing to another nursing unit. Creighton (1982) reports a case in which a nurse in obstetrics was assigned to an emergency room. A client entered the emergency room and complained of chest pain. He was given a markedly incorrect increased dosage of lidocaine by the obstetrical nurse. He died after cardiac arrest and subsequent irreversible brain damage. The nurse lost the malpractice lawsuit brought against her and the hospital.

A nurse who is floated should inform her supervisor of any lack of experience in the new nursing unit. The floated nurse should also request and be given orientation to the unit (Creighton, 1981).

The Children's Mercy Hospital
INCIDENT REPORT
*An incident is any happening which is
not consistent with routine operation
of the hospital or care of a particular
patient. It may be an accident or a
situation which might result in an
accident.*

Person(s) involved _____

_____

Complete as applicable if possible injury

□ Patient → □ Inpatient Diagnosis _____ Age _____
            □ Outpatient Who was supervising patient? _____

□ Employee → Department _____ Job title _____
             Length of time on job _____ Age _____ Home phone _____

□ Other → Home address & phone _____
          Reason for being at hospital _____

Exact location of incident _____ Date of incident _____ Time _____

Names & addresses} _____
of witnesses   } _____

INCIDENT FACTS _____
_____
_____
_____
_____
_____
_____
_____
_____
_____
                                    (Use reverse side if necessary.)

Was person involved seen by CMH physician because of incident?
                    □ No   □ Yes   Date _____ Time _____
Signature of person reporting _____ Date written _____

┌───┐
│ PHYSICIAN'S STATEMENT (Clinical information on patients must ALSO be charted.) │
│   │
│   Description of any injury _____   │
│   _____   │
│   │
│   Treatment given or recommended _____   │
│   _____   │
│   │
│   If employee involved, when is return to work permitted? _____ │
│   Signature of physician _____ Date _____ Time __ │
└───┘

If patient, parent, or nursing personnel involved, send to Nursing Supervisor. Send all
others to Administration.

(ADM 3/80)   8311-51

Fig. 17-3 Sample audit report.

The Children's Mercy Hospital
    INCIDENT REPORT

INCIDENT FACTS (continued from reverse side) _____
_____
_____
_____
_____
_____
_____
_____
_____
_____
_____
_____
_____
_____
_____
_____
_____
_____
_____

DO NOT WRITE BELOW THIS LINE
_____

Incident report number _____
Reviewers and dates of review

_____ __/__/__   _____ __/__/__

_____ __/__/__   _____ __/__/__

_____ __/__/__   _____ __/__/__

(ADM 3/80)   8311-51

Incident Reports

An incident report is filed in any unusual situation in which there is a possibility that a lawsuit might be filed. For example, if a nurse administers an incorrect dose of medication, a client falls out of bed, or an intravenous solution infiltrates the skin causing sloughing and scar formation, the nurse should complete an incident report. Most institutions provide a specific form for this purpose. The nurse records all the details of the incident, and the physician examines the client and gives his impression of any untoward effects that the error might have. Fig. 17-3 is a sample incident report.

Many nurses are reluctant to file incident reports because they believe such reports are detrimental to their employment record. Actually, incident reports are used by the institution administration for quality assurance and risk management. By reviewing incident reports, administrators can determine areas of client risk. For example, if a certain kind of problem has occurred repeatedly, educational methods can be used to prevent the problem in the future. In addition, the insurance carrier for a hospital or other institution relies on incident reports to assess liability and possible future claims.

Reporting Obligations

In some situations nurses are required to make a report to the appropriate authority. For example, most states require that if a child is a suspected victim of abuse, health care professionals must report their findings to the proper agency. A nurse may be involved in reporting other criminal activity as in cases of gunshot wounds, attempted suicide, or rape. Reporting of certain communicable diseases may also be required. Since what must be reported varies among states and provinces, the nurse should become familiar with the statutes in the area in which she practices.

Good Samaritan Laws

Good Samaritan laws have been enacted in almost every state and province to encourage health care professionals to assist in emergency situations. These laws limit liability and offer legal immunity for people who help in an emergency, providing they give the best possible care under the conditions of the emergency (Hemelt and Mackert, 1982). If a nurse stops at the scene of an automobile accident and gives emergency care as she has been taught (for example, using caution when moving the injured person in case there is a spinal injury, or applying pressure to stop hemorrhage), she would be acting within accepted standards given the fact that she did not have proper equipment.

Contracts

A contract is a written or verbal agreement between two people in which goods or services are exchanged. An oral contract is as binding as a written one but may be more difficult to prove. A breach of contract occurs if either party fails to carry out his agreed obligation.

When a nurse accepts a job in a particular hospital or health care agency, she enters into a contract with her employer. The basic understanding is that the nurse will perform her duties competently, adhering to the policies and procedures of the institution. In return her employer not only pays her for her services, but also furnishes the facilities and equipment in proper working order to enable her to provide efficient and competent care (Hemelt and Mackert, 1982).

Nurses also enter into contractual agreements with their clients. The nurse agrees to give competent care, and the client agrees to pay for the service. When a client signs an admission form on entering the hospital or agrees to nursing care in any health agency, the contract is initiated. Private duty nurses have specific written contracts with their clients.

Legal Issues in Practice Areas

Numerous possible legal liabilities exist in all areas of nursing practice. Any nurse who works in a specialized field should study the legal issues that pertain to her area of practice. Space does not permit a complete description of all legal liabilities, but a few issues involved in perinatal nursing, pediatric nursing, medical-surgical nursing, psychiatric nursing, and critical care nursing are discussed in the following sections.

Perinatal Nursing

The specialty of perinatal nursing involves care of women before, during, and immediately after pregnancy, as well as care of newborn infants. Many legal issues are involved in the care of a mother and her neonate. The Pregnant Patient's Bill of Rights is a set of guidelines for care during the perinatal period (see box).

Some of the ethical issues involved in contraceptive counseling are discussed in Chapter 14. From a legal standpoint, persons who receive sexual counseling or treatment for venereal disease have a right to privacy and confidentiality regarding these matters. However,

The Pregnant Patient's Bill of Rights

The Pregnant Patient has the right to participate in decisions involving her well-being and that of her unborn child, unless there is a clear-cut medical emergency that prevents her participation. In addition to the rights set forth in the American Hospital Association's "Patient's Bill of Rights" (which has also been adopted by the New York City Department of Health), the Pregnant Patient, because she represents *two* patients rather than one, should be recognized as having the additional rights listed below.

1. *The Pregnant Patient has the right,* prior to the administration of any drug or procedure, to be informed by the health professional caring for her of any potential direct or indirect effects, risks or hazards to herself or her unborn or newborn infant which may result from the use of a drug or procedure prescribed for or administered to her during pregnancy, labor, birth or lactation.

2. *The Pregnant Patient has the right,* prior to the proposed therapy, to be informed, not only of the benefits, risks and hazards of the proposed therapy, but also of known alternative therapy, such as available childbirth education classes which could help to prepare the Pregnant Patient physically and mentally to cope with the discomfort or stress of pregnancy and the experience of childbirth, thereby reducing or eliminating her need for drugs and obstetric intervention. She should be offered such information early in her pregnancy in order that she may make a reasoned decision.

3. *The Pregnant Patient has the right,* prior to the administration of any drug, to be informed by the health professional who is prescribing or administering the drug to her that any drug which she receives during pregnancy, labor and birth, no matter how or when the drug is taken or administered, may adversely affect her unborn baby, directly or indirectly, and that there is no drug or chemical which has been proven safe for the unborn child.

4. *The Pregnant Patient has the right,* if cesarean section is anticipated, to be informed prior to the administration of any drug, and preferably prior to her hospitalization, that minimizing her and, in turn, her baby's intake of nonessential preoperative medicine, will benefit her baby.

5. *The Pregnant Patient has the right,* prior to the administration of a drug or procedure, to be informed if there is *no* properly controlled follow-up research which has established the safety of the drug or procedure with regard to its direct and/or indirect effects on the physiological, mental and neurological development of the child exposed, via the mother, to the drug or procedure during pregnancy, labor, birth or lactation (this would apply to virtually all drugs and the vast majority of obstetric procedures).

6. *The Pregnant Patient has the right,* prior to the administration of any drug, to be informed of the brand name and generic name of the drug in order that she may advise the health professional of any past adverse reaction to the drug.

7. *The Pregnant Patient has the right* to determine for herself, without pressure from her attendant, whether she will accept the risks inherent in the proposed therapy or refuse a drug or procedure.

8. *The Pregnant Patient has the right* to know the name and qualifications of the individual administering a medication or procedure to her during labor or birth.

9. *The Pregnant Patient has the right* to be informed, prior to the administration of any procedure, whether that procedure is being administered to her for her or her baby's benefit (medically indicated) or as an elective procedure (for convenience or teaching purposes).

10. *The Pregnant Patient has the right* to be accompanied during the stress of labor and birth by someone she cares for, and to whom she looks for emotional comfort and encouragement.

11. *The Pregnant Patient has the right* after appropriate medical consultation to choose a position for labor and for birth which is least stressful to her baby and to herself.

12. *The Obstetric Patient has the right* to have her baby cared for at her bedside if her baby is normal, and to feed her baby according to her baby's needs rather than according to the hospital regimen.

13. *The Obstetric Patient has the right* to be informed in writing of the name of the person who actually delivered her baby and the professional qualifications of that person. This information should also be on the birth certificate.

14. *The Obstetric Patient has the right* to be informed if there is any known or indicated aspect of her or her baby's care or condition which may cause her or her baby later difficulty or problems.

Continued.

From Haire, D.B.: J. Nurse Midwife **20:**29, 1975.

The Pregnant Patient's Bill of Rights, cont'd

15. *The Obstetric Patient has the right* to have her and her baby's hospital medical records complete, accurate and legible and to have their records, including Nurses' Notes, retained by the hospital until the child reaches at least the age of majority, or, alternatively, to have the records offered to her before they are destroyed.

16. *The Obstetric Patient,* both during and after her hospital stay, has the right to have access to her complete hospital medical records, including Nurses' Notes, and to receive a copy upon payment of a reasonable fee and without incurring the expense of retaining an attorney.

It is the obstetric patient and her baby, not the health professional, who must sustain any trauma or injury resulting from the use of a drug or obstetric procedure. The observation of the rights listed above will not only permit the obstetric patient to participate in the decisions involving her and her baby's health care, but will help to protect the health professional and the hospital against litigation arising from resentment or misunderstanding on the part of the mother.

some states have passed laws requiring that parents of minors be informed if the minor seeks contraceptive information or treatment for venereal disease or if the minor girl becomes pregnant.

Infertility of couples who desire to have a child may pose legal questions that usually arise from the solution the couple chooses to solve their problem. One solution is the artificial insemination of a woman with sperm from a donor other than her husband. Because of the potential legal problems, the mother, her husband, and the donor must give written consent to the procedure. Preferably the husband and wife are not told the identity of the donor and vice versa.

Another solution to the problem of infertility is the use of a "surrogate mother." The husband donates sperm to be artificially inseminated into a woman who is not his wife. The woman bears the child and then relinquishes it to the husband and wife. Legal questions arise if the surrogate mother receives monetary compensation, since this might be defined as illegal "baby selling" (Annas, 1981). There may also be legal problems if the surrogate mother changes her mind and wants to keep the baby.

Certainly the most emotionally charged issue involved in the care of perinatal clients is abortion. Legal decisions about this issue have been made in legislative bodies and by the judicial process. One of the fundamental questions is when life begins, and the basic dilemma is which individual's rights are more important. If the fetus is a person, does it have a right to live, or should the woman's right to self-determination and privacy regarding her reproductive processes take precedence? There have been and probably will continue to be many legal changes regarding abortion. The nurse is obligated to be familiar with current laws affecting her practice in this area.

In most states and provinces, laws concerning abortion include provisions known as *conscience clauses.* These clauses allow nurses, physicians, and institutions to refuse to assist in abortions, without fear of reprisal, if it is against their ethical, moral, or religious principles (Harris, 1981). If a nurse is ethically or morally opposed to assisting in abortions, she should exercise her rights provided by conscience clauses. However, the nurse should never impose her values on her client (see Chapter 13).

Nurses have legal responsibilities regarding fetal monitoring during labor (Wiley, 1976). A claim of battery may be made if the nurse does not obtain the client's consent before attaching monitor leads. The nurse is also responsible for recognizing ominous fetal monitor patterns. If signs of fetal distress are noted, the nurse must notify the physician and prepare for emergency treatment such as an immediate cesarean section.

There are legal requirements in providing nursing care for newborns, such as properly identifying the infant-mother pair as soon as possible with fingerprints, footprints, and armbands or obtaining a sample for phenylketonuria (PKU) testing when required by law. Standards of care for the infant immediately after delivery include providing a clear airway, clamping the umbilical cord, and minimizing stress by drying the infant and keeping him warm. Resuscitation equipment must be available in the delivery room.

When a stillborn infant is delivered, the nurse must record all events surrounding the delivery. Although the atmosphere in a delivery room in this situation is disquieting, the nurse must complete legal requirements by careful documentation.

When an infant requiring intensive care is born, the

nurse has many legal responsibilities similar to those in other intensive care settings. Ethical problems involved in removing infants from ventilatory support are discussed in Chapter 14. There are legal questions as well; some view the withholding of treatment or nourishment as criminal homicide (Fost, 1982).

Iatrogenic disease caused by the treatment of a critically ill infant in a neonatal intensive care unit (NICU) may have legal consequences for those who have been involved in the infant's care. An iatrogenic disease is one resulting from treatment administered. For example, retrolental fibroplasia, a form of blindness caused by too much oxygen, is an iatrogenic disease. Frequent monitoring of the inspired oxygen concentration and frequent blood gas determinations are standards of care that must be met by nurses who work in an NICU.

BAPTISM

Parents of a seriously ill newborn may request that a minister or priest be called to baptize their infant. Roman Catholic parents might want their infant baptized by another Roman Catholic person if a priest is not available and the infant's death is imminent. A nurse may baptize an infant if his condition deteriorates, but she should determine that the parents wish to have the baby baptized. If the parents' religious beliefs do not include baptism and the nurse baptizes their infant, the act might be considered emotionally harmful to the parents.

Pediatric Nursing

Every state and province with child abuse legislation requires that suspected child abuse or neglect be reported. Health care professionals such as nurses are among those mandated to report suspected cases. To encourage persons to report such cases states and provinces provide legal immunity for the reporter if the report is made in good faith and without malice. A health care professional who does *not* report suspected child abuse or neglect may be held liable for civil or criminal legal action (Kreitzer, 1981).

As in all areas of nursing practice, negligence involving pediatric patients is possible. A $450,000 settlement was recently awarded in a New York case, *Beardsley v. Wyoming County Community Hospital*. A 6-year-old boy was taken to the hospital after a sledding accident. Although his prognosis was good following a splenectomy, the nurses administered D5W as his only intravenous fluid instead of alternating it with isotonic saline solution as ordered. Brain damage occurred, and although the boy's condition improved during the next 10 months, he was left with permanent residual damage. The monetary award was large because the boy had lost future earnings as a result of the nurses' negligent acts, which clearly did not meet appropriate standards of care. Regan (1981) suggests that monetary awards in future cases involving permanent injury to minors will probably be even higher.

A pediatric nurse is responsible for preventing a child in her care from accidentally harming himself. Cribs, which sometimes have a restraining device over the top, are designed to keep infants and toddlers from climbing out of bed and injuring themselves. All poisonous substances and sharp objects should be kept out of the reach of small children. Whenever possible, small children should be kept under constant surveillance to minimize opportunities for accidental harm.

Medical-Surgical Nursing

As in the case of pediatric clients, adults who are disoriented may require some form of restraint to prevent accidental self-injury. Side rails are available on most hospital beds to use with adult clients. Some disoriented elderly clients may also require belt restraints to prevent them from falling out of bed. If a client falls out of bed and injures himself, he may bring a lawsuit against the nurses and institution.

There are many other legal problems that can occur in the practice of medical-surgical nursing, such as those mentioned earlier in this chapter. Nurses who practice in this or any other area must be aware of the legal implications of their actions.

Critical Care Units

A nurse who works in a critical care setting is legally accountable for performing her duties as any well-trained critical care nurse would. Critical care nurses require additional training and ongoing in-service education to provide them with information regarding advances in care methods.

The staffing ratio in an intensive care setting should be one nurse for each client or at most 1:2½, depending on the severity of clients' conditions. The JCAH recommended these ratios because of the intensity of care required by such clients. They usually require careful observation and assessment of their condition and numerous treatment procedures, medications, or both. If a nurse is assigned to three or four intensive care clients and is unable to give appropriate care and a client suffers harm, the nurse would be liable for accepting the client assignment.

Possible legal problems for critical care nurses are associated with the use of electronic monitoring devices. No monitor can ever be considered totally reliable, and the nurse must not be completely dependent on it. There may also be electrical hazards. The equipment should be checked routinely by engineers to ensure that a client will not receive an electrical shock.

Psychiatric Nursing

The primary purpose for hospitalizing a client with mental illness is rehabilitation so that he may return to society as a useful and healthy citizen. Current principles of treatment suggest that a mentally ill client be given as much freedom as possible. One problem that arises from this freedom is the possibility that the client will slip away, or elope. If a client should be under close scrutiny because of his mental condition and the nurse fails to take due care to prevent his walking out of the health facility, the nurse and her employer would be held liable for any injuries the client sustains or inflicts as a result of his elopement.

Another concern for nurses who care for psychiatric clients is the possibility of client suicide. Obviously, if a client's history and hospital records indicate that he has suicidal tendencies, he must be kept under close surveillance.

Summary

The legal issues confronting practicing nurses today are many, but the nurse should view the law not with apprehension but as a helpful adjunct to defining nursing practice. Competent nursing care is an important part of all health care delivery systems. A nurse who is aware of legal rights and obligations will be better prepared to care for her clients.

Nursing standards of care serve to delineate and define appropriate nursing care. Some standards are stated in general terms such as those enacted in nursing practice statutes and those provided by the professional organizations of nurses. More specific standards are defined by a nurse's employing institution. If a nurse acts within the accepted standards of care, she reduces her chances of being involved in a malpractice lawsuit.

Some legal issues are involved in almost every branch of nursing, such as the necessity for informed consent, avoiding negligence, and the legal obligations involved in reporting unusual incidents. Some legal issues are confined to specific areas of nursing practice, such as conscience clauses for perinatal nurses asked to assist in abortions. However, regardless of the situation, nurses are responsible for knowing the laws that apply to their particular areas of nursing practice.

Any nurse who renders health care to clients must understand the legal significance of her acts. Knowledge of the law is necessary for all nurses in practice.

KEY CONCEPTS

✓ With the increased emphasis on client rights, a nurse in practice today must understand her legal obligations and responsibilities to her clients.

✓ The civil law system is concerned with the protection of a person's private rights, and the criminal law system deals with the rights of both individuals and society as a whole as defined by legislative statutes.

✓ Under the law, the practicing nurse must follow standards of care, which originate in nurse practice acts, the guidelines of professional organizations, and written policies and procedures of employing institutions.

✓ Both registered nurses and licensed practical nurses are licensed by the state or province in which they practice, based on educational requirements, the passing of an examination, and other criteria.

✓ A student nurse is expected to perform as a professional nurse, should be assigned only to tasks for which she is prepared, and should be carefully supervised.

✓ A tort is a civil wrong committed against a person or property, including unintentional torts such as negligence and intentional torts such as assault and battery.

✓ Nurses are responsible for performing all procedures correctly and exercising professional judgment as they carry out physician orders; otherwise they may be guilty of negligence.

✓ All clients are entitled to confidential health care and freedom from unauthorized release of information; otherwise the nurse may be guilty of invasion of privacy, slander, or libel.

✓ Assault is an act intended to coerce or provoke fear; nurses should act and speak carefully to avoid frightening, coercing, or physically intimidating clients.

✓ Battery is a willful, angry, or negligent touching of another's body or property in contact with the person; informed consent allows physical procedures to be carried out in a lawful manner.

✓ A nurse can be found guilty of malpractice if the following criteria are established: (1) the nurse (defendant) owed a duty to her client (plaintiff); (2) the nurse did not carry out that duty; (3) the client was injured; and (4) the client's injury resulted from the nurse's failure to carry out her duty.

✓ The nurse is responsible for confirming that informed consent has been given for any surgery or other medical procedure before the procedure is performed.

✓ Informed consent must meet the following criteria: (1) the person giving consent must be competent and of legal age; (2) the consent must be given voluntarily; (3) the person giving consent must thoroughly understand the procedure and its risks and benefits, as well as alternative procedures; and (4) the person giving consent has a right to have all of his questions answered to his satisfaction.

✓ In emergency situations informed consent is not necessary if it is impossible to obtain consent from either the client or an authorized person.

✓ Legal issues involving death include documenting all events surrounding the death, treating a deceased person with dignity (wrongful handling is grounds for a lawsuit), and obtaining consent for an autopsy from either the decedent (before death) or a close family member.

KEY CONCEPTS, *cont'd*

✓ A competent adult can legally give consent to donate specific organs, and the nurse may serve as the witness to his decision.

✓ Nurses may be witnesses for clients' wills, which must meet certain legal criteria.

✓ The nurse is obligated to follow the physician's order unless the nurse believes the order is in error or could be detrimental to the client, in which case the nurse must make a formal report explaining the refusal.

✓ Staffing standards have been set for the ratio of nurses to clients, and if the nurse is required to care for more clients than is reasonable, a formal protest should be made to nursing administration.

✓ The nurse must file an incident report in any unusual situation when there is a possibility of a lawsuit; such reports are also used for quality assurance and risk management.

✓ Depending on state and province laws, nurses are required to report child abuse; other possible criminal activities such as gunshot wounds, attempted suicide, or rape; and certain communicable diseases.

✓ Conscience clauses in most state and province laws allow any health care professional or institution to refuse to assist in abortions without fear of reprisal if it is against their ethical, moral, or religious principles.

✓ Nurses who practice in specialized areas such as critical care are legally accountable for performing specialized duties and therefore require additional training and ongoing in-service education.

REFERENCES

Annas, G.: Contracts to bear a child: compassion or commercialism? Harvey Lect., Hastings Center Report 11(2):23, 1981.

Cazalas, M.W.: Nursing and the law, ed. 3, Rockville, Md., 1978, Aspen Systems Corp.

Creighton, H.: Law every nurse should know, ed. 4, Philadelphia, 1981, W.B. Saunders Co.

Cushing, M.: Verbal no-code orders, Am. J. Nurs. 81:1215, 1981.

Fenner, K.: Ethics and law in nursing: professional perspectives, New York, 1980, Van Nostrand Reinhold Co., Inc.

Fost, N.: Putting hospitals on notice, Hosting Center Report, p. 5, August 1982.

Harris, C.H.: Legal and ethical aspects of maternity nursing. In Jensen, M., Benson, R., and Bobak, I., editors: Maternity care: the nurse and the family, St. Louis, 1981, The C.V. Mosby Co.

Hemelt, M.D., and Mackert, M.E.: Dynamics of law in nursing and health care, ed. 2, Reston, Va., 1982, Reston Publishing Co., Inc.

Horsley, J.E.: Short-staffing means increased liability for you, RN 44:73, 1981.

Kreitzer, M.: Legal aspects of child abuse: guidelines for the nurse, Nurs. Clin. North Am. 16(1):149, 1981.

Regan, W.A.: Nursing malpractice: a giant leap in damages, RN 44:69, 1981.

Rocereto, L.R., and Maleski, C.M.: The legal dimensions of nursing practice, New York, 1982, Springer Publishing Co., Inc.

Rothman, D.A., and Rothman, N.L.: The professional nurse and the law, Boston, 1977, Little, Brown & Co.

Wiley, J.: The nurse's legal responsibility in obstetric monitoring, J.O.G.N. 5(suppl.):77s, 1976.

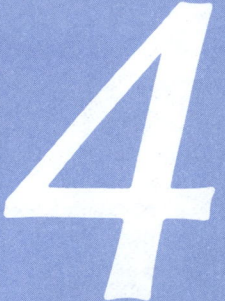

4

More than other health care professionals, nurses have the opportunity to address clients' needs on all levels, including psychosocial as well as physiological needs. Recognizing that clients are complex, multidimensional individuals, nurses by using the nursing process can provide health care in these areas through a holistic approach.

The five chapters in Unit 4 consider fundamental psychosocial needs nurses frequently encounter in practice. Illness or other problems may result in alterations in self-concept or body image or may adversely affect the client's sexual dimension. Similarly, illness may threaten the client's spirituality, or the client's spiritual resources may help in coping with the stresses of illness. Because psychosocial variables are culturally influenced, nursing care for ethnic or minority clients is based on an understanding of the client's cultural background. Finally, nursing care provided from a perspective including the client's family more fully assists both the client and the family in attaining their health goals.

Caring for Clients with Psychosocial Needs

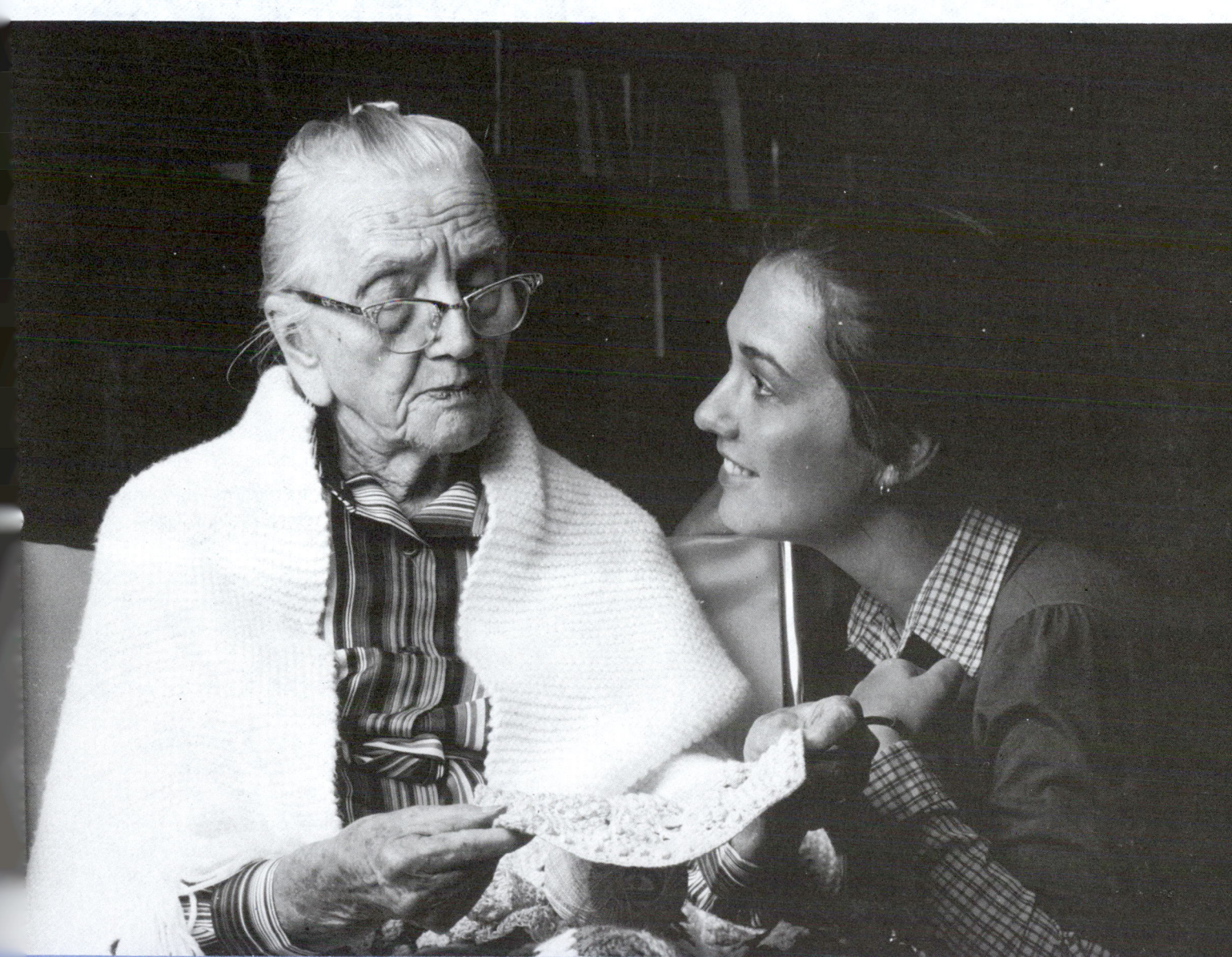

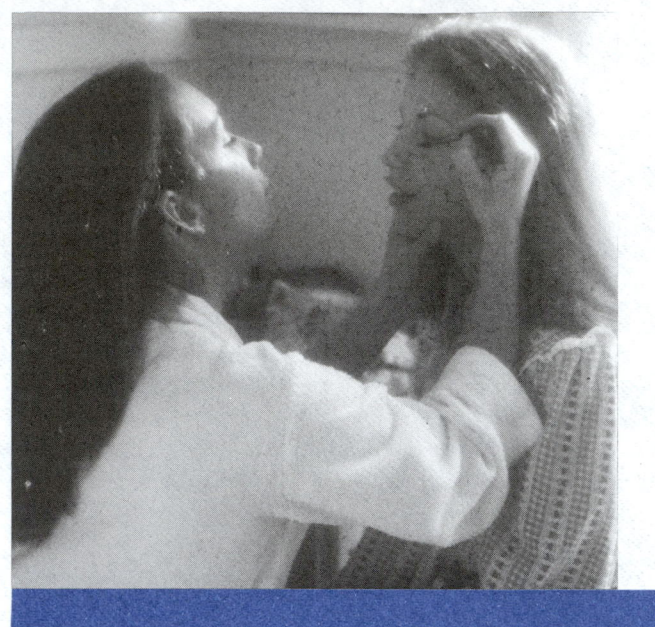

OBJECTIVES

Mastery of content in this chapter will enable the student to:

- Define the terms in the glossary.
- Describe how the self-concept develops by discussing Piaget's cognitive stages and Erikson's psychosocial stages.
- Discuss factors that influence each of the four components of self-concept: body image, self-esteem, roles, and identity.
- Describe the five processes of socialization.
- Identify stressors that affect each of the four components of self-concept.
- Explain the processes that can lead to role conflict, role ambiguity, and role strain.
- Discuss identity confusion as a developmental aspect of adolescence and as a problem of self-concept.
- Discuss ways in which the nurse's self-concept and nursing activities can affect the client's self-concept.
- Describe behaviors that may indicate each of the following: low self-esteem, disturbed body image, role strain, identity confusion, and depersonalization.
- List, for each of the four components of self-concept, at least two common nursing diagnoses in regard to alterations in self-concept.
- Describe the goals of care and specific nursing actions for each of the five levels of intervention for a client with an altered self-concept.

GLOSSARY

depersonalization Extreme form of identity confusion in which a person is unable to distinguish between inner and outer realities or between himself and others.

identity Component of self-concept; one's persisting consciousness of being oneself, separate and distinct from others.

identity confusion Form of altered self-concept in which a person does not maintain a clear consciousness of a consistent and continuous self.

imitation Process of socialization in which one acquires behaviors, knowledge, or skills from members of one's cultural group.

inhibition Process of socialization in which one learns to refrain from a behavior even when motivated to engage in that behavior.

reinforcement-extinction Process of socialization in which one learns to engage in certain behaviors (reinforcement) or to avoid certain behaviors (extinction).

role Set of behaviors by means of which a person participates in a social group.

role ambiguity State in which a person has unclear role expectations and feels unable to predict the outcomes of his behavior.

role conflict State in which a person experiences incongruent or incompatible expectations within one role or between two or more simultaneously held roles.

18 Self-Concept

role overload State in which a person experiences conflicting role priorities and must decide with which pressures to comply.

role strain Generalized state of frustration or anxiety produced by the stress of role conflict and ambiguity.

self-concept Complex integration of conscious and unconscious feelings, attitudes, and perceptions about one's identity, worth, roles, and physical being; how a person perceives and defines himself.

self-esteem Component of self-concept; a person's sense of self-worth.

self-ideal Aspirations, goals, values, and standards of behavior that a person considers ideal and strives to attain.

socialization Process by which a person, from infancy, acquires values, behaviors, skills, and roles from social norms and significant others.

A person's self-concept represents a complex integration of conscious and unconscious feelings, attitudes, and perceptions about his own worth, role, and physical being; it reflects his interpretations of past experiences, social interactions, and sensations. A person's self-concept is what he believes about himself as a separate and distinct entity; it is based in part on how he believes others see him (Cooley, 1956).

Self-concept is not the same as the self. The self includes the total subjective and objective qualities of a person as seen by himself and others. For example, the self includes the person's actual appearance, values, ideas, and knowledge, as well as the perceptions other persons have of the individual. Self-concept is the person's subjective image of the self—his perception of physical, emotional, and social attributes or qualities. The self-concept is a frame of reference for the individual that affects how the person deals with situations and relates to others. An individual's image of the self may or may not be accurate, and while the self may constantly undergo change, a person's self-concept is slow to change (Yamamoto, 1972). Discrepancies between the self and the self-concept may become a source of stress or conflict.

Hospitalization, illness, surgery, separation from family, and other health factors can affect various aspects of a person's self-concept. For example, amputation of an extremity results in an altered body image. The person's adaptation to the amputation includes integrating the bodily change into the concept of self in relation to the body—that is, body image. Chronic illness may affect a person's ability to provide financial support for his family, thereby affecting his sense of self-worth and his role within the family. These changes will also alter his self-concept. In each of these two examples, the altered self-concept would be readily apparent to a nurse. But many changes in clients' self-concepts may not be as apparent; therefore a nurse must understand how stressors affect self-concept and be able to recognize behaviors that show that a client is in need of nursing care directed toward assisting him with altered self-concepts.

The purpose of this chapter is to provide an overview of the development of self-concept, stressors affecting self-concept, and the role of the nurse in relation to the self-concepts of clients. To provide nursing care for a client with self-concept problems, the nurse uses the nursing process—assessing the client's condition, determining the nursing diagnosis, planning and implementing care, and evaluating care.

Development of Self-Concept

The development and maintenance of a self-concept constitute a complex process involving many variables. Of the major theories concerned with how the self-concept develops, those of Piaget and Erikson are perhaps most useful to the nurse. Erikson describes eight stages of psychosocial development, the completion of each of which is important to the evolution of a person's self-concept (Erikson, 1963). Piaget describes four stages of cognitive development (Piaget and Inhelder, 1969). These two theories do not conflict but rather represent different ways of looking at the development of self-concept.

Cognitive development involves the process of how a person patterns and organizes stimuli. A child progresses from a reflexive infant to an abstractly thinking adolescent through a schematic structuring of stimuli. Piaget defines "schema" as an organized form of behavior that has a definite purpose and that is associated with a particular mental representation of experiences and events. A child internalizes various events. Through assimilation, old schemata are used to solve new problems. The cognitive process of accommodation involves developing new schemata from old ones to solve new problems. The development of cognitive processes, according to Piaget, occurs in predictable ways, and everyone develops cognitively in similar patterns. Nurses can use Piaget's theory to examine the development of self-concept and also to plan nursing interventions for newborns, infants, children, and adolescents.

In each stage of psychosocial development, an individual faces certain tasks that, if not positively completed, may lead to psychological problems. Through social and cultural reinforcement, an individual learns the relevance of concepts, the cultural connotations of concepts, and the emotional significance of concepts. Erikson's theory demonstrates the influence of society on the development of self-concept. For example, an infant needs to develop a sense of trust if he is to be psychologically healthy. An infant who learns through parental reinforcement to trust his world will feel secure as an adult. Mistrust arises from uncertainty, frustration, discomfort, or physical harm. If a person does not develop a sense of trust as an infant, he may have difficulty with later psychosocial development. If he becomes ill as an adult, for example, he may experience a sense of physical and psychosocial vulnerability and a distrust of the environment, especially a hospital environment. With an insecure self-concept, he may have more difficulty with the changes caused by illness or therapy than the average person would have.

Piaget's stages of cognitive development and Erikson's stages of psychosocial development are discussed in more detail in Chapter 23.

Components of Self-Concept

A person's self-concept has four aspects: body image, self-esteem, roles, and identity. Each aspect develops from birth onward and reflects the changes that take place throughout the life span. Although these four components can be considered as separate aspects of a person's self-concept, they overlap and are interrelated. Thus, a person's self-concept can be described in terms of a continuum from strong to weak, or positive to negative, depending on the individual strengths of the four components.

Body Image

Body image is an individual's psychological experience of his body; it includes his feelings and attitudes toward his body. A person's self-concept is influenced by his view of his physical characteristics and physical abilities. The reverse is also true: a person's self-concept influences how he views his body.

Body image is affected by cognitive growth and by physical development. Any physical stimulus, whether originating inside or outside a person, affects the mental image or concept that person has of his body. Normal developmental changes, such as growth and aging, have a more apparent effect on a person's body image than on other aspects of self-concept. For example, a 2-year-old's body image is very different from an infant's, because of the ability to walk. This physical change, walking, depends on physical maturation. Somatic, behavioral, and topological elements or stimuli also play a part in the development and maturation of body image. Somatic elements include neurological, metabolic, endocrine, and hormonal factors. Hormonal changes occur during adolescence and in later stages of life (for example, menopause), influencing a person's body image. Aging involves a decrease in visual acuity, hearing, mobility, and perception, all of which may affect body image. Behavioral elements include experiences related to a person's cognitive, motor, and perceptual experiences and development. Topological stimuli are superficial sensations and physical characteristics of the body surface. Topological stimuli are particularly important during adolescence, when significant physical changes occur. During aging, topological stimuli are again important, as a person recognizes physical signs of old age.

Cultural and societal attitudes and values influence a person's body image. Youth, beauty, and wholeness are emphasized in American society, a fact that is apparent in television programs, movies, and advertisements. These attitudes and values affect how a person perceives his physical body, because body image is a combination of the ideal and the real.

Since a person's body image depends only partly on the reality of the body, people generally do not adapt quickly to changes in the physical body. As with the total self-concept, a physical change may not be incorporated into the image one has of one's body. Studies have shown, for example, that even people who have experienced significant weight loss do not readily perceive themselves as thin; in some cases such people continue dieting to an extreme in an effort to become thin, since they still have their old body images. Another example is normal aging. People often report that they do not feel different, but when they look in the mirror they are surprised by the older face or the gray hair.

Self-Esteem

Like body image, self-esteem is based on many internal and external factors. Self-esteem is an individual's sense of self-worth, an evaluation that an individual makes and maintains about himself. According to Erikson, the young child begins to develop a sense of usefulness by learning to act on his own initiative. Self-esteem is often related to a person's evaluation of his effectiveness at school, at work, within the family, and in other situations. Society and the family generally set the standards by which an individual evaluates himself.

Self-evaluation is an ongoing mental process. Self-

worth or self-esteem is a basic human need, according to Maslow's hierarchy (see Chapter 4). A person has an imperative need to feel competent and worthy of living. Self-esteem is thus involved in the enhancement and maintenance of self-concept. The value that a person feels he has is an important factor in psychosocial development and motivation (Gibson, 1980).

Self-esteem, although it depends on many factors, can be understood in terms of the relationship of a person's self-concept to his ideal self. The ideal self consists of the aspirations, goals, values, and standards of behavior that the person considers ideal and strives to attain. The ideal self originates in early childhood and develops throughout life; it is influenced by societal norms and the expectations and demands of parents and significant others. In general, a person whose self-concept comes close to matching his ideal self has a high level of self-esteem, whereas a person whose self-concept varies widely from his ideal self has a low level of self-esteem (Fig. 18-1).

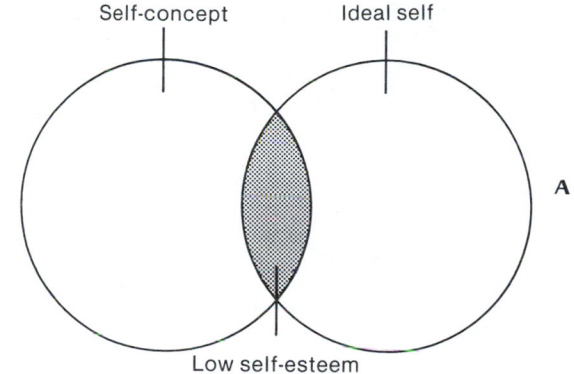

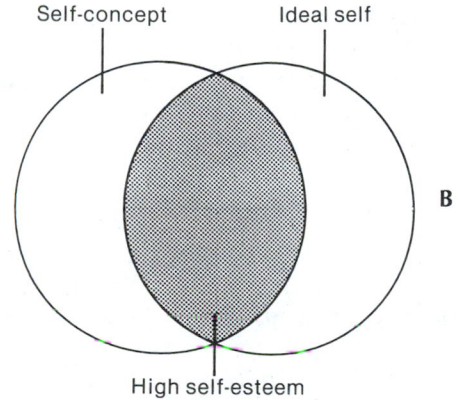

Fig. 18-1 **A,** Individual with a low level of self-esteem owing to a large discrepancy between self-concept and ideal self. **B,** Person with greater conformity of self-concept and ideal self and therefore with a high level of self-esteem.

Modified from Sundeen, S.J., et al.: Nurse-client interaction, ed. 2, St. Louis, 1981, The C.V. Mosby Co.

Studies have shown that extreme disparity between ideal self and self-concept is characteristic of many persons with mental illness.

Roles

A role is a set of behaviors by which a person participates in a social group. Each individual may have many roles. A woman may behave in one set of ways in the role of mother, in another set of ways as a career woman, and in a third set of ways as a daughter. Roles involve expectations or standards of behavior that have been accepted by society or the social group, such as family or community, in which one participates. A person's behavior is based on patterns established through the process of socialization. Socialization is the "acquisition of the requisite orientation for satisfactory functioning in a role" (Parsons, 1951). The process of socialization begins just after birth, when an infant responds to an adult and the adult responds to the behavior of the infant. Parsons (1951, 1972) considers the value-orientation patterns established in childhood to be a basic personality structure. The patterns are stable and change only minimally during adulthood. There are five methods through which the child learns behaviors that are sanctioned or approved by society:

1. *Reinforcement-extinction*—the process by which certain behaviors become common or are avoided, depending on whether they are reinforced or discouraged
2. *Inhibition*—the process by which a person learns to refrain from a behavior even when motivated to engage in the behavior
3. *Substitution*—replacement of one behavior by another that provides the same gratification
4. *Imitation*—the process by which one acquires knowledge, skills, or behaviors from members of one's social or cultural group
5. *Identification*—internalization of the values of a role model

During the socialization process a person generally develops the skills necessary for satisfactory functioning in many different roles. Unsuccessful socialization may lead to an inability to function acceptably according to society's values.

Brim and Wheeler (1966) differentiate between socialization of children and socialization of adults. Adults are more concerned with the actual behavior appropriate to roles than with learning the basic values implicit in roles. Adults are also expected to distinguish between ideal role expectations and realistic expectations. In addition, adults experience many roles and role expectations and increased role speci-

ficity. The self-other relationship is most important to adults. In other words, adults are concerned about their relationships with other persons in their lives. The success of relationships in various roles contributes to the adult's sense of well-being. In contrast, the I-me relationship predominates in children. The child learns about his own physical being and his immediate environment. Only after the child becomes comfortable with his physical self and has established trust in parents can he begin to socialize with other children.

An individual learns behaviors that are appropriate to a given role through interactions with people who hold beliefs about appropriate behaviors and who reward or punish the individual on the basis of those beliefs. To function effectively in a role, a person must know what the expected behavior and values are, must desire to conform to them, and must be able to meet the role requirements.

Roles involve three components: the individual, or actor; the behavior, or action; and the relationships between the individual and the behavior (Biddle and Thomas, 1966). Most individuals have more than one role. Common roles include mother or father, wife or husband, daughter or son, employee, friend, or boss. Each role involves meeting certain expectations of others. Fulfillment of these expectations leads to rewards; failure to comply with them leads to sanctions.

Identity

"Identity" is derived from the Latin word *idem*, which means "the same." Identity involves the persistent individuality and sameness of a person over time and in various circumstances; identity thus includes a level of consistency and continuity. It implies a consciousness of being oneself, distinct and separate from others.

Adolescence, Erikson's fifth stage of development, is a particularly crucial time for the development of identity. Adolescence is a time of physical changes, peer pressure, and preparation for future independence. If a person is unable to meet societal expectations and define himself, he experiences role diffusion, a form of identity confusion resulting from unclear roles. Identity is a complex, dynamic state. It includes a conscious sense of individuality, an unconscious striving for consistency in personal character, and maintenance of solidarity with the ideals of one's social group. An adolescent has an obvious need to belong and to be accepted by a peer group. The ability to form an identity is also related to cognitive development, for a person must be able to label himself and perceive labeling by others. A person with a sense of identity will feel integrated rather than diffuse.

During socialization, children experience the identification process and thereby learn culturally accepted behaviors and roles. A child identifies with parents, peers, teachers, culture heroes, and so on. To form an identity, he must have the ability to synthesize these learned behaviors into a coherent, consistent, and unique whole (Stuart and Sundeen, 1983). This synthesizing process is particularly characteristic of adolescence. However, a person's sense of identity is continually evolving and is influenced by his circumstances throughout life. The achievement of identity is necessary for involvement in intimate relationships, since much of a person's identity is expressed in relationships with others.

Sexual identity is a part of a person's general sense of identity. Sexual identity is the image a person has of himself or herself as a male or a female and the meaning that this has for the person. This image and its meaning depend on standards learned through the socialization process.

When a person behaves in ways that conform to his self-concept, he reinforces his sense of identity. But when a person behaves in ways that contradict his self-concept, he may experience anxiety and apprehension.

Stressors Affecting Self-Concept

A self-concept stressor is any factor or change, whether real or perceived, that threatens an individual's body image, self-esteem, roles, or sense of identity. Stressors challenge the adaptive capacities of a person. Stress is not unique to any one age group or to any cultural or economic group. Selye (1956) states that stress is "not the specific result of any one among our actions; nor is it a typical response to any one thing acting upon us from without; it is a common feature of all biological activities." Whether internal or external, the influencing factor affects an individual's equilibrium.

Different individuals react to the same situation with different degrees of stress. A variety of responses to stress may be observed, including anxiety, frustration, anger, inability to adjust to a situation, difficulty making decisions, and tension. An individual's perception of stress is an important factor that influences his response. A person does not have to understand a specific stressor in order to feel stress, as long as he perceives the stressor. Each person has learned a pattern of behavior that enables him to cope with or adapt to stressors. For example, some people apply problem-solving methods to stressful situations.

However, some people are immobilized by perceived threats and require help from other people. Adaptive patterns allow an individual to cope, but prolonged stress can deplete an individual's adaptive ability.

Stressors can affect a person's self-concept in any or all of its components. Hospitalization, illness, and surgery are common stressors that can have interrelated effects on self-concept. A physical change in the body leads to an altered body image, but the person's self-esteem and identity may also be affected. Certain chronic illnesses alter a person's roles, which may change his self-esteem and identity. The following example illustrates this interrelatedness of the four components of the self-concept. Assume that a man is injured in a car accident and that he experiences a loss of body function (paralysis of the legs and urinary incontinence) that causes an altered body image. The man had been a construction worker but can no longer function in his old job, resulting in an altered role. His self-esteem may be diminished because he no longer supports himself, and his identity will change in certain areas. Thus he will no longer have the same self-concept that he had before the accident. Because the self may change more quickly than the self-concept, he may experience a disparity between his self-concept and his reality, leading to stress and anxiety. His previous life experiences, his coping strategies, and his resources will influence how he adapts to his losses and changes.

A crisis is an experience of imbalance that occurs when a person cannot overcome obstacles with his usual methods of problem solving and adapting. During a self-concept crisis, as with other kinds of crises, supportive resources are often necessary to help the person learn new ways of coping with and responding to the event or situation.

The example of the paralyzed man involves a major crisis; this client requires help in adapting, and time is required in order for interventions to succeed. Rehabilitation and restoration of a positive self-concept do occur following traumatic events. An understanding of the relationships among a person's body image, self-esteem, roles, and identity is essential to the planning of appropriate nursing interventions.

Body-Image Stressors

Changes in the appearance or function of a body part or feature will require change in the person's body image. Changes in the appearance of the body, such as amputation or facial disfigurement, are obvious stressors affecting body image. Colostomy or ileostomy also alters the appearance and function of the body but the changes are not apparent when the person is dressed and active. Stressors that affect the body image through a change in function include renal disease and cardiac disease, in either of which the body no longer functions at an optimal level and the person is physically limited. Even the "normal" body changes resulting from aging are stressors that can affect a person's body image. Pregnancy affects body image, as does any significant weight gain or loss. Stressors affecting body image can be related to injuries from war or accidents, diseases involving sensorimotor change, physical alterations owing to surgical intervention, or toxic or metabolic disorders that may slowly alter a body function or require changes in such areas as diet and activity level.

The significance of a change in the appearance of the body or a loss of function varies among individuals and cultures. Paralysis caused by a war injury may be considered acceptable; the person may be treated as a hero and be praised for his bravery and strength, and governmental resources will be available to assist him in his rehabilitation. However, a young man who falls from a tree while drinking and suffers severe injuries and paralysis may receive a different response from society; people may be less accepting of his situation, and financial resources may be more difficult to obtain.

The significance of a loss of function or a change in appearance is affected by the individual's perception of the alteration, because body image consists of both ideal and real elements. For example, femininity is sometimes associated with the size of the breasts, and if a woman's body image incorporates this as the ideal, the loss of a breast by mastectomy may be a very significant alteration. Another consideration is the importance of body image within a person's self-concept. The greater the importance of body image, the greater the threat that a change in body image may be to the person's perception of self. In the example just mentioned, the woman's sexual identity may be affected by the loss of the breast.

Many people associate success with a specific body part or function. For example, an athletic person may consider his body and his physical activities to be the focus of his personal success. What happens if an accident occurs and he can never again participate in physical activities? How will he adapt or become rehabilitated? How does he revise long-accepted assumptions about himself and alter his life-style, including his sexual functioning? In order to regain a positive self-concept and maintain good health, he must adapt to the body-image stressor.

Studies have shown that after head and neck surgery people generally participate less in social interaction (Dropkin, 1979). A person who has had facial alterations may feel isolated, excluded, stigmatized, or helpless. The feeling of social isolation is often based in reality, because people are often afraid of embarrassing or offending a person who is in a wheelchair or who is badly burned or "deformed," and thus they avoid contact with the person. A person with an altered body image may fear rejection and isolation.

There have been and continue to be positive social changes with regard to illness and altered body image. The news media have increasingly presented positive stories about persons who have had major body-altering surgery. For example, accounts of a Canadian runner who was struck by a car and paralyzed showed this young man in a realistic but positive light. Recovery after mastectomy and procedures for performing breast self-examination have been presented on television. Movies have documented the amazing rehabilitation of young people after severe trauma. These stories presenting real people coping and adapting provide role models for persons undergoing unusual stressors, and for families, friends, and society. This social change may be helpful in eliminating much of the stigma associated with altered physical appearance for functioning, thereby reducing stressors to body image.

Self-help groups are available in most communities for persons who have had ostomies (United Ostomy Association), mastectomies (Reach to Recovery), or laryngectomies (Laryngectomy Club). Self-help groups assist people who are trying to lose weight, parents of children with spina bifida, and people with cancer. These groups provide a special kind of support. Someone who has experienced a particular stressor and who has adapted to it can be instrumental in helping a hospitalized client adapt to a body image change. Such a person can be a special role model, and his spouse or significant other can help the client's spouse assist in the adaptation.

Self-Esteem Stressors

Self-esteem is the sense of being competent and worthy. Self-esteem begins to develop in infancy, when perceived acceptance or rejection by parents is an important factor. Persons with high self-esteem are generally happier and more able to cope with demands and stressors than persons with low self-esteem (Gibson, 1980). Persons with low self-esteem tend to feel unloved and often experience depression and anxiety.

Many stressors may affect the self-esteem of the infant, toddler, preschooler, or adolescent. Inability to meet parental expectations, harsh criticism, inconsistent punishment, sibling rivalry, inability to emulate a successful sibling or parent, or repeated defeats may reduce the level of self-worth. Stressors affecting the self-esteem of adults include failures in relationships, divorce, and loss of a job.

Illness, surgery, or accidents that interrupt or change a person's life patterns may also decrease his feeling of self-worth. Chronic illnesses such as diabetes, arthritis, and cardiac dysfunction require changes in a person's accepted and long-assumed behavioral patterns. When a change is slow and progressive, the person sometimes has an opportunity for anticipatory mourning, and adaptation occurs along with the change. However, the more a chronic illness interferes with a person's ability to engage in activities that make him feel worthy or successful, the more it will affect his self-esteem.

An individual's evaluation of himself is based on relationships with others and on his activities. How an individual defines success or failure influences whether a change is a stressor in terms of his self-concept. Many people, for example, consider success at work to be important to a sense of achievement and worth. Chronic illness, surgery, or severe trauma may necessitate a change in a person's life work and thus may be a self-esteem stressor.

Societal standards and the responses of significant others also affect the significance of a stressor and its impact on self-esteem. Dyk and Sutherland (1956), in a classic study of ostomy patients, found that a husband generally accepted his wife's colostomy more readily than a wife accepted her husband's, apparently because society expects men to be strong, healthy, and working. Wives tended to view a colostomy as an indication that a man was now sick, in need of physical help, and unable to reenter the work force, even when the colostomy did not alter his ability to work.

Role Stressors

Throughout life a person undergoes numerous role changes. Both change within the same role and the adoption of new roles require the incorporation of new expectations and standards for behavior. Meleis (1975) identifies three categories of role transition: developmental, situational, and health-illness. Normal changes associated with growth and maturation result in developmental transitions. Situational transitions occur when one loses a parent, spouse, or close friend, moves, marries, or changes jobs. A health-illness transition is a movement from a state of health or well-being to one of illness. Any of these types of role transitions may threaten a person's self-concept. They may result in role conflict, role ambiguity, or role strain.

Role conflict is a lack of congruent or compatible role expectations (Broadwell, 1983). When a person is required to simultaneously assume two or more roles that have inconsistent, contradictory, or mutually exclusive expectations, role conflict may occur. For example, a woman's professional role may include the expectation that she make decisions on her own, while her role as a spouse may include the expectation that she share decision making equally with her husband; role conflict could result if she had to act in both roles simultaneously, such as if her job required her to relocate. The importance of each of the conflicting roles influences the degree of conflict the person experiences. A major role is a significant frame of reference; it influences how a person evaluates other role situations. Role conflict usually involves situations in which there is inconsistency between two or more expected and sanctioned behaviors and the person's major role does not eliminate this inconsistency.

There are four basic kinds of role conflict, which are distinguished according to the source of the conflicting expectations. Interpersonal conflict occurs when one or more other people have opposing or incompatible expectations for an individual in a particular role. For example, a woman's friends may have different expectations of how she should care for her children. Interrole conflict occurs when pressures or expectations associated with a role in one group oppose pressures or expectations associated with a role in another group. A man who compulsively works 10 to 12 hours a day at his job may have problems if his wife expects him to be home with the family. Person-role conflict occurs when role requirements violate the values of an individual. For example, a nurse who values the preservation of life will have conflict when faced with assisting a woman undergoing an abortion. Role overload is a conflict of priorities in which an individual is unable to decide with which pressures to comply. Role overload is a complex type of conflict involving both internal and external conflicts. A person may be expected to comply with the role expectations of one or more persons. He attempts to establish priorities; however, if it is impossible to deny any of the pressures, role overload develops. The expectations of the various roles become overwhelming, and the person does not have the physical, intellectual, economical, emotional, and other resources to adapt to or perform in them.

Role ambiguity involves unclear role expectations and an inability to predict the reactions of others to one's behavior (Broadwell, 1983). When there are unclear expectations, a person is unsure of what he is to do, how he is to do it, or both. Such a situation is often stressful and confusing. Role ambiguity is common in adolescence. Adolescents are pressured by parents, peers, and the media to assume adultlike roles. They may be expected to work, yet employment opportunities may be severely limited. Their parents may emphasize one set of expectations, yet not meet them themselves. For example, parents may demand that an adolescent not drink and drive, yet the adolescent may observe that they drink and drive themselves. Role ambiguity is also common in employment situations. In organizations that are complex, rapidly changing, or highly specialized, employees often become unsure of what is expected of them.

Role strain is a general term that incorporates role conflict and role ambiguity. Role strain may be expressed as a feeling of frustration resulting from the fact that a person feels inadequate or unsuited to a role. Role strain is often associated with sex role stereotypes (Stuart and Sundeen, 1983). Women in positions typically held by men may be perceived by others as less competent, less objective, or less knowledgeable than their male counterparts. Thus, many women in such situations feel that they must work harder and be better than average in order to compete. Men in typically female roles also encounter bias. In addition, a person's femininity or masculinity may be questioned, resulting in further stress.

Chapter 2 describes the sick role as an aspect of illness behavior. This role involves the expectations of others, and thus role strain may occur in association with the sick role. A person is expected to seek health care, to be ill only temporarily, to acknowledge that illness is undesirable, and to be dependent on health care providers. Role conflict may occur between any of these general societal expectations and the expectations of co-workers, family members, and others. For example, even though a person with a cardiac illness is expected to reduce his participation in physically stressful activities, friends may after a month or two expect the person to again participate in such activities, producing stress for the person.

The sick role may also involve role ambiguity. A person is expected to be dependent and yet, simultaneously, to participate actively so that he can be well and leave the sick role quickly. What then is expected of a chronically ill person? The sick role is supposed to be temporary, yet compliance with therapy may be necessary for the remainder of his life. At what point is the sick role no longer acceptable? How much dependence, submission, and undemanding behavior is required?

Clients who bring work to the hospital, keep in close contact with business associates, ask questions, and so on, may be considered "bad" clients by some health care workers. But then so are clients who will not help themselves, who are too dependent, or who do not resume social roles. In addition, sick role behaviors and expectations are based on societal standards. The standards adopted by health care providers may change more quickly than those accepted by clients, resulting in role strain.

Identity Stressors

A person's identity is affected by stressors throughout his lifetime. Adolescence, for example, is a critical period for the development of identity; many stressors during this stage may affect a person's sense of identity. Adolescence is a time of change, insecurity, and anxiety. The adolescent is trying to adjust to the physical and mental changes of his increasing maturity. He is required to prepare for a vocation, seek economic independence, form close relationships, and cope with emerging sexuality. Stressors may arise in any of these areas or as a result of conflicts between them.

An adult generally has a more stable identity and a more firmly held image of himself. Cultural and social, rather than personal, stressors may have more impact on an adult's identity. Social stressors may challenge an adult's values. Examples include finding oneself in the position of having to decide between career and marriage, cooperation and competition, or dependence and independence in a relationship (Stuart and Sundeen, 1983).

Menopause, retirement, decreasing physical abilities, and other factors associated with aging will also affect a person's sense of identity. Identity, like body image, is closely related to how one looks or what one can do. Changes in appearance and physical capabilities necessitate adaptation. Another potential stressor during this stage of life involves the question of whether a person has accomplished his life goals. Retirement may mean the loss of an important means of achievement and continued success. A person may begin to question who he is and what he has accomplished. Physical and emotional isolation may add additional stress as significant others die. Identity confusion, a form of altered self-concept in which a person does not maintain a clear, consistent, and continuous consciousness of personal identity, may result if he is unable to adapt to identity stressors. In extreme cases an individual may experience depersonalization, a state in which he is unable to distinguish between inner and outer realities or between self and others.

■ ■ ■ ■ ■

Thus a person's self-concept can be altered by stressors affecting body image, self-esteem, roles, or identity. Self-concept may also be affected by physical stressors, which can temporarily alter a person's perceptions or level of consciousness. Lack of oxygen, hyperventilation, biochemical imbalances, and sen-

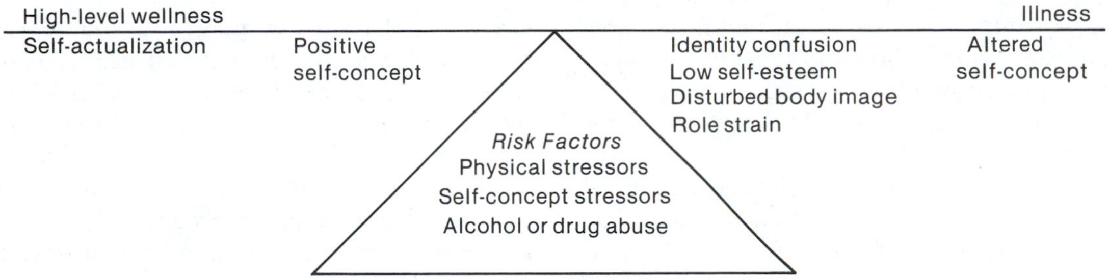

High-level wellness .... Illness

| Self-actualization | Positive self-concept | | Identity confusion | Altered self-concept |

Identity confusion
Low self-esteem
Disturbed body image
Role strain

Risk Factors
Physical stressors
Self-concept stressors
Alcohol or drug abuse

Fig. 18-2   Self-concept health-illness continuum.

sory deprivation, for example, will alter how one perceives the world and himself. Alcohol, drugs, and other toxic substances may also distort these perceptions.

Stressors that can potentially affect a person's self-concept are also risk factors in regard to the person's health. If a person is unable to adapt to such a stressor, his level of health may be lowered, and if the resulting identity confusion, low self-esteem, disturbed body image, or role conflict, strain, or ambiguity is not relieved, illness may result (Fig. 18-2).

Nurse's Effect on Client's Self-Concept

Impact of Nurse's Self-Concept

The nurse may be the first role model a client undergoing changes in self-concept encounters. The nurse's acceptance of a client with an altered self-concept may be the factor that stimulates positive rehabilitative results. In the case of a client whose physical appearance has changed and who must adapt to a new body image, both the client and his family may look to the nurse and observe her responses and reactions to the client's new situation. To be an effective role model, the nurse should acknowledge that she can have a significant impact on the client. The feelings and expectations of the nurse will be communicated both nonverbally and verbally to the client, his family, and his friends, and to other health care providers. Nursing plans that have been formulated to help a client with an altered self-concept can be either enhanced or defeated by the nurse's unconsciously communicated values and feelings. Thus the nurse should consider the following questions:

1. Can she identify her own feelings regarding health and illness?
2. Is she aware of her own personal reactions to stress, such as coping behaviors?
3. Does she recognize defense behaviors and coping behaviors in others?
4. What is her perception of her professional role?
5. Is she aware of her nonverbal communication?
6. Is she aware of her own values and of her own expectations in regard to people?
7. Is she capable of positively intervening on behalf of another person who has different values without trying to change or to judge the other person?

Nurses cannot deny that they have feelings, ideas, values, and expectations, and that they make judgments. In providing care, the nurse acts as a person who is separate and autonomous from others and who has her own self-concept, self-esteem, body image, roles, and identity. Her awareness and acceptance of herself can promote her understanding and acceptance of others. Every person makes decisions about himself, his environment, and other people on the basis of a personal frame of reference. As a professional the nurse must be prepared to work with other people who have their own frames of reference; she must develop an awareness of her own reactions to various situations and stressors.

A nurse's reaction to a client's illness, which is influenced by her own self-concept, can have a significant impact on the client's self-concept. A client with low self-esteem, for example, may be particularly sensitive to how a nurse involves him in his own therapy. If the nurse lacks self-confidence herself, she may be hesitant in making suggestions, thus inadvertently implying that the client might be unable to follow suggestions. She may insist that the client assume too much responsibility for his own care, thus frightening him. In either case the client's self-esteem may be additionally threatened, rather than strengthened. If, however, the nurse demonstrates confidence in the client's abilities and is self-confident herself, the client's sense of worth will be reinforced. A similar principle is operative in regard to identity: a nurse who is secure in her own identity can more readily accept and thus reinforce the client's identity, whereas a nurse who is not sure of her own identity may be unable to accept the client and may react to him as if he should be something or someone else, thus threatening his sense of identity.

The nurse's impact is most significant in the area of body image. A client who must adapt to a changed body image caused by illness or surgery needs support, as does the client's family. If the nurse feels, for example, that an ostomy or a mastectomy is a horrible thing, she should not express to the client that she feels terrible for him, but should talk with someone who has more experience in the care and rehabilitation of such clients. Meeting people who have had such surgery and who have recuperated and been rehabilitated can do wonders for a nurse's perspective. If a nurse feels insecure about her own body image, she is likely to react more strongly to changes in a client's physical appearance and functioning. Inadvertently making faces or avoiding a client are indications that a nurse is unable to cope with her own stress in regard to such physical changes. The self-concept of an incontinent client, for example, can be threatened by the perception that others find his situation unpleasant. Thus a nurse should be aware of her reactions, acknowledge them, and focus on the client. Otherwise the client may perceive the nurse's behavior as an attempt to isolate or reject him. The nurse should try to imagine what his feelings are, to imagine how she would feel if she were in his situation. If she can imagine how she would feel, then she can imagine what someone might do to ease her embarrassment, frustration, anger, or denial.

A nurse who works with someone undergoing body-image changes plays a major role in helping him adapt and cope. This role may not be easy, but it is rewarding to both the client and the nurse. The nurse can be the resource that the family and the client need in making this adjustment.

Impact of Nursing Activities

We all perceive some aspects of human experience as stressful, frightening, frustrating, anger provoking, or saddening. The stressors associated with illness and the treatment of illness affect an individual's self-concept in various ways. Clients need an environment that is safe, nonjudgmental, and supportive. Sultenfuss (1982) has specified three messages that should be conveyed from the nurse to the client to provide a therapeutic environment that does not threaten the client's self-concept:

1. Whatever the client communicates is normal and acceptable.
2. The communication is not threatening or frightening to the nurse.
3. The nurse will not reject or isolate the client because of anything he communicates.

Conveying these messages may sound like an easy task; however, consider them one at a time. The first message is that all communications are normal and acceptable. Is it all right if the client prefers relationships with someone of the same sex? Is it all right if the significant other is not a wife, husband, sister, or daughter? Is it all right if the client is looking forward to surgery? If the nurse, while providing care, implies that the client's values are in any way unacceptable, the client's self-esteem or sense of identity may be threatened. The second message is that the nurse does not feel threatened by the client's communications. Not reacting to anger with anger is an example. Clients who are angry may direct their anger toward nurses, other health care providers, or even their families. It is often difficult for the nurse not to react, to recognize that the client's anger may be related to loss of control or to an inability to act as usual. Reactions that reveal that the nurse is frightened or threatened can become stressors for the client's self-concept. To be able to convey the third message, the nurse must assess and evaluate her own actions and reactions. In addition, she must notice if other nurses or other health care personnel are avoiding a client. Isolation and rejection, real or imagined, will negatively affect the client's self-concept.

The nurse should be aware that many nursing and other health care activities in and of themselves can have an adverse effect on a client's self-concept, if the nurse does not take action to prevent this from happening. A hospitalized client, for example, almost always experiences role changes and lowered self-esteem as a result of his dependence on those who are providing care. In addition, physical examination of the client's body, drawing blood samples for laboratory analysis, and many other "routine" actions can threaten the client's body and his privacy. Because such nursing activities are far from routine for most clients, as is the health care environment itself, the client often feels alienated, out of place, and vulnerable, and these feelings affect how he views himself. The nurse can do much, however, to minimize these feelings and to assist the client in maintaining a positive self-concept. Encouraging visits by family members, for example, helps the client maintain his usual role within the family. Discussing all procedures with the client and encouraging his participation in the nursing care plan are examples of ways in which a nurse can respect the client's identity as a person who is capable of making decisions for himself; if he feels merely like a body being manipulated by health care professionals, he may suffer a loss of self-esteem. In general, the nurse's goal is to assist the client in carrying on as usual—as much as possible—with activities and relationships that support his self-concept. If the client's self-concept has depended on activities in which he is no longer able to participate, as in the case of an athlete who has experienced paralysis as a result of an injury, the nurse can help him adapt to this change through other kinds of activities that can assist him in rebuilding a strong self-concept.

The nurse's role and impact will be different with each client. Her primary role, perhaps, is as a role model. She provides an example for the client and his family. Her acceptance of the client as a human being who has ideas, feelings, and values, and who is worthy and whole despite illness or physical alterations, is important. The client's feelings of insecurity, fears of rejection, or loss of self-worth can be lessened through sensitive, knowledgeable nursing care.

Altered Self-Concept and the Nursing Process

Assessment

The nursing assessment should focus on the client's actual and potential self-concept stressors and on behaviors associated with an altered self-concept. The following are examples of stressors that may affect self-concept:

COMPONENT OF SELF-CONCEPT	EXAMPLES
Body image	Altered functioning after cerebrovascular accident
	Incontinence
	Arthritis
	Alteration or loss of body part (amputation, mastectomy, colostomy)
	Normal growth and developmental changes (aging, pregnancy)
Self-esteem	Loss of job
	Divorce or separation
	Repeated failures
	Unrealistic self-ideal
	Dependency on others
Roles	Incompatible role expectations
	Unclear role expectations
	Inability to adequately perform and cope with multiple roles
Identity	Tasks of adolescence
	Peer pressure
	Parent-child conflicts
	Sexual concerns
	Relationship concerns

TABLE 18-1

Behavior Associated with Alterations in Self-Concept

Alteration	Behavior	Examples
Low self-esteem, disturbed body image, role strain	Criticism of self and others	Ridicules self as "ugly," "no good," or "born loser"; self-pitying; may transform self-criticism into criticism of others (displacement)
	Denying oneself pleasure	Punishes self by avoiding desirable or pleasurable things such as favorite foods, social activities, or career opportunities
	Disturbed interpersonal relationships	Is cruel to or exploits others; overly dependent on others; withdrawal or isolation because of feelings of worthlessness
	Exaggerated self-importance	Attempts to compensate for low self-esteem by boasting about importance in one or more roles, such as his job
	Guilt	Punishes self for not meeting self-ideal; possibly expressed through nightmares or obsessions
	Unrealistic goals	Sets goals at unattainable levels and feels worthless when unable to meet them

Modified from Stuart, G.W., and Sundeen, S.J.: Principles and practice of psychiatric nursing, ed. 2, St. Louis, 1983, The C.V. Mosby Co.

Continued.

TABLE 18-1, cont'd

Behavior Associated with Alterations in Self-Concept

Alteration	Behavior	Examples
	Self-destructiveness	May engage in dangerous activities such as high-speed driving; may be accident prone; may consider or attempt suicide
	Physical manifestations	Psychosomatic illnesses, stress-related illnesses, substance abuse
	Polarized attitudes	Defensively perceives everything as good or bad, right or wrong
	Procrastination	Puts off activities and decisions because of ambivalence or insecurity
	Rejection of one's own capabilities	Neglects or rejects possibilities and capabilities because of low self-esteem; may speak of being continually bored
	Worrying	May be constantly concerned with upcoming situations, social interactions, or responsibilities
	Withdrawal from reality	If anxiety of self-rejection reaches an extreme, may withdraw from reality with hallucinations, delusions, and feelings of suspicion and paranoia
Identity confusion	Diffused time perspective	Sense of urgency combined with a failure to consider time when planning activities
	Diffused sense of industry	Inability to concentrate on work being performed
	Withdrawal from activities	Gradual withdrawal because of underlying despair or feelings of not belonging
	Escape behavior	Intense experiences such as alcohol or drug abuse, hard physical labor, or heavy exercise
	Substitute identity behavior	Readiness to join a club, group, or team and to allow the one role to substitute for personal identity
	Prejudice against others	Expressing bigotry toward others or establishing a scapegoat to strengthen one's own identity
	Rebellious behavior	Assuming a negative identity in terms of social norms
Depersonalization	Emotional passivity	Unable to feel pleasure; lack of spontaneity and animation; experiences world as dreamlike
	Distorted thinking	Confusion, time disorientation, memory and judgment impairments, loss of decision-making ability
	Social withdrawal	Feelings of alienation, insecurity, inferiority; heightened sense of isolation; incongruent or idiosyncratic communication

The nursing assessment also includes consideration of the client's previous coping behaviors, the nature of the stressors affecting him, the number and intensity of the stressors, and the client's internal and external resources. The client may perceive a threat to himself, for example, as being also a threat to a significant other. In addition, the nursing assessment should include the significant other if that person is to be a support and resource for the client.

Table 18-1 gives examples of behavior often associated with alterations in self-concept.

Nursing Diagnosis

On the basis of assessment data and observation of the client's behavior, the nurse determines the nursing diagnosis. The diagnosis should specify both the component of self-concept that is affected and the particular stressor to which the altered self-concept is related. Table 18-2 lists examples of such nursing diagnoses; they are grouped according to the component of self-concept that is involved.

Planning and Implementation

After determining the nursing diagnosis, the nurse plans care directed toward helping the client regain a healthy self-concept. Interventions center on helping the client adapt to the stressors that led to the altered self-concept and on supporting and reinforcing his development of coping methods.

In planning interventions, the nurse considers the client's present level of adaptation. The client's level of adaptation can be located on a continuum in each of the following five areas (Bernstein and Cope, 1976):

Active coping ↔ Passive surrender
Leading and co-managing treatment ↔ Resisting treatment
Loving exchange ↔ Rage
Awareness ↔ Denial
Adaptive defenses ↔ Maladaptive defenses

Planning should therefore take into account the client's position on each continuum. For example, a client may perceive his situation as overwhelming, and thus may passively surrender to circumstances rather than attempting to cope. The nursing care plan should include providing understanding and support as the client explores his self-concept and should permit the client's expression of feelings (crying, anger, depression). Clients need time to adapt to changes, and they need manageable, sequential steps to follow. Nurses must recognize a client's strengths and provide resources and education to help him turn limitations into strengths. Client education should be actively

---

TABLE 18-2

Examples of Nursing Diagnoses Involving Altered Self-Concept

Component of Self-Concept	Diagnoses
Body image	Altered body image related to fear of becoming obese Disturbed body image related to cerebrovascular accident Disturbed body image related to leukemia chemotherapy
Self-esteem	Low self-esteem related to death of spouse Low self-esteem related to fear of public speaking Low self-esteem related to overly high self-ideal
Roles	Role conflict related to incompatibility of newly assumed work and family roles Role strain related to incongruent cultural and personal expectations about aging
Identity	Identity confusion related to developmental crisis of adolescence Depersonalization and panic related to rejection by significant other Identity confusion related to unrealistic parental expectations Depersonalization related to drug or alcohol abuse

Modified from Stuart, G.W., and Sundeen, S.J.: Principles and practice of psychiatric nursing, ed. 2, St. Louis, 1983, The C.V. Mosby Co.

---

planned, and the client should be included throughout the planning phase.

The nurse should provide a therapeutic environment that supports the client through the stages of adaptation. Sultenfuss (1982) has identified four stages of adaptation: shock and panic, defensive retreat, acknowledgment, and adaptation. However, sometimes a person can adapt to a change in his body and integrate the change into his self-concept but still not accept the fact that a change has occurred. Clients often need a great deal of time to accept some changes.

In the case of a client who must adapt to an altered body image as a result of surgery or another physical change, a visit by a rehabilitated person is often helpful. However, the timing of such a visit is important, since the client may still be denying that the problem exists.

Text continued on p. 368.

TABLE 18-3

Approach to Nursing Interventions for Altered Self-Concept

Principle	Rationale	Nursing Actions
LEVEL ONE		
Goal: Expand the client's self-awareness		
Establish an open trusting relationship.	This reduces the threat that the nurse poses to the client and helps him to broaden and accept all aspects of his personality.	Offer unconditional acceptance.
		Listen to the client.
		Encourage discussion of his thoughts and feelings.
		Respond nonjudgmentally.
		Convey to the individual that he is a valued person who is responsible for himself and able to help himself.
Work with whatever resources the patient possesses.	Some resources, such as self-control and self-perception, are needed as a foundation for later nursing care.	Guidelines for the client with limited resources are as follows:
		1. Begin by confirming his identity.
		2. Provide support measures to reduce his level of anxiety.
		3. Approach him in an undemanding way.
		4. Accept and attempt to clarify any verbal or nonverbal communication.
		5. Prevent him from isolating himself.
		6. Help him establish a simple routine for himself.
		7. Help him set limits on inappropriate behavior.
		8. Orient him to reality.
		9. Reinforce appropriate behavior.
		10. Gradually increase activities and tasks that provide positive experiences for him.
		11. Assist him in personal hygiene and grooming.
		12. Encourage him to care for himself.
Maximize the client's participation in the therapeutic relationship.	Mutuality is necessary in order for the client to assume ultimate responsibility for his own behavior and coping responses.	Gradually increase the client's participation in decisions that affect his care.
		Convey to the client that he is a responsible individual.

Modified from Stuart, G.W., and Sundeen, S.J.: Principles and practice of psychiatric nursing, ed. 2, St. Louis, 1983, The C.V. Mosby Co.

TABLE 18-3, cont'd

Approach to Nursing Interventions for Altered Self-Concept

Principle	Rationale	Nursing Actions
LEVEL TWO		
Goal: Encourage the client's self-exploration		
Show interest in and accept the client's feelings and thoughts.	When the nurse shows interest in and accepts the client's feelings and thoughts, she is helping him to do so also.	Attend to and encourage the client's expression of his emotions, beliefs, behavior, and thoughts—verbally, nonverbally, symbolically, or directly.
		Utilize therapeutic communication skills and empathic responses.
		Note his use of logical and illogical thinking and his reported and observed emotional responses.
Help the client to clarify his concept of self and his relationships to others through self-disclosure.	Self-disclosure and understanding one's self-perceptions are prerequisites to bringing about future change; this may, in itself, bring about a reduction in anxiety.	Elicit his perceptions of his own strengths and weaknesses.
		Help him to describe his self-ideal.
		Identify his self-criticisms.
		Help him to describe how he believes he relates to other people and events.
Be aware and have control of your own feelings.	Self-awareness allows the nurse to model authentic behavior.	Be open to your own feelings.
		Accept both positive and negative feelings of your own.
		Therapeutic use of self:
		1. Share your own feelings with the client.
		2. Describe how another might have felt.
		3. Mirror your perception of the client's feelings.
Respond empathically, not sympathetically, emphasizing that the power to change lies with the client.	Sympathy can reinforce the client's self-pity; rather, the nurse should communicate that the client's life situation is subject to his own control.	Use empathic responses and monitor yourself for feelings of sympathy or pity.
		Reaffirm to the client that he is not helpless or powerless in the face of his problems.
		Convey verbally and behaviorally that the client is responsible for his own behavior, including his choice of maladaptive or adaptive coping responses.
		Discuss with him the scope of his choices, his areas of strength, and coping resources that are available to him.

Continued.

TABLE 18-3, cont'd

Approach to Nursing Interventions for Altered Self-Concept

Principle	Rationale	Nursing Actions
		Utilize the support systems of family and groups to facilitate the client's self-exploration.
		Assist the client in recognizing the nature of his conflict and the maladaptive ways in which he tries to cope with it.

LEVEL THREE

Goal: Assist the client in self-evaluation

Principle	Rationale	Nursing Actions
Help the client to clearly define the problem.	Only after the problem is accurately defined can alternative choices be proposed.	Identify relevant stressors with the client and ask for his appraisal of them.
		Clarify to the client that his beliefs influence both his feelings and his behaviors.
		Mutually identify faulty beliefs, misperceptions, distortions, illusions, and unrealistic goals.
		Mutually identify areas of strength.
		Place the concepts of success and failure in proper perspective.
		Explore with the client his use of coping resources.
Explore the client's adaptive and maladaptive coping responses to his problem.	Examination of client's choices made during coping will help define successful and unsuccessful responses.	Describe to the client how all coping responses are freely chosen and have both positive and negative consequences.
		Contrast adaptive and maladaptive responses.
		Mutually identify the disadvantages of the client's maladaptive coping responses.
		Mutually identify the advantages or "payoffs" of the client's maladaptive coping responses.
		Discuss how these payoffs have perpetuated the maladaptive response.

LEVEL FOUR

Goal: Assist the client in the formulation of realistic goals

Principle	Rationale	Nursing Actions
Help the client identify alternative solutions.	Only when all possible alternatives have been evaluated can change be effected.	Help the client understand that he can only change himself, not others.

Approach to Nursing Interventions for Altered Self-Concept

Principle	Rationale	Nursing Actions
		If the client holds inconsistent perceptions, help him to see that he can change the following:
		1. His beliefs or ideals, to bring them closer to reality. 2. His environment, to make it consistent with his beliefs
		If his self-concept is not consistent with his behavior, he can change the following:
		1. His behavior, to conform to his self-concept 2. The beliefs underlying his self-concept, to include his behavior 3. His self-ideal
		Mutually review how the client can use coping resources.
Help the client conceptualize his own realistic goals.	Goal setting that includes a clear definition of the expected change is necessary.	Encourage the client to formulate his own (not the nurse's) goals.
		Mutually discuss the emotional and practical consequences of each goal.
		Help the client clearly define the concrete change to be made.
		Encourage the client to enter new experiences for their growth potential.
		Utilize role rehearsal, role modeling, and role playing when appropriate.

LEVEL FIVE

Goal: Assist the client in becoming committed to his decision and in achieving his goals

Help the client take the necessary action to change maladaptive coping responses and maintain adaptive ones.	The ultimate objective in promoting the client's insight is to have him replace the maladaptive coping responses with more adaptive ones.	Provide opportunity for the client to experience success.
		Reinforce the strengths, skills, and healthy aspects of the client's personality.
		Assist the client in gaining the assistance he might need (vocational, financial, and social services).
		Use family and groups to enhance the client's self-esteem.
		Allow the client sufficient time to change.
		Provide the appropriate amount of support and positive reinforcement for the client to help him maintain his progress.

In providing care to a client who is experiencing stress that affects self-worth and identity, it is important that the nurse include activities in which the client will achieve success. Tasks should not be so difficult that the client cannot succeed. Ensuring a small success is better than risking a defeat at a larger task. Success is best achieved by providing sequential tasks.

The nurse should keep other nurses and other health care professionals up to date on the client's progress, because they can be involved in offering support and reinforcement for the client. If a body alteration is particularly severe, staff conferences are useful in helping nurses to handle their own feelings and emotions.

The specific nursing care plan for a client with an altered self-concept should be based on both short- and long-term goals of adaptation. For a client who is beginning to receive chemotherapy and who is experiencing body image stressors, for example, the short-term goals might include encouraging the client to describe the effects of the medication on his body and to express his feelings about his illness and treatment, and the long-term goal might be to help him to adapt successfully to and accept his new body image.

Interventions designed to help a client reach the long-term goal of adapting to changes in self-concept or attaining a positive self-concept are based on the premise that the client first develops insight and self-awareness concerning problems and stressors and then acts to solve the problems and cope with the stressors. This approach involves five specific levels of intervention (Stuart and Sundeen, 1983):

1. Increased self-awareness
2. Self-exploration
3. Self-evaluation
4. Formulation of realistic goals
5. Commitment to goals and achievement through action

Each level includes specific nursing goals and actions. The nurse helps the client proceed sequentially through the five levels. The extent of nursing actions at each level should be individualized, as should the planned time period for each level. If the alteration in self-concept is severe, the nurse should seek assistance from other professionals, such as mental health nurses, or should refer the client for specialized care. Table 18-3 describes in more detail the nursing interventions involved in each of the five levels.

Evaluation

The purpose of evaluation is to determine how well the client's outcomes have met the goals of nursing care. Desired outcomes include adequate social interaction, adequate self-care, acceptance of use of prosthetic devices, positive attitudes toward rehabilitation, movement toward independence, and return to preexisting roles at work or at home. The establishment of a therapeutic nurse-client relationship early in the rehabilitative process can help to get the client himself involved in evaluation.

The client's adaptation to major changes may take a year or longer, but the fact that this period is long does not signify maladaptation. The nurse should look for signs that the client has reduced some stressors, even though perhaps not all. Any person's reorganization of how he sees himself takes time. After all, a person's self-concept took years to develop to its preillness state, and additional change and development also require time.

Summary

The self-concept is a complex, dynamic entity. Many variables—including illness, hospitalization, and surgery—can affect any or all of the components of self-concept—self-worth, body image, identity, and roles. A person's self-concept is a combination of both the real self and the ideal self. The ideal self is based on social and cultural standards that an individual accepts and attempts to incorporate into his self-concept. A discrepancy between the real and the ideal can be a source of stress. The ideal provides standards by which a person judges himself. A positive self-concept is important to a person's developmental and cognitive growth throughout life, and numerous variables in each stage of life affect the self-concept.

The nurse's role in providing care for a client with a self-concept change depends on the severity of the alteration. Even an apparently minor loss of function, change in appearance, or role change can create a severe self-concept problem. Even a loss or change that is not apparent to others can result in an alteration in a client's self-esteem or identity. The nurse's own self-concept and her nursing actions can have positive or negative effects on a client's self-concept.

Everyone who is admitted to a hospital or seen by a health care provider should be assessed for stressors that may affect his self-concept in any of its components. Although most people can adapt to stressful situations, a client may need assistance in learning to cope with a new situation. Using the nursing process, the nurse identifies self-concept stressors and plans and implements care to encourage the client's self-awareness, self-exploration, and self-evaluation, which lead to the client's formulating realistic goals for coping with changes and then acting to achieve them.

KEY CONCEPTS

✓ The self-concept is an integrated set of conscious and unconscious feelings, attitudes, and perceptions about oneself.

✓ The components of the self-concept are body image, self-esteem, roles, and identity.

✓ The self-concept develops as a normal part of growth and maturation, and each developmental stage involves particular factors important to the development of a healthy, positive self-concept.

✓ Body image is influenced by cultural and societal values and attitudes as well as by an individual's perceptions of his body.

✓ Body-image stressors include changes in physical appearance or functioning caused by normal developmental changes or by illness.

✓ Self-esteem is a person's sense of self-worth; it depends on a person's self-ideal, which is influenced by societal values, and on the person's success in family, work, and other activities.

✓ Self-esteem stressors include illness (particularly chronic illness that involves changes in normal activities), surgery, and accidents, as well as the responses of other individuals to changes resulting from these events.

✓ Roles are learned through the process of socialization; they involve the expectations of others about how one should behave in particular positions (family member, employee, and so on).

✓ Role stressors include role conflict, role ambiguity, and role strain, any of which may originate in unclear or conflicting role expectations and may arise in or be aggravated by the effects of illness.

✓ Identity is a consistent and persistent sense of self as a person who is distinct from others; it develops throughout life.

✓ One's identity is particularly vulnerable during adolescence. Identity stressors during this time include the expectations of others to prepare for a career and independence, to cope with one's sexuality, and to make choices about relationships and roles; such stressors may lead to identity confusion or depersonalization.

✓ The nurse should be aware of how both her own self-concept and her nursing actions can affect a client's self-concept.

✓ A nursing assessment should include consideration of actual and potential self-concept stressors and observation for behaviors indicative of an altered self-concept.

✓ Nursing diagnoses in regard to an altered self-concept include changes in any or all of the four components of self-concept.

✓ Planning and implementation of nursing interventions for an altered self-concept involve expanding the client's self-awareness, encouraging self-exploration, aiding him in self-evaluation, helping him formulate goals in regard to adaptation, and assisting him in acting to achieve his goals.

REFERENCES

Bernstein, N.R., and Cope, O.: Emotional care of the facially burned and disfigured, Boston, 1976, Little, Brown & Co.

Biddle, B.J.: Role therapy: expectations, identities, and behaviors, New York, 1979, Academic Press, Inc.

Biddle, B.J., and Thomas, E.J., editors: Role theory: concepts and research, New York, 1966, John Wiley & Sons, Inc.

Brim, O.G., and Wheeler, S.: Socialization after childhood: two essays, New York, 1966, John Wiley & Sons, Inc.

Broadwell, D.C.: Validation of a role conflict, role ambiguity, and role predictability instrument, doctoral dissertation, Atlanta, 1983, Georgia State University.

Cooley, C.H.: Human nature and the social order, New York, 1956, The Free Press.

Dropkin, N.J.: Compliance in postoperative head and neck patients, Cancer Nurs. 2(5):379, 1979.

Dyk, R.B., and Sutherland, A.: Adaptation of the spouse and other family members to the colostomy patient, CA 9:123, 1956.

Erikson, E.H.: Childhood and society, New York, ed. 2, 1963, W.W. Norton & Co., Inc.

Gibson, D.E.: Reminiscence, self-esteem, and self-other satisfaction in adult male alcoholics, J. Psychiatr. Nurs., March 1980, p. 7.

Meleis, A.: Role insufficiency and role supplementation: a conceptual framework, Nurs. Res. 24:264, 1975.

Parsons, T.: Illness and the role of physician: a sociological perspective, Am. J. Orthopsychiatry 21:452, 1951.

Parsons, T.: Definitions of health and illness in light of American values and social structures. In Jaco, E.G., editor: Patients, physicians, and illness, 1972, ed. 2, New York, The Free Press.

Piaget, J., and Inhelder, B.: The psychology of the child, New York, 1969, Basic Books, Inc.

Seyle, H.: The stress of life, New York, 1956, McGraw-Hill Book Co.

Stuart, G.W., and Sundeen, S.J.: Principles and practice of psychiatric nursing, ed. 2, St. Louis, 1983, The C.V. Mosby Co.

Sultenfuss, S.R.: Psychosocial issues and therapeutic intervention. In Broadwell, D.C., and Jackson, B.S., editors: Principles of ostomy care, St. Louis, 1982, The C.V. Mosby Co.

Yamamoto, K.: The child and his image, Boston, 1972, Houghton Mifflin Co.

ADDITIONAL READINGS

Brundage, D.J., and Broadwell, D.C.: Altered body image. In Phipps, W.J., Long, B.C., and Woods, N.F., editors: Medical-surgical nursing: concepts and clinical practice, ed. 2, St. Louis, 1983, The C.V. Mosby Co.

Katchadourian, H.E., editor: Human sexuality, Berkeley, 1979, University of California Press.

Maslow, A.H.: Motivation and personality, New York, 1970, Harper & Row, Publishers, Inc.

Molla, P.M.: Self-concept in children with and without physical disability, J. Psychiatr. Nurs. 19(6):22, 1981.

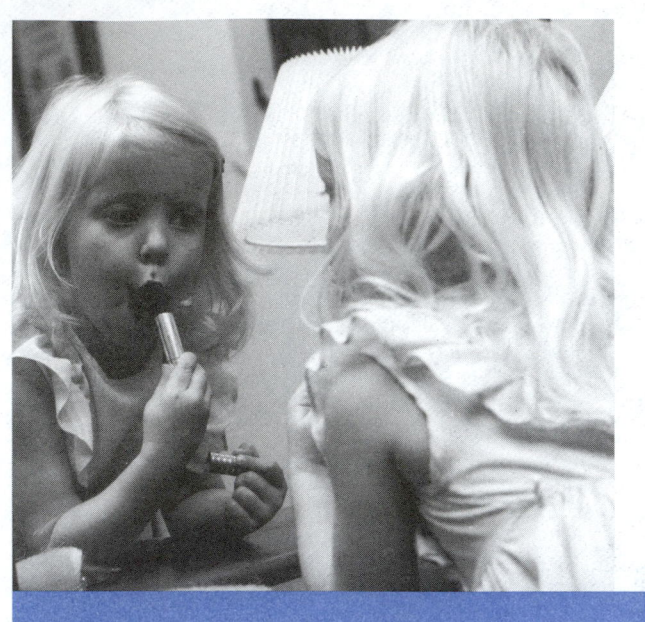

OBJECTIVES

Mastery of content in this chapter will enable the student to:

- Define the terms in the glossary.
- Discuss the nurse's role in maintaining or enhancing a client's sexual health.
- Describe variables that influence sexual preferences and behaviors.
- List and discuss the physical and psychological factors that influence feelings of sexuality.
- Describe physiological and psychological causes of sexual dysfunction.
- List interventions in the nursing plan for sexual health.
- Evaluate attainment of sexual health.
- Discuss resources for facilitating sexual health.

GLOSSARY

bisexual Sexual orientation involving erotic preferences for members of either sex.

contraception Means of preventing pregnancy, such as abstinence from coitus, use of spermicides or barriers, prevention of ovulation by hormone action, and sterilization.

female genitalia Female's external sex organs (vulva, mons veneris, labia majora, labia minora, clitoris, and vaginal opening) and internal sex organs (vagina, uterus, fallopian tubes, and ovaries).

follicular phase First part of the menstrual cycle, in which ovarian follicles grow to prepare for ovulation and the menstrual flow signifies that the uterus has shed its lining from the preceding cycle.

gender identity Awareness of being male or female that develops from infancy.

gender role Expression of one's maleness or femaleness to both oneself and others.

heterosexual Sexual orientation involving erotic preference for members of the opposite sex.

homosexual Sexual orientation involving erotic preference for members of one's own sex.

luteal phase Third and final phase of the menstrual cycle, in which the corpus luteum develops, preparing for implantation of the egg, and deteriorates if an egg is not implanted.

19 | *Sexuality*

male genitalia   Male external sex organs (penis and scrotum) and internal sex organs (testicles, epididymis, vas deferens, prostate gland, seminal vesicles, and Cowper's glands).

masturbation   Erotic self-stimulation by touching the genitals.

menarche   Onset of a girl's first menstruation, usually occurring between 11 and 15 years of age.

menopause   Natural cessation of menses by the ovaries; occurs in women between the ages of 45 and 60.

menstrual cycle   Recurring cycle of changes in the ovaries, uterus, and hormone levels, involving the development of an egg, ovulation, and implantation of the egg or sloughing of the corpus luteum.

menstruation   Time of menstrual flow during the menstrual cycle.

orgasm   Climax phase of sexual response, in which reflex muscular contractions occur and heart and respiratory rates peak.

ovulation   Second phase of the menstrual cycle, in which a mature egg is released from the ovary and moves down the fallopian tubes.

puberty   Developmental period of emotional and physical changes, including the development of secondary sex characteristics and the onset of menstruation and ejaculation.

secondary sex characteristics   Physical characteristics other than genitals that distinguish females from males, for example, the breasts.

sex   Classification of male or female based on many criteria, among them anatomical and chromosomal characteristics; refers also to biological aspects of sexuality and genital sexual activity.

sexual dysfunction   Inability or difficulty in sexual functioning caused by physiological or psychological factors or both.

sexual fantasy   Mental images of an erotic nature that may lead to sexual arousal.

sexual orientation   Clear, persistent desire of a person for one sex rather than the other.

sexual response cycle   Four phases of biological sexual response: excitement, plateau, orgasm, and resolution.

sexuality   Dynamic and diverse facet of the personality involving the biological, psychological, sociological, spiritual, and cultural dimensions, depending in part on the person's sense of sexual identity and affecting the person's values, attitudes, behaviors, and relationships with others.

sexually transmitted diseases (STDs)   Infectious diseases transmitted to any part of the body through contact with body fluids during sexual activities.

transsexual   Person whose gender identity is opposite his or her biological sex identity.

transvestism   Tendency to achieve psychic and sexual relief by dressing in clothing of the opposite sex.

Any attempt to make sense out of sexuality leads inevitably to a basic truth: human sexuality is incredibly dynamic and diverse. Sexuality begins to make sense, however, when it is viewed as part of the whole human experience. It is inextricably woven into the fabric out of which each of us is made. Knowledge about sexuality can give insight into the inner and social self. The expression of sexuality is one way in which a person reaches out to others.

Sexuality and sex are two different things. Sexuality is often described as a person's sense of being female or male. It has biological, psychological, social, and ethical components. Present from birth to death, it is a shaper of life experiences and in turn is shaped by those experiences. The word "sex" has a more limited meaning. It usually describes the biological aspects of sexuality such as genital sexual activity. Sex may be used for both pleasure and procreation. As a result of life's changes or by choice, sexual activity may be absent from a person's life for brief or prolonged periods of time.

Sexuality is not left behind when the client enters the health care system. Since sexuality touches all aspects of physical, mental, and social being, its presence in the health care setting should be acknowledged. Changes in health have a ripple effect in a person's life and inevitably lead to changes in sexuality. In recognition of this, contemporary definitions of health now include sexual health.

This chapter explores ways of incorporating information about health and sexuality into nursing practice. Clients have a right to compassionate and informed assistance in maintaining their sexual health, and nurses have a unique opportunity to help clients to maintain their sexual health and increase their sexual knowledge.

The definition of sexuality given previously provides the nurse with an outline of the sexual concerns that may confront her in the nurse-client relationship. Nurses encounter clients with biological, psychological, social, and ethical concerns involving sexuality in virtually all health care settings. Some clients ask specific questions about the effect of an illness, surgery, or medication on their sexual anatomy and sexual response. Others are too anxious or embarrassed to bring up their sexual concerns. In either case the nurse must be prepared to initiate an assessment of the client's concerns and plan an appropriate intervention.

Both nurses and clients have a role in learning to promote sexual health. Nurses can learn to create a relaxed and compassionate atmosphere for discussing sexual concerns. They can learn about sexual anatomy, sexual response and behavior, common sexual dysfunctions, and the effects of illness on sexuality. Clients can be encouraged to articulate their sexual concerns and questions. Everyone benefits when nurses learn to deal with sexuality as an integral part of the nursing process.

Concepts of Sexuality

The process by which people come to know themselves as females or males is not clearly understood. That a person is born with female or male genitalia and subsequently learns female or male social roles seems to be a key ingredient, yet this does not explain all of the variations of sexuality and sexual behavior. This diversity is more understandable when we remember that sexuality is intertwined with all aspects of self and of learning to be a person. The Sex Information and Education Council of the United States (1980) has defined sexuality in holistic terms as

a function of the total personality . . . concerned with the biological, psychological, sociological, spiritual and cultural variables of life which, by their effects on personality development and interpersonal relations, can in turn affect social structure.

Biological Identity

Biological differences between males and females are determined at conception. Female fetuses have received two X chromosomes, one from each parent, and male fetuses have received an X chromosome from the mother and a Y chromosome from the father. Initially the genitalia of the fetus are undifferentiated. It is not until the sex hormones begin to cue fetal tissues that the genitalia assume male or female characteristics. The male fetus is genetically programmed to produce testosterone, which causes the growth of some sexual parts and the inhibition of others, at about 7 weeks after conception. The corresponding sex hormone in females, estrogen, does not seem to be essential for the development of female genitalia. Thus, in the absence of significant amounts of testosterone, the female fetus continues to develop female reproductive anatomy. Hormones will continue to influence the individual at critical stages of fetal development and again at puberty. Barring any malfunction in the growth process, females will develop a cyclical menstrual cycle and female secondary sex characteristics. Males will develop a relatively constant production of sperm and male secondary sex characteristics (Perry and Whipple, 1981).

Gender Identity and Gender Role

As soon as an infant is born, the parents and the community into which it is born label it a girl or a boy. Perhaps the first words of the birthing helpers to the parent about the infant's sex start the development of the infant's gender role and gender identity. It is at birth, then, that the process that ultimately results in self-identification as female or male begins. When the use of amniocentesis informs the mother of the child's sex, she begins to adjust her thinking about the child's sexuality even before birth. As children begin to explore and understand their own bodies, they combine this information with the way society treats them to create an image of themselves as girls or boys. They accept that they will remain girls or boys and that changes in outward appearance will not alter their gender. This awareness is developing by the age of 3 years and is established by 5 to 7 years of age (Lion, 1982).

There has been much research and writing in the last decade on the origin of gender role behavior—the way people act as females and males. Social learning theorists believe that societal influences shape female and male behavior and are thus the primary source of a person's sense of femaleness or maleness. Since gender role behavior is encouraged by parents, peers, and the media, differences among individuals' sexual behavior develop.

Environmental factors alone do not satisfactorily explain the differences and similarities between female and male sexual behavior. Some researchers believe that sex hormones influence the development of fetal brain tissue, contributing to the differences in female and male sexual behavior. Most likely, as with other human behaviors, sexual behavior is a combination of many interacting biological and environmental factors.

For some people the inner sense of sexual identity does not match the biological body. Such people are known as transsexuals. A man may think of himself as a female in a male body, or a female may describe herself as a man trapped in a woman's body. There is no clear understanding of how this mismatch occurs. These people do not see their sexual identity as a matter of choice. Their identification of self as a sexual and social female or male is as clear and persistent, often from early childhood, as it is for people whose inner and outer identities match. Through counseling and perhaps rehabilitative sex reassignment surgery, such individuals may gain the relief they seek and deserve.

Sexual Orientation

Sexual orientation is the clear, persistent, erotic preference of a person for one sex or the other. The Kinsey studies of human sexuality showed a continuum between heterosexuality and homosexuality. Most people cluster near the heterosexual ("straight") end of the continuum, with a smaller percentage at the homosexual ("gay" or "lesbian") end, but some people are bisexual ("bi") and feel comfortable having sexual relations with either sex. It is not unusual for people to change their sexual orientation during their lifetime (Haeberle, 1978).

The origins of sexual orientation are still not understood. Biological theories describe heterosexuality and homosexuality in genetic terms, and thus as determined prenatally. Psychological theories have emphasized early learning experiences and cognitive processes as determining sexual orientation.

Homosexuality and transvestism are separate phenomena. Society sometimes thinks of homosexual men as somehow feminized and wishing to be like women, and of lesbians as desiring to be like men. This is a pervasive myth. Although there are some "effeminate"-behaving men and "masculine"-behaving women in the homosexual population, most homosexual men and women would define themselves as quite satisfied with their gender and social role. They simply have a persistent desire for their own sex. A transvestite is usually a heterosexual man who periodically dresses like a woman for psychic and sexual relief. Transvestites generally do this in private, and their behavior is sometimes kept secret even from the people closest to them.

Sexual Ethics

Since sexuality is linked to every aspect of living, any sexual decision involves personal, family, religious, and social standards of conduct. A person's ideas about ethical sexual conduct and emotions related to sexuality form the basis for sexual decision making. The spectrum of attitudes toward sexuality ranges from the traditional view of sex only within the marriage to an attitude that each individual must decide what is right. Sexual decisions that transgress a person's ethical code may result in internal conflict. The person may feel guilty or wrong and may even experience sexual dysfunction. He will either stop the behavior to reduce his negative feelings or adjust his ethical code to include the behavior.

There are several general approaches to ethical sexual decision making (Masters, Johnson, and Kolodny, 1982). In one approach sexual decisions are based solely on religion. Another approach views any sexual act between consenting adults in private as moral. Some people believe that moral sexuality is that which enhances personal growth and interpersonal relationships. Others believe that the morality of a sexual act must be decided on the basis of the situation in which it occurs. No matter what one believes about sexual ethics, some other thoughtful and moral person will have an opposing point of view.

The split between conservative and liberal thinking concerning sexuality does not seem to be diminishing. The debate over sexuality-related issues such as abortion, contraception, sexual variations, and premarital or extramarital intercourse continues. In the absence of a universally accepted moral code, it is important that each person make sexual decisions thoughtfully, with the best interests of the individual and the community in mind.

Attitudes toward Sexuality

Each person learns a set of behaviors that represent femininity or masculinity. Individuals reveal themselves as females or males by their gestures, mannerisms, clothing, vocabulary, and patterns of sexual activity. A person's attitudes toward these sexual feelings and behaviors change as the person grows older and passes through the life stages.

Nurses' and clients' attitudes toward sexuality and sexual behavior significantly affect how health care is provided. Attitudes can show themselves openly and dramatically. Clients may overhear disparaging remarks about their sexuality made by nurses or physicians. Nurses may refuse to deal with a client because of the client's sexual attitudes or behavior. On a more subtle level, the invasion of a client's privacy, lack of regard for a hospitalized client's need for time alone with a sexual partner, or even the way a nurse touches a client reflects attitudes toward sexuality.

Since good health includes sexual health, a client's sexuality should be a part of a health care program. Yet sexual assessment and interventions are not always included in health care. The area of sexuality can be emotionally loaded for both nurses and clients. Lack of information, conflicting value systems, anxiety, or guilt feelings of the client or nurse may cancel out the best intentions of nurses to promote sexual health. Clients may not bring up certain sexual concerns out of a fear that the nurse will be judgmental. Nurses may ignore clients' hints about sexual concerns because they are uncomfortable with the whole topic of sexuality. Such words as masturbation, homosexuality, abortion, and orgasm may have emotional overtones far out of proportion to the reality of the behavior.

Factors Influencing Attitudes

Biology and personality help to shape attitudes and behaviors, but other powerful factors are involved. Sexual attitudes can be the result of religious beliefs. A striking characteristic of contemporary religious thinking is the lack of agreement about sexual values and behavior. Not only are there differences among Catholic, Jewish, and Protestant teachings about sex, but within each faith there is often a lack of uniformity (Hogan, 1982). In addition, discrepancies exist between professed belief and actual behavior. People may publicly say they believe in a particular sexual value system but behave quite differently in private.

Society plays a powerful role in shaping sexual values and attitudes. Each social group has its own set of rules that guide the behavior of group members. These rules become an integral part of an individual's thinking. In the traditional, conservative value system the bias is toward sex as a reproductive function, and masturbation and sexual variations may be condemned because they do not serve the reproductive role. Sexual behavior is seen as serving to bind the couple closer together in the reproductive role. Sex strengthens the monogamous, heterosexual partnership and becomes the ultimate expression of love between the partners. This traditional view encompasses fixed roles for female and male sexual behavior.

A more individualistic morality became widespread in the 1960s and 1970s. Many people reevaluated their moral codes and came to see sexuality as a mode of self-expression. Many women asserted their right to control pregnancy and the expression of their sexual feelings. This "new morality" emphasized ownership of one's own body and feelings, free choice, and self-actualization.

Sexual bias may arise from the traditional nursing role. The historical image of the nurse is one of discipline, purity, and cleanliness. Because nurses had the right to touch hospitalized clients' bodies and carry out clients' personal hygiene, they were expected to suppress their own sexuality (Hogan, 1980a). Although these traditional attitudes have for the most part vanished from nursing practice, the bias involving traditional nursing roles may be evident to male nurses as they move into a historically female profession.

Clients' Sexual Attitudes

Each person has a sexual value system acquired over a lifetime of experiences. All people have personal beliefs and preferences concerning sexuality. These experiences either make it easy for a client to deal with sexual concerns in a health care setting or act as roadblocks. Some clients may be confused about their own sexual value system and thus experience ambiguous or distressing feelings when they deal with their sexuality.

The most common concern people have about their sexuality is whether their sexual attitudes, feelings, and actions are normal. Given the fact that society has not encouraged open talk about sexuality, such anxiety is understandable. Religion, society, the media, family, peers, and experience have all sent messages about sexual normalcy.

Clients may be concerned about how nursing interventions will affect their self-care abilities and sexual activities. This is most clear when dealing with masturbation and sexual fantasy. Traditionally there have been strong societal and religious prohibitions against both, especially for women. In most hospital settings, however, they are the only sexual outlets available to clients who feel well enough to engage in them. Yet the attitude of the nursing staff may prevent these activities. Nurses who do suggest fantasy or masturbation as part of an intervention may also bring the client into conflict with his personal beliefs and prohibitions.

Nurses' Attitudes toward Sexuality

Since health care professionals represent society, with its diverse sexual attitudes and behaviors, diversity is understandable and expected among health care professionals. A nurse can deal with her own attitudes by accepting their existence, exploring their sources, and finding ways to work with them. Professional behavior need not compromise the personal sexual ethics of nurse or client. Professional behavior must guarantee that the client is provided with the best health care possible without diminishing his sense of self-worth.

Nurses may find it difficult to be nonjudgmental about a client's sexuality when the client's orientation or values are different from their own. What seems strange or wrong to the nurse might seem normal and acceptable to the client. This is the result of the diversity of cultural and societal norms with which we live. Attempting to change a client's sexual attitudes and behaviors ignores the fundamental differences in attitudes among people. Promotion of sex education and honest examination of one's own sexual values and beliefs (see Chapter 13) can be helpful in reducing sexual bias. Such a process would emphasize the following for the nurse (Hogan, 1980b):

1. Awareness of beliefs, attitudes, and values about sexuality
2. Awareness of how beliefs and attitudes affect nursing practice
3. Knowledge of subject matter
4. Skill in assessment and intervention

Giving clients information about sexuality does not imply advocacy. Clients need accurate and honest information about how their illness may affect their sexuality and how sexuality can contribute to their wellness. Nurses need to provide that information so their own or clients' normal biases do not get in the way of the nursing process.

Sexual Anatomy and Physiology

Female Sex Organs

The female genitalia are comprised of external and internal sex organs. The external sex organs, referred

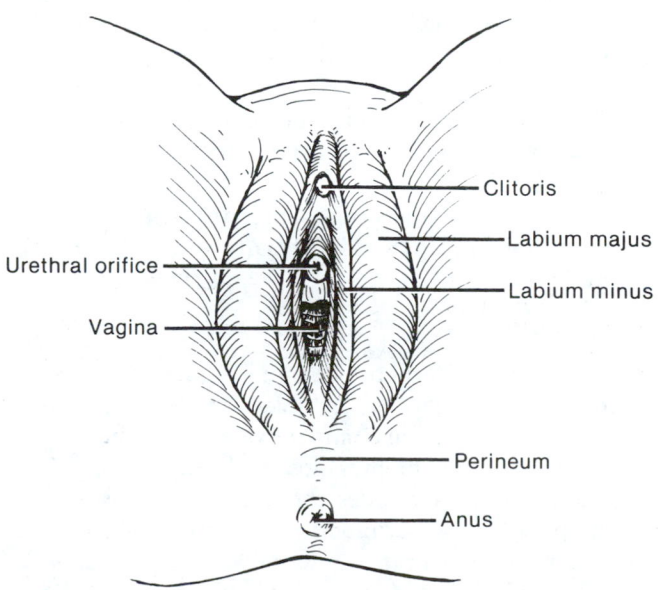

Fig. 19-1 External female sex organs.

Fig. 19-2 Internal female sex organs.

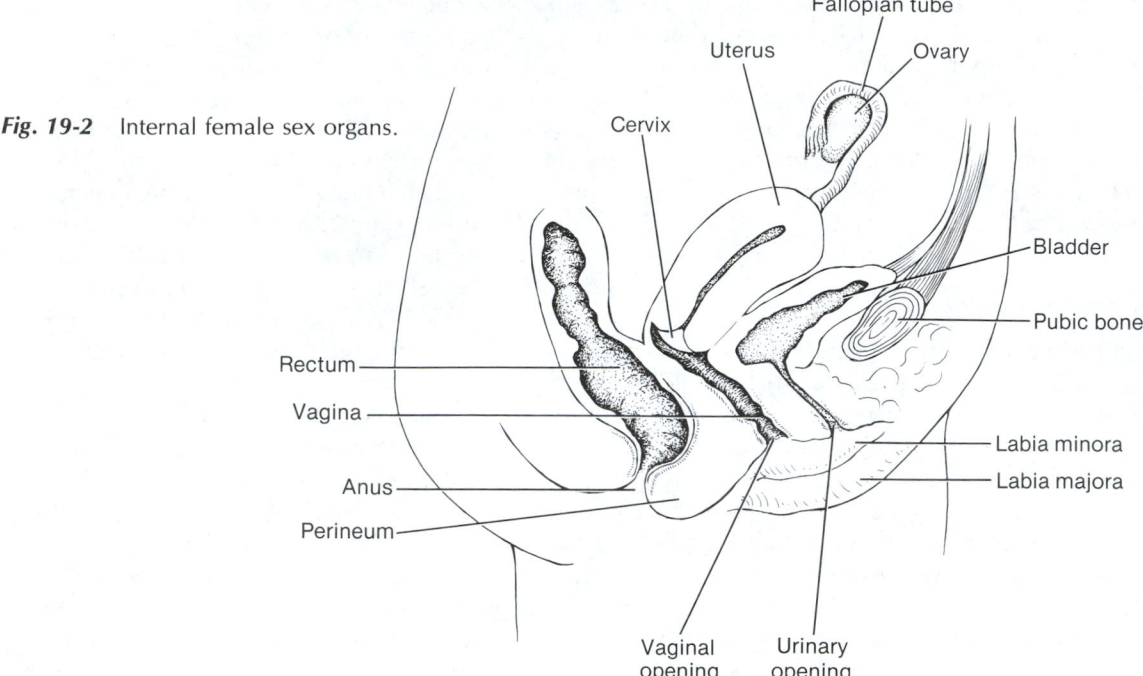

to collectively as the vulva, include the mons veneris, labia majora, labia minora, clitoris, and vaginal opening (Fig. 19-1). The vagina, uterus, fallopian tubes, and ovaries comprise the internal sex organs (Fig. 19-2).

VULVA

The mons veneris is a layer of fatty tissue that covers the pubic bone and is covered by pubic hair in the postpubescent female. The two labia majora are fatty folds of skin whose outer surfaces are covered with pubic hair and whose inner surfaces are smooth and hairless. The labia majora extend down from the mons veneris and form the outer boundaries of the vulva. They have sensory receptors that are sensitive to touch, pressure, pain, and temperature. The two labia minora, which are just inside the labia majora, are thin folds of pigmented skin that extend upward to form the clitoral hood. These inner folds possess many blood vessels and have many sensory nerve endings.

CLITORIS

When the clitoral hood is pulled back, the glans of the clitoris is revealed. It looks like a smooth, shiny pea. The clitoris has many nerve endings and is very sensitive to touch, pressure, and temperature. The clitoral hood also hides the clitoral shaft, which is composed of two cylinders of fibrous tissue (corpora cavernosa) that branch internally like an inverted **V** into two long extensions, the crura. The crura attach to the bony pelvis. A third cylinder (corpus spon-

giosum) divides into two vestibular bulbs that flank the vaginal opening.

INTROITUS

The vaginal opening, or introitus, is between the urethra and the anus. The hymen is a membranous fold of tissue that partially covers the introitus. It has no known function. It usually remains intact until the first intercourse.

The Bartholin's glands are two small ducts that open on the inner surface of the labia minora next to the vaginal opening. The Bartholin's glands secrete a small amount of lubricating fluid, but most of the vaginal lubrication for coitus comes from the walls of the vagina (Haeberle, 1978).

VAGINA

The vagina is a thin-walled, muscular organ that tilts upward at a 45-degree angle toward the small of the back (Masters, Johnson, and Kolodny, 1982). The walls of the vagina consist of a thin outer serosa, which is part of the membrane that lines the body cavity and covers its organs; a middle layer of smooth, involuntary muscle that is continuous with the muscle of the uterus; and an inner layer of moist mucous membrane called mucosa (Goldstein, 1976). The vagina serves as a passageway for menstrual flow and childbirth.

UTERUS

The uterus is a thick-walled muscular organ located between the urinary bladder and rectum. It is about

7.6 cm (3 inches) long and looks like a small pear turned upside down. The fallopian tubes enter the uterus on either side near the top (Haeberle, 1978). The wide upper part of the uterus is known as the body. The bottom part, called the cervix, protrudes into the vagina. The inner lining of the cervix contains many glands, which secrete varying amounts of mucus that plug the opening to the uterus. Changes in the cervical mucus indicate when ovulation is taking place. The mucus is more readily penetrable by sperm at the time of ovulation.

The uterus is composed of three layers: the thin external connective tissue layer called the perimetrium, the middle layer of smooth muscle called the myometrium, and the inner mucous membrane called the endometrium. Every month the endometrium thickens and prepares for possible implantation of a fertilized ovum. If no implantation occurs, the endometrium deteriorates and is discharged through the cervix and vagina during menstruation.

FALLOPIAN TUBES

The two fallopian tubes begin at the uterus and end in long fingerlike fimbriae near the ovaries. The chief function of the fallopian tubes is as a conduit for the passage of both egg and sperm so fertilization can take place. Fertilization usually occurs in the upper part of one of the fallopian tubes.

OVARIES

The two walnut-sized ovaries, one on each side of the uterus, have two functions. They produce eggs that are released into the fallopian tubes, and they secrete female hormones, including small amounts of androgen, directly into the bloodstream. The process of egg production begins in the female fetus and ends at birth. Every female is born with nearly 400,000 eggs, which remain in suspended development until puberty. Beginning at puberty one or several mature eggs are produced each month by either of the ovaries until both ovaries cease functioning following menopause.

BREASTS

The breasts are not a part of the external or internal sex organs but rather are considered secondary sex characteristics—physical characteristics other than genitals that distinguish females from males. The breasts are composed internally of fatty tissue and milk-producing glands. Variations in breast size are due mainly to the amount of adipose tissue around the milk glands. Breasts are often not symmetrical in size or shape. Visible changes in a woman's breasts occur in conjunction with her physical development. During adolescence both the fatty tissue and the glandular tissue develop markedly. With adulthood the breasts become conical or hemispherical. Breasts show some size variations at different phases of the menstrual cycle and when influenced by pregnancy, nursing, or birth control pills.

Each breast contains 15 to 20 lobes of glandular tissue, with each lobe drained by a duct opening onto the nipple surface. The lobes are surrounded by fatty and fibrous tissue, giving a soft consistency to the breast. The pink or brown pigment area surrounding the nipple is called the areola. The areola pigment and size vary from woman to woman. The nipples are pigmented and protuberant. Their size and shape vary among women. The nipples consist of smooth muscle fibers and a network of nerve endings that make them sensitive to touch and temperature.

Menstrual Cycle

Menstruation is the process by which the ovaries and the uterus prepare for the development and implantation of an egg. It is a cycle lasting an average of 28 days. Menarche, the onset of a girl's first menstruation, usually occurs between 11 and 15 years of age. Menopause, the cessation of menstruation, usually takes place between the ages of 45 and 50.

The menstrual cycle is best understood as a dynamic process involving the hypothalamus and pituitary gland (located in the brain), the ovaries, and the uterus (Fig. 19-3). Hormones travel through the bloodstream acting as chemical regulators of the menstrual cycle. The hypothalamus secretes gonadotropic-releasing hormone, which signals the pituitary gland to produce two hormones that act on the ovaries. Follicle-stimulating hormone (FSH) stimulates the saclike follicles of the ovaries to prepare for ovulation. Luteinizing hormone (LH) stimulates the release of an egg from a follicle and the development of the leftover follicle into the corpus luteum. The corpus luteum in turn produces the hormone progesterone. Once the organs involved in the cycle have been stimulated, they send chemical signals through the blood to the initiating gland to decrease the production of the stimulating hormone. In this way the cycle both stimulates and regulates itself.

The menstrual cycle can be divided into three phases: the follicular phase, ovulation, and the luteal phase. These phases involve the production of hormones, the development of an egg in the ovaries, and the development of the corpus luteum in the ovary, respectively. The corresponding phases for the uterus are the proliferative phase before ovulation and the secretory phase after ovulation. Although the average combined time of these phases is 28 days, it can range from 21 to 40 days. Activity occurs in two sites during

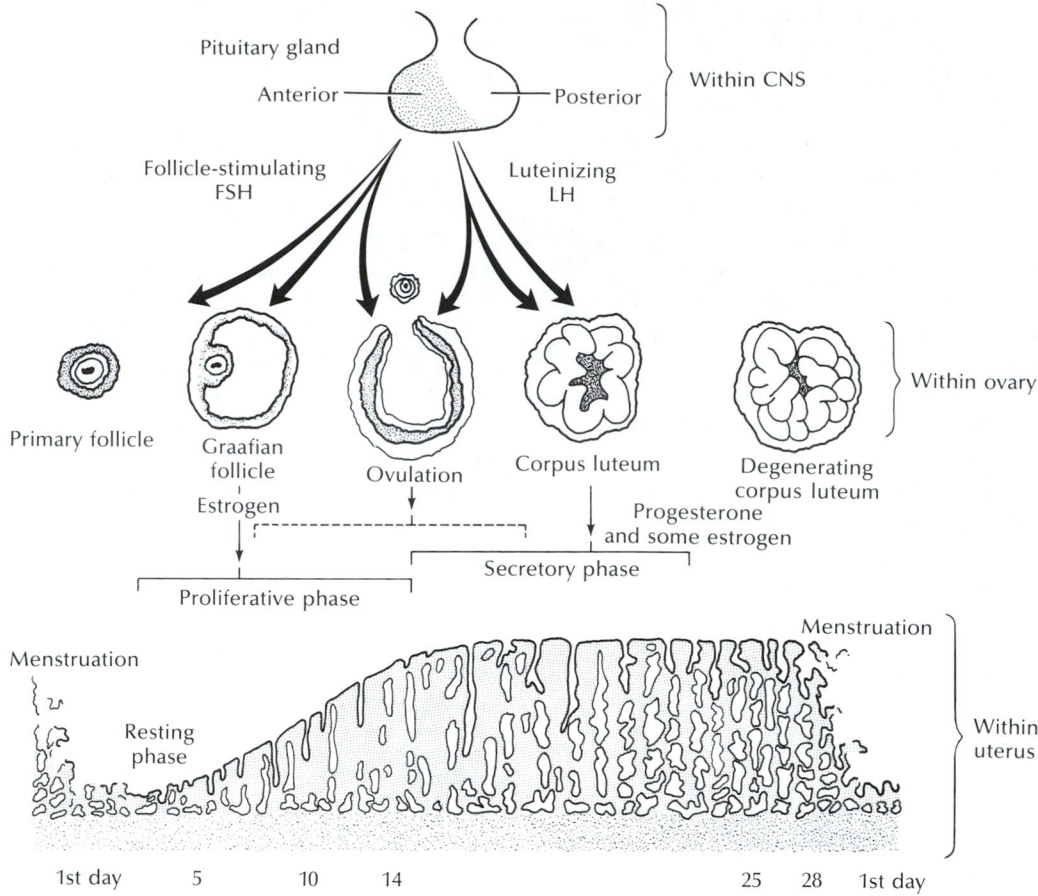

Fig. 19-3 Hormonal control of menstrual cycle.
From Jensen, M.D., et al.: Maternity care, ed. 2, St. Louis, 1981, The C.V. Mosby Co.

the cycle. In the ovaries follicular growth results in the expulsion of an egg and the development of the corpus luteum from the remaining follicle. In the uterus the endometrium thickens (proliferative phase) and, in the absence of a fertilized egg, sloughs off and passes out of the uterus as the menstrual flow (secretory phase).

During the follicular phase the pituitary gland, stimulated by the hypothalamus, releases FSH that in turn stimulates the growth of ovarian follicles. The follicles are clusters of cells surrounding an egg. The levels of estrogen and progesterone in the bloodstream during the follicular phase are low, and the uterus has shed its lining. The resulting menstrual flow of blood and bits of endometrial tissue lasts 3 to 6 days and amounts to 2 to 3 ounces (Masters, Johnson, and Kolodny, 1982). This flow signals the beginning of the new cycle. As follicular growth continues, increased estrogen production by the ovaries causes thickening of the uterine lining. The increased level of ovarian estrogen also stimulates the pituitary

gland to produce LH, which triggers the release of an egg.

Ovulation occurs about 14 days before the beginning of the next menstrual period. A mature follicle ruptures under the influence of the LH produced in the pituitary gland. The released egg begins its journey into and down the fallopian tube. At the mouth of the uterus, the cervical mucus responds to the increased levels of estrogen and becomes clear, stretchy, and slippery (Crooks and Baur, 1983).

The last phase of the menstrual cycle is the development of the corpus luteum from the follicle left behind after ovulation. The corpus luteum produces large amounts of estrogen and progesterone. It is the progesterone that causes thickening or proliferation of the endometrium as the uterus prepares to receive an egg. The progesterone also signals the hypothalamus to lower the output of the hormones triggering the production of LH and FSH in the pituitary gland. If a fertilized egg is not implanted in the uterus, the corpus luteum continues to deteriorate and estrogen and progesterone levels drop. The decrease in hormone production leads to sloughing of the uteral lining. As the hormone levels drop, the hypothalamus responds by stimulating the pituitary gland to produce FSH and LH, and a new cycle begins (Crooks and Baur, 1983).

SEX DURING MENSTRUATION

There is no physiological reason for a woman to abstain from sexual activity during menstruation. The uterine contractions during orgasm may even ease the discomfort of pelvic congestion and cramping. However, excessive menstrual flow or physical discomfort may discourage a woman from sex while she is menstruating. Cultural attitudes or other factors may also inhibit sexual activity during menstruation. If a couple does decide to abstain from genital sexual activity during menstruation, they can learn other ways of sharing intimacy until the woman is ready to resume sexual intercourse.

MENOPAUSE

One of the physiological responses to aging is the cessation of menstruation and fertility. Menopause takes place around 45 to 50 years of age. The ovaries cease production of estrogen and progesterone, although low levels of these hormones remain in the bloodstream from the continued activity of the adrenal glands. Each woman's body responds to menopause in its own way. For some women the only symptom is the disappearance of menstruation. Other women report headaches, "hot flashes," insomnia, and changes in breast and vaginal tissue. Hot flashes occur when the blood vessels rapidly dilate as a result of fluctuating hormone levels. The decrease in hormone levels also may affect the skin, breasts, and genitalia, causing the tissue to thin out. The resulting decrease in the length and elasticity of the vagina, as well as a decrease in vaginal lubrication, may make penetration uncomfortable or painful.

Menopause should not interfere with a woman's sexual capacity, and many women continue to be sexually active. Some women find that the lack of concern about pregnancy enhances their enjoyment of sex. Physical discomfort during penetration owing to reduced lubrication can be eased by using a water-based lubricant. A water-based lubricant is necessary so it can easily be removed with soap and water, thus removing a medium for bacterial growth and subsequent vaginitis and urethritis.

Male Sex Organs

The male sex organs produce sperm and hormones and provide a system for conveying sperm from the testicles to outside the body. The external male genitalia are the penis and scrotum. The male internal sex organs include the testicles, which produce hormones and sperm; the epididymis and vas deferens, a system of ducts that transport sperm; and the prostate gland, seminal vesicles, and Cowper's glands, whose secretions become part of the ejaculated semen (Fig. 19-4).

PENIS

The penis consists of the shaft, which is composed primarily of erectile tissue, and the glans, which has both erectile and sensory tissue. The penile shaft is comprised of three parallel tubes: two corpora cavernosa, which lie side by side, and beneath them a single corpus spongiosum, which surrounds the urethra. All three fibrous tubes of the penile shaft are spongelike. The large vascular spaces interposed between arteries and veins can become engorged with blood, causing the penis to become stiff and erect. The three tubes extend backward, each corpus cavernosum attaching to an arch of the pubic bone and the corpus spongiosum extending into the urethral bulb.

The anterior end of the corpus spongiosum fits over the corpora cavernosa and is called the glans. The glans resembles an acorn. The area where the glans arises abruptly from the shaft is called the corona, meaning crown. The glans and especially the corona, which contains many nerve endings, are the most sensitive parts of the penis. If the male is uncircumcised, the skin of the shaft continues forward and forms a loose-fitting hood over the glans. This hood is called the foreskin or prepuce. On the undersurface the glans is attached to the prepuce by a thin fold of skin called the frenulum, which is also very sensitive to touch. Circumcision is the removal of the foreskin.

SCROTUM

The scrotum is a thin, loose sac of skin that protects the two testicles. It is located at the base of the penis. The scrotum is divided into two compartments, each containing a testis, epididymis, and part of the vas deferens. The testis, epididymis, and parts of the vas deferens that are in the scrotum are considered internal organs even though they are outside the body cavity. The scrotum is responsive to temperature changes; cold temperatures cause it to contract, pulling the testicles closer to the body. The temperature in the scrotum is slightly lower than body temperature so sperm can be produced (Goldstein, 1976).

INTERNAL SEX ORGANS

The male internal sex organs are the testicles (or testes); the system of ducts called the epididymis, the

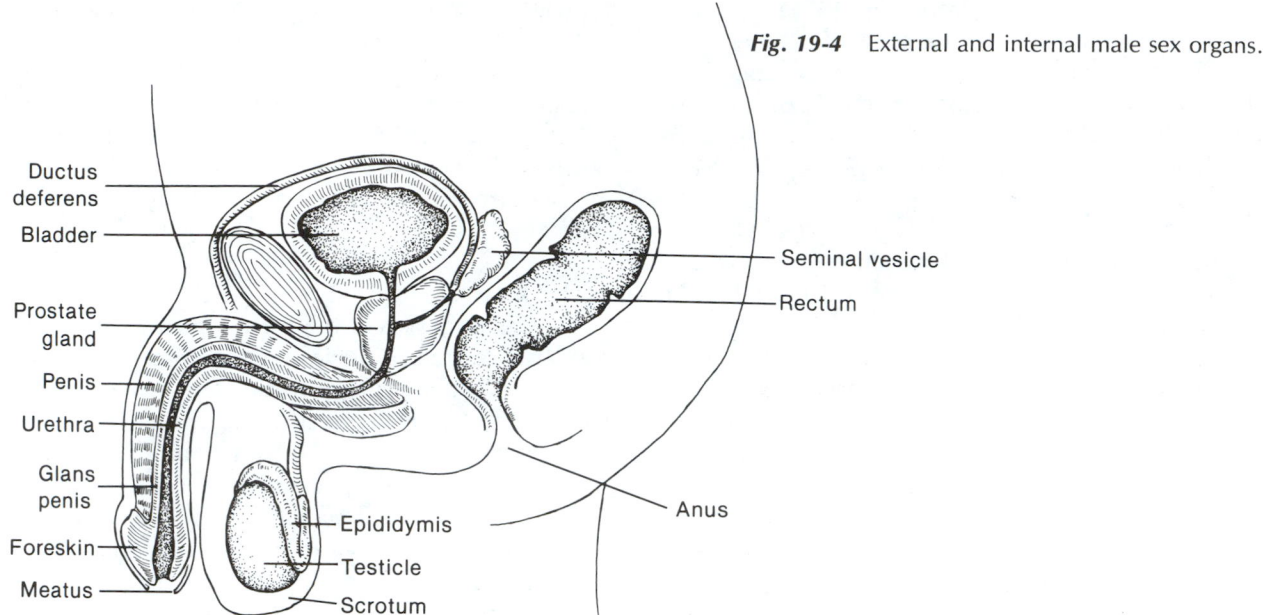

Fig. 19-4 External and internal male sex organs.

vas deferens, and the urethra; and some accessory organs (seminal vesicles, prostate gland, and bulbourethral glands). The left testicle usually hangs lower than the right. The testicles have two main functions: to produce sperm and to produce hormones. Sperm is produced in the seminiferous tubules inside each testicle. The hormones produced in the testicles are testosterone, estrogen, and androgen. Testosterone stimulates the growth and development of the genital organs and contributes to growth and development of bones and muscles. The function of the other hormones remains controversial.

The sperm drain into the epididymis, a duct that lies just outside the testicle. Sperm take 2 to 4 weeks to travel from the epididymis to the vas deferens. The vas deferens is a long tube from each testicle that goes up and out of the scrotum. It curves around the urinary bladder and then turns downward and opens into an enlargement 10 cm (4 inches) long called the ampulla. The ampulla is a reservoir for the sperm before they are discharged into the ejaculatory duct, which carries them through the prostate into the posterior urethra. The ejaculatory ducts result from the fusion of each seminal vesicle with the ampulla of its respective vas deferens. The urethra goes from the bladder to the penis tip and carries urine or semen.

The function of the seminal vesicles and prostate is to secrete seminal plasma. Their secretions serve primarily to dilute and carry the sperm. The secretions give the ejaculate its characteristic odor. The paired seminal vesicles, about 5 cm (2 inches) long, are glands secreting a portion of the ejaculate that contributes to the nutrition and reactivation of the sperm.

The prostate is about the size of a chestnut and is located beneath the bladder. The ejaculatory ducts and a portion of the urethra pass through it. The prostatic secretions unite with the sperm and nutrients passing into the urethra through the ejaculatory ducts. Even when a male is not ejaculating, small amounts of prostatic secretions are discharged into the urethra and eliminated in the urine.

The bulbourethral glands are pea-sized structures sometimes referred to as the Cowper's glands. They are located below the prostate on either side of the penile urethra. They secrete a clear, alkaline lubricating fluid that sometimes appears at the tip of the penis soon after sexual arousal. The function of this fluid is uncertain, but it is thought to neutralize the acidity of the urethra and make it a suitable environment for sperm.

Sexual Response

Sexual Response Cycle

Masters and Johnson (1966) have defined a sexual response cycle with four phases: excitement, plateau, orgasm, and resolution. These phases are the result of vasocongestion and myotonia, which are the basic physiological responses of sexual arousal (Tables 19-1 and 19-2). Vasocongestion is the pooling of blood in the genitals and female breasts during sexual arousal. In women this reaction leads to vaginal lubrication, tumescence of the clitoris and the labia minora and majora, and engorgement of the outer

TABLE 19-1

Comparison of Sexual Response Cycle in Younger and Older Women

Phase	Younger Women	Older Women
Excitement	Vaginal lubrication—"sweating" of vaginal walls Expansion of inner two thirds of vaginal barrel Increased sensitivity and engorgement of clitoris and labia Nipple erection and increase in breast size	Decrease in amount of vaginal lubrication Slower lubrication of vagina Slower reaction of clitoris to stimulation Much less engorgement of labia majora Only slight engorgement of labia minora Less enlargement of breast
Plateau	Retraction of clitoris under clitoral hood Formation of orgasmic platform—swelling of outer one third of vagina and labia minora Elevation of cervix and uterus—"tenting" effect "Sex skin": vivid color change in labia minora Areolar engorgement Increase in muscle tension and breathing	Orgasmic platform reduced by half Less expansive capacity of vaginal walls Loss of consistency of "sex skin" (labial color change) Less engorgement of areolae
Orgasm	Involuntary contractions of orgasmic platform, uterus, rectal and urethral sphincters, and other muscle groups Hyperventilation and increase in heart rate	Less tension from muscle contraction Less frequent rectal contractions Shortened vaginal contraction phase Shorter orgasm time
Resolution	Gradual relaxation of vaginal walls Rapid color change of labia minora Sweating reaction Breathing, heart beat, and muscle tension gradually return to normal Often ability to return to orgasm, since women do not experience a refractory period as men often do	Vaginal changes returning quickly to prearousal state Clitoral swelling lost Slower loss of nipple erection

third of the vagina (orgasmic platform). In men vasocongestion leads to erection of the penis. Myotonia, or neuromuscular tension, gradually increases throughout the body during the excitement and plateau phases. Myotonia peaks during orgasm, resulting in involuntary contractions of the woman's vagina and the man's vas deferens and urethra. Both women and men experience contractions of the arm and leg muscles, facial muscles, and gluteal muscles. Carpopedal spasms, or spastic contractions of the muscles of the hands and feet, may occur. After orgasm, both vasocongestion and myotonia return to prearousal levels.

The phases described by Masters and Johnson are not absolute. They are strongly influenced by psychological and environmental factors, and their timing and intensity vary from individual to individual.

EXCITEMENT

The excitement phase involves a gradual increase in sexual arousal. The earliest signs of sexual arousal are vaginal lubrication and penile erection. The vag-

inal barrel begins to elongate and increase in size, and the labia majora, nipples, and breasts become congested with blood. In men, the testicles become elevated and enlarged and the scrotum becomes elevated and thickened. In some men nipple erection and tumescense occur late in this phase.

PLATEAU

The responses of the excitement phase are heightened in the plateau phase. Vasocongestion and myotonia increase, as do heart rate, blood pressure, pulse rate, and respiration. In some women the breasts enlarge. The areolae become engorged, and a slight flush develops in the skin. There are marked color changes in the labia minora; as they swell, the color deepens from pink to a deep red. The clitoris moves upward and inward under the hood. The cervix and uterus pull back and up, causing a "tenting" of the cervical os while the vaginal barrel elongates.

In men the coronal ridge increases in circumference and deepens in color. The penis becomes congested and extends to its maximum size. The testicles enlarge

---

TABLE 19-2

Comparison of Sexual Response Cycle in Younger and Older Men

Phase	Younger Men	Older Men
Excitement	Penile erection Thickening and elevation of scrotum Moderate enlargement of testicles	Takes longer to attain an erection but can be maintained for long periods of time Less enlargement of scrotum Less elevation of testes
Plateau	Increase in size of glans (tip) of penis Glans may become intense in color Elevation and 50% increase in size of testicles Mucoid emission from Cowper's glands, possibly with sperm Increase in muscle tension and breathing	Less likely to have intensity of color change of glans Phase likely to be prolonged owing to better ejaculatory control Penis becomes fully erect just before ejaculation
Orgasm	Internal urinary sphincter closes Sensation of ejaculatory inevitability Contractions of vas deferens, seminal vesicles, prostate, and ejaculatory duct Relaxation of external bladder sphincter Contractions of urethral and rectal sphincter muscles Hyperventilation and increase in heart rate Ejaculation—sperm mostly in first part	Feeling of ejaculatory inevitability is eliminated Penile contractions are fewer in number and intensity Rectal contractions are less frequent Ejaculation lacks the same force and duration Less volume of semen
Resolution	Loss of penile erection Refractory period when continued stimulation is uncomfortable Sweating reaction Descent of testicles Breathing, heart rate, and muscle tension gradually return to prearousal level	Rapid loss of erection Refractory period (time it takes for stimulation to cause another erection) may be greatly extended Rapid descent of testicles

---

by 50% and elevate closer to the perineum. Drops of fluid secreted from the Cowper's glands may appear at the urethral opening (Goldstein, 1976).

ORGASM

Orgasm is the sudden release of the pooled blood and tension in the muscles at the climax of sexual excitement. It can be a highly pleasurable event involving the feeling of physiological and psychological release. A series of involuntary, reflex contractions, varying in intensity, occurs in the genitals and limbs. In women the outer one third of the vagina (orgasmic platform), uterine muscles, and anal sphincter contract rapidly. At the onset of ejaculation the internal bladder sphincter closes, preventing retrograde ejaculation into the bladder. Rhythmical contractions of the urethra, epididymis, seminal vesicles, prostate, and anal sphincter occur in men. The hands and feet may clutch and grasp. Heart rate, blood pressure, and respiratory rate all reach peak levels during orgasm. The clitoris and glans penis may be so sensitive at the

moment of orgasm that further stimulation is uncomfortable or painful.

RESOLUTION

Resolution involves a physiological and psychological return to an unaroused state. During the resolution phase there is a rapid loss of genital vasocongestion, nipple erection, and the sex flush. As vital signs return to normal, the palms or soles may start to sweat. The person experiences a feeling of relaxation.

In women the clitoris and vaginal barrel return to their prearousal state. The labia minora and majora fade to their usual pink color. All women have the capacity for multiple orgasms if they continue to receive effective sexual stimulation.

During the resolution phase there is a rapid loss of vasocongestion in the penis and scrotum. Immediately after orgasm most men experience reduced sensitivity to continued erotic stimulation. This so-called refractory period is a recovery time during which further orgasm or ejaculation is physiologically impossible. The refractory period is variable in duration and is a major difference in sexual response between the sexes. Most men are incapable of experiencing multiple orgasms in the same cycle. Women do not experience a refractory period.

AGING AND SEXUAL RESPONSE (Tables 19-1 and 19-2)

Given reasonably good health and the acceptance of sexual capacity, there is no reason why people cannot remain sexually active as long as they choose. Nonetheless, the aging process does have an effect on sexual behavior.

During the excitement phase older women often find that the vaginal barrel does not lubricate as much as before. The vaginal tissue becomes thinner and loses some of its elasticity. This is due to the change in estrogen level. There is less congestion in the labia minora, labia majora, and breasts. Older men usually take longer to achieve an erection, and the erection may be less full than in earlier years. There may be little testicular elevation, and the vasocongestion in the scrotum and testes is much less pronounced.

The plateau phase may be prolonged for both women and men. Women have decreased vasocongestion of the orgasmic platform. Men may have much better ejaculatory control.

The orgasm phase becomes shorter. The contractions of the orgasm may be fewer and more spasmodic and may even cause uncomfortable uterine contractions. Older women retain their ability to have multiple orgasms.

For men the sensation of ejaculatory inevitability may be less intense or gradually disappear from the orgasmic phase. The expulsive force of ejaculation decreases, as does the volume of seminal fluid expelled.

In both men and women the resolution period is quick. For men the erection is lost rapidly along with the rapid descent of the testicles. The refractory period may last several hours or even days.

Sexual Development

INFANCY

It appears that all the mechanisms of sexual response are present at birth. Signs of sexual arousal in infants have been observed even during birth. Vaginal lubrication, penile erection, and pelvic thrusting by infants indicate that sexual capacity is not limited to sexually mature adults. It must be emphasized that the aim and erotic content of adult sexuality are not a part of infant sexuality, which has pleasure and tension release as its aims.

CHILDHOOD

Children discover very early that genital touching can be pleasurable. They are also naturally and normally curious about their bodies and the bodies of others. Children may masturbate, and as with any other behavior, they need to learn when and where it is appropriate to do so. As children become more mobile and social, particularly at school age, it is not unusual for them to engage in some form of sex play with peers or siblings. Such play may range from "show-and-tell" or playing "doctor" to simulating intercourse. While there may be an element of gender role rehearsal for adult life in such play, its major focus for the child is just play. Through calm adult guidance children learn that their bodies are private, that people are in charge of their own bodies, and that there are appropriate times and places for touching the genitals. Masturbation continues to be the major sexual activity and, like hygiene activities and nudity, becomes private in later childhood.

PUBERTY

Puberty is a time of major emotional and physical change. Rising levels of sex hormones cause growth spurts, the development of secondary sex characteristics, and the onset of menstruation and ejaculation. Along with the physical changes go the tasks of entering the adult world of eroticized sexuality. This usually starts with hand-holding, dating, and greater interest in clothes in early adolescence. It is crucial that young people understand their own sexual value systems and decision-making processes, since they may face major sexual and contraception decisions during puberty.

The onset of puberty in girls is usually signaled by the development of the breasts. After an initial growth of breast tissue, the nipple and areola increase in size. This process, which is in part controlled by heredity, may begin as early as 8 years of age and may not be complete until the late teen years. Rising levels of estrogen are also beginning to affect the genitals. The uterus begins to enlarge, and increased vaginal lubrication occurs, either spontaneously or as a result of sexual arousal. The vagina lengthens, and pubic hair appears. Menarche, or the onset of the menstrual cycle, varies widely; it may occur as early as 8 years of age or not until 16 or later. Although the menstrual cycle is initially irregular and ovulation may not occur at first, girls who are sexually active need information about contraception.

Rising levels of testosterone in boys during puberty are signaled by an increase in size of the penis, testicles, prostate, and seminal vesicles. Both boys and girls may experience orgasm before puberty, but ejaculation in boys does not occur until the sex organs begin to mature, around the age of 12 or 14. About the time genital development takes place, pubic, facial, and body hair begins to grow. The voice changes as the larynx increases in size. This also occurs in girls, but in boys the more dramatic shifts or "cracking" of the voice may be a source of embarrassment. Boys must understand that, although they may not produce sperm with their first ejaculations, they will soon be fertile 24 hours a day. Boys entering puberty require information about contraception.

ADULTHOOD

A major task in adult sexuality is communicating one's sexual value system and negotiating sexual behavior with other adults. In the absence of any single, universally accepted cultural norm for adult sexual behavior, this can be a confusing process. Adults who choose to abstain from sex may experience pressure from those who are unable or unwilling to understand their choice. Single adults have the problem of finding appropriate sexual partners, avoiding sexually transmitted diseases, and establishing intimate relationships. People in relationships must deal with differences in sexual desire and changes in the feeling of love and closeness they have for each other. A person who is leaving a relationship often needs to relearn how to interact with others as a single person in social and sexual situations. One group with special needs that receives little public attention is adults who want to conceive but cannot. In a society that places great value on contraception and family planning, adults who cannot conceive are faced with emotional pain and frustration. They may experience a sense of failure as a woman or man and may feel that their bodies are somehow defective. They may direct every waking moment toward creating the right timing for conception. Most are in limbo until they either decide to adopt a child or accept that they will probably never have children.

OLDER ADULTHOOD

The capacity for sexuality is lifelong. Theoretically people can engage in sex as far into old age as they choose. However, older people face health concerns and societal attitudes that may make it difficult for them to continue sexual activity. Although declining physical abilities may make sex as they knew it painful or impossible, with sympathetic intervention they can experiment with and learn alternative ways of sexual expression. The decreasing vaginal lubrication that occurs with aging may make a supplemental lubricant necessary. Decreases in the fat pads that surround the clitoris may make it hypersensitive even to clothing rubbing on it. Cushions and bolsters can be used to support the limbs and torso in order to ease the strain on the body during sexual activity. An erect penis is not necessary for sexual pleasure. If erectile capacity is diminished or absent, men can be encouraged to continue to express their sexual feelings through touch, including with the flaccid penis.

Perhaps a more difficult obstacle for the elderly is the myth that sex is for the young. Some older people stop having sexual activity because they feel it is inappropriate for their age group. Hospitals, nursing homes, and other health care institutions may discourage sexual behavior among clients, although some nursing homes now give clients the opportunity and privacy to meet their needs for intimacy. Finding a partner may be a problem for some elderly persons. The need to touch, be touched, and be sexual must not be left out of the aging equation.

Problems Involving Sexuality

Personal and Emotional Conflicts

Ideally, sex is a natural, spontaneous act that passes easily through a number of recognizable physiological stages and culminates in one or more orgasms. Following sexual intercourse, there should be a period of "afterglow" in which both partners experience a sense of warmth, well-being, and closeness. In reality, this sequence of events is more the exception than the rule, as demonstrated by the number of self-help sexual enhancement books available in bookstores. Nurses can expect to encounter clients who have problems with one or more of the stages of sexual behavior, including the feeling of wanting sex, the physiology and emotions of having sex, and the feelings experienced after sex. Clients may unconciously provide the nurse with clues to their sexual problems. In such a case the nurse must act as a sleuth in helping the client define and deal with sexual problems.

FACTORS AFFECTING SEXUALITY

Sexual desire is an appetite that waxes and wanes. Furthermore, appetites vary among individuals: some people want and enjoy sex every day, whereas others want sex only once a month, and still others have no sexual desire and are quite comfortable with that fact. Sexual desire becomes an issue if the client simply wants to feel sexier more often, if the client believes it is necessary to measure up to some imagined cultural norm, or if a discrepancy in the sexual desires of the partners in a relationship appears to be causing conflict. Clients may bring up such sexual problems by saying that they "just don't feel turned on sexually" as they used to or that their partners seem demanding about sexual issues in the relationship.

The client should be assured that almost any change in one's environment or sense of self may lead to sexual changes, ranging from mild, transient emotional discomfort to a sexual dysfunction that requires professional counseling or therapy.

PHYSICAL FACTORS. There are physical reasons why a client may experience a decrease in sexual desire. Sexual activity may bring on pain or discomfort. Even imagining that sex could hurt can lessen one's sexual desire. Minor illness or simply feeling tired is a reason why a person may not feel sexual. Medications can affect sexual desire. Even the prescribing physician may not be able to predict the effects of a given medication on the client's sexual feelings and behavior. Poor body image, particularly when magnified by feelings of rejection or by body-altering surgery, can "turn off" clients sexually.

RELATIONSHIP FACTORS. Issues in a relationship can distract a person from wanting sex. Just as there is an ebb and flow of sexual appetite in an individual, so sexual desire ebbs and flows in a relationship. Couples often find after the initial glow of the relationship has faded that they are faced with major differences in their values or life-styles. The degree to which they still feel close to each other and interact on an intimate level will depend on their ability to negotiate and compromise. Thus, communication skills play a crucial role when dealing with sexual desire in a relationship. Decreased interest in sexual activity can result just from the anxiety of having to tell a partner what sexual behavior is acceptable or pleasurable.

LIFE-STYLE FACTORS. Life-style factors, such as the use or abuse of alcohol and the lack of time to devote to a relationship, can influence sexual desire. Traditionally associated with sexual behavior, particularly in advertisements, alcohol can induce a sense of well-being or seductiveness in the initial stages of sex. However, there is now ample evidence that alcohol's negative effects on sexuality far outweigh the euphoria it may initially produce. Finding the time for sexual activity is another life-style factor. Some clients do not know how to structure their working and home time to include sexual behavior. Working parents, for example, may feel so overburdened that they perceive sexual advances from a partner as one more demand on them. Such clients often describe their need to be alone to think and rest as more important than sex.

SELF-ESTEEM FACTORS. The client's level of self-esteem can also lead to personal and emotional conflicts involving sexuality. The degree of a client's sexual desire may depend on the client's sense of personal value and learned sexual skills. If sexual self-esteem has not been nurtured by encouraging the development of a strong sense of a sexual self and the learning of sexual skills, sexuality may bring forth negative feelings or lead to the suppression of sexual feelings. Sexual self-esteem can be lowered in many ways. Rape, incest, and physical or emotional abuse leave deep scars. Lowered sexual self-esteem can also result from lack of adequate sex education, negative role models, or attempts to live up to unrealistic personal or cultural expectations.

Sexual Dysfunction

The causes of sexual dysfunction may be physiological or psychological. Sometimes the cause of a dysfunction cannot be identified or is a combination of several factors. An estimated 10% to 20% of sexual dysfunctions are caused by physiological factors. In another 15% of cases, physiological problems contribute to the sexual dysfunction without being its sole cause. In most instances a sexual assessment should include a complete physical examination to identify or rule out physiological conditions that might be contributing to sexual dysfunction.

PSYCHOLOGICAL FACTORS

In many instances sexual dysfunction can be traced to a lack of knowledge about sexuality, ignorance of sexual techniques, or general misinformation about sexuality. For example, unsatisfactory lovemaking can be the result of a lack of information about sexual anatomy. This is hardly surprising in a society that generally places strong prohibitions on sexual behavior. Open discussion of sex, even between partners, traditionally has not been encouraged, and the unfortunate result has been feelings of distance or alienation.

Another psychological factor is the destructive belief that the ability to perform sexually is inherently developed by the time a person reaches adulthood. Sexual performance is often perceived as instinctual and mysteriously understood when a person "comes of age." Thus ignorance and silence about sexual matters prevail, since a person who lacks knowledge about sexual function seldom realizes that one needs to be taught this information. Myths and outright misinformation about sexuality add to the problem of a lack of knowledge for many individuals.

It is important for the nurse to understand how the phenomena of ignorance and avoidance of sexual issues have developed in our society. Human sexuality is a basic drive that is frequently accompanied by intense and conflicting emotions. Society has therefore developed standards for sexual behavior, which serve to minimize fears and confusion about how a person should act. Unfortunately, they can also create unrealistic expectations, demands, and restrictions that are internalized by individuals and become a part of their value systems.

The psychological forces that prevent violation of sexual rules in many cultures are guilt and anxiety. When guilt and anxiety become associated with early sexual learning, the person develops a pattern of inhibited sexual response and carries this through to adulthood. For instance, a woman may be actively discouraged from sexual stimulation in early childhood and as an adult may find that she not only has to learn to enjoy sexual stimulation, but also has to overcome negative feelings associated with her sexual self-concept.

Other sources of sexual anxiety, such as fear of failure, demand for performance, and rejection, can be destructive to sexual functioning. Anticipation of the inability to perform is a cause of erectile dysfunction and perhaps to some extent of orgasmic dysfunction. A person who has experienced an episode of failure will have an increased fear of its recurrence. Anticipatory anxiety related to sexual performance can start a self-defeating cycle of fear that escalates from a single failure into a state of serious chronic dysfunction. In "spectatoring," the phenomenon that maintains this cycle, one remains outside oneself and observes one's sexual responses. This results in poor performance, which then reconfirms one's anxieties and fear of failure (Masters and Johnson, 1970).

Fear of rejection by one's partner or an excessive need to please may also generate anxiety. To wish to give enjoyment and share pleasure with a partner is desirable and healthy. It is when this becomes a compulsive need to please, to perform, to serve, and to not disappoint that the emotion becomes dysfunctional.

Poor communication is frequently associated with sexual dysfunction. A person with communication problems may be unable to discuss sex and thus may have limited knowledge and restrictive standards of acceptable sexual behavior. In this self-defeating cycle, partners perpetuate ignorance, lack of understanding, and misinformation about their sexual and emotional needs. To communicate effectively about sex, they must openly share information about their interests, desires, and wishes. Negotiation and compromise result from effective communication patterns.

Other relationship issues often play a large part in sexual dysfunction. Anger, power struggles, and unresolved conflict within the relationship are important causes of sexual dissatisfaction that leads to dysfunc-

tion. Fear of pregnancy is a factor that may make it difficult for a woman to relax.

A history of sexual abuse may have an impact on sexual functioning. Anger, guilt, and a need for control are emotional sequelae to abuse and often underlie the development of sexual problems, including inhibited desire and avoidance of sexual contact. Researchers have begun to examine the variables associated with molestation that contribute to adult sexual adjustment. These include the person's age at the time of molestation, the frequency and duration of molestation, and the person's negative feelings associated with molestation. These findings help explain the variations in sexual functioning that exist among people with histories of abuse. Further investigation is needed to help us understand and effectively treat the population of abused persons who seek counseling for sexual difficulties (Livingston, McIntyre, and Fogel, 1984).

Tables 19-3 and 19-4 summarize the most common female and male sexual dysfunctions, their possible causes, and intervention strategies.

PHYSIOLOGICAL FACTORS

Orgasmic dysfunction in women is seldom caused by physiological factors. However, diabetes, alcoholism (Livingston and McIntyre, 1984), neurological problems, hormone deficiencies, and some pelvic disorders resulting from infections or surgery may impair or hinder orgasmic response. Vaginismus, or involuntary vaginal contraction, is most often caused by psychological factors, while dyspareunia, or painful intercourse, is more likely the result of poor vaginal lubrication caused by physical disorders such as infections, surgical scarring, diabetes, or use of drugs (for example, antihistamines, tranquilizers, or marijuana). Physiological causes for lack of sexual desire include hormone deficiencies, alcoholism, kidney failure, drug abuse, and severe chronic illness (Masters, Johnson, and Kolodny, 1982).

Physiological factors that may cause erectile dysfunction in men include neurological disorders such as spinal cord injury or multiple sclerosis, vascular insufficiency problems, hormonal deficiencies, and genital infections or injuries. Diabetes and alcoholism are the two most common physiological causes of erectile dysfunction. Both prescription medications and "street" drugs sometimes cause erection problems. Physiological problems rarely cause premature ejaculation, but delayed ejaculation is sometimes the result of neurological disorders. About 10% of cases of delayed ejaculation are due to drug and alcoholism (Livingston and McIntyre, 1984).

The distinction between physiological and psychological causes of sexual dysfunction is not always

TABLE 19-3

Common Female Sexual Dysfunctions

Description	Possible Causes	Interventions
Preorgasmic (primary orgasmic dysfunction): a woman who has never had an orgasm	Religious prohibitions Restrictive learning environment Fear of losing control Poor communication with partner Inadequate clitoral stimulation Excessive drug or alcohol use Past negative sexual experiences	Information on sexual prohibitions and restrictions Sensate focus exercises* Genital play Kegel exercises† Directed masturbation Nondemand intercourse Referral to a preorgasmic support group
Secondary orgasmic dysfunction: a woman who has experienced orgasm in the past but does not currently	Low sexual interest Attitude toward partner Causes listed for primary orgasmic dysfunction	Discussion of attitude toward partner Information on sexual prohibitions Sensate focus exercises* Nondemand intercourse Genital play Kegel exercises† Directed masturbation Partner communication
Vaginismus: a woman who experiences involuntary constriction of the outer one third of the vagina, making vaginal penetration impossible	Religious prohibitions Sexual prohibitions Experience of sexual assault Painful intercourse Painful pelvic examinations Alcohol abuse Traumatic early experiences with sex Fear of pregnancy, venereal disease, or cancer	Legitimization of existence of spasm Use of vaginal dilators in graduated sizes Kegel exercises† Improvement of partner communication
Dyspareunia: painful intercourse	Negative attitude toward partner Strong religious prohibitions Sexual prohibitions Genital sensitivity Physical problems (tears, infections, trauma, spasms, lack of lubrication) Roughness during intercourse Lack of arousal	Thorough and detailed examination of sex organs Treatment of physical problems Provision of sufficient lubrication Discussion of sexual attitudes Discussion of comfortable positions
Lack of desire: a woman who has lost interest in being sexual	Preorgasmia Strong negative emotions Illness Drug or alcohol use Avoidance response because of feeling sexually pressured Unresolved anger or fear Depression History of sexual abuse or incest Pain associated with intercourse	Discussion of attitude toward partner Information on sexual prohibitions and restrictions Sensate focus exercises* Kegel exercises† Genital play Resolution of any conflicts between partners

*Series of pleasurable touching exercises that are focused on sensual (not sexual) activities with a partner.
†Exercises for the pubococcygeus (PC) muscle to increase sensation and maintain muscle tone of the pelvic floor.

TABLE 19-4

Common Male Sexual Dysfunctions

Description	Possible Causes	Intervention
Primary erectile dysfunction: a male who cannot penetrate during sexual contact, has never been able to sustain an erection to the point of penetration, and may masturbate to ejaculation	Not well understood Extreme religious prohibitions Traumatic initial failure Performance anxiety and fears	Relieving pressure of goal-oriented sexual performance Discussing sexual prohibitions and restrictions Providing accurate information Sensate focus exercises Reducing "spectatoring" Restricting intercourse Encouraging female superior position with lubrication Encouraging options to intercourse, manual stimulation, oral/genital sex
Secondary erectile dysfunction: a male who cannot maintain or perhaps even experience an erection but has succeeded at penetration at least one time; has experienced erectile failure during at least 25% of his sexual opportunities	Interference with central nervous system caused by drugs, alcohol, stress, fatigue, diseases, or surgical procedures Performance anxiety Poor communication with partner Depression	Relieving pressure of goal-oriented sexual performance Discussing sexual prohibitions and restrictions Providing accurate information Sensate focus exercises Kegel exercises Reducing "spectatoring"
Premature ejaculation: a male who consistently ejaculates sooner than he would desire	Adolescent fast ejaculation patterning Failure to attend to internal cues of approaching ejaculation Lack of sensual self-awareness Performance anxiety	Providing accurate information Encouraging communication with partner Sensate focus exercises Kegel exercises Stop-start technique Encouraging different positions Retraining ejaculatory response Relieving pressure of performance anxiety Changing tempo of thrusting during intercourse
Delayed ejaculation: a male who cannot ejaculate during penetration	Religious restrictions Fear of impregnating Lack of physical interest Active dislike for partner Past traumatic sexual event Infidelity Punishment for masturbation as a child Excessive drug or alcohol use	Relieving pressure of goal-oriented sexual performance Discussing sexual prohibitions and restrictions Providing accurate information Sensate focus exercises Kegel exercises Encouraging communication with partner

clear. Physiological interventions sometimes clear up the problem. At other times there may be psychological concerns that have been masked by a physiological condition. It is important to monitor the client's progress carefully even when it seems that only a physiological condition is involved. An understanding of the possible psychological and physiological causes of sexual dysfunction is needed before the nurse can determine what further assessment and intervention is necessary in a given case.

Effects of Illness on Sexuality

Healthy sexuality involves all human dimensions, and illness can directly or indirectly influence any or all of these dimensions. While illness and the healing process do indeed influence established living patterns, the idea that health is a matter of degree rather than a matter of being either sick or well may be a new one for the client. Viewing sexuality in terms of a continuum rather than as being present or absent may also be a new concept for the client. The nurse's task is to help the client integrate the physical, psychological, and social systems during the course of the illness. The degree to which any nursing intervention involving sex is successful depends on the attitudes and beliefs of both nurse and client and their understanding of the effects of the illness and its treatment on sexual functioning.

The media's treatment of sexuality suggests that only the young and fit are sexual. Eroticized images and descriptions of ill or disabled people are rare. Because of this, most people seldom think about or imagine how ill people feel or behave sexually. A dynamic approach to total health care, however, considers all the ways in which an illness might affect a client's sexuality.

PHYSIOLOGICAL CHANGES AND CHRONIC ILLNESS

Sexual behavior depends on intact neural, vascular, and hormonal systems. The genitals and other soft body tissues that respond to sexual arousal require uninterrupted neural pathways and an adequate supply of blood. Hormones influence both sexual moods and physiological functioning in sexual expression. Joints and muscles must bend and stretch as the body gives expression to sexual feelings. Any change in any one of these systems can have a ripple effect on the others. To accommodate to changes in these systems, the client may have to learn new sexual behaviors. Changes in body functions and structures as a result of illness may not directly influence sexuality but may affect feelings of desirability and arousal. In this case it is the client's perception of self as sexually capable and sexually desirable that is being influenced.

Chronic illness interferes with sexuality because of the extended period of care and attention involved. A client may have no energy left for sexual feelings or activity. For a client with a highly debilitating illness, such as chronic lung disease, only very limited sexual activity may be possible. There are no therapies for reversing sexual impairment resulting from neurological or vascular disease (Unsain, Goodwin, and Schuster, 1982). Diseases such as diabetes not only necessitate changes in daily habits but also may lead to reduced sexual desire, lack of or change in orgasmic response, and erectile dysfunction. Chronic pain and limited range of movement present obstacles to sexual activity. To adjust to these limitations, the client must learn effective communication skills and be willing to experiment with new positions for sexual activity. The nurse has an essential role in facilitating these adjustments, particularly when the client's background does not encourage open discussion of sexual topics.

HOSPITALIZATION

Being hospitalized can have a powerful symbolic meaning to clients. Clients tend to think their situation is serious if a hospital is involved. The procedures of hospital health care may take on a mystery that is beyond a client's capacity to understand. The need to have some power over his life and the powerlessness of being hospitalized may become crucial issues for a hospitalized client. The client has left the home environment with its security and privacy and entered a much more public and intrusive environment. The hospital room is open to the nurse day and night, and privacy is represented only by a cubicle curtain. Hospital clothing is notoriously scant. Even carrying out activities of personal hygiene may be beyond the client's ability. Add to this the feelings of illness and anxiety, and it is no wonder that sexual behavior and feelings may diminish or vanish.

Nurses can assist clients in learning to meet sexual needs in the hospital setting. Simply acknowledging the openness of the setting lets a client know that the nurse understands. Knocking or signaling before entering the client's space is a basic courtesy and provides a needed sense of privacy. The use of a "do not disturb" sign offers the client some feeling of control over the privacy of his environment.

The effect of medications on sexual feelings and functioning is an enormously complex topic, simply because of the number of medications in use. Medications can interfere with sexual desire as well as all phases of the sexual response cycle. Three main issues are involved: whether the effects of a medication on sexual functioning are as described in the literature; whether the nurse and physician know about the effects; and whether the client has been informed of the effects. Radiotherapy and chemotherapy, particularly when they involve the pelvis or bowel, can also affect sexual functioning (Shipes and Lehr, 1982).

Surgery not only changes body structures and functions but also influences the client's body image (Dickman and Livingston, 1982). Surgical clients may experience loss of self-esteem and feelings of loss involving their masculinity or femininity (Lion, 1982). They may blame themselves for needing surgery and consider the surgical consequences their just punishment. Alteration or removal of the internal or external genitalia can make conventional and accustomed sexual activities uncomfortable or impossible. The client is then faced not only with the loss or alteration of body parts, but also with the potential of having to learn new sexual behaviors that may seem strange or repugnant. Prostatectomies, hysterectomies, mastectomies, and ostomies can be expected to create sexual problems for clients.

After a heart attack or heart surgery clients often have a decline in sexual activity (Lion, 1982). This is true even after they are evaluated as fit and able to resume normal activities of daily living. These clients typically fear having another attack or dying while masturbating or having intercourse. The client's partner is often anxious about initiating sex because of fear of contributing to another attack. Clearly, accurate and honest information is needed at every stage of the rehabilitation process. Such anxieties are cultivated through misunderstanding, misinformation, or lack of information on the client's part.

SEXUALLY TRANSMITTED DISEASES

Clients with sexually transmitted diseases (STDs) are seen in all health care settings. Health care literature and practice offer ample opportunity for the nurse to learn about illnesses and injuries that are directly related to sexual activities. The media have brought certain STDs to national attention, and through their efforts and those of public health agencies, information about and treatment of STDs are reaching an increasing number of people of all ages. Health care professionals also have an increased level of knowledge and treatment skill.

A major problem in dealing with STDs is finding and treating the people who have them. Sometimes people do not seek treatment because they are embarrassed about how they became infected. Some people may not even know they are infected because symptoms are absent or go unnoticed. Since sexual behavior may include the whole body rather than just the genitalia, many parts of the body are potential sites for an STD. The ears, mouth, throat, tongue, nose, and eyelids can be used for sexual pleasure. The entire surface of the skin can be thought of as having sexual potential. Although the perineum, anus, and rectum are rarely discussed in terms of sexual pleasuring, they are frequently included in sexual activity by both women and men. Furthermore, any contact with body fluids from another person around the head, an open lesion on the skin, the anus, or the genitals has the potential to transmit an STD.

Clients may be hesitant to talk about their sexual behavior if they feel it is "not normal," normal usually being whatever they believe society approves. Oral-genital sex, anal sex, or any sexual behavior that embarrasses the client may hinder the detection of an STD. Specific STDs of the throat and intestine can thus go undetected at great cost to the client.

The most valuable tool the nurse can develop for providing care in areas related to sexuality is communication skills. By questioning and talking with the client in a nonjudgmental manner that evokes trust, the nurse can pick up valuable clues about the presence of an STD that the client may have missed. The nurse can also begin to assess the client's attitudes toward sexuality and adjust the intervention to make it acceptable to the client's sexual value system.

Contraception

The ability to prevent a pregnancy or to plan the time between pregnancies should be part of a client's health care plan. An unwanted pregnancy can affect health on many levels. The health of the parent, the child, and ultimately the community in which they live depends on the presence of adequate physical, emotional, and financial resources to care for the child. A client who is burdened with an unwanted child often enters the health care system with stress-related complaints. The unwanted child may suffer neglect or even abuse.

Ways of preventing unwanted pregnancy have been developed. Each woman's right to choose if and when to become pregnant is generally acknowledged. It would seem then that it should be a simple process to match the desire to control pregnancy with an appropriate method of contraception. Yet the number of pregnancies among teenagers, abortions in all age groups, and unwanted children indicates that many sexually active people are not using contraceptive measures.

Factors Influencing Use of Contraception

The nurse considers three major factors when exploring why a client is not using contraception effectively: the client, the client's environment, and the appropriateness of the contraception technique (Fogel and Woods, 1981).

The first factor involves the client's ability to take meaningful action. For several reasons clients might not act in their own best interests in using contraception techniques. Some clients truly do not believe that they can control conception. Such clients often view themselves as controlled by events or people outside themselves. A client may also fail to use contraceptive measures because of a lack of knowledge about contraception or about the potential danger of a pregnancy to health or life-style. Shame, guilt, and denial can affect a client's ability to use contraception effectively. When a client uses contraception, he or she must acknowledge that sexual behavior is likely. This may be difficult for the client to admit. If the client has to deal with a pharmacist or health care provider to obtain contraceptives, the embarrassment or sense of personal risk may be too high for the client to act.

A second factor influencing the effective use of contraception is the client's environment. The client's family, community, or religion may disapprove of or prohibit contraception. A woman may have been reared in a family environment in which she was taught that sex for pleasure rather than procreation is wrong. A partner who is not knowledgeable about contraception or does not cooperate in its use increases the risk of contraception failure. People learn about contraception from peers, health care providers, or public health agencies. Good contraception education requires a health care system and an educational system that can deliver such education to the community. Not all communities can afford or support that kind of education.

Finally, the method of contraception must be appropriate for the client. The effectiveness of contraception is related to its safety, comfort, expense, availability, and ease of use. The nurse should remember in discussing contraception with clients that each method has a theoretical effectiveness and an actual effectiveness. The former is based on the ideal circumstances under which the method could be used. The latter considers all personal and environmental factors and may be considerably lower if the client does not use the method regularly or properly.

The decision to use or not use a contraceptive method must be made by the client. The nurse can play an effective role in the decision-making process by helping the client clarify values about contraception and by providing accurate information. The discussion between nurse and client might include questions such as the following:

1. How does the method work?
2. What are the risks involved in using the method?
3. How will it affect lovemaking?
4. Does the partner object to it?
5. Will it cause any discomfort?
6. Is it readily available and easy to use?
7. Will either partner feel embarrassed using it?
8. Are there other alternatives?

Contraception Methods

Some contraception methods do not require the help of a health care provider. Refraining from sexual contact or abstaining from sexual intercourse is 100% effective. Over-the-counter spermicidal products such as creams, jellies, foams, and sponges are put into the vagina before intercourse. They create a spermicide barrier between the uterus and ejaculated sperm. The female client must touch her genitals to use them. A rubber or condom is a thin rubber sheath that fits over the penis. It should have a reservoir at the tip to catch the ejaculant; otherwise the thin rubber might break. The condom requires that the client touch his penis. Both vaginal spermicides and condoms are most effective when the instructions are carefully followed. Their combined use has been found to be more effective in preventing pregnancy than the use of either alone.

Contraception methods that require the help or training of a health care provider include oral contraceptives (the "pill"), the intrauterine device (IUD), the diaphragm, and sterilization. Oral contraceptives prevent ovulation. The chemical content varies from manufacturer to manufacturer, and the directions for use must be carefully followed. IUDs are plastic devices inserted by a health care provider into the uterus through the cervical opening. They are shaped in rings, coils, or loops and may contain copper or be impregnated with progesterone. IUDs are long lasting and inexpensive after the initial cost of having one inserted. The diaphragm is a round rubber dome or cap, about 5 to 7 cm (2 to 3 inches) across, that has a flexible spring around the edge. It is used with a contraceptive cream or jelly and is inserted in the vagina so that it covers the cervical opening. It thus provides a physical as well as a spermicidal barrier. It also requires that the client touch her genitals each time it is used.

Sterilization has become more popular owing to improved surgical methods and increased societal approval. It is the most effective contraception method other than abstinence, and it is permanent. Female sterilization or tubal ligation involves cutting the fallopian tubes. It is done with a laparoscope through the abdominal wall, usually at the navel, or through the back of the vagina. The procedure involves only the fallopian tubes; no other part of the woman's sexual or hormonal system is affected. In male sterilization or vasectomy, the vas deferens that carries the sperm away from the testicles is cut and tied. Using a local anesthetic, the surgeon makes an opening in the scrotal sac and removes a segment of the vas deferens, tying off or cauterizing the ends to prevent them from rejoining. Since there are still sperm traveling up through the vas deferens, the client should be considered fertile for some time after the procedure. Sperm are usually absent from the ejaculant 6 to 8 weeks after the procedure (Crooks and Baur, 1983).

Contraceptive methods based on the menstrual cycle include the mucus method, the basal body temperature method, and the calendar method. Such methods are popular among clients who reject the idea of putting anything foreign into their bodies, who want a method with no side effects or health risks, or whose religious practices and beliefs prohibit the use of contraceptive agents. All three of the methods require that the client thoroughly understand the reproductive cycle of her body and be aware of the subtle signs and signals her body gives during the cycle. The mucus method is based on changes in the cervical mucus during menstruation. The client learns to recognize changes in the amount and consistency of her vaginal secretions. In the basal body temperature method the client records and plots changes in her body temperature to determine the time of ovulation. Basal body temperature drops slightly just before ovulation and rises slightly afterward. In the calendar or rhythm method the client charts the menstrual cycle with a calendar. By noting the first and last days of her cycle over a period of time, she can estimate her most fertile period.

Among the least effective methods are withdrawal and douching. Withdrawal is pulling the penis out of the vagina just before ejaculation. Since sperm may be present in the urethra even when there is no ejaculation, this method is not very effective. In addition, sperm can be carried into the vagina by the fingers, and thus even an ejaculation outside the vagina can potentially impregnate. Douching is also ineffective for contraception, since sperm move rapidly into the cervix after ejaculation and are quickly beyond the reach of the water from douching.

Sexuality and the Nursing Process

Assessment

Many nurses find that they are uncomfortable talking about sexuality with their clients, but they can reduce their discomfort with several methods. First, nurses should build a sound knowledge base and un-

derstanding of healthy sexuality and the most common sexual dysfunctions. The nurse must understand how sexual orientation, culture, and religious beliefs influence sexuality. Second, nurses can assess their own comfort level and limitations in discussing sexuality and sexual functioning (see Chapter 13). Finally, they can learn to recognize sexual problems that are outside the realm of their expertise and to refer the client for help.

Clients may use a variety of terms to describe their sexuality and sexual experiences. Nurses must be prepared to ask for explanations and clarifications if the terms used are unfamiliar (Dickman and Livingston, 1982). Nurses need to acknowledge their own values and belief systems concerning sexual functioning and not impose them on clients. The goal is to be non-judgmental, caring, and supportive.

SEXUAL HEALTH HISTORY

The nursing history is the first step in assessment. Every nursing history, whether taken in a clinic or hospital, should include a few sex-related questions to determine initially if the client has any sexual concerns. Examples of such questions are:

1. How has your illness (or impending surgery) affected your sex life?
2. How do you feel about the sexual part of your life?
3. It's not unusual for people with your condition to be experiencing some sexual problems. Has that been a concern to you at all?

If the client brings up sexual concerns, the nurse may want to take a more detailed sexual health history along with the nursing history. By including sexuality in the discussion, the nurse indicates that the client's sexual health is an important component of total health care.

A brief sexual history can be adapted to meet the client's needs. The nurse should assure the client of the confidentiality of the interview and explain why a sexual health history is included. It is helpful to let the client know how surgery, disease, and medications can affect sexual health.

A helpful guide for a brief sex history would include the following questions (Annon, 1975):

1. What does the client see as the sexual concerns?
2. When did these sexual concerns begin and how have they changed over time?
3. What does the client see as the cause of the concern?
4. What sorts of treatment has the client sought to help alleviate this concern?
5. How would the client like this concern to be resolved, and what are the client's goals for treatment?

INTERVIEW STRATEGIES

The nurse should ask the client to describe the problem as completely as possible so she can make a clear diagnosis. Several interview strategies can enhance both the nurse's and the client's comfort in discussing sexual issues (see also Chapter 15):

1. Use a warm and empathetic approach.
2. Allow plenty of time for the interview.
3. Assume that all clients are uncomfortable talking about their sexuality.
4. Listen carefully, and notice nonverbal cues of the client.
5. Use open-ended questions that encourage more than a yes-or-no response.
6. Adapt the interview to the client's life-style and attempt to overcome cultural and language barriers.
7. Have a rationale for each question and be willing to share this with the client.
8. Assume that all clients are sexually experienced unless they tell you otherwise.
9. Initiate the discussion with the topics that are least sensitive.
10. Avoid pressuring clients to respond to questions about their sexuality.

Some clients may be too embarrassed or not know how to ask the nurse sexual questions directly. Thus they may be very subtle in asking for information. The nurse must be aware of cues from the client that may indicate a question or problem in the area of sexuality. Such cues might include the following (Siemens and Brandzel, 1982):

1. Talking about going home from the hospital and being afraid of what their partner will think or expect of them
2. Asking direct easy questions and then seeming hesitant about the next question
3. Joking of a sexual nature
4. Asking questions that suggest concerns about achieving orgasm such as, "Could my clitoris be surgically moved down closer to my vagina?"
5. Making self-conscious comments such as, "Well, I'm just not as young as I used to be."
6. Using euphemisms such as, "I just want to be a good partner."
7. Looking down when asked a question about sexuality, blushing, and changing the topic
8. Asking questions about "normal" behavior such as, "Is it normal for a man to not ejaculate when he gets older?"

Observing and listening to clients' concerns about sexuality take practice. It is up to the nurse to clarify and paraphrase or ask questions that will help clients be more direct about sexual concerns.

PHYSICAL ASSESSMENT

The physical examination is important in the identification of sexual concerns or problems. The techniques of inspection and palpation are used in this examination (see also Chapter 29).

EXAMINATION OF WOMEN. Examination of a woman begins with inspection of the genitalia. The inspection includes the secondary sex characteristics: breast development, hair distribution, and the development of the external genitalia. The breasts are inspected to determine size, symmetry, contour, and appearance of the skin. Although often one breast is smaller than the other, the breasts usually are relatively symmetrical. Variations in breast contour may include the presence of masses, dimpling, or flattening. The color of the skin of the breasts, presence of thickened areas, and abnormalities of the venous pattern may be indicative of pathological processes. The nipples may be inverted, but this is usually not pathological. However, the direction in which the nipples are pointing may provide a clue to masses when there is asymmetry. Discharge from the nipples may indicate disease or may merely occur with the hormonal fluctuation of the menstrual cycle. Ulcerated areas and other nipple lesions require further exploration.

The external genitalia, including the labia majora and minora, mons, vulva, clitoris, urethral opening, and vaginal introitus, are examined before the internal pelvic examination. Inflammatory processes, ulcerations, congenital or surgical absence of structures, lesions, nodules, and discharge are noted. The labia minora, clitoris, and urethral opening can be inspected by separating the labia majora. While the labia are separated with the middle and index finger, the woman can be requested to strain down. Any bulging of the vaginal walls or gaping of the introitus is noted. The former may be indicative of cystocele and rectocele, and the latter of injury to the pubococcygeus muscle surrounding the vaginal outlet. Presence of surgical scarring, such as an episiotomy site, may also be noted at this time. This part of the examination affords the practitioner the opportunity to teach the woman Kegel's exercises if she does not already know how to do them (see box on p. 396).

During the physical examination, women can also be encouraged to examine their breasts each month. The conclusion of the menstrual period or a few days thereafter is the best time for this, since premenstrual engorgement of the breasts may cause them to be lumpy or tender. Because of the cyclical changes in the consistency of breast tissue, it is recommended that the self-examination be performed at a consistent point in the menstrual cycle. Breast self-examination is described in Chapter 29.

A pelvic examination is customarily performed as part of a total health assessment for women. It consists of two primary components: the speculum examination of the cervix and vagina and the manual palpation of the uterus and ovaries (see Chapter 29). The pelvic examination can be an educational experience for the woman, as well as an experience that validates her sexuality. The practitioner should avoid making an assumption about whether the woman is sexually active or with whom, as well as any assumption about her desire for fertility control. The examination should begin with the woman in a sitting position rather than in the lithotomy position (which usually causes poor eye contact and a feeling of inferiority). The woman should be offered a drape. Since some women prefer to see what is happening, the woman should be asked whether she would like a mirror. This often enables the woman to see her cervix or even her genitals for the first time. Many examiners use a lighted speculum to facilitate the woman's viewing of her own anatomy.

By explaining the steps of the examination, the examiner can validate the woman's sexuality and health. For example, the examiner might say "I'm going to look at your labia and clitoris now. . . they look very healthy." When preparing to insert the speculum, the examiner can inform the woman of any noise the speculum might make (plastic speculums are especially noisy) and also advise her of what will be done, for example, "Now I'm going to put two fingers in your vagina. I'm going to put the speculum into your vagina, and I'll open it up so you can see your cervix. Your vagina looks very healthy. Can you see your cervix?" Insertion of the speculum is facilitated by using warm tap water as a lubricant. Some practitioners advocate inserting the speculum blades at a slight oblique angle, whereas others prefer to insert the blades horizontally. The primary concern is avoiding painful pressure on the urethra. When removing the speculum, the practitioner closes the blades after the cervix is cleared to avoid pinching the cervix between the speculum blades.

The woman can participate in the bimanual examination. For example, she may wish to palpate her ovaries. This orientation to the pelvic examination affords many opportunities for teaching that sexuality is a wholesome, positive phenomenon.

EXAMINATION OF MEN. Inspection of the penis, scrotum, testicles, and breasts of the male is usually part of the general physical examination. As these structures are examined, the practitioner notes the hair distribution pattern over the axillary and pelvic areas.

The breasts are inspected for deviations in contour, symmetry, abnormalities in the skin, and irregularities of the nipple. Although breast cancers in men are rare, abnormal discharges or lesions should be noted and further addressed. The examiner looks for gynecomastia, an enlargement of breast tissue that often occurs during normal puberty as well as at other times during the life cycle.

Inspection of the penis includes observations of the skin for ulcers or lesions. The shaft is observed for deviations in shape and size or symmetry. The foreskin may be present in uncircumcised males, and the client may be asked to retract it to facilitate inspection of the glans area for the presence of lesions. Abnormalities of the glans and urethral meatus may also be noted, including deviations in the location of the urethra, ulcerations of the glans, and discharge from the urethral meatus.

The scrotal skin is inspected next for the presence of nodules or inflammation and to check contour. Usually the left testicle is somewhat lower in the scrotal sac than the right. Absence or atrophy of the testicles may also be identified by inspection. The penis, scrotal sac and contents, prostate gland, and rectum may be palpated. Usually the genitalia are examined with a gloved hand.

Explanations similar to those provided to women can be used when examining men. Some men may elect to use a mirror to see their genitals.

Kegel's Exercises for the Pubococcygeus Muscle

Sit on the toilet seat with your knees as far apart as possible. Start and stop the flow of urine. This will enable you to feel the pubococcygeus muscle.

Begin exercising this muscle gradually, at intervals throughout the day. The following exercises can be done each day:

1. Contracting the pubococcygeus muscle and holding for 3 seconds (this feels the same as it did when you stopped the flow of urine)
2. Contracting the pubococcygeus muscle rapidly
3. Breathing deeply and tightening the pubococcygeus muscle as you inhale
4. Bearing down, then relaxing, and as you relax, tightening the pubococcygeus muscle

Ten to 25 contractions each day is usually sufficient to maintain good muscle tone.

OTHER ASSESSMENT DATA

To fully evaluate the cause of a client's sexual difficulties, relevant historical and laboratory data are gathered. The client is queried about cardiovascular, respiratory, gastrointestinal, genitourinary, central nervous system, and endocrine functions, as well as the presence of intercurrent illnesses, use of prescription and nonprescription drugs, and habits such as use of alcohol. Sexual problems are often resolved when problems in other body systems, use of medications affecting sexual performance, and habits interfering with sexual appreciation or function are corrected with medical therapy.

Laboratory data useful in identifying the cause of a sexual dysfunction are obtained in a blood workup, including a complete blood count, thyroid function test, glucose tolerance test, and chemistry determinations. Vaginal cytology examinations, endocrine workups, electrocardiograms, and chest roentgenograms may reveal underlying conditions responsible for sexual problems (Woods, 1984).

Analysis and Diagnosis

After obtaining a thorough history, performing physical assessment, reviewing the literature, and consulting with appropriate people, the nurse must identify current problems relating to a client's sexual health and determine if the client is experiencing any specific sexual dysfunctions. With the diagnosis the nurse can plan interventions.

Planning and Intervention

PLISSIT MODEL

Annon's PLISSIT model (1975) provides the nurse with an intervention method for responding to clients'

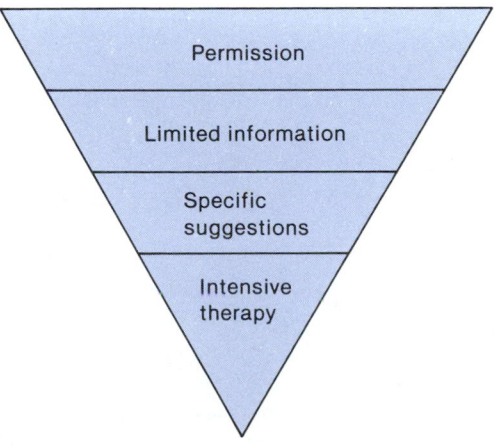

Fig. 19-5 PLISSIT model.

sexual concerns (Fig. 19-5). The model suggests four levels of intervention: *p*ermission, *li*mited *i*nformation, *s*pecific *s*uggestions, and *i*ntensive *t*herapy. The nurse can determine the levels at which she feels competent in responding and can make referrals beyond those levels. As Fig. 19-5 demonstrates, most clients need permission, fewer need limited information and specific suggestions, and only a small number need intensive therapy. The nurse can assist the client with most sexuality concerns through the first three levels of intervention.

Before attempting an intervention, the nurse must determine exactly what the client sees as the problem. When the nurse and client have a mutual understanding of the problem, the nurse may decide to respond using the PLISSIT model.

PERMISSION. Since many people do not discuss sexual matters with others, they may think that their feelings and behaviors are abnormal and may harbor feelings that they have a serious problem. Clients should be assured that their behaviors, thoughts, feelings, fantasies, or experiences are normal or common and that they are not crazy or deviant. For some, hearing from an authority that they are all right may alleviate the problem. For example, a nurse might say, "Masturbation is a normal form of sexual expression for women and men throughout their lives, regardless of whether they have a sexual partner or not," or "Women often experience a wide range of feelings in relation to being pregnant. Good for you for bringing up your concerns; let's sit down and talk about this."

LIMITED INFORMATION. A small amount of information can go a long way toward dispelling myths or easing a client's anxieties. Statistics, data, diagrams, or anatomical information can be very helpful. For example, a nurse could say, "For many men, feeling anxious or pressured about sexual performance causes them to have problems with achieving or maintaining an erection," or "As you can see in this diagram, the uterus lifts in the pelvis during sexual arousal. Perhaps the reason you experience internal pain with sexual intercourse is that you are not reaching a sufficient level of arousal."

SPECIFIC SUGGESTIONS. At the third level of intervention the nurse suggests a specific course of action for the client. Suggestions can take the form of books or articles, communication exercises, or new behaviors. The nurse may also refer the client to other agencies, support groups, or a sex therapist. An example of a specific suggestion is, "Would you be willing to spend some time in the next week telling your partner how you feel about having herpes? There is also a support group starting next month. I think you would find it helpful."

INTENSIVE THERAPY. Some sexual concerns are not alleviated by giving permission, limited information, or specific suggestions. In such a case the nurse should refer the client to an experienced therapist for more intensive therapy. Referral is appropriate whenever a client has a problem in an area the nurse knows nothing about or feels uncomfortable discussing.

EVALUATION

Evaluation is the final stage of the nursing process. At this time the nurse reassesses the client's level of health and the interventions used in order to determine which of the interventions were successful, which interventions should be modified, and which interventions were not helpful and need to be eliminated from the plan.

When the nurse and client have mutually identified the goals of intervention, evaluation is not difficult, since they are then able to determine whether an intervention has been appropriate and adequate to meet these goals. The client's verbal expression of satisfaction will indicate whether a nursing intervention has been helpful (Hogan, 1980a).

CASE STUDY

ASSESSMENT. Krista is a 27-year-old single woman who has an ongoing sexual relationship with a male partner. She has been hospitalized for 2 days recovering from pelvic inflammatory disease caused by a gonorrheal infection. On admission she was experiencing abdominal pain and low backache and had a fever. These symptoms have subsided as a result of massive intravenous doses of antibiotics.

This is her first hospitalization. She is mortified that she has a sex-related disease and is hesitant to share her feelings with the nursing staff for fear they will be judgmental. She has been found crying alone and says she is depressed because she does not know how she contracted gonorrhea. She does not know how to talk with her partner about this situation.

NURSING DIAGNOSIS
1. Lack of information about cause, treatment, and prevention of gonorrhea and pelvic inflammatory disease
2. Low sexual self-esteem
3. Difficulty in communicating with nursing staff and partner about sexual concerns

INTERVENTION*

1. Lack of information about prevention, etiology, and treatment of gonorrhea and pelvic inflammatory disease	P	Assure her that it is OK to ask questions about her disease process.
	LI	Explain the process of gonorrheal transmission.
		Teach signs and symptoms and complications of gonorrhea.
		Explain the course of treatment, medication regimen, and follow-up.
		Discuss the need for rest, especially after discharge from hospital.
		Reassure her that there will most likely be no sexual dysfunction as a result of this illness.
		Explain methods for prevention of reinfection.
	SS	Invite her partner to come in for information about STDs.
	IT	Make sure she has a list of community agencies where STD counseling is available.
2. Low sexual self-esteem	P	Assure her that it is OK to discuss all her feelings about herself as a sexual person.
		Emphasize that it is OK to have feelings of anxiety, anger, sadness, and depression when ill.
		Assure her that it is OK to ask questions about how gonorrhea might affect sexual functioning.
	LI	Discuss the psychological effects of having a STD on a person's feelings about sexuality.
		Explain the effects, if any, her medications will have on sexuality.
		Explain sexual self-esteem—feeling lovable and capable.
	SS	Give her positive feedback about your perception of her.

---

*Using PLISSIT model.

Encourage her to be as self-sufficient as possible in her own care.

Talk about her sexual expectations for when she goes home.

If masturbation is an acceptable part of her sexual behavior, encourage her to masturbate in the hospital. Make sure she has a "do not disturb" sign for her door.

Use role playing to help her say what she feels and wants.

IT If she desires, refer her to a sex therapist who can help her understand herself as a sexual person.

3. Difficulty in communicating with nursing staff and partner about sexual concerns

P Accept her attempt to initiate conversations about sexuality.

Praise her for bringing up the topic.

LI Explain that she is not alone wih these concerns.

Explain that communication skills are learned over time.

SS Teach basic communication skills.

Use role playing to teach her to talk with her partner about sex.

Discuss with her the specific conditions she needs for a satisfying sexual experience.

Talk about sensual options such as mutual massage and bathing with her partner.

If she wants, and the partner is willing, ask the partner to join these conversations.

IT Refer her to a sex therapist for further work if she chooses.

EVALUATION. On discharge from the hospital Krista is able to discuss how to protect herself from STDs. She reports feeling relieved after talking about her infection and her sexuality. She feels more comfortable, knowledgeable, and confident in her sexual awareness. As a result of the role playing, she is able to talk openly and honestly with her partner about her feelings regarding the illness and her sexuality. She leaves with a list of several community agencies that can provide her and her partner with counseling for sexual enhancement.

Summary

The nurse who provides care for a client with sexual concerns needs knowledge about sexuality, communication skills, and an understanding of the interaction between personal and cultural value systems. Knowledge about sexuality includes the effects of illness and treatment on sexual desire and sexual functioning. The client's sense of self as attractive, desirable, and sexual can be affected by illness and body changes resulting from surgery or disease. Aging, changes in life-style, and alterations in value system also affect a person's sexuality.

Nurses can learn to apply all stages of the nursing process in order to maintain or improve a client's sexual health. In this sense the nurse becomes a sex educator. Sex education will always be controversial because of the diversity of sexual values in our society. With sensitivity and insight, nurses can assist their clients in assuming responsibility for decisions about sexuality that will enhance their total health. Before counseling clients about sexuality, a nurse must examine her own sexual history and the belief system that guides her sexual behavior. In-service education programs, readings, and practice in talking about sexuality are valuable learning experiences for nurses.

✓ Because sexuality can involve a person's health in all dimensions, sexual concerns or problems should be addressed as a part of nursing care.

✓ Biological sex identity is determined genetically but may not correspond to a person's gender identity and gender role.

✓ Gender identity and gender role vary widely among individuals and result from the interaction of many biological and environmental factors.

✓ Sexual orientation, a person's erotic attraction to others, exists on a continuum between heterosexuality and homosexuality.

✓ Attitudes toward sexuality vary widely and are influenced by religious beliefs, society's values, the media, the family, and other factors.

✓ Nurses' attitudes toward sexuality also vary and may differ from the client's attitudes, and a nurse should be nonjudgmental about a client's sexual preferences and needs.

✓ Sexual stimulation varies among individuals but generally involves erotic fantasy and touching and the other senses.

✓ The range of sexual behavior includes manual stimulation, oral-genital stimulation, anal stimulation, and coitus.

✓ The four-phase sexual response cycle is a way of understanding the physiological changes of the sexual response during excitement, the plateau phase, orgasm, and resolution.

✓ Sexual development begins in infancy and involves some kind of sexual behavior in all developmental stages.

✓ The physiological sexual response changes with aging for both men and women, but aging need not lead to diminished sexuality.

✓ Clients' problems involving sexuality include personal and emotional conflicts, sexual dysfunctions, and the effects of illness on sexuality.

✓ Personal and emotional conflicts leading to sexual problems may originate in differences in sexual desires, physical factors, relationship problems, life-style factors, or low self-esteem.

✓ Specific sexual dysfunctions for both men and women result from psychological and physiological factors.

✓ Interventions for sexual dysfunctions depend on the condition and the client; interventions often include giving information, use of specific exercises, improving communication between partners, and specific techniques of the sexuality counselor.

✓ Sexuality is affected by physiological changes or chronic illness, hospitalization, and sexually transmitted diseases, and the nurse helps the client adapt to the situation and maintain healthy sexuality.

✓ Three general factors influence whether and how a client uses contraceptive methods: the client's personality and attitudes, the client's environment and possible conflicts with family or other attitudes, and the contraceptive method itself, which should match the client's needs.

✓ The nursing process can be applied to care for clients with sexual problems: assessment based on a physical examination and sexual history using special interview techniques, analysis and diagnosis of the sexual concern or dysfunction, planning and intervention such as that using the PLISSIT approach, and evaluation by the nurse and client of the extent to which sexual goals have been met.

REFERENCES

Annon, J.: The behavioral treatment of sexual problems. Vol. 1. Brief therapy, Honolulu, 1975, Enabling Systems, Inc.

Calderone, M., and Johnson, E.: The family book about sexuality, New York, 1981, Harper & Row Publishers, Inc.

Crooks, R., and Baur, K.: Our sexuality, Menlo Park, Calif., 1983, The Benjamin-Cummings Publishing Co., Inc.

Dickman, G., and Livingston, C.: Sex and the female ostomate, Los Angeles, 1982, United Ostomy Association, Inc.

Dickman, G., and Livingston, C.: Sexual variation. In Woods, N.F., editor: Human sexuality in health and illness, ed. 3, St. Louis, 1984, The C.V. Mosby Co.

Fogel, C., and Woods, N.F.: Health care of women, St. Louis, 1981, The C.V. Mosby Co.

Goldstein, B.: Human sexuality, New York, 1976, McGraw-Hill Book Co.

Haeberle, E.: The sex atlas, New York, 1978, The Seabury Press.

Hogan, R.: Human sexuality: a nursing perspective, New York, 1980a, Appleton-Century-Crofts.

Hogan, R.: Nursing and human sexuality, Nurs. Times 76:1296, 1980b.

Hogan, R.: Influences of culture on sexuality, Nurs. Clin. North Am. 17(3):365, 1982.

Kolodny, R., Masters, W., and Johnson, V. Textbook of sexual medicine, Boston, 1979, Little, Brown & Co.

Lion, E.M.: Human sexuality in nursing process, New York, 1982, John Wiley & Sons, Inc.

Livingston, C., and McIntyre, M.: Alcoholism and sexuality. In Woods, N.F., editor: Human sexuality in health and illness, ed. 3, St. Louis, 1984, The C.V. Mosby Co.

Livingston, C., McIntyre, M., and Fogel, C.: Sexual dysfunction: etiology and treatment. In Woods, N.F., editor: Human sexuality in health and illness, ed. 3, St. Louis, 1984, The C.V. Mosby Co.

Masters, W., and Johnson, V.: Human sexual response, Boston, 1966, Little, Brown & Co.

Masters, W., and Johnson, V.: Human sexual inadequacy, Boston, 1970, Little, Brown & Co.

Masters, W., Johnson, V., and Kolodny, R.: Human sexuality, Boston, 1982, Little, Brown & Co.

Perry, J., and Whipple, B.: Pelvic muscle strength of female ejaculators: evidence in support of a new theory of orgasm, J. Sex Res. 17(1):22, 1981.

Sex Information and Education Council of the United States: The SIECUS/New York University/Uppsala principles basic to education for sexuality, SIECUS Report 8:8, 1980.

Shipes, E., and Lehr, S.: Sexuality and the male cancer patient, Ca. Nurs. 5(5):375, 1982.

Siemens, S., and Brandzel, R.: Sexuality: nursing assessment and intervention, Philadelphia, 1982, J.B. Lippincott Co.

Unsain, I., Goodwin, M., and Schuster, E.: Diabetes and sexual functioning, Nurs. Clin. North Am. 17(3):387, 1982.

Woods, N.F.: Human sexuality in health and illness, ed. 3, St. Louis, 1984, The C.V. Mosby Co.

ADDITIONAL READINGS

Barbach, L.: For yourself, New York, 1975, Doubleday Publishing Co.

Barbach, L.: Women discover orgasms, New York, 1980, The Free Press.

Barbach, L.: For each other, Garden City, N.Y., 1982, Anchor Press/Doubleday.

Barbach, L., and Levine, L.: Shared intimacies: women's sexual experiences, Garden City, N.Y., 1981, Anchor Press/Doubleday.

Belliveau, F., and Richter, L.: Understanding human sexual inadequacy, New York, 1970, Bantam Books.

Dodson, B.: Liberating masturbation, New York, 1974, Body Sex Designs.

Elmassian, B., and Wilson, R.: Assessment and diagnosis of sexual problems, Nurse Pract. 7(6):13, 1982.

Federation of Feminist Women's Health Centers: A new view of a woman's body, New York, 1981, Simon & Schuster.

Friday, N.: My secret garden: women's sexual fantasies, New York, 1973, Pocket Books.

Green, R.: Human sexuality: a health practitioner's text, Baltimore, 1979, The William & Wilkins Co.

Kaplan, H.: The new sex therapy, New York, 1974, Bruner/Mazel.

Kaplan, J.: Disorders of sexual desire, New York, 1979, Simon & Schuster.

Kassorla, I.: Nice girls do, Los Angeles, 1980, Stratford Press.

Manley, M.: Taking a sexual history, Diabetes Educator 7(3):22, 1981.

Mims, F., and Swenson, M.: Sexuality: a nursing perspective, New York, 1980, McGraw-Hill Book Co.

Nass, G., et al.: Sexual choices, Monterey, Calif., 1981, Wadsworth Health Sciences Division.

O'Donnell, M., et al.: Lesbian health matters, Santa Cruz, Calif., 1979, Santa Cruz Women's Health Collective.

Silverstein, C., and White, E.: Joy of gay sex, New York, 1977, Crown Publishers, Inc.

Sisley, E., and Harris B.: Joy of lesbian sex, New York, 1977, Crown Publishers, Inc.

Zilbergeld, B.: Male sexuality, Boston, 1978, Little, Brown & Co.

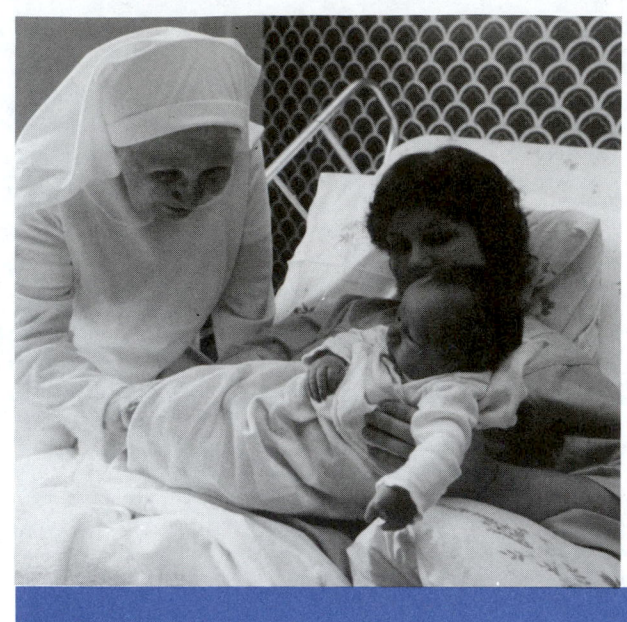

OBJECTIVES

Mastery of content in this chapter will enable the student to:

- Define spiritual health.
- Discuss the relationship of spiritual health to physiological and psychosocial health.
- Contrast spiritual and religious aspects of health.
- Assess components of spiritual health.
- Describe a spiritually healthy person.
- Describe the signs of unmet spiritual needs.
- List interventions in the nursing plan for spiritual care.
- Evaluate attainment of spiritual health.
- Identify resources that can help clients attain spiritual health.

GLOSSARY

spiritual health Awareness and openness to a Supreme Being, a presence with or in each person and in the world.

spiritual distress State of being out of harmony with a Supreme Being.

spirituality Spiritual dimension of a person, including the relationship with humanity, nature, and a Supreme Being.

religious Relating to specific practices, rites, and rituals of one's professed religion.

20 *Spiritual Health*

Human nature includes a spiritual component just as it encompasses physiological, psychological, and sociocultural components. Living fully requires spiritual health as well as mental and physical well-being. As with other dimensions of health, however, the perception of spiritual health is highly individualized, and spiritual health changes as other dimensions of health fluctuate.

The ultimate state of health would seem to be a delicate balance of all dimensions—physical, developmental, psychological, sociocultural, and spiritual. The spiritually alive person is alert to the meaning of life and the internal forces that motivate individuals toward goodness, beauty, and health. The spiritual dimension of nursing care may take on particular significance for the client who has a physical health problem. Clients who are physically unhealthy may not be able to manage their spiritual needs. The nurse giving holistic care seeks to determine all needs, including those considered within the spiritual realm. Just as the psychological or sociocultural needs may sometimes take precedence, so in certain situations, spiritual needs are of greatest concern to the client and the nurse.

According to Piles' study of spiritual care in nursing curricula (1980), the spiritual dimension has traditionally been considered part of the psychosocial dimension or the self-concept. In some nursing schools the spiritual aspect has been excluded from the definition of holistic care and from the curriculum. Although we have included spiritual health in this unit on psychosocial needs, we consider it a dimension separate from the self-concept. This chapter focuses on the Christian approach to spirituality but discusses the tenets of other major religions in regard to general health beliefs, birth, diet, health crises, and death.

Although in the past there was a dearth of material on the spiritual dimension of nursing care, nurses' need for information about applying standards of care in the spiritual realm has prompted authors and educators to address this topic in more depth.

In the last 10 years information about spiritual health has appeared increasingly in nursing literature. The monthly publication *The Nurses Lamp** encourages nurses to recognize and meet their client's spiritual needs.

The National Group for the Classification of Nursing Diagnoses has included spiritual diagnoses under the classification "spiritual distress"(Kim and Moritz, 1982). Several researchers have compiled descriptions of the practices of different religions to help nurses understand and provide for clients' religious practices.

Definition of Spiritual Health

Since the spiritual dimension of health should be considered in holistic care, it is helpful to have a working definition of spiritual health. Generally spiritual health can be considered an awareness and openness to a Supreme Being, a presence with or in each person

---

*Published by the Nurses Christian Fellowship, 223 Langdon St., Madison, Wisc.

and in the world. The response to this Supreme Being is faith or a belief system.

Meeks (1977) discusses belief systems and suggests the following specific questions for the individual's consideration in achieving high-level wellness:

1. What do I believe?
2. What gives meaning to my life?
3. How is my belief system working for me?
4. Is my behavior compatible with my belief system?
5. How does my belief system relate to my future?
6. Is there a relationship between my belief system and my health behavior?

Newman (1979) in her theory of nursing defines health as an expansion of consciousness; she mentions that studies of the brain have shown that some dimensions of consciousness have been neglected. The left hemisphere, usually predominant, is primarily responsible for the analytical, sequence-perceiving processes, while the right hemisphere, usually less dominant, is responsible for the synthesis-oriented, symbolic and intuitive modes. When both hemispheres are exercised, and when as much emphasis is placed on the symbolic and intuitive as on the analytical, consciousness develops more fully. Newman concludes that the expansion of consciousness is what life and therefore health are all about and that health can coexist with illness and even encompass it as a meaningful aspect.

In many belief systems, disease is viewed as part of a divine plan to test the individual's faith in a Supreme Being or to make him an example of patience or restitution. Thus one can find meaning in suffering. The goal of nursing, within this framework, is not simply to make people well or to prevent illness but to help those in health or illness to use the power within themselves as they evolve toward higher levels of consciousness. Newman's theory has profound implications for defining and sustaining spiritual health, for stimulating the right hemisphere of the brain, and for challenging the development of this facet of the personality and the spiritual dimension in nurses and their clients. Exploring with clients what is symbolic and spiritually supportive to them, providing the spiritual resources they request, and suggesting alternatives or sharing beliefs without imposing values are ways nurses can help clients find significance in suffering.

The spiritual dimension helps us find meaning in life, suffering, pain, illness, and death. It is this dimension that aids us in sustaining ourselves with significant symbols, words, objects, practices, and rituals. Spiritual distress, the state of being out of harmony with a Supreme Being, and realization of our limitations can thus be dealt with.

Relationship of Spiritual to Physiological and Psychosocial Dimensions of Health

The interrelatedness of the physiological, psychosocial, and spiritual dimensions is demonstrated by the great number of clients with psychosomatic diseases. The insistence of health care providers on a body-mind-spirit conceptual model of human nature results in their concern with the moral, ethical, and spiritual dimensions of personality and character development. Practitioners of holistic health care believe that each person has a spirit that coexists with the physical body and that can be thought of as the life spark that energizes the body. The nurse's goal in holistic health care is not simply to help a client be physically well, but to help the client achieve a balanced, dynamic integration of body, mind, and spirit. Holistic health care therefore includes meeting the client's physiological needs, promoting psychosocial relationships, and supporting the fulfillment of spiritual aspirations.

As a result of this threefold responsibility, nurses when dealing with clients and their families, and in their relationships with one another, should recognize that we are all spiritual beings with spiritual needs and aspirations. Nurses should realize the interdependence of the physiological, the psychosocial, and the spiritual aspects of development. Just as unexpressed anger and resentment can cause diseases referred to as psychosomatic, forms of spiritual distress such as guilt, irascibility, lack of forgiveness of self or others, and vindictiveness can lead to illness and suffering.

The client and family have a right to express their spiritual needs and to have them recognized and ministered to. As professionals, nurses have a right and responsibility to challenge spiritual growth in themselves and in others, just as they have obligations to foster physical health and promote psychosocial success.

Spiritual and Religious Aspects of Health

For the purposes of this chapter the word "spiritual" refers to an individual's relationship with a Supreme Being and the presence of that being in the world. Spirituality thus encompasses religion, which is specifically a person's affiliation with a denomination or sect. The word "religious" refers to the specific practices, rites, and rituals of a person's professed religion. Rites and rituals may enhance a person's spirituality but may not be recognized by the individual as essential to his relationship with the Supreme Being. The nurse should be aware of the client's general spiritual needs, which may be manifested in ways other than through specific religious practices, and should make it possible for the client to engage in his chosen practices. Information about the specific religious practices of different religions and sects is available from a number of sources. The following sections describe Hindu, Buddhist, Moslem, Jewish, and Christian beliefs and practices regarding birth, dietary restrictions, procedures in health crises, and death. It should be kept in mind that the spiritual dimension of health care, although it includes religious beliefs and rituals, is not limited to the practices and dogma of organized religions.

Beliefs about Health

Hindus believe that praying for health is the lowest form of prayer; thus they tend to dismiss or be unconcerned about bodily ills. The devotees of Buddhism have rich multireligious influences from Confucianism, Christianity, and Shintoism. Various branches and sects of Buddhism emphasize different practices; for example, the Theravada branch uses an intellectual approach, the Mahayana branch emphasizes involvement with humanity, and the Zen sect practices austerity. Followers of Hinduism and Buddhism usually accept modern medical science.

In Islam, the believer is considered to be a unique individual with an eternal soul. Moslems (Muslims) pray five times daily, facing Mecca. Older or more conservative Moslems may have a fatalistic view and may resist compliance with medical treatment.

Jews tend to believe in long life as reward for fidelity to God and observe Sabbath regulations, which may interfere with scheduled therapeutic procedures.

Christians generally regard themselves as children of God, redeemed by Christ and destined for eternal life. They seek to discern the will of God in life and suffering, but their beliefs generally do not conflict with modern medical practice.

Birth

No special birth ritual is required by Hinduism. Buddhist rites such as infant presentation, affirmation, confirmation, or ordination are performed in late childhood. According to Islamic doctrine, if abortion occurs after 130 days, the fetus is treated as a fully developed human being. Ritual circumcision is required by Orthodox and Conservative Jews on the eighth day after birth. Reform Jews favor ritual circumcision but do not consider it a religious impera-

tive. Among Jews a fetus is buried, not discarded.

Various forms of baptism are practiced by Christians. Both Episcopalians and Roman Catholics require infant baptism; the former do not baptize aborted fetuses and stillborn infants but the latter do. Baptists, Seventh-Day Adventists, Baha'i followers, and Mennonites are some of the religious groups that do not practice infant baptism. The form of baptism differs from sect to sect; for example, sprinkling is sufficient for the Orthodox Presbyterians, while the Pentacostals, Mormons, Baptists, and Church of Christ members require immersion.

Diet

Hindus have many dietary restrictions. Some sects are vegetarian, believing meat and intoxicants to be too stimulating to the senses. Some Buddhists also are vegetarians. Most members of the Buddhist religion practice moderation and do not use alcohol, tobacco, and drugs.

Eating pork is prohibited by Islam, and Ramadan, the ninth month of the Muhammedan or Muslim year (around June and July), is a period of daylight fasting. Orthodox and Conservative Jews strictly observe kosher dietary laws, which prohibit eating pork and shellfish and eating any meat with milk or milk products. Jews also have regulations about food preparation. Reform Jews do not observe kosher dietary laws.

Many Christian traditions have no dietary proscriptions. Some groups, such as Seventh-Day Adventists, Baptists, and Mormons, prohibit the use of alcohol, coffee, and tea; certain groups include tobacco with these prohibitions. Roman Catholics fast and abstain from meat on Ash Wednesday and Good Friday; some older Catholics continue to adhere to Friday abstinence. Armenian Catholics fast during Lent, and several branches of Christianity fast 1 to 6 hours before communion.

Health Crises

Hindus may view illness as the result of misuse of the body or as a consequence of sins committed in a previous life. However, they generally do not oppose medical treatment, considering its benefits at best transitory. Buddhist clients or their families may ask to have a Buddhist priest for counseling during illness. A family member usually remains with the sick person to care for physical and emotional needs.

Moslems use faith healing to provide psychological support rather than to treat the pathological condition involved. Family members are a great comfort to a Moslem and group prayer is strengthening, but there is no priest. The person submits to God's will in health and illness.

In Judaism it is required that the sick seek medical care. Rabbinical consultation is necessary before donation or transplantation of organs. Visiting the sick is considered a religious obligation for Jews.

Christians may want to receive communion from their minister or priest during illness; Roman Catholics may wish to receive several sacraments: reconciliation, the Eucharist, and anointing of the sick. Jehovah's Witnesses are generally opposed to blood transfusions. Some religious sects believe in faith healing and some in laying on of hands.

Death

To Hindus, death and rebirth are nearly synonymous. After death, certain rites are prescribed. The priest may tie a thread around the neck or wrist to indicate a blessing; he may pour water into the mouth. The family washes the body, which is then cremated. The family of a Buddhist may wish to have a priest called in at the time of death; last rite chanting is often practiced at the bedside.

Before death the Islamic client confesses sins and asks for forgiveness of the family. After death the family washes the body, then turns toward Mecca. As with Hindus, only relatives and friends touch the body. There is no autopsy unless required by law.

All Orthodox Jews and some Conservative Jews also oppose autopsy and cremation. Human remains are ritually cleansed by members of a ritual burial society, and burial is carried out as soon as possible.

Among Christians, no rituals are required before or after death by Christian Scientists, Church of Christ members, and Jehovah's Witnesses. Last rites are optional for Episcopalians and Lutherans but mandatory for Eastern Orthodox Christians and Roman Catholics. Additional restrictions may apply to cremation, autopsy, and burial of amputated parts or burial in consecrated ground.

■ ■ ■ ■ ■

The spiritual dimension of being involves more than adherence to religious dogma or practices. Spirituality includes an awareness of the influence of a Supreme Being as a direction and will in our lives. Being spiritually healthy means being energized or inspired by our relationship with the Supreme Being. Therefore living fully, valuing our potential and using our capacities, is a way of being spiritually healthy.

Spiritual Health and the Nursing Process

Assessment

Using Newman's definition of health as an expansion of consciousness, the nurse can assess a client's spiritual health by looking for evidence that spiritual motivation or aspiration assumes a significant importance in his life and behavior. Fish and Shelly (1978) refer to spiritual health as meaning and purpose in life and love and relatedness with other human beings. Brallier (1978) enumerates the characteristics of holistic health, and these can be understood as progressive or cumulative characteristics: realization of human potential, affirmation of the uniqueness and unlimited potential of each person, and achievement of a balanced dynamic integration of body, mind, and spirit.

Stoll (1979) suggests that when making a spiritual assessment the nurse include specific questions in the nursing history about the client's concept of a Supreme Being, the client's source of strength and hope, the significance of religious practices and rituals to the client, and the client's perceived relationships between spiritual beliefs and health. According to Lafferty (1979), positive spiritual health choices for clients seeking to improve their quality of life include meditation and prayer, value-oriented spiritual or religious discussion, reading a spiritual book or attending a religious or spiritual meeting, and developing a highly valued personal characteristic or eliminating a weak personal trait. These needs should be a part of the spiritual assessment.

Spiritual needs may be intensified in certain life situations, such as birth, death, a major health crisis, anxiety, apprehension, fear, newly diagnosed serious or chronic disease, isolation, and psychiatric episodes. It is often recommended that spiritual assessment be an extension of the psychosocial assessment and that it be pursued to the extent that the nurse intends to use the information for planning client and family care.

Determining who or what sustains the client will help in planning for spiritual health. The answers to the following questions about spiritual health will influence nursing care:

1. Who is the client's God?
2. What is the client's relationship with God?
3. How does the client express this spiritual relationship?
4. How does the client view himself?
5. Does the client act authentically and relate openly?

6. Does the client assume responsibility for behavior and its consequences?
7. To whom does the client relate among family and friends?
8. How does the client relate to health care personnel? To other clients? To the family? To strangers?
9. How have the client's diagnosis and therapy affected his self-concept? Emotional state? Will to live and cooperate with rehabilitation?

Spiritually healthy persons generally believe in a Supreme Being and view their ultimate welfare and peace in terms of their relationship to this being and the world at large. They are generally aware of their limitations as human beings but strive to act in accordance with their beliefs. They assume life's responsibilities with joy and cheerfulness.

Spiritually healthy persons relate in a loving manner to others. They are forgiving of injuries and are gentle and patient with others. They act justly and peacefully in their relationships. They exert a positive influence through their spiritual awareness of a larger meaningfulness in their lives and in the world.

As the nurse observes and analyzes the behaviors that demonstrate the client's level of spiritual health, it becomes obvious that the client's attitudes toward a Supreme Being, self, and others demonstrate the value the client places on spiritual health. Reactions to adversity, setbacks, delays in plans, aging, sickness, and suffering give clues to the client's spiritual values. As the nurse assesses the client's state of spiritual health, signs of unmet spiritual needs may emerge.

If the client demonstrates an incongruity between professed beliefs and actions, a nursing diagnosis of spiritual distress may be indicated. The client may express anger at the Supreme Being, a member of the pastoral care team, or the nurse. The client may question the meaning of life and suffering. Verbalizations about internal conflicts concerning beliefs and required treatment may demonstrate a spiritual need. For example, if a client believes his disease is a punishment for sinfulness, his cooperation with therapy will aggravate his guilt and prevent the restitution he believes necessary through suffering. If the client believes that eternal life follows temporal life, he may repudiate any attempt at treatment and rehabilitation, alienating both his family and health care personnel.

Observing the client's affect and attitude, behaviors, verbalizations, interpersonal relationships, and environment might give clues to spiritual needs. Therefore, spiritual assessment continues throughout all interactions with the client. Does the client receive visitors graciously or sullenly? Is the client's behavior toward other clients and health care personnel accepting and cooperative? Do the client's words and actions reflect the respect and reverence he has professed toward humanity? Are the client's spiritual values reflected in interactions with visitors? Do the client's get-well cards reflect appreciation of prayer and contain inspirational verse? Does the client receive religious cards? Is the client openly questioning the reason for his existence or suffering? Does the client seek spiritual assistance or admit an inability to continue his usual religious practices? Request for prayers may indicate a spiritual value or need. The client may ask the nurse about the moral implications of certain procedures in relation to beliefs about human life.

The conceptual model of human nature in physiological, psychosocial, and spiritual dimensions offers an additional approach to assessing spiritual needs. Questions such as the following can be derived from this model: To what extent have the client's physical disability and the therapeutic regimen altered his ability to maintain relationships with the Supreme Being and others? Are there moral or ethical implications of the diagnosis and treatment that conflict with the client's religious or spiritual values? Do the etiology, diagnosis, and treatment of the disease conflict with the client's belief system?

Nursing Diagnosis and Planning

The National Conference on the Classification of Nursing Diagnoses has defined spiritual distress and suggested etiologies and defining characteristics (see box on p. 408). The client's answers to questions in the nursing history, such as those posed in the preceding section on assessment, and the nurse's observations of the client's behaviors and interrelationships give clues to spiritual needs. However, clues must be validated and clarified before the nurse plans interventions. In the realm of spiritual care, the importance of the nurse's own spiritual aspirations, inspiration, and perception cannot be overemphasized. The nurse must remain aware of her responsibility to provide for clients' spiritual needs. To be attuned to spiritual aspects of care, a nurse should be aware of her own spiritual dimension and be comfortable in discussing spiritual matters. In addition, the nurse's perception of clues to the client's spiritual needs requires sensitivity, active listening, and responding to what is heard.

The nurse seeks validation from the client about a diagnosis of "spiritual distress." If the client concurs with the diagnosis, the nurse and the client together plan steps to meet this spiritual need. If the nurse has doubts about the client's ability to recognize his spiritual needs, consultation with the family may settle the question. If both the client and the family deny

Spiritual Distress (Distress of the Human Spirit)

DEFINITION

Distress of the human spirit is a disruption in the life principle that pervades a person's entire being and that integrates and transcends one's biologic and psychosocial nature.

ETIOLOGY

- Separation from religious and cultural ties
- Challenged belief and value system, e.g., result of moral or ethical implications of therapy or result of intense suffering

DEFINING CHARACTERISTICS

- Expresses concern with meaning of life and death and/or belief systems
- Anger toward God (as defined by the person)
- Questions meaning of suffering
- Verbalizes inner conflict about beliefs
- Verbalizes concern about relationship with deity
- Questions meaning for own existence
- Unable to choose or chooses not to participate in usual religious practices
- Seeks spiritual assistance
- Questions moral and ethical implications of therapeutic regimen
- Displacement of anger toward religious representatives
- Description of nightmares or sleep disturbances
- Alteration in behavior or mood evidenced by anger, crying, withdrawal, preoccupation, anxiety, hostility, apathy, etc.
- Regards illness as punishment
- Does not experience that God is forgiving
- Unable to accept self
- Engages in self-blame
- Denies responsibilities for problems
- Description of somatic complaints

From Kim, M.J., et al.: Pocket-guide of nursing diagnosis, St. Louis, 1984, The C.V. Mosby Co.

together to identify and meet all the needs of a client, including spiritual needs.

Dickenson (1975) suggests that ministry and spiritual care are inherent in nursing. She identifies the following factors in the nurse-client relationship that demonstrate the nurse's commitment to the client's spiritual health: support, self- and other-awareness, understanding, openness, and nonjudgmental acceptance. Several circumstances, however, may cause the nurse to be uncomfortable in providing spiritual care. One impediment may be the past role of spirituality or organized religion in the nurse's life. Perhaps an authoritarian upbringing has caused the nurse to rebel against the religious practices of her early years. Perhaps the nurse believes that religion or the spiritual dimension is a private matter for the client. Some nurses consider spiritual care, like client teaching, as something to be done only if and when time permits.

Some nurses feel unprepared to address the spiritual aspect of care with clients or have the misconception that spiritual needs should be left to the pastoral care department. A nurse may hesitate to include the spiritual dimension of care in planning because she feels unworthy to discuss such a topic. Yet spirituality is interrelated with other dimensions of being human and is shared by all human beings, and nurses should not feel that they need special educational or other preparation to consider the client's spiritual health when planning care. A concern for spirituality need not be confined to the pastoral care department, just as care directed toward the client's psychosocial health is not a specialized matter for psychiatrists only. In the spiritual dimension, as in other dimensions, the nurse is assisting the client toward a state of well-being and a sense of fulfillment.

Implementation

When the nurse identifies the client's spiritual needs and arrives at a diagnosis of spiritual distress, she plans to meet this need. Resources that may be included in implementing the plan are nursing interventions, family involvement, and counseling by the clergy. Other possible sources for spiritual care are members of the pastoral care department and nurses' support groups.

NURSING INTERVENTIONS

After having determined who and what sustains the client's spirituality, the nurse's responsibility is to support and enhance this belief system or find someone able to do so. If the client's image of the Supreme Being is negative, the nurse may choose to share her own concept of a Supreme Being. The nurse's sincer-

the existence of a spiritual need, the nurse should accept their decision. Possibly the client's minister, priest, or other spiritual adviser or a member of the pastoral care team has already recognized and ministered to the client's spiritual needs without the nurse's knowledge. Ideally the health care team works

ity, patience, and awareness of the client's spiritual distress will encourage the client to discuss his spiritual values. The nurse's own spirituality is a form of support as she challenges the client to clarify his beliefs about the Supreme Being, the spiritual dimension of life, and the meaning of suffering and pain.

How the client views himself is another area for intervention. If the nurse consistently treats the client as a unique individual with significant value and unlimited potential, the client's self-concept will be enhanced. The nurse should consider the client's wishes when scheduling activities and should provide the client with privacy and personal time for reflection on life.

Individuals at any point on the health-illness continuum have a need to be alone to interact with or be aware of a Supreme Being. Solitude may liberate the spirit and lead to true knowledge of self, peace and joy, and an appreciation of life on a more profound level. The nurse may help a hospitalized client gain from solitude through self-examination and redirection, a new perspective of his relationship with the Supreme Being, and a more positive self-concept.

If a client asks the nurse to pray for him or with him, it is appropriate to do so. Prayer can be offered aloud or in silence according to the client's wishes. Prayer has various purposes in different religions: praise, petition, thanksgiving, and reparation for sin. The client may want to praise God and offer thanks for blessings or to request health or freedom from pain. The client should be allowed time to express a particular need.

When the client asks the nurse for prayer or seems to need other spiritual support, the nurse should respond sincerely and genuinely. Different reactions may be appropriate for a client who is crying, who feels guilty, or who is experiencing a personal crisis. Some clients want to hold the nurse's hands when praying; others hold the palms upward in a posture of supplication. Raising or lowering the eyes indicates a disposition toward prayer. Standing, kneeling, and squatting are positions of prayer in different religious traditions. Nurses should follow the client's lead in this regard rather than their own religious backgrounds and practices.

INVOLVEMENT OF FAMILY AND FRIENDS

Relationships with others sustain a person's belief system. The love and support received from relatives and friends and the counsel from clergymen and spiritual advisors are encouragements to live better today than yesterday, more productively tomorrow than today. The nurse should urge family and friends to visit the client and demonstrate their love and concern. In some cases, working with or through family or friends

to provide the client's spiritual care is the most effective way to meet this need. Members of parish or church groups can be encouraged to send cards and assurance of prayers for recovery.

Including family members in a prayer service is a thoughtful gesture if this is appropriate to the client's religion and family members are comfortable participating. Reading favorite religious passages or prayerbooks may be requested and appreciated by the client and family. Such readings can be especially meaningful in expressing joy and praise and in putting into words needs for comfort and strength. Encouraging clients to keep significant symbols nearby can be a source of consolation and spiritual support. Since a visit to the hospital chapel or attendance at services can be important to the hospitalized client and family, a trip to the chapel or direction for finding the prayer room should be included when orienting the client and family to the medical facility.

ROLE OF THE CLERGY

Some hospitalized clients find a visit from their clergyman or spiritual adviser consoling. The nurse should ask clients if they would like to have their minister, priest, or spiritual adviser notified of their hospitalization. Ministers and pastors should be made welcome in nursing units. Keeping ministers informed of physiological and psychosocial, as well as spiritual, concerns, when requested by the client or family, helps in providing holistic health care. A willingness to cooperate with and facilitate the administration of sacraments, rites, and rituals of the client's religion shows respect for the client's spiritual values and needs.

Providing privacy for the client and his clergyman or spiritual adviser is a thoughtful and sensitive gesture. If the nurse is unsure about the proper routine in a client's religion, asking the minister, the family, or the client is appropriate. The nurse can adapt spiritual care to the client's religious tenets without sacrificing her personal beliefs.

OTHER RESOURCES

The nurse has other resources that can assist in facilitating her own and clients' spiritual health. Especially helpful are members of a hospital's pastoral care department, who can visit the client, administer sacraments or rites, and provide religious objects when requested. Taped meditations and televised religious services may also be available through the pastoral care department.

If a pastoral care representative is not a member of the client's religion, the client's or family's minister may be called to visit. In case of death, pastoral ministers can provide support to the family and friends.

They serve also as counselors and consultants for nursing personnel.

To sustain the nurse in her many roles, support systems such as prayer groups can be organized. Discussion groups can help nurses recognize their own spiritual needs so they can respect the client's right to do the same. Such groups can also focus on the responsible and appropriate application of the nursing process to spiritual needs.

Other organizations may provide further resources and support for nurses. The Nurses Christian Fellowship, for example, provides literature on interventions for spiritual needs and encourages nurses to seek help through prayer and discussion groups. A nurse's regular study of her religious beliefs can sensitize her to expressions of spiritual need and enrich her personal resources.

Religious practices that enhance spiritual and personal development can serve as resources for the nurse who highly values meeting client's spiritual needs as well as physiological and psychosocial needs.

Evaluation

Attainment of spiritual health can be considered a lifelong goal. However, to evaluate the effectiveness of nursing interventions in this dimension of health care, the nurse may compare the client's level of spiritual health with the behaviors and needs noted in the original assessment. The following questions may be helpful:

1. Is the client's belief system stronger?
2. Do the client's professed beliefs support and direct his actions and words?
3. Does the client derive peace and strength from spiritual resources (such as prayer and minister's visits) to face the rigors of treatment, rehabilitation, or impending death?
4. Does the client seem more in control and have a clearer self-concept because he has found meaning and purpose in life and suffering?
5. Is the client at ease in being alone? In having life's plans changed?
6. Is the client's behavior appropriate to the occasion?
7. Has reconciliation of differences, if any, taken place between the client and family members or others?
8. Are mutual respect and love obvious in the client's relationships with others?

It is helpful to consider how the client looks and feels when spiritual needs are met. The client should be experiencing emotions appropriate to the situation, developing a strong, realistic self-image and warm, open interpersonal relationships, and maintaining a sense of mission in life and confidence and trust in his Supreme Being.

A client whose spiritual needs are met will be peaceful regardless of illness and suffering. The client's calm countenance demonstrates that he has found answers to the questions of life and death, vulnerability, and pain. The spiritually healthy client will be a source of strength, hope, and inspiration for the nurse.

If the client is comfortable in expressing spiritual needs to the nurse or in sharing beliefs and religious resources, the nurse can assume that the psychological climate is encouraging verbalization of these needs. Does the nursing care plan schedule time for quiet, for prayer, for a visit to the chapel, and for attendance at services? Is provision for spiritual health considered as important as plans for medical and nursing care of a physiological or psychological illness?

Nurses can also evaluate their own personal spiritual health. Does the nurse plan time in her weekly schedule for activities supporting her faith and enriching the spiritual dimension of her life? Does the nurse's behavior reflect a positive self-image despite day-to-day problems? Do the nurse's responses to life and death mirror her convictions resulting from her spirituality?

Thus a nurse's evaluation of the attainment of spiritual health should include observation of the client's life situations, the nursing environment, and herself.

Summary

Nursing care that neglects the spiritual dimension cannot be called holistic. It overlooks a vital component of human nature, the spirit that nourishes and sustains the spark of life. To provide spiritual care the nurse must understand what spiritual health is and be able to recognize the spiritually healthy person. As with other dimensions of care, the norm is identified first for comparison during assessment. If spiritual needs are identified in the assessment, plans are made to intervene appropriately. In implementing the plan for spiritual care, nursing interventions are individualized according to the client's specific needs. The family's involvement and the ministrations of spiritual advisers are sought when indicated. Resources for facilitating client's spiritual care and for providing support for nurses are used as necessary. The rewards of meeting clients' spiritual needs include personal and professional fulfillment and enrichment.

KEY CONCEPTS

✓ Spiritual health is a state in which the person feels secure in a relationship with a Supreme Being, a presence with or in each person and in the world.

✓ To provide spiritual care in nursing, the nurse must understand what spiritual health is and be able to recognize the spiritually distressed person.

✓ Nurses should be aware of the client's general spiritual needs and facilitate the client's chosen practices.

✓ The spiritual dimension of care, although it may include religious beliefs and rituals, is not limited to the practices and dogma of organized religions.

✓ When making a spiritual assessment, the nurse includes questions about the client's concept of a Supreme Being, source of strength and hope, significance of religious practices and rituals, and perceived relationships between spiritual beliefs and health.

✓ The client's contradictory actions or attitudes may indicate that he is experiencing spiritual distress.

✓ To be attuned to spiritual aspects of care, nurses should be aware of their own spiritual dimension and be comfortable in discussing spiritual matters.

✓ The nurse should use available resources such as family members, clergy, and other members of the health care team to help the client maintain or regain a state of spiritual health.

REFERENCES

Brallier, L.W.: The nurse as holistic health practitioner, Nurs. Clin. North Am. 13(4):643, 1978.

Dickenson, S.C.: The search for spiritual meaning, Am. J. Nurs. 75(10):1789, 1975.

Fish, S., and Shelly, J.A.: Spiritual care: the nurse's role, Downers Grove, Ill., 1978, InterVarsity Press.

Kim, M.J., and Moritz, D.A., editors: Classification of nursing diagnoses, proceedings of the Third and Fourth National Conferences, New York, 1982, McGraw-Hill Book Co.

Lafferty, J.A.: Credo for wellness, Health Education 10(5):10, 1979.

Meeks, L.B.: The role of spiritual health in achieving high level wellness, Health Values: Achieving High Level Wellness 1(5):222, 1977.

Newman, M.: Theory development in nursing, Philadelphia, 1979, F.A. Davis Co.

Piles, C.L.: Spiritual care as part of the nursing curriculum: a descriptive study, Unpublished master's research project, St. Louis, 1980, St. Louis University School of Nursing.

Stoll, R.: Guidelines for spiritual assessment, Am. J. Nurs. 79(9):1574, 1979.

ADDITIONAL READINGS

Buys, S.A.M.: Discussion series sensitizes nurses to patient's spiritual needs, Hosp. Prog. 62(10):44, 1981.

Hoyman, H.S.: Models of human nature and their impact on health education, Nurs. Dig. 3(5):37, 1975.

Kasanof, D., Levy, J., and Striffler, R.C.: When religious belief affects therapy, Patient Care 8(19):99, 1974.

Pumphrey, J.B.: Recognizing your patient's spiritual needs, Nursing 77 7(12):64, 1977.

Shelly, J.A.: Spiritual care workbook: a companion to spiritual care; the nurse's role, Downers Grove Ill., 1978, InterVarsity Press.

Stallwood, J., and Stoll, R.: Spiritual dimensions of nursing practice. In Beland, I., and Passos, J., editors: Clinical nursing: pathophysiological and psychosocial approaches, ed. 3, New York, 1975, Macmillan, Inc.

Wheelock, R.D.: Unmet patient needs, Hospital Prog. 55(7):60, 1974.

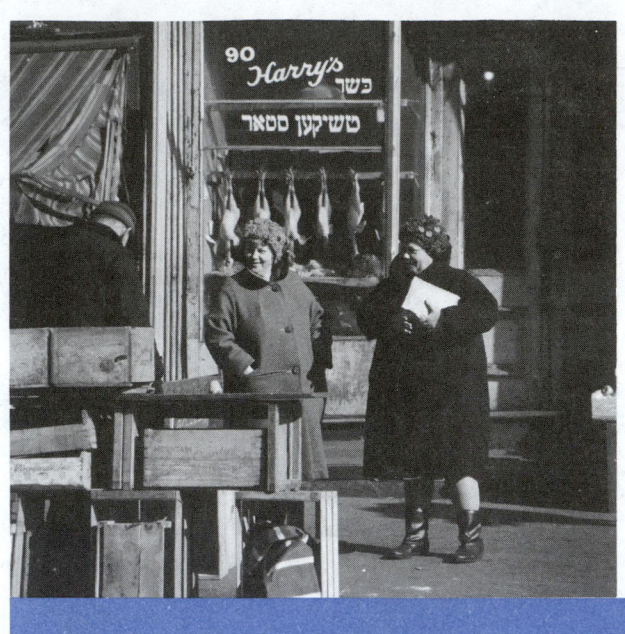

OBJECTIVES

Mastery of the content in this chapter will enable the student to:

- Define the terms in the glossary.
- Describe ways in which culture influences an individual.
- Discuss the relationship between ethnic nursing and holistic health.
- Explain how ethnocentrism can have negative effects on the nurse-client therapeutic relationship.
- Describe ways in which the nurse can overcome language barriers when providing care for ethnic minority clients.
- Describe forms of racism and potential effects on clients.
- Explain differences and similarities among ethnic cultural groups in terms of:

      Physiological susceptibility to disease
      Language
      Food and eating habits
      Time orientation
      Personal space and territoriality
      Attitudes toward the family
      Gender role behavior
      Emotional expression and pain reactions
      Emotional and mental health
      Health-illness beliefs and practices

- List general cultural characteristics of the four major ethnic minority groups in North America.
- Perform a cultural assessment with an ethnic minority client.
- List potential nursing diagnoses related to a client's ethnicity.
- Discuss several ways in which planning and implementation of nursing interventions can be adapted to a client's ethnicity.
- Explain the need for a nurse's self-evaluation when providing care to ethnic minority clients.

GLOSSARY

cultural assimilation Process by which members of an ethnic minority group lose cultural characteristics that distinguish them from the dominant cultural group.

cultural healer Member of an ethnic or cultural group who uses traditional methods of healing rather than modern scientific methods to provide health care for other members of the group, or members of another ethnic minority group.

culture Homogeneous, learned patterns of behavior, values, and attitudes shared by a group of people and passed from one generation to the next.

culture shock Disorder that occurs in response to transition from one setting to another; former behavior patterns are ineffective in such an unfamiliar situation and basic cues for social behavior are absent.

21 Culture, Ethnicity, and Nursing

dialect Variation of a language different from other forms of the same language in pronunciation, syntax, and word meanings; a dialect is usually shared by people in a geographical area or ethnic group.

dominant group Social group that controls the value system and the rewards in a society

ethnic stereotype Fixed concept or expectation about how members of an ethnic or cultural group act or think.

ethnicity Cultural group's sense of affiliation associated with the group's common social and cultural heritage.

ethnocentrism Tendency of members of one cultural group to view the members of other cultural groups in terms of the standards of behavior, attitudes, and values of their own group.

minority group Group of people who, because of physical or cultural characteristics, receive different and unequal treatment from others in the society; minority group members see themselves as recipients of collective discrimination.

personal space Culturally influenced set of attitudes and behaviors related to one's use of the physical space about oneself.

race Biological term for persons who share distinguishing physical features and genetic traits.

racism Any ethnocentric activity—cultural, individual, or institutional, deliberate or not—that is based on belief in the inherent superiority of a certain racial group over other groups and serves to maintain the oppression and subjugation of members of these groups.

Raza/Latina Term used instead of "Hispanic" or "Spanish origin" that accurately describes the many Indian and other ancestors of Puerto Ricans, Cubans, Mexicans/Chicanos, Spanish, and Central and South Americans.

subculture Large group of people who, although members of a larger cultural group (or in transition from one cultural identification to another), have shared characteristics that are not common to all members of the cultural group and that enable them to be thought of as a distinguishable subgroup.

*I*n a multicultural society, nurses will likely encounter clients from diverse cultures. To provide safe and personalized care, nurses must integrate clients' cultural backgrounds into the nursing process.

A person's cultural background primarily involves internalized collective standards of behavior, as well as shared values and attitudes. The standards of any cultural group, however, are not spelled out, and members of the cultural group may not even recognize them as standards, since many people assume that everyone in their cultural group shares the same standards and ideas. Thus one culture can seem odd to members of another culture. Culture involves what people consider appropriate behavior and the expectations of others regarding this behavior. A person's behavior is interpreted by others on the basis of cultural expectations.

Cultural and ethnic factors are significant in all persons, and thus nurses who seek to provide individualized total health care to clients need to understand the clients' cultural backgrounds. A nurse who provides care to a client who shares her cultural background may not be aware that she is responding to the client in cultural terms at all stages of the nursing

process, but when the same nurse seeks to provide care to a client of a different cultural or ethnic background, her lack of awareness may lead to less than fully effective care. For example, a middle-class, white nurse who holds the cultural value of punctuality may misinterpret the values of a Raza/Latina client who is an hour late for an appointment. The nurse may mistakenly believe that the client is resisting care, when actually this situation involves a difference in cultural attitudes toward time. The nurse is less effective in providing care, however, if such a lack of awareness leads to misunderstanding or misinterpretation. This example involves only one of many differences among various cultural and ethnic groups. Other such differences include physiological susceptibility to illness, use of verbal and nonverbal communication, food and eating habits, attitudes toward personal space, attitudes toward the family, forms of emotional expression, gender role behavior, reactions to pain, and health-illness beliefs and behavior.

Cultural background plays a major role in many aspects of life, leading to differences in how we interact with others and in the areas of politics, religion, economics, and so on. Cultural differences are particularly important to health care providers because of their roles in illness and the provision of health care. Culture influences how people perceive and react to illness, including how and when people seek health care and to whom they turn for care (see discussion of illness behaviors in Chapter 2).

For a nurse to successfully provide care for a client of a different cultural or ethnic background requires that effective intercultural communication take place between the nurse and the client. Such intercultural communication occurs when each attempts to understand the other person's point of view from his or her own cultural frame of reference. Effective intercultural communication is facilitated by the nurse's identification of areas of commonalities between nurse and client. After reaching a cultural understanding of the client, the nurse must consider cultural factors throughout the nursing process. Major nursing organizations have in the last decade emphasized the importance of considering cultural factors when delivering nursing care. According to the American Nurses' Association (1976), "Consideration of individual value systems and lifestyles should be included in the planning and health care for each client." A criterion applicable to baccalaureate nursing curriculum adopted by the National League for Nursing (1977) is that "the curriculum is based on the philosophy, purposes, and objectives of the program and recognizes the contribution of nursing and other disciplines toward meeting the health needs of a diverse and multicultural society."

Modesta Soberano Orque wishes to acknowledge the assistance and support of the following persons in making this chapter possible: Napoleon Bantayan, Thomas Ross Farnham, M.D., Carlota Mendoza, R.N., Maria Antonio Villamena, and Lynette Winegarden, R.N.

Culture and Ethnicity

The United States and Canada are commonly but erroneously believed to be "melting pots" of different cultures; that is, the dominant cultural group in each country is an assimilation of different cultures, primarily European. The U.S. population is approximately 83% white (U.S. Department of Commerce, 1983). According to the U.S. Department of State (1983), Canada is about 97% white. Yet culture is not the same as race. Whites in both countries include large European cultural groups such as French, German, and Italian populations. Nonwhite cultural groups include blacks, Asians, Native Americans, Hispanics (Raza/Latinas), and others. Although the idea of the "melting pot" suggests that these different cultural and racial backgrounds have been fused into a common culture shared by all, this apparent assimilation is often only superficial, involving aspects of shared language, styles of dress, and so on. In fact, many members of different cultural groups retain deeper characteristics of their cultures, including attitudes, values, and behavior patterns.

Concepts of Culture and Ethnicity

Culture has been defined as "the learned ways of acting and thinking which are transmitted by group members to other group members and which provide for each individual ready-made and tested solutions for vital problems" (Walter, 1952). Culture therefore includes diet, language and communication process, religion, art, history, family life processes, social groups' interactive patterns, value orientations, and healing beliefs and practices. Because culture is devised by people to solve human problems, it is universal; all people share in some culture. On the other hand, a culture of a certain people has qualities specific to that group. A cultural group thus has a particular pattern of behavior by which it can be distinguished from other groups. Culture is a *collective* pattern of a group, in which the individual participates to some extent. No two people with the same cultural background will share in the cultural pattern in exactly the same way because behaviors, attitudes, and values are learned individually as well as culturally.

Ethnicity, as defined by Werner (1979), is a group's "affiliation due to a shared linguistic, racial and/or cultural background." Inherent in this definition is the idea that members of an ethnic group have a similar cultural background or way of life.

The nurse and the client each have their own cultural life-styles. In some situations the nurses come from the white dominant group whereas clients belong to an ethnic minority group. The phrase "dominant group," as used here, means "a collectivity within a society which has preeminent authority to function as guardians and sustainers of the controlling value system and as prime allocators of rewards in the society" (Schermerhorn, 1970). In this chapter the terms "ethnic minority group" and "ethnic minority" are used synonymously with "minority group." Wirth (1945) defined minority as

a group of people who, because of their physical or cultural characteristics, are singled out from the others in the society in which they live for differential and unequal treatment, and who therefore regard themselves as objects of collective discrimination.

Thus the existence of a minority group in a society implies the existence of a corresponding majority group. Because members of the dominant group usually have higher social status and more privileges, minority group members are excluded from full participation in the life of the society.

Influences of Culture

Nurses providing care should consider all clients as individuals for the simple reason that each person is unique in terms of behavior, attitudes, values, and so on. But just as individuals are affected in many ways by family upbringing, personal experiences, genetic and biological factors, and other influences, so too are they influenced by the culture in which they were brought up and live.

How an individual is influenced, however, as well as the extent of the influence, depends on the individual. The cultural characteristics described later in this chapter are *group* characteristics of ethnic minorities. These characteristics may not be exhibited by every member of a cultural group. Any person, depending on personal experience, may have all, some, or none of these characteristics. A person never acquires a culture as a complete and absolute pattern. Instead, the person merely learns the prominent contours of a subculture. Differences among members of a cultural group are based on variables such as the following:

1. Age
2. Religion
3. Dialect(s) or language(s) spoken
4. Gender identity and roles
5. Socioeconomic background
6. Geographical location in the country of origin of the subcultural group with which the person ethnically identifies
7. Geographical location in the current country of residence of the subcultural group with which the person ethnically identifies

8. History of the subcultural group with which the person identifies in the country of origin
9. History of the subcultural group with which the person ethnically identifies in the current country of residence
10. Amount and type of contact of young people with older relatives who are the chief sources of traditional values
11. Degree of adoption of values in the current country of residence by the subcultural group with which the person ethnically identifies

Because culture influences different individuals' behaviors, values, and attitudes in various ways, the nurse must resist the temptation to stereotype the members of any cultural group. An ethnic stereotype is a fixed concept of how all members of an ethnic group act or think. A stereotype may be based on an accurate generalization of a particular ethnic group, yet a nurse's stereotyping of an ethnic minority client from that group may be inaccurate because what is generally true of a culture is not necessarily true of every individual in that culture. It has been shown, for example, that Italians are more likely to express pain vocally than most white Americans. A nurse providing care for a client of Italian background might therefore assume that this client is like many other Italians—a stereotype—and thus conclude that, since he has said nothing, he feels no pain. Because of the variables listed previously, however, this aspect of Italian culture may have had little influence on the individual client, who in fact may be experiencing pain. The nurse who stereotypes the client therefore is making a mistake in not encouraging the client to express his real feelings.

Stereotypes may or may not bear any relationship to reality. Stereotypes born out of racism, for example, generally are unrelated to reality, whereas some stereotypes, as in the preceding example of Italians, may be true of a cultural group but of many other people as well. In addition, stereotypes may be either positive or negative. An example of a positive stereotype is the belief that all clients of Japanese ancestry, being uncomplaining and cooperative, are "model" clients. A negative stereotype is the notion that all blacks are superstitious and lazy. Negative stereotypes clearly can create problems in dealing with a client, but so can positive stereotypes, because in both cases the nurse is considering not the individual client but her own image of the client.

The basic needs of all human beings, regardless of cultural background, are discussed in Chapter 4. *How* a person seeks to meet these needs is influenced by culture. The person's ethnic-cultural system can be understood as the totality of means by which the person meets needs.

Fig. 21-1 illustrates the influences of the ethnic-cultural system. In this framework the arrows arising from "basic human needs" are directed toward each component of the system (such as diet and religion), meaning that solutions to basic human needs lead to these cultural elements. Because basic human needs are universal, the components of the ethnic-cultural system are applicable to the client and to the nurse. A universal feature of the concept *basic human needs* seems to be its cyclical nature, representing people's continual adaptation to their environment. In the figure this notion is depicted by the circular arrows in the basic human needs section. Therefore, for any ethnic-cultural system, the degree to which basic human needs are reflected in each of these cultural components determines to a great extent the ethnic-cultural system's impact on how individuals meet these needs. Although all of these cultural components are present in any ethnic-cultural system, nuances of these components result in diversities between the ethnic-cultural systems of particular groups or individuals.

The components of the ethnic-cultural system have an impact on one another and on the entire system. Changes in the entire system are also reflected in the individual components. Thus in Fig. 21-1 the lines separating each of the components are equal and are dotted to show the interrelationships and interdependence of these factors. The nurse also needs to remember the interrelationships of the various cultural components and how they affect the client's care. For instance, because of his religious beliefs, a

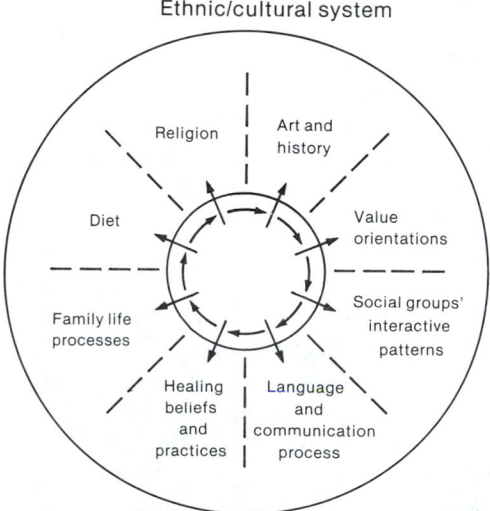

Fig. 21-1 Orque's ethnic-cultural system framework showing the components of the system applicable to the client or the nurse.

From Orque, M.S., Bloch, B., and Monrroy, L.S.A.: Ethnic nursing care: a multicultural approach, St. Louis, 1983, The C.V. Mosby Co.

Black Muslim might refuse to eat any pork product. In the initial client interview the nurse should give equal attention to the ethnic-cultural factors of diet and religion; later she can determine the relative importance of these factors in the client's care. For example, eating traditional Filipino foods during hospitalization might not be very important to a third-generation Filipino mother, but the influence of the Catholic religion on her views about family planning might be. Thus for this client the cultural factor of diet is less important than the cultural factor of religion, although for other clients the reverse might be true.

Orque's ethnic-cultural system framework provides the basis for Bloch's ethnic-cultural assessment guide, which will be discussed later.

Culture and Holistic Health

To give holistic care, nurses must be concerned not only with the client's ethnic-cultural system but also with the influences of the client's other dimensions on ethnic-cultural factors. The biological, psychological, and social dimensions greatly influence the ethnic-cultural system of either the client or the nurse.

The biological dimension includes all of the physiological life processes of a human organism. For example, in the physiological assessment of a black client, the nurse should be aware of differences between assessing black skin and assessing white skin. The nurse must also be knowledgeable about diseases to which blacks have greater susceptibility, as well as conditions to which they have extreme resistance. The psychological dimension includes the mental and behavioral processes and characteristics of individuals and groups. For example, the nurse must consider the influence of an ethnic minority client's self-concept on his interactions with non–ethnic minority health professionals. The social dimension includes all social institutions to which people belong. The nurse needs to be aware of the impact of institutional racism in health facilities on the care of ethnic minority clients and poor clients.

The interactions of the ethnic-cultural dimension with these other dimensions can be clearly illustrated by the socioeconomic influences on health care. Kosa and Zola (1975) divided U.S. society into three socioeconomic strata: the middle and upper classes, the blue-collar working class, and the poverty population. Although these strata may overlap, they may still be generally delineated in terms of their distinctive life-styles. These life-styles are influenced by or associated with the following factors:

1. Amount and source of resources (that is, income) available to members of each stratum

2. Their type of occupation and the prestige associated with each type
3. The type and value of their housing and neighborhood
4. Their level of knowledge and educational achievement
5. Their race or ethnic origin

The poverty population is the lowest of the three strata. In this class unemployment levels are typically high. Incomes and educational attainments of members tend to be low. According to Kosa and Zola, it is often believed that substantial proportions of the following U.S. population groups are included in this stratum:

1. The black, Puerto Rican, and Mexican American populations and other relatively poor ethnic minorities
2. The poor in large-city ghettos
3. The rural poor (residents of Appalachia or the Deep South)
4. Native Americans on reservations
5. The elderly
6. Migrant workers
7. The dependent poor

The life-style of members of the poverty population results in a significantly lower level of health. For example, in 1972 45% of Native American families reported yearly incomes of less than $6000, and 42% reported yearly incomes between $6000 and $8000. Almost one third of all Indian households were without adequate water and sewer and waste disposal systems. It is not surprising then that the incidence of tuberculosis among Indians is still about 10 times greater than that for all other races in the United States (U.S. Department of Health, Education and Welfare, 1978).

Not only do poor ethnic minorities have inadequate nutrition and housing, but they also have less access to quality personal health services than does the rest of the American population. Furthermore, cultural factors and the knowledge of how to use health services are also important in the relationship of these clients' socioeconomic backgrounds to their health status. Even when good health care is available, the poor do not generally avail themselves of this important resource to the extent that white-collar middle-class people do. The poor and the working class tend not to put a high priority on minor conditions, seeking medical treatment only at a relatively late stage. A possible explanation for this is that the poor are not assured of protection against economic hazards, especially those of a short-term nature. When the poor become sick, absence from employment is likely to result in economic consequences more severe than for middle-class employees. Compared with the poor population, middle-class people work in more protected jobs, are better educated, and are more likely to seek treatment for minor illnesses.

The nurse should also be aware of factors other than lack of finances and different value orientations that prevent ethnic minorities from procuring needed health care. Mosley (1977) identified some of these impediments:

1. The humiliation of a "means test" to establish medical indigence in order for the ethnic minority person to obtain so-called free care
2. Fragmentation of care through depersonalization and confusion of referrals to various medical specialty clinics
3. Operational features in the provision of the services, including inconvenient hours or location and unpleasant surroundings
4. Lack of communication, trust, and understanding between clients and personnel (Because of staff shortages, employees are usually unable to provide personalized care.)
5. Racial discrimination in provision of services (Some hospitals previously closed to ethnic minorities are still underutilized. Many hospitals still refuse to grant staff privileges to ethnic minority physicians.)
6. Lack of facilities and manpower (Most health personnel reside and practice in upper- and middle-class areas. They find the urban ghettos and slums and the remote rural areas where a large number of ethnic minorities reside unattractive. Hospitals also relocate in the suburbs to escape the blight of inner-city areas. Local politics often prevents the establishment of area-wide, centralized health facilities.)

In addition, the lack of bilingual health care personnel who are perceptive of clients' cultural backgrounds deters members of ethnic minority groups from seeking health care.

Clearly, then, cultural and ethnic factors are often interrelated with psychological, social, and economic factors. To provide holistic care to clients from varied cultural backgrounds, the nurse needs to understand how these factors interact for each client.

Ethnocentrism

Ethnocentrism is the tendency to view members of other cultural or ethnic groups in terms of the standards of behavior and values of a person's own group. Ethnocentrism is somewhat like egoism: egoism leads a person to react to others in purely personal, selfish terms, without accepting others as unique human beings with their own values and standards. Ethnocentrism leads a person to react to members of an-

other ethnic group without accepting or even considering cultural differences in values and standards. Because of our upbringing and education, however, most of us know when we are reacting egoistically, and we try to view the other in his or her own right. Yet often we are not aware of the similar ethnocentric reaction, because most often we tend to interact with others of the same cultural background, and thus we unconsciously judge other cultures by the standards of our own. An ethnocentric nurse, for example, might assume that everyone agrees that treatment should be based on scientific principles. If this nurse encounters a client from a different cultural background who believes in spiritual healing, she might consider the client silly, superstitious, or immature—an attitude the client would probably perceive. In such a case the client might be less cooperative with or reject nursing care, and in addition the nurse will have overlooked a potential resource for the client.

Both ethnocentrism and stereotyping may adversely affect client care. The nurse with either attitude fails to consider the client as an individual. In ethnocentrism the nurse assumes that the client should embrace her own values. In stereotyping the nurse assumes that the client automatically manifests *all* characteristics of his ethnic group. In either case the nurse cannot provide individualized holistic care to the client.

When ethnocentrism becomes pervasive, cultural racism can result. Racism is any ethnocentric activity—cultural, individual, or institutional, deliberate or not—that is based on the belief in the inherent superiority of a certain racial group over other groups and serves to maintain the oppression and subjugation of members of these groups. Racism can occur in cultural, individual, and institutional forms.

In the United States the major manifestation of cultural racism is the ethnocentric attitude that the white Anglo-Saxon Protestant cultural heritage is superior to cultural experiences of ethnic minority groups. However, some minority group members can also be culturally racist toward the certain members of the dominant cultural group and other ethnic minority groups, an attitude with which nurses must sometimes contend (Vigil, 1980). Aspects of both institutional and individual racism are involved in cultural racism. An example of individual racism is the belief of some white Anglo-Saxon Protestants that ethnic minorities are inferior to whites. Institutional racism is any institutional activity, intentional or unintentional, that by creating racial inequalities results in the oppression of ethnic minority groups. For example, institutional racism is reflected in the sometimes deplorable health status of nonwhites, which results from their inability to obtain good health care. Although racial segregation of clients in hospitals was officially ended with the passage of the Civil Rights Act of 1964, subtle discrimination still exists. Contemporary hospital rooms accommodate two to six clients, and hospital admitting clerks usually assign "compatible" clients to the same room. "Compatibility" often means that all clients in a room are the same race.

Racism can also be an unconscious phenomenon. A person may have learned racist attitudes from family members or other influences, and such attitudes may become manifest to ethnic group members even when the person has consciously rejected the attitudes. A nurse might unintentionally use a patronizing tone when speaking to a minority group client, even though she intends to convey empathy.

To avoid the problems of stereotyping, ethnocentrism, and racism, nurses must become aware of how their own values, standards of behavior, and attitudes differ from those of their clients. The values clarification process, described in Chapter 13, is an invaluable means of reaching this awareness. Similarly, nurses need to become sensitive to manifestations of institutional racism in order to work toward eliminating racial or ethnic inequalities.

Differences and Similarities among Ethnic-Cultural Groups

To provide individualized health care for ethnic group clients, nurses need to understand basic concepts of culture and the influence of culture. Nurses should also be aware of their own cultural background and the extent to which their culture has influenced their own values, behaviors, attitudes, and beliefs about health and illness. These elements are discussed in the preceding section. In addition, nurses require information about the cultural differences and similarities among the ethnic groups they are likely to encounter in nursing practice.

The process of recognizing commonalities between a nurse and a client is illustrated in Fig. 21-2. In this figure the two circles represent the respective ethnic-cultural systems of the client and the nurse. Each ethnic-cultural system includes the codification subsystem, which is a part of the language and communication process component. As shown in Fig. 21-1, the language and communication process is a key component of an ethnic-cultural system. Fig. 21-2 depicts the ethnic-cultural systems of the client and the nurse as existing side by side with an area of intersection joining them. This means that although the two ethnic-cultural systems coexist in the pluralistic American society, there are areas of similarities between these systems that the nurse and the client

could use to improve their intercultural communication.

In Fig. 21-2 the lines where the two circles intersect are cross hatched to denote that each ethnic-cultural system is expandable depending on either the client's or the nurse's ability to explore or develop further areas of commonality. It is also possible that both the nurse and the client could successfully determine or cultivate additional areas of shared experiences. For instance, a Cantonese-speaking Chinese client, through his repeated contacts with white nurses, might be encouraged to learn more conversational English in school. Similarly, white nurses, through frequent encounters with Cantonese-speaking Chinese clients, might become motivated to increase their abilities in medical conversational Cantonese.

Before nurses can successfully discover and cultivate areas of similarities, areas of difference between the nurse and the client should be explored. When aspects of the nurse's ethnic-cultural system are contrasted with those of the client along a continuum of minimal to maximal cultural differences, it is evident that the initial recognition of cultural diversities would facilitate the discovery of cultural similarities between the nurse and the client.

Areas of Difference and Similarity

Cultural groups vary in many ways, and several of these differences can be important for the nurse's understanding of the client and for the development of the nurse-client relationship. It is also important for the nurse to be aware of similarities among cultural groups requiring care. The following sections briefly describe some of the important areas of difference and similarity among certain ethnic minority groups. Later sections discuss certain dominant characteristics of various ethnic minority groups. In both discussions these descriptions are only generalizations:

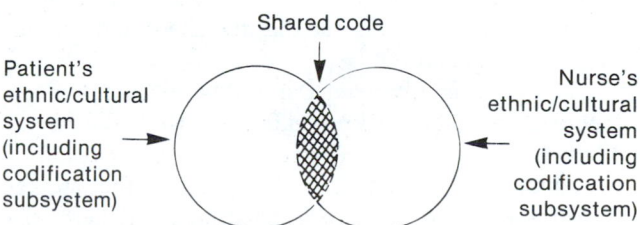

Fig. 21-2 Orque's intercultural communication model showing shared common coding between the client's ethnic-cultural system and the nurse's ethnic-cultural system.

Modified from Jensen, M., Benson, R., and Bobak, I.: Maternity care: the nurse and the family, ed. 2, St. Louis, 1981, The C.V. Mosby Co.

they are not true of all members of any ethnic minority group. As mentioned earlier, the influence of culture varies for each client, and therefore nursing care in this area, as in all other areas, should be individualized. Nonetheless, a general knowledge of cultural differences and similarities and particular cultural characteristics can help the nurse understand clients from diverse ethnic backgrounds.

LANGUAGE

Language differences are possibly the most important factor in providing nursing care to ethnic group clients, because they can affect all stages of the nursing process. Clear and effective communication is important when dealing with any client and is crucial if language differences create a cultural barrier between the nurse and the client. If the client does not speak the nurse's language, a translator is necessary. More often, however, the client speaks the nurse's language with limited ability or uses language with denotative or connotative meanings different from the nurse's meanings. For example, a client with limited language ability might know customary greetings such as "How are you?" or "Hello" but not understand health terms such as "pain" or "temperature" that are usually understood by lay persons in the dominant cultural group. Failure to communicate effectively with the client not only may cause unnecessary and cost delays in diagnosis and treatment but also may lead to tragic consequences. In one incident, for example, a white nurse failed to ascertain that the client truly understood preoperative instructions about washing the surgical site with povidone-iodine (Betadine). The non-English-speaking Asian client, throughout the time she was being instructed by the nurse, kept nodding and smiling when the nurse asked her, "Do you understand what I told you?" The nurse judged that the client understood the instructions. Much to the nurse's dismay, the client drank the whole bottle of povidone-iodine solution instead of washing with it. Fortunately the nurse discovered this error immediately, and appropriate medical measures were instituted to save the client's life. Thus a nurse should not readily assume that the client understands her communication.

Nurses urgently need the ability to communicate with clients who are limited in their use of the nurse's language, for when deprived of the most common medium of interaction with clients—the spoken word—nurses often become frustrated and ineffective in their interventions. Some nurses tend to avoid clients with whom they cannot communicate. Unfortunately, this creates a vicious circle of cultural misunderstandings between the nurse and the client. According to Muecke (1970) the nurse might behave toward the client in ways that could be misconstrued by the client:

1. The nurse shouts the same words louder. Raising the voice will not necessarily make the words more understandable, and such actions could also suggest hostility to the client.
2. The nurse focuses on the task rather than on the client. This might suggest that the nurse is more interested in doing the task than in concentrating on the client.
3. The nurse stops talking with the client altogether and starts doing things for him instead of with him. This might imply to the client that he is inferior.

The consequence of the nurse's actions is the painful isolation of the ethnic minority client in an unfamiliar milieu. Consequently, the client experiences cultural shock and may react by withdrawing, becoming hostile or belligerent, or being uncooperative.

Language differences can be bridged, however. The nurse can ask family members who are fluent in English to interpret for the client. In this way the family can also provide information about the client's background that could be valuable in holistic care. The health institution can also facilitate the search for an interpreter. For example, a list of bilingual or multilingual staff members and volunteers in a hospital might be kept in a central place such as the information desk.

Medical terms must be clearly explained to all clients, especially those with limited skills in the dominant language. Hospital jargon presents problems even for alert, oriented, adult clients who speak the dominant language. For example, many non–ethnic minority clients think that "force fluids" means "force urination" or "force elimination of fluids."

Differences in denotative meanings may exist between members of two different cultures, causing miscommunication. For instance, when a black youth says "That's bad" and means "That's good," a white adult might be confused. The black youth is speaking in an argot, or a special linguistic code of his cultural group. Another linguistic block to communication between ethnic groups comes from differences in connotative meanings for certain words, even when the denotative meanings are the same. For example, to a white person, "hospital" may mean a facility where modern health care is provided. Navajos, however, associate hospitals with death, since they believe that the ground and the building where any person dies become contaminated for an indeterminate period with evil spirits that will infect anyone who steps on this ground (Hall, 1963). Thus they avoid hospitals.

By giving special attention to the communication process, nurses can work to overcome language barriers with ethnic minority clients. Observing nonverbal behaviors, for example, can help clarify a client's communication, although nonverbal communication is also influenced by culture. Nurses can also learn how to phrase questions and statements to elicit information from clients whose ethnic background shapes their response. For example, when a Mexican American man is asked if he feels pain, he may simply say no if he believes that admitting pain is a sign he is not manly. The nurse might ask instead when he feels pain.

Finally, the nurse who practices in an area where many members of an ethnic minority live should attempt to learn the clients' language. No nurse can learn all the languages that may be encountered in practice, but it is possible for a nurse to learn one other language, such as Spanish. With languages that are more difficult, such as Vietnamese, the nurse can at least learn some basic terms. Many community health nurses have learned the languages of their clients, and nurses in other settings also should be aware of the problems that may arise because of language differences.

PHYSIOLOGICAL SUSCEPTIBILITY TO DISEASE

Because of genetic and life-style differences, some ethnic or racial groups are more susceptible to certain diseases than others. In general, ethnic groups with lower socioeconomic status are more susceptible to acquired diseases and conditions such as malnutrition and infections. Lactose intolerance is more prevalent among the ethnic minority groups discussed in the following sections, and skin cancer is less prevalent. Other conditions to which certain groups are susceptible follow.

HYPERTENSION. The incidence of hypertension is higher among blacks, as well as among Filipino and Japanese Americans eating traditional high-sodium diets, than among white Americans. The patterns of incidence in blacks are related to such factors as sex, age, and obesity.

SICKLE CELL ANEMIA. Sickle cell anemia is relatively common among blacks of West African descent. This is a genetic disease in which the red blood cells clump in the veins, leading to a pain crisis. Special counseling for parents of children with the disease, home treatment, and medical supervision are necessary interventions.

CANCER. Various ethnic and racial groups are more susceptible to different forms of cancer. Esophageal cancer, which is rare among whites, is the second leading cause of death for black men between 35 and 54 years of age. Stomach cancer is twice as prevalent in black men as in white men. Filipino Hawaiians have an incidence of liver cancer higher than that of any other ethnic group and twice as high as males of other races, possibly because of the diet of Filipino American workers on sugar plantations. Japanese Americans have a high incidence of cancer of the esophagus, stomach, liver, and biliary passage.

DIABETES. Diabetes mellitus has a significantly higher incidence among Raza/Latina (Hispanic) groups than in either blacks or whites. Diabetes is about twice as common among Filipino Hawaiians and Native Americans, particularly in the Southwest, as among whites. Nursing interventions may include dietary counseling based on knowledge of traditional foods and methods of preparation.

TUBERCULOSIS. Tuberculosis is associated with poor nutrition, poor sanitation, and crowded living conditions and thus has a higher incidence among ethnic groups with low socioeconomic status. Puerto Ricans in New York and Mexican Americans in the Southwest have high incidences. Tuberculosis is also more common among the elderly, recent immigrants from the Philippines, and South Vietnamese refugees entering North America.

COCCIDIOIDOMYCOSIS. Coccidioidomycosis is a fungous disease commonly found in migrant workers in arid or semiarid farming areas. This disease affects Filipino Americans and blacks approximately 10 times more often than other groups.

PARASITES. Intestinal parasites and other parasitic diseases are associated with poor health and sanitary conditions and thus tend to be more common among lower economic groups. Puerto Rican farm workers, Raza/Latina populations in New York and Los Angeles, and South Vietnamese refugees all have higher incidences of parasitic diseases.

DERMATOLOGICAL CONDITIONS. Keloid formation, an exaggerated skin healing process following trauma to the skin, is more common among blacks, as are conditions that cause hypopigmentation and hyperpigmentation. A mongolian spot, a blue pigmentation found in sacral and gluteal areas of some Raza/Latina and other ethnic minority group infants, is normal and harmless and usually fades and disappears in weeks or months.

For all ethnic groups skin color is an important factor in physiological assessment, but assessment of skin color depends more on the individual than on racial or genetic factors because individuals within any race vary widely in skin color. Color changes in dark-skinned clients must be determined differently from those in whites. For instance, in a dark-skinned person, pallor is the absence of the underlying red tones that normally give brown and black skin its glow. A black-complexioned person's skin will appear ashen gray, and a brown-skinned individual's skin will become yellow brown (Roach, 1977; Bloch and Hunter, 1981).

The nurse must also be aware of how skin color differences affect the self-concepts of Filipinos and Raza/Latinas. A Spanish colonial attitude that has persisted to the present is the preference by some Filipino and Raza/Latina families for the light-skinned child over the darker offspring. Many who are lighter in color claim to be either Spanish or white and seek to marry whites, often looking down on their own group to gain acceptance from whites (Simmons, 1974; Orque, Bloch, and Monrroy, 1983).

FOOD AND EATING HABITS

Food and eating habits vary widely among cultural groups, but in most these customs carry emotional and social significance. Therefore it is helpful for nurses to have a general understanding of the food habits of ethnic minority clients. In many cases family members can be permitted to bring special foods to hospitalized clients who are unhappy about hospital food. When teaching a client about dietary requirements related to specific illnesses, the nurse should be sensitive to cultural meanings of eating. In some ethnic minority groups, for example, being overweight symbolizes being loved and cared for by family members. In such a case an overweight client with diabetes who is merely told to lose weight may fail to comply with diet therapy because of cultural meanings. The nurse who is aware of cultural differences can resolve the problem by using communication techniques and by involving the client's family in the planning process.

Nurses should also be aware of their own cultural values related to food and eating, because these values influence their attitudes toward eating, including what foods are best, preferable methods of preparation, the appropriate times for eating, and how these factors are affected by illness. Only if the nurse identifies her own cultural values related to food can she be aware of a client's differences.

Nutritional factors for different ethnic-cultural groups are described in Chapter 38.

TIME ORIENTATION

The dominant white culture in the United States and Canada tends to be future oriented; that is, we think in terms of long-range goals, we are concerned with health care measures in the present to prevent the occurrence of illness in the future, and we generally prefer to plan ahead in making schedules, setting appointments, and organizing activities. Time orientation varies among different cultural groups, however, and a nurse who has an ethnocentric attitude toward time may find it difficult to understand and plan care for clients with a different time orientation. Many blacks, Raza/Latina persons, and Southern Europeans are oriented more to the present than the future. Such clients may not share the nurse's attitude toward matters related to time. An ethnic minority client may be late for an appointment not because of reluctance or lack of respect for the nurse but because he is less concerned about planning ahead to be on time than with the activity in which he is currently engaged. This time orientation difference may become important in health care measures such as long-term planning and explaining when medications should be taken. For example, if a client has not been regularly taking the medication prescribed to lower his blood pressure, teaching about the potential effects of hypertension should emphasize problems that might arise immediately rather than only the long-term problems, which because of time orientation differences may be less important to the client.

PERSONAL SPACE AND TERRITORIALITY

Territoriality is an attitude toward an area that a person has claimed and defends or reacts emotionally about when another encroaches on it. Personal space involves a person's set of behaviors and attitudes toward the space around himself. Both territoriality and personal space are influenced by culture, and thus different ethnic groups have varying norms related to the use of space.

Staff members and other clients frequently encroach on a client's territory in the hospital, which includes his room, bed, closet, and belongings. The nurse should try to respect the client's territory as much as possible, especially when performing nursing procedures. Even routine procedures should be explained to all clients, especially ethnic minority clients, to indicate to them that the nurse accepts them as persons. If a client has no critical problems, the nurse should tolerate visiting members of the extended family. This can remind the client of home, lessening the effects of isolation and shock from hospitalization.

Personal space is involved in many nursing activities, and the nurse should be sensitive about the ethnic minority client's attitudes toward personal space. For example, providing nursing care often involves touching the client, an action that has different meanings in different cultures and for different individuals. What is comforting to one client may be threatening to another. Standards of behavior vary also in terms of who, male or female, can touch the client, and where. The meaning of personal space also varies among cultures. Hall (1963) has studied the meaning of space and has identified different behaviors common in four different zones:

1. *Intimate zone* extending up to 1½ feet. Since this distance allows adults to have the most bodily contacts for perception of breath and odor, they do not find this acceptable in public places. Visual distortions are also present.
2. *Personal distance* extending from 1½ to 4 feet. This is an extension of the self that is like having a "bubble" of space surrounding the body. At this distance the voice may be moderate, the body odor may not be apparent, and visual distortion may have disappeared.
3. *Social distance* extending from 4 to 12 feet. This is reserved for impersonal business transactions. Perceptual information is much less detailed.
4. *Public distance* extending 12 feet or more. Individuals interact only impersonally. Communicators' voices must be projected, and subtle facial expressions may be lost.

These generalizations about the use of personal space are based on studying the behavior of white North Americans. Use of personal space varies among different individuals and ethnic groups. The extreme modesty practiced by members of some cultural groups and lower socioeconomic groups may prevent members from seeking preventive health care. Raza/Latina and Arab women, for example, are quite shy about physical exposure, especially when being examined by male physicians. Therefore these clients should be given the option of having female physicians and female nurses as their primary care providers.

ATTITUDES TOWARD THE FAMILY

Many chapters in this book discuss the importance of involving the client's family or significant others in all stages of the nursing process. Family behavior patterns vary among different cultural groups, however, and the nurse must be aware of such variations when involving the family in care. In most ethnic groups, for example, "the family" includes the entire extended family rather than only the nuclear family, as is typical in white middle-class culture. Because the family is often the principal source of support to a family member during illness, the nurse should involve the client's total family as much as possible and encourage the whole family to visit a hospital-

ized ethnic minority client. For any ethnic minority client, the nurse should consider the role of the client's family in making decisions about care and treatment.

The nurse should also be aware of specific differences in attitudes toward the family among ethnic groups. For example, Filipinos, Chinese Americans, and South Vietnamese tend to view mental illness as a stigma on the family's name and thus may seek professional care only when the family is no longer able to deal with the problem.

GENDER ROLE BEHAVIORS

The accepted norms for traditional gender role behaviors in other cultures may be significantly different from those in white North America. In some ethnic minority groups, for example, men are expected to appear strong, to hide their emotions, and to bear pain in silence; women may be expected to be quiet, modest, and passive. The husband may make decisions for the family, even decisions concerning the wife's health care. In some matriarchal cultures, on the other hand, the wife is responsible for much of a family's decision making. In providing family health care and when involving family members in the client's care, the nurse needs an awareness of variables in ethnic gender role behaviors in order to understand the specific behaviors of the client. For example, a white nurse may observe that a Chinese husband fails to give emotional support to his wife during her labor and delivery, a behavior the nurse may misinterpret unless she realizes that Asian men are usually embarrassed to express their emotions in public, that they consider childbirth solely "women's work," and that Asian women usually feel embarrassed and uncomfortable if their husbands participate in a function they consider their prerogative. Asian women have significant others, usually females, who can provide them with emotional support—mothers, in-laws, cousins, or close friends. In fact, in almost all non-Western cultures a female assistant is customarily available during pregnancy, labor and delivery, and the postnatal period to teach the woman how to mother and to provide her with emotional support. When these significant others are unavailable, the husband provides the wife with as much emotional support as he is able to give.

Understanding ethnic behavioral differences is crucial when the nurse provides client care involving the emotional and social dimensions. In the childbirth example here, the nurse who does not understand traditional behaviors of Asian men may mistakenly conclude that the husband and wife are in emotional conflict, a judgment that could lead to problems if the nurse plans care based on this assessment.

EMOTIONAL EXPRESSION AND PAIN REACTIONS

Because it is often important for the nurse to determine a client's emotional state, she needs to understand how patterns of emotional expression vary among ethnic minority groups. Chinese, Japanese, Filipinos, and American Indians generally do not openly express their feelings to persons outside the family. An inexperienced nurse, if she is expecting usual white North American expressions of feelings, may fail to notice that a client from one of these groups is undergoing emotional stress or conflict. Arabs, Jews, Raza/Latinas, and Italians tend to express their feelings in highly emotional ways. With a client from one of these cultural backgrounds an inexperienced nurse is likely to misinterpret facial expressions, gestures, weeping, and tones of voice and perhaps mistakenly assume the client is under great emotional duress.

The client's reaction to pain is similarly influenced by cultural background, and it is important for the nurse to be able to objectively evaluate a client's pain (see Chapter 37). To do so, nurses should be aware that their own attitudes about pain are culturally influenced. Even if clients from different cultural backgrounds perceive pain similarly, how they interpret and respond to the pain is shaped by cultural standards. This pattern is similar to the different forms of emotional expression in general. Clients of Jewish or Italian origin tend to be more vocal in expressing their pain, and white North Americans and the Irish tend to be more restrained and stoical in expressing their pain. As in other areas influenced by culture, nurses need to be aware of both their own cultural tendencies and those of their clients in order to assess needs and provide care throughout the nursing process.

EMOTIONAL AND MENTAL HEALTH

People from all ethnic minority groups can undergo the same emotional and mental stresses and conflicts as those in the dominant cultural group. One important difference arises, however, as a result of ethnic minority group members' experiences of prejudice and discrimination by the white dominant group. Often ethnic minority clients have formed defense mechanisms for relating to others from the dominant culture. Vander Zanden (1966) has described six patterns of behavior linked to these defense mechanisms: (1) acceptance, (2) aggression, (3) obsessive sensitivity, (4) efforts of ego enhancement, (5) self-hatred, and (6) assimilation. An ethnic minority person might simultaneously use more than one of these mechanisms.

Acceptance occurs when minority group members have acquiesced or have accommodated themselves to their disadvantaged status. Although covertly resentful, by internally accommodating the attitudes and expectations of the dominant group, the minority group member behaves in a good-natured or non-aggressive manner. Only a sensitive nurse can discern that this client's defense mechanism of agreeability may block genuine communication. For example, the client might fail to notify the nurse of some significant fact of his condition, forget to take medications, or miss appointments. Another manifestation of this defense mechanism is the minority group client's avoidance of situations in which he is likely to experience prejudice and discrimination. This defense mechanism often contributes to a reluctance to seek health care, since most health personnel belong to the white dominant group.

Aggression occurs when minority group members strike out against their subordinate status with hostile acts against members of the dominant group. Sometimes the minority group member expresses hostility indirectly by joking at the expense of the nurse or other clients. Sullenness or stubbornness and verbal hostility are more direct forms of expressing frustration.

When interacting with members of the dominant group, the minority group member may be hypersensitive to any signs of bigotry. The client may constantly observe the behaviors of the nurse for any evidence of prejudice. A client who detects bigotry may be less responsive to care or may not seek care. Studies have shown, for example, that families who missed clinic appointments reported more incidents of racial prejudice that involved hospital clerks, clinic nurses, social workers, and physicians.

As a defense mechanism, a minority group member may also seek to enhance his self-concept through compensatory behavior. An example of this type of behavior is the client's request for the most expensive room in the hospital or for a private duty nurse.

Acceptance of the dominant group's evaluation could lead a minority group member to develop unconscious self-hatred, usually accompanied by ambivalent feelings of inferiority. For example, a minority group client might apologize to a white nurse for the excited laughter and talk of members of his group during visiting hours.

Finally, one of the reactions of minority group members to white dominance is assimilation. Assimilation is the attempt by minority group members "to become socially and culturally fused with the dominant group" (Vander Zanden, 1966). For example, a Filipino man who anglicized his name during the 1930s in order to obtain a better job might now regret having done this, although at the time he was acutely aware that it was necessary for his economic survival.

HEALTH-ILLNESS BELIEFS AND PRACTICES

Chapter 2 discusses various health-illness beliefs and practices among different people. Beliefs and practices are influenced by many factors, including cultural background. Although all people have the same basic human needs, the means by which people seek to meet these needs are in part culturally determined, and thus the nurse should be aware of how members of ethnic minority groups may think and act in ways different from the dominant group.

Different cultural groups have a number of common health-illness beliefs and practices. For instance, in the black, Raza/Latina, Asian, and American Indian cultures, it is widely believed that health is the result of a balance in a person's relationship to nature. When this balance is disrupted, illness occurs. The Navajos, for example, use the Blessingway ceremony for those who are not in harmony with their environment (Wilson, 1983). Many lower-class black Americans believe that one can stay healthy by practicing moderation through proper diet, rest, and exercise (Snow, 1983).

Consistent with this view is the belief of Raza/Latinas, Filipinos, and South Vietnamese that the body has "hot" and "cold" areas. According to Abril (1977), this concept is derived from the Hippocratic theory of pathology, which states that illness is caused by an imbalance of the four humours: phlegm, blood, black bile, and yellow bile. Essentially the "hot and cold" concept views illness as stemming from an imbalance between hot and cold areas in the body. Diseases, as well as foods and herbs used for treatment, are classified as either "hot" or "cold" depending on their effects on the body. The practice prohibiting South Vietnamese, Filipino, and Raza/Latina mothers from bathing after delivery is also based on this belief.

The view that health is the result of a balanced interaction between human beings and nature is the crux of the yin and yang concept of the Chinese. The Chinese believe that yin and yang are opposing forces that move diametrically to maintain balance. Yang is characterized as positive, bright, warm (hot), and masculine. Yin is characterized as negative, dark, cold, and feminine. When the body is balanced, it contains both yin and yang. An excess of either will lead to illness. Again, "hot" and "cold" indicate status of health, not temperature or the spiciness of substances. Food and herbs are classified as "hot" and "cold" because they can be used to create the desired balance.

Ethnic minorities turn to cultural healers for a number of reasons. According to Harwood (1981), three general sets of reasons for using cultural healers apply to ethnic groups. First, nonmainstream health practitioners are used when Western medicine is too expensive or inconvenient to obtain. Members of particular ethnic minority groups may also experience special circumstances that make mainstream services unobtainable (such as the fear of deportation for illegal Mexican and Haitian immigrants). Second, cultural healers are often patronized when the client is dissatisfied with treatment provided by Western medicine. Specific instances that may lead to this form of behavior are when the recommended treatment modality is considered too drastic (such as surgery), when a chronic condition is refractory to standard therapy, and when a mainstream practitioner has communicated to the client either that he "doesn't know what's wrong" or that in his professional judgment nothing is wrong. Third, cultural healers are used for treating psychosocial problems. Examples vary from the "therapeutic women" among Italian Americans and the root workers patronized by some urban blacks to the more formally organized Haitian voodoo priests, Mexican *curanderos*, Navajo singers, and Puerto Rican *espiritistas*. The use of these healers may reflect the failure of the mainstream health care system to provide inexpensive and culturally appropriate psychosocial counseling to low-income groups, especially those who do not speak English.

According to Harwood (1981), use of cultural healers has implications for the mainstream health care delivery system. First, use of these healers sometimes makes medical diagnosis and treatment difficult. For instance, a hypertensive Chinese American client might be taking ginseng along with his antihypertension medications. However, because many Western physicians consider ginseng to be a tonic-stimulant, its use is contraindicated in hypertension (Campbell and Chang, 1973). Thus the health care professional must ask the client nonjudgmentally whether he is receiving therapy from a cultural healer. If the client is using a cultural healer, the health care provider should determine any contraindicated procedure and negotiate with the client and the healer changes necessary to maintain quality care for the client. Second, since cultural healers often complement the delivery of mainstream health care services, it behooves the health care provider to collaborate with the cultural healers in the client's care. Third, health care practitioners may adopt elements of the communication styles of cultural healers to enhance rapport with clients and thereby improve compliance with the health care regimen.

Because of poverty and discrimination, ethnic minorities often do not take advantage of preventive health services. For example, the California Department of Health Services (1979) reported that a random survey of 2-year-old children showed that whites are more likely to be immunized against disease than nonwhites. Specifically, only approximately 19% of white children were not immunized against measles, whereas the corresponding rates for black and Raza/Latina children were 36% and 39%, respectively. According to Lieberman (1974), however, "after acute environmental problems are . . . satisfactorily solved, patients are more willing to consider the preventive aspects of care being offered." Health professionals should therefore determine ways to improve the health care delivery system so that quality care will be available to all clients.

Cultural Groups in North America

The following sections briefly describe some of the major characteristics of four ethnic minority groups whose members nurses are likely to encounter in their practice—blacks, Raza/Latinas, American Indians, and Asians. The nurse must remember, however, that cultural background is only one of a number of influences on any person's values, beliefs, and behaviors; therefore the nurse must consider each client as an individual rather than stereotyping all clients of an ethnic minority group. On the other hand, a nurse who is unaware of culture differences may experience cultural conflict with clients.

One chapter cannot describe in detail the intraethnic variations within each of these four groups. For more discussion of these and other ethnic groups, the reader is referred to references and additional readings at the end of this chapter.

BLACKS

About 12% of the U.S. population is black. Important cultural characteristics of blacks include an orientation to the present rather than the future, an attitude toward scheduling and clock time more flexible than that of most nurses, and health beliefs and practices stemming from African origins. Many blacks, particularly in rural areas of the South, try traditional healing methods before seeking professional health care and may prefer to consult a folk healer, a spiritualist, and in some areas a voodoo priest or root doctor rather than a licensed professional. When a black client does seek medical or nursing care, it is important to learn what methods he is using to fight illness. The nurse should not discourage folk remedies unless they might interfere with therapy.

A major factor in providing health care for blacks is understanding the rhythmical and stylized dialect known as black English. Black English differs from standard English in pronunciation, syntax, and both denotative and connotative meanings of words. A nurse who is inexperienced in dealing with clients using black English may be unsure of a client's meaning or may feel frustrated when trying to communicate with him. The suggestions in the box apply not only to black clients but also to clients who speak in other languages or dialects, whose abilities to use the dominant language are limited, or whose language skills are good but whose values related to communication may be different from the nurse's.

Suggestions for Communicating with Clients Who Speak Other Languages

- Respect clients as individuals, regardless of how different their language skills and values are from your own. Do not judge clients' intellectual abilities or emotional states on the basis of how they use language.

- Do not treat ethnic minority group members differently from other clients, since such "special" treatment may be interpreted as patronizing.

- Do not assume that clients are angry, aggressive, or hostile if they speak more loudly or emotionally than most white clients.

- Use titles such as "Mr." or "Ms." unless you have established a first-name basis for the relationship.

- Do not attempt to use black English or any ethnic dialect with clients. This may be interpreted as making fun of clients or condescension.

- Do not attempt to impress ethnic minority clients by saying you have friends of the same ethnic or racial background.

- Be attentive to clients' nonverbal communications, which can help clarify what may seem confusing verbal communications.

- Make use of ethnic group preferences when giving care. Involve the extended family in communication, for example, or focus on oral rather than written teaching methods.

- Explain medical and nursing terms in simple, everyday words and be sure clients truly understand.

- If you do not understand what a client is saying, ask for clarification. Do not let your embarrassment at not understanding lead to the risks of misinformation.

Social factors to consider when providing care for black clients include differences in economic status, education, and social networks. Because the black population of the United States has a comparatively low income level, health care often has low priority, and clients may fail to comply with recommended therapies if they mean additional expense. Nurses must avoid blaming blacks for being on welfare, living in unhealthy conditions, or being less concerned about their health—behaviors that result more often from socioeconomic factors than from individual choice. The educational level of clients often depends on economic status as well, and nurses should consider the client's educational background as it is relevant in planning health teaching activities. Because the family and social network often have a major influence on the individual, nurses should make a point of involving the family and others in health care activities.

Psychological factors that deserve consideration include differences in self-concept, the impact of racism, and religious influences. Racial and ethnic identity, for example, may play an important role in self-esteem. The prevalence of racism in the United States may lead to anxiety and stress, which may in turn lead to paranoid behavior or suspicion on the part of some blacks. White nurses should realize that such behavior is not necessarily directed toward them as individuals. Finally, religion for many blacks promotes self-esteem and release of emotions, and spiritual resources can thus have a key role when a black client must adapt to illness.

RAZA/LATINA GROUPS

The term "Raza/Latina" refers to Puerto Ricans, Cubans, Mexicans/Chicanos, Central Americans, and South Americans. Many members of these groups prefer this term to such terms as "Spanish American," which is misleading because many Raza/Latina peoples are not solely of Spanish descent but are of mixed Indian and Spanish descent (mestizo) and often also have black ancestry. In the United States the fastest-growing minority group is the Raza/Latina.

Raza/Latina persons tend to be oriented to the present rather than the future. However, according to Romano, the abilities of Raza/Latinas to adapt and survive the many changes they encounter in the United States may mean that the time orientation of this group needs to be reevaluated (Murillo, 1978). In fact, Kluckhohn (1976) stated that the ability to "place a high value on change is future-oriented."

Some 85% to 90% of Raza/Latinas are Catholics and depend on spiritual resources in times of illness. They value modesty and privacy and tend to be self-conscious about physical examination and when dis-cussing birth control. Because many are tactful and polite, they may nod and seem to respond positively even when they do not understand the nurse because of limited skills in English. They often consider diseases to be a supernatural punishment, of magical origin, or caused by an imbalance of "hot" and "cold" in the body, and they may use folk methods or consult healers.

The family is the most important social unit for most Raza/Latina persons, and the family's needs generally take precedence over the individual's. The extended family may be large and can offer great support to the individual in illness. Children are very important in most Raza/Latina families, and child care is often provided by older siblings and members of the extended family.

Like some other ethnic minority groups, Raza/Latina people often live near each other in neighborhoods where cultural ties are strong and the Spanish language prevails. Many avoid hospitals and clinics outside their community, often because of language barriers. The nurse should not mistakenly assume, however, that all Raza/Latina peoples share a cultural unity; for example, Puerto Ricans and Cubans in the same area may not interact or get along well.

Not all Raza/Latinas identify with their cultural background; although many are proud of their origins, others deny their ethnicity and identify instead with whites. Because large numbers of Raza/Latinas are entering the United States, often with a loss of family support, culture shock is a particular problem. Culture shock is a reaction that occurs when, because of a change of culture, a person is forced to adapt to new forms of communication, customs, and values and attitudes of other people. The person often feels a strong sense of isolation, which lessens his ability to adapt and may result in self-concept problems. Seeking health care services can be especially stressful.

AMERICAN INDIANS

In 1980 there were approximately 1,420,400 American Indians, Eskimos, and Aleuts in the United States (U.S. Department of Commerce, 1981). About 270 Indian tribes live in 26 states (Farris, 1978). According to Statistics Canada (1983), there were approximately 413,380 American Indians residing in Canada in 1981. Because of a wide diversity among different Indian tribes and groups, one must be careful in generalizing about North American Indians. Nurses who practice in a geographical area where they encounter more than one tribe should become familiar with the cultural differences between the tribes.

Although the Indian Health Service, a division of the U.S. Public Health Service, was created in 1955 to provide health care services for Indians living on reservations, health care needs on reservations remain greater than in the general population. More recent legislation has focused on Indian management of health services in their own communities and has improved accessibility to health care for urban Indians as well as those on reservations.

The following are general characteristics of Indians maintaining traditional cultural heritage (Henderson and Primeaux, 1981):

1. Oriented toward living in the present rather than looking to the future
2. Task oriented—more concerned with finishing a task then with adhering to a schedule or to clock time
3. In harmony with nature, using environmental resources only as necessary
4. Generous and cooperative with others rather than competitive
5. Emphasizing extended families, often with three generations living together and the elders respected as family leaders

Nonverbal communication is important in many tribes, with moments of silence during conversation, eye contact, and body language cues. Traditional healing beliefs and practices are holistic, emphasizing total healing, mental and spiritual renewal, harmony with the environment, and health maintenance; healing methods are often ceremonial and guided by a medicine person. Many reservation Indians use traditional methods before seeking health care at a hospital or clinic. As previously mentioned, often Indians associate hospitals and clinics with disease and death, and thus they are reluctant to seek care. For example, pregnant Navajo women generally do not seek early prenatal care (Hall, 1963; Wilson, 1983).

Like many other ethnic groups, Indians maintain strong family ties, and family members provide support and assistance in times of illness. Decision making may be spread through the extended family, or a younger person may look to family elders for decisions regarding health care.

Indians often experience self-concept conflicts, since in recent decades the traditional tribal values have been confronted by the dominant white culture. Cultural conflict produces stress, and one result has been a greater suicide rate for American Indians; in the period between 1959 and 1970 it was one and a half times the overall U.S. rate (U.S. Department of Health, Education and Welfare, 1978). Violence and alcoholism, which are more common among American Indians than in the general U.S. population, may be attributed to the psychological stresses of cultural conflict and change. The alcoholism rate among American Indians is four to six times higher than the rate for the general U.S. population (U.S. Department of Health, Education and Welfare, 1978). Stress management is thus an important part of the health care needs of many North American Indians.

ASIAN AMERICANS

The four primary Asian ethnic groups in the United States are the Chinese (about 806,000), Japanese (about 701,000), Filipino (about 774,700), and Vietnamese (about 261,700) (U.S. Bureau of Census, 1983). According to the 1981 Canadian census, there were approximately 408,240 Chinese, 264,025 Japanese, and 121,445 Indochinese in Canada (Statistics Canada, 1983).

The Asian American groups vary widely in many respects and do not necessarily identify themselves collectively in terms of Asian heritage, although some similarities exist among these groups.

With Chinese American clients the nurse must be careful to avoid the stereotypes, promulgated by movies and television, of Chinese as inscrutable, sinister, or cunning. Discrimination against the Chinese has been strong in the United States, and as a result many Chinese Americans, particularly youths, may seem uncooperative or have feelings of powerlessness. Discrimination has led to the continued existence of Chinatowns. For the non-English-speaking Chinese, Chinatowns are the sole source of work opportunities. The elderly and retired workers live in these enclaves because they offer cheap (although often substandard) housing as well as access to Chinese restaurants and groceries. Chinatowns also serve as outlets for medical options: cultural healers, herbs, acupuncture, bone setting, and many patent Chinese medicines. The use of the traditional medicine system is particularly significant in that the most important health problem for low-income Chinese Americans is accessibility of health care services.

Traditional Chinese values and attitudes are related to the philosophies and religions of Confucianism, Taoism, and Buddhism, approaches to living too complex to be described here. In general, these perspectives stress holistic health and harmony between the self and the universe. Traditional values include self-respect, self-control, respect for elders, and family honor, loyalty, and pride. Health care is traditionally provided by herbalists, acupuncturists, and other cultural healers, but in many Chinese American communities Western medical services are found to be effective in reaching clients when they are provided by bilingual health care personnel. In communicating with Chinese American clients, the nurse must be careful to avoid inadvertently slighting personal or family dignity.

Japanese Americans value time and use it wisely, carefully following time schedules for medications and treatments. The Japanese, like the Chinese, have holistic concepts of health, and many supplement Western medical therapies with traditional remedies. Family support systems tend to be strong, but mental and some other illnesses carry a social or family stigma and may lead to social isolation. Racial discrimination against Japanese Americans, particularly the moving of Japanese Americans into concentration camps during World War II, has led to self-concept problems and cultural conflict, but many Japanese-American groups have adjusted well while maintaining their ethnic identity. Like some other ethnic minority persons (such as American Indians), many Japanese Americans are reluctant to seek health care outside their communities. It is particularly important that nurses avoid stereotyped images of Japanese American clients when they seem reticent and nonquestioning.

Filipino Americans often have a fatalistic view of life, accepting what happens as being the result of supernatural forces. This ethnic group is also strongly personalistic, encouraging warmth and friendship in social interaction. The family is highly valued along with interdependence rather than independence of family members. Filipino Americans generally emphasize social acceptance and avoid direct expression of anger. As a result of the Spanish colonization of the Philippines, the health beliefs and practices of many Filipino Americans involve a blend of native, Raza/Latina, and dominant American beliefs, and different cultural healers use different methods, although concepts of the supernatural are often incorporated. Because Filipino Americans like other ethnic minorities have experienced racism and discrimination, many have learned to use the defense mechanisms described earlier when interacting with members of the dominant white group. Because of the traditional fatalistic attitude, many Filipino Americans have considerable patience in times of illness and may endure pain with little noticeable response.

After the Vietnam War many South Vietnamese immigrated to the United States, and they have become a sizable ethnic group. The South Vietnamese are family centered and generally believe in an ordered universe controlled by spirits and deities, including the revered spirits of ancestors. Harmony in social interaction and duty to family are emphasized. Because most South Vietnamese entered the United States more recently than many other ethnic groups, and because many left Vietnam under traumatic conditions, mental and emotional illnesses are prevalent, including depression, anxiety, marital conflict, and psychosomatic illnesses.

Cultural Factors and the Nursing Process

When providing health care to ethnic clients, the nurse uses the nursing process approach as with all other clients. Because nurses are often from the dominant cultural group, however, and because providing effective holistic care requires forming a therapeutic relationship with the client, nurses must consider their clients' cultural values, behaviors, and attitudes at all stages of the nursing process. This consideration involves two kinds of awareness.

First, the nurse must be aware of her own culture because it has influenced her values, attitudes, and behaviors toward clients and toward health. The process of attaining cultural awareness begins with a values clarification approach as described in Chapter 13. By exploring her own values and understanding how they have been influenced by her culture, the nurse can objectively consider ways in which ethnic clients differ from herself and understand them better as individuals. A nurse who is aware of how her own values and attitudes are shaped by culture can avoid responding ethnocentrically or with prejudice to ethnic minority clients.

Second, the nurse needs to be aware of the client's cultural background and how it influences his behavior, values, and attitudes. In this way she can take into account the client's unique qualities, including both his assets, such as a strong family support system, and his potential problems, such as stress related to cultural conflict. Achieving this awareness of the client's ethnicity begins with study of the culture itself, careful observation, and an open mind toward cultural differences. In the first step of the nursing process, assessment, the nurse assesses the client's cultural characteristics as one factor related to actual or potential illness. This understanding is then applied throughout the nursing process.

Assessment

Bloch's ethnic-cultural assessment guide is a useful tool for the nurse who is assessing an ethnic minority client (Table 21-1). Data to be gathered relating to providing care for a particular ethnic minority client are divided into four sections: cultural, sociological, psychological, and biological/physiological. Not all areas of the guide apply to all ethnic groups or all individuals within an ethnic group; the nurse addresses each factor as it may be applicable to a given client. This information can be gathered during the interview along with standard nursing history data.

Text continued on p. 434.

TABLE 21-1

Bloch's Ethnic-Cultural Assessment Guide

Data Categories	Guideline Questions and Instructions	Data Collected
CULTURAL		
Ethnic origin	Does client identify with a particular ethnic group (e.g., Puerto Rican, African)?	
Race	What is client's racial background (e.g., black, Filipino, American Indian)?	
Place of birth	Where was client born?	
Relocations	Where has client lived (country, city)? During what years did he live there and for how long? Has he moved recently?	
Habits, customs, values, and beliefs	Describe habits, customs, values, and beliefs client holds or practices that affect his attitude toward birth, life, death, health and illness, time orientation, and health care system and health care providers. What is degree of belief and adherence by client to his overall cultural system?	
Behaviors valued by culture	How does client value privacy, courtesy, respect for elders, behaviors related to family roles and sex roles, and work ethics?	
Cultural sanctions and restrictions	*Sanctions*—What is accepted behavior by client's cultural group regarding expression of emotions and feelings, religious expressions, and response to illness and death?	
	Restrictions—Does client have any restrictions related to sexual matters, exposure of body parts, certain types of surgery (e.g., hysterectomy), discussion of dead relatives, and discussion of fears related to the unknown?	
Language and communication processes	What are some overall cultural characteristics of client's language and communication process?	
Language(s) and/or dialect(s) spoken	Which language(s) and/or dialect(s) does client speak most frequently? Where? At home or at work?	
Language barriers	Which language does client predominantly use in thinking? Does client need bilingual interpreter in nurse-patient interactions? Is client non-English-speaking or limited-English-speaking? Is client able to read and/or write in English?	
Communication process	What are rules (linguistics) and modes (style) of communication process (e.g., "honorific" concept of showing "respect or deference" to others using words only common to specific ethnic-cultural group)?	
	Is there need for variation in technique of communicating and interviewing to accommodate client's cultural background (e.g., tempo of conversation, eye and body contact, topic restrictions, norms of confidentiality, and style of explanation)?	
	Are there any conflicts in verbal and nonverbal interactions between client and nurse?	
	How does client's nonverbal communication process compare with that of other ethnic-cultural groups, and how does it affect client's response to nursing and medical care?	

Modified from Bloch, B.: Bloch's assessment guide for ethnic/cultural variations. In Orque, M.S., Bloch, B., and Monrroy, L.S.A.: Ethnic nursing care: a multicultural approach, St. Louis, 1983, The C.V. Mosby Co.

TABLE 21-1, cont'd

Bloch's Ethnic-Cultural Assessment Guide

Data Categories	Guideline Questions and Instructions	Data Collected
	Are there any variations between client's interethnic and interracial communication process or intracultural and intraracial communication process (e.g., ethnic minority client and white middle-class nurse, ethnic minority client and ethnic minority nurse; beliefs, attitudes, values, role variations, stereotyping [perception and prejudice])?	
Healing beliefs and practices Cultural healing system	To what cultural healing system does client predominantly adhere (e.g., Asian healing system, Raza/Latina *curanderismo*)? To what religious healing system does client predominantly adhere (e.g., Seventh Day Adventist, West African voodoo, Fundamentalist sect, Pentacostal)?	
Cultural health beliefs	Is illness explained by the germ theory or cause-effect relationship, presence of evil spirits, imbalance between "hot" and "cold" (yin and yang in Chinese culture), or disequilibrium between nature and man?	
	Is good health related to success, ability to work or fulfill roles, reward from God, or balance with nature?	
Cultural health practices	To what types of cultural healing practices does person from ethnic/cultural group adhere? Does he use healing remedies to cure *natural* illnesses caused by the external environment (e.g., massage to cure *empacho* [a ball of food clinging to stomach wall], wearing of talismans or charms for protection against illness)?	
Cultural healers	Does client rely on cultural healers (e.g., medicine men for American Indian, *curandero* for Raza/Latina, Chinese herbalist, hougan [voodoo priest], spiritualist, or minister for black American)?	
Nutritional variables or factors	What nutritional variables or factors are influenced by client's ethnic-cultural background?	
Characteristics of food preparation and consumption	What types of food preferences and restrictions, meaning of foods, style of food preparation and consumption, frequency of eating, time of eating, and eating utensils are culturally determined for client? Are there any religious influences on food preparation and consumption?	
Influences from external environment	What modifications if any in its food practices did client's ethnic group have to make in white dominant American society? Are there any adaptations of food customs and beliefs from rural setting to urban setting?	
Client education needs	What are some implications of diet planning and teaching to client who adheres to cultural practices concerning foods?	

SOCIOLOGICAL

Economic status	Who is principal wage earner in client's family? What is approximate total annual income of family? What impact does economic status have on life-style, place of residence, living conditions, and ability to obtain health services?	
Educational status	What is highest educational level obtained? Does client's educational background influence his ability to understand how to seek health services, literature on health care, client teaching	

Continued.

TABLE 21-1, cont'd

Bloch's Ethnic-Cultural Assessment Guide

Data Categories	Guideline Questions and Instructions	Data Collected
	experiences, and any written material client is exposed to in health care setting (e.g., admission forms, client care forms, teaching literature, and laboratory test forms)?	
	Does client's educational background cause him to feel inferior or superior to health care personnel in health care setting?	
Social network	What is client's social network (kinship, peer, and cultural healing networks)? How do they influence health or illness status of client?	
Family as supportive group	Does client's family feel need for continuous presence in client's clinical setting (is this an ethnic-cultural characteristic)? How is family valued during illness or death?	
	How does family participate in client's nursing care process (e.g., giving baths, feeding, using touch as support [cultural meaning], supportive presence)?	
	How does ethnic-cultural family structure influence client response to health or illness (e.g., roles, beliefs, strengths, weaknesses, and social class)?	
	Are there any key family roles characteristic of a specific ethnic-cultural group (e.g., grandmother in black and some American Indian families), and can these key persons be a resource for health personnel?	
	What role does family play in health promotion or cause of illness (e.g., would family be intermediary group in client interactions with health personnel and making decisions regarding his care)?	
Supportive institutions in ethnic-cultural community	What influence do ethnic-cultural institutions have on client receiving health services (i.e., institutions such as Organization of Migrant Workers, NAACP, Black Political Caucus, churches, schools, Urban League, community clinics)?	
Institutional racism	How does institutional racism in health facilities influence client's response to receiving health care?	
PSYCHOLOGICAL		
Self-concept (identity)	Does client show strong racial or cultural identity? How does this compare to that of other racial or cultural groups or to members of dominant society?	
	What factors in client's development helped to shape his self-concept (e.g., family, peers, society labels, external environment, institutions, racism)?	
	How does client deal with stereotypical behavior from health professionals	
	What is impact of racism on client from distinct ethnic-cultural group (e.g., social anxiety, noncompliance to health care process in clinical settings, avoidance of utilizing or participating in health care institutions)?	
	Does ethnic-cultural background have impact on how client relates to body image change resulting from illness or surgery (e.g., importance of appearance and roles in cultural group)?	

TABLE 21-1, cont'd

Bloch's Ethnic-Cultural Assessment Guide

Data Categories	Guideline Questions and Instructions	Data Collected
	Is there any adherence or identification with ethnic-cultural "group identity" (e.g., solidarity, "we" concept)?	
Mental and behavioral processes and characteristics of ethnic-cultural group	How does client relate to his external environment in clinical setting (e.g., fears, stress, and adaptive mechanisms characteristic of a specific ethnic-cultural group)? Are there any variations based on the life span?	
	What is client's ability to relate to persons (health personnel) outside his ethnic-cultural group? Is he withdrawn, verbally or nonverbally expressive, negative or positive, feeling mentally or physically inferior or superior?	
	How does client deal with feelings of loss of dignity and respect in clinical setting?	
Religious influences on psychological effects of health and illness	Does client's religion have a strong impact on how he relates to health and illness influences or outcomes (e.g., death or chronic illness, cause and effect of illness, or adherence to nursing and medical practices)?	
	Do religious beliefs, sacred practices, and talismans play a role in treatment of disease?	
	What is role of significant religious persons during health and illness (e.g., black ministers, Catholic priests, Buddhist monks, Islamic imams)?	
Psychological-cultural response to stress and discomfort of illness	Based on ethnic-cultural background, does client exhibit any variations in psychological response to pain or physical disability of disease processes?	

BIOLOGICAL/PHYSIOLOGICAL

(consideration of *norms* for different ethnic-cultural groups)

Data Categories	Guideline Questions and Instructions	Data Collected
Racial-anatomical characteristics	Does client have any distinct racial characteristics (e.g., skin color, hair texture and color, color of mucous membranes)? Does client have any variations in anatomical characteristics (e.g., body structure [height and weight] more prevalent for ethnic-cultural group, skeletal formation [pelvic shape, especially for obstetrical evaluation], facial shape and structure [nose, eye shape, facial contour], upper and lower extremities)?	
	How do client's racial and anatomical characteristics affect his self-concept and the way others relate to him?	
	Does variation in racial-anatomical characteristics affect physical evaluations and physical care, skin assessment based on color, and variations in hair care and hygienic practices?	
Growth and development patterns	Are there any distinct growth and development characteristics that vary with client's ethnic-cultural background (e.g., bone density, fat folds, motor ability)? What factors are important for nutritional assessment, neurological and motor assessment, assessment of bone deterioration in disease process or injury, evaluation of newborns, evaluation of intellectual status, or capacity in relationship to motor-sensory development in children? How do these differ in ethnic-cultural groups?	

Continued.

TABLE 21-1, cont'd

Bloch's Ethnic-Cultural Assessment Guide

Data Categories	Guideline Questions and Instructions	Data Collected
Variations in body systems	Are there any variations in body systems for client from distinct ethnic-cultural group (e.g., gastrointestinal disturbance with lactose intolerance in blacks, nutritional intake of cultural foods causing adverse effects on gastrointestinal tract and fluid and electrolyte system, and variations in chemical and hematological systems [certain blood types prevalent in particular ethnic-cultural groups])?	
Physiology of skin, hair, and mucous membranes	How does skin color variation influence assessment of skin color changes (e.g., jaundice, cyanosis, ecchymosis, erythema, and its relationship to disease processes)?	
	What are methods of assessing skin color changes (comparing variations and similarities between different ethnic groups)?	
	Are there conditions of hypopigmentation and hyperpigmentation (e.g., vitiligo, mongolian spots, albinism, discoloration caused by trauma)? Why would these be more striking in some ethnic groups?	
	Are there any skin conditions more prevalent in a distinct ethnic group (e.g., keloids in blacks)?	
	Is there any correlation between oral and skin pigmentation and their variations among distinct racial groups (e.g., leukoedema is normal occurrence in blacks)?	
	What are variations in hair texture and color among racially different groups? Ask client about preferred hair care methods or any racial-cultural restrictions (e.g., not washing "hot-combed" hair while in clinical setting, not cutting very long hair of Raza/Latina clients).	
	Are there any variations in skin care methods (e.g., using petrolatum jelly on black skin)?	
Diseases more prevalent among ethnic-cultural group	Are there any specific diseases or conditions that are more prevalent for a specific ethnic-cultural group (e.g., hypertension, sickle cell anemia, G-6-PD, lactose intolerance)?	
	Does client have any socioenvironmental diseases common among ethnic-cultural groups (e.g., lead paint poisoning, poor nutrition, tuberculosis resulting from overcrowding, alcoholism resulting from psychological despair and alienation from dominant society, rat bites, poor sanitation)?	
Diseases to which ethnic-cultural group has increased resistance	Are there any diseases to which client has increased resistance because of racial-cultural background (e.g., skin cancer in blacks)?	

Nursing Diagnosis

Nursing diagnoses for an ethnic client are similar to those for any client, with the addition of diagnoses specifically related to cultural differences. A diagnosis might involve potential problem areas during the client's interaction with the health care delivery system, such as the following:

1. Withdrawal related to cultural conflict and social isolation
2. Potential learning difficulties related to limited language skills in English
3. Stress and potential noncompliance with therapy related to perceived discrimination by members of nursing staff

4. Anxiety related to departure from traditional diet while hospitalized

A diagnosis might also involve the principal complaint of the client for which he is seeking health care, such as the following:

1. Altered self-concept related to culture shock on entering American school
2. Stress related to perceived discrimination by co-workers
3. Hypertension related to difficulty in following schedule of prescribed medication
4. Malnutrition related to low socioeconomic status

When determining nursing diagnoses for an ethnic minority client, the nurse should be as specific as possible in identifying the cultural variables involved in order to plan individualized nursing interventions for the client.

Planning and Implementation

When establishing the goals of care and planning specific interventions, the nurse again considers cultural variables as they relate to the individual client. The extended family should be involved in care, for example, if the family is the client's strongest support group. Cultural beliefs and practices can be incorporated into therapy. The client's educational level and language skills should be considered when planning teaching activities. Explanations of aspects of care usually not questioned by clients from the dominant cultural group may be required for an ethnic minority client to avoid confusion, misunderstanding, or cultural conflict. The nurse may have to alter her usual ways of interacting with clients to avoid offending or alienating a client with different attitudes toward social interaction and etiquette. An ethnic minority client who is modest and self-conscious about the body may need psychological preparation before some procedures and tests.

Given the diversity among individuals in an ethnic group, how can the nurse know what care the client will consider appropriate? One way is to involve the client and the family in planning care and to ask about their expectations. This should be done in every case, even if the nursing care cannot be modified. Because both the nurse and the client are likely to take many aspects of their cultures for granted, questions should be clear and explanations should be explicit.

Discussing cultural questions related to care with the client and family during the planning stage helps the nurse understand how cultural variables are re-lated to the client's health beliefs and practices, so that interventions can be individualized for the client. These questions can be based on Bloch's assessment guide and applied to specific interventions.

The keys to successful interventions with ethnic minority clients are communication and open-mindedness. In almost all cases the nurse will be able to adapt nursing interventions to avoid cultural conflicts with the client, once the client understands that the interventions the nurse is performing or suggesting maintain respect for his ethnicity and individuality.

Evaluation

The nurse evaluates the results of nursing care for ethnic clients as for all clients, determining the extent to which the goals of care have been met. Evaluation continues throughout the nursing process and should include feedback from the client and family. With an ethnic minority client, however, self-evaluation by the nurse is crucial as she increases skills for interacting with the client. The nurse should consider questions such as the following:

1. Am I open to understanding ways in which the client's values differ from mine?
2. Have I given sufficient attention to communicating with the client with limited language skills?
3. Have I successfully involved the client's family in the nursing process?
4. Am I incorporating the client's traditional beliefs and practices into nursing therapies?
5. Is my therapeutic relationship with the client grounded on respect for the client regardless of cultural differences?

Finally, nurses should evaluate their attitudes toward ethnic nursing care itself. Some nurses may believe that they should treat all clients the same and simply act naturally, but this attitude fails to acknowledge that cultural differences do exist and that there is no one "natural" human behavior. The nurse cannot act the same with all clients and still hope to deliver effective, individualized, holistic care. Sometimes inexperienced nurses are so self-conscious about cultural differences and so afraid of making a mistake that they impede the nursing process by not asking questions about areas of difference or by asking so many questions that they seem to pry into the client's personal life. The process of self-evaluation can help the nurse become more comfortable when providing care to ethnic minority clients.

Summary

The need for nurses to be sensitive toward culturally different clients is growing. Nurses are increasingly being challenged to learn about different cultures as they practice in a multicultural society. Ethnic nursing care is the nurse's effective integration of the client's ethnic-cultural background into nursing care, which is based on the nursing process. An ethnic-cultural system framework helps provide a holistic cultural perspective for the nurse. Awareness of ways in which clients with varying cultural backgrounds may differ from members of the dominant cultural group, the use of specific communication techniques, and cultural assessment are important if the nurse is to provide safe and effective individualized nursing care to all clients.

KEY CONCEPTS

✓ Cultural background affects a person's health in all dimensions, and therefore the nurse should consider the client's cultural background when planning care.

✓ Many ethnic and cultural groups in North America retain the cultural heritage of their original culture.

✓ How culture influences behaviors, attitudes, and values depends on many individual factors and thus is not the same for different members of a cultural group.

✓ Although the basic human needs are the same for all people, how a person seeks to meet those needs is influenced by culture.

✓ Ethnocentrism can impede the delivery of care to ethnic minority clients and when pervasive can become cultural racism.

✓ Stereotyping ethnic group members can lead to mistaken assumptions about an individual ethnic minority client.

✓ Cultural groups vary widely in susceptibility to disease, use of language, food and eating habits, time orientation, use of personal space and territoriality, attitudes toward the family, emotional expression and pain reactions, emotional and mental health, and health-illness beliefs and practices.

✓ The nurse should have an understanding of the general characteristics of the four major ethnic minority groups in North America—blacks, Raza/Latinas, American Indians, and Asian Americans—but should always individualize care rather than generalize about all clients in these groups.

✓ Before assessing the cultural background of a client, the nurse should assess how she is influenced by her own culture.

✓ Bloch's ethnic-cultural assessment guide is a useful tool for assessing the ethnic client's cultural background.

✓ The nursing diagnosis for an ethnic minority client should include potential problems in the client's interaction with the health care system and problems involving the effects of cultural conflict.

✓ The planning and implementation of nursing interventions should be adapted as much as possible to the client's cultural background.

✓ Evaluation should include the nurse's self-evaluation of attitudes and emotions toward ethnic nursing care.

REFERENCES

Abril, I.F.: Mexican American folk beliefs: how they affect health care, M.C.N. 1977:168, 1977.

American Nurses' Association: Code for nurses with interpretive statements, Kansas City, Mo., 1976, The Association.

Bloch, B., and Hunter, M.: Teaching physiological assessment of black persons, Nurse Educ. **6**:24, 1981.

California Department of Health Services: Two-year-old immunization survey, Berkeley, 1979, The Department.

Campbell, T., and Chang, B.: Health care of the Chinese in America, Nurs. Outlook **21**:245, 1973.

Farris, L.: The American Indian. In Clark, A., editor: Culture, childbearing, health professionals, Philadelphia, 1978, F.A. Davis Co.

Hall, E.T.: Proxemics: the study of man's spatial relations. In Goldstein, I., editor: Man's image in medicine and anthropology, New York, 1963, International Universities Press, Inc.

Harwood, A.: Ethnicity and medical care, Cambridge, Mass., 1981, Harvard University Press.

Henderson, G., and Primeaux, M.: The importance of folk medicine. In Henderson, G., and Primeaux, M., editors: Transcultural health care, Reading, Mass., 1981, Addison-Wesley Publishing Co., Inc.

Kosa, J., and Zola, I., editors: Poverty and health: a sociological analysis, rev. ed., Cambridge, Mass., 1975, Harvard University Press.

Lieberman, H.: Evaluating the duality of ambulatory pediatric care at a neighborhood center, Clin. Pediatr. **13**:52, 1974.

Kluckhohn, F.R.: Dominant and variant value orientations. In Brink, P.J., editor: Transcultural nursing: a book of readings, Englewood Cliffs, N.J., 1976, Prentice-Hall, Inc.

Mosley, D.Y.: Nursing students' perceptions of the urban poor, Pub. No. 23-1694, New York, 1977, National League for Nursing.

Muecke, M.A.: Overcoming the language barrier, Nurs. Outlook **18**:53, 1970.

Murillo, N.: The Mexican American family. In Martinez, R.A., editor: Hispanic culture and health care, St. Louis, 1978, The C.V. Mosby Co.

National League for Nursing: Criteria for the appraisal of baccalaureate and high degree programs in nursing, ed. 4, Pub. No. 15-1251, New York, 1977, The League.

Orque, M.S., Bloch, B., and Monrroy, L.S.A.: Ethnic nursing care, St. Louis, 1983, The C.V. Mosby Co.

Roach, L.B.: Color changes in dark skins, Nursing 77 **7**:48, 1977.

Schermerhorn, R.A.: Comparative ethnic relations: a framework for theory and research, New York, 1970, Random House, Inc.

Simmons, O.G.: Anglo-Americans and change: Mexican Americans in South Texas; a study in dominant-subordinate group relations, New York, 1974, Arno Press, Inc.

Snow, L.F.: Traditional health beliefs and practices among lower class black Americans, West. J. Med. **139**:821, 1983.

Statistics Canada, Census of Canada, Ottawa, 1981, Minister of Supplies and Services.

U.S. Department of Commerce, Bureau of Census: Current population reports: population characteristics, Series P-20, No. 374,

Population profile of the United States, 1981, Washington, D.C., 1982, U.S. Government Printing Office.

U.S. Department of Commerce, Bureau of Census: 1980 census of population: general population characteristics: United States summary, Washington D.C., 1983, U.S. Government Printing Office.

U.S. Department of Health, Education and Welfare: Indian health trends and services, Pub. No. (HSA) 78-12009, Washington D.C., 1978, U.S. Government Printing Office.

U.S. Department of State: Background notes, Canada, Pub. No. 7769, Washington D.C., 1983, U.S. Government Printing Office.

Vander Zanden, J.: American minority relations: the sociology of race and ethnic groups, ed. 2, New York, 1966, The Ronald Press Co.

Vigil, J.D.: From Indians to Chicanos: a sociocultural history, St. Louis, 1980, The C.V. Mosby Co.

Walter, P.A.: Race and culture relations, New York, 1952, McGraw-Hill, Inc.

Werner, E.E.: Cross-cultural child development: a view from the planet earth, Monterey, Calif., 1979, Brooks/Cole Publishing Co.

Wilson, U.: Nursing care of American Indian patients. In Orque, M.S., Bloch, B., and Monrroy, L.S.A.: Ethnic nursing care: a multicultural approach, St. Louis, 1983, The C.V. Mosby Co.

Wirth, L.: The problem of minority groups. In Linton, R., editor: The science of man in the world crisis, New York, 1945, Columbia University Press.

ADDITIONAL READINGS

Bauwens, E.E.: The anthropology of health, St. Louis, 1983, The C.V. Mosby Co.

Bloch, B.: Bloch's assessment guide for ethnic/cultural variations. In Orque, M.S., Bloch, B., and Monrroy, L.S.A.: Ethnic nursing care: a multicultural approach, St. Louis, 1983, The C.V. Mosby Co.

Branch, M.R., and Paxton, P.P.: Providing safe nursing care for ethnic people of color, New York, 1976, Appleton-Century-Crofts.

Brink, P.J., and Saunders, J.M.: Cultural shock: theoretical and applied. In Brink, P.J., editor: Transcultural nursing: a book of readings, Englewood Cliffs, N.J., 1976, Prentice-Hall, Inc.

Evaneshko, V., and Kay, M.: The ethnoscience research technique, West. J. Nurs. Res. **4**:49, 1982.

Fabrega, H.: Medical anthropology. In Siegel, B.J., editor: Biennial review of anthropology, Stanford, Calif., 1971, Stanford University Press.

Kleinman, A.: Patients and healers in the context of culture, Berkeley, 1980, University of California Press.

Leininger, M.: Transcultural nursing: concepts, theories and practices, New York, 1978, John Wiley & Sons, Inc.

Parsons, T.: The social system, Glencoe, N.Y., 1951, The Free Press.

Saunders, L.: Cultural difference and medical care: the case of the Spanish-speaking people of the Southwest, New York, Russell Sage Foundation.

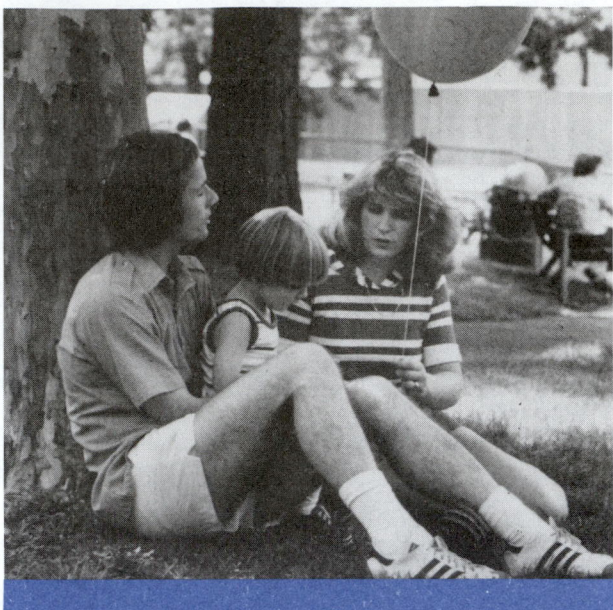

OBJECTIVES

Mastery of content in this chapter will enable the student to:

- Describe the importance of the family in terms of the health of individual members.
- Discuss how family members influence one another's health.
- Define the family in terms applicable to all family forms.
- Identify common concepts of the family held by clients.
- Describe five common family forms that nurses encounter in practice and discuss the relevant health concerns of each.
- Explain how the family's structure and pattern of functioning affect the health of family members.
- Describe what it means to view the family as an environment and explain how this perspective influences nursing practice.
- Define the concept of family health and discuss possible ways to assess or evaluate such health.
- Describe what it means to view the family as a single client and explain how this perspective influences nursing practice.

GLOSSARY

blended family   Family formed when parents bring together unrelated children from previous marriages.

communal family   Form of family comprised of unrelated adults rearing their children together in a communal living arrangement.

extended family   Form of family comprised of the nuclear family and all other relatives in both of the couple's families.

family   Group of interacting individuals comprising a basic unit of society; although concepts of what constitutes a family vary, the family usually has some degree of permanence, commitment, and attachment.

family as client   Nursing perspective in which the family is viewed as a unit of interacting members having attributes, functions, and goals separate from those of the individual family members; the nurse provides care to the family as a whole.

family as environment   Nursing perspective in which the family is viewed as the significant provider of physical, psychosocial, and emotional support to individual family members; the nurse provides care primarily to one of the family members.

family functions   Processes by which the family operates as a whole, including communication and manipulation of the environment for problem solving.

family health   Phenomenon that is more than the sum of the health of individual family members, including the achievement of satisfying family functioning and the attainment of family goals.

family of origin   Family into which a person is born, as distinct from the person's family of procreation.

family of procreation   Family a person forms through marriage and/or having children, as distinct from the person's family of origin.

family structure   Composition of the family organization of relationships among family members.

nuclear family   Form of family consisting of husband and wife and their children.

22 | *The Family*

Despite many challenges, such as the increasing divorce rate, the family remains a viable social unit within which individuals grow, develop, and seek health. The nurse therefore needs to be knowledgeable about the influence of the family on individual family members and their health. Twenty years ago many people predicted a decline in the influence families would have on their individual members. Rapid social change and a mobile population were anticipated to bring psychological as well as physical distancing of family members. However, although family members today may be geographically more distant from each other than in the past, research demonstrates the continuing presence of strong family ties and influence.

The 1980 White House Conference on Families reaffirmed the central role families play in many areas of life. Individuals receive substantial physical and emotional support from their families throughout life. Most adolescents in American society, for example, are not the primary providers of their own basic necessities but continue to seek material and psychological support from their families. Adolescents frequently rebel against their parents' values, yet they often acknowledge the importance of their parents' emotional support during times of stress.

For young married couples the influence of their families also remains strong. Gifts and economic and psychological support are exchanged between the couple and their parents, including assistance in areas such as providing transportation or child care. Support in such exchanges most commonly but not exclusively flows from the older to the younger family and is more frequent if both families feel an emotional closeness between them. Crises, including sudden illness, tend to increase the flow of these mutual exchanges. The benefits and obligations resulting from these exchanges are an important consideration in planning nursing care.

Although the elderly are often portrayed as isolated and alone, this is not the reality of most America's elderly. Families continue to provide significant support to their older members. More than two thirds of elderly persons see their children or communicate with them by telephone or letter at least once a week. Although financial support tends to flow from older parents to young families, affection and social support flow toward the elderly. Elderly people generally indicate that they desire and seek these exchanges with their younger family members, and most say they are satisfied with the number and kinds of exchanges they experience with their families.

The influence of family is important in American society, and the nurse must consider this influence in most interactions with clients. To ignore the family is to omit an important aspect of the client and to miss a possible resource for helping the client reach maximal health.

Family Influence and Health

The influence of family extends into the area of health. Family members influence one another's health beliefs, practices, and status. The family shapes early beliefs and values relative to health. Through the beliefs and values they instill, both parents have a strong influence on their child's later health practices. Health behavior reinforced in early life forms the basis on which the child develops long-lasting health habits. Interestingly, studies have shown that a client's use of prescribed medications is more closely related to family characteristics than to individual characteristics (Osteriveis, Bush, and Zukerman, 1979).

Another form of influence involves the perception of health and health problems. For example, mothers who have recently been ill are more sensitive to subjective indicators of ill health in their children. A mother with an upper respiratory infection who is experiencing malaise, anorexia, and shortness of breath may more quickly recognize similar symptoms in her child (for example, an increase in napping, picky eating, and avoidance of active play). She may therefore seek health care for the child earlier than if she herself were not ill.

The active participation of the father in family life has been shown to be associated with improved health care practices of all family members (Pratt, 1976). The reason for this association is unclear. The father may actually model and teach healthful behaviors, such as proper toothbrushing, or his general participation in family activities may provide encouragement and support to the children's mother in her teaching of the same behaviors. In either case the child's health practices are improved. The nurse should consider the father's influence in all phases of the nursing process to increase the potential avenues for improving the family's health.

The influence of family members on health is not only from parents to children. Children influence how parents perceive their own health. Also, at least in some mother-child pairs, if the child has acute illness the mother tends to have a heightened perception of her own health or illness. A similar influence on the father's perception of his own health seems likely. In families of children born with health problems, the parents are more likely to experience lowered self-esteem. All family members generally view their health within the context of other family members' health.

The wise nurse understands family members' influence on one another's health. In many situations the nurse incorporates the entire family into the nursing process, expanding avenues for intervention. This approach helps ensure that the interventions will be successful and have long-lasting effects. For example, the child may be the actual target of a school smoking prevention program. In recognition of the strong influence of parents' smoking, however, the nurse might first actively recruit the parents' participation in discussion sessions. A smoking cessation program for the parents might be developed to precede or run concurrently with the children's smoking prevention program. Even if active parental support cannot be obtained, student discussions can address parental smoking and its potential impact on their own behavior.

If the impact of the family is ignored, intervention opportunities may be lost. The mother who smokes but does not want her children to smoke might remain unaware of the effect of her own smoking on her children's smoking. The nurse has the opportunity to help her stop smoking or ask her children not to smoke.

In some cases the family's influence is in direct opposition to the objectives of nursing care for a family member. For example, a parent or sibling might be actively encouraging a young child to smoke. In this case the nurse planning a prevention program must consider whether the intervention will succeed within the current family climate. If the nurse's assessment shows that family members are promoting the child's smoking, the nurse adjusts the goals and interventions for the smoking prevention program. A new goal, for example, might be for siblings not to provide the child with cigarettes or tease the child if the child refuses to smoke. Implementation of nursing actions designed to reach these goals could then involve contact with the parents and siblings, as well as with the child. In any case, until the nurse assesses the family influence on a family member, this impact remains an unknown but possibly very important factor. Only after assessment and diagnosis can the nurse make plans to minimize negative family influences or to reinforce positive family influences in order to reach the desired health goals.

Incorporating the family into the nursing care plan is also important when illness, rather than health promotion, is the concern. Nursing care can accomplish much more in the rehabilitation of an elderly victim of a stroke, for example, if the care plan considers the family's life-style and patterns along with the client's needs. The nurse should incorporate medications and therapy into established family patterns when possible, rather than attempt to adjust family patterns for purposes of therapy. For example, if all family members have to be at work by 7 AM, the daily range of motion exercises that were performed in the morning in the hospital could be more consistently and effectively accomplished at home in the evening hours when family members can participate more easily.

To incorporate the family into the nursing process,

the nurse needs to understand different concepts of the family. Just what is a family? Who constitutes the family unit? What purposes do families fulfill? In what ways can the nurse view families to promote their health most effectively? How can family health be evaluated? All of these questions are addressed in the following sections.

Concept of Family

The practicing nurse often must consider who actually is a part of a client's family and to what extent the family can be incorporated into the nursing process. Nurses, like all people, have feelings and values deeply rooted in their own family experiences, which influence their ideas of what a family *should* be. Unless the nurse recognizes these values as her own rather than the client's, they may inhibit the nurse's understanding and acceptance of the client's perspective of his family.

Clients have widely varying concepts of family. Some clients consider the family to include only persons related by marriage, birth, or adoption. Other clients consider aunts, uncles, close friends, and cohabiting persons to be family. To accept all clients' concepts of family, the nurse can define the family as a group of interacting individuals comprising a basic unit of society (Fawcett, 1975). This definition is broad and flexible and recognizes widely divergent client conceptions of family as valid. It accepts differences in family structure and function arising from cultural and individual differences. Such an open perspective is useful to nurses because their clients have a wide variety of attitudes toward family.

Because a client may not be aware of his concept of family, the practicing nurse may need to ascertain the client's concept of his family. The nurse can simply ask the client, "Who do you consider your family?" or ask with whom he shares physical surroundings or strong emotional feelings. If the client is unable to express his concept of family, the nurse should observe with whom the client lives, spends time, and shares confidences and then ask the client to validate this observation: "Do you consider this person to be family or like family to you?"

The nurse's personal beliefs about the best composition of a family need not necessarily coincide with those of the client. The essential goal is to recognize and accept the client's view. The attitudes of many clients are based on commonly encountered family forms. The nurse should therefore be knowledgeable about these family forms and their health implications.

Family Forms

Family forms are patterns of people considered by family members to be included in a family. Although all families have some things in common, each family form has unique problems and resources in the nurse-client situation. Several common family forms are discussed in the following sections. The nurse working with families of several types should have an open perspective about what constitutes a family so as not to overlook potential family resources.

Nuclear Family

The nuclear family consists of the husband and wife and perhaps one or more children. For the children, this family is often referred to as their family of origin; for the parents, their family of procreation. Many couples in American society do not have reproduction as their primary goal, and childless families, occurring by choice as well as because of infertility, are often seen by the nurse for care. The presence or absence of children nonetheless does affect the family's health concerns. For example, routine immunizations and physical examination for children involve time and financial considerations for the family. When the nuclear family is not intact, the nurse can often help the family seek support from other sources, such as friends or the extended family, in times of illness.

Although the nuclear family is not necessarily the dominant American form of family, health care professionals often consider it to be the usual and ideal form. Because clients' concepts of the ideal family form vary, the nurse must be open to understanding other family forms as well.

Extended Family

The extended family includes relatives in addition to members of the nuclear family. Aunts, uncles, grandparents, and cousins are all part of the extended family. The extended family can be psychologically, as well as geographically, close or separated. The closer the extended family, the greater their influence on the client and the greater the importance of incorporating them into health care plans. Extended families often provide a larger range of experiences and talents, and therefore a more diverse support base, than can the nuclear family. At the birth of a child with a physical deformity, for example, the grandparents may be capable of providing comfort to the parents at a time when they feel extremely vulnerable and unable to give each other emotional support. Other relatives can be recruited to cook meals for the family in order to give the parents more time together or with their newborn child.

Single-Parent Family

Single-parent families are formed when one parent leaves the nuclear family as a result of death, divorce, or desertion. The circumstances of the separation influence its impact on the family. In the past, most single-parent families existed because of the death of one parent. Today such families are most commonly the result of divorce.

The proportion of children living in single-parent families increased from 9% in 1960 to 19% in 1978. A projected 25% of all children will live in single-parent families in 1990. The reduced financial resources accompanying the loss of one spouse significantly affect the health of single-parent families.

Specific health concerns of single-parent families include the following:

1. Adequate income to provide the essentials for a healthy life-style, including food, clothing, and recreation
2. Availability and access to medical care in the event of illness and child care arrangements during episodes of routine illness
3. Emotional health of all family members, particularly the children, because of the remaining parent's extra burden of accomplishing alone all the tasks of child rearing and nurturing

Blended Family

Blended families are formed when parents bring unrelated children from prior marriages into a new joint living situation as a result of remarriage or cohabitation. The nature of the prior living situations and rapidity with which the family members have had to adapt to changes influence their health. Multiple, rapid changes severely tax the family's coping resources. The stress experienced during the earlier family dissolution, the length of time in which each former family functioned with one parent, and the extent of the new family members' familiarity with one another also influence the blended family's coping capabilities.

Health concerns of blended families are currently being explored by researchers (Whiteside, 1982). Of primary interest is the mental health of family members during adjustment to the newly formed family pattern. This adjustment period can extend up to 2 years. The long-term impact of stress on the health of the individual family members and of the family as a whole during this extended adjustment period requires assessment. The nurse can assure families

that this period is a normal developmental phase and can help the family assess their resources to prevent or lessen stressful situations.

Communal Family

The communal family is not a recent development, as is often thought. Communal living reached a peak in number of members and rate of success in the 1840s. Although communal living may never again be that popular, economic pressures and shifting social attitudes could foster a substantial return to this form of family life. The membership of communal families varies. Members may share religious affiliation, economic commodities, ideology, goals of self-sufficiency, or desire for an extended family living arrangement.

The health concerns of communal families involve two major issues: the stability of relationships within the family and the nature of child-rearing practices. Stable relationships appear to bolster the mental health of family members; the concern with some communal families is that relationships are shifting or unstable so that less psychological and other support is provided to individual family members. The degree to which child rearing is shared between males and females also varies in different types of communes. In most communal living arrangements, however, females continue to provide the majority of child care. Specific child care practices vary from authoritarian to quite liberal. The nature of these practices is not as great a risk to children's emotional and mental health as are rapid changes in child-rearing practices that may occur if communal family membership changes rapidly. Changing membership can, on the other hand, expose the child to a wide range of supportive, loving adults.

Other Family Forms

The extent to which more loosely structured living arrangements are actual family forms is debatable. Some cohabiting, never married, heterosexual and homosexual couples define their relationships in family terms. Other couples with similar living arrangements do not. The difference may be each person's conscious intention to include the other as part of that person's family. In addition, some degree of permanence, commitment, and emotional attachment can be considered essential in establishing any family relationship (Miller and Janosik, 1980). The report of the White House Conference on Families (1980a and b) appears to substantiate this view, stressing commitment, support, fidelity, and responsibility as components of family ties. As with communal families, the health concerns with other family forms focus on the stability of family relationships and child-rearing practices.

Family Structure and Function

In addition to form, families have a structure and a pattern of functioning. Structure involves not only the ongoing membership in the family but also the organization and patterning of relationships among the individuals in a family. The processes by which the family as a whole operates comprise the family functioning. Nurses need to be aware of the family's structure and pattern of functioning in planning care for either a family member or the family as a whole.

An exceptionally flexible or rigid family structure may make it more difficult for a family to deal with a health problem. A rigid structure specifically dictates who is permitted to accomplish a given task. For example, the mother might be the only acceptable person to provide emotional support to the children, or the husband to provide financial support to the family. A change in the health status of the person responsible for a task places a burden on the family, because in a rigid structure no other person is available or acceptable to assume the task. The more essential the task, the greater the potential problems for the family. In working with rigidly structured families, the nurse's first intervention may be to show the family the benefits of a move toward more flexible patterns of action. Only after this is accomplished can specific alternative patterns be suggested by the nurse and considered by the family. If the mother who is the sole source of emotional support has an acute illness that requires hospitalization, the children will be without such support at a time when they need it most. The nurse's initial assessment might note changes in the children's behavior such as sleep disturbances, frequent crying, or regression to earlier patterns of behavior such as wetting or thumbsucking. Alternatively, the absence of emotional support from the father to the children, rather than the children's actual behavior, might be the first sign the nurse observes. An intervention based on a diagnosis of limited emotional support resulting from inflexible family structure might be to talk with the father about the children's needs, their current behavior, and how he could provide emotional support. The ages of the children would determine his specific actions.

A very rigid family structure may also severely limit the number of persons outside the immediate family who are allowed to assume family tasks. This rigidity often prevents a family from seeking or receiving necessary assistance. Such families may rebuke friends, neighbors, and health care professionals for "interfering." Although these families may openly recognize that they have needs that others can help them meet, they may feel it is wrong to accept assistance and therefore be unable to adjust to changes in task performance necessitated by health problems. Again, the initial nursing intervention might include discussions pointing toward the advantages of more flexible family structures. A family in which the husband has recently lost a limb may find work around the home a problem. If the family structure is too rigid, the wife may refuse to seek or accept outside help. If she attempts to take on additional tasks herself, she may become physically and emotionally exhausted, especially if she is unable to relinquish her usual tasks.

An extremely open structure can also present problems to the family facing a health concern. An underlying stability that otherwise would lead to automatic action during crisis or rapid change is often absent. The family often considers multiple alternatives, some of which are nonproductive and may lead to conflict and wasted time and energy. The efforts of one family member may duplicate the efforts of another. The family may seek outside assistance from numerous sources, which is ineffective without coordination. For example, the family may be receiving care from a member of the Visiting Nurses Association, a city public health nurse, and a private physician's nurse without telling each nurse about the involvement of the others. Confusion results when each family member attempts to act on the suggestions of a different nurse.

A moderately flexible structure is generally most beneficial to the family. Nursing interventions therefore may involve modulating the family pattern away from either extreme if that extreme is causing problems related to the health of an individual family member or the family as a whole. In general, however, the nurse attempts to work within the family structure when providing care rather than attempting to change the structure.

Family functioning involves the processes used by the family to achieve its goals. These processes include communication among family members, manipulation of the environment, and use of external resources (Miller and Janosik, 1980). Goals are more easily achieved when communication is clear and direct and when the family has control over their environment. Some families can exert their influence on the immediate environments of home, neighborhood, or school, yet other families may lack, or believe that they lack, control of these environments.

For example, one family may perceive the school environment to be within their control. If a child is about to be discharged from the hospital, they may have no problem discussing his diabetes with school personnel and arranging for special dietary and exercise requirements. After assessing this family the nurse may diagnose only the need for supportive intervention to affirm the family's actions. Another family may believe that the school environment is outside their control and thus feel helpless about making arrangements. The hospital nurse should diagnose this problem before the child's discharge. The plan might include referral to a public health nurse who can help the family gain their desired level of control over the school environment as it relates to the child's health. Referral to the school nurse is an alternative intervention. Evaluation includes not only the effectiveness of the family's goal achievement and processes they used to achieve their goal of control, but also their satisfaction with the process and outcome.

Many families mistakenly perceive their environment as uncontrollable. For example, the parents of a hospitalized preschooler may not recognize that they can control many aspects of the hospital routine unless the nurse points this out to them. They can make many decisions about what the child wears, what he eats, when he naps and sleeps, and how medications are administered. If the parents' goal is to maintain family routines during hospitalization, this is feasible with sensitive nursing support. The nurse attempts to provide any additional resources the family requires to manipulate their environment to the extent they desire. However, the resources available to the family promote effective family functioning only when present in forms the family can use. The nurse must therefore individualize all interventions to the family involved. For example, providing the phone number of a home health care agency may be useless to a family having no phone easily available to them. In summary, the nurse helps the family recognize and communicate their goals, evaluate their resources, and use problem-solving methods to obtain the necessary resources to achieve their goals.

As systems, families function to achieve goals. Health and many other family goals are inextricably tied. The reproductive, sexual, economic, and educational goals that were once considered the central goals of families no longer apply to all families. Although many families have these goals at various times during their development, providing psychological support to family members is now considered equally important by most families. The family remains the primary provider of such support, although individuals also receive support from other sources such as peer or professional groups (Croog, Lipson, and Levine, 1972).

Caplan (1975) suggests that the family has nine support functions for the individual family member (see boxed material). The emphasis on one or more functions varies from family to family. Within the same family individual members may differentially emphasize specific functions, and shifts in emphasis occur from time to time. Health problems are often a stimulus for such a shift. The nurse can help families provide these support functions to an individual member by assisting them in clarifying which functions have been altered or may in the future be altered by the health condition. The nurse assesses the extent of the family's achievement of the goals as well as their satisfaction with their means of reaching these goals. Intervention strategies help the family adjust their goals or the processes by which they attain them. For example, rehabilitation of a hemiplegic young adult after a traumatic accident may focus on the family function of providing feedback and guidance to help the individual continue to interact within society.

The nurse might assist the family to assess the current level of social interaction and specify what actions will increase the client's social interaction, such as movement back into a school or work setting. Structuring situations in the home that allow for successful social interactions enhances the young adult's self-esteem and gives him the confidence to participate beyond the family. These situations might include frequent satisfactory verbal interactions with family members, inviting one to two friends into the home

---

Support Functions of the Family

- Collects and disseminates information to family members
- Provides feedback to family members to guide them in interaction with the larger society
- Transmits to family members beliefs, values, attitudes, and coping mechanisms
- Guides family members in problem solving
- Provides practical services and concrete assistance such as financial aid
- Provides a safe, comfortable environment when family members need rest and recuperation
- Provides standards of behavior and attitudes against which family members can judge themselves
- Helps family members establish an identity and reinforces identity in times of stress
- Assists family members in controlling or working through negative emotions

for a brief visit, or role-playing potential stressful situations that the adult might encounter in future social interactions.

Just as the health status of family members influences the family's functioning, so does the family's functioning influence their own and society's perception of their health. When the family is satisfactorily meeting its goals, family members tend to perceive themselves and their family as healthy. Conversely, when they are not meeting their goals, families view themselves as unhealthy. Society tends to affirm these feelings, labeling families healthy or unhealthy. The constant stress resulting from inadequate functioning can also adversely affect an individual family member's health. Constant stress may disrupt cardiovascular function, blood pressure, and circulating neuroendocrine substances, and these disruptions are suspected precursors of poor health (see Chapter 5).

Family and Nursing

From a nursing perspective, the family can be approached in two different ways. The family can be seen as providing the environment within which the individual client strives for health or, alternatively, as a client itself. Viewing the entire family as a client means picturing the family as a system of interacting members, having attributes separate and different from those of the individual members. Which approach to use depends on the situation. If only one family member is receptive to nursing care, it is more realistic and practical to view the family as an environment. When all family members are involved in the day-to-day health care of one another, nursing intervention with one individual necessitates some change in the activities of the others. Therefore in such a situation it is more appropriate and efficient for the nurse to consider the family as the client.

In some cases the situation itself may determine which perspective is more appropriate. The family may be physically present but not greatly involved with the member who has sought nursing care. For example, a single, 25-year-old man lives at home with his parents and two younger siblings. He requests the assistance of the nurse in altering his diet and developing stress management techniques to help him cope with his borderline hypertension, which is thought to be related to his high sodium intake, a stressful job, and continuing expectations by his family for participation in their activities. The other family members have no health concerns. If the nurse viewed the family as the client's environment, she would focus on the client as an individual and might assess his knowledge of high-sodium foods, strategies for reducing the number of high-sodium foods in his diet, realistic opportunities to reduce the number and extent of perceived stressors in both his work and his family environments, and knowledge and skill in stress management skills such as relaxation or biofeedback techniques. Alternatively, if the nurse viewed the family unit as the client, the nurse would assess the family's current dietary patterns and their desire and resources for changing the patterns, demands on the hypertensive family member and potential for redistribution of the demand among other family members, and capabilities to support the hypertensive member's development and use of stress management techniques.

Family as Environment

Both approaches—family as environment and family as client—can be useful in providing effective nursing care. However, when only the individual is available for or receptive to care, the family can from a practical standpoint only be viewed as the client's environment. For example, the family of a young adult who lives away from the family and desires to maintain independence and distance can best be viewed as the environment. Similarly, in a situation involving an elderly person whose family is physically present but chooses not to become involved in health care, the family can realistically be treated as only a part of the client's environment.

When the nurse views the family as environment, her primary focus is on the health and development of an individual family member. Depending on the client's age, other environmental contexts might include school, work, or social groups. From an environmental perspective, the nurse assesses the extent to which the family provides the necessities for the individual to meet his basic human needs (see Chapter 4). These needs vary depending on the individual's developmental level and current situation. Subsequent chapters in this unit address these specific needs within a nursing context. If the family environment is not adequately fulfilling the client's needs, the nurse assists the client in altering the situation. Interventions focus on helping the client obtain the necessities from the family or helping the client seek and use alternative resources.

For example, an elderly client with a recent hip fracture is unable to prepare nutritious meals because of restricted mobility. The client lives alone, and the extended family does not function as a unified whole. Other family members say that they are unable to prepare meals three times a day for the client and that they cannot be called upon to intervene as a unit because of other demands on them. The nurse might suggest that on a rotating basis one family member prepare, freeze, and deliver to the client an entire week of individual packaged meals. The client could defrost these meals as needed. If the family is still unable or unwilling to provide such help, the nurse finds other resources for the client. Many cities have programs such as Meals on Wheels that prepare and deliver meals to shut-ins. The goal of the nursing intervention is to meet the client's nutritional needs.

The nurse must be aware that families provide more than just material essentials. When viewing the family as the client's environment, the nurse should also assess the family's ability to help the client meet psychological needs. Neighbors, friends, health professionals, and peer support groups are other environmental resources that can supplement family psychological support when it is inadequate to meet the needs of an individual. Regardless of the situation, when the nurse views the family as environment, the major focus is on the needs of the individual client. Assessment, diagnosis, planning, intervention, and evaluation will therefore concentrate on the individual's health.

Family as Client

A recent aproach to family nursing is to work with the family as a unit rather than individual members. The nurse inexperienced in family or small group dynamics may find this approach difficult. Working with the family as the client, however, has advantages when family members are closely tied and mutually receptive to nursing care. In closely interacting families, any nursing intervention with one member ultimately influences all members. By accepting the family as the client, the nurse recognizes and uses these reciprocal influences throughout the nursing process. The family unit rather than the individual is the primary focus of nursing care. For example, family patterns and traditions concerning meals, rather than an individual's nutritional needs, would receive the nurse's attention.

When the family unit is viewed as the client, the nurse can adopt a developmental perspective similar to that used with individuals. The developmental approach recognizes both the typical stages of family life and the variations of individual families.

Duvall (1977) hypothesizes that families pass through developmental stages, experiencing alternating periods of relative calm and conflict, in a process called the family life cycle. Duvall's framework addresses the traditional nuclear family. Her eight stages of family life and the tasks associated with each stage are as follows:

STAGE	TASK
1. Marital family	Establishing a marriage fulfilling to both partners and establishing relationships with members of each other's family
2. Childbearing family	Adjusting to parenthood and creating a home for the family
3. Preschool family	Nurturing children
4. School-age family	Educating and socializing the children and establishing social relationships with other families
5. Teenage family	Helping children balance freedom and responsibility
6. Launching family	Releasing children, redeveloping their own interests, and continuing to provide some support to children
7. Middle-aged family	Solidifying the marital relationship and maintaining links with other generations
8. Aging family	Adjusting to losses of job, spouse, and friends

More flexible developmental approaches view the family life cycle as heavily influenced by current sociocultural and personal expectations, the ages and developmental stages of individual family members, and prior family life experiences of the members. The term "family career" is often used in place of "family life cycle" in these approaches. They are more applicable to diverse family forms, some of which do not follow the life pattern outlined by Duvall.

Regardless of the specific framework, when the nurse views the whole family with a developmental perspective, the nursing process focuses on achievement of family tasks rather than, or in addition to, individual developmental tasks. In the Duvall framework, for example, a task of the middle-aged family is to solidify the marital relationship after children have moved away. For the family as a unit, this task is as crucial as the individual's achievement of a sense of generativity (see Chapter 23).

If the task of the individual and the task of the family demand conflicting actions, compromises must be made. For example, a middle-aged man experiencing depression may be able to meet individual needs by taking his grandson on weekend fishing trips but may along with his wife feel that this interferes with their rediscovery of interests as a couple. In such a case the nurse can help the couple evaluate their ability to meet both individual and family needs, perhaps by together making the fishing trip with the grandchild.

Consensus of all family members is one way to resolve these task conflicts. As another method to resolve conflict, the family can delegate responsibility for problem solving to one or more members of the family. The health implications of these methods of conflict resolution have not received much research. The most useful approach for the nurse appears to be helping families learn both methods and vary their use depending on the demands of the situation.

Providing nursing care to the family as a unit requires advanced study. Interested students are referred to Miller and Janosik (1980), who provide many case studies of the nursing process applied to the family as a whole. Whenever this approach is used, records of family structure, function, processes, communication, and problem solving must be kept by the nurse. The structure of the American health care system makes it difficult to provide effective nursing care to the family as a whole, since the system focuses on individual health. However, this focus may shift in the near future as more health care providers recognize the efficiency of caring for the entire family.

Evaluating the Family's Health

When the family receives nursing care as a client, the nurse must be able to measure the family's health as a basis for assessment and evaluation. Since the family as a whole is different from the individual family members, this measure of family health must be more than a summation of the health of all family members. The family's attainment of family development tasks may be one useful criterion. Litman (1974) includes successful family functioning, along with the health of individual family members, as a criterion for evaluation of family health. With this perspective the nurse assesses the family's functions, such as its ability to provide family members with values and codes of behavior, to guide family members in problem solving, and to give members practical service and concrete aid. If the family is dissatisfied with how it is functioning, the nurse determines a specific nursing diagnosis, plans interventions, implements these interventions with the family as a whole, and evaluates the family's change in functioning and their satisfaction with the new level of functioning.

Additional criteria for family health are whether family members have the opportunity to attain a satisfactory sense of identity and worth and whether the family's life-style minimizes risks and promotes active coping to achieve family goals (O'Brien, 1979). Since families vary in their specific goals, measures of family health must be flexible. If a practical, short-term family goal is a 2-week vacation at the beach, specific nursing interventions may be necessary if a 2-year-old, ventilator-dependent family member is to be included. In such a case the nurse assesses the emotional and physical support available to the family while away from their usual health care environment. Planning for emergencies might include providing a hospital in the vacation area with information about the child and perhaps even standing medical orders for use in an emergency. Another nursing intervention might be obtaining a portable electrical generator for use in case of power outage in the resort cabin. Evaluation before and after the vacation enables the nurse and family to know what else could have been done to improve the family's coping and to improve planning of similar future activities.

Few clinical measures of family health are currently available to the nurse, but this is an area of exciting and rapidly growing research. It seems reasonable that a true measure of family health will incorporate aspects of the health of all family members, as well as measurement of total family health. New research developments of family health criteria include determination of consensus and discrepancies between family members, use of family diaries addressing health concerns, and active coping efforts of family members.

Summary

Whether the family is viewed as the client's environment or as the client itself, the family assessment is an essential component of the nursing process. The family's influence on health is as significant now as ever, and each family member can influence the health of other family members. Since the concept of the family varies among different clients, the nurse begins the family assessment by assessing the client's attitude toward his own family.

Different family forms often have different health concerns and resources for resolving these concerns. The nurse assesses the family's structure and functioning to plan effective interventions when the family faces health problems. At times the family's structure and functioning may require alteration before the family can focus on a specific health problem.

The nurse can apply the nursing process whether the family is viewed as a highly significant environment within which the individual client seeks to maintain health or is viewed as the client itself. The most effective and appropriate approach depends on the situation. If the family is viewed as the client's environment, the nursing focus is on the individual family member's health. If the family as a whole is viewed as the client, the nurse focuses on the family's health, which is more than a summation of the health of individual family members. With either perspective the nurse maximizes therapeutic effectiveness by recognizing the family's influence and using its resources to promote both the individual's and the family's health.

KEY CONCEPTS

- ✓ The family has a significant impact on the lives of its members.
- ✓ Family members mutually influence one another's health beliefs, practices, and status.
- ✓ Because the concept of family is highly individual, the nurse should base nursing care on the client's attitude toward his family rather than on an inflexible definition of the family.
- ✓ Specific family forms tend to have typical family health problems with which the nurse should be familiar.
- ✓ The family's structure and functioning significantly influence the family's health and ability to respond to health problems.
- ✓ The nurse either can view the client's family as an important environment for the individual family member or can view the family unit as the client; the approach for any one family depends in part on the situation.
- ✓ Measures of the family's health involve more than a summation of individual family members' health.

REFERENCES

Caplan, G.: The family as a support system. In Caplan, G., and Killilea, M., editors: Support systems and mutual help: multidisciplinary explorations, New York, 1975, Grune & Stratton, Inc.

Croog, S., Lipson, A., and Levine, S.: Help patterns in severe illness: the roles of kin networks, nonfamily resources and institutions, J. Marriage Fam. **34**:34, 1972.

Duvall, E.M.: Marriage and family development, ed. 5, Philadelphia, 1977, J.B. Lippincott Co.

Fawcett, J.: The family as a living open system: an emerging conceptual framework for nursing, Int. Nurs. Rev. **22**:113, 1975.

Litman, T.: The family as a basic unit in health and medical care: a social behavioral overview, Soc. Sci. Med. **8**:495, 1974.

Miller, J., and Janosik, E.: Family focused care, New York, 1980, Gardner Press, Inc.

O'Brien, R.: A conceptualization of family health. In ANA Clinical and Scientific Sessions, Nashville, Tenn., Nov. 8-11, 1979, Kansas City, American Nurses' Association.

Osteriveis, M., Bush, P., and Zukerman, A.: Family context as a predictor of individual medication use, Soc. Sci. Med. **13**:287, 1979.

Pratt, L.: Family structure and effective health behavior: the energized family, Boston, 1976, Houghton Mifflin Co.

White House Conference on Families, Listening to America's Families: A summary of The Report to the President, Congress, and Families of the Nation, Washington D.C., November 1980.

White House Conference on Families, Listening to America's Families: The Report to the President, Congress and Families of the Nation, Washington, D.C., October 1980.

Whiteside, M.: Remarriage: a family developmental process, J. Marital Fam. Ther. **8**:59, 1982.

ADDITIONAL READINGS

American Nurses' Association Council of Nurse Researchers Conference: Nursing Science: Today and Beyond, Minneapolis, Sept. 22-24, 1983, Kansas City, The Association.

Carter, E., and McGoldrick, M.: The family life cycle: a framework for family therapy, New York, 1980, Gardner Press, Inc.

Mercer, R.: Nursing care for parents at risk, Thorofare, N.J., 1977, Slack, Inc.

5

Human growth and development involve many complex changes in all dimensions of a person throughout the life span. Only by understanding the normal ranges of growth and development within each developmental stage can the nurse assess the client's current status and intervene when necessary to promote continued healthy development. Each stage is associated with certain physiological and psychosocial health needs and risk factors, and the nurse's awareness of these elements is important when providing care for any kind of health problem. Similarly, each developmental stage involves unique resources and coping mechanisms the nurse can use to help clients adapt to the problems of illness. By incorporating a developmental perspective in nursing care, the nurse can more effectively address all the client's health needs. The chapters in Unit 5 promote this perspective by examining important theories of growth and development and appropriate health issues for each stage.

Growth and Development

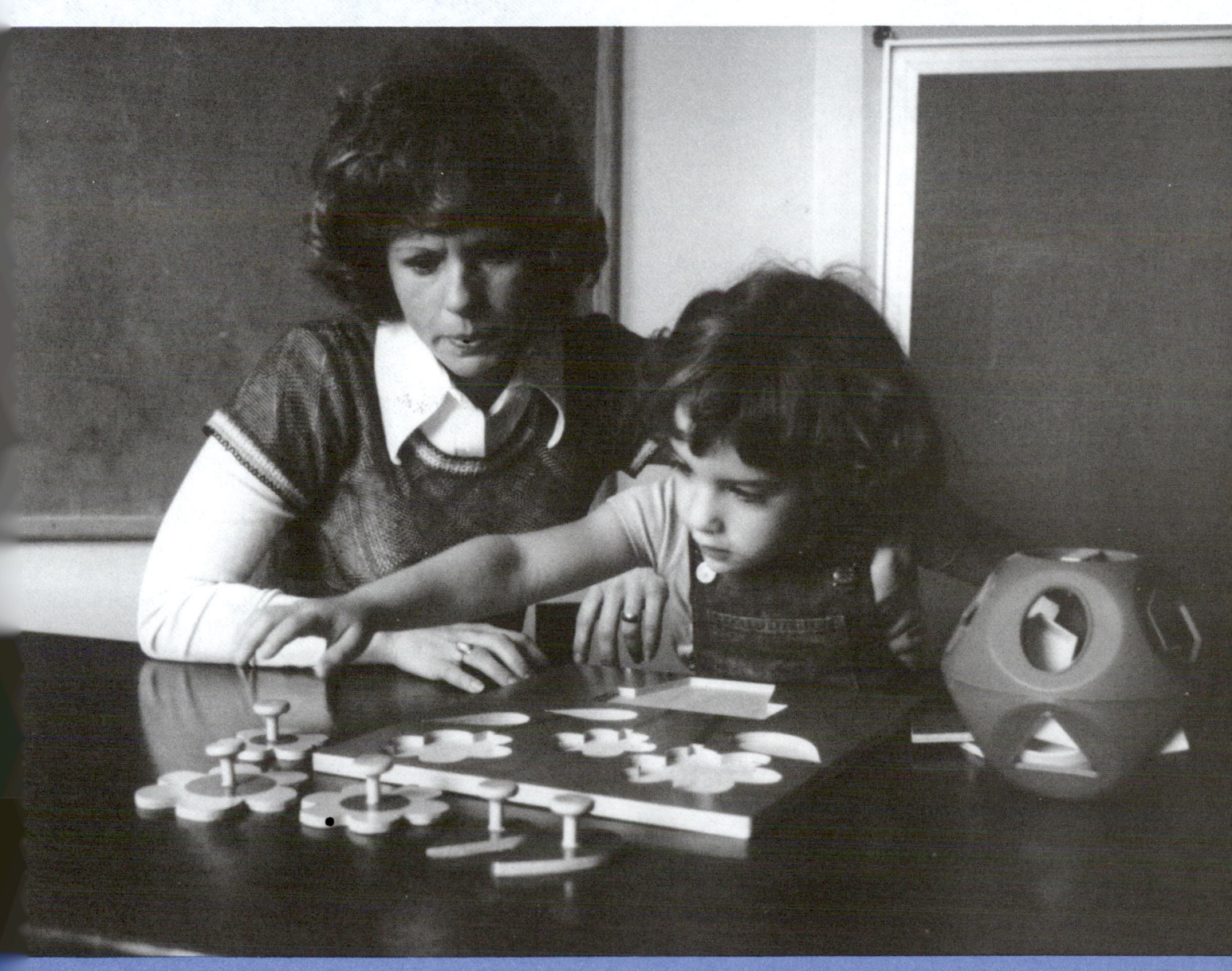

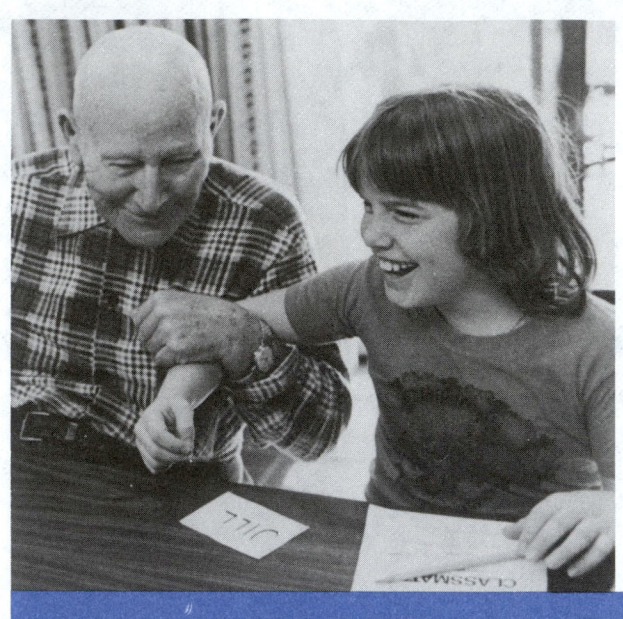

OBJECTIVES

Mastery of content in this chapter will enable the student to:

- Define the terms in the glossary.
- Describe three conceptual premises of commonalities in human development.
- Describe the six principles of growth and development related to the three conceptual premises.
- Discuss the major factors that influence growth and development.
- Compare and discuss the eight theories of development in their relation to nursing.

GLOSSARY

accommodation Process of responding to the environment through a new activity and thinking.

adolescence Stage of life from 12 to 21 years of age.

assimilation Process of incorporating new experiences into one's current activity or thinking.

critical period of development Specific time span during which the environment has its greatest impact on an individual's environment.

development Qualitative or observable aspects of the progressive changes an individual makes in adapting to the environment.

heredity Primary natural force influencing an individual's genetic development.

infancy Stage of life from 1 month to 1 year of age.

maturation Process of becoming fully developed and grown, involving the individual's biological ability and environmental opportunities to alter functions and learning.

neonate Stage of life from birth to 1 month of age.

older adult Stage of life from age 66 until death.

prenatal Stage of life from conception to birth.

preschooler Stage of life from 3 to 5 years of age.

school age Stage of life from 6 to 11 years of age.

toddlerhood Stage of life from 1 to 3 years of age.

young and middle adult Stage of life from 22 to 65 years of age.

23 Theoretical Perspectives of Growth and Development

Human growth and development are orderly, predictable processes that begin with conception and continue until death. Each person progresses through definite phases of growth and development during a lifetime, but the pace and behaviors of this progression are highly individual. An infant must learn to walk before he can run as a toddler, for example, but one infant may walk at 10 months and another may not develop the skill until 15 months of age. Both children progress through the same developmental phase and both demonstrate normal healthy behaviors, but each accomplishes the task at his own pace.

The individual's ability to progress through each developmental phase influences his level of health. The success or failure an individual experiences within a given phase affects his ability to complete subsequent phases. If the individual experiences repeated failures in his attempts to develop, inadequacies result that may threaten his health. If the individual experiences repeated successes, competencies result that help maintain and promote his health. A child who does not learn to walk by 18 or 20 months of age, for example, demonstrates delayed gross motor ability that slows exploration and manipulation of his environment, which are essential to his learning. A toddler who does walk by age 10 months is able to explore and find stimulation in his environment, thereby enhancing his learning.

Because nursing promotes the health of all individuals, of all ages, the nurse must (1) understand the growth and development process, (2) understand the theories and principles of growth and development, (3) be able to identify the various stages of growth and development, (4) be able to identify factors that influence an individual's developmental progress, and (5) assess the individual's ability to respond in a healthy manner to the process. Knowledge and understanding of these basic concepts provide the nurse with a foundation for delivering health care. A developmental approach allows the nurse to organize knowledge about human behavior into common patterns that can be applied with individual clients.

A developmental perspective helps the nurse understand *why* commonalities and variations exist and what influence they have on health. With this knowledge the nurse can intervene in a manner consistent with the client's unique needs and in the context of his general developmental level. For example, when planning care for a client 10 years of age, the nurse should know that nightly bed wetting, although considered normal at age 2, might be a symptom of a urinary tract infection, psychosocial problem, or parasitic infection for a 10-year-old.

This chapter discusses principles and concepts related to the growth and development process and to the application of these principles in health promotion and nursing roles. Subsequent chapters explore the stages of growth and development and the influence of family and other factors on these stages.

Definitions

Growth and development are synchronous processes, which are interdependent in the healthy individual. In time a person experiences both quantitative and qualitative changes.

Physical Growth

Physical growth is the quantitative or measurable aspect of an individual's increase in physical measurements (Waechter and Blake, 1976). Measurable growth indicators include height, weight, and the indices of dental, skeletal, and sexual age. Increases in these indicators demonstrate growth; for example, infants generally double their birth weight by 6 months of age and double their height by 36 months.

Age is an indicator of patterns of physical growth. Since most physical growth occurs before age 21 and in a definitive sequence, certain growth events can be expected at certain ages. Patterns or events that are out of sequence should alert the nurse to the need for intervention. For example, the nurse should know that the average female experiences a growth spurt that normally begins at approximately 9½ years of age, peaks at 12, and stops by 14. Synchronized with this growth spurt is the rapid sexual growth of puberty, beginning with breast budding at an average of 10 years, followed by the onset of menses at the average age of 12. Knowing this sequence of pubertal events allows the nurse to recognize deviations and take appropriate actions, such as referring a 17-year-old girl who has not menstruated for gynecological consultation.

Development

The qualitative or behavioral aspects of the individual's progressive adaptation to his environment are called development. An example of these qualitative changes is the increased functioning capacity that results from mastering several smaller skills. For instance, a significant qualitative and observable change for the toddler is saying "please" when asking for something. However, before the toddler develops this social skill, he must master several other skills: recognizing specific objects (such as a cookie), speaking coherently, and identifying sensations (such as appetite or hunger).

Maturation

Maturation is the process of becoming fully developed and grown. It involves the individual's biological dimension, alterations in function, and learning more mature behaviors. To mature, the individual may have to relinquish previous behaviors and learning, integrate new behaviors and learning into his existing behaviors, or accomplish both of these actions. The process of maturation influences the sequence and timing of the qualitative and quantitative changes associated with growth and development. For example, the infant relinquishes crawling for walking because it permits more extensive investigation of his environment and more learning. However, the infant cannot walk until he has developed the biological ability and structures to perform the action, that is, increased muscle cells and tone.

Critical Periods in Development

The stages of growth and development involve the concept of "critical periods of development." A critical period is a specific span of time during which the environment has its greatest impact on the individual (Sutterly and Donnelly, 1978). During these critical periods some form of sensory stimulation is necessary for developmental progression; without it, task completion is difficult or unattainable. For example, the toddler who has not been stimulated to learn to walk during a set time period may have difficulty learning to walk at another time. Delays in cognitive abilities eventually affect self-esteem as the individual is unable to keep pace with his peers. Consequently, this deficit in sensory stimulation in the environment has a potential cumulative effect that is detrimental to future development (Tackett and Hunsberger, 1981).

Therefore an individual's developmental progression depends on the timing and degree of stimulation, as well as his readiness to be stimulated by the environment. A stimulus that is provided too early may not be useful to the child. For example, an 18-month-old child cannot learn to write, regardless of the intensity of the stimuli, whereas a 6-year-old has the readiness and ability to learn to write if stimulated to do so.

Principles of Growth and Development

Growth and development involve certain commonalities that are true of all people. These commonalities are expressed by the following concepts:

1. An individual has adaptive potential for both qualitative and quantitative changes by receiving stimuli from and giving stimuli to his environment.
2. An individual derives his uniqueness from the interaction of heredity and environment.
3. The primary goal of development is achieving one's potential (self-realization or self-actualization).

The basic principles of growth and development follow:

1. *Development has direction,* proceeding in an orderly way and in a set sequence.
2. *Development is complex yet predictable,* occurring with a consistent pattern and chronology.

3. *Development is unique* to the individual and his genetic potential, and each individual tends to seek his maximal potential for development.
4. *Development occurs through conflict and adaptation,* and different aspects develop at different rates; this phenomenon creates periods of equilibrium and disequilibrium.
5. *Development involves challenges* for the individual, in the form of certain tasks specific to the individual's age and ability.
6. *Developmental tasks require practice and energy,* the focus of which varies with each developmental stage and task that is accomplished.

Stages of Growth and Development

Human growth and development are intricate, complex processes. Although these processes are continuous, they are often divided into stages organized by age group. While this chronological division is arbitrary, it is based on the timing and sequence of developmental tasks that the individual must accomplish in order to progress to another stage. The chronology of growth and development is listed in Table 23-1. These stages are discussed in more detail in subsequent chapters.

Prenatal Stage

The prenatal stage is the period from conception to birth. During this period the fetus grows and develops from a single cell to a complex physiological being. During the 9 months in utero all major organ systems develop, with some becoming functional before birth. The psychosocial being also begins to emerge during the gestation period.

Assessing the quality of the environment in which the fetus grows is an important step in ensuring good health in childhood. The nurse requires extensive knowledge of the many factors (such as heredity and maternal health and age) that influence gestational development. Application of this knowledge to the nursing process facilitates the provision of care. For example, understanding that rapid fetal brain growth occurs in the last trimester of pregnancy enables the nurse to focus on nutritional counseling of the expectant mother during this time.

Neonatal Stage

The neonatal stage is defined as the period from birth to 1 month of age. During this stage the new-born's physical functioning is mostly reflexive, and stabilization of major organ systems is the primary task. The newborn's behavior greatly influences the interaction between the newborn and his environment and care givers. For example, the average 2-week-old smiles spontaneously and is able to regard his mother's face. The impact of these reflexive behaviors is generally a surge of maternal feelings of love that prompt the mother to cuddle the baby.

Nurses can apply their knowledge of this stage of growth and development to promote newborn and parental health. If the nurse understands, for example, that the newborn's cry is generally a reflexive response to an unmet need (such as hunger), she can assist parents to identify ways to meet those needs, such as counseling the parents to feed their baby on demand rather than on a rigid schedule.

Infancy

Infancy is the period from 1 month to 1 year of age. Rapid physical growth and change characterize this stage. Psychosocial development, which is facilitated by the progression from reflexive to more purposeful behavior, advances. The interaction between the infant and his environment becomes greater and more meaningful. The infant who purposefully giggles and rolls over in response to his father's tickling is interacting more with his social environment and is receiving a greater response than when he merely smiled in response to a hug.

During this phase of growth and development the nurse can observe the individual's adaptive potential, since both qualitative and quantitative changes occur rapidly.

Toddlerhood

Toddlerhood is the stage that spans from 1 to 3 years of age. Physical growth and development decelerate somewhat from the rapid growth of infancy. By 2 years of age the physical growth rate has slowed. Psychosocially, the individuality of the child and his emerging personality become more apparent.

During this stage the nurse can see the complex nature of growth and development—they become more intricate, involve more elements, and entail more interaction with the environment. The child's physical and psychosocial skills stimulate reciprocal development. For example, the toddler can ask for a cookie or pull a chair over to the counter and climb up to get it himself, rather than pulling, pointing, or crying. Because of his expanding physical prowess and communicative ability, the toddler behaves in a more complex manner and has a greater impact on his environment.

TABLE 23-1

Chronology of Growth and Development

Stage	Age Span	Significant Behavioral Milestones
Prenatal	Conception to birth	Maternal physical and psychosocial adjustment to and progression through pregnancy
		Health and growth of fetus
Neonatal	Birth to 1 month	Infant attachment behaviors: rooting, sucking, grasping, clinging
		Visual fixation: objects, face
		Equality of body movements
Infancy	1 month to 1 year	Physical: lifts head, rolls, sits, crawls, pulls to stand, walks, grasps, rakes, transfers hand objects, uses pincer grasp
		Psychosocial: smiles, vocalizes, laughs, feeds self finger foods, says "Da-Da" and "Ma-Ma," plays peek-a-boo and pat-a-cake
Toddlerhood	1 to 3 years	Physical: walks well forward and backward, stoops and recovers, climbs, runs, jumps in place, throws overhand, voluntarily releases hand, uses spoon, drinks from cup, scribbles, builds two- then four-block tower
		Psychosocial: indicates wants by behaviors other than crying, increases vocabulary, imitates, helps with household chores, points to body parts, recognizes animals, engages in solitary play
Preschooler	3 through 5 years	Physical: rides tricycle, walks up then down stairs alternating feet, hops on one foot, tandem walks, draws circle, then cross, then triangle, dresses with assistance, then with supervision, then alone
		Psychosocial: knows first name, then age, then last name, engages in parallel play progressing to interaction play, uses plurals and three-word sentences progressing to complex sentences, follows directions, counts
School age	6 through 11 years	Physical: skips, skates, tumbles, tandem walks backward, prints progressing to script, ties knots, then bows
		Psychosocial: engages in interactive play with rules progressing to organized sports or activities, has significant peer relationships, enjoys hobbies, assumes complete responsibility for personal care
Adolescence	12 through 21 years	Physical: undergoes cognitive growth spurt, develops secondary sex characteristics, increases cognitive ability and formal operational thought
		Psychosocial: develops sense of identity and sex role, establishes independence, develops peer relationships with both sexes, develops life philosophy (values, beliefs), makes occupational decisions
Young and middle adulthood	22 through 65 years	Physical/cognitive: has established physical growth state and functioning, undergoes menopause, begins physical/physiological degeneration, refines formal operational abilities
		Psychosocial: develops self-sufficiency, pursues vocation/occupation, has intense interpersonal relationships (most frequently marriage and children)
Older adulthood	66 years until death	Physical/cognitive: has general slowing of physical and cognitive functioning
		Psychosocial: needs to establish highest degree of independence (self-sufficiency) physically possible by adapting environment to ability, reflects on life accomplishments, events, and experiences, continues interpersonal relationships

Preschool Stage

The stage of the preschool child extends from age 3 to the end of the fifth year. During this time, physical growth occurs at a slow, even pace, according to the individual child's pattern. The preschooler's personality and world expand rapidly as a result of increased physical and psychosocial skills. For example, the preschooler can now play *with* his neighborhood friends rather than *around* them. He can engage in this interactive type of play, which is distinct from earlier parallel or proximity play, because he has increased imaginative and physical skills and can share a common activity. The child's improved communication allows the nurse to learn more about him and his emerging personality as it is influenced by his increasing skills in all areas of development.

School-Age Stage

The school-age stage is age 6 through age 11. This time includes a portion of the prepubertal (or preadolescent) years, generally considered ages 10 to 12. Until the preadolescent growth spurt, the physical growth of a school-age child continues at his individual pace. Refinement of neuromuscular function is the major accomplishment of this stage. Rapid expansion of the school-age child's cognitive and social skills allows him to master a more complex and expanding environment. For example, the 9-year-old's increased abilities, his ability to engage in organized activities, and his desire to associate with peers allow him to pursue athletics and other activities.

During this stage the nurse can observe the individual's practice of skills and his energy investment as necessary for development; this is apparent in the school-age child's drive for achievement and mastery.

Adolescence

Adolescence begins at age 12 and extends through age 21. Physical growth is accelerated during this stage, including increases in all measurable indicators (height, weight, and dental, skeletal, and sexual age). The adolescent must mature to psychosocially emerge from this stage as an individual with a distinct identity.

This stage of life provides the nurse with an opportunity to observe (1) the adolescent in conflict, (2) how individuals develop coping behaviors, and (3) how individuals adapt to the conflicts present.

Young and Middle Adulthood

Young and middle adulthood spans the years from ages 22 to 65. Physical growth is complete at the onset of this stage with the individual having achieved his adult size and physical characteristics. Toward the end of this phase degenerative processes are occurring, often causing alterations in physical size and structure. The psychosocial processes involve increased and more intense relationships with other persons. Physical and psychosocial skills are refined and reshaped to allow the individual to proceed more effectively through this stage.

Observing individuals in this stage, the nurse learns about self-realization and how it is achieved, and about the adult maturational process. For example, the nurse may observe that some women achieve their potential by being homemakers, others by being working women, and still others by combining both roles. By recognizing that varied life-styles can provide potential and maturity, the nurse broadens her perspective on which to base care.

Older Adulthood

Older adulthood begins at age 65 and continues until death. No physical growth occurs during this stage, but rather a reversal process occurs in which body structures degenerate and functions slow. Psychosocial accomplishments and skills are varied and continue to be refined. Older adulthood is also a time for reflecting on life experiences and on the value of one's life and for making final alterations.

By observing individuals in this stage, the nurse learns the ways in which the end of life is approached, that is, with fear or acceptance. Nursing care can then be directed toward the individual's unique needs and responses. For example, a client who thinks only about what "might have been" will have more difficulty accepting death's imminence than one who believes he has accomplished his goals and contributed to his environment. Nursing care for the first individual would focus on helping him appreciate the value of his life. Nursing care for the second individual would focus on continued support.

Major Factors Influencing Growth and Development

The human being is a complex open system influenced by natural forces from within and by nurturing forces from the environment. The interaction between these forces ultimately affects the individual's development. In general, natural factors set the potential limits for an individual's development, while nurturing factors present opportunities for achieving that potential.

Forces of Nature

HEREDITY

The primary natural force influencing an individual's development is his genetic endowment, which is established at conception. The genetic endowment determines many aspects of the individual's physical and psychosocial being. Since the individual carries his unique genetic structure with him throughout life, this force affects all stages of development. For example, the same hereditary composition that determines an infant's sex, race, and hair color will also determine his physical growth and stature as an adolescent.

Heredity accounts in part for an individual's psychological uniqueness, as well as for the development of his physical characteristics. Research indicates that some behaviors are biologically inherited or influenced, particularly temperament (Thomas and Chess, 1977).

TEMPERAMENT

Temperament is defined as an individual's behavioral style. Three distinct temperaments have been documented: easy, slow to warm, and difficult (Table 23-2). Newborns have been found to demonstrate temperamental characteristics in the first weeks of life (Thomas and Chess, 1977). These behavioral characteristics influence subsequent interactions between the individual and his environment. A behavioral characteristic of a "difficult" individual is intense reactions such as anger. For example, because of his basic temperament, a "difficult" person may respond with anger to a request from a colleague to finish a report. His work environment, however, has taught him that overt expressions of anger are inappropriate.

Therefore he tempers his response to the colleague's request. If his response is not tempered and he becomes verbally hostile, he obviously affects his relationships in the work environment.

Understanding the variety of temperament characteristics and how they can affect the individual and his environment facilitates the nurse's ability to provide individualized care.

Forces of Nurturing

PSYCHOSOCIAL ENVIRONMENT

Family and peers are the most influential forces on an individual's psychosocial growth and development. The importance of these two factors should not be underestimated, for through family and peers an individual learns about himself, others, society, and the world in general.

FAMILY. The family is discussed in detail in Chapter 22. This section considers only the family's impact on the individual member. The family has a powerful influence on an individual's growth and development. The family's central purpose is the protection and promotion of family members (Duvall, 1977). Any interaction of the individual with other members of the family affects the individual and his developmental progression.

The family exerts its influence primarily through its universal functions, which include (1) helping the individual to survive, (2) providing security, (3) assisting the individual in his emotional and social development, (4) assisting the individual with maintenance of relationships, (5) teaching the individual about society and the world, and (6) assisting the

TABLE 23-2

Temperament and Personality Characteristics

Characteristic	Temperament		
	Easy	Slow to Warm	Difficult
Mood	Usually positive	Somewhat negative	Negative
Intensity of reaction to situations	Low to moderate	Low	High
Adaptability to new situations	Rapid	Slow	Slow
Regularity of body functions	Regular	Slow	Irregular
Reaction to new stimuli	Regular	Tendency to withdraw	Withdrawal
Activity level	Regular	Generally low	High

Modified from Thomas, A., and Chess, S.: Pediatr. Ann. **6**:26, 1977.

individual to learn roles and behaviors. The family molds the individual through its values, beliefs, customs, and expectations.

In addition, specific patterns and structures within the family influence the individual's growth and development. Each family establishes its own pattern of interaction and communication, based on assigned roles. For example, a 5-year-old girl may act coy and shy to get a toy from a male peer because this behavior works well with her older brother.

The individual's ordinal position in the family also influences development. Siblings expose the individual to a wider variety of skills and experiences, thereby promoting earlier and easier learning of motor, social, and language skills. However, the only child tends to have earlier intellectual development as a result of more frequent adult contact, whereas the youngest child with older siblings tends to be slower in language and social development because things are frequently done and said for him.

The sex of the individual also influences growth and development, primarily in terms of behavior. For example, boys tend to be more aggressive, physically and verbally, than girls, whereas girls usually exceed boys in verbal abilities and responsiveness to the peer group.

PEERS. An individual's peer group exerts the second greatest influence on development. Through and with the peer group the individual accomplishes a wide variety of developmental tasks, beginning in the early years and continuing throughout life. For example, a child cannot learn the skills of socialization without peers, the toddler must have age-mates if he is to learn to play, and the teenager needs peers in order to develop relationships.

The individual develops skills with peers in a manner distinctly different from that of the family; the individual also develops distinct styles of behavior for each group. Different styles of interacting are necessary because the patterns, structures, and functions of the two groups are different. For example, 8-year-olds learn to climb trees from peers (who may include siblings), not from parents. Once the skill has been mastered with peers, the child may proudly demonstrate it for his family.

Through the peer group an individual learns about success and failure, validates and challenges his thoughts, feelings, and concepts, and receives acceptance, support, and rejection as a unique person apart from his family. In addition, the peer group places demands, pressures, and expectations on the individual to adapt his behavior to achieve group purposes. Requests of the group are productive for the individual's development at some times, and nonproductive

at others. In general, interactions with peers leave lasting impressions.

The nurse should recognize and understand the importance of peers when providing care. This knowledge enables the nurse to assist the individual to use peer support and to balance the effect of peer influence.

LIFE EXPERIENCES

As the individual matures, he accumulates life experiences that enable him to progress developmentally by applying what has been learned to what needs to be learned. This learning process is the result of a series of steps. First, the individual must recognize and then master the task. In addition, the individual must master the skills and tasks of a developmental stage before progressing to the next stage, especially in closely related tasks and skills; for example, a toddler cannot climb if he has not learned to crawl as an infant.

Expertise in performing the assigned task follows mastery. This expertise expands the individual's capabilities within the environment. For example, the toddler who has learned to climb can push a chair to the countertop to reach the cookie jar or transfer his climbing expertise to the playground, which expands his environment.

Finally, these expert and expanded skills are integrated into the individual's whole functioning. Rather than focusing on a specific skill, the person uses his accumulated skills and experiences to develop a repertoire of effective behavior. For example, the preschooler who wants a cookie may use his past experiences of climbing and reaching (gross motor skills), opening and picking up (fine motor skills), and asking and saying please (language and socialization skills).

The nurse who recognizes the importance of life experiences in a person's development can individualize care by providing, modifying, or eliminating experiences.

HEALTH ENVIRONMENT

The individual's health affects not only his responsiveness to his environment but also the responsiveness of others to him. Of particular early importance are the prenatal environment, the nutritional state of the individual, and the adequacy of the individual's rest, sleep, exercise, and state of health.

PRENATAL HEALTH. The condition of the environment in which a fetus is conceived and grows affects the individual's future state of health. Both preconception and postconception factors influence fetal growth and development.

Factors that significantly affect the fetus's wellness and potential to grow, develop, and mature include the following:

1. Factors at conception
   a. Genetic
   b. Chromosomal
   c. Maternal age and health
   d. Blood incompatibilities
2. Maternal physical health during pregnancy
   a. Nutrition
   b. Substance use—drugs, alcohol, nicotine
   c. Weight gain
   d. Medical problems or previous conditions
3. Maternal psychosocial health during pregnancy
   a. Circumstances of conception and pregnancy
   b. Adjustment to pregnancy
   c. Past experiences, attitudes, and expectations
   d. Presence of support person(s)
4. Maternal use of prenatal health services
   a. Previous pregnancy history
   b. Degree of compliance with plan of care

The nurse promotes fetal growth and development through the assessment of prenatal factors and the promotion of maternal health. Good health in the prenatal stage is essential for the long-term health of the individual.

NUTRITION. The individual's nutritional state is significant in all stages of growth and development. Growth is regulated by dietary factors that have numerous effects. The adequacy of nutrients in the individual's diet influences whether and how physiological needs are met and subsequent growth and development (Whaley and Wong, 1983). Evidence of this effect is the fact that adequate brain growth is dependent on a balanced intake of nutrients, particularly fat. Without an adequate amount and balance of nutrients, deficits in height, weight, and developmental progression occur.

Knowledge about nutrition and its effects on growth and development is essential to all nursing care. Nutrition is a critical aspect of care for all individuals. Without this base, nursing's contribution is significantly reduced.

REST, SLEEP, AND EXERCISE. The individual's amount of rest, sleep, and exercise affect his growth and development. A balance between rest or sleep to provide the body with time to rejuvenate and exercise, the body's generating time, is similarly essential. An imbalance diminishes growth. The equilibrium reinforces physiological and psychological health. For example, a tired or overexerted child is cranky, fussy, and difficult to tolerate. A rested and relaxed child responds to his environment and its stimuli in a more pleasing, agreeable, and effective manner. Assisting individuals to achieve a balance between rest or sleep and exercise is an important nursing function. However, the nurse's recognition and understanding of the importance of such a balance must precede her ability to intervene in this area to promote health.

STATE OF HEALTH. The individual's current general state of health has an impact on subsequent developmental progression. Illness or injury has the potential for hampering growth and development. The nature and duration of the health problem influence its impact on developmental progress. For example, a 3-year-old who develops pneumonia may temporarily regress in his toilet training during the acute stage of the illness. A 3-year-old who is chronically ill may never develop bladder or bowel control because the nature of his illness physiologically prohibits control or leads to experiences (such as frequent hospitalizations) that disrupt the child's learning.

Individuals who experience the constant stress of a prolonged illness or injury may be unable to cope and to respond to the demands and tasks of their developmental stage (Whaley and Wong, 1983). In such situations the nurse's responsibility is twofold: to promote the individual's maximal health potential and, once that potential has been realized, to help the individual progress developmentally. For example, the nurse can help a chronically ill child remain free of acute respiratory infections by teaching the child and his family about the importance of good eating habits and obtaining adequate sleep and rest. Once the child achieves this relative level of health, the nurse can assist the child in completing his developmental tasks, such as toilet training, learning to share, or feeding and dressing himself.

LIVING ENVIRONMENT. Factors within the individual's everyday environment have an important effect on growth and development. Climate and season have been found to influence development. In particular, growth in height has been found to be faster in the spring and summer and growth in weight accelerates in the fall and winter. Warm or temperate climates may also influence the sanitary status of the environment, thereby affecting the individual's health.

Housing and the family's socioeconomic status have been found to influence growth and development. The more adequate and protective the housing and the higher the socioeconomic status, the greater the advantages and opportunities for growth and development. However, more does not necessarily mean better. The quality of a person's living environment may be more important than the quantity of socioeconomic resources when well-being is the goal.

Theories of Human Development

Since the beginning of this century, research into human growth and development has led to a number of different developmental theories. These theories vary in how humans are viewed and in what aspect of development is emphasized. Some theories view development as a continuous process, moving from the simple to the more complex. Others consider development as discontinuous, with alternating periods of relative equilibrium and disequilibrium. Different health care professionals often use different theoretical frameworks when providing care, which may complicate communication between health care providers. Therefore the nurse needs to be familiar with the more common theories to communicate effectively with other health professionals in planning, implementing, and evaluating coordinated health care. In addition, knowledge of various theories is essential for comprehensive nursing care because no one framework addresses all developmental areas of interest to nurses. The following sections review the most important developmental theories.

Freud's Psychoanalytic Theory

Sigmund Freud's theory of life development is called the psychoanalytic theory. Freud divides an individual's personality into three parts and hypothesizes five psychosexual stages of development. Freud's theory is based on analysis of clients with troubled behaviors.

According to Freud, the personality is composed of the id, the ego, and the superego. The id directs behaviors toward the goal of immediate gratification of needs. The newborn is ruled by the id. He cries and fusses until he feels the pleasure (gratification) he wants, that is, to be held, fed, or rocked. The superego is the individual's conscience. It is formed as the result of internalization of societal restrictions and demands. For example, the parental demand for a child to conform to certain expectations, such as telling the truth or sharing, leads to automatic learned behaviors on the part of the child. The ego represents the individual's conscious self, which has a compromising capacity. Dealing with the real world forces the individual to make a compromise between the permissiveness of the id and the restrictions of the superego. An example of the ego at work is the 16-year-old who wants to take his parents' car keys and go for a ride (id) but realizes that he may be placed on restriction and not be allowed to go to the weekend football game (superego); therefore he approaches his parents with his request to have the car to visit a friend for a specific length of time (ego).

Freud divides the mind into the conscious mind and the unconscious mind. The conscious mind includes all thoughts, feelings, or knowledge of which the individual is aware. The unconscious includes hidden thoughts, feelings, and desires, which may have been conscious at one time but are unconsciously repressed or consciously suppressed. Unconscious thoughts or feelings may emerge in dreams or in psychoanalysis.

TABLE 23-3

Freud's Stages of Development

Stage	Age (years)	Invested Body Zone	Significant Experiences
Oral	Birth-1	Mouth, lips, tongue	Sucking, rooting, feeding, weaning
Anal	2-3	Anal opening	Toilet training, holding on/letting go, exerting power and control by self
Phallic	4-5	Genitals	Genital manipulation, identification with same sex parent, developing gender characteristics
Latent	6-12	None hypothesized	Ego defense mechanisms, exhibits self-control behaviors, sex role and behaviors internalized
Genital	13 on	Genitals	Mature sexual identity, develops intimacy with others at varying levels of intensity

Modified from Hall, C.: A primer of freudian psychology, New York, 1954, The World Publishing Co.

Freud's theory of life development is based on a series of psychosexual stages through which an individual must pass. Specific developmental accomplishments must be attained in each stage, and at each stage psychic energy is invested in one primary body zone representing the developmental focus for that age. The specific body area changes from stage to stage and is the primary site for both expression and achievement of instinctual needs. Successful completion of each stage is necessary for subsequent stages to be entered without detrimental effects on future development. Table 23-3 presents a simplified view of Freud's stages of development.

Freud's psychoanalytic theory emphasizes the importance of early parent-child interactions and meeting instinctual needs. Alterations in health that involve these interactions, instincts, or invested body zones can have significant impact on the child's development. For example, an infant who has a cleft lip experiences interference in satisfying instinctual sucking needs and achieving oral gratification because of his inability to feed and suck effectively. The developing parent-infant bond may be hindered by the child's physical appearance.

Freud's theory of life development has several limitations: (1) it does not include all ages; (2) heavy emphasis is placed on physical and sexual development; (3) little emphasis is placed on adult behaviors and development; and (4) limited attention is given to cognitive and moral development. The theory cannot be easily applied to *normal* behavior, since it is based on data gathered from pathological behavior.

Despite its limitations, freudian theory is helpful in highlighting the importance of certain life experiences and early interactions that may have significant impact on later development. For example, the infant's need for oral stimulation should prompt the nurse to advise a new mother of her baby's need to suck more than when feeding. Knowing that a toddler wants to control his bowel movements enables the nurse to plan a gentle, positive program of toilet training that avoids a power struggle between the toddler and the mother and that is based on the toddler's physical and psychological readiness.

Erikson's Psychosocial Development Theory

Eric Erikson bases his theory of psychosocial development on the process of socialization. He views life development as a continuous struggle for an emotional-social equilibrium. While his theory acknowledges the presence of an id, an ego, and a superego as defined by freudian theory, Erikson's hypotheses emphasize ego development and learning to interact with the real world (Erikson, 1963). In addition, this theory places heavy emphasis on environmental influences and on the impact of parents, siblings, and extended family, as well as neighborhood, school, and society, on personality development.

According to Erikson the personality does not magically appear at a specific age; rather a person spends a lifetime constructing, shaping, and reshaping his personality. Psychological, social, biological, and environmental factors all influence the formation of the personality. Erikson defines stages of development during which specific tasks must be accomplished. These stages are similar to Freud's stages. The primary task of each stage has both positive and negative components, and the individual must satisfactorily balance the two components to progress developmentally. Through the achievement of these developmental tasks the individual resolves the conflict of the stage and attains an emotional-social equilibrium. However, Erikson stresses that the negative counterparts are never completely mastered and that they must be reexperienced periodically throughout life (Erikson, 1963). For example, a preschooler who has developed a trusting relationship (the basic task of infancy) continues to experience mistrust (the negative counterpart) when separated from his mother in the first week of nursery school. Concurrently, the mother must deal with her sense of guilt for creating feelings of mistrust in her child when she leaves him. The nurse who understands Erikson's theory and the delicate nature of the emotional-social equilibrium that must be achieved can facilitate the preschooler's and mother's coping through anticipatory guidance.

Erikson's stages of life development are summarized in the following paragraphs. Table 23-4 outlines all the stages and provides examples of stage mastery.

In stage I the conflict is *basic trust versus mistrust*. This stage occurs from birth to approximately 1 year of age. The newborn enters the world dependent on others for meeting his needs. If basic needs are met through a predictable and comforting relationship with the mother or other care giver, the infant develops a sense of trust. If needs are not met or are met only sporadically, the infant develops a sense of mistrust because he is never certain that expressed needs will be met.

Much of the foundation for psychosocial competence is developed during this stage. Without a sense of trust, peer and possibly intimate relationships will be difficult for the individual to sustain. Therefore the importance of a consistent, loving early care giver who is primarily responsible for the child cannot be overstated.

The conflict of stage II is *autonomy versus shame*

TABLE 23-4

Erikson's Stages of Development

Stage	Conflict	Developmental Task (sense to be achieved)	Approximate Age (years)	Behavior(s) Indicating Mastery
I	Trust versus mistrust	Trust	1	Separates from mother, explores environment, is not overly anxious or fretful
II	Autonomy versus shame and doubt	Autonomy	2-4	Feeds self, is toilet trained, has good control of gross motor function
III	Initiative versus guilt	Initiative	4-8	Adjusts to school and social spheres outside the home, plays cooperatively with peers
IV	Industry versus inferiority	Industry	8-12	Demonstrates school performance appropriate to age, follows instructions taking task to completion, participates in organized peer activities, is responsible for personal hygiene
V	Identity versus role confusion	Identity	13-20	Develops peer relationships with both sexes, defines goals in life, selects and prepares for vocation, gains independence from family
VI	Intimacy and solidarity versus isolation	Intimacy	20-30	Completes education, achieves economic independence through vocation, selects relationship partner and life-style, contributes to society (socially responsible)
VII	Generativity versus self-absorption and stagnation	Generativity	30-60	Stabilizes career, demonstrates concern for family and next generation, participates in community activities
VIII	Integrity versus despair	Integrity	60-death	Serves as counselor and advisor to younger generations, develops interests and abilities according to physical functioning, enjoys accomplishments

Modified from Erikson, E.: Childhood and society, New York, 1963, W.W. Norton & Co., Inc.

and doubt. Between the ages of 2 and 4 the child faces the task of developing a sense of autonomy. The child partially achieves this task by discovering the difference between independence and dependence. However, before a toddler can make this discrimination, he must have developed a sense of trust in the significant care giver; trusting allows the child to experience separateness of self and care giver.

In viewing themselves as separate beings, toddlers begin to explore their world. This exploration is made possible by increased physical abilities such as walking, climbing, and running. Toddlers quickly learn that their own behaviors influence their world and the people in that world. As an increasingly active contributor to the environment, the toddler effects changes that promote his sense of autonomy and independence.

Although exploration and independence are fun and challenging, they also present the child with unknowns that are sometimes frightening. Thus the toddler still needs and seeks closeness and dependence at times. The struggle of this stage involves balancing the behaviors that meet needs for both dependence and independence.

The conflict of stage III is *initiative versus guilt*. Between the ages of 4 and 8 years, children strive to set and achieve their own goals. To do this, they must master new skills and expand their world to include the school and neighborhood. They begin to assert themselves and their personalities more often at home and in environments outside the home.

Dependence needs continue throughout this phase, and children must continue to resolve the conflict between independence and dependence. Guilt feelings may arise when needs for dependence override needs for independence. The child's challenge is to achieve an equilibrium between wanting to stay near the family and familiar surroundings and wanting to reach out and assert or express individual feelings and behaviors. The child's developing physical, social, and language skills assist in the resolution of this phase, and play is the primary means of expression.

The conflict of stage IV is *industry versus inferiority*. This phase includes the middle school years, approximately ages 8 through 12. To achieve the task of developing a sense of industry rather than inferiority, children direct their energies toward physical, social, and cognitive skill competence (that is, industry). However, these skills are frequently underdeveloped or unequal to the situation, and a sense of inadequacy and inferiority results. Most school-age children experience periodic feelings of inferiority, but they are generally quick to recognize and use their competencies to handle these feelings, thereby avoiding long-term feelings of inadequacy.

During this phase of development a child becomes a productive group member. Eventually his capacity to contribute, collaborate, and work cooperatively in relationships toward a common goal becomes a measure of his success.

The conflict of stage V is *identity versus confusion*. Between 13 and 20 years of age, a person must leave childhood and become an adult. Adolescents must establish their own identity or be caught in confusion about their role in society and in social interactions. Intimate relationships must be established or social isolation may occur. Choices about sexuality must be made and the appropriate sexual behaviors mastered. Life-style and vocation decisions are necessary or the individual is adrift without goals.

This phase can be a chaotic one for the adolescent and those around him. While the adolescent's peer and social spheres are expanding, the expectations from others also increase. The individual must develop adult social and cognitive skills and establish

an equilibrium and emotional independence from his family.

In stage VI the conflict is *intimacy versus isolation*. Young adulthood, between 20 and 30 years of age, is the phase when the individual enters into reciprocal and successful love and work relationships or chooses to remain apart (isolated) from others in his environment. Allowing others to become close and share the physical and psychosocial aspects of his personality is the primary challenge. Most individuals in this phase choose to complete their education or training, build a career, select a significant other, and become involved with community and society. The person who is unable to make these choices and decisions becomes isolated from age-mates and work-mates, as well as society.

In stage VII the conflict is *generativity versus self-absorption*. Middle adulthood, ages 30 to 60, is a time when an individual is interested in establishing and guiding the next generation. An additional primary task in this phase is to ensure the continuation of one's work and life-style. Some individuals achieve a sense of generativity by rearing a family, others by promoting a cause, and still others by developing careers.

When the adult is unable to assume responsibility for promoting the future, he experiences a sense of stagnation. The individual who feels stagnant becomes self-absorbed and is unable to relate effectively to his world.

The conflict of stage VIII is *integrity versus despair*. During this stage the older adult, a person 60 or beyond, struggles to feel a sense of worth about his life and achievements. When the older adult feels his actions have been significant in his world, he has a sense of integrity. Frequently this feeling of worth is reinforced when others seek the person's leadership and guidance. Recognition by others that the older adult is wiser because of his experiences brings a sense of fulfillment. However, the individual who is unable to identify or accept his worth or who lacks the opportunity to act as an experienced person may feel despair and isolation.

Erikson's theory of life development emphasizes growth and development and conflict as an ongoing process. This is a realistic approach, since an individual's thoughts, feelings, and environment are seldom the same at all times. A person's ability to change and adapt behavior is important in maintaining control over his life. Erikson's theory addresses both what a person is attempting to achieve at a given time and what he wishes to avoid. With this theory the nurse can provide care directed toward the individual's particular stage of development. For example, the nurse who recognizes that a young school-age child is trying to establish a sense of initiative might encourage the child to enter an art contest at school if he likes drawing. At the same time the nurse encourages the child's parents to be supportive and positive, even if the outcome is not first prize.

The primary limitations of Erikson's theory are twofold. First, the age ranges for each stage are large, making it difficult to assign the completion of a task to a certain age. For example, the nurse cannot definitely determine that by age 20 an individual will have developed a sense of identity. The nurse can only recognize that this is the individual's goal. This age range variation may be particularly a problem for the adult stages because they are so broadly defined. Behavior patterns typical of the adult stages are also not as tangible or easily assessed as with the younger life cycle stages. Second, the task of one stage may overlap the next stage. For example, a child must have developed a degree of trust before he can initiate actions or behaviors reflective of his personality.

When using Erikson's theory in nursing practice, the nurse needs to recognize that achievement in a stage is not absolute. For example, the older adult who does not feel a sense of integrity is not necessarily consumed with despair. Also, a wide spectrum of behavioral patterns is available to the individual in achieving the positive portion of the stage. The key to progression through the stages is the individual's development of a balance between the two major conflicts of the stage. For example, an older person may feel unhappy about one aspect of his life but fulfilled about another. The nurse's role is to help the individual recognize both his assets and his liabilities and to build on his assets.

Maslow's Theory of Human Needs

Abraham Maslow developed a theory of growth and development based on a set of human needs. The stages of development are not divided by chronological age, since several of the needs may exist at one time (Brown and Murphy, 1981). However, ages when particular needs are most critical can be generally identified (Table 23-5).

Maslow views the most basic needs of human beings as physiological well-being and homeostasis. The needs are shaped by the human body's demand for food, water, shelter, and oxygen. Since the infant depends on others to provide these basic demands, infancy becomes the first stage in this theory. Movement into the next stage occurs once basic needs are met and the individual is physically able to proceed (Brown and Murphy, 1981).

In the second stage the need is for physical safety, which can be provided by clothing, a stable living

TABLE 23-5

Maslow's Hierarchy of Needs

Predominant Age of Need	Need
Infancy (birth-1½ years)	Physiological needs—food, warmth, shelter, oxygen, elimination
Toddler/preschool (2-5 years)	Physical safety—clothing, stable environment, rules and laws, freedom from fear, anxiety, and danger
Across all ages	Affection—parents, friends, family, relationships, community, country
School age and adolescence (6-19 years)	Self-esteem—control, respect, dignity, competence
Adolescence and adulthood (13 years and up)	Prestige—appreciation, importance, wisdom, motivation
Young to older adult	Self-actualization—contentment, satisfaction, homeostasis, fulfillment

Modified from Brown, M., and Murphy, M.: Ambulatory pediatrics for nurses, ed. 2, New York, 1981, McGraw-Hill Book Co.; and Maslow, A.: Toward a psychology of being, New York, 1968, Van Nostrand Reinhold Co., Inc.

environment, societal rules, and laws. Evidence of this developmental phase can be witnessed in all age groups, but the specific safety need varies. For example, the toddler who is expanding his physical world is more in need of a safe, stable living environment, such as a backyard in which to play, than is an older adult. The adult, on the other hand, has a greater need to live by the rules of the society and community.

The need for affection, love, and relationships dominates Maslow's third stage of development. This stage begins at birth, when a bond of affection is essential to well-being. The need for maternal love progresses to include the father, other family members, and friends. The love or affection developed broadens over the course of time to include relationships of varying depth, such as love of a spouse or an adult friend or even a feeling of belonging to a group. The object of love may be family, peers, or community.

The need for self-esteem is the fourth stage. The individual demonstrates a need to have control, respect, and competence. Infants and young children express this need by controlling parents with their responses. For example, the toddler quickly learns he can get a cookie if he asks and smiles rather than cries. Adults show this need by endeavoring to do well at work, thereby securing the respect of colleagues and feeling competent.

The fourth stage revolves around the need for prestige and is closely associated with the need for self-esteem. All human beings need to feel important and appreciated. This stage and the need for self-esteem are particularly motivating for adults.

The fifth and final phase in Maslow's theory is self-actualization. The individual has met all the other needs, is content with himself, and has developed an equilibrium within himself and with the environment.

Maslow's theory is useful to the nurse because it focuses on basic physical and psychosocial needs that are essential to human life. Recognizing the importance of these needs at certain times in the individual's life enables the nurse to facilitate their satisfaction. For example, a nurse who knows that all humans need love relationships can help the mother of a teenage girl understand the adolescent's desire for a steady boyfriend.

This theory also clearly demonstrates that development continues throughout life. It emphasizes continued meeting of needs rather than accomplishment of a state. However, several limitations exist: (1) self-actualization is a goal that is difficult to maintain; (2) the absence of specific age groups makes assessment of need satisfaction difficult; and (3) the complexities of the human being are not fully explained with an approach that centers on basic needs.

Piaget's Theory of Cognitive Development

Piaget's theory focuses on the development of cognition. Cognitive processes such as abstract reasoning, problem solving, and intellectual growth develop gradually through the childhood years and reach a stable operational phase in adolescence that is subsequently refined through the adult years.

According to Piaget, a variety of new experiences or stimuli must exist for learning to occur. The individual responds to these stimuli through assimilation and accommodation. Assimilation is the process in which a person incorporates new experiences into his current activity or thinking; that is, the individual adapts experiences for repeated use. For example, when the toddler sees a horse for the first time, he fits it into his current schema of four-legged animals and calls it a "doggie"; the experience and environ-

ment are adapted by the child. Accommodation is the process of responding to the environment through a new activity and thinking; that is, the individual himself adapts to the experience (Tackett and Hunsberger, 1981). For example, the toddler who wants a cookie asks his mother for one because he was punished last time for climbing the chair and taking it; the child changes himself to fit the experience and environment. The combination of these two processes allows the individual to organize his world by ordering and classifying his experiences. The result of this organization is adaptation or the balance between person and environment.

Using the processes of assimilation and accommodation, Piaget theorizes a sequence of intellectual development (Table 23-6). The first stage is the sensorimotor period, involving the first 2 years of life. During this period the infant moves from reflexive to symbolic behavior and uses his body extensively for expression and communication. The infant passes through six substages during this sensorimotor period:

1. *Substage 1.* This substage lasts from birth to 1 month of age and is characterized by primitive reflexes and random body movements (for example, the "startle" or Moro reflex) that usually result in the parent comforting the neonate.
2. *Substage 2.* This substage lasts from 1 to 4½ months of age and is characterized by habits of behavior learned by chance and repeated for pleasurable benefit (for example, crying to bring comfort or food). Repetitive reflex and random movements are the means of expression.
3. *Substage 3.* This substage lasts from 4½ to 9 months of age and is characterized by behaviors that are discovered accidentally and that are purposely repeated as a means for making the environment more interesting (for example, dropping food over the side of the high chair provokes a response in the mother or smearing it on the tray makes it look different; both actions change the environment and make it more interesting). Hand-eye coordination is essential.
4. *Substage 4.* This substage lasts from 9 to 12 months of age and is characterized by the coordination of more complex behaviors; perception begins to develop and the infant learns to avoid obstacles (for example, the child climbs down the stairs backward or learns that moving the toy out of the way is easier and faster than crawling around it).
5. *Substage 5.* This substage lasts from 12 to 18 months of age and is characterized by experimental behaviors. Different ways are discovered to achieve the desired results. Trial and error

TABLE 23-6

Piaget's Stages of Cognitive Development

Stage	Age (years)	Qualitative Change
Sensorimotor	Birth-2	Development proceeds from reflexive experience with the environment to controlled manipulations and ultimately to mental representations of the events.
Preoperational	2-7	Physical manipulation is no longer essential, but internal representations are extremely egocentric; solution of problems does not necessarily follow logical thought processes.
Concrete operations	7-11	Logical operations are developed and the child increasingly applies them to the solution of concrete problems; the child begins to understand relationships between objects.
Formal operations	11 and up	Logical operations can now be applied to solving hypothetical and verbal problems, as well as concrete problems.

and memory retention become evident as does beginning reasoning (for example, pointing, speaking, and whining all gain attention, but the child begins to realize that pointing achieves the desired result faster).

6. *Substage 6.* This substage lasts from 18 to 24 months of age and is characterized by symbolic thought and beginning ability to form mental images. The infant imitates others and learns the permanence of objects (for example, the child plays peek-a-boo and knows that a person will be there when his eyes open).

During the second period of cognitive development, the preoperational stage (from 2 to 7 years), the child sees things mainly from his own point of view. The child considers everything to be real and ascribes lifelike qualities to inanimate objects. Children in this cognitive period believe that they can make things happen just by thinking them and that the world exists for them alone. For example, the child who is hiding by turning his back and covering his eyes believes that he cannot be seen because he cannot see anyone. In this stage the child may appear quite illogical. By the end of this period the child learns to use language and memory and to understand past, present, and future events. The preoperational stage includes two substages:

1. *Substage 1.* Substage 1, from 2 to 4 years of age, is called the preconceptual phase. It is characterized by the ability to form mental images of unseen things. Play, language, and imitation are the primary tools for development of these images. Things are interpreted literally (for example, a child imagines cats and dogs falling from the sky when told, "It's raining cats and dogs").

2. *Substage 2.* Substage 2, from 4 to 7 years of age, is called the perceptual or intuitive stage. It is characterized by prelogical reasoning. At the end of this phase the child has become more social, is able to use language effectively to express himself, and is expanding experiences outside the home. Experiences and objects are judged by results and appearances (for example, when given a choice, a child will insist that a nickel is worth more than a dime because it is larger).

The third period of cognitive development occurs between 7 and 11 years of age and is called the concrete operations stage. Early in this period, thinking is based on the immediate, unanalyzed relationships between events in the environment and the child's point of view. The child cannot consider both whole and parts simultaneously but focuses only on the whole or the parts. For example, the 7-year-old child thinks it is unfair when he is not allowed to sleep over at a friend's house, failing to see the relationship between being denied the fun and the facts that it is a school night and the friend's younger brother is sick.

Toward the end of this stage, 9- to 11-year-old children demonstrate a greater reasoning ability and realism. According to Piaget, this stage of concrete operations allows children to realize that their way of thinking is not the only way, and now they are able to consider parts of the whole while maintaining a concept of the whole. Children at the end of this stage are able to consider a problem or event logically and arrive at a conclusion or solution. In the previous example, the 10-year-old child would not ask to spend the night at his friend's house, but rather would ask if his friend could sleep over on a weekend night.

Piaget's final stage of cognitive development begins

around 11 years of age and continues throughout life. This stage of formal operational thinking is characterized by logical reasoning. The individual develops the ability to use abstract logic, examine relationships, construct hypotheses, and test his thoughts through deductive reasoning. An example of this thought process is the adolescent's ability to consider multiple factors and decide whether to go to college or join the workforce.

Piaget's theory of cognitive development provides a well-defined framework for understanding intellectual abilities. The stages offer insight into how interactions are processed and interpreted based on the individual's skill. This approach is particularly useful to the nurse in providing care to children. For example, a nurse can explain to a toddler's mother that the child's thoughts at this age are egocentric, illogical, and literal and thus assist the mother to find more effective ways to communicate with the child. Similarly, recognizing that the school-age child is able to consider events logically in part or in their entirety should prompt the nurse to allow the 10-year-old child to give his own history in an acute care visit for a sore throat. Finally, recognizing the adolescent's ability to analyze problems systematically and arrive at solutions, the nurse counseling a teenage girl about birth control methods can discuss the advantages and disadvantages and allow the teenager to make the decision.

Piaget's theory is not without limitations, however. This theory deals only with cognition and does not take into account all psychosocial aspects of the personality. Furthermore, research shows that cognitive processes may be intermixed between stages and not as well defined or as universal as Piaget hypothesizes. When applying this theory in nursing situations, therefore, the nurse should assess the cognitive progression, as well as the psychosocial needs of the individual.

Havighurst's Theory of Developmental Tasks

Havighurst theorizes that learning is essential to life and that to understand growth and development one must understand learning and accept the premise that the human being continues to learn throughout his life (Havighurst, 1964). For example, a person learns to walk, to play, to develop relationships, to hold a job, to rear children, and to adjust to retirement. Furthermore, Havighurst postulates that learning is more difficult at some times than at others. Ultimately learning is responsible for the individual's patterns of behavior. All humans have the biological need to eat, for example, but feeding habits are learned and highly individualized.

Basic behaviors or actions that must be learned, such as walking, living with a spouse, or adjusting to changes associated with retirement, are described by Havighurst as developmental tasks. These developmental tasks are biological, social, and psychological and arise at a certain period in life. Successful achievement of the task leads to happiness and success with later tasks, and failure leads to unhappiness, disapproval by society, and difficulty with later tasks (Havighurst, 1964).

Developmental tasks originate in the individual's new or expanding physical and psychological resources and requirements. Some tasks arise strictly from physical maturation (for example, walking when legs and muscles are developed). Other tasks originate in societal or cultural expectations (for example, learning to add or read). Tasks come from within the individual through personal motives and aspirations or values (for example, becoming vice president of the firm because the individual desires it). Most developmental tasks involve a combination of these factors (for example, the child wins the spelling bee because he is expected to read and spell but also because he desires to be the best).

Similar to other theorists, Havighurst describes age periods during which the individual must normally accomplish the task in order to grow and develop. These stages and the primary tasks are described in Table 23-7.

Havighurst's approach is useful to the nurse because it describes specific accomplishments that the person must achieve, thereby facilitating goal-oriented nursing care. For example, a task of early adulthood is to take on civic responsibility. Knowledge of this task assists the nurse in helping the individual identify his feelings and accomplish this task in places such as his church, his child's school, or a political campaign. In addition, Havighurst's framework suggests that timing is important to learning. This provides the nurse with additional information on which to base care. For example, the nurse would not advise the mother of a 12-month-old infant to begin toilet training because the optimal physiological and psychological time for this learning is 24 to 30 months of age.

Havighurst's theory is limited by its overemphasis on learning and by the inflexible outcomes of learning (that is, success or failure with no adaptation). Since outcomes are socially and historically defined in this theory, it is somewhat outdated in defining tasks and choices. The theory does not address the multitude of other factors that can influence development (such as genetics, past experiences, and natural circumstances). Nursing care is generally based on human needs and individual differences, and encouraging constant success and excellence is not always realistic.

TABLE 23-7	

Havighurst's Development Tasks

Age Period	Tasks
Infancy and early childhood	Learn to walk, to take solid foods, to talk, to control elimination of body wastes, sex differences and sexual modesty, to relate emotionally to parents, siblings, and others, to distinguish right from wrong (develop a conscience); achieve physiological stability; form simple concepts of social and physical reality
Middle childhood	Learn physical skills necessary for ordinary games, to get along with age-mates, appropriate masculine or feminine social role; develop wholesome attitude toward self, skills in reading, writing, and calculating, concepts necessary for everyday living, morality, values, personal independence, attitudes toward social groups and institutions
Adolescence	Achieve mature relations with peers of both sexes, masculine or feminine social role, acceptance of one's body and image, emotional independence of parents and other adults, economic independence, selection and preparation for an occupation, preparation for marriage and family life, intellectual skills and concepts necessary for civic competence, socially responsible behavior, set of values and an ethical system
Early adulthood	Select a mate; learn to live with significant other; start family; rear children; manage a home; begin occupation; assume civic responsibility; identify with a social group
Middle age	Achieve adult civic and social responsibility; establish and maintain an economic standard of living; assist children to become responsible, happy adults; develop leisure activities; relate to spouse on a more intense basis; accept and adjust to physiological changes of middle age; adjust to and accept own aging parents
Later maturity	Accept and adjust to decreased physical strength and health; adjust to retirement, lower income, aging, and inevitable death of self and spouse; establish affiliation with age group; meet social and civic obligations; live in satisfactory physical environment

Modified from Havighurst, R.: Developmental tasks and education, ed. 2, New York, 1964, David McKay Co., Inc.

Havighurst's theory provides little room for the individual's adaptation or for relative degrees of success. For example, many adolescents today are not selecting occupations, going to college, or preparing for marriage but are postponing these decisions until young adulthood. Therefore the nurse needs to be aware that not all tasks defined by Havighurst apply to all adolescents. Developmental assessment must be individualized.

Social Learning Theory

Social learning theorists view human development as a process of learning and changing behavior. These theorists argue that, except for reflexes, there are no inborn structures that organize experiences and behaviors. Instead, specific behaviors are learned through a process of reinforcement. Furthermore, the theorists hypothesize that behaviors are drives that determine the individual's responses, are influenced by social cues, and must be reinforced. For example, a school-age child likes to win a fair contest. This desire to win motivates the child in many situations.

Social cues depend on the situation in which the child desires to win; that is, his friends may tease him for being a "brain" when he enters the science fair but support him when he misses a soccer goal. The child responds to the cues but not always in a consistent manner. The reinforcement the child receives for his response to the cues, along with his desire to win, determines which cues he will act on in the future and which responses will become extinct. The child in the previous example favors the support rather than the teasing and therefore focuses his desire to win on the soccer field and not at the science fair.

The concept of reinforcement is important in social learning theory. Reinforcements may be tangible (money, food, or toys) or abstract (praise, a smile, a frown, or verbal admonishment). The effectiveness of the reinforcement depends on the individual and the interaction. Furthermore, reinforcement may be positive or negative depending on the individual. For example, an apple might be a positive reward for one child who finishes his vegetables but no reward at all for another child, who prefers a cookie. Positive reinforcement generally increases a behavior and negative reinforcement causes extinction of the behavior.

Social learning theorists consider imitation another source of behavior. The individual imitates a person he views as valuable and worthy of imitation. If the imitation is reinforced, the behavior is continued. For example, the 4-year-old girl who is reinforced with laughs and smiles for dressing up in her mother's clothes is more likely to develop feminine characteristics and behaviors.

One limitation of the social learning theory is that little attention is given to the natural or inborn characteristics of the individual. The nurse frequently bases care on the individual's ability to direct his own destiny, and the simple pattern of reinforcement does not promote self-direction, since someone other than the individual must decide what behaviors to reinforce.

Social learning theory does have applications, however, particularly in situations where behaviors need to be changed. For example, the nurse can teach parents the principles of reinforcement for use in child rearing. Nursing care designed to help a client lose weight or stop smoking often employs these principles as well. The most important factor to remember in implementing such plans of care is that the individual must be motivated and capable of the behavior.

Kohlberg's Theory of Moral Development

Moral development is one component of psychosocial development; it involves the individual's establishment of a moral code that is consistent with society. Moral development depends on the child's ability to accept his social responsibility and to integrate personal principles of justice and fairness (Tackett and Hunsberger, 1981). For example, the 3-year-old child may tell his age-mate that they must share but may not have the ability himself to share consistently. In addition, the child's knowledge of right and wrong and behavioral expression of this knowledge must be founded on respect and regard for the integrity and rights of others. For example, the child who copies a friend's homework and does not admit his wrongdoing when the friend is accused and penalized has not developed a satisfactory moral code involving honesty and respect for others.

Kohlberg states that moral development follows the development of the ability to reason. According to this theory, moral development occurs in three levels, each of which has two stages (Table 23-8).

Level 1, preconventional or premoral morality, spans the approximate ages of 4 to 9 years. During this phase children perceive rules as absolute and unchangeable and are motivated primarily by a desire to avoid punishment or obtain a reward. This perception is congruent with the intellectual egocentricity and realism of children this age.

Stage 1 of the premoral level is characterized by this punishment-obedience orientation. For example, a 5-year-old child may initially refuse to dress himself for school but will do so if prompted because he wants to please his mother or avoid being scolded.

Stage 2 of the premoral level is naive hedonistic orientation in which the child does right to earn a favor or reward (Nelms and Mullins, 1982). The child at this stage begins to have some idea of reciprocal interaction but is primarily motivated to behave correctly for his own reward. For example, a young school-age child may bargain with his parents by saying, "I won't like you or hug you if you don't let me play in the snow."

The conventional morality level (ages 9 to 12) is based on the child's perception of rules that exist for the good of all. In stage 3 the child conforms to rules to please others and to garner approval. Internal standards begin to develop and behavior is group oriented. For example, a 10-year-old child generally asks permission to do things (sometimes to a fault) and expects all others to do the same.

Stage 4 occurs in the conventional morality level and is characterized by motives and standards that develop from a sense of conformity and to avoid censure from authority figures (Nelms and Mullins, 1982). For example, children in this stage view police as legitimate keepers of law and order. Therefore breaking the law by shoplifting seems immoral because they would have to answer to the police.

In the principled morality level (12 years and up) the individual accepts rules on the basis of his own judgment. The individual deals with moral issues in the abstract and accepts degrees of right or wrong when varying societal standards conflict.

In stage 5 the individual considers societal laws contracts between himself and society (for example, the individual will not rob others in society and others in society will not rob him). However, society's laws may be changed by mutual consent if they are deemed unjust. Stage 6 involves moral principles. This is an inner-directed phase that emphasizes doing what is morally right regardless of the circumstances. In this stage the individual has internalized moral standards.

Kohlberg's theory provides the nurse with a basis on which to assess the individual's moral development. By assessing the extent to which the individual has completed a level or stage, the nurse can help guide the individual, particularly if he is a child, toward a productive, wholesome life. If the individual encounters difficulty in a developmental stage, this theory may help both the individual and the nurse

TABLE 23-8

Kohlberg's Theory of Moral Development

Level and Stage	Age (years)	Characteristics
Level 1: Premoral	4-9	External control emphasized; behavior motivated by desire to receive reward or to avoid punishment
Stage 1: Obedience and punishment orientation	Probably 4-6	Good behavior to avoid punishment
Stage 2: Naive hedonistic orientation	Probably 6-9	Good behavior to reap a reward; beginning notion of reciprocity conforms to rules for own interest and social acceptance
Level 2: Conventional	9-12	Conforms to rules to please others; internal standards beginning to evolve; group-oriented concerns dictate to moral behaviors
Stage 3: "Good boy" orientation	Probably 9-10	Primary goal of pleasing others; conforms to rules to avoid negative reinforcement from care givers; gains a sense of what being "nice" is
Stage 4: Authority maintains morality	Probably 10-12	Conforms to avoid censure by legal authorities; perceives a need for social order
Level 3: Self-accepted moral principles	Adolescence throughout life	Deals with moral issues abstractly; experiences conflict between social standards; faces choices over questionable right or wrong
Stage 5: Contractual morality	Adolescence throughout life	Forms contracts with society in order to maintain morality; dysfunctional laws may be changed through an orderly process
Stage 6: Principles of conscience	Adolescence throughout life	Moral standards internalized by individual; need to do what is morally right, regardless of consequences

Modified from Kohlberg, L.: Stage and sequences: the cognitive-developmental approach to socialization. In Goslin, D.A., editor: Handbook of socialization theory and research, Chicago, 1969, Rand McNally & Co.; and Nelms, B., and Mullins, R.: Growth and development: a primary health care approach, Englewood Cliffs, N.J., 1982, Prentice-Hall, Inc.

understand the conflict. For example, the adolescent who is concerned about his friends' alcohol consumption but does not wish to alienate them by reporting their drinking may better understand this conflict by discussing with the nurse his moral beliefs and the dictates of his conscience. Such issues are excellent topics for teen groups or health education seminars because they help group members to explore their moral development.

The theory of moral development does have limitations, however. A person may be in several stages at once, and the ages assigned to the phases may be different for different individuals. The highest level of moral development is not necessarily more satisfactory for the individual and society than a lower phase of development (Nelms and Mullins, 1982). Finally, Kohlberg's theory focuses only on morality and does not address other psychosocial issues.

TABLE 23-9

Overview of Development Theories

Theory	Stages	Characteristics	Strengths	Limitations
Freudian psychoanalytical theory	Five age-related fixed stages	Basis of inner drives; psychosexual focus	Recognizes importance of instinctual needs; defines id, ego, superego as personality	Heavy emphasis on sexual behaviors; does not deal with adult development; based on data from psychiatric clients
Erikson's psychosocial development theory	Eight interdependent stages	Socialization focus; ongoing process throughout life directed toward balance; stages with positive and negative compoments that individual must balance	Recognizes role of social, biological, and environmental factors in development; relates specific tasks to appropriate age; well organized; includes all ages	Broad age ranges; does not include cognitive or moral development; tasks within stages are not absolute
Maslow's theory of human need	Six overlapping and variable need achievement levels	Human need focus; ongoing process directed toward homeostasis	Identifies human needs; recognizes physical and psychosocial aspects of person	Does not identify age chronologically, making assessment difficult; last stage/goal not generally attainable in absolute sense; does not fully explain the complex nature of human beings
Piaget's theory of cognitive development	Four major fixed stages; substages in first two major stages	Cognitive focus; defines process in terms of assimilation, accommodation, and adaptation	Accounts for heredity and environmental interaction; well defined; incorporates language concepts	Does not deal with psychosocial aspects; does not account for individual differences and variability in progression; strict hierarchical progress questionable
Havighurst's developmental tasks	Six fixed stages	Learning to develop is focus; ascribes a certain set of socially defined tasks to each age group	Specific definition of tasks needing completion; goal-oriented development; practical and organized by age; recognizes the importance of timing to development	Some tasks not reflective of changes in today's society; overemphasis on learning and somewhat inflexible in outcome (i.e., no adaptation); does not deal with cognition
Social learning theory	No stages	Based on drives, cues, responses, and reinforcement; behavior oriented; imitation major source of learned behavior	Achieves behavioral results; stimulus-response pattern well defined; applicable to all age groups without restraint	Does not recognize natural forces in humans; little recognition of psychosocial needs; little recognition of individuality and may not promote self-direction
Kohlberg's theory of moral development	Three levels and six stages that are overlapping and variable in regard to age	Follows a sequence corresponding to cognition; morality developed when cognitively prepared	Assigns order and definition to moral code development; serves as a basis for assessment of morality	Levels and stages are not absolute—variability probably does exist; final level difficult to achieve; does not address psychosocial issues

Selecting a Developmental Framework for Nursing

Providing nursing care to clients of all developmental stages is easier when the nurse bases her planning on a theoretical framework. An organized, systematic approach ensures that the client's needs are assessed and met by the care plan. If nursing care is delivered only as a series of isolated actions, one or more of the client's developmental needs may be overlooked. A developmental approach encourages organized care that is directed toward the client's current level of functioning to motivate self-direction and health promotion. For example, understanding an adolescent's need to become independent should prompt the nurse to establish a contract with a teenage client regarding the plan of care and its implementation.

The developmental approach also has advantages for the client. His current capabilities are used and he is actively involved in his own care. This total health is also promoted because the nurse is aware of his present developmental stage and the direction in which he is headed. Therefore the nurse can focus on health activities that promote task or development completion. For example, the nurse might encourage a young adult client to apply for a job promotion because both nurse and client recognize that he needs to establish his career, that he is motivated, and that he desires to succeed.

Although a developmental approach is expedient in nursing practice, no single theory addresses all needs relevant to nursing. All of these theories have advantages and disadvantages; the key to their importance in nursing practice is usefulness in guiding nursing assessment, diagnosis, planning, intervention, and evaluation of care. An ideal framework would be applicable to clients of all ages in a variety of settings and would consider the physical, psychosocial, and cognitive processes of the client. No one theory meets all these criteria. Therefore the nurse must combine the most useful aspects of several theories into a practical approach.

If the nurse integrates the various stage theories in a life span perspective, she can focus care on the aspect of development that demonstrates need. For example, nursing activities for a client with acute pneumonia would be based on meeting physical and psychosocial needs related to the illness. The nurse would concern herself with care that returns the client to a healthy state and that helps him deal with treatment, hospitalization, and recovery. Nursing care would not initially focus on promoting the client's career or deciding whether he should marry or move to a new community unless these were directly tied to the immediate concerns of the client.

A general age-stage developmental framework for nursing practice allows for individuality, even though most people share common experiences in the general developmental processes. Because individuals respond differently to common experiences and needs, movement within and between stages is highly individualized. Therefore the nurse should not rigidly apply the age stages of any developmental theory but rather should plan highly individualized care. Practicality and flexibility are the basis for successful nursing care.

Summary

Providing nursing care is a highly complex and individualized process. The nurse must first understand the individual and his growth and development. In addition, the nurse must assess the factors in the individual's life that have or will have influence on growth and development. Only then can the nurse and client make decisions about developmental needs and plan and implement nursing activities (interventions) that promote health.

This chapter has discussed the complexities of growth and development as interrelated processes that are influenced by multiple factors. The different developmental theories can be applied by the nurse in assessing the individual's strengths and weaknesses and in planning care accordingly.

In the following chapters a developmental approach is used to examine individually the different stages of growth and development. The physical, psychosocial, and cognitive dimensions of development are explored along with how developmental factors are relevant in the steps of the nursing process.

✓ Growth and development are orderly, predictable, interdependent processes that continue throughout the life span.

✓ People progress through similar stages of growth and development but at an individual pace and with individual behaviors.

✓ A person's ability to progress through each developmental stage influences the person's health in that stage and thereafter.

✓ A developmental perspective helps the nurse understand both commonalities and variations in each stage and their impact on the client's health.

✓ Development depends on progressive adaptation to the environment.

✓ Maturation is the process of altering previous functions and learning more mature behaviors, involving environmental opportunities and biological abilities.

✓ During critical periods of development a person faces certain tasks necessary for successful developmental progression.

✓ Development has direction, is complex but predictable, is unique for each individual, involves conflict and adaptation, presents challenges, and requires practice and energy.

✓ Growth and development can be understood in terms of different chronological stages involving tasks and changes.

✓ Growth and development are influenced by the inner forces of heredity and temperament and the outer forces of family, peers, life experiences, and elements in the person's environment.

✓ The developmental theories of Freud, Erikson, Piaget, Havighurst, Maslow, and Kohlberg help explain certain aspects of development and can be used by the nurse to form a perspective individualized for each client.

REFERENCES

Brown, M., and Murphy, M.: Ambulatory pediatrics for nurses, ed. 2, New York, 1981, McGraw-Hill Book Co.

Duvall, E.: Marriage and family development, Philadelphia, 1977, J.B. Lippincott Co.

Erikson, E.: Childhood and society, New York, 1963, W.W. Norton & Co., Inc.

Hall, C.: A primer of freudian psychology, New York, 1954, World Publishing Co.

Havighurst, R.: Developmental tasks and education, ed. 2, New York, 1964, David McKay Co., Inc.

Kohlberg, L.: Stages and sequence: the cognitive-developmental approach to socialization. In Goslin, D.A., editor: Handbook of socialization theory and research, Chicago, 1969, Rand McNally & Co.

Nelms, B., and Mullins, R.: Growth and development: a primary health care approach, Englewood Cliffs, 1982, Prentice-Hall, Inc.

Sutterly, D., and Donnelly, G.: Perspectives in human development: nursing throughout the life cycle, Philadelphia, 1973, J.B. Lippincott Co.

Tackett, J., and Hunsberger, M.: Family centered care of children and adolescents, Philadelphia, 1981, W.B. Saunders Co.

Thomas, A., and Chess, S.: Temperament and the parent-child interaction, Pediatr. Ann. 6:26, 1977.

Waechter, E., and Blake, F.: Nursing care of children, ed. 9, Philadelphia, 1976, J.B. Lippincott Co.

Whaley, L.D., and Wong, D.L.: Nursing care of infants and children, ed. 2, St. Louis, 1983, The C.V. Mosby Co.

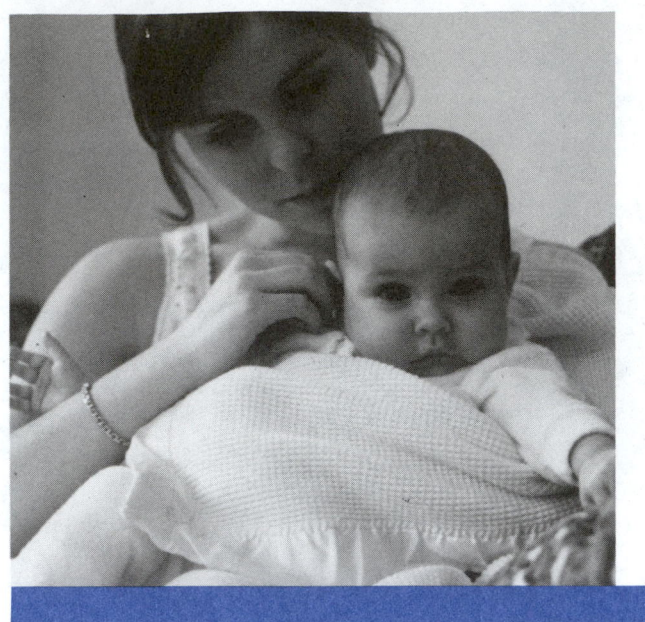

OBJECTIVES

Mastery of the content in this chapter will enable the student to:

- Define the terms in the glossary.
- Discuss teratogenic effects and ways in which the nurse can promote fetal health through prenatal education.
- Describe ways in which the nurse can provide support to the woman during pregnancy.
- Describe the physical growth characteristics of the unborn child, infant, and toddler.
- Identify physiological risk factors for the unborn child, infant, and toddler.
- Discuss physiological and psychosocial health concerns during the transition from intrauterine to extrauterine life.
- Identify factors important for normal cognitive development through infancy and toddlerhood.
- Explain the importance of parent-child attachment and list factors that may impede the attachment process.
- Describe variables that influence how the young child learns about and perceives his health status.
- Discuss ways in which the nurse can assist parents in promoting their child's health in all dimensions.

GLOSSARY

Apgar scale Assessment tool that rates the newborn's physiological status 1 to 5 minutes after birth.

attachment Initial psychosocial relationship that develops between parents and the neonate.

blastocyst Embryonic form that arises as a cavity within the morula, where cellular differentiation begins.

chromosomes Strands of DNA from the ovum and sperm that carry genes and thus determine genetic inheritance.

embyro Stage of human development from implantation of the fertilized ovum to the eighth week of intrauterine life.

fetus Stage of human development from the end of the embryonic period until birth.

lanugo Fine hair that normally covers the fetus after the fifth month of intrauterine life and is mostly shed by birth.

molding Overlapping and shaping of the soft skull bones during birth, usually resolved during the first few days of life.

morula Early stage of human development in which a solid mass of cells forms from the zygote approximately 3 days after fertilization.

placenta Organ surrounding the embryo and fetus through which pass nutrients and other substances from the mother and waste products from the fetus.

teratogenic Any chemical or physiological agent that may produce adverse effects in the embryo or fetus.

vernix caseosa Cheeselike substance that coats the skin of the fetus and newborn.

zygote Fertilized ovum created by the joining of the mother's ovum and father's sperm.

24 Unborn Child, Infant, and Young Child

Children are the future, and their health is the well-being of society. Understanding children and their growth and development is essential to promoting health and establishing healthful patterns for the entire life span. The nurse must have a clear understanding of what is normal or expected in the early developmental stages in order to guide and promote this normalcy and to prevent abnormalities as much as possible. For example, without the knowledge that the average 2½- to 3-year-old child is toilet trained, the nurse cannot promote learning of this skill at an appropriate earlier age.

Nursing practice that is based on principles of growth and development is organized and directed toward helping individuals adapt to changing internal and external conditions as they progress through life. This chapter considers the growth and development characteristics of the unborn child, the infant, the toddler, and the preschooler as related to nursing practice.

Unborn Child

From the moment of conception, human development proceeds at a rapid pace. The ovum and sperm each carry half the genetic material that guides many biochemical processes essential to the developing organism. Aberrations in the genes or chromosomes can be directly responsible for alterations in the individual's health, as in Down's syndrome. Other health problems result from environmental factors, such as fetal alcohol syndrome, which is induced by maternal alcoholism. Most intrauterine health problems are caused by a combination of genetic and environmental factors.

Intrauterine Life

Intrauterine life generally lasts 9 calendar or 10 lunar months. The organism's life begins when the ovum is penetrated by one sperm. The process of fertilization most often takes place in the fallopian tube, usually within 12 to 24 hours after the ovum is released from the ovary and sexual intercourse has occurred. The ovum and sperm fuse, and the material from both cell nuclei unite. The organism then has its full genetic complement in one pair of sex chromosomes and 22 pairs of autosomal chromosomes. The ovum and the sperm each contribute one chromosome to each pair. It is through this mechanism that genetically programmed diseases (such as Down's syndrome) and other genetically determined characteristics (such as eye color) are transmitted from parent to child.

The fertilized ovum, or zygote, passes through the fallopian tube to the uterus within 4 days. During this time the zygote continues to divide. By the third day a solid ball of cells, the morula, has formed. This solid ball soon develops a central cavity, or blastocyst. Even at this early stage the cells are beginning to differentiate in structure and function. Cells at one end of the blastocyst develop into the embryo, and those at the opposite end form the placenta. By day 4 the embryo has traveled through the fallopian tube into the uterus and is implanted in the uterine wall (Fig. 24-1).

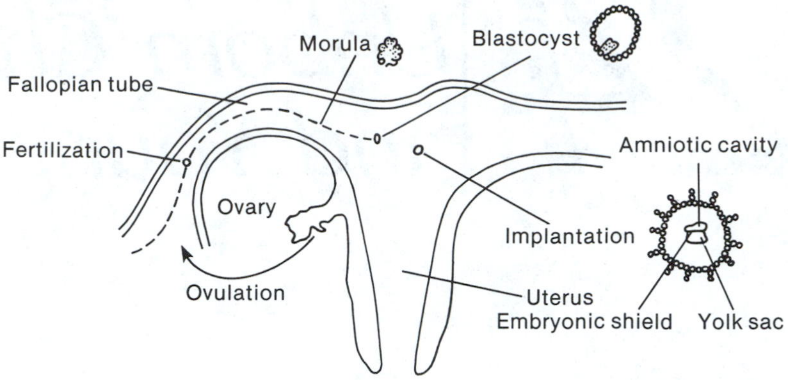

Fig. 24-1 The fertilization cycle.
From Nelms, B.C., and Mullins, R.G.: Growth and development: a primary health care approach, © 1982, p. 137. Reprinted by permission of Prentice-Hall, Inc., Englewood Cliffs, N.J.

Before implantation the embryo is relatively protected from the external environment. However, the organism is sensitive to changes in the immediate environment of the fallopian tube and uterus through which it travels. With implantation the embryo becomes more vulnerable to the larger maternal environment via exchange of materials through the placenta. The placenta produces essential hormones that help maintain the pregnancy and that permit transfer of material between the embryo and the mother, including oxygen, carbon dioxide, nutrients, and waste products. Since the placenta is extremely porous, noxious materials such as viruses and drugs can also pass from mother to child. The effect of noxious agents on the unborn child depends on the developmental stage in which exposure takes place. The extended period of gestation is frequently divided into three more limited time periods called trimesters. Because the embryo is in a different stage of development in each trimester, interference with the development process has different outcomes in each.

Physical Development

FIRST TRIMESTER

The first trimester is the first 3 calendar months. After implantation the fetal cells continue to differentiate and develop into essential organ systems. Differentiation involves changing cellular characteristics, whereas development involves changes in organ or other systems through a step or stage. These processes occur at different rates and times, and each organ is extremely vulnerable to environmental insult during its time of most rapid growth. Interference with growth can cause the congenital absence of an organ system or extensive structural or functional alterations. Fig. 24-2 shows the time periods for differentiation of major organ systems.

Since several organ systems are developing during the same time period, disruption of one system is often associated with disruption of others. The nurse should consider this simultaneous development when conducting the initial newborn nursing assessment, since the presence of one congenital defect frequently indicates the presence of others.

HEALTH CONCERNS. Agents capable of producing adverse effects in the fetus are called teratogens. Some teratogens produce defects only if the fetus is exposed to the agent at a critical time when the vulnerable organ is developing. One such teratogen is the rubella virus, which can cause abortion, stillbirth, or defects of the eyes, ears, and heart, primarily when exposure is in the first trimester. Other infectious agents such as those causing syphilis and herpes are also known to adversely affect fetal health.

Many drugs are teratogenic during the period of rapid organ growth (organogenesis) in the first trimester. Barbiturates, alcohol, hydantoin, anticonvulsants, and anticoagulants are only a few of the chemical agents associated with fetal abnormalities, and many others are under investigation (Stevenson, 1973). In addition, evidence is increasing that mothers who smoke deliver infants with lower birth weights than nonsmoking mothers.

With this knowledge of teratogenic effects the nurse can promote fetal health through prenatal education by encouraging the pregnant woman to avoid drug ingestion, smoking, and exposure to viral illnesses. The benefits of any drug needed to maintain the mother's health must be weighed against the potential harm to the fetus.

Pregnant women frequently consult the nurse regarding smoking and the use of over-the-counter drugs. The nurse should recommend abstinence from smoking and unnecessary drugs, explore life-style changes that can help the woman maintain abstinence, and teach the woman other, safer remedies to health problems. For example, nonpharmacological relaxation techniques are preferable to smoking or alcohol for relieving tension. The nurse also provides emotional support as the woman tries to implement new strategies.

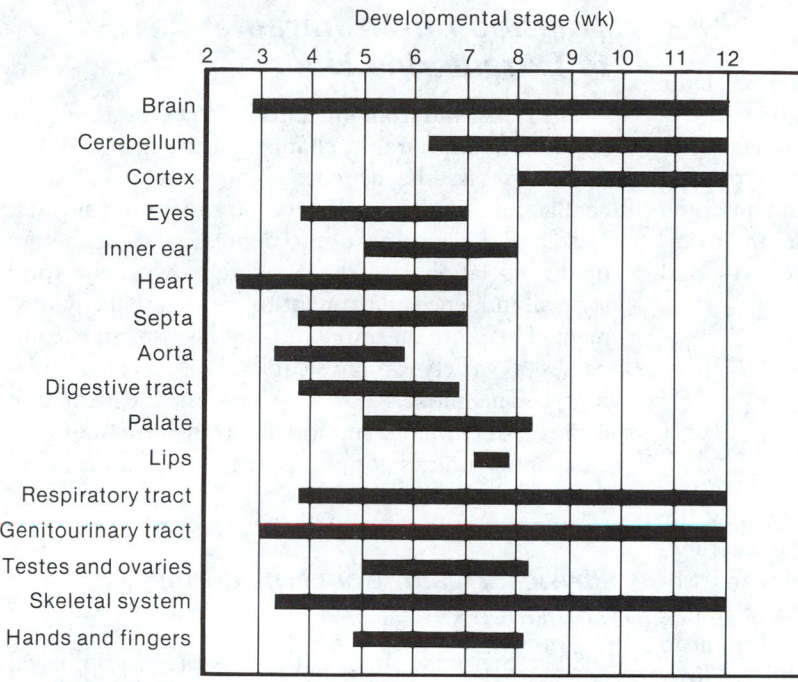

Fig. 24-2 Periods of organ differentiation.

From Whaley, L.F., and Wong, D.L.: Nursing care of infants and children, ed. 1, St. Louis, 1979, The C.V. Mosby Co.

SECOND TRIMESTER

The second trimester is the period from the third to the sixth prenatal months of life. Some organ systems continue their basic development during this time, and the functional capabilities of others are refined. By the end of the second trimester most organ systems are complete and capable of functioning. The fetus is therefore considered viable, or capable of life outside the uterus if given intensive environmental support. The fetus weighs about 0.7 kg (1½ pounds) and is approximately 30 cm (12 inches) long. Fingers and toes are differentiated, a rudimentary kidney functions, and the sex of the fetus is determinable.

The fetus is covered with vernix caseosa, a cheese-like substance that coats the skin. Lanugo, or fine hair, is present over most of the body. Both substances protect the thin, fragile skin and decrease in amount with further gestation. Prematurely born infants have greater amounts of these protective coverings than do full-term infants.

HEALTH CONCERNS. In the second trimester the fetal heartbeat becomes audible to stethoscope auscultation and the mother becomes aware of fetal movement. Both events are highly significant to the mother, since they provide tangible evidence of the pregnancy and reassure her that the fetus is alive. Therefore the nurse should focus on these events during prenatal care.

Changes in maternal behavior during this period include planning for the birth, concern for personal safety, and preoccupation with health and appear-ance. The nurse can help the woman adapt to such changes and plan for the impending birth. This is often a good time for education about gestational events and appropriate maternal rest and nutrition and for discussion of the birthing alternatives. In addition, the nurse's support and reassurance can help the expectant mother realize that every pregnancy is unique and that landmark events, such as fetal heartbeat, occur within a range of time rather than at an absolute time.

THIRD TRIMESTER

During the last 3 months of intrauterine life the fetus grows to approximately 50 cm (19 to 20 inches) in length. Subcutaneous fat is stored, and weight increases to between 3.2 and 3.4 kg (7 to 7½ pounds). The skin thickens, lanugo begins to disappear, and the fetal body becomes rounder and fuller.

A tremendous spurt in brain growth begins during the third trimester and lasts well into the first few years of postnatal life. The central nervous system has now established its total number of neurons and connections between neurons, and myelination of nerve fibers progresses at a rapid rate. Damage to the central nervous system during the third trimester can potentially alter later, higher-level cognitive functions. However, these alterations are not necessarily associated with the gross structural abnormalities of the central nervous system that result from damage in the first or second trimester (Dobbing, 1974). Exposure to noxious agents and the absence of essential nutrients are the most common causes of damage during this trimester. The nurse can teach the woman about these factors in prenatal education.

At the end of the third trimester the normal fetus is physically able to make the transition from intrauterine to extrauterine life. The cardiac system is capable of changing its circulation to end the bypassing of the lungs. The lungs are capable of maintaining the inflated state required for gas exchange, and primitive temperature maintenance systems, reflexes, and sensory organs are ready for use.

Cognitive Development

Relationships between prenatal events and cognitive development are difficult to establish. However, it is known that periods of anoxia during fetal life are associated with deficits in later cognitive functioning (Field, 1977). Some research shows an association between severely inadequate prenatal nutrition and subsequent lower brain weight, head circumference, and specific cognitive abilities. However, other studies show that, unless the malnutrition is severe and long term, the deficiencies can be averted by later supplemental nutrition. The effects of malnutrition on cognitive development are hard to prove because it is impossible to know what the cognitive abilities of the individual would have been if the malnutrition had not occurred. Until more is known, the prudent nurse intervenes to support adequate prenatal nutrition and prevent fetal anoxia. Interventions can include discussions of the four basic food groups, enrollment in a nutrition supplement program (Women, Infants, and Children [WIC] Program), and discussion of activities that may be associated with low blood oxygen levels.

Psychosocial Development

Little information is available about the relationship between prenatal experiences and the child's later psychosocial development. Some authorities believe that the biochemical environment of the uterus can significantly influence later psychosocial development. Because the biochemical environment is influenced by the mother's emotional state, the mother's emotional and physical states may have significant psychosocial consequences for the unborn child. Furthermore, the mother's emotional state may influence her behavior after childbirth, which in turn influences the child's psychosocial development. The nurse therefore assesses the family's response to the pregnancy and the sources of family stress so she can intervene to minimize potential adverse effects on the child's psychosocial development.

Transition from Intrauterine to Extrauterine Life

The transition from intrauterine to extrauterine life requires multiple rapid changes in the neonate. The nurse assesses the neonate's ability to make these changes and intervenes if necessary to ensure success. Gestational age, exposure to depressant drugs before or during labor, and the neonate's own behavioral style all influence adjustment to the external environment. Therefore the initial nursing assessment encompasses a variety of physical and psychosocial elements. The nurse's goal is to assess the neonate's current functioning, support his transition, and provide opportunities for the parents and the child to develop close emotional ties.

Physical Health Concerns during Transition

Since the nurse's first concern is the physiological functioning of the neonate's major organ systems, an immediate assessment of the neonate's condition is performed. Nursing care is then directed toward maintaining an open airway, stabilizing body temperature, and protecting the neonate from infection.

Patency of the neonate's airway is best ensured by removing naso-oropharyngeal secretions with a bulb syringe. Once the airway is open, the nurse directs efforts toward stabilization of body temperature. Wrapping the neonate in small, soft blankets usually provides adequate heat preservation. For neonates unable to sustain their body temperatures, Isolettes and incubators, which supply radiant heat, can be used. Proper handwashing helps protect the neonate from infection and should be performed before and between handling neonates. Friction is the most important element of the handwashing technique. Additional infection prevention measures include the instillation of antibiotics or 2 drops of 1% silver nitrate solution into the eyes to prevent *Neisseria gonorrhoeae* infections, which can be transmitted to the neonate during passage through an infected vaginal canal. A drying antiseptic agent, such as alcohol, should be applied daily to the umbilicus to prevent infection.

Most institutions require some form of immediate identification of the neonate. The nurse usually attaches identification bands to the mother and neonate and secures foot and hand prints for birth records. In addition, the nurse records the neonate's vital signs and measurements for the record.

The nurse is frequently responsible for performing an assessment of the neonate's physiological functioning at birth. The most widely used assessment tool

TABLE 24-1

Apgar Scoring

Sign	Score 0	Score 1	Score 2
Heart rate	Absent	Slow (below 100)	Over 100
Respiratory effort	Absent	Slow, irregular, hypoventilation	Good, crying lustily
Muscle tone	Flaccid	Some flexion of extremities	Active motion, well flexed
Reflex irritability	No response	Cry, some motion	Vigorous cry
Color	Blue, pale	Body pink, hands and feet blue	Completely pink

From Korones, S.: High-risk newborn infants: the basis for intensive nursing care, St. Louis, 1981, The C.V. Mosby Co.

is the Apgar scale, which rates five physiological characteristics. The newborn's heart rate, respiratory effort, muscle tone, reflex irritability, and color are rated to determine the overall status. The Apgar assessment is generally conducted at both 1 and 5 minutes after birth and may be repeated until the newborn's condition stabilizes. Table 24-1 outlines the scoring criteria of physiological functioning. A total score of 0 to 3 signifies severe distress, a score of 4 to 6 represents moderate difficulty, and a score of 7 to 10 indicates little difficulty in adjusting to extrauterine life.

The Apgar assessment is an organized approach to the evaluation of the neonate's transition from intrauterine life. The scale is widely accepted as a quick means of identifying neonates at highest risk for subsequent problems. The nurse can also use the Apgar score to determine areas that require further assessment and careful observation.

Psychosocial Concerns during Transition

After the immediate physical evaluation the nurse assesses the parents' and newborn's needs for close physical contact. Early parent-child interaction has been found to encourage later close parent-child attachment. Physical factors, such as the parents' fatigue, hunger, and health, and emotional factors, such as being happy about the birth and needing to be affectionate and to touch, see, and be close to the infant, are assessed. Merely placing the family together does not necessarily promote closeness or acquaintance. Both parent and neonate must be capable and desirous of exploring and responding to the other. Most healthy neonates are awake and alert for the first half hour after birth, and if the parents are receptive, this is an opportune time for parent-child acquaintance to begin. Close body contact, often including breast feeding, is a satisfying way for most families to start.

If immediate contact is not possible, the nurse incorporates such contact into the nursing care plan as early as feasible for both parents and neonate. This may mean bringing the newborn to an ill parent or bringing the parents to an ill or premature child. Attachment between parent and newborn occurs when both individuals elicit behaviors from each other that are reciprocal and complementary. Parental attachment behaviors include attentiveness and physical contact with the newborn. Neonate attachment behaviors involve maintaining contact with the parent. If there is prolonged separation, preterm and ill neonates and their parents have greater difficulty forming this attachment. The attachment process is further complicated if parents are unable to provide for the usual, anticipated infant care needs. The nurse should give the parents support throughout the early attachment process, for weeks or months if necessary, particularly if the newborn remains ill or separated from the parents.

Neonate

The neonatal period is the first 28 days of life. A comprehensive nursing assessment is performed as soon as the neonate's physiological functioning is stable, generally within a few hours after birth. At this time the nurse measures height, weight, head circumference, temperature, pulse, and respirations and observes general appearance, body functions, sensory capabilities, and responsiveness. In addition, the nurse coordinates screening tests and other laboratory tests as indicated by the neonate's state of health. Blood tests such as those for hypothyroidism and phenylketonuria (PKU) allow for early detection and treatment, thereby preventing permanent central nervous system damage. These and other screening tests are required by law in many states.

Assessment data provide baseline information and may reveal the need for nursing interventions. Sharing assessment knowledge with parents allows them to recognize and respond appropriately to the neonate's cues. This type of reciprocal interaction is basic to a satisfactory parent-child relationship.

Physical Development

The primary physical developmental goal of the neonate is stabilization of major body systems. This is characterized by functioning and behavior that are predominantly reflexive.

The average newborn weighs 3200 g (7 pounds, 1 ounce), is 50 cm (20 inches) in length, and has a head circumference of 35 cm (14 inches). Up to 10% of birth weight is lost in the first few days of life, primarily through fluid losses by respiration, urination, defecation, and decreased intake. Birth weight is regained by approximately the second week of life, and a gradual pattern of increase in weight, height, and head circumference is evident by 1 month. These increases average 4 to 7 ounces weight gain per week, 0.6 to 1.2 cm (½ to 1 inch) gain in length per month, and 2 cm increase in head circumference per month.

The neonate's heart rate gradually decreases from the fetal rate of 130 to 160 beats per minute to 120 to 140 beats per minute. Systole and diastole are of shorter duration, greater intensity, and higher pitch. The newborn's respiratory movements are primarily abdominal and vary in rate and rhythm. The average rate is between 30 and 50 respirations per minute. The axillary temperature ranges from 36.5° to 37° C and generally stabilizes within 24 hours after birth.

Normal physical characteristics include the continued presence of lanugo on the skin of the back, cyanosis of the hands and feet, especially during activity,

and a soft, protuberant abdomen. Skin color varies according to racial and genetic heritage. For example, mongolian spots (deeply pigmented areas across the sacrum and buttocks) are common in black, Asian, and Raza/Latina children. These spots fade spontaneously during the early preschool years. Molding, or overlapping of the soft skull bones, is common during birth. The bones readjust in a few weeks, producing the more rounded appearance of the neonatal skull. Linear breaks, sutures, and small diamond-shaped spaces, the fontanels, are palpable between the unfused skull bones. Fig. 24-3 illustrates the location of these landmarks. Both the anterior and the posterior fontanel are usually palpable at birth.

Normal behavioral characteristics of the newborn include periods of sucking, crying, sleeping, and activity. Movements are generally sporadic, but they are symmetrical and involve all four extremities. The relatively flexed position of intrauterine life continues as the neonate attempts to maintain an enclosed, secure feeling. Eye contact and eye movements should be assessed. Newborns normally watch the care giver's face, reflexively smile and respond to sensory stimuli, particularly the primary care giver's face, voice, and touch.

Neurological function is assessed by observing the neonate's level of activity, his alertness, irritability, and responsiveness to stimuli, and the presence and strength of reflexes. Normal reflexes include blinking

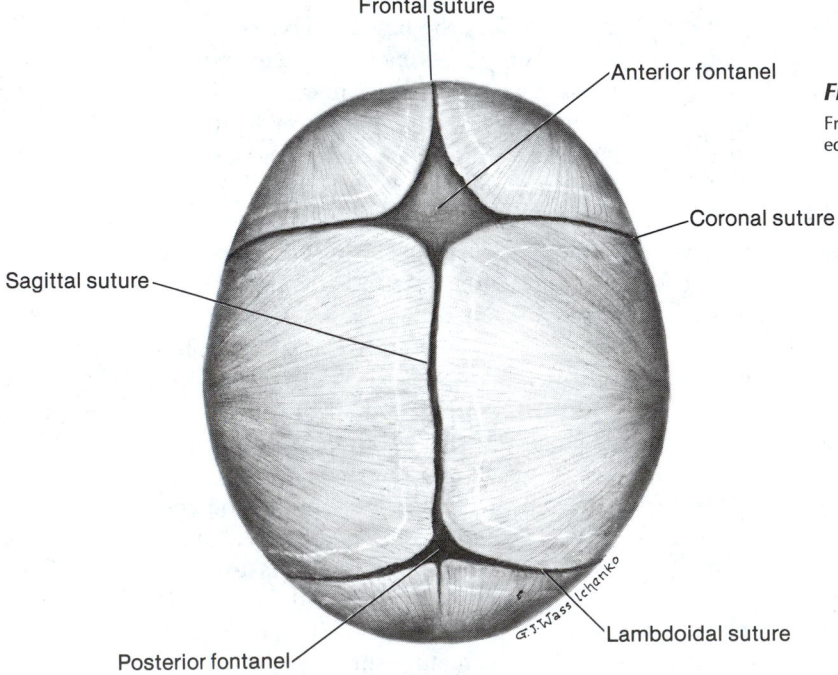

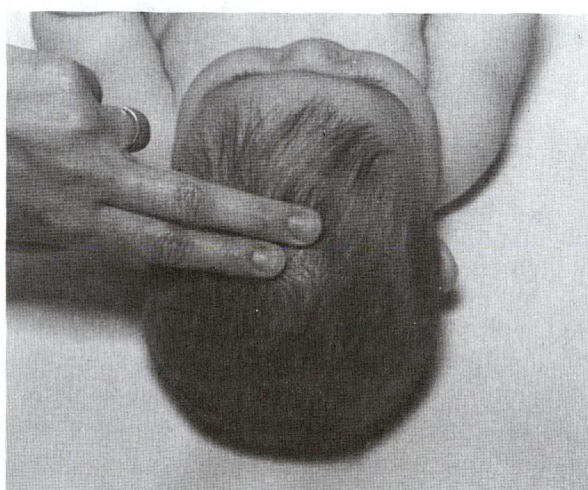

Fig. 24-3 Fontanels and suture lines.
From Whaley, L.F., and Wong, D.L.: Nursing care of infants and children, ed. 2, St. Louis, 1983, The C.V. Mosby Co.

in response to a bright light and startling in response to a sudden, loud noise. Table 24-2 lists other commonly evaluated neonatal reflexes. Their absence indicates possible trauma or central nervous system complications. Since the newborn is largely dependent on reflexes for responding to his environment, nursing assessment of these response characteristics is vital.

Cognitive Development

Early cognitive development begins with the neonate's innate behaviors, reflexes, and sensory func-

tions. During this time the newborn initiates reflex activities, assimilates new objects into behavior, and accommodates these behaviors to achieve what is desired. For example, the neonate learns to turn to the nipple. Although the infant behaves of his own volition, activities learned are limited to reflex and sensory function (Nelms and Mullins, 1982).

Sensory functions contribute to cognitive development in the newborn. At birth the newborn can focus on objects about 8 to 10 inches from the face and can perceive forms. A preference for the human face is apparent. Auditory and vestibular systems

---

TABLE 24-2

Infant Reflexes

Reflex	Stimulus	Response
Babinski	Using a blunt object, stroke lateral aspect of the plantar surface of foot from heel to toes.	Hyperextension or fanning of toes occurs. As myelinization is completed, the normal response becomes flexion (downward curling) of all toes; the positive (pathological) sign is hyperextension (dorsiflexion) of the great toe with or without fanning of the remaining toes.
Blinking	Shine a light suddenly at the infant's open eyes.	Eyelids close in response to light (disappears after first year).
Landau	Suspend infant carefully in prone position by supporting infant's abdomen with examiner's hand.	By 3 months of age the expected response consists of extension of head, trunk, and hips. Head is slightly above horizontal plane. (Reflex disappears by 2 years of age.)
Moro	With infant in supine position, gently support head and lift it a few centimeters off the surface. As soon as neck relaxes, suddenly release the head and let it drop back to the surface. *or* Produce sudden loud noise, or jar the table or crib suddenly.	Normal response is present at birth. The arms extend outward, the hands open, and then are brought together in midline. The legs flex slightly. Infant may cry. (Reflex usually disappears by 3 to 4 months.)
Neck righting	With infant in supine position turn head to one side.	Infant's trunk rotates in direction in which head is turned (appears at 4 to 6 months and disappears at 24 months).
Palmar grasp	With infant's head positioned in midline, place examiner's index fingers from ulnar side into infant's palm and press against palm.	Normal response is flexion of all fingers around examiner's fingers (present at birth and disappears by 4 months when infant is ready to reach).
Placing	Hold infant erect with the dorsum of one foot touching the undersurface of the examining table top.	Infant flexes hip and knee and places stimulated foot on top of the table (present at birth and disappears by 6 weeks or variable).
Plantar grasp	Place examiner's finger firmly across base of infant's toes.	Toes curl downward (present at birth and disappears by 10 to 12 months).
Rooting	Hold infant in supine position with head in midline and hands against chest. Stroke perioral skin at corner of mouth or cheek.	Infant opens mouth and turns head toward stimulated side (present at birth and disappears by 3 to 4 months [awake]; by 7 months [asleep]).

Modified from Chow, M., et al.: Handbook of pediatric primary care, ed. 2, Somerset, N.J., 1984, John Wiley & Sons, Inc.

function from birth. These sensory capabilities allow the neonate to elicit stimulation actively rather than simply receive stimuli passively. The nurse should teach the new mother the importance of providing sensory stimulation, such as talking to her baby and holding the newborn so that the baby can see her face. This allows the infant to seek or take in stimuli, thereby enhancing learning and promoting cognitive development.

Whether infant crying is the precursor of refined language is debatable. However, crying does elicit a response and care givers do discriminate among the various cry patterns of the neonate. Crying therefore has significance to both the newborn and the parents. For the neonate crying is a means of communication. Infants cry for a reason, although at times this reason is difficult to determine. Some babies cry because they are wet or hungry or want to be held; others cry just to make noise. An infant's crying may be frustrating for the parents if they cannot see an apparent cause. With the nurse's help, parents can learn to define their infant's cry patterns in order to take appropriate action when necessary.

Psychosocial Development

The first 28 days of life is a time when the parents and infants normally develop a deep attachment. Parent-child interactions during routine care enhance or detract from the attachment process. Feeding and brief periods of play consume much of the infant's waking hours. These interactive experiences provide a foundation from which later attachments form. The neonate is an active participant in the process.

If either the parent or the child experiences health complications after the birth, attachment may be compromised. The infant's behavioral cues may be weak or absent if the infant is ill. Care and care giving are less mutually satisfying. The tired, ill mother has difficulty interpreting and responding to her infant. Children with congenital anomalies, those who are too weak to be responsive to parental cues, and those who require special care all need supportive nursing care. For example, a child born with a heart defect may tire easily during feeding. He may rest frequently after several bursts of sucking and fall asleep after taking 1 to 1½ ounces. Such a child may awaken after 1½ hours, crying because he is hungry again. The mother, not understanding that this is a physiologically dictated sequence of events, may think the child is being fussy or that she is inadequate. Both infant and mother derive decreasing pleasure from feeding experiences. Attachment is not enhanced and may even be reduced unless intervention breaks the sequence of events.

Infant

Infancy follows the neonatal period and continues through the first year of life. Physical, cognitive, and psychosocial growth continues at a pace that is still rapid but somewhat slower than that set during the first 28 days of life.

Physical Development

Steady and proportional growth of the infant is more important than absolute growth values. Charts of normal age- and sex-related growth measurements enable the nurse to compare an infant's growth with norms for the child's age. With growth charts the nurse can also evaluate the infant's growth pattern by recording measurements of the weight, length, and head circumference at intervals. Repeated measurements that are recorded over time are the best way to identify growth problems. For example, an infant with a growth problem may be generally below the expected norms at all intervals or may experience an acute, brief interference with growth in any one or all of the parameters measured. Fig. 24-4 illustrates the growth patterns displayed in these two conditions.

NUTRITION

The quality and quantity of nutrition influence the infant's growth and development. The nurse's role in promoting good nutrition and dietary habits is to help parents select and provide a nutritionally adequate diet for their infant. The nurse therefore must have a sound knowledge base about nutrition. The nurse must also understand that nutrition is influenced by many variables (such as food preferences, being a slow eater, or having food allergies) and that no one diet is effective for all children or even for one age group.

FEEDING ALTERNATIVES. Supplying essential nutrients to the infant is a goal for the nurse and the parents. Since all nutrients necessary for growth during the first months of life are present in human milk, breast feeding is the current recommended feeding choice for infants. Because the breast milk contains essential nutrients of protein, fats, and carbohydrates, as well as immunoreactive proteins that bolster the infant's ability to resist infection, breast feeding is nutritionally sound. However, milk other than human milk may be used successfully for infant feeding. Commercially prepared formulas are popular because they are convenient, contain standard ingredients, and are fortified with vitamins and minerals. Whatever type of feeding is chosen by the parents, it is the

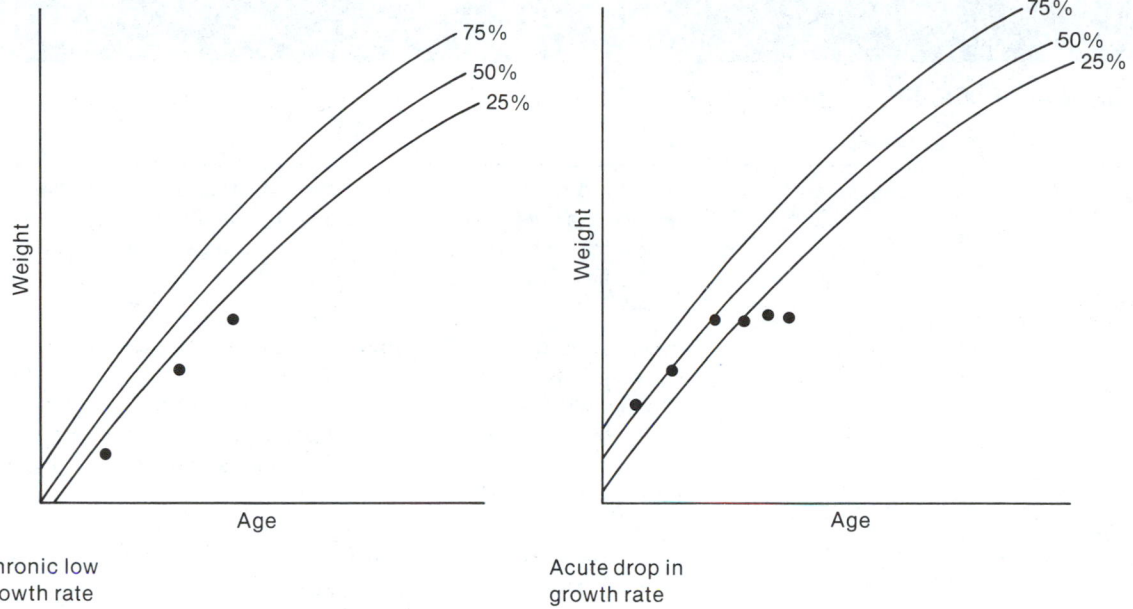

Fig. 24-4 Growth chart measurements.

nurse's responsibility to support and reassure them and help them feed the infant successfully.

The 1-month-old infant normally takes *approximately* 28 ounces of milk per day. This amount increases slightly during the first 6 months and drops to about 24 ounces per day by the end of the first year. Cereals, fruits, vegetables, and meats are increasingly important sources of nutrients during the second 6 months of life. The nurse must be aware, however, that the amount and frequency of feedings normally vary among infants. It is important for the nurse to teach parents about individual differences in feeding patterns. Table 24-3 provides feeding guidelines for the first year of life.

SUPPLEMENTATION. The need for dietary vitamin and mineral supplements is highly variable and depends on the specific diet of the infant. Full-term infants are born with some iron stores. The totally breast-fed infant absorbs adequate iron from breast milk during the first 4 to 6 months of life. After 6 months, iron-fortified cereal is generally considered an adequate supplemental source of iron. Because iron in formula is less readily absorbed than that in breast milk, formula-fed infants should receive iron-fortified formula throughout the first year. Adequate concentrations of fluoride to protect against dental caries are not available in human milk, and therefore fluoridated water or supplemental fluoride is generally recommended. The presence of fluoride in formula depends on the type of formula and the source of the water used in preparing the concentrated forms,

and supplementation may be necessary. In general, cow's milk is not recommended in the first year of life because of inadequate amounts of the essential nutrients, particularly fats and carbohydrates.

The association between overfeeding, infant obesity, and later adult obesity is still controversial. Recent studies do not unanimously suggest that overweight infants become obese adults without other contributing factors (Suskind, 1981). Early feeding experiences, however, may influence later eating habits. The nurse should therefore emphasize balanced nutrition and good dietary habits through feeding experiences mutually satisfying for the parents and infant.

Cognitive Development

The infant learns much by experiencing and manipulating the environment. The infant's developing motor skills and increasing mobility expand his environment and in combination with developing visual and auditory skills enhance cognitive development. For example, a 1-year-old infant can visually follow the path of a moving object. Improved visual acuity and eye-hand coordination allow grasping and exploration of objects. In addition, rudimentary color vision begins by 2 months of age and improves throughout the first year, making the environment more interesting to see and explore. The infant's hearing also progresses, allowing localization and discrimination of sounds. By 1 year of age the infant typically knows the meaning of several different sounds such as "Ma-Ma," "Da-Da," and "no."

TABLE 24-3

Guidelines for Feeding during the First Year

Age	Type of Feeding	Specific Recommendations
Birth-6 months	Breast feeding	This is most desirable complete diet for first half of year.* Infant requires supplements of fluoride (0.25 mg) regardless of the fluoride content of the local water supply, iron by 6 months of age, and vitamin D (400 units) if mother's diet is inadequate or if infant is not exposed to sufficient sunlight.
	Formula	Iron-fortified commercial formula is a complete food for the first half of the year.* Fluoride supplements (0.25 mg) are required when the concentration of fluoride in the drinking water is below 0.3 parts per million. Evaporated milk formula requires supplements of vitamin C, iron, and fluoride (in accordance with the fluoride content of the local water supply).
6-12 months	Solid foods	Solids may be added by 5 to 6 months of age; earlier introduction tends to contribute to overfeeding. First foods are strained, pureed, or finely mashed. "Finger foods" such as teething crackers, raw fruit, or vegetables can be introduced by 6 to 7 months. Chopped table food or commercially prepared junior foods can be started by 9 to 12 months. With the exception of cereal, the order of introducing foods is variable; a recommended sequence is weekly introduction of other foods, beginning with fruit, followed by vegetables, and then meat. Breast-fed infants require more high-protein foods than formula-fed infants. As the quantity of solids increases, the amount of formula should be limited to approximately 900 ml (30 ounces) daily.
	Cereal	Introduce commercially prepared iron-fortified infant cereals and administer daily until 18 months of age. Rice cereal is usually introduced first because of its low allergenic potential. Supplemental iron can be discontinued once cereal is given.
	Fruits and vegetables	Applesauce, bananas, and pears are usually well tolerated. Avoid fruits and vegetables marketed in cans that are not specifically designed for infants because of variable and sometimes high lead content and addition of salt, sugar, and preservatives. Offer fruit juice only from a cup, not a bottle, to reduce "nursing bottle caries."
	Meat, fish, and poultry	Avoid fatty meats. Prepare by baking, broiling, steaming, or poaching. Include organ meats such as liver, which has a high iron, vitamin A, and vitamin B complex content. If soup is given, be sure all ingredients are familiar to child's diet.
	Eggs and cheese	Serve egg yolk hard boiled and mashed, soft cooked, or poached. Introduce egg white in small quantities (1 teaspoon) toward end of first year to detect any allergic manifestation. Use cheese as a substitute for meat and as "finger food."

Modified from Whaley, L.D., and Wong, D.L.: Nursing care of infants and children, ed. 2, St. Louis, 1983, The C.V. Mosby Co.
*The American Academy of Pediatrics recommends breast-feeding or commercial formula feeding for up to 12 months of age. After 1 year whole cow's milk can be used.

Speech is an additional aspect of cognitive development. During the first year the infant proceeds from crying, cooing, and laughing to imitating sounds, comprehending the meaning of simple commands, and repeating words with knowledge of their meaning. By 12 months the infant begins to name objects in the environment. Such labeling is essential to later cognitive development.

The infant needs opportunities to develop and use the senses. Nurses have a responsibility to evaluate the appropriateness and adequacy of these opportunities. For example, an ill or hospitalized infant may lack the energy to interact with the environment, thereby slowing his cognitive development. On the other hand, continuous stimulation can overwhelm and confuse the infant. The individual infant needs to be stimulated according to his temperament, energy, and age capabilities. Visual, sensory, and tactile stimulation is as necessary for healthy development as food. The nurse uses stimulation strategies that maximize the infant's development while conserving his energy and orientation.

Psychosocial Development

During the first year the infant begins to differentiate himself from others as a separate being capable of acting on his own. Initially the infant is unaware of the boundaries of self, but through repeated experiences with the environment the infant learns where the self ends and the external world begins. This process of differentiation is slow, and the infant must occasionally experience brief frustrations along with more frequent and consistent satisfactions. As the infant determines his physical boundaries, he begins to respond to the presence of others. The 2- to 3-month-old infant begins to smile responsively rather than reflexively. Similarly, the infant can recognize differences in people when his sensory and cognitive capabilities improve. By 8 months of age most infants can differentiate a stranger from a familiar person, and they respond differently to the two. Close attachment to the primary care giver, most often a parent, is usually established by this age. The infant seeks out this person for support and comfort during times of stress. Finally, the ability to distinguish self from others allows the infant to interact and socialize more within his environment. By 9 months of age, for example, the infant is playing simple social games such as pat-a-cake and peek-a-boo. More complex interactive games such as hide-and-seek are possible by age 1.

The nurse assesses the availability and appropriateness of experiences that contribute to the infant's psychosocial development. Hospitalized infants may have difficulty establishing physical boundaries because of repeated bodily intrusions and painful sensations. Limiting these negative experiences and providing pleasurable sensations are nursing interventions that support early psychosocial development. Extended separations from parents complicate the attachment process and increase the number of care givers with whom the infant must interact. Unless the parents continue to provide the majority of care during hospitalization, the infant's needs will be satisfied inconsistently. These inconsistencies overwhelm the infant. Therefore, when feasible, the nurse should encourage the parents to provide routine daily care to their infant during hospitalization. When this is impossible, limiting the number of people providing daily care is advisable. The use of detailed nursing care plans for the infant's daily routine and needs can minimize inconsistencies.

Perception of Health

The foundation for a child's perception of his own health status is laid early in life. Internal body sensations as well as experiences with the outside world affect later self-perceptions. The nature of this influence and the value of nursing interventions to alter later perceptions are unknown. It is known, however, that parents tend to label infants who are ill in early life as more vulnerable than their siblings and that this labeling may later affect the child's perceptions of his own health. In addition, because infants and children depend on others for their health, the attitudes and experiences of care givers influence their later health attitudes and behaviors. The nurse has a responsibility to educate parents and other care givers about health promotion behaviors that will positively affect the child's perception of health and self.

Toddler

The toddler period ranges from approximately the first to the third year of life. Toddlerhood is characterized by increasing independence bolstered by greater physical mobility and cognitive abilities. The toddler is increasingly aware of his ability to control and is pleased with successful efforts with this new skill. This success leads the toddler to repeated attempts to control his environment. Unsuccessful attempts at control may result in negative behaviors and temper tantrums. These behaviors are most common when the parents thwart the initial independent action. Parents cite these as the most problematic behaviors during the toddler years and at times express frustration with trying to set consistent and firm limits while simultaneously enhancing independence in their child. Parents often seek the guidance of health care professionals for assistance in learning these essential parenting tasks.

Physical Development

Many general characteristics of physical development become obvious in the toddler years. The child now walks in an upright position with a broad-stanced gait, protuberant abdomen, and arms flung out to the side for balance. The gross motor skills continue to develop rapidly during the toddler years as evidenced by the ability to walk up and down stairs, kick a ball, jump, and stand on one foot for several seconds. By the end of the third year most toddlers can ride a tricycle and run well. Fine motor capabilities move from scribbling spontaneously to drawing circles and crosses accurately. By 3 years of age the child draws simple stick people and can usually stack a tower of small blocks. Improved mobility, the ability to undress, and development of sphincter control allow toilet training if the toddler has developed the necessary cognitive abilities. Parents often consult nurses for an assessment of their child's readiness for toilet training. The nurse needs to remind parents that patience, consistency, and a nonjudgmental attitude, in addition to the child's readiness, are essential components of successful training.

The cardiopulmonary system becomes stable in the toddler years. The heart and respiratory rates slow to 110 beats and 24 breaths per minute. Many health care professionals begin routine blood pressure measurement at age 3 to establish baseline values for the individual child. Standardized values for toddlers are still controversial, but normal readings are about 100/60 mm Hg.

The anterior fontanel generally closes between 12 and 18 months of age, ending the period of most rapid growth of the skull and brain. Routine measurement of head circumference is usually not continued past this age. After the skull bones fuse, increasing intracranial pressure is marked by headache, irritability, alterations in consciousness, and vomiting, rather than rapid increase in head circumference or bulging fontanels as before.

The rate of increase in both weight and length slows. By 2 years of age the child weighs four times his birth weight. Height during toddlerhood increases mainly as a result of increases in leg length. The slowed growth rates are accompanied by a decreased caloric need and smaller food intake, which leads some parents to worry about the adequacy of their child's dietary intake. The nurse can reassure the parents by confirming the child's continued proportional growth pattern with growth charts.

Most toddlers change from breast milk or formula to milk, consuming three to four glasses per day. Nutritional requirements are increasingly met by solid foods in the remaining three basic food groups. Since the consumption of more than a quart of milk per day decreases the child's appetite for these essential solid foods, the nurse should advise parents to limit milk intake to 28 ounces per day. The healthy toddler requires the daily intake of the foods in Table 24-4. Because parents frequently overestimate the size of a normal serving for their child, the nurse can reduce the parents' anxiety regarding inadequate intake by pointing out the normal serving size.

Children who are ill, are undergoing surgery, or have diseases involving ingestion, absorption, or utilization of nutrients require special dietary considerations. Alterations in the type of foods as well as calorie requirements may be necessary. Children on strict vegetarian diets also require careful plannning to ensure adequate, balanced intake.

Regardless of the child's health status, several basic principles of nutrition apply. Mealtime has psychosocial as well as physical significance. If the parents struggle to control the toddler's dietary intake, problem behaviors and conflicts may result. The nurse should encourage parents to offer a variety of nutritious foods at meals and provide only nutritious snacks between meals. Serving finger foods the toddler can eat by himself allows him to satisfy his drive for independence and need for control. Small *reasonable* servings allow the toddler to eat all of his meal.

Cognitive Development

The toddler moves from the sensorimotor to the preconceptual stage of cognitive development. In this

TABLE 24-4

Daily Dietary Requirements of the Healthy Toddler

Food	Number of Servings	Size of Serving
Milk	3-4	6-8 ounces
Meat	2-3	3 tablespoons
Vegetables and fruits	4	4 ounces
Cereals and breads	4 or more	½ slice of bread ½ cup rice or cereal

stage the child learns the permanency of objects, develops a memory of events, and begins to understand cause and effect. Thought has an egocentric focus, and the toddler is unable to assume the view of another. The toddler becomes increasingly capable of symbolic interaction and frequently expresses fantasy and magical thinking.

Since moral development is closely associated with cognitive ability, the moral development of a toddler is only beginning and is also egocentric. Toddlers do not understand concepts of right and wrong. However, they do grasp the fact that some behaviors bring pleasant results (positive reinforcement) and others elicit unpleasant results (negative reinforcement). Therefore, until the toddler achieves a higher level of cognitive function, he behaves simply to avoid the unpleasant and seek out the pleasant.

The 18-month-old child uses approximately 10 words. The 24-month-old child has a vocabulary of up to 300 words and is generally able to speak in short sentences. By 36 months most toddlers talk incessantly. They ask endless questions, can give their full name, follow and give simple commands, and use appropriate pronouns. Despite the wide vocabulary of older toddlers, most parents comment that their toddler's favorite word remains "no" until well into the third year.

Psychosocial Development

During toddlerhood the child develops increasing autonomy. Although toddlers are moving out to explore their immediate environment, they continue to return at periodic intervals for encouragement and the emotional support of parents. This process, called refueling, is illustrated by the toddler who can play alone in his bedroom but calls out at intervals to make sure that the parent is still in the house. Parents usually remain the most significant persons in the toddler's life.

The toddler is also capable of parallel play with others. Although two toddlers play in close proximity, true sharing or systematic turn taking is rare. The children play *next to* rather than *with* one another. Toddlers share toys inconsistently and rarely. Learning to control one's possessions, as well as oneself, is a primary task of toddlers; learning to share is a later development.

Since a toddler is extremely active yet unable to limit his own behavior, the parents must set limits. This inevitably causes conflict between the parent and child. Parents appreciate professional reassurance that this conflict lessens as the child grows older and internalizes behavior limits and that firm, consistent limit setting enhances this process.

Limit setting is extremely important for the toddler's safety. Automobile safety requires that the toddler remain in a car seat, even though he says (often loudly) that he would prefer to move freely about the car. Poisoning is another extreme hazard; the toddler's exploratory capabilities can lead him to open and taste noxious materials. The wise parent removes or locks up all possible poisons, including plants, cleaning materials, and drugs. In this way the parent creates a safer environment for the child's exploratory behavior.

Perception of Health

The toddler's perception of his own health is limited by his cognitive capabilities. The child increasingly recognizes internal body sensations but has difficulty pinpointing their location. Therefore the child often associates generalized responses with illness. The child who deviates radically from his usual pattern of eating, sleeping, or playing requires assessment to determine if these alterations are the result of illness.

During this stage the child begins to internalize the labels parents or health professionals give to the somatic states. That is, if the parents label particular sensations, such as abdominal discomfort, an "illness," the child begins to label related sensations similarly. At the same time the child observes and mimics the parents' health care practices. Health beliefs and practices are therefore being significantly shaped even in these early years.

Preschooler

The preschool years are a transition between toddlerhood and the school-age years. The period spans the ages between 3 and 5 to 6. Many people consider these the most intriguing years of parenting, since the child is less negative and can more accurately share his thoughts. Physical development continues to slow, and cognitive and psychosocial development is rapid.

Physical Development

Several aspects of physical development continue to stabilize in the preschool years. Heart and respiratory rates decrease only slightly to approximately 90 beats per minute and 24 breaths per minute. Blood pressure remains stable at about 90/60 mm Hg. Weight increases approximately 5 pounds per year, making the child's average weight about 45 pounds by age 5. Height increases less than 1 inch per year. Leg growth continues to account for most of the increase in height. Birth length is generally doubled by age 6, making the average height 42 inches. With this slowed growth pattern, nutritional needs remain relatively stable.

Large and fine muscle coordination improves. The preschooler runs well, walks up and down steps with ease, and learns to hop. By 6 years of age he can usually skip and throw and catch a ball. Improving fine motor skills allow intricate manipulations. The child can copy circles, crosses, squares, and triangles by 6 years of age. These skills make printing of letters and numbers possible.

The child needs opportunities to learn and practice these physical skills. Nursing care of both healthy and ill children includes an assessment of the availability of these opportunities. Although children with acute illnesses benefit from rest and exclusion from usual daily activities, children who have chronic conditions or who have been hospitalized for long periods need ongoing exposure to developmental opportunities. The parent and nurse weave these opportunities into the child's daily experiences, depending on the child's abilities, needs, and energy level.

Cognitive Development

The preschooler continues to master the preoperational stage of cognition. The continued egocentricity of early thinking makes it difficult to suggest acceptable alternatives to the preschooler. With maturation, experience, and the increasing use of symbolic thinking, the child becomes able to take the view of another and his thinking becomes less egocentric.

By 5 to 6 years of age, egocentric thinking is partially replaced by intuitive thought. The preschooler can increasingly solve a problem intuitively on the basis of only one aspect of a situation.

The preschooler's knowledge of the world remains closely linked to concrete experiences. Even the rich fantasy life of a preschooler is grounded in the child's perception of reality. The mixing of the two aspects by the child can become problematic; it leads to many childhood fears and may be misinterpreted by adults as lying when the child is actually presenting reality from his perspective.

Early causal thinking develops in the preschool years. Thought is transductive; that is, reasoning occurs from one particular to another. If two events are related in time or space, the child links them in a causal fashion. The hospitalized child, for example, may reason, "I cried last night, and that's why the nurse gave me the shot." As children near the age of 5, they begin to use or can be taught to use sets of rules to understand causation. The child then begins to reason from the general to the particular. This

forms the basis for more formal logical thought. The child can now reason, "I get a shot twice a day, and that's why I got one last night."

The preschooler's moral development expands to include a beginning understanding of behaviors considered socially right or wrong. The child continues to be motivated, however, by the wish to avoid punishment or the desire to obtain a reward. The primary difference between this stage of moral development and that of the toddler is that the preschooler is better able to identify the behaviors that elicit rewards or punishment and that he begins to label these behaviors right or wrong.

The child's improving language skills facilitate symbolic thought. Vocabulary increases greatly. By age 5 the child has more than 2000 words with which he can express himself. The child can name colors and body parts, and he can define familiar objects. However, the child may confuse phonetically similar words, such as "die" and "dye." Because of this limitation and literal interpretation of words, the preschooler may misunderstand things that are said to him. It is important for the nurse to assess whether the preschooler understands what is being told to him, especially when preparing him for treatment. Grammatical refinement also occurs during these years. The 5-year-old child uses longer sentences and appropriate adjectives.

Psychosocial Development

The preschooler continues to rely heavily on the support of parents or primary care givers for security, but he increasingly ventures out to initiate contact with other children and adults. The preschooler is less afraid of strangers and may ask a new adult acquaintance a seemingly unending stream of questions. The child seeks out experiences with peers and seems to enjoy this contact.

During times of stress or illness, however, the preschool child returns to a greater reliance on parents. This return to an earlier pattern of behavior, called regression, is not limited to the preschool years; it can occur anytime in a person's life. It occurs most often when people experience stress that they are unable to relieve with their prior coping behaviors. Regression involves stepping back to a more comfortable behavior, one that may have required less energy to maintain. Often these behaviors were helpful in the past, and the person consciously or unconsciously anticipates that they will help in the current situation. Regression is obvious in the preschooler because the regressive, dependent behavior contrasts markedly with the usual independent behavior. Parents are often confused and embarrassed by the child's regression and can benefit from the nurse's reassurance that this is a normal coping behavior for children under stress. The nurse should accept the regressive behavior of an ill child yet continue to help the child understand and gain control of the new situation. The nurse should provide experiences that the child can master with his current behaviors. These successes give the child the motivation and strength to return to his prior level of independent functioning.

Interactive play with peers begins in the preschool years. Parallel play moves to associative play, and, as the child nears school age, associative play becomes cooperative play. In associative play, children play with others in a similar activity, but there is very little organization or division of responsibility. As they develop, children engaged in cooperative play not only take turns but join efforts to produce desired outcomes. For example, preschoolers can work together to build a play store or take roles in a short play or skit. A sense of group initiative as well as self-initiative is developing during these play activities.

In many play activities the preschooler displays an awareness of social context. Sex role identification is strengthening, and children most often assume roles of persons of their own sex. Children frequently mimic or repeat social experiences they have had. This tendency is especially significant for the nurse working with hospitalized children. Through play the child may express questions, fears, anger, and misunderstanding regarding his illness and care. The nurse should be alert to the cues the child gives during spontaneous play and ensure that every child has the opportunity to play within his energy limits. The nurse can also use play to provide the child with new information or clear up misunderstandings. Play is not what the nurse does with preschoolers after all the work is done, *play is the work* of the nurse.

Perception of Health

Little research has explored the preschooler's perceptions of his own health. Although the parents' beliefs about the child's health are important in the child's developing sense of his health status, so are his bodily sensations and his ability to perform his usual daily activities. The preschooler is usually quite independent in washing, dressing, and feeding; alterations in this independence can influence his feelings about his own health.

Summary

The first 6 years of life is a time of dramatic strides in growth and development. Once fetal development has been completed, a newborn human being emerges whose abilities and physical capacities are primitive and reflexive. All physical and psychosocial needs of the newborn must be met by another person. During the first year, physical abilities and psychosocial skills increase. By 1 year of age the infant is becoming mobile, trusting, and able to influence his environment. Throughout the toddler years the individual grows in size, masters new physical skills, and gains a sense of self and independence. The toddler's world and opportunities expand as a result of his developmental progress. As the child approaches the end of the preschool years, his physical and emotional independence has increased. Cognitive skills have progressed dramatically, readying the child to enter a formal educational structure, which most societies provide for children of this age. With the transition from preschooler to school-age child, the child enters an exciting new phase. The school-age child lives in a rapidly expanding world; development continues through diverse and complex circumstances and experiences. The following chapter explores this continued development and its challenges for school-age children and adolescents.

KEY CONCEPTS

✓ Since the embryo and fetus grow and develop continuously through the intrauterine period, impairments in any body system may occur in utero.

✓ Health risks for the unborn child include genetic impairments and environmental factors (teratogens).

✓ Physiological health concerns during childbirth include adequate functioning of all systems and prevention of infection.

✓ A psychosocial health concern that begins at childbirth is the establishment of parent-child attachment.

✓ Physiological, cognitive, and psychosocial development continues throughout the neonate, infant, and toddler periods, and the nurse must be familiar with normal parameters in order to determine potential problems and promote normal development.

✓ The nurse recognizes that the child's perception of health and health behaviors begins early, and accordingly she assists both the parents and the child in establishing healthful patterns that will continue for the entire life span.

✓ The nurse educates the parents about risk factors and the child's health needs, provides emotional support to the parents in the prenatal period, and helps the parents understand the changes and needs of the developing child.

✓ Nursing interventions for an ill and hospitalized child encourage the child's continued cognitive and psychosocial development.

✓ Developmental assessment and nursing care are necessary to help the infant and child adapt to internal and external changes.

REFERENCES

Dobbing, J.: The later growth of the brain and its vulnerability, Pediatrics 53:2, 1974.

Field, T., et al., editors: Infants born at risk: behavior and development, New York, 1979, Spectrum Publications, Inc.

Nelms, B.C., and Mullins, R.: Growth and development: a primary health care approach, Englewood Cliffs, N.J., 1982, Prentice-Hall, Inc.

Stevenson, R.: The fetus and newborn infant: influences of the prenatal environment, St. Louis, 1973, The C.V. Mosby Co.

Suskind, R., editor: Textbook of pediatric nutrition, New York, 1981, Raven Press.

ADDITIONAL READINGS

Chow, M.P., et al.: Handbook of pediatric primary care, New York, 1979, John Wiley & Sons, Inc.

Conway, B.L.: Pediatric neurological nursing, Philadelphia, 1977, J.B. Lippincott Co.

Erickson, M.L.: Assessment and management of developmental changes in children, ed. 2, St. Louis, 1980, The C.V. Mosby Co.

Furstenberg, F.: Unplanned pregnancy: the social consequences of teenage pregnancy, New York, 1981, The Free Press.

Korones, S.: High-risk newborn infants: the basis for intensive nursing care, ed. 2, St. Louis, 1981, The C.V. Mosby Co.

Moore, M.L., and Galloway, K.: Newborn family and nurse, ed. 2, Philadelphia, 1981, W.B. Saunders Co.

Scipien, G., et al.: Comprehensive pediatric nursing, ed. 2, New York, 1979, McGraw-Hill, Inc.

Whaley, L.F., and Wong, D.L.: Nursing care of infants and children, ed. 2, St. Louis, 1983, The C.V. Mosby Co.

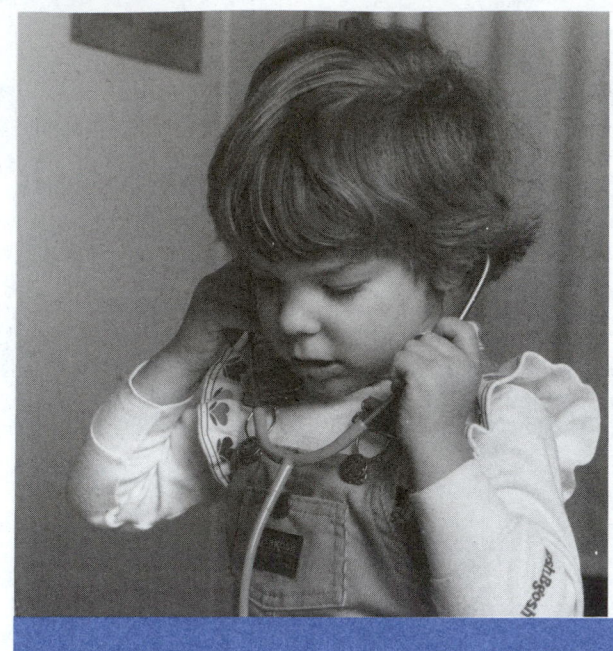

OBJECTIVES

Mastery of content in this chapter will enable the student to:

- Define the terms in the glossary.
- Describe the influence of the school environment on the cognitive and psychosocial development of the school-age child and adolescent.
- Discuss ways in which the nurse can help parents adjust to their child's developmental needs.
- Describe the normal physical changes that occur during the school-age years and adolescence.
- Discuss behaviors that reflect the cognitive development of the school-age child and adolescent.
- List nursing interventions for health concerns specific to the school-age child and adolescent.
- Compare and contrast the ways in which a school-age child and an adolescent develop moral values.
- Discuss the ways in which an adolescent gains a sexual, group, and personal identity.

GLOSSARY

abstract thought Final stage in the development of the cognitive thought processes that occurs between the ages of 12 and 15 years; it is characterized by adaptability, flexibility, the use of abstractions and generalizations, and logical problem solving based on observations.

concrete thought Stage in the development of cognitive thought processes that occurs in ages 7 to 11 years; it is characterized by increasingly logical and coherent thought, the ability to classify, sort, order, and organize facts, and an inability to generalize or think in abstractions.

estrogen Hormonal steroid compound that promotes the development of female secondary sex characteristics.

gonadotropic hormones Substances that are produced and secreted by the anterior pituitary gland and stimulate the function of the testes and ovaries.

menses Normal flow of blood, secretions, and tissue debris that occurs during menstruation, beginning on the first day of the menstrual cycle.

metacognition Act of reflecting on one's own thought processes.

puberty Beginning of the development of secondary sex characteristics.

syntax Arrangement of words as elements in a phrase, clause, or sentence.

testosterone Naturally occurring male sex hormone.

25 School-Age Child and Adolescent

School-age children and adolescents lead demanding, challenging lives. The developmental changes of individuals between ages 6 and 18 are diverse and span all areas of growth and development. Physical, psychosocial, cognitive, and moral skills are developed, expanded, refined, and synchronized so the individual may become an accepted and productive member of society. The environment in which the individual develops skills also expands and diversifies. Instead of being limited to family and close friends, it now may encompass the school, community, and church. Because of the expectations for development, the increasing skill and knowledge base, and environmental expansion, the individual may experience many difficulties and dilemmas in these stages. The nurse's responsibilites in caring for school-age children and adolescents are threefold. First, the nurse must have knowledge of the appropriate developmental stage for each age group in order to carry out assessment. For example, before assessing stage or task achievement of an adolescent, the nurse must know that adolescents normally strive to achieve a sense of identity while developing a moral code compatible with society. Second, the nurse needs to direct the school-age child or adolescent toward normal developmental behaviors, assisting the individual to maximize his abilities and use them to cope. By helping children and adolescents achieve the necessary developmental balance, the nurse promotes health. Table 25-1 provides an overview of developmental behaviors typical of school-age children and adolescents. Third, the nurse must involve the child or adolescent in charting an individual developmental course. Since school-age children have increased cognitive and social skills, they are better able to participate in their development. Not only can they describe their feelings about the changes brought by development, but they can think through these changes, eventually learning to solve problems on their own and achieve the outcomes they desire.

School-age children and adolescents must cope with changes involving all areas of development and frequently occurring at the same time. For example, the 6-year-old child must learn (1) to play with a group of children, following a set of rules, (2) to distinguish right from wrong, (3) to develop reasoning ability, and (4) to read and write. Because of the stress of these changes, a child may develop both physical and psychosocial health problems, for example, increased susceptibility to upper respiratory infections, school maladjustment, inadequate peer relationships, and learning disorders. The nurse's role is to help the child or adolescent avoid or minimize health problems.

School-Age Child

Calling the years between the ages of 6 and 12 the "school-age years" reflects a cultural bias, but this period usually does involve some type of schooling. Most cultures provide some systematic, structured learning experiences to assist children in becoming productive, functioning members of the society. For children in the United States and other industrialized countries, this means immersion in formal schooling. In some other cultures children acquire agricultural or hunting skills necessary for survival. These learning

Developmental Behaviors of School-Age Children and Adolescents

	School-Age Child	Adolescent
Interpersonal relations	Learns that parents can be wrong; continually appraises parent action and values; can sometimes be disillusioned with own parents and would like to trade them in or is certain he is adopted; learns to share some of his own thoughts only with peers; returns to parents and home for companionship, comfort, and security	Is ambivalent about expanding relationships; alternately believes parents are wonderful, wise, understanding, or deceitful, dishonest, stupid; has intense and unstable relationships with peers; has idealistic and shallow perception of world; strives for emotional independence
Fears	—	Worries about loss of identity (bodily, emotional) and failure (in school, career, friendship); is uncertain
Play	Gradually becomes more sensitive to others; shows superstitions, teasing, and insults in games; plays cooperatively—baseball, jacks, hopscotch; finds peers of the same sex and conformity to a group important; demonstrates hoarding by making collections	Develops skills in individual and group games, sports, and activities; joins clubs, groups, and sports teams; is part of a clique that involves peers of the same sex but shares activities with the opposite sex
Dependence	Rejects some ideas of parents and tries own ideas but usually returns to home base; reduces need for dependency by using rituals—bedtime, mealtime, bathtime; becomes responsible, reasonable, and dependable	Is highly ambivalent about wanting limits and needing freedom; discovers responsibility that comes with freedom; makes decisions on own
Morality	May cheat, especially in early years; thinks of own needs first and is out to satisfy them; can think of relationship between an act and its consequences; begins to develop an idea of what it means to live by a label (good boy, good girl, bad boy, bad girl); has a strict literal conscience; begins to be influenced morally by peer group with fixed rules and rituals; becomes concerned about right and wrong	Begins to see that own actions affect a large group of individuals rather than just self; begins logical thought about own principles, rights, and justice as compared with rest of community; establishes a moral code by internalizing principles
Self-image	Begins to see self as labeled by others (boy, girl, mean, nice, bully, cute, etc.); has increasing awareness of sexuality and reproduction, but is modest; is self-critical and anxious to do things right; recognizes individual differences	Learns through group contact; desires to be just like everyone else but more so; tries many different roles; worries excessively about body and bodily functions
Habits	Eating: eats with family and can sit through entire meal; has definite likes and dislikes, but may change suddenly; has rituals around mealtime—same location at table, same silverware, same food Bowels: needs no help from adults Sleeping: may spend night away from home Dressing: can decide on own clothing and dress self but may ask for help and then ignore it; can comb own hair Behavior: may develop annoying habits (i.e., hair twirling, nail biting)	Eating: tries many food fads; eats constantly because of worry over bodily functions, tries fad diets to correct specific problems; would rather eat with peers than family Sleeping: may be so wound up in activities that he sleeps very little; may have trouble going to bed and getting up in morning Dressing: conforms to peers in clothing, hair, makeup, jewelry

Modified from Brown, M.S., and Murphy, M.A.: Ambulatory pediatrics for nurses, ed. 2, New York, 1981, McGraw-Hill Book Co.

TABLE 25-1, cont'd

Developmental Behaviors of School-Age Children and Adolescents

	School-Age Child	Adolescent
Physical	Has increased gross motor ability: rides two-wheel bicycle, climbs trees; has increased manual dexterity, visual perception, and hand-eye coordination; can do multiple physical activities at one time (i.e., hold books, ride bicycle); has improved balance	Has completed major gross and fine motor development; expands experiences with physical capabilities
Cognitive	Is talkative; uses expressive language; begins to understand time and money; has increasing intellectual curiosity; develops favorite subjects to explore; can plan and see a project to completion	Develops adult intellectual skills and concepts; uses abstract logic: constructs hypotheses, and tests them through deductive reasoning

experiences can be interpreted as schooling and will be treated as such in this chapter. The provision of learning experiences that occurs in all cultures during later childhood and adolescence takes advantage of children's increasing physical, cognitive, and psychosocial abilities. Although some educational authorities advocate childhood learning programs, it is generally accepted that optimal learning occurs after, not before, 6 years of age.

The school or educational experience expands the child's world and is a transition from a life of relatively free play to a life of structured play, learning, and work. The school environment joins the home in influencing growth and development. This situation requires adjustment by both the parents and child. The child must learn to cope with the rules and expectations presented by school and peers. Parents must learn to allow their child to make decisions, accept responsibility, and learn from life's experiences.

The role of the nurse in this adjustment process is to promote health. The nurse can help the parents and child identify stresses before they occur and plan to minimize stress and the child's reaction to it. This intervention must include parent, child, and teacher for maximal success. Table 25-2 provides an overview of stresses commonly encountered by school-age children and appropriate nursing interventions.

Physical Development

HEIGHT AND WEIGHT

Gradual and steady physical growth and development occur between the ages of 6 and 12 years. Height increases 1 to 2 inches per year. Weight increase is more variable, averaging 3 to 6 pounds per year. Children generally take on a slimmer, more long-legged look.

Continued evaluation of the child's height and weight curve on a growth chart is essential. Alterations in growth provide a clue to the onset of many disease processes in childhood. Thus monitoring of growth indices, as well as vital signs, is an important tool of the nurse's assessment.

Until approximately ages 9 to 10, boys are an average of 1 inch taller and 2 pounds heavier than girls. Then girls begin a rapid growth period, and by age 12 girls are generally 2 pounds heavier and 1 inch taller than boys. The prepubertal physical changes and growth spurts can occur between 9 and 14 years for girls and 12 and 16 years for boys (Tanner, 1974). Until this time sexual growth and development of secondary sex characteristics, such as the growth of pubic hair, enlargement of the penis, and onset of menses, are minimal.

CARDIOVASCULAR FUNCTIONING

Cardiovascular functioning is refined and stabilized during the school-age years. The heart rate averages 65 to 90 beats per minute, the blood pressure normalizes at 110/70 mm Hg, and the respiratory rate stabilizes to 16 to 18 breaths per minute. Lung growth is minimal. However, by the end of this period the heart is six times the size it was at birth and has generally reached its adult size.

GROSS MOTOR COORDINATION

During the 7 years of the school-age period, children gain increasing control over their bodies. Strength doubles and large muscle coordination im-

TABLE 25-2

Potential School-Related Stresses

Age (years)	Stressor	Nursing Intervention
5-8	Adjusting to teacher's disciplinary approach	Promote parent-teacher-nurse communication through conferences aimed toward identifying expectations, encouraging parental involvement in school or classroom activities, and mediating in conflicts or difficult situations.
	Meeting teacher's behavioral expectations	Encourage communication between child and parent about school expectations, happenings, and adjustments
	Competing with peers for teacher's attention	Promote fair and equal treatment of children in the classroom. Discourage favoritism and performance comparisons and encourage appropriate individual attention and praise.
	Maintaining self-concept	Evaluate parent-child relationship for interaction problems that may transfer to classroom; communicate these to the teacher.
	Coping with hurtful honesty of peers	Promote close supervision of peer activities and behaviors. Discuss peer relationships, their nature, and characteristics with parents and teacher.
	Testing out new ideas and behaviors at home	Set limits on destructive or antisocial behaviors. Allow exploration of new behaviors and ideas with guidance.
	Coping with being away from home for extended period of time; adjusting to school rules and routines	Assist child to identify physical setup of school and daily routines in first few days.
8-10	Concentrating on cognitive pursuits; meeting cognitive expectations of school; meeting own and family's cognitive expectations to best of ability	Encourage communication about the child's performance between the parent, child, and teacher. Assist in identifying skills mastered and those in need of mastery. Assist in identifying early problems. Assess level of health, particularly sensory function, as it may relate to school difficulties. Accept the child and his performance and behaviors as individual when considered within the norm.
	Integrating peer values into behavior without interference with family values	Observe peer activities and interactions. Reinforce positive behaviors and performance. Provide education for parents and teachers regarding normal behaviors of age.
10-12	Assuming responsibility for own learning	Encourage the allocation of learning responsibilities and allow child to carry them out. Encourage the child's participation in identifying learning needs.
	Deriving satisfaction from own cognitive performance	Positively reinforce good performance and guide the child when performance is optimal; do not punish.

Modified from Laige, J.: The school age child and his family. In Hymovich, D., and Barnard, M., editors: Family health care: developmental and situational crises, New York, 1973, McGraw-Hill Book Co.; and McElroy, E., and Tackett, J.J.: Growth and development needs of the family with school age children: maintaining wellness. In Tackett, J.J., and Hunsberger, M., editors: Family centered care of children and adolescents, Philadelphia, 1981, W.B. Saunders Co.

Potential School-Related Stresses

Age (years)	Stressor	Nursing Intervention
	Participating in organized school or peer activity	Assist child in identifying school or peer group activity that he enjoys and in which he can potentially be successful. Assist parents in realizing need for extracurricular activities and encouraging the child's appropriate participation (i.e., avoid excessive demands to win and promote honest, fair play). Encourage teachers to recognize importance of after-school activities and avoid overloading children with homework.
	Beginning to develop a set of behavioral standards that reflect being in control and requiring little or no adult supervision	Promote good conduct through praise and example. Encourage parents to trust child, recognizing that not all behaviors will be "perfect."

proves. These developments make school-age children appear more skillful in their body movements. They can successfully participate in activities and games requiring coordinated muscle movements. Individual differences in the rate of mastering skills and ultimate skill achievement become apparent. The exposure to a variety of experiences, as well as innate ability, plays a role in the individual differences of motor skills.

FINE MOTOR COORDINATION

Fine motor coordination improves between the ages of 6 and 12 years. Most 6-year-old children can hold a pencil adeptly and print letters and words. By age 12 the child can make detailed drawings and write sentences in script. Painting, drawing, and model making provide vehicles for children to practice and improve their newly refined skills. Nurses should encourage children and have parents encourage their children to pursue these activities.

Assessment of a child's neurological development is often based on his fine motor coordination. Such assessment may include penmanship, stacking ability, and performance of sequential rapid, alternating movements such as touching the finger to the nose and then to the examiner's finger. Smooth movement without tremors is the normal response. Fine motor coordination is critical to success in the typical American school, where children must be able to hold pencils and crayons and use scissors and rulers. Teachers frequently ask the school nurse to conduct fine motor assessment of a child with questionable ability.

Nurses need to know what constitutes normal fine motor functioning in order to provide this initial neurological screening. The nurse should refer the child with deviations from normal function for a more thorough assessment.

NUTRITIONAL NEEDS

Nutritional requirements remain relatively stable in the school-age years. Children need to continue a balanced diet that includes the four basic food groups. Promotion of sound nutrition and good eating habits is an important part of the nurse's role. Nurses should encourage parents to provide a variety of foods for their children, in adequate amounts to support both growth and energy for play. Since play activities vary from day to day, energy requirements also vary. Children of this age do not usually eat a large amount of food at one time. Providing nutritious snacks is often the best way for a parent to ensure adequate nutritional intake for an active child. Small servings of fruit, vegetables, and high-protein foods should be made available to encourage nutritious snacking.

OTHER CHANGES

Other physical changes take place during the school-age years. A steady skeletal growth in the trunk and extremities occurs, and small and long bone ossification is present but not complete by age 12. Facial bones grow and remodel as indicated by the presence of frontal sinuses by age 8 or 9. Dental growth is prominent during the school-age years. By 10 years of age all primary teeth have been shed and

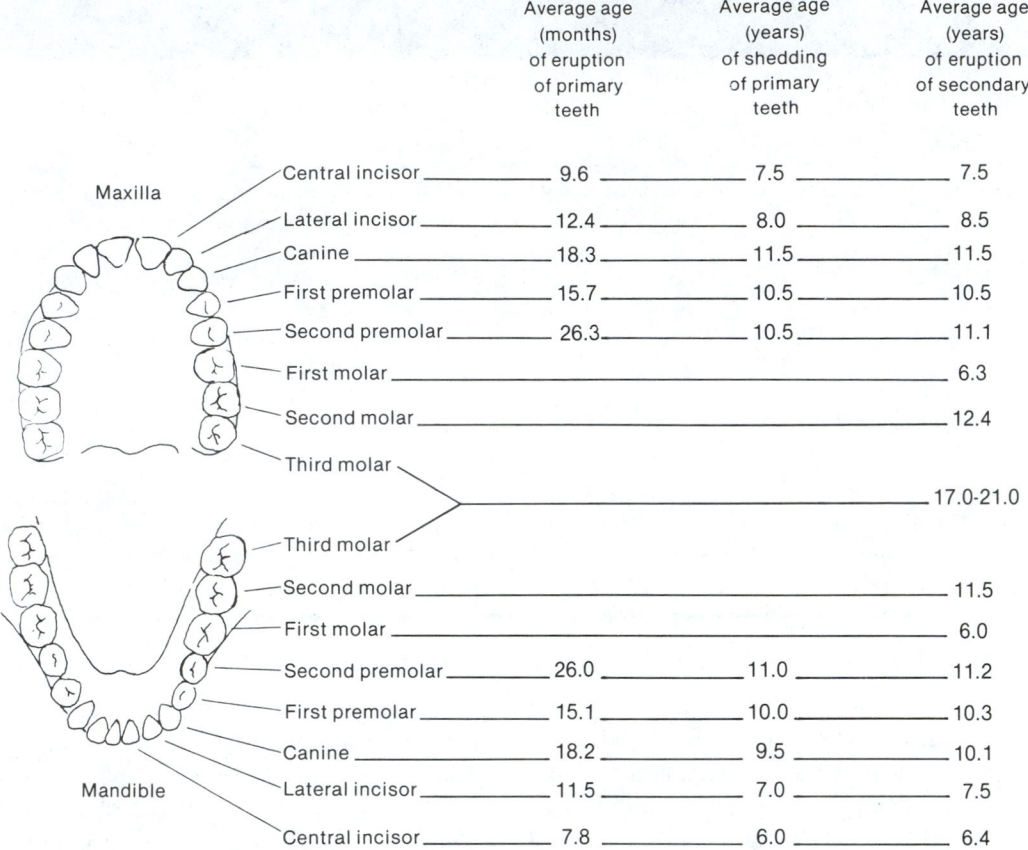

		Average age (months) of eruption of primary teeth	Average age (years) of shedding of primary teeth	Average age (years) of eruption of secondary teeth
Maxilla	Central incisor	9.6	7.5	7.5
	Lateral incisor	12.4	8.0	8.5
	Canine	18.3	11.5	11.5
	First premolar	15.7	10.5	10.5
	Second premolar	26.3	10.5	11.1
	First molar			6.3
	Second molar			12.4
	Third molar			17.0-21.0
	Third molar			
	Second molar			11.5
	First molar			6.0
	Second premolar	26.0	11.0	11.2
	First premolar	15.1	10.0	10.3
	Canine	18.2	9.5	10.1
Mandible	Lateral incisor	11.5	7.0	7.5
	Central incisor	7.8	6.0	6.4

Fig. 25-1 Sequence of eruption of secondary teeth.

From Whaley, L.F., and Wong, D.L.: Nursing care of infants and children, ed. 2, St. Louis, 1983, The C.V. Mosby Co.

the majority of permanent teeth have erupted. Fig. 25-1 illustrates the pattern and timing of dental shedding and eruption.

As skeletal growth progresses, overall body appearance and posture change. Earlier posture, which was characterized by a stoop-shouldered, slightly lordotic stance and prominent abdomen, changes to a more erect posture by the end of this period.

Eye shape alters as a result of skeletal growth. This improves visual acuity, and normal adult 20/20 vision is achievable. Screening for vision and hearing problems is easier, and results are more reliable because school-age children can more fully understand and cooperate with the test directions. The school nurse frequently assesses visual and auditory status of school-age children. Knowledge of normal functioning is essential as the basis for assessment.

Cognitive Development

Cognitive changes provide the school-age child with powerful capabilities for exploring, understand-ing, and communicating his understanding of the world. The ability to think abstractly, use past information, and plan for the future develops or improves during the years between 6 and 12. According to Piaget's theory, during these years children move toward the stage of formal operations, in which thought processes are abstract. Between the ages of 5 and 7, children learn to organize facts by classifying, sorting, and ordering. This process remains quite concrete, however, and is based on the child's perceptions. As experience increases, children consolidate their new skills and increasingly move from concrete thinking to inductive logic. Children can now group objects, identify general similarities and differences, and solve problems. By understanding principles of combination children can add, subtract, and count objects; this is evident in the common school-age pastime of collecting items such as stamps, rocks, or buttons. The manner in which the child groups items in a collection can serve as a clue to the child's understanding of objects and their uses.

Between the ages of 7 and 12, children become able

to carry out many cognitive processes without physically going through the motions or manipulating objects. Cognitive function extends beyond the child's past and potential concrete experiences. The child now considers the views of others, and his thinking is more socialized.

Children now begin metacognition, or thinking about their own thought processes. Metacognition allows one to plan and initiate strategies to improve one's learning processes. Some cognitive theorists consider metacognition the underlying principle responsible for cognitive growth (Siegler, 1978). The cognitive processes involved in short-term memory illustrate children's developing use of metacognition. Young children of 4 or 5 years are able to remember short lists of meaningful items. In a play situation, if given a list of items to obtain from a play store, the preschool child may aid his memory by repeating the list aloud to himself. If asked how he remembered the items, however, he is likely to be unable to respond. In contrast, school-age children *consciously* develop strategies for remembering the desired items. They may classify the items alphabetically or phonetically. If asked how they remembered, school-age children can describe their strategy. That is, they can think about their thinking, employing metacognitive processes. The use of metacognition allows school-age children to benefit from suggestions of ways to improve their cognitive strategies.

LANGUAGE DEVELOPMENT

Language development also continues in the school years. Children learn the language of both their peers and adults. Vocabulary increases with exposure to new words. Children are now less bound by the restrictions of their family's language. They become more aware of the rules of syntax, that is, the rules for linking words into phrases and sentences. School-age children can identify generalizations and exceptions to rules. They accept language as a means for representing the world in a subjective manner. They come to realize that words have arbitrary, rather than absolute, meanings. They can use different words for the same object or concept, and they understand that a single word may have multiple meanings.

UNDERSTANDING OF SPATIAL RELATIONSHIPS

During the school-age years the child's ability to understand spatial representation is refined. Children are now able to visualize various positions in space and evaluate how changes in position alter their perspective. For example, a 10-year-old can create a mental picture of how he would feel and where his body would be placed on a roller coaster making a 360-degree loop. In addition, children recognize that they, as well as objects, assume relative positions in space. These developing abilities are reflected by a child's increased ability to find his way around the neighborhood and read simple maps. Hospitalized children enjoy touring the facility, locating all of the departments to which they have been. The nurse accompanies the child to ensure his safety.

MORAL DEVELOPMENT

During the school-age years the child begins to show evidence of developing a moral code. Between the ages of 6 and 9 the child recognizes and labels behaviors as right or wrong, good or bad. This labeling is primarily influenced by the child's family and culture. Gradually the child applies these labels to his own behavior based on the pleasurable or unpleasurable consequences of an action. For example, the 5-year-old child labels taking a cookie without asking as bad. However, he will ask for the cookie only if the consequences are pleasurable (that is, he gets the cookie) and the unpleasurable (that is, receiving no cookie and possibly a scolding) is avoided.

As the child progresses through the school-age years, he becomes more concerned with activities that maintain and support society's norms. Peers, school, and society begin to influence the labeling of behaviors. The child between 9 and 12 is concerned with conformity, loyalty, and behavior that not only gains approval but helps others as well. The 11- or 12-year-old typically believes that obeying the rules and showing respect for authority are important.

Psychosocial Development

During the school-age years children are directing their energies toward increasing their skills. The child's psychosocial development is influenced by his physical and cognitive skill development. For example, improved fine motor capabilities, such as buttoning and tying, allow the school-age child to dress himself and take care of his personal needs. Most school-age children demand independence in activities of daily living because of their increased skill level. They develop strong preferences in how their needs are met. An adult's introduction or suggestion of new practices, styles of clothing, or food can meet with strong resistance, which is a reflection of the school-age child's need to maintain control and take the initiative in change. The nurse who recommends changes to parents or who attempts to implement changes in the school-age child's activities of daily living needs to consider the child's need for independence. The school-age child should be involved in any decisions about changes and the specific actions for implementing such changes.

PEER RELATIONSHIPS

Group, as well as personal, achievement becomes important to the school-age child and stimulates a sense of achievement. Successful outcomes are important in both physical and cognitive activities. Becoming a productive member of a peer group is important in this stage of development. Play increasingly involves peers and the pursuit of group goals. Although solitary activities are not eliminated, they are overshadowed by group play. Learning to contribute, collaborate, and work cooperatively toward a common goal becomes a measure of a child's success.

The school-age child prefers same-sex peers to opposite-sex peers. This strong gender identity is evidenced by the close network of same-sex companions a child maintains. In general both girls and boys view the opposite sex negatively. Peer influence becomes quite diverse during this stage of development. Mannerisms, clothing styles, and speech patterns are reinforced and influenced by contact with peers. Group identity increases as the school-age child approaches adolescence.

MORAL DEVELOPMENT

The need for a moral code and social rules becomes more evident to the school-age child as his cognitive ability and social experiences increase. For example, the 12-year-old child is able to consider what society would be like without rules because of his ability to reason logically and his experiences with group play employing rules. The child views rules as necessary principles of life, not just dictates from authorities. In the early school years, children strictly interpret and adhere to rules. As they develop, they make more flexible judgments and evaluate rules for applicability to a given situation. Late school-age children consider motivations, as well as the actual behavior, in making judgments of how their behavior will affect themselves and others. The ability to be flexible in applying rules and to take the perspective of others is essential in developing moral judgments. These abilities are present at times in earlier years, but they are more consistently displayed in later school years.

SELF-CONCEPT AND HEALTH

During the school-age years identity and self-concept are becoming stronger and more individualized. Behaviors are reinforced or altered by the child's experiences. A child's perception of his own wellness is based on readily observable facts, such as presence or absence of illness and adequacy of eating or sleeping. Functional ability is the standard by which a child judges his own health and the health of others.

Promotion of good health practices is a nursing responsibility. Programs directed toward health education are frequently organized and conducted in the school. The nurse's goal for such programs should be the development of behaviors that positively affect children's health status. Examples of program topics that encourage positive behaviors are dental health, good nutrition and eating habits, and treatment for a cold.

Specific Health Concerns

Accidents and injuries are a major health problem affecting school-age children. Motor vehicle accidents and accidents related to recreational activities or equipment are the leading causes of death or injury for school-age children. Nurses have a responsibility to promote health through accident prevention and safety education.

School-age children are also significantly affected by cancer, birth defects, influenza, and pneumonia (Department of Health, Education and Welfare, 1979). In this age group these problems have a relatively low mortality as compared with accidents, but a high morbidity.

School-age children face other significant health problems, including learning and school difficulties; behavioral disturbances; speech, hearing, or vision problems; and infectious diseases. To promote normal and healthy growth and development, the nurse must be aware of these risks and direct nursing actions toward their reduction.

Adolescent

Adolescence is the stage of development that marks the transition from childhood to adulthood. The term "adolescence" refers to the psychological maturation of the individual. Puberty is the biological maturation that makes reproduction possible (Tackett and Hunsberger, 1981).

The period of life between 13 and 18 years of age is characterized by a steady progression of physical, social, cognitive, psychological, and moral changes. The adaptations required by these changes push the adolescent to develop individualized coping mechanisms and styles of behaviors, which he will continue to use or adapt throughout life. Typical adolescent behaviors are outlined in Table 25-1.

During this stage of development an adolescent must establish his own identity, make major decisions regarding his life and vocation, develop and refine adult cognitive skills, and establish a code of morality by which all of these tasks are ordered. With so much to accomplish, it is little wonder that adolescents are frequently moody and difficult to live and work with.

The nurse's understanding of adolescents' developmental tasks provides a unique perspective for helping teenagers and their parents cope with the stresses of adolescence. Nursing activities, particularly education, can promote healthy development. They occur in a variety of settings and are directed toward the adolescent alone, the parents alone, or the adolescent and parent together. For example, the nurse can conduct seminars in a high school to provide practical suggestions for solving problems of concern to a large group of students, such as treating acne or making friends. Similarly, a group education program for parents on how to cope with teenage children would promote parental understanding and adolescent development. Programs such as these can occur in the school, a clinic, or a private office or in community groups. Regardless of the setting or topic, the nurse needs a basic understanding of adolescent growth and development before embarking on educational projects. In addition, the nurse must identify adolescents' need and desire to learn more about a specific topic or problem. Finally, involving the participants of the program in identifying the topic and developing the program produces more active, interested learners.

Physical Changes and Sexual Maturation

Physical changes occur rapidly during adolescence in both males and females. Sexual maturation occurs with the development of primary and secondary sexual characteristics. Primary characteristics are physical and hormonal changes that are necessary for reproduction, and secondary characteristics externally differentiate males from females. Four main focuses of the physical changes are summarized by Tanner (1974):

1. Increased growth rate of skeleton, muscle, and viscera
2. Sex-specific changes, such as changes in shoulder and hip width
3. Alteration in the distribution of muscle and fat
4. Development of the reproductive system and secondary sex characteristics

There is a wide variation in the timing of physical changes associated with puberty, and girls tend to begin their physical changes earlier than boys.

WEIGHT AND SKELETAL CHANGES

The majority of height and weight increases occur during the pubertal growth spurt, which generally precedes adult maturity by 1 to 2 years. The growth spurt for girls generally begins between the ages of 10 and 14. Height increases between 2 and 8 inches, and weight increases by 15 to 50 pounds. The male growth spurt usually takes place between the ages of 12 and 16. Height increases approximately 4 to 12 inches, and weight increases by 15 to 60 pounds. Fat becomes redistributed into adult proportions as height and weight increase, and gradually the adolescent torso takes on an adult appearance. Although individual differences and differences between the sexes do occur, growth generally follows a similar pattern for both sexes. The legs lengthen first, followed by widening of thighs, broadening of shoulders, and trunk growth. Hips then widen in females and shoulders continue to widen in males.

Personal growth curves continue to be meaningful in assessing physical development. The individual's progression along the curve, however, is more important than how closely measurements correspond to the norm. The nurse continues to chart growth measurements to evaluate growth changes in relation to past growth patterns.

EFFECTS OF PHYSICAL CHANGES ON PEER INTERACTION

Adolescents are sensitive about the physical changes that make them different from peers. For this reason they are generally interested in the normal pattern of growth, as well as in their personal growth curves. Consequently, the nurse should share this information to reassure adolescents that their own patterns are normal. If an adolescent deviates radically from the usual pattern, further assessment is necessary to identify the cause of the deviation. Weight extremes resulting from excessive or inadequate caloric intake are common nursing diagnoses during the adolescent years. Allowing the adolescent to see when and how the weight curve changed can be a first step in identifying the problem and implementing dietary changes.

PUBERTY

TIMING. Not only is there wide variation between the sexes as to when the physical changes of puberty begin, but there is also wide variation within the same sex. This variation is more pronounced in males (Tanner and Whitehouse, 1982). In American males the time of onset of pubertal changes appears to have a significant effect on psychosocial development. Early physical development has been found advantageous in later psychosocial interactions because early-developing males, who are more successful in group activities and peer relationships, gain an early sense of desirability that is maintained throughout later life. Less information is available about the impact of timing of physical development in females.

SEQUENCE. Despite the wide variation in timing, the sequence of pubertal growth changes is the same in

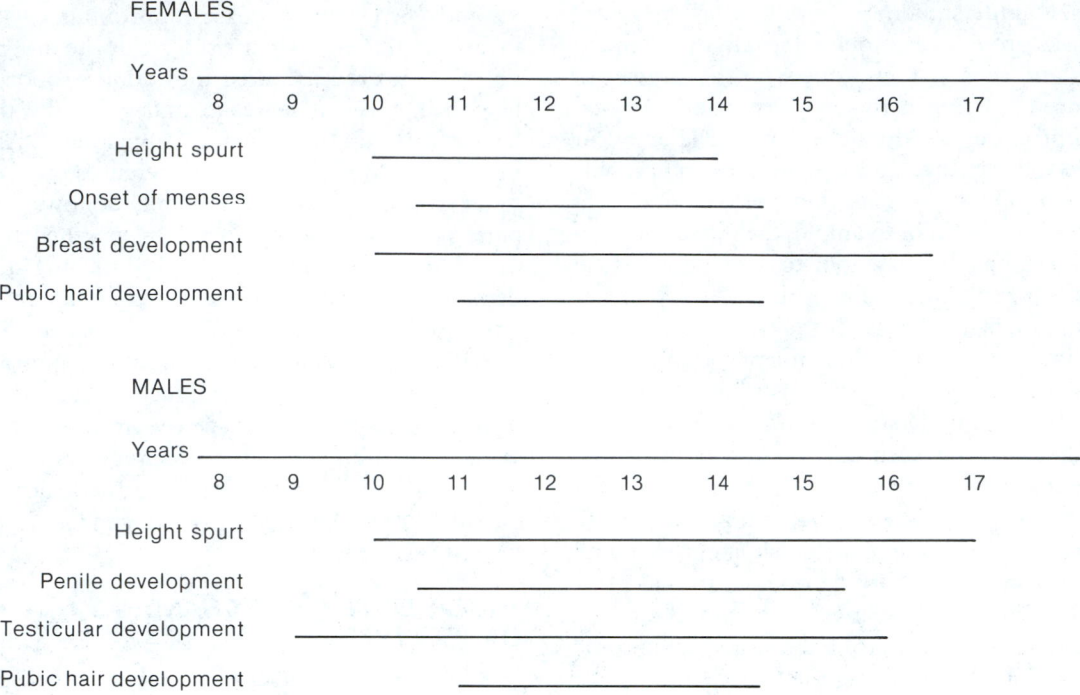

Fig. 25-2 Criteria for rating sexual maturity and growth.
Modified from Marshall, W., and Tanner, J.: Arch. Dis. Child. **45**:13, 1970.

most individuals. This stability is the basis of the most widely recognized and used systems for rating sexual maturity (Tanner and Whitehouse, 1982). Fig. 25-2 presents the criteria used in this categorization; the wide ranges of *normal* progression are stressed. As with increases in height and weight, the pattern of sexual changes is more significant than their time of onset. Large deviations from the normal time frames require investigation. For example, a 17-year-old girl who has not menstruated requires further assessment and referral. Being like one's peers is extremely important for adolescents. Any deviation in the timing of the physical changes can be extremely difficult for the adolescent to accept. The nurse therefore should provide emotional support for adolescents undergoing assessment of early or delayed puberty. Even adolescents whose physical changes are occurring at the normal times may seek confirmation of and reassurance about their normalcy.

HORMONAL CHANGES. In addition to the visible changes of puberty, invisible changes are also taking place. Among these are hormonal changes.

All pubertal events are created by hormonal changes within the body when the hypothalamus begins to produce releasing factors. The gonadotropic releasing hormones signal the pituitary to secrete gonadotropic hormones. The gonadotropic hormones stimulate ovarian cells to produce estrogen and testicular cells to produce testosterone. These hormones contribute to the development of secondary sex characteristics such as hair growth and voice changes and play an essential role in reproduction. The changing concentrations of these hormones are also linked to problems of concern to adolescents, such as acne and body odor. Understanding this hormonal physiology enables the nurse to educate and reassure adolescent clients.

▪ ▪ ▪ ▪ ▪

The physical changes that occur during adolescence are dramatic and rapid. They play a significant role in the concurrent psychosocial development of the adolescent. The presence of newly expanded cognitive abilities also influences psychosocial development.

Cognitive Development

School-age children can think logically about problems involving concrete situations. In adolescence the range of problems that can be addressed is extended, as is the ability to reason abstractly. Adolescents are capable of formal operations in which they must think about thinking and separate real from possible. This means that adolescents can use deductive reasoning even in situations beyond their concrete experiences.

Abstractions from hypothetical situations can be processed and understood. Adolescents can consider the logic of a problem, irrespective of its contents. They can solve even problems that require the simultaneous manipulation of several abstract concepts. Development of this ability is important in the adolescent's pursuit of an identity. For example, the newly acquired cognitive skills allow the teenager to decide which sex role behaviors are appropriate, effective, and comfortable, and to consider their potential impact on peers, family, and society. Being able to think logically about these behaviors and their outcomes encourages adolescents to develop their own thoughts and means of expressing sexual identity. In addition, a higher level of cognitive functioning makes the adolescent receptive to more detailed information regarding sexuality and sexual behaviors. For example, sex education for the adolescent can include an explanation of the physiology of the sexual changes, as well as a detailed outline of how birth control measures work to prevent normal physiological events.

However, having the potential to function at this cognitive level does not ensure corresponding performance. Both cognitive abilities and their performance vary greatly among adolescents. Indeed, an adolescent may perform at different cognitive levels in different situations. Past stimulation, experiences, and formal education in the use of logic and effective deductive strategies, as well as the individual situation, influence the expression of cognitive abilities.

LANGUAGE SKILLS

Language development is fairly complete by adolescence, although vocabularly continues to expand. The primary focus becomes the development of communication skills that can be employed effectively in various situations. The adolescent needs to be able to communicate thoughts, feelings, and facts to peers and to parents, teachers, and other persons of authority. The skills used in these diverse communication situations are varied. The adolescent must select the person with whom he wants to communicate, decide how much to say, and choose the way he will transmit the message. For example, the way a teenager tells his parents about a failing grade is not the same as the way he tells his friends. The adolescent develops different skills and styles of communication and learns how and when to use them most effectively. These diverse communication skills are used and refined throughout life.

MORAL DEVELOPMENT

The development of moral judgment depends heavily on cognitive and communication skills and peer interaction. Although moral development begins in early childhood, it is consolidated more fully in adolescence because of the presence of these skills. Adolescents learn to understand rules as cooperative agreements that can be modified to fit the situation, rather than as absolutes. Adolescents learn to apply rules by using their own judgment rather than simply to avoid punishment as in the earlier years.

Kohlberg (1964) explains moral development in terms of a number of stages, summarized in Table 23-8. Adolescents can achieve the highest level of moral judgment presented in this system; at this level morality is derived from individual principles of conscience. Adolescents judge themselves by internalized ideals; this often leads to conflict between personal and group values. Group values become less significant in later adolescence.

As with other cognitive abilities, not all adolescents attain the same level of moral development. There is, however, a general forward movement through the stages of moral development, and the sequence of the stages is similar for all individuals even when the time of achievement varies.

Psychosocial Development

As adulthood approaches, teenagers must establish intimate relationships or remain socially isolated. An emotional independence from and equilibrium with their families must be established, and they must adjust to and master their own sexuality.

Adolescence is a time when identity is consolidated. In addition, choices about vocation and life-style must be made. Evolving from all these tasks is a sexual, group, and personal identity that is unique to the individual.

SEXUAL IDENTITY

Achievement of sexual identity is enhanced by the physical changes of puberty. The physical evidence of being a mature male or female encourages the development of masculine and feminine behaviors. If these physical changes involve deviations, the person is more likely to develop sexual identity problems. Adolescents are dependent on these physical clues because they want assurance of maleness or femaleness and because they do not wish to be different from peers. Without the physical characteristics of maleness or femaleness, the process of achieving sexual identity is difficult. Additional influences on the development of sexual identity are cultural attitudes and expectations of sex role behavior and the role models available to the adolescent. The masculine and feminine behaviors teenagers see and the expectations they perceive for behaving as a man or woman affect how they express sexuality. The adolescent has mastered sexuality when he feels comfortable with his sexual behaviors, choices, and relationships.

GROUP IDENTITY

Adolescents seek a group identity because of needs for esteem and acceptance. Similarity in dress or speech is common in teenage groups. Popularity remains a major concern of adolescents. Trends in the desire for popularity have not changed much in recent years. Females of middle-class status, more than any other group, regard popularity as particularly important. Conforming to group activities, being friendly, being oneself, and having a good personality are considered by teenagers to be the most important factors in gaining popularity (Padin, Lerner, and Spiro, 1981). Popularity with the opposite sex as well as with same-sex peers becomes important during adolescence. The strong need for group identity seems in conflict at times with the adolescent's striving for personal identity. It is as though the adolescent requires a close bond with peers so he can later redefine himself against this group identity.

FAMILY RELATIONSHIPS

The movement toward stronger peer relationships is contrasted with the adolescent's movement away from parents. Although financial independence for adolescents is not the norm in American society, many adolescents work part-time, using their income to bolster their independence. The adolescent has more control over purchases and social activities if the parents are not the only financial resource.

Some adolescents and their families have more difficulty during these years than others. The differences can be a result of the number, extent, and nature of the adolescent's usual cyclical movements from periods of independence to relative dependence. Adolescents need to make choices, act independently, and experience the consequences of their actions. This testing, however, is best done against a firm, supportive, family foundation. The family needs to allow independence while providing a haven in which adolescents can contemplate their actions. Families that are unable to provide this support complicate the adolescent's movement toward identity formation.

PERSONAL IDENTITY

One component of personal identity involves selecting an occupational or vocational direction in life. Because of society's changing needs, adolescents must be somewhat future oriented in making these choices. However, because the jobs that will be available or that adolescents will find rewarding 10 or 20 years in the future are not clear, selecting a livelihood is a complicated task. The nurse should provide emotional support to adolescents during this process and should help them select courses of action that promote self-satisfaction and identity.

An additional part of an adolescent's personal identity is his perception of his health. This component is of specific interest to health care providers. Healthy adolescents evaluate their own health according to their feelings of well-being, ability to function normally, and absence of symptoms. Interventions to improve the adolescent's health perception might therefore concentrate on these areas. Health problems that cause severe or long-term alteration of these factors may permanently alter the adolescent's self-identity.

Specific Health Concerns

Several issues are of particular concern in the adolescent years. The leading cause of death in adolescence remains accidents (Shen, 1980), with motor vehicle accidents being the most common. Such accidents are often associated with alcohol or drug abuse, depression, and generalized feelings of stress. Nurses can help educate adolescents to recognize these factors in themselves and their peers; educational interventions can reduce the potential for accidents.

Another area of concern to adolescent health is the formation of healthy habits of daily living. Emphasis on exercise, sleep, nutrition, and stress reduction habits is increasing. It is the nurse's responsibility to recognize the importance of these habits and to identify ways to adapt them to the individual adolescent. To do this the nurse must assess what habits are positive and negative for the individual, as well as the person's attitude about health. Both accidents and the formation of healthy habits have psychological as well as physical components and effects. Extensive and long-term follow-up is required if individualized interventions are to be successful. The nurse needs to be aware of the prevalence of these problems and make assessments accordingly.

Sexual experimentation is common among adolescents. Peer pressures, physiological and emotional changes, and societal expectations all contribute to early heterosexual and homosexual relations among adolescents. The nurse's responsibility is to provide adolescents and their families with sex education and counseling. The degree of sexual activity among teenagers may not change significantly but the degree of informed, consenting participation can. Two prominent consequences of adolescent sexual activity are sexually transmitted disease and pregnancy.

Sexually transmitted diseases are the most common communicable diseases among adolescents. The combined incidence of gonorrhea, syphilis, and genital herpes simplex has increased to over 12 million cases a year. Nurses should encourage early recognition and prompt reporting and treatment in order to reduce this incidence.

Adolescent pregnancy is a major concern in American society. The physical, educational, and psychosocial consequences to the mother have received much investigation. Low–birth weight infants, higher school dropout rates, and later social isolation are all cited as negative consequences of adolescent pregnancy. The nurse working with pregnant adolescents will be confronted with these and other problems. The adolescent male may also experience problems related to teenage pregnancy. Early marriage, higher school dropout rates, and relative social isolation from peers are potential problems.

Summary

In the school-age and adolescent years the individual grows and develops significantly. At the beginning of the school-age years the child is a slightly egocentric, inquisitive, reality-oriented person whose physical and cognitive abilities do not always measure up to his psychosocial needs and desires. By age 12, the child has become intellectually and physically adept, has established a social sphere, has begun to develop a moral code, and has started to mature sexually.

Further developmental advances are made during the adolescent years. By age 18, most adolescents have made the transition to adulthood. They are well on their way to becoming socially responsible, productive human beings, capable of sustaining interpersonal relationships and a vocation and demonstrating formal cognitive abilities and moral judgment, all with a firmly developed individual identity.

A nurse may have the responsibility of guiding and counseling individuals through the school-age and adolescent stages, which are particularly challenging because of the diversity and simultaneous development of changes in all spheres. Being able to examine and assess all components of these and other developmental stages is an essential skill of nursing.

KEY CONCEPTS

✓ A developmental task of the school-age child is the formation of an identity.

✓ The prepubertal growth spurt usually affects girls at an earlier age than boys.

✓ Changes in a child's growth pattern may indicate the onset of disease.

✓ During the school-age years, a child gains the muscle strength and coordination needed to participate in complex gross and fine motor activities.

✓ The school-age child develops the ability to think abstractly, reflect on his own thought processes, and plan for the future.

✓ During the school-age years, the child learns the rules of language development.

✓ The school-age child develops a sense of what is morally right and wrong and respects the role of authority.

✓ The extent to which the school-age child develops physically and cognitively will influence his psychosocial development.

✓ The school-age child has the need to exert control and make his own decisions.

✓ The school-age child learns to develop cognitively and psychosocially through peer relationships.

✓ The adolescent must adapt to significant stressors in order to gain a sense of identity and achieve psychological maturity.

✓ During adolescence primary and secondary sexual characteristics develop.

✓ The adolescent becomes concerned about patterns of growth because he fears being different from his peers.

✓ There is wide variation among members of the same sex as to when physical changes of puberty occur.

✓ Physical changes of puberty are linked to hormonal changes.

✓ The adolescent is capable of abstract thought and deductive reasoning.

✓ Although the adolescent's use of language is well developed, he must acquire effective communication skills.

✓ The adolescent's sense of right and wrong evolves from his application of moral rules to daily decision making.

✓ The formation of a meaningful identity rests on an adolescent's needs for normal physical development, acceptance from peers, independence from the family, and choice of a future occupation.

✓ Sexually transmitted diseases are the most common communicable diseases among adolescents.

REFERENCES

Department of Health, Education, and Welfare: Healthy people, Washington D.C., 1979, U.S. Government Printing Office.

Kohlberg, L.: Development of moral character and moral ideology. In Hoffman, M.L., and Hoffman, L.N.W., editors: Review of child development research, vol. I, New York, 1964, Russell Sage Foundation.

Padin, M., Lerner, R., and Spiro, A.: Stability of body attitudes and self esteem in late adolescence, Adolescence 61:371, 1981.

Shen, J., editor: The clinical practice of adolescent medicine, New York, 1980, Appleton-Century-Crofts.

Siegler, R.: Children's thinking: what develops? Hillsdale, N.J., 1978, Lawrence Erlbaum Associates, Inc.

Tackett, J.J., and Hunsberger, M., editors: Family centered care of children and adolescents, Philadelphia, 1981, W.B. Saunders Co.

Tanner, J.M.: Sequence and tempo in the somatic changes of puberty. In Grumbach, M.M., et al., editors: Control of the onset of puberty, New York, 1974, John Wiley & Sons, Inc.

Tanner, J.M., and Whitehouse, R.H.: Atlas of children's growth: normal variation and growth diseases, New York, 1982, Academic Press, Inc.

ADDITIONAL READINGS

Brown, M.S., and Murphy, M.A.: Ambulatory pediatrics for nurses, ed. 2, New York, 1981, McGraw-Hill Book Co.

Chow, M., et al.: Handbook of pediatric primary care, New York, 1979, John Wiley & Sons, Inc.

Laige, J.: The school aged child and his family. In Hymovich, D. and Barnard, M., editors: Family health care: developmental and situational crises, New York, 1973, McGraw-Hill Book Co.

Marshall, W., and Tanner, J.: Variations in the patterns of pubertal changes in girls, Arch. Dis. Child. 44:291, 1969.

Marshall, W., and Tanner, J.: Variations in the patterns of pubertal changes in boys, Arch. Dis. Child. 45:13, 1970.

Whaley, L.F., and Wong, D.L.: Nursing care of infants and children, ed. 2, St. Louis, 1983, The C.V. Mosby Co.

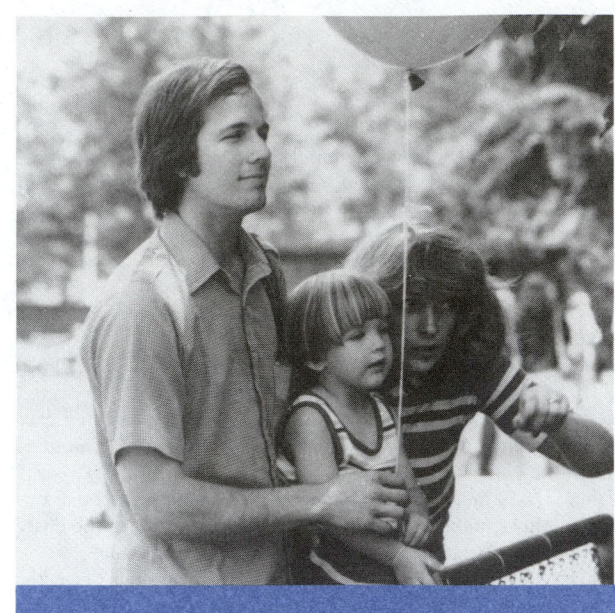

OBJECTIVES

Mastery of content in this chapter will enable the student to:

- Define the terms in the glossary.
- Discuss developmental theories of the young and middle adult.
- List and discuss the major life events of the young and middle adult and the childbearing family.
- Describe the developmental tasks of the young adult, the childbearing family, and the middle adult.
- Discuss the significance of the family in the life of the adult.
- Describe the normal physiological changes in young and middle adulthood and in pregnancy.
- Discuss the cognitive and psychosocial changes occurring during the adult years.
- Describe the health concerns of the young adult, the childbearing family, and the middle adult.

GLOSSARY

climacteric Physiological developmental change that occurs in the male reproductive system between the ages of 45 and 60.

family stress Stress related to the individual's roles, relationships, or functions within the family.

infertility Man's, woman's, or couple's involuntary inability to conceive.

lactation Process and period in which the mother produces milk for the infant.

maturity State of adulthood in which the person has attained independence with a balanced development in cognitive, psychomotor, and emotional dimensions.

morning sickness Pregnant woman's symptoms of nausea and vomiting related to changes in serum hormone levels.

orgasmic maturity Physiological maturity of the reproductive system enabling the individual to complete the adult sexual response cycle.

proactive decision Decision made by an individual directed at attaining a goal.

puerperium Period of approximately 6 weeks after childbirth during which the woman's reproductive system is in transition to the nonpregnant state.

reactive decision Decision made by an individual in response to the influence of others.

26 Young and Middle Adult

Young and middle adulthood is a period of challenges, rewards, and crises. Adults have the challenge of entering the workforce, the reward of a job well done, and the crises associated with caring for parents and rearing a family or remaining single. Many adults have responsibility for persons at each end of the age continuum; an adult may be supporting his own family while having to care for older parents or in-laws.

Adult development involves orderly and sequential changes in characteristics and attitudes. Developmental changes are sequential in the sense that earlier characteristics help to shape subsequent behavior and characteristics (Beck, Rawlins, and Williams, 1984). As the person progresses through life, he continues to evolve and change. The changes experienced by the young adult include the natural processes of maturation and socialization. The young adult passes through alternating periods of stability and change. During periods of stability the person makes certain choices in his life and builds a structure around them. In periods of change the individual reevaluates these choices and considers new alternatives (Levinson et al., 1978).

Young adulthood is the period between the early twenties and the late thirties or early forties. During this time the person increasingly separates from his family of origin, establishes career goals, and decides whether to marry and begin his own family or remain single. The young adult is active and must adapt to new experiences.

The person's entry into middle age depends on various events that generally signify transition into this time of life. The middle adult years are commonly understood to include the 45- to 65-year-old group, with the years from 40 to 45 considered the midlife transition (Levinson et al., 1978).

The midlife transition occurs when a person becomes aware that changes in reproductive and physical abilities signify the beginning of another stage in life. During this transition period the individual may reappraise his goals in life and add new goals.

From 1970 to 1981 the U.S. population increased by 25 million. Of the 166 million people over 18 years old, the 45- to 64-year-old group is the largest, followed by the 25- to 34-year-old group. The median age of the population of Canada and the United States has been rising slowly but consistently over the last decade and is now 30.3 years in the United States. This is important information for nurses, who are providing care for more young and middle adults than ever before both in the community and in hospitals. By understanding the characteristics of these developmental periods and their special concerns, the nurse can focus on the special physical, psychological, social, and health needs of clients in these age groups.

Maturity and Adulthood

A person can be said to have reached maturity when he has attained a balance of growth in intellectual, psychomotor, and emotional areas. The mature individual feels comfortable with the abilities, knowledge, and responses he has developed over the years. This background of experience serves the person well in dealing with new situations and in carrying out day-to-day activities.

A mature person looks at the world with a broad perspective, based on a blend of insight, emotion, and imagination. He takes on problems that can be solved but recognizes and learns to live with unsolvable problems.

The mature person is open to suggestions and can accept constructive criticism without a major loss of self-esteem. The mature person weighs other persons' input and recommendations when making a decision, but is not overly influenced or intimidated by others. Above all, the mature person develops by learning from his own and other's experiences.

Other characteristics of the mature person are related to interpersonal communication and behavior. The mature person acknowledges both accomplishments and shortcomings. When he makes mistakes, his ego is not crushed and he does not transfer blame to others. He draws on his life circumstances and background as sources of information for self-reflection and self-awareness.

The pleasure principle—the drive for immediate gratification of a need—so dominant in infancy and early childhood is much less active in the behavior of the mature adult. In fact, it is the ability to set long-range goals and direct energy toward a distant objective that is often the crucial element in a person's self-actualization. An intrinsic belief system and persistent striving toward a goal enable the person to relate to the world in a consistent, mature manner.

All societies evolve or change with time. Sometimes changes come abruptly and with force. When that occurs, as in modern times, the transition into full adulthood and toward maturity is made more difficult in many ways. Revolutionary changes can alter commonly held beliefs and challenge the value of many traditional behaviors. The stresses inherent in developing maturity and judgment are greatly increased in times of change. High levels of stress can have adverse effects on a person's health status. The nurse can help a young or middle adult maintain health by understanding that finding a place in society is a developmental task in this stage of life. The nurse can teach and assist the person to cope with the stress of a changing society.

Young Adult

Theories of Young Adulthood

Many theorists have attempted to describe the phases of young adulthood and the related developmental tasks. The works of three theorists are par-

ticularly valuable in understanding this developmental period as related to health care.

LEVINSON'S THEORY

Levinson has identified four phases of young adult development (Levinson et al., 1978). First is the early adult transition (ages 18 to 20). During this transition the person may physically separate from his family as by going away to school, desires emotional and financial independence and freedom in decision making, develops an adult identity, and explores career and family goals. The second phase is the entrance into the adult world (ages 21 to 27). In this phase the young adult continues to explore alternative careers and life-styles. He may obtain his own apartment, change jobs, and make tentative commitments such as planning for engagement or marriage. In the second phase the young adult begins to develop a foundation for his life activities and plans lifetime goals. The third phase is a period of transition (ages 28 to 32). Many young adults, mindful of the "biological clock," view this as a critical turning point for marriage and the beginning of a family. During this time the young adult may modify his life activity. This transition period may be stressful for some young adults who do not feel they have achieved some of their goals. The last phase is settling down (ages 33 to 39). During this phase the person experiences greater stability, commitments to self and family, career advancement, productivity, and termination of a mentor relationship (Beck, Rawlins, and Williams, 1984; Levinson et al., 1978).

DIEKELMANN'S THEORY

A second theory for young adult development has been developed by Diekelmann (1976), a nurse. Diekelmann proposes that the young adult experiences five developmental tasks. First, the young adult achieves independence from parental controls. Second, he begins to develop strong friendships and intimate relationships outside the family. Third, he establishes a personal set of values, some of which he obtains from his parents and peer group. Fourth, he develops a sense of personal identity. Last, he prepares for his life work and develops the capacity for intimacy (Diekelmann, 1976; Stanhope and Lancaster, 1984).

GOULD'S THEORY

Gould (1978) maintains that adults must learn to stop thinking in terms of childhood irrationalities that limit their lives. When a person abandons false assumptions such as the belief that his parents will always be available for financial support and decision making and that the world is a fair and undemanding place, adulthood begins. This maturational process occurs in four phases. In the first phase (ages 16 to 22), the young adult leaves his parents and establishes independence. In the second stage, "I'm nobody's baby now" (ages 22 to 28), the individual tests and challenges the idea that he will have the same values as his parents. Life skills are refined. The individual thinks and plans, values common sense, and accepts being sometimes wrong. In general, the individual can accept the outcomes of daily living. In the third phase, "opening up to what's inside" (ages 28 to 34), the person's life experiences lead him to see that life is not always simple and controllable. A period of reexamination of self begins. Finally, in the fourth phase, the premidlife decade (ages 35 to 45), the person acts on the basis of a new personal vision. The person must be able to accept that death is inevitable. Many persons must learn that it is possible to live without a partner. In addition, because of life circumstances, especially for women, it is important for the person to learn to anticipate change and to develop interests beyond the family. Gould points out that the outcome of the difficult premidlife decade is frequently enormous personal growth for the individual.

■　■　■　■　■

These theories provide the nurse with a basis for understanding the life events and developmental tasks of the young adult. Each young adult, however, brings unique characteristics and needs to this developmental stage. Clients in this developmental stage present challenges to nurses who themselves are young adults and who are coping with the demands of this period. Young adult nurses must be careful to recognize the needs of their young adult clients even if they themselves are not experiencing the same challenges and events.

Physiological Development

Unlike the adolescent, the young adult experiences few maturational changes in body shape or physical structures. The exception to this is the pregnant or lactating woman. The physical, cognitive, and psychosocial changes and the health concerns of the pregnant woman and the childbearing family are extensive and are detailed in a later section.

Young adults are usually quite active, experience severe illnesses less commonly than other age groups, tend to ignore physical symptoms, and often postpone seeking health care. The physical features of young adults begin to change as they approach middle age (see Table 23-1, p. 456). Unless the client has an illness, the physical assessment findings are generally within normal limits.

Nonetheless, clients in this developmental stage

may benefit from a personal life-style assessment (see box on p. 514). The personal life-style assessment developed by Stanhope and Lancaster (1984) can help the nurse and the client identify habits that can increase the risk for cardiac, malignant, pulmonary, renal, or other chronic diseases.

Cognitive Development

Rational thinking habits increase steadily through the young and middle adult years. Formal and informal educational experiences, general life experiences, and occupational opportunities dramatically increase the individual's conceptual and problem-solving skills, as well as motor skills. A rich, stimulating environment for the growing and maturing adult encourages the development of full creative potential. Research has shown that creative potential is greatest in the years between 35 and 40. Creativity in the years between 40 and 50 is comparable to that between 20 and 30. The IQ measurements of young and middle adults remain stable as long as they continue to use their verbal and other cognitive skills. Learning occurs, but not as quickly when high-level psychomotor ability is needed.

Identifying a preferred occupational area is a major task of the young adult. When a person knows his skills, talents, and personality characteristics, occupational choices are easier and the person is generally more satisfied with his choices. In the young and middle adult years, job satisfaction has been found to be a major factor in achievement and responsibility.

An understanding of how young adults learn assists the nurse as she develops teaching plans for the client. The adult comes to the teaching-learning situation with a background of unique life experiences. The nurse therefore always views a young adult, like other clients, as a unique individual. The adult's compliance with a particular regimen being taught, such as medications, treatments, or life-style changes, involves a decision-making process. The teaching process should present the client with as much information as he needs to make a decision to comply with the prescribed course. The nurse should be available to answer questions as the young adult makes his choices.

Because the young adult is continually evolving and adjusting to changes in his home, workplace, and personal life, his decision-making process ideally should be flexible. The more secure the young adult is in his roles, the more flexible and open to change he is. The insecure person tends to be more rigid in his decisions. The nurse therefore encourages open-minded, flexible decision making by helping the young adult cope with stresses that may affect his sense of security.

Personal Life-Style Assessment

Directions: Write your response to each of the items using a maximum of three sentences. Record your answer based on your immediate reaction; do not contemplate items for a lengthy period.

PHYSICAL DIMENSIONS

Describe your habits in a typical week as related to the following activities:

1. Sleep	7. Alcoholic intake	12. Foot and nail care
2. Rest periods	8. Medications	13. Work, job
3. Exercise	9. Skin care	14. Work, home
4. Hair care	10. Elimination	15. Diet
5. Dental care	11. Sex	16. Medical checkup
6. Smoking		

How long do you expect to live?

PSYCHOSOCIAL AND/OR SPIRITUAL DIMENSIONS

Describe your habits in a typical week as related to the following activities:

1. Reading for pleasure	6. Community activities for pleasure
2. Reading for intellectual stimulation	7. Community activities for service
3. Meditation	8. Recreational activities
4. Interaction with friends	9. Hobbies
5. Interaction with family	10. Sports

COPING MECHANISMS

How do you handle stress on the job? At home?

What is your personal motto for life? (Eat, drink, and be merry; do unto others as you would have them do unto you, etc.)

What kind of actions by others make you angry? How do you handle the anger?

What goal do you have for this year? How do you plan to meet it?

What goals do you have for the next 5 years? How do you plan to meet them?

Are you satisfied with your present financial status?

What kind of things cause you the greatest anxiety?

How would you describe your relationship with your spouse or most significant other? Your children? Your in-laws and other relatives? Your parents?

What do you consider to be your life task?

On a scale from 1 to 10, how would you rate your present state of health (1—least healthy to 10—most healthy). How does your life-style contribute to or detract from your present state of health?

From Stanhope, M., and Lancaster, J.: Community health nursing: process and practice for promoting health, St. Louis, 1984, The C.V. Mosby Co.

The nurse should determine whether the young adult is making proactive or reactive decisions. In proactive decision making the choices made are goal directed. In reactive decision making the choices are made in response to the influence of others. Everyone makes both proactive and reactive decisions (Beck, Rawlins, and Williams, 1984). However, when a person is secure in his role, values, knowledge, and beliefs, he tends to make more proactive decisions.

Psychosocial Development

The emotional health of the young adult is correlated with the individual's ability to address and resolve personal and social tasks. Certain patterns or trends are relatively predictable. Between the ages of 23 to 28 the person refines his self-perception and ability for intimacy. From ages 29 to 34 the person directs enormous energy toward achievement and mastery of the world around him. The years from 35 to 43 are a time of vigorous examination of life goals and relationships. Alterations are made in the adult's personal, social, and occupational lives. Often the stresses of this reexamination result in a "midlife crisis" whose outcome is changes in marital partner, life-style, and occupation.

In the young adult years the person generally gives more attention to occupational and social pursuits.

During this period the individual attempts to improve his socioeconomic status. Upward mobility is possible through career choices. However, many career choices require special educational preparation, and success may depend on family or social associations. Career and personal counseling can help the individual identify career choices and set realistic goals. The nurse who works with adults can make appropriate referrals when problems involving socioeconomic status and career or educational issues become apparent.

Ethnic factors and sex differences also have a sociological and psychological influence in an adult's life. A frank understanding of the expectations and limitations imposed by social stereotyping or on the basis of ethnicity, race, or gender enables the adult to understand and cope with boundaries he may experience in interactions with others. The individual can choose to remain within the prescribed expectations of his society or to relate to the society in his own unique way. Support from the nurse, access to information, anticipatory guidance, and appropriate referrals open a world of possibilities for achievement of the adult's full potential. Because health is not merely the absence of disease but involves wellness in all human dimensions, the holistic, humanistic nurse acknowledges the importance of the young adult's psychosocial needs as well as those in other dimensions.

The young adult must make three major decisions: a career, whether to marry, and whether to become a parent. Although each individual makes these decisions based on individual factors, the nurse should understand the general principles involved in these aspects of psychosocial development in order to assess the young adult's psychosocial status.

CAREER

Many adults devote a major portion of their energy and interest to their chosen career. Therefore a successful vocational adjustment is important in the lives of most men and women. Successful employment not only ensures economic security but also leads to friendships, social activities, and support from co-workers. In addition, in North America a person's occupation and achievements are major determinants of social status and self-esteem (Kaluger and Kaluger, 1979).

The women's movement and the escalating cost of living have made two-career marriages increasingly common. The two-career marriage has benefits as well as liabilities. In addition to increasing the family's financial base, the woman who works outside the home is able to expand her friendships, activities, and interests. Stresses may occur in a two-career family, however, as when one partner desires to change to a job in a different city. The other partner may not want to relinquish a job or may have limited employment opportunities in the new city.

Tensions may also result when one partner's job requires the expenditure of physical, mental, or emotional energy beyond business hours. The other spouse may feel that this additional business time is infringing on the couple's time together. With a couple who have children, the spouse at home may resent having primary responsibility for the children after completing a full day's work.

The male and female stereotypes of the past are decreasing. Men are becoming more involved in child rearing and homemaking duties. Women are becoming active in house and automobile maintenance. The major principle for avoiding stress in a two-career family is that neither partner can assume all responsibilities. For some families a solution may be to limit recreational expenses and instead hire someone to do routine housework. Others may set up an equal division of house, shopping, and cooking duties.

SEXUALITY

The development of the secondary sexual characteristics occurs during the adolescent years (see Chapter 25). Physical development is accompanied by the ability to perform sexual acts. The young adult usually has emotional maturity to complement the physical ability and is therefore able to develop mature sexual relationships.

ORGASMIC MATURITY. Masters and Johnson (1970) have contributed much important information about the physiology of the adult sexual response. Orgasmic maturity in sexual response occurs in four phases: excitement, plateau, orgasm, and resolution (see Chapter 19).

More important than either the individual's type or frequency of sexual intercourse is the psychodynamic aspect of sexual activity. The person's psychological beliefs and expectations give feelings of pleasure and satisfaction to the young as well as the middle adult. To maintain total wellness, adults should be encouraged to explore various aspects of their sexuality (see Chapter 19).

CHILDBEARING CYCLE. Conception, birth, and lactation are the major phases of the childbearing cycle. However, the changes of childbearing are far more extensive and complex. The nurse can assist the couple to prepare for this cycle through health teaching in such areas as nutrition, anatomy, and physiology and discussions of feelings and attitudes toward childbearing and child rearing. Education such as Lamaze classes can prepare the couple to participate in the birthing process. The LaLeche League, a support group for nursing mothers, offers practical advice about breast feeding.

The personal and social changes occurring in the lives of the couple following the birth of a baby cannot be underestimated. The nursing assessment of the couple's response to the birthing experience and parent-child bonding are detailed in a later section of the chapter.

FAMILY

SINGLEHOOD. The social pressure to get married is not as great as it once was. Today it is socially acceptable for a young adult to leave home and live in an apartment or to own a home without first marrying. In the period between 1970 and 1975, one in four persons between the ages of 25 and 34 was unmarried (Kaluger and Kaluger, 1979).

Another cause for the increased single population is the expanding career opportunities for women. Women enter the job market with greater career potential and have greater opportunities for financial independence. Today's young woman does not have to depend on a husband to pay for housing, travel, or further education.

It is also becoming more socially acceptable for single individuals to live together outside of marriage. In North America an estimated 2% to 3% of two-income households are singles living together. Similarly, it has become more socially acceptable for married couples to separate or divorce if they find their marital situation unsatisfactory.

Many factors influence the choice of singlehood or marriage (Table 26-1). Neither singlehood nor marriage is totally stress free, but the problems common in both can usually be resolved by the individual or couple alone or with the assistance of a counselor.

TABLE 26-1

Factors Influencing Choice of Singlehood or Marriage

Singlehood		Marriage	
Pushes Toward	**Pulls Toward**	**Pushes Toward**	**Pulls Toward**
Limitations (suffocating one-to-one relationships, feeling trapped, monotony)	Career opportunities and mobility	Financial security	Parental influence
	Variety of experiences	Influence from mass media	Desire for children
Obstacles to self-development and self-expression	Self-sufficiency and self-expression	Expectation of partners	Peer pressure
			Romantic image of marriage
Boredom, unhappiness, and anger	Sexual availability and variety	Unhappy home life	Love (physical attraction, emotional attachment)
	Exciting life-style and experience	Interpersonal and personal reasons	
Role playing and conformity to expectations	Freedom to change and experiment	Fear of independence	Security, social status, prestige
Poor communication with mate	Mobility	Loneliness	Social stability
Feelings of sexual frustration	Sustaining friendships	Alternatives that did not seem feasible	
Limited friends, isolation, loneliness	Support groups such as men's and women's groups, group living arrangements, specialized groups	Social and cultural influences	
Limitation of mobility and available experience		Regular sex	
Influence of and participation in women's movement and other social movements		Guilt over singlehood	

Modified from Stein, P.J.: Family Coordinator **24**:4, 1975.

MARRIAGE. Every couple's relationship is unique. While there are no rules that guarantee a successful marriage, some guidelines are useful for building a happy marriage. Before marriage the couple ideally should complete five tasks. First, they should make certain that their emotions are based on love rather than simply physical or sexual attraction. Early in a relationship, each is physically or sexually attracted to the other, but these feelings do not necessarily provide a basis for a marriage or other long-term commitment. When one or both partners begin to think of the other as "a person I need to be with" or "a friend and a lover," the relationship may be progressing beyond physical and sexual attraction.

Second, both partners should explore their motivation for wanting to marry. Is the desire to marry a result of family and social pressure? Do they wish to marry because they hear the "biological clock" ticking? Does the man desire marriage because having a wife is good for his career?

Third, the couple contemplating marriage should focus on developing clear communication. Several questions should be discussed. If both partners want children, how many and when? How are finances to be managed, and will both partners participate in financial decisions and management? If either partner has an ill or elderly parent, how will the married couple cope with the inevitable future needs of the parent? What are the career goals of both partners before and after children? If the future husband wants his wife to quit her job and remain home with the children, does that goal complement his wife's plans? How does the couple anticipate the resolution of common marital stressors, such as financial pressures, household chores, and job pressure?

Fourth, the couple who plans marriage should understand that any annoying behavior patterns and habits are unlikely to change after marriage. The person who is compulsive is likely to remain so after marriage. Likewise, the disorganized individual also retains this behavior.

Last, the couple should determine their compatibility in important beliefs and values. For example, if one partner places a high value on fidelity and the other does not, their marriage is headed for conflict. Religious values and needs, such as church affiliations, should also be considered.

Stages of Marriage. Like an individual life, a marriage relationship generally passes through developmental stages.

The *establishment stage* begins at the wedding and continues as the couple attempts to function as a dyad. They learn patterns of sexual expression and how to live intimately with each other. They must learn styles of conflict resolution, decision making, and role patterns. In addition, each partner may experience a sense of loss of individuality and self in the transition from "me" to "we." Together the married partners help each other achieve seven goals:

1. Seeking mutual self-growth and well-being
2. Practicing open communication techniques
3. Being tolerant of each other
4. Responding appropriately to each other's moods
5. Being kind and issue centered during arguments
6. Being each other's best friend
7. Bargaining openly regarding duties, obligations, and privileges

The *family orientation stage* is directed toward childbearing and child-rearing activities. Parenting roles must be defined and practiced. Self-concept, financial, and commitment stresses may occur. Nurturing and socialization needs of the children can put pressure on the couple's intimate relationship. Each parent's image of the "perfect parent" may conflict with reality. Parent-child relationships can become stressful as the child pulls away and experiments.

A couple who cannot or chooses not to have children may direct their energies to their careers or to participation in the lives of other families with children.

In the middle adult years, as children depart from the household, the family enters the *postparental family stage*. Time and financial demands on the parents decrease, and they face the task of redefining their own relationship. Plans for retirement and moving to a smaller home or apartment are made. It is a time to reassess life. As grandchildren arrive, grandparenting styles must be chosen.

Dyad Responsibility of the Married Couple. When establishing a household and family, the married couple has important work to do as a team. They have the following tasks:

1. Establishing an intimate relationship
2. Deciding on and working toward material and economic goals
3. Establishing guidelines for power and decision-making issues
4. Setting standards for extrafamily interactions
5. Finding companionship with other couples for a social life
6. Choosing mores, values, and ideologies acceptable to both

These major tasks of adults require considerable maturity and self-esteem. When faced and carried out, however, they provide the foundation for a stable relationship.

Growth in marriage extends over many years. Success in solving the formidable problems that occur in any marriage offers marital partners insight into each other.

PARENTHOOD. The availability of contraception makes it easier for today's couples to decide when to start a family. One factor influencing that decision is the reason for wanting a child. Social pressures may encourage a couple to have a child or may influence them to limit the number of children they have. Economic considerations frequently enter into the decision-making process, since having and bringing up children is expensive. The later average age for first marriages and postponed pregnancies because of career goals mean that general health status and age are also considerations in decisions about parenthood (see Chapter 22).

Nurses are often involved in teaching and counseling clients about contraception. Providing information and guidance about the decision making necessary for responsible parenting is also a valuable service.

Phases of Parenthood. Parenthood is a process during which the parent assumes several roles. The psychological adjustment to parenting begins with the adoption of a parental self-image. A nurturing role emerges to meet the needs of the newborn. The authoritative role is added as the toddler begins to test the world around him and the parent must offer guidance.

Through the later school years and adolescence the parent functions in an integrative role, permitting the freedom for personal growth while offering safety and guidance.

In the departure phase the parent must relinquish the parent role as the young person is launched into adulthood. At this time parent and child must establish a new relationship as fellow adults.

HALLMARKS OF EMOTIONAL HEALTH

Most young adults have the physical and emotional resources and support systems to meet the many challenges, tasks, and responsibilities they face. During a psychosocial assessment of a young adult, the nurse can assess for 10 hallmarks of emotional health (see boxed material), which indicate that the young adult has successfully matured in this developmental stage.

Health Concerns

PHYSIOLOGICAL CONCERNS

The average young adult is active and without major health problems. However, the young adult's fast-paced life-style may put him at risk for the development of illnesses or disabilities during his middle or older adult years. In addition, infertility is a problem for many young adults.

RISK FACTORS. Risk factors for the young adult's health originate in the community, life-style, and family history. Stanhope and Lancaster (1984) have identified five community factors that present risks: (1) violent death and injury, (2) substance abuse, (3) unwanted pregnancies, (4) sexually transmitted diseases, and (5) environmental or occupational factors. Life-style habits such as smoking, stress, lack of exercise, and poor personal hygiene also increase the risk of future illness, as does family history of cardiovascular, renal, endocrine, or neoplastic disease.

Community Factors. Violence is the greatest cause of mortality and morbidity in the young adult population. Death and injury can occur from physical assaults, motor vehicle or other accidents, and suicide attempts. Recent statistics show that homicides account for approximately 10% of deaths, motor vehicle accidents for 48.7 deaths per 100,000, and suicides for 32.5 deaths per 100,000 in the 20- to 48-year-old group (Stanhope and Lancaster, 1984).

Substance abuse, the use of alcohol or drugs, directly or indirectly contributes to mortality and morbidity in young adults. Even if an intoxicated young adult is not severely injured in a motor vehicle accident he has caused, the accident may well result in death or permanent disability to another young adult.

Ten Hallmarks of Emotional Health

- A sense of meaning and direction in life
- Successful negotiation through transitions
- Absence of feelings of being cheated or disappointed by life
- Attainment of several long-term goals
- Satisfaction with personal growth and development
- When married, feelings of mutual love for partner; when single, satisfaction with social interactions
- Satisfaction with friendships
- Generally cheerful attitude
- Not sensitive to criticism
- No unrealistic fears

Modified from Stanhope, M., and Lancaster, J.: Community health nursing: process and practice for promoting health, St. Louis, 1984, The C.V. Mosby Co.

Dependence on stimulant or depressant drugs can result in death. Overdose of a stimulant drug ("upper") can stress the cardiovascular and nervous systems to the extent that death occurs. The use of depressants ("downers") can lead to an accidental or intentional overdose and death.

It is a misconception that drug abuse occurs only among adolescents. Cocaine is increasingly used by young adults who have families and responsible jobs. Chapter 45 discusses the many physiological and psychosocial problems that may result from substance abuse.

A young adult who has recovered from substance abuse is still at risk for long-term effects that surface in middle or older adult years. These include hepatitis, cardiovascular and pulmonary disease, chromosome damage, hepatic cirrhosis, and recurrent infections (Stanhope and Lancaster, 1984).

Unwanted pregnancies, although more common among adolescents, can also have long-term physical and emotional effects if they occur in the young adult years. For example, a 25-year-old woman with an unplanned pregnancy may choose to terminate the pregnancy. If she is unable to resolve her feelings about the loss, she may require long-term counseling. Another woman may choose to have the baby and give it up for adoption, but similarly be unable to accept the loss. Still another may decide to keep the child but, because of the emotional, financial, and other burdens, suffer severe emotional stress, lose weight, and find herself unable to cope.

Sexually transmitted diseases include syphilis, gonorrhea, genital herpes, and acquired immune deficiency syndrome (AIDS). These diseases may occur in any sexually active person. Recently there has been a decrease in sexual promiscuity. Many young adults are seeking to establish meaningful relationships before engaging in sexual activity.

Sexually transmitted diseases have immediate effects such as infection, discharge, and discomfort. They may also lead to chronic disorders as with genital herpes; infertility, which is a common sequela of gonorrhea; or even death as with AIDS.

A common *environmental or occupational risk factor* is exposure to airborne particles, which may cause lung diseases and cancer. Such lung diseases include silicosis from inhalation of talcum and silicon dust, pneumoconiosis from inhalation of coal dust, and emphysema from inhalation of smoke. Cancers resulting from occupational exposures may involve the lung, liver, brain, blood, or skin (Table 26-2).

Life-Style. Life-style habits, particularly those that activate the stress response (see Chapter 5), have been documented to increase the risk of illness.

Smoking is a well-documented risk factor for pulmonary, cardiac, and vascular diseases. The inhaled cigarette pollutants increase the risk of lung cancer, emphysema, and chronic bronchitis. The nicotine in tobacco is a vasoconstrictor that acts on the coronary arteries, increasing the risk of angina, myocardial infarction, and coronary artery disease. Nicotine also causes peripheral vasoconstriction and may lead to vascular problems such as Raynaud's disease or Buerger's disease.

Prolonged *stress* increases wear and tear on the body's adaptive capacities. Stress-related diseases such as ulcers, emotional disorders, and infections can occur (see Chapter 5).

Exercise patterns can affect a person's present and future health status. Research has demonstrated that exercise producing a sustained increase in pulse rate for 15 to 20 minutes three times a week improves cardiopulmonary function by decreasing blood pressure and heart rate. In addition, exercise decreases fatigability, insomnia, tension, and irritability.

TABLE 26-2

Occupational Hazards Associated with Cancers

Occupational Chemical	Cancer
Asbestos	Mesothelioma (pleural and peritoneal) Lung
Vinyl chloride (plastics)	Liver (hemangiosarcoma) (200 times at risk) Brain (4 times at risk) Lung (2 times at risk)
Benzene	Leukemia, predominantly acute myelogenous
Bischloromethane ether	Oat cell carcinoma
Chromium	Nasal or paranasal sinus, lung, larynx
Arsenic	Lung
Coal tar pitch, coke oven emissions	Lung, larynx, skin
Iron oxide	Lung, larynx
Nickel	Lung
Petroleum distillates	Lung, larynx

From Stanhope, M., and Lancaster, J.: Community health nursing: process and practice for promoting health, St. Louis, 1984, The C.V. Mosby Co.

Personal hygiene habits can be risk factors. Sharing eating utensils with a person who has a contagious illness obviously increases the risk of illness. Poor dental hygiene increases the risk of periodontal disease. These diseases—gingivitis, or inflammation of the gums, and periodontitis, or loss of tooth support—can be avoided through routine brushing and flossing (see Chapter 35).

A *familial history* of a disease may put a young adult at risk for developing the disease in his middle or older adult years. For example, a young man whose father and paternal grandfather had a myocardial infarction in their fifth decade of life has a risk for a future myocardial infarction. As noted in Chapter 7, the presence of certain chronic illnesses in the family increases the family members' risk of developing a disease. This family risk is distinct from hereditary disease.

INFERTILITY. Infertility is the involuntary reduction in one's reproductive ability. Most health professionals define it as the inability to conceive after a year or more of regular sexual intercourse (Fogel and Woods, 1981). An estimated 10% to 15% of all couples are infertile. About half of the couples who are evaluated and treated in major infertility clinics, however, become pregnant (Fogel and Woods, 1981). In about 10% to 20% of couples the cause of the infertility is unknown and the couple will remain infertile. The remaining 30% have the cause of their infertility diagnosed, but they remain infertile owing to endometriosis, blocked fallopian tubes, or decreased sperm motility.

Infertility occurs in both men and women. Infertility in women can result from endocrine or nutritional imbalances, lack of ovulation, congenital abnormalities, or infections. The following outline details causes of infertility in women*:

1. Tubal obstruction or dysfunction
   a. Pelvic inflammatory disease
   b. Tuberculosis
   c. Puerperal infection
   d. Endometriosis
   e. Congenital anomalies
   f. Peritonitis (from ruptured appendix or viscus from surgery)
2. Ovulation factors
   a. Anovulation
   b. Inadequate corpus luteum
   c. Amenorrhea with low estrogen production
   d. Production of pathological ova

e. Ovarian tumors, Stein-Leventhal syndrome
   f. Ovarian endometriosis
   g. Genetic absence of follicular tissue
3. Uterine factors
   a. Myomas, polyps
   b. Developmental anomalies of the endometrial cavity
   c. Synechiae
   d. Congenital absence of uterus
   e. Endometritis
   f. Endometriosis
   g. Insufficient transformation of endometrium
   h. Neoplasms
   i. Infections
   j. Pelvic inflammatory disease
4. Cervical factors
   a. Obstruction or stenosis of cervix from surgery or neoplasms
   b. Destruction of endocervical glands from surgery
   c. Chronic cervicitis
   d. Inadequate cervical mucus
5. Vaginal factors
   a. Congenital absence of vagina
   b. Imperforate hymen
   c. Vaginismus
   d. Vaginitis
   e. Hyperacidity of vaginal secretions

In men infertility is due to interference with the development of sperm, decreased motility of sperm, obstruction in transport of sperm from the testicles to the urethra, and interference with ejaculation of the sperm. The following outline details causes of infertility in men*:

1. Decreased production of spermatozoa
   a. Varicocele
   b. Testicular failure
   c. Endocrine disorders
   d. Cryptorchidism
   e. Other causes—stress, smoking, heat, systemic infections
2. Abnormal semen
   a. Low volume
   b. Necrospermia and agglutination
   c. High viscosity
   d. Autoimmunity
3. Ductal obstructions
   a. Epididymis, postinfection
   b. Congenital absence of vas deferens
   c. Postvasectomy
   d. Ejaculatory duct, postinfection

---

*Modified from Fogel, C.I., and Woods, N.F.: Health care of women: a nursing perspective, St. Louis, 1981, The C.V. Mosby Co.

*Modified from Fogel, C.I., and Woods, N.F.: Health care of women: a nursing perspective, St. Louis, 1981, The C.V. Mosby Co.

4. Failure to transport spermatozoa to vagina
   a. Ejaculatory disturbances
   b. Hypospadias
   c. Sexual problems such as impotence

For some infertile couples, the nurse may be the first resource identified. Particularly in a community or clinic setting where the nurse-client relationship has developed over an extended period, the couple may feel more comfortable discussing their fertility problems with the nurse. To effectively intervene with a couple who have a fertility problem, the nurse should be familiar with fertility centers to which the couple can be referred.

PSYCHOSOCIAL CONCERNS

The psychosocial health concerns of the young adult often are related to stress, such as job stress or family stress. As noted in Chapter 5, stress can be valuable in motivating a client to change and move ahead. However, if the stress is prolonged and the client is unable to adapt to the stressor, health problems can develop.

JOB STRESS. Job stress can occur every day or from time to time. Most young adults are able to handle day-to-day crises. Situational job stress may occur when a new boss enters the workplace, a deadline is approaching, or the worker is given new responsibilities. Job stress also occurs when a person becomes dissatisfied with his job or responsibilities. Because individuals perceive jobs differently, the types of job stressors vary from client to client.

FAMILY STRESS. Family stressors can occur at any time in family life. Family life has peaks, when everyone in the family works together, and valleys, when everyone appears to pull apart.

As with all groups, each family has certain predictable roles or jobs for members. These roles enable the family to function and be an effective part of society. One necessary role is the family leader. In most families one parent is the leader or both parents act as co-leaders. In single-parent families the one parent or occasionally a member of the extended family is the family leader.

Communication within the family is both formal and informal. Family members often share common mannerisms for nonverbal messages. The openness of communication varies from family to family. Many communication skills are learned behaviors and are handed down from generation to generation. A nurse can observe a family's communication patterns for clues to improve interviews, health teaching, and health counseling with family members.

Achievement expectations depend on family task and goal performance roles. Each family has its own definitions of who does what both inside and outside the family boundaries. Individual members who attempt to redefine these levels of task and goal performance can expect a response from the family, who may be either supportive or nonsupportive.

In some situations, family stressors are the result of *marital dissatisfaction*. This dissatisfaction can have multiple causes (see boxed material below). As with other stressors, some marital stressors can be resolved but others cannot.

Family stress may also occur in the *step-family*. The high number of divorces and remarriages has greatly increased the number of new family units. Traditionally known as step-families, these new family groups warrant the attention of the nurse who is concerned with health maintenance and health promotion.

A nurse's anticipatory guidance to step-family members reduces feelings of isolation, fear, and stress. The nurse teaches the family members that feelings of grief and loss are to be expected and are actually a healthy response to a major life event. Bargaining with God, self, and other family members can be expected as new family ties and traditions are established. Bargaining is a difficult process, and the in-

---

Factors Influencing Marital Dissatisfaction

- Money: insufficient income to meet primary needs for food, shelter, and clothing; inability of the couple to agree on the use of money available
- Sex: inability to achieve a mutually satisfying level of sexual intimacy; unplanned pregnancy or sterility of one partner
- In-laws: inability to integrate differing family roles and communication patterns
- Recreation: incongruent use of leisure time and resources
- Friends: inability to establish new couple-centered friendships; differing expectations regarding role or choice of friends
- Addictive substances: health, personality, and other changes caused by chemical abuse
- Religion/culture: inability to resolve difficulties stemming from differing religious and cultural values, beliefs, and behaviors
- Children: inability to develop mutually satisfactory childbearing and child-rearing goals

dividual reaches out for strength from others (see Chapter 46).

Step-family members develop new community and friendship networks and a unique family identity. Integration occurs as the individual family members accept the new family identity and functioning.

Stress is also common in *single-parent families*. The single parent often experiences stress related to being the sole wage earner, disciplinarian, problem solver, and decision maker. The single parent needs a support system that can provide advice, financial support, and a respite from day-to-day decision making.

■ ■ ■ ■ ■

A nurse with insight comes to understand her own family of origin and can tolerate the different lifestyles of clients. Meeting the health needs of the individual and the family is the focus of nursing. The nurse who accepts the realities of diversity is able to help clients achieve health goals within the context of many social choices.

Pregnant Woman and Childbearing Family

A developmental task for most young adult couples is the decision to begin a family. Although the physiological changes of pregnancy and childbirth occur only in the woman, the cognitive and psychosocial changes and the health concerns affect the entire childbearing family, including the husband, siblings, and grandparents.

PHYSIOLOGICAL CHANGES

The woman who is anticipating becoming pregnant benefits from maintaining good health practices, such as a balanced diet, exercise, dental checkups, avoidance of alcohol, and cessation of smoking before conception. A woman who is trying to become pregnant should not attempt a weight reduction diet. The physiological changes and needs of the pregnant woman vary with each trimester.

FIRST TRIMESTER. Some of the physiological changes of the first trimester occur in all women, while others affect only certain women. The nurse must be familiar with these physiological changes, their cause, and helpful interventions for the pregnant woman (Table 26-3).

During this period there are no signs of pregnancy observable by others. If a woman frequently has morning sickness, however, her family, friends, and co-workers may be able to guess that she is pregnant.

The newly pregnant woman needs routine prenatal care. The first visit includes a pelvic examination.

After the thirteenth week of pregnancy, pelvic examinations are not done. Instead the physician or certified nurse-midwife measures fetal growth by palpating the abdomen to determine the size of the uterine fundus.

SECOND TRIMESTER. In the second trimester the growth of the uterus and fetus results in some of the physical signs of pregnancy (Table 26-4). Morning sickness has usually disappeared, and the woman's energy level is restored if her nutritional intake has caught up with her metabolic demands. The urinary frequency ceases and she is able to sleep through the night.

If this is the woman's first pregnancy, she may be able to see and feel the enlarged uterus. In second and subsequent pregnancies the woman may be "showing" by the beginning of the second trimester.

THIRD TRIMESTER. During the third trimester there is an increase in Braxton-Hicks contractions, fatigue, and urinary frequency. The uterus continues to grow (Table 26-5). Close to the time of the onset of labor, the woman may experience a burst of energy during which she cleans the house and prepares for the baby by shopping for baby clothes, food, and diapers. This period is called "nesting." Many experts in obstetrics and seasoned veterans of pregnancy believe that "nesting" indicates a rapidly approaching time of delivery.

PUERPERIUM. The puerperium is a period of approximately 6 weeks following delivery. During this time the uterus involutes, returning to approximate prepregnancy size. In addition, the uterine lining regenerates. The top layer of lining is sloughed off and the endometrium reforms. The sloughed-off layer, referred to as "lochia," is excreted via the vagina. Lochial discharge is present in all women who have delivered a fetus, whether the delivery is vaginal or via caesarian section. Lochia is also present when the woman has delivered a stillborn infant.

There are three stages of lochia. First is *lochia rubra*, a bright red to pink drainage that may contain small clots and lasts from delivery to the fourth or fifth postpartum day. Lochia increases with nursing because sucking on the breasts causes uterine contraction. Physical activity also increases lochia because of the effect of gravity. *Lochia serosa* is a pink to brownish discharge lasting from about the fifth postpartum day to 2 weeks postpartum. Occasionally the new mother may note a return of bright red discharge. She should not be alarmed if this is just occasional spotting and does not fully saturate a menstrual pad. *Lochia alba*, a white to yellow discharge,

TABLE 26-3

Physiological Changes in the First Trimester

Symptom	Cause	Appropriate Nursing Interventions
Amenorrhea (one or two missed periods)	Fertilization of the egg by the sperm	
Positive pregnancy test done at home or in laboratory	Presence of human chorionic gonadotropin (HCG) in first voided urine specimen of day	Instruct woman to obtain prenatal care, avoid all medications, avoid alcohol intake, and maintain good nutritional habits.
Morning sickness—nausea and/or vomiting from sixth week to end of fourth month; may occur in the morning, evening, or all day long	Increased serum hormone levels	Instruct client to eat dry crackers, cold fluids, such as ice and popsicles, and small frequent meals to reduce nausea. Have client inform her doctor if prolonged vomiting results in a weight loss of 5 or more pounds, abdominal pain, or tenderness (Fogel and Woods, 1981).
Breast enlargement and tenderness; nipples darkened and enlarged	Increased estrogen levels	Instruct woman to wear a supportive bra at all times, even while asleep. Application of ice packs will decrease tenderness.
Urinary frequency	Pressure of uterus on bladder	Reassure client that frequency decreases as the enlarging uterus moves from the pelvis upward to the abdominal region. Prepare client for return of frequency as the head of the fetus moves into the pelvis in the middle to late third trimester.
Fatigue	Hormonal increases Increased nutritional demands on the woman Decreased nutritional intake resulting from morning sickness	Ensure that client has proper nutrition, sleep patterns, and rest periods to help decrease fatigue.
Chadwick's sign on pelvic examination (6-8 weeks): bluish violet hue of mucous membranes of the vulva, vagina, and cervix	Vascular congestion	Instruct client to have prenatal pelvic examination to confirm changes in the cervix.

Data from Jones, D.A., Lepley, M.K., and Bates, B.A.: Health assessment across the life span, New York, 1984, McGraw-Hill Book Co.

begins after the brown discharge and may last anywhere from 2 to 6 weeks.

Breast changes occur about the third or fourth postpartum day. The breast becomes firm and tender, indicating that milk is available for the infant. The tenderness is relieved by nursing. The mother should be instructed to begin nursing slowly, usually starting with 2 minutes a side and working up to 10 minutes. The woman should also be instructed to alternate the beginning side at each nursing period because the infant sucks more vigorously at the beginning of the nursing period. If the same breast is used initially each time, the nipple will quickly become sore and cracked. A maximal period of 10 minutes a side is recommended, since a hungry infant can drain a breast in about 5 minutes.

The greater the quantity of milk consumed, the greater the quantity of milk produced. When the mother decides to decrease the number of breast feedings or the infant's needs decrease, the quantity of milk production decreases. Unfortunately, the demand and supply system of lactation is not foolproof,

TABLE 26-4

Physiological Changes in the Second Trimester

Symptom	Cause	Appropriate Nursing Interventions
INSPECTION		
Integument: pigmented nipple and breast, hyperpigmentation of abdominal line (linea nigra), mottling of cheeks or forehead (chloasma or "mask of pregnancy"), local or generalized pruritus	Melanocyte-stimulating hormone	Reassure client that skin color changes are normal and temporary. Instruct client to avoid hot baths and use of lotions, which can dry skin and increase itching.
Mouth: hypertrophy of gums (pregnancy epulis), causing gingival swelling and bleeding	Proliferation of interdental papillary blood vessels, resulting in local inflammation and hyperplasia	Teach client good "flossing" technique. Instruct client to get routine dental checkups during second trimester.
Lungs: increased respiratory rate	Increase in oxygen consumption by 20%	
Abdomen: heartburn	Increased hydrochloric acid, decreased gastric mobility, and esophogeal reflux	Instruct client to avoid foods that precipitate heartburn. Check with her physician about use of antacids. Have client sleep in high Fowler's position.
Genitalia: pelvic examination not routinely performed from the first prenatal visit until the last month of pregnancy to avoid trauma to the developing fetus and placenta		
PALPATION		
Neck: enlarged thyroid, goiter of pregnancy	Response of thyroid to increased metabolic demands	Reassure client that this is a normal finding in some women.
Breasts: hyperplasia and tenderness	Gradual development of glandular tissue	Instruct client to increase her bra size as needed.
Abdomen: increasing size of uterine fundus—at level of symphysis at 9 weeks, at intra-abdominal organs at 12 weeks, between symphysis and umbilicus at 16 weeks, at umbilicus at 20-22 weeks	Growth of fetus	Reinforce nutrition. Enroll client and partner in childbirth preparation classes.
Sensation of movement or gaslike movements (quickening)	Fetal motion	Instruct client to notify physician if these movements are absent or decline.
Braxton-Hicks contractions	Expanding uterus and preparation of uterus for labor	Instruct client that these are irregular short contractions, not early labor, and will continue periodically throughout the pregnancy. Instruct client to notify her physician if contractions become regular and increased in frequency and duration.
Fetal heartbeat heard with Doppler or Fetoscope; rate of 120-140 beats per minute, with points of maximal intensity determined by fetal position		Allow mother to hear heartbeat.

Data from Jones, D.A., Lepley, M.J., and Baker, B.A.: Health assessment across the life span, New York, 1984, McGraw-Hill Book Co.

and the woman's breasts may become engorged and painful. Aspirin, if not contraindicated, may decrease the pain. Warm, moist compresses on the breast increase circulation to the breast and reduce engorgement. Manual expression of the milk also relieves engorgement.

The nursing mother must care for her breasts. She should wear a good supportive bra, which may be needed round the clock if her breasts are tender. The mother should be instructed to clean the nipple region with water and a mild soap before each feeding. After nursing, the nipples should be exposed to the air to dry thoroughly. If it is impractical for the mother to expose her breasts to the air for 10 to 15 minutes after every nursing period (every 3 to 4 hours), she can try drying her breasts with a blow dryer set on a *cool* setting and held 12 inches from the breast. If the mother notices nipple cracking, she should use nipple shields for the first few minutes of nursing when the infant's suck is the strongest.

TABLE 26-5

Physiological Changes in the Third Trimester

Symptom	Cause	Appropriate Nursing Interventions
Lungs: dyspnea	Pressure of fetus against diaphragm, decreasing lung expansion	Instruct client to sit upright. Use of two pillows at night may ease breathing during sleep.
Heart: cardiac displacement with counterclockwise rotation and lateral upward displacement of heart	Elevation of diaphragm by enlarging uterus, displacing heart	Reassure client that these are temporary changes.
Increased pulse rate and palpitations	Increased metabolic rate and increased plasma blood volume	
Breasts: increased colostrum, the precursor of true milk	Preparation of breasts for lactation	Instruct client to express colostrum to prevent clogged milk ducts. If client chooses to breast feed, instruct her to "toughen" her nipples using lanolin cream and vigorous drying with a towel after bathing. This will decrease the risk of cracked nipples during the initial nursing phase.
Abdomen: fundus at xiphoid at 36 weeks; baby's head down by ninth month as determined by palpation; mother may feel that baby has "dropped" and that pressure on xiphoid, diaphragm, and stomach is relieved	Descent of baby's head into pelvis (engagement), which may occur at any point from thirty-sixth week to onset of labor	Reassure client of baby's growth. Reassure client that baby can be safely repositioned in utero if needed. Reassure client that her pregnancy is coming to an end.
Elimination system: increased urinary frequency, constipation	Pressure on bladder from enlarged fetus; pressure and displacement of colon and decreased gastric motility	Instruct client to reduce fluid intake after 8 PM and increase roughage in diet.
Extremities: pedal edema (increased in hot, humid weather)	Fluid retention and decreased venous return	Unless edema is accompanied by elevated blood pressure and protein in urine, reassure client that this is normal. Instruct her to elevate her feet whenever possible.
Musculoskeletal system: waddling gait	Altered center of gravity in pregnancy	Instruct client to wear low, comfortable shoes. High heels may cause her to lose her balance and fall.

Data from Jones, D.A., Lepley, M.K., and Baker, B.A.: Health assessment across the life span, New York, 1981, McGraw-Hill Book Co.

Finally, the nursing mother requires a balanced diet, with an additional 500 to 750 calories depending on the infant's milk requirements. Fluid intake must be increased by 2500 to 3000 ml, with further increases during the hot summer months.

■ ■ ■ ■ ■

Multiple physiological changes occur in pregnancy and the puerperium, and there are concurrent changes in role, responsibility, and body image. The expectant father also needs knowledge and emotional support and requires the 9 months to prepare for his responsibilities.

COGNITIVE CHANGES

The cognitive changes during pregnancy affect both parents and occur gradually or quickly. The cognitive changes primarily involve sensory perception and needs for education.

SENSORY PERCEPTION. The pregnant woman generally experiences changes in sensory perception. Temporary changes occur in visual and hearing acuity, taste, and smell. Many pregnant women frequently stroke the abdomen, possibly because of a change in the sensation of touch or other sensory need. The woman may be using the sensation of touch to initiate bonding with her child (Jones, Lepley, and Baker, 1984).

NEEDS FOR EDUCATION. The entire childbearing family needs education about pregnancy, labor, delivery, breastfeeding, and integration of the newborn into the family structure.

Childbirth classes help the parents plan for the birth of the child. Such classes focus on the normal physiological changes of pregnancy and the processes of labor and delivery. The classes prepare the expectant parents for natural childbirth or childbirth with anesthesia. Other types of classes may emphasize newer advances in obstetrics, such as birthing rooms.

Many health care centers also have sibling preparation classes. These classes explain to children in the family, at their level of comprehension, the processes of pregnancy, birth, and integration of the baby into the family structure.

PSYCHOSOCIAL CHANGES

Like the cognitive changes of pregnancy, psychosocial changes may occur at various times during the 9 months of pregnancy and in the puerperium. The major categories of psychosocial changes involve body image, role, sexuality, coping mechanisms, and stresses during the puerperium.

BODY IMAGE. Although the physical changes of pregnancy are not obvious to others until the second trimester, the woman generally perceives changes in her body during the first 3 months.

One change that some women consider positive is an increase in breast size, which may make the woman feel more feminine and sexually appealing. Also, because she is pregnant, the woman may take extra time with her hygiene and grooming, trying new hairstyles and makeup.

The woman who is having difficulty with morning sickness and fatigue may have a poor body image. She may be too tired and ill to care about her appearance. Her major goal is often just getting through the phase of morning sickness and fatigue.

Most women, particularly those who are pregnant for the first time, enjoy the second trimester. They are beginning to "show" and start planning their maternity wardrobe. Their energy level has returned to normal and they have a general feeling of well-being. Because they are able to feel the baby move and hear the heartbeat, the baby becomes real to them and they are able to fantasize about the infant's features.

During the third trimester the fetus grows more rapidly. Toward the end of the pregnancy the woman may feel big, awkward, and unattractive. It is important that her family and support group help the pregnant woman feel more attractive. For example, her husband may bring home flowers or be more attentive. This may also be a good time for the woman to buy a comfortable nightgown and robe for the postpartum period. If she plans to breast feed the infant, she should select a nightgown that can easily accommodate breast feeding. She should also be counseled not to anticipate wearing her prepregnancy clothes home from the hospital. Because the uterus takes time to involute completely, she will need to wear loose clothing for a bit longer.

ROLE CHANGES. As the pregnancy advances, both partners think about their role changes. It is normal for expectant parents to feel ambivalent about the upcoming event and to wonder if this is the right time to begin a family. Both partners may also be concerned about their ability to be parents. They may observe the interactions between parents and children in their friends' families and wonder if they can cope. The nurse can help the future parents overcome their insecurities about parenting by emphasizing that the infant and the parent grow together, learning about each other's habits, moods, and behaviors. The major dreads for first-time parents are the "terrible two's" and toilet training. However, since no woman has given birth to a 2-year-old, the parents have time to prepare for these developmental tasks.

Another role change can involve the choice to remain employed or to stay home after the baby's birth. This is no longer solely a woman's decision. An increasing number of men are becoming househusbands. This is occurring because some wives make more money than their husbands and therefore need to remain in the workforce. In addition, a husband may be laid off or become unemployed near the time of the child's birth.

SEXUALITY. Pregnancy does not alter a woman's basic sexual response, nor is sexual activity harmful to a normally developing fetus. Often the pregnant woman and her partner need to be reassured about these facts.

However, the woman's perception of her body image influences her desire for sexual activity. Some women may feel more attractive and sexually desirable. Others perceive the changes in their bodies as unattractive. A woman may desire cuddling and holding rather than sexual intercourse (Jones, Lepley, and Baker, 1984).

COPING MECHANISMS. Pregnancy requires many adjustments. The pregnant woman and her partner need to remember that, while childbirth and child rearing are wonderful, they are also stressful. Many times the partners are unable to cope with a particular stressor such as finding new housing, preparing the nursery, or participating in childbirth classes.

The nurse can help parents overcome these stresses by selecting nursing interventions to reduce stress and cope with situational crises (see Chapter 5). A vacation or merely a good night's sleep during the third trimester can be a good way to reduce stress.

STRESSES DURING THE PUERPERIUM. It is not uncommon for the new mother to bring the baby home from the hospital, place him in his crib, sit down, and wonder, "Now what do I do?" A visiting nurse can help the new parents during the transition from hospital to home. Many child-care books are available that can help prepare parents for their baby's needs and for their own emotional and social adjustments. A new mother needs to know, for example, that on a rainy day when the baby has rarely stopped crying, she may also find relief in a good cry. The mother can hand the baby to her husband as he walks in the door from work and take a long bath with a glass of wine. Neither of these behaviors indicates poor parenting. On the contrary, they may be good coping practices.

A second stressor during the puerperium may be the mother's return to work. She may feel guilt, worry, relief, or a sense of freedom. Even when a return to work is necessary, as in the case of a single parent, the mother has mixed emotions about leaving her child. She should be assured that there is no evidence that children have better emotional health and social skills if a parent remains at home.

HEALTH CONCERNS

The pregnant woman and her partner have many health questions. Will the pregnancy be normal? Will the baby be normal? Where will the baby be born? The majority of the health needs related to pregnancy can be met with proper prenatal care.

PRENATAL CARE. Prenatal care is routine examination of the pregnant woman by an obstetrician, a nurse practitioner, or a certified nurse-midwife. During the prenatal visit the pregnant woman's weight and blood pressure are monitored, her urine is checked for glucose, acetone, and protein, and the fundus is measured. Regular health care can address common health concerns such as preeclampsia, eclampsia, excessive weight gain, and the high-risk infant.

Preeclampsia is an abnormal condition of pregnancy characterized by the onset of acute hypertension after the twenty-fourth week of gestation. The classic triad of preeclampsia includes hypertension, proteinuria, and edema.

Eclampsia is a complication of pregnancy characterized by grand mal seizures, coma, hypertension, proteinuria, and edema. A client with eclampsia requires bed rest, quiet, and parenteral administration of magnesium sulfate. The symptoms of preeclampsia and eclampsia are reversed when the fetus is delivered.

Excessive weight gain increases the woman's risk for salt and water retention, which may result in hypertension. Depending on the pregnant woman's body build and prepregnancy weight and the fetal growth, the ideal weight gain is 9 to 13 kg (19 to 30 pounds). Rapid weight gain with edema after the twenty-fourth week of pregnancy can indicate the development of preeclampsia.

Rapid weight gain with corresponding rapid growth of the uterus can also indicate a possible multiple birth. Diagnostic tests, such as ultrasonography, can confirm the presence of multiple fetuses.

The high-risk infant is a neonate, regardless of birth weight, size, or gestational age, who, because of preconceptual, prenatal, natal, or postnatal conditions or circumstances that interfere with the normal birth process or impede adjustment to extrauterine growth and development, has a greater than average chance of morbidity or mortality, especially within the first 28 days of life.

Middle Adult

In middle adulthood from age 45 to 65, the adult makes lasting contributions through involvement with others. Personal and career achievements have often already been experienced and the person has socioeconomic stability. Many find particular joy in assisting their children and other young people to become productive and responsible adults. This is also a period of helping aging parents progress through the later years of life. Using leisure time in satisfying and creative ways is a challenge that, if met satisfactorily, will enable the individual to prepare for retirement.

Both men and women must adjust to inevitable biological changes. As in adolescence, the middle-aged adult uses considerable energy to adapt his self-concept and body image to physiological realities and changes in physical appearance. High self-esteem, a favorable body image, and a positive attitude toward physiological changes are fostered when the adult engages in positive health behaviors. Physical exercise, a balanced diet, adequate sleep, and good hygiene practices promote a vigorous, healthy body. Such health habits also support the body during the time when stressors place the individual at risk for acute and chronic illness.

Theories of Middle Adulthood

ERIKSON'S THEORY

According to Erikson's developmental theory, the primary developmental task of the middle years, the seventh stage of life, is to achieve generativity. Generativity is the willingness to care for and guide others. The middle adult can achieve generativity with his own children or the children of close friends, or through guidance in social interactions with the next generation. If the middle adult fails to achieve generativity, stagnation occurs, which is manifested by the person's excessive concern with himself or destructive behavior toward his children and the community.

HAVIGHURST'S THEORY

Havighurst's developmental theory has been summarized in terms of the following seven developmental tasks for the middle adult (Beck, Rawlins, and Williams, 1984):
1. Achieving adult civic social responsibility
2. Establishing and maintaining a standard of living
3. Helping teenage children become responsible and happy adults
4. Developing leisure activities
5. Relating to one's spouse as a person

6. Accepting and adjusting to the physiological changes of middle age
7. Adjusting to aging parents

Other theorists have supported Havighurst's model. In this perspective the middle adult can be viewed as healthy in the psychosocial dimension if he is successfully meeting the seven tasks. Currently the responsibility of the middle adult to the older adult parent is receiving more recognition than in the past.

BUHLER'S THEORY

Another theorist, Buhler, emphasizes goal formation and achievement during the middle adult years. The ability to achieve one's goals depends on four factors: the satisfaction of needs, the ability to expand creatively, personal adjustment to limitations, and consistency in the inner self. The middle-aged adult who believes that the majority of his life goals have not been achieved may be depressed, even to the point of suicide (Beck, Rawlins, and Williams, 1984).

Physiological Changes

Major physiological changes occur between the ages of 45 and 65. Table 26-6 summarizes these normal developmental changes, as noted on physical assessment.

The most visible changes are graying of the hair, wrinkling of the skin, and thickening of the waist. Balding commonly begins during the middle years, but it may also occur in the young adult. Often these physiological changes have an impact on the person's self-concept and body image. The most significant physiological changes during middle age are menopause in women and the climacteric in men.

MENOPAUSE

Menstruation and ovulation occur in a cyclical rhythm in the female body from adolescence into middle adulthood. Menopause is the disruption of this cycle, primarily because of the inability of the neurohumoral system to maintain its periodic stimulation of the endocrine system. The ovaries no longer produce estrogen and progesterone, and the blood level of these hormones drops markedly. Menopause typically occurs between the ages of 45 and 60. It is often preceded by a period of irregular cycles. Menopausal symptoms may be mild or quite dramatic. The range of physical manifestations includes "hot flashes," breast pain, headaches, and heart palpitations. Psychological symptoms such as depression, anxiety, and irritability can also occur. In some women these symptoms begin before the cessation of the menses, but in others they occur at the same time as or even

Physiological Changes in the Middle Adult as Found during Physical Assessment

Body System	Findings
Integument	Intact; appropriate distribution of pigmentation; slow progressive decrease in skin turgor; graying and loss of hair (Baldness patterns in males are established by age 55. Hair loss after this time might have other causes.)
Head and neck	Symmetry of scalp, skull, and face; normal accessory organs of vision
Eyes	Visual acuity by Snellen chart <20/50; pupillary reaction to light and accommodation; normal visual fields and extraocular movements; normal retinal structures
Ears	Normal auditory structures and acuity
Nose, sinuses, and throat	Patent nares and intact sinuses, mouth, and pharynx; trachea at midline; lateral thyroid lobes nonpalpable
Thorax and lungs	Anterior-posterior (A-P) diameter increased; respiratory rate 16 to 21 breaths per minute and regular; ratio of respiratory rate to heart 1:4; normal tactile fremitus, resonance, and breath sounds heard throughout
Heart and vascular system	Normal heart sounds: systole—$S_1<S_2$ at the base, diastole—$S_1>S_2$ at the apex; point of maximal impulse at fifth intercostal space in the midclavicular line and 2 cm or less in diameter Vital signs: temperature 36.7° to 37.6° C (97° to 99.6° F); pulse 60-100 (conditioned athlete $\cong$ 50); blood pressure: systolic—95-140 mm Hg, diastolic—60-90 mm Hg; all pulses palpable
Breasts	Decreased size owing to decreased muscle mass; normal nipples
Abdomen	No tenderness or organomegaly; decreased strength of abdominal muscles
Female reproductive system	Change in menstrual cycle and in duration and quantity of menstrual flow; "hot flashes"; change in cervical mucosa
Male reproductive system	Normal penis and scrotum; prostatic enlargement in some individuals
Musculoskeletal system	Decreased muscle mass; pathological fractures owing to osteoporosis; decreased range of joint motion
Neurological system	Appropriate affect, appearance, and behavior, lucidity and appropriate level of cognitive ability; intact cranial nerves; adequate motor responses; responsive sensory system

several years after the cessation of menses. Still other women remain entirely free of symptoms. The nurse can encourage the client to describe her own response to the menopausal experience. Referral to a physician is indicated when the client says that her symptoms are interfering with her activities of daily living or have become an unmanageable psychological stressor.

CLIMACTERIC

The climacteric or andropause, so named because of the decreased level of androgens, occurs in men in their late forties or early fifties. Throughout this period and thereafter, a man is still capable of producing fertile sperm and fathering a child. After the male climacteric, however, penile erection is less firm, ejac-ulation is less frequent, and the refractory period is longer (Beck, Rawlins, and Williams, 1984).

Cognitive Changes

Changes in the cognitive function of middle adults are rare except in the presence of illness or trauma. The middle adult is able to continue learning new skills and information. Some middle-aged adults enter educational or vocational programs to prepare themselves for entering the job market or changing jobs.

When caring for a middle-aged adult, the nurse must remember that his level of cognitive function is usually unchanged. Therefore, he is able to participate fully in health education or health promotion programs.

Psychosocial Changes

The psychosocial changes in the middle adult may involve expected events, such as children moving away from home, or unexpected events, such as a marital separation or the death of a spouse. These changes may result in stress that can affect the middle adult's overall level of health.

CAREER TRANSITION

Career changes may occur by choice or as a result of changes in the workplace or society as a whole. In recent decades middle-aged adults are more often changing occupations because after a long period in the same field they find themselves bored with their present employment. In some cases technological advances or other changes force the middle-aged adult to seek a new job. Such changes, particularly when unanticipated, may result in stress that can affect the person's health, as well as family relationships, self-concept, and other dimensions.

SEXUALITY

The onset of menopause can affect the middle-aged woman's sexual health. Because of the cessation of ovulation and the inability to conceive, the woman may desire more sexual activity with her partner because pregnancy is no longer a possibility. On the other hand, while menopause does not decrease libido or sexual response, the menopausal woman may feel less sexually attractive and may not be eager to participate in regular sexual intercourse or may feel stress in her sexual relationship with her partner.

The middle-aged man may notice changes in the strength of his erection and a decrease in his ability to experience repeated orgasms. However, sexual responses remain unchanged and the ability to fertilize an egg still exists. Like the middle-aged woman, the man may experience stresses related to sexual changes or a conflict between his sexual needs and self-perceptions and social attitudes or expectations.

MARITAL CHANGES

Marital changes that may occur during middle age include death of a spouse, separation, divorce, and the choice of remarrying or remaining single. A client who is widowed, separated, or divorced goes through a period of grief and loss in which it is necessary to adapt to the change in marital status (see Chapter 46).

If the single middle adult decides to marry, the stressors of marriage are similar to those for the young adult. In addition, the couple may have to cope with the social expectations and pressures related to middle-age marriage.

FAMILY TRANSITIONS

The departure of the last child from the home of the middle-aged parents may or may not be a stressor. Many parents welcome freedom from child-rearing responsibilities, whereas others feel lonely or directionless because of this change. Eventually the parents usually reassess their marriage and are able to resolve conflicts and plan future goals. Occasionally this readjustment phase may lead to marital conflicts for which no resolution can be achieved and which result in separation and divorce (Beck, Rawlins, and Williams, 1984).

CARE OF THE AGING PARENTS

The increasing life span in the United States and Canada has led to increased numbers of older adults in the population. Therefore there are greater numbers of middle-aged adults who must address the personal and social issues confronting their aging parents.

Housing, employment, health, and economic realities have altered the traditional social expectations between generations in families. The middle-aged adult and the older adult parent may have conflicting priorities related to their relationship. Negotiations and compromises are useful in defining and resolving such problems. Nurses deal with both middle and older adults in the community, long-term care facilities, and hospitals. The nurse can help identify the health needs of both groups and can assist the multigenerational family in determining the health and community resources available to them as they make decisions and plans.

Health Concerns
PHYSIOLOGICAL CONCERNS

STRESS. Because the middle-aged adult is experiencing physiological changes and faces certain health realities, his perception of health and health behaviors are often important factors in maintaining health. Today's complex world makes individuals more prone to stress-related illnesses such as heart attacks, hypertension, migraine headaches, ulcers, colitis, autoimmune disease, backache, tension, arthritis, and cancer.

When the middle-aged adult seeks health care, the nurse's focus on the goal of wellness can guide the client to evaluate his health behaviors, life-style, and environment. Attention to risk factors that can be altered to improve the client's health can add years to the client's life and increase the quality of life. The nurse can encourage the client to use the social readjustment scale (see Chapter 5) or other guide to assess his risk for stress-related illnesses. Any change in the life of the individual or his family can be stressful. A nurse can use a self-assessment tool to help the client evaluate his health status and develop positive health behaviors.

ASSESSING LEVELS OF WELLNESS. The nurse must be able to assess the health status of the middle adult client. Such assessment offers direction for planning nursing care and is useful in evaluating the effectiveness of nursing interventions. Table 26-6, showing the physiological changes of the middle-aged adult, can also be used as a guide for physical assessment, along with other standard assessment techniques (see Chapter 7).

FORMING POSITIVE HEALTH HABITS. A habit is a person's usual practice or manner of behavior. This behavior pattern is reinforced by frequent repetition until it becomes the individual's customary way of behaving. Some habits support health, such as exercise and brushing and flossing the teeth each day. Other habits involve risk factors to health, such as smoking or eating foods with little or no nutritional value.

In the assessment phase of the nursing process the nurse frequently obtains data indicating both positive and negative health behaviors of the client. In the planning, implementation, and evaluation phases the nurse then helps the client maintain habits that protect his health and offers healthier alternatives to poor habits.

Health teaching and health counseling are often directed at improving health habits (see Chapter 16). The more fully the nurse understands the dynamics of behavior and habits, the more successfully she can work with the client to bring about or reinforce health-promoting behaviors (see boxed material).

The nurse's role in helping the client form positive health habits is that of teacher and facilitator. By providing information about how the body functions and how habits are formed and changed, the nurse raises the client's level of knowledge regarding the potential impact of his behaviors on his health. No person can change a habit for another person. The client has control of and is responsible for his own behavior. The nurse can explain psychological principles of changing a habit and offer information about health risks. The nurse can also offer positive reinforcement (such as praise and rewards) for behaviors and decisions that are health directed. Such reinforcement increases the likelihood that the behavior will be repeated. Ultimately, however, it is the client who

---

Dynamics of Behavior and Habits

- Habits are frequently repeated behaviors.
- The more often a behavior is repeated, the more likely that it will be repeated thereafter.
- Habits can be a stress reduction mechanism for the individual (for example, nail biting) but may be simultaneously detrimental to health (for example, alcohol consumption).
- Habits often meet some basic need for the person.
- Changing a habit requires a significant motivation by the client. Changing the habit must provide greater pleasure or satisfaction than the habit itself.
- Any change in habits or behavior patterns creates stress.

---

decides which behaviors will become habits of daily living.

PSYCHOSOCIAL CONCERNS

Two common psychosocial health concerns of the middle adult are anxiety and depression.

ANXIETY. Adults often experience anxiety in response to physiological and psychosocial changes that show they are entering middle age. Such anxiety can motivate the adult to rethink life goals and can stimulate productivity. For some adults, however, this anxiety precipitates psychosomatic illness and preoccupation with death. In this case the middle adult views his life as half or more over and thinks in terms of the time he has left to live (Beck, Rawlins, and Williams, 1984).

Clearly the presence of a life-threatening illness, marital transition, or job stressor increases the anxiety of the client and his family. The nurse may need to use crisis intervention or stress management techniques to help the client adapt to the changes of the middle adult years (see Chapter 5).

DEPRESSION. Depression is common among adults after entrance into the middle years and may have many causes. The risk factors for depression are listed in Table 26-7. Menopause is no longer believed to be a sole cause of depression. Depression that occurs during the middle years, often referred to as agitated depression, is characterized by moderate to high anxiety, bizarre physical complaints, and paranoid ideation. Depression may be worsened by the abuse of alcohol or other substances. The nurse may need to

From Beck, C.M., Rawlins, R.P., and Williams, S.R.: Mental health–psychiatric nursing: a holistic life-cycle approach, St. Louis, 1984, The C.V. Mosby Co.

TABLE 26-7	

Risk Factors for Depression in the Middle Years

Risk Factor	Characteristics
Sex	Female
Age	Declines for women after early fifties; increases for men after late fifties
Social isolation	Absence of intimate, confiding relationships following a change in the nature of the relationship with parents, children, and spouse
Losses	Parental deprivation or loss of a mother before age 14; other losses during midlife such as job loss, career difficulties, marital problems, and physical changes; departure of last child from home
Family history	History of depression in the family of origin

refer a severely depressed middle-aged client for specialized psychological therapy.

Health Promotion for Young and Middle Adults

Community health programs for young and middle adults are designed to prevent illness and promote health, as well as to detect disease in the early stages. Nurses can make valuable contributions to community health by taking an active part in the planning of screening and teaching programs.

Family planning, birthing, and parenting skills are some program topics in which adults might be interested. Health screening for diabetes, hypertension, eye disease, and cancer is a good opportunity for the nurse to perform assessment and provide health teaching and health counseling.

Health education programs can promote changes in behavior and life-style. The nurse as health teacher offers the client information that will enable him to make good decisions regarding his health practices. With health counseling the nurse and client design a plan of action that addresses the client's health and well-being. Through objective problem solving the nurse assists the client to grow and change.

Regardless of the age of family members and the structure of the family, they face certain health tasks. The nurse as health teacher and health counselor understands the autonomy of the family and supports it while promoting family health.

Nursing roles include community-centered care, hospital-based acute care, and care of the chronically ill. Participation in community health programs for the adult or family often requires the full extent of nursing roles and skills.

Summary

Transitional periods and developmental tasks of the young and middle adult and family members can be a source of stress and conflict that can threaten health. Often several family members are facing different developmental issues at the same time, increasing the strain on the family.

The nurse who understands the interrelationship of physiological, cognitive, and psychosocial needs, and their influence on overall health, assesses life changes as a part of the nursing history of a young or middle adult. Anticipatory guidance can provide the client with insight into the normal life cycle events within a family. The nurse can inform the client about the normal growth and development patterns of young and middle adulthood. In addition, the nurse providing care for the young or middle adult may teach the client about marriage stages and the challenges, conflicts, and stresses associated with marriage.

With an understanding of the norms and common problems faced by others in the same developmental period, young adult and middle-aged clients are better able to put health-related events into perspective. When the client experiences more complex difficulties, the nurse can refer the client for the appropriate professional counseling.

KEY CONCEPTS

✓ Adult development involves orderly and sequential changes in characteristics and attitudes that adults experience over a period of time.

✓ Many changes experienced by the young adult are related to the natural process of maturation and socialization.

✓ Maturity is reached when the young adult attains a balance of growth in the intellectual, psychomotor, and emotional areas.

✓ The young adult is in a stable period of physical development, except for the changes related to pregnancy.

✓ Cognitive development continues throughout the young and middle adult years.

✓ The emotional health of the young adult is correlated with his ability to address and resolve personal and social problems.

✓ The young adult must choose career and decide whether to remain single or marry and begin a family.

✓ The pregnant woman needs to understand the physiological changes occurring in each trimester.

✓ The cognitive and psychosocial changes and health concerns during pregnancy and the puerperium affect the parents, the siblings, and often the extended family.

✓ Prenatal care reduces maternal and fetal mortality and morbidity.

✓ Midlife transition begins when a person becomes aware that physiological and psychosocial changes signify passage to another state in life.

✓ Erikson, Havighurst, and Buhler have described the primary developmental tasks of the middle adult.

✓ Two significant physiological changes of the middle years are menopause in women and the climacteric in men.

✓ Cognitive changes are rare in middle age except in cases of illness or physical trauma.

✓ Psychosocial changes for the middle adult may be related to career transition, sexuality, marital changes, family transition, and care of the aging parent.

✓ The health concerns of the middle adult commonly involve stress-related illnesses, health assessment, and adoption of positive health habits.

REFERENCES

Beck, C.M., Rawlins, R.P., and Williams, S.R.: Mental health–psychiatric nursing: a holistic life-cycle approach, St. Louis, 1984, The C.V. Mosby Co.

Diekelmann, N.L.: The young adult: the choice is health or illness, Am. J. Nurs. 76:1276, 1976.

Fogel, C.I., and Woods, N.F.: Health care of women: a nursing perspective, St. Louis, 1981, The C.V. Mosby Co.

Gould, R.: Transformations, New York, 1978, Simon & Schuster, Inc.

Jones, D.A., Lepley, M.K., and Baker, B.A.: Health assessment across the life span, New York, 1984, McGraw-Hill Book Co.

Kaluger, G., and Kaluger, M.F.: Human development: the span of life, ed. 3, St. Louis, 1984, The C.V. Mosby Co.

Levinson, D., et al.: The seasons of a man's life, New York, 1978, Alfred A. Knopf, Inc.

Masters, W.H., and Johnson, V.E.: Human sexual response, Boston, 1970, Little, Brown & Co.

Stanhope, M., and Lancaster, J.: Community health nursing: process and practice for promoting health, St. Louis, 1984, The C.V. Mosby Co.

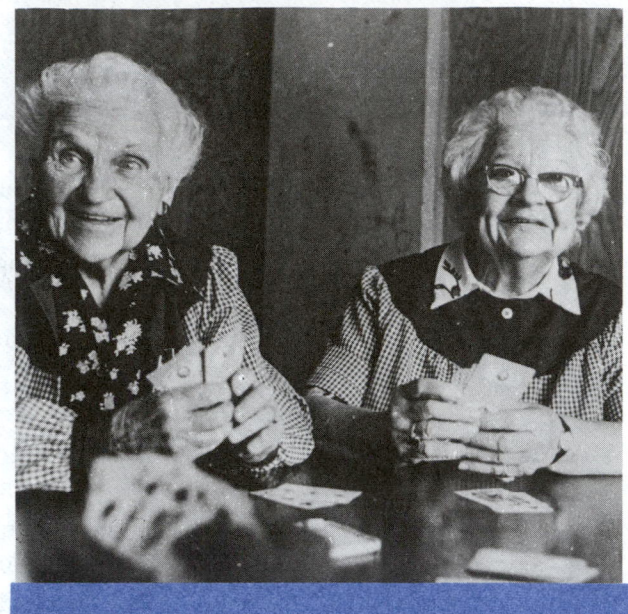

OBJECTIVES

Mastery of content in this chapter will enable the student to:

- Define the terms in the glossary.
- Describe common myths and stereotypes about the older adult.
- Discuss the four physiological theories of aging.
- Discuss the three psychosocial theories of aging.
- State and discuss the developmental tasks of the older adult.
- Describe the physiological changes of aging.
- Discuss the specific cognitive changes of dementia and organic brain syndrome found in some older adults.
- Discuss the psychosocial changes related to retirement, social isolation, sexuality, housing, and death to which the older adult must adjust.
- Discuss the physical and psychosocial health concerns of the older adult and the related nursing interventions.
- Discuss nurses' attitudes toward older adults.
- Describe community and institutional health care services available to the older adult.

GLOSSARY

ageism Attitude that disadvantages, separates, and stigmatizes older adults on the basis of age-related characteristics.

Alzheimer's disease Disease of the brain parenchyma that causes a gradual and progressive decline in cognitive functioning.

attitudinal isolation Social isolation that occurs because of the older adult's personal or cultural values.

behavioral isolation Social isolation that occurs because of the older adult's socially unacceptable behaviors.

confabulation Defense mechanism in which the person fabricates experiences or situations and often recounts them in a detailed and plausible way in order to fill in and cover up gaps in memory.

dementia Irreversible mental state characterized by decreased intellectual function, changes in personality, impaired judgment, and often changes in affect as a result of permanently altered cerebral metabolism.

geographical isolation Social isolation of the older adult resulting from urban crime, institutional barriers, and distance from family.

geriatrics Branch of health care dealing with the physiology and psychology of aging and with the diagnosis and treatment of illnesses affecting the aged.

Korsakoff's syndrome Psychosis characterized by disorientation of time, place, and person, amnesia for recent events, and confabulation.

27 Older Adult

organic brain syndrome   Any psychological or behavioral abnormality associated with transient or permanent brain dysfunction caused by a disturbance of the physiological functioning of brain tissue.

presbyacusis   Condition that affects the client's ability to hear high-pitched sounds and sibilant consonants such as "s," "sh," and "ch."

presbyopia   Decline in the ability of the eyes to accommodate for close and detailed work.

presentational isolation   Social isolation that occurs because of the older adult's socially unacceptable appearance or presentation of self to others.

reality orientation   Therapeutic modality for restoring an individual's sense of the present.

reminiscence   Recalling the past for the purpose of assigning new meaning to past experiences.

resocialization   Technique that assists the older adult to expand his social network within his community.

respite care   Short-term health services to the dependent older adult either in his home or in an institutional setting.

sundowning   Phenomenon in which the restlessness, confusion, and wanderings of the older adult increase with approaching darkness.

Wernicke's syndrome   Illness occurring with advanced stages of vitamin B_1 depletion and accompanied by nystagmus, papillary abnormalities, ataxia, tremor, and stupor.

The older adult is in the last developmental stage of the human life span. Traditionally this developmental stage begins after retirement, usually between 65 and 75 years of age. No other population group is increasing as rapidly as the older adults. Because of this population growth, health care professionals must focus on identifying and meeting the needs of the older adult. Older adults are seeking greater participation in the identification, definition, and resolution of health and social issues affecting them. In addition to increasing longevity, a greater incidence of chronic health problems, technological advances, and contemporary economic, social, ethical, and health issues have prompted health care professionals to focus on improving the quality of life for older adults as well as its duration (Stanhope and Lancaster, 1984).

The increased life expectancy and decreased birth rate have resulted in a "graying" population. Demographers project a continuing increase in the older adult population well into the next century (Table 27-1). The life expectancy for persons born in 1980 is 70 years for men and 78.7 years for women (Department of Health and Human Services, 1981). The older adult population is expanding in all cultural and ethnic groups in the United States and Canada. In the United States blacks comprise approximately 8% of persons 65 years and older. This percentage is expected to increase to 11% by 2000 (Stanhope and Lancaster, 1984). Asians and Pacific islanders account for 6% of the older adult population, and Native Americans and Hispanics account for 4% (Office of Human Development Services, 1981). The

TABLE 27-1

Population Growth and Projections for Older Adults

Year	Total Number (in millions)	Percent of Total Population
1900	3.0	4.1
1940	9.0	6.8
1980	25.5	11.3
1990	30.2	12.1
2000	32.4	12.2
2010	35.4	12.6
2020	45.6	15.4
2030	55.8	18.2

From Office of Human Development Services: Facts about older Americans, 1980-81, Washington, D.C., Department of Health and Human Services.

greatest percentages of the older population reside in the Sunbelt states such as Florida, Arizona, and California.

Nursing care of older adults poses special challenges because of the diversity in clients' physical, cognitive, and psychosocial health. Older adults vary in their level of function and productivity as members of society. Many older adults are physically active, alert and intelligent, socially engaging, and productive members of their communities. On the other end of the scale are older adults who have lost the physical capacity to care for themselves, are confused or withdrawn, and are unable to make decisions concerning their needs.

Before making any health assessment the nurse should be aware of the normal expected findings of physical and psychosocial assessment for an older adult and should consider the normal changes of aging. A comparison of expected and actual findings prevents the nurse from focusing on abnormal assessment data. In other words, the nurse should not assume that all older adults have signs, symptoms, or behaviors representative of the lower end of the health continuum. By remembering that each older adult is an individual, the nurse can avoid stereotyping this age group.

Myths and Stereotypes

In recent years a health speciality area has been developed for the older adult. Geriatrics is the branch of health care dealing with the physiology and psychology of aging and with the diagnosis and treatment of diseases affecting the aged. Although research concerning the health needs of older adults has increased greatly, many myths and stereotypes about this age group persist. Some of these stereotypes depict the elderly as people who lack understanding, have difficulty remembering, are rigid, spend most of their time drowsing, and are unpleasant to others. Furthermore, the elderly are often stereotyped as ill, crippled, hard of hearing, and bald.

Many people believe that a majority of the elderly are institutionalized. In fact, only about 5% of the elderly population is in institutional settings (Public Health Service, 1976-1977).

While the financial constraints on the elderly are significant, 85% of persons 65 years and older have incomes above the poverty level (Office of Human Development Services, 1981). However, the incomes of most elderly persons are fixed or do not rise as quickly as inflationary increases in the cost of food, housing, utilities, and health care.

Many people incorrectly believe that the elderly have decreased learning ability. As a result, health care professionals often fail to provide health education opportunities for the elderly, since they wrongly assume that older clients cannot learn to care for themselves (Stanhope and Lancaster, 1984).

There are many misconceptions concerning older adults and sex. Older adults are thought to be without sexual desire for a variety of reasons (see the boxed material opposite). In reality the older adult still experiences sexual drive and activity, although these are altered owing to physiological changes and sociocultural expectations. Health problems and medications may also alter sexual activity, as may changes in the availability of a mate, privacy, and living arrangements.

Our society values attractiveness, energy, and youth. As people age, their contributions become less appreciated. It is as if, after leaving the workforce at some arbitrarily selected age, an individual no longer possesses worth for the society.

These feelings have led to the concept of ageism, which is discrimination against people because of increasing age, just as racism and sexism are forms of discrimination because of skin color and gender. However, unlike sexists or racists, who will not experience a change in their skin color or gender, ageists are usually dimly aware that someday they too will be old. This produces some uneasiness and anxiety. The differences between young people and old people that many in the younger generation boast about will come home to them when they too become old.

Unfortunately, when we allow a youth image to dominate society, we lose touch with the most diver-

> ## Common Myths and Misconceptions about Sex and Aging
>
> - Sex does not matter in old age. The later years are supposed to be (and usually are) sexless.
> - Interest in sex is abnormal for older people.
> - Remarriage after the loss of a spouse should be discouraged.
> - It is all right for older men to seek younger women as sex partners, but it is ridiculous for older women to be sexually involved with younger men.
> - Older people should be separated according to sex in institutions to avoid problems for the staff and criticism by families and the community.
> - Emission of semen during sexual activity weakens men and therefore should be avoided in old age.
> - Masturbation is a childish activity that should not continue after adolescence.

sified segment of our population. Older adults have a unique perspective on many social, economic, and technological developments. In the past 100 years we have gone from riding in horse-drawn carriages to space shuttle flights. Older adults may have seen the two world wars, the Spanish Civil War, the Korean War, and the Vietnam War and must now live with the threat of nuclear war. In regard to the health care system, older adults have lived from the era of the family doctor into the age of specialization. They have seen the establishment of the United States' first national health insurance, the Medicare and Medicaid systems. It should be clear that older adults are unique and valuable to society, even though society fails to take full advantage of their potential. The dramatic increases in the numbers of older adults, however, may mean a change in their impact on society.

A nurse may enter the profession with certain preconceptions about older adults. To provide correct and individualized nursing care for these clients, she may first need to clarify her values about the elderly (see Chapter 13). The nurse must learn to distinguish between myth and reality and be able to identify her clients' strengths and limitations.

Theories of Aging

Aging is a complex biopsychosocial process. Different theorists have attempted to describe the aging process with frameworks that explain the physiolog-

ical or psychosocial changes occurring with advancing age. The aging process begins with conception and terminates with death, and many changes occur in the intervening years.

Physiological Theories

GENETIC THEORY

The genetic theory of aging states that the life span of a human is programmed within the genes. Some researchers believe that the life span is programmed in the DNA molecule before birth. Thus an individual inherits his family's tendencies for short or long life. Cells die and are replaced according to the DNA coding system set up at the time of conception. Studies done with animals in the 1970s yielded evidence that the loss of DNA from aging cells reduces the production of RNA by DNA molecules, thus leading to cell impairment. Current and future research will determine whether these cellular programming changes are the result of evolutionary phenomena or physiological changes that occur with advancing age (Forbes and Fitzsimmons, 1981).

STRESS THEORY

The stress theory of aging has also been referred to as the wear-and-tear theory. This theory postulates that nongenetic factors are important in the pathogenesis of aging and death (Groër and Shekleton, 1983.) Natural changes occur in the body over the lifetime of an individual. Cells are continually dying and being replaced in order for the body to maintain itself. As we age, the ability to replace the worn-out and discarded cells is lessened by the stresses experienced over a lifetime. These stresses and their effects vary depending on the individual's personality, coping mechanisms, occupation, and life-style. Because of physiological changes involved in the process of aging, the older adult needs more time than the younger person to adapt to a stressful situation (Forbes and Fitzsimmons, 1981).

IMMUNOLOGICAL THEORY

Theorists have speculated on several erratic cellular mechanisms capable of precipitating attacks on various tissues through autoaggression or immunodeficiencies. These mechanisms occur with greater frequency in aging and may explain the adult onset of chronic conditions such as diabetes mellitus, valvular heart disease, and arthritis (Ebersole and Hess, 1981).

Psychosocial Theories

In the past, psychosocial theories of development have focused primarily on the child and the adolescent. There are theories about certain aspects of psychosocial aging, but there is no adequate evidence to support a single theory. Researchers have demonstrated that genetic endowment is not the primary determinant of longevity; life-style, personality, and environmental factors also influence longevity (Murray, Huelskoetter, and O'Driscoll, 1980).

DISENGAGEMENT THEORY

The disengagement theory formulated by Cummings and Henry (1961) postulates that aging people withdraw from customary roles and engage in more introspective, self-focused activities. This theory includes four basic concepts: (1) the aging person and society mutually withdraw from each other; (2) disengagement is biologically and psychologically intrinsic and inevitable; (3) disengagement is considered necessary for successful aging; and (4) disengagement is beneficial for both the elderly and society (Maddox, 1974).

ACTIVITY THEORY

The activity theory disagrees with the disengagement theory and holds that the continuation of middle-adult activities is the criterion of successful aging. Most members of the aging population maintain a high level of activity. The individual's level of activity is influenced by past life-style and by present social and economic forces. According to this perspective, the maintenance of optimal physical, mental, and social activity is necessary for successful aging (Havighurst, 1963).

CONTINUITY THEORY

The continuity theory of aging is also referred to as the developmental theory. Neugarten (1964) noted that as people age their personality traits remain the same and their behavior becomes more predictable. The older adult continues to be capable of developing

support relationships to help him meet his psychological and social needs.

■ ■ ■ ■ ■

The theories of aging described here demonstrate that aging is not a simple progression and that there is no one universally accepted theory that can predict and explain the complexities of the older adult. The nurse must be aware of the uncertainties about the aging process, the scientific attempts to explain these phenomena, and the myriad of environmental factors that play a part in this process.

Growth and Development

As in the other stages of life, the older adult has specific developmental tasks. These are described by Burnside (1979), Duvall (1971), and Havighurst (1953) and include seven major categories (see the boxed material on this page).

First, the older adult must adjust to the physical changes of aging. As each body system ages, changes in appearance and system functioning occur. These changes are not associated with a disease state but are the normal changes anticipated with an older adult. The normal structural and functional changes associated with aging are described in the following section on physiological development.

Second, the older adult is commonly retired from full-time employment and therefore must adjust to boredom, decreased socialization, and reduced income. However, since retirement is usually anticipated, the person may be able to plan ahead to participate in consultation or volunteer activities. The majority of older adults, while above the poverty level, are on fixed incomes and find it difficult to meet their basic needs because of rising costs.

Third, the majority of older adults are faced with the death of their spouse, their friends, and in some instances their children. This loss is often difficult to resolve. Assisting the older adult through the grieving process enables him to adjust to the loss (see Chapter 46). When the grieving process has ended, the surviving spouse, friend, or parent may need help to identify other resources to fill the void left by the deceased.

Fourth, although the process of aging is inevitable, it is often difficult for the older adult to perceive himself as an aging person. Some older adults may demonstrate their inability to cope with aging by denying their upcoming retirement, requesting that their grandchildren not call them "Grandma" or "Grandpa," or choosing to live like a young or middle adult. The inability to accept the realities of aging is

---

Developmental Tasks of the Older Adult

- Adjusting to decreasing health and physical strength
- Adjusting to retirement and reduced income
- Adjusting to the death of a spouse
- Accepting oneself as an aging person
- Maintaining satisfactory living arrangements
- Realigning relationships with adult children
- Finding meaning in life

different from merely remaining active and can pose a threat to the client's level of health if he exceeds his physical limitations.

Fifth, an older adult may be required to change his living arrangements. For example, physical impairments may necessitate relocation to a smaller home with all the rooms on one floor. Severe health problems may require the older adult to live with his children or other relatives or friends for a time or perhaps permanently. A change in an older client's living arrangements may require an extended period of adjustment during which he needs assistance and support from health care professionals and his family.

Sixth, the older adult often needs to redefine his relationship with his adult children. The issues of role reversal, dependence, conflict, guilt, and loss require recognition and resolution. Frequently the adult children must cope with guilt feelings if they feel that they should have "come sooner" or made the older adult move into their home. Often adult children must realize that the behaviors of the older adult are symptoms rather than inherent meanness, stubbornness, or cantankerousness.

Last, the older adult must learn to acquire new activities and interests to maintain the quality of life. A person who has remained active throughout his adult life may find it relatively easy to meet new people and acquire new interests, because the social skills are already present. However, the older adult who has always been somewhat introverted, with socialization occurring only through his employment and family, may have difficulty meeting new people during his retirement, since he has not acquired the social and communication skills that would help him increase his social contacts.

These seven developmental tasks are common to many older adults. How an older adult adjusts to the changes of aging, however, depends on the individual. For some the adaptation and adjustment are easy and without stress. For others, each developmental task presents a major stress for which nursing intervention is needed.

Physiological Changes

The older adult's concept of his health generally depends on how well he functions. Therefore older adults actively engaged in activities of daily living consider themselves healthy, and those whose activities are limited by physical, emotional, or social impairments may perceive themselves as ill.

The physiological changes that occur with advancing age vary with each client. Table 27-2 describes the general types of physiological changes that can be anticipated with older adults.

The physiological changes of aging are not pathological processes. They occur in all persons but take place at different rates and depend on accompanying circumstances in an individual's life. The nurse should become knowledgeable about these changes in order to provide care correctly for the older adult and to assist the older adult in adapting to the changes.

The nurse assessing the older adult client should also consider the potential for sensory changes that may influence her data gathering. For example, if the client has problems with visual function that result from cataracts, or hearing impairments that result from nerve deafness, the nurse must consider these deficits in choosing communication techniques. If a client is unable to pick up on the nurse's visual or auditory cues, the assessment data may be inaccurate or misleading. For example, if a client has difficulty hearing the nurse's questions, his inappropriate response may lead the nurse to believe that he is confused.

General Survey

In an initial inspection of the older adult, the nurse may observe facial wrinkles, gray hair, loss of tissue on the extremities, and an increase in tissue and fat in the truncal region. Older clients are often encountered during a health fair or a health promotion or illness prevention program, such as hypertension screening, rather than in an institutional setting.

INTEGUMENTARY SYSTEM

The skin loses resilience and moisture, taking on the characteristic dryness of old age. The epithelial layer thins, and elastic collagen fibers shrink and become rigid. Wrinkles of the face and neck reflect lifetime patterns of muscle activity and facial expressions, the pull of gravity on tissue, and diminished elasticity.

Spots and lesions may also be present on the skin. Smooth, brown, irregularly shaped spots (age spots or senile lentigo) initially appear on the backs of the hands and on the forearms. Small, round, red or brown "cherry angiomas" may be found on the trunk. Seborrheic lesions or keratosis may appear as irregular, round or oval, brown, watery lesions.

HEAD AND NECK

The facial features of the older adult become more pronounced as a result of the loss of fat and skin elasticity. The facial features may appear asymmetrical because of missing teeth or improperly fitting dentures. In addition, changes in voice pitch (usually

TABLE 27-2

Normal Physical Changes of Aging

System	Normal Findings
Integumentary	
Skin color	Spotty pigmentation in areas exposed to the sun; pallor even in the absence of anemia
Moisture	Dry, scaly
Temperature	Extremities cooler; perspiration decreased
Texture	Decreased elasticity; wrinkles; folding; sagging
Fat distribution	Decreased on extremities; increased on abdomen
Hair	Thinning and graying on scalp; axillary and pubic hair and hair on extremities may be decreased; facial hair in men decreased; chin and upper lip hair may be present in women
Nails	Decreased growth rate
Head and neck	
Head	Nasal and facial bones sharp and angular; loss of eyebrow hair in women; men's eyebrows become bushier
Eyes	Decreased visual acuity; decreased accommodation; reduced adaptation to darkness; sensitivity to glare
Ears	Decreased pitch discrimination; diminished light reflex; diminished hearing acuity
Nose and sinuses	Increased nasal hair; decreased sense of smell
Mouth and pharynx	Use of bridges or dentures; decreased sense of taste; atrophy of the papillae of the lateral edges of the tongue
Neck	Thyroid gland nodular; slight tracheal deviation resulting from muscle atrophy
Thorax and lungs	Increased anterior-posterior diameter; increased chest rigidity; increased respiratory rate with decreased lung expansion
Heart and vascular	Significant increase in systolic pressure with slight increase in diastolic pressure; changes in heart rate at rest are usually not significant; peripheral pulses easily palpated; pedal pulses weaker and lower extremities colder, especially at night
Breasts	Diminished breast tissue
Gastrointestinal	Decreased salivary secretions, which make swallowing more difficult; decreased peristalsis; decreased production of digestive enzymes: hydrochloric acid, pepsin, and pancreatic enzymes; constipation
Reproductive	
Female	Decreased estrogen; decreased uterine size; decreased secretions; atrophy of epithelial lining of the vagina; decreased frequency of intercourse
Male	Decreased testosterone; decreased frequency of intercourse; decreased sperm count; decreased testicular size
Urinary	Decreased renal filtration and renal efficiency; subsequent loss of protein from kidney; nocturia in both men and women
Female	Urgency and stress incontinence resulting from decrease in perineal muscle tone
Male	Frequent urination resulting from prostatic enlargement
Musculoskeletal	Decreased muscle mass and strength; bone demineralization (more pronounced in women); shortening of trunk as a result of intervertebral space narrowing; decreased joint mobility; decreased range of joint motion
Neurological	Decreased rate of voluntary or automatic reflexes; decreased ability to respond to multiple stimuli; insomnia, shorter sleeping periods

Modified from Ebersole, P., and Hess, P.: Toward healthy aging: human needs and nursing response, St. Louis, 1981, The C.V. Mosby Co.

a rise) occur as a result of decline in power and range.

The older adult's visual acuity declines. This may be the result of retinal damage, a reduction in pupillary diameter, a reduction in opacity of the lens, or loss of lens elasticity. Presbyopia, a decline in the ability of the eyes to accommodate for close and detailed work, is commonly present. Presbyopia begins early in the fourth decade and continues throughout life. The older adult also has a reduced ability to see in darkness.

Auditory changes are subtle and may first be noted as difficulty hearing speech. Age-related changes in auditory acuity are called presbyacusis. Presbyacusis affects the client's ability to hear high-pitched sound and sibilant consonants such as "s," "sh," and "ch." The assessment of the older client's hearing is best accomplished using a 202 8Hz frequency tuning fork to screen for high-frequency losses (Forbes and Fitzsimmons, 1981).

Taste buds atrophy and lose efficiency. The older adult is able to discern salt, sweet, sour, and bitter tastes but less acutely. As a result, he may heavily season his food. His sense of smell is also decreased, further reducing his ability to taste.

THORAX AND LUNGS

Because of changes in the musculoskeletal system, the configuration of the thorax sometimes changes. There is an increase in the anterior-posterior diameter. Kyphosis is a subtle, progressive change in the vertebral structure that is permanent when accompanied by osteoporosis. Calcification of the costal cartilage can cause decreased mobility of the ribs (Forbes and Fitzsimmons, 1981).

Decreased muscle mass and muscle tone lead to decreased lung expansion. The decreased elasticity of the lung alveoli results in emphysematous changes in the lungs, and hyperresonance is present on percussion. If kyphosis or chronic obstructive lung disease is present, breath sounds are distant.

HEART AND VASCULAR SYSTEM

Decreased contractile strength of the myocardium results in a decreased cardiac output. The decrease is significant when the older adult is mentally or physically stressed by anxiety, excitement, illness, or strenuous activity. The body tries to compensate for decreased cardiac output by increasing the heart rate during exercise. However, after exercise it takes longer for the client's rate to return to the baseline rate.

Frequently the older adult's baseline blood pressure rises. This is the result of vascular changes and the accumulation of sclerotic plaques along the walls of the vessels.

Peripheral pulses are palpable but frequently weaker in the lower extremities. The lower extremities are cold, particularly at night, which may necessitate wearing socks to bed.

BREASTS

Decreased muscle mass, muscle tone, and elasticity result in decreased breast size in older women. In addition, the breasts sag.

GASTROINTESTINAL SYSTEM AND ABDOMEN

The aging process leads to an increase in the amount of tissue in the trunk and abdomen. As a result, the abdomen increases in size. Because muscle tone and elasticity are decreased, it also becomes more protuberant.

The older adult also experiences changes in gastrointestinal function. Some of these may be slight, such as the sudden development of intolerance to certain foods. Because of decreased peristalsis the older adult experiences a delayed gastric emptying and may be unable to consume large meals. Decreased peristalsis also affects emptying of the colon, resulting in constipation.

REPRODUCTIVE SYSTEM

Changes in the structure and function of the reproductive system occur as the result of hormonal alterations. Female menopause is related to a reduced responsiveness of the ovaries to pituitary hormones and a resultant decrease in estrogen and progesterone levels. In males there is no definite cessation of fertility associated with aging. Spermatogenesis begins to decline during the fourth decade but continues into the ninth. Most men experience a climacteric, or "male menopause," but this condition may result from underlying illness.

The changes in reproductive structure and function do not affect libido. A decline in the frequency of sexual activity can be a result of illness, death of a sexual partner, decreased socialization, or loss of sexual interest.

URINARY SYSTEM

Hypertrophy of the prostate gland may develop in older men. The hypertrophy enlarges the gland, and pressure is displaced to the neck of the bladder. As a result, the older man may experience an increase in frequency, voiding small amounts of urine. In addition, prostatic hypertrophy can result in difficulty initiating and maintaining a stream.

Older women, particularly those who have had children, can experience stress incontinence, in which an involuntary release of urine occurs when the woman coughs, sneezes, or lifts an object. This is a result of a weakening of the perineal and bladder muscles. In addition, older women notice an urgency in voiding.

MUSCULOSKELETAL SYSTEM

The older adult who exercises regularly does not lose as much bone and muscle mass or tone as those who are inactive. Muscle fibers are reduced in size, and muscle strength diminishes in proportion to the decline in muscle mass.

The postmenopausal woman has a greater rate of bone demineralization than does the older man. Women who maintain their calcium intake throughout their adult life and into menopause experience less bone demineralization than those who do not.

NEUROLOGICAL SYSTEM

The number of neurons in the nervous system begins to decrease at about the middle of the second decade (Ebersole and Hess, 1981). These neurons do not regenerate, and decrease or damage in neurons can lead to functional changes. The changes can affect the special senses described earlier. In addition, the client may experience a decreased sense of balance or uncoordinated motor responses.

The sleep-wake cycle is also influenced by the brain. Characteristically, older adults do not sleep through the night. This disruption has three causes. First, the sleep cycle is shortened. Second, sleep disruption can be the result of frequent bladder emptying, pain, or psychological upsets. Third, the older adult may be taking medication that affects his sleep-wake cycle.

■ ■ ■ ■ ■

The physiological changes of aging described here are common and can be anticipated. Some older clients may experience all of these changes, and others may experience only a few. The body continually changes with age, but how these changes affect the client depend on the individual's level of health, lifestyle, stressors, and environmental conditions.

Cognitive Changes

Much of the psychological and emotional trauma of old age arises from the misconception that older adults always have cognitive impairments—that all elderly people are senile. Gerontologists have documented that the structural and physiological changes occurring in the brain during the aging process do not necessarily affect the older adult's adaptive and functional abilities (Ebersole and Hess, 1981).

Neurophysiological cellular changes vary among individuals, and even with obvious cellular loss some older adults do not demonstrate mental deterioration. Furthermore, some clients with significant cerebral cell loss respond well to therapy and regain function.

Occasionally when cerebral dysfunction is present, the client's preexisting behavioral tendencies are magnified. Therefore a person who has engaged in compulsive behaviors during his young and middle adult years becomes more compulsive during his older years. Certain specific cognitive changes occur in the older adult when cerebral dysfunction or trauma is present. It is helpful for the nurse to understand these cognitive changes so she can help clients maintain optimal functioning.

Dementia

Dementia is an irreversible mental state characterized by decreased intellectual function, personality change, impairment of judgment, and emotional changes that result from permanently altered cerebral metabolism (Smith and Kingsbourne, 1977).

Dementia has three basic components (Ebersole and Hess, 1981). First, cognitive impairments may indicate memory loss (usually involving recent events), personality changes, and decreased problem-solving ability. Second, neuropathological impairments may result in changes in body functioning, such as ambulation, hygiene activities, elimination, and other activities of daily living. Third, the cognitive and neuropathological changes may lead to immobility, infection, or trauma.

When caring for an older adult who is depressed, the nurse should not assume that he has dementia, although he may exhibit all the clinical manifestations of it. The client who does not have dementia can be encouraged to become involved in his community. He can also safely live alone if he chooses.

Organic Brain Syndrome

Organic brain syndrome, also referred to as organic mental disorder, is any psychological or behavioral abnormality associated with transient or permanent brain dysfunction caused by a disturbance of the physiological functioning of brain tissue. Some organic brain syndromes are acute and potentially reversible, whereas others are chronic with irreversible cerebral impairments. All clients with organic brain syndromes have impairments in attention span, learning, and memory. In addition, some clients have hallucinations, delusions, aphasias, emotional lability, and depression.

ACUTE DISORDERS

Acute disorders of the organic brain syndrome are potentially reversible. Acute disorders have many causes, including toxins such as lead, diseases, metabolic imbalances, drugs, malnutrition, trauma (especially head injuries), infections, neoplasms, overwhelming stress such as that caused by abrupt translocation or loss, and severe depression. According to Ebersole and Hess (1981), at least 21% of cases of acute organic brain syndrome are misdiagnosed as chronic organic brain disorders.

CHRONIC DISORDERS

Chronic brain disorders are irreversible and usually progressive. However, with careful and supportive nursing management, clients with chronic brain disorders can remain in their homes.

ALZHEIMER'S DISEASE. Alzheimer's disease affects the brain parenchyma. The disease has a gradual course with a progressive decline in cognitive functioning. Three stages of the disease have been described (see the boxed material below) (Hayter, 1974).

Nursing management of clients with Alzheimer's disease is complex. The limited mobility of these clients increases their risk for the hazards of immobility. Therefore the nurse must continually meet the client's physical needs (see Chapter 31). The client's confusion usually increases at night, and he may wander through his home, or, if hospitalized, through the nursing division. As the client progresses through the three stages, communication becomes increasingly difficult. The client may easily misperceive his environment and feel threatened. The typical behavioral responses of the client with Alzheimer's disease who feels threatened include aggressive gestures or acts, increased voice volume, restlessness, agitation, and hostility (Bartol, 1979). The nursing care plan is individualized to help the client with Alzheimer's disease use his capacities to the maximum (see the boxed material below).

VASCULAR DISORDERS. Vascular brain disorders are the result of arteriosclerotic changes in the brain that ultimately affect its functioning. Arteriosclerotic dementia has several distinguishing characteristics: periods of remission, preservation of personality, insight, lability of emotion, and epileptoid attacks. Vas-

---

Three Stages of Alzheimer's Disease

FIRST STAGE (2 TO 4 YEARS)

- Memory loss
- Poor judgment
- Lack of spontaneity
- Time disorientation
- Blaming others for difficulties encountered
- Moodiness
- Hypochondriasis

SECOND STAGE (FEW MONTHS)

- Restlessness at night
- Increased memory loss
- Inability to recognize and interpret environment accurately
- Sensory impressions dulled
- Movement and gait disturbances

THIRD STAGE

- Irritability
- Seizures
- Disorientation in all spheres
- Illogical or incoherent communication
- Coma
- Death

Modified from Hayter, J.: Am. J. Nurs. **74:**1460, 1974.

Comprehensive Nursing Care Objectives for the Client with Alzheimer's Disease

- Keep ambulatory as long as possible.
- Protect from physical injuries.
- Maintain daily exercise program.
- Maintain optimal nutritional status.
- Maintain integrity of gums and mucous membranes to preserve dental function.
- Assess and evaluate the need for psychotropic medications.
- Provide cognitive stimuli.
- Provide regular social interaction.
- Maintain self-esteem through involvement with activities of daily living.
- Maintain reality orientation.
- Maintain a structured milieu.
- Avoid unnecessary translocation.
- Maintain nonverbal and verbal communication patterns.
- Modify negative behavior through behavior modification.
- Provide ongoing support for family members.
- Protect from infection.
- Prevent the hazards of immobility.

Modified from Bartol, M.: J. Gerontol. Nurs. **5:**21, 1979.

cular brain disorders may result from the following sources:

1. Arteriosclerotic plaques blocking cerebral circulation
2. Cerebrovascular accident (stroke)
3. Systemic emboli lodging in cerebrovascular pathways
4. Transient ischemic attacks
5. Decreased cerebral circulation resulting from decreased cardiac output or rupture of cerebral aneurysm
6. Severe hypertension

The client with cognitive impairment resulting from a vascular disorder usually has a history of hypertension, diabetes mellitus, blackouts, falls, or seizures. In addition, some physical impairment, such as hemiplegia or hemiparesis, is usually present. The nursing management of clients with vascular brain disorders is similar to that described in the boxed material on p. 543.

SUBSTANCE ABUSE AND COGNITIVE IMPAIRMENT.

Long-term abuse of alcohol and drugs can affect cognitive functioning. After 15 to 20 years of alcohol abuse, tolerance for drinking declines. Prolonged use of large amounts of alcohol creates cerebral, cerebellar, sensory, and peripheral nervous system damage. With chronic alcoholism many clients also have vitamin B_1 deficiency. A prolonged deficiency can cause neuropathy, myopathy, and encephalopathy, exhibited as Wernicke's syndrome or Korsakoff's syndrome. Wernicke's syndrome is present in more advanced stages of vitamin B_1 depletion and is characterized by nystagmus, pupillary abnormalities, ataxia, tremor, and stupor. Korsakoff's syndrome is a psychosis characterized by disorientation of time, place, and person, amnesia for recent events, and confabulation. Confabulation is a defense mechanism in which the person fabricates experiences or situations and recounts them in a detailed and plausible way in order to fill in and cover up gaps in memory.

The exact effects of prolonged drug abuse on the older adult have not been clearly described, but cognitive impairments may occur that are similar to those associated with alcohol abuse. In addition, a drug overdose may cause cerebral impairment. In this case the cognitive impairment may be the result of decreases in oxygen supply and its delivery to the brain.

■ ■ ■ ■ ■

The nurse who cares for the older adult with cognitive impairments is challenged both to meet the physical needs of the client and to improve or maintain his present state of cognitive functioning. To achieve these objectives, the nurse may use three types of interventions: reality orientation, resocialization, and remotivation. These are described later in the chapter.

Psychosocial Changes

The older adult must adapt to many psychosocial changes that occur with aging. Although these changes vary among clients, there are some psychosocial changes common to the majority of older adults.

Retirement

Retirement in our society often carries associations of passivity and seclusion and thus often leads to psychosocial stresses. These stresses include role changes with the spouse or family and the problems of social isolation (see the next section).

The mandatory retirement age varies depending on the individual's circumstance. For example, the mandatory retirement age in a state civil service job may be 65, whereas a federal employee may not be required to retire until he is 70 years old. In private industry the mandatory retirement age is usually between 62 and 70. An increasing number of companies are developing early retirement plans to provide opportunities for advancement of younger employees. One popular program is the "30 and out" plan, which allows workers to retire with full pension, and in some cases large bonuses, after 30 years of employment.

Preretirement planning is advisable during middle age and is essential in late middle age (see Chapter 26). People who plan retirement activities before actually retiring generally make a better adjustment. For example, an individual may plan to become active in volunteer work, remodeling projects in the home, traveling, or other activities.

Retirement also has an impact on the homemaker who does not work outside the home. Tension can occur between the retired spouse and the homemaker if the retired person sits around the house for a prolonged period of time. Tension occurs because of role changes in the relationship and because the homemaker may feel that her workload is increased.

The most powerful factors that influence the retired person's satisfaction with life are health status, the option to continue working, and sufficient income. Men who retire unwillingly are at risk for alcoholism, depression, and suicide (Ebersole and Hess, 1981).

The nurse can help clients and their families prepare for retirement. The nurse can generally assist most effectively those clients with whom she has had a long-term relationship, as in a community or outpatient setting.

The counseling of older adults for retirement should focus on six issues (Diekelman, 1978). First, what provisions have the client and family made for retirement income? Will these financial resources be sufficient to meet housing, entertainment, food, energy, clothing, health care, and unanticipated needs? For how long will these resources meet the needs—5 years, 10 years, or indefinitely?

Second, what postretirement activities are available? On what abilities, skills, and interests can the client draw? Will any of these be a source of income?

Third, what living arrangements may be needed? Is the present house too large, difficult, or expensive to maintain? Relocation should be given careful consideration. Ideally the client should spend several months in the new location before making a permanent commitment.

Fourth, what preparations have been made for role changes? Have the marriage partners discussed how they will spend their time together? Will they divide household tasks, spend more time with grandchildren, or become involved in volunteer or community activities?

Fifth, what provisions have been made to meet health care needs? How will the retired couple meet their exercise, nutrition, and other health needs?

Last, how will the retired person attend to his legal affairs? Estate planning, education in legal affairs, and ability to cope with bureaucratic procedures are essential in the later years. Community colleges, offices on aging, and legal aid services for the elderly may provide guidance in these matters.

Social Isolation

Many older adults experience social isolation, which increases as they advance in years. There are four types of social isolation: attitudinal, presentational, behavioral, and geographical. Some older adults may be affected by all four types, and others may be affected by only one (Ebersole and Hess, 1981).

Attitudinal isolation occurs because of personal or cultural values. Ageism is a prevailing attitude that stigmatizes the older adult because of certain characteristics. It is a negative bias against and rejection of people of advanced age. Therefore attitudinal social isolation occurs when the older adult is not as easily accepted into social interactions or relationships because of society's bias toward the aged. Attitudinal isolation can be particularly damaging to the older adult because a vicious circle may result: as the older adult is increasingly rejected, his self-esteem

may diminish, leading to fewer attempts to form social relationships and thus to even greater social isolation.

Presentational isolation results from the person's unacceptable appearance or other factors involved in how he presents himself to others. Factors contributing to presentation isolation are body image, hygiene, or visible signs of illness or functional loss (Ebersole and Hess, 1981). The person becomes isolated either because of the rejection of others as a result of these factors or because he seeks little interaction as a result of self-consciousness related to these factors.

Behavioral isolation results from the person's unacceptable behaviors. In all age groups and particularly with the older adult, socially unacceptable behaviors cause other people to withdraw. Behaviors commonly associated with behavioral isolation of the older adult include confusion, behaviors associated with organic brain syndrome, alcoholism, eccentricity, and incontinence. The nurse can use behavior modification techniques to help decrease the frequency of these behaviors in the older adult (Ebersole and Hess, 1981).

Geographical isolation occurs because of (1) distance from family, (2) urban crime, and (3) institutional barriers.

In today's mobile society it is common for children to live great distances from their parents. As the parents grow older, begin to have physical limitations, or experience the death of a spouse, the opportunity to visit their children decreases, leading to further isolation.

In urban areas a high crime rate can deter the older adult from socializing for fear of being mugged. If the older adult lives in a high-crime area, he may be unwilling to leave his home, since it might be vandalized or robbed while he is out visiting friends.

One type of institutional barrier is a lack of easy access for wheelchair-dependent older adults or those who require the use of walkers, canes, or crutches. In addition, when an older adult requires institutional care, he becomes segregated from friends and family outside the institution. His social interaction depends largely on those who come to the extended care or nursing home facility to visit him.

A client who is alone is not necessarily lonely; many people, including older adults, enjoy being alone. Nurses need to determine if clients who are alone are lonely or have merely chosen to be alone. The effects of loneliness and social isolation vary depending on how the person is able to meet basic human needs. Fig. 27-1 shows the relationship of basic human needs to loneliness and social isolation. Loneliness is often associated with poor health, dissatisfaction with

| Feelings related to hierarchical loneliness and isolation | | **Factors** |

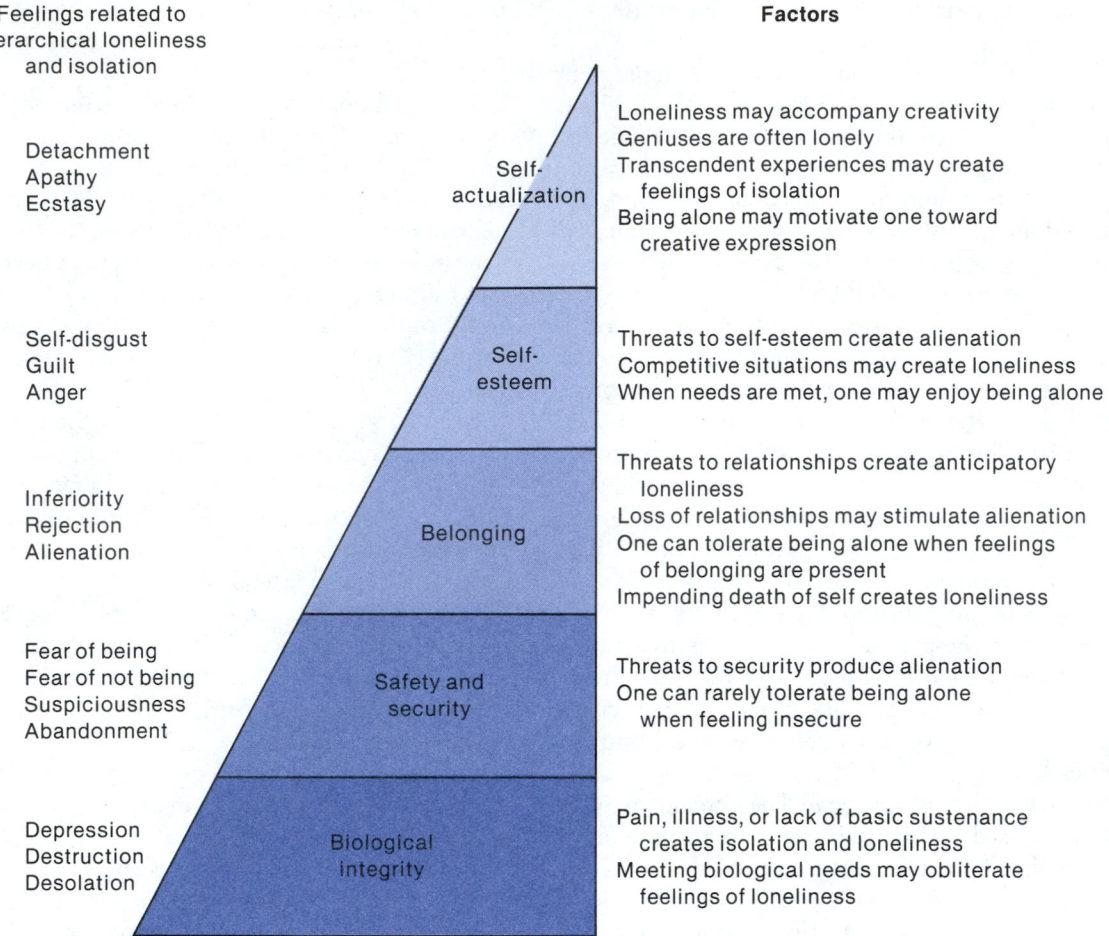

Feelings related to hierarchical loneliness and isolation		**Factors**
Detachment Apathy Ecstasy	Self-actualization	Loneliness may accompany creativity Geniuses are often lonely Transcendent experiences may create feelings of isolation Being alone may motivate one toward creative expression
Self-disgust Guilt Anger	Self-esteem	Threats to self-esteem create alienation Competitive situations may create loneliness When needs are met, one may enjoy being alone
Inferiority Rejection Alienation	Belonging	Threats to relationships create anticipatory loneliness Loss of relationships may stimulate alienation One can tolerate being alone when feelings of belonging are present Impending death of self creates loneliness
Fear of being Fear of not being Suspiciousness Abandonment	Safety and security	Threats to security produce alienation One can rarely tolerate being alone when feeling insecure
Depression Destruction Desolation	Biological integrity	Pain, illness, or lack of basic sustenance creates isolation and loneliness Meeting biological needs may obliterate feelings of loneliness

Fig. 27-1 Loneliness in relation to Maslow's hierarchy of needs.

From Ebersole, P., and Hess, P.: Toward healthy aging: human needs and nursing response, St. Louis, 1981, The C.V. Mosby Co.

housing and other environmental factors, and the loss of a spouse.

The nurse can assist the lonely older adult in rebuilding a social network. One method is through outreach programs designed to make contact with isolated older adults. The program may be planned to meet the nutritional needs of older adults, such as Meals on Wheels; socialization needs, such as daily telephone calls by volunteers; or need for activities, such as outings to a play, symphony performance, or park. In addition, the nurse can investigate formal or informal networks within the older adult's community (Table 27-3). These networks increase the older adult's opportunity to meet people with similar activities, interests, and needs.

Sexuality

Sexuality has been increasingly recognized as an important concern in the care of older adults. The older adult, whether healthy and active or frail, has the need to express sexual feelings. Sexuality is linked with a person's identity and validates the person's belief that he can give to others and have the gift appreciated. Sexuality involves love, warmth, sharing, and touching between people, not just the physical act of intercourse.

When caring for the older adult, the nurse must ensure that nursing care is also directed toward helping the client maintain sexual health. Sexual health is the integration of somatic, emotional, intellectual, and social aspects of sexual being in ways that are positively enriching and that enhance personality, communication, and love (Woods, 1983).

To help the older adult achieve or maintain sexual health, the nurse needs to understand the physical changes in sexual response. The knowledge of sexual changes described in Table 27-4, as well as the physical changes in male and female genitalia, enables the

TABLE 27-3

Formal and Informal Contacts Increasing the Social Networks of the Older Adult

Formal	Informal
Church	Neighbors
Grandparenting	Maids, waitresses in small hotels
Foster Grandparents	
Vista	Beauty salons, restaurants, bars, service personnel, shops
Peace Corps	
Retired Senior Volunteer Program	
National Retired Teachers Association	Psychological withdrawal—dreams, fantasies, hallucinations, daydreams
Unions	Fictive kin—soap operas
Friends of the Library	Interest in celebrities
Volunteers	Laundromats
Public school	Sports
Senior centers	Old people bus
Title VII nutrition sites	Special tours
Involved in social issues for seniors	Education, arts, and crafts courses
	Trailer courts
	Retirement communities
	Pets
	Plants
	Dancing
	Physicians' office
	Clinics
	Lobby gazers
	Vicarious participation
	Surrogate families— nurses, aides
	Nursing home—social corridor
	General social touching
	Radio shows
	Nostalgia
	Phone lines

From Ebersole, P., and Hess. P.: Toward healthy aging: human needs and nursing response, St. Louis, 1981, The C.V. Mosby Co.

nurse to educate the older adult client about actual or anticipated changes in sexual functioning.

As discussed earlier, the libido does not decrease, but the frequency of sexual activity may decline. The older woman who does not understand the physical changes affecting sexual activity may become concerned that her sex life is approaching its natural conclusion with the onset of menopause. The older man may feel similarly when he discovers a change in the firmness of his erection, has a decreased need for ejaculation with each orgasm, or has an extended recovery period between episodes of intercourse.

In addition to the physical changes affecting sexual functioning, many older adults may be taking drugs that depress sexual activity, such as antihypertensives, antidepressants, sedatives and tranquilizers, or hypnotics. In addition, certain drugs increase libido in older adults. Phenothiazines increase sexual desire in women, and levodopa has a similar effect in men (Woods, 1983).

The nurse's role in assisting the older adult to achieve sexual health is twofold. First, the nurse may be a counselor to one or both sexual partners, describing different methods for sexual satisfaction. Second, the nurse may be a consultant to help other nurses and health care professionals understand the sexual behavior and needs of older adults.

Not all nurses feel comfortable in counseling clients about their sexual health. The nurse need not feel obligated to carry out such counseling activities. However, the nurse should recognize when the client requires assistance to understand the physical changes in sexual function, to resume sexual activity after an illness, or to adapt to the sexual changes resulting from medication. If the nurse is uncomfortable in discussing sexuality, she should seek the assistance of another nurse or health care professional.

The nursing student needs to recognize that her knowledge of clients' sexual needs will increase with her professional growth. As she gains information about human sexuality, she will be able to incorporate this information into the nursing care plan (see Chapter 19).

Housing and Environment

Changes in social roles, family responsibilities, and health status influence the older client's choice of living arrangements. Some older adults choose to live in a multigenerational household with family members. Others prefer to live in their own home or apartment in a multigenerational neighborhood or community. The so-called leisure or retirement communities provide the older person with living and social opportunities in a one-generational setting. Federally subsidized housing, where available, offers older adults individual apartments with communal social and in some cases eating arrangements. The types of housing most appropriate for the older adult depend on his level of independence (Fig. 27-2).

In assisting the older adult with his housing needs, the nurse should assess the client's activity level and restrictions, his financial status, accessibility of public transportation and community activities, environmental hazards, and support systems. In addition, the

TABLE 27-4

Physical Changes in Sexual Response in the Older Adult

Phase	Female	Male
Excitation	Diminished vaginal lubrication (1 to 3 minutes may be required for adequate amounts to appear); diminished flattening and separation of labia majora; disappearance of elevation of labia majora; decreased vasocongestion of labia minora; decreased elastic expansion of vagina (depth and breadth); slower and less prominent uterine elevation or tenting; decreased muscle tension	Less intense and slower erection (but can be maintained longer without ejaculation); less vasocongestion of scrotal sac; less pronounced elevation and congestion of testicles; decreased muscle tension
Plateau	Decreased capacity for vasocongestion; decreased areolar engorgement; labial color change less evident; less intense swelling or orgasmic platform; decreased secretions of Bartholin's glands	Nipple erection and sexual flush less often; no color change at coronal ridge of penis; decrease or absence of secretory activity (lubrication) by Cowper's gland before ejaculation
Orgasm	Fewer contractions of orgasmic platform; rectal sphincter contractions with severe tension only	Fewer penile contractions; fewer rectal sphincter contractions; decreased force of ejaculation with decreased amount of semen (if long ejaculation, seepage of semen occurs)
Resolution	Observably slower subsidence of nipple erection; quicker subsidence of vasocongestion of clitoris and orgasmic platform	Slow subsidence of vasocongestion of nipples and scrotum; loss of erection and descent of testicles shortly after ejaculation; refractory time extended (time required before another erection ranges from several to 24 hours, occasionally longer)

Modified from Ebersole, P., and Hess, P.: Toward healthy aging: human needs and nursing response, St. Louis, 1981, The C.V. Mosby Co.

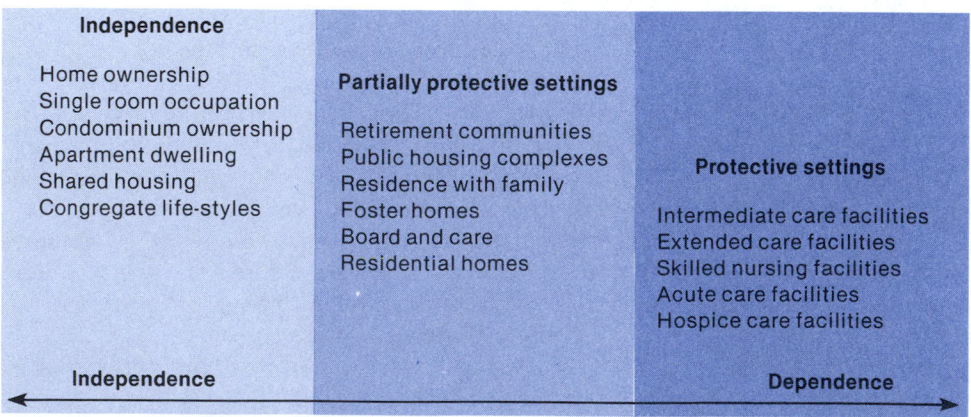

Fig. 27-2 Continuum of housing security.

From Ebersole, P., and Hess, P.: Toward healthy aging: human needs and
nursing response, St. Louis, 1981, The C.V. Mosby Co.

nurse should help the client determine how long the housing arrangement will be appropriate. For example, an older adult with recently diagnosed mild angina may not be able to live in a second-floor apartment longer than 1 year, and he should be advised to find a first-floor living arrangement.

Housing and the environment as a whole are important because they can have a major impact on the health of the older adult. The environment can support or hinder physical and social functioning, enhance or drain the individual's energy, and complement or tax existing physical changes such as vision and hearing. For example, red, orange, and yellow are the colors easiest for the elderly to see. Pastels fade and cannot be distinguished. Green, blue, violet, white, and dark colors are the most difficult to see. Some older adults in health care settings can have difficulty finding their room door, but painting the door frame a brighter color to contrast with the wall allows the older person to distinguish the door at a distance and find the room. Painting a stripe along the bottom of a wall makes the boundaries of a hall or room visible. The glare of highly polished floors should be eliminated.

Furniture should be comfortable and address the arthritic problems of the elderly. It should be easy to get into and out of, should not be too low or overstuffed, and should provide back support. A dining room chair should be tested for comfort during meals and height in relation to the table. The nurse should caution the elderly client to examine all furniture carefully for size, comfort, and functional capacity before purchasing.

The nurse has the challenge of assessing the individual environmental needs of older adults in both the home and institutional setting. The nurse can modify the environment to increase the independence and functional ability, and thus the quality of life, for older adults.

Death

Birth and death are universal yet individually unique events in the human life span. Death of the young or middle-aged person is often viewed as tragic because life goals are uncompleted. A common misconception is that the death of an older adult is always a blessing and the culmination of a full and rich life. Many dying older adults still have life goals, and they are not emotionally prepared to die. Families and friends are often unable to cope with the process of dying and the subsequent loss of a loved one.

With appropriate knowledge and skills the nurse can help make the dying process a time of fullfillment and growth and a completion of life governed by the individual with the support, understanding, and assistance of those around him. Chapter 46 describes the work of Kübler-Ross and the five stages of dying: denial, anger, bargaining, depression, and acceptance. Chapter 46 also describes nursing interventions for the dying client and his family.

Health Concerns

Older adults particularly value good health. A state of wellness provides the individual with energy, vitality, and a zest of life.

The nurse is in a unique position to establish health maintenance programs that promote the older adult's wellness. Nurses possess many skills that can be put into action at sites where the elderly congregate. Senior citizens' centers, churches, schools, shopping malls, supermarkets, libraries, and hospital lobbies can be used to conduct screening tests and present information to older adults on specific health topics. Using innovative, creative approaches, the nurse can include health promotion activities in health assessments for older adults.

Physiological Health Diagnoses

Approximately 80% of adults over the age of 65 have at least one chronic health problem. The effect of the chronic health problem on mobility and independence depends on the individual client. The nurse should be familiar with certain chronic health problems that are common in the older adult population.

CARDIOVASCULAR PROBLEMS

The cardiovascular problems most frequently associated with aging are hypertension, angina pectoris, myocardial infarction, and cerebrovascular accident.

Hypertension is diagnosed when repeated blood pressure measurements of 95 mm Hg diastolic and 160 mm Hg systolic are present. The risk factors for hypertension include smoking, obesity, lack of exercise, and stress. Blacks are at a greater risk than whites, and men are at greater risk than women. Treatment of hypertension includes weight reduction, decreased salt intake, exercise, stress management, and drugs (Stanhope and Lancaster, 1984).

Angina pectoris is a coronary artery disease in which chest pain is induced by exercise or stress. The risk factors for angina include family history of heart disease, obesity, hyperlipidemia, smoking, and stress. The treatment varies but usually includes vasodilator therapy, an exercise program, smoking cessation, weight reduction, and stress management.

Myocardial infarction (heart attack) is a disease in which one portion of the coronary artery or the entire artery becomes occluded, thus depriving the myocardium of its oxygen and blood supply. Myocardial ischemia then occurs. Risk factors include a family history of cardiac disease, angina pectoris, diabetes mellitus, smoking, obesity, hypertension, hyperlipidemia, lack of exercise, and stress. The treatment of a myocardial infarction involves hospitalization, followed by a rehabilitation period in which habits are modified. These modifications include weight reduction, exercise, smoking cessation, dietary changes, and stress management.

Cerebrovascular accident (stroke) occurs when the vessels supplying blood to a certain portion of the brain become occluded, resulting in decreased circulation to that area. Risk factors for cerebrovascular accident include hypertension, hyperlipidemia, diabetes mellitus, and family history of cardiovascular disease.

CANCER

Malignant neoplasms are the second most common cause of death among older adults. Along with early detection and treatment, the nurse can develop programs to decrease the older adult's risk for cancer. Examples of such programs include smoking cessation, teaching clients to perform breast self-examinations (see Chapter 29), encouraging clients to have routine Pap smears, and educating clients about the seven danger signals of cancer.

ARTHRITIS

Approximately 44% of older adults have arthritis. It is more common in women than in men (Stanhope and Lancaster, 1984). The degree to which the mobility of the older adult with arthritis is affected depends on the extent of the disease and the joints affected. Arthritis has no cure, but recently developed pharmacological agents can decrease joint pain and swelling and therefore increase range of joint motion.

SENSORY IMPAIRMENTS

The older adult usually experiences changes in vision, hearing, taste, and smell. Frequently these changes are the result of the normal aging process. The nurse can help the older adult client identify resources to help correct visual and auditory problems (see Chapter 44). Seasonings can make food more palatable for the older adult.

DENTAL PROBLEMS

Dental problems are common in older adults. When they are present, there can also be changes in the client's taste and a decrease in nutritional intake. Be-

TABLE 27-5	
Mortality of Older Adults, 1978	
Disease	**Percent**
Heart disease	44
Malignant neoplasms	19
Cerebrovascular disease	12
Influenza and pneumonia	3

Modified from Office of Human Development Services: Facts about older Americans, 1980-81, Washington, D.C., 1981, Department of Health and Human Services.

cause of missing teeth or poorly fitting dentures, the older adult may restrict his diet to soft foods.

The nurse can help prevent dental and gum disease through health education. In addition to teaching the older adult to maintain routine dental care, the nurse can teach specific measures to reduce the risk of gum disease, such as proper brushing and flossing techniques (see Chapter 35). The nurse can help the client with ill-fitting dentures or other dental problems identify resources in the community that provide dental services to older adults at reduced rates.

Mortality

The four major causes of death in older adults are heart disease, malignant neoplasms, cerebrovascular disease, and influenza and pneumonia (Table 27-5).

Health screenings and health fairs can identify older adults at risk for fatal illnesses or illnesses that will impair their present level of functioning, so that illness prevention activities can be initiated. In addition, the older adult, especially one with a chronic disease, should be encouraged to obtain a yearly flu shot. If an older adult has a history of pneumococcal pneumonia, he should be encouraged to get a Pneumovax vaccination, which provides lifelong immunity against pneumococcal pneumonia.

Drug Effects

As a group, adults over 65 are the greatest users of prescription medications. The most frequently prescribed medications are for heart and vascular disease, hypertension, depression, diabetes mellitus, respiratory diseases, and gastrointestinal disorders (Ebersole and Hess, 1981).

Many medications may interact with one another, either potentiating or negating the effect of another drug. In addition, some medications increase confusion, affect balance, or cause dizziness, nausea, or vomiting. Some older adults are unwilling to take prescribed drugs because of the side effects.

Sedatives and tranquilizers may increase nighttime confusion. In this phenomenon, referred to as sundowning, the older adult may experience increased restlessness, confusion, and an urge to wander with approaching darkness. Sundowning is difficult for family members to cope with, and they may be unable to sleep for fear that the older adult will wander away and come to harm. In a hospital setting, nurses are frequently forced to use Posey restraints to prevent the older adult from wandering.

Nutrition

Minimal nutritional needs for the older adult are the same as those of younger adults except that greater amounts of calcium, vitamin C, and vitamin A are required. Total caloric intake usually declines in response to illness and changes in metabolic rate and physical activity. Nutritional needs of the older adult are described in Chapter 38.

Exercise

The older adult should be encouraged to maintain a pattern of physical exercise and activity. Before beginning an exercise program the client should have a complete physical examination, which may include a stress cardiogram or stress test. This provides information about the person's cardiovascular function during periods of sustained exercise.

Before the older adult begins an exercise program, the nurse should assess his activity tolerance and plan a program that meets his physical needs while allowing for any physical impairments (see Chapter 30).

■　■　■　■　■

Most older adults are interested in their health and are capable of taking charge of their lives. Their major goals are to remain independent for as long as possible and to prevent disability. Initial screenings by nurses establish baseline data that can be used to determine the individual's level of wellness, identify health needs, and design health maintenance programs for preventing later problems.

Nursing students will find it very challenging to test their knowledge base and nursing skills while participating in screening sessions. Under the direction of an instructor, students may present seminars or demonstrations on nutrition, arthritis, hypertension, foot and skin care, Heimlich's maneuver, medications, and exercise. Other topics, such as consumer affairs, safety precautions, and Medicare reimburse-

ment policies, are also of interest to the elderly. Nurses can significantly improve the quality of life and health of the elderly by health promotion, teaching, advising, and counseling, in addition to their traditional role of providing care during illness. The use of self-help strategies is appropriate for the aging population because of their limited financial and social resources. Many older adults monitor their own or their spouse's blood pressure, shop at health food stores, attend health fairs, plan meals around a special diet, and care for a spouse with a chronic disease. The self-help network of older adults is extensive and can be found in many settings. For example, while shopping in the supermarket, older adults may exchange information about the best physician for cataract surgery, the hospital that provides the best nursing care and treatment, and what nursing homes to stay away from. They have their own "gray grapevine" of consumer information about health care for the elderly.

As part of any health screening, the nurse should encourage the older adult to complete a stress inventory scale and discuss it with the nurse. Individuals at high risk for illness resulting from stress should receive health teaching from the nurse. The nurse needs to be knowledgeable about relaxation and stress reduction techniques and must assist the client in selecting and learning the best one for his life-style.

Psychosocial Health Concerns

Psychosocial health concerns vary widely among older adults. Many role transitions occur between middle age and older adulthood. Because of these changes, the cognitive and social changes, and the physical effects of aging, many older adults require nursing assistance to maintain psychosocial health.

Interventions for the psychosocial health of the older adult resemble those used with other age groups (see Unit 4). However, some interventions are more crucial for the older adult who is experiencing social isolation, cognitive impairment, or other psychosocial health problems. These interventions include therapeutic communication, touch, reality orientation, resocialization, reminiscence, and interventions to improve body image.

THERAPEUTIC COMMUNICATION

With therapeutic communication the nurse perceives, reacts to, and respects the client's uniqueness. The nurse who communicates effectively with an older adult client will be accepted as one who shares a genuine concern for his welfare.

The nurse cannot simply walk into a client's environment and immediately establish a therapeutic relationship. She must first be knowledgeable and skilled in different communication techniques. The student nurse can practice these techniques with other students (see Chapter 16).

TOUCH

Touch is the first sense to become functional. Throughout the life span, touch provides knowledge about others. In all cultures, gently touching another person conveys affection and friendliness. Often older adults who are victims of social isolation are deprived of the touching and holding that were important parts of their earlier lives.

Touch is a therapeutic tool that nurses can use to help meet the comfort needs of the older adult. Touch can provide sensory stimulation, reduce anxiety, orient the person to reality, relieve physiological and emotional pain, and give comfort during the dying process (Barnett, 1972).

An older adult who is isolated, dependent, or ill, who fears death, or who lacks self-esteem has a greater need for touch. The client may invite the nurse's touch by reaching for her hand. Too often elderly men are misunderstood and wrongly accused of sexual advances when they demonstrate this need for touch. The nurse should recognize that the older adult client may be suffering from touch deprivation. Nurses should be careful not to touch clients in a condescending way, however, such as with a pat on the head or a gentle pinch of the shoulder. Touch should convey respect and sensitivity for the client. Because the client may have an unmet need for intimacy, the nurse should not be surprised if the client reciprocates with touch.

REALITY ORIENTATION

Reality orientation was described by Folsom in 1973. It is a communication modality used for making the client aware of time, place, and person. The major purposes of reality orientation include (1) restoring the client's sense of reality, (2) improving the client's level of awareness, (3) promoting socialization, (4) elevating the client to his maximal level of independent functioning, and (5) minimizing confusion, disorientation, and physical regression.

The nurse can use reality orientation techniques in any setting. Anytime an older adult experiences a change in environment, surgery, illness, or emotional stress, such as the death of a spouse or a friend, he is at risk for becoming disoriented. Environmental changes, such as the bright lights and lack of windows in intensive care and specialized units in a hospital, often lead to disorientation and confusion. The client's environment and the nursing personnel are constantly changing in the hospital and the client's immediate environment is unstable, making coping and adaptation difficult. It is no wonder that many older clients lose track of time and become confused while in the hospital. The problem is compounded by tranquilizers, sleeping medication, anesthesia, and restraints that immobilize the client and take away his dignity.

The nurse should anticipate disorientation and confusion as a consequence of hospitalization, relocation, surgery, loss, or illness and incorporate reality orientation interventions into the client's nursing care plan. These interventions are based on seven principles (see the boxed material opposite). Consistent use of the techniques of reality orientation helps to reorient the older adult to his surroundings.

RESOCIALIZATION

Resocialization is an intervention that assists the older adult to expand his social network within his community. Resocialization is especially beneficial to older adults whose previous social interaction depended on their employment. Once they retire, these adults find themselves without people with whom to socialize. Similarly, resocialization is important for older adults whose spouse or close friends have died.

The key in using resocialization is to know the resources available to the client within his own community. Many older adults are eager to participate in senior citizen groups, foster grandparent programs, or volunteer work in their local hospitals. However, they may not know how to make the initial contact. The nurse can provide the older adult with the name of the person to contact or can get in touch with the agency herself. For resocialization to be effective, the nurse and the client must work together.

DEVELOPING SECONDARY RELATIONSHIPS. Just as socialization is important for older adults at risk for social isolation, secondary relationships are important for older adults who still maintain their primary relationships. For many older adult clients, family and friends continue to provide long-term support. However, it is important that the older adult develop reliable secondary relationships with peers, thus providing a social group that is not bound by the emotions frequently experienced in families. For example, a group of elderly persons in a day-care center gain enjoyment from socializing with their peers and with young staff members. They share experiences and concerns but are not related to one another except by common feelings or ideas.

The nurse can help the elderly form secondary relationships by holding discussions of topics of mutual interest at day-care centers, nutrition program sites,

Guidelines for Reality Orientation

REALISM

- Use reality information such as time, date, place, and name in all conversational content.
- Refer to clocks and other reality orientation props when necessary.
- Do not reinforce delusions or hallucinations.
- Direct persons back to reality-oriented endeavors if they begin to ramble in conversation or to talk unrealistically.
- If persons begin to show erratic behavior, such as picking at clothes, give them purposeful things to do.

INDEPENDENCE

- Express confidence in the person's ability to be self-directing.
- Encourage persons to perform tasks and make decisions alone, assisting them only when necessary.
- Make sure the person has whatever aids are needed, such as glasses, dentures, and hearing aids, and that these are in working order.
- Provide bowel and bladder training when necessary.
- Provide speech or physical therapy when necessary.
- Reduce medication to a minimum.

INDIVIDUALIZATION

- Keep reality orientation classes small to permit attention to individual needs.
- Allow the person to keep familiar treasures and objects.
- Encourage the person to maintain meaningful object relationships.

REINFORCEMENT

- Watch for small changes in behavior that indicate progress, and reward these behaviors.
- Reward persons for correct behavior with verbal praise, touch, or smiles.
- Reinforce achievement with increased responsibility.
- Encourage any special talents or interests.

REPETITION

- Repeat information, directions, statements, and questions as necessary.
- Be patient and allow time for a response or reply.
- Give people clues to the answer when asking question; if they are unable to answer, tell them the correct response and let them repeat it.

CLARITY

- Enunciate clearly and speak slowly to be sure the person understands.
- Reword statements and questions if necessary.
- Give concise directions in clear, simple, short statements.

CONSISTENCY

- Maintain continuity in the care of the person.
- Adhere to scheduling.
- Use the same personnel whenever possible.

From Beck, C.M., Rowlins, R.P., and Williams, S.R.: Mental health—psychiatric nursing: a holistic life-cycle approach, St. Louis, 1984, The C.V. Mosby Co.

or long-term care centers. For example, older clients with arthritis may benefit from discussing ways to maintain activity. The older adult appreciates information that is accurate, logically organized, and relevant to health needs. The following are some guidelines for conducting discussion sessions:

1. Select a small, quiet room that is well lit and has comfortable furniture. Be sure to consider any visual, hearing, or musculoskeletal impairments.
2. Keep meetings short enough to promote learning while not becoming exhausting (20 minutes).
3. Choose participants who are able to learn and participate in discussions.
4. Consider the older adults' sensory deficits when choosing content and visual aids (for example, brightly colored posters with large print).
5. Present only one topic for discussion at each meeting.
6. Make it clear to clients that participation in the group is voluntary.

Establishing peer group meetings for the older adult allows the participants to develop secondary relationships independently. The older adult learns to share ideas and solve problems without dwelling on physical ailments or feelings of hopelessness.

REMINISCENCE

Reminiscence is recalling the past for the purpose of assigning new meanings to past experiences (Beck, Rowlins, and Williams, 1984). Reminiscing is an

TABLE 27-6

Reminiscence Group Strategies

	Cognitively Impaired	Psychologically Disturbed	Depressed
Patient selection	No more than five members; age cohorts; both sexes	10 members; varied ages; both sexes	Eight to 10 members; those with similar problems, for example, grieving, retired; both sexes
Structure	Consistent place and time; frequent, 30-minute meetings; coleaders	Consistent place and time; biweekly, 1-hour meetings; one leader consistently	Varied meeting places; weekly, 1-hour meeting; variable leadership
Process	Connect specific events, things, and places common to group.	Connect members through shared feelings and survival strategies.	Focus members on successful coping during life span; encourage mutuality.
Goals	To stimulate memory, enhance identity, raise self-esteem, increase socialization skills	To recognize feelings and meaning of suppressed conflicts, enlarge coping strategies, integrate self-view, promote universality	To reduce feelngs of hopelessness, restore personal control, increase affectual responsiveness, develop a sense of integrity and acceptance of life as lived, promote caring between members
Nurse's function	Provide a comfortable, mildly stimulating environment. Select props that will stimulate memories. Assist members by giving specific information, reminders and clues. Give praise and recognition for any participation.	Establish a private meeting and a closed group. Plan to focus on specific developmental stages or critical life events. Accept and validate all expressions of feeling. Clarify multiple meanings of events. Reduce anxiety.	Provide a comfortable, stimulating environment. Appeal to sensory memories. Focus members' attention on evidence of caring and sharing. Demonstrate a caring attitude. Allow time to complain.

From Ebersole, P., and Hess, P.: Toward healthy aging: human needs and nursing response, St. Louis, 1981, The C.V. Mosby Co.

adaptive function of the older adult. As a therapeutic technique, reminiscence is an elaboration of the natural way older adults revive their past in an attempt to make order and meaning and reconcile conflicts and disappointments as they prepare to let go of their human existence (Butler, 1963).

Reminiscence can be used for cognitively impaired, psychologically disturbed, or depressed older adults. The nurse organizes the group and selects strategies for reminiscence by adapting the size of the group, the group's structure, process, and goals, and her own activities to meet the needs of group members. Table 27-6 details the primary techniques of reminiscence.

BODY IMAGE INTERVENTIONS

The way an older adult presents himself has a significant impact on his body image and feelings of isolation. Certain physical characteristics of old age are socially desirable, such as slimness and distinguished-looking gray hair. Other features are also impressive, such as a lined face that displays character or wrinkled hands that convey a lifetime of hard work. Too often, however, society envisions elderly people as incapacitated, deaf, obese, or shrunken in stature. When an older adult is hospitalized or has an acute or chronic illness, the related physical dependence makes it difficult for the person to maintain his body image. A nurse who has stereotyped views about the appearance of older adults may give little attention to grooming or hygiene activities.

Consequences of illness and aging that can threaten the older adult's body image include invasive diagnostic procedures, pain, surgery, prostheses, loss of sensation in a body part, skin changes, dependence on life-sustaining medication, denture odor, loss of scalp hair, and incontinence.

The nurse has a direct influence on the older adult client's appearance. The nurse must consider the importance to the older adult client of maintaining a pleasant appearance and presenting a socially acceptable image. It takes little effort for the nurse to assist the client in combing matted hair, cleaning stained dentures, shaving an unkempt beard, or changing urine-stained clothing. The older adult does not choose to have an objectionable appearance. The nurse should also be sensitive to odors in the client's environment. Nurses commonly lose awareness of objectionable odors after constant exposure to them. Odors created by urine-stained linen, a full bedpan, and certain illnesses often surround the older adult. By controlling sources of offending odors, the nurse may prevent family members and friends from shortening their visits or not coming at all because of these factors.

Nurses' Attitudes Toward Older Adults

Why is it important for nurses to assess their attitudes toward aging? How do nurses' attitudes influence the nursing care they provide? How can nurses foster positive attitudes toward the aged? These are important questions for the nurse to examine. Negative attitudes displayed by the nurse toward older adult clients may result in a reduction in the older adults' sense of security, adequacy, and well-being. Furthermore, such attitudes may lead to a decline in the quality of care. Clients in long-term care facilities present a special challenge for the nurse. Such clients are often considered losers by themselves or society or both. How can the nurse promote the independence and self-esteem of a client who feels he has lost everything and life is not worth living?

Clearly the nurse must examine and clarify her own attitudes and values toward the older adult client to provide the most effective care. Research has shown that a nurse's age, level of education, employment experience, and type of agency where employed influence whether the nurse holds negative stereotypes about older adults. The nurse's personal experiences with older adults such as family members also affect her attitudes when caring for older adults. Chapter 13 discusses techniques to assist the nurse in clarifying personal and professional values. If the nurse cannot change her negative attitudes, she should work in health care settings that do not involve care for older adults, such as children's hospitals or obstetric units.

Nurses who work with older adults must collect complete and accurate assessment data, including the client's strengths and resources as well as his limitations. For example, the nurse should consider the client's hobbies, work history, and methods of dealing with stress. Information about such resources helps the nurse engage in meaningful and purposeful interactions with the client. The client will sense the nurse's interest in him as a unique individual.

The nurse's interventions should attempt to incorporate the client's accustomed routines or rituals. The older adult often feels more secure when he can continue familiar rituals while hospitalized or living in an institution. For example, if the nurse learns that the client follows certain practices at bedtime, including these practices in the nursing care plan will alleviate the client's anxiety in unfamiliar surroundings and provide him with the opportunity to remain independent.

The specialty of geriatric nursing has expanded to provide nurses with creative approaches for maximizing the potential of the older adult client. With the knowledge that is now available regarding the unique needs and problems of the elderly, nurses working in geriatrics can better maintain their clients' physical abilities and create an environment for psychosocial health.

Community and Institutional Health Care Services

The health care services that are generally available are described in Chapter 3. However, there are five types of services that are used more frequently by the older population than by others.

Home Care

Home health care services and homemaker services prevent or delay institutionalization for older adults who need assistance with self-care and activities of daily living. These agencies may be governmental, private, or voluntary.

Home health care is covered by Medicare and health insurance carriers. Care is provided by professional nursing staff or nonprofessional staff, such as homemaker aides.

Hospice

The hospice is a community resource for the terminally ill. A hospice can be an independent unit within the community or may be contained within an institutional setting. Clients seeking hospice care include those with cancer, end-stage renal, cardiovascular, or pulmonary disease, or degenerative neuromuscular disease. The hospice program focuses on meeting the needs of the dying client and his family. The hospice provides pain control and maintains the client's quality of life. The hospice does not institute life support or other measures to prolong the life of the terminally ill.

Day Care

Day care is an institutional program that provides an alternative to institutionalization. A day-care center offers health services for a client who is able to remain at home during the evening and night. In addition, day care often enables the client's family or other caretaker to maintain employment and other activities (Stanhope and Lancaster, 1984).

Respite Care

Respite care is a form of short-term health service provided to the dependent older adult in his home or an institutional setting. Respite care enables the permanent caretaker to be away from the home, for example, to go on vacation or just to have a rest from the responsibilities of caring for a dependent older adult.

Respite care can be a valuable resource for a person whose ill or dependent parent lives with his family. With such services the adult child is able to care for his parent but can also have time alone with his spouse and children.

Long-Term Care

Situations of declining health, decreased physical and human resources, and increased dependence may necessitate the older adult's institutionalization in a long-term care facility. Such a facility provides extended residential, intermediate, or specialized nursing care, medical care, and personal and psychosocial services.

The decision for institutional care is not easy, and the family requires a great deal of support. In addition, the family may need the nurse's help in locating the proper facility to meet the needs of the client. When possible the facility chosen should be close to the client's and family's home to provide accessibility for visits.

Summary

Nursing care for the older adult is both a challenging and a rewarding experience. The older adult must learn to adapt to physical, cognitive, and social changes. The degree of these changes varies from one person to another. Likewise, adaptive capacities are different for each client.

Nurses must develop care plans to meet the individual needs of the older adult, while trying to maintain an optimal level of physical and cognitive function. The nurse also incorporates family and community resources to assist in the care of the older adult.

The older adult's level of independence depends on his physical health, cognitive abilities, and social support network. When any of these areas are absent or dysfunctional, the older adult's ability to maintain his independence decreases and he needs more extensive health care services.

KEY CONCEPTS

✓ Myths and stereotypes portray the elderly as ill, rigid in thinking, institutionalized, poor, unable to learn, and without sexual needs.

✓ Physiological and biological theories of aging rely on physiological explanations for the aging process; these include the genetic theory, free radical theory, stress theory, and immunological theory.

✓ The psychosocial theories of aging, which include the disengagement, activity, and continuity theories, attempt to describe the effects of life-style, personality, and environmental factors on longevity.

✓ The older adult must adjust to physical changes in all body systems.

✓ The older adult must adjust to retirement.

✓ The death of a spouse, a friend, or children affect adaptation to aging.

✓ Many older adults have difficulty perceiving themselves as old.

✓ Some older adults require a change in living arrangements.

✓ Realignment of relationships between older adults and their children is necessary.

✓ The older adult must acquire new activities and interests to maintain the quality of his life.

✓ Physiological changes are a normal part of aging and not the result of an illness.

✓ Structural and physiological changes that occur in the brain during the aging process do not necessarily impair the older adult's adaptation and functional ability.

✓ Cerebral dysfunction can magnify preexisting behavioral tendencies.

✓ Characteristics of dementia include decreased intellectual function, personality change, impaired judgment, and change in affect.

✓ Organic brain syndrome includes acute, potentially reversible disorders and chronic, irreversible, progressive disorders.

✓ Classic symptoms of active and chronic organic brain syndromes include decreases in attention span, learning, and memory. Some clients have hallucinations, delusions, aphasias, emotional lability, and depression.

✓ Chronic organic brain disorders include Alzheimer's disease and vascular disorders.

✓ Cognitive impairment can result from chemical substance abuse.

✓ Psychosocial changes affecting the older adult include retirement, social isolation, change in housing, death, and sexual changes.

✓ Sexuality is linked with a person's identity and validates the person's belief that he can give to others and have the gift appreciated.

✓ In addition to physical changes, drugs prescribed for the older adult may affect sexual functioning.

✓ Changes in social roles, family responsibility, and health status influence the choice of living arrangements appropriate for the older adult.

✓ The older adult and his family require nursing interventions to help them cope with the dying process.

KEY CONCEPTS, *cont'd*

✓ The major health problems of the older adult include hypertension, angina pectoris, myocardial infarction, cerebrovascular accident, cancer, arthritis, sensory impairments, and dental problems.

✓ The four leading causes of death in the older population are heart disease, malignant neoplasms, cerebrovascular disease, and influenza and pneumonia.

✓ Nursing interventions for psychosocial problems should be individualized; they include the technique of therapeutic communication, touch, reality orientation, resocialization, and reminiscence.

✓ A nurse's attitudes toward older adults affect the quality and level of care she delivers to that population.

✓ Health care services for older adults are available in the community and institutional settings.

REFERENCES

Barnett, K.: A survey of the current utilization of touch by health team personnel with hospitalized patients, Int. J. Nurs. Stud. 9:195, 1972.

Bartol, M.: Dialogue with dementia: non-verbal communication in patients with Alzheimer's disease, J. Gerontol. Nurs. 5:21, 1979.

Beck, C.M., Rowlins, R.P., and Williams, S.R.: Mental health—psychiatric nursing: a holistic life-cycle approach, St. Louis, 1984, The C.V. Mosby Co.

Burnside, I.M.: Transition to later life: developmental theories and research. In Burnside, I.M., Ebersole, P., and Monea, H.E., editors: Psychosocial caring through the life span, New York, 1979, McGraw-Hill Book Co.

Butler, R.: Life review: an interpretation of reminiscence in the aged, Psychiatry 26:65, 1963.

Cummings, E., and Henry, W.E.: Growing old: the process of disengagement, New York, 1961, Basic Books, Inc.

Department of Health and Human Services: Final report: the 1981 White House Conference on Aging, Washington, D.C., 1981, The Department.

Diekelman, N.: Pre-retirement counseling, Am. J. Nurs. 78:1337, 1978.

Duvall, E.M.: Family development, ed. 4, Philadelphia, 1971, J.B. Lippincott Co.

Ebersole, P., and Hess, P.: Toward healthy aging: human needs and nursing response, St. Louis, 1981, The C.V. Mosby Co.

Forbes, E.J., and Fitzsimmons, V.M.: The older adult: a process for wellness, St. Louis, 1981, The C.V. Mosby Co.

Groër, M.W., and Shekleton, M.T.: Basic pathophysiology: a conceptual approach, ed. 2, St. Louis, 1983, The C.V. Mosby Co.

Havighurst, R.J.: Human development and education, New York, 1953, David McKay Co., Inc.

Havighurst, R.J.: Successful aging. In Williams, R.H., Tibbits, C., and Donahue, W., editors: Process of aging, vol. 1, New York, 1963, Atherton Press.

Hayter, J.: Patients who have Alzheimer's disease, Am. J. Nurs. 74:1460, 1974.

Maddox, G.L.: Disengagement theory: a critical evaluation, Gerontologist 4:80, 1974.

Murray, R.B., Huelskoetter, M.M.W., and O'Driscoll, D.L.: The nursing process in later maturity, Englewood Cliffs, N.J., 1980, Prentice-Hall, Inc.

Neugarten, B.L.: Personality in middle and late life, New York, 1964, Atherton Press.

Office of Human Development Services: Need for long-term care: information and issues, Washington, D.C., 1981, Department of Health and Human Services.

Public Health Service: Health United States, 1976-1977, Washington, D.C., 1976-1977, Health Resources Administration, National Center for Health Statistics, Department of Health, Education and Welfare.

Smith, W.L., and Kingsbourne, M., editors: Aging and dementia, New York, 1977, Spectrum Publications.

Stanhope, M., and Lancaster, J.: Community health nursing: process and practice for promoting health, St. Louis, 1984, The C.V. Mosby Co.

Woods, N.F.: Human sexuality in health and illness, ed. 3, St. Louis, 1983, The C.V. Mosby Co.

ADDITIONAL READINGS

Isaacs, B.: The evaluation of drugs in Alzheimer's disease, Age Aging 8:115, 1979.

Palmore, E.: Facts on aging, Gerontologist 17:315, 1977.

6

The components of nursing care in all settings involve many kinds of skills. Some nursing skills are used more commonly with particular illnesses or health conditions, but other skills are essential in the care of most clients. The six chapters in Unit 6 consider the most often required nursing skills. Measurements of vital signs and physical assessment are carried out, often at repeated intervals, for all clients with physiological illness. Skills related to maintaining correct body alignment and joint motion, as well as those for preventing or minimizing the hazards of immobility, are important for clients whose mobility is affected by illness. Finally, the nurse's skills in administering medications and preventing or controlling infection in the health care agency or home are essential when providing care for clients with many different health needs.

Skills Essential
to Nursing Practice

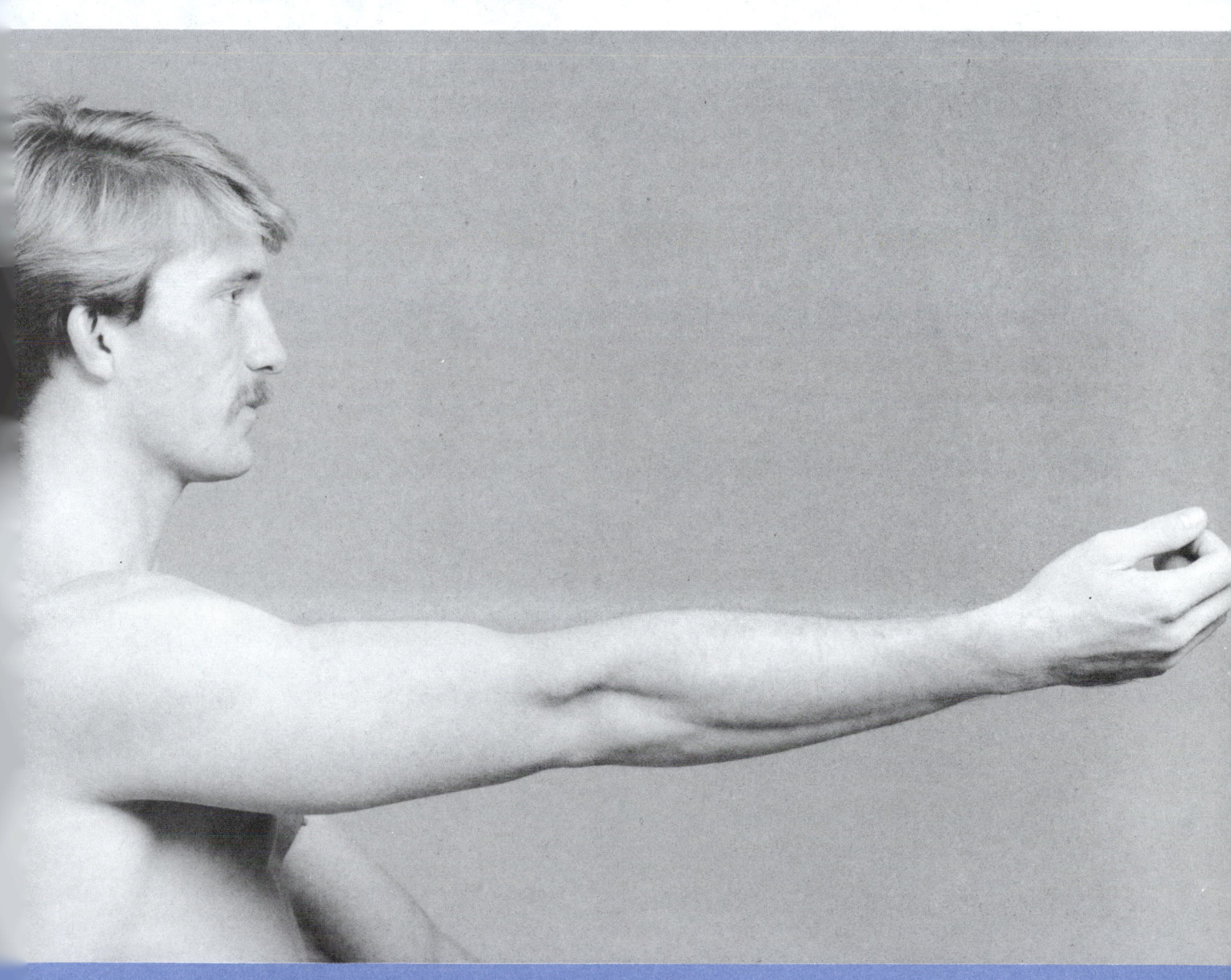

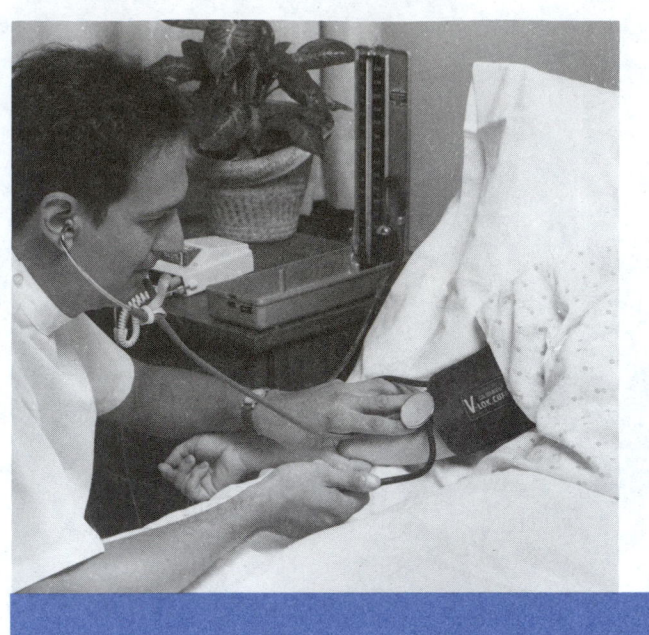

OBJECTIVES

Mastery of content in this chapter will enable the student to:

- Define the terms in the glossary.
- Accurately assess a client's oral, rectal, and axillary temperatures.
- Accurately assess a client's pulse, respirations, and blood pressure.
- Discuss the relationship between physiological function and measurement of vital signs.
- Identify normal vital sign values for an adult and an infant.
- Describe variables that alter vital sign values.
- Discuss the nurse's responsibility to ensure accurate vital sign measurements.
- Accurately record and report vital sign measurements.

GLOSSARY

anoxia Condition characterized by a relative or total lack of oxygen; may be local or systemic.

bradycardia Slower than normal heart rate; heart contracts fewer than 60 times per minute.

calorie Amount of heat required to raise 1 gram of water 1° centigrade at atmospheric pressure; a kilocalorie or large calorie, used to represent energy values of food, is 1000 times as large as the small calorie, the unit used in physics to describe energy exchange in the body.

centigrade Denotes a temperature scale in which 0° is the freezing point of water and 100° is the boiling point of water at sea level; also called Celsius.

costal Of or referring to the ribs.

cyanosis Bluish discoloration of the skin and mucous membranes caused by an excess of deoxygenated hemoglobin in the blood or a structural defect in hemoglobin.

diaphoresis Secretion of sweat, especially profuse secretion associated with an elevated body temperature, physical exertion, or emotional stress.

diurnal Daily.

eupnea Normal respiration that is quiet, effortless, and rhythmical.

febrile Pertaining to or characterized by an elevated body temperature.

hematocrit Measure of the packed cell volume of red cells, expressed as a percentage of the total blood volume.

hemodynamics Study of the circulation of the blood.

hemorrhage External or internal loss of a large amount of blood in a short period of time.

hypercarbia Greater than normal amounts of carbon dioxide in the blood; also called hypercapnia.

hypertension Disorder characterized by an elevated blood pressure persistently exceeding 150/90 mm Hg.

28 Assessment of Vital Signs

hyperthermia Higher than normal body temperature.

hypotension Abnormal lowering of blood pressure, which is inadequate for normal perfusion and oxygenation of tissues.

hypothermia Abnormal lowering of body temperature below 93° F or 35° C, usually caused by prolonged exposure to cold.

hypoventilation Reduction in the volume of air that enters the lung for gas exchange; oxygen exchange is insufficient to meet metabolic demands of the body.

insensible water loss Loss of fluid from the body by evaporation, as normally occurs during respiration.

orthostatic hypotension Abnormally low blood pressure occurring when a person stands up.

pyrogen Any substance that causes a rise in body temperature, as in the case of bacterial toxins.

tachycardia Rapid regular heart rate ranging between 100 and 150 beats per minute.

thermoregulation Internal control of body temperature.

tidal volume Amount of air inhaled and exhaled during normal ventilation.

vital signs Temperature, pulse, respirations, and blood pressure.

The vital signs—temperature, pulse, respirations, and blood pressure—are indicators of a person's health status. Numerous factors such as the temperature of the environment, physical exertion, and the effects of illness cause vital signs to change, sometimes beyond a person's normal range. Measurement of vital signs provides data that can be used to determine a client's usual state of health (baseline data), as well as his response to physical and psychological stress and medical and nursing therapy. An alteration from a client's normal vital signs may signal the need for medical or nursing intervention.

A nurse measures vital signs many times in the course of a career. When a client comes to a clinic, physician's office, or hospital or is seen by a nurse at home, measurement of vital signs is a routine part of the complete physical assessment (see Chapter 29). They may also be measured separately as part of a review of the client's condition. Vital signs are a quick and efficient way of monitoring a client's condition or identifying the presence of problems. The basic skills required to measure vital signs are simple but should not be taken for granted. The nurse should not consider the procedure routine and dull or the findings isolated or insignificant. In conjunction with other physiological measurements, vital signs are the basis for clinical problem solving. When the nurse learns the physiological variables that influence vital signs and recognizes the relationship of vital sign changes to other physical assessment findings, she will be able to make precise determinations of the client's health problems. Careful measurement techniques ensure accurate findings.

Incorporating Vital Signs into Practice

While providing care to clients, the nurse encounters many situations requiring vital sign measurement. The process of taking vital signs is therefore not routine but rather an individualized approach to assessment. The nurse's judgment is critical in determining the need for and frequency of vital sign measurement.

The following guidelines help the nurse to incorporate vital sign measurement into nursing practice:

1. *The nurse should know the client's normal range of vital signs.* The client's normal values serve as a baseline for comparison with the nurse's subsequent findings. The clinic record or hospital chart contains the client's vital sign values during a time of relative physical stability. If the client enters the emergency room without a record or comes to the clinic for the first time, the normal values for clients in the same age range are used as the baseline data.

2. *The nurse should know the client's medical history and the therapy and medications he is receiving.* Some illnesses or treatments have predictable effects on vital signs.

3. *The nurse should control environmental factors that may influence vital sign values.* Measuring a pulse after the client exercises or experiences an emotional upset or checking the client's temperature in a warm, humid room may yield values that are not true indicators of the client's condition.

4. *In a hospital environment or extended care setting, the nurse assigned to the client should measure his vital signs.* Throughout the course of a shift, the nurse makes observations of the client's condition. Vital signs provide important information about the client's state of health. The nurse assigned to a client is the best one to collect vital signs, interpret their significance, and make decisions about the client's care.

5. *The nurse decides the frequency of vital sign assessment.* In the hospital the physician orders a minimum frequency of vital sign measurements for each client, but the nurse is responsible for determining if more frequent assessments are required. If a client's physical condition begins to deteriorate, the nurse implements more frequent vital sign monitoring, perhaps as often as every 5 to 10 minutes. After a client returns from surgery or a major diagnostic examination such as cardiac catheterization, frequent measurements are taken until the client's vital signs stabilize to the before-procedure range. The collection of data as a basis for determining changes and trends is useful in making therapeutic decisions.

6. *The nurse makes certain that equipment is functional and appropriate.* The equipment used to measure vital signs must work properly to ensure that measurements are accurate. Unless a blood pressure cuff is the appropriate size, for example, readings will be inaccurate.

7. *The nurse uses an organized, systematic approach to measure vital signs.* Vital signs are not checked haphazardly. In a hospital setting a nurse may be assigned to several clients. Running back and forth between different clients' rooms to collect vital signs is poor practice. The nurse must establish and maintain a systematic method. For example, many nurses measure a client's temperature first. By using a glass thermometer, the nurse can observe the temperature while checking pulse, respirations, and blood pressure.

8. *The nurse verifies and communicates significant changes in the vital signs.* Baseline measurements provide data enabling the nurse to recognize fluctuations in vital signs. The nurse who is familiar with a client's vital signs will be able to recognize abnormalities. When a value is abnormal, a fellow nurse or a physician should repeat the vital sign measurement to verify it. A physician should be notified immediately when abnormal signs are assessed.

When to Take Vital Signs

- On the client's admission to a hospital or an extended care facility
- In a hospital on a routine schedule according to a physician's order
- During a client's visit to a clinic or physician's office
- Before and after any surgical procedure
- Before and after any invasive diagnostic procedure
- Before and after the administration of medications that affect cardiovascular and respiratory function
- Whenever the client's general physical condition suddenly worsens (as with loss of consciousness or increased intensity of pain)
- Before nursing interventions that may influence any one of the vital signs (such as before ambulating a client previously on bed rest or before a client performs range of motion exercises)
- Whenever the client reports to the nurse any nonspecific symptoms of physical distress (such as feeling "funny" or "different")

Vital signs provide physiological data that the nurse uses in practice and are the most frequently collected form of assessment data. Knowledge of the physiological mechanisms reflected by each vital sign and of the causes and clinical implications of abnormalities helps the nurse initiate specific interventions. For example, a nurse knows that the volume of blood in the cardiovascular system directly influences blood pressure. A client in hemorrhagic shock loses an excessive amount of blood and therefore has a drop in blood pressure. The nurse further knows that a continued drop in blood pressure can be fatal. The nurse initiates interventions to restore the client's blood pressure, such as administering fluids and blood and controlling the loss of blood.

Vital signs assist the nurse in performing routine care measures as well as critical care interventions. The boxed material opposite outlines when the nurse should assess vital signs. For example, the client's pulse indicates his tolerance for exercise or his need for pain medication. The client's respiratory rate may reveal his need to be repositioned so he can breathe more easily.

Body Temperature

In health, the body's tissues and cells function best within a relatively narrow temperature range. Despite extremes in environmental conditions and physical activity, regulatory mechanisms keep the temperature of the inside of the body or "core" relatively constant. Even when a nude person is exposed to temperatures as low as 13° C (55° F) or as high as 60° C (140° F) in dry air, the core temperature remains stable.

In contrast, the body's surface temperature rises and falls with the temperature of the environment. Skin temperature may fluctuate between 20° C (68° F) and 40° C (104° F) without damage. The skin is the principal site of heat loss from the body. Humans can control body temperature by adding or removing clothing, seeking shelter, taking a cool or warm bath, or adjusting the temperature of a room. The measures humans use to control the body's surface temperature help support the more complex internal controls of thermoregulation.

Normal Body Temperature

No single temperature is normal for all people. However, for healthy adults the average temperature is 37° C (98.6° F) when measured orally. Axillary temperatures are usually a few tenths of a degree lower than oral readings, and rectal temperatures are

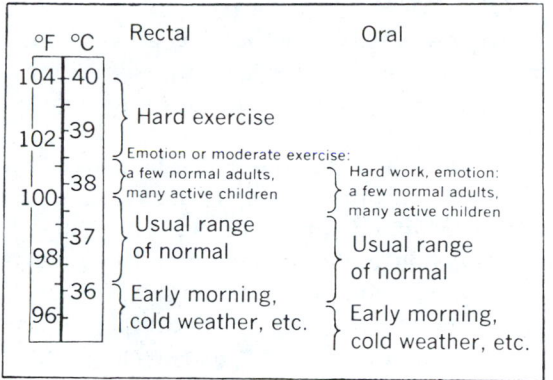

Fig. 28-1 Ranges of rectal and oral temperatures found in normal persons.

From Mountcastle, V.B.: Medical physiology, vol. 2, ed. 14, St. Louis, 1980, The C.V. Mosby Co.

a few tenths of a degree higher. The oral temperature is a reliable measurement of the body's core temperature; however, the rectal temperature is believed to be more accurate because of the rectum's greater proximity to pelvic viscera. For clinical practice it is important to know the normal temperature range and when a temperature is febrile (above normal) or below normal. The temperature range for a normal active adult is greater than might be expected. Fig. 28-1 shows the temperature ranges commonly found in normal healthy adults. Exercise, climatic conditions, and emotional reactions are variables that affect body temperature. If an adult client is confined to bed in a room at a comfortable temperature, body temperature below 36° C (97° F) or above 38° C (100° F) is considered abnormal.

Physiology of Body Temperature

The intricate balance of body temperature levels results from a coordination of various body systems. *For the body temperature to remain constant, the heat produced in the body must equal the heat lost to the environment.* Chemical energy made available by the combustion of carbohydrates, proteins, and fats in body tissues is converted into heat, which is lost to the environment by convection, radiation, conduction, and evaporation. The internal core temperature may vary from 35° C (95° F) to 41° C (105° F) depending on conditions, but in a healthy person the temperature will return to its resting level near 37° C (98.6° F) by thermoregulation. A nurse therefore applies knowledge of the processes of heat production and heat loss in promoting a client's temperature regulation.

HEAT PRODUCTION

Heat is produced in the body as a by-product of metabolism. Food is the primary fuel source for metabolism. Although the amount of heat produced is greater when a person is active, heat production is a constant process. In the quiet, resting person, most of the heat is generated in the body core: the trunk, viscera, and brain. During work the principal site of heat production is the musculature. Thermoregulation allows the body to maintain a fairly constant core temperature regardless of where heat production occurs. Hormones enter the bloodstream to regulate heat production by facilitating the breakdown of food elements and promoting their use for energy.

BASAL METABOLIC RATE. The intake of carbohydrates, fats, and proteins results in a synthesis of the important enzyme adenosine triphosphate (ATP). ATP is the energy source for major cellular functions. The chemical breakdown of ATP's high-energy phosphate bonds releases 8000 calories (cal) or 8 kilocalories (kcal) for each mole of ATP. The basal metabolic rate (BMR) is a measurement of the rate of energy use in the body during absolute rest. The metabolic rate is based in part on a person's oxygen consumption. Metabolism is calculated in terms of kilocalories per square meter of body surface. A man between 20 and 30 years of age has a BMR of 39.5 kcal/m^2/hr (Mountcastle, 1980). An adolescent's BMR is higher, ranging from 43 to 46 kcal/m^2/hr. An older adult (70 to 80 years) has a BMR of 33 to 35 kcal/m^2/hr. Women tend to have slightly lower BMRs than men of the same age. In addition to food ingestion, a person's metabolic rate is influenced by exercise, hormonal factors, and activity of the sympathetic nervous system.

MUSCLE ACTIVITY. Exercise has a dramatic effect on the body's heat production. As exercise levels increase, the amount of energy or muscular work created increases. The energy of muscular work comes from the oxidation of foods, primarily carbohydrates and fat. Under conditions of *moderate work,* such as the everyday work of nurses, salesclerks, and assembly line workers, the average hourly energy expenditure is about three times the BMR. Under conditions of *heavy work,* which includes manual labor such as mining, farming, and jobs in heavy industry, the average hourly energy expenditure is four to eight times the BMR. Even activities such as shifting from a bed to a chair, dressing, and walking down a hallway can elevate the metabolic rate. For clients whose energy reserves are minimal and whose body temperatures are already elevated, any form of physical exertion can increase heat production and body temperature.

Shivering of skeletal muscle is another mechanism for temperature regulation. If the body temperature becomes too low, shivering increases body heat production. The tone of skeletal muscles throughout the body increases. During maximum shivering, body heat production may be four to five times greater than normal (Guyton, 1981).

A client's surface temperature may fall even though he has a fever. Shivering in such a situation causes the body temperature to rise further. The nurse often administers medications that reduce shivering to prevent a fever from becoming dangerously high.

THYROID HORMONE SECRETION. The thyroid gland releases two hormones, thyroxine and triiodothyronine, which increase basal metabolism by promoting the breakdown of glucose and fat. These hormones are not released constantly into the circulation; thyroid-stimulating hormone (TSH), secreted by the anterior pituitary gland, regulates their release according to metabolic demands.

Thyroid hormones promote oxidative metabolism in tissues such as those of the liver, heart, skeletal muscles, and kidneys. Thyroxine has a slower effect than triiodothyronine in causing oxidative metabolism. The thyroid hormones must be present for the normal increase in heat production under normal temperature conditions. However, neither thyroxine nor triiodothyronine assists in temperature regulation when a person is exposed to cold temperatures.

SYMPATHETIC STIMULATION. Stimulation of the sympathetic nervous system by the chemical mediators norepinephrine and epinephrine increases the body's metabolic rate. Both epinephrine and norepinephrine stimulate muscle and liver cells to break down glycogen. As glycogen is metabolized, glucose is made available to the cells as a source of energy. The release of epinephrine and norepinephrine occurs primarily when the body's glucose level falls below normal.

HEAT LOSS

As the body is producing heat, it is also losing heat. A balance between heat loss and heat production maintains the body's temperature at a stable level. If heat loss is excessive, however, the body temperature will fall below normal. Because of the skin's structure and exposure to the environment, a person normally loses heat continuously. Heat is lost through four basic processes: radiation, conduction, convection, and evaporation. If these heat loss mechanisms are impaired, the body temperature will rise significantly. By understanding these mechanisms, the nurse learns to control heat loss to the environment.

RADIATION. The human body continuously gives off infrared heat rays. If a person stands nude in a room at normal room temperature, approximately 60% of his total heat loss occurs through radiation. Heat rays are also given off by other objects such as the sun, light bulbs, and even the walls of a room. The body absorbs this radiated heat, which may cause an overall increase in body temperature. If the temperature of the body is greater than that of the environment, a greater amount of heat is radiated from the body than toward it.

The amount of heat loss through radiation can be reduced by covering the body with clothing, especially dark, closely woven clothes. Heat radiates through clothing that is loosely woven and lightweight. Dark skin absorbs more solar heat than white skin. This may explain different behavioral methods of temperature regulation among different races in different climates.

CONDUCTION. Conduction is the flow of heat from one object to another with which it is in contact. Heat loss through conduction is normally minimal. However, if a nude person sits on a chair, there is rapid heat conduction until the chair's surface temperature begins to rise. When the chair and skin surface reach the same temperature, conductive heat loss ceases.

There also may be a loss of heat by conduction to air and water. If the air immediately adjacent to the skin is cooler than the skin's surface, the body's heat will warm the air. When the temperature of the air next to the skin equals skin temperature, there is no further loss of body heat by conduction. Wearing several layers of clothing helps create layers of warmed air surrounding the body, which ultimately keeps the person warm and reduces heat loss.

Conduction of heat through water is a more important form of heat loss because water can absorb far more heat than air can. Heat is also conducted more easily through water. The body cannot create a warm "insulation zone" of water next to the skin as it does in the air. The rate of heat loss from the skin can be quite high. Water used to bathe clients should be above body temperature (37.7° to 40.5° C [100° to 115° F] for adults; 37.7° to 40.5° C [100° to 105° F] for children). However, if a client's temperature is abnormally elevated, the nurse can lower the client's fever by bathing him with water that is warm but still below body temperature. The water will absorb heat. Cold water is not used because of the danger of lowering the client's temperature too quickly.

Heat is conducted from the internal organs to the skin. An obese person can tolerate cold better than a thin person because of his thicker layer of insulating fat. Women tend to have a thicker layer of subcutaneous fat than men, which provides greater insulation between the skin and deeper tissues and thus reduces heat loss.

A person can gain heat from conduction when the skin surface is exposed to warmer air or water. This is not a source of heat production and thus usually has a minimal effect on overall heat balance, except in cases of extreme temperatures.

CONVECTION. A warm layer of air usually exists close to the skin's surface. The heated air may rise from the skin and pass to the cooler air by natural convection. Convection depends on the temperatures of the skin and air and the air velocity.

Increasing room ventilation by opening windows or using fans increases heat loss by forced convection. When a person walks or runs, convective heat loss is increased. When a person walks briskly or stamps his feet in cold temperatures, loss of heat by convection is greater than the heat gain from muscular activity.

If a person's body comes in contact with both cold water and air, heat loss from the body increases dramatically. Together the water and air remove essentially all of the heat that reaches the skin's surface from the body core. Therefore the nurse avoids bathing clients in a drafty room and keeps body parts covered that are not being bathed.

Convective heat transfer from the bloodstream to the skin is controlled by the sympathetic nervous system. For each liter of blood at 37° C (98.6° F) in the body core that flows to the skin and returns to the core at 36° C (96.8° F) the body loses 1 kcal of heat (Mountcastle, 1980). In cold temperatures, vasoconstriction prevents convective loss to the arms and legs and the skin of the trunk. In warm temperatures exercise causes blood flow to the skin to increase heat loss 10 fold for efficient heat transfer.

EVAPORATION. For each gram of water that evaporates from the body surface, approximately 0.6 kcal of heat is lost (Mountcastle, 1980). Evaporation is an efficient mechanism for heat loss even when the environmental temperature exceeds that of the skin. To be effective in such a case, however, evaporative heat loss must exceed metabolic heat production and heat absorbed by radiation and convection.

The body always loses some heat by evaporation. Normally this insensible water loss occurs from the skin and lungs. Even though the skin appears dry, water is diffusing through the outer skin layers and evaporating. The drying effect from evaporation can cause skin scaling and itching, as well as drying of the nares and pharynx.

The body does not control insensible water loss through evaporation for the purpose of temperature regulation. However, the body does control sweating, which significantly increases heat loss by evaporation.

Mechanisms of Temperature Control

The balance between heat loss and heat production is the result of various internal control mechanisms. Information about changes in body temperature travels to the central nervous system via nerve impulses. The temperature control center then gives feedback information to the organs to initiate temperature control responses. When the illness alters any of the integrated body systems, the result is a body temperature that may be either too hot or too cold.

NEURAL CONTROL

The hypothalamus, located between the cerebral hemispheres, is the primary center for integrating the physical and chemical processes of heat production and loss. The hypothalamus is the body's thermostat, capable of sensing minute changes in body temperature. When nerve cells in the hypothalamus become heated beyond a set point, impulses are sent out to initiate a reduction in body temperature. The body breaks into a sweat, blood vessels dilate, and heat production is inhibited. If the hypothalamus senses that the body's temperature is too low, signals are sent out for thyroxine release, vasoconstriction, and muscle shivering. Lesions or trauma to the hypothalamus can cause serious alterations in temperature control.

SKIN IN TEMPERATURE REGULATION

The skin has three roles in temperature regulation. First, it insulates the body. The skin, subcutaneous tissue, and fat keep heat inside the body. When blood flow between the skin's layers is reduced, the skin alone is an excellent insulator. Persons with more body fat have better natural insulation than those who are slim and muscular.

The way the skin controls body temperature is similar to the way an automobile radiator controls engine temperature. The engine of an automobile generates a great deal of heat. Water is pumped through the engine's system to collect the heat and carry it to the radiator, which transfers the heat from the water to the outside air. The engine's temperature thus stays within safe limits to prevent damage from overheating. In the human body the internal organs produce heat, and at times during exercise or increased sympathetic stimulation the amount of heat produced is greater than normal body core temperatures. Blood flows from the internal organs, carrying heat to the body surface. The skin is well supplied with blood vessels. In the most exposed areas of the body—the hands, feet, and ears—blood can flow directly from arteries to veins, bypassing capillaries. Blood flow through the more vascular areas of the skin may vary from barely present to as much as 30% of the cardiac output (Guyton, 1981). Heat is transferred from the blood, through vessel walls, to the skin's surface and is lost to the environment through the various heat loss mechanisms. The body's core temperature remains within safe limits.

The degree of vasoconstriction of the arteriovenous system determines the amount of blood flow and heat loss to the skin. If the core temperature must be lowered, the hypothalamus inhibits sympathetic impulses, blood vessels dilate, and more blood reaches the skin's surface. On a hot, humid day the blood vessels in the hands are dilated and easily visible. In contrast, if the core temperature becomes too low, the hypothalamus initiates vasoconstriction and blood flow to the skin lessens. Thus body heat is conserved.

The skin's third role is that of temperature sensor. The skin is well supplied with heat and cold receptors. Since the cold receptors are more plentiful, however, the skin functions primarily to detect cold surface temperatures. When the skin becomes chilled, its sensors send information to the hypothalamus, which initiates three reflexes: shivering to increase body heat production, inhibition of sweating, and vasoconstriction of blood vessels.

SWEAT GLAND SECRETION

Sweat glands are located deep beneath the dermal layer of the skin. They secrete sweat, a watery solution containing high concentrations of sodium and chloride, which passes through tiny ducts on the skin's surface. The glands are innervated by sympathetic nerve fibers. Acetylcholine is a primary mediator for nerve impulses reaching the sweat glands. However, epinephrine and norepinephrine may also stimulate sweat glands. Impulses from the hypothalamus travel via autonomic nerve pathways to the spinal cord and then to sweat glands throughout the skin's surface. When the body's temperature rises, sweat glands release sweat, which eventually evaporates from the skin's surface to facilitate heat loss. When temperatures are cold, the hypothalamus inhibits sweat gland secretion. When skin disease interferes with sweating, exposure to, and especially exercise in, the heat can cause dangerously high body temperature. Persons with impaired sweating must dampen their skin and clothing even during normal sedentary activity.

Factors That Affect Body Temperature

The nurse must be aware of the factors that affect body temperature in order to assess temperature variations and evaluate the significance of deviations from normal.

AGE

At birth the newborn leaves a warm, relatively constant environment and enters one in which temperatures fluctuate widely. The immature physiological mechanisms of infants are not capable of maintaining stable body temperatures. The infant's temperature may change drastically according to changes in its environment. Extra care is therefore needed to protect the newborn. Clothing must be adequate and exposure to temperature extremes must be avoided. When protected from environmental extremes, the newborn's body temperature is maintained within the range of 35.5° to 37.5° C (96° to 99.5° F) as measured rectally.

Temperature regulation continues to be labile until a child reaches puberty. Children commonly have transient temperature elevations after relatively slight exertion in warm weather.

The normal temperature range gradually drops as an individual approaches old age. A temperature of 35° C (95° F) orally is not unusual for an elderly person in cold weather. Older adults are particularly sensitive to temperature extremes because of a deterioration in the mechanisms of thermoregulation, such as poor vasomotor control and reduced basal metabolism.

EXERCISE

An earlier section describes how muscle activity increases heat production. Any form of exercise can increase body temperature. After severe prolonged exercise, such as long-distance running, body temperatures may temporarily reach levels as high as 39° to 41° C (103.2° to 105.8° F) (Petersdorf, 1980).

HORMONAL INFLUENCES

Women generally experience greater fluctuations in body temperature than men. Hormonal variations during the menstrual cycle are responsible for body temperature fluctuations. Progesterone levels rise and fall cyclically during a menstrual cycle. Before a menstrual cycle, progesterone levels are low and the body temperature falls a few tenths of a degree Fahrenheit below the baseline level. The lower temperature persists until ovulation occurs. At ovulation, greater amounts of progesterone enter the circulation and raise the body temperature to previous baseline levels or higher. Plotting out temperature variations during the menstrual cycle to determine when ovulation occurs is a form of birth control.

DIURNAL VARIATIONS

Body temperatures normally change throughout the day. Usually the temperature is at its lowest point between 1 and 4 AM (Fig. 28-2). During the day, body temperatures rise steadily, peaking around 4 to 6 PM. Then the temperature gradually falls to its minimum level early in the morning. At one time temperature variations were believed to be due solely to the greater daytime activity. However, the temperature pattern is not automatically reversed in people who work during the night and sleep during the day. It takes approximately 1 to 3 weeks for the cycle to reverse. Daily patterns of hormonal variation contribute to the cause of diurnal temperature variations. Each client exhibits different patterns, which the nurse assesses to analyze temperature variations.

STRESS

Physical and emotional stress increases body temperature through hormonal and neural stimulation. The client who is fearful or anxious about entering a hospital or a physician's office may register a higher than normal temperature. The nurse can obtain a more accurate temperature reading by waiting until the client's emotional stress subsides.

ENVIRONMENT

Environment influences body temperature. If a client's temperature is assessed in a very warm room or if he has just been outside on a cold blustery day, the nurse can expect to see a temperature variation.

Although the human body is capable of surviving temperature extremes, precautions are needed to avoid injury. The limit of heat that a person can tolerate depends largely on whether the heat is dry or wet. If the air is completely dry and air currents are adequate to promote evaporation from the body, a person can tolerate a temperature of 65.5° C (150° F) for several hours without serious effects. In contrast, if the humidity is 100%, the body temperature rises when the environmental temperature rises above 34.4° C (94° F). If a person is performing strenuous work in humid conditions, the critical environmental temperature can be as low as 29.4° C (85° F) (Guyton, 1981).

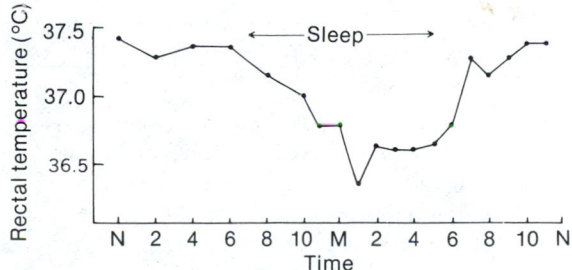

Fig. 28-2 Twenty-four-hour temperature cycle (circadian rhythm). Temperature chart (average for 7 days) of normal man confined to bed.

From Mountcastle, V.B.: Medical physiology, vol. 2, ed. 14, St. Louis, 1980, The C.V. Mosby Co.

The body's exposure to temperatures below freezing may result in freezing of the skin's surface, or frostbite. Exposed parts of the body such as fingers, toes, and earlobes are more susceptible to frostbite. If frostbitten areas are rewarmed immediately with warm water (43.3° C [110° F]), permanent damage may be averted.

Nature of Fever

A fever is a body temperature above 38° C (100° F) under resting conditions. Brain abnormalities caused by tumors or trauma may interfere with the ability of the hypothalamus to regulate temperatures. The presence of certain disease processes alters the "set point" or internal core temperature set by the hypothalamus. Bacteria and degenerating body tissues secrete pyrogens, substances that increase the set point. Once the set point is raised, the body acts to produce and conserve heat. It may take several hours for the body temperature to reach the new set point. During this time the person experiences chills and feels cold even though his temperature may already be high. During chills, vasoconstriction, shivering, piloerection (upright projection of body hairs and "goose bumps" designed to conserve heat), and sympathetic stimulation occur. Once the body temperature reaches the new hypothalamic setting, the chills subside and the person feels neither cold nor hot.

When a fever develops, the body's metabolism increases tremendously and the person needs adequate nourishment. As a result of the increased metabolism, the body's oxygen consumption rises. If the client with a fever already has cardiac or respiratory problems, the stress of a febrile episode may be overwhelming. The client who suffers a prolonged elevation in body temperature will become seriously weakened as a result of an exhaustion of the body's energy stores and the increased work of breathing.

The signs and symptoms of fever are simply the reflections of the body's attempt to conserve and produce heat. The client may initially feel cold and may seek warmth by putting on more clothing, bundling up in blankets, or even using heating pads. The skin is cool and pale as a result of vasoconstriction. Extensive shivering may occur during episodes of chills. The nurse should attempt to keep a client with chills comfortably warm. Although his temperature is rising, cooling the body during a chill is inappropriate, since it will merely aggravate shivering and increase discomfort.

When the chill subsides, excess covering or clothing should be removed to prevent unnecessary warming. The client's temperature should be monitored. An elevated temperature should be documented in the client's record and reported to the physician immediately. The physician may order diagnostic tests to determine the cause of the fever. Often antipyretic drugs are administered to reduce the body's temperature. However, recent studies suggest that not treating a low-grade fever is beneficial. A fever is an important part of the body's immune response, and premature treatment of low-grade fevers may impair the body's ability to fight infection.

A prolonged temperature elevation places the client at risk of becoming dehydrated. Fluids are needed to replace those lost as a result of increased metabolism. The client who has difficulty meeting increased oxygen demands often becomes restless and even disoriented. In children, convulsions are a fairly common but dangerous side effect of high fever. Prolonged high temperatures can result in irreversible brain damage.

After the cause of a fever is removed, the hypothalamic set point drops. The body begins to initiate heat loss mechanisms. The skin becomes warm and flushed as a result of vasodilation. Diaphoresis, or excessive sweating, acts to further lower the body's temperature. The client becomes more alert and has renewed energy.

Nursing Measures for the Client with a Fever

- Provide fluids (at least 3 liters per day for a client with normal cardiac and renal function) to replace fluids lost through insensible water loss, sweating, and increased metabolism.
- Bathe the client with tepid water to reduce body's surface temperature by promoting convection and evaporation of heat.
- Provide oral hygiene, since oral mucous membranes dry easily as a result of dehydration.
- Reduce external covering on the client's body to promote heat loss through radiation and conduction. Do not induce chilling.
- Keep clothing and bed linen dry to increase heat loss through conduction and convection.
- Provide well-balanced meals to meet increased metabolic needs.
- Reduce frequency of activities that increase oxygen demands, such as excessive turning and ambulation.
- Provide supplemental oxygen therapy as ordered to improve oxygen delivery to body cells.
- Monitor pulse and respirations, which may increase as a result of an elevated metabolic rate.

The three common types of fever differ according to the pattern of body temperature elevation. In an *intermittent* fever the body temperature rises at some point during the day but returns to normal within 24 hours. An intermittent fever commonly "spikes" or reaches its highest point in the late afternoon or evening. A *remittent* fever remains elevated for a day or more. Throughout the course of the fever there are marked variations in temperature. A *relapsing* fever is characterized by periods of fever lasting a few days, alternating with several days of normal body temperature.

The boxed material opposite summarizes the principles of caring for the client with an elevated temperature. The nurse initiates measures to support whatever heat loss or heat conservation responses the body initiates. The nurse administers nutritional and fluid supplements to replace losses resulting from increased metabolic needs.

Assessment of Body Temperature

SITES

There are three sites for measuring body temperature: the mouth, rectum, and axilla. Each site has advantages and disadvantages (Table 28-1).

MOUTH. The mouth is the most convenient and acceptable site for temperature measurement. The nurse's primary consideration in measuring an oral temperature is the client's safety. Table 28-1 summarizes situations in which oral thermometer insertion is contraindicated.

Oral temperatures can be affected by a number of variables. The nurse should wait 20 minutes to measure oral temperature after the client has ingested hot or cold liquids or food or has been smoking. An oral thermometer should not be used if the client is receiving continuous oxygen therapy. Cooled oxygen will lower the reading, and temporary removal of the oxygen mask for an oral temperature measurement seriously reduces arterial oxygen levels (Felton, 1978). If a client is receiving oxygen, rectal or axillary temperature measurement is best.

RECTUM. Rectal temperature measurements are most useful when the client is unable to use an oral thermometer. A rectal thermometer should always be used for infants and children, although it is difficult for an infant or child to lie still the necessary 2 to 4 minutes. A rectal thermometer is not used for newborns because of the risk of injuring the rectal mucosa. A rectal reading is considered to be the most reliably accurate because there are a minimum of factors that can alter the results. A rectal temperature is usually a few tenths of a degree higher than an oral temperature. Even within the rectum there are variations of 0.1° to 0.9° C, depending on the position of the thermometer (Mountcastle, 1980). The lowest rectal temperatures register in the parts of the rectal wall closest to the veins carrying cooler blood from the legs and buttocks.

AXILLA. The axilla is the safest site for temperature measurement, especially for newborns. However, it takes significantly longer to determine an axillary temperature than an oral or rectal temperature. In addition, keeping the thermometer in position un-

---

TABLE 28-1

Selection of Sites for Temperature Measurement

Site	Advantages	Disadvantages
Mouth	Most accessible site; more comfortable for client	Should not be used for clients who could be injured by thermometer, who are unable to hold thermometer properly, or who might bite down on thermometer: infants or small children, confused or unconscious clients, clients who have had oral surgery, clients with trauma to face or mouth, clients experiencing oral pain, clients who breathe only with mouth open, clients with history of convulsions, clients experiencing a shaking chill
Rectum	Thought to provide most reliable measurement	Should not be used for clients after rectal surgery, clients who have a rectal disorder such as tumor or hemorrhoids, or clients who cannot be positioned for proper thermometer placement such as those in traction
Axilla	Safest method because noninvasive	Least accurate

Fig. 28-3 Comparison of Fahrenheit and centigrade calibrations.

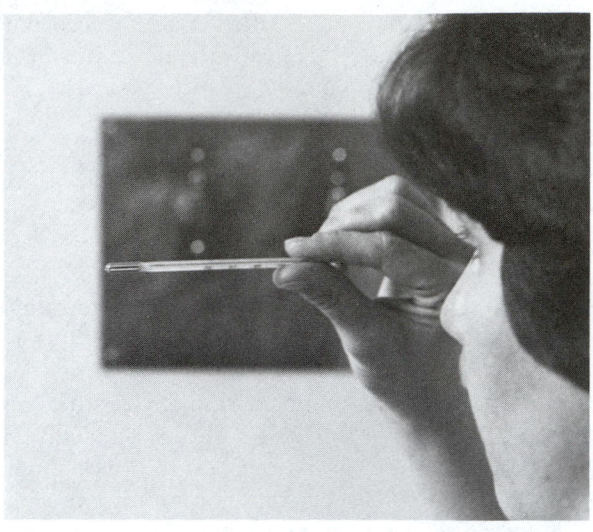

Fig. 28-4 The nurse reads a glass thermometer by holding it horizontal at eye level.

derneath the client's axilla for the necessary length of time is difficult. The nurse must hold the thermometer in place during the entire measurement period. The axillary temperature is usually 0.6° C (1° F) lower than the oral temperature.

TYPE OF THERMOMETER

Three types of thermometer are available for determining body temperature: mercury in glass, electronic, and disposable.

MERCURY-IN-GLASS THERMOMETERS. The mercury-in-glass thermometer is the type most familiar to clients. The thermometer consists of a glass tube that is sealed at one end and has a mercury-filled bulb at the other. Exposure of the bulb to heat causes the mercury to expand and rise in the enclosed tube. The length of the thermometer is marked with either Fahrenheit or centigrade calibrations (Fig. 28-3). The farthest point reached by the mercury in the tube is the temperature reading. The mercury will not fluctuate or fall unless the thermometer is shaken vigorously.

A mercury thermometer is read by holding it with the fingertips horizontally at eye level, with the bulb pointed to the left (Fig. 28-4). *The bulb should not be touched;* touching it might bring the fingers into contact with the client's body secretions. The thermometer is rotated slowly until the column of silver mercury appears. The calibrated line at the end of the mercury column is the temperature reading.

Three types of glass thermometers are the oral, the stubby, and the rectal. The oral thermometer is slender, allowing for greater exposure of the bulb against the blood vessels in the mouth. Most manufacturers paint the tip blue to distinguish the thermometer as an oral type. The stubby thermometer is shorter and thicker than the oral type. It can be used to measure temperature at any site. The rectal thermometer has a blunt end designed to prevent trauma during rectal insertion. A rectal thermometer is recognized by its red tip.

The time delay for recordings and the easy breakability are major disadvantages of mercury-in-glass thermometers. Advantages of these thermometers are the low price, wide availability, and reliable accuracy.

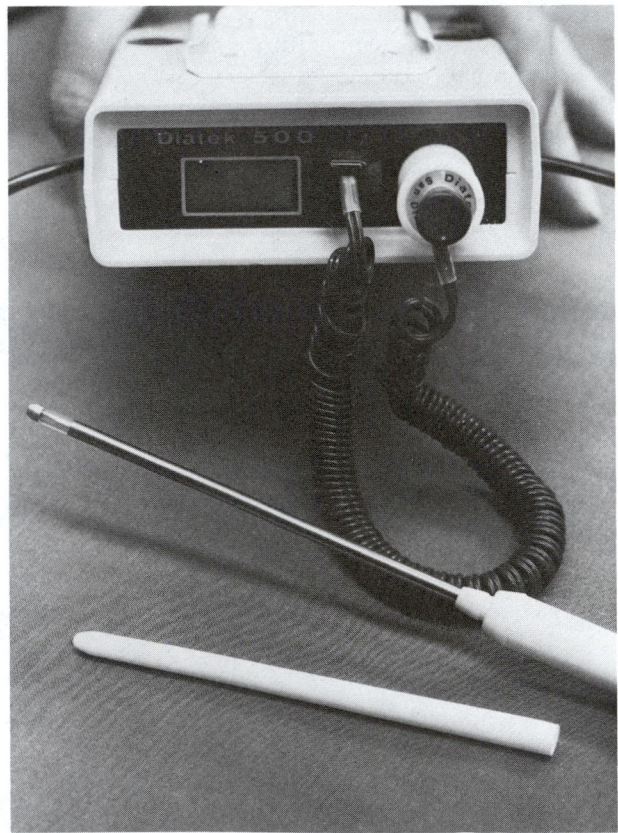

Fig. 28-5 Electronic thermometer.

PROCEDURE 28-1

Oral Temperature Measurement

STEPS	RATIONALE
1. Hold the tip of the thermometer in your fingertips.	This prevents contamination of the bulb to be inserted into the client's mouth.
2. If the thermometer is stored in a disinfectant solution, rinse it in cold water before using.	Rinsing removes potentially irritating disinfectant. Hot water might cause mercury to expand and break the bulb.
3. Wipe the thermometer from the bulb end toward the fingers in a rotating manner. Dispose of the tissue.	Rotating friction helps remove microorganisms. Wiping toward fingers prevents contamination of bulb end.
4. Read the mercury level.	Mercury is to be below 35.5° C (96° F). The thermometer reading must be below the client's actual temperature before use.
5. If the mercury is above the desired level, shake the thermometer down. Grasp the tip of the thermometer securely and stand away from any solid objects. Sharply flick the wrist downward as though you were cracking a whip. Continue until the reading is at the appropriate level.	Brisk shaking lowers the mercury level in the glass tube. Standing in an open spot prevents breakage of the thermometer.
6. Ask the client to open his mouth and gently place the thermometer in the sublingual pocket (under the tongue) lateral to the center of the lower jaw.	Heat from superficial blood vessels under the tongue produces the temperature reading.
7. Ask the client to hold the thermometer with lips closed.	The lips hold the thermometer in the proper position during recording.
8. Leave the thermometer in place 3 to 8 minutes according to agency policy.	Studies disagree as to proper length of time for recording. Nichols and Kucha (1972) recommend 8 minutes for oral glass thermometers. Graves and Markarian (1980) found that glass thermometers kept in place for 8 minutes recorded values on the average only 0.07° F higher than those kept in for 3 minutes. Therefore they recommend 3 minutes as more practical.
9. Carefully remove the thermometer.	
10. Wipe off any secretions with a soft tissue. Wipe in a rotating fashion from the tip to the bulb. Dispose of the tissue.	Wiping prevents contact of microorganisms with nurse's hands. The tip is the area of least contamination and the bulb is the area of greatest contamination.
11. Read the thermometer.	
12. Store the thermometer in its container after shaking it down again.	Proper storage prevents breakage.
13. Record the client's temperature on the proper chart or flowsheet.	Vital signs should be recorded immediately before they are forgotten.

ELECTRONIC THERMOMETERS. Many health care institutions use electronic thermometers. The electronic thermometer consists of a battery-powered display unit, a thin wire cord, and a temperature-sensitive probe, which is covered by a disposable plastic probe to prevent the transmission of infection (Fig. 28-5). Separate probes are available for oral and rectal use. Within only a few seconds of insertion a reading appears on the display unit, after which the probe is withdrawn and the probe cover discarded. Temperature readings appear in Fahrenheit or centigrade or both.

An electronic thermometer is not necessarily more accurate than a glass thermometer. For example, the variables that alter oral temperature measurements affect all types of thermometers. An electronic ther-

PROCEDURE 28-2

Rectal Temperature Measurement

STEPS	RATIONALE

Follow steps 1 through 5 of the oral temperature procedure (p. 573), using a rectal thermometer.

6. Draw curtains around the client's bed or close the room door. Keep the client's upper body and lower extremities covered.

This maintains the client's privacy and minimizes embarrassment.

7. Ask an adult client to roll over onto his side, assuming the Sims' position with upper leg flexed. Move aside bed linen to expose only the anal area. A child may lie in a prone position.

This provides optimal exposure of anal area for correct thermometer placement.

8. Squeeze a liberal amount of water-soluble lubricant onto a tissue. Dip the thermometer's bulb end into the lubricant, covering 2.5 to 3.5 cm (1 to 1½ inches) for an adult or 1.2 to 2.5 cm (½ to 1 inch) for an infant or child.

Inserting the thermometer into the lubricant container would contaminate all the unused lubricant. Lubrication minimizes trauma to the rectal mucosa during insertion.

9. Put a disposable glove on your dominant hand.

This step is optional. It helps reduce contact with microorganisms.

10. With your nondominant hand raise the client's upper buttock to expose the anus. While an infant lies prone on a bed or on your lap, gently retract both buttocks with your fingers.

Raising the buttocks fully exposes the anus.

11. Gently insert the thermometer into the anus in the direction of the umbilicus. Insert 1.2 cm (½ inch) for an infant and 3.5 cm (1½ inches) for an adult.

Proper insertion ensures adequate exposure to blood vessels in the rectal wall.

12. Do not force the thermometer. Ask the client to take a deep breath and blow out, and insert the thermometer as the client breathes deeply. If you feel resistance, withdraw the thermometer immediately.

Gentle insertion prevents trauma to mucosa or breakage of the thermometer. Taking a deep breath helps to relax the anal sphincter.

13. Hold the thermometer in place 2 to 4 minutes according to agency's policy. You may have to hold an infant's legs.

Holding the thermometer prevents injury to the client.

14. Remove the thermometer.

15. Wipe any secretions off with a tissue. Wipe down in a rotating fashion from the tip to the bulb. Dispose of the tissue.

Wiping prevents nurse's contact with microorganisms. The tip is the area of least contamination and the bulb is the area of greatest contamination.

16. Wipe the client's anal area to remove lubricant or feces.

This provides for the client's comfort.

17. Read the thermometer.

18. Help the client return to a more comfortable position.

This restores the client's comfort.

19. Wash the thermometer in lukewarm soapy water and then rinse with cool water.

Washing mechanically removes organic material that otherwise might be a source of infection.

20. Dry the thermometer and return it to its container after shaking it down.

Proper storage prevents breakage.

21. Remove the glove by pulling it off at the wrist, turning it inside out. Discard the glove in the proper receptable.

Avoidance of contact with the glove's outer surface minimizes spread of microorganisms.

22. Wash hands.

Washing prevents contamination.

23. Record the client's temperature in the proper chart or flowsheet. Signify a rectal reading by the capital letter R.

Vital signs should be recorded immediately after measurement. The R prevents later confusion with oral or axillary measurements.

PROCEDURE 28-3

Axillary Temperature Measurement

STEPS	RATIONALE
Follow steps 1 through 5 of the oral temperature procedure, using an oral or stubby thermometer.	
6. Move clothing or gown away from the client's shoulder and arm.	This provides optimal exposure of the axilla.
7. Insert the thermometer into the center of the axilla, lower the client's arm over the thermometer, and place the client's forearm across his chest.	This maintains proper position of the thermometer against blood vessels in axilla.
8. Leave the thermometer in place for 10 minutes or as long as recommended by agency. Gently hold a child's arm in place.	Movement can cause displacement of the thermometer.
Follow steps 9 through 12 of the oral temperature procedure.	
13. Record the client's temperature on the proper chart or flowsheet. Signify an axillary reading by the capital letter *A*.	Vital signs should be recorded immediately after measurement. The *A* prevents later confusion with oral or rectal measurements.

mometer may be more inaccurate because the sensor probe is inserted for a shorter time.

The greatest advantage of electronic thermometers is the saving in time. They can be inserted immediately, readings appear within seconds, and they are easy to read. Because of the shortened measurement time the client's discomfort is minimized.

DISPOSABLE THERMOMETERS. Some institutions use disposable, single-use thermometers. These are thin strips of plastic with chemically impregnated paper. They are used only for oral temperatures and are inserted in the same way as an oral glass or electronic thermometer. The chemical dots on the thermometer change color to reflect the temperature reading. Only 45 seconds is needed to record a temperature.

TAKING A TEMPERATURE

In measuring body temperature in any site, the following basic principles should be followed carefully to maintain the client's safety and ensure accuracy in measurement:
1. The most appropriate site for measuring the client's temperature is assessed.
2. All necessary equipment is assembled to ensure an uninterrupted procedure—thermometer, soft tissue, lubricant (rectal use only), pen or pencil, and record or worksheet.
3. The hands are washed using medically aseptic technique (see Chapter 34) to prevent the spread of infection.
4. The client is positioned properly and the purpose and method for the procedure are explained.

To simplify the discussion of temperature measurement, the use of mercury-in-glass thermometers in the three sites is explained in Procedures 28-1, 28-2, and 28-3.

CONVERSION OF TEMPERATURE READINGS

Institutions vary with regard to the temperature scales they use. Nurses generally do not have to concern themselves with temperature conversions, since each institution uses thermometers with the preferred scale. Many thermometers have dual scales. When it is necessary to convert temperature readings, the following formulas can be used:

To convert Fahrenheit to centigrade, subtract 32° from the Fahrenheit reading and multiply the result by $\frac{5}{9}$.

$$C = (F - 32°) \times \tfrac{5}{9}$$

To convert centigrade to Fahrenheit, multiply the centigrade reading by $\frac{9}{5}$ and add 32° to the product.

$$F = (\tfrac{9}{5} \times C) + 32°$$

Pulse

Blood flows through the body in a continuous circuit. The heart is a pulsatile pump, ejecting blood intermittently into the arterial system. Approximately 60 to 70 ml of blood enters the aorta with each ventricular contraction (stroke volume). With each stroke volume ejection the walls of the aorta distend, creating a pulse wave that travels rapidly toward the distal ends of the arteries. The pulse wave moves 15 times faster through the aorta and 100 times faster through the small arteries than the ejected volume of blood (Guyton, 1981). When a pulse wave reaches a peripheral artery, it can be palpated by pressing the artery lightly against underlying bone or muscle.

Assessment of Cardiovascular Function

Assessing the pulse provides valuable data for determining the integrity of the cardiovascular system. The pulse rate is an indirect measurement of cardiac output. The volume of blood pumped by the heart during 1 minute is the cardiac output. In an adult the heart normally pumps 5000 ml of blood per minute throughout the circulation. The cardiac output (CO) is the product of the ventricle's stroke volume (SV) and the heart rate (HR) per minute: CO = HR × SV. When factors alter either heart rate or stroke volume, the other component attempts to compensate to maintain a stable cardiac output. For example, the stroke volume of a well-trained athlete is greater than normal, and thus the heart rate is slower.

An abnormally slow, rapid, or irregular pulse can indicate the heart's inability to deliver an adequate cardiac output. The pulse can thus be a sensitive indicator of cardiovascular malfunction.

The nurse commonly assesses the radial or apical pulse or both during routine assessment of vital signs. The radial pulse, located along the radial or thumb side of the inner wrist, is the most accessible pulse for assessment. Assessment of other pulse sites such as the brachial or femoral (see Chapter 29) is unnecessary unless a complete physical assessment is conducted or there are indications of impaired peripheral blood flow.

The nurse assesses the apical pulse by auscultating heart sounds (see Chapter 29). If the radial pulse is inaccessible because of a dressing, cast, or other encumberance, the apical pulse is assessed instead. When a client has a history of cardiovascular disease and displays symptoms of cardiac alterations, the apical pulse is the most accurate for assessing heart function. If an assessment of the radial pulse reveals ab-

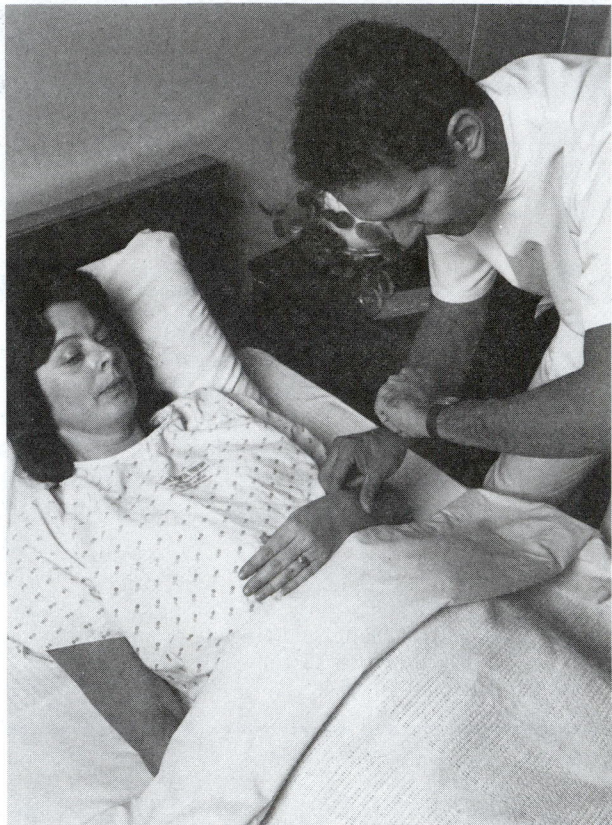

Fig. 28-6 Placing the client's relaxed hand over the lower chest allows the nurse to assess the client's pulse and respirations simultaneously.

normalities, the findings should be confirmed by checking the apical pulse. The apical pulse is the best site for assessing an infant's or young child's heart rate.

Pulse Assessment

The middle three fingers of the hand are used to palpate a pulse (Fig. 28-6). The tips are the most sensitive parts of the fingers for detecting the pulsation of the arterial wall. Beginning students sometimes apply excessive pressure over the artery and totally obliterate the pulse. It often helps to imagine the anatomical position of the artery when attempting to locate it. If the pulse is not easily located on one side, the other can be tried. The client's extremity should be kept in a relaxed position to permit full exposure of an artery. For assessment of the radial artery, the client's wrist should be extended and relaxed. This position ensures that the artery lies superficially above the radius. Procedure 28-4 outlines pulse assessment.

PROCEDURE 28-4

Radial Pulse Assessment

STEPS	RATIONALE
1. Use a wristwatch with a second hand.	
2. Wash hands.	Washing reduces chances of transmitting microorganisms.
3. Explain the purpose and method of procedure to the client.	Explanations relieve the client's anxiety and facilitate his cooperation during the procedure.
4. Have the client assume a supine or sitting position. If the client is supine, place his arm across his lower chest with wrist extended and palm down. If the client is sitting, bend his elbow 90 degrees and support his lower arm on the chair or on the examiner's arm. Extend his wrist with palm down.	Proper positioning fully exposes the radial artery for palpation.
5. Place the first three fingers of your hand along the radial artery and lightly compress against the radius.	The fingertips are most sensitive to vibration. Do not palpate with the thumb or you may feel your own pulse accidentally.
6. Obliterate the pulse initially, and then relax pressure so the pulse is easily palpable.	A pulse is more accurately assessed with moderate pressure. Too much pressure occludes the pulse, and too little prevents the examiner from feeling the pulse with regularity.
7. When the pulse can be felt regularly, use the watch's second hand and begin to count the rate, starting with zero, and then 1, and so on.	The rate is determined accurately only after the assessor is assured that the pulse can be palpated. Timing should begin with zero. The count of 1 is the first beat felt after timing begins.
8. If the pulse is regular, count for 15 seconds and multiply the total by 4.	A regular rate can be accurately assessed in 15 seconds.
9. If the pulse is irregular, count for a full minute.	The longer time ensures an accurate count.
10. Assess the rhythm and strength of the pulse and the elasticity of the arterial wall.	Assessing these factors provides complete assessment of pulse character.
11. Assist the client to a comfortable position.	
12. Record characteristics of pulse in medical record or flowsheets.	Vital signs should be recorded immediately.

RATE

Before measuring a client's pulse, the nurse should know his baseline heart rate for comparison. At birth an infant's rate ranges from 100 to 160 beats per minute. The pulse rate slows with age. At age 4 the average pulse rate is 80 to 120 beats per minute. By adolescence the rate varies between 60 to 100 beats per minute and remains so throughout adulthood.

The nurse should determine whether the client is receiving any medications that may affect heart rate or contraction. The pulse should be assessed before such medications are administered. The client should be at rest during measurement of the pulse because physical activity increases the heart rate. It may be necessary to wait 10 to 15 minutes after activity before measuring the pulse.

Some practitioners prefer to make baseline measurements of the pulse rate as the client assumes a sitting, standing, and lying position. Postural changes cause changes in pulse rate because of alterations in blood volume and sympathetic activity. The heart rate typically increases when a person moves from a lying to a sitting or standing position.

Table 28-2 summarizes factors that can alter the pulse rate. Any form of physical exercise increases the heart rate. However, in the case of a well-trained

TABLE 28-2

Factors That Influence Pulse Rates

Factor	Effect
Exercise	Short term: increased rate Long term: strengthened heart muscle, resulting in lower than normal rate at rest and a quicker return to resting rate after exercise
Fever, heat	Increased rate
Acute pain, anxiety	Increased rate because of sympathetic stimulation
Unrelieved severe pain	Decreased rate because of parasympathetic stimulation
Medications	
Digitalis	Decreased rate
Atropine	Increased rate
Hemorrhage (loss of blood)	Increased rate
Postural changes	
Lying	Decreased rate
Standing or sitting	Increased rate

athlete, the long-term benefit of exercise is a strong heart muscle and slower heart rate. An athlete's heart is capable of producing a greater stroke volume with each contraction. Thus the heart rate slows to maintain a constant cardiac output. An athlete's heart rate may be below 60 beats per minute. Acute pain, anxiety, and medications that cause sympathetic nervous system stimulation increase the heart's rate. The heart rate slows as a result of parasympathetic stimulation and drugs that slow conduction of electrical impulses through the heart.

Tachycardia is an abnormally elevated heart rate, above 100 beats per minute. Bradycardia is a rate below 60 beats per minute. The apical pulse should be assessed if bradycardia or tachycardia is detected in another pulse site.

RHYTHM

Successive beats of the heart normally occur at regular intervals. If an interval is interrupted by an early or late beat or if a beat is missed, the individual has an abnormal rhythm or arrhythmia (see Chapter 29). An arrhythmia threatens the heart's ability to function properly, particularly if it occurs repetitively. The nurse assesses an arrhythmia by noting an interruption in the successive pulse waves. If an arrhythmia is present, the regularity of its occurrence should be assessed. To confirm the presence of an arrhythmia, the physician may order an electrocardiogram.

The nurse may also measure the client's apical pulse in conjunction with the radial pulse to determine if a pulse deficit exists (see Chapter 29). This is particularly important when the nurse notes an arrhythmia. When there is a pulse deficit, the radial pulse is generally slower than the apical. This phenomenon reflects an inefficient contraction of the heart, which fails to transmit a pulse wave to the arterial system.

STRENGTH

The strength or amplitude of a pulse reflects the volume of blood ejected against the arterial wall with each heart contraction. Assessing the pulse strength is a subjective process and requires considerable practice. Normally the pulse strength remains the same with each heartbeat. A normal pulse is full, easily palpable, and not easily obliterated by the assessor's fingers. A bounding pulse is easily palpated and difficult to obliterate. A weak pulse is difficult to palpate and easy for the assessor to lose during palpation. The weak pulse is thready and often rapid. Some institutions use a classification system for pulse strength (see Chapter 29).

ELASTICITY

A normal artery feels straight, smooth, round, and elastic when palpated. Certain conditions change the quality of the arterial wall. For example, in arteriosclerosis the vessel walls harden and become cordlike, and the artery becomes torturous and twisted.

The elasticity or expansibility of an artery does not affect the pulse rate, rhythm, or strength. However, elasticity does reflect the general status of the peripheral vascular system.

EQUALITY

Pulses on both sides of the peripheral vascular system should be assessed. The nurse assesses both radial pulses to compare the characteristics of each. A local interruption of blood flow, such as a clot, is one condition that may cause variations between pulse sites.

Respiration

Oxygenation is the most basic of human physical needs. Human survival depends on the ability of oxygen (O_2) to reach body cells and for carbon dioxide (CO_2) to be removed from the cells. Respiration involves two distinctly different processes: *external res-*

piration, or the movement of air between the environment and the lungs, and *internal respiration,* or the movement of oxygen at the cellular level between hemoglobin and single cells. External respiration further involves four complex but interrelated processes: *ventilation,* the mechanical movement of air to and from the lungs, *conduction,* the movement of air through the airways of the lungs, *diffusion,* movement of O_2 and CO_2 between alveoli and red blood cells, and *perfusion,* distribution of blood through the pulmonary capillaries.

The nurse can directly assess only the process of external respiration, specifically by assessing ventilation. The rate, depth, and rhythm of ventilatory movements indicate the quality and efficiency of the respiratory process. Before measuring clients' respirations, the nurse should understand the physiological mechanisms of breathing.

Control of Respiration

Breathing is a relatively passive process. People seldom think about the mechanisms involved in moving air in and out of the lungs. The respiratory center in the brainstem is responsible for the involuntary control of respirations. Adults normally breathe in a smooth, uninterrupted pattern of 12 to 20 breaths per minute. Ventilation is regulated by levels of CO_2, O_2, and pH in the arterial blood. The most important factor in the control of ventilation is the Pco_2 of arterial blood. An elevation in the Pco_2 causes the respiratory center to initiate an increased rate and depth of breathing. The increased ventilatory effort removes excess CO_2 during exhalation. Hypercarbia, a chronic excess of CO_2 in the arterial blood, can eventually depress ventilation.

Chemoreceptors (carotid and aortic bodies) located in the periphery are sensitive to hypoxia, or low levels of arterial O_2. If arterial oxygen levels fall, the chemoreceptors signal the respiratory center to increase the rate and depth of ventilation. Hypoxia is usually unimportant in the control of ventilation. However, in clients with chronic lung disease such as emphysema or bronchitis, the hypoxic drive to increase ventilation is very important. These persons have chronic hypercarbia and thus have lost the normal stimulus for ventilation. A low level of arterial O_2 is the only stimulus that allows a client with chronic lung disease to breathe.

Mechanics of Breathing

Normal breathing is relatively passive, but muscular work is involved in moving the lung and chest wall. Inspiration is a more active process than expi-

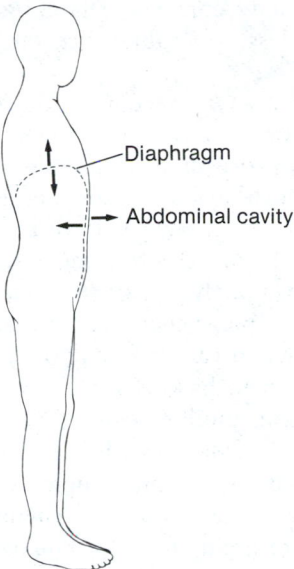

Fig. 28-7 On inspiration the diaphragm contracts, pushing the abdominal organs down and forward. The diaphragm relaxes on expiration, allowing the abdominal organs to return to their original position.

ration. During inspiration a considerable amount of muscular activity moves air into the lungs. The diaphragm is a thin, dome-shaped muscle inserted into the lower ribs. Impulses from the respiratory center travel via the phrenic nerve to the diaphragm. As the diaphragm contracts, the abdominal organs move downward and forward, increasing the vertical dimension of the chest cavity. At the same time the ribs lift upward and outward to facilitate the transverse expansion of the lungs. Fig. 28-7 demonstrates how diaphragmatic movement affects the size of the chest cavity. On expiration the diaphragm relaxes and the abdominal organs return to their original positions. The elastic lung and chest wall also return to a relaxed state. Little energy is required to move air out of the lungs. Only during exercise, voluntary hyperventilation (increased ventilation), and certain disease states does expiration become an active process.

The assessment of respirations relies on the nurse's recognition of normal thoracic and abdominal movements. During quiet breathing the chest wall gently rises and falls. Contraction of the intercostal muscles between the ribs or of the accessory muscles in the neck and shoulders is not visible. Passive breathing is more diaphragmatic as the abdominal cavity slowly rises and falls.

When breathing requires greater effort, rib (costal) movement increases. The intercostal and accessory muscles work actively to move air in and out. The shoulders may rise and fall, and the accessory muscles in the neck visibly contract. Diaphragmatic movement becomes less noticeable as costal breathing increases.

The nurse learns to recognize the situations in which passive or active breathing is to be expected. The respiratory process may be impaired by a number of conditions such as diseases of lung tissue, alterations in the O_2-carrying capacity of blood cells, and impairment in the muscles that move the chest wall. Each condition directly affects the character of ventilation. For example, a client with a reduced number of red blood cells breathes faster to increase O_2 delivery. A client who has pain in the chest wall voluntarily splints, or inhibits ventilatory movement on the painful side, and thus breathes less deeply. A careful assessment of respirations coupled with the physical assessment of the thorax (see Chapter 29) helps reveal the client's ability for adequate oxygenation of body cells.

Assessment of Respirations

Respirations are the easiest of all vital signs to assess, but they are often the most haphazardly measured. Sometimes a nurse merely estimates the client's respiratory rate. When physicians request vital signs, they are generally more concerned about temperature, pulse, and blood pressure measurements. However, the nurse should not underestimate the significance of assessing respirations. Recognition of a sudden change in the character of a client's respirations is important, as in the following situation:

Immediately after surgery Mr. Troy's respirations are 16 per minute, regular, and shallow. The client 30 minutes later begins to complain of abdominal pain near the area of surgery. The nurse's assessment reveals respirations at 32 per minute, regular, and labored. Obviously the client's physical status has changed. Although it is likely that other vital sign measurements have also changed, the significance of Mr. Troy's respiratory status should not be ignored.

It is important to assess the client's respirations when he is at rest. If the client is anxious or fearful or has just completed exercising, the respirations will likely be increased in both rate and depth. A skillful nurse does not let the client know that she is assessing his respiratory rate. If the client is aware of the nurse's intentions, he may consciously alter his rate and depth of breathing. One way to assess respiratory rates inconspicuously, if the client's chest movements can be observed adequately, is by counting respirations immediately after measuring the pulse rate, with the nurse's hand still placed on the client's wrist (see Fig. 28-6). To avoid startling or arousing an infant, respirations should be the first vital sign assessed. The rapid rise and fall of a young child's chest wall are easily observed.

The nurse should always assess respirations care-

Assessment of Respirations

STEPS	RATIONALE
1. Use a wristwatch with a second hand.	
2. Place the client's arm in a relaxed position across his abdomen or lower chest, or place your hand directly over the client's upper abdomen.	This position is used during assessment of the pulse. The client's or nurse's hand rises and falls during the respiratory cycle.
3. Observe a complete respiratory cycle (one inspiration and one expiration).	
4. For an adult count the number of respirations in 30 seconds and multiply by 2. For an infant or young child count respirations for a full minute.	The respiratory rate is equivalent to the number of respirations per minute. Young infants and children breathe in an irregular rhythm.
5. If an adult's respirations have an irregular rhythm or are abnormally slow or fast, count for a full minute.	Accurate interpretation requires assessment for at least 1 minute.
6. While counting, note whether depth is shallow, normal, or deep and whether rhythm is normal or one of the altered patterns.	The character of ventilatory movements may reveal specific alterations or disease states.
7. Record the results on a chart or flowsheet.	Vital signs should be recorded immediately.

fully to avoid overlooking signs that may be relevant to a client's physiological needs. When assessing a client's respirations, the nurse should keep in mind (1) the client's normal ventilatory pattern, (2) the influence any disease or illness has on respiratory function, (3) the relationship between respiratory and cardiovascular function, and (4) the influence of various therapies on respirations.

The objective measurements that comprise an assessment of a client's respiratory status include the rate and depth of breathing and the rhythm of ventilatory movements. The specific technique for assessing respirations is shown in Procedure 28-5.

RATE

The respiratory rate varies with age. A newborn infant breathes at a rate of 30 to 60 respirations per minute. As the child grows older, the respiratory rate gradually slows. A 2-year-old child takes 20 to 30 breaths per minute. A 6-year-old has a respiratory rate of 18 to 26 breaths per minute. Among adults normal rates vary from 12 to 20 respirations per minute. With advancing age, respiratory rates again increase.

A number of factors influence the rate of respiration. During and after any form of physical exercise, respirations increase to meet the body's greater oxygen needs. An elevation in body temperature causing an increase in the body's metabolic rate likewise elevates the respiratory rate. Pain and anxiety also typically increase respirations. The long-term effects of smoking may cause changes in the lung's airways, resulting in an increased respiratory rate. Drugs that depress central nervous system function lead to a lowering of the respiratory rate. Certain disorders of the brainstem impair the respiratory control center and inhibit respirations.

DEPTH

The depth of respirations can best be gauged by observing the degree of excursion or movement in the chest wall. The nurse subjectively describes ventilatory movements as shallow, normal, or deep. Chapter 29 describes a more objective means of measuring chest excursions by palpation of chest wall movement. This technique can be used if the nurse observes that chest excursion is unusually shallow.

During a normal relaxed breath (tidal breath) a person takes in 500 cc of air. The diaphragm moves approximately 1 cm ($\frac{4}{10}$ inch), and the ribs retract upward from the body's midline approximately 1.2 to 2.5 cm ($\frac{1}{2}$ to 1 inch). A deep respiration involves a full expansion of the lungs with full exhalation. Respirations are shallow when only a small quantity of air passes through the lungs and ventilatory move-

ment is almost imperceptible. The student can recognize normal relaxed breathing by watching a friend or noting her own breathing.

Body position influences depth of respiration. When a person stands or sits erect, the thoracic cage is unencumbered and free to rise and fall fully. A stooped posture or a slumped position impairs full ventilatory movement. The nurse can intervene to help a client assume positions that maximize ventilation.

Certain drugs also reflect the depth of respirations. Narcotics in particular characteristically depress the client's ability to increase the volume of air inspired. Monitoring respirations is one of the nurse's major responsibilities after narcotic administration.

Exercise increases the depth of respirations. Certain emotional states such as fear or anxiety also increase respiratory depth.

The capacity of the lungs to take in air varies depending on sex and age. Full capacity is determined by taking as deep a breath as possible and then blowing it all the way out. The amount of air exhaled after a full inspiration is the lung's vital capacity. Men tend to have a greater vital capacity than women of the same age. Infants and young children have smaller vital capacities than adolescents and adults. With advancing age the lung loses its elasticity, and the capacity for forcible exhalation declines. Nursing care may focus on increasing the client's efforts to breathe deeply. The nurse's knowledge of the client's normal capacity to move air is helpful in planning realistic therapy.

RHYTHM

Normal breathing is regular and uninterrupted. A regular interval occurs after each respiratory cycle. Infants tend to breathe less regularly. The young child may breathe slowly for a few seconds and then suddenly breathe more rapidly.

While assessing respirations, the nurse estimates the time interval after each respiratory cycle. Respiration is either regular or irregular in rhythm. Cheyne-Stokes respiration (see Table 28-3) is a serious alteration in ventilatory rhythm. The condition results from injury to the brain's respiratory center and frequently signals imminent death. A more common type of rhythm alteration is seen when a person consciously holds his breath before diving into water or lifting a heavy object.

Sighing should not be confused with abnormal ventilatory rhythm. Periodically throughout the day a person takes deep breaths, or sighs. A sigh is a protective physiological mechanism that expands small airways and alveoli not used during a normal tidal breath and prevents their collapse.

TABLE 28-3

Alterations in Respiration

Term	Description
Bradypnea	Rate of breathing is abnormally slow but regular.
Tachypnea	Rate of breathing is abnormally rapid.
Hyperpnea	Respirations are increased in depth and rate. This occurs normally with exercise.
Apnea	Respirations cease. Persistent cessation is called respiratory arrest.
Hyperventilation	The rate of ventilation exceeds normal metabolic requirements for exchange of respiratory gases. The rate and depth of respirations increase. There is an excessive intake of O_2 and blowing off of CO_2.
Hypoventilation	The volume of air entering the lungs is insufficient for the body's metabolic needs. The respiratory rate is below normal and the depth of ventilation is depressed.
Cheyne-Stokes respiration	Respiratory rhythm is irregular, characterized by alternating periods of apnea and hyperventilation. The respiratory cycle begins with slow, shallow breaths that gradually increase to abnormal depth and rapidity. Gradually breathing slows and becomes shallower, climaxing in a 10- to 20-second period of apnea before respiration resumes.
Kussmaul respiration	Respirations are abnormally deep but regular, similar to hyperventilation. This is characteristic of clients with diabetic ketoacidosis.
Dyspnea	Breathing is difficult and is characterized by an increased effort to inhale and exhale. The person actively uses intercostal and accessory muscles to breathe.

GENERAL RESPIRATORY CHARACTER

While assessing the three objective qualities of rate, depth, and rhythm, the nurse also observes factors related to the general character of a client's respirations.

Depending on the level of oxygenation, respiratory alterations may cause changes in skin color and level of consciousness. The nail beds, lips, and skin may take on a bluish or cyanotic appearance when arterial oxygen levels are reduced (see Chapter 29). As oxygenation decreases, a person typically becomes more restless and anxious and tries harder to breathe.

When a client uses more effort to breathe, he is dyspneic. In this condition the client actively uses his accessory muscles in the chest and neck to breathe. A dyspneic client usually reports feeling short of breath.

Sounds of breathing may indicate a respiratory disorder. Inflammation or stricture of the trachea or larynx causes an obstruction to airflow. As a client inhales, air passing the obstruction creates a harsh crowing sound or respiratory stridor, which can easily be heard without a stethoscope. Chapter 29 describes in detail the normal and abnormal breath sounds that can be heard by auscultation with a stethoscope. Vesicular and bronchovesicular sounds are produced as air normally passes through the airways. Abnormal sounds such as crackles and wheezes are the product of air passing through moisture or an airway stricture.

Respiratory alterations may cause any number of changes in the features or characteristics of breathing. Table 28-3 describes several common respiratory alterations.

Blood Pressure

To cause blood to flow throughout the circulatory system, the heart pumps blood into the arteries under high pressure. Blood pressure is the force exerted by the blood against a vessel wall. The standard unit for measuring blood pressure is millimeters of mercury (mm Hg). The measurement indicates the height to which the blood pressure can raise a column of mercury.

During a normal cardiac cycle (see Chapter 29) blood pressure reaches a peak that is followed by a trough. The peak or maximum pressure occurs during systole as the left ventricle pumps blood into the aorta. The normal systolic blood pressure in a healthy adult is 120 mm Hg. The trough occurs during diastole as the ventricles relax. Diastolic pressure is the minimal pressure exerted against the arterial walls at all times. The average diastolic blood pressure in a normal adult is 80 mm Hg. The nurse records blood pressure with the systolic reading before the diastolic, for example, 120/80. The difference between systolic and diastolic pressure is the pulse pressure. Thus, if the blood pressure is 120/80, the pulse pressure is 40 mm Hg.

Physiology of Arterial Blood Pressure

Blood pressure reflects the interrelationships of various hemodynamic factors: cardiac output, peripheral vascular resistance, blood volume, blood viscosity, and elasticity of arteries. Each factor significantly affects the others. For example, a reduction in arterial elasticity increases peripheral vascular resistance. The following are variables associated with increased blood pressure:

1. Increased cardiac output
2. Increased peripheral vascular resistance
3. Increased blood volume
4. Increased blood viscosity
5. Decreased arterial elasticity

Variables associated with decreased blood pressure include the following:

1. Decreased cardiac output
2. Decreased peripheral vascular resistance
3. Decreased blood volume
4. Decreased blood viscosity
5. Increased arterial elasticity

The complex control of the cardiovascular system normally prevents any single factor from permanently changing the blood pressure. For example, if blood volume falls, the body compensates with increased peripheral resistance to maintain the blood pressure at a normal level. A knowledge of the hemodynamic variables improves the nurse's ability to assess blood pressure alterations.

The blood pressure (BP) is a product of the cardiac output (CO) and peripheral vascular resistance (R): BP = CO × R. Whenever volume increases in an enclosed space, the pressure in that space rises. Thus, as the cardiac output increases, more blood is pumped against the arterial walls, causing an elevation in blood pressure. Exercise temporarily elevates blood pressure as the demand for cardiac output increases.

The size of arteries and arterioles changes to adjust blood flow to the needs of local tissues. The smaller the lumen of a vessel, the greater its peripheral vascular resistance to blood flow. When blood flow to a major organ falls sharply, peripheral arteries vasoconstrict to shunt blood to the major vessels supplying the organ. Arterial pressure rises to push blood through vessels that have become narrowed. As resistance rises, so too does arterial blood pressure. In contrast, as vessels dilate and vascular resistance falls, the blood pressure drops.

The volume of blood circulating within the vascular system affects blood pressure. Most adults have a circulating blood volume of 5000 ml. Normally the blood volume remains constant. However, if volume increases, more pressure is exerted within the arterial walls. The rapid, uncontrolled infusion of intravenous fluids is a typical cause of elevated blood pressure. When circulating blood volume falls, as in the case of hemorrhage or dehydration, the blood pressure falls.

The term "viscosity" refers to the thickness of blood. The hematocrit, or the percentage of red blood cells in the blood, determines blood viscosity. A greater viscosity increases the difficulty with which the blood flows through small blood vessels. When the hematocrit rises and blood flow slows, pressure builds within the arterial system as the heart continues to maintain its cardiac output. In polycythemia, a condition characterized by an increased hematocrit, a client's blood pressure is elevated.

Normally the walls of an artery are elastic and easily distensible. As pressure within the arteries increases, the diameter of vessel walls also increases. Arterial distensibility prevents wide fluctuations in blood pressure. For example, if the volume ejected by the heart suddenly increases, the arteries can distend and absorb much of the increase in pressure. However, in certain diseases such as arteriosclerosis the vessel walls lose their elasticity and are replaced by fibrous tissue that cannot stretch well. With a reduced elasticity there is greater resistance to blood flow. As a result, when the left ventricle ejects its stroke volume, the vessels no longer yield to the pressure. Instead, a given volume of blood is forced through the rigid arterial walls, and the pressure rises. Systolic pressure is more significantly elevated than diastolic pressure as a result of reduced arterial elasticity.

Factors Influencing Blood Pressure

A number of factors, as described in the following paragraphs, influence blood pressure. The nurse's understanding of these factors ensures a more accurate interpretation of clients' blood pressures. A single abnormally high (hypertensive) or low (hypotensive) reading is not a sufficient basis for concluding that a problem exists. Blood pressure readings taken on at least three separate visits or days should be averaged to confirm the presence of an abnormality. A client is hypertensive if his blood pressure is consistently greater than 140 mm Hg systolic and 90 mm Hg diastolic. A hypotensive reading is a systolic value below 90 mm Hg.

AGE

The normal blood pressure level varies throughout life. At birth an infant's blood pressure is 60 to 80 mm Hg systolic. With advancing age the blood pressure rises. Normal blood pressures for a variety of ages follow:

AGE	ARTERIAL PRESSURE (mm Hg)	
Newborn (3000 g [6.6 pounds])	Systolic	50-52
	Diastolic	25-30
	Mean	35-40
4 years	85/60	
6 years	95/62	
10 years	100/65	
12 years	108/67	
16 years	118/75	
Adult	120/80	

SYMPATHETIC NERVE STIMULATION

Anxiety, fear, pain, and emotional stress initiate sympathetic stimulation, causing blood pressure to rise. Sympathetic stimulation increases the heart rate, which in turn increases the cardiac output and the peripheral vascular resistance through vasoconstriction.

SEX

Through childhood there is no difference in blood pressure levels between boys and girls. After puberty, males have higher readings as a result of hormonal variations. When a woman reaches menopause, however, her blood pressure tends to be higher than that of a man of the same age.

MEDICATIONS

A number of medications can directly or indirectly affect blood pressure. Antihypertensive medications have the specific effect of lowering blood pressure. They act by relaxing vascular smooth muscle, inhibiting sympathetic stimulation, and changing the heart rate. After administration of an antihypertensive drug, the nurse assesses the client's blood pressure at a time that coincides with the drug's onset of action.

Diuretics are commonly used medications that lower blood pressure by reducing circulating fluid volume. A diuretic reduces the reabsorption of sodium and water by the kidneys. As a result, more urine is excreted and less water is retained in the vascular system.

Narcotics normally do not affect blood pressure unless a client receives an overdose. High doses of narcotics eventually result in shock and lowered blood pressure.

DIURNAL VARIATION

Blood pressure levels vacillate over the course of a day. The blood pressure is typically lowest in the early morning. It gradually rises during the morning and afternoon, peaking in late afternoon or evening. No two persons have the same pattern or degree of variation. The student may find it interesting to have a friend check her blood pressure at intervals during 24 hours.

TABLE 28-4

Conditions Causing Alterations in Blood Pressure

Condition	Effect	Cause
Hemorrhage	Lowers pressure	Decreased blood volume
Increased intracranial pressure	Raises pressure	Disturbance in cardiovascular control mechanisms in brainstem
Acute pain	Raises pressure	Increased vasomotor tone and peripheral vascular resistance as a result of sympathetic stimulation
Chronic renal failure	Raises pressure	Increased blood volume resulting from increased retention of sodium and water; release of renin, a vasopressor that increases peripheral vascular resistance
Essential hypertension	Raises pressure	Increased peripheral vascular resistance resulting from progressive thickening of arterial walls
General anesthesia	Lowers pressure	Decreased vasomotor tone resulting from depression of vasomotor center in brainstem

Variations in Blood Pressure

A number of conditions can result in blood pressure changes. Table 28-4 summarizes typical alterations a nurse might observe. The most common alteration in blood pressure is hypertension, an often asymptomatic disorder characterized by blood pressure persistently exceeding 150 mm Hg systolic or 90 mm Hg diastolic. Essential hypertension (hypertension of unknown cause) accounts for over 90% of the cases of high blood pressure in the United States. The condition is more prevalent in older persons and in blacks. Factors that have been linked to essential hypertension include heredity, cigarette smoking, high cholesterol levels in the diet, and caffeine and alcohol ingestion.

Hypertension causes thickening and loss of elasticity in the arterial walls. Peripheral vascular resistance increases within the affected vessels. Blood flow to vital organs such as the heart, brain, and kidneys decreases. A hypertensive person may die of heart failure, kidney failure, or a cerebrovascular accident (stroke) if hypertension remains uncontrolled.

When planning therapy for a client with hypertension, the nurse must know the client's normal blood pressure level. Repeated measurements over several hours or days usually reveal the client's normal range. The nurse bases judgments regarding medication administration and nursing therapy on the client's normal reading rather than the average reading for healthy persons of the same age and sex. For example, if the client's normal pressure is in the range of 150 to 160/90 mm Hg, the nurse who measures his blood pressure at 160/90 mm Hg will not report it to the physician as abnormal. If the client does not know his normal blood pressure, the nurse should inform him after assessing it. A client with hypertension is more motivated to comply with therapy if he knows how well his pressure is controlled.

Blood Pressure Equipment

Before assessing blood pressure the nurse must become comfortable in using a sphygmomanometer and stethoscope.

SPHYGMOMANOMETER

A sphygmomanometer is comprised of a pressure manometer, an occlusive cloth cuff that encloses an inflatable rubber bladder, and a pressure bulb with a release valve to inflate the cuff (Fig. 28-8).

The two types of manometers are the aneroid and the mercury. The aneroid manometer has a glass-enclosed circular gauge containing a needle that registers millimeter calibrations. A metal bellows within the gauge expands and collapses in response to pressure variations in the inflated cuff. Since metal parts in the aneroid model are subject to temperature expansion or contraction, the aneroid instrument is less reliable than the mercury type. Before using the aneroid model, the nurse must be sure that the needle points to zero and the manometer is correctly calibrated. An aneroid manometer should be recalibrated against a perfectly working mercury manometer at least once a year. Aneroid manometers have the advantages of being lightweight, portable, and compact.

Mercury manometers are the more accurate type of sphygmomanometer. Repeated calibrations are not necessary. The mercury manometer is an upright tube containing mercury. Pressure created by the inflation of the compression cuff moves the column of mercury upward against the force of gravity. Millimeter calibrations mark the height of the mercury column. To ensure accurate readings, the mercury column should always be at zero when the cuff is deflated and it should fall freely as pressure is released. Deviations indicate that the manometer is malfunctioning. Mercury manometers are wall mounted or portable. Ac-

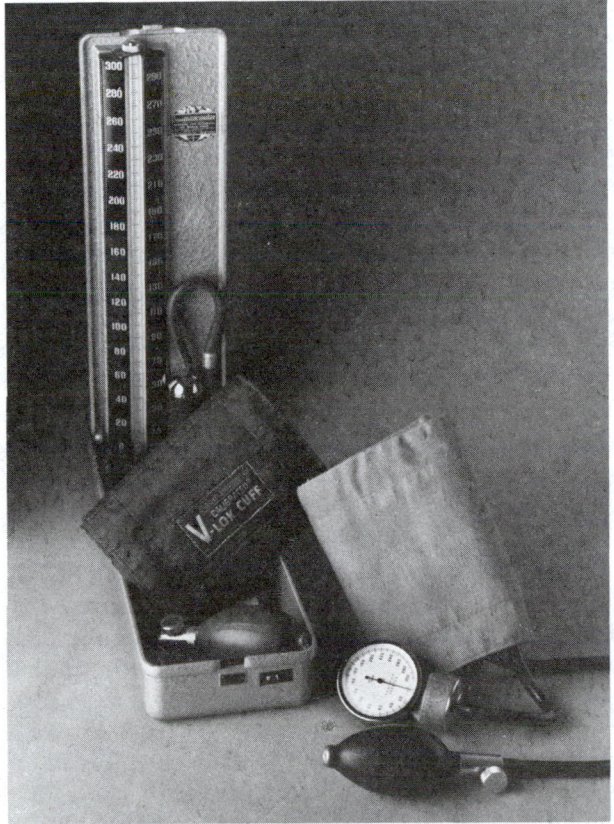

Fig. 28-8 A sphygmomanometer is comprised of a pressure manometer, a cloth cuff with a rubber bladder, and a pressure bulb. Mercury manometer is at left, and aneroid manometer at right.

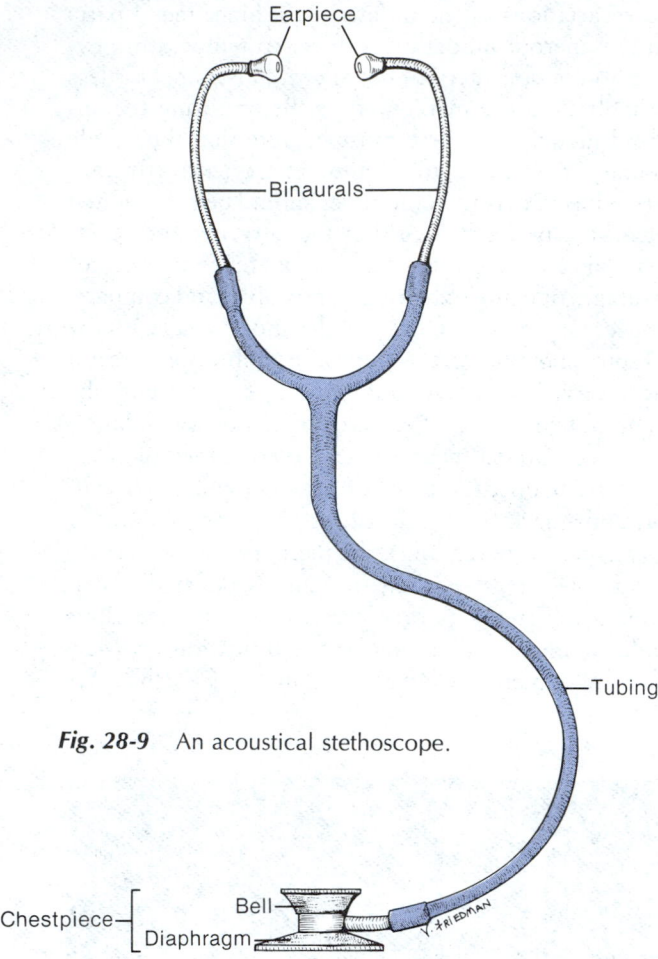

Earpiece

Binaurals

Tubing

Fig. 28-9 An acoustical stethoscope.

Chestpiece — Bell

Diaphragm

comes too tightly closed, the deflation of the pressure cuff will be difficult to regulate. The pressure bulb is made of a tough rubber and should be free of leaks.

STETHOSCOPE

The acoustical stethoscope is the instrument most commonly used for auscultation. Usually sound waves originating from an internal organ reach the body's surface and are dissipated into the air. Unless the sounds are of a high amplitude, the unassisted ear cannot hear them clearly. The stethoscope is a closed cylinder that prevents the dissipation of sound waves as they reach the body's surface and amplifies them for the examiner (Fig. 28-9). The four major parts of the stethoscope are the earpieces, binaurals, plastic or rubber tubing, and chestpiece. The nurse uses a stethoscope extensively in her practice and therefore should invest in a well-made instrument.

The earpieces should fit snugly and comfortably in the nurse's ears. The binaurals should be angled and strong enough that the earpieces stay firmly in the ears without causing discomfort. To ensure the best reception of sound, the earpieces follow the contour of the ear canal. For most persons, therefore, the earpieces should point toward the face as the stethoscope is put on.

The rubber or plastic tubing should be flexible and 30 to 40 cm (12 to 18 inches) in length. Longer tubing decreases the transmission of sound waves through the stethoscope. The tubing should be thick walled to help eliminate transmission of extraneous noises when the tubing rubs against other surfaces.

The chestpiece should include a bell and a diaphragm. The diaphragm is the circular, flat-surfaced portion of the chestpiece and has a thin plastic disk on the end. It transmits high-pitched sounds such as bowel and lung sounds best. To receive full amplification of sound through the diaphragm, the examiner holds it firmly against the skin. The bell transmits low-pitched sounds such as heart and vascular sounds. The bell is held lightly against the skin (Fig. 28-10). Compressing the bell against the client's skin reduces sound amplification. The bell and diaphragm are rotated into position on the chestpiece depending on which part the nurse chooses to use. The diaphragm or bell must be in proper position during use in order for the nurse to hear sounds through the stethoscope.

Assessment of Blood Pressure

Arterial blood pressure may be measured either directly or indirectly. The direct method requires the insertion of a thin catheter into a client's artery. Tubing connects the catheter with electronic monitoring

curate readings are obtained only by looking at the meniscus of the mercury at eye level. Looking up or down at the mercury results in measurement distortions.

Cuffs for measurement are available in several sizes (newborn to extra large). Ideally the width of the inflatable bladder within the cuff should be 40% of the circumference (or 20% wider than the diameter) of the midpoint of the limb on which the cuff is to be used (American Heart Association, 1980). For an average adult arm a bladder 12 to 14 cm (4.8 to 5.6 inches) wide is satisfactory. The length of the bladder should be approximately twice the recommended width. A bladder of this length nearly encircles the arm and minimizes the risk of misapplication. An improperly fitting cuff produces inaccurate blood pressure readings. A cuff that is too wide causes falsely low readings, and a narrow cuff can cause falsely high readings.

Before using a sphygmomanometer the nurse should manipulate the parts of the pressure bulb and release valve. The valve should be clean and freely adjustable in either direction. If a valve sticks or be-

equipment. The monitor displays a constant arterial pressure reading. Because of the risk of sudden blood loss from an artery, direct monitoring is used only in an intensive care setting.

The indirect method requires use of the sphygmomanometer. The nurse may choose to use either of two indirect techniques: auscultation and palpation. Assessing the blood pressure indirectly by auscultation is the most widely used technique.

AUSCULTATION

The best environment for blood pressure measurement by auscultation is a quiet room at a comfortable temperature. Although the client may lie or stand, sitting is the preferred position. In most cases blood pressure readings obtained with the client in the supine, sitting, and standing positions are similar. In some clients, however, blood pressure changes with position. The nurse may compare sitting and standing blood pressure readings to determine whether a change occurs. Orthostatic hypotension, or the lowering of blood pressure when the client moves from a sitting to a standing position, results from reduced blood volume and is a side effect of antihypertensive medications. The client's blood pressure should always be measured before administering such medications.

The client's position should be the same during each measurement to permit a meaningful comparison of values. The nurse should attempt to control factors such as pain, anxiety, exposure to cold, exertion, and eating or smoking before the assessment, since they can cause artificially high readings.

During a client's initial assessment the nurse should measure the blood pressure in both arms. Normally there is a difference of 5 to 10 mm Hg between the arms. In subsequent assessments the blood pressure should be measured in the arm with the higher pressure. Pressure differences greater than 10 mm Hg indicate conditions such as aortic stenosis or an arterial occlusion in the arm with the lower pressure.

When the client is positioned comfortably, any constricting clothing that interferes with cuff or stethoscope application should be removed. A loose-fitting gown is ideal. The nurse should relax while assessing the client's blood pressure, since a look of concern might cause the client undue anxiety.

The nurse asks the client his normal blood pressure. If the client does not know, the nurse informs him of her findings. This is a good opportunity to educate a client about normal blood pressure and the dangers of hypertension. Procedure 28-6 describes blood pressure auscultation.

Indirect measurement of arterial blood pressure works on a basic principle of pressure. The external

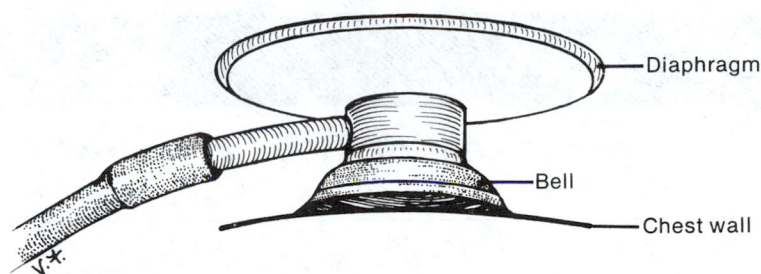

Fig. 28-10 Chestpiece with bell and diaphragm.

application of pressure beyond that which keeps a vessel open causes the vessel to close. For example, in a client with a normal blood pressure of 120/80 mm Hg, blood flows freely through the brachial artery at a systolic pressure of 120 mm Hg. Inflation of the cuff gradually applies pressure to tissues surrounding the brachial artery. When the cuff pressure exceeds 120 mm Hg, the artery collapses, blood flow ceases, and auscultation reveals an absence of sounds. When the cuff pressure is released, the point on the manometer at which sounds reappear through auscultation is the client's systolic pressure.

Korotkoff, a Russian surgeon, first described the sounds heard over an artery during cuff deflation in 1905. The first Korotkoff sound is a clear rhythmical tapping that gradually increases in intensity. *The systolic blood pressure is recorded as the point at which the first sound appears.* As the cuff pressure continues to decrease, a murmur or swishing sound appears. This second Korotkoff sound occurs as the vessel distends with blood, creating vibrations in the vessel wall. The third Korotkoff sound is crisper and more intense. At this phase the vessel remains open in systole but obliterates in diastole. The muffling of this sound marks the fourth Korotkoff sound. At this point the cuff pressure falls below the intraluminal pressure within the vessel. The final or fifth Korotkoff sound is actually an absence of sound. Institutions vary as to the final sound to use in recording the diastolic blood pressure. *In adults the diastolic pressure is usually considered to be the point at which Korotkoff sounds disappear.* However, many physicians prefer recording both the fourth and fifth sounds. Often Korotkoff sounds do not disappear in a child before the manometer reaches 0 mm Hg. *For this reason many clinicians use the appearance of the fourth sound, or muffling of Korotkoff sounds, to indicate the diastolic pressure in children.*

When the sound has ceased, the nurse deflates the cuff rapidly and removes it from the client's arm. If the nurse is unsure of a reading, a colleague should check the pressure.

PROCEDURE 28-6

Assessment of Blood Pressure by Auscultation

STEPS	RATIONALE
1. Assemble the sphygmomanometer and stethoscope.	
2. Determine the proper cuff size.	The proper cuff size is necessary so the correct amount of pressure is applied over the artery.
3. Wash your hands.	Washing removes microorganisms to prevent transmission to the client.
4. Explain the purpose of the procedure.	Explanations reassure the client.
5. Assist the client to a comfortable sitting position, with arm slightly flexed, forearm supported at heart level, and palm turned up.	Having the arm above heart level would produce a false low reading. This position facilitates cuff application.
6. Expose the upper arm fully.	Exposing the upper arm ensures proper cuff application.
7. Palpate the brachial artery. Position the cuff 2.5 cm (1 inch) above the site of brachial artery pulsation (antecubital space).	
8. Center the arrows marked on the cuff over the brachial artery.	Inflating the bladder directly over the brachial artery ensures that proper pressure is applied during inflation.
9. Be sure the cuff is fully deflated. Wrap the cuff evenly and snugly around the upper arm.	This ensures that proper pressure will be applied over the artery.
10. Be sure the manometer is positioned at eye level.	Eye level placement ensures accurate reading of mercury level.
11. If you do not know the client's normal systolic pressure, palpate the radial artery and inflate the cuff to a pressure 30 mm Hg above the point at which radial pulsation disappears. Deflate the cuff and wait 30 seconds.	This determines the maximal inflation point and prevents ausculatory gap. The 30-second delay prevents venous congestion and falsely high readings.
12. Place the stethoscope earpieces in the ears and be sure sounds are clear, not muffled.	Each earpiece should follow the angle of the examiner's ear canal to facilitate hearing.
13. Relocate the brachial artery and place the diaphragm (or the bell) of the stethoscope over it.	Proper stethoscope placement ensures optimal sound reception. The American Heart Association recommends use of the bell for hearing the low-pitched Korotkoff sounds clearly.

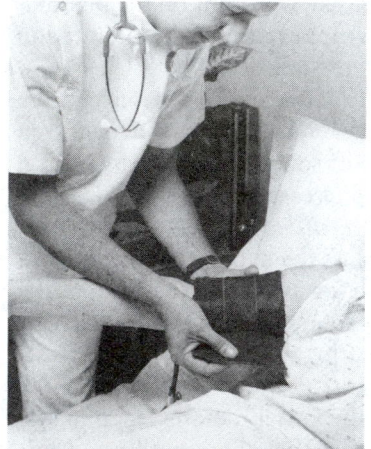

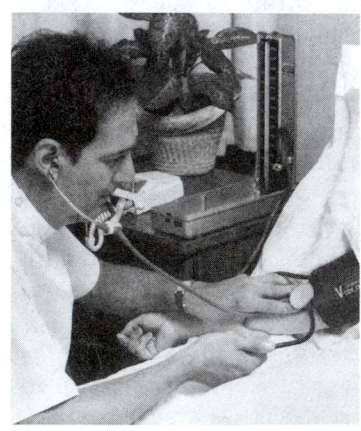

Assessment of Blood Pressure by Auscultation

STEPS	RATIONALE
14. Close the valve of the pressure bulb clockwise until tight.	Tightening the valve prevents air leak during inflation.
15. Inflate the cuff to 30 mm Hg above the client's normal systolic level.	Proper cuff inflation ensures accurate pressure measurement.
16. Slowly release the valve, allowing the mercury to fall at a rate of 2 to 3 mm Hg per second.	Too rapid or slow decline in the mercury level may lead to an inaccurate reading.
17. Note the point on the manometer at which the first clear sound is heard.	The first Korotkoff sound indicates the systolic pressure.
18. Continue to deflate the cuff gradually, noting the point at which a muffled or dampened sound appears.	The fourth Korotkoff sound may be recorded as the diastolic pressure in adults with hypertension. The American Heart Association recommends it as the indication of diastolic pressure in children.
19. Continue cuff deflation, noting the point on the manometer at which sound disappears.	The American Heart Association recommends recording the fifth Korotkoff sound as the diastolic pressure in adults.
20. Deflate the cuff rapidly and remove it from the client's arm unless you need to repeat the measurement.	Continuous cuff inflation causes arterial occlusion, resulting in numbness and tingling of the client's arm.
21. If repeating the procedure, wait 30 seconds.	The delay prevents venous congestion and falsely high readings.
22. Fold the cuff and store it properly.	Proper maintenance of supplies contributes to instrument accuracy.
23. Assist the client to the position he prefers and cover his upper arm.	This maintains the client's comfort.
24. Record findings on the medical record or flowsheet.	Vital signs should be recorded immediately.

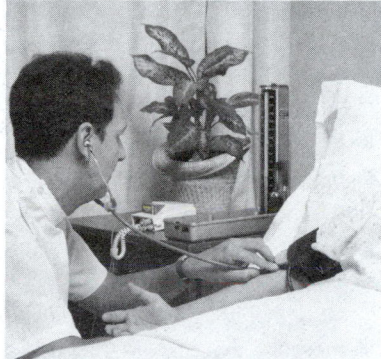

TABLE 28-5

Common Mistakes in Blood Pressure Assessment

Error	Effect
Bladder or cuff too wide	False low reading
Bladder or cuff too narrow	False high reading
Cuff wrapped too loosely	False high reading
Deflating cuff too slowly	False high diastolic reading
Deflating cuff too quickly	False low systolic and false high diastolic reading
Stethoscope that fits poorly or impairment of the examiner's hearing, causing sounds to be muffled	False low systolic and false high diastolic reading
Inaccurate inflation level	False low systolic reading
Multiple examiners using different Korotkoff sounds	Inaccurate interpretation of systolic and diastolic readings

The American Heart Association (1980) recommends recording two numbers for a blood pressure measurement: the points on the manometer when the first sound is heard for systolic and when the fifth sound is heard for diastolic. Some institutions recommend recording the point when the fourth sound is heard as well, especially for clients with hypertension. The numbers are divided by slashed lines (for example, 120/80 or 120/100/80), and the arm used to measure the blood pressure is noted (for example, RA 130/70).

There are several possibilities for error if the auscultation procedure is not followed correctly. Table 28-5 summarizes common mistakes in measurement.

ASSESSMENT OF BLOOD PRESSURE IN CHILDREN

Because of a child's small arm size and tendency to be anxious or restless during an examination, auscultation of blood pressure can be a problem in children. Korotkoff sounds are difficult to hear in infants because of the sound's low frequency and amplitude.

The same criteria for cuff size in adults apply to cuffs for children. The inflatable bladder must completely or nearly completely encircle the extremity.

When pressure is being assessed, an infant or child under 5 years of age should lie supine with the arms supported at heart level. Older children may sit. It is important to have the child relaxed and calm. A delay of at least 15 minutes before taking a reading is recommended to allow the child to recover from recent activity or apprehension.

The nurse uses the same technique of auscultation that is employed in adults. In an infant the auscultatory sounds may be too faint to hear. In such a case ultrasonic stethoscopes capable of detecting low-frequency sounds are very useful. If an ultrasonic stethoscope is unavailable, an indirect method called the flush method can be used to measure blood pressure. In this method a cuff is placed on the infant's wrist or ankle. The nurse raises the infant's extremity and compresses the hand or foot distal to the cuff in a firmly wrapped elastic bandage. When the extremity is compressed, the nurse lowers it to heart level and inflates the cuff to 200 mm Hg. The nurse quickly removes the bandage and lowers the manometer pressure at a rate not exceeding 5 mm Hg per second. The mean or average blood pressure is denoted by the appearance of a flush or return of color in the infant's hand or foot. This measurement is more accurate when it is performed in a well-lit room so the nurse can clearly observe the flush. The flush technique has the potential for increasing an infant's discomfort or restlessness and thus may cause a false high reading.

PALPATION

The indirect palpation technique is useful for clients whose arterial pulsations are too weak to create Korotkoff sounds. Severe blood loss and weakened myocardial contractility are examples of conditions that result in blood pressures too low to auscultate accurately.

The blood pressure cuff is applied in the same manner as in the auscultation method. The radial artery is palpated throughout the procedure instead of using a stethoscope. When the cuff is inflated to the desired level, the valve is released and the mercury is allowed to fall 2 mm Hg per second. As soon as the radial pulse is again palpable, the manometer reading is noted. This reading is the systolic blood pressure. The diastolic pressure is difficult to determine by palpation. A subtle change in sensation, usually in the form of a thin snapping vibration, marks the diastolic level. When the palpation technique is used, the systolic value and the manner in which it was measured are recorded.

The palpation technique is used along with auscultation in some instances. In some clients, particularly hypertensive ones, the sounds usually heard over the brachial artery when the cuff pressure is high disappear as pressure is reduced and then reappear at a lower level. This temporary disappearance of sound is the *auscultatory gap*. It typically occurs between the first and second Korotkoff sounds. The gap in sound may cover a range of 40 mm Hg and thus may cause an underestimation of systolic pressure or overestimation of diastolic pressure. The examiner must be certain to inflate the cuff high enough to hear the true systolic pressure before the auscultatory gap. Palpation of the radial artery helps determine how high to inflate the cuff. The examiner inflates the cuff 30 mm Hg above the pressure at which the radial pulse was palpated. The range of pressures in which the auscultatory gap occurs is recorded (for example, "BP 180/94 with an auscultatory gap from 180 to 160").

ASSESSMENT OF BLOOD PRESSURE IN LOWER EXTREMITIES

Occasionally dressings, casts, intravenous catheters, or other devices make the upper extremities inaccessible, and blood pressure must be measured in the lower extremities. Also, in clients with certain blood pressure abnormalities it is helpful to compare upper extremity blood pressure with that in the legs. The popliteal artery, located behind the knee in the popliteal space, is the site for auscultation. The cuff must be wide and long enough to allow for the larger girth of the thigh. The cuff is positioned with the bladder over the posterior aspect of the midthigh. Placing the client in a prone position is best. If such a position is impossible, the client should be asked to flex his knee slightly for easier access to the artery. The procedure is the same as with brachial artery auscultation. Systolic pressure in the legs is usually higher by 10 to 40 mm Hg than in the brachial artery, but the diastolic pressure is essentially the same.

Coin-Operated Sphygmomanometer

Coin-operated computerized machines for measuring blood pressure are now available in public places. These machines have appeared as a result of greater public interest in health maintenance, and the nurse should be generally familiar with them so she can answer clients' questions and offer information.

The consumer sits in front of the machine. His arm rests within the inflatable cuff, which contains a pressure sensor. The cuff fits over the clothing. A visual display informs the user of his blood pressure in 60 to 90 seconds, a considerably longer time than with the manual method.

The American Heart Association (1980) does not recommend using coin-operated sphygmomanometers because of their questionable accuracy. Often the machines are placed in areas where environmental noise is high, which may interfere with the computer's function. Improper cuff placement is a common problem. Furthermore, many of the machines do not have educational material available to encourage follow-up visits to a physician.

The National High Blood Pressure Education Program Coordinating Committee (1980) points out the following advantages of home and coin-operated sphygmomanometers:

1. Readily available blood pressure measurement helps motivate clients receiving antihypertensive medication to maintain the therapeutic regimen.
2. Measurement of blood pressure at home, at work, or in public places may encourage involvement of client and family in the treatment program.
3. Promotion and accessibility of machines can reinforce the importance of blood pressure measurement.
4. Multiple measurements outside health care settings assist in treatment decisions and in evaluating efficacy of prescribed therapy for hypertension.

The committee notes two concerns:

1. Availability of blood pressure devices in public places may cause clients to become overly conscious of their blood pressures and to misinterpret the results.
2. A blood pressure reading without an explanation of its significance and limitations of reading is a questionable public service.

The nurse has the responsibility to advise clients of the possible inaccuracies in coin-operated sphygmomanometers. A client whose blood pressure has been reported to be high by a machine should be encouraged to see his physician to confirm the blood pressure reading. Using coin-operated devices is probably better than not having blood pressure checked at all; however, the client must understand the meaning and implications of the readings.

Reporting and Recording Vital Signs

The measurement of vital signs is useless unless values are appropriately recorded and abnormalities are reported. In the hospital setting physicians often prescribe values beyond which vital signs should be reported to them. A typical order is, "Call physician

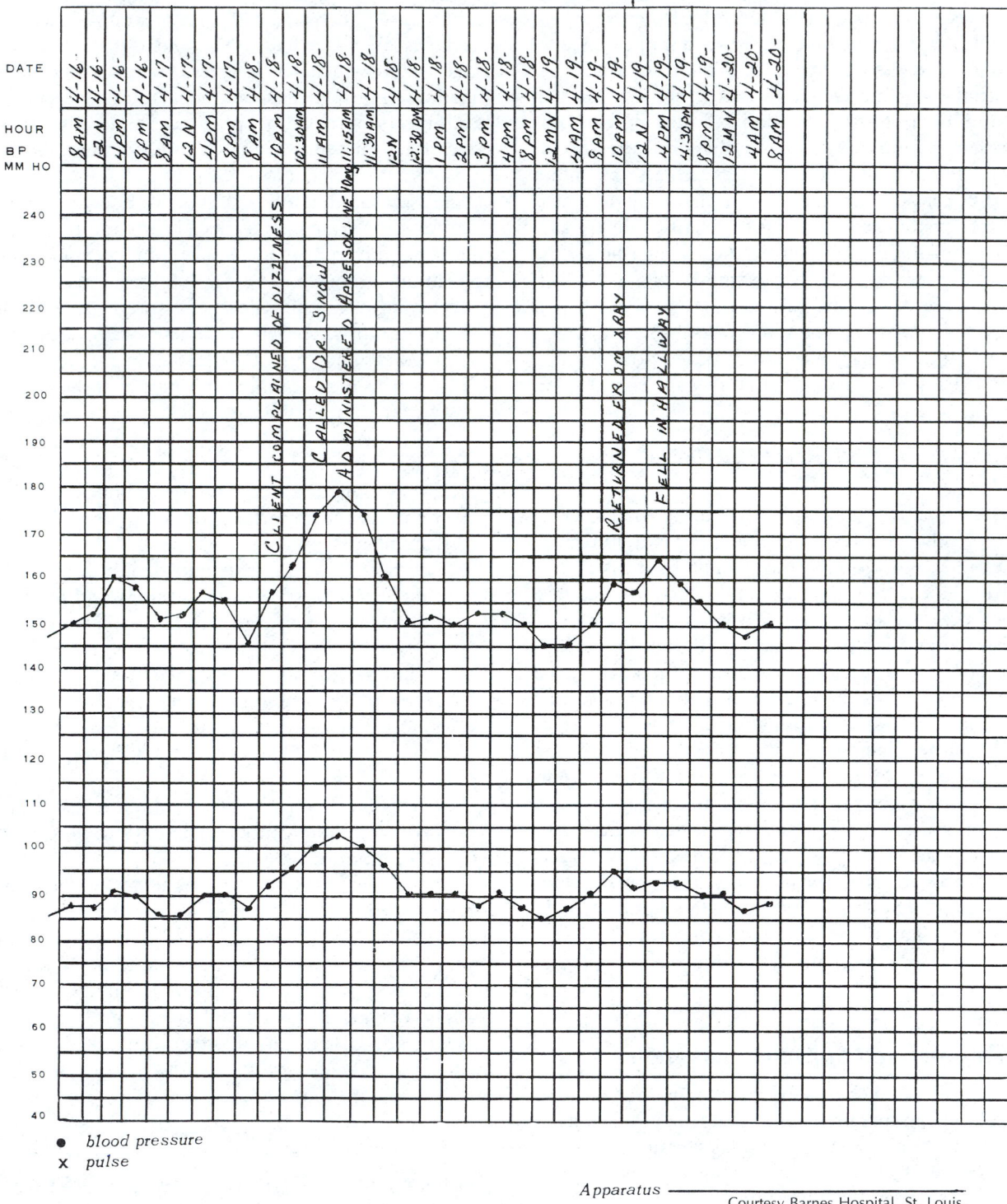

Fig. 28-11 Sample blood pressure chart for 4 days of measurement, showing systolic pressure *(top line)* and diastolic pressure *(bottom line)*. Note the diurnal variation over the first 2 days. On the third and fourth days assessment was made more frequently because of the client's report of symptoms, the observed rise in pressure, and the administration of antihypertensive medication.

if systolic ≥160 mm Hg and diastolic ≥100 mm Hg.''

Graphs on which vital sign values can be charted simplify recording. Fig. 28-11 shows a sample form. Additional significant information, such as symptoms precipitating vital sign measurements (for example, chest pain, dizziness, and flushing) and abnormalities in the vital signs, is recorded in the nurse's progress notes. The nurse documents any interventions initiated as a result of vital sign measurement. Whenever a significant change in the client's vital signs is assessed, it is reported immediately to the appropriate personnel.

Summary

Vital sign measurements are a basic series of physiological assessments that reflect a client's health status. The nurse uses these data in making clinical decisions. Various physical and psychological factors can create changes in vital signs. However, if the nurse knows the physiological nature of each vital sign, reasons for any variations from normal, and the clinical implication of abnormal values, she can make accurate judgments regarding the need for intervention.

The nurse is frequently the health care provider who has the greatest contact with clients. Therefore it is the nurse who decides the need for and frequency of vital sign assessment. Assessment of vital signs is not simply a routine chore but rather an integral part of a nurse's practice. The nurse will be more successful in incorporating vital sign measurement into practice by following certain guidelines, such as knowing a client's normal range of vital signs and using a systematic assessment approach.

Before measuring any vital sign, the nurse should understand the physiological controls governing it. For example, body temperature is a balance between heat loss and heat production, and blood pressure is a product of cardiac output and peripheral vascular resistance. Each physiological control is influenced by certain variables such as age, physical exercise, or hormonal changes. When the nurse understands the effects of these variables, she is better prepared to anticipate normal variations in vital signs. A nurse cannot recognize abnormalities without first knowing what is normal.

Basic principles apply in the procedures for assessing vital signs accurately. Good medical aseptic technique should be used. The client should be placed in the most comfortable position that is suitable for measurements. Procedures should be explained to the client to reduce anxiety. The nurse should not rush through an assessment and should not estimate values. All characteristics of a vital sign are assessed. Results are recorded promptly and accurately.

Assessment of vital signs is among the easiest of physical assessments. A deliberate, knowledgeable approach to measurement ensures accurate, complete results.

KEY CONCEPTS

✓ Vital signs may be measured as part of a complete physical examination or more commonly in a review of the client's condition.

✓ The nurse assesses vital sign changes in conjunction with other physical assessment findings.

✓ The nurse uses her own judgment in determining the frequency of vital sign measurement.

✓ Knowledge of the factors that influence vital signs assists the nurse in interpreting abnormal values.

✓ Vital signs are a basis for evaluating a client's response to nursing interventions.

✓ Assessment of vital signs yields the most accurate values when the client is inactive and the environment is controlled for the client's comfort.

✓ Normally, heat production balances heat loss to maintain body temperature.

✓ The nurse assists the client in maintaining body temperature by initiating interventions that promote heat loss or heat production.

✓ The oral route is the most accessible and acceptable site for temperature measurement, but the rectal temperature most accurately reflects the body's core temperature.

✓ Characteristics of a pulse reflect the status of a client's cardiovascular function.

✓ The pulse of a normal healthy adult is strong, full, and rhythmical and averages 80 beats per minute.

✓ The nurse assesses the presence and character of peripheral pulses to determine the adequacy of local blood flow.

✓ Assessment of respirations involves observation of ventilatory movements.

✓ Blood pressure levels reflect the relationship among several hemodynamic variables, and alterations in blood pressure can indicate altered health status.

✓ Blood pressure can be measured by either the auscultation or the palpation method.

✓ Changes in any vital sign can influence characteristics of the other vital signs.

REFERENCES

American Heart Association: Statement on automated blood pressure machines of the coin operated type, Dallas, 1979, The Association.

American Heart Association: Recommendations for human blood pressure determination by sphygmomanometers, Dallas, 1980, The Association.

Felton, C.L.: Hypoxemia and oral temperatures, Am. J. Nurs. 78:57, 1978.

Graves, R.P., and Markarian, M.F.: Three minute time intervals when using an oral mercury-in-glass thermometer with or without J-temp sheaths, Nurs. Res. 29:323, 1980.

Guyton, A.C.: Textbook of medical physiology, ed. 6, Philadelphia, 1981, W.B. Saunders Co.

Mountcastle, V.B.: Medical physiology, vol. 2, ed. 14, St. Louis, 1980, The C.V. Mosby Co.

National High Blood Pressure Education Program: Statement on blood pressure measurement devices used by consumers, Bethesda, Md., 1980, U.S. National Heart, Lung and Blood Institute.

Nichols, G.A., and Kucha, D.H.: Taking adult temperatures: oral measurement, Am. J. Nurs. 72:1090, 1972.

Petersdorf, R.C.: Disturbances of heat regulation. In Isselbacher, K.J., et al., editors: Harrison's principles of internal medicine, ed. 9, New York, 1980, McGraw-Hill Book Co.

ADDITIONAL READINGS

Adelman, E.M.: When the patient's blood pressure falls what does it mean? What should you do? Nursing 80 10:26, 1980.

Blainey, C.G.: Site selection in taking body temperatures, Am. J. Nurs. 74:1859, 1974.

Electronic thermometers, the better alternative? Health Devices 12:18, 1982.

Erickson, R.: Oral temperature differences in relation to thermometer and technique, Nurs. Res. 29:157, 1980.

Flynn, J.B., and Moore, P.V.: Coin operated sphygmomanometers, Am. J. Nurs. 81:533, 1981.

Porth, C.M., and Kaylor, L.E.: Temperature regulation in the newborn, Am. J. Nurs. 78:1691, 1978.

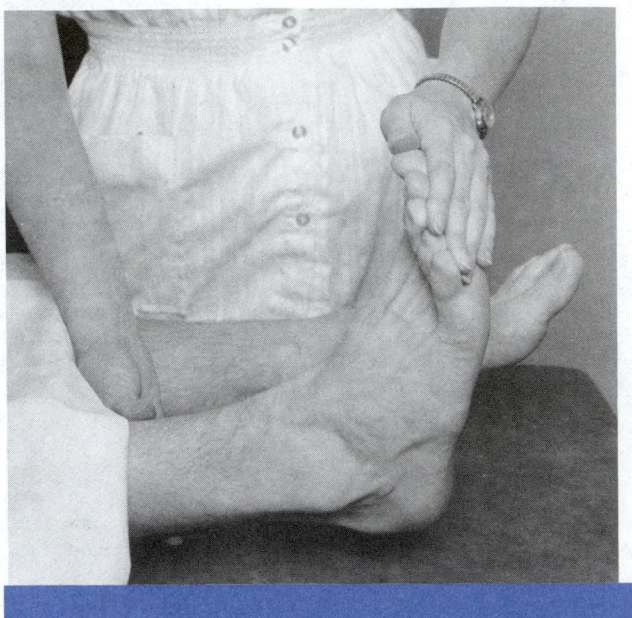

OBJECTIVES

Mastery of content in this chapter will enable the student to:

- Define the terms in the glossary.
- Discuss the purposes of physical assessment.
- Describe the techniques used with each of the physical assessment skills.
- Describe the proper position for the client during each phase of the examination.
- List techniques used to promote the client's physical and psychological comfort during an examination.
- Make needed environmental preparations before an examination.
- Use physical assessment skills during the performance of routine nursing care measures.
- Conduct physical assessments in an organized and proper fashion.
- Discuss ways to incorporate health teaching into the examination process.
- Describe physical measurements made in assessment of each body system.
- Summarize assessment findings on a physical examination form.

GLOSSARY

accommodation reflex Adjustment of the eyes for near vision, comprised of pupillary constriction, convergence of the visual axes, and increased convexity of the lens.

acromegaly Chronic metabolic condition caused by overproduction of growth hormone and characterized by gradual, marked enlargement and elongation of bones of the face, jaw, and extremities.

alopecia Partial or complete loss of hair; baldness.

anthropometry Measurement of various body parts to determine nutritional and caloric status, muscular development, brain growth, and other parameters.

atrophy Wasting or diminution of size or physiological activity of a part of the body caused by disease or other influences.

bilirubin Orange-yellow pigment of bile formed principally by the breakdown of hemoglobin in red blood cells.

borborygmus Audible abdominal sound produced by hyperactive intestinal peristalsis.

bruit Abnormal sound or murmur heard while auscultating an organ, gland, or artery.

buccal Of or pertaining to the inside of the cheek or the gum next to the cheek.

carcinoma Malignant epithelial neoplasm that tends to invade surrounding tissue and spread to distant regions of the body.

cirrhosis Chronic degenerative disease of the liver.

consensual light reflex Constriction of the pupil of one eye when the other eye is illuminated.

crackle Fine bubbling sound heard on auscultation of the lung; produced by air entering distal airways and alveoli, which contain serous secretions.

dorsal Pertaining to the back or posterior.

edema Abnormal accumulation of fluid in interstitial spaces of tissues.

emphysematous Of or pertaining to emphysema, an abnormal condition of the lungs, characterized by overinflation and destructive changes of alveolar walls.

exophthalmos Abnormal protrusion of one or both eyeballs.

friction rub Dry grating sound heard during auscultation, caused by rubbing of tissue surfaces.

gait Manner or style of walking, including rhythm, cadence, and speed.

glaucoma Abnormal condition of elevated pressure within the anterior chamber of the eye caused by obstructed outflow of aqueous humor.

gurgle Abnormal coarse sound heard during auscultation of the lung; produced by air entering large mucus-containing airways.

29 The Physical Examination

hirsutism   Excessive body hair in a masculine distribution caused by heredity, hormonal dysfunction, or medication.

hyperpigmentation   Unusual darkening of the skin.

integument   Skin and its appendages: hair, nails, and sweat and sebaceous glands.

jaundice   Yellow discoloration of the skin, mucous membranes, and sclera, caused by greater than normal amounts of bilirubin in the blood.

malabsorption syndrome   Set of symptoms resulting from disorders in the intestinal absorption of nutrients, characterized by anorexia, weight loss, bloating of the abdomen, and muscle cramps.

malignant tumor   Neoplasm that is anaplastic and invasive and that spreads to other body tissues.

melanin   Black or dark brown pigment that occurs naturally in the skin, hair, and iris.

ophthalmic   Of or pertaining to the eye.

pallor   Unnatural paleness or absence of color in the skin.

palpebra   Portion of the conjunctiva that lines the inner surface of the eyelids; it is thick, opaque, and highly vascular.

PERRLA   Acronym for "pupils equal, round, reactive to light, accommodative"; the acronym is recorded in the physical examination if eye and pupil assessment is normal.

pigmentation   Organic coloring material, such as melanin, that gives color to the skin.

pleura   Delicate serous membrane enclosing the lung.

pleural cavity   Cavity within the thorax that contains the lungs.

point of maximal impulse (PMI)   Point where the heartbeat can most easily be palpated through the chest wall.

ptosis   Abnormal condition of one or both upper eyelids in which the eyelid droops, caused by weakness of the levator muscle or paralysis of the third cranial nerve.

rigidity   Condition of stiffness or inflexibility, as in muscle rigidity.

Rinne's test   Method of assessing auditory acuity useful in distinguishing conductive from sensorineural hearing loss.

sebaceous gland   One of the small organs in the dermis that secretes an oily substance (sebum) on the skin's surface and in the hair.

serous fluid   Clear fluid that reduces friction between structures covered by serous membranes, such as the lung.

sign   Objective finding perceived by an examiner, such as a fever, rash, abnormal reflex, or abnormal breath sound.

spasm   Involuntary muscle contraction of sudden onset.

systemic Of or pertaining to the whole body rather than to a localized area.

tracheostomy Opening through the neck into the trachea with an indwelling tube inserted; created surgically to produce an airway.

turgor Normal resiliency of the skin caused by the outward pressure of the cells and interstitial fluid.

uremia Presence of excessive amounts of urea and other nitrogenous wastes in the blood; occurs in renal failure.

ventral Of or pertaining to an anterior position, toward the abdomen.

vitiligo Benign acquired skin disease consisting of irregular patches of various sizes totally lacking in pigment; exposed areas of skin are most affected.

There is much to be learned about a client's physical condition. Some clients come to the physician's office, neighborhood clinic, or hospital with specific information to share about alterations in health status. Other clients may not be aware that they have physical or psychological abnormalities. The nurse uses every contact with the client to gather information pertinent to the client's welfare. A careful, detailed scrutiny of the body parts can help to reveal the nature and extent of any abnormalities. During a physical examination the skills of physical assessment become tools providing the nurse with the means to make intelligent and precise clinical judgments.

As the nurse becomes experienced in physical assessment, the practice of nursing becomes more rewarding because the nurse is better able to work as part of a decision-making team with the physician. Using the techniques of physical assessment makes the nurse more aware of a client's condition. The nurse learns to assess the same clinical variables the physician measures at the client's bedside or in a clinic or office setting. The accuracy and validity of a nurse's physical assessment have significant impact on the physician's choice of therapy. Continuity in health care management is improved when the nurse is able to make ongoing, objective, and comprehensive assessments.

Purposes of Physical Examination

A physical examination involves a comprehensive assessment of a client's overall physical condition and of each body system. The process of physical assessment entails the actual measurement of a body part's integrity and function. A complete physical examination is performed in the following situations:

1. For routine screening to promote preventive health care
2. As a requisite for eligibility for health insurance, military service, or a new job
3. During admission to a hospital

The nurse uses physical assessment skills for several purposes:

1. To expand and enrich the client's data base
2. To enable nursing management of a greater variety of client problems
3. To evaluate the effectiveness of nursing care
4. To develop a level of credibility in promoting the nurse-client relationship

Data Base

The nurse gathers thorough and detailed information about the client's health status with the nursing health history (see Chapter 7). However, a client may be unaware of a physical problem, so a thorough assessment of physical status is necessary. Even if a history is complete, a physical assessment reveals information that refutes, confirms, or supplements the existing data base. For example, the client may tell the nurse, "I've been having this terrible pain across the lower part of my back." The nurse may ask several questions to clarify the nature of the client's pain. However, unless the nurse sees the severe bruise across the client's back, the symptom of pain could suggest any of a number of ailments.

No one assessment finding can conclusively reveal the nature of an abnormality. Dryness of the tongue and mucous membranes is not alone indicative of dehydration. Further assessment is required for a definitive diagnosis. The nurse thus learns to group significant findings into patterns of data. In addition, each abnormal finding leads the nurse to ask questions about what additional information may be needed. A nurse who observes swelling of the client's ankles will decide what further areas need to be assessed: Skin color? Pulses? Movement of the extremity? As more data are collected, the nurse is able to identify the client's problems more easily.

The information gathered during an initial physical assessment provides a baseline of the client's functional abilities. The baseline is not necessarily a normal group of physical findings but rather the pattern of findings the nurse identifies when first assessing the client. During the client's subsequent hospital stay or clinic visit, the nurse repeats the assessment of pertinent physical variables. Any findings that differ from the baseline data suggest a change in the client's condition. For example, an initial examination may reveal the client's heart rate to be 84 beats per minute and regular with the blood pressure at 116/78 mm Hg. The same client undergoes extensive surgery and 1 day later is found by the nurse to have an irregular pulse of 112 beats per minute, with a blood pressure of 100/68 mm Hg. The nurse's assessment indicates a significant change in the client's condition, necessitating immediate action. Another example involves a client who has decreased range of motion in the knee following an injury. After the application of heat packs and the initiation of exercise, the nurse reassesses the knee's range of motion and finds improvement from the baseline level.

The nurse monitors the progress of a client's disease and response to therapy through physical assessment. Continued collection of data confirms existing medical and nursing diagnoses and promotes the identification of new problems.

Management of Client Problems

Any part of a physical examination may reveal information that can be used to plan the client's care. The nurse uses examination skills in making judgments about clients' problems and their management. For example, the nurse in a hospital observes the condition of the client's skin while bathing the client. A community health nurse measures the visual acuity of a diabetic client to assess for complications of the disease. The industrial nurse examines a client's wound suffered during a work-related accident.

After physical assessment (a part of the first stage of the nursing process), the nurse determines the nursing diagnosis (the second stage), and then plans the nursing measures to manage the client's problems (the third stage). Observing dry skin over the client's extremities alerts the nurse to avoid the use of soap during subsequent baths. The nurse teaches the client with diminishing visual acuity the importance of seeing an ophthalmologist regularly. The industrial nurse carefully cleans the client's wound to prevent infection. The nurse incorporates physical findings into nursing care and also notifies the physician of any findings that require medical diagnosis or intervention, such as the presence of skin lesions, decreased visual acuity, and active bleeding from a wound.

Performing the mechanics of physical assessment is relatively simple. The more difficult challenge lies in relating findings to the decision-making process that follows. Knowledge of anatomy, physiology, and pathology complements the nurse's physical assessment skills, enabling the nurse to make accurate nursing diagnoses and implement appropriate nursing therapies.

Evaluation of Nursing Care

Each nurse is made accountable for her actions through evaluating the results of nursing care, the final stage of the nursing process. Physical assessment skills provide a dimension that enhances the evaluation of nursing measures through the monitoring of physiological outcomes of care (see Chapter 11). Two examples may clarify this: The nurse determines that a client suffering pulmonary congestion will benefit from deep breathing exercises and coughing to remove secretions. A client who is forced to remain in bed for a prolonged time may need elastic stockings applied to promote circulation in his legs. In each example the nurse uses physical assessment skills to evaluate the efficacy of the interventions. By auscultating the lungs, the nurse is able to determine whether pulmonary congestion was alleviated. Inspection of the skin's color and palpation of distal pulses inform the nurse as to whether the elastic stockings are too tight.

Physical assessment skills offer the means to make detailed objective measurements. It is helpful to know when the client with difficulty breathing feels that the lungs are less congested. However, the improved character of breath sounds as heard with a stethoscope provides more relevant findings. The nurse relies less on assumption and second guessing when physical assessment is used to evaluate effectiveness of nursing care.

Credibility between Nurse and Client

The nurse gains the client's trust through competency. As the client witnesses the nurse's actions, trust can be either won or lost on the basis of the nurse's skills. The client appreciates the attentive nurse who painstakingly inspects the condition of a wound, gently palpates a painful abdomen, or listens to the lungs to be assured that everything is normal. When the nurse's findings complement those of the physician, the client realizes that the nurse is a professional. Performing a physical examination is an important action for the nurse in establishing a meaningful relationship with the client.

Integration of Physical Assessment with Nursing Care

Nurses in community agencies, screening clinics, schools, and private practice typically perform complete physical examinations. The nurse caring for clients in a hospital or nursing home is more likely to perform only parts of a physical examination at any given time. In all settings physical examination should be integrated with the nurse's routine care. For example, as the client is bathed, the nurse has the opportunity to inspect all body parts. While assisting a client walking down the hallway, the nurse is able to assess the client's gait and lower leg strength. During meals the nurse observes the client's dexterity in using eating utensils and the ability to swallow foods.

The nurse uses all senses when working with the client. The nurse's eyes, ears, hands, nose, and even taste assess the client as he interacts with the environment. As the nurse cultivates these senses, every minute spent with the client becomes useful. Findings gathered through the nurse's senses are made meaningful by association to previous experience and the nurse's own knowledge. For example, the nurse learns to recognize the difference between a distended abdomen and one that is rotund from obesity. Practice enables the nurse to recognize subtle differences between sounds heard with a stethoscope. Using the skills of physical assessment during the administration of nursing care helps the nurse gain expertise and confidence with these skills.

Skills of Physical Assessment

Chapter 7 briefly introduces the skills of inspection, palpation, percussion, and auscultation. This chapter provides a more detailed description of those skills, the additional skill of olfaction, and each skill's application in the physical examination.

Inspection

The nurse inspects or visually examines the client to detect significant physical signs. The nurse first learns to recognize normal physical characteristics before attempting to distinguish abnormal findings. Experience is needed to recognize normal variations among clients, as well as ranges of normal in an individual client.

Inspection is a simple technique, yet it is the most underused. Often a nurse hurries through an examination without taking the time to inspect the client thoroughly. For example, in a quick examination the nurse might fail to detect a rash under a client's arm.

The quality of the inspection depends on the observer's astuteness and willingness to spend time doing a thorough job.

Good lighting and exposure of the body part are essential for inspection. Each area is inspected for size, shape, color, symmetry, position, and abnormalities, such as lesions of the skin or mouth. If possible, each area inspected is compared with the same area on the opposite side of the body.

When body cavities are inspected, an additional source of light is required. A simple penlight can be used to inspect the oral cavity. An examination light is used to illuminate the vaginal canal.

The nurse who uses careful scrutiny during inspection will gain a wealth of information about the client. The resultant findings raise further questions requiring more in-depth examination. Palpation is often used with or after visual inspection.

Palpation

Further assessment of body parts is made through the sense of touch. The hands can make delicate and sensitive measurements of specific physical signs, so palpation is used to examine all accessible parts of the body (Table 29-1). The nurse uses different parts of the hand to detect such characteristics as texture, temperature, and the perception of movement.

TABLE 29-1

Palpation

Area of Body Examined	Criteria Measured by Palpation
Skin	Temperature, moisture, texture, turgor and elasticity, tenderness, thickness
Organs (e.g., liver, intestine)	Size, shape, presence of tenderness, presence or absence of masses, vibration of voice sounds (lung)
Glands (e.g., thyroid, lymph)	Swelling, symmetry, mobility
Blood vessels (e.g., carotid or femoral artery)	Pulse amplitude, elasticity, pulse rate, pulse rhythm
Muscles	Size, shape, tone, presence of tenderness, presence of spasm or rigidity
Bones	Symmetry, shape, presence of deformity, presence of tenderness

It is important for the client to be relaxed and positioned comfortably. A client's muscle tension during palpation impairs the assessor's ability to use this technique effectively. For example, tension of the abdominal muscles makes palpation of underlying organs impossible and mimics muscle rigidity. Asking the client to take slow deep breaths will enhance muscle relaxation. Tender areas are palpated last. The nurse can ask the client to point out the more sensitive areas and can note any nonverbal signs of discomfort.

The client will appreciate warm hands, short fingernails, and a gentle approach. Tactile pressure is applied in a slow, gentle, deliberate manner. Light palpation of structures such as the abdomen is done primarily to determine areas of tenderness. The nurse's hand is placed on the part to be examined and depressed about 1 cm (½ inch). Any tender areas found are examined further. The sensation of touch is best preserved with a light intermittent pressure. Heavy prolonged pressure causes a loss of sensitivity in the nurse's hand (Fig. 29-1).

The most sensitive parts of the hand, the pads of the fingertips, are used to assess texture, shape, size, consistency, and pulsatility (Fig. 29-2, *A*). Temperature is best measured using the dorsum or back of the hand (Fig. 29-2, *B*) and fingers, where the examiner's skin is thinnest. The palm of the hand (Fig. 29-2, *C*) is more sensitive to vibration. The nurse measures position, consistency, and turgor by lightly grasping the body part with the fingertips (Fig. 29-2, *D*).

After light palpation has been applied, deeper palpation is used to examine the condition of organs, such as those in the abdomen. The nurse depresses the area being examined approximately 2 cm (1 inch). Caution is the rule. A student nurse should not attempt deep palpation without the assistance of a qual-

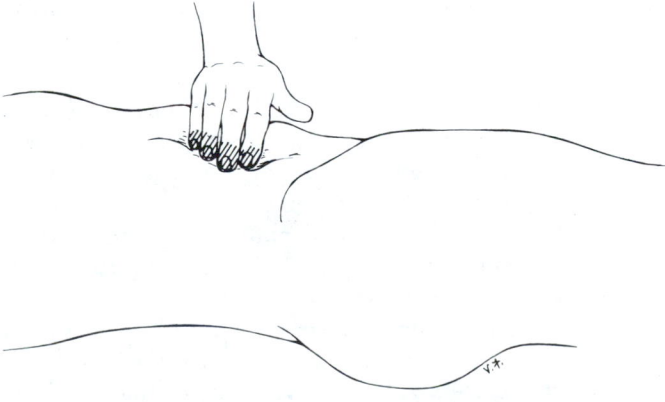

Fig. 29-1 During light palpation the nurse uses gentle pressure to depress the underlying body part. If the nurse detects areas of tenderness, the area is examined further.

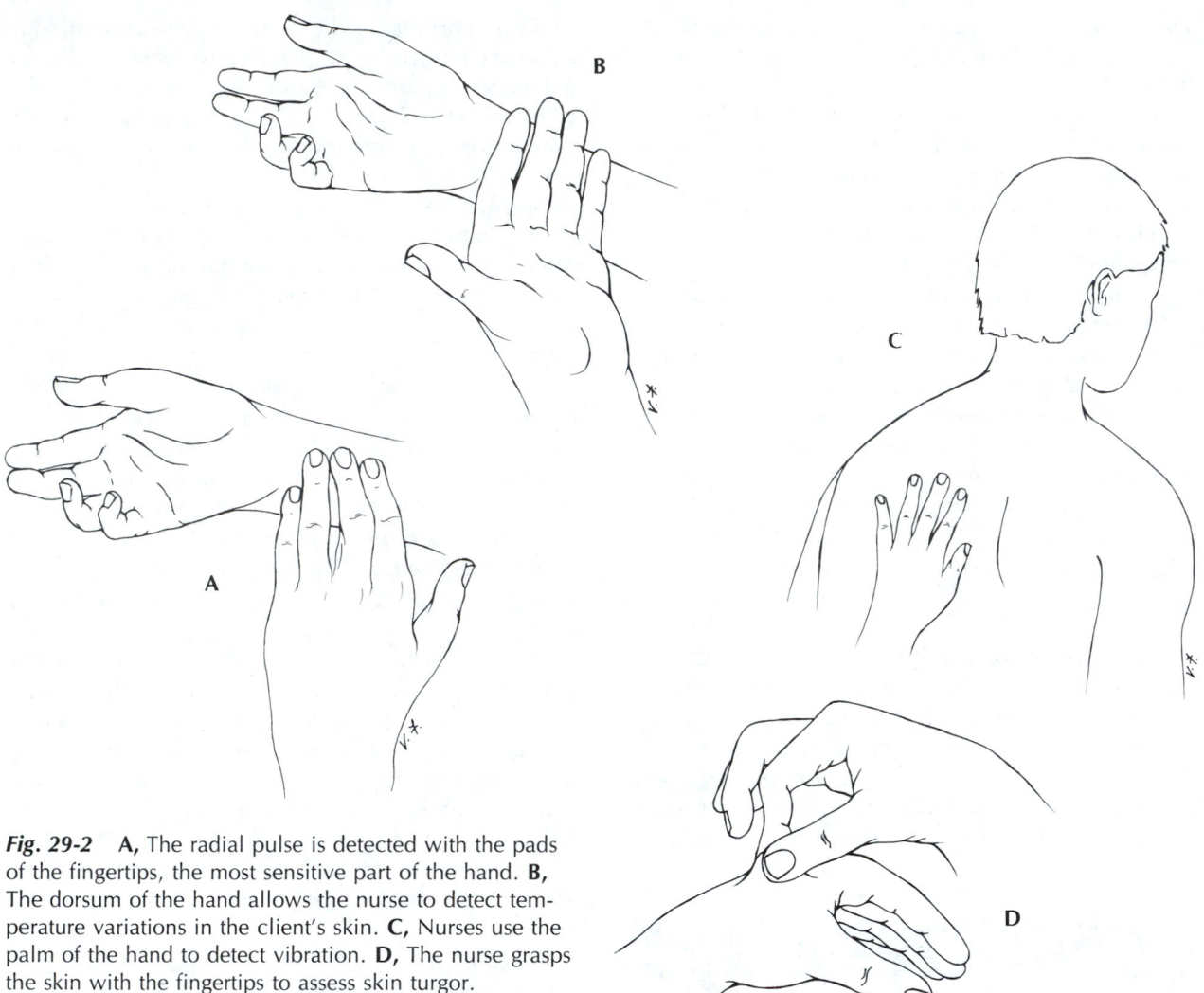

Fig. 29-2 **A,** The radial pulse is detected with the pads of the fingertips, the most sensitive part of the hand. **B,** The dorsum of the hand allows the nurse to detect temperature variations in the client's skin. **C,** Nurses use the palm of the hand to detect vibration. **D,** The nurse grasps the skin with the fingertips to assess skin turgor.

ified instructor, since deep prolonged pressure could cause internal injury. Deep palpation may be applied with one hand or both hands (bimanually) (Fig. 29-3). Each nurse develops an individual technique. When the nurse is using bimanual palpation, one hand (called the sensing hand) is relaxed and placed lightly over the client's skin. The other hand (active hand) applies pressure to the sensing hand. The lower hand does not exert pressure directly and thus retains the sensitivity needed to detect organ characteristics.

The nurse must not use palpation without giving careful consideration to the client and his condition. If the client is reported to have a fractured rib, extreme care is used when locating the painful area. A vital artery is not palpated with pressure sufficient to obstruct blood flow. The nurse must consider the area of the body being examined and the reason for using palpation, and must have the ability to discriminate and interpret the significance of what is being sensed.

Percussion

Percussion is the physical assessment skill that requires the most dexterity. Through percussion the location, size, and density of an underlying structure are determined. Percussion helps to verify abnormalities assessed through palpation and auscultation. For example, if the nurse hears abnormal breath sounds while auscultating the lungs, percussion may rule out the presence of fluid in the lungs. When the examiner strikes the body's surface with a finger, vibration and sound are produced. This vibration is transmitted through the body tissues, and the character of the sound heard depends on the density of the underlying tissue. For example, the normal lung transmits sounds with high intensity and low pitch, whereas the more solid liver transmits a high-pitched sound of soft intensity. By knowing how various densities influence sound, the nurse is able to locate organs or masses, map their boundaries, and determine their size. An

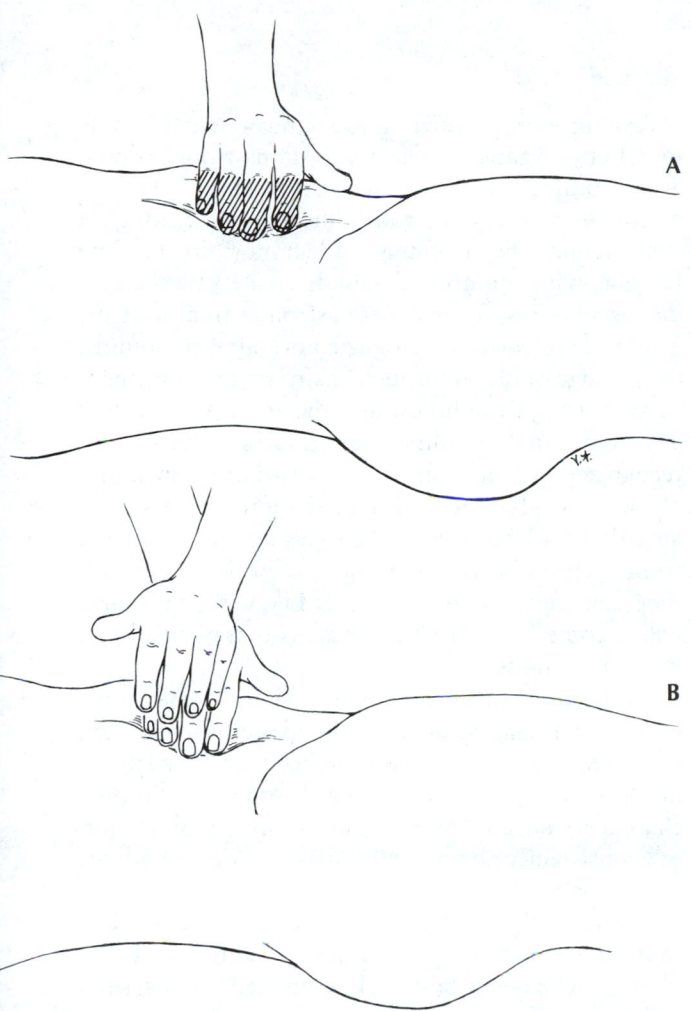

abnormal sound suggests the presence of a mass or substance such as fluid within an organ or body cavity.

There are two methods of percussion: direct and indirect. The direct method involves striking the body surface directly with the fingers. Typically one or two fingers are used. The indirect technique is performed by placing the middle finger of the examiner's nondominant hand (called the pleximeter) firmly against the body surface. With palm and fingers remaining off the skin, the tip of the middle finger of the dominant hand (called the plexor) strikes the base of the distal joint of the pleximeter (Fig. 29-4). The examiner uses a quick, sharp stroke with the plexor finger, keeping the forearm stationary (Fig. 29-5). The wrist must remain relaxed to deliver the proper blow. If the blow is not sharp, if the pleximeter is held loosely, or if the palm rests on the body surface, the sound is dampened or softened, preventing transmission of sound to underlying structures. The same force must be applied to each area so an accurate comparison of sounds can be made. A light, quick blow usually produces the clearest sound.

Percussion produces five types of sounds: tympany, resonance, hyperresonance, dullness, and flatness. Each sound is typically created by certain types of underlying tissues. Each sound is judged by its inten-

Fig. 29-3   **A,** During deep palpation the nurse depresses the underlying tissues approximately 2 cm (1 inch). Deep palpation allows the nurse to assess the condition of underlying organs. **B,** Position of hands for bimanual palpation. The underlying sensing hand detects the condition of underlying tissues and organs.

Fig. 29-4   To perform indirect percussion the nurse places the middle finger of the nondominant hand against the body's surface. The tip of the middle finger of the dominant hand strikes the tip of the middle finger of the nondominant hand.

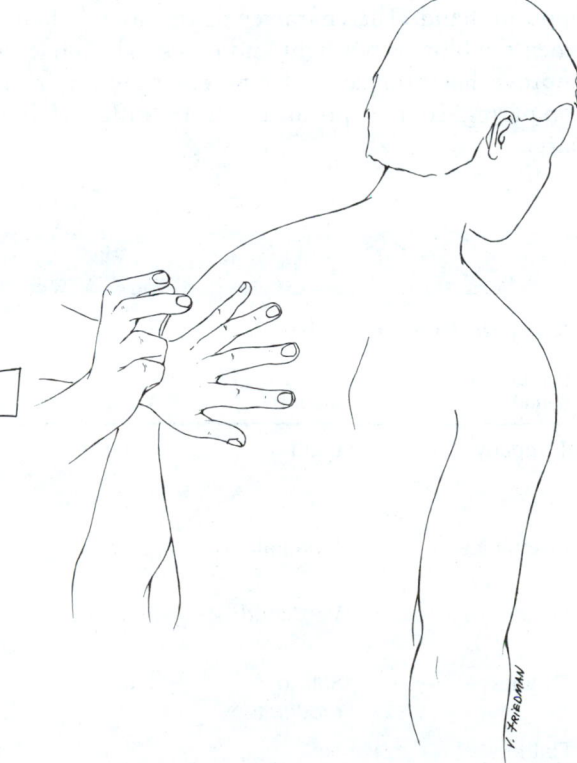

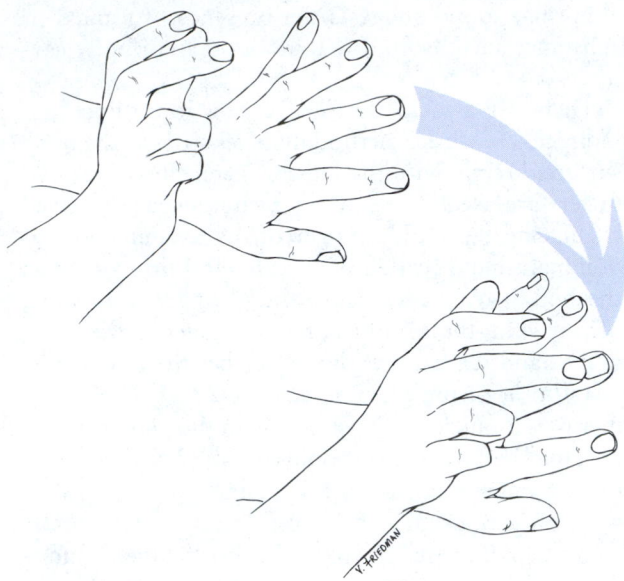

Fig. 29-5 A quick light wrist action ensures a clear sound during percussion.

sity, pitch, duration, and quality. Table 29-2 summarizes characteristics of percussion sounds.

Becoming proficient in percussion takes considerable practice. The nurse should practice flexing the wrist by keeping the forearm stationary. The hand could be placed on the surface of a table and the middle finger struck with the middle finger of the opposite hand. The character of the sound changes when the blow is not light and quick. The nurse can improve her proficiency by practicing on a friend, comparing sounds produced from different body parts.

Auscultation

Auscultation is listening to sounds created in various body organs to detect variations from normal. Some sounds can be heard with the unassisted ear, although most sounds can be heard only through a stethoscope. The beginning student must first become familiar with the normal sounds created by the cardiovascular, respiratory, and gastrointestinal systems. The student learns to recognize normal heart sounds, the passage of blood through an artery, the movement of air through the lungs, and the sounds of normal gastrointestinal motility. Abnormal sounds can be recognized only after the normal variations in sound are learned. The nurse becomes more successful in auscultation by knowing the types of sounds arising from each body structure and the location in which they can most easily be heard. Likewise, the nurse will become familiar with the areas that normally do not emit sounds.

To become proficient in auscultation the nurse needs good hearing acuity, a good stethoscope, and knowledge of how to use a stethoscope properly. A nurse with any type of hearing disorder should purchase a stethoscope with greater sound amplification or consistently have colleagues validate findings through auscultation.

Chapter 28 describes the parts of the acoustical stethoscope and the general use of the bell and diaphragm. The bell is best for low-pitched sounds, such as heart and vascular sounds, and the diaphragm is best for high-pitched sounds, such as bowel and lung sounds.

A nurse must become familiar with the stethoscope before attempting to use it with a client. It would be helpful to practice using the stethoscope with a friend.

TABLE 29-2

Sounds Produced by Percussion

Percussion Sound	Intensity	Pitch	Duration	Quality	Anatomical Location Where Examiner Hears Sounds
Tympany	Loud	High	Moderate	Drumlike	Enclosed air-containing space: gastric air bubble, puffed-out cheek
Resonance	Moderate to loud	Low	Long	Hollow	Normal lung
Hyperresonance	Very loud	Very low	Longer than resonance	Booming	Emphysematous lung
Dullness	Soft to moderate	High	Moderate	Thudlike	Liver
Flatness	Soft	High	Short	Flat	Muscle

A number of extraneous sounds created by movement of the tubing or chestpiece will interfere with auscultation of body organ sounds. By deliberately producing these sounds, the nurse can learn to recognize and disregard them during the actual examination. The boxed material below presents a number of exercises to help the nurse become more familiar with using a stethoscope.

Exercises to Increase Familiarity with the Stethoscope

1. Place the earpieces in your ears with the tips of the earpieces turned toward the face. *Lightly* blow into the stethoscope's diaphragm. Again place the earpieces in your ears, this time with the ends turned toward the back of the head. *Lightly* blow into the stethoscope's diaphragm. The earpiece should follow the contour of the ear canal. Comparing amplification of sounds with the earpieces in both directions helps you learn what fit is best for you. Once you have learned the right fit for the loudest amplification, wear the stethoscope the same way each time.

2. Put on the stethoscope and *lightly* blow into the diaphragm. If the sound is barely audible, *lightly* blow into the bell. Sound is carried through only one part of the chestpiece at a time. If the sound is greatly amplified through the diaphragm, the diaphragm is in position for use. If the sound is barely audible through the diaphragm, the bell is in position for use.

3. Put on the stethoscope and place the diaphragm over a friend's arm. Move the diaphragm lightly over the hair on the arm. The bristling sound created by rubbing of hair against the diaphragm mimics a sound heard in the lungs. The diaphragm should be held firmly and stationary to eliminate extraneous sounds.

4. Place the diaphragm over the anterior part of your chest. Ask a friend to speak in a normal conversational tone. Environmental noise seriously detracts from hearing the noise created by body organs. Whenever a stethoscope is used, both the client and the examiner should remain quiet.

5. Place the stethoscope on and gently tap the tubing. It is often difficult to avoid stretching or movement of the stethoscope's tubing. The examiner should be in a position so that the tubing hangs free. Moving or touching the tubing creates extraneous sounds.

The four characteristics of sound are frequency or pitch, intensity or loudness, quality, and duration. The *frequency* of a vibration is the number of wave cycles generated per second by the vibrating object. The higher the frequency, the higher the pitch of a sound and vice versa. *Loudness* of a sound is the amplitude of the sound wave produced by a vibrating object. A high-energy sound wave creates high amplitudes, resulting in a loud noise. Auscultated sounds are described as either loud or soft. *Quality* is used to distinguish sounds of similar frequency and loudness arising from different sources. Terms such as blowing, swishing, or gurgling describe the quality of a sound. A sound varies in *duration* or length according to the number of continuous vibrations. Vibrations are diminished or dampened by frictional resistance. Layers of soft tissue dampen the duration of sounds coming from deep internal organs. Duration of sound is either short, medium, or long. With practice the nurse learns the normal four characteristics for each type of sound auscultated. For example, a normal breath sound heard over most of the lung is low pitched, soft in intensity, and blowing in quality, with the inspiratory sound lasting longer than the expiratory sound.

Auscultation requires much concentration, practice, and application of knowledge. The nurse must consider the part of the body to be auscultated. What causes the sounds to be produced? For example, the first heart sound is caused by closure of the mitral valve. Where can the sound best be heard? The heart sound is best auscultated at the fifth intercostal space along the midclavicular line. How is the sound heard normally? The first heart sound has the quality of a loud "lub," while the second sound is a "dub." Once the nurse understands the nature of auscultated sounds, she is better prepared to recognize abnormal sounds and their origins.

Olfaction

Certain alterations in body function create characteristic body odors (Table 29-3). The sense of smell helps the nurse detect abnormalities that cannot be recognized by any other means. For example, a client with a cast is expected to experience discomfort as a result of the nature of the injury. However, the nurse who notes a strong odor to the cast will suspect that the client's discomfort may also be related to a wound infection. The client's discomfort alone would not reveal the presence of an infection. Findings from olfaction matched with findings from other assessment skills allow the nurse to detect serious abnormalities.

TABLE 29-3

Assessment of Characteristic Odors

Odor	Site or Source	Potential Causes
Alcohol	Oral cavity	Ingestion of alcohol
Ammonia	Urine	Urinary tract infection
Body	Skin, particularly in areas where body parts rub together (under arms, beneath breasts)	Poor hygiene, excess perspiration (hyperhidrosis), foul-smelling perspiration (bromhidrosis)
Fecal	Wound site Vomitus Rectal area	Wound abscess Bowel obstruction Fecal incontinence
Foul-smelling stools in infant	Stool	Malabsorption syndrome
Halitosis	Oral cavity	Poor dental and oral hygiene, gum disease
Sweet fruity, ketones	Oral cavity	Diabetic acidosis
Stale urine	Skin	Uremic acidosis
Sweet, heavy, thick	Draining wound	*Pseudomonas* (bacterial) infection
Musty	Casted body part	Infection inside cast
Fetid sweet	Tracheostomy or mucous secretions	Infection of bronchial tree (*Pseudomonas* bacteria)

Olfactory sensations are difficult to describe. The more experience the nurse has in working with clients, the more familiar she will become with certain odors. If a nurse notices an unfamiliar odor and is unsure of its source, she should ask a colleague to confirm this assessment.

Preparation for Examination

No portion of a physical examination should be conducted haphazardly. Poor preparation can easily result in incomplete or inaccurate findings. The nurse must take time to make the necessary arrangements to prepare a client properly. The environment must be suitable for the examination, and all needed equipment must be available. The client should be physically and psychologically prepared so that the nurse can conduct the examination smoothly with little interruption. The nurse assists the client to assume proper positions throughout the examination so that body parts are easily accessible and the client remains comfortable. Each aspect of this preparation ensures that the examination will be carried out efficiently.

Preparation of Environment

The physical examination is performed in privacy. In the hospital the client frequently is examined in his room. If the client is in a semiprivate room, the room curtains or dividers around the client's bed should be closed to ensure privacy.

An examination room that is well equipped for all necessary procedures is preferable. Adequate lighting is needed for proper illumination of body parts. Ideally an examination room is soundproofed to the extent that the client is comfortable discussing his illness with the nurse. The nurse should eliminate any sources of extraneous noise such as a television or radio and take precautions to prevent interruptions from other health care personnel during the examination.

Examination tables are relatively high and narrow. The client should be carefully assisted to avoid falling while getting on and off the table. A confused, combative, or uncooperative client should not be left on the table without supervision.

Examination tables are often hard and uncomfortable. During parts of the examination when the client lies supine, the head of the table can be raised about 30 degrees. The client may also be given a small pillow. When examining a client in bed, the nurse can

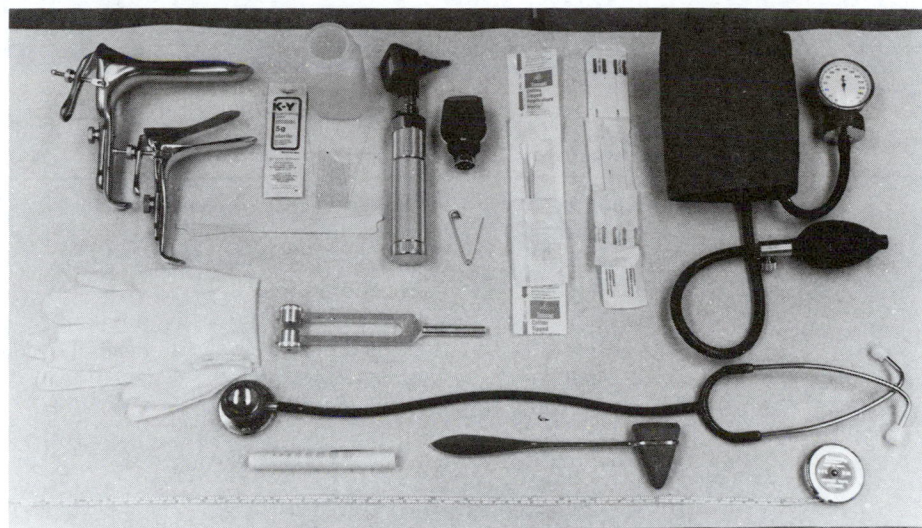

Fig. 29-6 Equipment used during a physical examination. Clockwise from upper right: Sphygmomanometer, stethoscope, tape measure, reflex hammer, penlight, disposable gloves, vaginal speculums, cervical spatula, petrolatum jelly, specimen container and slides, otoscope, ophthalmoscope attachment, safety pin, cotton tip swabs, and tongue blades.

raise the bed in order to reach the client's body parts more easily.

Preparation of Equipment

The client does not want the examination to be prolonged unnecessarily, so the nurse has all equipment ready and available before the examination begins (Fig. 29-6). If possible, the equipment to be used should be kept warm. The diaphragm of the stethoscope may be briskly rubbed between the hands before it is applied to the client's skin. Warm water should be run over the vaginal speculum. A most important piece of equipment, the examiner's hands, should also be warmed. All equipment must be checked to see that it functions properly. The ophthalmoscope and otoscope require a good battery and light bulb. Equipment typically used for physical assessment is listed in the box at right.

Physical Preparation of Client

The client's physical comfort is vital to the success of the examination. Before starting, the examiner should ask the client if he needs to use the toilet. An empty bladder and bowel facilitate examination of the abdomen, genitalia, and rectum. This is a good time to collect any needed urine or fecal specimens. The examiner should explain to the client the proper method for collecting specimens and be sure each specimen is properly labeled.

Equipment and Supplies for Physical Assessment

- Blood pressure cuff
- Cotton applicators
- Disposable pad
- Drapes
- Eye chart (e.g., Snellen chart)
- Flashlight and spotlight
- Forms (e.g., physical, laboratory)
- Gloves (sterile or clean)
- Gown for client
- Lubricant
- Ophthalmoscope
- Otoscope
- Papanicolaou smear slides
- Paper towels
- Percussion hammer
- Safety pin
- Scale with height measurement rod
- Specimen containers and microscope slides
- Stethoscope
- Swabs or sponge forceps
- Tape measure
- Thermometer
- Tissues
- Tongue depressor
- Tuning fork
- Vaginal speculum
- Wristwatch with second hand

TABLE 29-4

Positions for Examination

Position		Areas Assessed	Rationale	Limitations
Sitting		Head and neck, back, posterior thorax and lungs, anterior thorax and lungs, breasts, axilla, heart, vital signs, and upper extremities	Sitting upright provides full expansion of lungs and provides better visualization of symmetry of upper body parts.	A physically weakened client may be unable to sit. Use supine position with head of bed elevated instead.
Supine		Head and neck, anterior thorax and lungs, breasts, axilla, heart, abdomen, extremities, pulses	This is the most normally relaxed position. It prevents contracture of abdominal muscles and provides easy access to pulse sites.	If client becomes short of breath easily, examiner may need to raise head of bed.
Dorsal recumbent		Head and neck, anterior thorax and lungs, breasts, axilla, heart	Certain clients with painful disorders are more comfortable with knees flexed.	Position is not used for abdominal assessment since it promotes contracture of abdominal muscles.
Lithotomy		Female genitalia and genital tract	This position provides maximal exposure of genitalia and facilitates insertion of vaginal speculum.	This is an embarrassing and uncomfortable position, so minimize time the client spends in this position. Keep client well draped. A client with severe arthritis or other joint deformity may be unable to assume this position.
Sims'		Rectum	Flexion of hip and knee improves exposure of rectal area.	Joint deformities may hinder the client's ability to bend hip and knee.
Prone		Musculoskeletal	This position is used only to assess extension of the hip joint.	This position is intolerable for a client with respiratory difficulties.

Physical preparation involves being sure the client is dressed and draped properly. A client in the hospital will most likely be wearing only a simple gown. An outpatient will have to undress. If the examination is to be limited to certain body systems, it may be unnecessary for the client to undress completely. The client should be given privacy during undressing and plenty of time to finish. Walking into the room as the client undresses will create considerable embarrassment.

Drapes and gowns are made of linen or disposable paper. Once the client has undressed and donned the gown, he should sit or lie down on the examination table with the drape over the lap or lower trunk. The examiner should make sure the client stays warm by eliminating drafts, controlling room temperature, and providing warm blankets. Seriously ill and elderly clients are more susceptible to chilling. The examiner should ascertain that the client is comfortable. The client may become more relaxed if he is offered a pillow, sip of water, or tissue.

POSITIONING

During the examination the client will be asked to assume certain positions to facilitate various parts of the assessment. Table 29-4 lists the preferred positions for each part of the examination and contains figures illustrating these positions. The client's ability to assume a position will depend upon his physical strength and degree of wellness. Many of the positions, such as the lithotomy and knee-chest, are embarrassing and uncomfortable. It is therefore important to keep the client in those positions no longer than necessary. The examiner should explain the position to be assumed and assist the client to the proper position. The drapes should be adjusted to be sure that the area to be examined is accessible and that no body part is unnecessarily exposed. More than one position can be assumed for the same part of an examination (for example, supine and sitting for assessment of the anterior thorax), so the nurse first chooses the position that provides greater accessibility and accuracy in assessing body parts (sitting for anterior thorax). However, if the client is too weak or is physically unable to assume a position, the nurse may choose an alternative position.

Psychological Preparation of Client

Having one's body examined by another person can be a highly stressful experience. The possibility that the examiner will find something abnormal creates anxiety. The client is easily embarrassed when he is forced to answer sensitive questions about bodily functions or when body parts are exposed and examined. The elimination of the client's anxiety may be the nurse's highest priority before the examination. A thorough explanation of what will be done and how lets the client know what to expect and prepares him with the knowledge needed to cooperate in the examination (Fig. 29-7). The nurse conducting a complete examination first tells the client in general terms what is to be done. For example,

Ms. Bryce, I am going to do a complete physical examination so that I can have a good idea of whether you have any health problems. As we go along, I will explain to you exactly what I will be doing. Feel free to ask any questions. If you become uncomfortable, please tell me.

Then as examination of each body system is begun, the examiner explains actions in detail. For example,

As I examine your breasts, I want you to relax lying down. First, I want to be sure I do not see anything unusual in the color, size, or shape of your breasts. Then I will gently use my hands to feel for any nodules or masses.

Simple explanations are used when describing actions. Complicated terminology may confuse the client and add to his fears. Each part of the examination is explained to avoid surprises. The examiner's demeanor should be professional, yet tone of voice and facial expression should be relaxed to put the client at ease. The client should be encouraged to mention any discomfort experienced during the assessment.

When the client and examiner are of opposite sexes, it is helpful to have a third person of the client's sex present in the room. Having a third person is particularly helpful when examination of the sexual organs is required. The presence of a third person assures the client that the examiner will behave in an ethical manner, and the third person acts as a witness to the examiner's proper conduct.

Throughout the examination the client's emotional responses are monitored. Does his facial expression convey fear or concern? Does he exhibit body movements suggesting anxiety, such as frequently pulling the drape around his body or tensing up as the examiner touches his body? The examiner must remain calm and explain each step of the assessment clearly. It may become necessary to stop the examination and ask if the client feels anxious, afraid, or uncomfortable. The client should not be forced to continue. Postponement of the examination until a later time may be advantageous, since accuracy may be greater when the client can cooperate and relax. If the client's fears are the result of misconceptions, the examiner attempts to clarify the purpose of the examination and how it is to be performed.

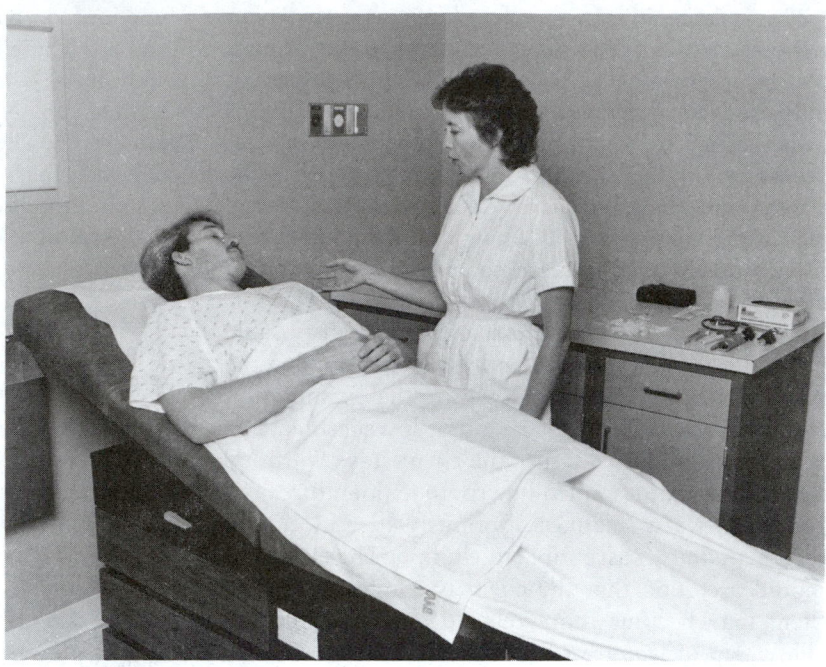

Fig. 29-7 The nurse explains the purpose and steps of the physical examination to the client.

Organization of the Examination

The extent of an examination depends on its purpose. A client who comes to the clinic with symptoms of a severe chest cold will not routinely require a neurological assessment. A client returning from surgery for a fractured leg will require assessment of circulatory and musculoskeletal function rather than a breast examination. When a client is admitted to the hospital, a complete examination is usually performed. Clients with specific symptoms or needs often require only portions of an examination.

The performance of a complete examination follows the nursing history (see Chapter 7). The nurse uses information from the history to focus attention on specific parts of the examination. For example, if the client's history revealed symptoms of abdominal discomfort, the nurse gives special scrutiny in the abdominal assessment. Findings from the history generally reveal a pattern of related signs and symptoms. The physical examination supplements information from the history to confirm or refute the data.

Each nurse develops a personal system for conducting a physical examination. Whatever the system chosen, the nurse must be sure that it is well organized so important assessments are not forgotten or deleted. A commonly used system is one organized by the "head-to-toe" orientation. The examiner begins with an assessment of the head and neck area, progressing methodically down the body to incorporate all body systems. Using a head-to-toe approach helps the nurse anticipate the order of systems to assess.

As each body system is assessed, the nurse compares both sides of the body for symmetry. Both sides of the face are inspected for symmetry of expression, the lungs' breath sounds are auscultated bilaterally, and both sides of the abdomen are percussed and palpated for presence of masses. A degree of asymmetry is normal; for example, the biceps muscle in the client's dominant arm may be more developed than the same muscle in the nondominant arm.

Certain priorities must be considered with respect to the client's condition during the examination. If the client is seriously ill, systems of the body that are most at risk for being abnormal are assessed first. For example, the cardiovascular status of a client with severe chest pain is carefully monitored. If the client exhibits fatigue, rest periods are provided between the assessments. If part of the examination is not critical, it should be deferred until the client is rested. Painful procedures should be performed near the end of the examination.

While performing the examination, the nurse records the results on the assessment form in specific anatomical terms. Using scientific terminology ensures that any professional who reads the findings of the examination will have the same understanding. Fig. 29-8 illustrates the planes of the body to describe anatomical positions. Using common medical abbreviations helps to make the nurse's notes brief and concise.

The nurse uses a physical assessment form (Fig. 29-9) to record assessment findings. The form is organized in the same sequence as the examination is con-

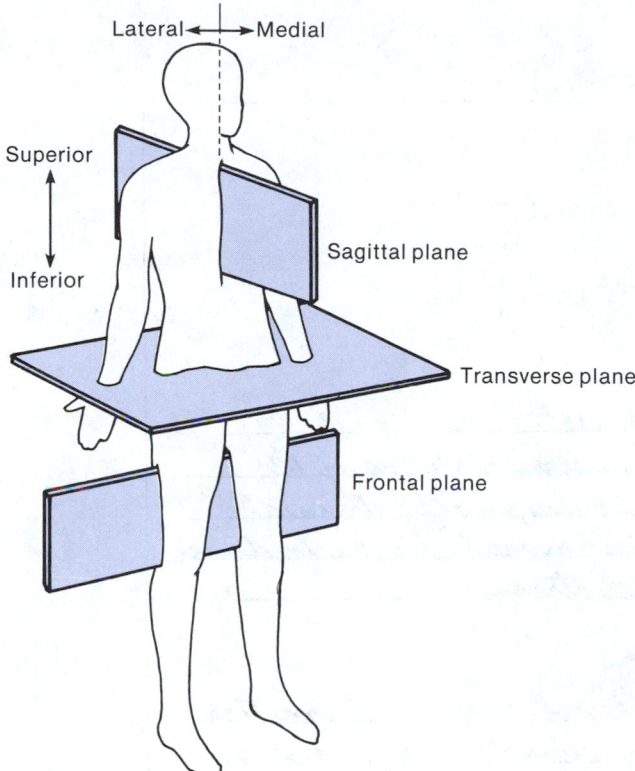

Lateral ← | → Medial

Superior

Inferior

Sagittal plane

Transverse plane

Frontal plane

Fig. 29-8 The nurse describes assessment findings in terms of their anatomical position within specific body planes.

ducted. Results of assessments and other key findings are recorded in quick notes during the examination to keep the client from waiting too long. Complete observations can be recorded at the end of the examination. If a client seems uncomfortable or anxious during this recording, either the recording should be stopped or the findings explained.

The Examination

The physical examination is composed of individual assessments for each body system. Each assessment incorporates the skills of inspection, palpation, auscultation, and percussion as appropriate.

General Survey

From the time the nurse first encounters the client, assessment begins. During the nursing history the nurse makes mental notes of the client's behaviors and appearance, which later are recorded as data for the general survey. The survey is the preliminary portion of the examination during which the client's height and weight, vital signs, and general appearance

are recorded. If any abnormalities or signs of problems are revealed during the survey, the nurse more closely scrutinizes the affected body systems later during the examination.

Most nurses prefer measuring vital signs before assessing the individual body systems, because positioning or moving the client during the examination could interfere with the accurate recording of temperature, pulse, respirations, and blood pressure. However, it is also appropriate for the nurse to measure specific vital signs during the body systems assessment. For example, the pulse can be assessed during examination of the peripheral pulses or the heart, and respirations during examination of the thorax. Body temperature is always measured during the general survey.

Before measuring the client's height and weight, the nurse asks the client what he weighs and how tall he is. A discrepancy between the client's perceptions and actual height and weight may provide a clue to the client's body image. The client's response usually reveals how satisfied the client is with weight and size. A discussion of height and weight allows the nurse to determine whether there have been recent weight gains or losses. A sudden change in weight can indicate the presence of serious disease. If a client is retaining fluids, his weight may change as much as 5 pounds in a day. If there has been a significant weight gain or loss, the client is asked how much weight was gained or lost, over what period of time, and whether the change in weight was the result of changes in dietary habits or appetite. During the examination distribution of body fat is noted. Generalized fat distribution is characteristic of simple obesity.

The client is always weighed at the same time, on the same scale and wearing the same clothes. In a hospital setting it is fairly easy to weigh the client at the same time each day, usually before breakfast. In a clinic or office setting, however, weighing the client at the same time for each visit is difficult. The same scale should be used to ensure accuracy of measurement. The measurement of weight varies greatly depending on the amount of clothing the client wears. In a hospital the client is weighed in the same type of gown. In the clinic the client should remove shoes and coat and be weighed in street clothes if a gown is not to be worn.

Clients capable of bearing their own weight use a standing scale. The client stands on a platform as the weight is indicated on a numerical scale (Fig. 29-10). A paper towel is placed on the platform so the client's feet remain clean.

The nurse uses a stretcher scale for clients unable to bear weight. The client lies on the stretcher and the scale underneath records the weight. Stretcher

PHYSICAL EXAMINATION FORMAT

Height *5'7"*   Weight *195 lbs*

BP *138/74*   Pulse *82 reg.* Temp. *98⁸*   Resp. *18*

General survey *Mildly obese male, appears stated age of 63; appropriate affect when questioned, neatly dressed, maintains hygiene, posturing reveals slight lordosis, in no apparent physical distress*

Integument:

Skin: *Color normal in face, trunk, upper extremities. Paleness in lower legs. Skin warm, dry, reduced turgor, no edema. 1-2 cm tan nodules along outer surface right hand, nontender, no drainage, appear to be warts.*

Hair: *Slight balding of forehead, skin dry, thin. Decreased growth of hair over lower legs.*

Nails: *Pink, good capillary return, normal thickness.*

Head, Eyes, Ears, Nose, and Throat (HEENT):

Head: *No tenderness, masses or lesions*

Eyes: *PERRLA Reads newspaper print without difficulty, 20/20 with glasses. OS-some tearing and inflammation of conjunctiva. Sclera and lids normal. OD- unremarkable fundus - disc visualized - no lesions or hemorrhages of macula visualized.*

Ears: *Bilaterally, no drainage, no tenderness on palpation. Canal with excess cerumen, TM light reflex. Bright clear landmarks; hearing acuity normal bilaterally. Weber no lateralization, Rinne + AC/BC*

Fig. 29-9 Physical examination format.

Nose: Symmetrical, mucosa pink, clear discharge noted in right nares, no lesions or edema

Sinuses: Nontender

Mouth: Upper and lower dentures. Lips symmetrical, pink, dry, without lesions. Gums pink, moist, with area of roughness noted on R upper aspect. Tongue without abnormalities. Palate and pharynx pink, smooth, with clear mucous drainage along posterior pharynx.

Neck: Supple, good ROM, lymph nodes nonpalpable bilaterally, thyroid nonpalpabal, trachea midline, carotid pulse strong, regular, without bruits.

Thorax: Symmetrical, AP diameter 1:2, without retractions or deformities. Respirations regular. Excursion 5-6 cm anteriorly and posteriorly. Normal tactile and vocal fremitus bilaterally. Vesicular breath sounds auscultated over all fields, slightly decreased intensity over anterior R and L lower lobes.

Heart: PMI 5th ICS 1 cm to R of MCL. No pulsations or vibrations. Rate 82; normal S_1, S_2 without murmurs.

Vascular: Pulses 3+ and equal bilaterally, regular rate and rhythm.

Breasts: Breasts symmetrical, without palpable lesions. Nipple and areola without drainage, lesions, or edema. Lymph nodes nonpalpable.

Abdomen: Convex and symmetrical, with 6 cm scar in RUQ. Without lesions or varicosities. Bowel sounds audible in all 4 quadrants. Abdomen soft, nontender, without palpable masses. Without CVA tenderness. Liver nonpalpable.

Genitalia: Decreased pubic hair distribution.

Penis: Circumcised, without discharge, lesions, or edema.

Fig. 29-9, cont'd Physical examination format.

Continued.

Scrotum: *Testes descended, without tenderness or masses. Erythematous rash noted on undersurface of scrotal sac, without drainage. Without hernia.*

Rectal: *Rectal wall smooth, without masses or tenderness. Prostate nontender, firm, slightly enlarged.*

Musculoskeletal: *Lordotic posture, ambulates with broad base of support. Without obvious deformities. Gross ROM normal in all extremities except R knee: flexion 100° with onset of pain, hyperextends and internally rotates 0°. Knee joint tender to palpation with moderate swelling. Normal muscle strength and tone in all extremities.*

Neurological:

Mental status: *Patient alert and oriented, responds appropriately to questions. Recalls recent and past events. Asks pertinent questions about condition. Tests for abstract thinking, association, and judgment deferred. Cranial nerves intact.*

Sensory: *Able to distinguish sharp from dull at all points tested. Able to distinguish vibratory sensation on upper extremities. Decreased vibration sensation on R knee. Position sense intact in upper and lower extremities.*

Coordination: *Normal Romberg. Tests for coordinated movement deferred.*

Reflexes:

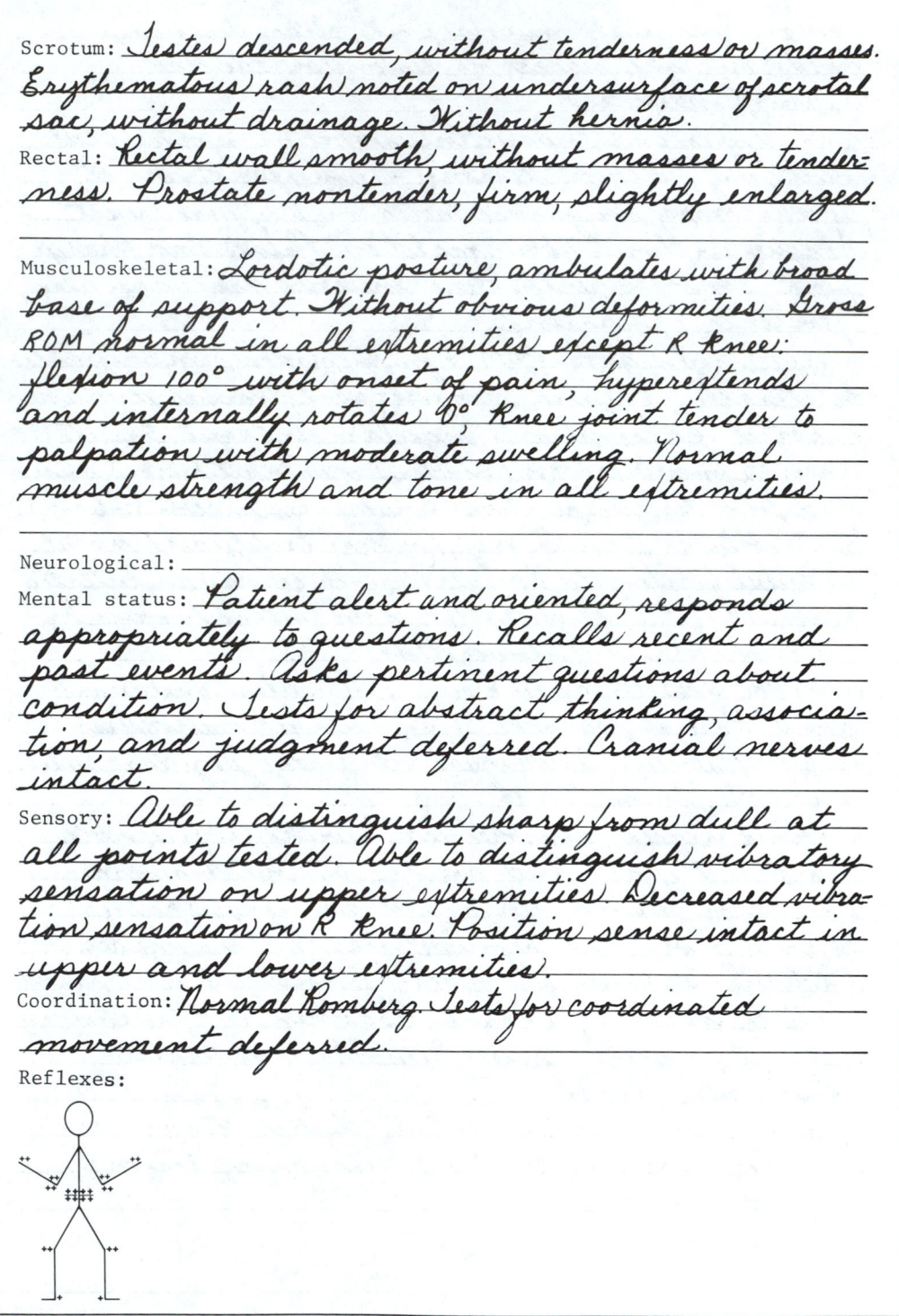

Fig. 29-9, cont'd Physical examination format.

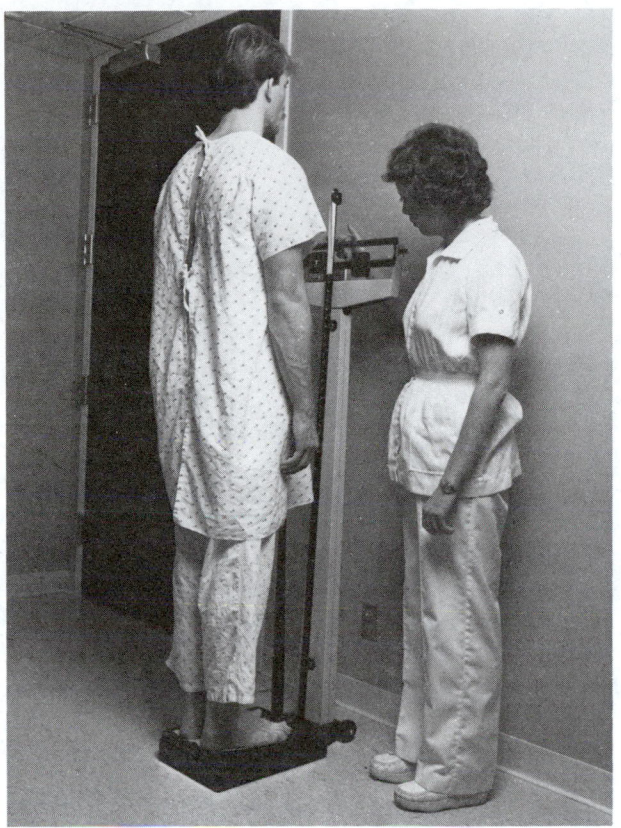

Fig. 29-10 The client stands on the scale as the nurse adjusts the balance.

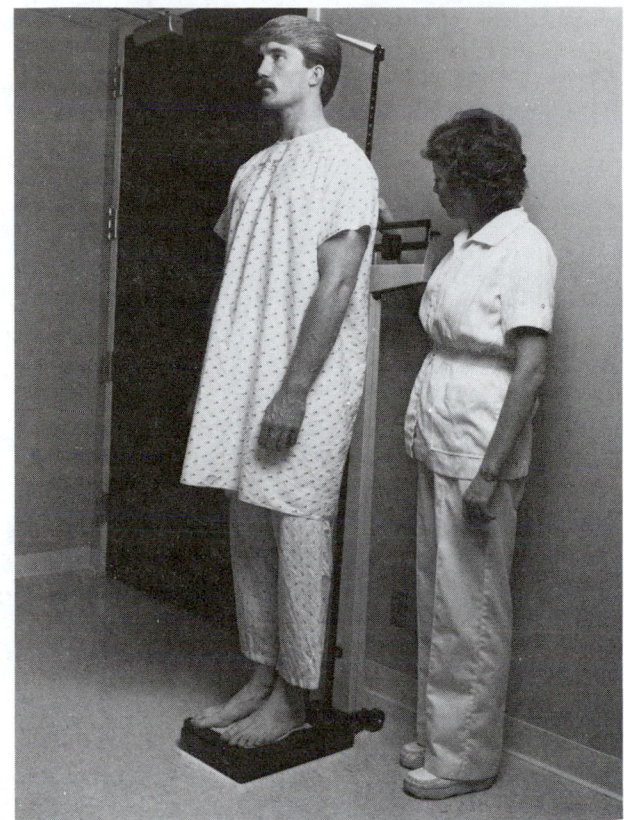

Fig. 29-11 The client stands erect to permit an accurate measurement of height.

scales can be elevated so clients may be transferred easily from bed to scale.

A table model scale is used to weigh an infant, who is usually unclothed. Most of these scales have basketlike containers that hold the infant. The nurse must be sure to protect the child from falling out of the scale.

Height is measured using a special attachment on a standing scale (Fig. 29-11). The client should remove shoes and stand as straight as possible, exercising good posture. For clients who have poor balance or are physically weakened, special scales are available that allow the client to hold on to the scale.

To measure the length of an infant who cannot stand, the nurse places the child supine on a hard, flat surface, such as a table or countertop. The infant's knees are extended and the soles of the feet are supported upright, and then the child is measured from the soles of the feet to the vertex of the head.

An older child's height can be measured by simply having him stand straight against a wall, with the heels, back, and head touching the wall. A flat object (such as a cardboard tablet) is placed on the child's

head and the point on the wall perpendicular to the tablet is marked. The distance from the point on the wall to the floor is the child's height.

Growth charts have been developed based on the average height and weight of selected populations. Because of variations in cultural trends, economic standards, and health habits, growth charts are subjective standards of measurement. However, growth charts do provide a general guideline to assess a client's nutritional status and physical development.

The nurse assesses the client's general appearance through a head-to-toe series of observations. The experienced nurse is able to sum up the client's condition with little or no conversation. Statements such as "The client is in no acute distress" or "The client appears ill" are summations frequently used to record the nurse's general impressions. Information is gained from the general features and characteristics of illness, for example, the gait of Parkinson's disease and the facial appearance of a depressed client. Fig. 29-12 offers guidelines for assessing the client's general appearance.

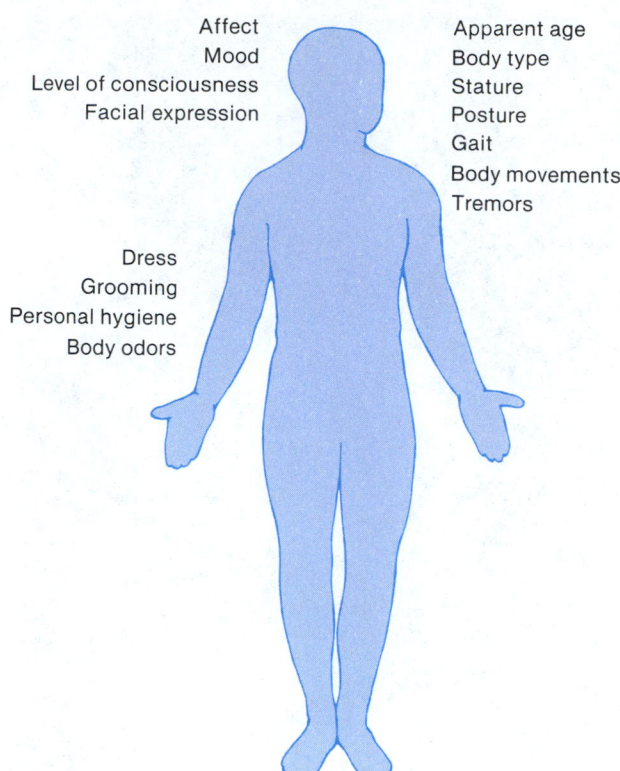

Affect
Mood
Level of consciousness
Facial expression

Apparent age
Body type
Stature
Posture
Gait
Body movements
Tremors

Dress
Grooming
Personal hygiene
Body odors

Fig. 29-12 Criteria to assess in general survey.

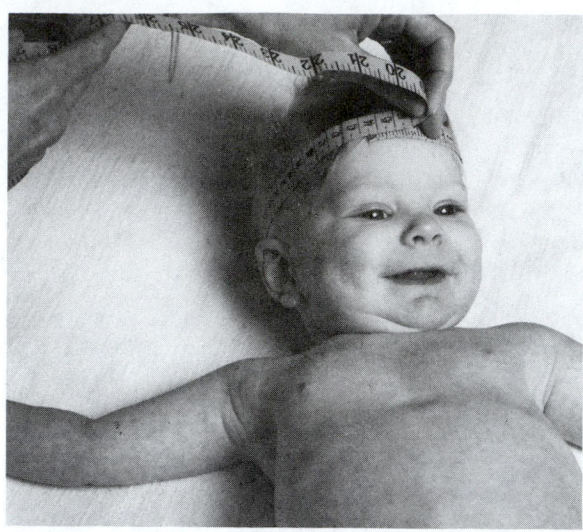

Fig. 29-13 The nurse measures a child's head circumference by placing the tape measure anteriorly over the lower forehead and posteriorly over the prominent occipital bone.

Anthropometry

Anthropometry is gradually coming into common use as a series of assessment techniques. Anthropometry is comparative measurements of the human body and its parts. Height and weight, skinfold thickness, and circumference of the arm, chest, and head are common measurements. A person's nutritional status and overall growth and development can be estimated by anthropometric technique.

Skinfold thickness is a simple and practical way of measuring body fat. Skinfold measurements reveal subcutaneous fat and reflect a person's general caloric status. A pair of calibrated calipers measures skinfold thickness. The best sites for measurement are the upper abdomen, subscapular area, and deltoid triceps behind the upper arm. A fold of skin is grasped so that both sides run parallel. The nurse must not pinch bone or muscle. The calipers are then applied using constant pressure. Standards of obesity have been developed on minimum skinfold thickness (Table 29-5).

Measurement of head circumference is an indirect means of estimating brain growth. This is of particular interest during infancy, since a child's brain development is complete by 1 year of age. The infant lies supine and a measuring tape is placed around the head. The point of greatest circumference is anteriorly over the lower forehead, just above the supraorbital ridges, and posteriorly over the prominent part of the occipital bone (Fig. 29-13). Normal measurements of head circumference are 31 to 37 cm (12.4 to 14.8 inches) at birth. Lower circumference values are cause for concern.

The measurement of arm circumference is an indicator of muscular development. Abnormalities suggest that the client's protein and caloric intake is inadequate. Usually the examiner measures the circumference of the left arm at its midpoint. The measuring tape should be taut but not to the extent of compressing underlying muscle. A circumference of 29.3 cm (11.7 inches) for males and 28.5 cm (11.4 inches) for females is normal.

Integument

The skin or integumentary system serves the important functions of providing the body's external protection, regulating body temperature, and acting as a sensory organ for pain, temperature, and touch. Assessment of the integumentary system includes the skin, hair, scalp, and nails. The nurse may take the time initially to observe all skin surfaces or may assess the skin gradually as other body systems are examined. The nurse uses assessment findings to determine the type of hygiene measures required to maintain integrity of the integument. Adequate nutrition and hydration become goals of therapy if the nurse identifies alterations in the integument's status (see Chap-

TABLE 29-5

Percentiles for Triceps Skinfold for Whites of the United States, Health and Nutrition Examination Survey I of 1971 to 1974

		Triceps Skinfold Percentiles (mm^2)														
Age Group	n	5	10	25	50	75	90	95	n	5	10	25	50	75	90	95
		Males								Females						
1-1.9	228	6	7	8	10	12	14	16	204	6	7	8	10	12	14	16
2-2.9	223	6	7	8	10	12	14	15	208	6	8	9	10	12	15	16
3-3.9	220	6	7	8	10	11	14	15	208	7	8	9	11	12	14	15
4-4.9	230	6	6	8	9	11	12	14	208	7	8	8	10	12	14	16
5-5.9	214	6	6	8	9	11	14	15	219	6	7	8	10	12	15	18
6-6.9	117	5	6	7	8	10	13	16	118	6	6	8	10	12	14	16
7-7.9	122	5	6	7	9	12	15	17	126	6	7	9	11	13	16	18
8-8.9	117	5	6	7	8	10	13	16	118	6	8	9	12	15	18	24
9-9.9	121	6	6	7	10	13	17	18	125	8	8	10	13	16	20	22
10-10.9	146	6	6	8	10	14	18	21	152	7	8	10	12	17	23	27
11-11.9	122	6	6	8	11	16	20	24	117	7	8	10	13	18	24	28
12-12.9	153	6	6	8	11	14	22	28	129	8	9	11	14	18	23	27
13-13.9	134	5	5	7	10	14	22	26	151	8	8	12	15	21	26	30
14-14.9	131	4	5	7	9	14	21	24	141	9	10	13	16	21	26	28
15-15.9	128	4	5	6	8	11	18	24	117	8	10	12	17	21	25	32
16-16.9	131	4	5	6	8	12	16	22	142	10	12	15	18	22	26	31
17-17.9	133	5	5	6	8	12	16	19	114	10	12	13	19	24	30	37
18-18.9	91	4	5	6	9	13	20	24	109	10	12	15	18	22	26	30
19-24.9	531	4	5	7	10	15	20	22	1060	10	11	14	18	24	30	34
25-34.9	971	5	6	8	12	16	20	24	1987	10	12	16	21	27	34	37
35-44.9	806	5	6	8	12	16	20	23	1614	12	14	18	23	29	35	38
45-54.9	898	6	6	8	12	15	20	25	1047	12	16	20	25	30	36	40
55-64.9	734	5	6	8	11	14	19	22	809	12	16	20	25	31	36	38
65-74.9	1503	4	6	8	11	15	19	22	1670	12	14	18	24	29	34	36

From Frisancho, A.R.: Am. J. Clin. Nutr. **34**:2540, 1981.

ter 35). Two physical assessment skills, inspection and palpation, are used to measure the integument's function and integrity.

SKIN

The skin is a mirror that reflects an individual's general health and well-being. Any break or disruption of the skin signals a person's predisposition to infection. In addition, the lines and curves of the face can help to reveal a person's emotional health.

Certain skin changes, both normal and abnormal, are common to specific age groups. The infant commonly exhibits skin rashes from allergies to solid foods. As the child grows older, he is prone to certain specific skin changes; for example, with the onset of adolescence facial acne is a common finding. The adult notices skin changes representative of advancing age, such as loss of hair on the scalp and a diminishing firmness in skin tissue. The elderly person develops an overall wrinkling of the skin with decreased elas-

ticity or turgor and a significant reduction in the quantity of hair covering the extremities and axillary and pubic areas.

Adequate illumination of the skin is mandatory during assessment. The examination begins with inspection of the skin's color, moisture, temperature, texture, and turgor. The presence of edema and any lesions should be noted. If abnormalities are seen, findings from palpation will complement the data base. Fig. 29-14 illustrates a normal cross section of the skin's layers and structure.

COLOR. Skin color varies from body part to body part and from person to person. Table 29-6 lists common variations in skin color. Normal skin pigmentation ranges in tone from ivory to deep brown. For a person who works extensively outside, the exposed areas of the body such as the face and arms will be more pigmented than the rest of the body. For clients with dark pigmented skin it is more difficult to note

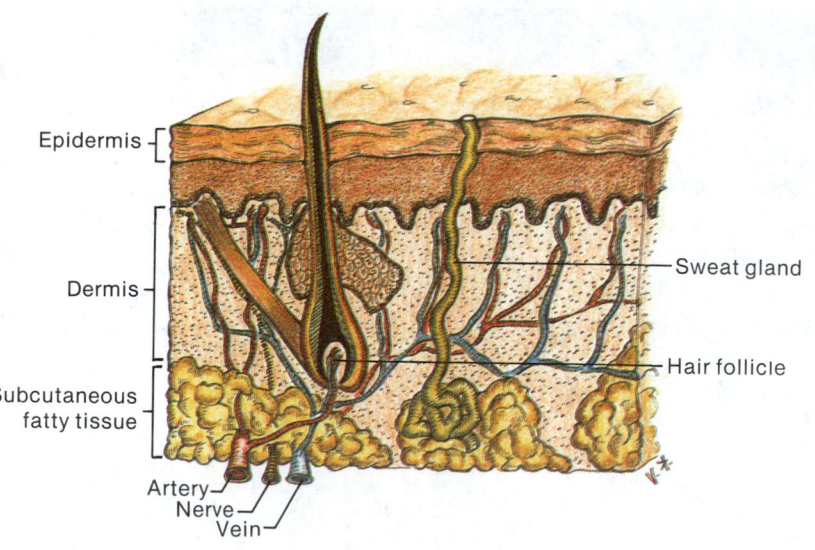

Epidermis

Dermis

Subcutaneous
fatty tissue

Sweat gland

Hair follicle

Artery
Nerve
Vein

Fig. 29-14 A cross section of the skin reveals three layers: epidermis, dermis, and subcutaneous fatty tissue.

changes such as pallor, cyanosis, or jaundice.

The nurse learns to focus inspection on areas of abnormal pigmentation and on sites where abnormalities are more easily identified. For example, pallor is most easily perceived in the buccal mucosa of the mouth, particularly in individuals with dark skin. Cyanosis is more readily seen in areas of least pigmentation: lips, nail beds, palpebral conjunctiva, and palms. The sclera is the best site to inspect for presence of jaundice.

The inexperienced nurse may find it helpful to ask the client if he has noticed changes in skin coloring. The client usually knows his body best. Asking the client is more useful when the client's skin coloring is different from that of the nurse.

TABLE 29-6

Skin Color Variations

Color	Condition	Causes	Assessment Locations
Bluish (cyanosis)	Increased amount of deoxygenated hemoglobin; associated with hypoxia	Heart or lung disease, cold environment	Nail beds, lips, mouth, skin (severe cases)
Pallor (decrease in color)	Reduced amount of oxyhemoglobin	Anemia	Face, conjunctiva, nail beds
	Reduced visibility of oxyhemoglobin resulting from decreased blood flow	Shock	Skin, nail beds, conjunctiva, lips
	Congenital or autoimmune condition causing lack of pigment	Vitiligo	Patchy areas on skin
Yellow-orange (jaundice)	Increased deposition of bilirubin in tissues	Liver disease, destruction of red blood cells	Sclera, mucous membranes, skin
Red (erythema)	Increased visibility of oxyhemoglobin caused by dilation or increased blood flow	Fever, direct trauma, blushing, alcohol intake	Face; area of trauma
Tan-brown	Increased amount of melanin	Suntan, pregnancy	Areas exposed to sun; face, areola, nipples

MOISTURE. The hydration of skin and mucous membranes helps to reveal body fluid imbalances, changes in the integument's environment, and regulation of body temperature. Excessively dry skin may indicate dehydration or the use of excessive amounts of soap during bathing. The client should be asked about the amount and type of soap used for bathing. Perspiration reveals the body's attempt to promote heat loss. A dry tongue can be a sign of dehydration or mouth breathing.

The fingertips are used to feel moisture on the skin. What appears to be thin and watery may be thick and oily. If there are any lesions oozing fluid, the color, odor, amount, and consistency are noted.

TEMPERATURE. The temperature of the skin depends on the amount of blood circulating through the dermis. An increased or decreased skin temperature thus reflects an increase or decrease in blood flow. Temperature is more accurately assessed by palpating the skin with the dorsum or back of the hand. Skin temperature may be the same throughout the body or may vary in one area, such as the localized warmth at an infected wound site or the coldness of fingers resulting from reduced blood flow. Assessment of skin temperature is a basic assessment whenever the client is at risk of having impaired circulation, for example, after application of a cast or tight bandage or after vascular surgery.

TEXTURE. The character of the skin's surface and the feel of deeper portions are its texture. The nurse determines whether the client's skin is smooth or rough by stroking it lightly with her fingertips. The texture of the skin is not normally uniform throughout. Localized changes may be found as the result of trauma or lesions. When irregularities in texture are found, the nurse asks the client if he has experienced any recent injury to the skin. Deep palpation of the skin may reveal irregularities such as localized areas of hardness, commonly caused by repeated intramuscular or subcutaneous injections. If the client is a diabetic or is receiving vitamin B$_{12}$ or iron injections, these hardened areas are a common finding.

TURGOR. Turgor is the skin's elasticity. Elasticity may be diminished by edema or dehydration. Normally the skin loses its elasticity with age.

To assess the skin's turgor, a fold of skin on the back of the client's hand or forearm is grasped with the fingertips and released (Fig. 29-15). The nurse notes the ease with which the skin moves and the speed at which it returns to place. Normally the skin snaps back immediately to its resting position. The client with poor skin turgor does not have a resilience

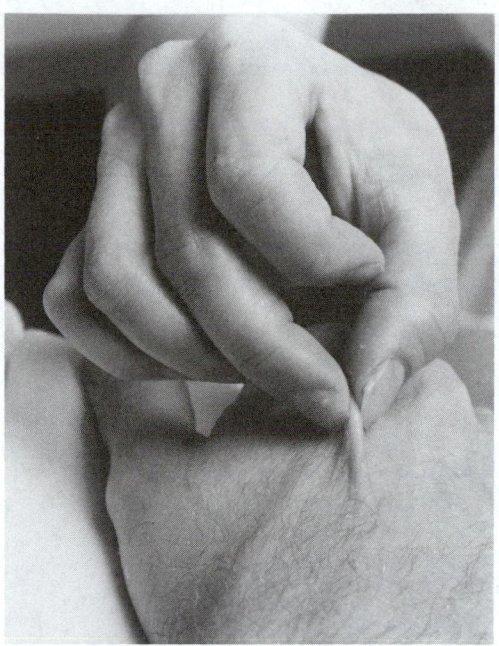

Fig. 29-15 Assessment for skin turgor.

to the normal wear and tear on the skin. A decrease in turgor predisposes the client to skin breakdown.

LESIONS. Whenever a lesion is detected, it is inspected for color, location, size, type (Table 29-7), grouping (for example, clustered or linear), and distribution (localized or generalized). Palpation determines the lesion's mobility, contour (flat, raised, or depressed), and consistency (soft or hard). Certain types of lesions present a characteristic pattern. For example, a tumor is usually hard, localized, and immobile. Primary lesions such as macules and nodules arise from some stimulus to the skin. Secondary lesions such as ulcers occur as alterations in primary lesions.

Once a lesion is identified, it is closely inspected with good illumination. The lesion is palpated gently, covering its entire area. If the lesion is moist or draining fluid, gloves are worn during palpation, since contact with drainage could spread infectious organisms.

It is helpful to ask the client if he has noticed any lesions of the skin and whether a lesion has recently changed in character. Cancerous lesions frequently undergo changes in color and size. Any abnormal lesions are reported to the client's physician because further examination may be required.

EDEMA. Areas of the skin become swollen or edematous as a result of accumulation of fluid in the tissues. Direct trauma and impairment of venous return are two common causes for edema. Edematous areas should be inspected for location, color, and shape.

TABLE 29-7

Skin Lesions

	Lesion	Size (cm)	Description	Example
	Primary			
	Macule	<1	Flat, nonpalpable, change in skin color	Freckle, petechia
	Papule	<0.5	Palpable, circumscribed; solid elevation in skin	Elevated nevus
	Nodule	0.5-2	Elevated solid mass; deeper and firmer than papule	Wart
	Tumor	>1-2	Solid mass; may extend deep through subcutaneous tissue	Epithelioma
	Wheal	Varies	Elevated area of superficial localized edema; irregularly shaped	Hive, mosquito bite
	Vesicle	<0.5	Circumscribed elevation of skin filled with serous fluid	Herpes simplex, chickenpox
	Pustule	Varies	Similar to vesicle; lesion filled with pus	Acne, staphylococcal infection

TABLE 29-7 , cont'd

Skin Lesions

	Lesion	Size (cm)	Description	Example
	Secondary			
	Ulcer	Varies	Deep loss of skin surface; may extend to dermis; frequently bleeds and scars	Venous stasis ulcer
	Atrophy	Varies	Thinning of skin with loss of normal skin furrow; shiny and translucent skin	Arterial insufficiency

For the client with dependent edema caused by poor venous return, typical sites of edema are the feet, ankles, and sacrum. The formation of edema separates the skin's surface from the pigmented and vascular layers, masking skin color. Often the skin becomes stretched and takes on a shiny appearance. The nurse palpates areas of edema to determine mobility, consistency, and tenderness. When pressure from the examiner's finger leaves an indentation in the edematous area, it is called pitting edema. To check the degree of pitting edema the nurse presses the edematous area firmly with the thumb for 5 seconds. The depth of the pitting determines the degree of edema. For each centimeter in depth, the nurse records a plus sign (1 cm equals 1+ edema, 2 cm equal 2+ edema, and so on).

HAIR

Two types of hair cover the body: terminal hair (long, coarse, thick hair that is easily visible on the scalp, axilla, and pubic areas) and vellus hair (small, soft, tiny hairs covering the whole body except for palms and soles). The nurse is concerned primarily with assessing the distribution, thickness, texture, and lubrication of hair. In addition, the nurse inspects for the presence of pediculosis (lice) and other vermin.

Much of the information gathered about characteristics of hair growth comes from the client. In addition, the nurse needs to be aware of the normal distribution of hair growth in males and females.

Both sexes have the fine vellus hair covering the body in addition to scalp hair, eyebrows, and eyelashes. With the onset of puberty, a change in the amount and distribution of hair growth occurs. Clients with hormone disorders may experience an unusual distribution and growth of hair. Females with hirsutism have hair growth on the upper lip, chin, and cheeks, with vellus hair becoming coarser over the body. A change in hair growth can have damaging effects on the client's body image and emotional well-being.

Changes may occur in the thickness, texture, and lubrication of scalp hair. A number of disturbances in body function, such as a febrile illness and general anesthesia, can result in hair loss. Scalp disease can also cause loss of hair. Baldness (alopecia) or thinning of the hair is usually related to genetic tendencies. The hair is normally lubricated from the oil of sebaceous glands located within the hair follicle. Excessively oily hair is associated with androgen hormone stimulation. Dry brittle hair occurs with aging and with excessive use of shampoo or other chemical agents. Poor nutrition often causes development of dry, coarse, discolored hair.

The amount of hair covering the extremities may be reduced as a result of arterial insufficiency. This is most commonly seen over the client's lower extremities. In females loss of hair should not be confused with shaven legs.

The nurse makes a general inspection of hair follicles on the scalp and pubic areas to determine the presence of lice or other vermin. There are three types of lice: *Pediculus humanus* var. *capitis* or head lice, *Pediculus corporis* or body lice, and *Pediculus pubis*

TABLE 29-8

Abnormalities of the Nail Bed

	Type	Description	Causes
	Normal nail		
	Clubbing	Change in the angle between nail and nail base, so eventually the angle is greater than 180 degrees; nail bed softens, with nail flattening; fingertips often enlarged	Chronic lack of oxygen: heart disease, pulmonary disease
	Beau's lines	Transverse depressions in the nails, indicative that nail growth was temporarily disturbed; grows out over several months	Systemic illness, such as severe infection; injury to the nail
	Koilonychia (spoon nail)	Concave curves	Iron deficiency anemia; syphilis; use of strong detergents
	Splinter hemorrhages	Red or brown linear streaks in the nail bed	Minor trauma; subacute bacterial endocarditis; trichinosis
	Paronychia	Inflammation of skin at base of nail	Local infection; trauma

or crab lice. Head and crab lice tend to attach their eggs to a person's hair. The tiny eggs look like oval particles of dandruff. The lice themselves are difficult to see. Head and body lice are very small with grayish white bodies. Crab lice have red legs. The nurse also looks for bites or pustular eruptions in the hair follicles and in areas where skin surfaces meet, such as behind the ears and in the groin. The discovery of lice warrants immediate attention. The nurse instructs the client on proper treatment (see Chapter 35) and explores the possible sources of lice. Lice are most commonly spread by direct contact with infested clothing or people.

SCALP

The scalp is inspected for lesions after any wigs or hairpieces are removed. It is wise to first ask the client if he has noticed anything unusual about the scalp or hair. Lesions can easily go unnoticed in a thick growth of hair. The scalp is inspected for contour and the presence of lesions. Carefully separating the hair at various locations allows the nurse to take a thorough look at the scalp. Any lesion is assessed using the same guidelines that were described in the discussion of skin lesions. If lumps or bruises are found, the client should be asked if he has experienced recent trauma to the head. Moles on the scalp are not unusual. The nurse should warn the client that combing or brushing can cause a mole to bleed. Scaliness or dryness of the scalp is frequently caused by dandruff or psoriasis.

NAILS

The nails can reflect an individual's general state of health. Normally the nails are transparent, smooth, and convex, with pink nail beds and translucent white tips. In black clients a brown or black pigmentation is normally present between the fingernail and nail base. Nails normally grow at a constant rate. Direct injury or generalized disease can impair nail growth.

The nails are inspected for color, thickness, shape, and curvature. The color of nails is a good indicator of blood oxygenation. A bluish or purplish cast to the nail bed occurs with cyanosis; white pallor is the result of anemia. Thin nails can be a sign of nutritional deficiency. Changes in the shape and curvature of nails are indications of systemic disease (Table 29-8). Palpation of the nails assesses adequacy of circulation or capillary refill. To palpate, the nurse gently grasps the client's finger and observes the color of the nail bed. Next, gentle, firm pressure is applied with the thumb to the nail bed quickly and released. As the pressure is applied, the nail bed appears white or blanched; however, the pink color should return immediately upon release of pressure. Failure of the pinkness to return promptly indicates circulatory insufficiency.

Head and Neck

An examination of the head and neck reviews the integrity of anatomical structures including the head, eyes, ears, nose, mouth, pharynx, and neck (lymph nodes, carotid arteries, thyroid gland, and trachea). The carotid arteries can also be assessed during the assessment of arteries. The nurse needs to have a good understanding of each anatomical area and its normal physiological function. Assessment of the head and neck uses the skills of inspection, palpation, and auscultation, with inspection and palpation often used simultaneously.

HEAD

The nurse inspects the client's head, noting the size, shape, and contour. Normally, the skull is generally round with prominences in the frontal area anteriorly and the occipital area posteriorly. Local skull deformities are typically caused by trauma. In infants a large head (see previous discussion of anthropometry) may result from congenital anomalies or the accumulation of cerebrospinal fluid in the ventricles (hydrocephalus). Adults may have large-sized heads as a result of excessive growth hormone secretion (acromegaly).

EYES

The eyes are perceived by most people as vital to life since they allow one to interact freely in the environment and to watch the miracles of life. Often vision is taken for granted. Nurses should recommend that clients under the age of 40 have a complete eye examination every 3 to 5 years. If the client has a family history of eye disease, diabetes, or hypertension, the nurse should suggest more frequent examinations. After the age of 40, eye examinations should be performed every 2 years, particularly to screen for glaucoma.

The nurse should be familiar with the typical symptoms of eye disease. During the examination, the client is asked if he has experienced any of the following:

1. Pain
2. Photophobia (sensitivity to light)
3. Burning
4. Itching
5. Excess tearing or crusting
6. Diplopia (double vision)
7. Blurred vision
8. Spots or floaters
9. Flashing lights
10. Halos around lights

Assessment of visual symptoms may lead to the identification of specific eye disorders. If the client acknowledges the presence of any of these symptoms, the physician must be notified.

Examination of the eye focuses on the assessment

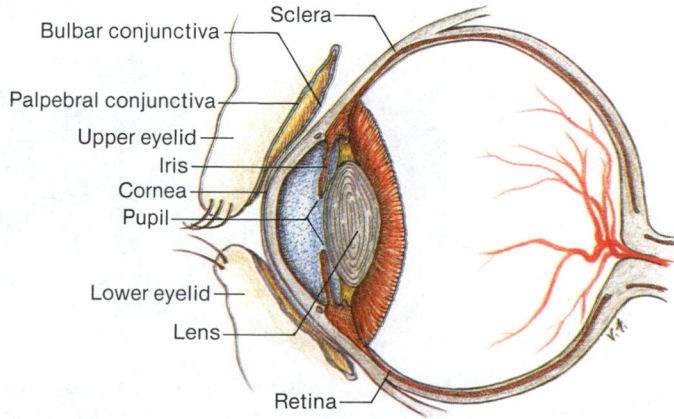

Fig. 29-16 Cross section of the eye.

of visual acuity, visual field, extraocular movements, and external and internal eye structures. Fig. 29-16 is a cross section of external and internal eye structures.

VISUAL ACUITY. The nurse makes a cursory assessment of the client's visual acuity by having him read any available print, such as a newspaper or magazine. There must be adequate lighting. If the client normally wears glasses, the glasses should be worn as he reads. If the client has difficulty reading, the nurse tests further by asking him to use each eye separately. An opaque index card is used to cover one eye at a time; the client should not cover the eye with his hand. The client with severe visual impairment should be asked to count the nurse's upraised fingers. Assessment of a client's visual acuity may reveal a change in acuity or the need for further examination. It also informs the nurse of the amount of assistance the client may need to perform activities of daily living, such as bathing and eating. The client's ability to read printed educational materials is also determined during the eye examination.

If a more accurate assessment of visual acuity is required, a Snellen eye chart may be used. The client wears his glasses, but not if the glasses are intended only for reading. The nurse positions the client 20 feet from the chart. The client reads the smallest line of print possible three times; once with both eyes, then with each eye separately while the opposite eye is covered with the opaque card (Fig. 29-17). The client is successful when he is able to read more than half the letters or figures in the line. The visual acuity score is recorded in two numbers. The Snellen chart has standardized numbers at the end of each line of the chart. The numerator is the number 20 or the standard distance the client stands from the chart. The denominator is the distance from which the normal eye can read the chart. Normal vision is 20/20. The larger the denominator, the poorer the client's visual acuity. For example, a client with 20/200 vision can read a letter 20 feet away that a normal person could read 200 feet away. For clients who are unable to read, the E chart is used (Fig. 29-18). Instead of reading letters, the client tells the examiner which direction each E is pointing. Children use Snellen charts that have images of familiar objects.

VISUAL FIELD. Normally, a person looking straight ahead can see objects to the right, left, upper, and lower directions of the visual field. Clients with visual field alterations have a portion of their visual fields blacked out. Optic nerve damage or retinal disorders are common causes.

The nurse determines whether the client's visual fields are intact by asking the client to look straight

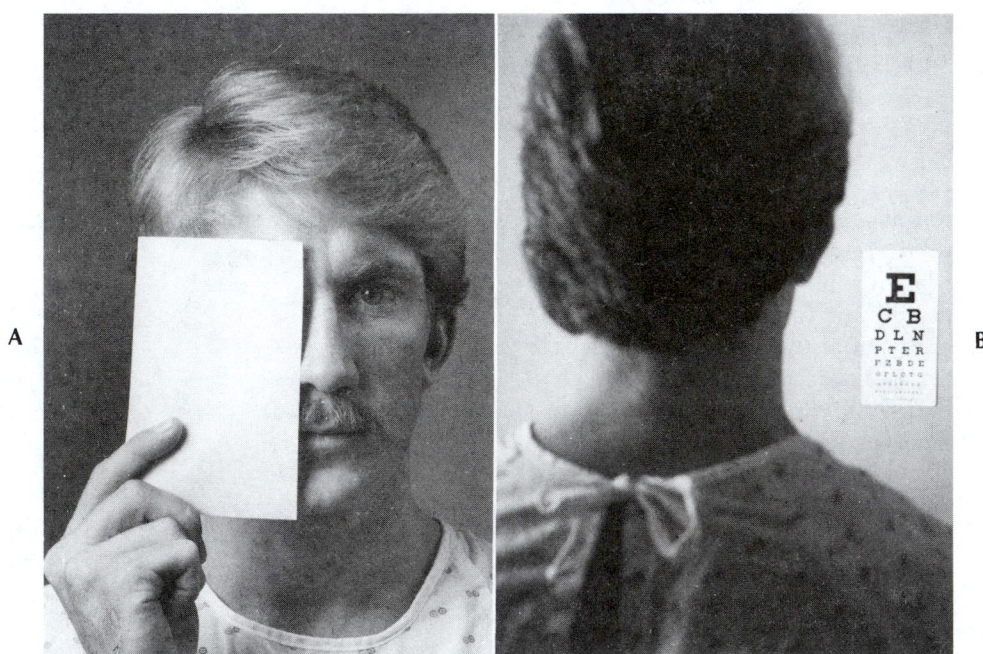

Fig. 29-17 Assessment of visual acuity. **A,** The client holds an opaque index card over one eye. The nurse assesses each eye separately for visual acuity. **B,** The client stands 20 feet away while reading the Snellen chart. The procedure is repeated for the other eye.

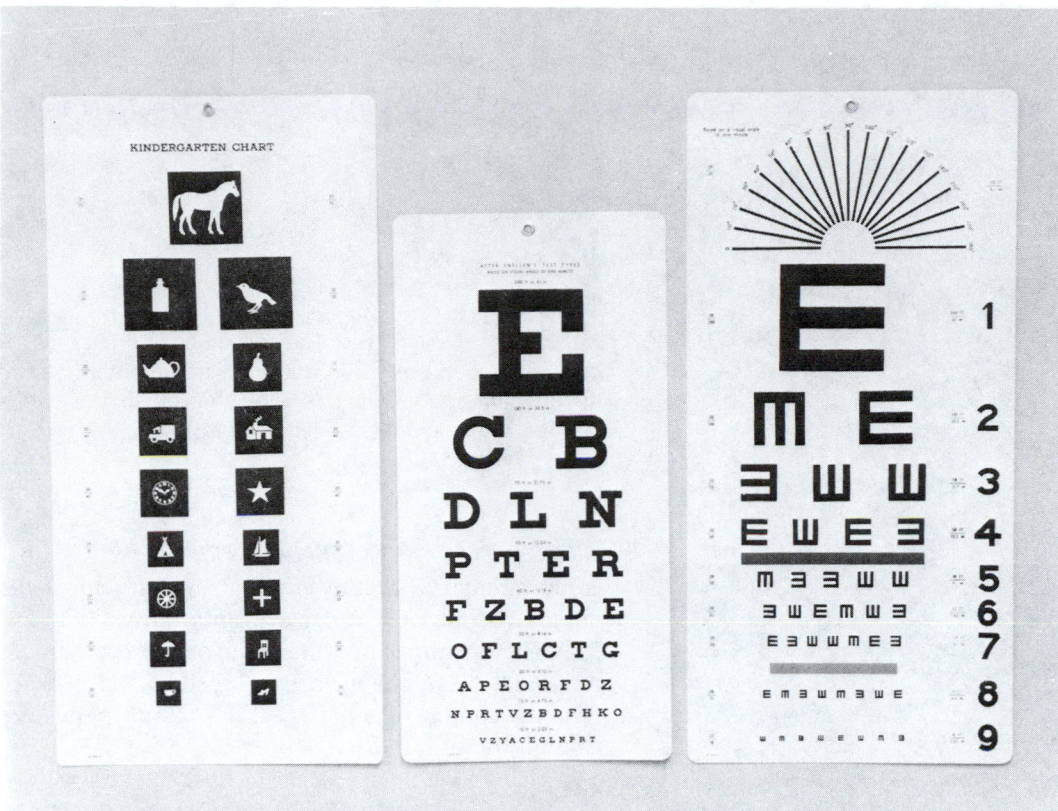

Fig. 29-18 Three types of Snellen charts. Left to right: children's chart, standard Snellen chart, and a Snellen E chart for clients who are unable to read.

ahead and introducing a moving object (the nurse's finger) into the client's field of vision. This allows the nurse to identify whether the client is able to see peripherally to the main line of vision.

To test a client's visual fields the nurse has the client stand 2 feet away, facing her. The nurse's eyes should be close to eye level with those of the client. The client gently closes or covers one eye and looks at the nurse's eye directly opposite. The nurse closes the other eye so that the field of vision is superimposed on that of the client. The nurse moves a finger outside the field of vision, then slowly brings it back into the visual field. The client is asked to tell when he sees it. If the nurse sees the finger before the client does, this indicates that a portion of the client's visual field is reduced. This procedure is repeated for each field of vision.

A client with visual field impairment requires a detailed eye examination by an ophthalmologist.

EXTRAOCULAR MOVEMENTS. Six small muscles guide the movement of each eye. Both eyes move parallel to each other in each direction of gaze. As the client looks straight ahead toward the nurse, he

should follow the movement of the nurse's finger through the eight cardinal gazes (Fig. 29-19). The finger is kept at a comfortable distance (6 to 12 inches) from the client (Fig. 29-20, *A*). The client looks to the right, to the left, up, down, and diagonally up and down to the left and right. The examiner's finger stays within the normal field of vision (Fig. 29-20, *B*). The client should not move or turn his head. As the client gazes in each direction, the nurse moves the finger slowly and smoothly. This is not a test to determine if the client can follow a rapidly moving finger.

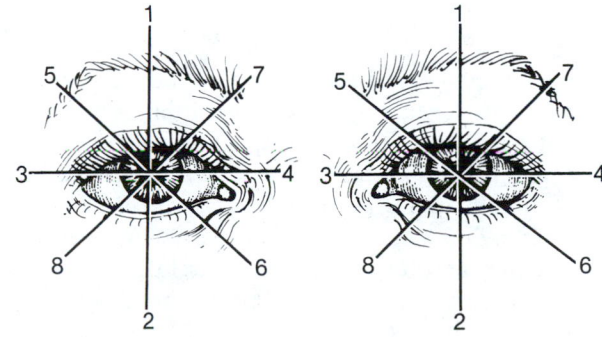

Fig. 29-19 The eight directions of gaze. The nurse directs the client to follow the movement of the nurse's finger through each of the gazes.

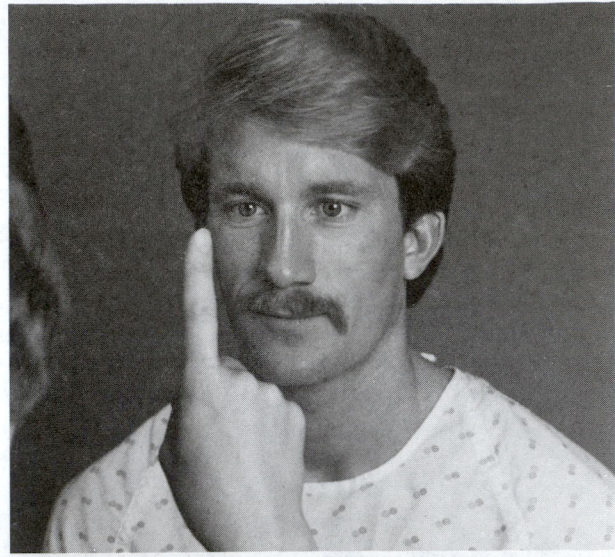

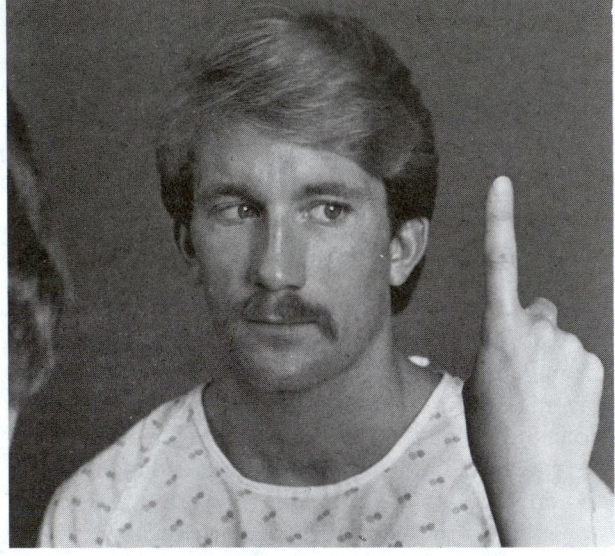

Fig. 29-20 **A,** To test extraocular movement the client begins by looking straight ahead at the examiner's finger. **B,** The client follows movement of the nurse's finger through each of the eight cardinal gazes.

The nurse observes for parallel eye movement, the position of the upper eyelid in relation to the iris, and the presence of abnormal movements such as nystagmus. With nystagmus there is a fine rhythmical oscillation of the eyes. The nurse can often initiate nystagmus in a client with normal eye movement by having him gaze to the far left or right. As the eyes move through each direction of gaze, the upper eyelid only covers the iris slightly.

Disturbances in eye movement reflect local injury to eye muscles and supporting structures or a disorder of the cranial nerves innervating the muscles.

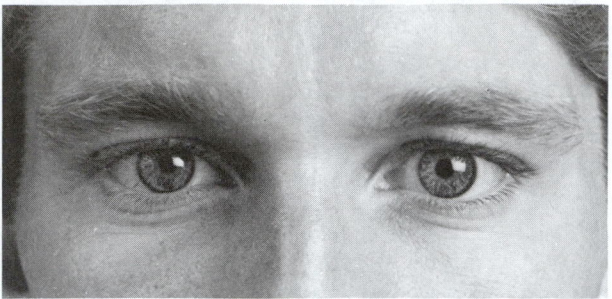

Fig. 29-21 Normal eyes. The sclerae and corneas are clear. The open eyelids do not fall over the pupils, and the lid margins rest flush against each eyeball. The eyelashes turn out and away from each eyeball.

ASSESSMENT OF EXTERNAL STRUCTURES. To become familiar with the external eye structures the nurse can first look at her eyes in a mirror (Fig. 29-21). The position and alignment of the eyes should be noted. Next, the eyebrows, eyelids, lacrimal apparatus, conjunctivae, sclerae, irises, and pupils are carefully scrutinized.

Position and Alignment. The nurse stands directly in front of the client at eye level and asks the client to look at the nurse's face. First the eyes' position and alignment are noted. The eyes are normally parallel to each other. Bulging of the eyes (exophthalmos) is usually caused by a thyroid disorder. If the eyes appear crossed or gaze in different directions, this is called strabismus. Strabismus is caused by neuromuscular alterations or an inherited defect in eye position.

Eyebrows. Normally the eyebrows are symmetrical. The eyebrows are inspected for quantity of hair and movement. A loss or absence of hair is indicative of hormonal disturbances. If a flaking of skin is seen around the brows, the client should be asked if he has experienced chronic irritation of the eye. Frequently a form of dandruff affects the eyebrows, with particles of skin entering and irritating the eyelids. If the client is unable to move the eyebrows, paralysis of the facial nerve exists.

Eyelids. When the eyes are open in a normal position, the lids do not cover the pupil and sclera cannot be seen above the iris. The lids are also close to the eyeball. An abnormal drooping of the lid over the pupil is called ptosis (pronounced "toe-sis"); it is caused by edema or impairment of the third cranial nerve. Defects in the position of the lid margins may be observed. Frequently elderly clients have lid margins that turn out or in. A disruption of the lid margin may lead to irritation of the conjunctiva.

The eyelids should be inspected further for color, edema, and the presence of lesions. Normally the lids are the same color as the client's skin. Redness of the lids is indicative of inflammation or infection. Heart and kidney failure and allergies can create edema of the eyelids, which impairs the ability of the lids to close. If lesions are present, they are inspected for typical characteristics in addition to the presence of discomfort or drainage.

Any disorder of the eyelid can impair the eye's external protection. The surface of the eye should be properly lubricated with tears.

Lacrimal Apparatus. The anterior surface of the eye, comprised of the sensitive cornea and conjunctiva, is moistened or lubricated by tears secreted from the lacrimal gland (Fig. 29-22). The gland is located in the upper outer wall of the anterior part of the orbit. Tears flow from the gland across the eye's surface to the lacrimal duct, which is located in the nasal corner or inner canthus of the eye. The lacrimal gland can be the site of tumors, infections, and abscesses. The area of the gland is inspected for edema and redness and palpated gently to detect tenderness. Normally the gland cannot be felt.

The nasolacrimal duct may become obstructed, blocking the flow of tears. The client will complain of excess tearing. The nurse looks for evidence of edema in the inner canthus. Mild palpation of the duct at the lower eyelid just inside the orbital rim may cause a regurgitation of tears.

Conjunctivae and Sclerae. The conjunctiva has two portions. The bulbar conjunctiva covers the exposed surface of the eyeball up to the outer edge of the cornea. The palpebral conjunctiva is the delicate membrane lining the eyelids. Normally the conjunctiva is transparent, enabling the examiner to view the tiny underlying blood vessel. It is the presence of blood vessels that gives the palpebral conjunctiva its light pink color. The sclera is seen under the bulbar conjunctiva and normally has the color of white porcelain.

Care must be taken when inspecting the conjunctiva. For adequate exposure the eyelids must be retracted without placing pressure directly on the eyeball. The lower lid is gently depressed with the thumb pressed against the bony orbit and the client is asked to look up (Fig. 29-23). Many clients begin to blink, making the examination difficult. Often the client can depress the eyelid to facilitate examination. The conjunctiva's color and the presence of edema or lesions are noted. A pale conjunctiva results from anemia,

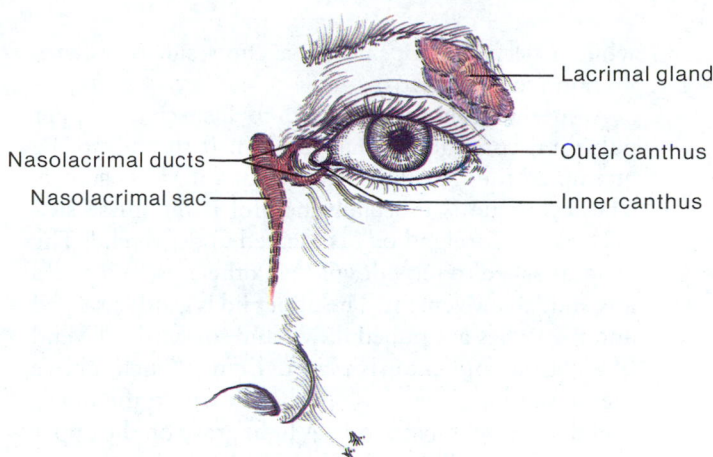

Fig. 29-22 The lacrimal apparatus secretes and drains tears, which moisten and lubricate eye structures.

Labels: Lacrimal gland, Outer canthus, Inner canthus, Nasolacrimal ducts, Nasolacrimal sac

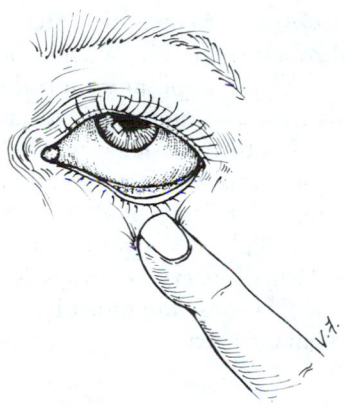

Fig. 29-23 Technique for retracting lower eyelid.

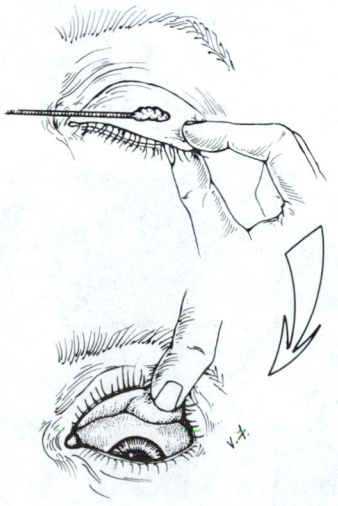

Fig. 29-24 Technique for inspecting upper palpebral conjunctiva.

while a fiery red appearance is the result of inflammation (conjunctivitis).

A special technique is used to inspect the upper palpebral conjunctiva (Fig. 29-24). It should not be attempted the first time without qualified assistance. The technique is especially helpful if the nurse suspects that a foreign body is located under the lid. The client is asked to look down, relax the eyes, and avoid any sudden movement. The upper lid is gently grasped and the lashes are pulled down and forward. The end of a cotton applicator is placed 1 cm (½ inch) above the lid margin. The nurse pushes down on the upper eyelid, turning it inside out. A light grasp on the upper lashes keeps the lid inverted. After inspection the eyelashes are gently pulled forward and the client is instructed to look up. The eyelid will return to its normal position.

If a foreign body appears to be embedded in the eye, one *must not attempt to remove it*. A physician should be notified immediately.

Pupils and Irises. Light enters the internal structures of the eye through the pupil. When a beam of light is shined through the pupil and onto the retina, the third cranial nerve is stimulated and innervates the muscles of the iris to constrict. Any abnormality existing along the pathway from the retina across the nerve pathways to the iris will alter the ability of the pupils to react to light. Changes in intracranial pressure, lesions along the nerve pathways, locally applied ophthalmic medications, and direct trauma to the eye may alter pupillary reaction.

The nurse observes the pupils for size, shape, equality, accommodation, and reaction to light. The pupils are normally round and equal in size. Dilated or constricted pupils can result from neurological disorders or the effect of eye medications. The surrounding iris is inspected for the presence of defects along its margins. Pupillary reflexes include those to light and accommodation. Pupillary reflexes should be tested in a dimly lit room, but not one so dark that the examiner cannot see the client's pupils clearly. As the client looks straight ahead, the nurse takes a penlight and brings it from the side of the client's face, directing the light onto the pupil (Fig. 29-25, *A*). If the client looks at the light there will be a false reaction to accommodation. The pupil that is directly illuminated constricts and the opposite pupil contracts consensually (Fig. 29-25, *B*). The nurse observes the quickness of the reflex.

To test accommodation, the examiner holds a finger approximately 10 to 15 cm (4 to 6 inches) from the client's nose. The client is asked to gaze at the finger and then at the wall in the distance. The pupils normally constrict when looking at the examiner's finger and dilate when looking at the wall.

OPHTHALMOSCOPIC EXAMINATION OF INTERNAL EYE STRUCTURES. The internal eye cannot be observed without an instrument to illuminate the eye structures. The ophthalmoscope is the instrument used to inspect the fundus, which includes the retina, choroid, optic nerve disc, macula, fovea centralis, and retinal vessels. Clients who are in greatest need of an

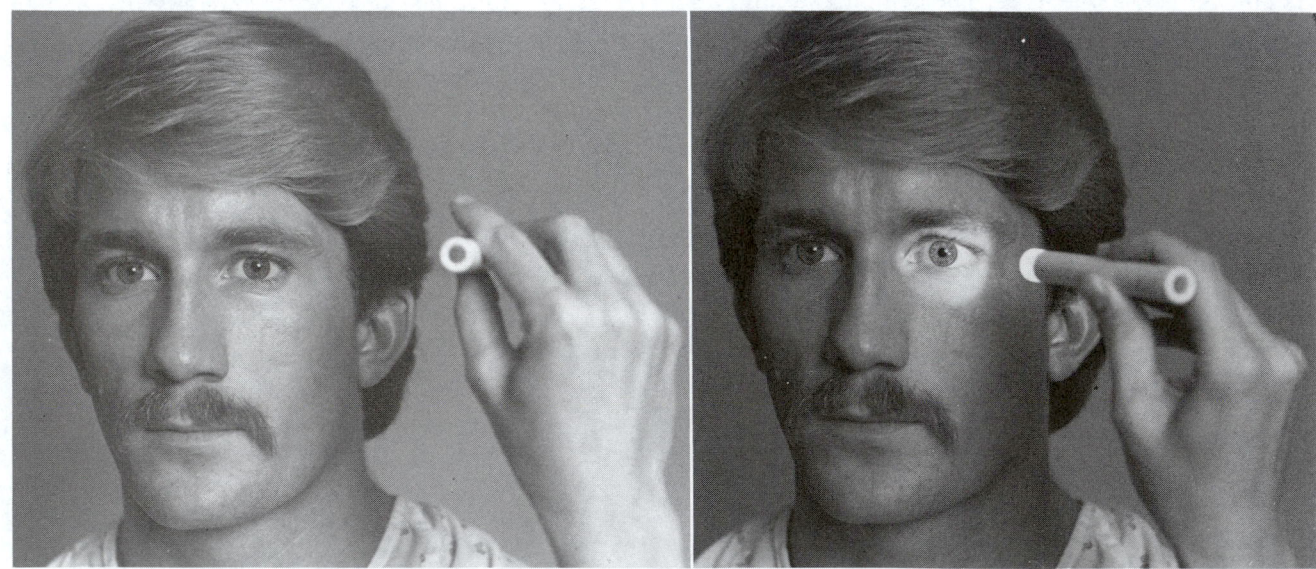

Fig. 29-25   A, To check pupil reflexes, first hold the penlight to the side of the client's face. **B,** Illumination of the pupil causes pupillary constriction.

examination of the fundus are those with diabetes, hypertension, and intracranial disorders.

The nurse must become comfortable in knowing how to handle the ophthalmoscope and must be able to recognize the normal appearance of the fundus. The direct ophthalmoscope has a battery tube light source, two dials or disks, and a keyhole viewer (Fig. 29-26). The dial at the top of the battery tube changes the light image. Five light patterns are available, but the large white light is used for general examination. The disk at the top controls the choice of lens. The lens disk rotates clockwise for selection of a variety of lenses.

The nurse should practice holding the ophthalmoscope in each hand, using the index finger to rotate the lens disk. The examiner turns the white light on, sets the lens setting to 0, and looks through the keyhole, focusing on near objects such as the palm of the hand. Reading the newspaper with the ophthalmoscope is useful practice. During actual examination the examiner keeps both eyes open while looking through the keyhole.

The examination is performed in a darkened room. The examiner and client sit in comfortable positions facing each other with their eyes at the same height. The ophthalmoscope's light is switched on and the lens rotated to 0. The index finger is kept on the lens

disk in order to refocus the ophthalmoscope during the examination.

The examiner's right hand and eye are used to examine the client's right eye, and the left hand and eye are used for the client's left eye. The client is asked to gaze straight ahead over the examiner's shoulder throughout the examination.

The ophthalmoscope is held firmly against the face (Fig. 29-27). At a distance of approximately 25 cm (10 inches) from the client and lateral to his line of vision, the examiner shines the light on the pupil. A bright orange glow in the pupil, called the red reflex, can then be seen. The light from the ophthalmoscope causes the pupil to constrict. The light is slowly moved in toward the pupil, while the examiner keeps it focused on the red reflex (Fig. 29-28). The examiner must relax and keep both eyes open. As the light approaches the pupil, the examiner will begin to see structures of the fundus. Rotating the lens disk allows the examiner to bring the internal structures into focus. The examiner inspects the size, color, and clarity of the disc, integrity of vessels, presence of retinal lesions, and appearance of the macula and fovea (Fig. 29-29). Normally the following are observed:

1. A clear, yellow optic nerve disc
2. Reddish pink retina
3. Light red arteries and dark red veins
4. A 3:2 vein to artery ratio in size proportion
5. The avascular macula

If any abnormalities are observed, the client should be examined by an ophthalmologist. The client's fundus should not be illuminated for extended periods. The bright light of the ophthalmoscope is very irritating and can cause discomfort and tearing. During

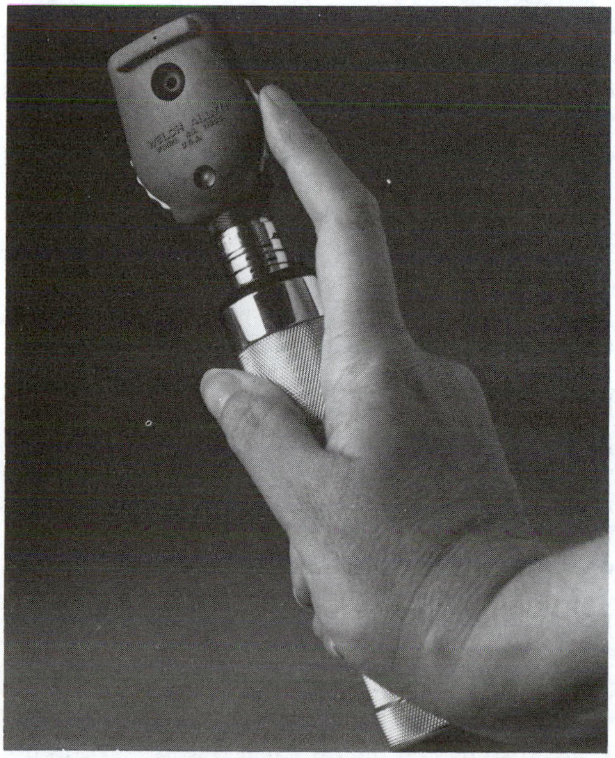

Fig. 29-26 An ophthalmoscope.

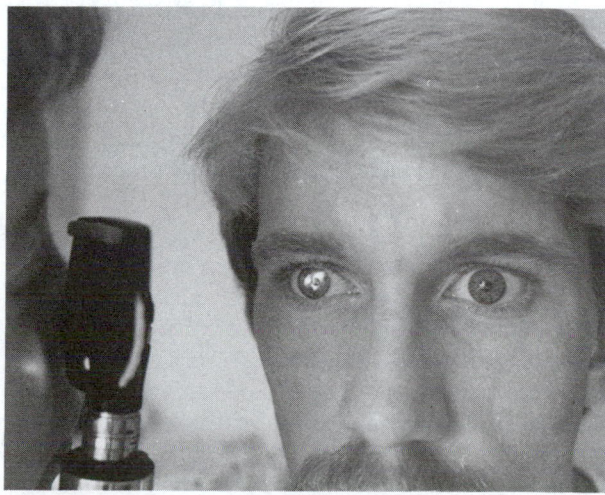

Fig. 29-27 The ophthalmoscope's light illuminates the pupil. The nurse looks for an orange glow or "red reflex."

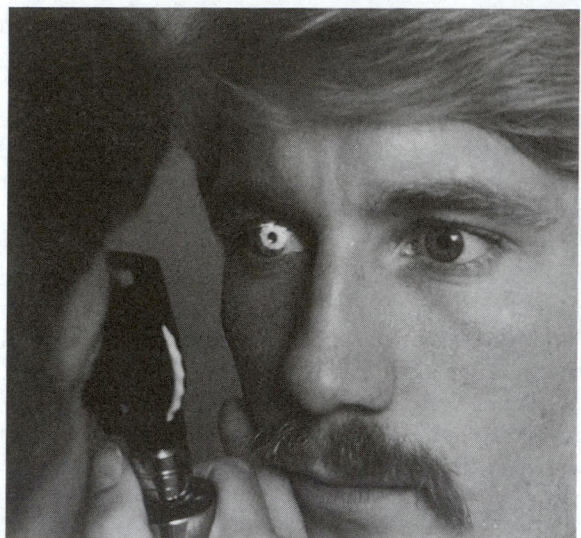

Fig. 29-28 To visualize internal eye structures, the nurse moves in toward the pupil with the light focused on the red reflex.

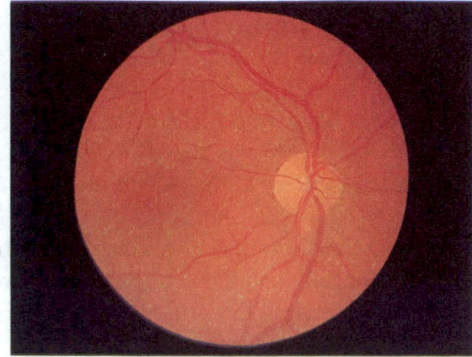

Fig. 29-29 Normal fundus.

From Malasanos, L., et al.: Health assessment, ed. 2, St. Louis, 1981, The C.V. Mosby Co.

the examination the client should be encouraged to mention any discomfort.

EARS

The ears are relatively easy structures to assess because of their accessibility. The nurse inspects the condition of outer and middle ear structures, palpates external structures, and assesses the client's hearing acuity (Fig. 29-30). Disorders of the ear are the result of one of four types of problems: mechanical dysfunction (blockage by ear wax or foreign body), trauma (foreign bodies, noise exposure), neurological disorders (auditory nerve damage), and acute illnesses (viral infection). The nurse considers each potential type of problem while making observations. During the assessment the nurse asks the client if he has experienced ear pain, itching, discharge, tinnitus (ringing in the ears), or change in hearing ability. Each symptom helps to determine the nature of the client's problem.

AURICLES. The nurse looks at the auricles' placement, size, and symmetry (Fig. 29-31). The auricles are normally level with each other. The upper point of attachment to the head is in a straight line with the lateral canthus of the eye. Low-set ears are a sign of congenital abnormality. The auricle is gently palpated for the presence of lesions. If the client complains of pain or if the ear appears inflamed, the auricle is pulled and the tragus pressed. If palpating the external ear increases the client's pain, an external ear infection is probably present. The nurse should

observe closely for the presence of discharge from the ear, and the size of the external auditory meatus should be noted. A yellow or greenish discharge is a sign of infection. The meatus should not be swollen or occluded.

EAR CANALS AND EARDRUMS. The deeper structures of the external and middle ear can be observed only with the use of an otoscope. A special ear speculum attaches to the battery tube of the ophthalmoscope (Fig. 29-32). Speculums are made in different sizes to conform to the size of clients' ear canals (Fig. 29-33). For best visualization the largest speculum that fits comfortably into the ear canal should be used.

Before inserting the speculum, the examiner checks for foreign bodies in the opening of the auditory canal. Children commonly place objects in their ears. It is very important that the client avoid moving the head during the examination, lest damage be inflicted to the canal and tympanic membrane. Infants and young children often need to be restrained. For best results the parent should be asked to hold the child. Infants should lie supine with their heads turned to one side and their arms held securely at their sides. Young children can sit on their parent's lap with their legs held between the parent's knees.

To insert the speculum properly, the nurse asks the client to tip the head slightly to the opposite shoulder. Pulling the auricle upward and backward in the adult helps to straighten the ear canal (Fig. 29-34). In infants the auricle is pulled backward and downward,

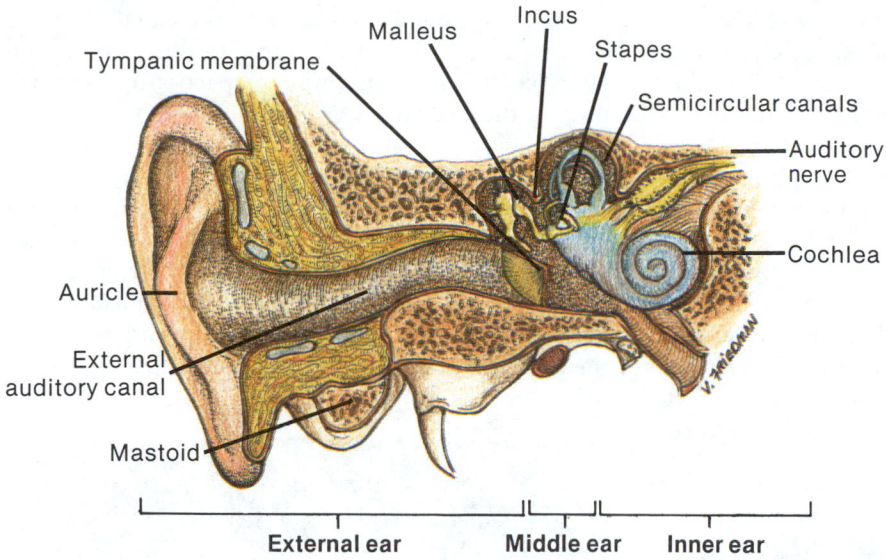

Fig. 29-30 Ear structures. The external ear consists of the auricle and external auditory canal. Middle ear structures include the tympanic membrane and bony ossicles (malleus, incus, and stapes). The semicircular canal, cochlea, and auditory nerve are the inner ear structures.

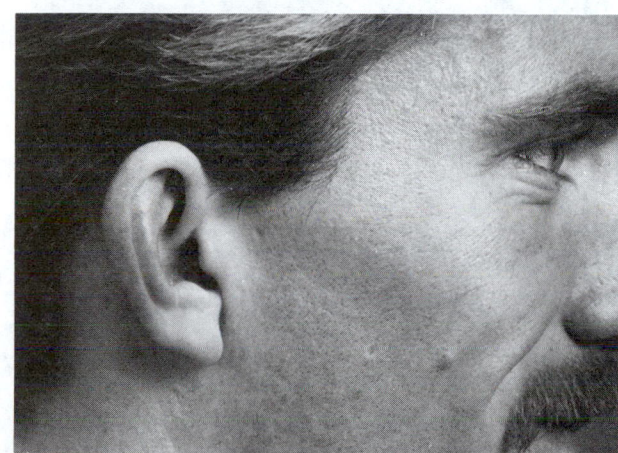

Fig. 29-31 The upper edge of the auricle is normally in alignment with the lateral canthus of the eye.

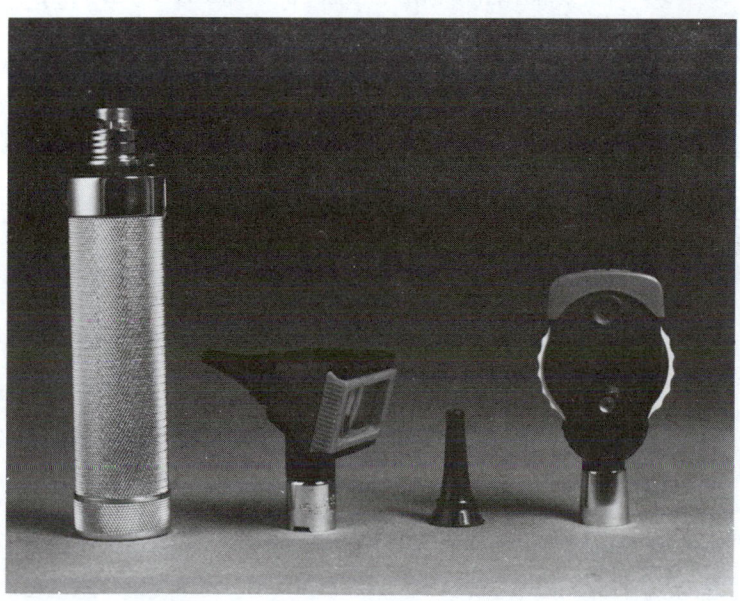

Fig. 29-32 Battery tube with ophthalmoscope and otoscope attachments.

and in older children the auricle is pulled backward and upward. The nurse inserts the speculum, taking care not to abrade the lining of the canal. The skin of the canal is very thin and sensitive to any minor trauma. Some nurses choose to hold the otoscope upside down so they can use a hand to brace against the client's head and prevent sudden movement of the otoscope.

The nurse identifies the presence of cerumen (ear wax) and observes for lesions, foreign bodies, or discharge in the canal. A reddened canal is a sign of inflammation. During the examination the examiner asks the client how the ear canal is normally cleaned. The examiner should caution the client on the danger

of inserting pointed objects into the canal. The use of cotton-tipped applicators to clean the ears should be avoided, since this causes impaction of cerumen deep in the ear canal.

The light from the otoscope allows clear visualization of the eardrum (tympanic membrane). The nurse must be familiar with the common anatomical landmarks and their appearance (Fig. 29-35). The otoscope is slowly moved to see the entire drum and its periphery. The normal eardrum is a translucent or pearly gray. Since the eardrum is angled away from the ear canal, the light from the otoscope appears as

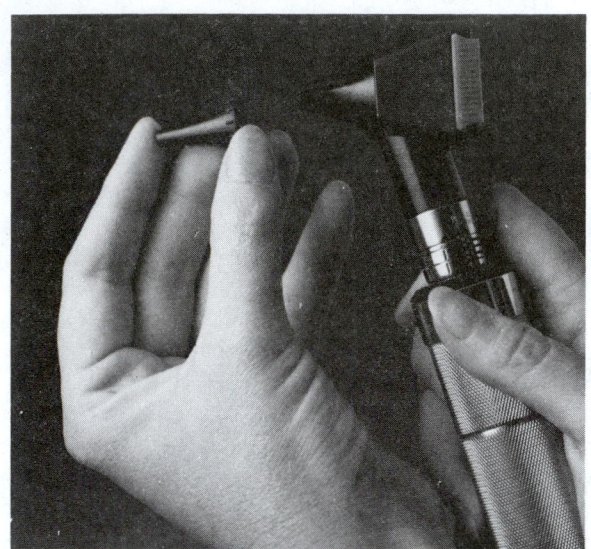

Fig. 29-33 The otoscope has different sized speculums to fit the client's ear canal.

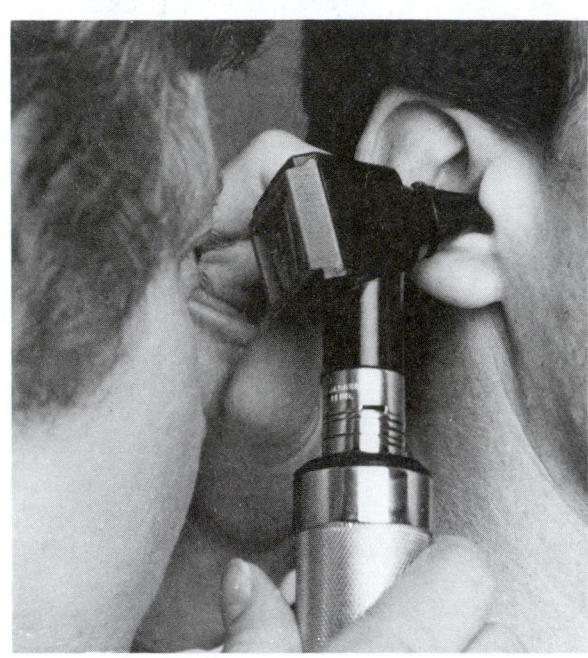

Fig. 29-34 In an adult, pulling the auricle upward and backward straightens the ear canal for easier otoscope placement.

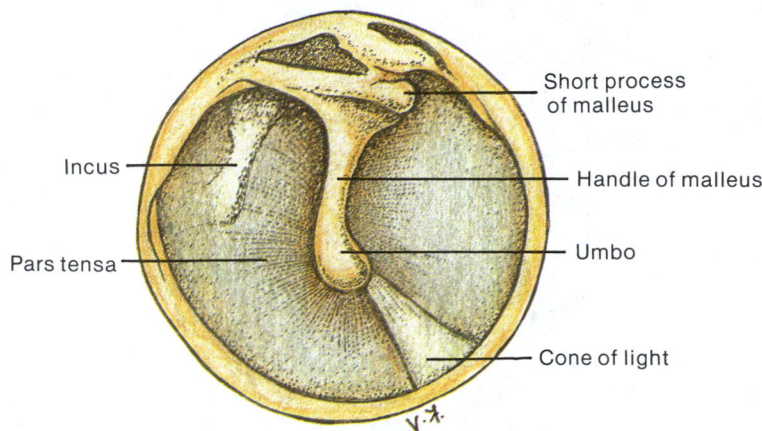

Incus —
Pars tensa —
Short process of malleus
Handle of malleus
Umbo
Cone of light

Fig. 29-35 Normal tympanic membrane.

PROCEDURE 29-1

Tuning Fork Tests

TEST AND STEPS	*RATIONALE*

WEBER'S TEST (LATERALIZATION OF SOUND)

1. Hold the fork at its base and strike it against the palm of the hand or the knuckle.
2. Place the base of the vibrating fork on the top of the client's head.
3. Ask the client where sound is heard.

A client with normal hearing hears sound equally in both ears or in midline of head. In conduction deafness, air conduction is blocked. Vibrating fork transmits sound through bone directly to inner ear structures. Sound is heard best in affected ear.

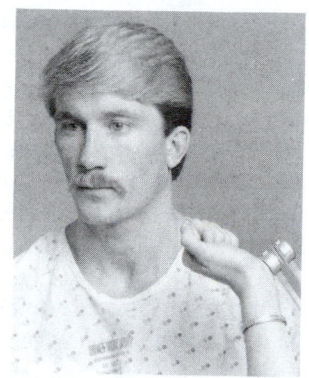

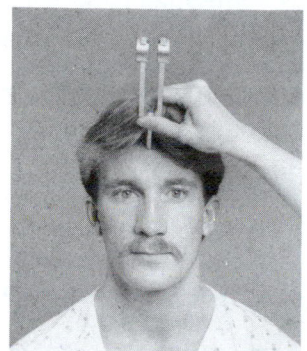

RINNE'S TEST (COMPARISON OF AIR AND BONE CONDUCTION)

1. Strike the tuning fork against the palm of the hand or the knuckle.
2. Place the vibrating fork on the mastoid process.
3. Ask the client to inform you when sound is no longer heard.
4. Immediately place the vibrating fork close to the external ear meatus.
5. Ask the client to inform you if sound can be heard.

Normally, hearing through air conduction is better than through bone conduction (positive Rinne). In conduction deafness sounds through bone conduction can be heard after air conduction sounds become inaudible (negative Rinne).

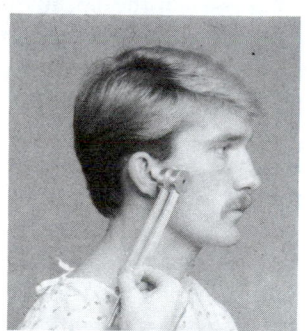

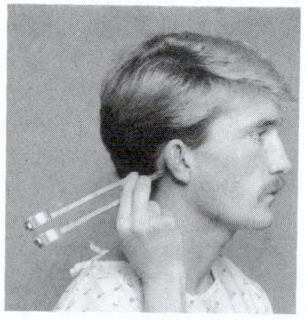

a cone shape rather than a circle. The umbo is near the center of the drum, behind which is the attachment of the malleus. A knoblike structure at the top of the drum is created by the underlying short process of the malleus. The examiner should check carefully to be sure there are no tears or breaks in the eardrum's membrane.

HEARING ACUITY. Often the nurse can tell from the client's response to conversation or from his requests to the nurse to repeat statements whether a hearing loss is present. There are three types of hearing loss: conduction, sensorineural, and mixed. A conduction loss involves an interruption of sound waves as they travel from the outer ear to the cochlea of the inner ear, because they are not transmitted through the outer and middle ear structures. Examples of causes of conduction hearing loss are a swelling of the auditory canal or a tear in the eardrum. A sensorineural loss involves the inner ear, the auditory nerve, or the hearing center of the brain. Sound is conducted through the outer and middle ear structures, but the continued transmission of sound becomes interrupted at some point beyond the bony ossicles. A mixed loss involves a combination of conduction and sensorineural loss.

Some clients are more at risk for developing hearing loss. The industrial nurse is keenly aware of clients who work in environments where noise levels are high, and such clients may be seen in other settings as well. The client must be asked if he spends a large amount of time or works around loud noises. Sensorineural loss is a common occurrence in the elderly. Certain medications (for example, antibiotics and aspirin) also can cause hearing disorders.

A simple assessment can be performed to screen for hearing loss. One ear is tested at a time. The client is asked to occlude one ear or the nurse can occlude it with her finger. The nurse stands approximately 30 cm (1 foot) away, exhales fully, and softly whispers numbers toward the unoccluded ear. The nurse must cover her mouth or ask the client to close his eyes to prevent lip reading. If necessary, the nurse can gradually increase voice intensity until the client correctly repeats the numbers. Use of consecutive numbers should be avoided so the client will not anticipate the number. A ticking watch may be used, but the spoken word allows for more accuracy and control in testing.

Use of a tuning fork is a more refined test for determining the nature of a hearing loss. By tapping the tuning fork against the palm, the examiner creates a vibrating column that emits sound waves. Placement of the fork either in front of the auricle or on the mastoid process behind the ear allows for the testing of air and bone conduction. Placement of the fork on the top of the client's head tests for lateralization of sound. Procedure 29-1 describes the Weber and Rinne tuning fork tests.

If hearing acuity is impaired, the client is referred to a physician for further examination. The nurse takes precautions to ensure effective communication with the client. Standing on the side of the client's good ear, speaking in a clear normal tone of voice, and facing the client so he can see the speaker's lips and face are simple means to improve the client's hearing of conversation (see Chapter 44). Effective communication may become a priority in obtaining cooperation and information from the client during the examination.

NOSE AND SINUSES

The integrity of the nose and sinuses is assessed by means of inspection and palpation. It is useful to know if the client's nursing history indicates allergies, nasal obstruction, epistaxis (nosebleeds), discharge, frequent colds, or postnasal drip.

NOSE. While inspecting the nose, the nurse observes for asymmetry, inflammation, or deformity. Recent trauma may have caused edema and discoloration. If swelling or deformities exist, the nose is palpated gently for tenderness, swelling, and underlying deviations.

The nasal mucosa and septum are further inspected. The mucosa and septum can be grossly examined by illuminating each nostril with a penlight. A nasal speculum is required for closer inspection and adequate visualization of the deeper turbinates.

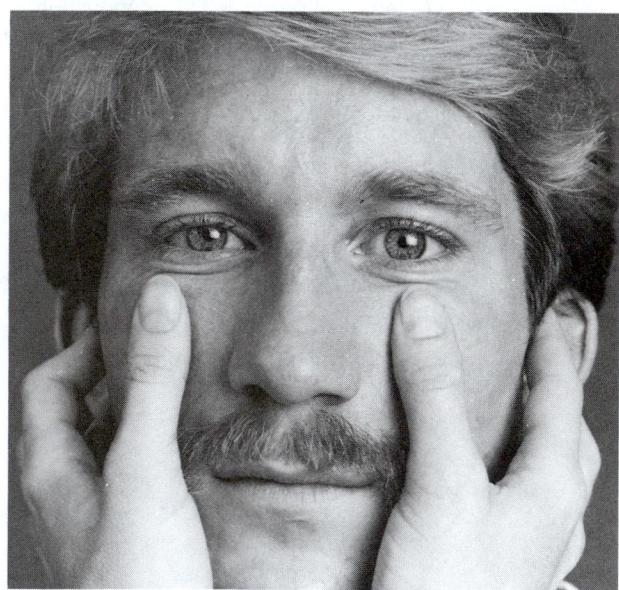

Fig. 29-36 Palpation of maxillary sinuses.

The anterior end of the nose is observed first. The mucosa is inspected for its color, presence of lesions, discharge, swelling, and evidence of bleeding. Normal mucosa is pink. Discharge resulting from sinus irritation is generally clear and watery. A sinus infection results in yellowish or greenish discharge. A pale mucosa with clear discharge is a sign of allergy. For the client with a nasogastric tube, the nurse routinely checks for local excoriation of the nares, characterized by redness and sloughing of the skin.

The client tips his head back slightly to give the examiner a clearer view of the septum and turbinates. The septum is inspected for deviation, lesions, and superficial blood vessels. A deviated septum can obstruct breathing and interfere with passage of a nasogastric tube.

SINUSES.

The examination of the sinuses is limited to palpation. In cases of allergies or infection, the interior of the sinuses becomes inflamed and swollen. The most effective way to assess for tenderness is by externally palpating the frontal and maxillary facial areas (Fig. 29-36). Gentle upward pressure elicits tenderness easily and reveals the severity of sinus irritation. Pressure should not be applied to the eyes. Fig. 29-37 is a cross section of the nasal sinus cavities.

MOUTH AND PHARYNX

As in the case of the integument, the oral cavity can reveal information about the client's overall health. Too frequently the nurse hurries through an assessment of the mouth and pharynx. Oral hygiene is a vital part of many clients' care plans, for example, clients who suffer dehydration, are restricted from drinking or eating, have experienced facial trauma or surgery, or require use of an oral airway. The oral cavity functions as a sensory organ for taste and pain responses and a motor system for chewing, swallowing, and speech. Numerous physiological alterations can cause disorders of the mouth and pharynx, so the nurse should take the time to examine all structures with care.

For this examination a penlight and tongue depressor or single gauze square are needed. At times a clean glove is used to palpate lesions. The examiner is seated facing the client at eye level.

MOUTH.

A client who wears dentures should be asked to remove them and offered a paper towel and denture cup. This is a good time to ask whether the client has noticed any pain in the mouth or gums.

The lips are inspected for color, texture, hydration, contour, and the presence of lesions. As the client opens his mouth to semifullness, the nurse views the lips from end to end. Normally the lips are pink, moist, symmetrical, and smooth (Fig. 29-38).

To view the inner oral mucosa, the nurse has the client open the mouth slightly and gently pull the lower lip away from the teeth (Fig. 29-39, *A*). This process is repeated for the upper lip (Fig. 29-39, *B*). The mucosa is inspected for color, hydration, texture, and the presence of lesions, such as ulcers, abrasions, or cysts.

For adequate visualization of the buccal mucosa a tongue depressor or gauze square is used to retract the lips (Fig. 29-40). The penlight illuminates the more posterior portion of the mucosa. The client should open the mouth wide so the nurse can note the mucosa's color, texture, and hydration. Normally the mucosa is a glistening pink. Hyperpigmentation is seen in 10% of whites after the age of 50 and up to 90% of blacks by the same age. For clients with normal pigmentation the buccal mucosa is a good site to inspect for jaundice or pallor. The appearance of

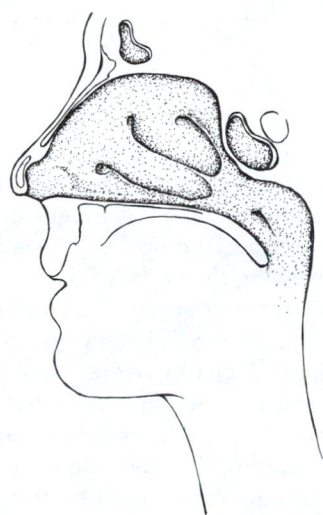

Fig. 29-37 Cross section of nasal sinuses.

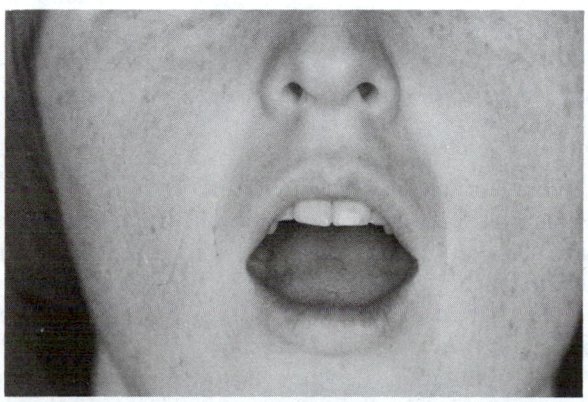

Fig. 29-38 The lips are normally pink, symmetrical, smooth, and moist.

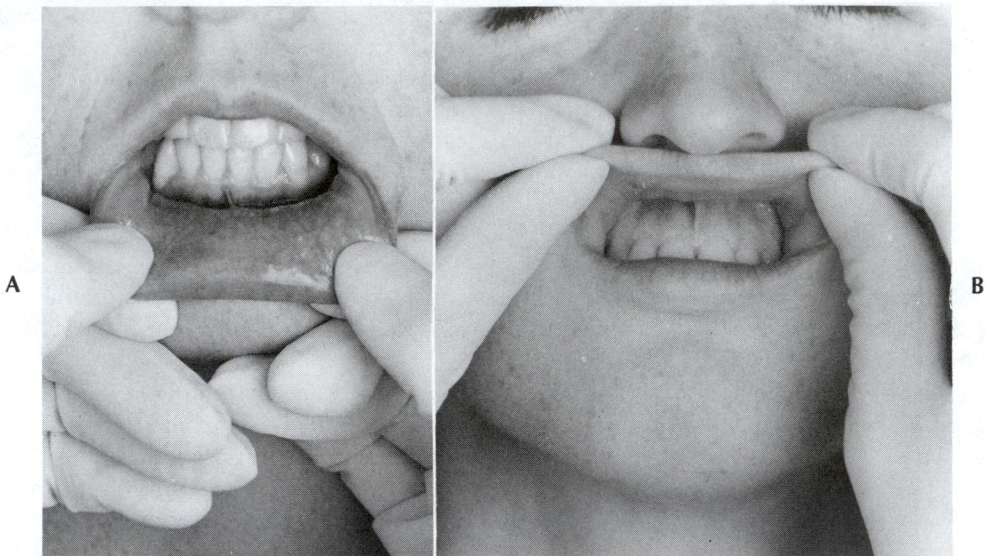

Fig. 29-39 **A,** Inspection of inner oral mucosa of lower lip. **B,** Inspection of upper lip mucosa.

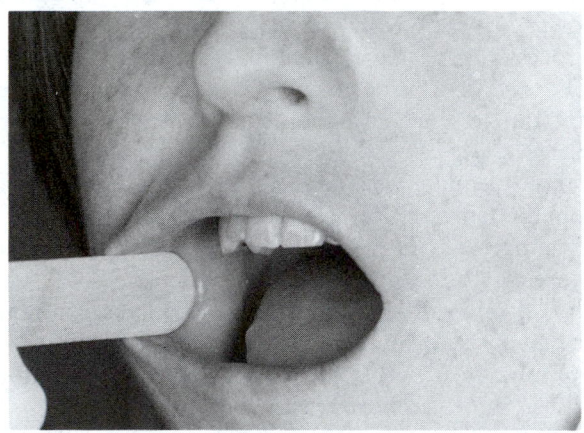

Fig. 29-40 Retraction of the lips permits visualization of the buccal mucosa.

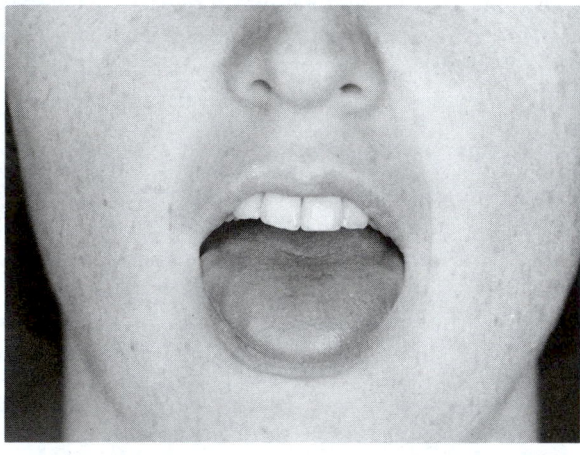

Fig. 29-41 The client protrudes the tongue for adequate visualization.

thick white patches (leukoplakia) can be seen in heavy smokers and alcoholics. The presence of leukoplakia should be reported, since it can also be a precancerous lesion.

The gums or gingivae are examined for color, edema, retraction, bleeding, and lesions. Healthy gums are pink, moist, and smooth. If a client wears dentures, any irregularity or lesion of the gums can create discomfort and significantly impair the ability to chew. Inadequate nutrition is a common problem for clients with ill-fitting dentures.

The quality of a client's dental hygiene is easily determined by inspecting the teeth. The client should open the lips and clench the teeth. The position and alignment of teeth are noted. To examine the posterior surface of the teeth the nurse has the client open the mouth with lips relaxed. A tongue depressor may be needed to retract the lips and cheeks, especially when one is viewing the molars. The presence of dental caries and extraction sites and the teeth's color should be noted. Normal, healthy teeth are smooth, white, and shiny. A chalky white discoloration of the enamel is an early indication that caries is forming. Brown or black discolorations indicate advanced caries. While examining the teeth the nurse can ask the client what techniques are used to clean them. This is a good opportunity for client education.

Tongue. The tongue is carefully inspected on all sides, and the floor of the mouth is checked. The client first relaxes the mouth and sticks the tongue out halfway (Fig. 29-41). If the client is forced to protrude the tongue too far, the gag reflex may be elicited. Using the penlight for illumination, the nurse examines the tongue for color, size, position, texture, and the presence of coating or lesions. The number of papillae (taste buds) varies throughout life. The tongue should appear medium red in color with smooth lateral margins and free mobility. When the tongue protrudes, it lies in the midline. The dorsum of the tongue should not be exceptionally smooth.

The tongue is highly vascular, particularly on the undersurface. Extra care is taken to inspect the undersurface, a common site of origin for oral cancer lesions. The client lifts the tongue to permit adequate inspection (Fig. 29-42). If nodules or cysts are noted, the nurse palpates them to determine size, tenderness, consistency, and mobility. The area under the tongue is also a site for oral cancer. Varicosities (swollen, tortuous veins) may be seen. Varicosities rarely cause problems; they are common in the elderly.

Palate. The client should extend the head backward, holding the mouth open so the nurse can inspect the hard and soft palates (Fig. 29-43). The hard palate or roof of the mouth is located anteriorly. The soft palate extends posteriorly toward the pharynx. The palates are observed for color, shape, and the presence of extra bony prominences or defects. It is common to visualize a bony growth or exostosis between the two palates.

PHARYNX. An examination of the pharyngeal structures is performed primarily to rule out the presence of infection, inflammation, or lesions. The method used to expose the pharynx should be explained. The client tips the head back slightly, opens the mouth wide, and says "ah." The nurse places the tip of a tongue depressor on the middle third of the tongue, taking care not to press the lower lip against the teeth. If the tongue depressor is placed too far anteriorly, the posterior part of the tongue mounds up, obstructing the view. The gag reflex is elicited whenever the tongue depressor touches the posterior tongue.

With the aid of a penlight, the nurse first inspects the uvula and soft palate (Fig. 29-44). Both structures, which are innervated by the tenth cranial nerve (vagus), should rise centrally as the client says "ah." The anterior and posterior pillars are examined and the presence or absence of tonsillar tissue is noted. The posterior pharynx is the last structure to view. Normally pharyngeal structures are pink and well hydrated. Any edema, petechiae (small hemorrhages),

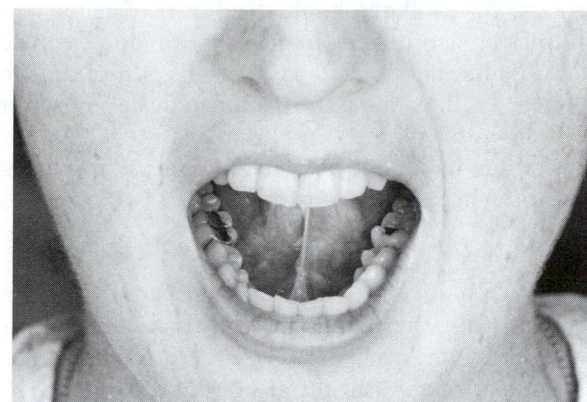

Fig. 29-42 The undersurface of the tongue is highly vascular.

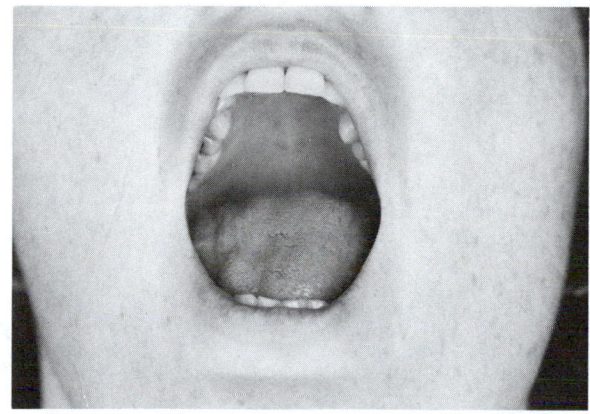

Fig. 29-43 The hard palate is located anteriorly in the roof of the mouth.

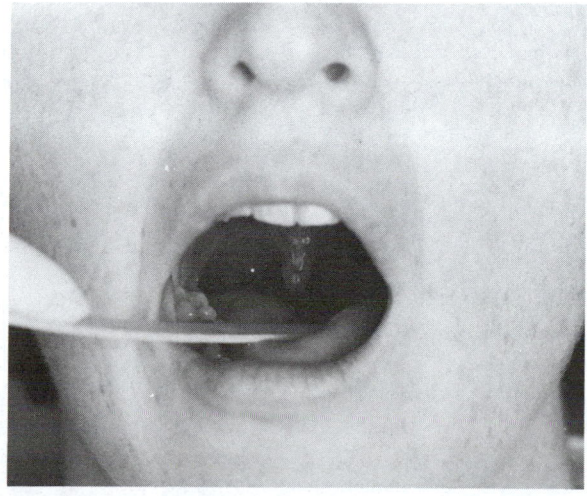

Fig. 29-44 A tongue depressor allows the nurse to visualize the uvula and posterior soft palate.

lesions, or exudate should be noted. Clients with chronic sinus problems frequently exhibit a clear exudate that drains along the wall of the posterior pharynx. Any yellow or green exudate indicates infection. A client with a typical sore throat has a reddened and edematous uvula and tonsillar pillars with the possible presence of yellow exudate.

NECK

The lymph nodes of the head, the carotid arteries, jugular veins, thyroid gland, and trachea are all located within the neck (Fig. 29-45). Many nurses defer assessment of the carotid arteries and jugular veins until the cardiovascular assessment is performed. The nurse with an understanding of normal anatomical locations is better prepared to examine neck structures. The different structures within the neck are inspected and palpated. The skill of auscultation is also used.

The examination is best performed with the client sitting. The client raises the chin and tilts the head backward. The neck is inspected for asymmetry, edema, masses, or scars. If any masses are seen, they should be palpated to determine size, shape, tenderness, consistency, and mobility.

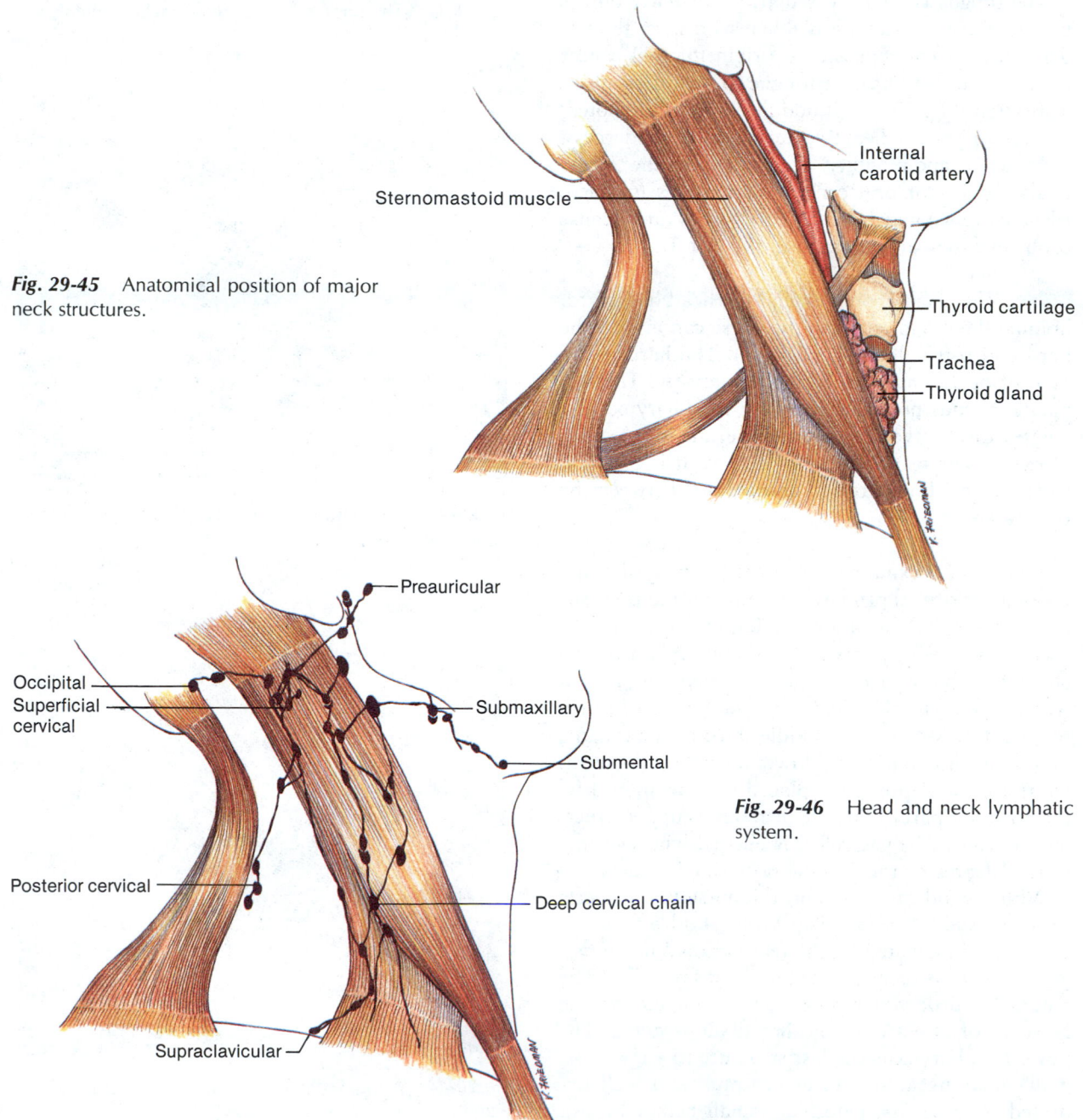

Fig. 29-45 Anatomical position of major neck structures.

Labels (Fig. 29-45): Sternomastoid muscle; Internal carotid artery; Thyroid cartilage; Trachea; Thyroid gland

Fig. 29-46 Head and neck lymphatic system.

Labels (Fig. 29-46): Preauricular; Occipital; Superficial cervical; Submaxillary; Submental; Posterior cervical; Deep cervical chain; Supraclavicular

LYMPH NODES. An extensive system of lymph nodes collects lymph from the head, ears, nose, cheeks, and lips. Fig. 29-46 illustrates the location of each major lymphatic center in the head and neck.

A methodical approach is used to examine the lymph nodes in order to avoid overlooking any single node or chain. Both sides of the neck must be inspected and compared. During palpation the nurse stands behind or to the side of the client for easy access to all nodes. Using the pads of the middle three fingers of each hand, the nurse palpates gently in a rotary motion over the nodes (Fig. 29-47). If excessive pressure is applied, small nodes are missed and palpable nodes are obliterated.

The lymph nodes serve as collecting sites for the drainage of lymphatic fluid. The nodes become enlarged from localized and systemic infection. It is not unusual for a lymph node to remain permanently enlarged after serious infection; such enlarged nodes are usually nontender. The lymph nodes can also become the site of malignant tumors. A malignancy is classically hard, immobile, irregularly shaped, and often nontender.

THYROID GLAND. The thyroid gland lies in the anterior lower neck, in front of and to both sides of the trachea. The gland is fixed to the trachea with the isthmus overlying the trachea and connecting the two irregular, cone-shaped lobes (Fig. 29-48). The nurse assesses the thyroid gland by inspection and palpation.

The examiner stands in front of the client and inspects the area of the lower neck overlying the thyroid gland for visible masses and symmetry. The client should extend the neck and swallow, with the nurse noting whether these maneuvers cause a bulging of the gland. It may be easier for the client to swallow if he has a glass of water. Normally the thyroid cannot be visualized.

To palpate the gland, the examiner stands either in front of or behind the client. For the posterior approach the client is instructed to lower the chin to relax the neck muscles. Both of the nurse's hands are placed around the neck with the fingertips overlying the lower trachea (Fig. 29-49). The thyroid isthmus is palpated and the client asked to swallow. Any enlargement of the isthmus as it rises should be noted. To examine each lobe, the nurse has the client turn the head slightly toward the side being examined (Fig. 29-50). For example, during examination of the left lobe the client lowers the chin and turns the head slightly to the left. The examiner's right hand gently displaces the thyroid to the left while the left hand palpates the lobe. This procedure is repeated for the right lobe. Normally the thyroid gland is not enlarged; however, in extremely thin individuals the thyroid is more easily palpable. Enlargement is a manifestation of thyroid dysfunction. Masses or nodules can be signs of malignant disease.

The anterior approach follows the same maneuvers as the posterior approach. The nurse uses the index and middle fingers of the dominant hand to palpate the isthmus as the client swallows. Then, with the client's head turned alternately to each side, the nurse displaces each lobe and palpates with the other hand.

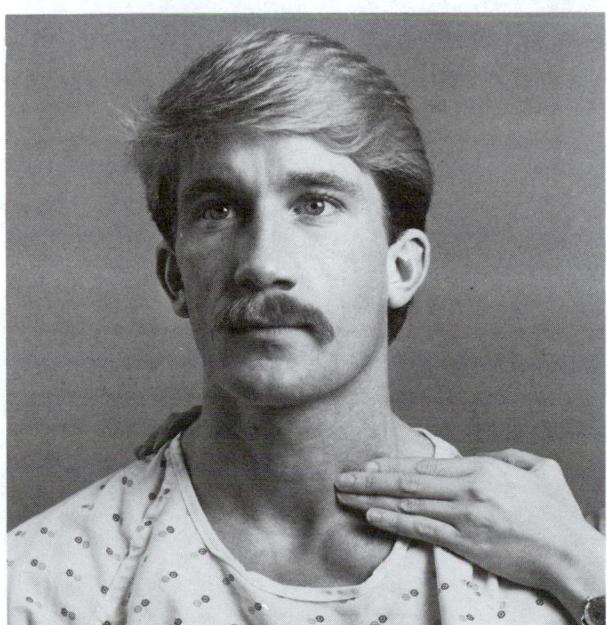

Fig. 29-47 Palpation of cervical lymph nodes.

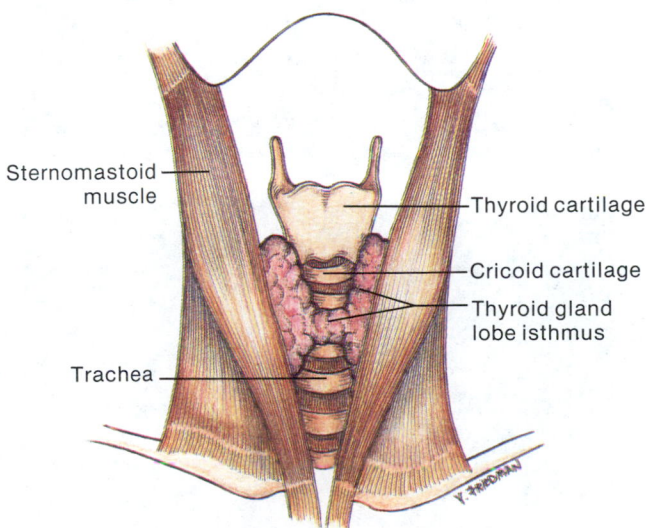

Sternomastoid muscle

Trachea

Thyroid cartilage

Cricoid cartilage

Thyroid gland lobe isthmus

Fig. 29-48 The thyroid gland lies anteriorly in the neck. It is fixed to both sides of the trachea with the isthmus overlying the trachea.

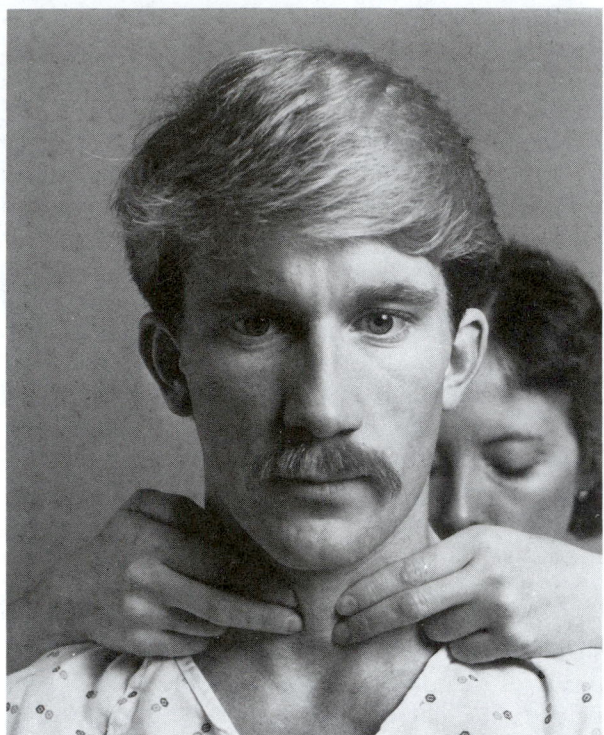

Fig. 29-49 Posterior approach for palpation of the thyroid gland.

TRACHEA. The trachea is a part of the upper airway that can be directly palpated. It is normally located in the midline above the suprasternal notch. Masses in the neck or mediastinum and pulmonary abnormalities can cause the trachea to be displaced laterally. The client may sit or lie down during the palpation. The position of the trachea is determined by palpating at the suprasternal notch, slipping the thumb and index fingers to each side (Fig. 29-51). Forceful pressure must not be applied to the trachea because this may elicit a cough.

Thorax and Lungs

The lungs are enclosed within the bony rib cage and muscular thoracic wall. These structures allow the lungs to move air into and out of the airways in the process of ventilation. Oxygen entering the lungs reaches the alveoli to be diffused across pulmonary capillaries by way of respiration. The lungs serve two important physiological functions, the oxygenation of circulating blood and the maintenance of acid-base balance. Physical assessment of the thorax and lungs takes into consideration the vital ventilatory and respiratory roles of the lungs. If the lungs are affected by disease, other body systems will reflect alterations.

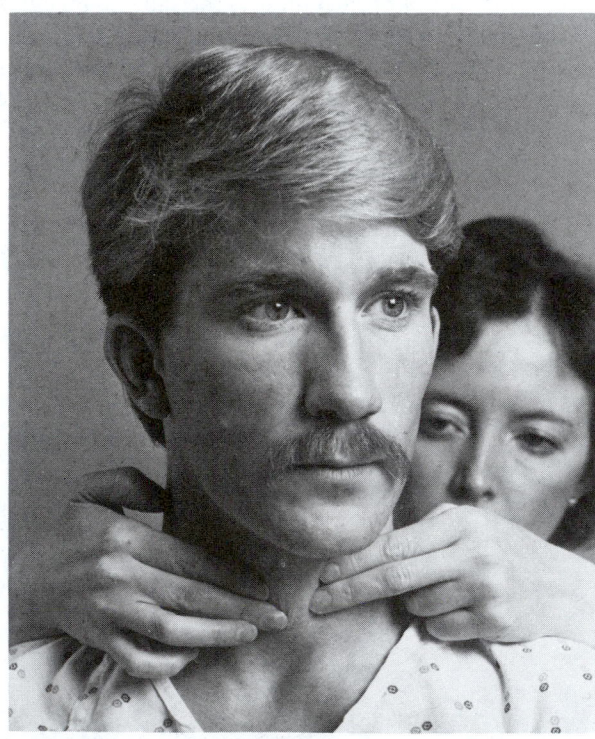

Fig. 29-50 The nurse palpates each thyroid lobe by having the client lower his chin and turn his head toward the side being examined.

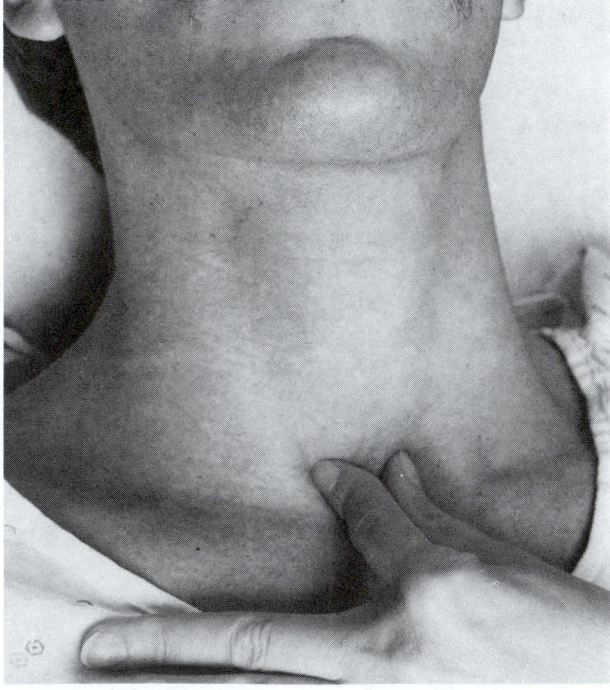

Fig. 29-51 The nurse palpates the trachea just above the suprasternal notch.

Fig. 29-52 Anterior chest landmarks. From left, midsternal line, left midclavicular line (vertical line intersecting the midpoint of the clavicle), and left anterior axillary line (vertical line along anterior axillary fold).

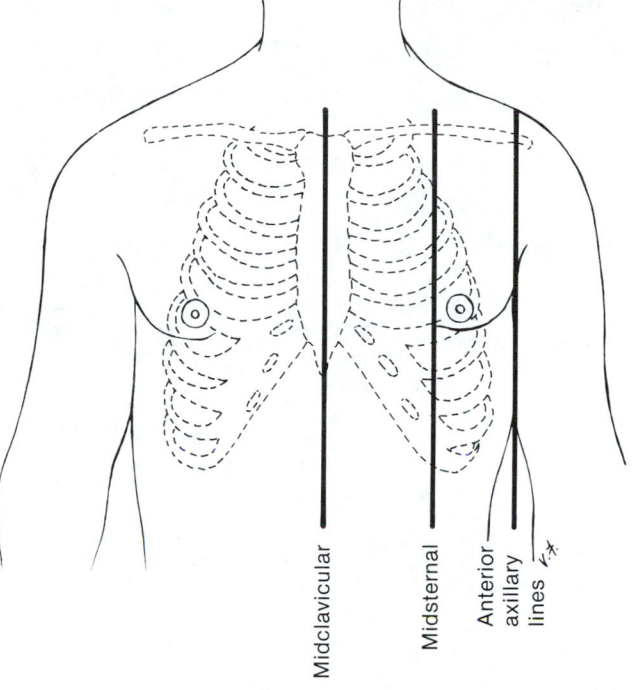

Fig. 29-53 Lateral chest landmarks. From left, posterior axillary line, midaxillary line, and anterior axillary line.

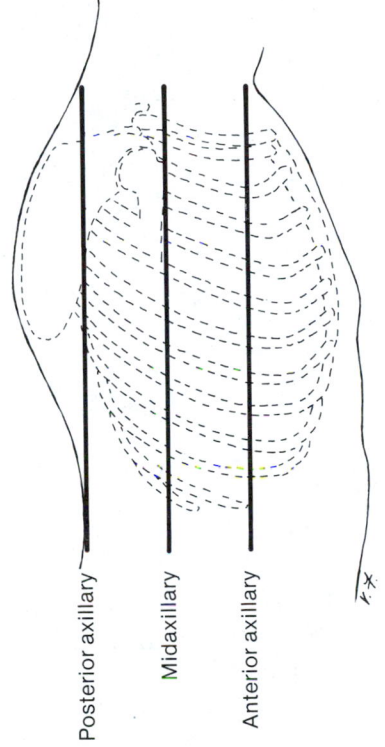

Fig. 29-54 Posterior chest landmarks. Center line is vertebral line along spinous processes. Lines to left and right are left and right scapular lines (vertical lines along tips of scapulae).

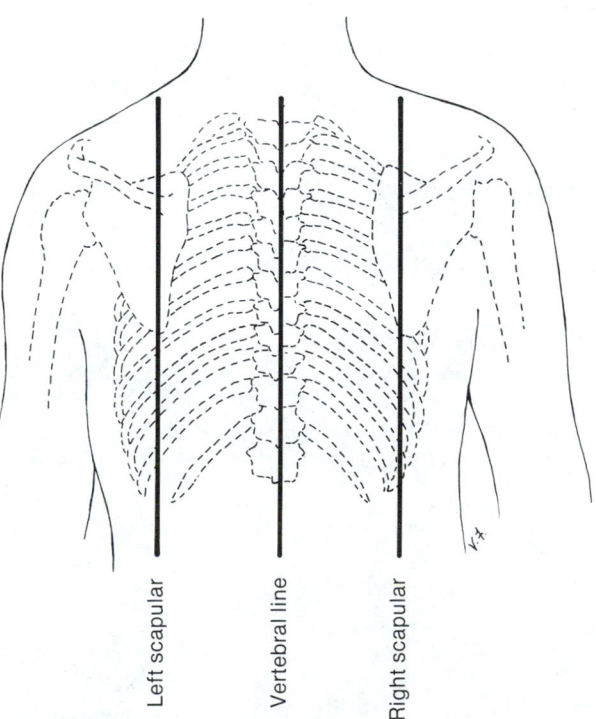

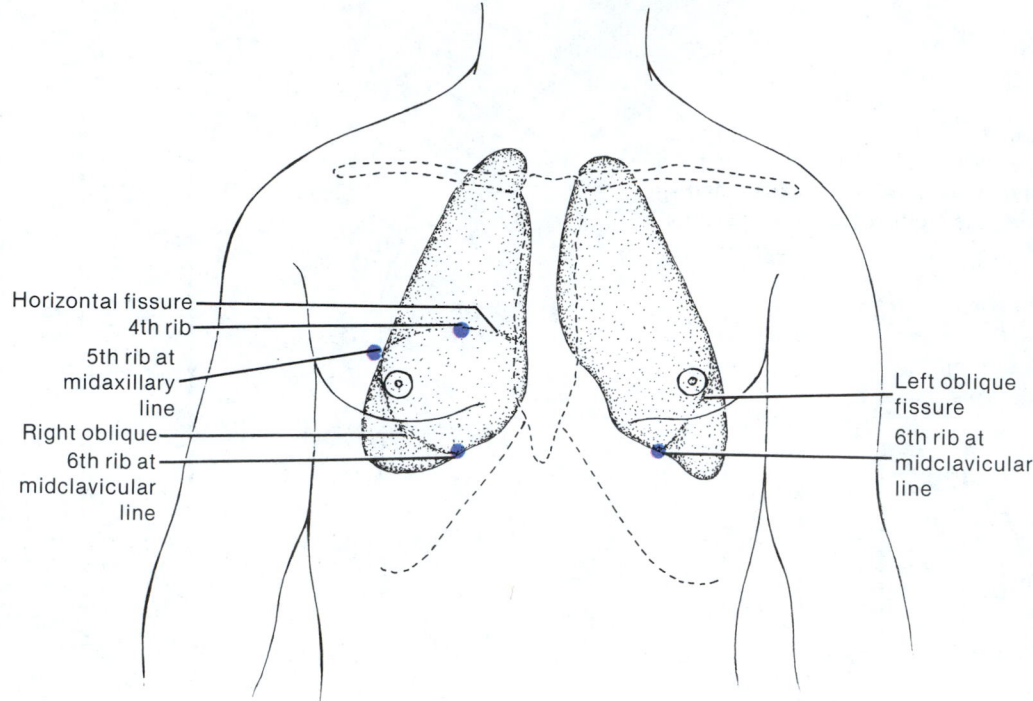

Fig. 29-55 Anterior position of lung lobes in relation to anatomical landmarks.

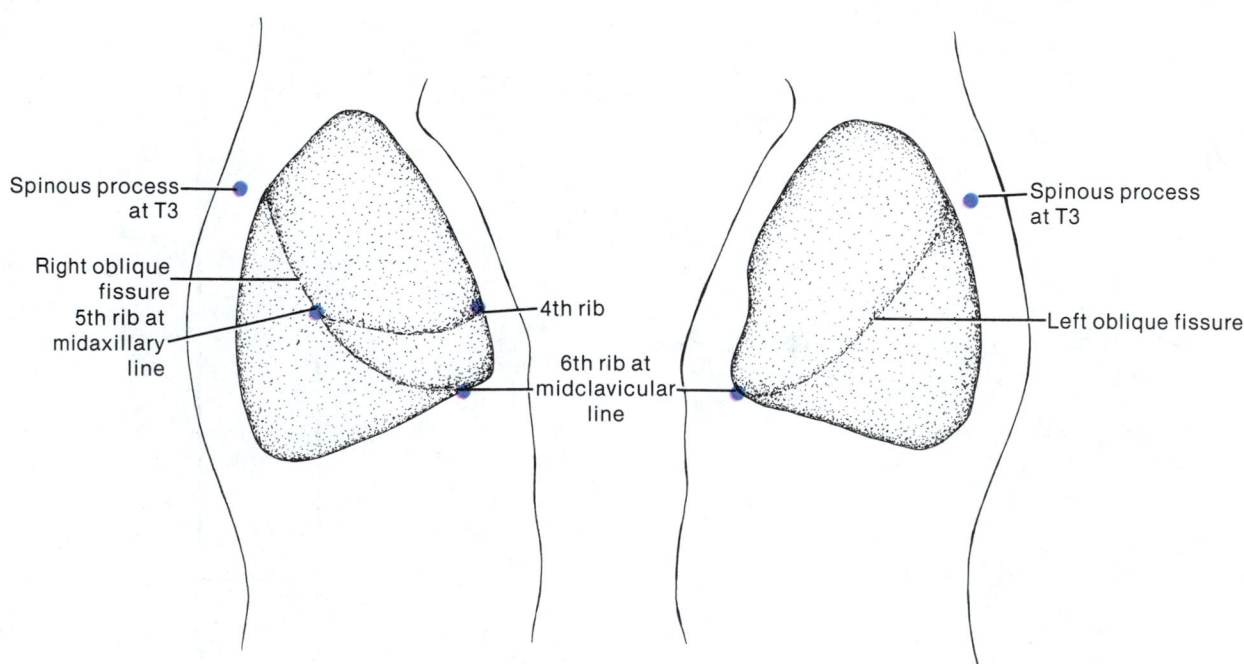

Fig. 29-56 Lateral position of lung lobes in relation to anatomical landmarks.

For example, reduced oxygenation can cause changes in a person's mental alertness because of the brain's sensitivity to lowered oxygen levels. Evidence of cyanosis may be seen in the skin or mucous membranes when oxygenation becomes inadequate. The alert nurse uses the data from all body systems to determine the nature of pulmonary alterations.

Pulmonary disease can arise acutely or exist as a chronic, long-term health problem. Nurses in all health care settings have opportunities to screen clients early for pulmonary disorders, as well as to assess the course of any chronic pulmonary disability. Information from the nursing history helps the nurse analyze the significance of pulmonary assessment findings.

Before assessing the thorax and lungs, the nurse must be familiar with the landmarks of the chest. These landmarks help the nurse describe the location of findings and use assessment skills correctly. For example, by knowing the position of underlying organs in relation to the landmarks, the nurse can anticipate where to percuss or auscultate the chest wall. The landmarks are a series of imaginary lines and easily identifiable anatomical landmarks such as the ribs and spine.

The lungs and thorax are assessed anteriorly, laterally (on both sides), and posteriorly. Anteriorly, the examiner refers to the midsternal, midclavicular, and anterior axillary lines in recording localized findings (Fig. 29-52). Laterally, key landmarks are the anterior, posterior, and midaxillary lines (Fig. 29-53). The vertebral line, arising along the spinous processes, and the scapular line, extending vertically along the scapula's tip, are the posterior landmarks (Fig. 29-54).

During the examination the nurse should keep a mental image of the location of the lobes of the lung (Fig. 29-55). Locating the position of each rib is critical to visualizing what lobe of the lung is being assessed. The angle of Louis, at the junction between the manubrium and the body of the sternum, is the starting point for locating the ribs anteriorly. Knowing that the second rib extends from the angle makes it easy to locate and palpate the intercostal spaces (between the ribs) in succession. The spinous process of the third thoracic vertebra and the fourth, fifth, and sixth ribs serve to locate the lung's lobes laterally. The lower lobes project laterally and anteriorly (Fig. 29-56). Posteriorly the tip or inferior margin of the scapula lies approximately at the level of the seventh rib (Fig. 29-57). Once the seventh rib is identified, the examiner can count upward to locate the third thoracic vertebra and align it with the inner borders of the scapula to locate the posterior lobes.

All the skills of physical assessment are used during examination of the lungs and thorax. The nurse learns

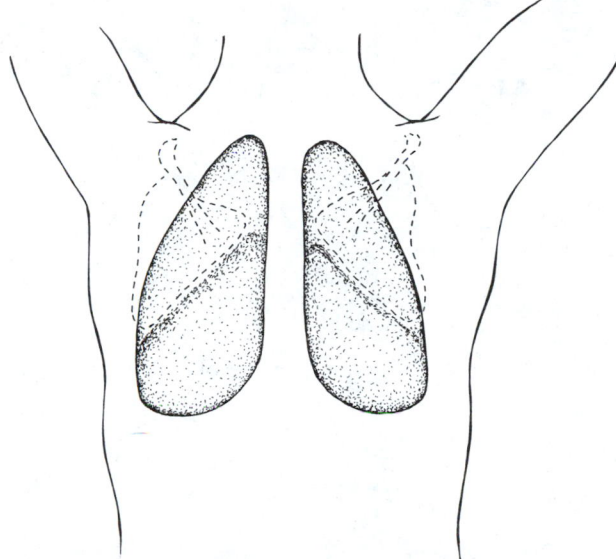

Fig. 29-57 Posterior position of lung lobes in relation to anatomical landmarks.

to use these skills especially for clients at risk for developing pulmonary complications, such as the client confined to bed rest who cannot expand the lungs fully, the client with chest or abdominal pain that impairs deep breathing, or the client with a history of a chronic cough.

POSTERIOR THORAX

The examination begins with inspection of the posterior thorax. The client is in a sitting position with the top gown removed. The nurse cannot properly inspect the thorax if the client lies on his side. Both sides of the thorax must be compared during the assessment.

The shape of the client's chest is noted. Normally the chest contour is symmetrical and the chest is twice as wide as it is deep (anteroposterior diameter in a 1:2 ratio) (Fig. 29-58). A small infant has a 1:1 ratio, with the chest having an almost round shape. Abnormal contours are caused by congenital and postural alterations. Chronic lung disease is characterized by a barrel-shaped chest (anteroposterior to lateral diameter becomes 1:1).

Standing at a midline position behind the client, the nurse looks for deformities, position of the spine, slope of the ribs, retraction of the intercostal spaces on inspiration, and bulging of the intercostal spaces on expiration. The scapulae normally are symmetrical and closely attached to the thoracic wall. The spine normally is straight without lateral deviation. Posteriorly, the ribs tend to slope across and down. The ribs and intercostal spaces are easier to see in a thin person. Normally no bulging or active movement oc-

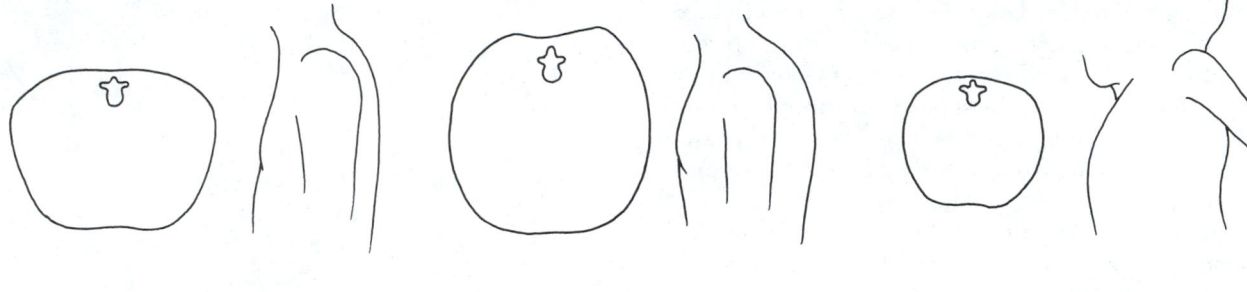

| Normal adult | Barrel chest | Normal infant |

Fig. 29-58   Anteroposterior diameter of normal chest, barrel chest, and infant's chest.

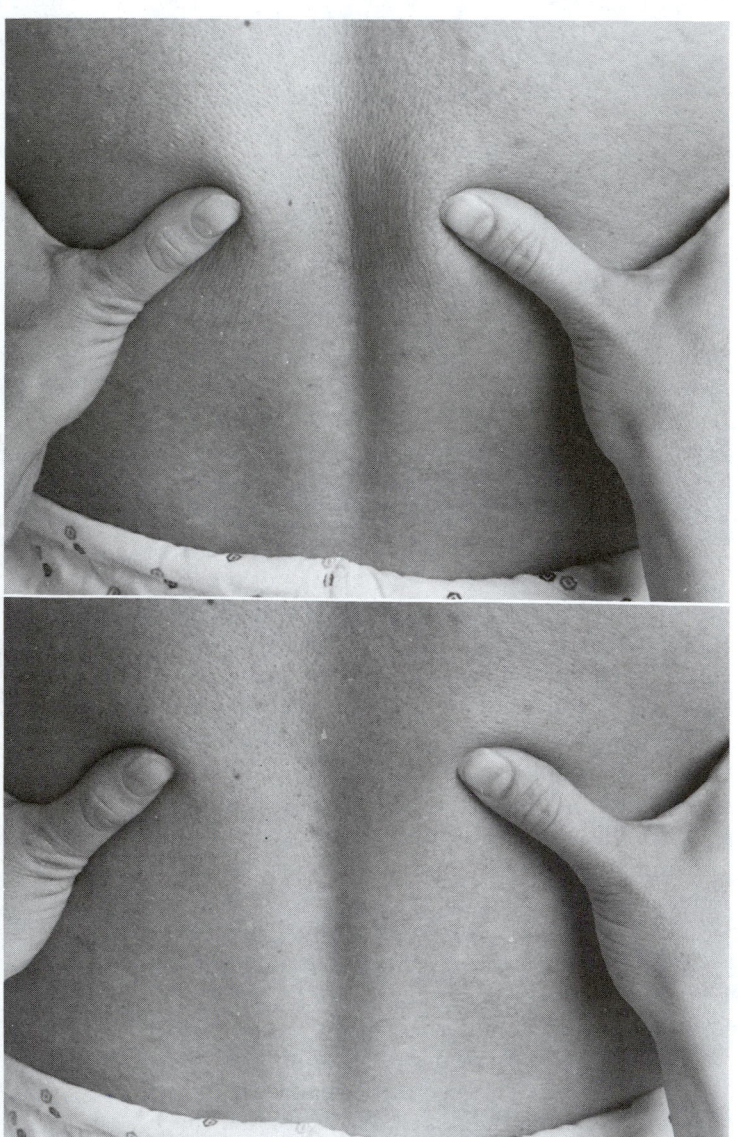

A

B

Fig. 29-59   **A,** Position of nurse's hands for palpation of posterior thorax excursion. **B,** As the client inhales, the movement of chest excursion separates the nurse's thumbs.

curs within the intercostal spaces during breathing. The presence of bulging indicates that the client is using great effort to breathe.

The nurse may also inspect the posterior thorax to determine the rate and rhythm of breathing (see Chapter 28). The thorax as a whole is observed. The entire thorax normally expands and relaxes regularly with equality of movement.

Palpation of the posterior thorax assesses further characteristics and confirms or supplements assessment findings. The chest is palpated to detect lumps or masses, identify areas of tenderness, measure chest excursion, and elicit tactile fremitus.

If a suspicious mass or swollen area is detected, it is palpated for size, shape, and the typical qualities of a lesion. When pain or tenderness is elicited, deep palpation is not used, since deep palpation of a fractured rib segment could displace the bone fragment inward against vital organs.

Chest excursion is a part of this examination that is easy to practice with a friend. The benefit of this assessment is to determine the depth of a client's breathing. It is therefore necessary to be able to judge normal excursion. Likewise, it is helpful to know the client's normal excursion. Pain, postural deformity, and fatigue are just some of the conditions that can reduce chest excursion.

The nurse stands behind the client and places her hands on the lower portion of each rib cage. The hands are parallel, with the thumbs approximately 2 inches apart pointing toward the spine and the fingers pointing laterally. The hands are pressed toward the client's spine so that a small fold of skin appears between the thumbs. The nurse does not slide her hands over the client's skin. After exhalation the client takes a deep breath and the movement of the examiner's thumbs is noted. Normally the thumbs are separated 3 to 5 cm (1½ to 2 inches) during excursion. The nurse can also feel the symmetry of respiratory movement during excursion. The two sides of the thorax should expand equally (Fig. 29-59).

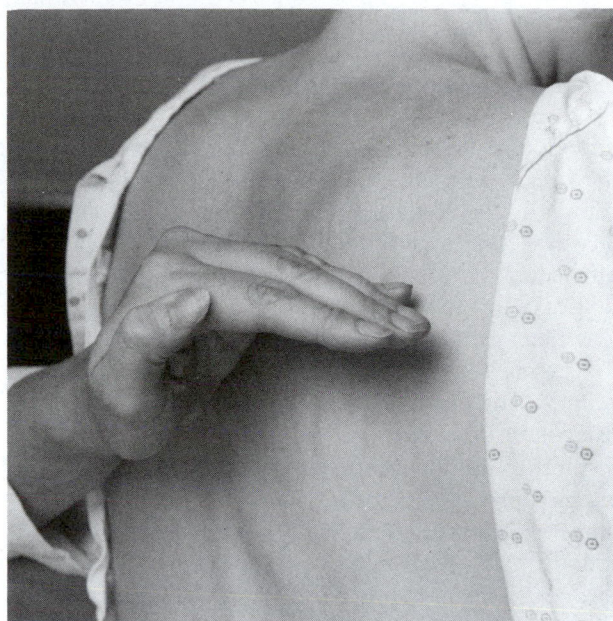

Fig. 29-60 The nurse uses the outer surface of the palm of the hand to palpate for fremitus.

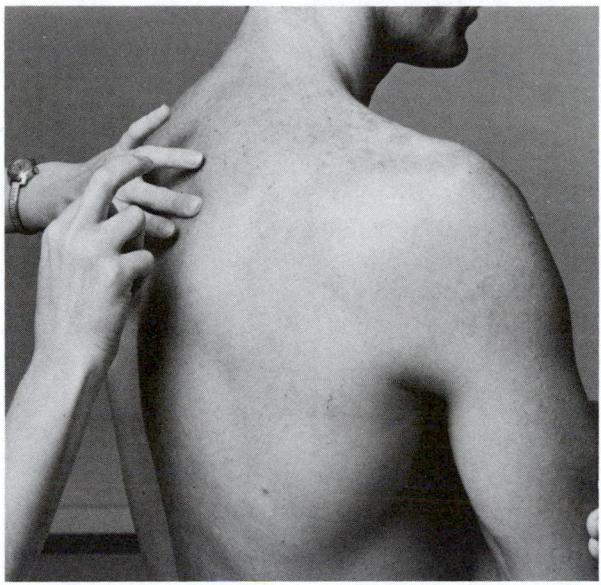

Fig. 29-61 Position of client for percussion of posterior chest wall.

During speech the sound created by the vocal cords is transmitted through the lung to the chest wall. The sound waves create vibrations that can be palpated externally. These vibrations are called tactile or vocal fremitus. The accumulation of mucous secretions, the collapse of lung tissue, or the presence of lung lesions can block the vibrations from reaching the chest wall.

To palpate for fremitus, the examiner places the ball or lower palm of the hand on symmetrical areas of the thorax (Fig. 29-60). The client is asked to say "99." Normally there is a faint vibration as the client speaks. Both sides of the thorax are compared, moving from top to bottom. Only one hand is used to ensure accuracy. If the fremitus is faint, it may be necessary to ask the client to speak louder or lower the tone of voice. Symmetry of fremitus is normal. Vibrations are strongest at the top near the level of the tracheal bifurcation. It is easy to assess for fremitus in a crying infant, since strong vibrations can be felt through the chest wall.

Percussion of the chest wall determines whether underlying lung tissue is air filled, fluid filled, or solid. The client folds the arms forward across the chest (Fig. 29-61). This position separates the scapulae further to expose more lung to assessment. Using the indirect technique, the nurse percusses in the intercostal spaces over symmetrical areas of the lung. Fig. 29-62 shows how following a systematic pattern starting posteriorly and then moving laterally and anteriorly allows the examiner to compare percussion notes for all lung lobes. Resonance, the sound created

by air-filled lungs, is normally heard over the posterior thorax. The chest is normally more resonant in the child than in the adult. If the nurse percusses over the scapulae, ribs, spine, or any area that is fluid filled, the percussion note will sound dull. The presence of a lung mass causes a flat sound. An examiner may percuss over a bony area to compare sounds to be assured that resonance is what is being identified.

Auscultation can be used to assess the movement of air through the tracheobronchial tree. Normally air flows through the airways in an unobstructed pattern. Recognizing the sounds created by normal airflow allows the nurse to detect sounds caused by the presence of mucus or obstruction in the airways. In addition, auscultation assesses the lung's condition.

In an adult the diaphragm of the stethoscope is placed over the posterior chest wall between the ribs (Fig. 29-63). The bell works best in a child because of the small chest (Fig. 29-64). The client should take slow deep breaths with the mouth slightly open. If the client breathes too rapidly, he may become faint. The examiner listens to an entire inspiration and expiration at each position of the stethoscope. If sounds are faint, as in the case of the obese client, the client should be asked to breathe harder and faster temporarily. Breath sounds are much louder in children because of the thinness of the chest wall. The same systematic pattern should be used during percussion, comparing the right and left sides. An inexperienced student may attempt to auscultate all of the left side and then return to the right side. This is incorrect.

The assessor must compare the sounds in one region on one side of the body with sounds in the same region on the opposite side. It is impossible to remember the quality of all sounds noted on one side of the body and then compare with the other side.

The nurse auscultates for normal breath sounds and abnormal or *adventitious* sounds. Normal breath sounds differ in character depending on the area of the lungs being auscultated. Sounds normally heard over the posterior thorax include bronchovesicular and vesicular sounds. Bronchovesicular sounds are medium-pitched sounds of medium intensity nor-

mally heard posteriorly between the scapulae. The sounds have a blowing quality, with the inspiratory phase equal to the expiratory phase. The character of bronchovesicular sounds is related to the larger underlying airways. Vesicular sounds are heard over the lungs' periphery (except over the scapula). The sounds are created by air moving through the smaller airways. Vesicular sounds are soft, breezy, and low pitched, and the inspiratory phase is about three times longer than the expiratory phase.

It takes considerable practice, on self or a friend, to learn to recognize and differentiate normal breath sounds. The primary features to assess include quality, pitch, intensity, and the comparative length of inspiratory and expiratory phases.

Once proficient at detecting normal sounds, the nurse will become better able to detect adventitious sounds. Abnormal sounds result from air passing through moisture, mucus, or narrowed airways or from an inflammation between the lung's pleural linings. Adventitious sounds often occur superimposed over normal sounds. The four types of adventitious sounds include crackles (also referred to as rales), gurgles or rhonchi, wheezes, and pleural friction rub. Each sound is caused by a specific entity and is characterized by typical auditory features (Table 29-9).

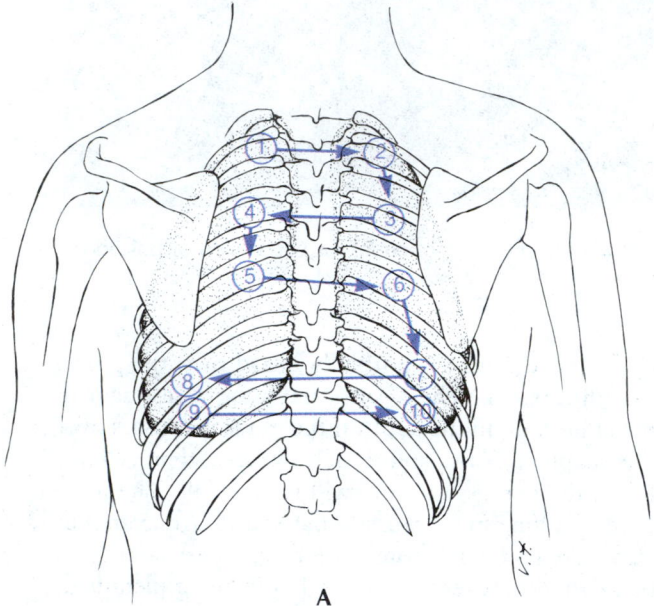

A

Fig. 29-62 The nurse follows a systematic pattern (posterior-lateral-anterior) when comparing percussion notes. The same pattern can be used during auscultation.

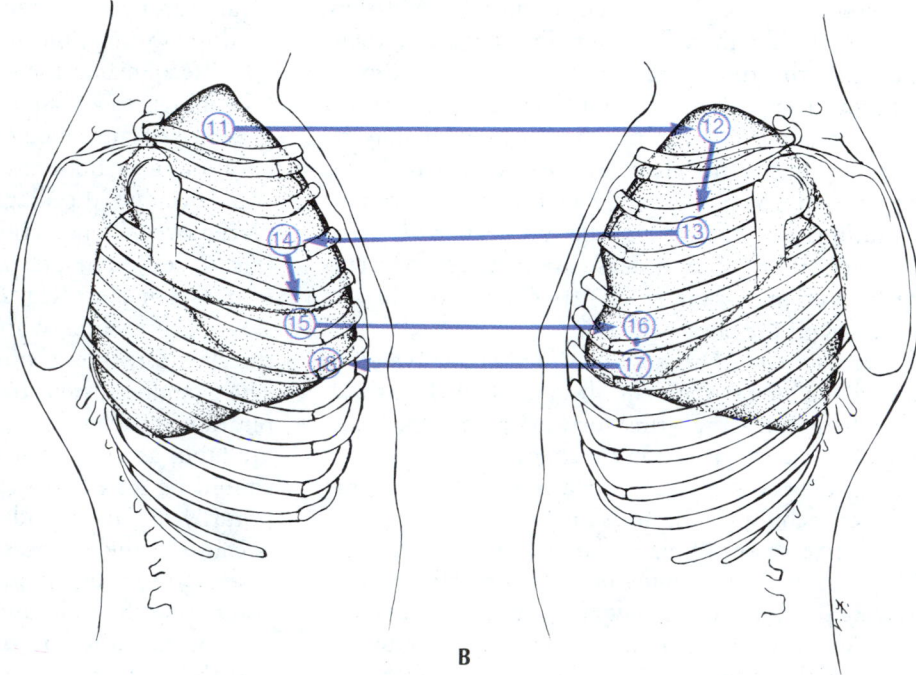

B

The nurse should learn to describe in simple terms the abnormal sounds that are heard, rather than being overly concerned with using the proper label. Many nurses and even physicians differ as to the terms used to label lung sounds. The location of the sounds, as well as their specific characteristics, should be noted, as should the absence of breath sounds (found in clients with collapsed or surgically removed lobes).

If previous percussion revealed abnormalities in tactile fremitus, it is helpful to auscultate for whispered voice sounds. The stethoscope is placed over the same locations used to assess breath sounds. The client says "99" or "eee" in a normal tone of voice. Normally the sounds are muffled, with "eee" sounding like "aaa." Next the client should whisper "99." The client's voice is normally heard faintly and indistinctly. Some lung abnormalities may cause voice sounds to become clear and distinct.

LATERAL THORAX

The client remains sitting during examination of the lateral chest. Usually the nurse simply extends the assessment of the posterior thorax to the lateral sides of the chest. The client is asked to raise his arms up straight in the air (Fig. 29-65). This position improves access to lateral thoracic structures. If the client tires,

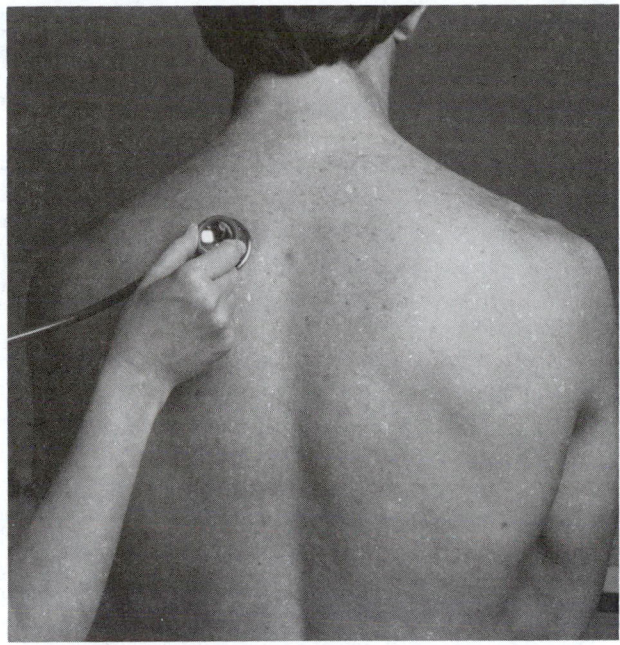

Fig. 29-63 In an adult the nurse uses the diaphragm of the stethoscope to auscultate breath sounds.

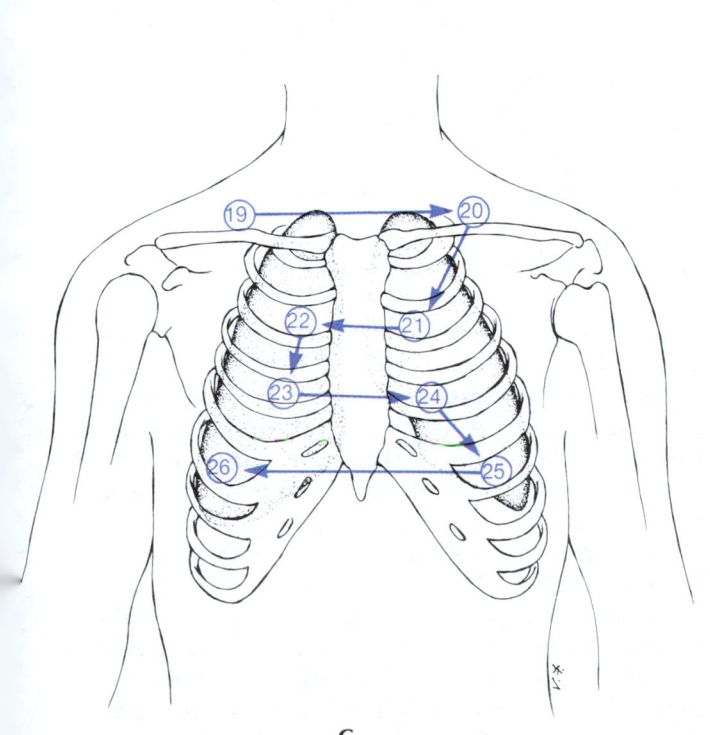

C

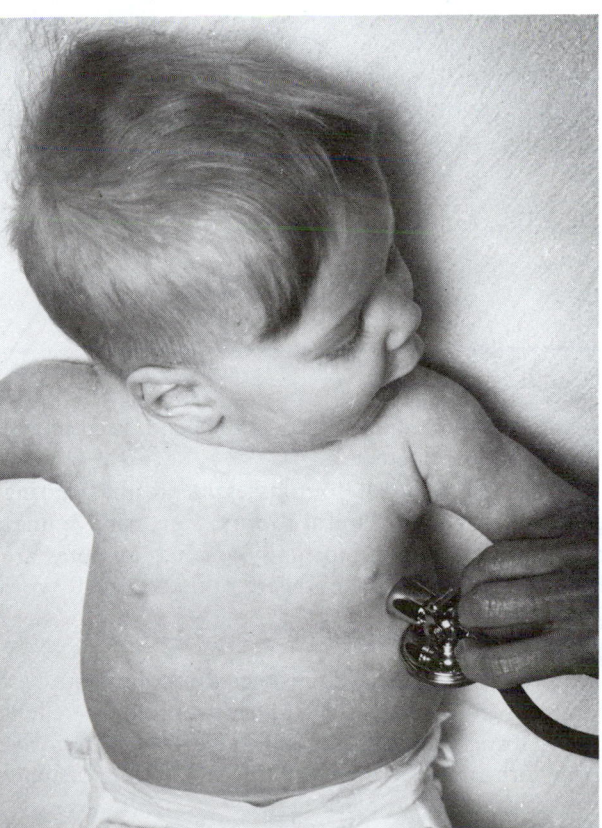

Fig. 29-64 An infant's breath sounds can best be auscultated with the bell of a stethoscope.

TABLE 29-9

Adventitious Sounds

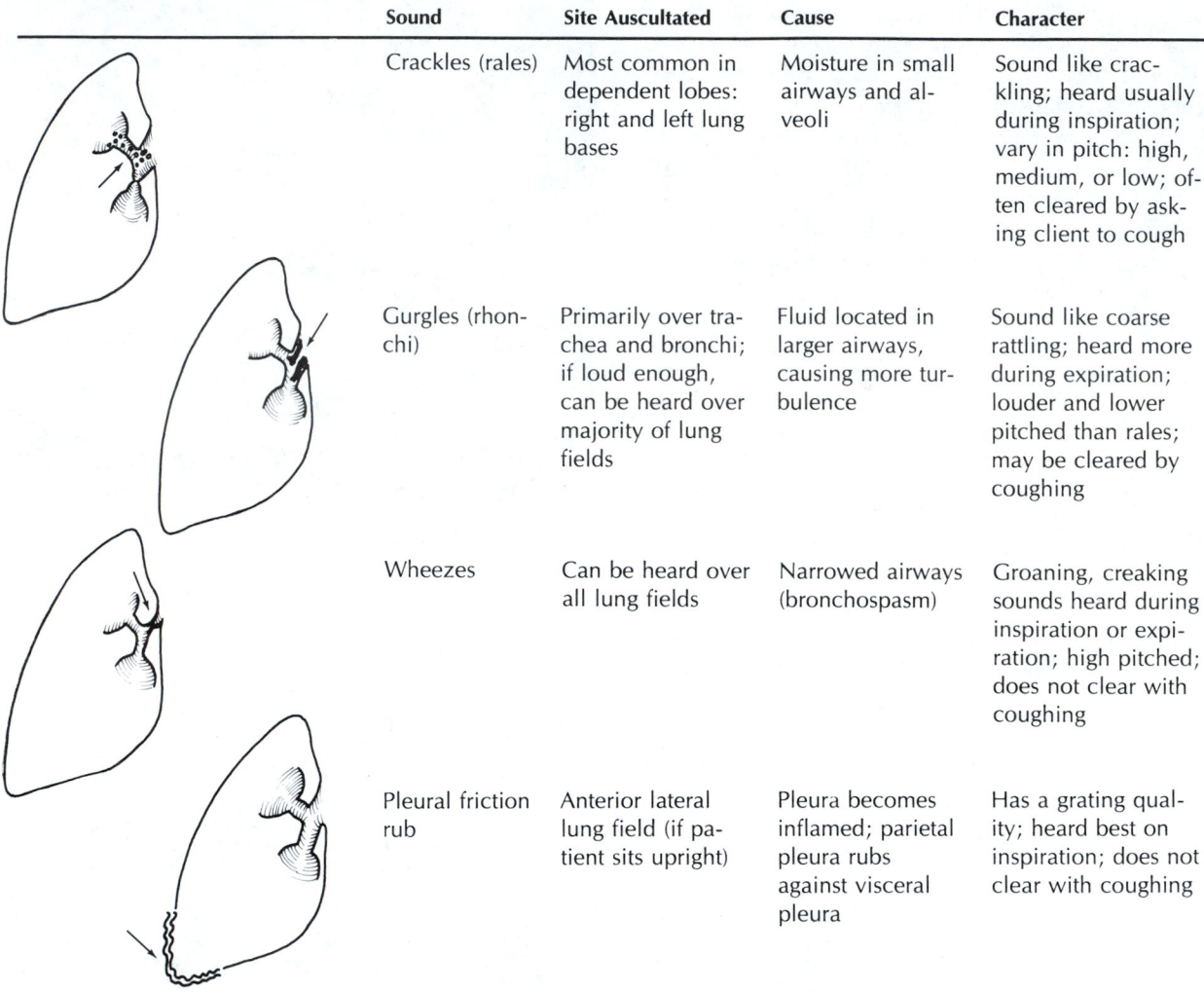

	Sound	Site Auscultated	Cause	Character
	Crackles (rales)	Most common in dependent lobes: right and left lung bases	Moisture in small airways and alveoli	Sound like crackling; heard usually during inspiration; vary in pitch: high, medium, or low; often cleared by asking client to cough
	Gurgles (rhonchi)	Primarily over trachea and bronchi; if loud enough, can be heard over majority of lung fields	Fluid located in larger airways, causing more turbulence	Sound like coarse rattling; heard more during expiration; louder and lower pitched than rales; may be cleared by coughing
	Wheezes	Can be heard over all lung fields	Narrowed airways (bronchospasm)	Groaning, creaking sounds heard during inspiration or expiration; high pitched; does not clear with coughing
	Pleural friction rub	Anterior lateral lung field (if patient sits upright)	Pleura becomes inflamed; parietal pleura rubs against visceral pleura	Has a grating quality; heard best on inspiration; does not clear with coughing

he can rest the hands on top of the head, keeping the upper arms abducted.

The nurse uses all four assessment skills during examination of the lateral thorax. Excursion cannot be assessed laterally. Normally, percussion notes are resonant and breath sounds are of the vesicular type.

ANTERIOR THORAX

The anterior thorax is inspected for the same features observed for in the posterior thorax. The client is still sitting to ensure full lung expansion. Anteriorly, the width of the costal angle is noted; it is usually greater than 90 degrees.

The accessory muscles of breathing—the sternomastoids and trapezius in the neck and the abdominal muscles—are observed. Breathing is usually a passive activity with little effort required to ventilate. When the client is forced to use effort to ventilate, the accessory muscles come into play and can be seen contracting.

The respiratory rate and rhythm are more often assessed anteriorly. The male client's respirations are usually diaphragmatic, while the female's are more costal. In other words, during respiration, the male normally moves his ribs less than the female. The male's abdominal muscles are more prominent as they move slowly in and out.

The examiner palpates anteriorly for areas of abnormality, tenderness, chest excursion, and tactile fremitus. To measure chest excursion anteriorly, the nurse places the hands on the lateral rib cage with the thumbs approximately 5 cm (2 inches) apart and

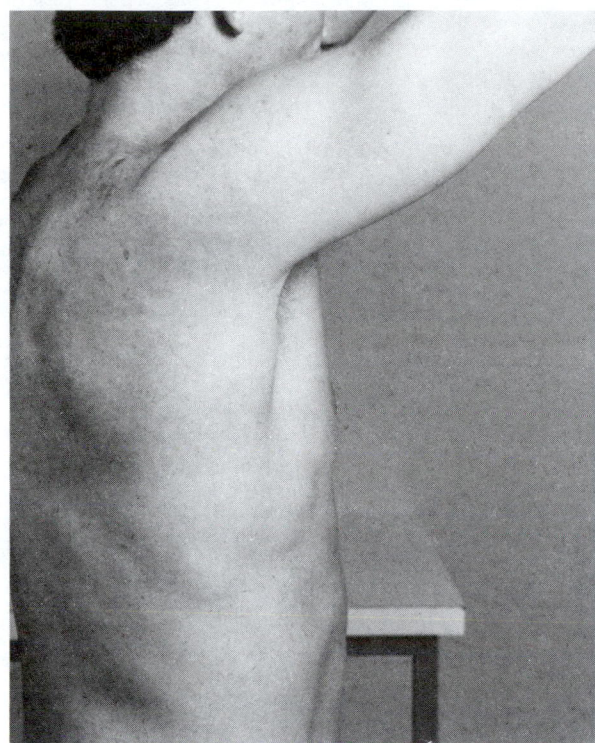

Fig. 29-65 Lifting of the client's arms improves access to lateral thoracic structures.

angled along each costal margin. The thumbs are pushed toward the client's midline to create a fold of skin between the thumbs (Fig. 29-66, *A*). As the client inhales deeply, the thumbs should normally separate approximately 3 to 5 cm (1½ to 2 inches), with each side expanding equally (Fig. 29-66, *B*).

Tactile fremitus is again elicited over the chest wall. The anterior findings differ from the posterior findings as a result of the presence of the heart and the female breast tissue. Fremitus is decreased over the precordium (area over the heart and lower thorax). The nurse will not be able to sense vibrations over breast tissue; therefore it is necessary to retract the breasts gently during palpation. If the breasts are large, this portion of the examination may be omitted.

Percussion of the anterior thorax again follows a systematic pattern. It is important for the nurse to imagine the location of all internal organs that are accessible to examination anteriorly. The underlying liver, heart, and stomach create percussion notes characteristically different from those of the lung (Fig. 29-67). Percussion may be conducted with the client in a sitting or lying position; however, the procedure is easier for the examiner if the client lies down. The examiner starts above the clavicles and moves across and then down. The female breasts are displaced as

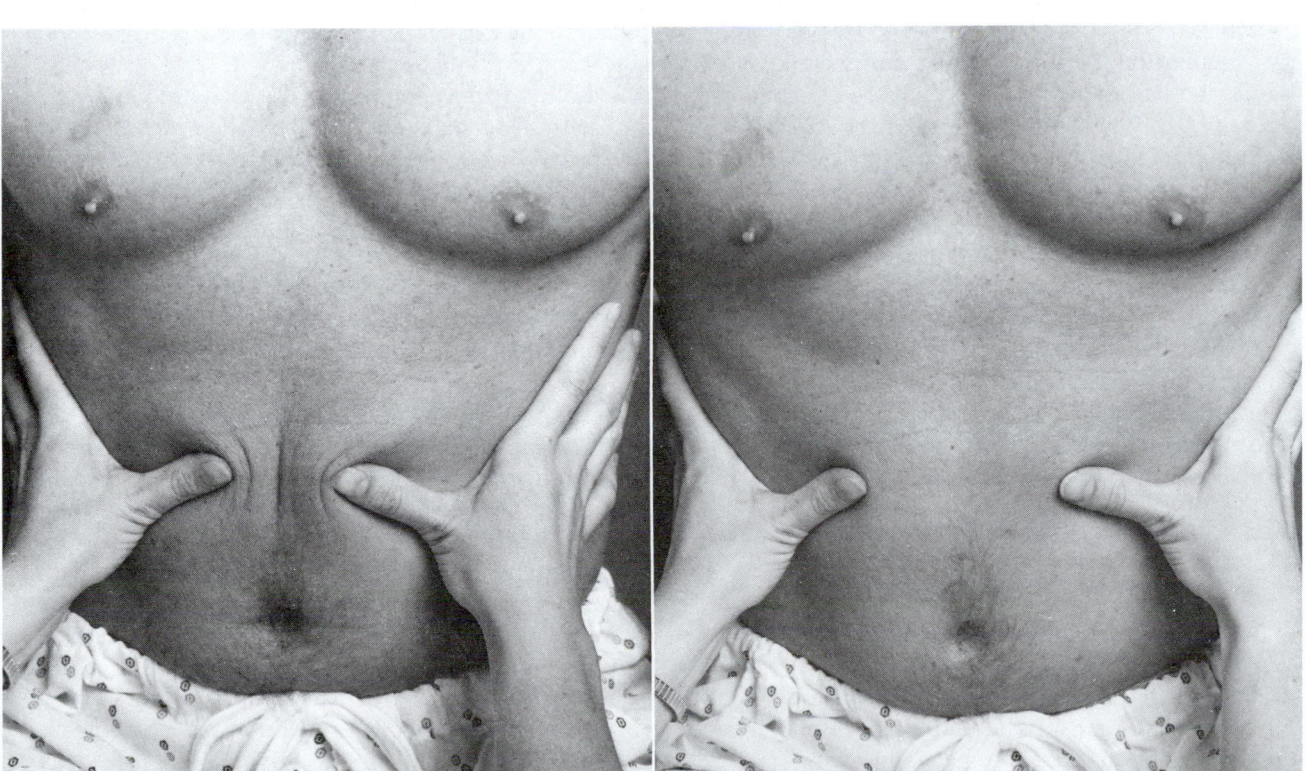

Fig. 29-66 **A,** Position of nurse's hands before excursion of the anterior chest wall. **B,** As the client inhales, the nurse's hands normally separate 3 to 5 cm (1½ to 2 inches).

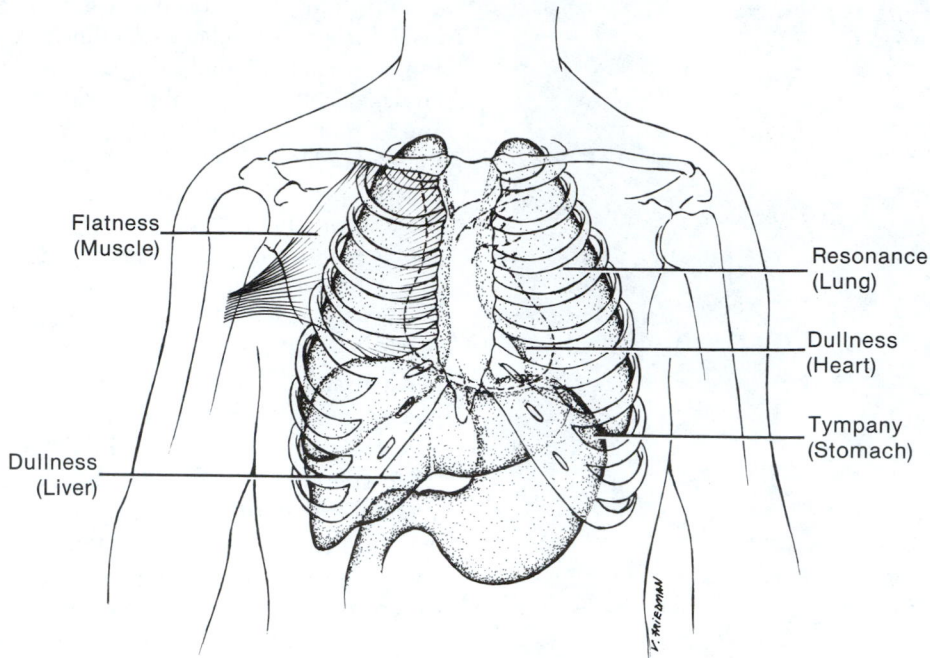

Fig. 29-67 Variations in percussion notes in normal thorax and upper abdomen.

needed. The normal lung is resonant. As the examiner proceeds downward, the areas of heart and liver dullness and the tympanic gastric air bubble will be detectable.

Auscultation of the anterior thorax follows the same pattern as percussion (Fig. 29-68). The client should sit if possible to maximize chest expansion. In addition to bronchovesicular and vesicular sounds, there is a normal breath sound that can be heard anteriorly. This bronchial sound is loud and high pitched. It has a hollow quality with expiration lasting longer than inspiration (3:2 ratio). It is normally heard only over the trachea.

When auscultating for adventitious sounds, the nurse should pay particular attention to the lower lobes. Static mucous secretions accumulate more in dependent areas of the lung, so the lower lobes are usually the first site for crackles to be detected (see Table 29-9).

Heart and Vascular System

The nurse cannot assess the heart's function without examining the integrity of the vascular system as well. The two systems work together in delivering blood to the organs, tissues, and cells. An alteration in heart function is likely to be manifested by changes in the peripheral vascular system. For example, if the heart rate is irregular, the assessor will palpate an irregular arterial pulse.

The cardiovascular nursing history provides data enabling the nurse to anticipate and be more observant of physical abnormalities. Particular attention is given to the existence of underlying heart disease and the identification of cardiac risk factors (smoking, alcohol use, and poor eating and exercise patterns).

The nurse may choose to begin centrally with the heart and then move peripherally to the vascular system or vice versa. Whatever method chosen should be an organized one. If a complete examination is being performed, it is easy to move from an examination of the thorax to the heart. The client is already in a suitable position and the chest is exposed for examination.

HEART

Assessment of heart (cardiac) function is performed through the anterior thorax. The nurse forms a mental image of the heart's exact location. In the adult the heart is located in the center of the chest (precordium) behind and to the left of the sternum, with a small section of the right atrium extending to the sternum's right (Fig. 29-69). The base of the heart is the upper portion and the apex is the bottom tip. The surface of the right ventricle comprises most of the heart's anterior surface. A section of the left ventricle shapes the left anterior side of the apex. The apex actually touches the anterior chest wall at approximately the fifth intercostal space along the midclavicular line, known as the point of maximal impulse

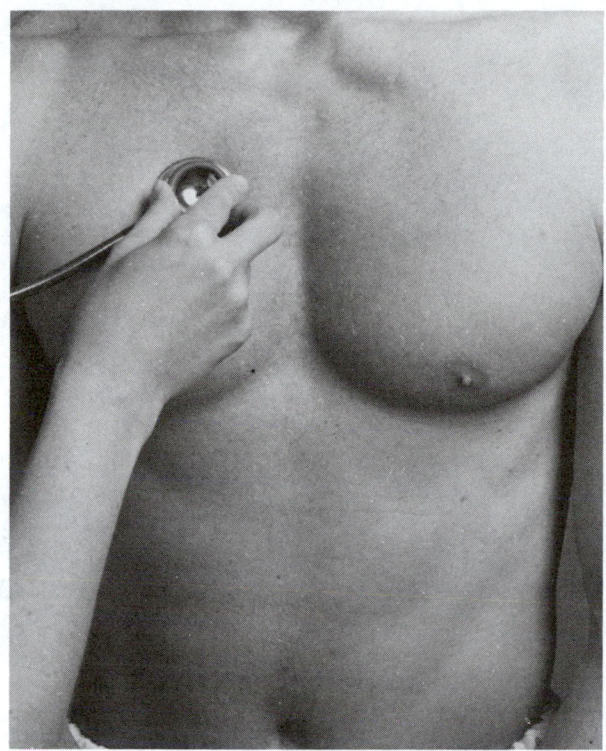

Fig. 29-68 Auscultation of anterior chest wall.

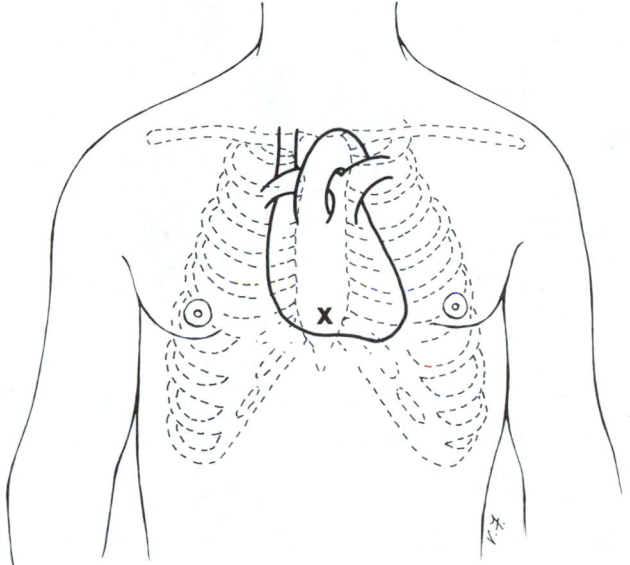

Fig. 29-69 Anatomical position of heart in relation to sternum and ribs.

(PMI). Only the right atrium, right ventricle, and left ventricle are directly accessible to examination.

An infant's heart is positioned more horizontally and has a larger diameter in comparison with the total chest diameter than in an adult. The apex of the heart in an infant is at the third or fourth intercostal space, just to the left of the midclavicular line. By the age of 7 a child's PMI is in the same location as the adult's.

To understand the significance of assessment findings, the nurse must first understand timing in relation to the cardiac cycle (Fig. 29-70). The heart normally pumps blood through its four chambers in a methodical, even sequence. As the blood flows through each chamber, certain events occur; valves open and close, pressures within chambers rise and fall, and chambers contract. Each event creates a physiological sign that can be detected by an examiner. Both the right and left sides of the heart function in a coordinated fashion. Blood flows from the right atrium to the right ventricle and from the left atrium to the left ventricle by way of the atrioventricular valves. The tricuspid valve separates the right atrium and ventricle, and the mitral valve separates the left atrium and ventricle. Blood passes from the right ventricle through the pulmonic valve to the pulmonary artery. Similarly, blood leaves the left ventricle through the aortic valve into the aorta.

As the nurse assesses heart function, it is helpful to imagine the events of the cardiac cycle. Events occurring on the left side of the heart have the most dramatic effect on assessment findings. Pressure is greatest on the left side so longer and louder sounds are created. Events on the left side slightly precede those on the right. While the left ventricle is at rest (diastolic phase), the pressure in the left atrium exceeds that in the ventricle, creating a pressure gradient that moves blood through the opened mitral valve. During ventricular filling, pressure rises in the ventricle to exceed the pressure in the left atrium. Just before the ventricle contracts, the mitral valve closes to prevent regurgitation of blood back into the atrium. The closure of the mitral valve creates the first heart sound (S_1). The ventricular pressure builds, causing the aortic valve to open as the ventricle contracts (systolic phase). Blood flows into the aorta, elevating aortic pressure. When the ventricle empties, pressure within the chamber falls. To prevent regurgitation from the aorta back into the left ventricle, the aortic valve closes, creating the second heart sound (S_2). As ventricular pressure continues to fall, it drops below that of the left atrium. The mitral valve reopens to again allow ventricular filling. The rapid filling of the ventricle may create a third heart sound (S_3), heard more often in children and young adults.

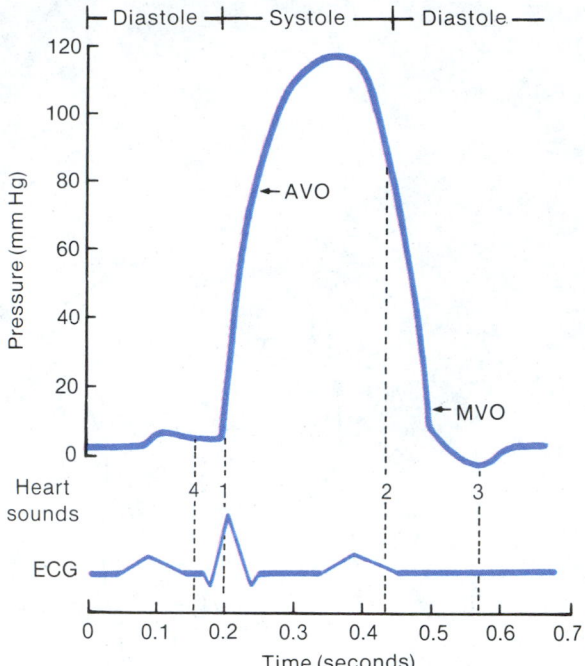

Fig. 29-70 Cardiac cycle.

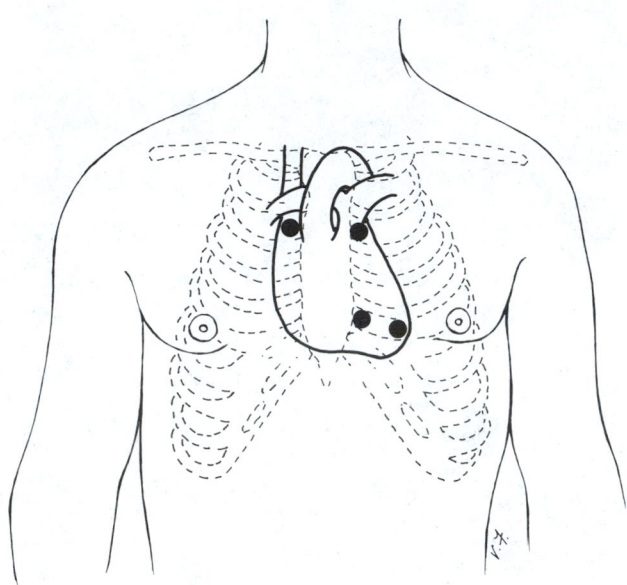

Fig. 29-71 Anatomical sites for assessment of cardiac function.

When the atria contract to enhance ventricular filling, a fourth heart sound (S_4) is produced. The S_4 is not normally heard in adults.

A knowledge of events in the cardiac cycle will help the nurse associate findings with the heart's function, so the presence of abnormal signs will become more meaningful.

The examination begins with the client supine or with the upper body slightly elevated, since clients with heart disease frequently suffer shortness of breath while lying flat. The nurse stands on the client's right side. The client must refrain from talking, especially during auscultation of heart sounds. The nurse must always be sensitive to the client's reaction during an examination; the client with a healthy cardiac history will especially become alarmed if the nurse shows concern about findings of the examination.

INSPECTION AND PALPATION. The two skills of inspection and palpation are used simultaneously. The examination proceeds in an orderly fashion, with the nurse directing attention to the anatomical sites that are best suited for assessment of cardiac function. The angle of Louis lies between the sternal body and manubrium and can be felt as a prominence on the sternum. The nurse can slip the fingers down each side of the angle until she is able to feel the second intercostal spaces (Fig. 29-71, *upper left dot*). The

second intercostal space on the right is the aortic area, and the left second intercostal space is the pulmonic area. Deeper palpation is required to feel the spaces in obese clients or those with well-developed chest muscles.

The aortic and pulmonic areas are inspected for pulsations. Viewing these areas at an angle to the side improves the likelihood of detecting pulsations. Pulsations may arise from abnormalities in major vessels of the heart or improper valve closure. The ball of the hand is used to palpate vibrations. Pulsations are more easily felt with the fingertips. If a vibration or pulsation is palpated, its occurrence is timed in relation to systole or diastole by auscultating heart sounds simultaneously (see auscultation section opposite).

Inspection and palpation continue over the other anatomical sites. Once the pulmonic area is located (Fig. 29-71, *upper right dot*), the nurse simply moves the fingers down two to three intercostal spaces on the left to the tricuspid area (Fig. 29-71, *lower left dot*). To find the apical area (Fig. 29-71, *lower right dot*), the nurse locates the fifth intercostal space just to the left of the sternum and moves the fingers laterally to the left midclavicular line (LMCL). Some examiners are able to locate the apical area with the palm of the hand, while others use their fingertips. Normally, the apical impulse, or PMI, is a light tap felt in an area 1 to 2 cm (½ inch) in diameter (Fig.

29-72). If the nurse is unable to find the PMI with the client in the supine position, the client is asked to roll onto the left side. This maneuver moves the heart closer to the chest wall. The heart's size can be estimated with the client lying supine by noting the diameter of the PMI and its position relative to the midclavicular line. In cases of serious heart disease, the cardiac muscle enlarges, with the PMI found to the left of the midclavicular line.

The PMI of an infant can usually be found near the third or fourth intercostal space. It is easy to palpate the child's PMI because of the thin chest wall.

The final area to inspect and palpate is the epigastric area at the tip of the sternum. In normal clients the pulsation of the abdominal aorta may be seen and felt here.

PERCUSSION. Percussion is used rarely during assessment of the adult's heart. Skilled examiners may be able to percuss the heart's borders to determine size. Chest x-ray studies are much more efficient in determining heart size.

In infants percussion can more easily detect the heart's borders because of the heart's proximity to the chest wall. It is particularly important in children with congenital defects whose hearts may be enlarged or malpositioned.

AUSCULTATION. Auscultation of the heart is performed to detect normal heart sounds, extra heart sounds, and murmurs. The nursing student should first become skilled at recognizing normal heart sounds. This is easier said than done, because heart sounds are of low intensity and human ears are protected from loud noises by a masking phenomenon, which lowers receptivity to faint sounds. Concentration is important in detecting heart sounds, and all sources of room noise should be eliminated. The nurse should practice with a healthy friend who has a chest wall thin enough to transmit sound clearly. The examination should begin with the nurse using the diaphragm of the stethoscope. The friend should hold his breath temporarily or breathe slowly so that the nurse can listen with minimal interference, since breath sounds make detection of heart sounds difficult. The nurse can listen over each auscultatory site but should not try to auscultate over bone.

When beginning with a client, the nurse should explain the procedure to relieve the client's anxiety. If it takes several seconds to hear the heart sounds, the nurse should explain why so the client will not worry that something is wrong. It will be necessary to lift the female client's left breast to listen better to the chest wall.

The nurse's aim is to identify the first and second

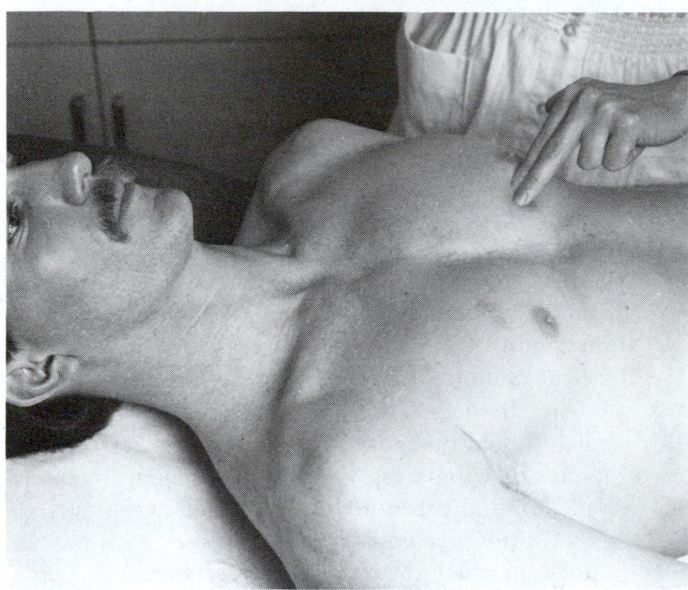

Fig. 29-72   Palpation of point of maximal impulse at the fifth intercostal space along the left midclavicular line.

heart sounds (S_1 and S_2). At normal slow rates, S_1 is low pitched and dull in quality, sounding like a "lub." S_1 is heard best at the apex. The first sound precedes the short systolic phase of heart contraction. If the nurse has difficulty detecting S_1, she may be able to identify it by timing it in relation to the carotid pulse (see later vascular section). S_1 occurs just before the carotid pulsation at systole.

S_2 is heard best at the aortic area. The sound is higher pitched and shorter than S_1. S_2 creates the sound of "dub." Many examiners learn to cue first into the sound of S_2 at the aortic site. By slowly inching the stethoscope diagonally toward the apex and keeping the sound in focus, the nurse will note that S_2 begins to diminish in sound (Fig. 29-73). S_1 becomes slightly louder, and soon both heart sounds can be heard as "lub-dub."

The nurse should practice identifying S_1 and S_2 with the bell of the stethoscope (Fig. 29-74). The bell is designed to pick up lower-pitched sounds such as heart sounds. The bell should not be pressed too firmly against the chest wall, or transmission of sounds is destroyed. A light touch ensures proper sound reception.

During a normal examination the nurse should not move back and forth between the aortic and apical areas. A systematic approach should be used; the nurse can start with the aortic area and move to the pulmonic, tricuspid, and apical areas, or the reverse sequence can be followed. Whichever method is used, the nurse should follow it consistently to be sure all sites are assessed.

Because of their thin chest walls, children have louder heart sounds than adults. The sounds are also of a higher pitch and shorter duration.

Once the nurse feels comfortable in hearing S_1 and S_2, the heart rate and rhythm can be identified. Each combination of S_1 and S_2 or "lub-dub" counts as one heartbeat. The first time a client is assessed the rate is counted for a full minute. If the rate is regular, meaning that the intervals between each beat are equal, the next count may be taken for 30 seconds and multiplied by 2. If any irregularity is detected, the rate should be counted for a full minute.

Once the heart rate and rhythm are assessed, the nurse should pay attention to the character of heart sounds by comparing S_1 and S_2. The intensity, pitch, and duration are noted. Some examiners prefer to concentrate first on only one sound at each auscultatory site; then they repeat the assessment sequence to note the character of S_2. As the nurse becomes proficient, she can analyze both sounds while progressing through each auscultation site. Normal findings are:

Aortic area: S_2 at its loudest, louder than S_1
Pulmonary area: S_2 louder than S_1
Tricuspic area: S_2 softer than S_1
Apical: S_2 softer than S_1

Arrhythmias. Failure of the heart to beat at regular successive intervals is an arrhythmia. Arrhythmias interfere with the heart's ability to empty properly. For example, if the ventricles contract prematurely before filling is completed, the cardiac output is insufficient. Certain arrhythmias can be life threatening. Table 29-10 summarizes common types of arrhythmias.

A common irregularity that does not threaten cardiac output is that which occurs during a respiratory cycle. The nurse can auscultate the apical pulse until a regular rhythm is noted, then ask the client to take a deep inspiration. The pulse rate increases at the peak of inspiration. As the client exhales, the pulse rate declines. This phenomenon, called sinus arrhythmia, is common in children and young adults. Blood becomes trapped momentarily in lungs as the person deeply inhales. As a result, the heart's stroke volume falls. To compensate for a reduced stroke volume, the heart rate momentarily accelerates to maintain cardiac output. During expiration blood reaches the heart, a normal stroke volume returns, and the heart's rate slows. Sinus arrhythmia is less likely to occur as the client takes slow passive breaths.

When the heart rhythm is irregular, apical and radial pulse rates are compared to determine if a pulse deficit exists (Fig. 29-75). In a pulse deficit the radial pulse is generally slower than the apical, since ineffective contractions fail to transmit pulse waves to the periphery. The nurse may assess for a pulse deficit in one of two ways: (1) A radial pulse is measured for 1 minute and then an apical pulse immediately assessed for 1 minute. The rates are then compared. (2) A colleague can assess the apical pulse as the nurse simultaneously measures the client's radial pulse. Any difference in pulse rate is reported to the physician immediately.

Extra Heart Sounds. The experienced nurse learns to perceive extra heart sounds. S_3 and S_4 are low-pitched sounds heard best with the bell of the stethoscope. Both sounds occur during the diastolic phase of the cardiac cycle.

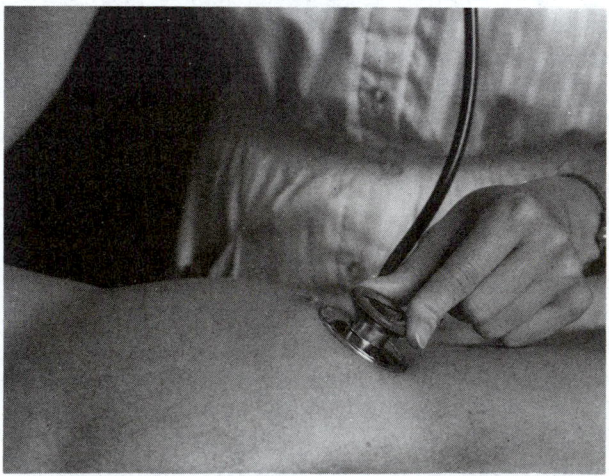

Fig. 29-73 Auscultation of heart sounds at the point of maximal impulse using diaphragm of stethoscope.

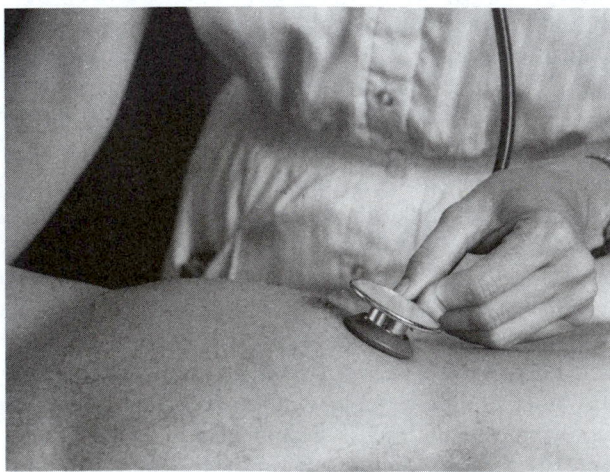

Fig. 29-74 The bell of the stethoscope is applied lightly to the chest wall to detect low-pitched heart sounds.

TABLE 29-10		

Common Types of Arrhythmias

Condition	Definition	Cause
Sinus arrhythmia	The pulse rate changes during respiration. The pulse rate increases at the peak of inspiration and declines during exhalation.	Blood is momentarily trapped in the lungs during inspiration, causing a fall in the heart's stroke volume.
Sinus tachycardia	The pulse rhythm is regular, but the rate is accelerated at greater than 100 beats/minute.	Exercise, emotional stress, and caffeine or alcohol ingestion are common factors that cause increased firing of the sinoatrial node.
Sinus bradycardia	Pulse rhythm is regular but the rate is slower than normal at 40-60 beats/ minute.	The sinoatrial node fires less frequently. This is common in well-conditioned athletes.
Premature ventricular contraction	Premature beat occurs before regularly expected heart contraction.	The ventricle contracts prematurely as a result of electrical impulse bypassing the normal conduction pathway.

Often one can hear extra sounds more easily with the client on his left side. S_3 is heard best at the apical site. S_3 occurs right after S_2 to create the sound "lub-dub-ee" or "ken-tuc-*ky*" (S_1, S_2, S_3). The sound of S_3 is normal in children up to adolescence but can be a sign of heart failure in adults.

S_4 is also heard best at the apical site. The sound occurs near the very end of diastole, just before S_1. The sound can be very confusing to a beginning student. S_4 creates the sound pattern "dee-lub-dub" or "*Ten*-nes-see" (S_4, S_1, S_2). S_4 is heard in many healthy elderly clients; however, it can be a sign of hypertension.

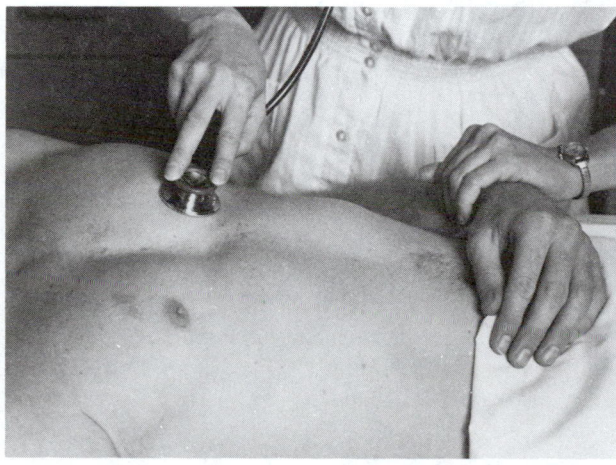

Fig. 29-75   The nurse auscultates heart sounds for 1 minute and then palpates the radial pulse to detect a pulse deficit.

MURMURS. The beginning student should not be overly concerned with identifying heart murmurs. However, it is helpful to understand what they are and their implications to the client's health. Murmurs are blowing or "whooshing" sounds created by changes in blood flow through the heart or by abnormalities in valve closure. Murmurs can indicate an impairment of the heart to pump blood effectively. In contrast, certain murmurs are asymptomatic and cause the client no problems. Murmurs are relatively common in children.

VASCULAR SYSTEM

The peripheral vascular system provides the channels for carrying oxygenated blood pumped from the heart to the cells of the body and to return deoxygenated blood through the veins back to the heart. The nurse assesses the capability of the heart to maintain normal blood flow by measuring the client's blood pressure (see Chapter 28). The status of a client's blood pressure also reflects the overall integrity of the arterial system. Inelastic narrowed arterioles create an abnormal elevation in blood pressure.

The nurse makes a more detailed assessment of the vascular system by assessing the integrity of arteries and veins accessible to examination. In addition the nurse notes the condition of the extremities perfused by the vascular system. If an abnormality interferes with arterial perfusion or venous return, changes are reflected in the skin and tissues of the affected extremities.

An experienced nurse is able to integrate the examination of the vascular system with the assessment of the head and neck, skin, and musculoskeletal system. For example, when palpating cervical lymph nodes, the nurse may also palpate the carotid artery. When the skin is inspected, the nurse will learn to look for signs of arterial and venous insufficiency. The vascular system is discussed separately to ensure that all aspects of the examination are learned. However, the client will appreciate the efforts of the nurse who is able to minimize the length of an examination and still acquire the necessary information.

To examine the vascular system the nurse uses the skills of inspection, palpation, and auscultation.

ARTERIES. When the left ventricle pumps blood into the aorta, pressure waves are transmitted throughout the arterial system. The pressure waves are manifested as pulses that are palpable in arteries close to the skin or overlying bone. The nurse must be familiar with the normal anatomical sites where pulses are palpable.

The carotid artery supplies oxygenated blood to the head and neck (Fig. 29-76). The artery is protected by the overlying sternocleidomastoid muscle. (The muscle gets its name from its attachment to the sternum inferiorly and mastoid bone superiorly.) Although there are two carotid arteries, one on each side of the neck, an occlusion of one artery can result in serious brain damage because these arteries are the only source of arterial blood to the brain.

In the upper extremities the primary artery is the brachial, which channels blood to the radial and ulnar arteries of the forearm and hand. If circulation in the brachial artery becomes compromised, the hands will not receive adequate circulation. If circulation in either the radial or the ulnar artery becomes impaired, the hand will still receive adequate perfusion. The interconnection between the radial and ulnar arteries affords a safeguard against arterial occlusion (Fig. 29-77).

The femoral artery is the primary artery in the leg, delivering blood to the popliteal, posterior tibial, and dorsalis pedis arteries (Fig. 29-78). The foot is protected from local arterial occlusion by an interconnection between the posterior tibial and dorsalis pedis arteries.

Examination of Carotid Arteries. To examine the carotid arteries, the nurse has the client assume a sitting position. *One carotid artery is examined at a time.* If both arteries were to be occluded during palpation, the client could lose consciousness as a result of inadequate circulation to the brain. *The carotids must*

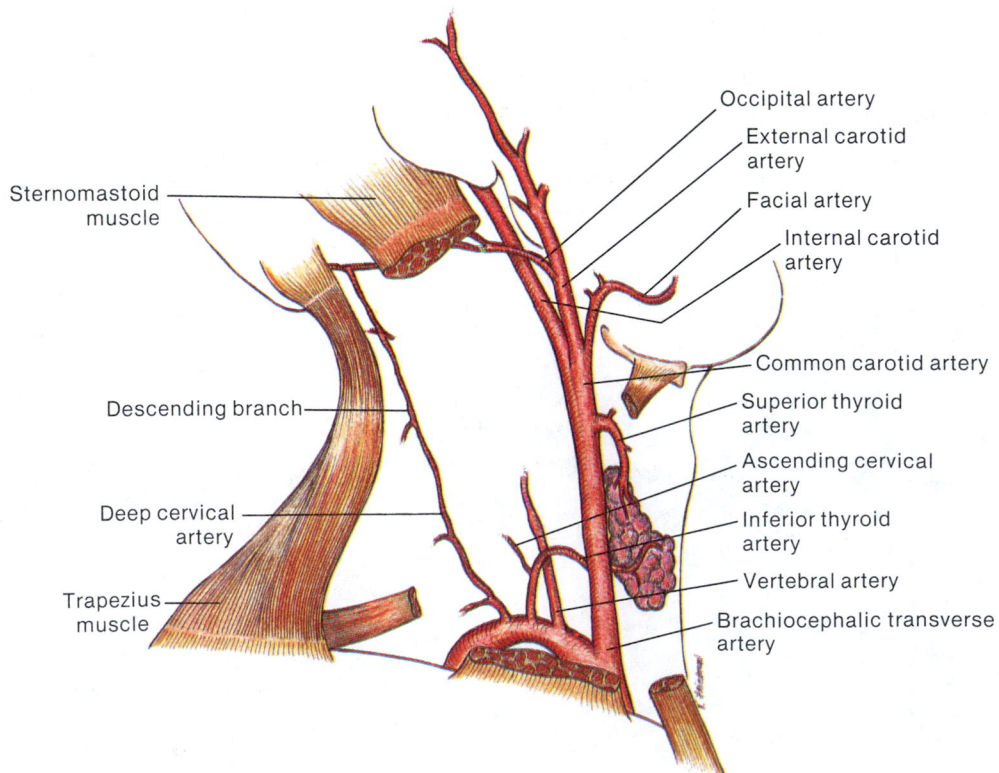

Fig. 29-76 Anatomical position of carotid artery.

Sternomastoid muscle

Descending branch

Deep cervical artery

Trapezius muscle

Occipital artery

External carotid artery

Facial artery

Internal carotid artery

Common carotid artery

Superior thyroid artery

Ascending cervical artery

Inferior thyroid artery

Vertebral artery

Brachiocephalic transverse artery

not be vigorously palpated or massaged. The carotid sinus is in the upper third of the neck. Its stimulation can cause a reflex drop in heart rate and blood pressure.

The neck is inspected for obvious pulsation of the artery. Sometimes the wave of the pulse can actually be seen. The carotid is the only site for assessing the quality of a pulse wave. Only an experienced assessor can evaluate the quality of the wave in relation to systole and diastole of the cardiac cycle.

To palpate the pulse, the nurse slides the index and middle fingers around the medial edge of the sternocleidomastoid muscle. The client should turn his head slightly toward the side examined (Fig. 29-79). This maneuver permits better access to the artery. The nurse palpates gently to avoid occlusion of circulation.

The normal carotid pulse is localized rather than diffuse. A strong pulse, the carotid has a thrusting quality. As the client breathes, no change occurs during either inspiration or expiration. Rotation of the neck or a shift from a sitting to a supine position does not change the carotid's quality. Both carotid arteries should be equal in pulse rate, rhythm, and strength and be equally elastic.

The carotid is the only pulse that is auscultated (Fig. 29-80). A common problem in the elderly population is the development of narrowing of the carotid artery lumen. When the lumen of a blood vessel is narrowed, its blood flow is disturbed. As blood passes through the narrowed section, a turbulence is created, causing a blowing or swishing sound. The blowing sound is called a bruit (pronounced "brew-ee") (Fig.

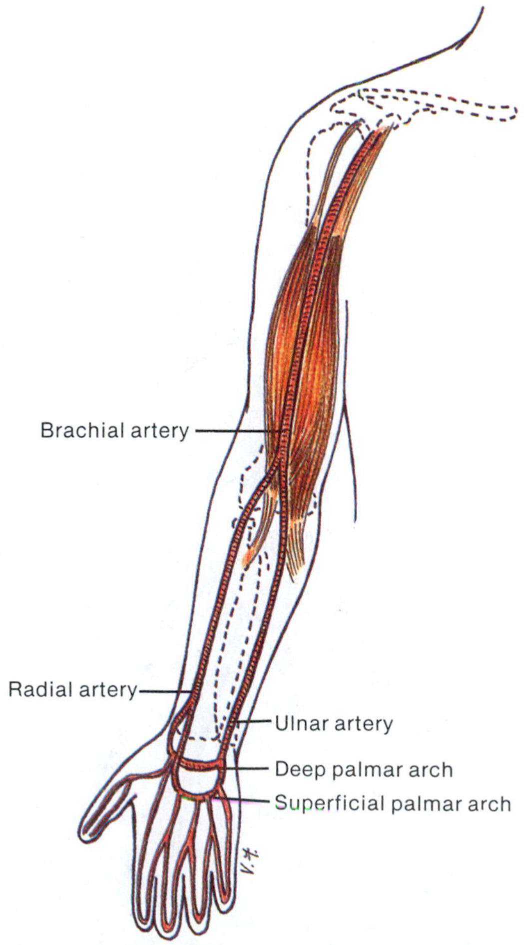

Brachial artery

Radial artery

Ulnar artery

Deep palmar arch

Superficial palmar arch

Fig. 29-77 Anatomical positions of brachial, radial, and ulnar arteries.

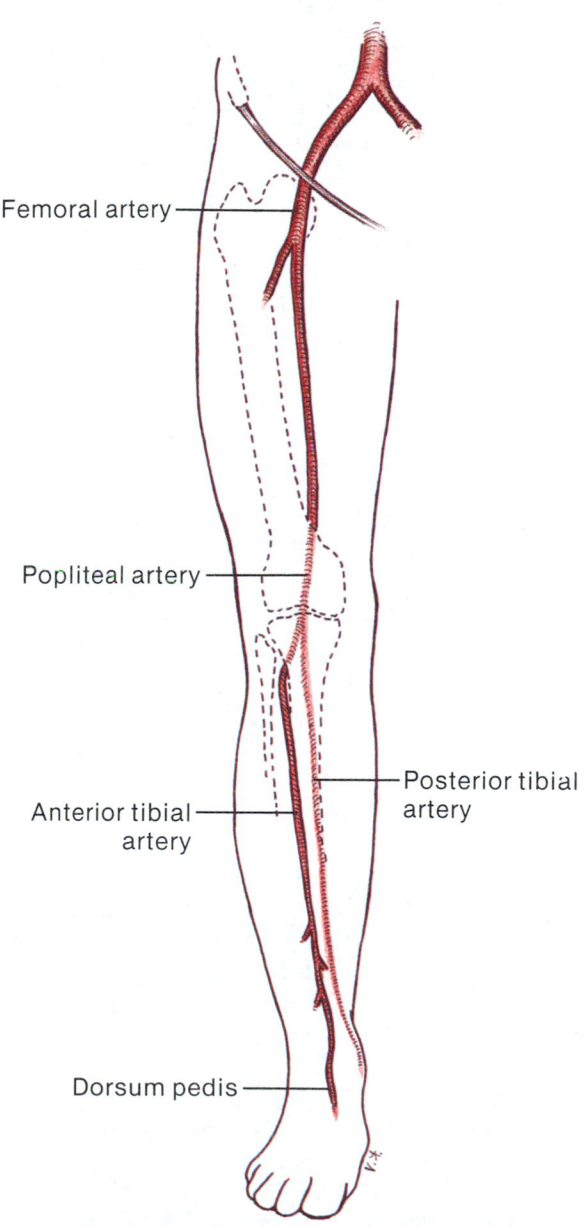

Femoral artery

Popliteal artery

Anterior tibial artery

Posterior tibial artery

Dorsum pedis

Fig. 29-78 Anatomical position of femoral, popliteal, dorsalis pedis, and posterior tibial arteries.

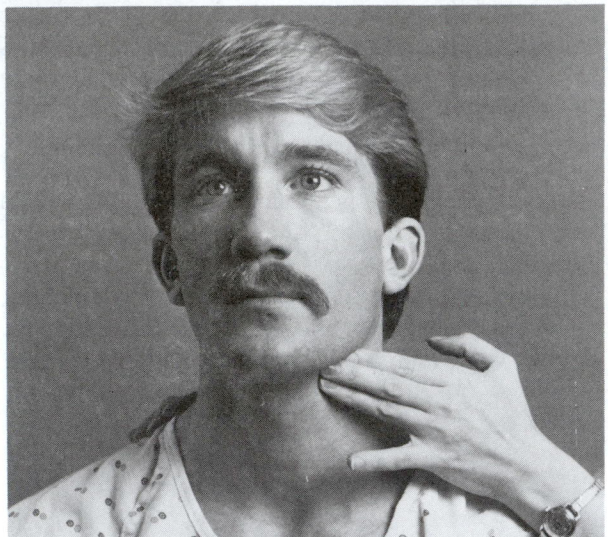

Fig. 29-79 Palpation of internal carotid artery along margin of sternomastoid muscle.

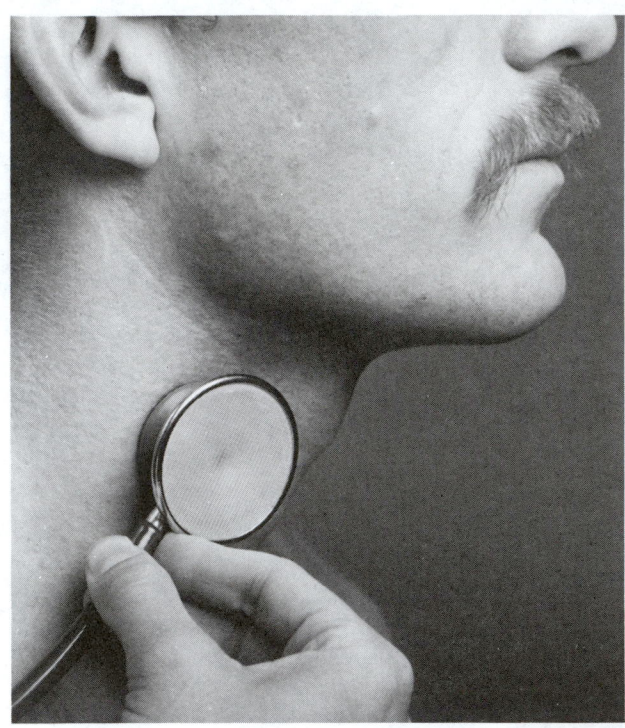

Fig. 29-80 Auscultation for a carotid bruit.

29-81). The diaphragm of the stethoscope is placed over the carotid artery. Normally no sound is heard. Both arteries are compared for the presence of bruits.

VEINS. The most accessible veins to examine are the internal and external jugular in the neck. Both jugular veins drain blood from the head and neck into the inferior vena cava. The jugular veins lie superficially and can easily be seen when they are distended. Distention commonly occurs with the client in a supine position.

The venous systems of the upper and lower extremities are also examined. Within the legs the great saphenous vein lies anteriorly and superficially, draining blood into the deeper femoral vein. Smaller saphenous veins lie posteriorly along the back of the leg to join deeper veins at the popliteal space.

Examination of Jugular Veins. The jugular veins are inspected to measure venous pressures. Venous pressure is influenced by blood volume, the capacity of the right atrium to receive blood and send it to the right ventricle, and the ability of the right ventricle to contract and force blood into the pulmonary artery. Any factor resulting in greater blood volume within the venous system results in an elevated venous pressure.

The nurse can visualize venous pressure by inspecting the jugular veins. In the supine position a client's jugular veins are normally distended. However, as the client's head is elevated, the effect of gravity enhances venous emptying, making it more difficult to visualize the veins. Therefore the client should recline with his head elevated approximately 30 degrees. The level of

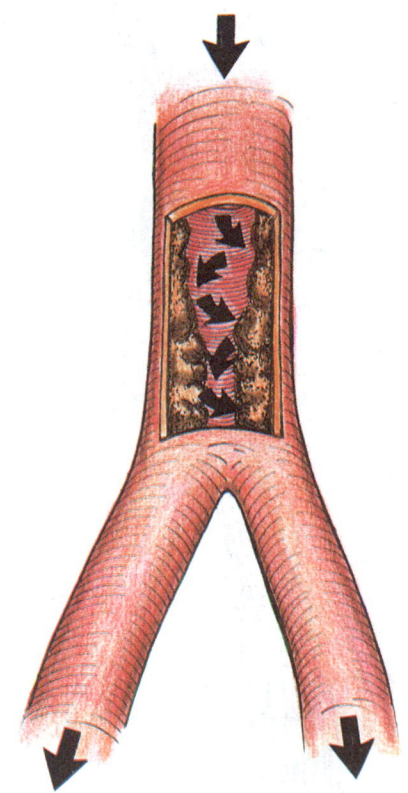

Fig. 29-81 Occlusion or narrowing of the carotid artery disrupts normal blood flow. The resultant turbulence creates a sound (bruit) that the nurse can auscultate.

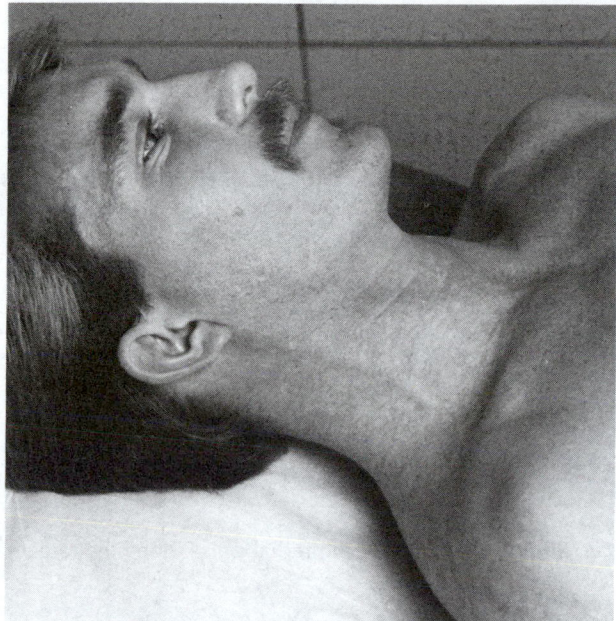

Fig. 29-82 When a client lies supine, the jugular veins distend and become visible.

TABLE 29-11

Indicators for Assessing Local Blood Flow

Indicator	Rationale
Systemic diseases (arteriosclerosis, atherosclerosis, diabetes)	Disease results in changes in the integrity of the walls of arteries and smaller blood vessels.
Coagulation disorders (thrombosis, embolus)	Blood clot causes mechanical obstruction to blood flow.
Local trauma or surgery (contusion, fracture, vascular surgery)	Direct manipulation of vessels or localized edema impairs blood flow.
Application of constricting devices (casts, dressings, elastic bandages, restraints)	Constriction causes a tourniquet effect, impairing blood flow to areas below site of constriction.

venous pressure is found by first finding the highest visible point of the jugular vein. The height of the vein's distention in relation to the sternal angle is measured. The vertical distance between the sternal angle and the highest point of jugular venous distention is the venous pressure (Fig. 29-82). Pressures higher than 3 cm are considered elevated, a cardinal sign of heart disease.

EXAMINATION OF PERIPHERAL ARTERIES AND VEINS.
When inspecting the vascular system peripherally, the nurse assesses the adequacy of blood flow to the extremities. Table 29-11 summarizes a number of factors that may impair circulation to the hands or feet. Altered blood vessel integrity, mechanical obstruction to blood flow, and any overlying constriction on vessel walls reduce perfusion of peripheral tissues. An alert nurse locates and palpates pulses at or below expected sites of circulatory impairment.

The condition of the extremities is observed (Table 29-12). The color of skin and nail beds indicates the degree of perfusion. The temperature of extremities reveals the presence of arterial or venous insufficiency. Specific skin changes are characteristic of arterial and venous alterations. Swelling of hands and feet can be a sign of vascular problems.

Peripheral Arteries. Regardless of the site, each peripheral artery is palpated for the following characteristics:

1. Elasticity of the vessel wall
2. Rate and rhythm of pulse
3. Strength of pulse
4. Type of pulse
5. Equality of pulses

The wall of an artery is normally elastic, making it easily palpable. After the artery is depressed, it will spring back to shape when pressure is released. An abnormal artery may be described as hard, inelastic, or calcified.

As is the case with heart rate, the peripheral pulse rate is measured for 1 minute. Usually only the radial artery is chosen as the site to determine pulse rate when the nurse measures vital signs (see Chapter 28). With palpation the nurse will normally feel the pulse wave at regular intervals. When an interval is interrupted by an early, late, or missed beat, the pulse rhythm is irregular.

The strength of a pulse is a measurement of the force in which blood is ejected against the arterial wall. An increased cardiac output results in a strong pulse. Exercise, fever, and emotional stress are factors that may cause a strong pulse. Some examiners use a scale rating from 0 (zero) to 4 + for the strength of a pulse:

0   No pulse is palpable.
1 +   Pulse is difficult to palpate, weak and thready in character, and easy to obliterate.
2 +   Pulse is difficult to palpate, and light pressure will locate pulse. Discriminating touch senses that it is stronger than 1.

TABLE 29-12

Signs of Venous and Arterial Insufficiency

Assessment Criterion	Venous	Arterial
Color	Normal or cyanotic	Pale; worsened by elevation of extremity; dusky red when extremity lowered
Temperature	Normal	Cool (blood flow blocked to extremity)
Pulse	Normal	Decreased or absent
Edema	Often marked	Absent or mild
Skin changes	Thin, shiny skin; decreased hair growth; nails thickened	Brown pigmentation around ankles

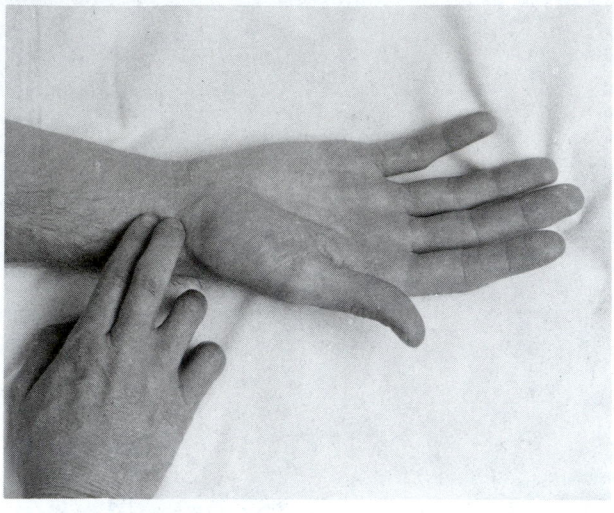

Fig. 29-83 Palpation of the radial pulse along the radial side of the forearm.

3+ This is normal pulse, easy to palpate and not easily obliterated.

4+ Strong pulse is easily palpated, seems to bound against fingertips, and cannot be obliterated.

The type of a pulse describes the nature of the pulse wave. Only an experienced examiner can recognize specific pulse types. One example is the *water hammer pulse,* which causes a knocklike sensation, with a sudden increase in strength followed by a sudden fall in strength.

All peripheral pulses are measured for equality and symmetry. The left radial pulse is compared with that of the right, the left brachial pulse is compared with the left radial, and so on. An inequality may indicate a localized obstruction or an abnormally positioned artery.

The nurse should practice locating all pulses either on self or on a friend. To locate pulses in the arm, the nurse has the client sit or lie down. The radial pulse is found along the radial side of the forearm, at the wrist. In a thin individual a groove is formed lateral to the flexor tendon of the wrist. The radial pulse can be felt with light palpation in the groove (Fig. 29-83).

The *ulnar pulse* is on the opposite side of the wrist and tends to feel less prominent than the radial pulse (Fig. 29-84). An examiner palpates the ulnar pulse only when arterial insufficiency to the hand is expected.

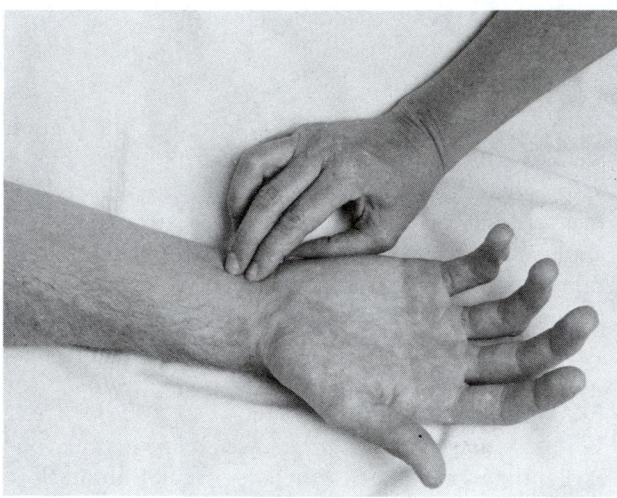

Fig. 29-84 Palpation of the ulnar pulse.

To palpate the *brachial pulse,* the nurse finds the groove between the biceps and triceps muscle above the elbow at the antecubital fossa (Fig. 29-85). The artery runs along the medial side of the extended arm. The nurse palpates the artery with the fingertips of the first three fingers in the muscle groove.

The *femoral pulse* is found best with the client lying down with inguinal area exposed (Fig. 29-86). The femoral artery runs below the inguinal ligament, midway between the symphysis pubis and the anterosuperior iliac spine. Deep palpation may be required to feel the pulse. Bimanual palpation is effective in obese clients. The nurse places the fingertips of both hands on opposite sides of the pulse site. A pulsatile sensation can be felt as the fingertips are pushed apart by the arterial pulsation.

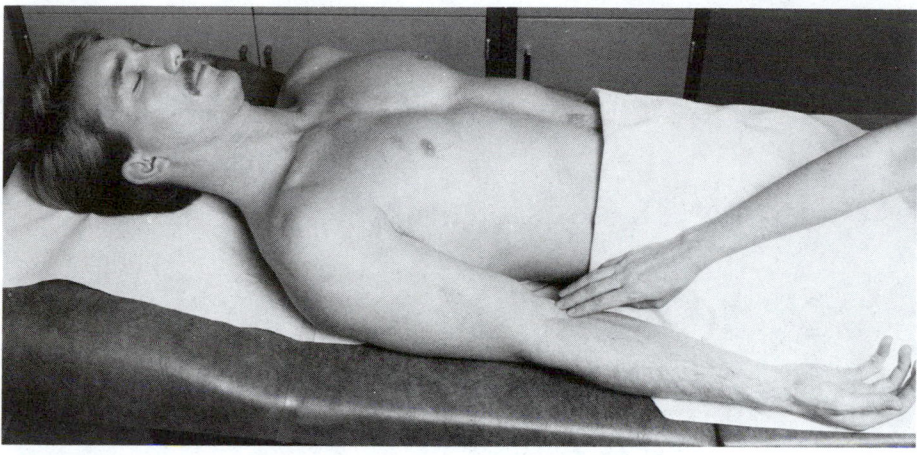

Fig. 29-85 The nurse palpates the brachial pulse by placing fingertips in the groove between the biceps and triceps muscles.

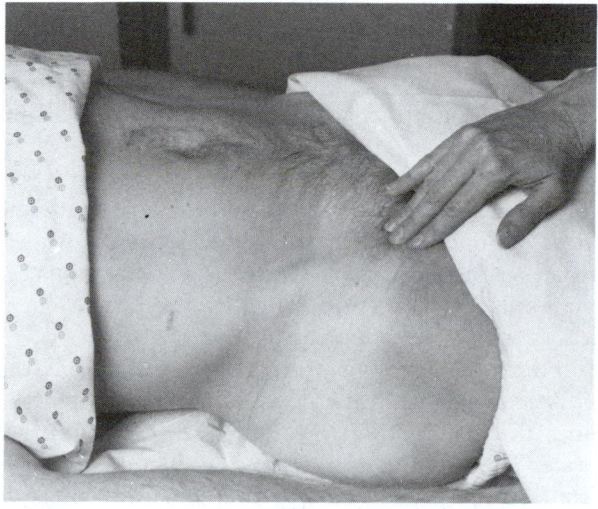

Fig. 29-86 The femoral pulse is usually palpated at the inguinal area midway between the symphysis pubis and anterosuperior iliac spine.

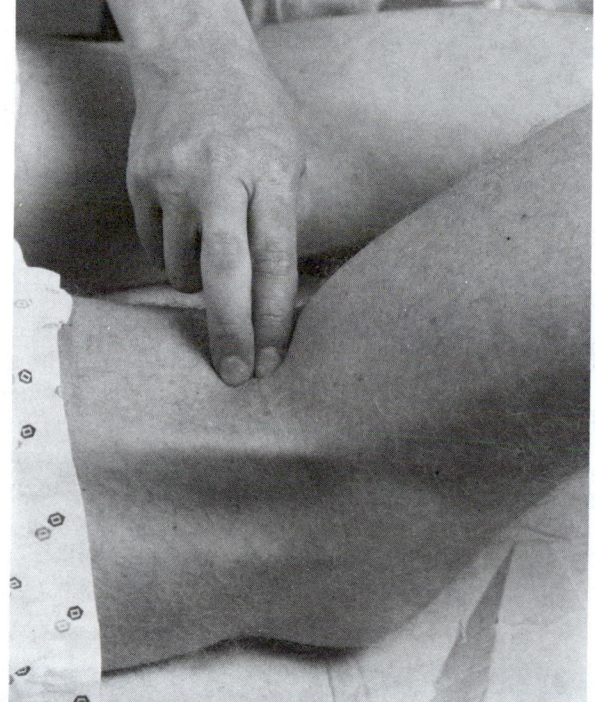

Fig. 29-87 The client lies with knee slightly flexed to give the nurse access to the popliteal pulse.

The *popliteal pulse* is found behind the knee (Fig. 29-87). The client should slightly flex the knee with the foot resting on the examination table. The client may also assume a prone position with the knee slightly flexed. The client is instructed to keep leg muscles relaxed. The nurse palpates with the fingers of both hands deeply into the popliteal fossa, just lateral to the midline. The popliteal is one of the more difficult pulses to locate.

With the client's foot relaxed the nurse locates the *dorsalis pedis pulse*. The artery runs along the top of the foot in a line with the groove between the extensor tendons of the great toe and first toe (Fig. 29-88).

Often an examiner finds the pulse by placing the fingertips between the great and first toe and slowly inching up the foot. This pulse may be congenitally absent.

The *posterior tibial pulse* is found on the inner side of each ankle (Fig. 29-89). The nurse places the fingers behind and below the client's medial malleolus (ankle bone). The artery is easily located with the client's foot relaxed and slightly extended.

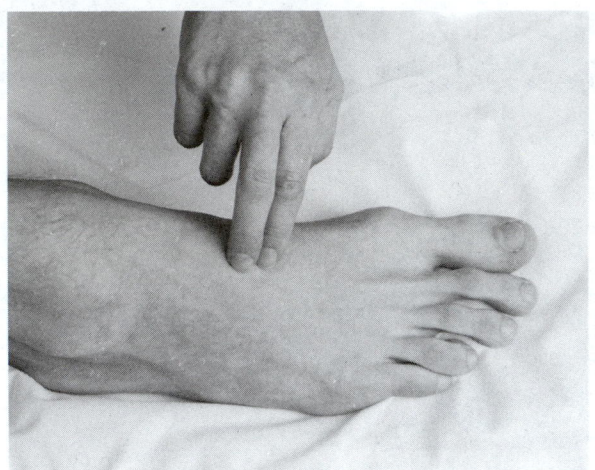

Fig. 29-88 The dorsalis pedis pulse is palpated at a point along a line with the groove between the extensor tendons of the great and first toes.

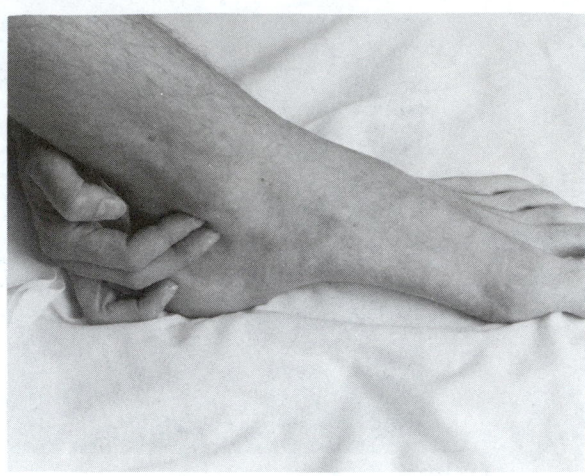

Fig. 29-89 Palpation of posterior tibial pulse below the medial malleolus.

Breasts

It is important to examine the breasts of both the female and the male client. A small amount of glandular tissue, a potential site for the growth of cancer cells, is located in the male breast. In contrast, the majority of the female breast is glandular tissue.

FEMALE BREASTS

The breasts are often a sensual part of a woman's body and are also a common site for disease. Breast cancer is the leading cause of death among women between the ages of 30 to 45 (American Cancer Society, 1978). Early detection is the key to achieving a cure. Most breast masses are found by clients themselves. All women should perform monthly breast self-examinations. Women with a family history of breast cancer should be examined yearly by a physician in addition to performing monthly self-examination.

A breast self-examination is quickly and easily performed. As the nurse assesses the client's breasts, she takes the opportunity to teach the client how to perform a self-examination. The breast examination uses the skills of inspection and palpation. The client learns to adapt these skills for use at home.

If the client already performs self-examinations, the nurse can ask what method she uses and when she does the examination in relation to her menstrual cycle. The best time for a self-examination is on the last day of the menstrual period, when the breast is no longer swollen or tender from hormone elevations. If the woman is postmenopausal, she should check her breasts the same time each month. The pregnant

---

TABLE 29-13

Normal Changes in the Female Breast During a Woman's Life Span

Age of Occurrence	Normal Characteristics
Puberty (10-12 years)	Breast buds appear. Nipples darken. Areola diameter enlarges. One breast may grow more rapidly than the other.
Young adulthood (20-30 years)	Breasts reach full (nonpregnant) size. Shape is generally symmetrical. Breasts may be unequal in size.
Pregnancy	Breast size gradually enlarges two to three times the previous size. Nipples enlarge and may become erect. Areola darkens. Superficial veins become prominent. A yellowish fluid (colostrum) may be expelled from the nipple.
Menopause	Breasts shrink. Tissue becomes softer, sometimes flabby.

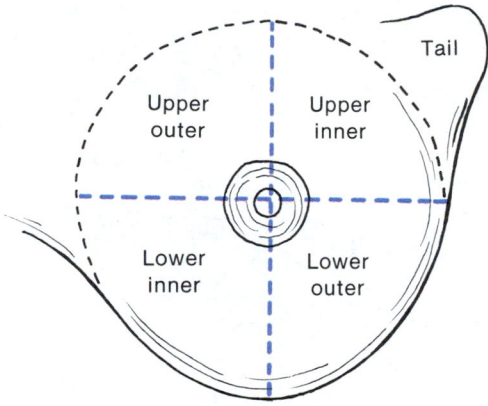

Fig. 29-90 The nurse localizes assessment findings by dividing each breast into four quadrants and an axillary tail.

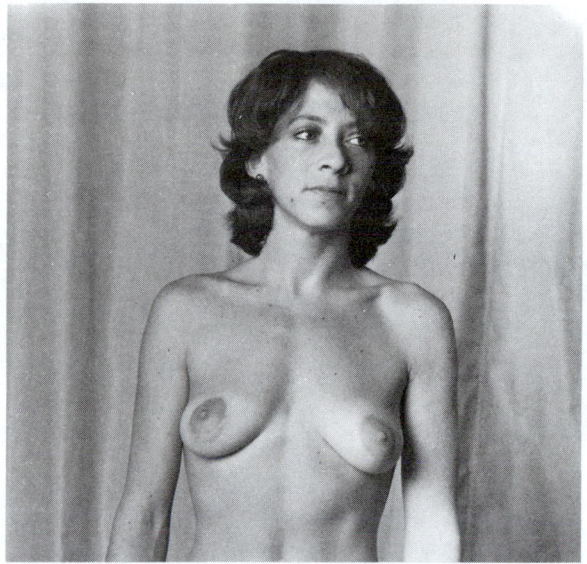

Fig. 29-91 With the client's arms at her sides, inspect the breasts for size, symmetry, contour, shape, and presence of retraction or dimpling.

woman also must check her breasts on a routine monthly basis.

The client's history should alert the nurse to any signs of breast disease and normal developmental changes. Because of its glandular structure, the breast undergoes many changes during a woman's life span (Table 29-13). Before or during the examination the nurse can ask the client if she has noticed pain or tenderness in the breast, discharge from the nipple, or a change in the size of the breast. If the client has noticed a lump or mass, she should be asked to point it out.

INSPECTION. The client is asked to remove the top gown or drape to allow simultaneous visualization of both breasts. The client may assume a standing or sitting position with arms at her sides. If possible, the nurse places a mirror in front of the client during inspection so she can see what to look for when performing a self-examination. To recognize abnormalities, the client must be familiar with the normal appearance of her breasts.

The nurse describes observations or findings in relation to imaginary lines that divide the breast into four quadrants and a tail. The lines cross at the center of the nipple (Fig. 29-90). Each tail extends outward from the upper outer quadrant.

The breasts are inspected for size and symmetry (Fig. 29-91). It is not unusual for one breast to be larger. However, a difference in size may be caused by inflammation or presence of a mass. The breasts usually extend in area from the third to the sixth ribs. The nipple is usually at the level of the fourth intercostal space. As the woman becomes older, the ligaments supporting the breast tissue weaken, causing the breasts to sag and the nipples to lower.

The nurse observes the contour or shape of the breasts and notes any masses, retraction, or flattening. Retraction or dimpling results from invasion of underlying ligaments by tumors. The ligaments become fibrotic and pull the overlying skin inward toward the tumor. The presence of edema also changes the breasts' contour. To bring out the presence of retraction, the nurse asks the client to raise her arms above her head or press her hands against her hips (Fig. 29-92). Each maneuver causes a contraction of the pectoral muscles, which will accentuate the presence of retraction.

The overlying skin is carefully inspected for color and venous pattern. The breasts normally are the color of surrounding skin surfaces. Venous patterns are more easily seen in thin clients or pregnant women. The presence of edema or inflammation is noted. The client herself may be the best person to identify changes. For women with large breasts the nurse should be sure to look carefully at the undersurface, a common site for redness and excoriation caused by rubbing of skin surfaces.

The normal areolae and nipples of a white female are pink, becoming brown with pregnancy. In dark-skinned clients the nipple is darker than other skin surfaces. Pregnancy causes an even darker color to develop. The nipple and areola are inspected for size and shape. A slight asymmetry is not unusual. The nurse also observes the direction in which the nipples point. Normally they point in symmetrical directions. If the nipple has recently become inverted or turned inward, this may indicate an underlying growth. The

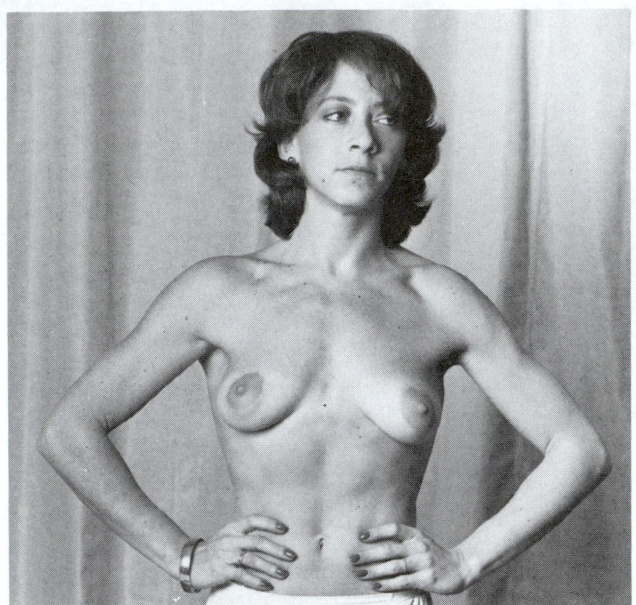

Fig. 29-92 Pressing hands against hips contracts pectoral muscles. This maneuver accentuates any existing tissue retraction.

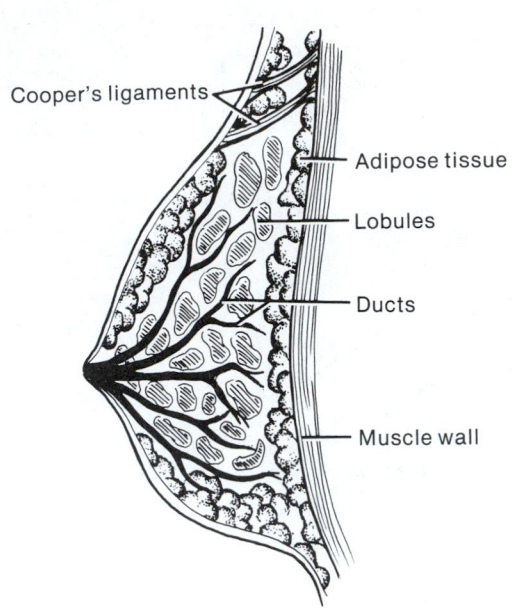

Fig. 29-93 Cross section of breast tissue.

Cooper's ligaments
Adipose tissue
Lobules
Ducts
Muscle wall

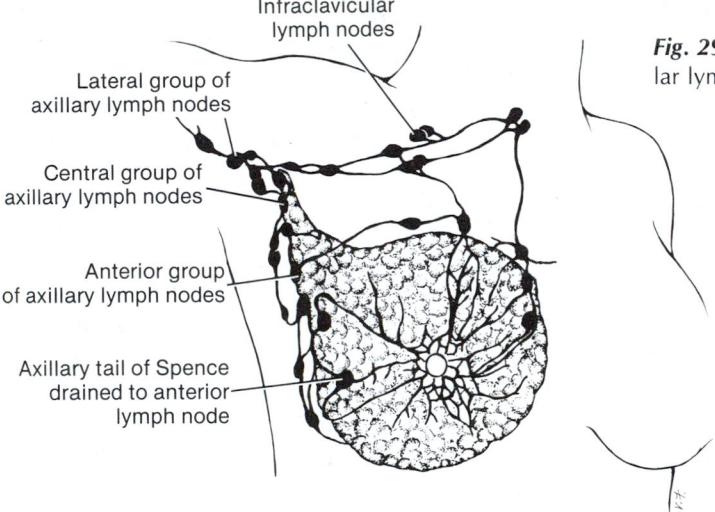

Infraclavicular lymph nodes

Lateral group of axillary lymph nodes

Central group of axillary lymph nodes

Anterior group of axillary lymph nodes

Axillary tail of Spence drained to anterior lymph node

Fig. 29-94 Anatomical position of axillary and clavicular lymph nodes.

presence of rashes or ulcerations is not normal. Any bleeding or discharge from the nipple is noted. The color of a discharge may range from clear yellow to green.

As the nurse inspects the breasts, she explains to the client what she is looking for. The client must be taught the significance of abnormal signs or symptoms.

PALPATION. Palpation allows the nurse to determine the condition of underlying breast tissue and lymph nodes. Breast tissue consists of glandular tissue, fi-

brous supportive ligaments, and fat (Fig. 29-93). Glandular tissue is organized into lobes that end in ducts opening onto the nipple's surface. The largest portion of glandular tissue is located in the upper outer quadrant and tail of each breast. Suspensory ligaments connect to skin and fascia underlying the breast to support the breast and maintain its upright position. Fatty tissue is located superficially and to the sides of the breast.

A large proportion of lymph from the breasts drains into axillary lymph nodes. If cancerous lesions metastasize or spread, the lymph nodes commonly be-

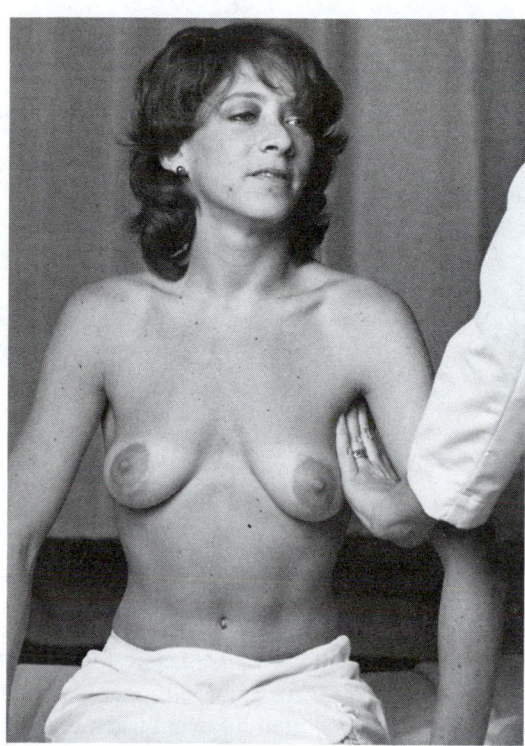

Fig. 29-95 The nurse supports the client's arm and palpates axillary lymph nodes.

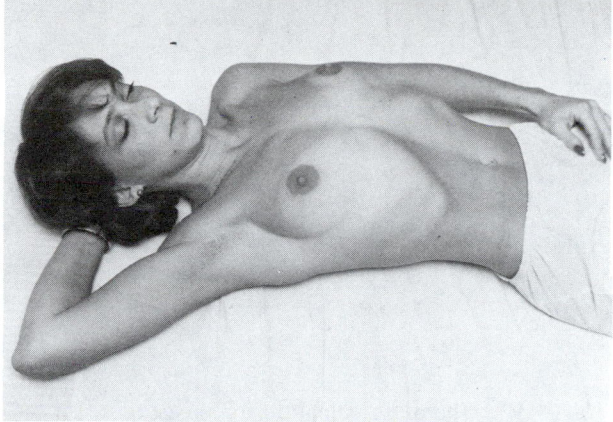

Fig. 29-96 The client lies flat with arm abducted and hand under head to help flatten breast tissue evenly over the chest wall.

come involved. The nurse becomes knowledgeable about the location of supraclavicular, infraclavicular, and axillary nodes (Fig. 29-94). A tumor of one breast may involve nodes on the opposite side as well as those on the same side.

The lymph nodes are palpated while the client is in a sitting position. Easy access is gained to the axillary nodes with the client's arms at her sides and muscles relaxed (Fig. 29-95). To gain the necessary muscle relaxation, the nurse abducts and supports the client's right arm with the left hand. The axillary nodes are palpated with the fingertips of the nurse's right hand, using a gentle circular motion. Four areas of the axilla are palpated: (1) the edge of the pectoralis major muscle along the anterior axillary line, (2) the chest wall in the midaxillary area, (3) the upper part of the humerus, and (4) the anterior edge of the latissimus dorsi muscle along the posterior axillary line. Normally lymph nodes are not palpable. A palpable node feels like a small mass that may be hard, tender, and immobile. The supraclavicular and infraclavicular nodes are palpated as the nurse stands at the client's right side. The procedure is reversed for the client's left side.

It may be difficult for the client to learn to palpate for lymph nodes. Lying down with the arm abducted makes the area more accessible. The client is instructed to use her left hand for the right axillary and

clavicular areas. The nurse can take the client's fingertips and move them in the proper circular fashion. The client then uses her right hand to palpate left-sided nodes.

Palpation of breast tissue is best performed with the client lying supine. This position allows the breast tissue to flatten evenly against the client's chest wall (Fig. 29-96). The client should raise her hand and place it behind the neck to further stretch and position breast tissue evenly. Often the examiner places a small pillow or towel under the client's shoulder blade to further position breast tissue.

The consistency of normal breast tissue varies widely. Only with practice can the nurse become adept at recognizing all variations. The breasts of a young client are firm and elastic. In an older client the tissue may feel stringy and nodular. The client's familiarity with the texture of her own breasts is most important; this is gained through monthly self-examination.

If the client complains of a mass, the nurse should start examining the opposite breast first to ensure an objective comparison of normal and abnormal tissue. The pads of the first three fingers are used to compress breast tissue gently against the chest wall. Palpation is performed in a rotary motion using an organized approach. Some examiners start in the upper outer quadrant, where tumors develop most frequently (Fig. 29-97). After the entire quadrant is palpated, the nurse moves systematically to the lower outer, lower inner, and upper inner quadrants. Another method is to proceed in and out, starting at the nipple. This pattern of palpation appears like the spokes of a wheel. Whatever pattern of examination the nurse uses, she must be sure to cover the entire breast and tail. Attention is directed to any areas of tenderness.

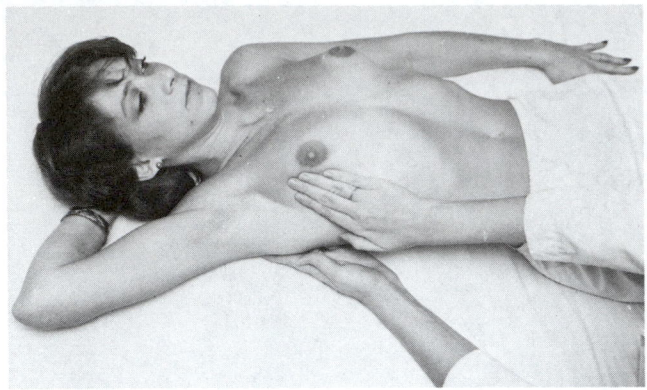

Fig. 29-97 The nurse palpates each breast quadrant using a rotary motion of the fingertips.

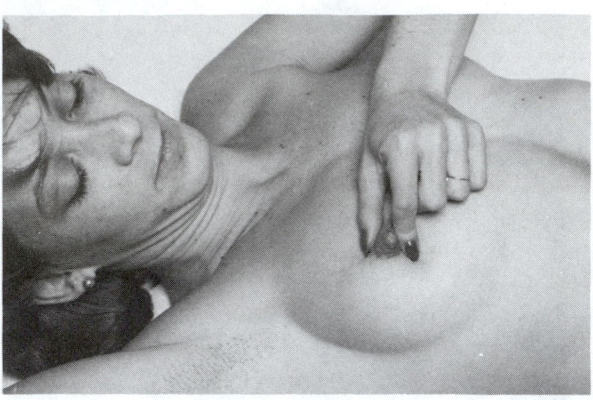

Fig. 29-98 The client palpates the nipple for presence of discharge.

When palpating large pendulous breasts, the nurse uses a bimanual technique. The inferior portion of the breast is supported in one hand while the nurse uses the other hand to palpate breast tissue against the supporting hand.

During palpation the nurse notes the consistency of breast tissue. The lobular feel of glandular tissue is normal. The lower edge of each breast may feel firm and hard. This is the normal inframammary ridge and not a tumor. It may be helpful to move the client's hand so she can feel normal tissue variations. Abnormal masses are palpated to determine the following:

1. Location in relation to quadrants
2. Size in centimeters
3. Shape (for example, round or discoid)
4. Consistency (soft, firm, or hard)
5. Tenderness
6. Mobility
7. Discreteness (whether boundaries of mass are easily detected)

Cancerous lesions are hard, fixed, nontender, and irregular in shape.

Special attention is given to palpating the nipple and areola. The entire surface is gently palpated. The thumb and index finger compress the nipple, and the nurse notes any discharge. As the nurse examines the nipple and areola, the nipple may become erect with wrinkling of the areola. These changes are normal.

Once the nurse has completed the examination, the client can demonstrate self-palpation (Fig. 29-98). Observing the client's technique helps the nurse emphasize the importance of a systematic approach. The client is urged to see her physician if she discovers any abnormal mass during routine monthly self-examination.

MALE BREASTS

Examination of the male breast is relatively easy. The nipple and areola are inspected for nodules, edema, and ulceration. An enlarged male breast may result from obesity or glandular enlargement. Fatty tissue feels soft, whereas glandular tissue is firm. Any masses are palpated for the same characteristics as in the female breast. Since male breast cancer is relatively rare, routine self-examinations are unnecessary.

Abdomen

The abdominal examination can be complex owing to the multiple organs located within the abdominal cavity. A thorough nursing history will help in the interpretation of physical signs. For example, if the client complains of abdominal pain, the pain may be caused by alterations in any number of organs, such as the stomach, intestines, pancreas, or bladder. By previously acquiring specific historical data, the nurse can localize symptoms more efficiently during the examination.

A mental image of underlying abdominal organs facilitates the nurse's ability to assess the abdomen (Fig. 29-99). Two systems of landmarks map out the abdominal region. In both systems the xiphoid process (tip of the sternum) marks the upper boundary of the abdominal region. The symphysis pubis delineates the lowermost boundary. One system divides the abdomen into quadrants by two imaginary lines crossing at the umbilicus (Fig. 29-100, *A*). The second system divides the abdomen into nine sections (Fig. 29-100, *B*). It is generally easier to learn the position of each abdominal organ in relation to one of the four quadrants. Assessment findings are recorded in relation to the quadrants.

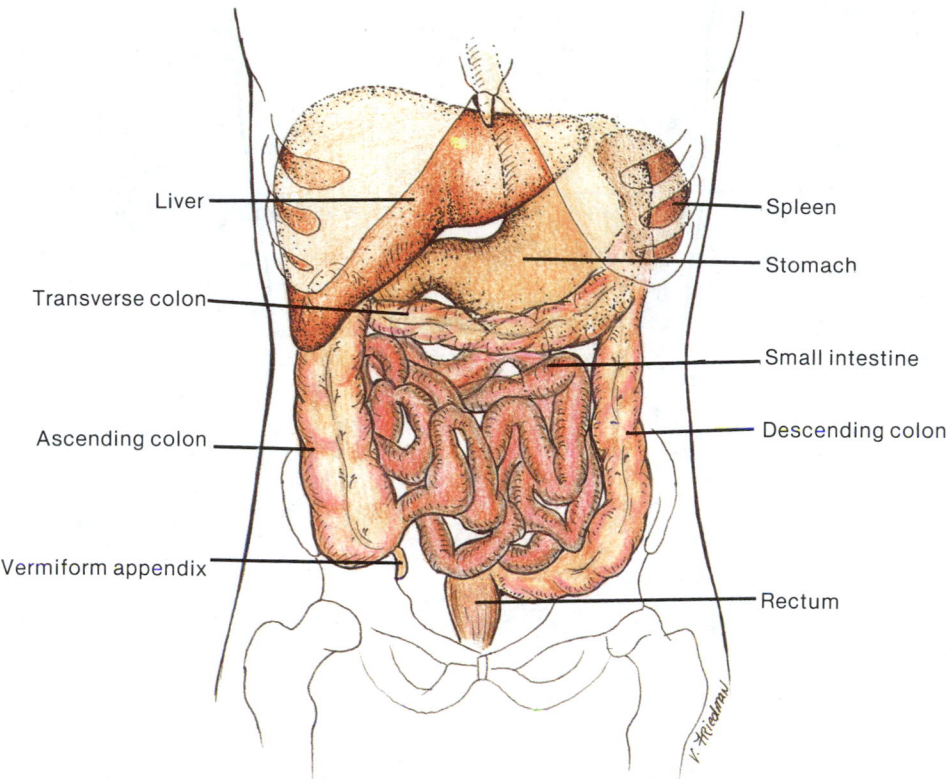

Liver — Spleen — Stomach

Transverse colon — Small intestine

Ascending colon — Descending colon

Vermiform appendix — Rectum

Fig. 29-99 Position of underlying abdominal organs in relation to anatomical landmarks.

The examiner must not forget to include an assessment of abdominal organs that lie posteriorly. The kidneys are protected by the lower ribs and heavy back muscles. The costovertebral angle is a landmark used during palpation of the kidney (Fig. 29-101).

In preparing the client for an abdominal examination, it is important that he be able to relax. A tightening of abdominal muscles will hinder the nurse's accuracy with palpation. To help the client relax, the nurse can ask if he needs to empty his bladder. The room should be warm and the client's upper chest and legs draped. The client lies supine with arms down at his sides (Fig. 29-102). If the nurse allows the client to place his arms under his head, there is a tendency to tighten abdominal muscles. The client is offered small pillows to place under his head and knees. It is helpful for the nurse to warm her hands and stethoscope. Maintaining a conversation except during auscultation distracts the client from the assessment. The examination is done slowly and calmly. If the client reports pain, he should point tender areas out. Tender areas are assessed last and approached cautiously.

An abdominal assessment is routine for any client in the hospital setting who has had abdominal surgery or who has undergone invasive tests involving ab-

dominal organs. The order of an abdominal examination differs slightly from previous assessments. The nurse begins with inspection, then follows with auscultation. It is important to ausculate before palpation and percussion, since palpation and percussion may alter the frequency and character of bowel sounds.

INSPECTION

The nurse stands on the client's right side and inspects the abdomen, then sits to look across the abdomen's surface. Standing helps detect abnormal shadows and movement. The sitting position provides a horizontal view allowing for detection of abnormal protuberances.

The skin of the abdomen's surface is inspected, noting scars, venous patterns, lesions, and striae (stretch marks). The presence of artificial openings may indicate drainage sites resulting from surgery (see Chapter 48) or the presence of an ostomy (see Chapters 39 and 40). Scars reveal evidence of past trauma or surgery that may have created permanent changes in underlying organ anatomy. Normally, venous patterns are faint except in the very thin client. Any lesions are observed for characteristics previously described in the skin assessment section. Striae result from stretching of tissue by obesity or pregnancy.

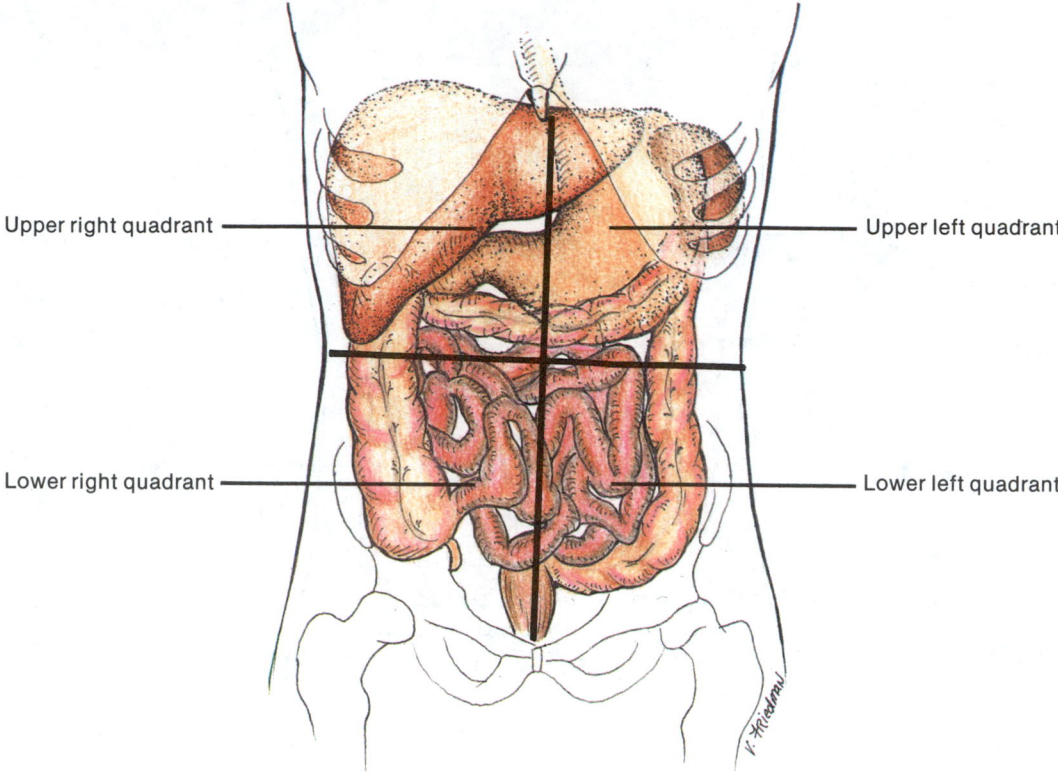

Upper right quadrant

Upper left quadrant

Lower right quadrant

Lower left quadrant

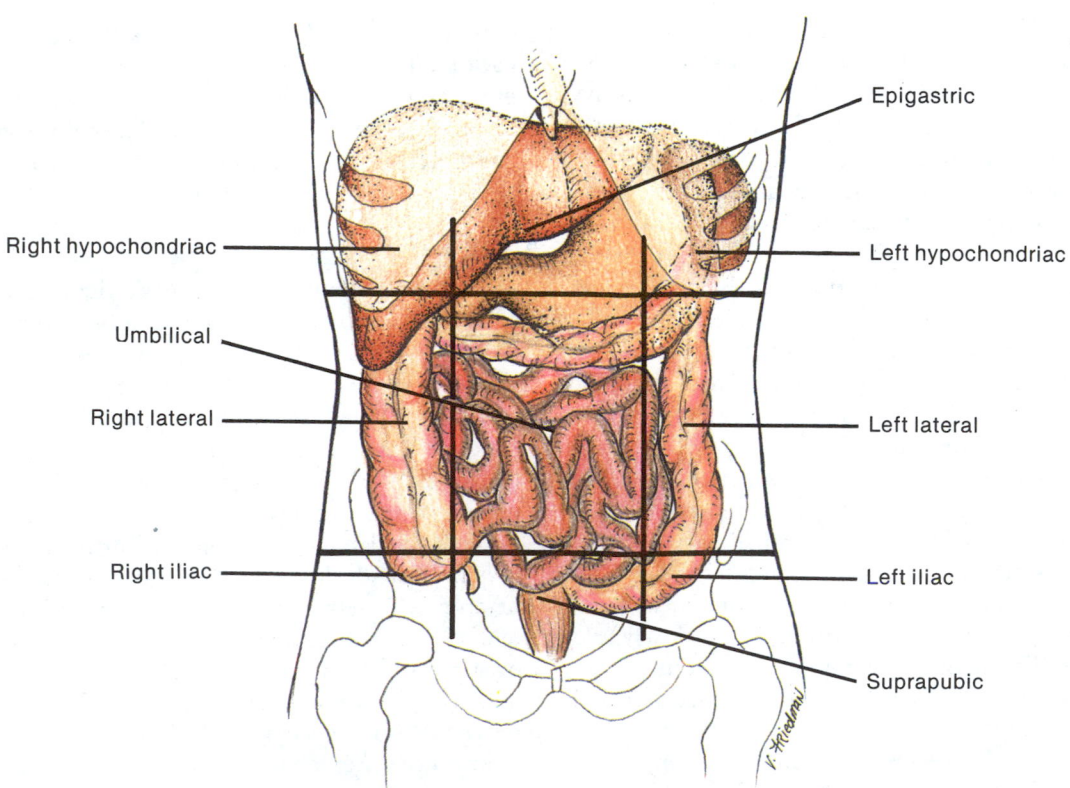

Epigastric

Right hypochondriac

Left hypochondriac

Umbilical

Right lateral

Left lateral

Right iliac

Left iliac

Suprapubic

Fig. 29-100 **A,** Division of abdomen into quadrants. **B,** Division of abdomen into nine anatomical sections.

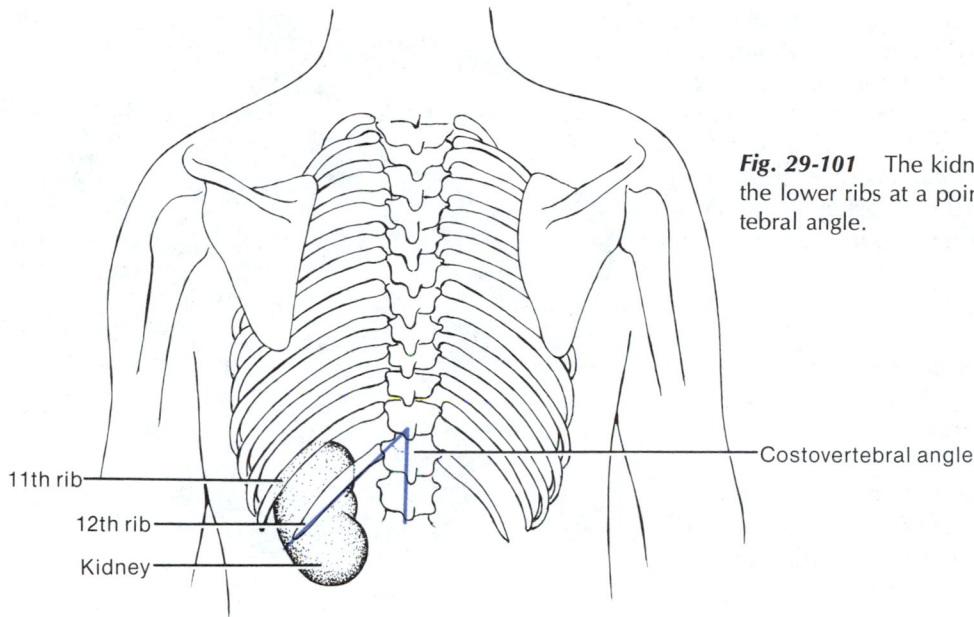

Fig. 29-101 The kidneys normally lie behind the lower ribs at a point even with the costovertebral angle.

11th rib

12th rib

Kidney

Costovertebral angle

The shape and symmetry of the abdomen are noted, as is the presence of any masses. A flat abdomen forms a horizontal plane from the xiphoid process to the symphysis pubis. A round abdomen protrudes in a convex sphere from the horizontal plane. Women's abdomens tend to appear more convex than men's as a result of excess fat or poor muscle tone. A concave abdomen appears to sink into the muscular wall. The presence of masses on only one side or asymmetry is abnormal and can be indicative of an underlying pathological condition.

Distention is an abnormality in shape that is frequently seen in the hospital and clinic setting. Intestinal gas, tumor, or fluid in the abdominal cavity may cause distention. When distention is generalized, the entire abdomen protrudes. The skin often appears taut as if it were stretched over the abdomen. When gas causes distention, the flanks do not bulge. However, if fluid is the source of the problem, the flanks will bulge. The client should be asked to roll onto his side. A protuberance forms on the dependent side if fluid is the cause of the distention. The nurse asks the client if his abdomen feels unusually tight. The feeling of fullness after a heavy meal can cause temporary distention. The nurse must be careful not to confuse distention with obesity. In obesity the abdomen is large, rolls of adipose tissue are often present along the flanks, and the client does not complain of tightness in the abdomen. The source of distention can be further clarified using palpation and percussion.

The abdomen is next inspected for movement. The nurse should remember that males breathe abdominally whereas females breathe more costally. If the client has severe pain, respiratory movement is diminished and the client tightens abdominal muscles to guard against the pain. On closer inspection the nurse may see peristaltic movement and aortic pulsation by looking across the abdomen from the side to detect movement. It may take several minutes to see a peristaltic wave. In contrast, aortic pulsations occur with each beat of systole and appear in the midline above the umbilicus (epigastric area).

The final portion of inspection involves observation of the umbilicus, noting the position, shape, color, and any presence of discharge or a protruding mass.

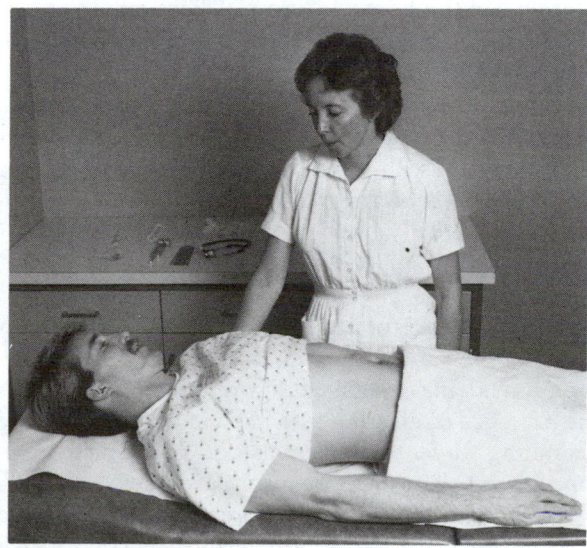

Fig. 29-102 During the abdominal assessment the nurse helps the client relax.

Normally, the umbilicus is a flat or concave hemisphere, positioned midway between the xiphoid process and symphysis pubis. The color is the same as that of the surrounding skin. The presence of underlying masses can cause displacement of the umbilicus. Hernias (protrusion of abdominal organs through the muscle wall) cause upward protrusion of the umbilicus. Normally, no discharge is emitted from the umbilical area.

AUSCULTATION

The nurse auscultates the abdomen to listen to the bowel sounds of intestinal motility and to detect vascular sounds. The diaphragm of the stethoscope is placed over each of the four quadrants (Fig. 29-103). Normally, air and fluid move through the intestines, creating soft gurgling or bubbling sounds in each quadrant. The sounds do not occur with regularity. It normally takes 5 to 20 seconds to hear a bowel sound; however, it may take as long as a minute. Each sound lasts about ½ second. The best time to auscultate bowel sounds is between meals. Sounds are generally described as normal or audible, absent, hyperactive, or hypoactive.

It takes practice to recognize the different qualities of sounds. The nurse must listen 3 to 5 minutes before deciding that bowel sounds are absent. Absent sounds indicate a cessation of gastric motility.

Hyperactive sounds are loud, "growling"-type sounds called borborygmi, which indicate increased gastric motility. Inflammation of the bowel, excess ingestion of laxatives, and reaction of the intestines to certain foods cause increased motility. Often hyperactive sounds are so loud the nurse does not need a stethoscope to hear them. Borborygmi may also be heard when the stomach "growls" because of hunger.

The thoracic aorta runs midline through the abdomen before branching into the femoral arteries. Narrowing of the aorta may cause abnormal bruits. The bell of the stethoscope is used to detect the blowing-type sounds. In some cases the nurse may also be able to hear renal artery bruits by placing the stethoscope posteriorly over the costovertebral angle.

PERCUSSION

As in the case of the thoracic examination, percussion of the abdomen is used to map out underlying organs and masses. In addition, percussion reveals the presence of air in the stomach and intestines. The beginning student will use this skill in a limited fashion. Practice is needed to ensure accuracy.

The position of underlying organs must be kept in mind. For general orientation the nurse percusses each of the four quadrants to discriminate between the sounds of dullness and tympany. Tympany predom-

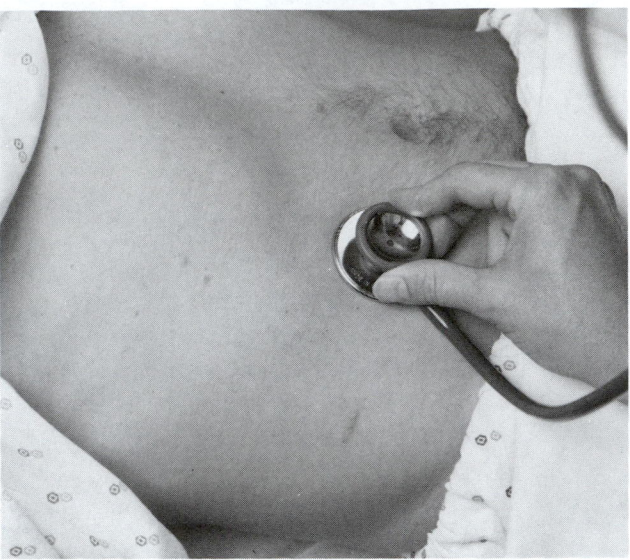

Fig. 29-103 Auscultation for bowel and vascular sounds.

inates as a result of air existing within the stomach and intestines.

Percussion allows the nurse to identify borders of the liver. The nurse starts at the right iliac crest and percusses upward along the midclavicular line (Fig. 29-104). The percussion note changes from tympanic to dull at the liver's lower border. Usually the border is at the right costal margin. The upper border is found by percussing down from the clavicle. The nurse also percusses in the intercostal spaces. This time the note changes from resonant to dull. The liver's upper border is usually found in the fifth, sixth, or seventh intercostal space. The distance between the points where dullness is percussed should be 6 to 12 cm (2½ to 5 inches). With liver disease the liver enlarges.

The kidneys are percussed to rule out the presence of inflammation. The client may sit or stand upright. The nurse may use direct or indirect percussion (Fig. 29-105). The nurse strikes the client firmly with the ulnar surface of the closed fist along each costovertebral angle at the scapular lines. If the client's kidneys are inflamed, tenderness is easily elicited during percussion. Normally the client feels no discomfort.

PALPATION

With palpation, the beginning nursing student is primarily concerned with detecting areas of abdominal tenderness and noting the quality of any abnormal distention or mass. As the nurse becomes more skilled, she learns how to palpate for the presence of specific organs such as the liver, spleen, and kidney.

The abdomen is lightly palpated over each quad-

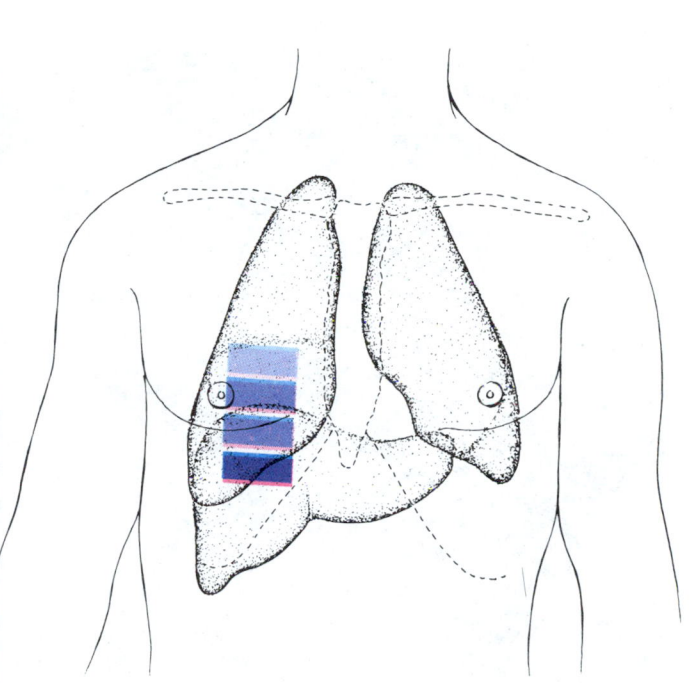

Fig. 29-104 To locate the liver borders the nurse percusses downward noting the changing sound from resonance (lung) to dullness (liver).

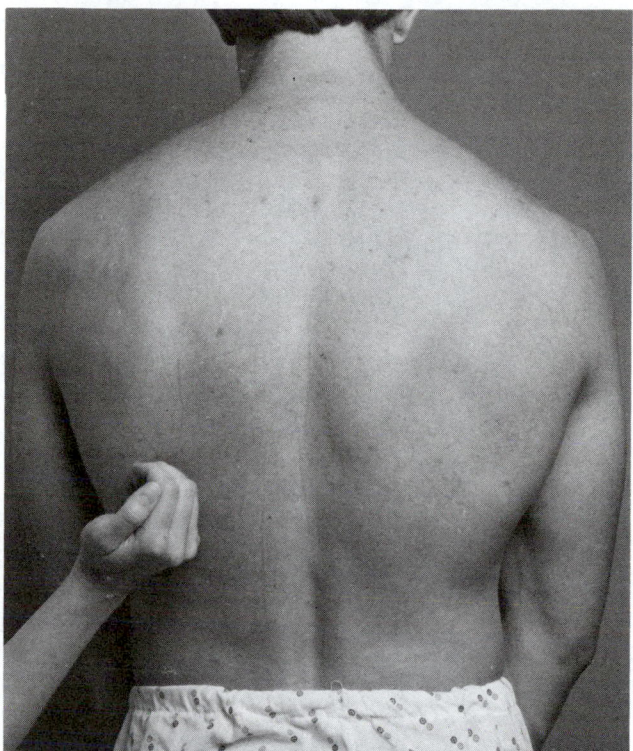

Fig. 29-105 Percussion for kidney tenderness along costovertebral angle.

rant. The skin is depressed approximately 1.3 cm (½ inch). The nurse must avoid quick jabs and use smooth coordinated movements (Fig. 29-106). If the client is ticklish, the nurse can place his hand under hers until he is able to tolerate the touch of the hand. The nurse feels for muscle tone, abdominal stiffness, or masses and must watch the client's face for signs of discomfort. If the nurse palpates a sensitive area, guarding, a voluntary tightening of underlying abdominal muscles, may occur. One organ the nurse can usually detect with light palpation is the bladder. Normally the bladder lies below the symphysis pubis. If the bladder becomes distended, the nurse can palpate the top of its dome just below the umbilicus and above the symphysis pubis.

With experience the nurse can perform deep palpation (Fig. 29-107). A qualified examiner must assist until the nurse becomes skilled in the technique. Short fingernails are a must; one or two hands may be used. It is particularly important for the client to be relaxed as the hands are depressed approximately 2.5 to 7.5 cm (1 to 3 inches) into the abdomen. Deep palpation is never used over a surgical incision or over extremely tender organs. It is also unwise to use deep palpation on abnormal masses.

Each quadrant is surveyed systematically. If a deep mass is located, the nurse notes all of its character-

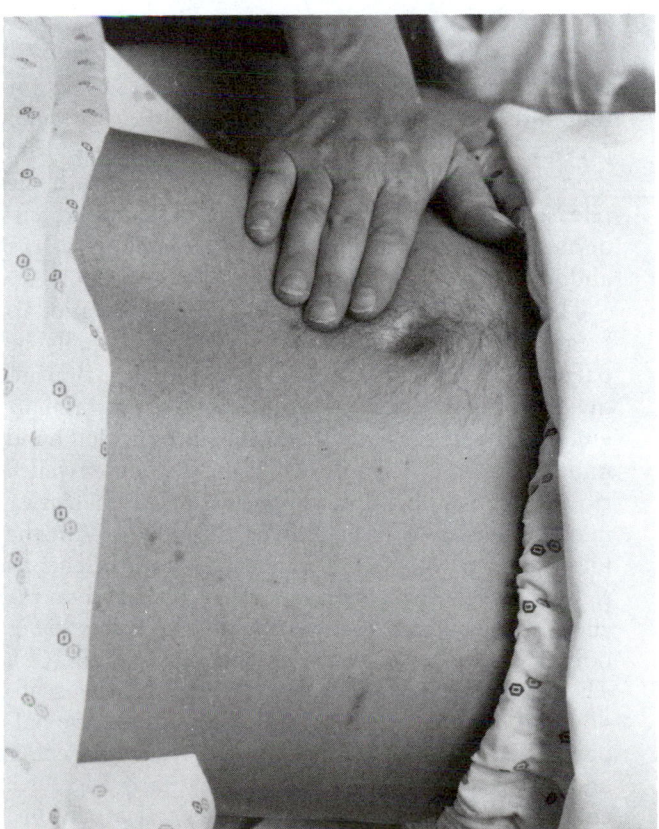

Fig. 29-106 Light palpation of the abdomen.

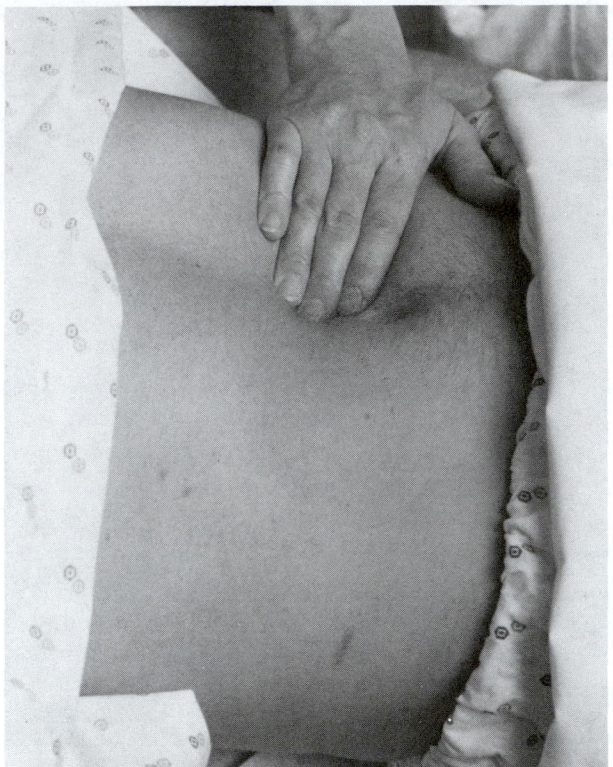

Fig. 29-107 Deep palpation of the abdomen.

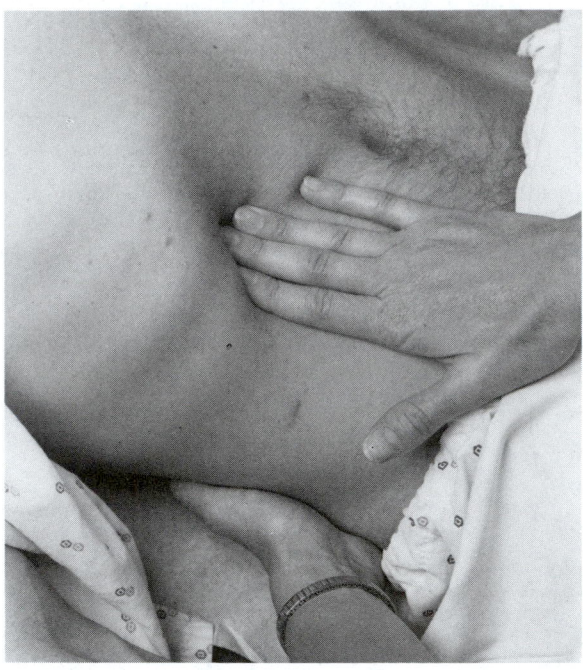

Fig. 29-108 The nurse's left hand is placed under the client's posterior thorax at the twelfth rib. The nurse's right hand palpates in and up to feel the liver's edge.

istics. If tenderness is found, the examiner checks for rebound tenderness. With this test the examiner presses her hand deeply into the involved area and then lets go quickly. If pain is aggravated with the release of the hand, the test is positive. Rebound tenderness occurs in clients with inflammation of the abdominal cavity (peritonitis).

The nurse uses deep palpation in an attempt to locate the liver's edge. The liver cannot usually be palpated in a normal adult. However, in a thin individual the liver's edge may be felt at the costal margin. To palpate the liver, the nurse places her left hand under the client's right posterior thorax at the twelfth rib and then applies upward pressure. This maneuver makes it easier to feel the liver anteriorly. With the fingers of her right hand pointing toward the client's right costal margin, the nurse places her hand on the client's right upper quadrant below the liver's lower border, then presses gently in and up (Fig. 29-108). The client should take a deep breath, using his abdominal muscles. As the client inhales, the nurse palpates the liver's edge. The normal liver is nontender and has a regular contour with a sharp edge. An enlarged liver may be indicative of several conditions. If the nurse palpates a hard nodular margin, she suspects carcinoma. A smooth, nontender, enlarged liver

is a sign of cirrhosis. Hepatitis causes the liver to feel smooth and tender on palpation. If the liver's edge cannot be palpated, the client should not be forced to undergo repeated maneuvers.

Female Genitalia and Rectum

An examination of the genital area is viewed with uncertainty by many women. The young adolescent will likely be fearful of the unknown. A woman's cultural background may contribute to her apprehension. The lithotomy position assumed during the examination is often a source of embarrassment. The nurse uses a calm, reassuring, and attentive approach. The client's comfort is most important in the way she is positioned and draped. Each portion of the examination is explained in advance so the client can anticipate the nurse's moves. Any delays that might aggravate the client's embarrassment are to be avoided.

The examination is relatively simple and should be a part of each woman's preventive health care, since uterine and vaginal cancer has a high incidence rate. All women over the age of 20 are advised to have a yearly examination.

The client may be seen by the nurse for the specific

purpose of having a complete examination of the female reproductive organs, or the nurse performing routine hygiene measures or preparing to insert a urinary catheter may use the opportunity to examine the external genitalia.

The nursing history should include data collected in the following areas: menstrual history, onset of menopause, obstetrical history describing each pregnancy, current and past contraceptive practices, history of genitourinary problems, and use of hormone medications.

PREPARING THE CLIENT

If the client is having a complete examination, the following special equipment will be needed:

1. Examination table with stirrups
2. Vaginal speculum
3. Adjustable light source
4. Sink
5. Lubricant
6. Clean disposable gloves
7. Glass microscopic slides
8. Sponge forceps or swabs
9. Wooden spatulas
10. Specimen bottles with fixative solution

All equipment must be ready before the examination begins.

Often it will be necessary to collect a urine specimen. If this is the only examination to be performed, the client should empty her bladder before the examination begins. An empty bladder will help the client relax during the examination.

If a vaginal examination is to be performed, the client should be placed in a lithotomy position. This position is most practical, since it allows full visualization of the genital area. The client lies on her back, the thighs are flexed and abducted, the knees are flexed, and the feet rest in stirrups (Fig. 29-109).

A square drape or sheet is given to the client. She holds one corner over her sternum, the adjacent corners fall over each knee, and the fourth corner covers the perineum. Once the examination begins, the drape over the perineum is lifted.

If the nurse wishes to examine only the external genitalia, she helps the client assume the lithotomy position in bed or on the examination table. The client flexes her knees perpendicular to the bed and is then asked to relax her thighs, allowing each leg to abduct to the side. The client's head may be elevated for comfort. A woman suffering pain or deformity of the joints may be unable to assume a lithotomy position. In this situation it may be necessary to have the client abduct only one leg or to have another nurse assist in separating the client's thighs.

The male examiner should always have a female in

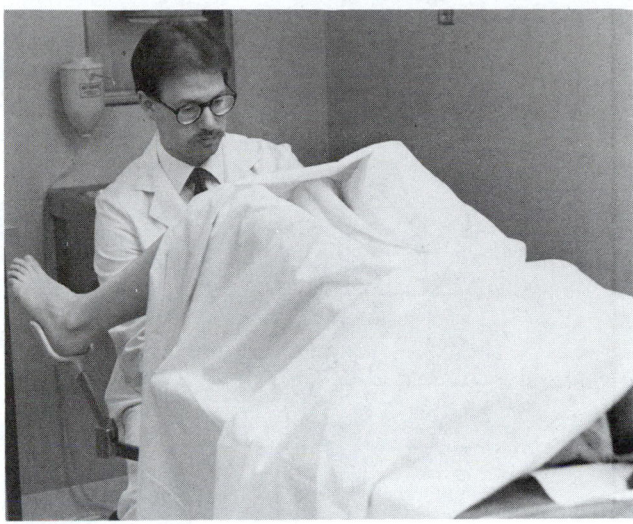

Fig. 29-109 Position of client for genital examination.

attendance during the examination. A female examiner may prefer to work alone but should have a female attendant if the client is particularly anxious or emotionally unstable.

EXTERNAL GENITALIA

The perineal area must be well illuminated. Both hands are gloved for the examination to facilitate the assessment and prevent the spread of infection.

The perineum is extremely sensitive and tender; the area is not touched suddenly without warning the client. It is best to touch the neighboring thigh first before advancing to the perineum.

The quantity and distribution of hair growth are inspected. Hair grows in a triangle over the female perineum, with the base of the triangle near the upper border of the pubic bone. The sides of triangular hair growth cover the outer surfaces of the labia majora.

The skin of the perineum is slightly darker than the skin of the rest of the body. The mucous membranes appear dark pink and moist.

The labia majora are usually plump and well formed in a normal adult female. After childbirth the labia majora are separated, causing the labia minora to become more prominent. When a woman reaches menopause, the labia majora become thinned. With advancing age they become atrophied. The labia majora are normally without inflammation, edema, lesions, or lacerations.

To inspect the remaining external structures, the nurse with her nondominant hand gently places the thumb and index finger inside the labia minora, and retracts the tissues outward (Fig. 29-110). The nurse should be sure to have a firm hold to avoid repeated retraction against the sensitive tissues. The clitoris,

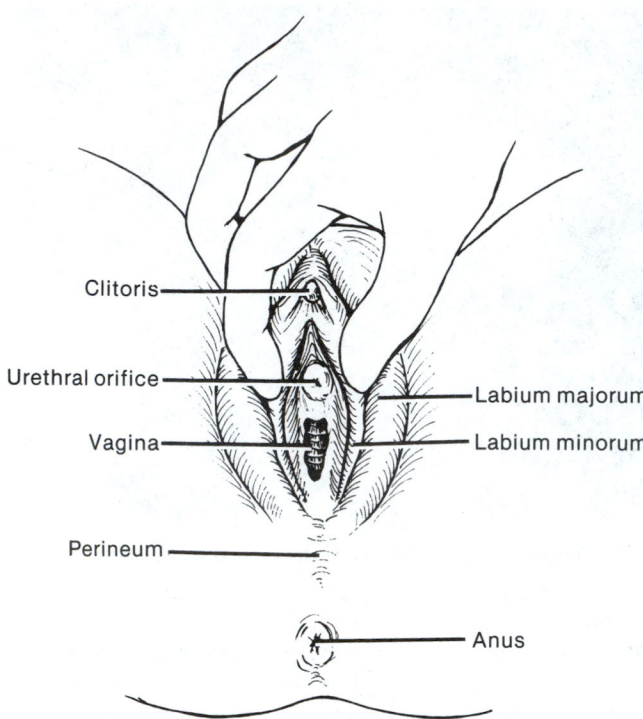

Fig. 29-110   Female external genitalia.

Labeled on figure: Clitoris, Urethral orifice, Vagina, Perineum, Anus, Labium majorum, Labium minorum

labia minora, urethral orifice, hymen, and vaginal orifice are then examined, paying particular attention to any discharge, inflammation, edema, ulceration, or lesions.

The size of the clitoris is variable; however, it should not exceed 2 cm (8/10 inch) in length or 1 cm (4/10 inch) in width. If inflamed, the clitoris will be a bright cherry red. In young women it is a common site for syphilitic lesions or chancres, which appear as small open ulcers that drain serous material. Elderly women may have malignant changes that result in dry, scaly, nodular lesions.

The labia minora are normally thinner than the labia majora. It is not unusual for one side to be larger. In the female who is a virgin, the labia normally lie together. As a result of childbirth or intercourse they tend to gape more and fall to the sides.

The urethral orifice is carefully observed for inflammation. The urethra is often difficult to locate. The inexperienced nurse frequently mistakes the vaginal orifice for the urethra. The urethra is a small slit or pinhole opening just above the vaginal canal. In women who have had several childbirths, the opening to the vaginal canal often extends upward, interfering with the view of the urethra.

There are minute openings of the Skene's gland around the urethra. If the nurse suspects inflammation, she checks for urethral discharge. The nurse gently places her index finger in the vaginal orifice

and milks the urethra gently from inside outward. Drainage will be manually expressed if inflammation is present. If drainage is found, the nurse changes her gloves for the remainder of the examination.

While inspecting the vaginal orifice or introitus, the examiner notices the condition of the hymen, which is just inside the introitus. In the virgin the hymen may restrict the opening of the vagina. Only remnants of the hymen remain after sexual intercourse.

If inflammation and edema are found near the posterior end of the introitus, Bartholin's glands may be infected. The glands cannot normally be palpated. To attempt palpation the nurse places her thumb and index finger between the labia majora and introitus and palpates one side at a time.

Often there is a loss of support of the vaginal outlet. A portion of the vaginal wall and bladder may prolapse or fall into the introitus. The client is asked to strain downward as if she were voiding. If the client lacks adequate muscular support, the vaginal walls will bulge, blocking the introitus opening.

The nurse may also inspect the anus at this time, looking for the presence of lesions and hemorrhoids (enlargement of blood vessels around the anus).

SPECULUM EXAMINATION OF INTERNAL GENITALIA

The speculum consists of two blades: the top, which is movable, and the bottom, which is fixed. The blades are attached by a thumbscrew that can be adjusted to open or close the blades. Beginning students are unlikely to perform a speculum examination, since the procedure requires considerable practice. One must not attempt the procedure without supervision by an experienced examiner, since incorrect use of the speculum can cause trauma to vaginal tissues. During the examination, specimens are collected for testing for the presence of cervical and vaginal cancer (Papanicolaou [Pap] smears).

A speculum is required for the examination of the vaginal walls and cervix. First, the proper size speculum is selected. The smallest size will fit the virginal female. If the women is sexually active, a medium-sized speculum is best. For women who have had children, the examiner uses a medium to large speculum. The nurse must learn to feel comfortable in handling the speculum.

Before the examination begins, the speculum blades are warmed in warm running water. Water is the ideal lubricant: commercially prepared lubricants interfere with Pap smear studies. The nurse sits on a stool facing the client's perineum. The adjustable light is placed over the examiner's shoulder, directed toward the examination site.

If the nurse is right handed, she holds the speculum

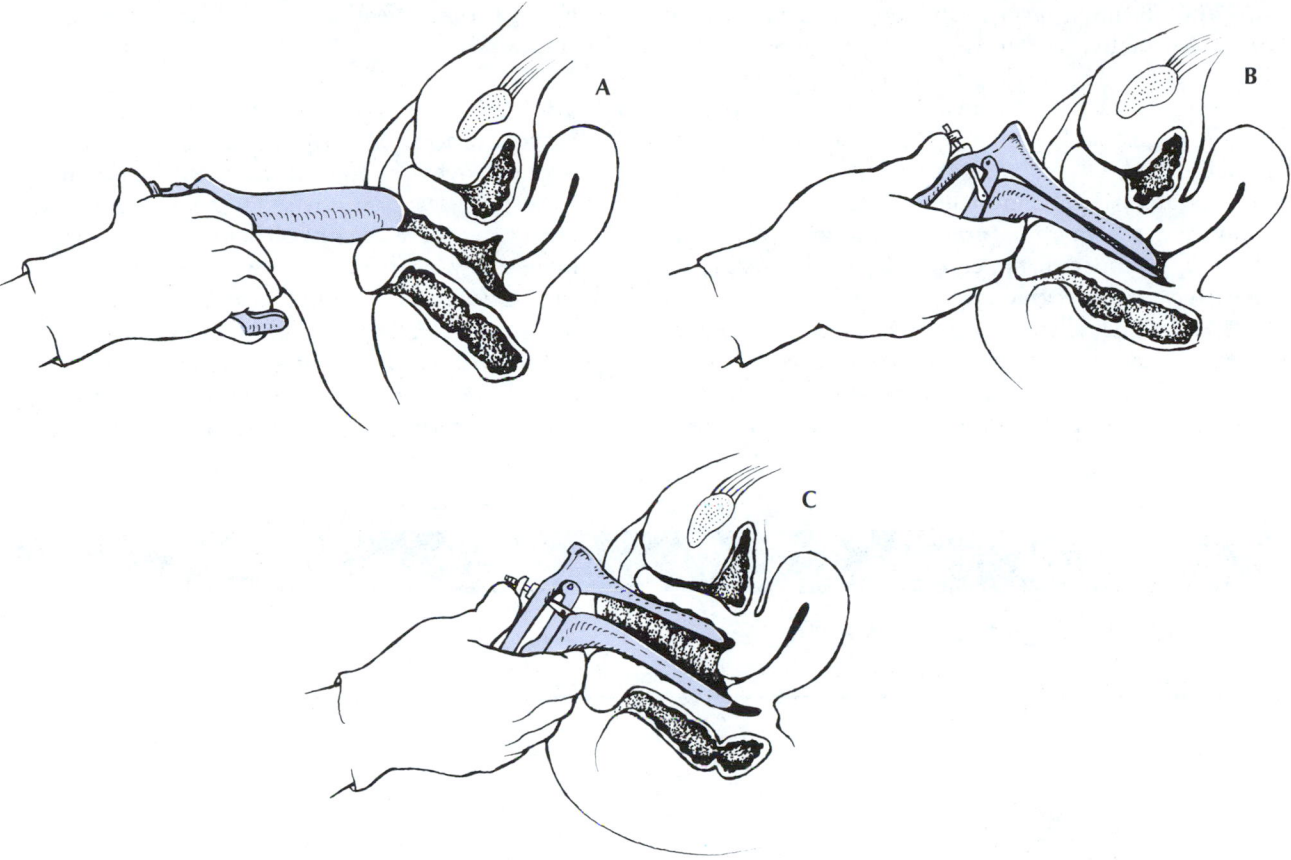

Fig. 29-111 Insertion of vaginal speculum. **A,** Speculum is introduced at oblique angle. **B,** Speculum is inserted downward at a 45-degree angle to table. **C,** Blades are opened after full insertion.

in her right hand. The nurse explains to the client what is about to happen. If the woman has never been examined, two fingers are gently inserted into the vagina to explore for abnormalities (Fig. 29-111). Then with two fingers the nurse presses down on the perineal body just inside the introitus. After checking to be sure the speculum blades are closed, the nurse introduces the closed speculum obliquely (rotated 50 degrees counterclockwise from the vertical position) past her fingers. The speculum is inserted downward at a 45-degree angle toward the examination table to avoid trauma to the urethra (this maneuver corresponds with the normal downward slope of the vaginal canal). Care is taken to avoid pulling the pubic hair or pinching the labia.

After the wide portions of the blades have passed the introitus, the speculum is rotated so the blades are horizontal. The blades are opened slowly after full insertion and the speculum is moved to visualize the cervix. When the cervix is in full view, the blades are locked in the open position.

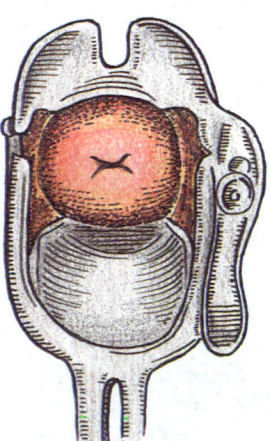

Fig. 29-112 Appearance of cervix through vaginal speculum.

CERVIX. The nurse inspects the cervix and its opening or os. Normally, the cervix is a glistening pink color (Fig. 29-112). The cervical diameter is approximately 2.5 to 3 cm (1 to 1²/₁₀ inches) in a normal young female. In an elderly woman the cervix is smaller. The presence of discharge, lacerations, ulcerations, or lesions is abnormal. Cancerous lesions tend to bleed easily and the margins are difficult to identify. A bluish appearance of the cervix (Chadwick's sign) is an early sign of pregnancy.

The os is usually small and closed in the female who has had no children. Childbirth causes the os to be larger with a slight curvature. Any discharge is examined carefully for color, odor, quantity, and consistency. Chronic infections yield thick, malodorous discharges.

PAP SMEAR. A Papanicolaou smear is a screening test for cervical cancer. Women who are sexually active and women over the age of 20 who do not have symptoms of disease are advised to have annual tests until two smears are negative. Thereafter, tests are to be done every 3 years until the age of 65. Women at risk for cervical cancer should have annual checkups.

The smear samples are easily collected while the speculum remains in the vaginal canal. As indicated in Table 29-14, the examiner collects cells from three sites: the endocervical area, the outer cervix, and the

---

TABLE 29-14

Methods for Obtaining Pap Smears

	Location	Technique
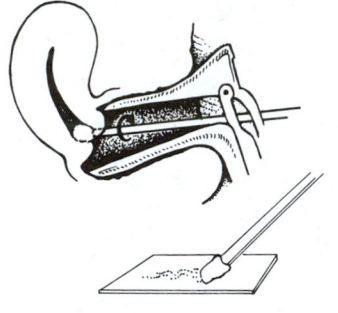	Endocervical	Use a cotton swab or applicator. Gently insert swab through the cervical os. Rotate the swab 360 degrees. Apply cells and secretions to glass slide. Apply fixative solution and label slide.
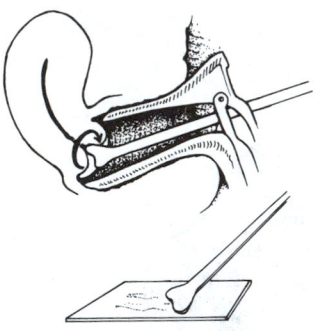	Outer cervix	Use the wooden Ayre spatula. Place tip of longer arm in cervical os. Rotate spatula, scraping the outer surface of the cervix. Apply cells to glass slide. Apply fixative solution and label slide.
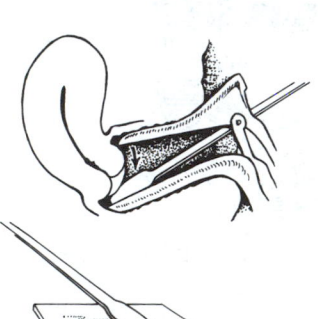	Vaginal pool	Rotate spatula, inserting handle into vagina. Place handle on vaginal floor. Apply cells and secretions to glass slide. Apply fixative and label slide.

vaginal pool. After each specimen is obtained, the nurse prepares each slide with the fixative solution. The specimens are labeled with the client's name and the source of the specimen.

VAGINA. The vaginal walls are viewed more easily as the speculum is withdrawn. As the speculum leaves the cervix, the thumbscrew is loosened but the blades are kept open with the thumb. During withdrawal the nurse inspects the vaginal wall's texture, color, and support. Any discharge or lesions are noted. The color is normally pink throughout. Females commonly acquire yeast infections, which cause a thick, white, patchy, curdlike discharge that clings to the vaginal walls.

The nurse closes the blades gradually as the speculum is removed to avoid excess stretching and pinching of the mucosa. The blades should be closed comletely as the speculum emerges from the introitus.

PALPATION OF ORGANS

The final phase of the examination is the assessment of the internal reproductive organs by means of palpation. The examiner requires extensive practice to recognize the normal size, shape, and consistency of internal organs.

The examiner stands facing the client. The index and middle fingers of the dominant hand are liberally lubricated, then gently inserted into the vagina. The thumb is kept abducted and the remaining fingers are flexed into the palm of the hand. The fingers are gently moved downward posteriorly. The nurse will be able to feel the cervix, which is easily palpable. The cervix will feel like a firm, smooth, rounded button. The os is the depression felt in the middle of the cervix.

More experienced examiners proceed to bimanual palpation. The fingers of the dominant hand remain in the vagina. The other hand is placed over the abdomen midway between the umbilicus and symphysis pubis. When the examiner presses down firmly on the client's abdomen, the internal organs are depressed against the examiner's dominant hand. Depending on the placement of the outside hand, the examiner can palpate the uterus and ovaries. Each organ is checked for position, size, shape, consistency, unusual tenderness, and the presence of masses.

RECTAL EXAMINATION

After the genital examination is a good time to perform the rectal examination. First the perianal area is inspected for lesions, discoloration, inflammation, and hemorrhoids. Any lesions are described in detail. Next, the rectal wall is palpated. The gloved index finger is relubricated as needed. The client is instructed to bear down as though she were having a bowel movement. She should be cautioned that she will feel as though she must pass a bowel movement. As the anal sphincter relaxes, the nurse's fingertip is gently inserted into the anal canal and her finger directed toward the client's umbilicus.

Each side of the rectal wall is palpated systematically, noting any nodules or irregularities. The client is asked if she feels any tenderness. When the finger is advanced to its full extent, the client is asked to bear down. Higher lesions will descend against the fingertips. The client is encouraged to relax as much as possible. Sphincter tone is tested by instructing the client to tighten the muscles around the examining finger. The nurse gently withdraws her finger. The stool on the glove can be tested for microscopic evidence of blood (see Chapter 40).

When the nurse has finished examining the genitalia, she cleanses the perineum and anal area to remove any moisture or drainage. The client is helped to a normal sitting position and her lower torso is covered with a drape. The client should feel comfortable before the examination is continued.

Male Genitalia and Rectum

An examination of the male genitalia considers the integrity of the external genitalia, the inguinal ring and canal, and the prostate gland. Because the incidence of sexually transmitted disease in adolescents and young adults is high, an assessment of the genitalia should be a routine part of any health maintenance examination for this age group. If this is the only assessment to be performed on a client, the nurse must be sure to collect a nursing history that includes a review of urinary function, a sexual history, and a discussion of sexually transmitted disease.

An examination of the genitalia creates the same anxiety and concern for a male as for a female. Because today's society emphasizes sexuality and because often the client partly equates healthy sexuality with normal reproductive organs, the male who has alterations in genitourinary function may feel that his sexuality is threatened. The client may also feel uncomfortable about having a female nurse examine him.

The female nurse must learn to relax during the male client's genital examination, since her anxiety would make the procedure highly embarrassing for both herself and the client. If the female nurse feels uncomfortable, she should ask a male nurse or male physician to perform the examination. Unless the nurse feels good about her own sexuality, she will have difficulty helping the client explore health-related problems. The nurse should not discuss the client's sexual activity during the examination, since

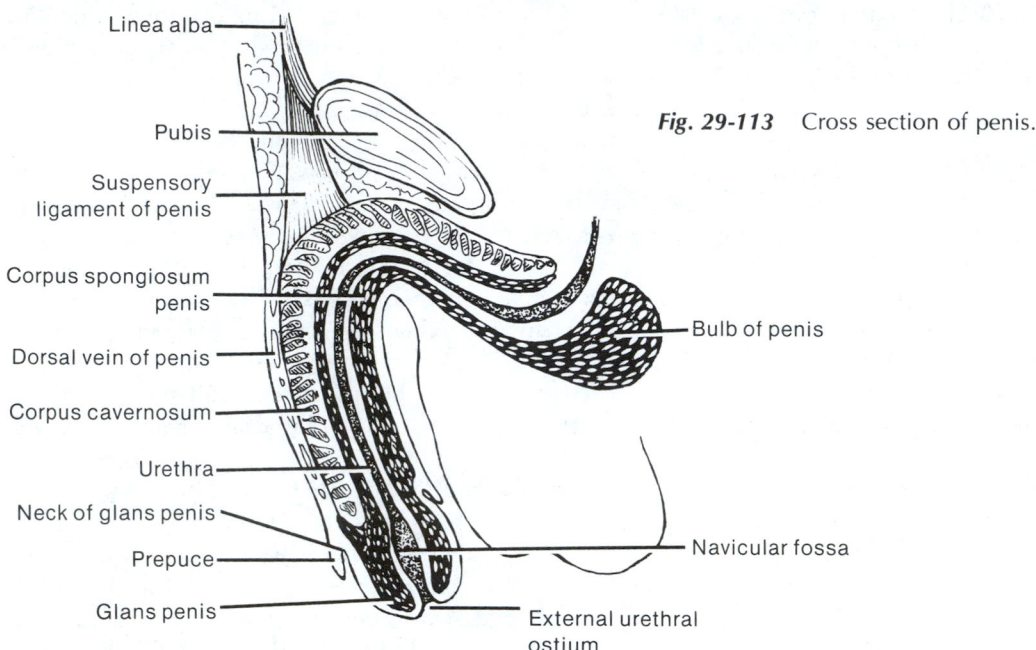

Linea alba
Pubis
Suspensory ligament of penis
Corpus spongiosum penis
Dorsal vein of penis
Corpus cavernosum
Urethra
Neck of glans penis
Prepuce
Glans penis
Bulb of penis
Navicular fossa
External urethral ostium

Fig. 29-113 Cross section of penis.

the client might perceive this discussion as evaluative or judgmental.

The client's modesty must be preserved. The genitalia are gently manipulated to avoid causing discomfort. The nurse can help him relax by explaining each step of the examination and by moving through each step of the assessment quickly. The examination begins with the client lying supine with the chest, abdomen, and lower legs draped. Inspection and palpation are the assessment skills used.

PENIS

The nurse observes the structures comprising the penis: the shaft, corona, prepuce (foreskin), glans, and urethral meatus (Fig. 29-113). The penile structures should not be excessively manipulated or an erection may be elicited.

In uncircumcised males the foreskin is retracted to reveal the glans and urethral meatus. The meatus should be positioned at the tip of the glans. In some congenital conditions the meatus is displaced along the penile shaft. The urethral meatus is observed for discharge, lesions, edema, and inflammation. The glans is carefully checked around its entire circumference for lesions. The area between the foreskin and glans is a common site for venereal lesions. A small amount of a thick white secretion between the glans and foreskin is normal. If there is evidence of abnormal discharge or inflamed lesions, gloves are applied. Any lesion is palpated gently to note tenderness, size, consistency, and shape. When inspection of the glans is completed, the foreskin is pulled down to its original position.

The nurse continues to inspect the entire shaft of the penis, including the undersurface, looking for any lesions, scars, or areas of edema. A client who has been lying in bed for a prolonged period of time may develop dependent edema in the shaft. The shaft is palpated between the thumb and first two fingers to detect any localized areas of hardness.

SCROTUM

The nurse must be particularly cautious while inspecting and palpating the scrotum, since the structures that lie within the scrotal sac are very sensitive.

The scrotum is a saclike structure divided internally into two halves. Each half contains a testicle, epididymis, and the vas deferens, which travels upward into the inguinal ring. It is normal to find the left testicle lower than the right. The nurse inspects the scrotum's size, shape, and symmetry while observing for lesions or edema. The scrotum is gently lifted to view the posterior surface. The scrotal skin is usually loose; a tightening of the skin may reveal edema. The scrotum's size normally changes with temperature variations as its dartos muscle contracts in cold and relaxes in warm temperature.

The underlying testicles are normally ovoid and approximately 2 cm (½ to 1 inch) in diameter. The testicles and epididymis are gently palpated between the nurse's thumb and first two fingers. The size, shape, and consistency of the organs are noted. The testicles feel smooth and firm. The epididymis is resilient. In the elderly client the testicles decrease in size and are less firm in palpation. The client should be asked about any unusual tenderness. The nurse continues palpating the vas deferens separately as it forms the spermatic cord toward the inguinal ring, noting the presence of nodules or swelling.

INGUINAL RING AND CANAL

The external inguinal ring provides the opening for the spermatic cord to pass into the inguinal canal. The canal forms a passage through the abdominal wall, a potential site for hernia formation. A hernia is protrusion of a portion of intestine through the inguinal wall or canal. An intestinal loop may even enter the scrotum. The client stands during this portion of the examination.

Both inguinal areas are inspected for signs of obvious bulging. During inspection the client is asked to strain or bear down. The maneuver will help make a hernia more visible.

A bulge may not be visible. To be assured that a hernia is not present, the nurse palpates the inguinal ring and canal (Fig. 29-114). Using the right index finger, the nurse gently invaginates the loose scrotal skin on the right side, starting at a point low on the scrotum. The finger follows the spermatic cord up to the inguinal ring. The tip of the finger may enter the inguinal canal but force must not be applied. Once the finger reaches the farthest point along the canal, the nurse asks the client to cough and strain down. If the client has a hernia, it will protrude against the

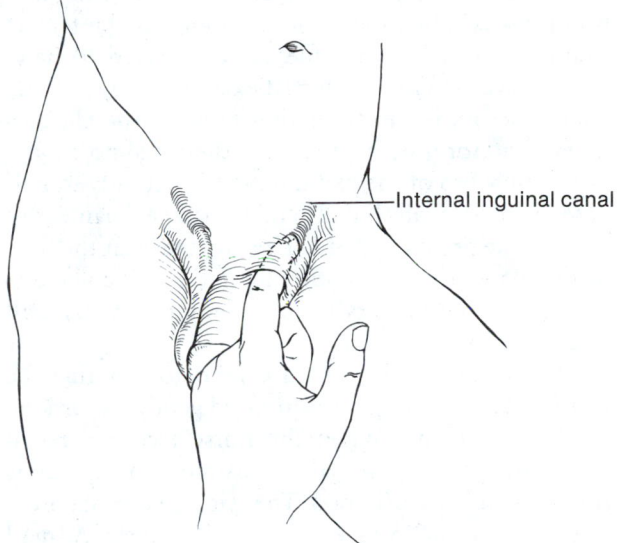

Fig. 29-114 Invagination of the loose scrotal skin allows for palpation of inguinal ring and canal.

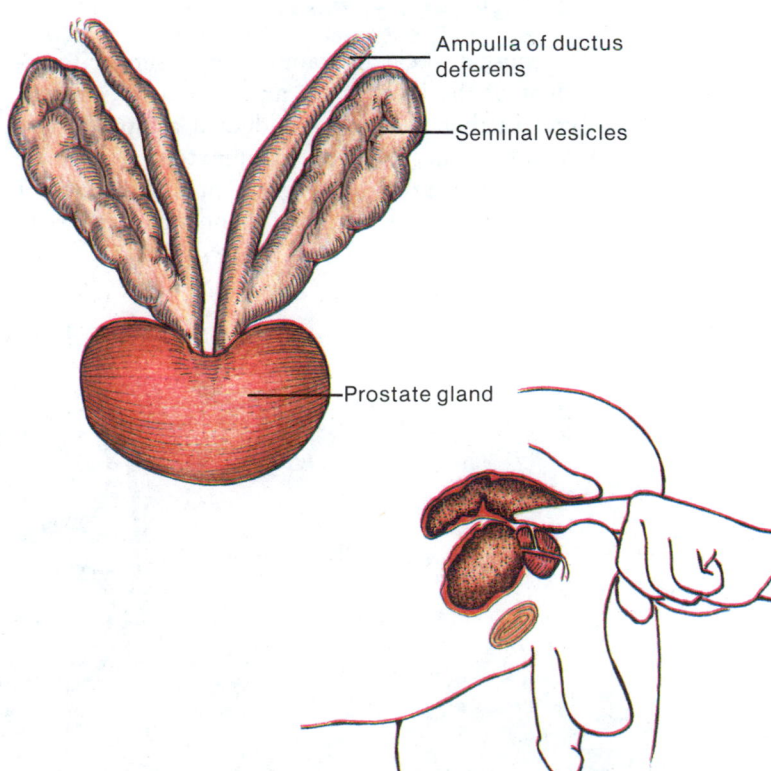

Fig. 29-115 Palpation of the prostate gland during the rectal examination.

examining finger. The nurse repeats the procedure on the client's left side using her left index finger.

RECTAL EXAMINATION

The procedure for a male client's rectal examination follows much the same technique as the female examination. However, the client is asked to bend over forward with his hips flexed and upper body resting across the examination table. If the client is nonambulatory, he may assume the Sims' position.

The purpose of the examination is not only to palpate the rectal walls but also to determine the integrity of the male prostate gland. The prostate is at the base of the bladder surrounding the urethra. The gland is only a few centimeters from the anterior rectal wall (Fig. 29-115).

Gloves and a lubricant are used to examine the rectum. The index finger is inserted gently toward the client's umbilicus. When the nurse feels the rectal wall, she palpates for the prostate. The gland is rounded and heart shaped. The size of a normal prostate varies from 2.5 to 4 cm (1 to 1½ inches). A small groove divides the gland into two lobes. The gland normally feels firm, without bogginess or tenderness. Hardness or nodules are abnormal.

The examination of the rectal walls then continues. It is important to palpate all sides of the wall for evidence of abnormalities.

Musculoskeletal System

The musculoskeletal examination is similar to assessment of the integument and peripheral vascular systems in that it can be conducted at appropriate times during the complete examination. The nurse can easily integrate this portion of her assessment with other nursing care as the client walks, moves in bed, feeds himself, rises from a chair, or practices range of motion exercises. The assessment of musculoskeletal function focuses primarily on determination of range of joint motion, muscle strength and tone, and the condition of joints and muscles. The appropriate portions of the examination are incorporated into those assessments previously described. For example, while inspecting the posterior thorax, the nurse might also assess the curvature and range of motion of the spine.

Assessment of musculoskeletal integrity is especially important when the client reports pain or loss of function in a joint or muscle. The nurse can question the client about whether he has suffered recent trauma or has bone or joint disease. Frequently muscular disorders are manifestations of neurological disease. For this reason a neurological assessment (see p. 686) is often conducted simultaneously. For example, a muscle may be damaged from direct injury or become weakened as a result of loss of nerve innervation.

As the nurse measures the status of the client's musculoskeletal function, she should also consider the client's ability to perform the activities of daily living. Any limitations affect the methods of care implemented by a nurse. The client with musculoskeletal alterations may require greater assistance with performing activities of daily living. In addition, the client may need to be educated in alternative ways to maintain mobility (for example, crutch walking).

It is important to review the anatomy of bone and muscle placement and joint structure. Joints vary in their degree of mobility. Some, as in the knee, are freely movable (Fig. 29-116). The spinal vertebrae are examples of slightly movable joints. An understanding of muscle and bone structure enhances the nurse's perception of the nature of musculoskeletal problems.

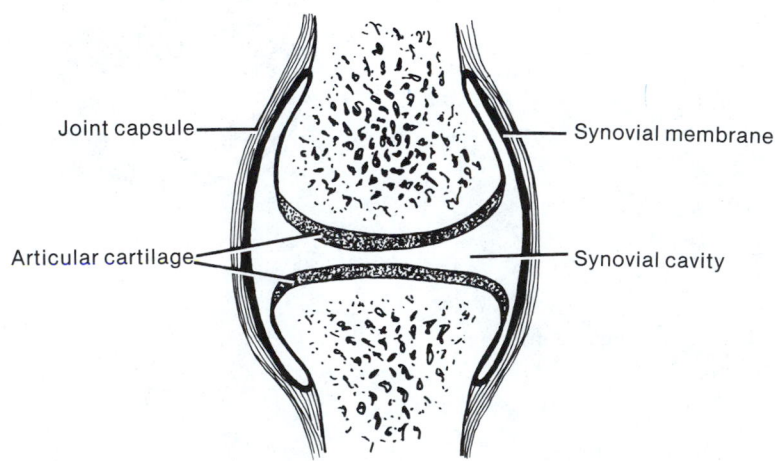

Fig. 29-116 Joint capsule with synovial membranes and cavity.

The examination uses the skills of inspection and palpation. The muscles and joints should be exposed and free to move. Depending on the muscle groups being assessed the client assumes a sitting, supine, prone, or standing position.

GENERAL INSPECTION

Initially the nurse observes the client's gait and posture. As the client walks into the examination room, the nurse's assessment of musculoskeletal function begins. When the client is unaware of the nature of the nurse's observations, his gait is more natural. Later a more formal test involves having the client walk in a straight line away from the nurse and then return. The nurse looks for foot dragging, limping, shuffling, and the position of the trunk in relation to the legs. Normally the client walks with arms swinging freely at his sides and the head and face leading the body.

The normal standing posture is an upright stance with parallel alignment of the hips and shoulders (Fig. 29-117). Looking sideways at the client, the nurse can note the normal cervical, thoracic, and lumbar curves. The head is held erect. As the client sits, some degree of rounding of the shoulders is normal. Common postural abnormalities include kyphosis, lordosis, and scoliosis (Fig. 29-118). Kyphosis or hunchback is an exaggeration of the posterior curvature of the thoracic spine. Lordosis or swayback is an increased lumbar curvature. A lateral spinal curvature is called scoliosis.

During a general inspection the nurse looks for symmetry of joints, muscles, and extremity length and the presence of any obvious musculoskeletal deformities. A general review will allow pinpointing of areas requiring specialized assessment.

RANGE OF JOINT MOTION

The nurse asks the client to put each joint through its full range of motion. If the client is weakened by illness, the nurse assesses range of motion passively by gently supporting and moving the extremities through their range of movement. The nurse must learn the correct terminology for the movements the joints are capable of making (Table 29-15). It is also helpful to practice range of motion of one's own joints to learn the limits of mobility. The same body parts are compared for equality in movement.

As the nurse assesses the client's range of motion, she does not force a joint into a painful position. The nurse must know what each joint's normal range is and the extent to which the client's joints can be moved (Table 29-16). Ideally, the client's normal range is assessed to determine a baseline for assessing later change (see Chapter 30).

A goniometer measures the precise degree of motion in a particular joint and is used primarily in clients who have a suspected reduction in joint movement. The instrument has two flexible arms with a

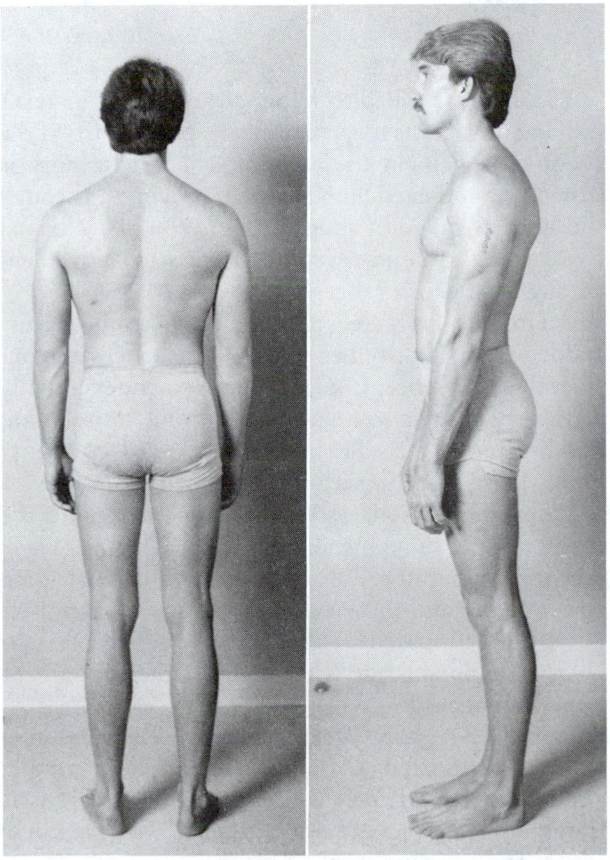

Fig. 29-117 **A,** Normal standing position. Client's hips and shoulders are aligned in parallel. **B,** Viewing the client sideways allows the nurse to observe the cervical, thoracic, and lumbar curves.

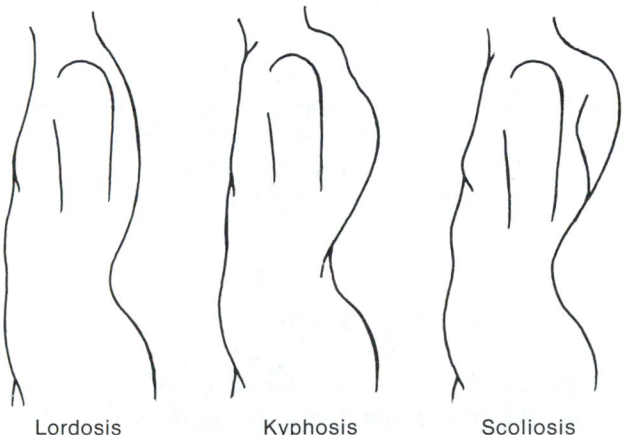

Lordosis   Kyphosis   Scoliosis

Fig. 29-118 Common postural abnormalities.

TABLE 29-15

Terminology for Normal Range of Motion Positions

Term	Range of Motion	Examples of Joints
Flexion	Movement decreasing the angle between two adjoining bones; bending of a limb	Elbow, fingers, knee
Extension	Movement increasing the angle between two adjoining bones	Elbow, knee, fingers
Hyperextension	Movement of a body part beyond its normal resting extended position	Head
Pronation	Movement of a body part so front or ventral surface faces downward	Hand, forearm
Supination	Movement of a body part so front or ventral surface faces upward	Hand, forearm
Abduction	Movement of an extremity away from the midline of the body	Leg, arm, fingers
Adduction	Movement of an extremity toward the midline of the body	Leg, arm, fingers
Internal rotation	Rotation of a joint inward	Knee, hip
External rotation	Rotation of a joint outward	Knee, hip
Eversion	Turning of the body part away from the midline	Foot
Inversion	Turning of the body part toward the midline	Foot
Dorsiflexion	Flexion of the toes and foot upward	Foot
Plantar flexion	Bending of the toes and foot downward	Foot

180-degree protractor in the center. The center of the protractor is positioned at the center of the joint being measured (Fig. 29-119, *A*). The arms extend along the body parts on each side of the protractor. A measurement is taken of the joint angle before moving the joint. After taking the joint through a full range of motion, the nurse measures the angle again to determine the degree of movement (Fig. 29-119, *B*). The reading is compared with the normal degree of joint movement.

While putting each joint through its range of motion, the nurse makes a number of basic observations. She notes any stiffness or instability in the joint during movement (Fig. 29-120). The nurse can palpate any unusual movement of the joints during range of motion. Each joint is observed for evidence of swelling or deformity. If a joint appears swollen and inflamed, the nurse may be able to detect warmth in the tissue by palpation. The surrounding tissues are inspected for muscle atrophy (decrease in size of muscle mass) and skin changes.

MUSCLE TONE AND STRENGTH

The nurse may assess muscle strength and tone during the measurement of range of motion. Tone is the slight muscular resistance felt by the examiner as the relaxed extremity is passively moved through its range of motion. Experience is needed to detect variations in muscle tone.

The client is asked to allow an extremity to relax or hang limp. This is often difficult, particularly if the client feels pain in the extremity. The extremity is supported and each limb grasped, moving it through the normal range of motion (Fig. 29-121). Normal tone causes a mild, even resistance to movement through the entire range.

If a muscle has increased tone or hypertonicity, any sudden passive movement of a joint is met with considerable resistance. Continued movement eventually causes the muscle to relax. A hypotonic muscle that has little tone feels flabby. The involved extremity hangs loosely in a position determined by gravity.

When the nurse is assessing muscle strength, the client must assume a stable position. The client will perform a number of maneuvers demonstrating strength of major muscle groups. Symmetrical muscle pairs are compared. The upper extremity on the client's dominant side is normally stronger than the nondominant side.

Each muscle group is examined. The client assumes a position of strength (Fig. 29-122). The examiner applies a gradual increase in pressure to a muscle group, for example, extension of the elbow. The client resists the pressure applied by the examiner by attempting to move against resistance, for example, flexion of the elbow. The client maintains resistance until instructed to stop. As the examiner varies the amount of pressure applied, the joint moves. Table

TABLE 29-16

Normal Range of Motion

Body Part	Motion	Measurement
Jaw	Open and close jaw. Move jaw side to side. Move jaw forward.	Able to insert three fingers Bottom side teeth overlapping top side teeth Top teeth behind lower teeth
Neck	Touch chin to sternum. Extend neck with chin pointing toward ceiling. Bend neck laterally, ear toward shoulder. Rotate neck with ear toward chest.	Flexion 70-90 degrees Hyperextension 55 degrees Lateral bending 35 degrees Rotation 70 degrees to the left and right
Spine	Bend forward at the waist. Bend backward. Bend to each side.	Flexion 75 degrees Extension 30 degrees Lateral bending 35 degrees
Shoulder	Abduct arm straight up. Adduct arm toward midline of trunk. Abduct arm straight horizontally to floor; bring arm backward toward spine and forward across chest. Flex or elevate forward with arm straight. Extend backward with arm straight.	Abduction 180 degrees Adduction 45 degrees Horizontal extension 45 degrees Horizontal flexion 130 degrees Flexion 180 degrees Extension 60 degrees
Elbow	Extend lower arm to normal extreme. Flex lower arm towards biceps. Hyperextend arm beyond normal resting point. Supinate lower arm. Pronate lower arm.	Extension 150 degrees Flexion 150 degrees Hyperextension up to 10 degrees Supination 90 degrees Pronation 90 degrees
Wrist	Flex wrist toward lower arm. Extend wrist backward. Deviate wrist laterally toward radius. Deviate wrist laterally toward ulna.	Flexion 80-90 degrees Extension 70 degrees Radial deviation 20 degrees Ulnar deviation 30-50 degrees
Fingers	Flex fingers into a fist and then extend them flat. Spread fingers apart. Cross fingers together. Oppose fingers: touch each fingertip with thumb.	Flexion 80-100 degrees (varies with joint) Extension up to 45 degrees Abduction 20 degrees between fingers Adduction (fingers will touch) Includes abduction, rotation, and flexion
Hip	Raise leg with knee straight. Raise leg with knee flexed. Lying prone, extend leg straight back. Abduct partially flexed leg outward. Adduct partially flexed leg inward. Flex knee and swing foot away from midline. Flex knee and swing foot toward midline.	Flexion 90 degrees Flexion 110-120 degrees Extension 30 degrees Abduction 45-50 degrees Adduction 20-30 degrees Internal rotation 35-40 degrees External rotation 45 degrees
Knee	Flex knee with calf touching thigh. Extend knee beyond normal point of extension. Rotate knee and lower leg toward midline.	Flexion 130 degrees Hyperextension 15 degrees Internal rotation 10 degrees
Ankle	Dorsiflex foot with toes pointing toward head. Plantar flex foot with toes pointing down. Turn foot away from midline. Turn foot toward midline.	Dorsiflexion 20 degrees Plantar flexion 45 degrees Eversion 20 degrees Inversion 30 degrees
Toes	Curl toes under foot. Raise toes to point upward. Spread toes apart.	Flexion 35-60 degrees (varies with joints) Extension up to 90 degrees (varies with joints) Varies

A   B

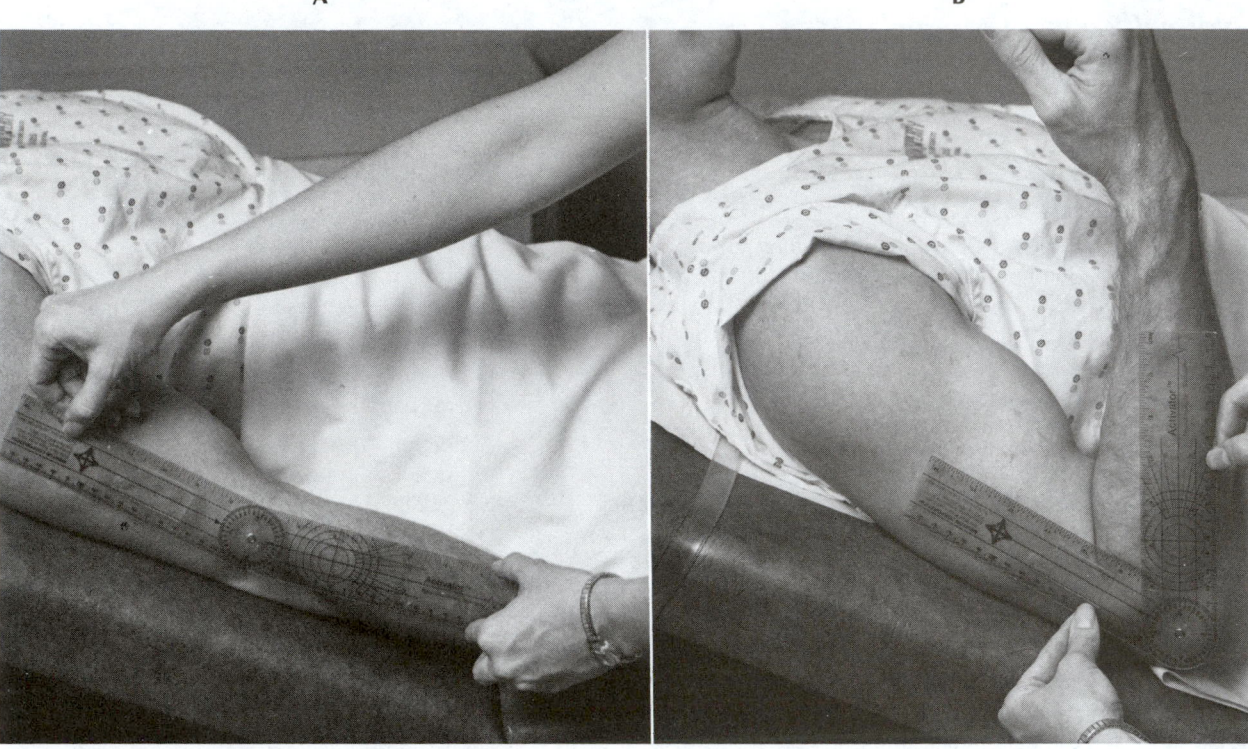

Fig. 29-119 **A,** The nurse positions the goniometer at the center of the elbow with the arms extending along the client's upper and lower arms. **B,** After the client flexes his arm the goniometer measures the degree of joint flexion.

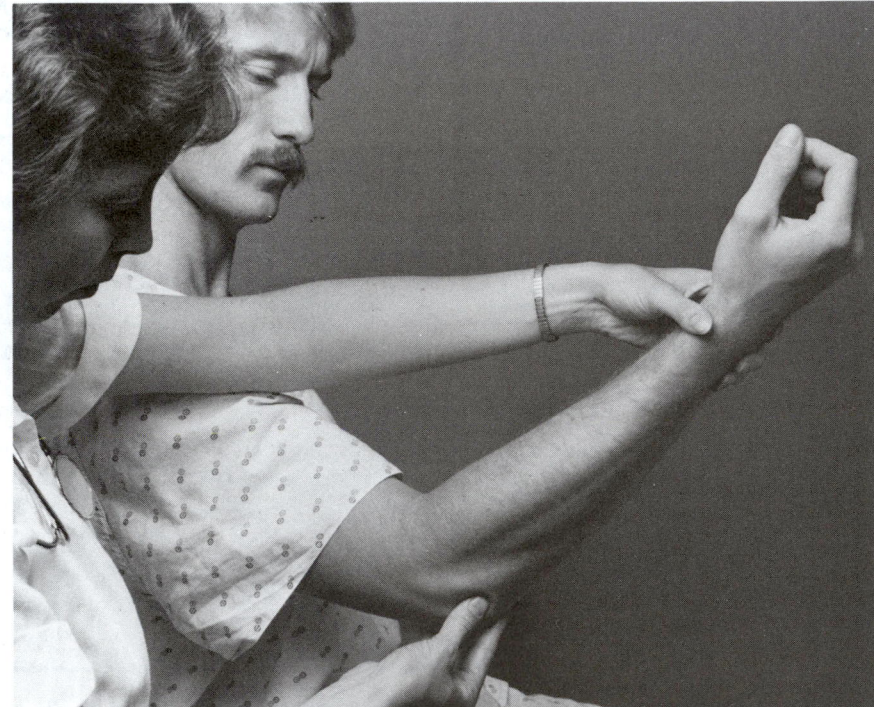

Fig. 29-120 The nurse palpates joint stability as the client moves the arm through its range of motion.

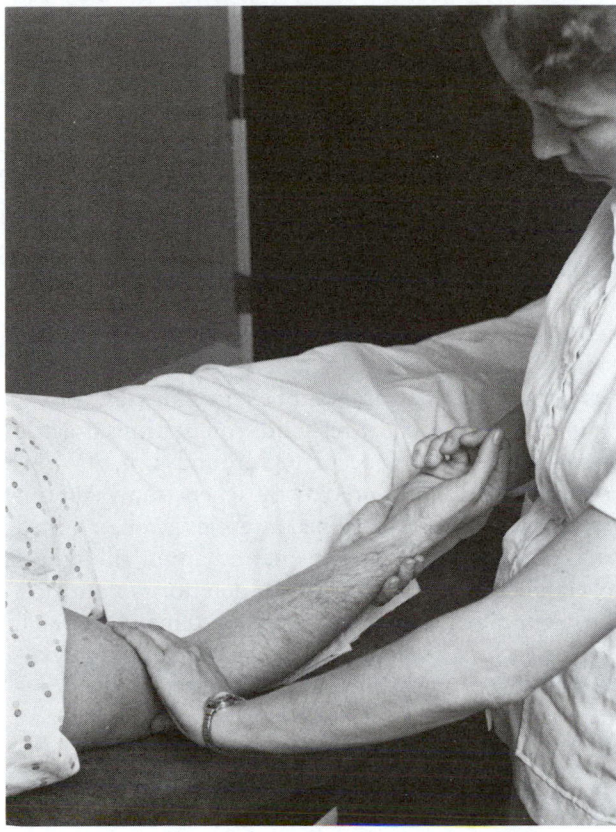

Fig. 29-121 The nurse palpates muscle tone while moving the extremity passively.

TABLE 29-17

Maneuvers to Assess Muscle Strength

Muscle Group	Maneuver
Neck (sternocleido-mastoid)	Place hand firmly against client's upper jaw. Ask client to turn head laterally against resistance.
Shoulder (trapezius)	Place hand over midline of client's shoulder, exerting firm pressure. Have client raise shoulders against resistance.
Elbow	
Biceps	Pull down on forearm as client attempts to flex arm.
Triceps	As client's arm is flexed, apply pressure against the forearm. Ask the client to straighten his arm.
Hip	
Quadriceps	When the client is sitting, apply downward pressure to the thigh. Ask the client to raise the leg up from table.
Gastrocnemius	With client sitting hold the skin of his flexed leg. Ask the client to straighten the leg against resistance.

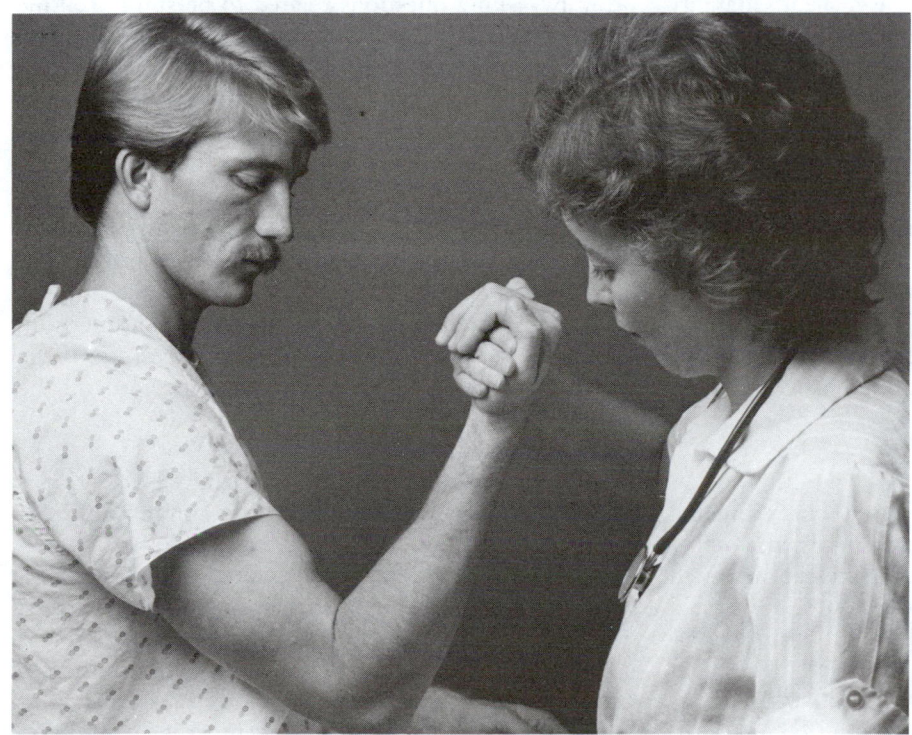

Fig. 29-122 Testing a client's muscle strength.

29-17 describes a number of maneuvers for measuring muscle strength.

If a weakness is identified, the muscle's size is compared to its opposite counterpart by measuring with a tape measure the muscle body's circumference. A muscle that has atrophied or become reduced in size may feel soft and boggy when palpated.

Neurological System

The neurological system is responsible for many functions, including the initiation and coordination of movement, reception and perception of sensory stimuli, organization of thought processes, control of speech, and storage of memory. A close integration exists between the neurological system and all other body systems. For example, urine production relies in part on the adequacy of blood flow to the kidneys, and the size of arterioles supplying the kidneys is under neural control.

An assessment of neurological function alone can be quite time consuming. An efficient nurse integrates neurological measurements with other parts of the physical examination. Cranial nerve function can be tested during the survey of the head and neck. Mental and emotional status is observed as the nursing history is collected. Reflexes are measured while the musculoskeletal system is assessed.

A number of variables must be considered when deciding how extensive the examination should be. The client's level of consciousness influences his ability to follow directions. The client's physical status influences assessment. For example, a client's inability to walk makes a detailed assessment of coordination difficult. The client's chief complaint also helps determine the need for a thorough neurological assessment. If the client complains of headache or a recent loss of function in an extremity, a complete neurological review is mandatory. Complaints relating to abdominal pain or breathing difficulties require only a brief screening of neurological function.

Before attempting to integrate a neurological assessment with other examinations, one must be familiar with its major categories: mental and emotional status, cranial nerve function, sensory function, motor function, and reflexes.

MENTAL AND EMOTIONAL STATUS

A great deal can be learned about the client's mental capacities and emotional state by simply interacting with him. Although mental function may be measured by grouping a number of tests together, the skilled nurse subtly poses questions throughout an examination to gather necessary data and observes the client at all times to detect the appropriateness of emotions and the ideas or thoughts expressed.

An alteration in mental or emotional status may reflect a disturbance in cerebral functioning. The cerebral cortex controls and integrates functions measured in the assessment. Primary brain disorders, drug effects, and metabolic changes are examples of alterations leading to changes in mental and emotional status.

LEVEL OF CONSCIOUSNESS.

The levels of consciousness exist along a continuum from full awakeness, alertness, and cooperation to unresponsiveness to any form of external stimuli. A person's consciousness is his level of awareness of environmental stimuli. A fully conscious client responds to questions quickly and perceives events occurring around him. As consciousness becomes altered, the client may demonstrate irritability, a shortened attention span, a dulled perception of the environment, and an unwillingness to cooperate. As consciousness deteriorates further, the client may become disoriented and may be unable to recall who or where he is or the time of day. Eventually a client may be unable to follow simple commands such as "Squeeze my fingers" or "Move your toes." At this lowered level of consciousness, the client often is responsive only to painful stimuli. Applying firm pressure with the thumb over the sternum or root of the fingernail will elicit a response from the client. A client who is unresponsive to verbal and painful stimuli is comatose.

If the client's consciousness seems to be impaired, the nurse asks questions that are short and to the point. The nurse checks the client's level of orientation by asking questions related to person ("Tell me your name." "Tell me who I am."), place ("What is the name of this place?" "Tell me where you are."), and time ("What day is this? What month? What year?").

The client's ability to understand and answer the examiner's questions will have a direct effect on the nurse's ability to perform a complete examination. The client must be aroused to his full alertness before the assessment can be conducted. When the nurse is uncertain whether the client understands a question, she must rephrase it or ask a similar question. If the client becomes irritable or confused, portions of the examination that require client feedback should be skipped or delayed.

Many conditions can alter a client's level of consciousness. Fever and pain are two common physiological alterations that can create confusion, disorientation, and irritability, depending on their severity. A client who is experiencing severe emotional stress, such as the loss of a loved one, may be confused and disoriented. Disturbed levels of consciousness are also common in disorders of other body systems such as diabetic coma, liver failure, hemorrhage, and hypoxia, in which either the release of metabolic wastes or the lack of oxygen impairs neurological function.

BEHAVIOR AND APPEARANCE. The client's behaviors, moods, hygiene, grooming, and choice of dress reveal pertinent information about his mental status. Many observations of behavior and appearance are made during the initial general survey.

The nurse must be perceptive of the client's mannerisms and actions during the entire physical assessment. The nurse notes whether the client responds appropriately to directions and observes his mood throughout the examination. The nurse notices the manner of the client's speech and his level of participation in the examination procedures.

The client's appearance reflects how he feels about himself. His personal hygiene, such as unkempt hair, a dirty body, or broken dirty fingernails, should be noted. The nurse observes the cleanliness, fit, and state of repair of the client's clothes. (Poorly fitted clothes may be a symptom of a person's poverty rather than inappropriate apparel.) Also the nurse can observe whether the client's choice of clothing is appropriate to the setting or type of weather. Because there are many styles and fads of clothing in our society, the nurse must be careful to avoid judging the client simply by what he wears. Yet a deterioration in a client's appearance may result from a poor self-image or an inability to attend to the process of grooming.

INTELLECTUAL FUNCTION. A person's intellectual function includes memory (recent, immediate, and past), knowledge, abstract thinking, association, and judgment. Each aspect of intellectual function is tested through a specific assessment technique. However, because the client's cultural and educational background has a significant bearing on his ability to respond to the test questions, the nurse should not ask questions related to concepts or ideas with which the client is unfamiliar.

MEMORY. It is easy to assess a client's memory of past events by having him recall such things as previous medical history, family history, a birthday, or an anniversary. Of course, the nurse must have access to a previous medical record or be able to confer with a family member to validate the client's accuracy. If the client was seen on a previous day, his memory of past events may be tested by asking if he remembers a conversation that took place. The nurse tests immediate recall by having the client repeat a series of numbers, for example, "Repeat these numbers after me: 7, 4, 1, 8, 6" or "Repeat the following series of numbers backwards: 6, 1, 4, 3." Normally an individual is able to repeat a series of five to eight digits

forward and four to six digits backward. Recent memory measures the ability of the client to remember events occurring the same day. One might ask the client to recall instructions given earlier during the assessment or to relate what his physician explained to him previously. The client's memory should be casually tested; he must not be made uncomfortable or threatened by questions.

KNOWLEDGE. The nurse can assess the client's knowledge by asking him what he knows about his illness or the reason for being hospitalized. By assessing a client's knowledge, the nurse determines the client's ability to learn or understand. If there is an opportunity to teach the client information, the nurse can test his mental status by asking for feedback during a follow-up visit.

ABSTRACT THINKING. Interpreting abstract ideas or concepts reflects the capacity for abstract thinking. A higher level of intellectual functioning is required for an individual to explain such phrases as "A stitch in time saves nine" or "Don't count your chickens before they're hatched." The nurse notes if the client's explanations are relevant and concrete. The client with altered mentation will likely interpret the phrase literally or merely rephrase the words.

ASSOCIATION. Another higher level of intellectual function involves finding similarities or associations between concepts: a dog is to a beagle as a cat is to a Siamese. The nurse names related concepts and asks the client to identify their associations. It is sufficient to use simple concepts.

JUDGMENT. Judgment requires a comparison and evaluation of facts and ideas to understand their relationships and to form appropriate conclusions. The nurse attempts to measure the client's ability to make logical decisions. By assessing judgment the nurse also measures the client's ability to organize thought processes. The nurse may choose to ask the client why he decided to seek health care or how he plans to adjust to his limitations when he returns home following his illness. A simpler test would involve asking the client what he would do if placed in a situation such as being locked out of his home or suddenly becoming ill when alone at home.

CRANIAL NERVE FUNCTION

Many of the measurements used to assess the integrity of organs within the head and neck also assess cranial nerve function. The 12 cranial nerves are assessed in order of their number. A dysfunction in any one nerve reflects an alteration at some point along the cranial nerve's distribution. The cranial nerve as-

TABLE 29-18

Cranial Nerve Function and Assessment

Number	Name	Type	Function	Method of Assessment
I	Olfactory	Sensory	Sense of smell	Ask client to identify different nonirritating aromas such as coffee, vanilla.
II	Optic	Sensory	Vision	Use Snellen chart; ask client to read printed material.
III	Oculomotor	Motor	Extraocular eye movement	Assess directions of gaze.
			Pupil constriction and dilation	Measure pupil reaction to light reflex.
IV	Trochlear	Motor	Upward and downward movement of eyeball	Assess directions of gaze.
V	Trigeminal	Sensory and motor	Sensory nerve to skin of face	Assess corneal reflex. Measure sensation of light, pain, and touch across skin of face.
			Motor nerve to muscles of jaw	Assess client's ability to clench teeth.
VI	Abducens	Motor	Lateral movement of eyeballs	Assess directions of gaze.
VII	Facial	Sensory and motor	Facial expression	Ask client to smile, frown, puff out cheeks, raise and lower eyebrows.
			Taste	Have client identify salty or sweet tastes on front of tongue.
VIII	Auditory	Sensory	Hearing	Assess client's ability to hear spoken word.
IX	Glossopharyngeal	Sensory and motor	Taste	Ask client to identify sour, salty, or sweet taste on back of tongue.
			Ability to swallow	Use tongue blade to elicit gag reflex.
			Movement of tongue	Ask client to move tongue.
X	Vagus	Sensory and motor	Sensation of pharynx	Ask client to say "ah". Observe palate and pharynx move.
			Ability to swallow	Use tongue blade to elicit gag reflex.
			Movement of vocal cords	Assess client's speech for hoarseness.
XI	Spinal accessory	Motor	Movement of head and shoulders	Ask client to shrug shoulders and turn head against examiner's passive resistance.
XII	Hypoglossal	Motor	Position of tongue	Ask client to stick out his tongue to the midline.

TABLE 29-19

Assessment of Sensory Nerve Function

Sensory Function	Equipment	Method	Precautions
Pain	Safety pin	Ask client to tell you when he feels a dull or sharp sensation. Alternately apply the pointed and blunt ends of the pin to the skin's surface. Note areas of numbness or increased sensitivity.	Areas where skin is thickened, such as heel or sole of foot, may be less sensitive to pain.
Temperature	Two test tubes, one filled with hot water, the other with cold	Touch the client's skin with the tube. Ask the client to identify hot versus cold sensation.	May omit test if pain sensation is normal.
Light touch	Cotton ball or cotton-tip applicator	Apply a light wisp of the cotton to different points along the skin surface. Ask the client to tell you when he feels a sensation.	Apply along areas where the client's skin is thin or more sensitive, i.e., face, neck, inner aspect of arms, or top of feet and hands.
Vibration	Tuning fork	Apply vibrating fork to distal interphalangeal joint of fingers and interphalangeal joint of the great toe.	Be sure the client feels vibration and not merely pressure. Have him tell you when the vibration stops.
Position		Grasp the client's finger, holding it by its sides with your thumb and index finger. Alternate moving the finger up and down. Ask the client to tell you whether the finger is up or down. Repeat procedure with the toes.	Avoid rubbing adjacent appendages as the finger or toe is moved.
Two-point discrimination	Two safety pins	Lightly apply the points of two safety pins simultaneously to the skin's surface. Ask the client if he feels one or two pinpricks.	Apply pins to same anatomical site by fingertips, palm of hand, or upper arms. Minimal distance at which a client can discriminate two points varies (normally 2 or 3 mm on fingertips).

sessment becomes easy once the nurse is familiar with the nerve's normal functions. In order to remember the order of the 12 nerves this simple phrase can be used: "On old Olympus' towering tops a Finn and German viewed some hops." The first letter of each word in the phrase is the same as the first letter of the names of the cranial nerves (Table 29-18).

SENSORY FUNCTION

The sensory pathways of the central nervous system conduct sensations of pain, temperature, position, vibration, and crude and finely localized touch. Different nerve pathways relay the various types of sensations. For most clients a quick screening of sensory function is sufficient. However, the client who has symptoms of altered or decreased sensation, motor impairment, or paralysis requires a more extensive examination.

Normally a client has sensory responses to all stimuli tested. Sensations along the body's surface are felt equally on both sides of the face, trunk, and extremities. All sensory testing is performed with the client's eyes closed so he is unable to see when or where a stimulus strikes the skin (Table 29-19). Stimuli are applied in a random, unpredictable order to maintain the client's attention. The client should say when he perceives the particular stimulus. The nurse compares symmetrical areas of the body as she applies stimuli to the arms, trunk, and legs.

MOTOR FUNCTION

An assessment of motor function includes the same measurements made during the musculoskeletal examination. In addition, cerebellar function is determined. The cerebellum coordinates muscular activity, maintains balance, and helps control posture.

COORDINATION. It is difficult for the nurse to explain to the client the tests used to measure coordination. To avoid confusion the nurse simply demonstrates each assessment maneuver and then has the client repeat it after determining that the client's mobility is normal so that he is physically able to make the necessary movements. The nurse observes the smoothness and balance of movements tested.

Performing rapid, rhythmical, alternating movements demonstrates coordination in the upper extremities. First, the client pats his hand against his thigh as fast as he can while he is in a sitting position. The client should be able to strike the thigh rapidly and evenly without hesitation. Next the client alternately strikes the thigh with the hand supinated and then pronated. The speed and symmetry of movement are noted. An additional maneuver for upper extremity coordination involves touching each finger with

the thumb of the same hand in rapid sequence. The client's dominant hand is slightly less awkward when performing this movement.

A final measurement of upper extremity coordination involves the point-to-point test. The nurse stands in front of the client holding her index finger 2 feet in front of the client's face. She asks the client to touch her finger with his index finger and then to touch his nose alternately. The client moves his finger back and forth repeatedly. The nurse looks for any tremor of the hand or awkwardness in movement. The test may be repeated with the client's eyes closed.

Lower extremity coordination is tested with the client in a supine position. The nurse places her hand at the ball of the client's foot. The client taps the nurse's hand with his foot as quickly as possible. Each foot is tested for speed and smoothness. The feet do not move as rapidly or evenly as the hands.

A final test involves having the client sit with his eyes closed and place the heel of his foot on the opposite knee. The client then slides his heel down the opposite leg to his foot. This maneuver normally is performed evenly without the heel sliding off the leg.

BALANCE. To assess the client's general balance, the nurse has him stand with his feet together and his

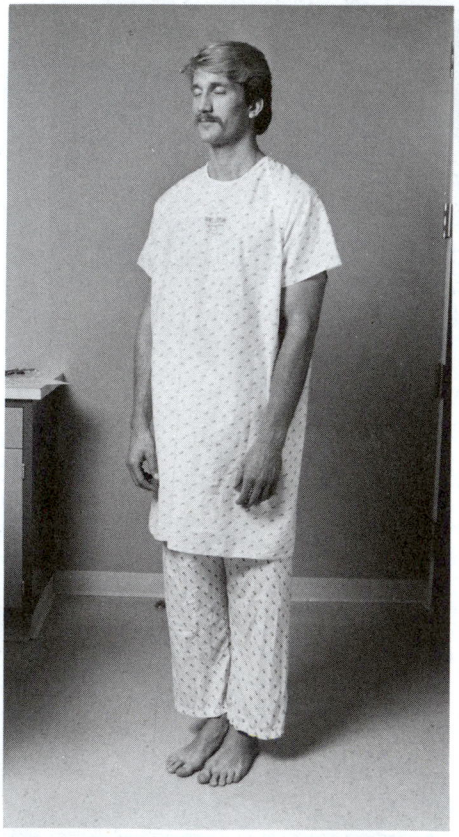

Fig. 29-123 Position of the client for a Romberg test.

eyes closed (Fig. 29-123). The nurse observes the client for presence of swaying, while protecting his safety by standing at his side in anticipation of a fall. Slight swaying is normal in an elderly client. The client normally does not have to break his stance. The test for balance is called the Romberg test.

REFLEXES

Eliciting reflex reactions allows the nurse to assess the integrity of sensory and motor pathways of the reflex arc and specific spinal cord segments. The assessment of reflexes does not determine higher neural center functioning. Fig. 29-124 traces the pathway of the reflex arc. When the muscle and tendon are stretched, nerve impulses travel along afferent nerve pathways to the dorsal horn of the spinal cord segment. Impulses synapse and travel to the efferent motor neuron in the spinal cord. A motor nerve then sends the impulses back to the muscle, causing the reflex response.

The two categories of normal reflexes are deep tendon reflexes, elicited by mildly stretching a muscle and tapping a tendon, and cutaneous reflexes, elicited by stimulating the skin superficially. Reflexes are graded as follows:

0   No response
1+ Low normal or diminished response
2+ Normal
3+ Brisker than normal; may not indicate disease
4+ Hyperactive and very brisk; often associated with spinal cord disorders

When reflexes are being assessed, the client should relax as much as possible to avoid voluntary movement or tensing of muscles. The nurse positions the client's limbs to slightly stretch the muscle being tested. The reflex hammer is held loosely between the nurse's thumb and fingers so it can swing freely and tap the tendon briskly. The nurse compares the symmetry of the reflex from one side of the body to the other (Figs. 29-125 and 29-126). Often practitioners use stick figures to record reflexes. Table 29-20 summarizes common deep tendon and cutaneous reflexes.

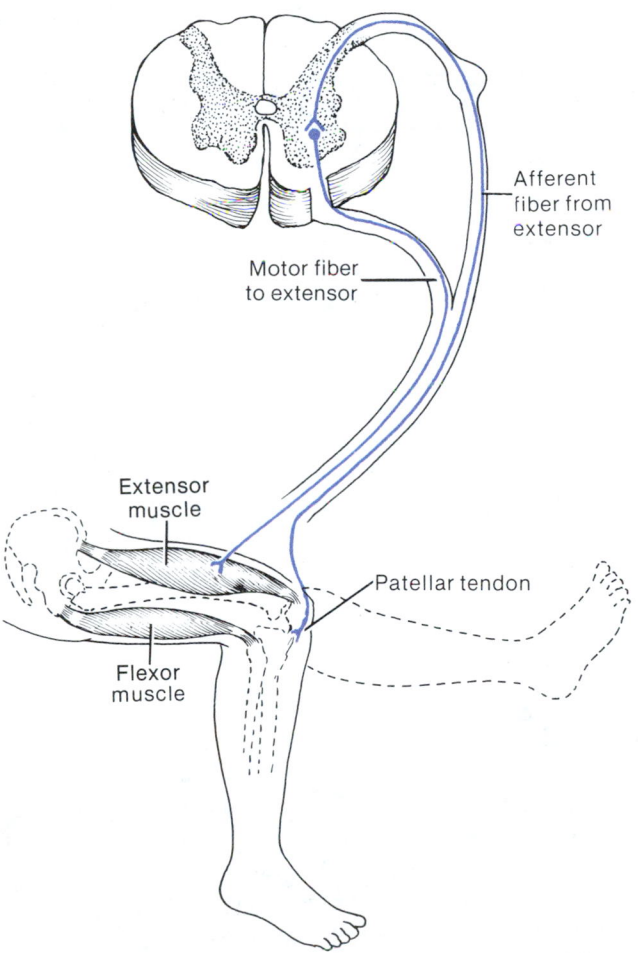

Fig. 29-124 Pathway of reflex arc.

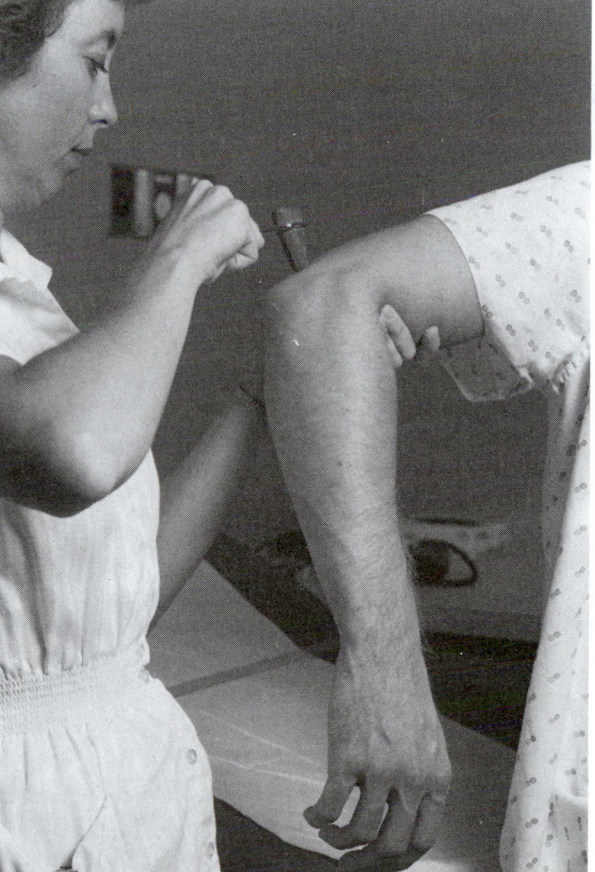

Fig. 29-125 The nurse supports the upper arm to allow for relaxation of the triceps muscle. The reflex hammer strikes the triceps tendon causing elbow extension.

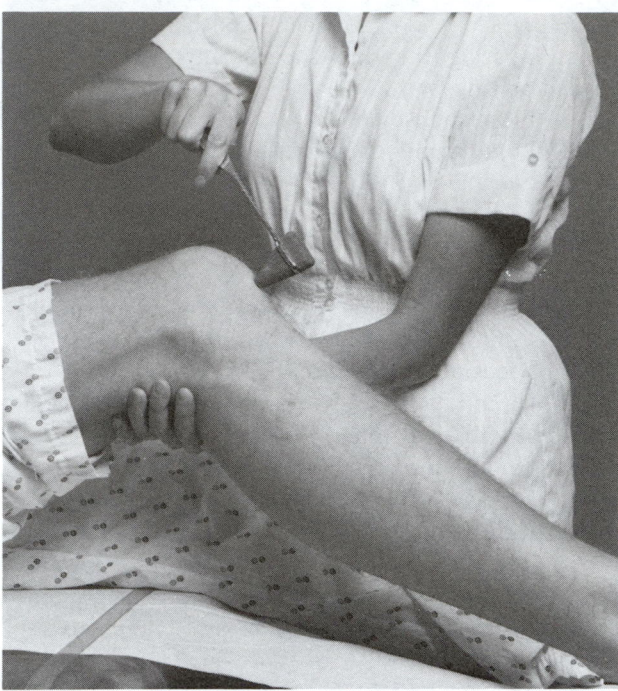

Fig. 29-126   Position for eliciting patellar tendon reflex. The lower leg normally extends.

After the Examination

After completing the assessment the nurse assists the client in dressing if necessary. The hospitalized client may need help in returning to bed and assuming a comfortable position. When the client is comfortable, it is helpful to share with him a summary of the assessment findings. If the findings have revealed serious abnormalities such as a tumor or highly irregular heart rate, the client's physician should be consulted before any findings are revealed. It is the physician's responsibility to make definitive medical diagnoses. The nurse can explain that she has found a "growth or lesion," which the physician will examine.

One of the nurse's responsibilities after the examination is to clean the examination area. The nurse stores all reusable equipment and disposes of supplies and equipment that cannot be reused. If the client's bedside was the site for the examination, the nurse clears away soiled items from the bedside table and makes sure the client's bed linen is dry and clean. The client may appreciate a clean gown and the opportunity to wash his face and hands.

TABLE 29-20

Assessment of Common Reflexes

Type	Procedure	Normal Reflex
Deep tendon reflexes		
Biceps	Flex the client's arm at the elbow with palms down. Place your thumb in the antecubital fossa at the base of the biceps tendon. Strike the thumb with the reflex hammer	Flexion of arm at elbow
Triceps	Flex the client's elbow, holding the arm across the chest, or hold the upper arm horizontally and allow the lower arm to go limp. Strike the triceps tendon just above the elbow.	Extension at elbow
Patellar	Have the client sit with his legs hanging freely over the side of the bed or chair or have the client lie supine and support his knee in a flexed position. Briskly tap the patellar tendon just below the patella.	Extension of lower leg at knee
Plantar	Have the client lie supine with legs straight and feet relaxed. Take the handle end of the reflex hammer and stroke the lateral aspect of the sole from the heel to the ball of the foot, curving across the ball.	Flexion of toes
Cutaneous reflexes		
Gluteal	Have the client assume a side-lying position. Spread apart the client's buttocks and lightly stimulate the perineal area with a cotton applicator.	Contraction of anal sphincter
Abdominal	Have the client stand or lie supine. Stroke the abdominal skin with the base of a cotton applicator over the lateral borders of the rectus abdominis muscle toward the midline. Repeat the test in each abdominal quadrant.	Contraction of rectus abdominis muscle with pulling of umbilicus toward the stimulated side

After completing the examination the nurse checks to be sure her recording of the assessment is complete. If she delayed making any entries in the assessment form, she does so at this time to avoid forgetting any important information. If entries were made periodically during the examination, they are reviewed for accuracy and thoroughness. Significant findings are communicated to appropriate medical and nursing personnel, either verbally or in the client's written care plan.

Often the client needs a number of ancillary examinations such as x-ray examination, laboratory tests, or ultrasonography after a physical examination. The tests provide additional screening information to rule out the presence of abnormalities and they help in the diagnosis of specific abnormalities found during the examination. Unit 8 describes ancillary tests in detail.

Summary

The physical examination is a vital part of the nurse's arsenal of assessment tools. Through the assessment the nurse is able to make insightful clinical decisions that contribute to the client's health management. Each body system is reviewed following a methodical sequence of observations and measurements. The nurse may conduct a total physical examination or may integrate portions of the examination into routine nursing care measures.

Information gathered during physical assessment supplements data obtained in the nursing history and from ongoing nurse-client interactions. As a result of more thorough data gathering, the nurse is able to make nursing diagnoses with greater precision. There-fore the client's plan of care becomes more individualized and comprehensive. Physical assessment findings also reveal whether specific nursing measures were successful in managing client problems. As the nurse becomes adept in physical assessment, clients recognize her professional competence.

Before attempting physical assessment, the nurse must become familiar with the principles and techniques of inspection, palpation, percussion, and auscultation. In addition, the nurse can use her sense of smell to detect certain abnormalities. Considerable practice is required before each skill is performed accurately and efficiently. A working knowledge of anatomy and physiology complements physical assessment skills.

Before an examination begins, the nurse takes the necessary steps to prepare the client and the setting. Measures are taken to ensure the client's privacy and psychological and physical comfort. The examination is not initiated haphazardly. The client becomes an active participant as the nurse carefully explains each step of the examination. A calm, gentle approach facilitates the client's cooperation during many of the examination procedures.

It is important that the examination be conducted in an organized fashion. Each system review entails numerous observations. A "helter skelter" approach will lead the nurse to forget essential measurements. Basic principles for a thorough examination include comparing both sides of the body for symmetry, completing each system before moving to the next, using each skill as appropriate, and recognizing which observations have priority for a client.

The physical assessment form provides a summary of the relevant observations to make in a complete physical examination.

KEY CONCEPTS

✓ The physical examination involves a comprehensive assessment of all body systems, whereas a physical assessment entails the measurement of a specific body part's function and integrity.

✓ Baseline assessment findings reflect the client's functional abilities when the nurse first assesses the client and serves as the basis for comparison with subsequent assessment findings.

✓ Physical assessment provides data the nurse can use in making nursing diagnoses and implementing nursing therapies.

✓ Assessment data can be used to evaluate the physiological outcomes of nursing care.

✓ Physical assessment of a child or infant requires the nurse to apply principles of physical growth and development.

✓ The nurse can use time more efficiently by integrating physical assessment with routine nursing care.

✓ Inspection requires good lighting, full exposure of the body part, and a careful comparison of the part with its counterpart on the opposite side of the body.

✓ Palpation involves the use of different parts of the hand to detect different types of physical characteristics.

✓ For a body part to be palpated correctly, the client must fully relax.

✓ Percussion is the detection of differences in density of underlying tissues by listening to sounds produced while striking the body's surface.

✓ Through the skill of auscultation the nurse assesses the character of sounds created in various body organs.

✓ A good stethoscope should have earpieces that fit snugly, a flexible thick-walled tubing of the proper length, and a chestpiece with a bell and diaphragm.

✓ Correct use of a stethoscope involves holding the diaphragm firmly against the skin and applying the bell lightly against the skin's surface.

✓ A physical examination should be performed only after proper preparation of the environment and equipment, and after preparing the client physically and psychologically.

✓ Throughout the examination the nurse should keep the client warm, comfortable, and informed of each step of the assessment process.

✓ The client assumes various positions during the physical examination to provide greater accessibility of body parts and increase accuracy in assessment.

✓ The nurse should use a systematic approach whenever conducting a physical assessment.

✓ When assessing a client who is seriously ill, the nurse concentrates on the body systems most likely to be affected.

✓ Information from the nursing history helps the nurse focus attention on specific parts of the examination.

✓ During the initial general survey the nurse assesses the client's vital signs, height and weight, and general appearance.

✓ When assessing a client's weight, the nurse should ask if the client has recently experienced a significant change in weight.

✓ Findings from the skin assessment may determine a client's need for better nutrition and hydration, as well as improved hygiene.

✓ Changes in the distribution of hair may be due to hormonal and circulation alterations.

✓ After the age of 40 a person should have an eye examination every 2 years.

✓ The pupillary light reflex should be checked in a dimly lit room.

✓ A client should be warned against moving during examination of ear structures with an otoscope.

✓ Examination of the oral cavity is a basic part of the nurse's assessment before administering oral hygiene.

KEY CONCEPTS, cont'd

✓ An enlarged lymph node may be the sign of localized or systemic infection or a malignant growth.

✓ A nurse's accuracy in assessing the thorax, heart, and abdomen is enhanced by creating a mental image of internal organs in relation to external anatomical landmarks.

✓ During assessment of the thorax the nurse compares both sides moving from top to bottom.

✓ The nurse uses the diaphragm of the stethoscope to auscultate breath sounds in an adult, but the bell amplifies sounds best in a child.

✓ The apical pulse is more easily auscultated at the point of maximal impulse, along the fifth intercostal space at the midclavicular line.

✓ When assessing heart sounds, the nurse imagines events occurring during the cardiac cycle.

✓ The carotid arteries should never be palpated simultaneously.

✓ When it is difficult to palpate a peripheral pulse, the nurse assesses circulatory adequacy by noting color, temperature, skin changes, and the presence of edema in the extremities.

✓ While examining a woman's breasts the nurse explains the techniques for regular breast self-examinations.

✓ The best time for a breast self-examination is on the last day of each menstrual period, or on the same day each month for pregnant and postmenopausal women.

✓ The abdominal assessment differs from other portions of the examination in that auscultation follows inspection.

✓ If the client and nurse are of opposite sexes, a nurse of the same sex as the client should be present during examination of the genitalia.

✓ Examination of female and male genitalia requires gentle palpation of body parts.

✓ Assessment of musculoskeletal function can easily be conducted while observing the client ambulate or participate in other active movements.

✓ The nurse assesses the client's mental and emotional status by interacting with the client throughout the examination.

✓ At the end of the examination the nurse provides for the client's comfort and then completes a detailed review of physical assessment findings.

REFERENCE

American Cancer Society: 1979 cancer facts and figures, New York, 1978, The Society.

ADDITIONAL READINGS

Bates, B.: A guide to physical examination, ed. 2, Philadelphia, 1979, J.B. Lippincott Co.

Block, G.J., et al.: Health assessment for professional nursing, New York, 1981, Appleton-Century-Crofts.

Burger, D.: Breast self-examination, Am. J. Nurs. 79:1088, 1979.

Norman, S.: The pupil check, Am. J. Nurs. 82:588, 1982.

Reynolds, J.I., and Logsdon, J.B.: Assessing your patients' mental status, Nursing 79 9:26, 1979.

Sana, J.M., and Judge, R.D.: Physical assessment skills for nursing practice, ed. 2, Boston, Little, Brown, & Co.

Schweiger, J.L., et al.: Oral assessment: how to do it, Am. J. Nurs. 80:654, 1980.

Smith, C.: Abdominal assessment a blending of science and art, Nursing 81 **11**:42, 1981.

Visich, M.A.: Breath and heart sounds, Nursing 81 **11**:64, 1981.

OBJECTIVES

Mastery of content in this chapter will enable the student to:

- Define the terms in the glossary.
- Describe the roles of the skeleton, skeletal muscles, and nervous system in the regulation of movement.
- Describe normal body alignment for standing, sitting, and lying down.
- Discuss the physiological influences on body alignment and joint mobility.
- Discuss the pathological influences on body alignment and joint mobility.
- Assess for alterations in body alignment and joint mobility.
- State the correct nursing diagnoses for impaired body alignment and joint mobility.
- Write nursing care plans for impaired body alignment and joint mobility.
- Describe the correct procedures for lifting.
- Describe the positioning techniques for the supported Fowler's position, supine position, prone position, side-lying position, and Sims' position.
- Describe the procedure for assisting a client to move up in bed.
- Describe the procedure for moving a helpless client up in bed.
- Describe the procedure for repositioning a helpless client.
- Describe the procedure for assisting a client to a sitting position.
- Describe the procedure for assisting a client to a sitting position at the side of the bed.
- Describe the procedure for transferring a client from bed to chair.
- Describe the procedure for a three-person carry.
- Describe complete range of joint motion exercises.
- List the types of mechanical devices used for walking.
- Describe how to measure a client for crutches.
- Describe crutch safety.
- Describe the five crutch gaits.
- Describe how to get into a chair with crutches.
- Evaluate the nursing plan for maintaining body alignment and joint mobility.

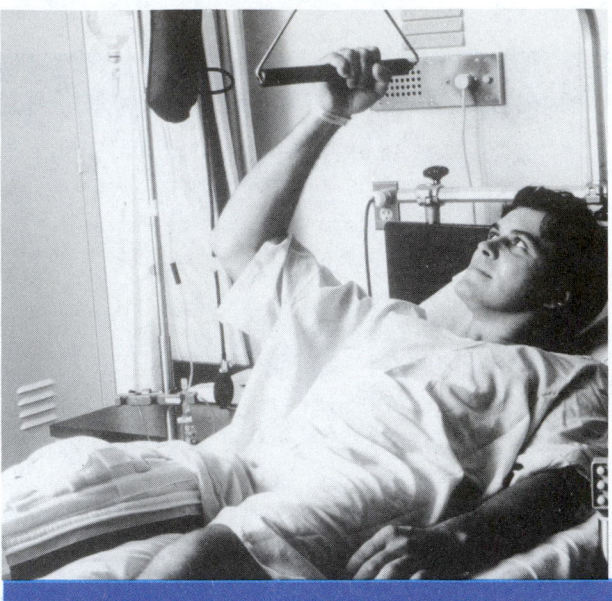

GLOSSARY

Achilles tendon Thickest and strongest tendon in the body.

activity tolerance Kind and amount of exercise or work that a person is able to perform.

antagonistic muscles Group of muscles that work together to bring about movement at the joint.

antigravity muscles Muscles involved with stabilization of joints by opposing the effect of gravity on the body.

body mechanics Coordinated efforts of the musculoskeletal and nervous systems to maintain proper balance, posture, and body alignment.

cartilage Nonvascular, supporting connective tissue located mainly in the joints and in the thorax, trachea, layrnx, nose, and ear.

cartilaginous joint Slightly movable, highly elastic cartilage that unites bony surfaces.

cerebellum Portion of the brain located in the posterior cranial fossa behind the brainstem.

crutch gait Gait assumed by a person on crutches by alternately bearing weight on one or both legs and on the crutches.

exercise Performance of any physical activity for the purpose of conditioning the body, improving health, or maintaining fitness or as a therapeutic measure.

fibrous joint Tough layer of fibrous connective tissue that binds bones firmly together.

flat bones Bones providing for structural contours of the skeleton.

30 | *Body Mechanics*

footboard   Board placed perpendicular to the mattress, parallel to and touching the plantar surface of the client's foot, and used to maintain dorsiflexion of the feet.

fracture   Breakage of bone caused by violence to the body; disruption of bone tissue continuity.

friction   Effect of rubbing or the resistance that a moving body meets from the surface on which it moves; a force that occurs in a direction to oppose movement.

gravity   Heaviness of an object resulting from the universal effect of the attraction of a planetary body.

hand rolls   Maintaining the thumb slightly adducted and in opposition to the fingers.

hand-wrist splints   Splints individually molded for the client to maintain proper alignment of the thumb, slight adduction of the wrist, and slight dorsiflexion.

irregular bones   Bones of the vertebral column and some bones of the skull.

isometric contraction   Increased muscle tension without muscle shortening.

isotonic contraction   Increased muscle tension resulting in muscle contraction and muscle shortening.

joints   Connections between bones; classified according to structure and degree of mobility.

ligaments   White, shiny, flexible bands of fibrous tissues binding joints together and connecting various bones and cartilage.

long bones   Bones that contribute to height of the person or length of an extremity such as the arm or length of a portion of an extremity such as the hand.

muscle tone   Normal state of balanced muscle tension.

myoneural junction   Point at which impulses traveling along motor nerves are transferred to muscle fibers.

neurotransmitter   Chemical that transfers the electrical impulse from the nerve fiber to the muscle fiber.

pathological fractures   Fractures resulting from weakened bone tissue; frequently caused by osteoporosis or neoplasms.

posture   Position of the body in relation to the surrounding space.

proprioception   Sensation achieved through stimuli originating from within the body regarding spatial position and muscular activity.

proprioceptors   Nerve endings located in muscles, tendons, and joints that respond to stimuli originating from within the body regarding spatial position or movement.

restraints   Devices used in the immobilization of clients, especially confused, elderly, and disoriented clients.

sandbags Sand-filled, plastic tubes that shape to body contour to maintain body alignment.

short bones Bones occurring in clusters and usually permitting movement of the extremities.

skeletal muscle Parallel striated fibers under voluntary control.

skeleton Supporting framework for the body, comprising 206 bones that protect delicate structures, provide attachments for muscles, allow body movement, serve as major reservoirs of blood, and produce red blood cells.

synergistic muscles Muscles contracting together to accomplish the same movement.

synostotic joint Joint in which bones are joined by bones and there is no movement between the bones.

synovial joint Joint in which freely movable, contiguous bony surfaces are covered by articular cartilage and connected by ligaments lined with synovial membrane.

tendons White, glistening fibrous bands of tissue that connect muscle to bone.

weight Force exerted on a body by the gravity of the earth.

Clinical nursing requires the nurse to incorporate knowledge and skills into practice. One such component of knowledge and skill is body mechanics. Body mechanics is a broad term used to describe coordinated efforts of the musculoskeletal and nervous systems as the person moves, lifts, bends, assumes a standing, sitting, or lying posture, and completes activities of daily living.

Many nursing activities, such as lifting a client, transferring a client from bed to chair, or positioning an immobilized client, require muscle exertion by the nurse. To reduce the risk of injury to both the client and the nurse when transferring a client, the nurse must be knowledgeable about and practice proper body mechanics.

Body mechanics includes knowing how and why certain muscle groups are used. The nurse also needs to understand the regulation of movement: basically, how coordinated body movement involves integrated functioning of the skeletal system, skeletal muscle, and nervous system. In addition, certain muscle groups are used primarily for movement and others primarily for posture.

This chapter describes how and why movement is regulated; the basics of the integrated functions of the skeleton, skeletal muscles, and nervous systems; posture and body alignment; and joint mobility. The chapter focus is on body alignment and joint mobility. Immobility and its impact on the client are introduced; a detailed description of the hazards of immobility appears in Chapter 31.

Regulation of Movement

Coordinated body movement involves the integrated functioning of the skeletal system, skeletal muscle, and nervous system. Because these three systems cooperate so closely in the mechanical support of the body, they can be considered almost a single functional unit. The skeleton and the skeletal muscles contribute to the shape of the body in both its length and width, and to the individual distribution of fat that determines the type of body construction (Strand, 1978). In addition, the skeletal system provides the body support structures for movement, and the muscles provide the necessary strength. The nervous system permits the initiation of and voluntary control of movement.

Skeletal System

The skeleton is the supporting framework for the body and is comprised of 206 bones. There are four types of bones in the skeleton: long, short, flat, and irregular. *Long bones* contribute to height (such as the femur, fibula, and tibia in the leg) and length (such as the phalanges of the fingers and the toes). *Short bones* occur in clusters and, when combined with ligaments and cartilage, usually permit movement of the extremities. Two examples of short bones are carpal bones in the foot and the patella in the knee. *Flat bones* provide structural contour, such as bones in the skull and the ribs in the thorax. *Irregular bones* make up the vertebral column and some bones of the skull, such as the mandible.

In addition to providing the supporting structure of the body, the skeleton has four other functions. First, the skeleton provides attachments for muscles and ligaments. These attachments allow movement of parts of the skeleton, such as opening and closing the mouth or extending an arm or a leg. Second, the skeleton protects vital organs; for example, the skull protects the brain, and the ribs protect the heart and lungs. Third, bones assist in the regulation of calcium balance. Bones are able to store calcium and release it to the circulation as needed. The regulation of calcium balance is controlled by the parathyroid hormone. Fourth, the internal structure of the bones contains bone marrow, participates in red blood cell production, and acts as a reservoir for blood. Although the last two functions are indirectly related to movement, they should not be overlooked when assessing a client's strength and mobility.

Clients with altered calcium regulation and metabolism are at risk for developing pathological fractures, which can occur in all types of bone but are most commonly found in the ribs and weight-bearing bones. These fractures result from weakened bone tissue and are frequently caused by osteoporosis or neoplasms. Osteoporosis, which results from increased bone resorption of calcium and decreased bone formation, is frequently observed in postmenopausal women, immobilized clients, and clients receiving long-term steroid therapy. Neoplasms result from primary bone tumors and metastases from primary cancers, such as those of the lung, breast, or prostate. Osteoporosis and bone neoplasms weaken the structure of the bone so that fractures may result from simple weight bearing. Pathological fractures can easily occur during activities of daily living, such as when a postmenopausal woman receiving steroid therapy fractures her hip as she descends stairs. In like manner, spontaneous rib fractures can occur during coughing.

Clients with altered bone marrow function or diminished red blood cell production are usually weakened and fatigue easily. The weakness and fatigue not only increase the immobility of these clients but place them at risk of falling. Both falling and immobilization result in trauma to the musculoskeletal system, and the nurse must identify these risks early in assessment of the client's mobility and body alignment.

CHARACTERISTICS OF BONE

The characteristics of bone include firmness, rigidity, and elasticity. Firmness results from inorganic salts such as calcium and phosphate that are laid down in the bone matrix. Firmness is related to the bone's rigidity, which is necessary to keep long bones straight and enables them to withstand weight bearing. In addition, bones have a degree of elasticity and skeletal flexibility that changes with age.

The composition of the skeleton changes throughout the life span. The newborn has a large amount of cartilage and is highly flexible but is unable to support weight. The toddler's bones are more pliable than those of an elderly person and are able to withstand some falls better. For example, a toddler who falls down a few stairs might have some minor bruises and fright but probably would not sustain injury to his skeletal system. However, a 65-year-old man could fall down those same stairs and fracture his hip.

Discussion of the skeletal system's role in the regulation of movement would be incomplete without a brief summary of the role of joints, ligaments, tendons, and cartilage.

JOINTS

A joint is any one of the connections between bones. Each joint is classified according to its struc-

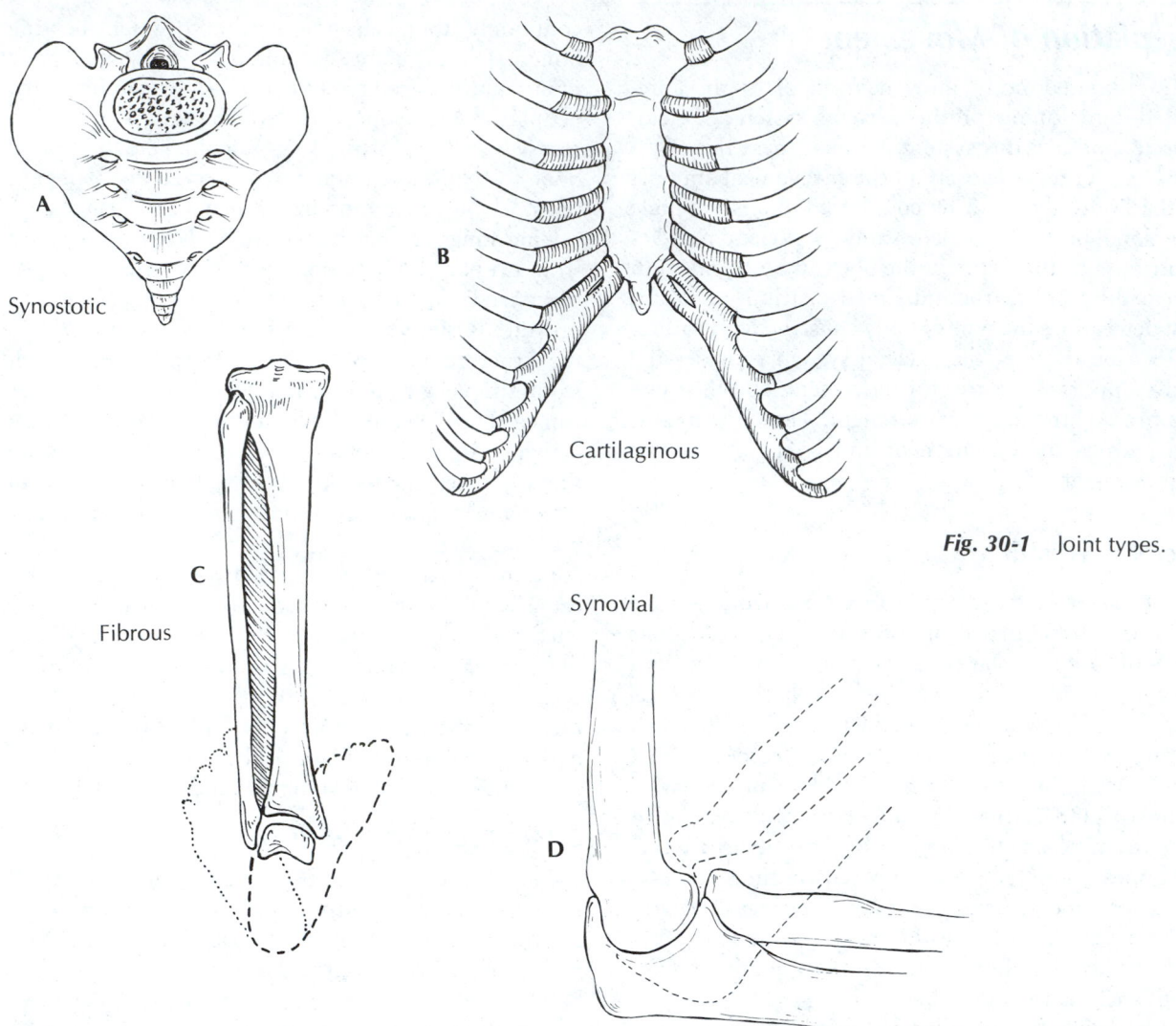

A — Synostotic

B — Cartilaginous

C — Fibrous

D — Synovial

Fig. 30-1 Joint types.

ture and degree of mobility. There are four classifications of joints: synostotic, cartilaginous, fibrous, and synovial.

The *synostotic joint* occurs when bones are joined by bones. No movement is associated with this type of joint, and the bony tissue that forms between the bones provides strength and stability. The classic example of this type of joint is the sacrum, in which vertebrae are joined together (Fig. 30-1, *A*).

The *cartilaginous or synchondrodial joint* has little movement but is elastic and uses cartilage to unite body surfaces. Cartilaginous joints are found when bones are exposed to a constant pressure, such as the costosternal joints between the sternum and the ribs (Fig. 30-1, *B*).

The *fibrous or syndesmodial joint* has a tough layer of fibrous connective tissue that binds bones firmly together. Because of the flexibility of connective tissue, some movement of the joint is permitted. For example, the connective tissue between the tibia and

fibula joins the bones in a fibrous joint at their distal ends, where they provide a socket for the upper part of the talar bones of the foot (Strand, 1978). Together these bones and connective tissues form the ankle joint, which permits the plantar and dorsal flexion of the foot (Fig. 30-1, *C*).

The *synovial or true joint* is a freely movable joint in which contiguous bony surfaces are covered by articular cartilage and are connected by ligaments lined with a synovial membrane. The joining of the humeral radius and ulna by cartilage and ligaments forms a pivotal joint (Fig. 30-1, *D*). Other types of synovial joints are the ball-and-socket joints, such as the hip joint, and the hinge joints, such as the interphalangeal joints of the fingers.

LIGAMENTS

Ligaments are white, shiny, flexible bands of fibrous tissue binding joints together and connecting various bones and cartilages. Ligaments are elastic

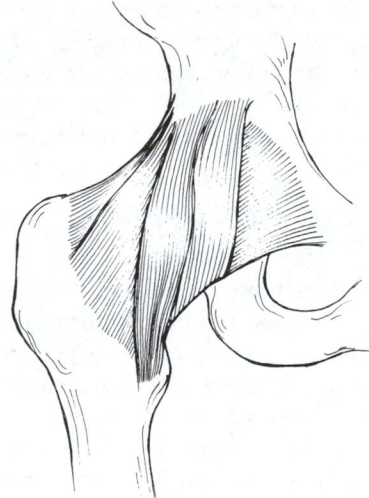

Fig. 30-2 Ligaments of the hip joint.

and aid joint flexibility and support (Fig. 30-2). In addition, in some areas of the body ligaments have a protective function. For example, the ligaments between the vertebral bodies, the nonelastic ligaments and the ligamentum flavum, prevent damage to the spinal cord during movement of the back.

TENDONS

Tendons are white, glistening, fibrous bands of tissue that connect muscle to bone. Tendons are strong, flexible, and inelastic and occur in various lengths and thicknesses. The Achilles tendon (tendo calcaneus) is the thickest and strongest tendon in the body. It begins near the middle of the posterior of the leg and attaches the gastrocnemius and soleus muscles in the calf to the calcaneal bone in the back of the foot (Fig. 30-3).

CARTILAGE

Cartilage is nonvascular, supporting connective tissue located chiefly in the joints and in the thorax, trachea, larynx, nose, and ear. The fetus has a large amount of temporary cartilage, which is replaced by bone during infancy. Permanent cartilage is unossified except in advanced age and certain diseases such as osteoarthritis.

Joints, ligaments, tendons, and cartilage permit strength and flexibility of the skeleton. Strength enables the skeletal system to support the body. Flexibility is demonstrated through range of joint motion, which is discussed in a later section of this chapter. However, the strength and flexibility of the skeleton do not result entirely from these four structures; adequate skeletal muscle is also necessary.

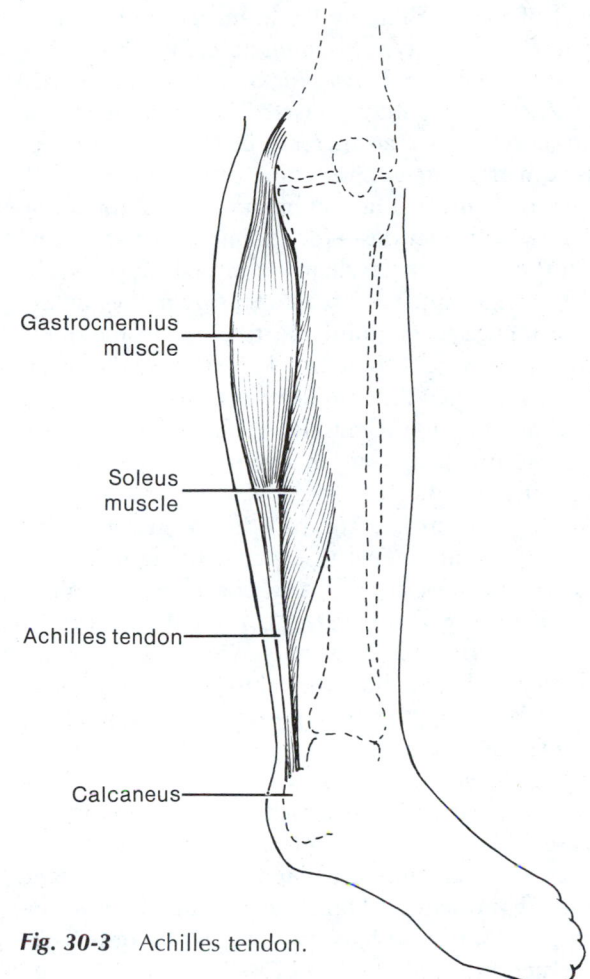

Fig. 30-3 Achilles tendon.

Skeletal Muscle

The movement of bones and joints involve active processes that must be carefully integrated to achieve coordination. The skeletal muscles, because of their ability to contract and relax alternately, are the working elements of movement. The contractile elements of the skeletal muscle are enhanced by its anatomical structure and attachment to the skeleton.

Skeletal muscle is composed of parallel striated fibers under voluntary control. Each muscle is covered by a fibrous sheath and is divided into fibers containing myofibrils. The myofibrils in turn are made up of thick filaments that contain myosin and thin filaments that contain actin. Actin and myosin are proteins needed for muscle contraction and relaxation.

Muscle contraction follows a stimulus from an electrochemical impulse that travels from the nerve to the muscle across the myoneural junction. The electrochemical impulse causes the thin actin-containing filaments to shorten, thus contracting the muscle. Removal of the stimulus results in muscle relaxation.

There are two types of muscle contractions: isotonic and isometric. In *isotonic* contraction, increased muscle tension results in muscle shortening. *Isometric* contraction causes an increase in muscle tension or muscle work but no shortening of the muscle. Voluntary movement is a combination of isotonic and isometric contractions—for example, what occurs when the nurse lifts a client up in bed. Initially, the client's weight causes increased tension in the muscles of the nurse's arms until the tension (isometric) is equal to the weight to be lifted and the weight of the lower arm. When this equilibrium is reached, continued stimulation to the muscles results in muscle shortening (isotonic), bending the elbow, and the client is lifted off the bed.

Although isometric contractions do not result in muscle shortening, energy expenditure is increased. This type of muscle work is comparable to having a car in neutral with the driver continually depressing the accelerator and racing the engine. The driver is not going anywhere but is certainly expending a large amount of energy. It is important for the nurse to recognize the energy expenditure associated with isometric exercises because these exercises are contraindicated in some illnesses such as cardiopulmonary disease.

Each skeletal muscle is capable of isometric and isotonic contractions. Some skeletal muscles are concerned primarily with movement, while others are concerned primarily with posture.

MUSCLES CONCERNED WITH MOVEMENT

The muscles concerned primarily with movement are located near the skeletal region where movement is caused by leverage. Leverage occurs when specific bones, such as the humerus, ulna, and radius, and the associated joints, such as the elbow joint, act together as a lever. Thus the force applied to one end of the bone to lift a weight at another point tends to rotate the bone in the direction opposite that of the applied force. The muscles that attach to the bones of leverage provide the necessary strength to move the object.

Leverage is characteristic of the movements of the upper extremities. The arm muscles are parallel to one another and extend the full length of the bones. The long parallel muscles provide strength and work together with the bones and joints to enable the person to lift an object with the arms.

MUSCLES CONCERNED WITH POSTURE

Muscles associated primarily with maintaining posture are short and featherlike in appearance because they converge obliquely at a common tendon. Muscles of the lower extremities, the trunk, the neck, and the back are concerned primarily with posture. These muscle groups work together to stabilize and support body weight when the person is standing or sitting. It is the work of these muscles that allows the individual to maintain a sitting or standing posture for a period of time.

MUSCLE REGULATION OF POSTURE AND MOVEMENT

Posture and movement can be reflections of an individual's personality and mood. For example, an individual with a dramatic personality gestures with the hands to illustrate an idea, and a person who is fatigued or depressed may slouch.

Posture and movement are also dependent on the skeleton and the shape and development of the skeletal muscles. Coordination and regulation of different muscle groups depend on muscle tone and the activity of antagonistic, synergistic, and antigravity muscles.

This section introduces the student to the muscle components necessary for movement and posture and describes how the nervous system regulates movement and how the skeletal muscles and nerves interact to achieve voluntary coordinated movement.

MUSCLE TONE. Muscle tone or tonus is the normal state of balanced muscle tension. The tension is achieved by alternate contraction and relaxation of neighboring fibers of a specific muscle group. Muscle tone enables a body part to be maintained in a functioning position without muscle fatigue. In addition, muscle tone promotes venous return to the heart, as is the case with the muscles of the legs. The continuous contraction and relaxation of the muscle fibers act as a pump to propel the venous blood toward the heart.

Muscle tone is achieved through continual use of the muscles. Activities of daily living require muscle action and help to maintain muscle tone. When a client is immobilized or experiences prolonged bed rest, his activity level and thus his muscle tone decrease. A nurse caring for an immobilized client institutes nursing interventions designed to reduce the hazards of immobility on the musculoskeletal system, as well as the other systems of the body (Chapter 31).

MUSCLE GROUPS. The antagonistic, synergistic, and antigravity muscle groups are coordinated by the nervous system and work together to maintain posture and initiate movement.

Antagonistic muscles work together to bring about movement at the joint. During movement the active mover muscle contracts while its antagonist relaxes. For example, when flexing the arm, the active mover, the biceps brachii, contracts and its antagonist, the triceps brachii, relaxes. During extension of the arm the active mover, now the triceps brachii, contracts and the new antagonist, the biceps brachii, relaxes.

Synergistic muscles contract together to accomplish the same movement. When the arm is flexed, the strength of the contraction of the biceps brachii is increased by contraction of the synergistic muscle, the brachialis. Thus with synergistic muscle activity there are now two active movers, the biceps brachii and the brachialis, that contract while the antagonistic muscle, the triceps brachii, relaxes.

Antigravity muscles are specifically involved with the stabilization of joints. These muscles continuously oppose the effect of gravity on the body and permit the person to maintain an upright or sitting posture (Strand, 1978). In an adult the antigravity muscles are the extensors of the leg, the gluteus maximus, the quadriceps femoris, the soleus muscles, and the muscles of the back.

Skeletal muscles support posture and carry out voluntary movement. The muscles are attached to the skeleton by tendons, which provide strength and permit motion. The movement of the extremities is voluntary and requires coordination from the nervous system.

Nervous System

Movement and posture are regulated by the nervous system. The major voluntary motor area, located in the cerebral cortex, is the precentral gyrus or motor strip. A majority of motor fibers descend from the motor strip and cross at the level of the medulla. Thus the motor fibers from the right motor strip initiate voluntary movement for the left side of the body, and the opposite is true for movement on the right side of the body.

When voluntary movement is initiated, impulses descend from the motor stip to the spinal cord by way of the corticospinal tract. An impulse leaves the spinal cord through efferent motor nerves and travels through nerves to the muscles, where movement occurs. The impulse is propelled by synapses, which keep the impulse traveling in one direction. In addition, a majority of motor fibers are encased in a myelin sheath and are called myelinated fibers. Along the myelinated fibers is a series of indentations known as Ranvier's nodes. These nodes increase impulse transmission because the impulse is able to jump from node to node.

The transmission of the impulse from the nervous system to the musculoskeletal system is an electrochemical event and requires a neurotransmitter. Basically, neurotransmitters are chemicals that transfer the electric impulse from the nerve across the myoneural junction to the muscle. When the neurotransmitter reaches the muscle, it stimulates the muscle and movement occurs. The body contains several neurotransmitters; a common one is acetylcholine.

Movement can be impaired by disorders that alter neurotransmitter production, transfer across the synaptic cleft, or activation of muscle activity. One illness, myasthenia gravis, is believed to result from a deficit in the neurotransmitter acetylcholine at the myoneural junction.

The maintenance of posture is also regulated by the nervous system and requires support from the musculoskeletal system. Posture, usually considered in terms of sitting or standing, is the position of the body in relation to the surrounding space. It is maintained by coordination of the muscles that move the limbs, by proprioception, and by a sense of balance.

PROPRIOCEPTION

Proprioception is achieved through stimuli originating from within the body regarding spatial position and muscular activity. Proprioception in the body is monitored by proprioceptors, which are any nerve endings located in muscles, tendons, and joints.

As a person carries out activities of daily living, proprioceptors are continuously monitoring muscle activity and body position. For example, the proprioceptors on the soles of the foot contribute to correct posture while standing or walking. In standing there is continuous pressure on the bottom of the feet. The proprioceptors monitor the pressure, communicating this information through the nervous system to the antigravity muscles. The standing person remains upright until deciding to change position. As a person walks, the proprioceptors on the bottom of the feet monitor pressure changes. Thus when the bottom of the moving foot comes in contact with the walking surface, the individual automatically moves the stationary foot forward. The proprioceptors allow people to walk without having to watch their feet.

BALANCE

When standing, running, lifting, or performing activities of daily living, a person must have adequate balance or he will fall. Balance is assisted through control by the nervous system, specifically by the cerebellum and the inner ear. The cerebellum is the portion of the brain located in the posterior cranial fossa behind the brainstem. The major function of the cerebellum is to coordinate all voluntary movement, particularly highly skilled movements such as those required in golf and skiing (Strand, 1978). In addition, the cerebellum assists in balance, such as permitting a person to stand on one foot with eyes closed (Romberg test of cerebellar function; see Chapter 29).

Within the inner ear are the semicircular canals, three fluid-filled structures that assist in maintaining balance. The fluid within the canals has a certain inertia, and when the head is suddenly rotated in one direction, the fluid within the canal in the same direction remains stationary for a moment while the canal turns with the head. This allows a person to change position suddenly without losing balance.

Impairment of Movement

Smooth, coordinated, and purposeful movement is the result of the integration of structure and function of the skeleton, skeletal muscle, and nervous system. When any part of these is damaged or destroyed, movement is impaired. The skeleton can be damaged by fractured bones or joints and torn ligaments, tendons, and cartilage. Disease affecting the composition of bone, such as osteoporosis or neoplasms, restricts movement. Muscle abnormalities, such as muscular dystrophy, decrease muscle strength and mobility. Diseases of the nervous system, such as multiple sclerosis, or damage to the nervous system, such as a spinal cord injury, restricts voluntary motor activity. Each of these diseases or injuries that reduce movement increases the risk for actual or potential impairment of body alignment or joint mobility. Assessment of these impairments is presented in a later section.

Overview of Body Mechanics

Body mechanics is the coordinated efforts of the musculoskeletal and the nervous systems to maintain proper balance, posture, and body alignment during lifting, bending, moving, and performing activities of daily living. Proper body mechanics reduces the risk of injury to the musculoskeletal system. Body mechanics also facilitates body movement, so that a person is able to carry out a physical activity without using excessive muscle energy.

It is crucial for nursing students early in their education to be aware of correct body mechanics. Clinical nursing requires a strong theoretical knowledge base, coordinated psychomotor skills, and physical endurance. Nurses assist clients to turn, walk, and increase their activity. On occasion a nurse is faced with a client who is physically unable to move and must be positioned and transferred by the nurse. The best self-protection for the nurse while administering care is to consistently and habitually incorporate the principles of sound body mechanics into practice, thus reducing the risk of musculoskeletal injury.

Body mechanics is concerned with three areas: body alignment, body balance, and coordinated body movement.

Body Alignment

Body alignment refers to the condition of the joints, tendons, ligaments, and muscles in various body positions. Whether a person is standing, sitting, or lying down, there are correct and incorrect body alignments. Correct body alignment reduces strain on the joints, tendons, ligaments, and muscles and is associated with adequate muscle tone.

The assessment section in this chapter describes how to assess body alignment in a client who is standing, sitting, or lying down and how to identify abnormalities. The intervention section of the chapter details nursing procedures commonly used for maintaining or restoring correct body alignment.

Body Balance

Proper body alignment contributes to body balance. When the body is improperly balanced, the center of gravity is displaced, increasing the force of gravity and the possibility of falling. Body balance is achieved when there is a wide base of support, the center of gravity is within the base of support, and a vertical line falls from the center of gravity through the base of support (see Fig. 30-5).

Body balance is also enhanced by posture. The better the posture, the greater the balance. Clinical nursing activities require the nurse to maintain proper body alignment, which can be improved by two simple techniques. First, the base of support can easily be widened by separating the feet at a comfortable distance. Spreading the feet too far, however, can lead to discomfort and instability. Second, balance is increased by bringing the center of gravity closer to the base of support by bending the knees and flexing the hips until the person is squatting and still maintaining proper back alignment.

Coordinated Body Movement

The nurse uses a variety of muscle groups for each nursing activity, such as walking during nursing rounds, administering medications, lifting and transferring clients, and moving objects. The physical forces of weight and friction can influence body movement. Correctly used, these forces increase the nurse's efficiency. Incorrect use can impair the nurse's ability to lift, transfer, and position clients.

WEIGHT

Weight is the force exerted on a body by gravity. Gravity is the heaviness of an object, resulting from the universal effect of the attraction between any body of matter and a planetary body. The force of the attraction depends on the relative masses of the bodies and the distance between them. In addition, each object has a center of gravity. When an object is lifted, the lifter must be able to overcome the object's weight and have knowledge of the location of its center of gravity. In symmetrical objects the center of gravity is located at the exact center of the object. For example, the center of gravity of a perfect cube is its geometrical center. Since people are not geometrically perfect, their centers of gravity are usually at 55% to 57% of standing height and are located in the midline.

The force of weight is always directed downward, which is why an unbalanced object falls. This fact has great clinical significance for the nurse. Clients who are unsteady fall because, as their centers of gravity become unbalanced, the downward force of their weight eventually causes them to fall over, fall out of bed, or fall out of the chair. Therefore the nurse needs to design nursing interventions that protect such clients from falling and ensure their safety (Chapter 34).

FRICTION

Friction is a force that occurs in a direction to oppose movement. As the nurse turns, transfers, or moves a client up in bed, friction must be overcome. A nurse can reduce friction by following some basic principles.

First, the greater the surface area of the object to be moved, the greater the friction. Nurses are able to use this principle when moving a client up in bed. If the client is unable to assist in the procedure, the client's arms should be placed across the chest. This decreases the client's surface area and reduces friction.

Second, a passive or immobilized client produces greater friction to movement. Thus, whenever possible, the nurse should use some of the client's strength and mobility when lifting, transferring, or moving the client up in bed. This can be effected by (1) a preliminary explanation of the procedure and the client's responsibility and (2) establishing when the client is to become active. For example, in moving a client up in bed, the total procedure is explained and the client is instructed to push with the feet on the count of three. Thus the client knows what is being done, what to do, and when. As a result, the client and nurse work together, and because the client is active, friction is reduced.

Third, friction can be reduced by pulling rather than pushing a client. Pulling tends to have an upward component and decreases the pressure between the client and the bed or the chair. The use of a plastic liner under a pull sheet reduces friction because the object is more easily moved along a smooth surface.

Principles of Body Mechanics

Proper body mechanics is as important to the nurse and client as proper nutrition; it has the potential for affecting the nurse's and the client's level of wellness. Correct body mechanics is necessary to health promotion, as well as the prevention of disability.

Health promotion activities that involve physical exercise incorporate basic principles of body mechanics. Proper exercising increases the work and strength of certain muscle groups. The runner gradually reconditions skeletal muscles, the muscles of respiration, and the cardiac muscles. The weight lifter increases muscle mass while using proper body mechanics to lift the weight. The ballet dancer uses correct muscle groups to perform such movements as jumps and spins safely.

Incorporating principles of body mechanics also prevents disability. Through lecture, discussion, and demonstration, the nurse teaches colleagues as well as clients' families how to lift, transfer, or position clients properly. A nurse who is teaching a client's family how to transfer the client from bed to chair can increase and reinforce the family's knowledge by consistently demonstrating proper body mechanics.

Whether the nurse is moving an immobilized client, assisting a client from the bed to the chair, or teaching a client how to carry out activities of daily living efficiently, knowledge of basic principles of body mechanics is crucial. The nurse also incorporates knowledge of physiological and pathological influences on body alignment and mobility. The boxed material on p. 706 lists principles that are useful for a variety of nursing settings and all age groups of clients.

Physiological Influences on Body Alignment and Mobility

Throughout the life cycle the body's appearance and functioning undergo normal change. The greatest impact of the physiological changes on the musculoskeletal system is observed in childhood and old age.

Infant

The newborn infant's spine is flexed and lacks the anteroposterior curves of the adult. The first spinal curve occurs when the infant extends the neck from

Principles of Body Mechanics

- The wider the base of support and the lower the center of gravity, the greater the stability of the nurse.
- The equilibrium of an object is maintained as long as the line of gravity passes through its base of support.
- When the line of gravity shifts outside the base of support, the amount of energy required to maintain equilibrium is increased.
- Equilibrium is maintained with least effort when the base of support is broadened in the direction in which movement occurs.
- Stooping with hips and knees flexed and the trunk in good alignment distributes the work load among the largest and strongest muscle groups and helps to prevent back strain.
- The stronger the muscle group, the greater the work it can perform safely.
- The use of a larger number of muscle groups for an activity distributes the work load.
- Facing the direction of movement prevents abnormal twisting of spine.
- Pushing, pulling, or sliding an object on a surface requires less force than lifting an object, since lifting involves moving the weight of the object against the pull of gravity.
- Moving an object by rolling, turning, or pivoting requires less effort than lifting the object, since momentum and leverage are used to advantage.
- The use of a lever when lifting an object reduces the amount of weight lifted.
- The less the friction between the object moved and surface on which it is moved, the less the force required to move it.
- Moving an object on a level surface requires less effort than moving the same object on an inclined surface, because the pull of gravity is less on a level surface.
- Working with materials which rest on a surface at a good working level requires less effort than lifting them above the working surface.
- Contraction of stabilizing muscles preparatory to activity helps to prevent ligaments and joints from strain and injury. *INTERNAL GIRDLE*
- Dividing balanced activity between arms and legs protects the back from strain.
- Variety of position and activity helps to maintain good muscle tone and prevent fatigue.
- Alternating periods of rest and activity help to prevent fatigue.

From Winters, M.: Protective body mechanics in daily life and nursing, Philadelphia, 1952, W.B. Saunders Co.

PULL IN ABDOMEN + TUCK IN HIPS BEFORE YOU LIFT SOMEONE PROTECTS VISCERA, INTERNAL GIRDLE

the prone position. As growth and stability increase, the infant is able to sit upright and stand, and, as a result, the thoracic spine straightens and the normal curve of the lumbar spine begins to appear (Daniels and Worthingham, 1977).

The infant's musculoskeletal system is flexible. On observation, the infant's extremities are flexed and the joints have complete range of joint motion. As the newborn matures, the musculoskeletal system becomes stronger and the infant is able to resist movement and reach out and grasp objects (Chapter 24). The strengthening of the muscles enables the infant to pull from a sitting to a standing position. Because this event frequently occurs before the child is able to figure out how to sit down again, the baby becomes unhappy and cries.

As the baby grows, musculoskeletal development permits the child to support his weight to stand alone and to walk. The baby's posture is awkward because the head and upper trunk are carried forward. Since the body weight is not evenly distributed along a line of gravity, the child is off balance and falls easily.

Toddler

After the first year of life the infant enters the toddler stage (see Chapter 24). Anyone who observes children who have just begun to walk can easily understand why they are called toddlers: they toddle along. The toddler's posture—slightly swaybacked with a protruding abdomen—is awkward. As the child walks, the legs and feet are usually far apart and the feet are slightly everted. Toward the end of the toddler stage the posture appears less awkward, the curves in the cervical and lumbar vertebrae are accentuated, and the foot eversion disappears (Daniels and Worthingham, 1977).

Child

By the third year of life the child's body is slimmer, taller, and better balanced. The abdominal protrusion is decreased, the feet are not as far apart, and the arms and legs have increased in length. In addition, the child appears more coordinated so that the patterns of walking, running, or climbing stairs are similar to the adult's.

From the third year through beginning adolescence the musculoskeletal system continues to develop. The long bones in the arms and legs grow in length. Muscles, ligaments, and tendons become stronger, resulting in improved posture and increased muscle strength. Greater coordination enables the child to perform tasks that require fine motor skills, such as writing, drawing, building, or other creative activities (see Chapter 25).

Adolescent

The adolescent experiences major changes in body shape and functioning (see Chapter 25). This developmental stage is usually initiated by a tremendous growth spurt. Growth is frequently uneven; the long bones may grow very quickly but the growth of the appropriate muscle groups may be slower, or there can be rapid muscle development without appropriate long bone growth. As a result the adolescent may be awkward and appear uncoordinated.

Adolescent girls usually grow and develop earlier than boys. The girl's shape develops curves. The hips widen; fat is deposited in the upper arms, thighs, and buttocks; and the breasts begin to grow.

The boy's changes in shape are usually the result of long bone growth and increased muscle mass. Legs become longer and hips narrower. Muscular development increases in the chest, arms, shoulders, and upper legs.

Postural problems, common during this developmental stage, are frequently caused by the emotional stress of growing up rather than by an abnormality of the musculoskeletal system. For example, teenage girls frequently walk with stooped shoulders to hide the discrepancy between their height and the height of teenage boys. Teenagers' discomfort with their new body shapes is probably another cause of poor posture.

Adult

The adult who has correct posture and body alignment feels good, looks good, and generally appears self-confident. In addition, the healthy adult has the necessary musculoskeletal development and coordination to carry out activities of daily living and other desired tasks (see Chapter 26).

Normal changes in posture and body alignment in adulthood occur mainly in pregnant women. These changes result from the body's adaptive response to weight gain and the growing fetus. The center of gravity shifts toward the anterior (Fig. 30-4). The pregnant woman leans back and is slightly swaybacked. She may complain of backaches, particularly in the later stages of pregnancy.

Elderly Adult

The aging process results in changes in the musculoskeletal system (see Chapter 27). Degenerative joint changes may decrease range of joint motion. Skeletal muscle mass and strength may be reduced. Changes in the structure of the bone matrix may result in brittle, fragile bones (Hudson, 1983). Elderly adults, especially women, commonly have a greater flexion of the cervical vertebrae.

The elderly person walks more slowly and appears less coordinated. The older person may also take smaller steps, keeping the feet closer together, which decreases the base of support. Thus body balance is unstable, and the individual is at greater risk for falls and injuries.

■ ■ ■ ■ ■

Because a nurse may deliver care to a variety of clients in different age groups, the nurse should in-

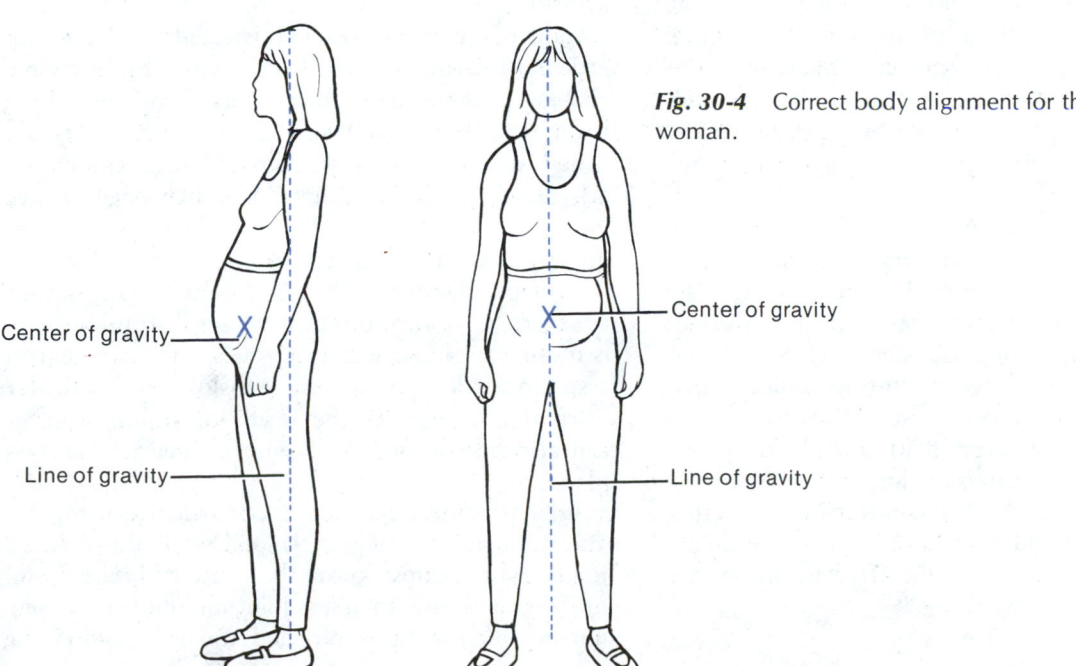

Center of gravity

Line of gravity

Center of gravity

Line of gravity

Fig. 30-4 Correct body alignment for the pregnant woman.

corporate the principles of growth and development into nursing care plans. For example, when caring for an elderly person, the nurse should request help from another person when transferring the client from bed to chair because the elderly individual moves more slowly and loses his balance more easily. However, the nurse may not need help to transfer a younger adult of the same height and weight as the elderly client because the younger adult has greater balance and coordination.

Pathological Influences on Body Alignment and Mobility

A variety of pathological conditions affect body alignment and joint mobility. Although a complete description of each condition is beyond the scope of the chapter, the student needs knowledge about musculoskeletal disorders. Through tables and summaries this section provides baseline information about these pathological influences, which are broken down into six categories: postural abnormalities, pathophysiological mechanisms affecting bone formation, altered joint mobility, impaired muscle development, damage to the central nervous system, and direct trauma to the musculoskeletal system. A subsequent section on intervention describes in detail the nursing procedures used to maintain or restore body alignment and joint mobility.

Postural Abnormalities

Congenital or acquired postural abnormalities affect the efficiency of the musculoskeletal system, as well as body alignment, balance, and appearance. During physical assessment the nurse observes body alignment and range of joint motion (see Chapter 29). Postural abnormalities impair either alignment or mobility or both.

The nurse requires some knowledge about the characteristics, causes, and treatment of the common postural abnormalities (Table 30-1). The nurse uses this baseline knowledge first to improve the client's body alignment during lifting, transfer, and positioning. Second, because some postural abnormalities affect range of joint motion, the nurse maintains range of joint motion in the affected joint and utilizes the client's range in the remaining joints. Last, the nurse is able to design nursing interventions to strengthen affected muscle and joint groups, improve the client's posture, and adequately use the affected and the unaffected muscle groups.

Pathophysiological Mechanisms Affecting Bone Formation

The skeleton provides the structural support for the body, protects soft tissues and organs, and is the anchoring site for the origin and insertion of muscles. In addition, the bone affects calcium metabolism and blood formation in the body. The functional activities of bone cells include modeling, remodeling, and repairing. Modeling involves the growth processes that allow the bones of the newborn to develop into the large, identically shaped bones of the adult. Modeling is dependent on dietary and physiological factors. Remodeling occurs in both the growing and the full-grown skeleton and involves coupling of the constantly occurring processes of bone resorption and formation. Repair is the cellular process that occurs in response to a fracture (Groër and Shekleton, 1983).

Nurses care for clients who have actual or potential alterations in the modeling, remodeling, or repair of bone. Table 30-2 describes disorders that are the result of abnormal bone modeling or remodeling. A later section on direct trauma to the musculoskeletal system describes the repair of bones.

Altered Joint Mobility

Joint mobility can be altered by inflammation, degeneration, or articular disruption. Arthritis is an inflammation of the joints characterized by swelling and pain. It can result from a direct inflammatory reaction in the joint tissue such as gouty arthritis, an infectious process such as septic arthritis, or an immune-mediated inflammatory process such as rheumatoid arthritis.

Joint degeneration is demonstrated by changes in articular cartilage combined with hypertrophic changes at the articular bone ends (Groër and Shekleton, 1983). Synovial and cartilaginous joints are equally affected, and degenerative changes commonly affect weight-bearing joints. Although degenerative joint disease is not caused by inflammation, it is frequently termed osteoarthritis.

Articular disruption may be as mild as a sprain or as severe as dislocation. In articular disruption there is trauma to the articular capsules, such as a tear in a sprain, or a separation in a dislocation. Articular disruption is usually the result of trauma, but it can also be congenital, as with congenital hip dysplasia.

Inflammation, degeneration, or articular disruption alters the degree of joint mobility of the affected joints. Nurses must know the cause of limited joint mobility and how to assess joint mobility and design nursing interventions directed toward maintaining

TABLE 30-1

Postural Abnormalities

Abnormality	Description	Cause	Treatment
Torticollis	The head is inclined to the affected side, in which the sternocleidomastoid muscle is contracted	Congenital or acquired	Surgery, heat, support, or immobilization depending on the cause and severity
Lordosis	Exaggeration of the anterior convex curve of the lumbar spine	Congenital; temporary as with pregnancy	Based on cause; frequently treated with spine-stretching exercises
Kyphosis	Increased convexity in the curvature of the thoracic spine	Congenital; rickets; tuberculosis of the spine	Based on cause and severity; includes spine-stretching exercises, sleeping without pillows, using a bed board, bracing, and spinal fusion
Kypholordosis	Combination of kyphosis and lordosis		Based on cause; similar to methods used in kyphosis or lordosis
Scoliosis	Lateral curvature of the spine, unequal heights of hips and shoulders	Congenital; poliomyelitis; spastic paralysis; unequal leg length	Based on cause and severity; immobilization and surgery
Kyphoscoliosis	Abnormal anterorposterior and lateral curvature of the spine	Congenital; poliomyelitis; cor pulmonale	Based on cause and severity; immobilization and surgery
Congenital hip dysplasia	Hip instability with limited abduction of the hips and, occasionally, adduction contractures; head of the femur does not articulate with the acetabulum because of abnormal shallowness of the acetabulum	Congenital; more common with breech deliveries	Maintaining continuous abduction of the thigh so that the head of the femur presses into the center of the acetabulum; abduction splints, casting, or surgery
Knock-knee (genu valgum)	Legs curved inward so that the knees knock together as the person walks	Congenital; rickets	Knee braces and surgery if not corrected by growth
Bowlegs (genu varum)	One or both legs bent outward at the knee; normal until 2-3 years of age	Congenital; rickets	Slowing the rate of curving if not corrected by growth; in the case of rickets, vitamin D, calcium, and phosphorus intake increased to normal ranges
Clubfoot	95%: medial deviation and plantar flexion of the foot (equinovarus); the remaining 5%: lateral deviation and dorsiflexion (calcaneovalgus)	Congenital	Based on the degree and rigidity of the deformity; casts, splints such as the Denis Browne splint, and surgery
Foot-drop	Characterized by dorsiflexion, inability to invert the foot because of peroneal nerve damage	Congenital; trauma; improper position of the immobilized client	Cannot be corrected
Pigeon-toes	Internal rotation of the forefoot or the entire foot, common in infants	Congenital; habitual	Corrected by growth or by wearing reversed shoes

TABLE 30-2

Pathophysiological Mechanisms Affecting Bone Formation

Disorder	Cause and Characteristics
Marfan's syndrome	This congenital, autosomal dominant trait is characterized by excessive longitudinal growth in the cartilage of all epiphyseal plates. The affected person is tall and thin with excessively long extremities, muscular underdevelopment, joint hypermobility, and a risk of cardiovascular disease.
Achondroplastic dwarfism	Fifty percent of individuals with this congenital, autosomal dominant trait die in utero or during the first year of life. Growth of the cartilage in the epiphyses of the long bones and skull is altered, resulting in premature ossification and decreased skeletal development. Dwarfism is characterized by bulging forehead, short and thick extremities, and a near-normal trunk.
Osteogenesis imperfecta	This inherited, autosomal dominant trait results in defective development of the connective tissue. Bones are brittle or fragile and are fractured with the slightest trauma.
Osteopetrosis	This inherited, autosomal recessive trait results in a failure or inhibition of resorption of calcified cartilage and fibrous bone. Bone density is increased and multiple fractures are common.
Osteoporosis	In osteoporosis an absolute loss of bone volume is caused by an alteration in the normal ratio of bone formation to resorption. This mechanism can result from (1) hormonal changes such as menopause, (2) disease or immobilization, (3) steroids, or (4) aging. Pathological fractures develop easily.
Osteomalacia	Osteomalacia is characterized by a loss of calcification of the matrix with decreased bone density. It is caused by a decreased amount of calcium and phosphorus available in the blood for bone mineralization. Bones become weak and soft, eventually resulting in fractures.
Rickets	Rickets is a name for the condition of osteomalacia that occurs in children, usually as a result of a deficiency in vitamin D, calcium, and phosphorus. The disease is characterized by abnormal bone formation such as bowleg.
Paget's disease (osteitis deformans)	This disease of unknown etiology affects middle-aged and elderly persons and is characterized by excessive bone destruction and unorganized repair, which cause bone pain, bowing of lower limbs, and pathological fractures.

Data from Groër, M.W., and Shekleton, M.E.: Basic pathophysiology: a conceptual approach, ed. 2, St. Louis, 1983, The C.V. Mosby Co.

and improving a client's range of joint motion. Chapter 29 describes the assessment of range of joint motion. The section on intervention in this chapter provides the student with a step-by-step procedure for maintaining range of joint motion.

Impaired Muscle Development

Inadequate development of the skeletal muscles affects body alignment, balance, and mobility. The muscular dystrophies are the most common developmental impairments of skeletal muscles (Table 30-3). Muscular dystrophies are a group of genetically transmitted diseases characterized by progressive pathological changes in the skeletal muscles, resulting in muscle wasting and weakness (Groër and Shekleton, 1983).

Damage to the Central Nervous System

Damage to any component of the central nervous system that regulates voluntary movement results in impaired body alignment and mobility. The motor strip in the cerebrum can be damaged by trauma from a head injury, ischemia from a cerebrovascular accident (stroke), or bacterial infection from meningitis. The amount of voluntary motor impairment is directly related to the amount of destruction of the motor strip. For example, in the case of a person with a right-sided cerebral hemorrhage with complete necrosis, destruction of the right motor strip and left-sided hemiplegia are consequences. However, a person with a right-sided head injury will have cerebral edema and damage (but not destruction) of the motor strip, and with extensive physical therapy, voluntary movement gradually returns to the left side.

TABLE 30-3

Muscular Dystrophies

	Inheritance	Age at Onset	Major Clinical Features	Course
Duchenne type	X-linked recessive	Early childhood	Symmetrical weakness; initially pelvifemoral; weakness shoulder girdle later and then trunk muscles; "pseudohypertrophy" of calves; reduced intelligence	Progressive; inability to walk by puberty; death by age 20
Becker type	X-linked recessive	Second decade	Milder variant of Duchenne type	"Benign"; ability to walk into adult life
Facioscapulohumeral	Autosomal dominant	Childhood to late adult life	Usually facial weakness first; scapular weakness; humeral weakness	"Benign"; course not progressive
Limb-girdle	Autosomal recessive	Variable onset first to sixth decade	Two variants: (1) pelvifemoral weakness, (2) shoulder girdle weakness	Variable progression; disability within 20 years
Distal myopathy	Autosomal dominant	Middle to late adult life	Weakness of small muscles, hands; weakness of tibialis anterior; weakness of gastrocnemius	Slow progression
Ocular myopathy	?Autosomal dominant	Variable	Group of syndromes all having weakness of extraocular muscles initially; sometimes involvement of face, neck, limbs	Rarely progressive

From Robbins, S., and Cottran, R.: Pathologic basis of disease, Philadelphia, 1979, W.B. Saunders Co.

Because voluntary motor fibers descend from the motor strip in the cerebrum down the spinal cord, trauma to the spinal cord also impairs mobility. The most comon trauma is transection of the spinal cord in which motor fibers are cut and there is a complete bilateral loss of voluntary motor control below the level of the trauma. Spinal cord trauma frequently results from diving or automobile accidents or gunshot or knife wounds to the neck and back.

Direct Trauma to the Musculoskeletal System

Direct trauma to the musculoskeletal system can result in bruises, contusions, sprains, and fractures. The more severe fractures are the focus of the discussion in this section. A fracture is a disruption of bone tissue continuity. Fractures most commonly result from direct external trauma, but they can also occur as a consequence of some deformity of the bone, as with pathological fractures of osteoporosis, Paget's disease, and osteogenesis imperfecta.

As the fracture heals, the bone undertakes the repair process. During repair the fractured bone initiates a cellular process that results in bone formation. Young children are able to form new bone more easily than adults and, as a result, have few complications after a bone fracture. Treatment includes positioning the fractured bone in proper alignment and immobilizing it to promote the normal healing process and to restore function. Immobilization results in a certain amount of muscle atrophy, loss of tone, and joint stiffness. The nurse designs a program of exercises to restore full joint mobility and muscle strength gradually to the affected area.

Any acquired or congenital condition that affects the structure of the musculoskeletal or nervous system impairs to some degree the person's body alignment or joint mobility. The impairment can be temporary or permanent. Regardless of the duration of the impairment, the nursing care plan includes interventions that maintain the present level of alignment and joint mobility, as well as interventions designed to increase the client's level of motor function.

Based on data collected during assessment, the nurse determines the client's care plan. When assessing a client's body alignment and joint mobility, the nurse also evaluates the client's ability to perform activities of daily living.

Assessment

The nursing assessment of a client's body alignment and joint mobility is usually conducted during the complete physical assessment. In this section on assessment and subsequent sections on the components of the nursing care plan, the content is divided into two categories: body alignment and joint mobility. This division is intended to help the student assess the client, diagnose problems, and plan, deliver, and evaluate nursing care. However, the student should be aware that body alignment and joint mobility are closely related.

Body Alignment

The assessment of a client's body alignment can be carried out with the client standing, sitting, or lying down. This assessment has six objectives:
1. Determining normal physiological changes in body alignment resulting from growth and development
2. Identifying deviations in body alignment caused by poor posture

3. Providing an opportunity for the client to observe his posture
4. Identifying learning needs of the client for maintaining correct body alignment
5. Identifying the presence of trauma, muscle damage, or nerve dysfunction
6. Obtaining information concerning other factors that contribute to poor alignment, such as fatigue, malnutrition, and psychological problems

The first step in assessing body alignment is to put the client at ease so he does not assume unnatural or rigid positions. When assessing body alignment of an immobilized or unconscious client, all pillows and positioning supports should be removed from the bed and the client placed in the supine position.

STANDING

The nurse should focus assessment of body alignment for the standing client on the following points:
1. The head is erect and midline.
2. When observed posteriorly, the shoulders and hips are straight and parallel.
3. When observed posteriorly, the vertebral column is straight.
4. When the client is observed laterally, the head is erect and the spinal curves are aligned in a reversed **S** pattern. The cervical vertebrae are anteriorly convex, the thoracic vertebrae are posteriorly convex, and the lumbar vertebrae are anteriorly convex.
5. When observed laterally, the abdomen is com-

Fig. 30-5 Correct body alignment when standing.

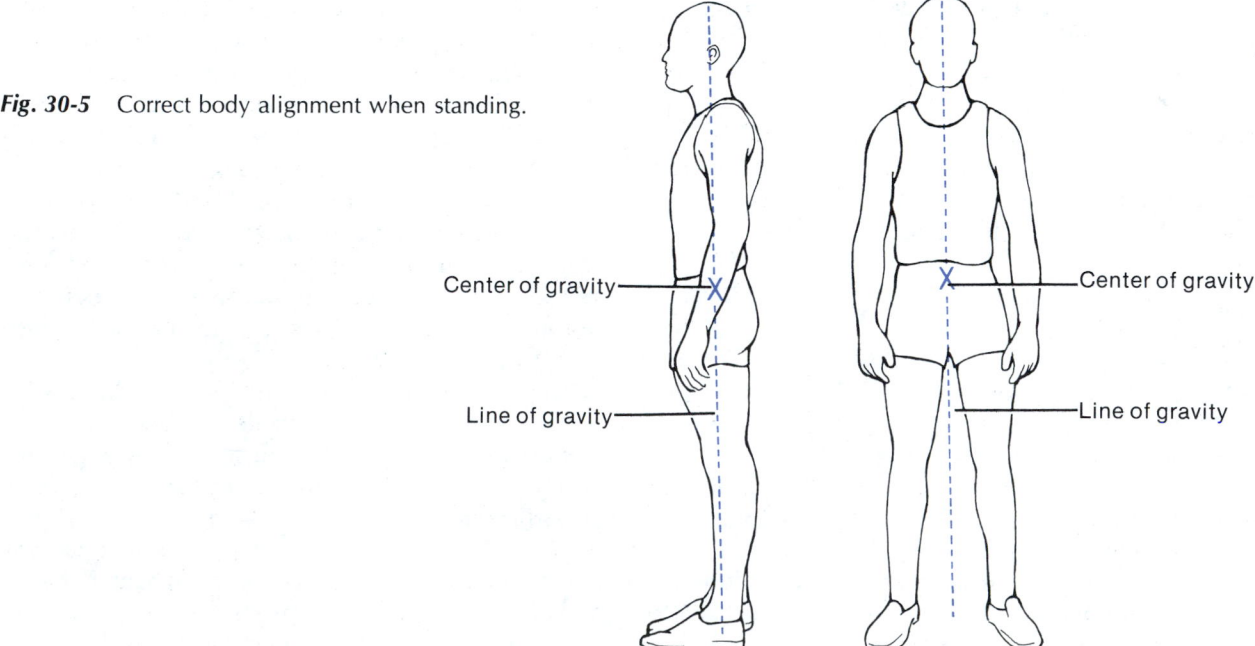

Center of gravity

Line of gravity

Center of gravity

Line of gravity

fortably tucked in and the knees and ankles are slightly flexed. The person appears comfortable and does not seem conscious of the flexion of knees or ankles.

6. The client's arms are comfortably at the sides.
7. The feet are placed slightly apart to achieve a base of support, and the toes are pointed forward.
8. When the client is viewed anteriorly, the center of gravity is in the midline, and the line of gravity is from the middle of the forehead to a midpoint between the feet. Laterally the line of gravity runs vertically from the middle of the skull to the posterior third of the foot (Fig. 30-5).

SITTING

The nurse assesses the alignment of the sitting client by the following observations:
1. The head is erect, and the neck and vertebral column are in straight alignment.
2. The body weight is evenly distributed on the buttocks and thighs.
3. The thighs are parallel and in a horizontal plane.
4. Both feet are supported on the floor. With clients of short stature, a footstool is used and the ankles are comfortably flexed.
5. A 2 to 4 cm (1- to 2-inch) space is maintained between the edge of the seat and the popliteal space on the posterior surface of the knee. This space ensures that there is no pressure on the popliteal artery or nerve to decrease circulation or impair nerve function.
6. The client's forearms are supported on the armrest, in the lap, or on a table in front of the chair (Fig. 30-6).

It is particularly important to assess alignment when sitting if the client has muscle weakness, muscle paralysis, or nerve damage. Because of these alterations, the client has diminished sensation in the affected area and is unable to perceive pressure or decreased circulation. Proper alignment while sitting reduces the risk of musculoskeletal system damage in such a client.

LYING DOWN

People who are conscious have voluntary muscle control and normal perception of pressure. As a result they usually assume the position of comfort when lying down. Because their range of motion, sensation, and circulation are within normal limits, they change positions when they perceive muscle strain and decreased circulation.

The assessment of a client's body alignment while lying down requires that the client be placed in the lateral position with all pillows and positioning supports removed from the bed (Fig. 30-7). The client's body should be supported by an adequate mattress. The vertebrae should be in straight alignment without any observable curves. This assessment provides baseline data concerning the client's body alignment.

Clients at risk of damage to the musculoskeletal system when they are lying down include clients with impaired mobility, such as those in traction or with arthritis; clients with decreased sensation, such as those with hemiparesis resulting from a stroke; clients with impaired circulation, such as those with diabetes; and clients with lack of voluntary muscle control, such as those with spinal cord injuries.

When a nursing assessment indicates that a client is at risk for damage to the musculoskeletal system while lying down, nursing interventions are directed toward maintaining proper body alignment while rotating the client. The discussion and detailed procedures for the semi-Fowler's, supine, prone, lateral, and Sims' positions are presented in the intervention section of this chapter.

Mobility

The assessment of a client's mobility enables the nurse to determine the client's coordination and bal-

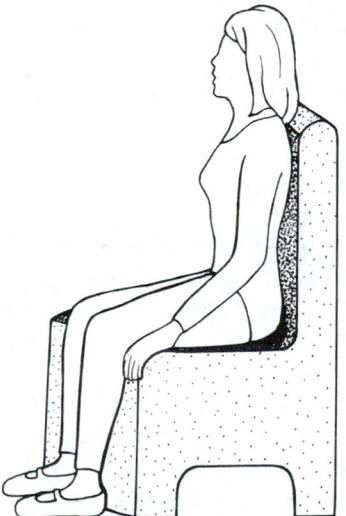

Fig. 30-6 Correct body alignment when sitting.

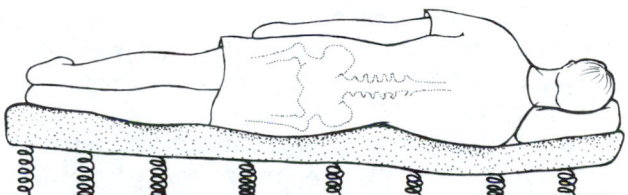

Fig. 30-7 Correct body alignment when lying down.

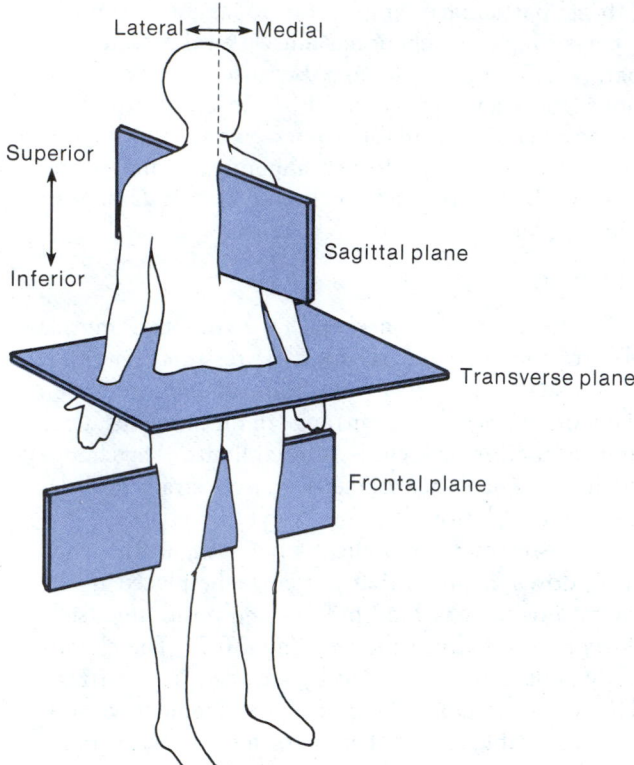

Lateral ← → Medial

Superior ↕ Inferior

Sagittal plane

Transverse plane

Frontal plane

Fig. 30-8 Planes of body.

TABLE 30-4

Joint Movements in Each of the Three Planes

Plane	Joint Movement	Examples of Joint
Sagittal	Flexion	Elbow, fingers, knee
	Extension	Elbow, fingers, knee
	Hyperextension	Head, hip
Frontal	Abduction	Leg, arm, fingers
	Adduction	Leg, arm, fingers,
	Eversion	Foot
	Inversion	Foot
Transverse	Pronation	Hand, forearm
	Supination	Hand, forearm
	Internal rotation	Knee, hip
	External rotation	Knee, hip
	Dorsiflexion	Foot
	Plantar flexion	Foot

ance while walking, the client's ability to carry out activities of daily living, and the client's ability to participate in an exercise program. The assessment of mobility has three components: range of joint motion, gait, and exercise.

RANGE OF JOINT MOTION

Range of joint motion is the maximal amount of movement possible at a joint in one of the three planes of the body: sagittal, frontal, and transverse (Fig. 30-8). The *sagittal plane* is a line that passes through the body from front to back, dividing the body into a left and a right side. The *frontal plane* passes through the body from side to side and divides the body into front and back. The *transverse plane* is a horizontal line that divides the body into upper and lower portions (Bilger and Greene, 1973).

Chapter 29 describes the terminology for normal range of joint motion positions (see Table 29-15), details the normal range of joint motion (see Table 29-16), and discusses the basis for assessment of range of joint motion.

Joint mobility in each of the planes is limited in direction by ligaments, muscles, and the construction of the joint. However, there are joint movements that are specific to each plane (Table 30-4).

The nurse, assessing range of joint motion, collects data to answer these questions: Is any stiffness or instability palpated in the joint during movement? Does any joint appear swollen or inflamed? Does any joint feel warm to the touch? Does the client experience pain on movement? Is there any limitation of movement; if so, how much? Does the muscle mass surrounding each joint appear to be within a normal range? Is joint movement equal on both sides of the body?

Clients whose joint mobility is restricted because of illness, disability, or trauma require exercise of their joints to reduce the hazards of immobility. These exercises, performed by the nurse, are called passive range of joint motion exercises. The nurse takes each affected joint through its complete range of joint motion. Since passive exercises are specific nursing interventions, they are detailed and illustrated in the intervention section of this chapter.

GAIT

Gait is the second area to evaluate in the assessment of a client's mobility. Gait is the manner or style of walking, including rhythm, cadence, and speed. Assessing a client's gait allows the nurse to draw conclusions about the client's balance, posture, and ability to walk without assistance.

Initially the nurse observes the overall appearance of the walking client. Normally, the adult posture is well aligned; that is, the head is erect and the vertebrae are straight. Knees and feet point forward, and arms are at the sides with the elbows flexed. The arms swing freely in alternation with leg swings.

TABLE 30-5

Physiological Effects of Exercise on Major Body Systems

System	Effects
Cardiovascular	Increased cardiac output from a resting value of 5 liters/minute to a maximum of 35 liters/minute in trained athlete*; strengthening of the cardiac muscle; increased heart rate; increased venous return; dilation of skeletal muscle arterioles (localized hyperemia)
Respiratory	Increased respiratory rate; increased depth of respiration; increased alveolar ventilation reaching as high as 120 liters/minute†
Metabolic	Increased use of circulatory glucose and fatty acids; increased breakdown of muscle and liver glycogen stores into glucose; increased triglyceride breakdown; increased use of fatty acids for body fuel; increased metabolic rate; increased production of body heat
Musculoskeletal	Increased muscle tone; increased muscle size; increased strength; maintenance of joint mobility

*Data from Vander, R.J., Sherman, J.H., and Luccano, D.S.: Human physiology: the mechanisms of body function, New York, 1979, McGraw-Hill Book Co.
†Data fom Guyton, A.C.: Function of the human body, ed. 4, Philadelphia, 1974, W.B. Saunders Co.

The actual activity of walking takes place in a four-phase sequence: heel strike, stance, push-off, and swing (Daniels and Worthingham, 1977). During *heel strike* the foot is approximately at a right angle to the leg. The knee is extended but not locked, in readiness for slight flexion as the body weight is shifted forward into the stance phase. During *stance* the trunk is maintained in a vertical position with the head and neck properly aligned. At *push-off* there is plantar flexion of the foot and hyperextension of the metatarsophalangeal joints of the toes. During *swing* the foot easily clears the floor with good alignment. The rhythm of movement is unchanged and remains coordinated.

EXERCISE

Exercise is the performance of any physical activity for the purpose of conditioning the body, improving health, or maintaining fitness or as a means of therapy for correcting a deformity or restoring the overall body to a maximal state of health. When a person exercises, physiological changes occur in body systems (Table 30-5).

CARDIOVASCULAR SYSTEM. To sustain the increased skeletal muscle activity during exercise, the blood supply delivered to the muscles must be increased, which is achieved by an increased cardiac output. Initially the heart rate increases during exercise. The contractile force of the cardiac muscle of the left ventricle increases, as does the volume of blood ejected (stroke volume). Increases in heart rate and stroke volume increase the cardiac output.

In addition to the increased cardiac output, the dilation of the arterioles within the skeletal muscles increases delivery of blood and oxygen to the muscle tissue. The person's body surface becomes warm and red as the result of the localized hyperemia from arteriolar dilation.

RESPIRATORY SYSTEM. The increased physiological activity during exercise requires an increased supply of oxygen (O_2) for delivery to body tissues. In order to have an increased amount of O_2 available for delivery, the person must increase the amount of O_2 inhaled. First, the body has an ability to increase the depth of respiration, which results in an increased tidal volume. Tidal volume is the amount of air inhaled and exhaled. Increased tidal volume results in more O_2 inhaled. Second, the respiratory rate quickens during exercise. Third, the increased tidal volumes and respiratory rate cause increased alveolar ventilation. The measurement of alveolar ventilation is determined by multiplying the respiratory rate by the tidal volume. Thus, increasing both rate and tidal volume increases the alveolar ventilation. Last, the increased respiratory rate increases the excretion of carbon dioxide (CO_2). During exercise the body's metabolic activity increases, and CO_2 is formed as a waste product. The increased respiratory rate allows the person to "blow off" excess CO_2, which helps to maintain the body's acid-base balance.

METABOLIC SYSTEM. Exercise requires the body to mobilize fuel to provide the energy required for muscle contraction. Three major fuels are used by exercising muscle: circulatory glucose, circulatory fatty acids, and stored glycogen. To make these three fuels available for use, the overall metabolic activity of the body increases, producing more body heat and waste products such as the CO_2 previously mentioned.

MUSCULOSKELETAL SYSTEM. Exercise affects the functioning and strength of the musculoskeletal system. During exercise the muscle tone, size, and strength increase. As a result the person is able to exercise longer with each strengthening of the muscles. Joint mobility is also maintained because the exercise itself requires movement of body parts.

The overall effect of exercise on physiological functioning is improvement. All systems become stronger and function more efficiently. In nursing, certain interventions are directed toward exercise. However, nurses frequently care for clients whose mobility is somewhat or completely restricted and, as a result, develop nursing therapies designed to reduce the hazards of immobility (see Chapter 31).

Activity Tolerance

The nurse's assessment of the client's energy level includes the physiological effects of exercise and activity tolerance. Activity tolerance is the kind and amount of exercise or work that a person is able to perform. The assessment of activity tolerance is necessary when planning any activity such as walking, range of joint motion, or activities of daily living for clients with acute or chronic illness. In addition, knowledge of the client's activity tolerance is needed to plan other nursing therapies inside or outside the home. For example, when a client with chronic pulmonary disease fatigues easily, the nursing care is designed to incorporate frequent rest periods so that routine hygiene care does not leave the individual exhausted for the remainder of the day.

Activity tolerance assessment includes data from the client's physiological, emotional, and developmental domains (see boxed material). This assessment provides the nurse with baseline data about the client's activity patterns and activity tolerance (Gordon, 1976). In addition, this assessment is applicable in all clinical settings and is quickly completed.

The client who experiences changes in physiological function on exercise, such as dyspnea or chest pain, will not tolerate activity as well as the client who remains free of dyspnea or chest pain. Likewise, the weak or debilitated client is unable to sustain activity over a period of time because the greater the energy needed to complete the activity, the faster muscle fatigue and generalized weakness are experienced.

People who are depressed, worried, or anxious are frequently unable to tolerate exercise. Depressed clients are usually not motivated to participate in activity. Clients who are worried or anxious fatigue easily because they expend a great deal of energy in worry and anxiety. Thus they may experience physical and emotional exhaustion.

Developmental changes also affect activity tolerance. As the infant grows and enters the toddler stage, the activity level increases and the need for sleep declines. The child entering nursery school, preschool, or the primary grades expends mental energy in learning and may require more rest after school before being able to play strenuously. The adolescent going through puberty may require more rest because much of the body's energy resources is expended for the growth spurt and hormone changes.

The pregnant woman has fluctuations in her energy tolerance. During the first trimester she may experience increased fatigue. Hormonal changes and fetal development utilize body energy, and the woman may be unable or unmotivated to carry out physical activities. The second trimester of a normal pregnancy usually results in a return of activity tolerance to the prepregnancy state. In fact some women actually note that their activity tolerance is greater during this period. During the last trimester fetal development con-

---

Assessment of Activity Tolerance

PHYSIOLOGICAL

- Frequency of illness or surgery during past 12 months
- Types of illnesses or surgery during past 12 months
- Cardiopulmonary status
- Musculoskeletal status
- Sleep patterns
- Presence of pain, pain control
- Vital signs, range
- Exercise activity and pattern
- Abnormality in laboratory studies, such as decreased arterial oxygen concentration (PaO_2), decreased hemoglobin

EMOTIONAL

- Mood
- Motivation
- Chemical addictions, such as drugs, alcohol, nicotine
- Self-image

DEVELOPMENTAL

- Age
- Sex
- Pregnancy
- Change in muscle mass resulting from developmental changes
- Changes in skeletal system because of developmental changes

sumes a great deal of the mother's energy. In addition, because of the size and location of the fetus, the pregnant woman's ability to take a deep breath is decreased and a reduced amount of O_2 is available for physical activities.

As the person grows older, the body changes, the muscle mass is reduced, the posture changes, and the composition of the bones is altered. As a result, activity tolerance changes. The individual may still exercise but instead of running 2 miles a day, for example, he now rides a bike for 1 mile every other day.

Mobility and alignment are intertwined; the person with poor body alignment may experience reduced mobility. The nurse, identifying nursing diagnoses that reflect actual or potential changes in the client's body alignment or mobility, is able to design nursing strategies that reduce or prevent hazards resulting from poor body alignment or limited joint mobility.

Nursing Diagnosis

Nursing diagnoses in this chapter are divided into two sections: diagnoses commonly associated with altered body alignment and those associated with altered joint mobility. This section and the subsequent sections on planning, implementing, and evaluating follow this format to help the student plan, deliver, and evaluate appropriate nursing care. However, it is important that the student realize that these nursing diagnoses—as well as those representing other dimensions of the client—are closely related. In addition, the diagnoses described are only a representative

---

TABLE 30-6

Examples of Nursing Diagnoses Related to Altered Body Alignment

Nursing Diagnosis	Etiology	Assessment Findings
Potential for poor standing alignment related to pregnancy	Center of gravity moved anteriorly because of increased size of fetus (see Fig. 30-4)	Slightly backward tilt; increased anterior concavity of lumbar vertebrae; frequent complaints of low back pain; inability to wear high-heeled shoes without experiencing back pain
Abnormal sitting posture related to kyphosis	Prior history of rickets or tuberculosis of the spine; congenital malformation	Increased anterior convexity of cervical vertebrae when observed laterally; vertebrae not in straight alignment when observed posteriorly; head and neck not erect
Impaired body alignment related to loss of bone volume	Overall mechanism osteoporosis caused by hormonal changes, immobilization, long-term steroid therapy, or aging	History of pathological fractures; inability to assume correct standing, sitting, or supine alignment; unsteady gait
Impaired body alignment related to inadequate muscle development or muscle mass	Muscular dystrophy; immobilization; catabolic illness such as severe infection or neoplasm	Decreased muscle tone; muscle atrophy; muscle weakness; inability to support correct body alignment when standing or sitting
Impaired body alignment related to the absence of nerve innervation	Cerebrovascular accident; head trauma; neurosurgery; spinal cord trauma	Absence of sensation and movement in affected extremities; decreased muscle tone in affected extremities; muscle atrophy in affected extremities; inability to support extremity; inability to support body alignment when standing, sitting, or lying down
Impaired body alignment related to immobilization	Fractured bones; central nervous system trauma or dysfunction; surgery	Inability to maintain body alignment; limited active range of joint motion; presence of a cast or traction; decreased sensation and movement to an extremity; decreased muscle tone; muscle atrophy

sampling. The student is encouraged to use these diagnoses for clients' nursing care plans but should also use them as guidelines for developing individualized nursing diagnoses.

Body Alignment

Alterations in body alignment can result from developmental changes, postural abnormalities, abnormalities in bone formation, impaired muscle development, damage to the central nervous system, and direct trauma to the musculoskeletal system (Table 30-6). Altered body alignment as a result of developmental changes is usually temporary and does not result in impaired physiological functioning. For example, the pregnant woman's low back pain subsides with rest and after delivery of the baby. The adolescent whose posture is poor usually outgrows discomfort with an adult body and improved posture.

Postural abnormalities significantly impair body alignment, and body alignment remains poor until the postural abnormality is corrected, if possible. The nurse who cares for a client with altered body alignment related to a postural abnormality develops a plan of care directed toward preventing any future body alignment problems. For example, if the client has mild kyphosis, the nurse may be able to prevent further spinal curvature by instructing the client to use a bed board and sleep without pillows.

Impairment of body alignment related to a loss of bone volume can involve all age groups. The impairment may be short-term, as with a client who is temporarily immobilized in traction, or long-term, as with a postmenopausal woman who has osteoporosis. Again, the nurse directs nursing care toward maintaining body alignment and reducing any future impairments.

Clients with impaired body alignment related to inadequate muscle development or muscle mass can also experience both long-term and short-term impairments. Clients with inadequate muscle development are frequently those with a muscle disease such as muscular dystrophy. In such cases nurses direct their care toward maximal use of muscle groups and achievement of optimal body alignment for each individual. Inadequate muscle mass can be long-term as with degenerative neuromuscular diseases; however, it can also be short-term. For example, a college student develops a severe systemic infection and is hospitalized for 1 month. During the first 3 weeks of hospitalization he may be quite ill and bedridden. Because of catabolic illness, infection, and bed rest, some of his protein-rich muscle mass is used by the body for fuel and some of his muscle mass de-

creases because of the disease. Nursing care is designed to increase his muscle mass by exercising his muscle groups and increasing his dietary protein intake.

Impaired body alignment related to the absence of nerve innervation is permanent, since nerves are unable to regenerate. Thus nursing interventions are aimed at retaining the client's maximal alignment and reducing any future decrease in body alignment.

Impairment in body alignment related to immobility depends on the reason for immobilization. Immobilization of a fractured extremity certainly has different implications from spinal immobilization following spinal cord trauma. Immobilized extremities usually do not have the overall physiological and emotional consequences present with total immobilization. As with other nursing diagnoses associated with impaired body alignment, impaired alignment related to immobilization requires the nurse to reduce further alterations (see Chapter 31).

Joint Mobility

The nursing diagnoses presented in this section are examples related to temporary or localized changes in joint mobility (Table 30-7). Other nursing diagnoses related to immobility are described in Chapter 31. The nursing diagnoses related to altered joint mobility and immobilization are separated because clients frequently have diminished joint mobility without complete immobilization and it is important for the student nurse to differentiate between the two.

As with impairment of body alignment, altered joint mobility can be related to developmental changes, postural abnormalities, abnormalities in bone formation, impaired muscle development, damage to the central nervous system, and direct trauma to the musculoskeletal system.

Decreased joint mobility related to aging is usually slow and progressive. The limitations in joint mobility may originate as local changes and gradually result in generalized limitations on range of joint mobility. The nursing care plan is directed toward maintaining the present level of function and increasing joint mobility.

Impaired joint mobility related to postural abnormalities can be congenital as with congenital hip dysplasia or acquired as with the development of a joint contracture. The cause of the impairment determines the goal of nursing action. In the care of a client with congenital hip dysplasia the appropriate intervention is to maintain adduction of the hip, while the goal of care for a joint contracture is to maintain the present level of mobility.

TABLE 30-7

Examples of Nursing Diagnoses Related to Altered Joint Mobility

Nursing Diagnosis	Etiology	Assessment Findings
Decreased joint mobility related to aging	Neurological, such as a cerebrovascular accident; skeletal, such as a pathological fracture	Unsteady gait; history of falling; use of adaptive devices to increase joint mobility; hemiplegia; hemiparesis; osteoporosis
Impaired joint mobility related to foot-drop	Neurological; iatrogenic, such as the result of improper positioning	Foot continuously in plantar flexion; decreased range of joint motion
Limited joint mobility related to joint inflammation	Arthritis	Decreased range of joint motion; joint tender to touch; joint feels warm; joint reddened; pain on movement
Decreased joint mobility related to degeneration of weight-bearing joints	Degenerative joint diseases	Inability to withstand weight bearing; reduced range of joint motion; degenerative joint changes observed on x-ray studies
Impaired joint mobility related to trauma to musculoskeletal system	Trauma to skeleton, joint, muscle, tendon, or ligament	Decreased range of joint movement; pain on movement; abnormal positioning of extremity

Impaired joint mobility related to a loss of bone volume frequently involves elderly clients and is a long-term impairment. The bone loss increases the client's risk for degenerative joint changes. As a result, as the bone loss continues, the bony structure of the weight-bearing joints disintegrates and mobility decreases.

Inadequate muscle development and absence of nerve innervation have a secondary effect on joint mobility. Joint mobility is impaired because the person lacks the muscle development, strength, or voluntary ability to move the joint. Nursing should direct care toward prevention of permanent reductions in joint mobility.

Limitations in joint mobility related to immobilization depend on the cause or purpose of immobilization. As with congenital hip dysplasia the hips are in continuous adduction. The purpose of the treatment is to press the head of the femur into the center of the acetabulum, thus making the cavity larger to support the femur head. The leg of the client with a fractured femur is immobilized in a cast to promote proper alignment while the fracture heals.

The nursing diagnoses described in this section acquaint the student with the various types of impaired body alignment and mobility. After the nurse correctly identifies the nursing diagnosis, a plan of care is developed.

Planning

Body Alignment

The nurse caring for a client with impaired body alignment develops a nursing care plan with goals that are individualized to the client's needs, his level of impairment, and the cause of the impairment. However, the following general goals apply to most age groups and health care settings:

1. Maintaining proper body alignment
2. Restoring proper body alignment or returning client to optimal level of body alignment
3. Reducing injuries to the musculoskeletal system resulting from impaired alignment
4. Decreasing muscle strain
5. Preventing deformities or complications to the skin and musculoskeletal system

The primary nursing goal is to maintain proper body alignment. Frequently this goal is included in the nursing care plan before any impairments are observed. Maintaining body alignment is especially important in clients with actual or potential limitations in mobility. For example, a comatose client should be positioned with pillows and the position changed at least every 2 hours to reduce the risk of poor alignment and future injury to the skin and musculoskeletal system.

The nursing assessment and nursing diagnoses serve as a basis for designing the plan of care. Planning care for clients with altered body alignment is frequently an independent nursing function; physicians rarely order specific body positions except after surgery, anesthesia, or trauma to the central nervous system.

Joint Mobility

Impaired joint mobility affects all age groups, and the impairments can be localized or generalized to include all joints. In addition, the impairment can be short-term, such as limited wrist mobility resulting from a fracture; progressive, such as decreased joint mobility related to rheumatoid arthritis; or permanent, such as foot-drop.

The nursing care plan for reduced joint mobility—like impaired body alignment—includes goals that are individualized to the client's need, his limitation of joint mobility, and the cause of the limited joint mobility. However, the following general goals can be individualized to most age groups and health care settings:

1. Preserving full range of joint motion
2. Maintaining each joint's present range of mobility
3. Preventing contractures
4. Maintaining client's ability to complete activities of daily living

The primary nursing goal is the preservation of full range of joint motion. This is particularly important in clients who have limitations of overall mobility such as the client with a spinal cord injury, the client who is comatose, or the client who has had a stroke.

Whenever a client has an illness or injury that prevents any of the activities necessary for physical independence, it is the nurse's responsibility to plan measures that prevent or decrease the limitation of joint mobility. Clients should have varying amounts and types of activities. Whenever possible they should be encouraged to engage in some self-help activity such as bathing, feeding, or dressing.

If a client is incapable of self-care, frequently the nurse must develop a plan to help the client meet individual needs. When joint mobility is reduced, the nurse develops the client's present joint mobility to its optimal state. Unless contraindicated, passive range of joint motion exercises are included in the nursing care. Passive range of joint motion exercises and the adaptive devices to increase mobility are described in the section on implementation of joint mobility measures.

Implementation

Body Alignment

To maintain proper body alignment the nurse correctly lifts the client, uses proper positioning techniques, and safely transfers clients from bed to chair or bed to stretcher. The procedures described in this section incorporate principles of body mechanics that are needed to maintain or restore body alignment.

LIFTING TECHNIQUES

The rate of injuries in occupational settings has increased in recent years, and more than half of these injuries are back injuries that are the direct result of improper lifting and bending techniques (Owens, 1980). The most common type of back injury is strain on the lumbar muscle group, which includes the muscles surrounding the lumbar vertebrae. Muscle injury to these areas affects the person's ability to bend forward, backward, and side to side. In addition, the ability to rotate the hips and lower back is decreased.

The nurse is at risk for injury to the lumbar muscles in lifting, transferring, or positioning the immobilized client. Before lifting, the nurse should assess ability to lift the client or object by determining the following basic lifting criteria:

1. *Position of weight.* The weight of the object to be lifted should be as close to the lifter as possible. Positioning the object in such a manner utilizes the lifting force of the nurse because the object to be lifted is in the same plane as the nurse.
2. *Height of the object.* The best height for lifting vertically is slightly above the level of the middle finger of a person with the arm hanging at the side (Owens, 1980). This is approximately 2 feet off the ground and is closer to the lifter's center of gravity.
3. *Body position.* When the lifter's body position will vary with different lifting tasks, a general rule is applicable to most lifting situations: the body is positioned so that multiple muscle groups are able to work together in a synchronized manner.
4. *Maximum weight.* Each nurse should know the maximum weight that is safe to carry—safe for the nurse as well as the client. An object is excessively heavy if its weight is 35% or more of a person's body weight. Therefore a nurse who weighs 130 pounds should not try independently to lift an immobilized 100-pound woman. Although the nurse may be able to lift the woman successfully, there is a risk of drop-

PROCEDURE 30-1

Proper Lifting

STEPS	RATIONALE
1. Assess the basic four lifting measures: position of weight, height of object, body position, and maximum weight. Determine if you are able to do it yourself or if you require help.	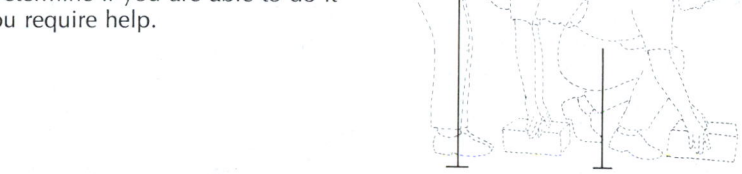
2. Come close to the object to be moved.	This increases body balance during the lift.
3. Enlarge your base of support.	This maintains better body balance, thus reducing the risk of falling.
4. Lower your center of gravity to the object to be lifted.	This increases body balance and enables muscle groups to work together in a synchronized manner.
5. Maintain proper alignment of the head and neck with the vertebrae.	This reduces the risk of injury to the lumbar vertebrae and muscle groups.

ping the client or causing injury to the nurse's back.

Thus the nurse determines the right position of the weight, the right height of the object, correct body position of the lifter, and the maximum weight that can be lifted before actually lifting.

In lifting, the nurse should follow a procedure designed to protect the musculoskeletal system (Procedure 30-1). First the nurse's entire body is brought close to the object to be lifted. Second, the feet are slightly apart. Third, with the head erect and the neck and vertebrae in proper alignment, the nurse's center of gravity is lowered toward the object to be lifted.

Lifting an object from a high shelf increases risks to the lifter because it is more difficult to maintain body balance. To reach an object overhead, people frequently stand on tiptoe with their feet together, thereby decreasing their base of support, elevating their center of gravity, and ultimately decreasing their balance.

The nurse who must lift an object from a high shelf should (1) use a safe, stable step stool or ladder for elevation; (2) stand as close to the shelf as possible; and (3) quickly transfer the weight of the object from the shelf to her arms and over her base of support. These three principles maintain the lifter's base of support and align the weight of the object close to the individual's center of gravity.

POSITIONING TECHNIQUES

Clients with impaired nervous, skeletal, or muscular system functioning and increased weakness and fatigability frequently require assistance from the nurse to attain proper body alignment while lying in bed or while in a sitting position. A variety of devices are available for the nurse to use in maintaining good body alignment for clients while they are being positioned (Table 30-8).

Pillows are readily available in most hospitals or extended care facilities; however, when the client is at home, the pillow supply is limited. Before using any pillow, the nurse should determine if it is the proper size. A thick pillow under the client's head may increase cervical flexion. A thin pillow under body prominences may be inadequate to protect the underlying skin and tissue from damage caused by pressure. When additional pillows are unavailable or if pillows are an improper size, the nurse can fold sheets, blankets, or towels for positioning aids.

A *footboard* is placed perpendicular to the mattress, parallel to and touching the plantar surfaces of the client's feet (Fig. 30-9). The goal of the footboard is to prevent foot-drop by maintaining the feet in dorsiflexion. After placing a footboard on the bed, the nurse needs to evaluate the board's position and determine correct placement, since a small client's feet may not reach the board.

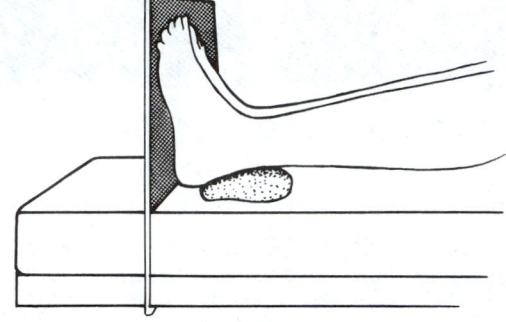

Fig. 30-9   Footboard.

TABLE 30-8

Devices Used for Proper Positioning

Device	Uses
Pillow	Provides support of body or extremity; elevates a body part; splints incisional area to reduce postoperative pain during activity or coughing and deep breathing
Footboard	Maintains feet in dorsal flexion
Trochanter roll (see Fig. 30-10)	Prevents external rotation of legs when the client is in the supine position
Sandbag	Provides support and shape to the body contours; immobilizes an extremity; maintains specific body alignment
Hand roll	Maintains the thumb slightly adducted and in opposition to the fingers; maintains fingers in a slightly flexed position
Hand-wrist splint	Individually molded for the client to maintain proper alignment of the thumb; slightly adducted in apposition to the fingers; maintains the wrist in slight dorsal flexion
Trapeze bar	Enables the client to raise trunk from the bed; enables the client to transfer from bed to wheelchair; allows the client to perform exercises that strengthen upper arms
Restraint	Reduces or limits body movement; protects the client from injury
Side rail	Allows the weak client to roll from side to side or to sit up in bed
Bed board	Provides additional support to the mattress and improves vertebral alignment

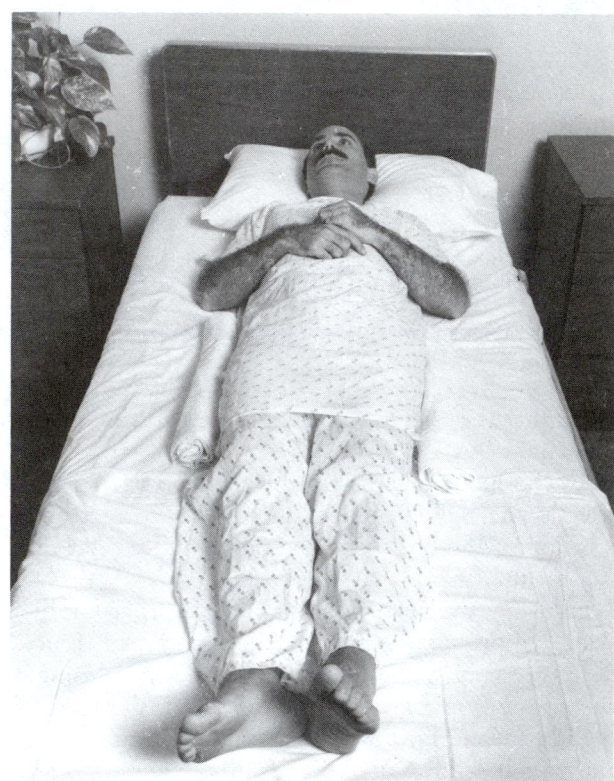

Fig. 30-10   Trochanter roll.

The *trochanter roll* is used to prevent external rotation of the legs when the client is in the supine position. To form a trochanter roll, a cotton bath blanket is folded lengthwise to a width that will extend from the greater trochanter of the femur to the lower border of the popliteal space (Fig. 30-10). The blanket is placed under the client's buttocks and then rolled counterclockwise until the thigh is in the neutral position or in inward rotation. When the correct alignment of the hip is achieved, the patella faces directly upward.

Sandbags are sand-filled plastic tubes that can be shaped to body contours. Sandbags can be used in place of or in addition to trochanter rolls. They immobilize an extremity or maintain a body alignment.

Hand rolls maintain the thumb in slight adduction and in opposition to the fingers. The major goal of a hand roll is to maintain the hand, thumb, and fingers in a functional position. Hand rolls can be made by folding a washcloth in half, rolling it lengthwise, and securing the roll with tape. The roll is placed against

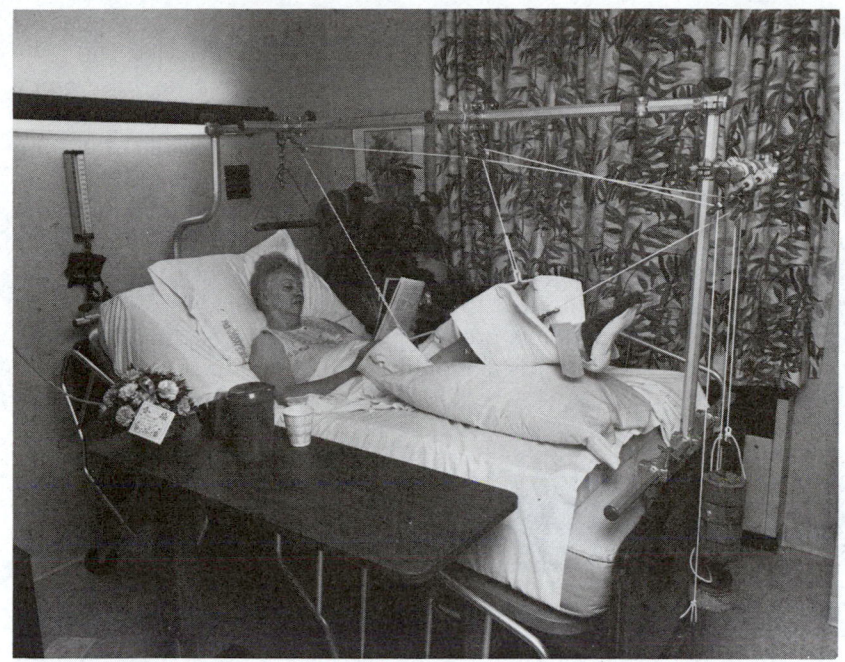

Fig. 30-11 Trapeze bar for a client in traction.

the palmar surface of the client's hand. The nurse evaluates the position of the hand roll to make sure the hand is indeed in a functional position. If washcloths are in short supply, a hand roll can be made by placing a roll of Kerlix against the palmar surface of the client's hand.

Hand-wrist splints are individually molded for the client to maintain proper alignment of the thumb (slight adduction) and the wrist (slight dorsiflexion). These splints should be used only for the client for whom the splint was made.

The *trapeze bar* descends from a securely fastened overhead bar that is attached to the bed frame. The trapeze allows the client to pull with upper extremities to raise the trunk off the bed, to assist in transfer from bed to wheelchair, or to perform upper arm strengthening exercises (Fig. 30-11).

Restraints are devices used to immobilize clients, especially confused, elderly, or disoriented clients. A common jacket restraint is the Posey bed jacket (Fig. 30-12). When placing the jacket on the client, the nurse laps one side of the jacket over the other on the client's back (Fig. 30-13). The ties are placed under the loop on the jacket and secured to the bed frame. Restraints should *never* be tied to the bedside rails because the client may be injured if a side rail is lowered with the restraint in place. (See Chapter 34 for safety principles in using restraints.)

Side rails, bars positioned along the sides of the length of the bed, ensure client safety (see Chapter 34) and are also useful for increasing mobility. In

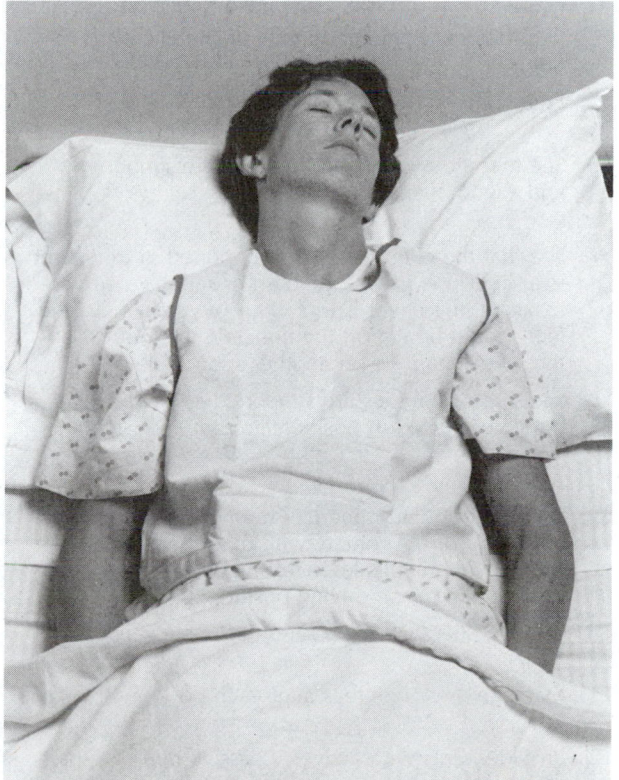

Fig. 30-12 Posey bed jacket restraint.

addition, they allow the weak client to roll from side to side or sit up in bed.

Bed boards are plywood boards placed under the entire surface area of a mattress. They are useful for increasing back support and alignment, especially with a soft mattress.

All of these devices, except the hand and wrist splints, are readily available for use in a hospital or community setting. Hand-wrist splints are especially designed to mold to the contour of the client's hand, and they are most commonly used to increase function in a client with limited mobility related to ner-

vous system dysfunction such as the client with hemiplegia after a cerebrovascular accident (stroke).

Although each of the procedures for positioning clients has specific guidelines, there are some general guidelines the nurse should follow for all clients who require positioning assistance (Procedure 30-2).

These guidelines help to reduce the risk of injury to the musculoskeletal system when the client is in a sitting position or lying in bed. When joints are unsupported, their alignment is impaired. Likewise, if the joints are not positioned in a slightly flexed position, their mobility is decreased. The support and

---

PROCEDURE 30-2

Ensuring Proper Positioning

STEPS	RATIONALE
1. Raise the level of the bed to a comfortable working height.	This raises the level of work toward the nurse's center of gravity.
2. Determine what equipment is needed. Organize the work area. Remove obstacles.	This provides for safe, organized positioning.
3. Tell the client what you are doing and what he can do to help.	This enables the nurse to use the client's mobility and strength, if possible.
4. Determine if you will need help, and if so, get help before beginning to change the client's position.	This provides the nurse with the opportunity to assess her ability to move the client independently and ensures her safety and that of the client.
5. Place one pillow beneath the client's head.	A pillow provides support to the head without causing flexion, hyperextension, or lateral flexion of the neck.
6. See that elbows, knees, and hips are supported and slightly flexed.	This ensures proper alignment when these joints are supported. Flexion prevents prolonged hyperextension, which could impair joint mobility.
7. See that the client's feet are supported. If the client is in bed, provide a footboard or sandbags, if necessary. If the client is in a chair or wheelchair, the feet should be flat on the floor, on the footrest of the wheelchair, or on another support device.	Support maintains dorsal flexion and helps to prevent foot-drop.
8. See that extremities are supported and, whenever possible, placed in positions for free movement.	Support reduces the risk of joint dislocation, particularly in instances when there is underlying nerve damage, as after a stroke. Allowing the extremity to move freely assists in maintaining joint mobility.
9. See that bony prominences are not permitted to remain in direct contact with other body parts, such as the client's knee resting on the thigh of the other leg in the side-lying position.	Pressure increases the risk of skin breakdown and damage to the musculoskeletal system.
10. Change client's body position at least every 2 hours.	This removes pressure from the dependent body tissues and reduces the risk of the formation of pressure sores.
11. Massage pressure areas after each position change.	Massage increases blood supply to the pressure areas and reduces risk of pressure sores.
12. Provide joints with active or passive range of joint motion at least twice a day.	This maintains joint mobility and reduces risk of joint contractures.

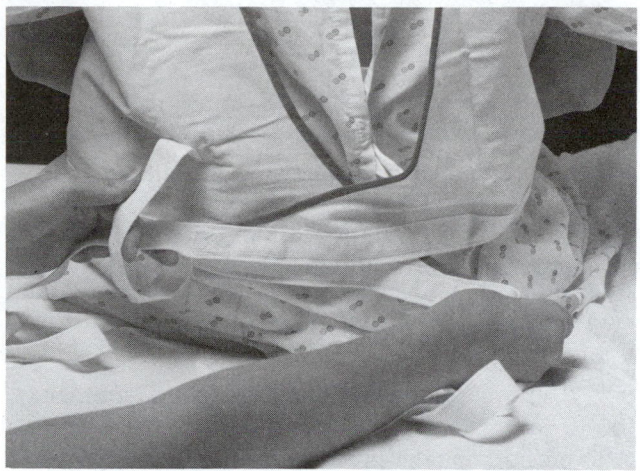

Fig. 30-13 Placing a Posey jacket restraint on a client.

flexion of the client's joints are directed to returning or maintaining the client's optimal mobility and to reducing the risk of injury to the musculoskeletal system. During client positioning, the nurse must also determine the presence of pressure points. When actual or potential pressure areas exist, nursing interventions involve removing the pressure, changing the position, or massaging pressure areas. These interventions are aimed at decreasing the risk for the development of pressure sores and further trauma to the musculoskeletal system.

The supported Fowler's, supine, prone, side-lying, and Sims' positions are described in the next sections. Each step of the procedure and its rationale are included, along with nursing guidelines. The step-by-step procedures are written for positioning those clients who are immobilized or have limited voluntary motor control. Clients who have complete mobility,

---

PROCEDURE 30-3

Supported Fowler's Position

USE: Fowler's position improves cardiac output and ventilation and assists in urinary or bowel elimination. In addition, the Fowler's position makes it easier for the bedridden client to eat, socialize, read, or watch television.

STEPS	RATIONALE
1. Elevate the head of the bed 45 to 60 degrees.	This increases comfort, improves breathing, and increases the client's opportunity to socialize, relax, or watch television.
2. Allow the head to rest against the mattress or on a very small pillow.	This prevents flexion contracture of the cervical vertebrae.
3. If a large pillow is used, turn it lengthwise to support the client's upper back, shoulders, and head.	This prevents flexion contracture of the cervical vertebrae and maintains vertebral alignment.
4. Use pillows to support the arms and hands if the client does not have voluntary control or use of arms and hands.	This prevents shoulder dislocation from the effect of downward gravitational pull of unsupported arms, promotes circulation by preventing venous pooling, reduces edema in the hands or arms, and prevents flexion contractures of the wrist.
5. Position pillow at lower back.	This supports lumbar vertebrae and decreases flexion of the vertebrae.
6. Place a small pillow or roll under the thighs. If lower extremities are paralyzed or if the client is unable to control lower extremities, use a trochanter roll in addition to the pillow placed under the thighs.	This prevents hyperextension of the knees and occlusion of the popliteal artery from pressure from body weight. The trochanter roll prevents external rotation of the legs.
7. Place a small pillow or roll under the ankle region.	This prevents prolonged pressure on the heels from the bed.
8. Place a footboard at bottom of the client's feet.	Footboard maintains dorsal flexion and prevents footdrop.

motor control, and sensory perceptions and who are conscious and oriented usually change position frequently and assume a position of comfort.

SUPPORTED FOWLER'S POSITION. In the supported Fowler's position the head of the client's bed is elevated 45 to 60 degrees and the client's knees are slightly elevated without pressure to restrict circulation to the lower legs (Procedure 30-3). Proper alignment of the body when the client is in this position requires support that maintains comfort and reduces the risk of damage to body systems. The angle of head and knee elevation and the length of time the client should remain in the Fowler's position are influenced by the type of illness and the client's overall condition. The supports must permit flexion of the hips and knees and proper alignment of the normal curves in the cervical, thoracic, and lumbar vertebrae.

The following are common trouble areas for the client in the Fowler's position:

1. Increased cervical flexion because the pillow at the head is too thick and the client's head thrusts forward
2. Extension of knees, allowing the client to slide to the foot of the bed
3. Pressure on the posterior aspect of the knee, decreasing circulation to the feet
4. Externally rotation of hips
5. Arms dangling unsupported at the client's sides
6. Feet unsupported
7. Unprotected pressure points at the sacrum and heels

After positioning the client, the nurse should reassess the client in the Fowler's position to determine if any of these problems exist.

PROCEDURE 30-4

Supine Position

USE: The dorsal recumbent or supine position is required following spinal surgery and some spinal anesthesia. In addition, this is an alternative position for an immobilized client.

STEPS	RATIONALE
1. Place a pillow under the upper shoulders, neck, and head, unless contraindicated following some spinal surgery or anesthesia.	This maintains correct alignment and prevents flexion contracture of cervical vertebrae and hyperextension of cervical vertebrae.
2. Place a small pillow or roll under the lumbar spine.	This provides support to lumbar vertebrae, especially when a firm mattress is being used, and reduces flexion of lumbar vertebrae.
3. When necessary, place trochanter rolls or sandbags parallel to the lateral surface of the client's thighs.	This reduces external rotation of the legs.
4. Place a small pillow or roll under upper leg to flex the knee slightly.	This prevents hyperextension of the knee and improves circulation by reducing pressure from the bed on the popliteal artery.
5. Place a small pillow or roll under the ankle to elevate the heels.	Raising the heels from the surface of the bed reduces pressure on the heels.
6. Place a footboard against the bottom of the client's feet.	This maintains dorsal flexion and prevents foot-drop.
7. Place pillows under the forearms, maintaining upper arms parallel to the client's body.	This reduces internal rotation of the shoulders and prevents extension of the elbows.
8. Have the client grasp hand rolls or towels or use hand splints when available.	This reduces extension of fingers and abduction of thumb and maintains thumb slightly adducted and in opposition to the fingers.

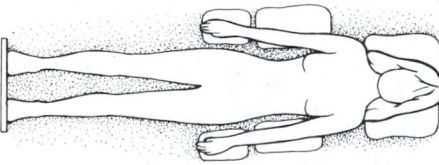
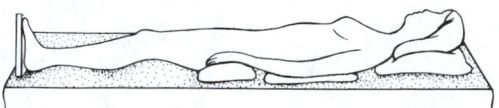

SUPINE POSITION. The supine position, in which the client rests on the back, is also called the dorsal recumbent position (Procedure 30-4). In the supine position the relationship of body parts is essentially the same as in good standing alignment except that the body is in the horizontal plane. Pillows, trochanter rolls, and hand rolls or arm splints are used to increase comfort and to reduce injury to the skin or musculoskeletal system.

The mattress should be firm enough to support the cervical, thoracic, and lumbar vertebrae. The shoulders are supported and the elbows are slightly flexed to control shoulder rotation. A foot support is used to prevent foot-drop, maintain proper alignment, and provide freedom of movement for the feet.

As with the previous position, there are some common trouble areas for the supine position:

1. Pillow at the head too thick, increasing cervical flexion
2. Head flat on the mattress
3. Shoulders unsupported and internally rotated
4. Elbows extended
5. Thumb not in opposition to the fingers
6. Hips externally rotated
7. Unsupported feet
8. Unprotected pressure points at the lumbar vertebrae, elbows, and heels

If any of these problems occur after positioning the client in the supine position, the nurse should correct them immediately.

PRONE POSITION. The client assuming the prone position is lying face down (Procedure 30-5). The pillow under the client's head should be of a thickness that prevents cervical flexion and maintains alignment of the lumbar spine. Placing a pillow under the client's lower leg permits dorsal flexion of the ankles and some knee flexion, which promotes relaxation. If a pillow is unavailable, the client's ankles should be in dorsiflexion over the end of the mattress. Body alignment is poor when the ankles are continuously in plantar flexion and the lumbar spine remains in hyperextension.

As with other positions the nurse should assess for and correct any of the following potential trouble points:

1. Neck hyperextension
2. Hyperextension of lumbar spine
3. Plantar flexion
4. Unprotected pressure points at the chin, elbows, hips, knees

---

PROCEDURE 30-5

Prone Position

USE: The primary therapeutic use of the prone position is as an alternative position for a client who is immobilized or on prolonged bed rest.

STEPS	RATIONALE
1. Turn client's head to one side and support with a small pillow. When excessive drainage from the mouth is present, the pillow may be contraindicated.	This reduces flexion or hyperextension of the cervical vertebrae.
2. Place a small pillow under the client's belly below the level of the diaphragm.	This reduces pressure on the breasts in some female clients, decreases hyperextension of lumbar vertebrae, and improves breathing by reducing pressure on the diaphragm from the mattress.
3. Position the client toward the foot of the bed so the feet hang over the mattress, or support the lower legs with a pillow to elevate the toes.	This prevents foot-drop and reduces external rotation of the legs and pressure on the toes from the mattress.

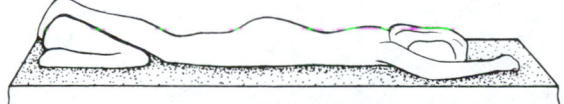
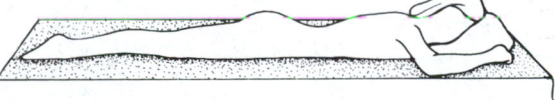

SIDE-LYING POSITION. In the side-lying (or lateral) position the client is resting on the side, with the major portion of body weight on the dependent hip and shoulder (Procedure 30-6). When the client is positioned in the side-lying position, the trunk alignment should be the same as in good standing position. For example, the structural curves of the spine should be maintained, the head should be supported in line with the midline of the trunk, and rotation of the spine should be avoided, especially in the helpless client (Bilger and Greene, 1973).

The following trouble points are commonly observed in clients in the side-lying position:

1. Lateral flexion of the neck
2. Spinal curves out of normal alignment
3. Shoulder and hip joints internally rotated, adducted, or unsupported
4. Lack of support for feet
5. Lack of protection for pressure points at the ilium, knees, and ankles

SIMS' POSITION. The Sims' position differs from the side-lying position in the distribution of the client's weight (Procedure 30-7). In the Sims' position the

---

PROCEDURE 30-6

Side-Lying (Lateral) Position

USE: The side-lying position removes pressure from the bony prominences on the back.

STEPS	RATIONALE
1. Place a pillow under the client's head and neck.	This (1) maintains alignment, (2) reduces lateral flexion of the neck, and (3) decreases muscle strain on the major neck muscle (sternocleidomastoid).
2. Both arms are slightly flexed: the uppermost arm is supported by a pillow that is placed under the forearm, and the other arm is supported by the mattress.	This decreases internal rotation and adduction of shoulder, preventing dislocation of the shoulder. Supporting both arms in a slightly flexed position protects the joints, and it also improves ventilation because the chest is able to expand more easily.
3. Place one or two pillows under the uppermost leg. Pillows should be placed the distance from the groin to the foot.	This prevents internal rotation and adduction of the thigh and reduces pressure to the bony prominences of the leg from the mattress.
4. Place supports, such as sandbags and footboard, at the client's feet.	This prevents foot-drop.
5. Place rolled pillow parallel to client's back.	This maintains support and alignment of the vertebrae and prevents (1) the client from rolling back out of alignment and (2) rotation of the spine.

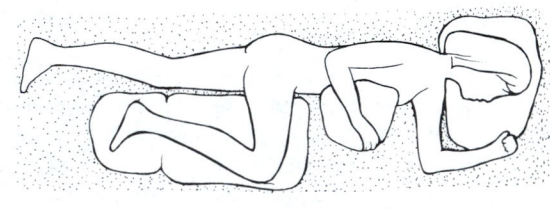

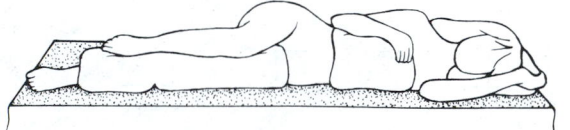

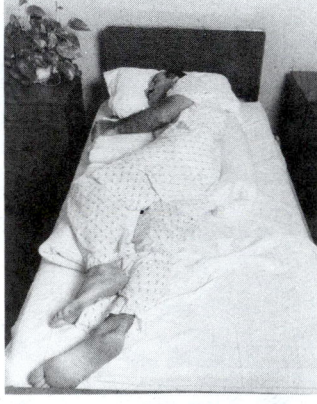

client's weight is placed on the anterior ilium and the humerus and clavicle.

Trouble points commonly observed in clients in the Sims' position include the following:

1. Lateral flexion of the neck
2. Internal rotation, adduction, or lack of support to the shoulders and hips
3. Lack of support for the feet
4. Lack of protection for pressure points at the ilium, humerus, clavicle, knees, and ankles

CHANGING THE CLIENT'S POSITION. Correct positioning of clients is crucial for maintaining proper body alignment. Any client whose mobility is decreased is at risk for developing contractures, postural abnormalities, and pressure sores. The nurse has the primary responsibility to minimize this risk, which is done by positioning clients in one of the positions presented here every 2 hours (see Chapter 31).

PROCEDURE 30-7

Sims' (Semiprone) Position

USE: Sims' position is frequently used for the unconscious client to increase drainage of mucus from the mouth; in addition, this position provides an alternative position for the client who is immobilized or on bed rest.

STEPS	RATIONALE
1. Turn the client's head to the side and place a small pillow underneath.	This maintains proper alignment and prevents lateral flexion of the neck.
2. Place a pillow under the flexed arm; the pillow should go from the hand to elbow.	This prevents internal rotation of the shoulder.
3. Place a pillow under the flexed leg. The pillow should go from the knee to the foot.	This prevents internal rotation of the hip and adduction of the leg and reduces pressure on the knees and ankle from the mattress.
4. Place sandbags parallel to the plantar surface of the foot.	This prevents foot-drop.

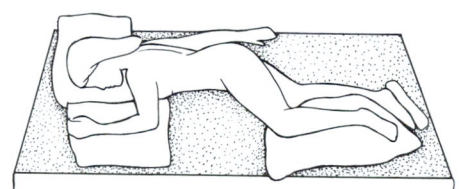

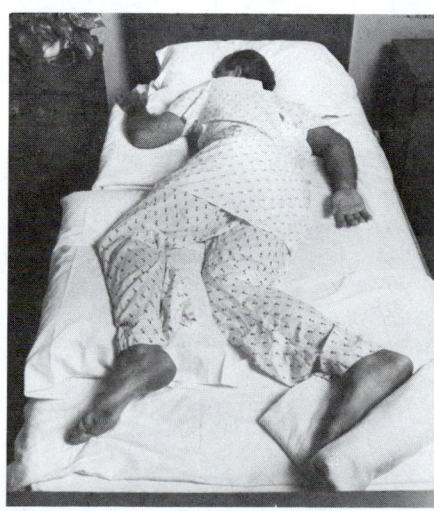

TRANSFER TECHNIQUES

Nurses frequently encounter semihelpless, helpless, or immobilized clients whose position must be changed, who must be moved up in bed, or who must be transferred from bed to chair or bed to stretcher. The nurse learns body mechanics early in the educational process. Proper use of body mechanics enables the nurse to move, lift, or transfer clients safely and also protects the nurse from injury to the musculoskeletal sytem.

Nurses use many transferring techniques. This section details the procedures for the most common techniques. However, the nurse follows some general guidelines in any transfer procedure:

1. Raising the side rail on the side of the bed opposite the nurse to prevent the client from falling out of bed on that side
2. Elevating the level of the bed to a comfortable height
3. Assessing the client's mobility and strength to determine what assistance he can offer during transfer
4. Explaining the procedure and specifically describing what is expected of the client

Clients who are experiencing pain may require some analgesia before movement to minimize discomfort and to provide relaxation. The nurse who is attempting transfer or moving techniques for the first time should request help to reduce the risk of injury to both client and nurse. The nurse should also recognize personal strength and its limits. Moving a completely immobilized client alone is difficult and, in some cases, impossible and dangerous.

After moving, lifting, or transferring procedures, the nurse should always assess the client's body alignment and correct any trouble points. Mechanical devices, such as a Hoyer lift used to transfer immobilized clients, are described in Chapter 31.

MOVING A CLIENT IN BED. Clients require varying levels of assistance to move up in bed or to the side-lying position or to sit up at the side of the bed. For example, a young, healthy, postpartum woman may require assistance to support her as she sits at the side of the bed for the first time, while the elderly man 1 day after an appendectomy may lack strength and require assistance from one or more nurses to sit at the side of his bed.

How then does the nurse determine what the client is able to do alone and how many people are needed to help move the client in bed? First the nurse assesses the client to determine if the illness precludes exertion, as with cardiovascular disease. Next, the nurse determines if the client comprehends what is expected. For example, a client recently medicated for postoperative pain may be too lethargic to understand instruction, and to ensure his safety, two nurses are needed to move him in bed. Third, the nurse determines the comfort level of the client. Fourth, the nurse evaluates her knowledge of the procedure and her strength. Last is the determination of whether the client is too heavy or too immobile for the nurse to complete the procedure alone. In doubtful cases the nurse should always request assistance from another person. Procedures 30-8 through 30-12 describe the procedures commonly used in moving clients in bed and transferring them to a sitting position at the side of the bed.

Assisting a Client to Move Up in Bed (One or Two Nurses)

STEPS	RATIONALE
1. Face the head of the bed. (If two nurses assist the client, each nurse stands at one side of the bed and follows the procedure.)	Facing the direction of movement prevents twisting of the nurse's body when moving the client.
2. Place feet apart with the foot nearest the bed behind the other foot.	A wide base of support increases the nurse's balance. One foot behind the other foot allows the nurse to transfer her body weight as the client is moved up in bed.
3. If possible, ask the client to flex the knees, bringing the feet as close to the buttocks as possible.	This enables the client to use the femoral muscles during the process of actually moving up in bed
4. Instruct client to flex the neck, tilting the chin toward the chest.	This prevents hyperextension of the neck when moving the client to the head of the bed.
5. Ask the client to assist in moving by (1) using the trapeze bar if available or (2) pushing on the bed surface.	The client uses the upper extremity muscles to elevate the trunk and reduce friction when moving up in bed.
6. Ask the client with limited upper extremity strength or mobility to place the arms across the chest.	This prevents friction from dragging the arms across the bed surface during the move.
7. Flex your knees and hips, thus bringing your forearms closer to the level of the bed.	This increases your balance and strength by bringing the center of gravity closer to the client, the "object" to be moved.
8. Place the arm that is closer to the head of the bed under the client's shoulder and the other arm under the thighs (see Fig. 33-20).	This prevents trauma to the client's musculoskeletal system because the shoulder and hip joints are supported, and it evenly distributes the client's weight.
9. Instruct the client to move up in bed on the count of three.	This prepares the client for the actual move, thus reinforcing the client's assistance in moving up in bed.
10. On the count of three, rock and shift your weight from the back leg to the front leg, and at the same time the client pushes with the heels and elevates the trunk.	Rocking enables the nurse to improve her balance and overcome inertia. The shifting of the nurse's weight counteracts the client's weight. When the client pushes with the heels and lifts the trunk, friction is reduced.
11. Reassess the client's body alignment and pressure point areas. If poor body alignment or pressure points are present, use nursing interventions to reduce the risk of damage to the musculoskeletal system.	Proper body alignment increases the client's comfort, promotes rest, and reduces the hazards of immobility (see Chapter 31).

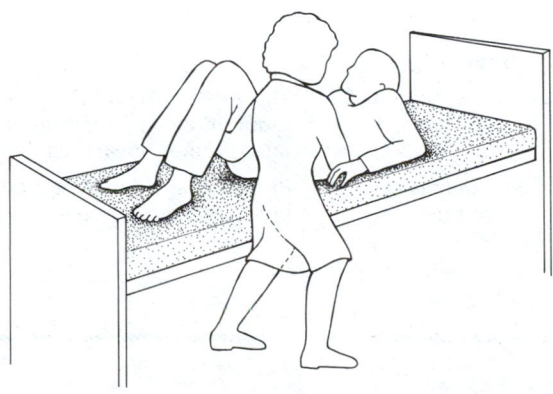

Moving a Helpless Client Up in Bed (One Nurse)

STEPS	RATIONALE
1. Place the client in the supine position with the head of the bed flat and all pillows removed from the bed. Stand on one side of the bed.	This maintains the client in the supine position and enables the nurse to easily assess body alignment throughout the move and to administer any additional care, such as suctioning or hygiene needs, which may be needed during the procedure. Placing the head of the bed to the flat position reduces the gravitational pull on the client's upper body. Removing all pillows from the bed reduces interference from equipment during the procedure.
2. Begin at the client's feet. Face the foot of the bed at a 45-degree angle and slide the client's legs diagonally toward the head of the bed.	Positioning is begun at the client's legs because they are the least weight to be supported, facing the direction of movement ensures proper balance for the nurse, and the diagonal motion permits pull in the direction of the force.
3. Move parallel to the client's hips and flex your knees and hips as needed to bring your arms level with the client's hips.	This maintains the nurse's proper alignment, brings her closest to the "object" to be moved, and lowers her center of gravity as necessary.
4. Slide the client's hips diagonally toward the head of the bed. If available, a pull sheet may be useful. (A pull sheet is usually a full-sized bath blanket or sheet that is folded to extend the distance from the client's shoulders to 2 inches below the popliteal space. When moving the client, use the sheet to pull the client or a portion of the client's body.)	This aligns the client's hips and feet.
5. Move parallel to the client's head and shoulders, and flex your knees and hips as needed to bring your arms level with the client's body.	This maintains the nurse's proper alignment, brings her closer to the "object" to be moved, and lowers her center of gravity as necessary.
6. Slide the arm closer to the head of the bed under the client's head and neck, with the hand reaching under and supporting the far shoulder.	This supports the head and neck, maintaining their proper alignment during transfer. Placement of the nurse's hand on the client's far shoulder supports that joint during movement.
7. Place the other arm under the client's chest.	This supports the client's body weight and reduces friction during movement.
8. Slide the client's trunk, shoulders, head, and neck diagonally toward the head of the bed.	This realigns the body on one side of the bed.
9. Elevate the side rail next to the client. Move to the other side and elevate side rail, switching sides of the bed until the client is at the desired height.	This protects the client from falling out of bed.
10. Center the client in the bed, moving the body in the same three sections.	This protects the client from falling and provides ample room on either side of the client for turning, positioning, or other nursing care activities.
11. Reassess the client's body alignment and pressure point areas. If poor body alignment or pressure points are present, use nursing interventions to reduce risk of damage to the musculoskeletal system.	Proper body alignment increases the client's comfort, promotes rest, and reduces the hazards of immobility.

PROCEDURE 30-10

Repositioning a Helpless Client

STEPS	RATIONALE
1. Lower the head of the bed, if elevated, to the flat position.	This reduces gravitational pull on the client's upper body.
2. Remove all pillows and devices used in the previous position.	This reduces interference during repositioning.
3. Face the client, move close to the bed, and assume a broad stance with one foot in front of the other.	This prevents twisting of the nurse's body, brings her center of gravity close to the object to be moved, and increases balance.
4. Place your upper arm under the client's shoulders while supporting the cervical vertebrae and head.	This supports alignment of the shoulders and prevents flexion or hyperextension of the head and neck during repositioning.
5. Place your outer arm under the client's thighs.	This supports alignment of the hip and evenly distributes the client's body weight.
6. Rock in the direction of movement; that is, if you are turning the client to the side, rock away from the bed; if you are moving the client toward center of the bed, rock toward the bed.	Rocking overcomes inertia and makes use of the nurse's body weight in the direction of movement.
7. Assess for any reddened pressure points from previous position.	Early identification of pressure points reduces the risk of formation of pressure sores.
8. Massage pressure points.	This increases circulation to tissues and muscles.
9. Place client in the supine, prone, side-lying, or Sims' position (see Procedures 30-3 through 30-6), and evaluate for proper alignment.	Rotation of positions reduces the risk of damage to the musculoskeletal system from immobility.

PROCEDURE 30-11

Assisting the Client to a Sitting Position

STEPS	RATIONALE
1. Place client in a supine position.	This enables the nurse to continually assess the client's body alignment and to administer additional care, such as suctioning or hygiene needs.
2. Remove all pillows from the bed.	This decreases interference while sitting the client up in bed.
3. Face the head of the bed.	This reduces twisting of the nurse's body when moving the client.
4. Place the feet apart with the foot nearer the bed behind the other foot.	This improves the nurse's balance and allows her to transfer her body weight as the client is moved to a sitting position.
5. Place hand farther from the client under the shoulders, supporting the client's head and cervical vertebrae.	This maintains alignment of the head and cervical vertebrae and allows for even lifting of the client's upper trunk.
6. Place the other hand on the bed surface.	This provides support and balance.

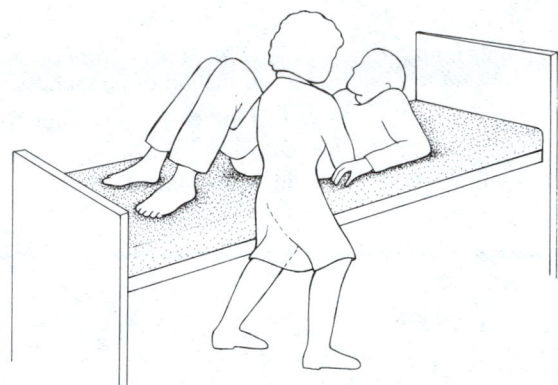

STEPS	RATIONALE
7. Raise the client to a sitting position by shifting your weight from the front leg to the back leg.	This improves the nurse's balance, overcomes inertia, and transfers the weight in the direction in which the client is moved.
8. Push against the bed and arm that was placed on the bed surface.	This divides the activity of raising the client to a sitting position between the nurse's arms and legs and protects the back from strain. By bracing one hand against the mattress and pushing against it as the nurse lifts the client, part of the weight that would be lifted by the back muscles is transferred through the arms onto the mattress (Bilger and Greene, 1973).

PROCEDURE 30-12

Assisting the Client to a Sitting Position on the Side of the Bed

STEPS	RATIONALE
1. Place client in the side-lying position, facing you on the side of the bed that the client will be sitting on.	This prepares the client to move to the side of the bed and protects the client from falling.
2. Raise the head of the bed to the highest level or the highest level that the client is able to tolerate.	This decreases the amount of work needed by client and nurse to raise the client in the sitting position.
3. Stand opposite the client's hips.	This places the nurse's center of gravity nearer the client.
4. Turn on a diagonal so that you are facing the client and the far corner of the foot of the bed.	This reduces twisting of the nurse's body because the nurse is facing the direction of movement.
5. Place feet apart with the foot closer to the head of the bed in front of the other foot.	This increases balance and allows the nurse to transfer weight as the client is brought to a sitting position at the side of the bed.
6. Place the arm nearer the head of the bed under the client's shoulders, supporting the head and neck.	This maintains alignment of the head and neck as the nurse brings the client to the sitting position.
7. Place the other arm over the client's thighs.	This supports the hip and prevents the client from falling backward during the procedure.
8. Move the client's lower legs and feet over the side of the bed.	This decreases friction and resistance during the procedure.
9. Pivot toward your rear leg, allowing the client's upper legs to swing downward.	This allows gravity to descend the client's legs.
10. At the same time, shift your weight to your rear leg and elevate the client.	This allows the nurse to transfer weight in the direction of motion.
11. Remain in front of the client until the client regains balance.	This reduces risk of falling.
12. Lower the level of the bed until the client's feet touch the floor.	This supports the client's feet in dorsal flexion and allows the client to easily stand at the side of the bed.

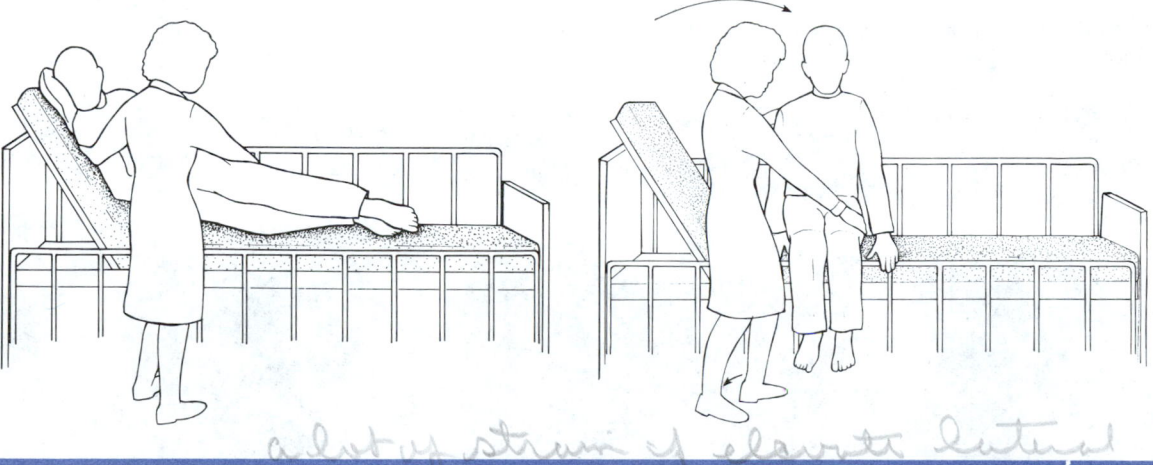

TRANSFERRING A CLIENT FROM BED TO CHAIR.
The transfer of a client from bed to chair by one nurse requires assistance from the client and should not be attempted with clients who are unable to assist or to comprehend the nurse's instructions (Procedure 30-13). As with other procedures the nurse explains it to the client before attempting the transfer. The environment is also prepared, with obstacles moved out of the way. The chair is placed next to the bed with the back of the chair in the same plane as the head of the bed. Placement of the chair allows the nurse to pivot with the client and to transfer the client's weight quickly to the chair.

A safe transfer is the first priority. The nurse who is doubtful about her strength or the client's ability to help should request assistance from another person before beginning the procedure. The client should be allowed to stand at the side of the bed for a minute so he can quickly be lowered back into it in case of dizziness or fainting.

PROCEDURE 30-13

Transferring from Bed to Chair

STEPS	RATIONALE
1. Assist client to a sitting position on the side of the bed. Have chair in position with back of chair parallel to head of bed.	
2. Spread your feet apart.	This ensures balance with a wide base of support.
3. Flex your hip and knees, aligning your knees with the client's.	Flexion of knees and hips lowers the nurse's center of gravity to the object to be raised; aligning knees with the client's allows for stabilization of the knees when the client stands.
4. Straighten your hips and legs.	This uses correct body mechanics to raise client to a standing position.
5. Pivot on the foot that is farther from the chair, moving the client directly in front of the chair.	This maintains support of the client while allowing adequate space for the client to move.
6. Instruct the client to use the armrests on the chair for support.	This increases client's stability.
7. Flex your hips and knees while lowering the client into the chair.	This prevents injury to the nurse resulting from poor body mechanics.
8. Assess the client for proper alignment for a sitting position.	See Fig. 30-6.

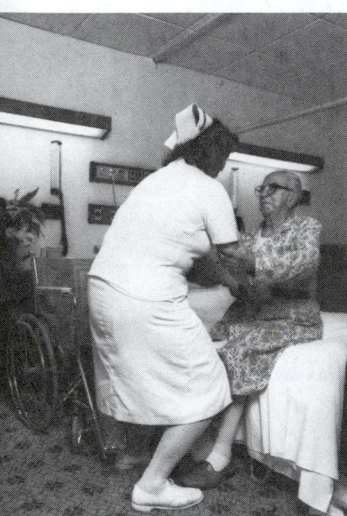 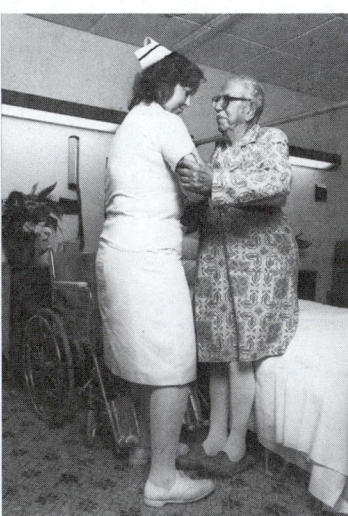 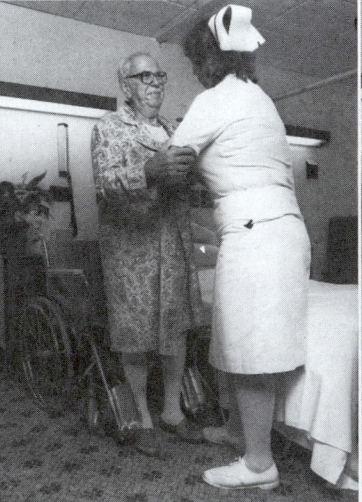 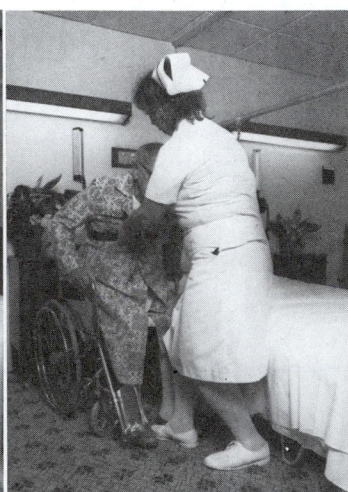

TRANSFERRING A CLIENT FROM BED TO STRETCHER. An immobilized client who must be transferred from bed to stretcher or bed to bed requires a three-person carry (Procedure 30-14). This transfer technique is best implemented when all personnel who are doing the lifting are of a similar height. If their centers of gravity are within the same plane, they can lift as a balanced unit.

Caution is used when the client to be transferred has trauma to the spinal cord. If a client with a spinal cord injury must be moved, the three-person carry is used and spinal alignment is maintained during the transfer.

The client should be prepared for the transfer and, whenever possible, asked to help, for example, by folding his arms over his chest. The environment should be free from obstacles, and any unnecessary equipment should be removed from the bed. The stretcher should be placed at a right angle to the bed so the lifters can pivot toward the stretcher and transfer the client quickly.

As with all procedures, safety is the priority. Safety is increased in the three-person carry if all the lifters work together. Therefore one person should assume the leadership role and direct the other two.

PROCEDURE 30-14

Three-Person Carry

STEPS	RATIONALE
1. The three nurses stand side by side and face the side of the client's bed.	This prevents twisting of the nurse's body.
2. Each person assumes responsibility for one of these three areas: (1) head and shoulders, (2) hips, and (3) thighs and ankles.	This distributes the client's body weight.
3. Each assumes a wide base of support with the foot closer to the stretcher in front, knees slightly flexed.	This increases balance and lowers the center of gravity of the lifters.
4. The lifters' arms are placed under the client's head and shoulders, hips, and thighs and ankles, with their fingers securely around the other side of the client's body.	This distributes client's weight over the lifters' forearms.
5. The lifters roll the client toward their chests.	This moves the workload over the lifters' base of support.
6. On the count of three, the client is lifted and held against the nurses' chests.	This enables the lifters to work together and safely lift the client.
7. On the second count of three, the nurses step back and pivot toward the stretcher, moving forward if needed.	This transfers the weight toward the stretcher.
8. The nurses gently lower the client onto the stretcher by flexing their knees and hips until their elbows are level with edge of the stretcher.	This maintains alignment of the nurses during transfer.
9. The nurses assess the client's body alignment, place safety straps across the client, and raise the side rails.	This reduces risk of injury from poor alignment or falling.

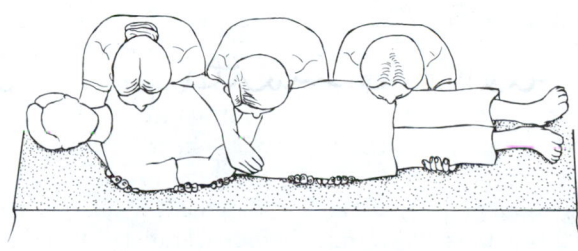

Joint Mobility

To ensure adequate joint mobility the nurse can teach the client about range of joint motion exercises. When the client does not have voluntary motor control, the nurse institutes passive range of motion exercises. Joint mobility is also increased when clients walk. Occasonally clients need to use mechanical devices such as crutches to increase the ability to walk.

Range of Joint Motion Exercises

Clients with restricted mobility are unable to perform some or all range of joint motion exercises independently. This limitation can be identified in clients in whom one extremity has limited movement or in completely immobilized clients. When caring for clients with actual or potential impaired mobility, the nurse designs interventions directed toward maintaining maximal joint mobility. One such nursing intervention is range of joint motion exercises.

To ensure that clients routinely receive these exercises, the nurse should schedule them at specific times, perhaps along with another nursing activity, such as during the client's bath. This method enables the nurse to systematically assess and improve the client's range of joint motion. In addition, the activity of bathing or receiving a bed bath usually requires that the extremities and joints are put through complete range of motion.

Range of joint motion exercises may be completely active (the client is able to move all joints through their range of motion unassisted), or completely passive (the client is unable to move independently and the nurse moves each joint through its range of motion), or somewhere in between. With a weak client, for example, the nurse may merely provide support while the client performs most of the movement, or the client may be able to move some joints actively while the nurse passively moves others. The nurse first assesses the client's ability to engage in active range of motion exercises and the need for support from the nurse. As a general principle, exercises should be as active as the client's health and mobility allow.

Contractures may develop in joints that are not moved periodically through their range of motion. A contracture is a permanent shortening of a muscle and the eventual shortening of associated ligaments and tendons. If a contracture occurs because the joint is immobilized for a long period of time, the person will not be able to use the joint normally and it may become fixed in one position.

Unless contraindicated, the nursing plan should include moving the extremities through as nearly full range of joint motion as possible. Passive range of

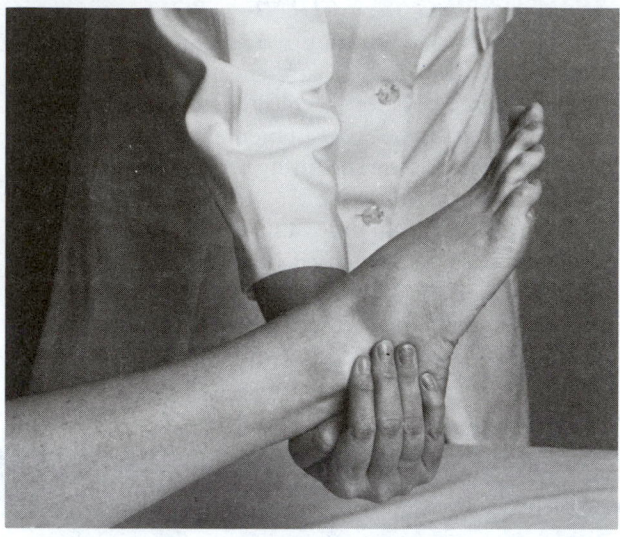

Fig. 30-14 Using a cupped hand to support a joint.

joint motion exercises should be initiated as soon as the individual loses the ability to move the extremity or joint. Movements are carried out slowly and smoothly and should not cause pain. Each movement should be repeated five times during the exercise period.

When performing passive range of joint motion exercises, the nurse stands at the side of the bed closest to the joint being exercised. If an extremity is to be moved or lifted, the nurse places a cupped hand under the joint to support it (Fig. 30-14), supports the joint by holding the adjacent distal and proximal areas (Fig. 30-15), or supports the joint with one hand and cradles the distal portion of the extremity with the remaining arm (Fig. 30-16).

The following sections describe the specific movements for the major joints in the body. Table 30-9 details range of joint motion for each area and illustrates the motion of each joint.

NECK

Range of joint motion for the neck is permitted by the flexibility of the cervical vertebrae and the pivotal connection between the head and neck. Unless contraindicated because of spinal surgery, spinal cord trauma, or other central nervous system trauma, range of joint motion exercises should be performed by clients with limited neck mobility. When flexion contracture of the neck occurs, the client's neck is permanently flexed with his chin close to or actually touching his chest. Ultimately, the client's total body alignment is altered, the visual field is changed, and the overall level of independent functioning is decreased.

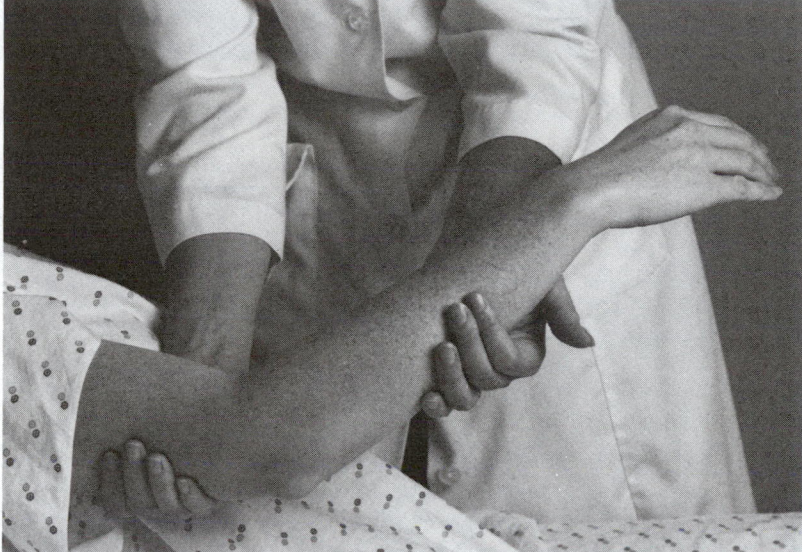

Fig. 30-15 Supporting the joint by holding the distal and proximal areas adjacent to the joint.

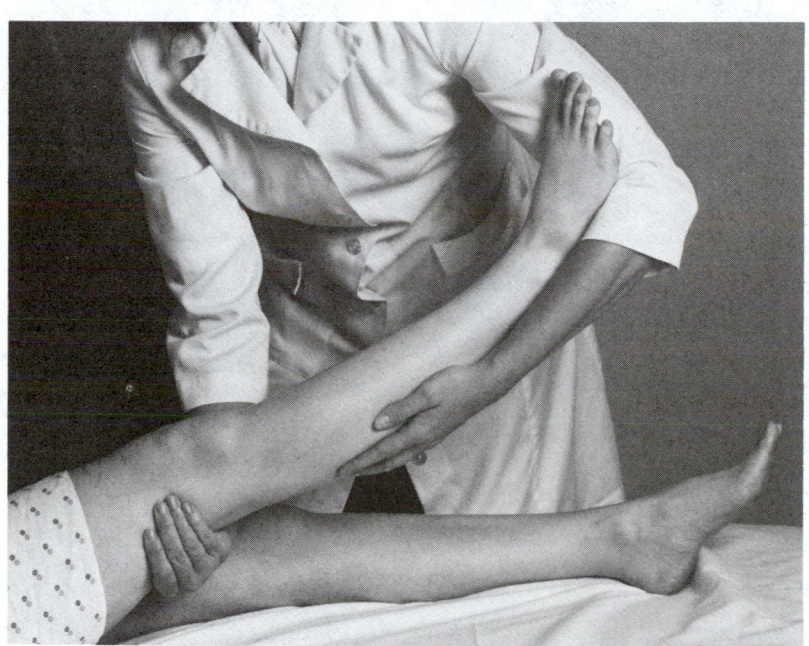

Fig. 30-16 Cradling the distal portion of an extremity.

SHOULDER

One feature of the shoulder that sets it apart from other joints in the body is that the strongest muscle controlling it, the deltoid, is in complete elongation in the normal position of rest. No other muscle exerts its full strength if it begins a movement when in complete elongation. Thus, exercising the shoulder effectively increases the power of the deltoid and range of joint motion; to accomplish this, the shoulder must first be abducted (Bilger and Greene, 1973).

The goal of action in the shoulder is full range of motion. Shoulder movements include flexion, exten-sion, hyperextension, abduction, adduction, internal and external rotation, and circumduction. It is important that the full range of motion in the shoulder be maintained or regained to avoid pain.

When caring for a client with limited voluntary control of the shoulder, the nurse should design interventions to place and support the shoulder in the adducted position. This can be achieved with slings when the client is standing or sitting or pillows when the client is in bed. Supporting and positioning the shoulder prevent pain, joint dislocation, and further changes in body alignment.

Text continued on p. 745.

TABLE 30-9

Range of Joint Motion Exercises

Body Part	Type of Joint	Type of Movement	Range (degrees)	Primary Muscles	
Neck, cervical spine	Pivotal	Flexion: bring chin to rest on the chest	45	Sternocleidomastoid	
		Extension: return head to erect position	45	Trapezius	
		Hyperextension: bend head back as far as possible	10	Trapezius	
		Lateral flexion: tilt head as far as possible toward each shoulder	40-45	Sternocleidomastoid	
		Rotation: turn head as far as possible to the right and to the left	180	Sternocleidomastoid, trapezius	
Shoulder	Ball and socket	Flexion: raise arm from side position forward to a position above the head	180	Coracobrachialis, biceps brachii, deltoid, pectoralis major	
		Extension: return the arm to position at side of the body	180	Latissimus dorsi, teres major, triceps brachii	
		Hyperextension: move arm behind the body, keeping elbow straight	45-60	Latissimus dorsi, teres major, deltoid	
		Abduction: raise arm to the side to a position above the head with palm away from the head	180	Deltoid, supraspinatus	
		Adduction: lower arm sideways and across the body as far as possible	320	Pectoralis major	

T A B L E 30 - 9, cont'd

Range of Joint Motion Exercises

Body Part	Type of Joint	Type of Movement	Range (degrees)	Primary Muscles	
		Internal rotation: with elbow flexed, rotate the shoulder by moving the arm until the thumb is turned inward and toward the back	90	Pectoralis major, latissimus dorsi, teres major, subscapularis	
		External rotation: with elbow flexed, move arm until thumb is upward and lateral to the head	90	Infraspinatus, teres major, deltoid	
		Circumduction: move the arm in a full circle. Circumduction is a combination of all movements of the ball-and-socket joint	360	Deltoid, coracobrachialis, latissimus dorsi, teres major	
Elbow	Hinge joint	Flexion: bend the elbow so that the lower arm moves toward its shoulder joint and the hand is level with the shoulder	150	Biceps brachii, brachialis, brachioradialis	
		Extension: straighten elbow by lowering hand	150	Triceps brachii	
		Hyperextension: bend the lower arm back as far as possible	10-20	Triceps brachii	
Forearm	Pivotal	Supination: turn lower arm and hand so that palm is up	70-90	Supinator, biceps brachii	
		Pronation: turn lower arm so that palm is down	70-90	Pronator teres, pronator quadratus	
Wrist	Condyloid	Flexion: move palm toward inner aspect of the forearm	80-90	Flexor carpi ulnaris, flexor carpi radialis	
		Extension: move fingers so that fingers, hands, and forearm are in the same plane	80-90	Extensor carpi ulnaris, extensor carpi radialis brevis, extensor carpi radialis longus	

Continued.

T A B L E 30 - 9, cont'd

Range of Joint Motion Exercises

Body Part	Type of Joint	Type of Movement	Range (degrees)	Primary Muscles
		Hyperextension: bring dorsal surface of hand back as far as possible	80-90	Extensor carpi radialis brevis, extensor carpi radialis longus, extensor carpi ulnaris
		Abduction (radial flexion): bend the wrist medially toward the thumb	Up to 30	Flexor carpi radialis, extensor carpi radialis brevis, extensor carpi radialis longus
		Adduction (ulnar flexion): bend the wrist laterally toward fifth finger	30-50	Flexor carpi ulnaris, extensor carpi ulnaris
Fingers	Condyloid hinge	Flexion: make a fist	90	Lumbricales, interosseus volaris, interosseus dorsalis
		Extension: straighten fingers	90	Extensor digiti quinti proprius, extensor digitorum communis, extensor indicis proprius
		Hyperextension: bend fingers back as far as possible	30-60	
		Abduction: spread fingers apart	30	Interosseus dorsalis
		Adduction: bring fingers together	30	Interosseus volaris
Thumb	Saddle	Flexion: move thumb across palmar surface of hand	90	Flexor pollicis brevis
		Extension: move thumb straight away from hand	90	Extensor pollicis longus, extensor pollicis brevis

Range of Joint Motion Exercises

Body Part	Type of Joint	Type of Movement	Range (degrees)	Primary Muscles	
		Abduction: extend thumb laterally (usually done when placing fingers in abduction and adduction)	30	Abductor pollicis brevis	
		Adduction: move thumb back toward hand	30	Adductor pollicis obliquus, adductor pollicis transversus	
		Opposition: touch thumb to each finger of the same hand		Opponeus pollicis, opponeus digiti minimi	
Hip	Ball and socket	Flexion: move the leg forward and up	90-120	Psoas major, iliacus, iliopsoas, sartorius	
		Extension: move leg back beside the other leg	90-120	Gluteus maximus, semitendinosus, semimembranosus	
		Hyperextension: move leg behind body	30-50	Gluteus maximus, semitendinosus, semimembranosus	
		Abduction: move leg laterally away from body	30-50	Gluteus medius, gluteus minimus	
		Adduction: move leg back toward medial position and beyond if possible	30-50	Adductor longus, adductor brevis, adductor magnus	

Continued.

TABLE 30-9, cont'd

Range of Joint Motion Exercises

Body Part	Type of Joint	Type of Movement	Range (degrees)	Primary Muscles	
		Internal rotation: turn foot and leg toward the other leg	90	Gluteus medius, gluteus minimus, tensor fasciae latae	
		External rotation: turn foot and leg away from the other leg	90	Obturatorius internus, obturatorius externus	
		Circumduction: move leg in a circle		Psoas major, gluteus maximus, gluteus medius, adductor magnus	
Knee	Hinge joint	Flexion: bring heel back toward back of thigh	120-130	Biceps femoris, semitendinosus, semimembranosus, sartorius	
		Extension: return leg to the floor	120-130	Rectus femoris, vastus lateralis, vastus medialis, vastus intermedius	
Ankle	Hinge joint	Dorsal flexion: move foot so that toes are pointed upward	20-30	Tibialis anterior	
		Plantar flexion: move foot so that toes are pointed downward	45-50	Gastrocnemius, soleus	
Foot	Gliding	Inversion: turn sole of foot medially	10 or less	Tibialis anterior, tibialis posterior	
		Eversion: turn sole of the foot laterally	10 or less	Peroneus longus, peroneus brevis	

TABLE 30-9, cont'd

Range of Joint Motion Exercises

Body Part	Type of Joint	Type of Movement	Range (degrees)	Primary Muscles	
Toes	Condyloid	Flexion: curl toes downward	30-60	Flexor digitorum, lumbricalis pedis, flexor hallucis brevis	
		Extension: straighten toes	30-60	Extensor digitorum longus, extensor digitorum brevis, extensor hallucis longus	
		Abduction: spread toes apart	15 or less	Abductor hallucis, interosseus dorsalis	
		Adduction: bring toes together	15 or less	Adductor hallucis, interosseus plantaris	

ELBOW

The elbow functions optimally at an angle of approximately 90 degrees. An elbow fixed in full extension is very disabling and limits the client's independence. If the elbow becomes contracted in any position, active or passive range of joint motion exercises usually result in increased stiffness.

The normal elbow joint movements include flexion, extension, and hyperextension. The nurse should not force the elbow joint beyond its capacity. The elbow joint is particularly likely to develop pain because of limited mobility, and unlike the shoulder joint, increasing the range of motion will not relieve the pain (Bilger and Greene, 1973).

FOREARM

Most functions of the hand are best carried out with the forearm in moderate pronation. When the forearm is fixed in a position of full supination, the client is quite disabled. For optimal functioning the forearm must be able to rotate from supination to pronation (Bilger and Greene, 1973).

WRIST

The primary function of the wrist is to place the hand in slight dorsal flexion, the position of functioning. Therefore full range of joint motion in the wrist is not as great a priority as maintaining the wrist in a functional position. When the wrist is fixed in even a slightly flexed position, the person's grasp is weakened. In the immobilized client the functional position of the wrist can be achieved by using hand and splint rolls.

FINGERS AND THUMB

The range of motion in the fingers and the thumb enables the client to perform activities of daily living as well as activities requiring fine motor skills such as carpentry, needlework, drawing, or painting.

The functional position of the fingers and thumb is slight flexion of the thumb in opposition to the fingers. In clients with restricted mobility, hand rolls will help to maintain this functional position.

HIP

Since the lower extremities are concerned chiefly with locomotion and weight bearing, the stability of the hip joint may be more important than its overall mobility (Bilger and Greene, 1973). For example, if one hip has no mobility but is fixed in a neutral position and fully extended, it is possible for the client to walk without a significant limp.

Contractures fix the hip in positions of deformity. Excessive abduction makes the affected leg appear too long, whereas excessive adduction makes the affected leg appear too short; in either case the client has limited locomotion and walks with an obvious limp. Flexion contractures result in lordosis when the person is standing. Internal and external rotation contractures cause an unacceptable, unbalanced gait (Bilger and Greene, 1973).

KNEE

A primary function of the knee is stability, which is achieved by range of joint motion, ligaments, and muscles. However, the knees cannot remain stable under weight-bearing conditions unless there is adequate quadriceps power, which maintains the knee in full extension. Range of joint motion exercises should include pulling the knee into full extension.

A stiff knee can result in serious disability, the degree of which depends on the position in which the knee is stiffened. If the knee is fixed in full extension, the person must sit with leg thrust straight out in front. When the knee is flexed, the person limps while walking. The greater the flexion, the greater the limp. Complete flexion contractures prevent the person from walking without a walker or crutches.

If it is impossible to prevent knee stiffness, the nurse should try to ensure that the knee becomes fixed in a position of slight flexion, 10 to 20 degrees. This permits walking without an excessive limp or sitting without excessive forward thrust of the leg at the knee (Bilger and Greene, 1973).

ANKLE AND FOOT

During walking, movement of the ankle joint is minimal; however, the joint must be stabilized and able to bear weight or the person will fall. If joint mobility is diminished, the nurse should maintain the joint in a position in which walking can be carried out with a forward rolling motion from the heel onto the forefoot.

When the person relaxes as in sleep or in a coma, the foot relaxes and assumes a position of plantar flexion. This results from relaxation of the gastrocnemius and soleus muscles, which maintain dorsiflexion. If the foot remains in plantar flexion without support, these two muscles shorten and the dorsiflexion muscles try to compensate by overstretching. As a result the foot becomes fixed in plantar flexion (footdrop), which impairs the client's ability to walk.

Inversion and eversion must also be avoided in order to allow the foot to rest flat on the floor (see Table 30-9). The foot must be flat on the floor to allow weight bearing and proper walking.

TOES

Excessive flexion of the toes results in a clawing. When this is a permanent deformity, the foot is unable to rest flat on the floor. Flexion contractures are the most common foot deformity associated with reduced joint mobility.

Adequate range of joint motion gives the client the necessary mobility to carry out activities of daily living, to exercise, and to engage in relaxing activities. In addition, adequate range of motion in the lower extremities allows the client to walk.

Walking

In the normal walking posture the head is erect, the cervical, thoracic, and lumbar vertebrae are aligned, the hips and knees have appropriate flexion, and the arms swing freely in alternation with the legs. Illness or trauma can reduce the person's activity tolerance so that assistance in walking is required. In addition, temporary or permanent damage to the musculoskeletal and nervous systems may necessitate use of a mechanical device for walking.

ASSISTING A CLIENT TO WALK

Like the other procedures presented in this section, assisting the client to walk requires preparation. First, the nurse assesses the client's activity tolerance, strength, presence of pain, coordination, and balance to determine the exact type of assistance needed. For example, a 26-year-old woman who is 12 hours postpartum may need one nurse to help her walk. This assistance is usually a precaution in case the new mother becomes dizzy or unsteady on her feet. A 52-year-old man 1 day after an appendectomy may require two nurses. Older clients, clients with a more severe illness or who have had surgery, and heavy clients usually require walking assistance from two people.

Second, the nurse explains how far the client should try to walk, who is going to help, when the walk will take place, and why walking is important. In addition, the nurse and client determine how much independence the client can assume.

Third, the nurse double-checks the environment to be sure there are no obstacles in the client's path—that the chairs, over-the-bed table, and wheelchair are out of the way so the client does not need to expend any energy walking an obstacle course.

Fourth, before the client begins to walk, resting points should be established in case the client's activity tolerance is less than was estimated or the client becomes dizzy. When a client has been in bed for a day or two, a 10-foot distance from the bed to the bathroom can rapidly drain his energy.

Fifth, the client should be assisted to a position of sitting at the side of the bed and should rest for 1 to 2 minutes before standing up. Likewise, after standing, the client should remain stationary for a minute or two before moving. It is important to allow the client to stabilize before walking; if the client becomes dizzy, the bed is still nearby and the nurse can quickly ease him back to bed. The longer the period of immobility the greater the physiological changes, especially the changes in circulation; when the person stands, blood pressure may drop (see Chapter 31). Various methods are used for walking a client. The next sections describe one- and two-nurse methods.

ONE NURSE. The nurse should provide support at the waist so the client's center of gravity remains midline. This can be achieved when the nurse places both hands at the client's waist or uses a walking belt. A walking belt is a leather belt that encircles the client's waist and has handles attached for the nurse to hold while the client walks. Clients should not lean to one side because their center of gravity is no longer midline, which distorts their balance, and their risk of falling is increased.

The client who at any point appears unsteady or complains of dizziness should be returned to bed or a chair, whichever is closer. If the client faints or begins to fall, the nurse should assume a wide base of support with one foot in front of the other, thus supporting the client's body weight. Then the nurse gently lowers the client to the floor, protecting the head. Although lowering a client to the floor is not difficult, the student should practice this technique with a friend or classmate before attempting it in a clinical setting.

Occasionally clients with hemiplegia (one-sided paralysis) or hemiparesis (one-sided weakness) need assistance to walk. The nurse always stands on the client's affected side and supports the client by holding her arm around the client's waist and her other arm around the inferior aspect of the client's upper arm so that the nurse's hand is supporting the client's axilla. Providing support by holding the client's arm is incorrect because, if the client should faint or fall, the nurse cannot easily support his weight and lower him to the floor. In addition, if the client falls with the nurse holding his arm, his shoulder joint may be dislocated.

A nurse who has even the slightest doubt about her strength and ability to ambulate a client alone should request help. The two-nurse method helps to distribute the client's weight evenly.

TWO NURSES. The nurses stand on either side of the client. Each nurse's near arm is around the client's waist, and her other arm is around the inferior aspect of the client's arm so that both nurses' hands are supporting the client's axillae.

A second method requires that the nurses and client be of similar height. The nurses stand on either side of the client with their near arms slipped under the client's arms toward the back. The nurses then grasp each other's arms. The client's arms are placed over the nurses' shoulders, and the nurses stabilize the client's hands with their free hands. This technique is very effective with weakened or heavy clients.

MECHANICAL DEVICES USED FOR WALKING

Walkers are extremely light, movable devices, about waist high, made of metal tubing. They have four widely placed, sturdy legs. The client holds the handgrips on the upper bars, takes a step, moves the walker forward, and takes another step (Fig. 30-17).

Canes are lightweight, easily movable devices about waist high, made of wood or metal. Two common types of canes are the single straight-legged cane and the quad cane (Fig. 30-18). The single straight-legged cane is more common and is used to support and balance a client with decreased leg strength. This cane should be kept on the stronger side of the body. First, for maximum support when walking, the client places the cane forward 15 to 25 cm (6 to 10 inches), keeping body weight on both legs. Second, the weaker leg is moved forward to the cane so the body weight is divided between the cane and the stronger leg. Third, the stronger leg is advanced past the cane so the weaker leg and the body weight are supported by the cane and weaker leg. During walking, the client continually repeats these three steps. The client must be taught that two points of support, such as both feet or one foot and the cane, are present at all times.

The quad cane provides the most support and is used when there is partial or complete leg paralysis or some hemiplegia. The same three steps used with the straight-legged cane are taught to the client.

Crutches are often needed to increase a client's mobility. The use of crutches may be temporary such as

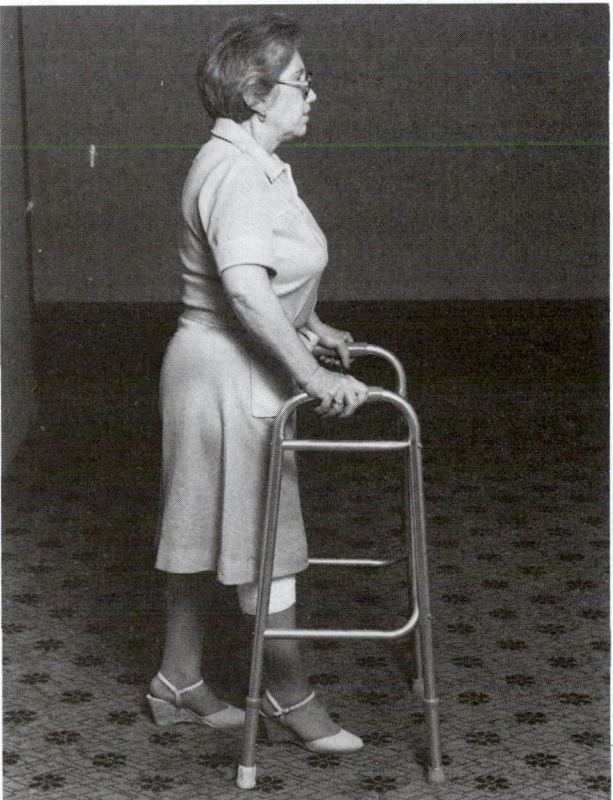

Fig. 30-17 Client using a walker.

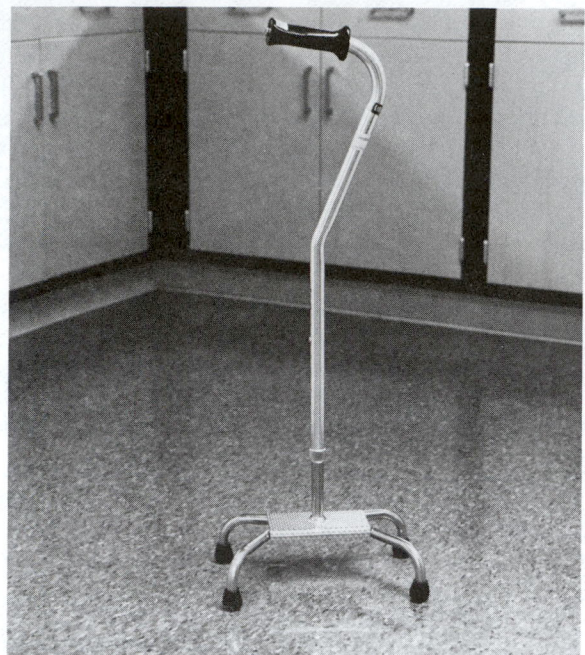

Fig. 30-18 Quad cane.

following ligament damage to the knee. Crutches may be needed permanently, for example, by the client with paralysis of the lower extremities. A crutch is a wooden or metal staff. There are two types of crutches, the double adjustable Lofstrand or forearm crutch (Fig. 30-19), and the axillary wooden crutch (used in Figs. 30-20 through 30-29). The forearm crutch has a handgrip and a metal band that fits around the client's forearm. Both the metal band and the handgrip are adjusted to fit the client's height. The axillary crutch has a padded curved surface at the top, which fits under the axilla. A handgrip in the form of a crossbar is held at the level of the palms to support the body. It is important that crutches be measured for the appropriate length and that clients be taught how to use their crutches safely, how to achieve a stable gait, how to ascend and descend stairs, and how to rise from a sitting position.

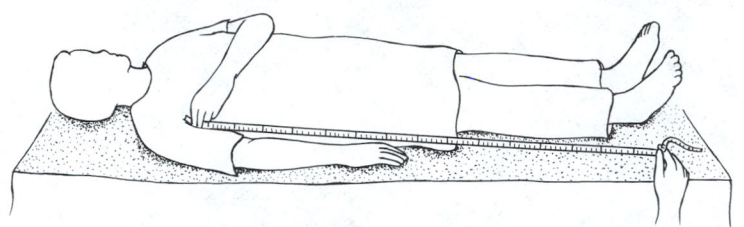

Fig. 30-20 Measuring crutch length.

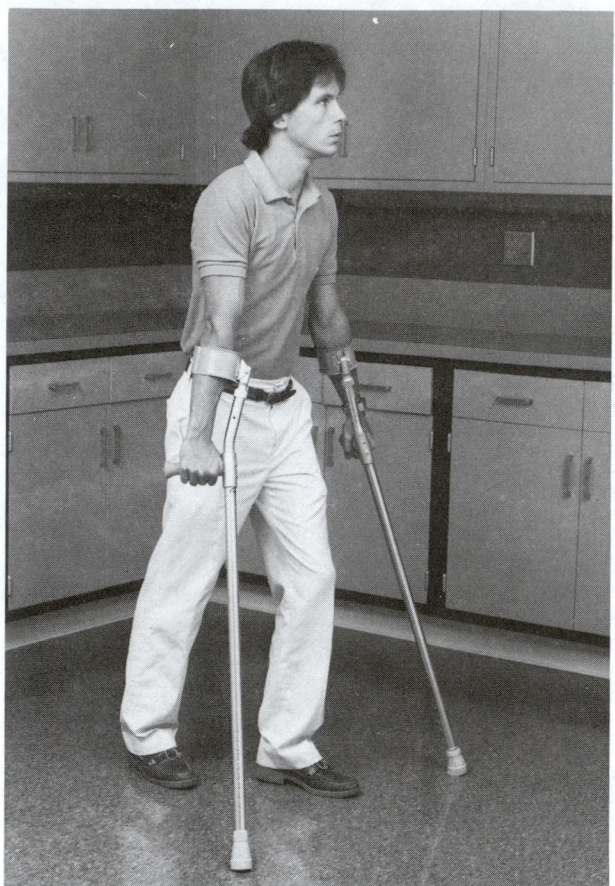

Fig. 30-19 Double adjustable Lofstrand or forearm crutch.

MEASURING FOR CRUTCHES. The axillary crutch is the more common crutch used. Measurements include three areas: the client's height, the angle of elbow flexion, and the distance between the crutch pad and the axilla. When crutches are fitted, the length of the crutch should be from three to four finger widths from the axilla to a point 15 cm (6 inches) lateral to the client's heel (Sine et al., 1981) (Fig. 30-20).

It is important that the handgrips be positioned so the client's body weight is not supported by the axillae. Pressure on the axillae increases risk to underlying nerves, which could result in partial paralysis of the arm. Correct position of the handgrips is determined with the client upright, supporting his weight by the handgrips with his elbows slightly flexed (20 to 25 degrees). Elbow flexion is verified with a goniometer (Fig. 30-21). When the height and placement of the handgrips have been determined, the nurse should again verify that the distance between the crutch pad and the client's axilla is three to four finger widths (Fig. 30-22).

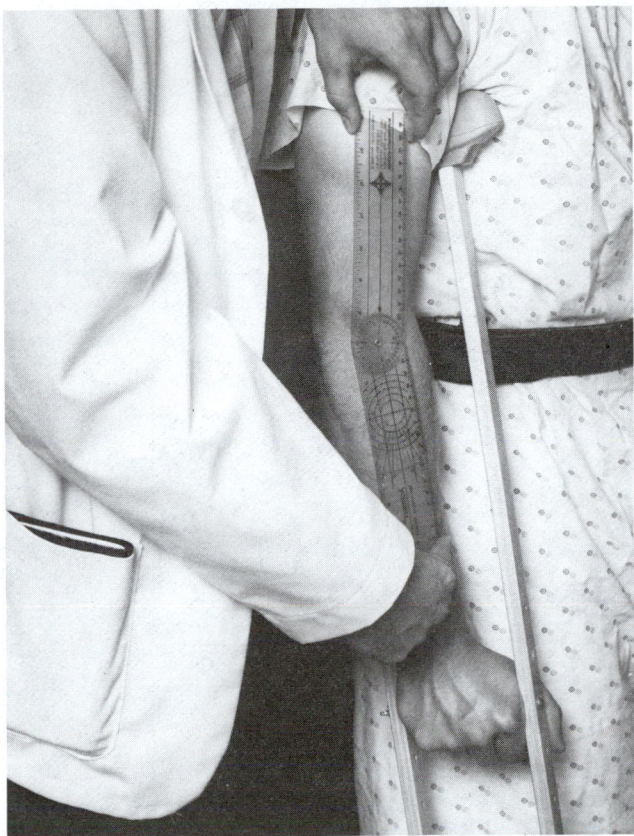

Fig. 30-21 Verifying correct elbow flexion with crutches. Measurement is obtained with a goniometer.

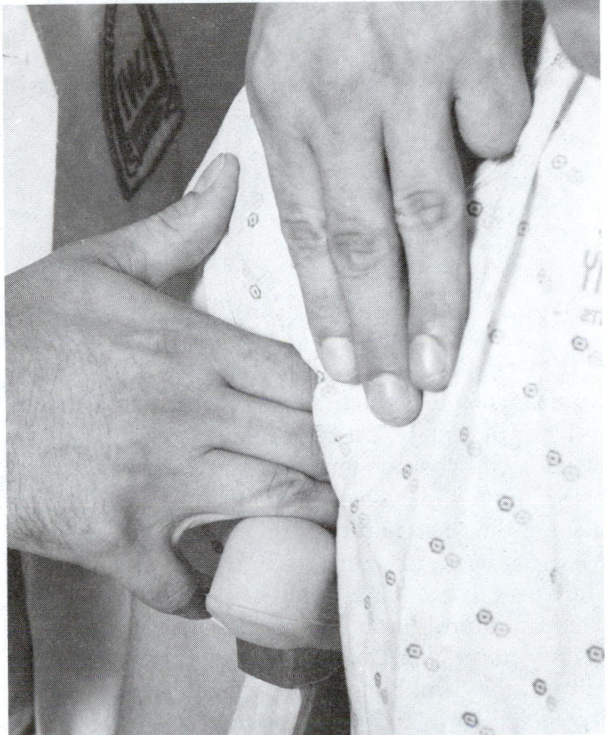

Fig. 30-22 Verifying correct distance between crutch pads and axilla.

CRUTCH SAFETY. Before being allowed to walk independently with crutches, the client should be taught the following safety guidelines:

1. Clients with axillary crutches must be aware of the dangers of pressure on the axilla. Therefore they must not use crutches that fit improperly or lean on their crutches to support their body weight.
2. Crutch-dependent clients should be taught to inspect the crutch tips routinely. The rubber tips should be securely attached to the crutches. When the tips are worn, they should be replaced immediately. Rubber crutch tips increase surface friction and prevent the crutches from slipping.
3. Crutch tips should remain dry. If the tips become wet, the client should dry them off. Water decreases surface friction and increases the risk that the crutches will slip.
4. The structure of the crutches should also be routinely inspected. Cracks in a wooden crutch decrease the crutch's ability to support the client's

weight. Bends in aluminum crutches can alter the client's body alignment, increasing the risk of further damage to the musculoskeletal system.
5. Clients should be given a list of medical suppliers in their community. This allows the clients to obtain repairs, new rubber tips, handgrips, and crutch pads.
6. Crutch-dependent clients should always have spare crutches and tips on hand.

CRUTCH GAIT. The crutch gait is the gait assumed by a person on crutches by alternately bearing weight on one or both legs and on the crutches. The gait selected by the nurse is determined by her assessment of the client's physical and functional abilities and the disease or injury that resulted in the need for crutches. This section summarizes the basic crutch stance and the four standard gaits: four-point alternating gait, three-point alternating gait, two-point gait, and swing-through gait.

The basic crutch stance is the *tripod position,*

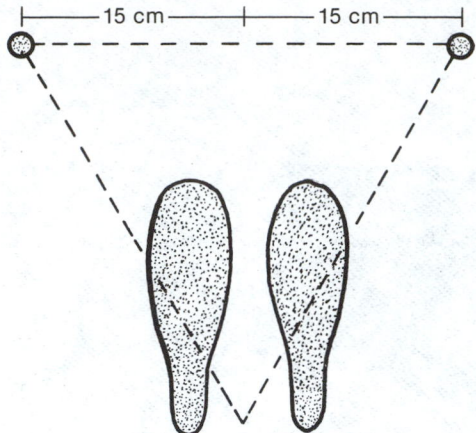

Fig. 30-23 Tripod position, the basic crutch stance.

formed when the crutches are placed 15 cm (6 inches) in front of and 15 cm to the side of each foot (Fig. 30-23). This position improves the client's balance by providing a wider base of support. The body alignment of the client in the tripod position includes erect head and neck, straight vertebrae, and extended hips and knees. No weight should be borne by the axillae. The tripod position is used before crutch walking.

Four-point alternating or *four-point gait* gives stability to the client but requires weight bearing on both legs. Each leg is moved alternately with each crutch so that three points of support are on the floor at all times (Fig. 30-24).

Three-point alternating or *three-point gait* requires the client to bear all of the weight on one foot. In a three-point gait, weight is borne on the uninvolved leg (Fig. 30-25, *A*), then on both crutches (Fig. 30-25, *B*), and the sequence is repeated. The affected leg does not touch the ground during the early phase of the three-point gait. Gradually the client progresses to touchdown and full weight bearing on the affected leg.

The *two-point gait* requires at least partial weight bearing on each foot (Fig. 30-26). The client moves each crutch at the same time as the opposing leg, so the crutch movements are similar to arm motion during normal walking.

The *swing-through* or *swing-to gait* is frequently used by paraplegics who wear weight-supporting braces on their legs. With weight placed on the supported legs, the client places the crutches one stride in front and then swings to or through the cruches while they support the client's weight.

CRUTCH WALKING ON STAIRS. When ascending stairs on crutches, the client usually uses a modified three-point gait (Fig. 30-27). First the client stands at the bottom of the stairs and transfers the body weight

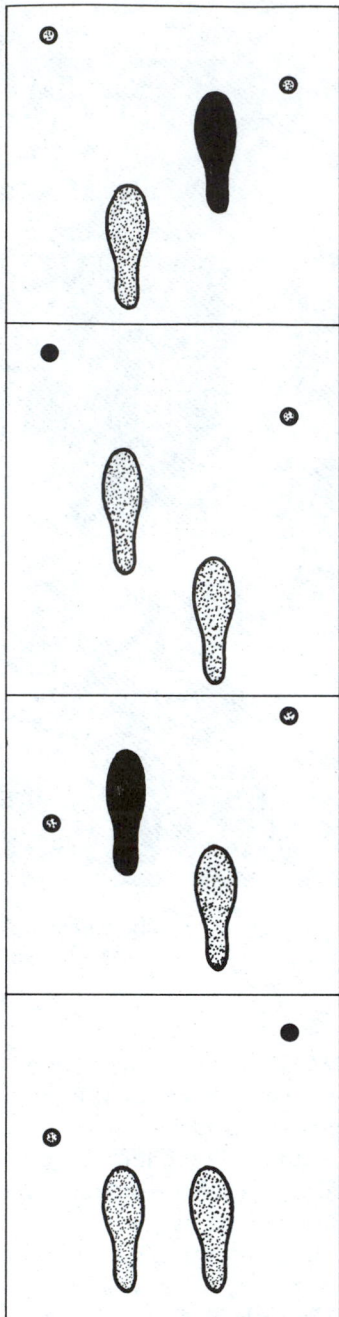

Fig. 30-24 Four-point alternating gait.

to the crutches. Second, the unaffected leg is advanced between the crutches to the stairs. The client then shifts weight from the crutches to the unaffected leg. Last, the client aligns both crutches on the stairs. This sequence is repeated until the person reaches the top of the stairs.

To descend the stairs (Fig. 30-28), a three-phase sequence is also used. First, the client transfers body weight to the unaffected leg. Second, the crutches are placed on the stair and the client begins to transfer

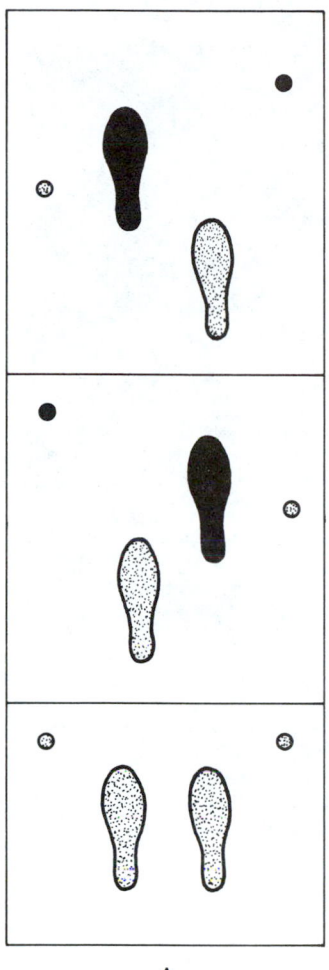

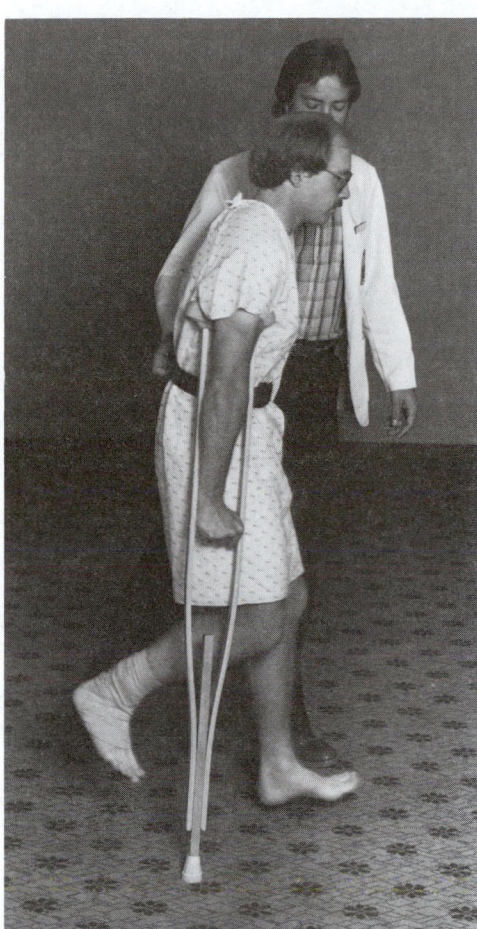

A   B

Fig. 30-25 **A,** Three-point alternating gait, with weight borne on the uninvolved leg. Dot indicates unaffected leg. **B,** Weight borne on both crutches.

body weight to the crutches, moving the affected leg forward. Last, the unaffected leg is moved to the stairs with the crutches. Again, the client repeats the sequence until reaching the bottom of the stairs.

Since in most cases clients will need to use crutches for some time, they should be adequately taught to use crutches on stairs before discharge. This instruction applies to all crutch-dependent clients, not only those who have stairs in their homes.

SITTING IN A CHAIR WITH CRUTCHES. As with crutch walking and crutch walking up and down stairs, the procedure for sitting in a chair involves phases and requires the client to transfer weight. First, the client gets positioned at the center front of the chair with the posterior aspect of the legs touching the chair. Second, the client holds both crutches in the hand opposite the affected leg. If both legs are affected, as with a paraplegic who wears weight-supporting braces, the crutches are held in the hand on the client's stronger side. With both crutches in one hand the client supports body weight on the unaffected leg and crutches (Fig. 30-29). While still holding the crutches, the client grasps the arm of the chair

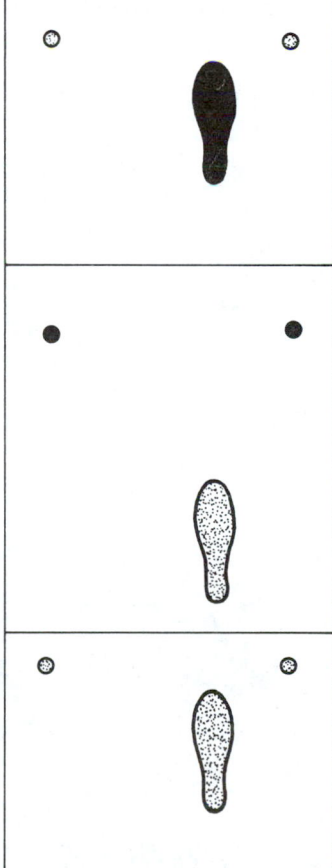

Fig. 30-26 Two-point gait.

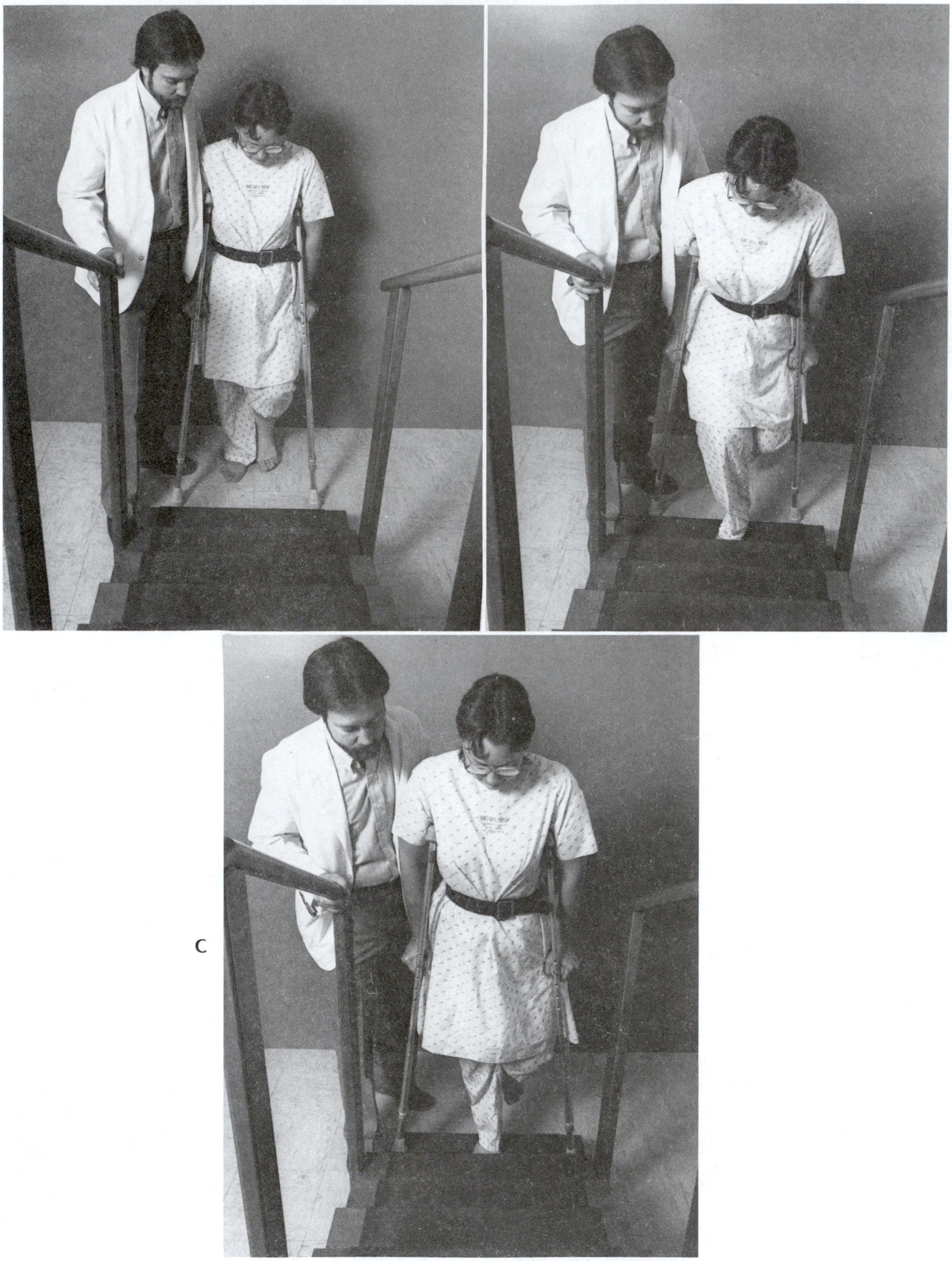

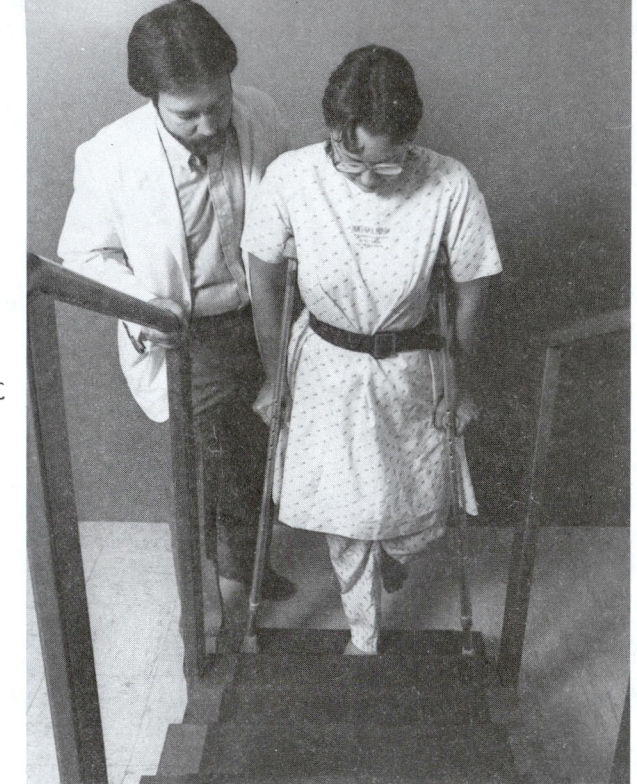

Fig. 30-27 Ascending stairs. **A,** Weight is placed on crutches. **B,** Weight is transferred from crutches to unaffected leg on the stairs. **C,** Crutches are aligned with unaffected leg on the stairs.

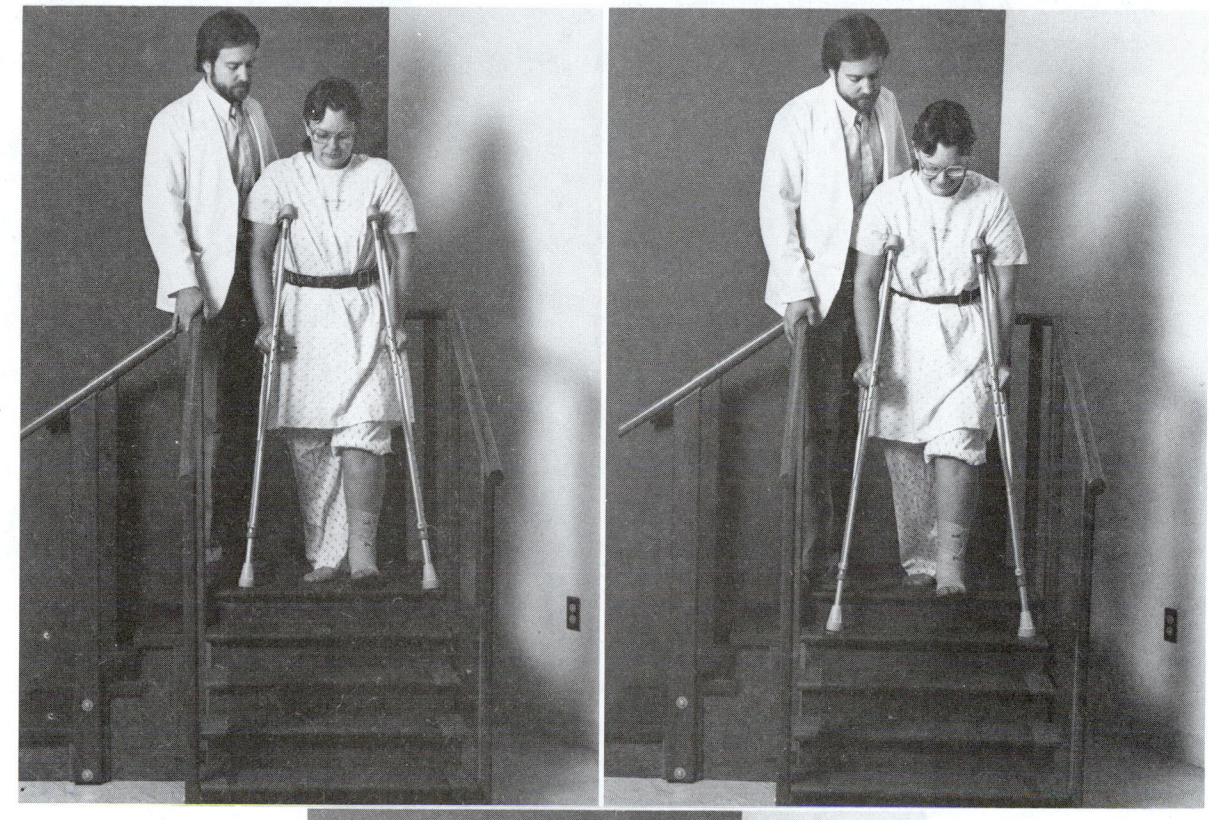

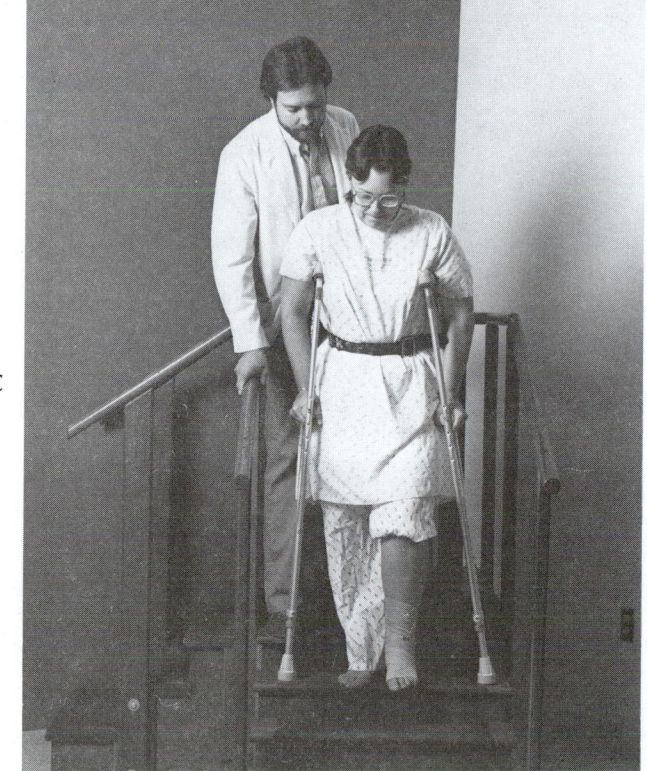

Fig. 30-28 Descending stairs. **A,** Body weight on unaffected leg. **B,** Body weight transferred to crutches. **C,** Unaffected leg aligned on stairs with crutches.

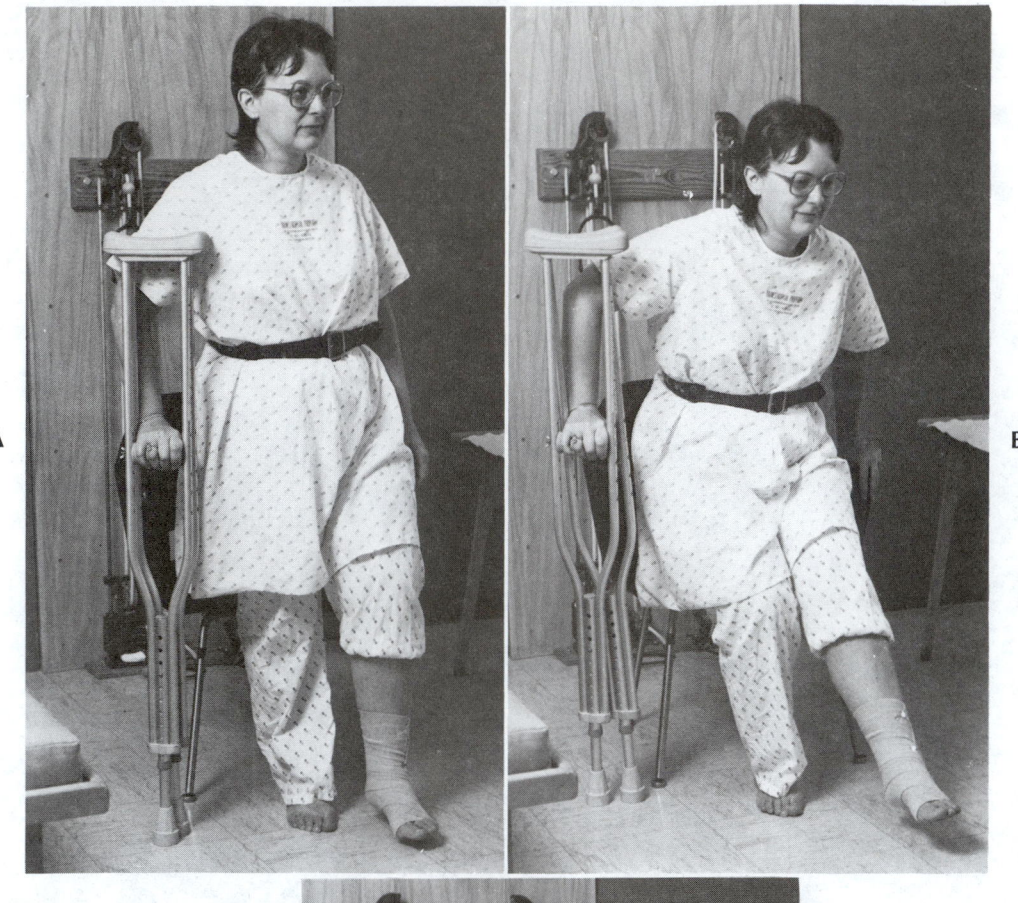

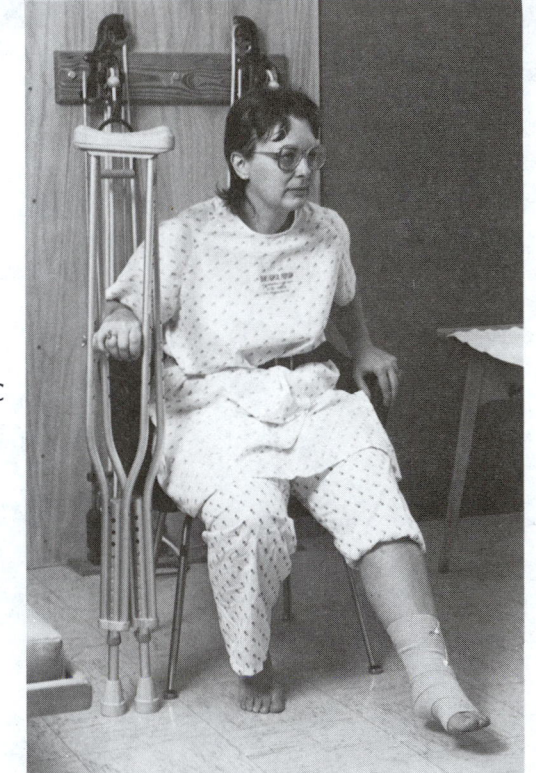

Fig. 30-29 Sitting in a chair. **A,** Both crutches are held by one hand. Client transfers her weight to the crutches and the unaffected leg. **B,** Client grasps arm of the chair with free hand and begins to lower herself into the chair. **C,** Client completely lowers herself into the chair.

with the remaining hand and lowers the body into the chair. To stand, the procedure is reversed, and the client when fully erect should assume the tripod position before beginning to walk.

■ ■ ■ ■ ■

The interventions designed to maintain the client's body alignment and joint mobility use the principles of body mechanics. The nurse also uses body mechanics to avoid self-injury when lifting and transfering clients. When positioning a client, the nurse employs principles of body mechanics to reduce or prevent injury to the client's musculoskeletal system, since the nurse is responsible for protecting clients from damage caused by limitation of movement. This and other hazards of immobility are discussed in Chapter 31.

Evaluation

The evaluation of nursing care for clients with altered body alignment or joint mobility is easily presented in one section because nursing strategies to improve body alignment usually also improve joint mobility and vice versa.

The desired outcome is the restoration of normal body alignment and joint mobility. If that is unrealistic, the nurse measures the success of nursing care against the client's achievement of his maximal joint mobility and body alignment. Successful outcomes can include the following:

1. Improved body alignment and joint mobility
2. Normal muscle tone
3. Absence of muscle strain
4. Absence of joint contracture or deformities
5. No skin breakdown; intact pressure points
6. Increased activity level
7. Increased level of independence in completing activities of daily living

Maintaining good body alignment and joint mobility increases a client's level of independence and overall mobility. A client with inadequate joint mobility must receive assistance to carry out activities of daily living. The best approach to problems with body alignment and joint mobility is prevention, which begins early in the health care plan.

Summary

The nurse incorporates knowledge of the physiology of movement and the principles of body mechanics to transfer and position clients safely, as well as to assist clients to use walkers and crutches safely. Through the use of the nursing process, the nurse develops a nursing care plan for clients with potential or actual alterations in body alignment. The alteration may be temporary, as in the case of a pregnant woman, or permanent, as in the case of the client with a cerebrovascular accident (stroke).

Correct body mechanics protects the nurse and the client from injuries to the musculoskeletal system. For example, by employing the principles of body mechanics the nurse can transfer a client from bed to chair without self-injury or injury to the client.

Occasionally, clients with impaired body alignment have restricted mobility or are totally immobilized. Immobilization affects all aspects of the client's life. The next chapter describes the hazards of immobility and teaches the nursing student to apply the principles of body mechanics while reducing these hazards.

KEY CONCEPTS

✓The term "body mechanics" describes the coordinated efforts of the musculoskeletal and nervous systems as the person moves, lifts, bends, assumes a standing, sitting, or lying position, and completes activities of daily living.

✓Coordinated body movement requires the integrated functioning of the skeletal system, skeletal muscles, and nervous system.

✓The skeleton provides the bony support structure for movement, for the attachment of ligaments and muscles, for protection of vital organs, for some of the regulation of calcium, and for red blood cell production.

✓The nervous system provides the initiation and voluntary control of movement.

✓A joint is a connection between bones and can be one of four types: synostotic, cartilaginous, fibrous, or synovial.

✓ Ligaments bind joints together and connect bones and cartilages.

✓ Tendons connect muscle to bone.

✓ Cartilage is nonvascular, supportive connective tissue located chiefly in the joints and in the thorax, trachea, larynx, nose, and ear.

✓ Muscle contraction is the result of an electrochemical impulse that is transmitted from the nerve to the muscle; two types of contraction are possible, isotonic and isometric.

✓ Muscles primarily associated with movement are located near the skeletal region where movement results from leverage, which is characteristic of the movements of the upper extremities.

✓ Muscles primarily associated with posture are located in the lower extremities, the trunk, the neck, and the back.

✓ Coordination and regulation of different muscle groups depend on muscle tone and the activity of antagonistic, synergistic, and antigravity muscles.

✓ The motor strip in the cerebral cortex controls voluntary movement.

✓ The transfer of an impulse from the nerve fiber to a muscle requires a neurotransmitter.

✓ Proprioceptors are nerve endings, in muscles, tendons, and joints, that respond to stimuli originating from within the body regarding spatial position or movement.

✓ Balance is assisted through nervous system control by the cerebellum and inner ear.

✓ Body alignment is the condition of the joints, tendons, ligaments, and muscles in various body positions.

✓ Body balance is achieved when there is a wide base of support, the center of gravity falls within the base of support, and a vertical line falls from the center of gravity through the base of support.

✓ Coordinated body movement can be influenced by physical forces of weight, friction, and leverage.

✓ Developmental stages influence body alignment and mobility; the greatest impact of physiological changes on the musculoskeletal system is observed in children and older adults.

✓ Pathological conditions that affect body alignment and mobility include postural abnormalities, altered bone formation, altered joint mobility, impaired muscle development, damage to the central nervous system, and direct trauma to the musculoskeletal system.

✓ The assessment of a client's body alignment determines normal physiological changes and deviations in alignment; allows the client to observe posture; identifies learning needs of the client as well as the presence of trauma, damage, or dysfunction; and provides other information concerning a client's body alignment.

✓ Assessment of a client's mobility enables the nurse to determine the client's coordination, balance, and ability to complete activities of daily living and makes it possible to evaluate or plan the client's exercise program.

✓ Range of joint motion is the maximal movement possible at a joint in one of the three planes of the body: sagittal, frontal, and transverse.

KEY CONCEPTS, *cont'd*

✓ Assessing gait allows the nurse to draw some conclusions about the client's balance, posture, and ability to walk without assistance.

✓ The nurse's assessment of the client's energy level includes the physiological effects of exercise and the client's activity tolerance.

✓ Activity tolerance is affected by developmental and pathological changes.

✓ When lifting or transferring a client, the nurse considers the basic four principles of lifting: position of weight, height of object, body position, and maximal weight.

✓ Clients with impaired body alignment require nursing interventions to maintain them in the supported Fowler's, supine, prone, side-lying, and Sims' positions.

✓ Transfer techniques require the nurse to use correct body mechanics to move the client in bed, from bed to chair, and from bed to stretcher.

✓ Range of joint motion exercises include one or all of the body joints.

✓ The nurse can cup the joint to be moved, hold the distal and proximal areas adjacent to the joint, or cradle the distal portion of the extremity.

✓ Interventions for a client with impaired joint mobility also entail helping the client to walk with one or two nurses.

✓ Mechanical devices to promote walking include canes and walkers, which require specific nursing interventions.

REFERENCES

Bilger, A.J., and Greene, E.H.: Winger's protective body mechanics: a manual for nurses, New York, 1973, Springer Publishing Co., Inc.

Daniels, L., and Worthingham, C.: Therapeutic exercise for body alignment and function, ed. 2, Philadelphia, 1977, W.B. Saunders Co.

Gordon, M.: Assessing activity tolerance, Am. J. Nurs. 76:72, 1976.

Groër, M.W., and Shekleton, M.E.: Basic pathophysiology: a conceptual approach, ed. 2, St. Louis, 1983, The C.V. Mosby Co.

Hudson, M.F.: Safeguard your elderly patient's health through accurate physical assessment, Nursing 83 (Can. ed.) 13(11):58, 1983.

Owens, B.D.: How to avoid that aching back, Am. J. Nurs. 80:984, 1980.

Sine, R.D., et al.: Basic rehabilitation techniques: a self-instructional guide, ed. 2, Rockville, Md., 1981, Aspen Systems Corp.

Strand, F.L.: Physiology: a regulary systems approach, New York, 1978, Macmillan, Inc.

ADDITIONAL READINGS

Rantz, M.F., and Courtial, D.: Lifting, moving, and transferring patients, ed. 2, St. Louis, 1981, The C.V. Mosby Co.

Winters, M.: Protected body mechanics in daily life and nursing, Philadelphia, 1952, W.B. Saunders Co.

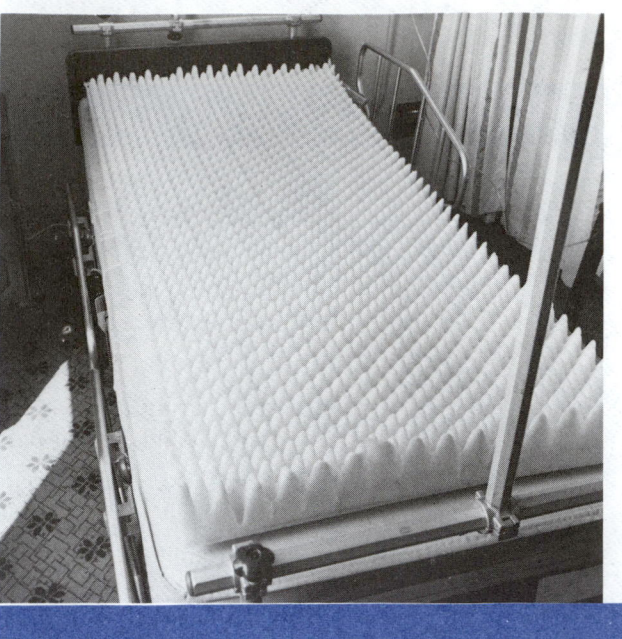

OBJECTIVES

Mastery of content in this chapter will enable the student to:

- Define the terms in the glossary.
- Describe mobility and immobility.
- Discuss the benefits and hazards of bed rest.
- Identify changes in metabolic rate associated with immobility.
- Describe altered protein metabolism.
- Describe fluid changes associated with immobility.
- Describe the alterations in exchange of nutrients associated with immobility.
- Describe the alterations in gastrointestinal functioning associated with immobility.
- Describe the alterations in respiratory function associated with immobility.
- Discuss the mechanism of orthostatic hypotension.
- Describe how immobilization increases cardiac workload.
- Describe the mechanism of thrombus formation.
- Describe the musculoskeletal changes associated with immobility.
- List the classes of decubitus ulcers.
- Discuss the factors that contribute to decubitus ulcer formation.
- Discuss the effects of immobilization on urinary and bowel elimination.
- Describe the psychosocial effects of immobilization.
- Describe the developmental effects of immobilization.
- Complete a nursing assessment of an immobilized client.
- List at least 15 nursing diagnoses associated with immobility.
- Develop a nursing care plan for an immobilized client.
- List appropriate nursing interventions for an immobilized client.
- State evaluation criteria for the immobilized client.

GLOSSARY

anemia   Disorder characterized by a decrease in hemoglobin in the blood.

bed rest   Placement of the client in bed for therapeutic reasons for a prescribed period.

bone resorption   Destruction of bone cells and release of calcium into the blood.

decubitus ulcer   Inflammation, sore, or ulcer in the skin over a bony prominence.

depression   Abdominal emotional state characterized by exaggerated or inappropriate feelings of sadness, melancholy, dejection, worthlessness, emptiness, and hopelessness.

immobility   Inability to move about freely, caused by any condition in which movement is impaired or therapeutically restricted.

ischemia   Decreased blood supply to a body part, such as skin tissue, or to an organ, such as the heart.

negative nitrogen balance   Condition occurring when the body excretes more nitrogen than it takes in.

renal calculus   Calcium stone in the renal pelvis.

thrombus   Accumulation of platelets, fibrin, clotting factors, and the cellular elements of the blood attached to the interior wall of a vein or artery, sometimes occluding the lumen of the vessel.

31 | *Hazards of Immobility*

hysical mobility is important in our society. A client's work, social interaction, development, and relaxation depend on his ability to move his body parts freely. In addition, movement of body parts or the entire body is essential for maintenance of the client's total well-being, including physiological, psychosocial, and developmental dimensions.

Movement serves many purposes, such as expression of an emotion with a nonverbal gesture, self-defense, satisfaction of basic needs, the activities of daily living, and recreational activities. To maintain normal physical mobility, the nervous, muscular, and skeletal systems of the body must be intact and functioning (see Chapter 30).

When a body part or the entire body is immobilized for a time, secondary disabilities may develop in one or several body systems. The greater the degree of immobility and the longer the immobilization, the greater is the risk for the development of disabilities.

The body's regulation of movement is discussed in Chapter 30. Immobility is described separately here because the many hazards to the immobilized or partially immobilized client require a different and potentially more extensive nursing care plan.

Changes in the client's mobility may result from many types of health problems. Clients with certain illnesses or injuries become immobilized but return to mobility with rehabilitation. Other clients, such as those with spinal cord injuries and certain degenerative conditions such as multiple sclerosis, may experience a sudden or gradual shift from mobility to long-term or permanent immobility. A third group of clients are not actually immobilized by an illness or injury but are placed on bed rest or restricted ambulation for therapeutic reasons. All these groups face similar hazards related to immobility.

Both immobility and the return of mobility influence the client's physiological, psychosocial, and developmental dimensions. The nurse uses the nursing process to meet the client's needs in all dimensions related to altered mobility. Commonly used procedures to reduce the hazards of immobility are presented in detail in this chapter.

Mobility

Mobility is a person's ability to move about freely. Mobility is often essential to the client's perception of his health. For example, a client whose left leg is immobilized in a cast may be unable to carry out the activities of daily living independently and as a result may view himself as ill. Mobility and immobility are best understood as the endpoints of a continuum, with many degrees of partial immobility in between.

Complete Mobility

Complete, unrestricted mobility requires voluntary motor and complete sensory control of all body regions. Nurses in most health care settings see completely mobile clients, including women who have had an uncomplicated normal delivery of a newborn, many preoperative clients, and clients admitted for diagnostic tests. Other clients are capable of mobility but have been placed on bed rest because of an illness such as a myocardial infarction. These clients can develop health problems as a consequence of their bed rest.

Complete mobility has many benefits for the client's physiological and psychosocial well-being. Complete mobility offers the client an opportunity to achieve his needs and goals independently and to maintain social interaction and usual roles.

Partial Mobility

Clients who are partially mobile usually have a motor or sensory alteration in a region of the body or a therapeutic restriction. For example, the client with a broken leg has restricted mobility because of a cast or traction. A paraplegic immobilized in a wheelchair as a result of a spinal cord injury may maintain independence but has lost mobility of his lower extremities because of the loss of motor and sensory control.

A partial loss of mobility may be temporary or permanent. Temporary losses may result from reversible trauma to the musculoskeletal system such as joint dislocations, fractured bones, or sprains. Permanent losses of mobility are usually caused by irreversible neurological impairments, such as hemiplegia resulting from a cerebrovascular accident (stroke) or paraplegia resulting from a spinal cord injury. In addition, inflammatory processes such as poliomyelitis and Guillain-Barré syndrome can leave the client with a temporary or permanent impairment of mobility because the sensory and motor tracts of the nervous system are affected.

In some instances the restriction of mobility is beneficial for the client's recovery. This is particularly true with trauma to the musculoskeletal system. Immobilization of the affected area allows the extremity to heal in the proper alignment. With muscle sprains, immobilization reduces trauma and allows the muscles to heal. With trauma to the spinal cord, early immobilization prevents further neurological damage and preserves the client's remaining sensory and motor function.

The hazards associated with partial mobility depend on the degree and duration of immobilization. For example, a client whose fractured arm is set in a cast for 6 weeks may experience muscle weakness and a reduced ability to carry out activities of daily living. However, these hazards are temporary and disappear shortly after the client is able to move his arm again. In contrast, a client with a fractured femur who is placed in traction for a month is more susceptible to the hazards of immobility. The client with permanent partial loss of mobility is continually at risk for the hazards of immobility and needs to be taught early in his rehabilitation how to reduce these hazards.

Immobility

Immobility occurs when the client cannot move about freely because of any condition that impairs movement. Some clients move back and forth on the mobility-immobility continuum, but in other cases, as with an unconscious client, the client's immobility is absolute and continues for an indefinite period.

Four conditions may result in immobility. First, physical inactivity, such as bed rest, is manifested by a reduction in body movement. Second, physical restriction or limitation of movement, as by a cast, is manifested by an imposed reduction of movement. Third, restriction in changes in body position and posture results in a loss of the body's ability to adapt to such changes. For example, a client on prolonged bed rest may be unable to maintain his blood pressure when he sits up suddenly. Fourth, sensory deprivation causes a reduction in the stimulus to move and is manifested by even greater physical inactivity. For example, a client with hemiplegia does not perceive pressure in the region of paralysis and as a result does not change his body position to relieve the pressure (Spencer, Valbona, and Carter, 1965). The degree of a client's immobility depends on how many of these four conditions are present (Groër and Shekleton, 1983).

Another factor influencing the degree of immobility is the duration of the immobile state. For example, a client with a severed spinal cord has permanent immobility below the level of the trauma, whereas a client with torn ligaments in his knee experiences temporary immobility until the ligaments are repaired and healing occurs. Regardless of the cause, immobility has multiple negative effects on all body systems.

Bed Rest

Bed rest is an intervention in which the client is restricted to bed for therapeutic reasons for a prescribed period of time. Bed rest has different meanings among nurses, physicians, and other health care professionals. For example, one professional may assume that the order for bed rest allows the client bedside commode privileges, whereas another may expect the client to use a bedpan. Therefore nurses should clarify with physicians specifically what is meant by bed rest orders.

Objectives of Bed Rest

Bed rest can have several therapeutic advantages. First, it reduces physical activity and the oxygen needs of body tissues, which is beneficial for clients with recent myocardial infarction because the myocardium and body tissues do not compete for available oxygen. Bed rest also reduces pain and in some cases the need for large doses of analgesics. Allowing the newly postoperative client as much bed rest as possible will help to reduce incisional pain. The nurse should organize the postoperative client's care plan to provide for 1- to 2-hour periods of bed rest throughout the first few postoperative days. Even if the postoperative client is required to turn, cough, and deep breathe every 2 hours and walk from his bed to a chair (Chapter 47), he can still benefit from bed rest.

Bed rest allows ill or debilitated clients an opportunity to rest and in some instances regain their strength. Although febrile clients may be too weak or exhausted to sit in a chair, when the febrile state is over these clients can gradually tolerate more activity and require fewer periods of bed rest.

Finally, bed rest can benefit clients psychologically. Overworked and exhausted clients frequently require periods of uninterrupted rest, relaxation, and sleep.

Bed rest has physiological and emotional benefits only if the client finds it restful. Clients who are resistant to bed rest may actually expend more energy in fighting bed rest than they would if allowed to move from bed to chair. Therefore the nurse must continually assess and evaluate her client's physical and emotional responses to bed rest.

Clients with a wide variety of conditions are placed on bed rest. The box on the right lists conditions often requiring bed rest. The list is not all inclusive and does not apply to all clients with these conditions. However, clients with acute myocardial infarctions, neurological injuries, and extensive lower-extremity fractures are routinely placed on bed rest. The duration of bed rest depends on the illness or injury and the client's prior state of health.

Hazards of Bed Rest

The hazards associated with bed rest affect the client in all dimensions. A client's response to prolonged bed rest is influenced by psychosocial and developmental factors, prior physical and emotional health, the reason for bed rest, and the duration of bed rest.

Many clients on bed rest have intact motor and sensory tracts and can perceive pressure to the skin and muscles. As a result, they may be able to change position independently, and their skin may be less

---

Conditions Requiring Bed Rest

CARDIOVASCULAR CONDITIONS
- Acute myocardial infarction
- Postoperative cardiovascular surgery
- Congestive heart failure

NEUROLOGICAL CONDITIONS
- Head injuries
- Neurosurgery
- Spinal cord trauma
- Degenerative neurological conditions such as myasthenia gravis

MUSCULOSKELETAL CONDITIONS
- Muscle strains and sprains in lower extremities
- Torn ligaments in lower extremities
- Fracture in lower extremities

INFECTIOUS PROCESSES
- Hepatitis
- Glomerulonephritis

CANCER
- During chemotherapy
- During radiation
- Terminal phase

---

susceptible to the hazards of immobility than the skin of clients whose immobility results from other impairments and conditions. Nonetheless, clients on bed rest, like other immobile clients, must be continually assessed.

Response of the Client to Altered Mobility

The effects of immobility are systemic and functional and result from a lack of activity. No body system is immune to the effects of immobility. Experiments have shown that healthy people who are immobilized for a prolonged time receive the same effects as those whose immobility results from illness.

Frequently the effects of immobility occur gradually. The greater the extent and the longer the duration of immobility, the more pronounced are the consequences.

The boxed material on p. 762 lists the effects of immobility in all dimensions. This list is only a gen-

Effects of Immobility in all Dimensions

PHYSIOLOGICAL

- Metabolic
  - Fluid and electrolyte changes
  - Bone demineralization
  - Altered exchange of nutrients and gases
  - Altered gastrointestinal functioning
- Respiratory
  - Decreased lung expansion
  - Pooling of secretions
- Cardiovascular
  - Orthostatic hypotension
  - Increased cardiac workload
  - Thrombus formation
- Musculoskeletal
  - Decreased endurance
  - Decreased muscle mass
  - Atrophy
  - Decreased stability
  - Contracture formation
  - Osteoporosis
- Skin
  - Decubitus ulcer formation
- Elimination
  - Renal calculi
  - Stasis of urine
  - Kidney infection
  - Fecal impaction

PSYCHOSOCIAL

- Depression
- Behavioral changes
- Change in sleep-wake cycles
- Decreased coping abilities
- Decreased problem-solving abilities
- Decreased interest in surroundings
- Increased isolation
- Sensory deprivation

DEVELOPMENTAL

- Young
  - Retardation of developmental stages
- Elderly
  - Increased rate of dependence
  - Increased rate of loss of system functions

eralization, however, and does not apply to all clients in all situations. Immobility can affect different physiological systems simultaneously or separately. A client may not show any physiological effects of immobility whereas emotionally he appears depressed and intellectually he has decreased problem-solving abilities.

Physiological Responses

Each body system is at risk for impairments resulting from immobility. The severity of the impairment depends on the client's age and overall health and the degree of immobility. Elderly clients with chronic illness develop pronounced effects of immobility more quickly than younger clients. The following sections detail the effects of immobility on each body system.

METABOLIC CHANGES

Immobility disrupts normal metabolic equilibrium in the following ways: reduced metabolic rate, tissue atrophy and protein catabolism, fluid and electrolyte imbalances, bone demineralization, alterations in the exchange of nutrients, and gastrointestinal disturbances (Olson, 1967).

DECREASED METABOLIC RATE. Bed rest or reduced activity results in a decrease in the client's basal metabolic rate (BMR). The BMR is the amount of energy used in a unit of time by a fasting, resting subject to maintain vital functions.

The client's metabolic rate falls in response to the decreased energy requirement of the body cells, which is directly related to cellular oxygen demands. However, immobilized clients experiencing an infection may have an elevated metabolic rate because infection usually causes fever, which increases tissue oxygen requirements. In addition, immobilized clients with wounds often have an increased metabolic rate to promote wound healing. Febrile or traumatized immobilized clients commonly have tissue atrophy and protein catabolism, which further alter their metabolic equilibrium.

TISSUE ATROPHY AND PROTEIN CATABOLISM. During immobilization, anabolic processes are decreased and catabolic processes are increased. This alteration is further potentiated by fever or conditions that increase the body's metabolic demands.

Anabolic processes are constructive metabolic activities that convert simple substances into more complex compounds, as in the conversion of amino acids into muscle mass. *Catabolic processes* are metabolic activities that break down body structures to produce energy, as in the breakdown of protein stores to provide glucose for the body's energy requirements.

If the rate of catabolism exceeds anabolism for a prolonged time, the body excretes more nitrogen than it takes in and a state of negative nitrogen balance occurs. During periods of immobility, urinary excretion of nitrogen increases with the negative nitrogen balance. This increased nitrogen excretion has been shown to occur on the fifth or sixth day of immo-

Conditions Associated with Negative Nitrogen Balance in Immobilization

- Poor nutrition before immobilization
- Alcohol or drug abuse
- Preexisting gastrointestinal disorder
- Preexisting kidney disorder
- Trauma
- Burns
- Fever
- Cancer
- Infection in one or more body systems
- Coma
- Surgery
- Anorexia
- Restrictions on food-seeking activities, such as traction

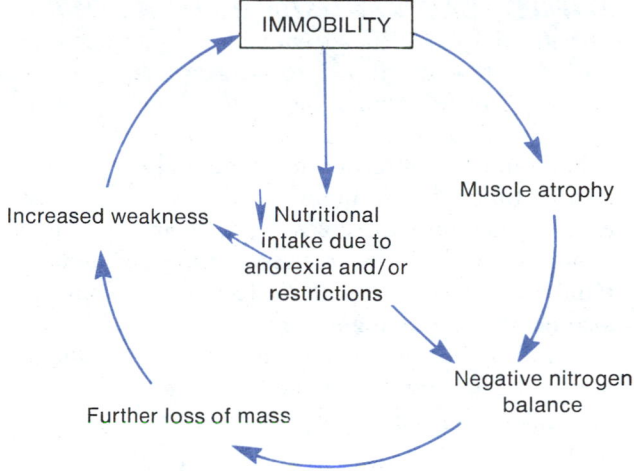

Fig. 31-1 Factors contributing to negative nitrogen balance associated with immobility.

From Groër, M.M., and Shekleton, M.E.: Basic pathophysiology: a conceptual approach, ed. 2, St. Louis, 1983, The C.V. Mosby Co.

bilization in healthy subjects (Groër and Shekleton, 1983). The nitrogen loss reflects the depletion of muscle mass. Certain pathological states and factors accelerate the rate of protein depletion and thus the development of negative nitrogen balance (see boxed material above).

Immobilized clients with trauma, fever, chronic illness, or poor nutritional status are at risk for further impairments in nutritional status and for negative nitrogen imbalance. Poor nutritional and negative nitrogen imbalance compound the muscle wasting and loss of strength that occur in immobility, thus resulting a vicious circle of impaired nutrition and immobility (Fig. 31-1).

The major consequence of negative nitrogen balance is an inadequate supply of nitrogen for protein synthesis, which promotes the rebuilding of muscle mass and wound healing. When body protein stores are catabolized, protein is excreted in the urine, leading to hypoalbuminemia, which in turn can result in fluid and electrolyte imbalances.

FLUID AND ELECTROLYTE IMBALANCES. When the body's protein stores become depleted, serum protein concentrations decrease, altering normal fluid pressures (see Chapter 43). In addition, fluid shifts from the intravascular to the interstitial compartments in the dependent areas of the body, resulting in edema. Venous stasis leads to an increase in hydrostatic pressure (Groër and Shekleton, 1983).

The immobilized client can develop any of the electrolyte disturbances described in Chapter 42. The type of imbalance present depends on the client's age, previous level of health, and renal function. Hypercalcemia resulting from bone demineralization is a common electrolyte disturbance in immobilized clients.

BONE DEMINERALIZATION. Bone demineralization occurs during immobilization, resulting in disuse osteoporosis. Bone demineralization is believed to be caused by two factors: decreased muscle activity and decreased weight-bearing activity. The immobilized client's muscle activity is limited, and there is no weight-bearing by the long bones in the lower extremities. With increased bone demineralization, calcium resorption causes calcium to enter the blood, resulting in hypercalcemia. Hypercalcemia and disuse osteoporosis affect the musculoskeletal and elimination systems.

ALTERATIONS IN EXCHANGE OF NUTRIENTS. Because of decreased protein and caloric intake and altered cardiovascular and respiratory functioning, the exchange of nutrients at the cellular level is decreased. The cells do not receive adequate glucose, amino acids, and fats or the necessary oxygen to carry out metabolic activities.

In addition, the pressure exerted on body tissues because of immobilization decreases local circulation to the tissues. If the pressure exists longer than 2 hours, tissues are completely deprived of needed nutrients and oxygen, and cells begin to die. This sequence of events contributes to the development of decubitus ulcers.

ALTERED GASTROINTESTINAL FUNCTIONING.
The inactivity associated with immobility decreases the rate at which food products are digested (see Chapter 38). Abdominal bloating, nausea, epigastric burning, and food regurgitation may result.

Food intake is a second factor that alters gastrointestinal function. An immobilized client may experience a pronounced decrease in food intake if he is unable to feed himself, unless nursing personnel or family members assist with his feeding. Appetite may also be affected by immobilization.

The changes in gastrointestinal functioning and the associated inactivity ultimately affect bowel elimination, often resulting in constipation or fecal impaction.

RESPIRATORY CHANGES

Respiratory problems occurring with prolonged immobility are due to four major factors: decreased hemoglobin, decreased lung expansion, generalized muscle weakness, and stasis of secretions.

The altered metabolism results in a decrease in the number of red blood cells, which contain hemoglobin. Hemoglobin transports oxygen from the alveoli in the lungs to the tissues (see Chapter 41). Decreased hemoglobin results in anemia. When anemia is present, the oxygen-carrying capacity of the blood is reduced and the amount of oxygen available to the tissues is decreased. Initially the body tries to adapt

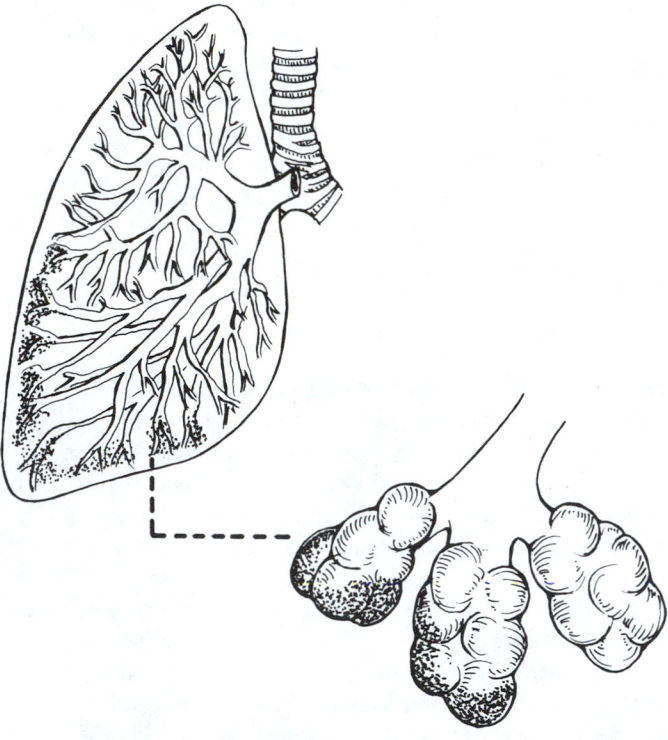

Fig. 31-2 Pooling of secretions in the dependent regions of the lungs in the supine position.

to the decreased hemoglobin by increasing the heart rate, but this is a short-term adaptive response and ultimately increases cardiac workload.

Immobilization also decreases lung expansion because of the pressure exerted by the mattress on the dependent lung region. Decreased lung expansion leads to a decrease in the rate of the exchange of respiratory gases between the lungs and the circulating blood volume and an increase in the pooling of respiratory secretions.

Normally, blood is oxygenated in the pulmonary circulation when it comes in contact with the oxygen-filled alveoli. The carbon dioxide waste product is carried by the blood to the lungs and is exhaled during expiration. When lung expansion is decreased, the surface area of expanded lung tissue through which the respiratory gases are exchanged is also decreased, resulting in a reduction of gas exchange. Therefore less oxygen is available for the blood. Carbon dioxide is retained and respiratory acidosis develops (see Chapter 42).

With decreased lung expansion and immobilization, secretions stagnate or pool in the dependent region of the lungs (Fig. 31-2). Such pooling does not occur in healthy subjects immobilized in experimental studies, but persons who smoke or who have a chronic lung condition or a cough are at risk for pooling. Pooling of secretions is dangerous for immobilized clients. The secretions allow bacteria to grow, which may lead to hypostatic bronchopneumonia.

The immobilized client with an underlying disease may also experience generalized muscle weakness, which ultimately affects the muscles of respiration and the muscles needed to cough. Lung expansion declines further and coughing becomes weaker. These two factors increase the distribution of mucus around the bronchi, particularly when the client is in a supine, prone, or lateral position. Fig. 31-3 demonstrates gravity's effect on mucus distribution within a bronchus. When the client is in a horizontal position, mucus accumulates in the dependent regions of the bronchial tube. Because mucus is an excellent medium for bacterial growth, hypostatic bronchopneumonia may result.

CARDIOVASCULAR CHANGES

The cardiovascular system is also affected by immobility. The three major changes are orthostatic hypotension, increased cardiac workload, and thrombus formation (Olson, 1967).

ORTHOSTATIC HYPOTENSION. Orthostatic or postural hypotension is a drop of 15 mm Hg or more in blood pressure when the client rises from a sitting

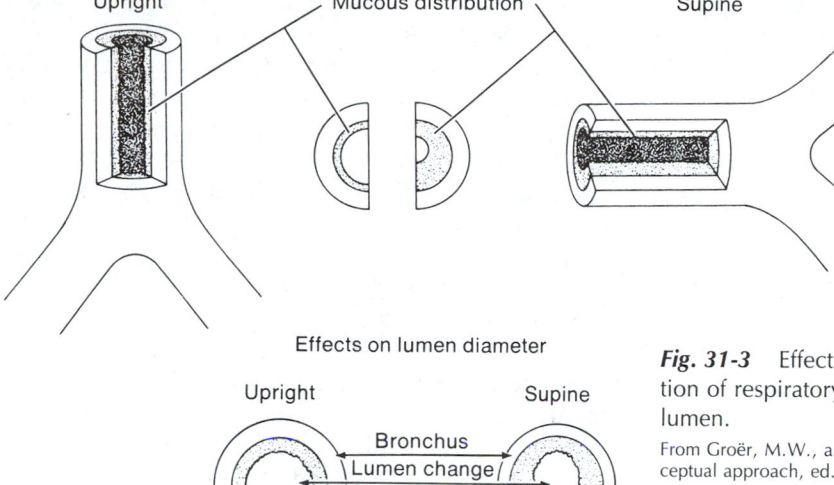

Upright   Mucous distribution   Supine

Effects on lumen diameter

Upright   Supine

Bronchus
Lumen change
Mucus

Fig. 31-3 Effect of recumbency and gravity on distribution of respiratory tract and diameter of bronchiolar lumen.

From Groër, M.W., and Shekleton, M.E.: Basic pathophysiology: a conceptual approach, ed. 2, St. Louis, 1983, The C.V. Mosby Co.

to a standing position. Immobilized clients and those on prolonged bed rest are at risk for orthostatic hypotension because the ability of the autonomic nervous system to equalize the blood supply is diminished in a person who has been recumbent for a prolonged period.

Normally the baroreceptor reflexes elicit an immediate sympathetic response to the decreased arterial blood pressure that occurs when a person stands up. This sympathetic response causes peripheral vasoconstriction, which prevents the pooling of blood in the lower extremities and maintains arterial blood pressure.

In an immobilized client the absence or reduction of peripheral vasoconstriction allows a pooling of venous blood in the lower extremities. This in turn decreases venous return to the heart, leading to a decreased cardiac output and lower blood pressure. As a result the client becomes dizzy on rising and may even faint.

Prolonged immobility also decreases muscle tone, contributing to orthostatic hypotension. Decreased muscle tone in the legs reduces the muscular pump's action on the great veins in the lower extremities. Venous return to the heart is decreased, resulting in hypotension.

Although orthostatic hypotension cannot be prevented, its effects can be minimized. The later section on intervention details nursing measures helpful in reducing postural effects on blood pressure.

INCREASED CARDIAC WORKLOAD. An immobilized client in a horizontal position has an increased cardiac workload. In this position blood that normally pools in the lower extremities is mobilized and increases the venous return to the heart. As a result

the heart must increase its stroke volume. The overall workload of the heart is increased, and the resting pulse rate rises, which further contributes to the workload.

In immobile clients the workload of the heart is further increased by the Valsalva maneuver. The Valsalva maneuver is any forced expiratory effort against a closed airway, as when a person holds his breath and tightens his muscles in a concerted, strenuous effort to move a heavy object or to change position in bed. Clients on bed rest tend to use the Valsalva maneuver when employing their arms and upper trunk muscles to move in bed. When the held breath is released, intrathoracic pressure falls and the venous return to the heart increases, which in turn increases heart rate. Clients with cardiac illness should be discouraged or prevented from doing the Valsalva maneuver because it can precipitate cardiac arrest.

THROMBUS FORMATION. Thrombus formation is another major hazard to the cardiovascular system resulting from immobility. A thrombus is an accumulation of platelets, fibrin, clotting factors, and the cellular elements of the blood attached to the interior wall of a vein or an artery, sometimes occluding the lumen of the vessel (Fig. 31-4). Thrombi form because immobility increases venous stasis, hypercoagulability, and external pressure against the veins (Olson, 1967). The venous stasis is the result of decreased muscular contraction, which promotes venous return. The hypercoagulability occurs when material released from the platelets and increased calcium (from the effect of immobilization on the skeleton) activate prothrombin, which in turn forms thrombin. Thrombin converts fibrinogen to fibrin, and the blood becomes thicker and more prone to coagulation. The external

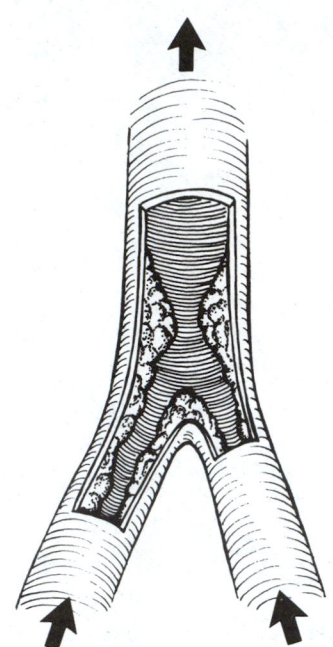

Fig. 31-4 Thrombus formation in a vessel.

pressure against the veins is the result of improper body alignment. For example, the use of supports under the client's knees in the high Fowler's position restricts circulation to the lower leg and foot, increasing the risk of thrombus formation because of the venous stasis and hypercoagulability of the blood.

In addition to the central circulation, immobility affects the peripheral circulation. As a result of pressure on the skin and underlying surfaces, tissue capillaries become ischemic and are destroyed. These effects are discussed in the later section on the skin.

MUSCULOSKELETAL CHANGES

The effects of immobility on the musculoskeletal system can include permanent impairment of mobility. Immobility can cause gradual changes in both the muscles and the skeleton. Chapter 30 reviews the physiology and regulation of movement and the interrelationships of muscular and skeletal function.

MUSCULAR ALTERATIONS. Restricted mobility affects the client's muscles in four ways: loss of endurance, decreased muscle mass, atrophy, and decreased stability. *Loss of endurance* results primarily from decreased functional capacity of the muscles associated with disuse. The diminished functional capacity of muscles used only infrequently and for nonstrenuous activity is characterized by decreased muscle mass, atrophy, and decreased stability (Groër and Shekleton, 1983).

Decreased muscle mass and subsequent decreases in strength are directly related to disuse and the nutritional alterations associated with immobility. The increased catabolism and reduced anabolism result in a reduction in both cell size and available cellular energy. The condition of decreased muscle mass is frequently referred to as muscular atrophy.

Muscular atrophy resulting from immobilization is observable and measurable. For example, the calf muscles in a leg that has been in a cast for 6 weeks appear, and can be measured to be, smaller than before immobilization.

The antigravity muscles in the legs appear to be the most affected by immobilization, lending support to the theory that the normal stresses of gravity are important in maintaining function, development, and therefore mobility (Groër and Shekleton, 1983). Immobility reduces muscle tone, leading to atrophy, decreased muscle mass, and reduced endurance.

Reduced muscle endurance for physical activity results from both changes in the muscles and altered cardiovascular functioning. Immobility increases the cardiac workload, and heart rate and cardiac output may actually fall, further decreasing muscular endurance.

The manifestations of these muscular effects include weakness, fatigability, and tachycardia. If the immobilized client does not participate in some type of exercise plan, the loss of endurance will lead to greater reduction in physical activity, thus increasing the loss of endurance in a vicious circle.

In addition, the immobilized client experiences decreased physical stability. Immobility disrupts muscular stability and reduces the client's ability to move steadily. Such clients are at risk for losing their balance when changing position. Previously immobilized clients also may have difficulty in maintaining equilibrium while in an upright, weight-bearing position because of the changes in the muscles and skeleton.

SKELETAL ALTERATIONS. Immobilization causes two major alterations in the skeletal system: joint contractures and osteoporosis. Joint contractures involve both the muscles and the skeletal system.

Contractures. A joint contracture is an abnormal and usually permanent condition of a joint, characterized by flexion and fixation and caused by disuse, atrophy, and shortening of muscle fibers. When a contracture occurs, the muscle cannot maintain the normal full range of joint motion. Unfortunately, contractures usually leave the joint in a nonfunctional position. One such condition is permanent flexion of the elbow joint (Fig. 31-5). A client with this type of contracture is unable to use the arm to carry out activities of daily living.

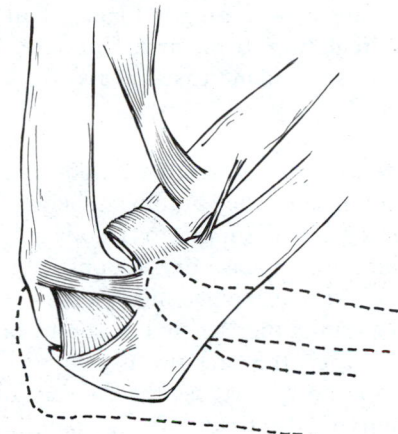

Fig. 31-5 Contracture of the elbow resulting in permanent flexion of the joint. Normally the elbow is able to extend to a 90-degree angle *(dotted line)* and to a 180-degree angle (not illustrated).

A second common contracture is foot-drop (Fig. 31-6). Foot-drop results in the foot being permanently fixed in plantar flexion (see Chapter 30). Ambulation is difficult with the foot in this position. If foot-drop occurs in both feet, the client is unable to walk without the aid of adaptation devices.

Nursing care for partially or completely immobilized clients is directed toward the prevention of contractures. Contractures can be reduced or prevented by active or passive range of joint motion exercises, proper body alignment, and positioning aids (see Chapter 30).

Osteoporosis. Marked reductions in skeletal mass, referred to as disuse osteoporosis, routinely accompany prolonged immobilization or paralysis (Hulley et al., 1971). The processes of bone formation and resorption (destruction of bone cells) are normally maintained in balance. Immobility, however, causes bone resorption to be relatively greater. Since bone resorption causes the release of calcium into the blood, immobilized clients are also hypercalcemic. Calcium is also excreted in large quantities in the urine, which predisposes the immobilized client to renal calculi.

The link between disuse osteoporosis and immobility is twofold. Both immobilization and non-weight-bearing activities increase the rate of bone resorption.

The nurse can help reduce disuse osteoporosis by performing passive exercises for the immobilized client. It is frequently impossible for an immobilized client to carry out weight-bearing activities.

When the immobilized client is able to become more mobile, the nurse plans a gradual increase in

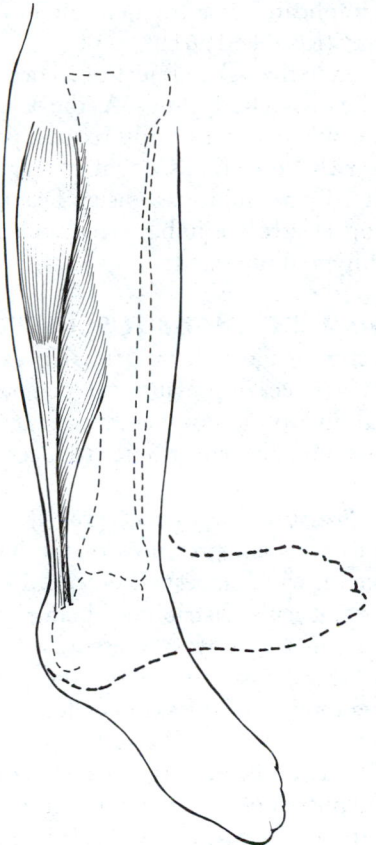

Fig. 31-6 Foot-drop. Ankle is fixed in plantar flexion.

activity. The use of gradually increasing exercises helps the client increase his activity tolerance and muscle strength. Other nursing interventions are described later in the section on the nursing process.

SKIN CHANGES

Immobilization has little effect on the skin of a healthy person but has devastating effects on the elderly and on sensory- or motor-impaired clients. The effect of immobility on the skin is compounded by the impaired body metabolism and negative nitrogen balance. Any break in the skin's integrity is difficult to heal, which may lead to further immobilization. This skin effect is referred to as a bedsore, pressure sore, or decubitus ulcer.

A decubitus ulcer is an inflammation, sore, or ulcer in the skin over a bony prominence. Decubitus ulcers have long been recognized as a hazard for debilitated and immobilized clients. Since they interfere with the skin, the body's first line of defense against the entry of bacteria and other pathogens, the client is at risk for systemic infection. They prolong morbidity and interfere with the rehabilitation and maintenance of the client confined to a chair or bed, and they have also been implicated as a frequent major factor leading to death (Kosiak, 1961).

In addition to the risk of infection, a decubitus ulcer increases the loss of body fluids. As the decubitus ulcer invades the subcutaneous body tissues, protein- and electrolyte-rich body fluids begin to exit at the decubitus site. If the fluid loss is significant, the client can develop electrolyte imbalances such as hypokalemia and hypoalbuminenia.

MECHANISM OF DECUBITUS ULCER FORMATION. Decubitus ulcers form primarily as a result of pressure. The effect of pressure can be potentiated by an unequal distribution of weight over the body. Reactive hyperemia also contributes to ulcer formation.

Effects of Pressure. Because of gravity, a person is subjected to constant pressures of the body against any surface on which it rests (Berecek, 1975a). If the pressure is unevenly distributed, being greater on a certain part of the body, a pressure gradient is increased on those tissues receiving the pressure. The cellular metabolism of the skin is altered at the point of pressure.

Normally tissue metabolism depends on receiving oxygen and nutrients from the blood supply and eliminating metabolites and carbon dioxide. Any factor that interferes with this process clearly affects cellular metabolism and, as a result, the function or actual life of the cell.

Pressure affects cellular metabolism by decreasing or obliterating tissue circulation. Subsequently, tissue metabolism is changed. Pathological changes begin to occur 1 to 2 hours after the reduction in tissue circulation (Berecek, 1975a).

Distribution of Weight over the Body. When a client is lying in bed or sitting in a chair, the weight of the body is heavily placed on certain bony prominences. The body surfaces subjected to the greatest weight or pressure are those at greatest risk for decubitus ulcer formation. Researchers have shown that, in people with normal body weight, the following body regions receive the greatest pressures (Linden et al., 1965):

POSITION	POINTS OF PRESSURE
Sitting	Ischial tuberosities, sacrum
Supine	Back of skull, elbows, sacrum, ischial tuberosities, heels
Prone	Elbows, knees, toes
Side-lying	Knees, greater trochanters

The longer the pressure is applied, the greater is the risk of skin breakdown. Leaving an immobilized client in a single position for longer than 2 hours decreases circulation to the area, interferes with cellular metabolism, and increases the risk of skin breakdown.

Reactive Hyperemia. When the blood supply to the tissues is diminished, they become ischemic. Ischemia is a decreased blood supply to a body part, in this case the skin. A compensatory response of the tissues to ischemia is reactive hyperemia, an increased blood flow. This permits the ischemic tissue to be flooded with blood when the pressure is removed. The increased blood flow increases the delivery of oxygen and nutrients to the tissue. The metabolic debt resulting from pressure can then be met, healthy equilibrium restored, and necrosis of the compressed tissue avoided (Berecek, 1975a). Reactive hyperemia is a compensatory response and is effective only if the pressure is removed before the damage begins in the critical period between 1 and 2 hours.

CLASSIFICATION AND PROGRESSION OF DECUBITUS ULCERS. Decubitus ulcer formation may occur initially in the superficial layers of the skin. The ulcer that is first seen as an area of erythema can progress rapidly to penetrate the underlying tissues and can even extend so deep that bony surfaces are exposed. Deep sores do not originate in the skin but are considered to result from a process that begins in deep tissues and spreads to the surface (Berecek, 1975a). The visible surface area of a decubitus ulcer is like the tip of an iceberg: there is more tissue necrosis below the skin surface.

Guttmann (1955) defined the following stages in the development of a decubitus ulcer:

I. Reddening of the skin, which disappears when the pressure is relieved
II. Superficial circulatory and tissue damage; reddening and edema that do not disappear; induration of the superficial tissue
III. Destruction of the subcutaneous layers; necrotic cells; destruction of the underlying capillary bed
IV. Advanced destruction of subcutaneous capillaries and muscle mass; if deep enough, exposure of underlying bone

The initial stage is transient circulation disturbances. The pressure is sufficient to cause reddening of the skin, which disappears when the pressure is relieved (Fig. 31-7, A). The second stage is definite, superficial circulatory and tissue damage. In this stage reddening and edema of the affected area do not disappear on decompression and result in induration of the tissue. The superficial layers of the skin may be excoriated or blistered, or, if the deep layers of the

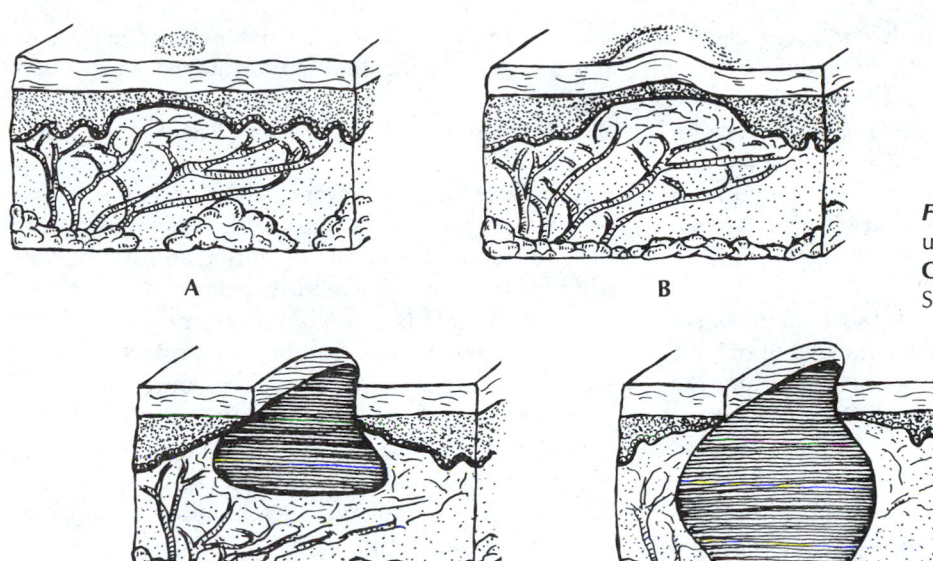

Fig. 31-7 **A,** Stage I decubitus ulcer. **B,** Stage II decubitus ulcer. **C,** Stage III decubitus ulcer. **D,** Stage IV decubitus ulcer.

skin are involved, there may be superficial necrosis and ulcer formation (Fig. 31-7, *B*). Last is the stage of deep, penetrating necrosis. The destruction involves subcutaneous tissues and includes fascia, muscles, and bone (Fig. 31-7, *C*). Deep penetrating ulcers may develop over the sacrum, ischial tuberosities, and trochanters. These ulcers may even penetrate to the bone (Fig. 31-7, *D*). Major decubitus ulcers can result in bone erosion and, if an infection is present, osteomyelitis.

FACTORS CONTRIBUTING TO THE FORMATION OF DECUBITUS ULCERS. Although decubitus ulcers are caused primarily by pressure, other factors may contribute to their formation. These include shearing force, moisture, poor nutrition, anemia, and infection.

Shearing force is the pressure exerted when a client is moved or repositioned in bed by being lifted or when he is allowed to slide down in bed (Fig. 31-8). With a shearing force the skin adheres to the surface of the bed while the layers of subcutaneous tissue and even the bones slide in the direction of body movement. The underlying tissue capillaries are compressed and severed by the pressure.

The presence of *moisture* on the skin increases the risk of ulcer formation. The moisture can be due to perspiration, incontinence of urine or feces, wound drainage, or vomitus. Moisture reduces the skin's resistance to other physical factors, such as pressure or shearing force, increasing the potential for ulcer formation. The susceptibility to decubitus ulcers increases proportionally with the duration of skin moisture.

The immobilized client, who is unable to meet his own hygiene needs, depends on the nurse to maintain his skin integrity. The nurse must therefore incorporate a hygiene routine into the plan of care, including removal of skin bacteria that would increase the risk of decubitus ulcer formation if left to grow.

Clients with *poor nutrition* often experience serious weight loss, muscle atrophy, and decreases in subcutaneous tissue and muscle mass (see Chapter 38). Because of these changes, less tissue is present to serve as padding between the skin and the underlying bone. Therefore the effects of pressure are increased on the remaining tissue.

Fig. 31-8 Shearing force.

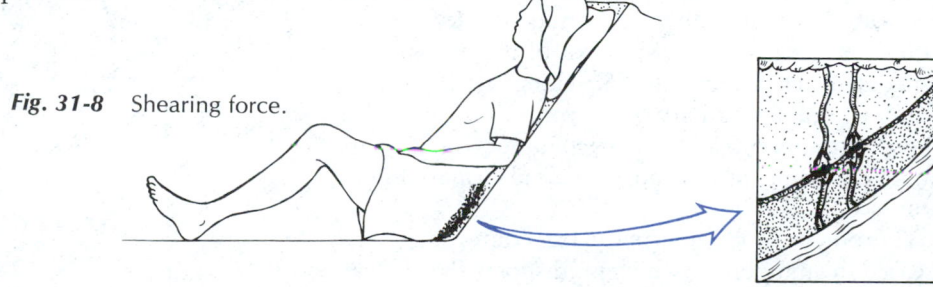

Poor nutritional status can also alter the client's fluid and electrolyte balance. In clients with severe protein loss, hypoalbuminemia leads to a shift of fluid from the extracellular fluid volume to the tissues, resulting in edema. In addition, clients with poor nutritional status generally have impaired wound healing. When a break in the skin occurs, limited nutritional resources are available to promote healing.

Clients with *anemia* are at risk for decubitus ulcer formation because the decreased hemoglobin reduces the oxygen-carrying capacity of the blood and the amount of oxygen available to the tissues. The anemia also alters cellular metabolism and impairs wound healing.

Infection results from the presence of bacteria within the body. When an infection is present, the metabolic demands and therefore the oxygen and nutritional demands of the body increase. In addition, the fever that usually accompanies the infection increases skin moisture, which further predisposes a client to skin breakdown.

ELIMINATION CHANGES

URINARY ELIMINATION.
The client's urinary elimination is altered by immobilization. Urine retention, renal calculi, and urinary tract infection may result. The anatomy of the kidney is such that, in the upright position, urine flows out of the renal pelvis and into the ureter and bladder in accordance with gravitational forces (Olson, 1967). However, when the person is immobilized, the kidney and ureters are on a level plane and urine formed by the kidney must be expressed into the bladder against gravity. Because the peristaltic contractions of the ureters are insufficient to overcome gravity, the renal pelvis may fill before urine is expressed into the ureters (Fig. 31-9). This condition results in urinary stasis, which can increase the development of renal calculi and infection.

Renal calculi are calcium stones that lodge in the renal pelvis and pass through the ureters. The stones are not a direct result of immobility but rather a consequence of the high level of urinary calcium associated with the recumbent position. Research has shown that urinary calcium increases begin after 2 days of immobility and reach a maximal level in the fifth week (Dietrick, 1948). Most of these stones are composed of calcium salts. Calcium salt deposition is influenced by urinary stasis infection, increased phosphate concentration, urine alkalinity, altered citric acid/calcium ratio, and decreased urine production.

The potential for a urinary tract infection is increased by immobility, which predisposes the kidneys to urinary stasis. This in turn enables bacteria to grow in the stagnant urine. In addition, stagnant urine permits the accumulation of deposits within the renal pelvis, resulting in the formation of renal calculi (Fig. 31-10).

Phosphate concentration in the urine is increased because of the effect of immobility on the skeleton. Disuse osteoporosis occurring during immobility thus affects the calcium/phosphorus balance.

Because immobilization reduces metabolic activity, fewer acid products of metabolism are formed to be excreted, causing the pH to rise. However, the citric acid concentration remains unchanged by immobility. The alkalinity of the urine and the altered ratio between citric acid and calcium concentrations favoring the calcium level enhance precipitation of calcium salts within the urine.

Urine formation is usually decreased in immobilized clients because of two factors. The immobilized client's fluid intake is generally decreased because he must depend on others for oral fluids (see Chapter 42). Also, since the cardiac output is decreased when a person is recumbent, renal blood flow is diminished and urinary output declines. The urine is frequently more concentrated, with a greater ratio of particulate matter to fluid. This greater concentration also increases the risk of calculus formation.

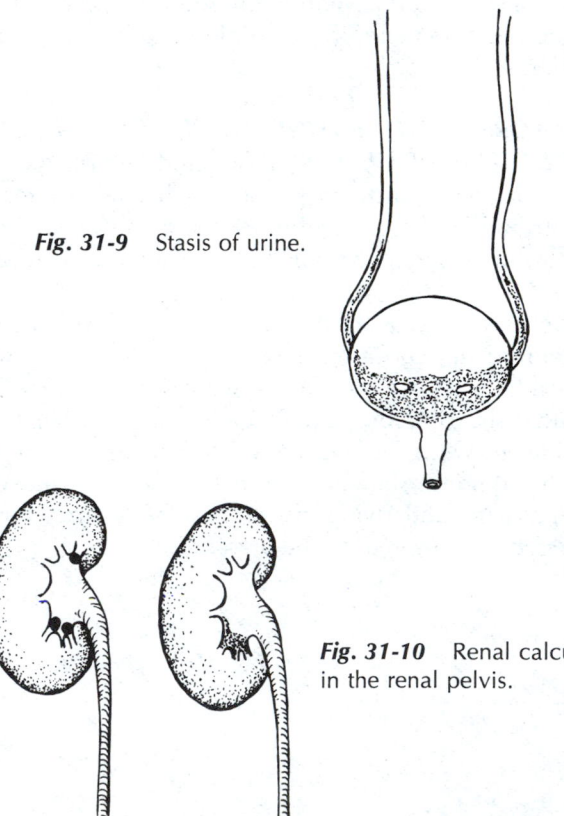

Fig. 31-9 Stasis of urine.

Fig. 31-10 Renal calculi in the renal pelvis.

Urinary tract infections result from bacteria in one or more structures of the urinary tract. Most of these infections are caused by gram-negative bacteria, especially *Escherichia coli (E. coli)* or species of *Klebsiella, Proteus, Pseudomonas,* or *Enterobacter.* Common types of urinary tract infections are cystitis, pyelonephritis, and urethritis (see Chapter 39). During immobilization, urinary tract infections frequently result from three causes: incorrect perineal care, indwelling catheter, and urinary reflex.

Incorrect perineal care is a major cause of infection, particularly among women who have fecal incontinence. Because of the proximity of the female urethra to the anal region, in an incontinent woman *E. coli* bacteria may enter the urinary tract by way of the urethra, resulting in an infection. Correct perineal care can reduce the risk of infection.

Another cause of urinary tract infections in immobilized clients is an indwelling urinary catheter. An indwelling catheter provides a pathway for bacteria to ascend into the bladder and kidney, causing pyelonephritis.

Urinary tract infections can be the result of reflux urine in noncatheterized clients. Because the bladder is unable to empty completely, urine backs up into the ureters. If the bladder is allowed to overfill, it becomes distended and urine can back up into the renal pelvis, resulting in pyelonephritis. The bladder of an immobilized client should be palpated to detect distention. If distention is present, it may be relieved with the insertion of a sterile catheter or emptied by the Cridé method (see Chapter 39).

BOWEL ELIMINATION. Bowel elimination is also affected by immobilization. The most common alteration is constipation. Constipation does not result directly from immobility but rather from weakened abdominal and perineal muscles and decreased gastric mobility, which are effects of immobilization (Groër and Shekleton, 1983). In addition, immobility may cause a decrease in the client's expulsive power and defecation reflex, contributing to constipation.

The lack of exercise weakens abdominal and perineal muscles and thereby interferes with the mechanical processes necessary for bowel elimination. As a result the client is unable to assist with the elimination process and retains some or all fecal contents (Olson, 1967).

The loss of the defecation reflex as a consequence of immobility is related to several factors. Primarily the immobilized client may be forced to suppress the need to defecate because no one is available to assist him onto the bedpan. Postponing defecation when the stimulus is present may produce an inhibition of colonic motility and a weakening of the gastrocolic reflex (Olson, 1967).

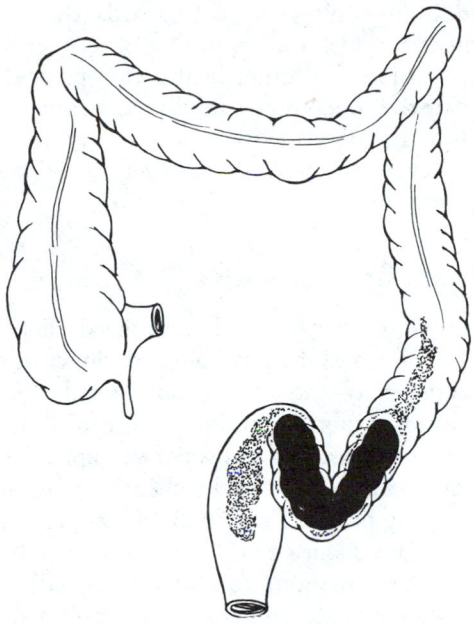

Fig. 31-11 Fecal impaction with liquid stool passing around the impaction.

The nursing care plan should be designed to prevent constipation. Uncorrected constipation can lead to fecal impaction, an accumulation of hardened fecal material in the rectum or sigmoid colon. When fecal material remains in the bowel, water is continually reabsorbed from it through the intestinal wall, and the fecal contents become increasingly drier and harder. In fact, the stool may become so hard that, although the person continually has the urge to defecate, he may be unable to expel the stool.

An early sign of an impaction is the frequent passage of liquid stool. This is not diarrhea; the liquid stool is merely passing around the area of impaction (Fig. 31-11). An untreated impaction can lead to a mechanical bowel obstruction that may completely or partially occlude the intestinal lumen, blocking normal propulsions of liquid and gas. The resulting fluid stasis within the intestine produces distention and increases the intraluminal pressure. Finally, intestinal function becomes depressed, dehydration occurs, and absorption ceases, resulting in fluid and electrolyte imbalance (see Chapter 40).

■ ■ ■ ■ ■

Immobility presents hazards for every system of the body. The type and degree of impairment depend on the duration of immobility, the reason for immobilization, and the client's overall level of health. Through the nursing process the nurse designs therapies whose overall goal is to reduce the hazards of immobility for the body's physiological functioning.

In addition to physiological hazards, the immobilized client is at risk for impairments in other dimensions. As nurses and other health care professionals investigate the effects of immobility, data are gathered about how the decreased level of activity affects the whole client, and nurses can then anticipate the client's total needs.

Psychosocial Responses

The nurse caring for an immobilized client must meet needs beyond the physiological dimension. Immobilization may lead to emotional, intellectual, and sociocultural responses, and nursing care should address these psychosocial needs. For example, the nurse must anticipate changes in the client's mood, behavior, or coping patterns and intervene appropriately.

Changes in a client's emotional status usually occur gradually, and without careful nursing assessment they may go unobserved by nursing personnel. While all the adaptive coping mechanisms described in Chapter 5 can occur in the immobilized client, four emotional alterations are most common: depression, behavioral changes, changes in the sleep-wake cycle, and reduced functioning of coping mechanisms.

DEPRESSION

Depression is an abnormal emotional state characterized by exaggerated feelings of sadness, melancholy, dejection, worthlessness, emptiness, and hopelessness out of proportion to reality. The clinical manifestations range from a slight lack of motivation and inability to concentrate to physiological alterations and severe emotional dysfunction.

The immobilized client is at risk for becoming depressed because of changes in role, self-concept, and other factors. Depression can result from worrying about present and future levels of health, finances, and family needs. Because immobilization removes the client from his daily routine, he has more time to worry about his disability and level of health. This can quickly increase the client's depression, causing him to become more withdrawn.

Assessing the client's behavioral changes continually throughout the period of restricted mobility helps the nurse identify changes in the client's self-concept (see Chapter 18). The nurse learns to recognize early signs of depression and to develop nursing interventions that will help the client adapt to his restricted mobility and thus decrease his depression.

BEHAVIORAL CHANGES

The behavioral changes resulting from immobilization vary widely depending on the individual client.

Moreover, changes in behavior may differ from day to day for an individual client.

Common behavioral changes include hostility, belligerence, giddiness, withdrawal, confusion, and anxiety. Early in the nursing process the nurse should interview the client's family and friends concerning his normal behavioral patterns in order to gain baseline data about his usual behaviors. If the nurse later observes any unexpected behavior, she can intervene to reduce the effects of immobilization on the client's behavioral patterns.

CHANGES IN SLEEP-WAKE CYCLE

The immobilized client requires round-the-clock nursing care. Because of the physiological hazards, the client cannot be allowed to sleep for 8 hours without having his position changed or other nursing care performed. Disruption of the client's normal sleeping pattern can further potentiate the client's behavioral changes. Nursing interventions should be used to ensure that the client receives sufficient sleep.

The client who is on bed rest and is able to change his position during sleep does not require continuous physical nursing care. Unless other treatment activities are required during the night, the nursing care plan for the physiologically stable client on bed rest can provide for uninterrupted sleep.

DECREASED COPING ABILITIES

Long-term immobility or bed rest can affect the client's usual coping patterns. For example, the client who formerly used problem-solving cognitive activities as a means of adapting to stress may be unable to make decisions or participate even minimally in his nursing care. Such a client may withdraw and become passive. The passive client allows nurses to care for him and is not interested in increasing his independence or involvement in his care.

Early in the care of an immobilized client the nurse should determine what the client normally does to handle stress. She then designs a nursing care plan that will allow the client to continue to use these coping abilities or help him develop new ones.

■　■　■　■　■

The psychosocial changes in the client resulting from immobilization are often difficult to recognize and to resolve with interventions. The chapters on stress adaptation (Chapter 5) and self-concept (Chapter 18) describe assessment methods for identifying changes in the client's psychosocial status. In addition, the chapter on grieving (Chapter 46) discusses the complex emotions of a client who has experienced a functional loss.

Developmental Effects

The developmental changes associated with immobility tend to be greater with clients at each end of the life span: the young and the elderly. The immobilized young or middle adult may experience few if any developmental changes.

The infant, toddler, or preschooler is usually immobilized because of trauma or the need to correct a congenital skeletal abnormality. Immobilization can retard the child's motor skill development and intellectual development.

Nurses caring for immobilized children should plan activities for the child that provide physical and psychosocial stimuli. Other activities focus on the specific effects of immobilization. For example, the parents of a 1-year-old with immobilized lower extremities resulting from congenital hip dysplasia need to be reassured that the delay in their child's walking is temporary and that, following a period of muscle strengthening exercises, the child's motor development will progress.

Immobilization of elderly clients increases their physical dependence on others and accelerates the functional losses in physiological systems. Usually immobilization of an elderly client results from a degenerative disease such as osteoarthritis, neurological trauma such as a cerebrovascular accident (stroke), or the presence of a chronic illness such as cardiopulmonary disease. For some clients immobilization occurs gradually and progressively, whereas for others, especially those who have had a stroke, the immobilization is sudden.

When providing nursing care for an elderly client, the nurse should develop a nursing care plan that encourages the client to perform as many self-care activities as possible, thereby maintaining the client's highest level of mobility.

■ ■ ■ ■ ■

Bed rest and immobilization have beneficial effects and when used appropriately can help restore the client's previous level of wellness. However, any restriction in mobility is accompanied by many potential hazards that affect the client in all dimensions. If the nurse does not intervene appropriately, the effects of immobility can rapidly worsen, increasing the client's disability and the duration and cost of his health care. The nurse continually assesses immobilized clients to minimize these hazards.

Assessment

The nursing assessment includes the client's present mobility and potential effects of immobility.

Assessment of Mobility

Assessment of the client's mobility focuses on range of joint motion, muscle strength, and gait and posture. Perhaps the best way for the nurse to assess these is to observe the client carrying out activities of daily living. As the client meets his hygiene needs, such as combing his hair, brushing his teeth, and bathing, the nurse can determine his range of joint motion. Table 30-9 describes the normal range of movement for all joints in the body.

Observation of the client during activities of daily living also enables the nurse to estimate the client's fatigability and muscle strength. These assessment data assist the nurse in developing a nursing care plan that encourages the client to maintain his present level of mobility by increasing his energy level or his overall muscle strength.

Finally, observing the client's posture and gait helps the nurse determine what type of assistance the client may require to change positions or transfer from bed to chair. This information helps the nurse assess the client's overall level of mobility and coordination.

Specific assessments for range of joint motion, muscle strength, and posture and gait are described in Chapter 30, along with nursing diagnoses and interventions for impaired mobility. The remaining sections of this chapter focus on the nursing process for clients with actual or potential effects of immobility.

Assessment for the Hazards of Immobility

The nurse assesses the immobilized client for the hazards of immobility by performing a head-to-toe physical assessment (see Chapter 29). In addition, the nursing assessment should focus on certain physiological areas, as well as the client's psychosocial and developmental dimensions.

PHYSIOLOGICAL ASSESSMENT

The physiological hazards of immobility that may be identified during a nursing assessment are summarized in Table 31-1.

METABOLIC SYSTEM. When assessing the client's metabolic functioning, the nurse uses anthropometric measurements to evaluate muscle atrophy, intake and output records and laboratory data to evaluate fluid and electrolyte status, assessment of wound healing to evaluate alterations in the exchange of nutrients, and the client's food intake and elimination patterns to determine altered gastrointestinal functioning.

Anthropometric measurements include height, weight, mid–upper arm circumference, and triceps skinfold measurements. Ideally, this assessment

TABLE 31-1

Physiological Hazards of Immobility

System	Assessment Techniques	Abnormal Findings
Metabolic	Inspection	Muscle atrophy
	Anthropometric measurements (mid–upper arm circumference, triceps skinfold measurement)	Decreased amount of subcutaneous fat
	Palpation	Generalized edema owing to hypoalbuminemia
	Inspection	Slowed wound healing
Respiratory	Inspection	Asymmetrical chest wall movement
	Auscultation	Presence of rales, rhonchi, wheezes
Cardiovascular	Auscultation	Orthostatic hypotension
	Auscultation and palpation	Increased heart rate; presence of third heart sound; weak peripheral pulses
Musculoskeletal	Inspection and palpation	Increased diameter in calf or thigh
	Palpation	Restricted joint motion
Skin	Inspection	Break in skin integrity
Elimination	Inspection	Decreased urine output, concentrated urine

should be done early in the period of immobilization and should be repeated at 3-week intervals. A decrease in mid–upper arm circumference, measured in centimeters, or triceps skinfold, measured in millimeters, indicates a decline in muscle mass (Blackburn, 1977). This decline, along with decreased serum protein and decreased white cell count, can indicate that the client is breaking down more protein than he is building up. As a result he may be at risk for severe negative nitrogen imbalance. Measurements of the mid–upper arm circumference and triceps skinfold provide baseline information about the client's amount of subcutaneous fat, which may be lost during immobilization.

The client's intake and output measurements assist the nurse in determining if a fluid imbalance exists. Dehydration and edema can increase the speed of skin breakdown in an immobilized client. Laboratory tests, specifically measurement of serum electrolytes and calcium, can also indicate the presence of an electrolyte imbalance.

If an immobilized client has a wound, the speed of healing indicates how well nutrients are being delivered to the tissues for use. The normal progression of wound healing indicates that the metabolic needs of the injured tissues are being met.

Anorexia occurs commonly in immobilized clients. The nurse should assess the client's food intake before the tray is removed from the bedside to determine how much the client is actually eating. Nutritional imbalances can be avoided if the nurse learns the client's dietary patterns and food preferences early in his immobilization.

RESPIRATORY SYSTEM. A respiratory assessment should be performed every 2 hours for clients with restricted activity patterns. The nurse should inspect chest wall movements during the full inspiratory-expiratory cycle. If a client has an atelectatic area, the chest movement may be asymmetrical. In addition, the nurse should auscultate the entire lung region to identify regions of diminished breath sounds, rales, rhonchi, or wheezes. Auscultation should focus on the dependent lung fields, since pulmonary secretions tend to gravitate to these lower regions. A complete respiratory assessment identifies the presence of secretions and can be used to determine the nursing interventions necessary to maintain optimal respiratory function.

CARDIOVASCULAR SYSTEM. The cardiovascular nursing assessment of the immobilized client includes blood pressure monitoring, evaluation of apical and peripheral pulses, and observation of the venous system. Because of the risk for orthostatic hypotension, the client's blood pressure should be measured, particularly when changing from recumbency to a sitting or standing position. In this way the client's ability to tolerate postural changes can be assessed.

The nurse also needs to assess the apical and peripheral pulses. Recumbency increases cardiac workload and results in an increased pulse rate. In some clients, particularly the elderly, the heart may not be able to tolerate the increased workload, and a form of cardiac failure may develop. The presence of a third heart sound, heard at the apex, can be an early indication of congestive heart failure. Monitoring the client's peripheral pulses allows the nurse to evaluate the heart's ability to pump the blood throughout the body. The absence of a peripheral pulse, particularly one that was previously present, should be documented and reported to the client's physician.

The presence of edema may indicate the heart's inability to handle the increased workload. Because edema moves to dependent body regions, assessment of the immobilized client should include the sacrum, legs, and feet. If the client's heart is unable to tolerate the increased cardiac workload, the peripheral body regions, such as the hands, feet, nose, and earlobes, will be colder than the central body regions.

Finally, the nurse assesses the client's venous system because deep vein thrombosis is a hazard of restricted mobility. A dislodged thrombus, called an embolus, may travel through the circulatory system to the client's lungs or brain and impair that organ's circulation. Emboli to the lungs or the brain pose a threat to the client's life.

To assess for the presence of a deep vein thrombosis, the nurse should remove the client's elastic stockings once every 8 hours and observe the calves for redness, warmth, and tenderness. In addition, calf circumference should be measured daily. To do this the nurse marks a point on each of the client's calves 10 cm from his midpatella. The circumference is measured each day using the mark as a reference point for placement of the tape measure. One-sided increases in calf diameter can be an early indication of thrombosis. Since deep vein thrombosis can also occur in the thigh, thigh circumference measurements should be taken daily if the client is prone to thrombosis. In many clients, deep vein thrombosis can be prevented by exercise and the application of elastic stockings. Both procedures are detailed in the intervention section later in the chapter.

MUSCULOSKELETAL SYSTEM. The major musculoskeletal abnormalities that may be identified during the nursing assessment include decreased muscle tone, loss of muscle mass, contractures, and osteoporosis. The anthropometric measurements described earlier may indicate losses in muscle tone and muscle mass.

Range of joint motion exercises assist in preventing contractures from developing or worsening. Range of joint motion is measured with a goniometer (see Chapter 30).

Disuse osteoporosis cannot be identified by means of physical assessment. However, postmenopausal women and persons with increased serum and urine calcium levels are at greater risk for bone demineralization. The risk of disuse osteoporosis should be considered when planning nursing interventions; for example, rib percussion and vibration should be done cautiously with a client with probable disuse osteoporosis, because of the risk of rib fracture.

SKIN. The nurse must continually assess the client's skin for signs of breakdown. The skin should be observed each time the client is turned or hygiene measures are performed. At the minimum the client's skin should be assessed every 2 hours.

In addition, the nurse should be alert for risk factors that can increase the client's potential for skin breakdown. First, the nurse assesses the client's position to determine whether a shearing force exists. If it does, the client's position should be changed immediately. Second, the nurse assesses the client's skin for any moisture such as excreta or perspiration, which increases the chance of skin breakdown. Third, the nurse assesses all possible pressure points to determine whether they are adequately protected. Chapter 30 describes the correct body alignments for the Fowler's, supine, prone, side-lying, and Sims' positions and the pressure points that can increase the risk of skin breakdown. Last, the nurse assesses the client's nutritional status and looks for evidence of infection, since these are risk factors for skin breakdown.

ELIMINATION SYSTEM. The client's elimination status should be evaluated on each shift, and the total intake and output should be evaluated every 24 hours. The nurse should determine that the client is receiving the correct amount and type of fluids orally or parenterally (see Chapter 42).

Inadequate fluid and electrolyte balances or intake and output can increase the client's risk for renal impairment, ranging from recurrent infections to kidney failure. These conditions decrease the client's overall level of mobility and increase the duration and cost of care.

Assessment of the client's elimination status should also include the frequency and consistency of bowel movements. Accurate assessment enables the nurse to intervene before fecal impaction occurs.

Psychosocial Assessment

Changes in the client's psychosocial status usually occur slowly and are often overlooked by health care personnel. The nurse should observe for inappropriate changes in the client's emotional status. If the client seems depressed, the nurse should observe him for several days before concluding that his depression is abnormal. Everyone becomes depressed at some time, especially hospitalized and immobilized clients, but not all depression requires nursing intervention. The client's depression may be due to boredom or isolation and may be alleviated by increasing bedside activities and occupational therapy.

The nurse also observes for behavioral changes, such as the cooperative client who becomes argumentative or the modest client who begins to expose himself repeatedly. The nurse should try to determine the reasons for such behavioral alterations in order to identify specific nursing therapies that can minimize or resolve the problems.

Unexplained changes in the client's sleep-wake cycle must be identified and corrected. Most such disruptions can be prevented or minimized, such as those occurring because of nursing activities, a noisy environment, or discomfort or pain. Disruptions in the sleep-wake cycle may also occur because of medications such as analgesics, sleeping pills, or cardiovascular drugs.

Finally, the nurse should observe for changes in the client's use of his normal coping mechanisms to adapt to his immobilization (see Chapter 5). Decreasing coping ability may cause the client to become disoriented, confused, or depressed or to experience other behavioral changes.

Because these psychosocial changes usually occur gradually, the nurse should observe the client's behavior on a daily basis. If behavioral changes do occur, the nurse should determine the causes and evaluate the changes as short- or long-term. Identifying the cause helps the nurse design appropriate nursing interventions to resolve the problem.

Developmental Assessment

Assessment of the immobilized client should include developmental considerations to ensure that all the client's needs are identified. With a young child the nurse determines whether the child is able to meet developmental tasks and is progressing normally. The child's development may regress or be slowed because of immobilization. By identifying a child's overall developmental needs, the nurse can design nursing therapies to maintain the child's normal development. When developmental delays are temporary, the nurse may also need to assure the parents.

Developmental assessment is as important with the geriatric client as with the young child. The nursing assessment enables the nurse to determine the elderly client's ability to meet his needs independently and to adapt to developmental changes, such as declining physical functioning and altered family and peer relationships. A decline in the client's developmental functioning needs prompt investigation to determine why the change has occurred and what can be done to restore the client to his optimal level of function.

Nursing Diagnosis

An immobilized client may have one or more of many problems related to the immobility. Common nursing diagnoses in all dimensions are listed in the box on p. 777. These nursing diagnoses are only a representative sample. The individualized nursing care plan is based on the specific nursing diagnoses for the immobilized client.

Many alterations in physiological functioning are related to immobility, and impaired functioning in one system may also affect another system. For example, urinary stasis can quickly lead to a kidney infection, which produces fever and sweating. The resulting increase skin moisture may then increase the potential for skin breakdown. Therefore the nursing diagnosis of "impaired urinary elimination related to infection" should lead the nurse to consider the additional nursing diagnosis of "potential impairment in skin integrity related to increased moisture."

Too often the physiological dimension is the sole focus of nursing care for immobilized clients and the psychosocial and developmental dimensions are neglected. Yet these dimensions can be equally important in the client's health. For example, during immobilization the client's social interaction and stimuli are decreased. Ultimately the client becomes isolated, withdrawn, and bored. Such clients may frequently use the nurse's call bell to request minor physical attention, when their real need is greater socialization and contact with other people.

Immobilization of a family member changes the family's structure and functioning. For example, if the father is immobilized in traction because of an injury, his role in the family is changed. He is unable to participate in decision making or social activities, and his contributions to the family's income may be decreased. The family's response to this change may lead to problems. The children may resent the fact that their father is unable to attend their sports and school activities. Their mother may be frustrated because she must make many of the family's decisions. Any change in family structure of functioning usually results in stress and anxiety for all family members.

Examples of Nursing Diagnoses Associated with Impaired Mobility

PHYSIOLOGICAL
Metabolic

- Decreased muscle mass related to decreased metabolic rate
- Decreased body proteins related to decreased protein intake
- Fluid volume deficit related to decreased fluid intake
- Fluid volume overload related to electrolyte and protein imbalances
- Decreased body mass related to decreased intake of nutrients

Respiratory

- Altered exchange of oxygen related to decreased lung expansion
- Altered exchange of oxygen related to airway secretions
- Altered airway clearance related to impaired cough

Cardiovascular

- Alterations in cardic output related to sudden postural changes
- Increased cardiac workload related to recumbency
- Impaired venous circulation related to thrombus formation

Musculoskeletal

- Reduced activity tolerance related to muscle weakness
- Limited range of joint motion related to contracture formation
- Limited weight-bearing ability related to bone demineralization

Skin

- Impaired skin integrity related to immobility
- Impaired skin integrity related to poor nutrition
- Impaired skin integrity related to infection
- Impaired skin integrity related to pressure
- Impaired skin integrity related to presence of decubitus ulcer

Elimination

- Impaired urinary elimination related to urinary stasis
- Impaired urinary elimination related to renal calculi
- Impaired urinary elimination related to infection
- Impaired urinary elimination related to decreased fluid intake
- Impaired bowel elimination related to inactivity
- Impaired bowel elimination related to dietary changes
- Impaired bowel elimination related to fecal impaction

PSYCHOSOCIAL

- Altered coping patterns related to reduced activity
- Altered sleep-wake cycle related to nursing care activities
- Decreased problem-solving abilities related to immobilization
- Increased social isolation related to immobilization
- Alterations in behavior and mood related to decreased activity
- Altered relationships with family members related to immobilization
- Sensory deprivation related to social isolation

DEVELOPMENTAL

- Potential delayed cognitive development related to reduced opportunities for stimulation (toddler)
- Decreased ability to develop a sense of individual identity related to the social isolation of immobilization (adolescent)
- Potential maturational crisis in assuming responsibilities related to loss of employment during immobilization (young adult)
- Decrease ability to meet independence needs related to progressive functional losses (elderly client)

General Nursing Goals for the Immobilized Client

PHYSIOLOGICAL
Metabolic

- Maintain caloric intake.
- Maintain fluid balance.
- Prevent muscle wasting.

Respiratory

- Maintain patent airway.
- Maintain lung expansion.
- Prevent stasis of pulmonary secretions.

Cardiovascular

- Maintain cardiac output during postural changes.
- Reduce cardiac workload.
- Promote venous return.

Musculoskeletal

- Maintain present level of range of joint motion.
- Increase activity tolerance.
- Increase tolerance to weight-bearing activities.

Skin

- Maintain skin integrity.
- Reduce the duration of pressure.
- Prevent contact of the skin with moisture.

Elimination

- Maintain proper fluid intake.
- Prevent bladder distention.
- Prevent bowel impaction.

PSYCHOSOCIAL

- Promote client's "normal" coping patterns.
- Maintain client's sleep-wake pattern.
- Promote socialization.
- Increase contact with family or significant others.
- Provide adequate stimuli to maintain client's orientation.

DEVELOPMENTAL

- Increase client's ability to complete activities of daily living.
- Promote physical and mental stimulation.

Nursing diagnoses for health needs in developmental areas reflect changes from normal activities of the client's developmental stage. Unit 5 details the developmental tasks and potential stresses for each stage. Immobility may disrupt the client's abilities to meet any of those needs or to adapt to stresses. Immobility may, for example, precipitate a developmental crisis if the client is unable to resolve problems and continue to mature.

Planning

The overall goal of the nursing care plan for the client with restricted mobility is to prevent the hazards of immobility. The box at left lists the goals of nursing care for all the client's dimensions. To achieve these goals, the nurse develops specific interventions for each health need. Throughout the period of immobility, the nurse is continually planning nursing care, delivering nursing therapies, evaluating the client's responses, and reassessing the client's health needs.

Clients with impaired mobility are often unable to carry out the activities of daily living without the assistance of nurses or other health care professionals. For example, a client with bilateral arm casts cannot feed himself, and therefore someone must assist him with feeding to meet his caloric and nutritional needs. A client immobilized with his leg in traction cannot meet his hygiene, elimination, or exercise needs, and therefore the nursing care plan is designed to provide the client with the necessary assistance to achieve these basic needs.

The nursing care plan for the immobilized client would be incomplete if the nurse did not include measures for gradually increasing the client's mobility status (see the boxed material at right). Clients whose mobility has been restricted require a progressive plan for restoring mobility. Because immobilization decreases muscle strength and physical endurance, leading to fatigue with movement, activities are planned to gradually increase the client's activity tolerance, muscle strength, and physical endurance. With such a plan the client gradually assumes greater independence for carrying out activities of daily living. Eventually the client achieves his highest level of mobility.

Implementation

Nursing interventions for the completely or partially immobilized client focus on preventing the hazards of immobility. Interventions should therefore be directed toward needs in all the client's dimensions.

> ### General Nursing Goals for Increasing a Client's Mobility Status
>
> - Increase time periods when the client is out of bed.
> - Increase the distance the client walks.
> - Increase the frequency of the client's walks.
> - Promote flexibility exercises.
> - Promote independent completion of self-care activities.
> - Increase exercise activities.

Metabolic System

The immobilized client requires a high-protein, high-caloric diet with vitamin C supplements. The protein is needed to repair injured tissue and to rebuild depleted protein stores. A high calorie intake provides the body with the necessary fuel to meet current metabolic needs and to replace subcutaneous tissue that may have been destroyed. Supplementation with vitamin C is necessary for replacement of protein stores.

If the client is unable to eat, nutrition must be provided parenterally or enterally. Enteral feedings include the delivery of high-protein, high-calorie, vitamin-, mineral-, and electrolyte-complete solutions through a nasogastric, gastrostomy, or jejunostomy tube (see Chapter 38). Total parenteral nutrition is the delivery of nutritional supplements through a central intravenous catheter (see Chapter 42). The specific nursing interventions for enteral and parenteral nutrition are detailed in Chapters 38 and 42.

Respiratory System

Nursing interventions for the respiratory system are aimed at promoting expansion of the chest and lungs, preventing stasis of pulmonary secretions, maintaining a patent airway, and promoting adequate exchange of respiratory gases.

PROMOTING EXPANSION OF THE CHEST AND LUNGS

The effects of bed rest and immobility on expansion of the lungs and chest are described in an earlier section of this chapter. The nurse can counteract reduced chest expansion with several interventions. First, changing the position of the client every 2 hours allows the dependent lung to reexpand. This maintains the elastic recoil property of the lungs and clears the dependent lung of pulmonary secretions.

The nurse should encourage the client to deep breathe and cough every 1 to 2 hours. Alert clients can be taught to deep breathe or yawn every hour. This action expands all lobes of the lungs and prevents atelectasis. Coughing reduces the stasis of pulmonary secretions. For unconscious clients with an artificial airway in place, the nurse can expand the chest and lungs by using an Ambu bag (see Chapter 41).

The nurse uses discretion when administering postoperative pain medication. These medications can depress the respiratory center so the rate of respiration or expansion of the lungs is decreased. The nurse should ask a postoperative client who has received pain medication to deep breathe and cough at the peak effect of the analgesic, 20 to 30 minutes after administration. This reduces the respiratory depressant action of the drug.

If abdominal binders and rib supports are required, they should be removed every 2 hours to allow the client to breathe deeply. Removal may be contraindicated, however, for the newly postoperative or post-trauma client.

PREVENTING STASIS OF PULMONARY SECRETIONS

Stagnant secretions accumulating in the bronchi and lungs of the immobilized or bedridden client may lead to the growth of bacteria and the subsequent development of pneumonia. Despite the nurse's interventions to prevent pulmonary secretions, such secretions do develop.

The stagnation of secretions can be reduced by changing the client's position every 2 hours. This change rotates the dependent lung, mobilizing the secretions.

Perhaps the best method for preventing pulmonary secretions is *chest physiotherapy*. This is the use of positioning techniques to drain secretions from specific segments of the bronchi and the lungs into the trachea, from which the client expels the secretions by coughing. The respiratory assessment findings identify the areas of the lungs that require chest physiotherapy. Clients are then placed in appropriate positions to promote drainage of pulmonary secretions from affected areas. The nurse uses pillows and slant boards to position clients properly and cupping, clapping, and vibrating techniques to dislodge and mobilize secretions. Chest physiotherapy is a precise procedure requiring specific nursing skills. The complete step-by-step procedure is presented in Chapter 41.

MAINTAINING A PATENT AIRWAY

Immobilized clients and those on bed rest are generally in a weakened condition. If the weakness progresses, the client's cough reflex gradually becomes inefficient. If the client is too weak or unable to cough up his secretions, the nurse must maintain a patent airway by using suctioning techniques. The stasis of secretions in the lungs may be life threatening for an immobilized client because hypostatic bronchopneumonia can easily develop. Assessment findings that may indicate this condition include productive cough with greenish yellow sputum, fever, and pain on breathing. Dislodging and mobilizing the stagnant secretions reduce the risk of pneumonia.

In the immobilized client an obstructed airway is usually the result of a mucus plug. The nurse can implement the following therapies to maintain the patent airway.

First, the nurse can ask the client to deep breathe and cough every 1 to 2 hours. The nurse instructs the client to take in three deep breaths and cough with the third exhalation. This produces a more forceful, productive cough without greatly fatiguing the client.

Second, the nurse may use nasotracheal or orotracheal suction to remove secretions in the upper airways of a weakened client unable to cough productively. This procedure must be performed aseptically. The nurse places a suction catheter in the client's nose or through his mouth and applies suction to remove secretions that have accumulated in the upper airways (see Chapter 41).

Third, the nurse can maintain a patent airway by suctioning secretions from an artificial airway such as an endotracheal or tracheal tube. The nurse inserts a catheter into the artificial airway in a sterile procedure. Through suctioning, pulmonary secretions are removed from both the upper and lower airways (see Chapter 41).

Cardiovascular System

The effects of bed rest or immobilization on the cardiovascular system include orthostatic hypotension, increased cardiac workload, and thrombus formation. Nursing therapies are designed to minimize or prevent these three alterations.

REDUCING ORTHOSTATIC HYPOTENSION

The causative factors and effects of orthostatic hypotension are described in an earlier section. Nursing interventions can assist in reducing orthostatic hypotension.

First, interventions are directed toward maintaining muscle tone, as by leg exercises and the application of elastic stockings. When muscle tone is maintained, venous return to the heart is increased and stasis of blood in the lower extremities is prevented.

The nurse should encourage the client to get out of bed as soon as possible, even if the move is only

to a nearby chair. This activity assists in maintaining muscle tone and promotes venous return to the heart. The client should be moved out of bed gradually. To document any orthostatic changes, the nurse measures baseline blood pressure with the client in the supine position. The nurse then raises the client to a high Fowler's position and measures the blood pressure again to detect any lowering of pressure. The client is left in the high Fowler's position for a few moments to allow his body to adapt to any drop in blood pressure. The nurse continually assesses the client for signs of dizziness, lightheadedness, or seeing spots.

The next step is having the client sit at the side of the bed with his feet on the floor. The client is told that he should lie down if he feels dizzy or faint. The client sits for a few minutes, and if no dizziness or weakness occurs, he stands up at the bedside for a minute before beginning to walk. If he should become dizzy or weak, he can be lowered quickly and safely to his bed. If the client experiences no dizziness, the nurse assists him to a chair. Gradually increasing the frequency and duration of the client's ambulation helps overcome any orthostatic hypotension and muscle fatigue resulting from bed rest or immobilization.

REDUCING CARDIAC WORKLOAD

The nurse designs interventions to reduce cardiac workload, which is increased by immobility. The nurse's primary intervention is discouraging the client from using the Valsalva maneuver.

The nurse can provide the alert, partially immobilized client with an overhead trapeze bar that allows the client to change position without increasing intrathoracic pressure. The nurse teaches the client not to hold his breath but to use pursed lip breathing when changing position (see Chapter 41).

The nurse intervenes to prevent constipation in the inactive client (see Chapter 40). This reduces use of the Valsalva maneuver, which may be employed by the constipated client when straining to evacuate a stool.

PREVENTION OF THROMBUS FORMATION

Inactivity increases venous stasis, hypercoagulability, and external pressure against the veins, which in turn increase the risk of deep vein thrombosis. Three nursing measures can minimize the potential for thrombus formation.

First, the nurse positions the client properly to prevent pressure on the posterior region of the knee and deep veins of the legs. Chapter 30 includes the detailed procedures for placing clients in the high Fowler's, supine, prone, Sims', and side-lying positions.

Second, the nurse incorporates routine exercises

PROCEDURE 31-1

Applying Elastic Stockings

STEPS	RATIONALE	
1. Remove elastic stockings at least twice a day.	This enables the nurse to cleanse and assess the skin and vessels of the legs.	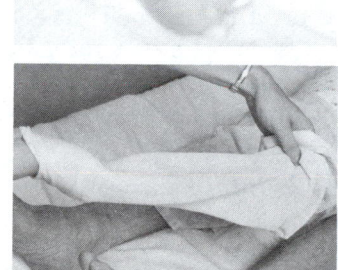
2. After the legs have been cleansed, apply a small amount of talcum powder to each leg and foot.	Talcum powder reduces friction and allows for easier application of the stocking.	
3. Turn elastic stocking inside out by placing one hand into the sock, holding the toe of the sock with your other hand, and pulling.	This allows easier application of the stocking.	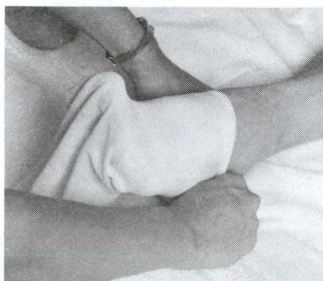
4. Place the client's toe into the foot of the elastic stocking, making sure that the sock is smooth.	Wrinkles in the sock can impede circulation to the lower region of the extremity.	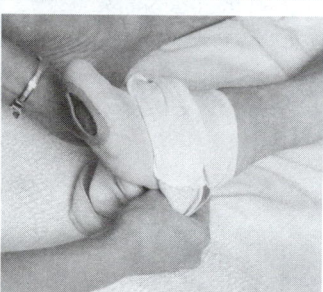
5. Slide the remaining portion of the sock over the client's foot, being sure that his toes are covered. The sock will now be right side out.	If the toes remain uncovered, they will become constricted by the elastic and their circulation can be reduced.	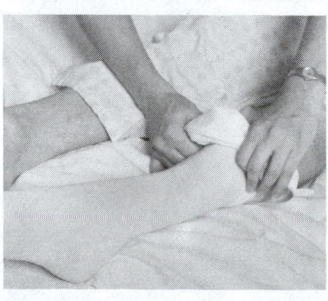
6. Slide the sock up over the client's calf until the sock is completely extended. Be sure the sock is smooth and no ridges are present.	Ridges impede venous return and can counteract the overall purpose of the elastic stocking.	
7. Instruct the client not to roll his socks partially down.	Rolling the sock partially down will have a constricting effect and impede venous return.	

into the client's care plan. If the client does not have voluntary control of his extremities, the nurse performs passive range of joint motion exercises (see Chapter 30). The nurse can perform such exercises while bathing the client and can assess the venous system at the same time.

Third, the use of elastic stockings reduces the risk of thrombus formation. Elastic stockings are available in toe-to-knee and toe-to-midthigh sizes. They promote venous return by maintaining pressure on the muscles of the lower extremities. Elastic stockings should be removed and reapplied at least twice a day, and the nurse should make sure the stockings are clean and dry (Procedure 31-1).

If the nurse suspects deep vein thrombosis, she should report it immediately. The leg should be elevated with no pressure on the area of thrombosis. The client, family, and nursing personnel should be instructed *not* to massage the region.

Musculoskeletal System

The immobilized client must receive some type of exercise to prevent excessive muscle wasting and atrophy and joint contractures. The total amount of activity required to prevent physical disuse syndromes is only about 2 hours in a 24-hour period, but this activity must be scheduled so the client does not remain inactive for more than 1 hour at a time.

If the client is unable to move a portion or all of his body, the nurse must perform passive range of joint motion exercises for all immobilized joints while bathing the client, and at least two or three more times throughout the day. If one extremity is paralyzed, the client can be taught to put each joint independently through its range of motion.

Some orthopedic and neurological conditions require more frequent passive range of motion exercises to restore the injured joint or extremity to maximal function. Clients with such conditions may use automatic equipment for passive range of joint motion exercises (Fig. 31-12). The equipment extends an extremity to a prescribed angle for a prescribed period. This method is beneficial when the client must gradually increase the degree and duration of extension to achieve optimal functioning of the affected area.

Clients on bed rest should have active range of joint motion exercises incorporated into the daily schedule (see Chapter 30). The client can perform these exercises during the activities of daily living. Table 31-2 describes the joint movements that occur with various daily activities.

Passive and active range of joint motion exercises maintain the functioning of the musculoskeletal system. The nurse should also plan interventions for the gradual return of mobility in clients who will be able to resume their preillness activity patterns.

The best nursing intervention is establishment of a progressive exercise program individualized to the client's level of health, age, weight, chronicity of ill-

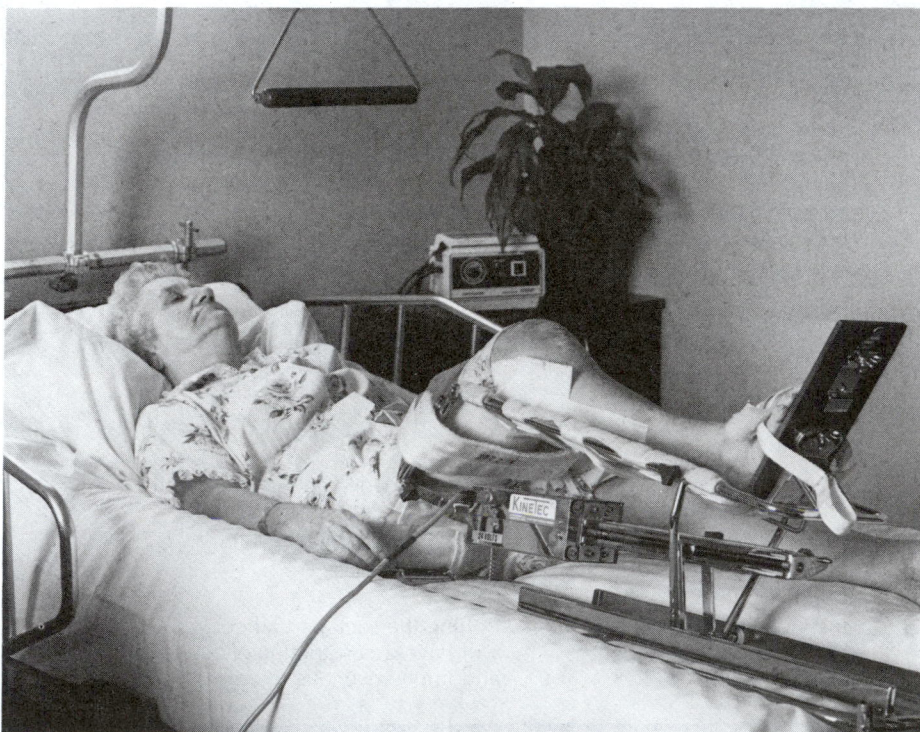

Fig. 31-12 Automatic range of joint motion exercises.

TABLE 31-2

Incorporating Active Range of Joint Motion Exercises into Activities of Daily Living

Joint Exercised	Activity of Daily Living	Movement
Neck	Nodding head yes	Flexion
	Shaking head no	Rotation
	Moving right ear to right shoulder	Lateral flexion
	Moving left ear to left shoulder	Lateral flexion
Shoulder	Reaching to turn on overhead light	Extension
	Reaching to bedside stand for book	Extension
	Scratching back	Hyperextension
	Rotating shoulders toward chest	Abduction
	Rotating shoulders toward back	Adduction
Elbow	Eating, bathing, shaving, grooming	Flexion, extension
Wrist	Eating, bathing, shaving, grooming	Flexion, extension, hyperextension, abduction, adduction
Fingers and thumb	All activities requiring fine motor coordination, e.g., writing, eating, hobbies	Flexion, extension, abduction, adduction, opposition
Hip	Walking	Flexion, extension, hyperextension
	Moving to side-lying position	Flexion, extension, abduction
	Moving from side-lying position	Extension, adduction
	Rolling feet inward	Internal rotation
	Rolling feet outward	External rotation
Knee	Walking	Flexion, extension
	Moving to and from a side-lying position	Flexion, extension
Ankle	Walking	Dorsiflexion, plantar flexion
	Moving toe toward head of bed	Dorsiflexion
	Moving toe toward foot of bed	Plantar flexion
Toes	Walking	Extension, hyperextension
	Wiggling toes	Abduction, adduction

ness, and motivation. A progressive exercise program gradually increases the client's physical activity to reverse the deconditioning associated with bed rest (Winslow and Weber, 1980).

Progressive exercise programs are used for clients with musculoskeletal, neurological, cardiopulmonary, renal, and other chronic diseases. Before beginning the program the client should perform flexibility exercises unless they are contraindicated. Initially the client stands erect with feet slightly apart. Then, while maintaining hip and knee extension, he moves the upper body from side to side (Fig. 31-13, *A*). Ideally, the maximum range is a lateral flexion of 45 degrees. The client then rotates his trunk 360 degrees (Fig. 31-13, *B*). Finally, the client stands erect, flexes the waist 90 degrees, brings himself upright, and hyperextends his upper body 30 degrees (Fig. 31-13, *C*). No client should be encouraged to do these flexibility exercises until he is physiologically stable and can tolerate easy activities such as sitting, standing, and walking to a

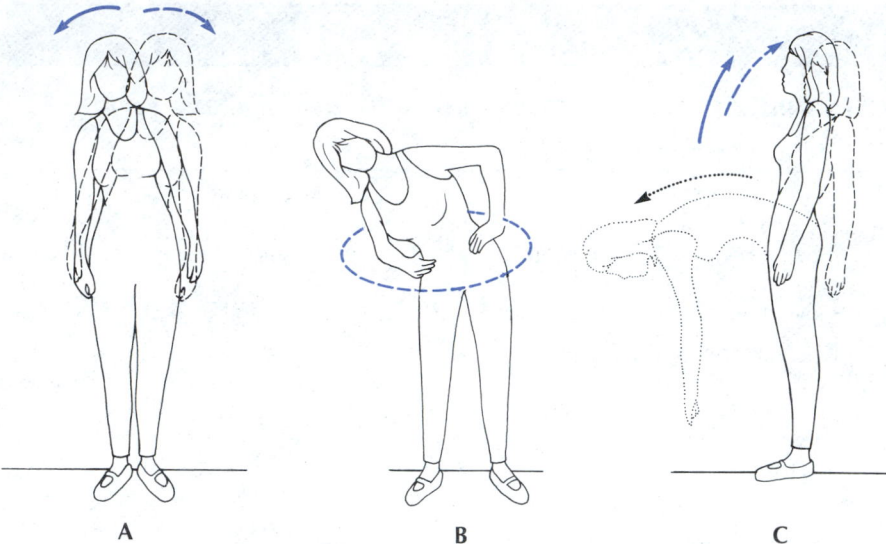

Fig. 31-13 Flexibility exercises. **A,** Flexing upper body from side to side. **B,** Rotation of trunk 360 degrees. **C,** Hyperextension of upper body.

chair. The first two flexibility exercises can be performed while the client is sitting. Flexibility exercises help to alleviate the stiffness associated with bed rest.

When a client begins flexibility and progressive exercises, he should be encouraged not to push himself and to stop and report any pain or dizziness. The nurse should use baseline assessments of the client's vital signs, skin color, presence of pain, and fatigability to monitor the client's tolerance to the activity throughout the exercise period.

The nursing interventions described in this section are designed to prevent musculoskeletal problems associated with immobility. These include decreased muscle mass, muscle atrophy, decreased endurance, contractures, and disuse osteoporosis. Maintaining proper functioning of the musculoskeletal system also reduces the effects of immobility on the skin.

Skin

As discussed previously, the major risk to the skin from restricted mobility is the formation of decubitus ulcers. Nursing interventions therefore focus on the prevention or treatment of decubitus ulcers.

PREVENTING DECUBITUS ULCERS

The first step in the prevention of decubitus ulcers is to assess the client's risk factors, as outlined previously. The nurse then reduces environmental factors that can accelerate decubitus ulcer formation, such as high room temperature, moisture, or wrinkled bed linen.

The nursing care plan includes interventions to reduce pressure to the skin, thereby decreasing the risk of decubitus ulcer formation. The immobilized client's position should be changed every 2 hours around the clock.

After the client is turned, the nurse should massage all areas that received pressure. Massaging the pressure points improves circulation and delivers oxygen and nutrients to the region to correct the metabolic debt created by the pressure. Fig. 31-14 illustrates the potential pressure points for clients in the Fowler's, prone, supine, and side-lying positions. When the client is repositioned, the nurse checks to see that all pressure points are protected. As noted in Chapter 30, the nurse protects pressure points by using flotation pads, sheepskin, and trochanter rolls and pillows (see boxed material below).

Nursing Interventions to Prevent Decubitus Ulcers

- Assess for pressure points every 1 to 2 hours.
- Rotate client's position every 1 to 2 hours.
- Massage reddened pressure points.
- Maintain smooth bed linens.
- Keep client's skin dry.
- Reposition the client properly.
- Use mechanical devices properly to reduce pressure.

The nurse also uses three types of mechanical devices to prevent or treat decubitus ulcers: devices that support specific pressure areas of the body, such as the heels, sacra, buttocks, and elbows; devices that aid in turning or moving the client; and devices that support the entire body in such a way that pressure is either minimized or equalized (Table 31-3) (Berecek, 1975b).

DEVICES TO SUPPORT SPECIFIC PRESSURE AREAS. Devices that help support pressure areas are used to minimize the effect of immobilization on specific body parts. The devices described in this section reduce pressure by dispersing it over a larger area or lifting specific body parts from the bed or chair.

Flotation Pads. Flotation pads are constructed of Silastic, silicone, or polyvinyl chloride and are very pliable. Because the consistency of the pad is similar to fat, the pad serves as a layer of artificial fat to protect bony surfaces. The flotation pad also disperses pressure over a larger area, lessening supracapillary pressures (Berecek, 1975b).

Sheepskin. Sheepskins are widely used and work best against the client's bare skin. Sheepskins have four distinct advantages. First, the sheepskin is a resilient substance that disperses pressure over a greater body surface. Second, if the client slides over the sheepskin, friction and shearing forces are reduced. Third, moisture is absorbed and dissipated by the spongelike qualities of the wool. Last, sheepskin is economical and can be laundered. Sheepskins are available in various sizes and are contoured to accommodate the rounded surfaces of heels and elbows (Berecek, 1975b).

Pillows and Trochanter Rolls. Pillows and trochanter rolls lift the potential pressure area off the mattress. For example, a small pillow or trochanter roll under a client's ankles lifts the heels off the bed, reducing pressure in that area. Pillows also separate two points of pressure. For example, when a client is in the side-lying position, a pillow under the uppermost leg prevents pressure from the upper knee on the lowermost leg.

DEVICES USED IN TURNING A CLIENT. Devices that help turn an immobilized client are used when long-term immobilization is anticipated. Usually these clients have severe musculoskeletal trauma or damage to the central nervous system.

CircOlectric Bed. The CircOlectric bed is an electronically controlled bed that can be vertically rotated

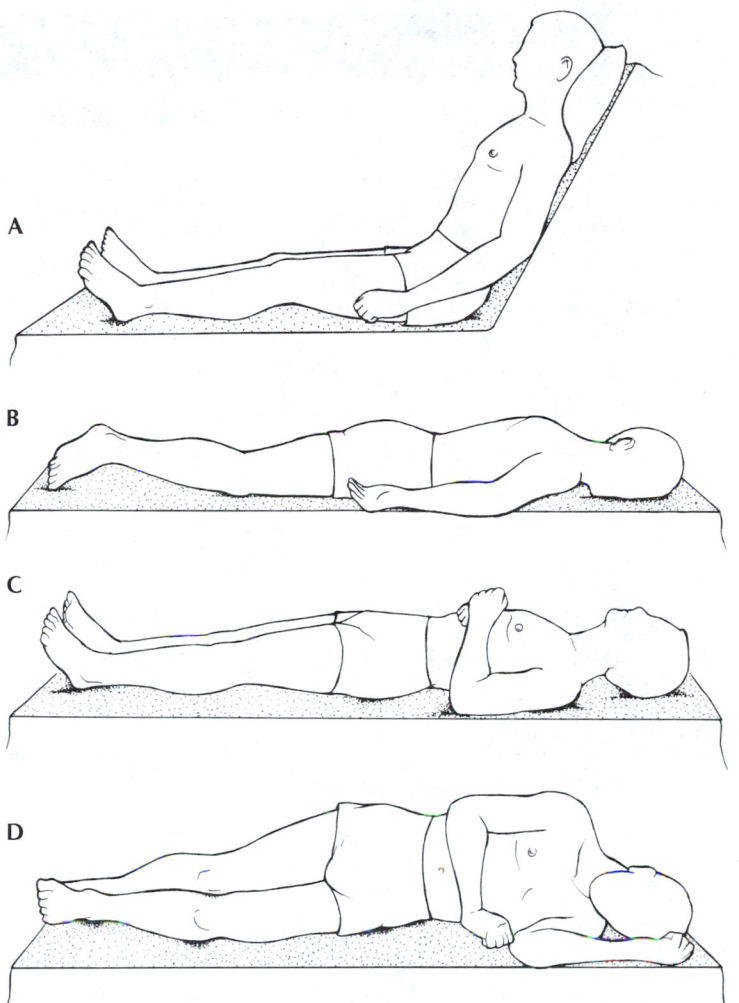

Fig. 31-14 Pressure points *(shaded areas)* for clients in the, **A,** high Fowler's, **B,** prone, **C,** supine, and, **D,** side-lying positions.

210 degrees and permits turning the client from the prone to the supine position. The pressure points that occur in these positions still require protection. This bed is beneficial for clients whose extremities or vertebrae must remain in continuous alignment.

Guttman Bed. The Guttman bed allows the client to be rotated from left to right and back to the supine position. It is used for clients with spinal cord injuries who require spinal immobilization.

Rotokinetic Treatment Table. The Rotokinetic treatment table is a bed that rotates the client 270 degrees every 3 minutes from the extreme left lateral position to the extreme right lateral position. The bed is most useful for clients with recent spinal cord injuries. It is designed to reduce the hazards of immobility and permit optimal nursing care of the immobilized client.

TABLE 31-3

Mechanical Devices Used to Prevent or Treat Decubitus Ulcers

Purpose	Device	Effects
To support pressure areas of the body	Flotation pads	Disperse pressure to a specific body area over a larger area
	Sheepskin	Disperses pressure over a greater body surface, reduces friction, absorbs moisture
	Pillows and trochanter rolls	Lift the pressure site off the mattress, separate two points of pressure
To aid turning a client	CircOlectric bed	Rotates client vertically from prone to supine positions
	Guttman bed	Rotates client from prone to supine positions and side to side
	Rotokinetic treatment table	Rotates client continuously
	Stryker wedge turning frame	Rotates client horizontally from prone to supine positions
To minimize or equalize pressure	Alternating air mattress	Alternates pressure points by alternating inflation and deflation of a series of air cells every 3 to 7 seconds
	Water mattress	Disperses and evenly distributes client's body weight over the mattress
	Clinitron bed	Decreases pressure and eliminates shearing, friction, and maceration; disperses and evenly distributes client's weight through fluidization (gentle flow of temperature-controlled air forced upward through mass of fine ceramic microspheres so client floats on dry fluid)
	Egg crate mattress	Disperses and evenly distributes client's body weight over the mattress

Stryker Wedge Turning Frame. The Stryker frame promotes turning the client from the supine to prone positions. Unlike the CircOlectric bed, which turns the client vertically, the Stryker turning frame is used for horizontal turning.

DEVICES TO MINIMIZE OR EQUALIZE PRESSURE. Beds designed to minimize or equalize body pressure points function according to two principles. The surface of the bed may be designed to alter points of pressure against the body surface at regular time in-

tervals. The surface of the bed also molds itself to the client's body to distribute the weight of the body over a wider area, preventing concentration of pressure over bony prominences, which impedes circulation (Berecek, 1975b).

Alternating Air Mattresses. Alternating air mattresses are constructed of polyvinyl air cells arranged horizontally or vertically. The mattress is attached to a pump that alternately inflates and deflates a series of air cells every 3 to 7 seconds, thereby continually altering the points of pressure. The nurse should use only one sheet between the air mattress and the client, since additional sheets, sheepskins, or absorbent pads decrease the effectiveness of the mattress.

Water Mattresses. Water mattresses are designed to disperse and evenly distribute the client's weight over the mattress. Water beds have proved effective for reducing skin breakdown, but some clients have experienced hallucinations, nightmares, disorientation, and depression on these beds. In addition, nursing measures, such as bathing, catheterization, or dressing changes, are more difficult.

Clinitron Bed. The Clinitron bed is designed to distribute a client's weight evenly over the mattress. The bed minimizes pressure and eliminates shear, friction, and maceration through the principle of fluidization. Fluidization is created by forcing a gentle flow of temperature-controlled air upward through a mass of fine ceramic microspheres. The client floats on a dry fluid, and the contact pressure of the client's body to the mattress surface is maintained at 11 mm Hg or less.

Egg Crate Mattress. The egg crate mattress is a foam rubber pad that rests on the regular bed mattress. The foam rubber peaks help to disperse and evenly distribute the client's weight, decreasing pressure points.

■ ■ ■ ■ ■

Prevention is the key to the problem of decubitus ulcers. Frequent complete nursing assessments of a client's skin can quickly identify pressure points at risk for decubitus ulcer formation. If an ulcer does form, the nurse continues to use preventive interventions to minimize the ulcer and prevent new ulcers from forming. In addition, the nurse uses a variety of skin care techniques to promote healing of the ulcer.

TREATMENT OF DECUBITUS ULCERS

CARING FOR THE SKIN. Of primary importance in the treatment of decubitus ulcers is the cleanliness of the ulcer area and all skin surfaces. Maintaining cleanliness may be extremely difficult with incontinent, feverish, or confused clients.

Moisture in and around an area of skin breakdown can cause further ulceration and infection. Many products are available for the care of decubitus ulcers (Table 31-4). The nurse should clean the affected area with an antiseptic solution at least every 2 hours and more often if the client is diaphoretic or incontinent. The antiseptic agent prevents the growth or further development of microorganisms. Caution is needed because antiseptics can damage tissue unprotected by the dermis and may inactivate certain medications.

The ulcer should be thoroughly rinsed with saline after cleaning to minimize the effect of the antiseptic on the tissue (Fowler, 1982).

An ulcer that has necrotic tissue or eschar or shows signs of sloughing must be debrided. Eschar is the scab or dry crust that results from excoriation of the skin. Sloughing is the shedding of dead tissue as the result of skin ulceration. Debridement is the removal of necrotic tissue so healthy tissue can regenerate.

For reddened areas or skin breaks, skin care products that lubricate and protect the skin, stimulate circulation, and promote wound healing are recommended. When the ulcer bed is pink with granulation tissue throughout, a dressing is indicated to promote healing. A clean, moist environment promotes migration of epithelial cells across the ulcer surface (Fowler, 1982).

REVITALIZING THE BODY. Protein and hemoglobin levels are important considerations in the treatment of decubitus ulcers. A client can lose as much as 50 g of protein a day from an open, weeping decubitus ulcer. This is a sizable amount of the normal daily requirement of 60 g for women and 70 g for men (Kavchak-Keyes, 1977b).

Increased protein intake, two to four times normal, helps to rebuild epidermal tissue. An increased caloric intake, at least one and one half times normal, helps to replace subcutaneous tissue. Increased intake of vitamin C promotes protein synthesis (Kavchak-Keyes, 1977b).

A low hemoglobin level decreases the delivery of oxygen to the tissues and causes further debilitation. Whenever possible, the client's hemoglobin should be maintained at 12 g/100 ml.

■ ■ ■ ■ ■

Nursing care of the immobilized client must address the prevention of decubitus ulcers. In 1979 it was estimated that the presence of a decubitus ulcer could increase hospital costs by $15,000. In addition, a decubitus ulcer can slow the rehabilitation of clients with central nervous system damage. When a client with a spinal cord injury develops a decubitus ulcer on his lower extremities, he must be confined to bed and not allowed up in a wheelchair because of the effect of pressure from the wheelchair on the ulcer. Preventing decubitus ulcers saves the client both time and money and permits a quick return to maximal mobility.

Elimination System

Nursing interventions for maintaining optimal urinary functioning are directed toward keeping the client well hydrated without causing bladder disten-

TABLE 31-4

Decubitus Skin Care Products

Type	Purpose	Ulcer Assessment
CLEANSING AGENTS		
Antiseptic agents (hydrogen peroxide, povidone-iodine, hypochlorite solution)	Reduction of microorganisms	Necrotic debris present
Physiologic saline or water	Cleansing	Ulcer with pink granulation bed, no necrotic debris
Chemical enzymatic agents*		
Travase Ointment	Proteolysis	Eschar
Collagenase ointment	Collagenolysis	Sloughing
Elase Ointment	Fibrinolysis	Sloughing
Absorption-granulation aids		
Granulex	Mild debriding action to stimulate granulation tissue	No necrotic debris
Debrisan	Absorption of tissue fluid	Secretions, no necrotic debris
Bard Absorption Dressing	Absorption of tissue fluid, provides moist environment	No necrotic debris
WOUND COVERINGS		
Gauze	Packing	Debridement of loose debris
Absorbent sponges	Wicking of drainage	Absorption, packing
Nontransparent occlusive dressing	Maintenance of moist environment	No necrotic debris
Semipermeable transparent adhesive film	Maintenance of moist environment	No necrotic debris

Modified from Fowler, E.: J. Gerontol. Nurs. **8**:680, 1982.
*Discontinue use when the ulcer bed is pink with granulation tissue.

tion and the reflux of urine into the ureters and in some instances the renal pelvis.

Adequate hydration helps prevent renal calculi and urinary tract infections. The client should void large amounts of dilute urine. If the client is also incontinent, the nurse should modify the care plan so the client's increased urinary output does not cause skin breakdown.

To prevent bladder distention, the nurse must assess the frequency and amount of urinary output. A client who continually dribbles urine and whose bladder is distended has overflow incontinence. If the immobilized client does not have voluntary control of bladder elimination, the nurse may be required to insert a straight catheter or an indwelling Foley catheter in order to alleviate and prevent bladder distention (see Chapter 39).

The nurse must also record the frequency and consistency of bowel movements. If a client is unable to maintain normal bowel patterns, the physician may order administration of stool softeners, cathartics, or enemas (see Chapter 40).

Psychosocial Problems

The nursing assessment can identify the effects of prolonged immobilization on the client's psychosocial dimension. People who have a tendency toward depression or mood swings are at greater risk for developing these changes during bed rest or immobilization.

First, the nurse should anticipate changes in the client's psychosocial status before they develop in order to intervene with preventive nursing measures.

The nurse can provide routine and informal socialization for the client. Nursing activities can be planned to give the client opportunities to talk and interact with the staff. If possible the client should be placed in a room with other clients who are mobile and interactive. If the client must remain in a private room, staff members should be asked to visit the client at least once a day.

Second, the nurse provides stimuli to maintain the client's orientation and entertain the client. A daily newspaper helps the client keep track of current events and the movement of time. Bedside chats at appropriate moments orient the client to the schedule of nursing activities, meals, and visiting hours. Books from the hospital library help occupy the client when he is alone. If the client's condition permits, he can participate in craft activities. Radio and television may provide the client with stimulation and help to pass the time.

Third, clients should be encouraged to wear their glasses or artificial teeth and to shave or apply makeup. These are normal activities through which people maintain body image. Assisting a client to maintain body image can alleviate the depression resulting from immobilization.

Fourth, the client should be involved in his care whenever possible. For example, the nurse should allow the client to determine when he would like his bed made. Some clients rest better during the night when fresh sheets are put on in the evening rather than in the morning. The client should be encouraged to perform as much self-care as possible. Hygiene and grooming articles should be kept within easy reach so the client can attend to his own needs.

Fifth, nursing care between 10 PM and 7 AM should be scheduled to minimize interruptions of the client's sleep. This may involve administering medications and assessing vital signs at times when the client must be turned or receive special skin care.

Last, the nurse should observe the client for failure to cope with his restricted mobility. If the nursing care plan is not improving the client's coping patterns, outside assistance may be required from a clinical nurse specialist, counselor, social worker, clergyman, or other consultant. Recommendations of these consultants should be incorporated into the plan of care.

Developmental Changes

Ideally, immobilized clients continue normal development. However, this goal is unrealistic for the very young or the very old. Nursing interventions can help in this area.

First, particularly with a young child, nursing care should stimulate the client mentally as well as phys-

ically. Play activities can be incorporated into the nursing care plan for children. Puzzles, for example, can help develop fine motor skills, and reading can help the child learn and develop cognitively. An immobilized child should be placed in a room with children of the same age who are not immobilized unless a contagious disease is present. Nursing activities, such as dressing changes, cast care, and care of traction, can be designed to require participation of the child. The nurse must recognize extreme changes from the child's normal behavioral patterns. If these behavioral changes continue, the nurse should seek a consultation from a clinical nurse specialist, counselor, or other health care professional whose specialty is treating children.

Immobilization or restricted mobility of the elderly presents different nursing problems than with any other age group. Elderly clients usually have one or

---

Physiological Evaluation Criteria for the Immobilized Client

METABOLIC SYSTEM

- No decrease in muscle mass
- Normal serum protein levels
- Fluid and electrolyte balance
- Preimmobilization weight

RESPIRATORY SYSTEM

- Absence of pulmonary secretions
- Absence of indicators of respiratory tract infection, such as productive cough, fever, pleuritic chest pain.

CARDIOVASCULAR SYSTEM

- Absence of orthostatic hypotension
- No increase in resting pulse rate
- Absence of deep vein thrombosis

MUSCULOSKELETAL SYSTEM

- Return of preimmobilization activity tolerance
- Complete range of joint motion
- Complete weight bearing

SKIN

- Absence of decubitus ulcers

ELIMINATION SYSTEM

- Absence of signs of kidney infection, such as frequency, burning, hesitation, fever, flank pain
- Absence of constipation
- Absence of fecal impaction

more chronic illnesses. Because of their age and the presence of chronic illness, the elderly are at high risk for the hazards of immobility. Once a chronically ill elderly client has been immobilized, he is unlikely to regain his previous functional abilities.

Inactive elderly clients are at greater risk for confusion, depression, and disorientation, which result from immobilization, chronic illnesses, medications, and the aging process itself. Therefore the elderly require nursing interventions designed to orient them to the day, date, and time. A calendar and a clock with a large dial should be in the client's room at all times. The calendar should be marked so the client can immediately identify the day and date. Chapter 27 describes other nursing measures to assist elderly clients in meeting their developmental needs.

Nursing care should be planned to allow the elderly immobilized client to perform as many activities of daily living as possible. If the client did his own grooming before his mobility was restricted, he should be encouraged to continue grooming activities unless contraindicated.

The nurse should always remember that the elderly client is extremely susceptible to all the hazards of immobility. A nursing care plan for an elderly client with limited mobility should be designed to prevent or minimize these hazards, rather than allowing problems to develop and then treating them. The frail elderly client may need his position changed every hour instead of every 2 hours, and he may need more frequent range of joint motion exercises. Not only are the elderly more susceptible to the hazards of immobility, but the consequences of immobility appear more quickly and become severe more rapidly.

Evaluation

Since the overall goal of care for the immobilized client is to prevent or minimize the hazards of immobility, the evaluation of nursing care is based on the presence or absence of the consequences of immobility and the client's response to nursing interventions.

If none of the physiological effects of immobility is present, the client's systems are functioning optimally (see boxed material on p. 789). Such a client can return to mobility with no physiological consequences. This ideal state is difficult to achieve and usually occurs in the previously healthy child or young adult.

Psychosocial Evaluation Criteria for the Immobilized Client

- Preimmobilization coping patterns
- Use of new coping patterns when necessary
- Minimal disruption in sleep-wake cycle
- Minimal and short-term behavioral changes
- Social and family interactions
- No indication of sensory deprivation

Evaluation of nursing care in the psychosocial dimension is based on the client's responses to interventions (see boxed material above). Ideally, the client who has been immobilized is able to maintain social interaction, interests, and coping patterns. This goal is easily achieved when immobilization is short-term. As immobilization continues, however, the client's coping strategies may cease to be successful.

The evaluation criteria for the developmental dimension are no measurable decline in the client's functioning or delay in development. These are difficult to attain for immobilized elderly clients, but a well-designed nursing care plan can minimize the developmental consequences of immobilization.

Summary

Immobilization can adversely affect the client in all dimensions. Although in some cases immobilization is necessary to promote wound healing, proper skeletal alignment, or rest after an illness, it involves many hazards and risks. Nursing care seeks to prevent adverse effects from occurring and to minimize them when they do occur. Using the nursing process, the nurse assesses physiological, psychosocial, and developmental health needs, diagnoses actual or potential problems related to immobilization, and plans and delivers nursing care to meet the client's needs and prevent or resolve problems. Because the effects of immobility can be extensive, nursing care for immobilized clients remains a challenging area.

KEY CONCEPTS

✓ Normal physical mobility depends on intact and functioning nervous and musculoskeletal systems.

✓ The risk of disabilities related to immobilization depends on the extent and duration of the immobilization.

✓ Immobility may result from illness or trauma or may be prescribed for therapeutic reasons but in any case presents hazards in the physiological, psychological, and developmental dimensions.

✓ Decubitus ulcers are one of the most common physiological hazards of immobility, but the nurse can take actions to prevent or treat them.

✓ Psychosocial effects of immobility include depression, behavioral changes, changes in the sleep-wake cycle, decreased coping abilities, and developmental effects.

✓ The nurse uses the nursing process to provide care for clients experiencing or at risk for the adverse effects of immobility.

✓ Assessment focuses on range of joint motion, musculoskeletal status, and complete physical examination for potential adverse effects in all body systems, as well as psychosocial and developmental effects.

✓ After identifying nursing diagnoses, the nurse plans and implements interventions to prevent or minimize the hazards and complications of immobilization.

✓ Interventions address the client's psychosocial and developmental needs that result from immobilization.

✓ The primary evaluation criterion for nursing care in the developmental dimension for immobilized clients is the prevention of any measurable decline in the client's functioning or delay in development.

REFERENCES

Berecek, K.H.: Etiology of decubitus ulcers, Nurs. Clin. North Am. 10:157, 1975a.

Berecek, K.H.: Treatment of decubitus ulcers, Nurs. Clin. North Am. 10:171, 1975b.

Blackburn, G.L., et al.: Nutritional and metabolic assessment of the hospitalized patient, J. Parenteral Enteral Nutr. 1:11, 1977.

Deitrick, J., et al.: Effects of immobilization upon various metabolic and physiologic functions of normal men, Am. J. Med. 4:3, 1948.

DiMascio, S.: Debrisan for decubitus ulcers, Am. J. Nurs. 79:684, 1979.

Fowler, E.: Pressure sores: a deadly nuisance, J. Gerontol. Nurs. 12:680, 1982.

Groër, M.W., and Shekleton, M.E.: Basic pathophysiology: a conceptual approach, ed. 2, St. Louis, 1983, The C.V. Mosby Co.

Guttman, L.: The problem of treatment of pressure sores in patients with spinal paraplegia, Br. J. Plast. Surg. 8:196, 1955.

Hulley, S.B., et al.: The effect of supplemental oral phosphate on the bone mineral changes during prolonged bed rest, J. Clin. Invest. 50:2506, 1971.

Kavchak-Keyes, M.A.: Four proven steps for preventing decubitus ulcers, Nursing 77 7:58, 1977a.

Kavchak-Keyes, M.A.: Treating decubitus ulcers using four proven steps, Nursing 77 7:44, 1977b.

Kosiak, M.: Etiology of decubitus ulcers, Arch. Phys. Med. Rehab. 42:19, 1961.

Linden, O., et al.: Pressure distribution on the surface of the human body, Arch. Phys. Med. Rehab. 46:378, 1965.

Olson, E.V.: The hazards of immobility, Am. J. Nurs. 67:779, 1967.

Spencer, W., Valbona, C., and Carter, R.: Physiologic concepts of immobilization, J. Phys. Med. Rehab. 46:89, 1965.

Winslow, E.H., and Weber, T.M.: Progressive exercises to combat hazards of bedrest, Am. J. Nurs. 80:440, 1980.

ADDITIONAL READINGS

Byrne, N., and Feld, M.: Overcoming the red menace: preventing and treating decubitus ulcers, Nursing 84 14:55, 1984.

Feustel, D.E.: Pressure sore prevention: age, there is the rub, Nursing 82 12:78, 1982.

Goldberg, W.G., and Fitzpatrick, J.J.: Movement with the aged, Nurs. Res. 29:339, 1980.

Stewart, A.F., et al.: Calcium homeostasis in immobilization: an example of resorptive hypercalciuria, N. Engl. J. Med. 306:1136, 1982.

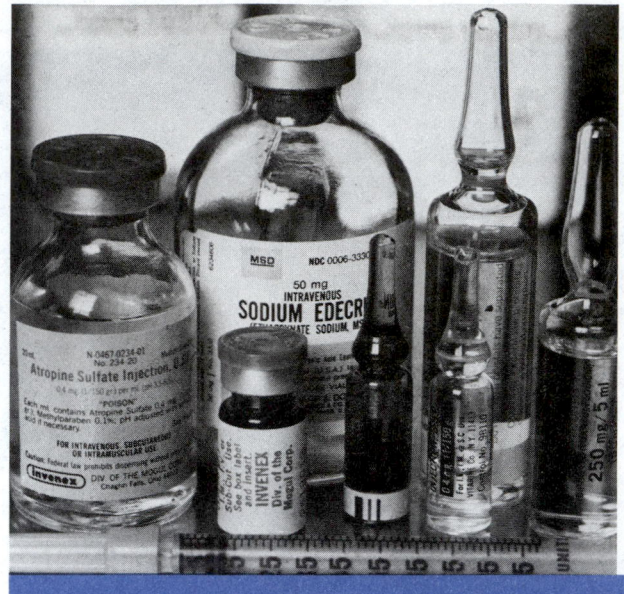

OBJECTIVES

Mastery of content in this chapter will enable the student to:

- Define the terms in the glossary.
- Distinguish between different types of drug names.
- Discuss the nurse's legal responsibilities in drug prescription and administration.
- Describe the physiological mechanisms of drug action.
- Discuss the factors influencing absorption, distribution, metabolism, and excretion of medications.
- Differentiate among toxic, idiosyncratic, allergic, and side effects of drugs.
- Discuss factors unique to an individual that influence drug actions.
- Describe factors to consider in choosing routes of drug administration.
- Correctly calculate a prescribed drug dosage.
- Differentiate between the types of drug orders.
- Discuss factors to include in assessing a client's needs for and response to drug therapy.
- List the "five rights" of drug administration.
- Correctly prepare and administer:
  An oral preparation
  A subcutaneous injection
  An intramuscular injection
  An intradermal injection
  Topical skin preparations
  Eye drops and ointments
  Ear drops
  Nose drops
  Vaginal instillations
  Rectal suppositories

GLOSSARY

ampule Small sterile glass or plastic container that usually contains a single dose of solution to be administered parenterally.

anaphylactic reaction Severe and sometimes fatal systemic hypersensitivity reaction to a sensitizing substance, for example, a drug, venom, foods, or a chemical.

aspirate Withdraw fluid or air into the barrel of a syringe or a suction device.

biotransformation Process by which living organisms metabolize or modify the chemical structure of drugs.

compatibility Ability of two or more drugs to be administered at the same time without causing undesired side effects or changing the therapeutic effects of the drugs.

detoxify Remove the toxic quality of a substance; the liver acts to detoxify chemicals in drug compounds.

diluent Agent that makes a solution or mixture thinner or more liquid by admixture.

drug abuse Use of a drug to obtain effects for which it is not prescribed; may lead to physical, social, and psychological harm.

drug addiction Condition characterized by an overwhelming desire to continue taking a drug to which one has become habituated through repeated use; physiological symptoms occur when the regular use of the drug is discontinued.

32 Administration of Medications

drug dependence   Psychological or physiological reliance on a chemical agent.

formulary   Listing of drugs and information about them used by health practitioners to prescribe appropriate therapy.

half-life   Time required for elimination processes to reduce the blood concentration of a drug by half.

infusion   Introduction of a substance, such as a fluid, drug, electrolyte, or nutrient, directly into a vein by means of gravity flow.

injection   Act of forcing a liquid into the body by means of a syringe.

instillation   Procedure in which a fluid is slowly introduced into a cavity or passage of the body (for example, rectum) and allowed to remain for a specific length of time before being withdrawn or drained.

intra-arterial   Within an artery.

intra-articular   Within a joint.

intracardiac   Within the myocardium.

intradermal injection   Form of injection in which the solution is introduced into the dermis of the skin.

intramuscular (IM) injection   Form of injection in which the solution is introduced into the body of a muscle.

intrathecal   Within the spine.

intravenous (IV) injection   Form of injection in which the solution is introduced into a vein.

irrigation   Process of washing out a body cavity or wounded area with a stream of fluid.

over-the-counter drug   Drug available to a consumer without a prescription.

parenteral   Not in or through the digestive system; typically refers to administering medications by injection.

portal system   Network of veins that drains blood from the abdominal portion of the gastrointestinal tract, the spleen, the pancreas, and the gallbladder to the liver.

potentiation   Synergistic action in which the effect of two drugs given simultaneously is greater than the effect of the drugs given separately.

prescription   Authorized order for medication, therapy, or a therapeutic device.

subcutaneous injection   Form of injection in which the solution is introduced into subcutaneous tissues.

synergistic agent   Substance that augments or adds to the activity of another substance or agent.

topical   Pertaining to a drug or treatment applied to the surface of a part of the body.

vial   Glass container with a metal-enclosed rubber seal.

The safe and accurate administration of medications is one of the nurse's most important responsibilities. Drugs are a primary means of therapy for clients with health alterations, but any drug has the potential for causing harmful effects when administered improperly to a client. The nurse is responsible for understanding a drug's effects, administering the drug correctly, and monitoring the client's response.

Often a client must rely on the administration of medications to ensure his well-being. The client may have to take several medications at a time or take medications only when specific symptoms develop. It is important for the nurse to help clients understand the medications they receive so they can self-administer medications safely.

The safe administration of medications requires more than just a knowledge of a specific drug's action. The nurse must also understand the client's previous health problems and the nature of his present disorder to determine whether a particular medication should be given. The nurse's judgment is critical in assuming responsibility and accountability for proper drug administration.

Drug Nomenclature and Forms

The nurse encounters drugs under a variety of different nomenclatures or names. The nurse must be careful to obtain the exact name and spelling for a particular drug.

Names

A drug's *chemical name* is most meaningful to the chemist who develops and tests different drugs. The chemical name provides an exact description of the drug's composition. An example of a chemical name is acetylsalicylic acid, which is commonly known as aspirin.

The *generic name* is given by the manufacturer who first develops the drug. Protected by law, the generic name is given before a drug receives official approval. All manufacturers list drugs by their licensed generic names. Aspirin is an example of a generic name.

Federal legislation in 1962 mandated that there be one *official name* for each drug. The official name is the name under which a drug is listed in official publications such as the *United States Pharmacopeia* (USP). Often a drug's generic name becomes its official name, as with aspirin.

The *trade name, brand name,* or *proprietary name* is the name under which a manufacturer markets a drug. All drugs with a given generic and official name must have the same chemical structure, but a drug's trade name identifies the company responsible for the drug's manufacture. A generic drug thus may have many different trade names. The trade name has the symbol ® at the upper right of the name, indicating that the manufacturer has registered the drug. So that lay persons will recognize trade names readily, manufacturers choose names that are easy to pronounce, spell, and remember. Since many companies may produce the same drug, similarities in trade names can be confusing. Most hospital and clinic pharmacies attempt to dispense medications with the same trade names consistently so nurses can become familiar with the drugs. Table 32-1 lists examples of the different drug names.

Classification

Nurses learn to categorize drugs with similar characteristics by their *class.* Drug classification indicates the effect of the drug on a body system (for example, central nervous system depressant), the symptoms the drug relieves (for example, anti-inflammatory), or the drug's desired effect (for example, tranquilizer). Each class contains drugs that are prescribed for similar types of health problems. The physical and chemical

TABLE 32-1	

Examples of Drug Names

Official	Generic	Chemical	Trade
Sodium pentobarbital	Pentobarbital	Sodium 5-ethyl-5-(1-methylbutyl) barbiturate	Nembutal, Nembutal Sodium
Tetracycline	Tetracycline	4-(Dimethylamino)-1,4,4a,5,5a,6,11,12a-octahydro-3,6,10,12,12a pentahydroxy-6-methyl-1, 11-dioxo-2-naphthacenecarboxamide	Achromycin, Panmycin, Tetracyn V
Aspirin	Aspirin	Acetylsalicylic acid	Bufferin, Ecotrin, Empirin Analgesic

composition of drugs within a class is not necessarily the same. A drug may also be part of more than one class. For example, aspirin is an analgesic, an antipyretic, and an anti-inflammatory drug.

Since learning specific information about every medication is almost impossible, nurses should learn the general characteristics of drugs in each class. Each class has certain nursing implications for proper administration and monitoring of drug effects. For example, nursing implications related to diuretic administration include monitoring intake and output, weighing the client daily, assessing the development of edema in body tissues, and monitoring serum electrolyte levels. The nursing implications for all drugs within a class provide guidelines for safe and effective client care.

Drug Forms

Drugs are available in a variety of forms or preparations. The form of the drug determines its route of administration. For example, a capsule is taken orally and a solution may be given intravenously. The composition of a drug is designed to enhance its absorption and metabolism within the body. Many drugs are available in several forms. For example, acetaminophen (Tylenol) comes in tablets, capsules, pediatric elixirs, and suppositories. Whenever administering a medication, the nurse must be certain to give the medication in the proper form. Table 32-2 lists common forms of medications.

Drug Legislation and Standards

When a client receives a medication, he should be able to assume that it will produce its desired beneficial effect, that it will not cause direct harm, and that the nurse will administer it correctly. For the consumer's safety and benefit, federal and state legislation governs the production, distribution, prescription, and administration of drugs. Controls on the use of pharmacologically active substances range from individual institutional policies to strict federal laws.

Legislation and Control

In the United States drug legislation began with the Pure Food and Drug Act of 1906. The act focused attention on the purity of food but also set official standards for drugs. Manufacturers were required to label drugs accurately and to ensure that the strength and purity of drugs conformed to their claims. Since that time federal law has extended and refined governmental controls on drug sales and distribution, drug testing, naming and labeling, and the regulation of controlled substances. Tables 32-3 and 32-4 provide a brief review of drug legislation in the United States and Canada.

State drug laws must conform with federal legislation. States can also impose additional controls, including control of substances not regulated by the federal government. For example, states vary with regard to the legal sale and use of alcoholic beverages. Some states set the legal drinking age at 21, while others designate age 18. States also set different regulations for punishment of persons found driving while intoxicated or for illicit use of controlled drugs.

Governmental bodies at the local level also regulate use of alcohol and tobacco. It is not unusual while traveling through the United States to find a "dry" town or county that prohibits sale of alcoholic beverages.

Health care institutions establish individual policies that must conform to federal, state, and local regu-

TABLE 32-2

Forms of Medications

Form	Description
Capsule	Solid dosage form for oral use; medication in a powder, liquid, or oil form and encased by a gelatin shell; capsule colored to aid in product identification
Elixir	Clear fluid containing water and alcohol; designed for oral use; usually has a sweetener added
Extract	Concentrated drug form made by removing the active portion of a drug from its other components; for example, a fluid extract is a drug made into a solution from a vegetable source
Glycerite	Solution of drug combined with glycerin for external use; contains at least 50% glycerin
Liniment	Preparation usually containing alcohol, oil, or soapy emollient that is applied to the skin
Lotion	Drug in liquid suspension that is applied externally to protect the skin
Ointment (salve)	Semisolid, externally applied preparation, usually containing one or more drugs
Paste	Semisolid preparation, thicker and stiffer than an ointment; absorbed through the skin more slowly than an ointment
Pill	Solid dosage form containing one or more drugs, shaped into globules, ovoids, or oblong shapes; true pills rarely used, since they have been replaced by tablets
Solution	Liquid preparation that may be used orally, parenterally, or externally; can also be instilled into a body organ or cavity, e.g., bladder irrigations; contains water with one or more dissolved compounds; must be sterile if for parenteral use
Suppository	Solid dosage form mixed with gelatin and shaped in the form of a pellet for insertion into a body cavity (rectum or vagina); melts when it reaches body temperature, releasing the drug for absorption
Suspension	Finely divided drug particles that are dispersed in a liquid medium; when suspension left standing, particles settle to the bottom of the container; commonly an oral medication and is not to be given intravenously
Syrup	Medication dissolved in a concentrated sugar solution; may contain flavoring to make drug more palatable
Tablet	Powdered dosage form compressed into hard disks or cylinders; in addition to primary drug, contains binders (adhesive to allow powder to stick together), disintegrators (to promote tablet dissolution), lubricants (for ease of manufacturing), and fillers (for convenient tablet size)
Enteric-coated	Tablet for oral use coated with materials that do not dissolve in the stomach; coatings dissolve in the intestine where medication is absorbed
Tincture	Alcohol or water-alcohol drug solution
Troche (lozenge)	Flat, round dosage form containing drug, flavoring, sugar, and mucilage; dissolves in mouth to release drug

lations. The size of an institution, the types of services it provides, and the types of professional personnel it employs influence the policies for drug control, distribution, and administration. Institutional policies are often more restrictive than governmental controls. An institution is concerned primarily with preventing health problems that result from drug use. For example, a common institutional policy is the automatic discontinuation of antibiotic therapy after a set number of days. Although a physician may reorder an antibiotic, this policy helps to control unnecessarily prolonged drug therapy, which may lead to sensitivity or toxic reactions.

Federal, state, and local legislation governs nursing practice, including the administration of medications. State nurse practice acts define and set limits on the scope of a nurse's professional functions and responsibilities. These acts are joint policy statements made by nursing, medical, and hospital associations in a state. Institutions and agencies may interpret specific actions allowed under the acts, but they cannot modify, expand, or restrict the act's intent. The nurse practice acts protect the public from unskilled, undereducated, and unlicensed nurses.

Nurses must become familiar with regulations affecting drug use in the area where they practice. When

TABLE 32-3

Federal Drug Laws in the United States

Date	Title of Law	Provisions
1906	Pure Food and Drug Act	Designated official standards for drugs (*United States Pharmacopeia* and *The National Formulary*); specified standards for drug labeling
1912	Sherley Amendment	Prohibited manufacturers from making fraudulent claims regarding drug efficacy and therapeutic effects
1914	Harrison Narcotic Act	Legally classified drugs believed to be habit forming as narcotics; regulated importation, manufacture, sale, and use of narcotic substances
1938	Federal Food, Drug, and Cosmetic Act	Added the *Homeopathic Pharmacopeia of the United States* as a third drug standard; required that a drug preparation be approved as safe by the Food and Drug Administration (FDA) before marketing; further outlined criteria for drug labeling
1945	Amendment to the Food and Drug Act	Provided for certification of biological products used as drugs (for example, insulin or antibiotics) on a batch basis; allowed for direct supervision and inspection of drug production
1952	Durham-Humphrey Amendment	Distinguished between prescription ("legend") and nonprescription drugs
1962	Kefauver-Harris Amendment	Authorized the FDA to supervise drug production in order to ensure safety and efficacy and to establish official drug names; specified greater controls on investigational drugs
1970	Comprehensive Drug Abuse Prevention and Control Act (Controlled Substances Act)	Set strict controls on manufacture and distribution of controlled drugs (possession of controlled substances unlawful without a prescription); established government programs to promote prevention and treatment of drug dependence

TABLE 32-4

Canadian Drug Legislation

Date	Title of Law	Provisions
1908	Proprietary or Patent Medicine Act	Set standards to protect consumers from unsafe and ineffective nonprescription drugs
1953	Canadian Food and Drug Act	Prohibited sale of contaminated, unsafe drugs and of improperly labeled drugs; designated official standards (*Pharmacopoeia Internationalis, The British Pharmacopoeia, The Canadian Formulary*); defined certain controlled drugs; prohibited advertising of prescription and controlled drugs to the general public; set standards for labeling
1961	Canadian Narcotic Control Act	Restricted sale, possession, and use of narcotics; set guidelines for reporting loss or theft of narcotics; set standards for labeling and record keeping

moving from one state to another, a nurse may discover significant differences in the laws governing drug use. For example, laws vary concerning who may prescribe medications and administer drugs intravenously. In the past, only physicians prescribed medications, although it was not unusual for a nurse to request that a client receive a medication. For example, a nurse might say, "Mrs. Jones has had an upset stomach; can she have some Amphojel?" Several states* have recognized the expanding role of the nurse and have revised nurse practice acts to include prescribing of medications. In most cases this privilege is limited to licensed nurse practitioners.

Administering medications directly into a vein is a responsibility many nurses now assume. Because the intravenous injection of medications may cause serious adverse effects, previously only physicians were allowed to give such injections. Nurses who perform this function must be qualified through proper training, education, and experience.

The nurse is responsible for following legal provisions in administering controlled substances. Controlled substances can be dispensed only with a prescription. Violations of the Controlled Substances Act are punishable by fines, imprisonment, and loss of nurse licensure. Hospitals and other health care institutions have policies for the proper storage and distribution of controlled substances. All narcotics must be double locked in a secure container or cabinet. The nurse uses a special record form when dispensing a drug from the locked container. This form has columns for recording the client's name, the date, the time of administration, the name of the drug, the dosage, and the signature of the nurse dispensing the drug. The form is organized in such a way that the nurse can keep an accurate count of the amount of narcotics used and remaining (Fig. 32-1). If a discrepancy occurs, the nurse investigates immediately and reports the loss to the appropriate personnel.

If a nurse administers only part of a premeasured dose of a controlled substance, a second nurse must witness the disposal of the unused portion. For example, if a client's medication order is for 75 mg of Demerol and the nurse has only a 100 mg ampule, the nurse must discard the extra 25 mg as another nurse looks on. The unused portion of the drug must be accounted for on the record form.

The nurse in charge carries a set of keys for the narcotics cabinet. This accessibility to the drugs is limited to authorized personnel. During an institution's change of shift, a nurse going off duty and the

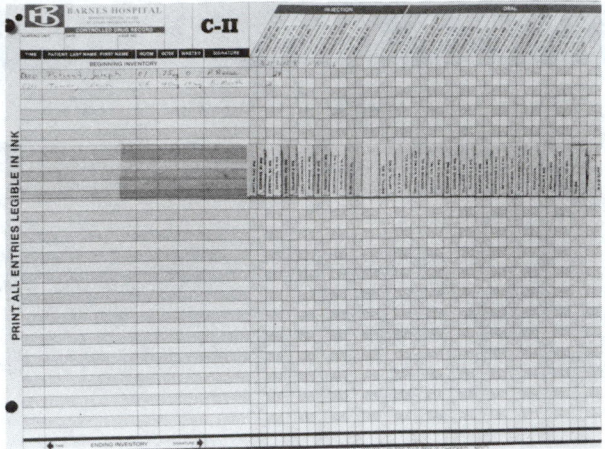

Fig. 32-1 The nurse uses a special form for documenting the dispensing of controlled substances. The law requires recording of the client's name, time of drug administration, type and dosage of drug, and signature of the nurse administering the medication.

nurse replacing her inventory the controlled substances. The nurse arriving on duty counts the number of narcotics remaining, and the other nurse compares that number with the number on the record form. Both nurses sign the form to indicate that the count is correct.

Nontherapeutic Drug Use

Despite legislative controls, some people use drugs for purposes other than their proper purpose. The indiscriminate use of drugs poses serious health problems for the user, his family, and the community. In the past, the misuse or abuse of medications was related to their therapeutic qualities, such as the relief of pain or reduction in anxiety. Today, factors such as peer pressure, curiosity, and the pursuit of pleasure are motivators for drug use. Problems with drug use are not limited to heroin, cocaine, and other "hard" drugs. Millions of people in the United States and Canada consume alcohol daily. It takes only a few minutes of watching television, with its frequent advertisements for pain relievers, decongestants, and antacids, to realize that our society is drug conscious. Table 32-5 lists common terms associated with nontherapeutic use of drugs.

The nurse has an ethical and legal responsibility to understand the problems of persons who use drugs improperly. When caring for clients with suspected drug problems, the nurse must be aware of her own values and attitudes about clients who willfully use potentially harmful substances. The nurse cannot de-

---

*Alaska, Arizona, Idaho, Maine, Maryland, Michigan, Mississippi, Nevada, New Hampshire, New Mexico, North Carolina, Oregon, South Dakota, Tennessee, Utah, Vermont, and Washington.

TABLE 32-5

Terms Associated with the Nontherapeutic Use of Drugs

Term	Definition	Example
Abuse	Use of a chemical substance for nontherapeutic purposes that do not comply with cultural or social standards	A worker ingests alcohol while on the job.
Addiction	Inability to control a drive or craving for a chemical substance	Activities of daily living, e.g., work, socializing with friends, or caring for children, are interrupted by the use of drugs.
Drug dependence	Reliance on the continual use of a substance	A person uses a chemical substance continually throughout a day, often to deal with stressors or problems.
Physical dependence	State characterized by physiological changes that result from frequent use of a chemical substance; failure to take the drug on which one depends leads to withdrawal symptoms	A person experiences lethargy, reduced mental capacity, and inability to make judgments.
Psychological dependence	State characterized by an emotional reliance on a drug to attain a sense of well-being	A person may have a mild desire or intense craving for the drug. Feelings of guilt or shame are resolved by taking more drugs.
Tolerance	State developing with the continual ingestion of a chemical substance in which it eventually becomes necessary to increase the dose to produce the same effects achieved from previous doses	Persons taking opiates, e.g., morphine or codeine, must continually increase the dosage to feel euphoria and freedom from discomfort.

velop a therapeutic relationship with a client if her personal values interfere with her acceptance of the client or understanding of the client's needs. Being familiar with the physical, psychological, and social changes resulting from drug abuse allows the nurse to identify clients with drug problems. For example, a client with a drug problem enters an acute care setting for treatment of a medical problem such as diabetes. Unless the nurse or physician recognizes the drug problem, the client's physical condition can become seriously compromised.

The nurse must have up-to-date information about trends in substance abuse and their legal implications. Nurses see clients with drug problems in a variety of health settings. The nurse has the opportunity to be a key figure in counseling and educating clients about the risks of drug abuse. Chapter 45 describes in detail the nature of health problems related to chemical dependence.

Drug Standards

In 1906, as a result of the Pure Food and Drug Act, the U.S. government set standards for drug quality and purity. Official publications—the *United States Pharmacopeia* (USP) and the *National Formulary*—set standards for drug strength, quality, purity, packaging, safety, labeling, and dosage form. In Canada the *British Pharmacopoeia* (BP) sets similar standards. Physicians, nurses, and pharmacists depend on these standards to ensure that clients receive pure drugs in safe and effective dosages. Drugs originate from plant, animal, and mineral sources or are synthetically produced. For drugs in different forms to produce a predictable effect, there must be uniform standards regulating production and quality.

PURITY

Ideally a drug contains only chemical agents that have therapeutic effects. Unfortunately, most medications also contain some form of contaminant such as solvents, fillers, dyes, waxes, or inks. Pharmaceutical manufacturers must meet standards for the type and concentration of extraneous substances that are allowed in drug products.

POTENCY

The strength or potency of a medication depends on the concentration of active drug in the preparation. Chemical assay or analysis measures the concentration of various ingredients in a medication. If the active ingredient is unknown, pharmaceutical laboratories test the drug on animals. Accepted standards are used to measure the effect on the laboratory animal.

BIOAVAILABILITY

The bioavailability of drugs is a standard recently established by scientists, drug manufacturers, and the government. A drug's bioavailability is its ability to be released from its dosage form, dissolved, absorbed, and transported by the body to its site of action. Scientists measure bioavailability by determining blood or tissue concentrations of a drug at a specified time after administration.

EFFICACY

Objective interpretation of a drug's effectiveness is difficult. Comparing the clinical progress of clients receiving actual drugs with those receiving placebos provides a long-term view of drug efficacy. Animal studies can also provide information on drug efficacy.

SAFETY

Long-term studies help to reveal the incidence and severity of undesirable medication effects. Official drug publications list the most common side effects, as well as the rare toxic effects, of a medication. It may take a considerable time before an investigator knows that a specific drug is absolutely safe. Therefore a complete evaluation of drug safety is not always possible before a new drug reaches the market.

Nature of Drug Actions

Drugs act to produce therapeutically useful effects on a human organism. A drug does not create a function in a tissue or organ but rather *alters* physiological functions within the body. Drugs may protect cells from the influence of other chemical agents, may promote cell function, or may accelerate or slow cell processes.

Mechanisms of Action

Drugs produce their actions in one of three ways: altering body fluids, altering cell membranes, or interacting with receptor sites.

A drug can exert its effect by altering the chemical properties of a body fluid. For example, an antacid such as aluminum hydroxide gel (Amphojel) neutralizes the stomach's acid contents. Other drugs specifically alter the pH of urine.

Some drugs, such as general anesthetic gases, interact with cell membranes. Cell membranes contain a lipid substance that attracts certain lipid-soluble medications. As the drug dissolves in the lipid-containing cell membrane, the properties of the cells are altered, leading to the drug's action.

The most common mechanism of drug action is the binding of drugs to a cell's receptor sites. Specific molecules in cells interact with drugs having a similar three-dimensional shape or chemical structure. The phenomenon is like fitting a key into a lock. When cellular sites match in such a way as to cause chemical bonding, the drug locks into the site and has the desired effect. Cell receptors are usually proteins and nucleic acids. The stronger the bond between drug and receptor site, the more biologically active is the drug.

Receptors localize drug effects. Each tissue or cell in the body possesses a unique group of receptors. For example, receptors in the myocardial cells respond to digitalis preparations, and thus the drug digoxin can increase cardiac contractility. Cells in other tissues such as the kidney or lung do not respond to digoxin because of a difference in receptors.

Pharmacokinetics

Pharmacokinetics is the study of how drugs enter the body, reach their site of action, are metabolized, and exit from the body. The nurse uses knowledge of pharmacokinetics in timing drug administration, selecting the route of administration, judging the client's risk for alterations in drug action, and observing the client's response to medications.

ABSORPTION

A drug is not effective unless it reaches its site of action. Most medications, except for those applied topically, must enter the systemic circulation to exert their therapeutic effects. Factors influencing drug absorption include route of administration, ability of the drug to dissolve, and conditions at the site of absorption.

The nurse administers drugs by several routes, such as oral ingestion, rectal administration, and various parenteral routes (skin, inhalation, intravenous administration). Each route has a different influence on drug absorption, depending on the physical structure of the tissues. The skin is relatively impermeable to chemicals, making absorption slow. The mucous membranes and respiratory airways allow for quick drug absorption because of the high vascularity of mucosal and alveolar-capillary surfaces. Since orally administered drugs must pass through the gastrointestinal tract to be absorbed, the overall rate of absorption may be slow. Intravenous injection produces more rapid absorption than either topical or oral administration, since the intravenous route provides immediate access to the systemic circulation.

The ability of an oral medication to dissolve once it is ingested depends largely on its form or preparation. Solutions and suspensions already in a liquid state are absorbed more readily than tablets or capsules. Solid dosage forms must first disintegrate to expose large surface areas of the chemical to gastric and intestinal secretions. Manufacturers add disintegrators and chemical buffers to drugs to speed dissolution. Drugs that are acidic pass through the gastric mucosa rapidly. Drugs that are basic are not absorbed before reaching the small intestine.

Conditions at the site of absorption influence how easily medications enter the systemic circulation. When the skin becomes abraded, topically applied substances can easily penetrate the dermis and underlying tissues. Topical substances that are normally prescribed for their local effect can cause serious reactions when absorbed through the skin's layers. The formation of edema in mucous membranes slows drug absorption, since medications take longer to diffuse to blood vessels. The absorption of parenterally administered medications depends on the blood supply of the tissues into which the drug is injected. Since muscles have a richer blood supply than subcutaneous tissues, a drug given intramuscularly is absorbed more quickly than one injected subcutaneously. In some instances a delayed subcutaneous absorption is preferable to produce long-lasting drug effects. If a client's tissue perfusion is poor, as in the case of circulatory shock, the intravenous route is best. Intravenous administration provides the most rapid and dependable action, since the drug enters the bloodstream directly.

Oral medications are absorbed more easily when administered between meals. When the stomach is filled with food, the contents are emptied slowly into the duodenum, thus slowing drug absorption. Certain foods and antacids cause drugs to bind into complexes that cannot pass through the gastrointestinal tract lining. For example, milk interferes with the absorption of iron and tetracycline. Some drugs are destroyed by the increased acidity of gastric contents and protein digestion during a meal. For example,

insulin is a protein molecule that is digested when taken orally. Enteric coatings resist dissolution in gastric juices and prevent certain medications from being digested in the upper gastrointestinal tract. The coating also protects the stomach lining from irritation by the medication. The enteric coating dissolves when the medication reaches the basic environment of the intestines.

The nurse often has little choice concerning the route by which to administer a medication. However, knowledge of factors that alter or impair drug absorption helps the nurse administer drugs correctly. Neither food nor antacid drugs should be given within 2 hours before and 1 hour after an orally administered medication. If a person normally eats three meals a day (7 to 8 AM, 12 to 1 PM, 6 to 7 PM), the best administration times are 9 to 10 AM, 2 to 4 PM, and 8 to 10 PM. However, some clients take multiple medications, making such a medication schedule difficult to follow. If a drug (such as aspirin or iron) irritates a client's gastrointestinal tract, it should be administered immediately after a meal. Before administering a drug by injection, the nurse assesses for local factors that may impair drug absorption. The nurse chooses injection sites carefully, avoiding sites of bruising, scarring, or swelling.

DISTRIBUTION

When a drug has become absorbed, it travels to its sites of action, metabolism, and excretion. Drugs travel more easily through certain types of tissues. A medication passes more easily from interstitial to intravascular spaces than between body compartments; for example, drugs pass more easily from cerebrospinal fluid to brain or from intra-articular (joint capsule) to intravascular space. Blood vessels are readily permeable to most dissolved substances unless the drug particles are large or bound to serum proteins. Since drugs move freely from blood vessel to interstitial fluids, the concentration of a drug at a specific site depends on (1) the number of blood vessels in the tissues, (2) the degree of local vasodilation or vasoconstriction, and (3) the rate of blood flow to a tissue site.

Any factor that affects circulatory dynamics within a tissue will affect drug distribution by the vascular route. Exercise, warming, and chilling alter local circulation. For example, if a client applies a warm compress to an intramuscular injection site, the resultant vasodilation increases drug distribution. Changes in the heart's stroke volume, blood pressure, and blood volume may impair or enhance general circulation. When a client's blood pressure drops, perfusion to the kidneys falls and distribution of a medication to the renal system becomes impaired.

Not all drugs cross cell membranes easily. Cells that secrete milk, tears, saliva, sweat, bile, and gastric and intestinal juices are impermeable to some medications. Few drugs are distributed evenly throughout the body, and the tissue to be treated by the medication may not receive the highest concentration of the drug.

METABOLISM

After a drug reaches its site of action, it becomes metabolized into an inactive form that is more easily excreted. Biotransformation occurs under the influence of enzymes that detoxify, degrade, and remove biologically active chemicals. Most biotransformation occurs within the liver, although the lung, kidney, blood, and intestines also metabolize drugs.

The liver is especially important, since its specialized structure oxidizes and transforms many toxic substances. Chemicals ingested with foods cross over the intestinal mucosa to enter the portal circulation. The liver degrades many harmful chemicals before they become distributed to the tissues.

If a client has an alteration in function of organs that participate in drug metabolism, he is at risk for drug toxicity. Liver disease can result in a potentially harmful buildup of drugs within the body. Clients with hepatic dysfunction therefore receive low doses of medications. Even a small sedative dose of a barbiturate may cause a client with liver disease to lapse into a hepatic coma.

EXCRETION

Once drugs are metabolized, they exit the body through the kidneys, liver, bowel, lungs, and exocrine glands. The chemical makeup of a drug determines the organ of excretion. Gaseous and volatile compounds such as ether, nitrous oxide, and alcohol exit through the lungs. Alcohol diffuses easily from the blood to the lungs to be exhaled. Deep breathing and coughing (see Chapter 47) help the postoperative client eliminate anesthetic gases more rapidly.

The exocrine glands excrete lipid-soluble drugs. Since drugs that enter the saliva cause a foul taste, good oral hygiene is necessary. When medications exit through sweat glands, a client's skin may become irritated. The skin may also acquire an odor because of drug excretion. The nurse assists the client in good hygiene practices (see Chapter 35) to promote cleanliness and skin integrity. If a drug exits through the mammary glands, there is a risk that a nursing infant will absorb the chemicals. Mothers should minimize drug use while nursing.

The gastrointestinal tract is another route for drug excretion. Many drugs enter the hepatic circulation to be broken down by the liver and excreted into the bile. Once the chemicals enter the intestines through the biliary tract, there is the chance that they will be reabsorbed by the intestines. This process of enterohepatic circulation results in a gradual elimination of drugs. Factors that increase peristalsis, such as laxatives and enemas, accelerate drug excretion through the feces, while factors that slow peristalsis, such as inactivity and improper diet, may prolong a drug's effects.

The kidneys are the main organs for drug excretion. Some drugs escape extensive metabolism and exit unchanged in the urine. Other drugs must undergo biotransformation in the liver before being excreted by the kidney. If a client's renal function declines, he is at risk for drug toxicity. If the kidney cannot adequately excrete a drug, it may be necessary to reduce the dosage. Maintenance of a normal fluid intake in the client with normal renal function ensures proper elimination of drugs by preventing toxic drug buildup.

Types of Drug Action

Because of its chemical makeup and physiological action, a drug may produce more than one effect.

DESIRED ACTION

A drug's desired action is the expected or predictable physiological response it causes. Each drug has a desired or therapeutic effect for which it is prescribed. For example, the nurse administers codeine phosphate to create analgesia and gives theophylline to dilate narrowed respiratory bronchioles.

SIDE EFFECTS

Predictably a drug will cause other, secondary effects. Side effects may be harmless or injurious. In the example of codeine phosphate, a client may also experience constipation. Theophylline has the potential for causing headache and dizziness. If the side effects are serious enough to negate the beneficial effects of a drug's therapeutic action, the physician may discontinue the drug.

TOXIC EFFECTS

After prolonged intake of high doses of medication, or when a drug accumulates in the blood because of impaired metabolism or excretion, toxic effects develop. Excess amounts of a drug within a person's body may have lethal effects depending on the drug's action. For example, morphine, a narcotic analgesic, relieves pain by depressing the central nervous system.

However, toxic levels of morphine cause severe respiratory depression and death.

IDIOSYNCRATIC REACTIONS

Medications may cause unpredictable effects such as an idiosyncratic reaction in which a person overreacts or underreacts to a drug or has a reaction different from normal. It is impossible to predict which clients will have an idiosyncratic response. An example is the effect that may result from succinylcholine administration. The drug is used to paralyze the respiratory muscles in order to facilitate the insertion of an endotracheal tube (see Chapter 41) before the introduction of a general anesthetic. Most people have an enzyme (pseudocholinesterase) that destroys succinylcholine, thus making the drug short acting. The small percent of the population that does not have this enzyme is at risk for being paralyzed for several hours after succinylcholine administration.

ALLERGIC REACTIONS

Another unpredictable response to a drug is the allergic reaction, which comprises 5% to 10% of all drug reactions. A client can become sensitized immunologically to the initial dose of a medication. With repeated administration the client develops an allergic response to the drug, its chemical preservatives, or a metabolite. The drug or chemical acts as an antigen, triggering the release of the body's antibodies.

A client's allergic reaction may be mild or severe. Allergic symptoms vary, depending on the individual and the drug. Among the different classes of drugs, antibiotics cause a high incidence of allergic reactions. Common, mild allergy symptoms are summarized in Table 32-6. Severe or anaphylactic reactions are characterized by sudden constriction of bronchiolar muscles, edema of the pharynx and larynx, and severe wheezing and shortness of breath. The client may also become severely hypotensive, necessitating emergency resuscitation measures.

A client with a known history of an allergy to a medication should wear an identification bracelet or medal. This alerts nurses and physicians to the client's drug allergies if he is unconscious when receiving medical care.

DRUG INTERACTIONS

When one drug modifies the action of another drug, a drug interaction occurs. Drug interactions are common in individuals taking multiple medications. A drug may either potentiate or diminish the action of other drugs. A drug may also alter the way in which another drug is absorbed, metabolized, or eliminated from the body, therefore changing the actual concentration of the second drug. For example, if one drug slows the absorption of another drug, as in the case of antacids affecting iron, the concentration of the second drug falls and it does not produce its desired effect. When one drug increases the absorption or reduces the elimination of another drug, a potentiation effect is produced. The second drug will be present in a higher concentration than anticipated.

When two drugs act *synergistically,* the effect of the two drugs combined is greater than the effect that would be expected if the individual effects of the two drugs acting alone were added together. Alcohol is a central nervous system depressant that commonly has a synergistic effect on medications such as antihistamines, sedative-hypnotics, antianxiety drugs, antidepressants, and narcotic analgesics. Even with low doses of these medications, the ingestion of alcohol will aggravate drowsiness. If the client receives high doses of the medications, alcohol can aggravate respiratory depression.

A drug interaction is not always undesirable. Often a physician orders combination drug therapy to create a drug interaction for the client's therapeutic benefit. For example, a client with moderate hypertension typically receives several drugs, such as diuretics and vasodilators, that act together to keep the blood pressure at a desirable level.

TABLE 32-6

Mild Allergic Reactions

Symptom	Description
Urticaria (hives)	Raised, irregularly shaped skin eruptions with varying sizes and shapes; eruptions have reddened margins and pale centers
Eczema (rash)	Small raised vesicles that are usually reddened; often distributed over a person's entire body
Pruritus	Itching of the skin; accompanies most rashes
Rhinitis	Inflammation of mucous membranes lining the nose, causing swelling and a clear watery discharge
Wheezing	Constriction of smooth muscles surrounding bronchioles that decreases diameter of airways; occurs primarily on inspiration because of severely narrowed airways; development of edema in pharynx and larynx that further obstructs airflow

Factors Influencing Drug Actions

Because of differences in the manner in which drugs act and their types of action, there is considerable variability in clients' responses to medications. Other factors separate from characteristics of the medication also influence drug actions. A nurse soon discovers that a client may not respond in the same way to each successive dose of a medication. Likewise, the same drug dosage may cause very different responses in different clients. Drug actions are influenced by genetic differences, physiological variables, environmental conditions, and psychological factors.

GENETIC DIFFERENCES

A person's genetic makeup affects the manner in which biotransformation of drugs occurs. Metabolic patterns are often similar within families. Genetic factors determine whether naturally occurring enzymes are present to assist in drug degradation. As a result, members of a family may share a sensitivity to a medication.

A pregnant woman risks injuring her unborn child by taking medications. The risk is greatest during the first trimester of pregnancy. Physicians are cautious in prescribing medications for women who may be pregnant. Nurses should instruct pregnant women to avoid self-medication with nonprescription drugs.

PHYSIOLOGICAL VARIABLES

The client's *sex* affects the response to drugs. Hormonal differences between males and females alter the metabolism of certain drugs. Hormones and drugs compete with each other in biotransformation since they are degraded by the same metabolic processes. Diurnal variations in estrogen secretion may be responsible for the cyclic fluctuations in drug reactions that women experience.

A person's *age* has a direct effect on drug action. Infants lack many of the enzymes necessary for normal drug metabolism. Infants and children also require dosages lower than those adults can tolerate.

A number of physiological changes accompanying the aging process influence the client's response to drug therapy (Table 32-7). Body systems undergo functional and structural changes that alter the influence of drugs. The nurse initiates actions that minimize a drug's harmful effects and promote the client's remaining functional capacities.

Body weight affects a client's response to medications. There is a direct relationship between the amount of drug administered and the amount of body tissue in which it is distributed. In obese clients a lower concentration of drug accumulates in the body tissues that are the target for drug action. The less a client weighs, the greater is the concentration of a drug in tissues and the more powerful are the drug's effects. When administering potent drugs such as cardiovascular and antihypertensive agents and narcotic analgesics, physicians often calculate dosages on the basis of the client's body weight. In the case of children who have little body fat, the body surface area (BSA) is the basis for dosage calculation.

If a client's *nutritional status* is poor, proper cell function for the biotransformation of drugs cannot occur. Like all body functions, drug metabolism relies on adequate nutrition for enzyme and protein formation. Most drugs bind with proteins before being distributed to their sites of action.

Any *disease state* that impairs the function of organs responsible for normal pharmacokinetics also impairs drug action. Altered skin integrity, reduced gastrointestinal absorption or motility, and impaired renal or hepatic function are just some of the disease-related conditions that can reduce a drug's efficacy or place a client at risk for drug toxicity.

ENVIRONMENTAL CONDITIONS

A client's exposure to severe physical and emotional *stress* triggers a hormonal response that eventually may interfere with drug metabolism. Ionizing *radiation* creates a similar effect by altering the rate of enzyme activity.

Exposure to *heat and cold* can affect responses to drugs. Hypertensive clients receive vasodilators to control their blood pressure. In hot weather it often becomes necessary to reduce vasodilator dosages, since the temperature adds to the medication's effects. Cold weather tends to promote vasoconstriction, necessitating an increase in vasodilator dosage.

A client's reaction to a medication may vary depending on the *setting* in which he takes a drug. Clients in protective isolation often receive less pain relief from an analgesic than clients who are hospitalized in a room where they can be visited by family members. Similarly, when a person drinks alcohol alone, he may only become sleepy. However, drinking with a group of friends can cause the person to become playful and outgoing.

PSYCHOLOGICAL FACTORS

A number of psychological factors influence a client's use of drugs and his response to a medication. A person's *attitude* about drugs may stem from early experiences of familial influences. Seeing a parent use medications frequently may cause a child to accept drugs as a normal part of life.

The *meaning* or significance a drug or drug taking has for a client also influences his response to therapy. A drug may serve as a means for a person to overcome feelings of insecurity. In this situation the client de-

TABLE 32-7

Influence of Drug Actions in the Elderly

Body System	Physiological Change	Drug Action/ Client Response	Nursing Interventions
Gastrointestinal tract			
Oral cavity	Loss of elasticity in oral mucosa, which becomes dry and easily abraded	Greater sensitivity to drugs that cause dryness of mouth; susceptibility to gum disease and dental caries	Rinse oral cavity frequently with tepid clear water. Floss daily. Brush gently. Use substitute saliva.
Esophagus	Delayed esophageal clearance because of weakened contractions and failure of lower esophageal sphincter to relax	Difficulty swallowing large tablets or capsules; tissue erosion caused by drugs such as aspirin and uncoated potassium chloride	Position client upright. Administer full glass of permitted liquid with drug. Crush tablets and mix with food (if gastric pH does not affect absorption).
Stomach	Decrease in gastric acidity and peristalsis	Potentiation of irritating effects of highly acidic drugs (e.g., aspirin)	Have client drink full glass of water and take medication with nonfat snack to reduce gastric distress.
Large intestine	Reduced colon muscle tone; loss of defecation reflex	Slowing of drug excretion; overuse and abuse of laxatives by client	Provide normal fluid intake. Instruct client to eat bulk-forming foods and avoid use of constipating drugs.
Skin and vasculature	Reduced subcutaneous skin fold thickness in extremities (less body fat); reduced elasticity in skin and vasculature	Client's blood vessels fragile; client prone to easy bleeding following an injection	Avoid using veins in hand for intravenous injections. Apply pressure to injection sites following drug administration. Observe injection sites for bleeding.
Liver	Reduced liver size; decline in hepatic blood flow	Longer biotransformation time; longer than normal duration of drug action; greater risk for drug sensitivity and toxicity	Monitor for signs of liver impairment (jaundice, pruritus, dark urine). Question dosages for clients with known liver disease.
Kidney	Reduced glomerular filtration; decreased tubular function and renal blood flow	Risk of drug accumulation and toxicity	Prevent urinary retention (use free-flowing catheters, observe frequency of urination). Monitor for signs of renal impairment (reduced output, difficulty urinating). Question dosages for clients with renal disease.

pends on drugs as a means of coping with life. In contrast, if a client resents his physical condition, his anger and hostility may result in adverse reactions to medications. Often medications provide a sense of security. The regular use of over-the-counter drugs such as vitamins, laxatives, and aspirin gives many people a sense of control over their health.

The *nurse's behavior* when administering a drug can have a significant impact on the client's response to a medication. If the nurse conveys to the client a sense that the medication can be helpful, it is more likely the drug will have a positive effect. If the nurse seems uncaring when the client experiences discomfort, the medication she administers may prove relatively ineffective.

Drug Dose Responses

After the nurse administers a drug, it begins to undergo absorption, distribution, metabolism, and excretion. Except when administered intravenously, drugs take time to enter the bloodstream. The quantity and distribution of a drug in different body compartments change constantly.

When a physician prescribes a medication, the goal is to achieve a constant blood level within a safe therapeutic range. Repeated doses are required to achieve a constant therapeutic concentration of a medication, since a portion of a drug is always being excreted. For example, after oral administration the drug enters the gastrointestinal tract and begins to dissolve in the stomach. During dissolution a portion of the drug passes through the gastrointestinal mucosa to enter the bloodstream. As the process of absorption con-

tinues, the serum drug concentration increases. The drug continues to dissolve and absorption continues until all of the medication leaves the gastrointestinal tract. When absorption ceases, only metabolism, excretion, and distribution continue. The highest serum concentration (peak concentration) of the drug usually occurs just before the last of the drug is absorbed. After peaking, the serum drug concentration falls progressively (Fig. 32-2). With intravenous drug infusions, the peak concentration occurs much more quickly, but the serum level also begins to fall immediately.

All drugs have a serum half-life. This is the time it takes for excretion processes to lower the serum drug concentration by half. To maintain a therapeutic plateau, the client must receive regular fixed dosages. After an initial medication dose the client receives each successive dose when the previous dose reaches its half-life (Fig. 32-3). In this way an almost constant therapeutic drug concentration is maintained.

It is very important for the client and nurse to follow regular dosage schedules and adhere to prescribed doses and dosage intervals. Knowledge of the time intervals of drug action also helps the nurse to anticipate a drug's effect:

Onset of drug action   Period of time it takes after a drug is administered for it to produce a response

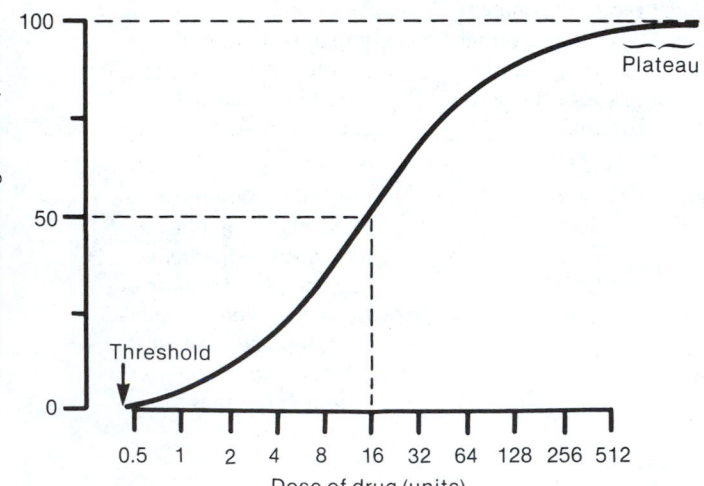

Fig. 32-2 Drug dose response curve.

From Clark, S., and Queener, J.: Pharmacological basis of nursing practice, St. Louis, 1982, The C.V. Mosby Co.

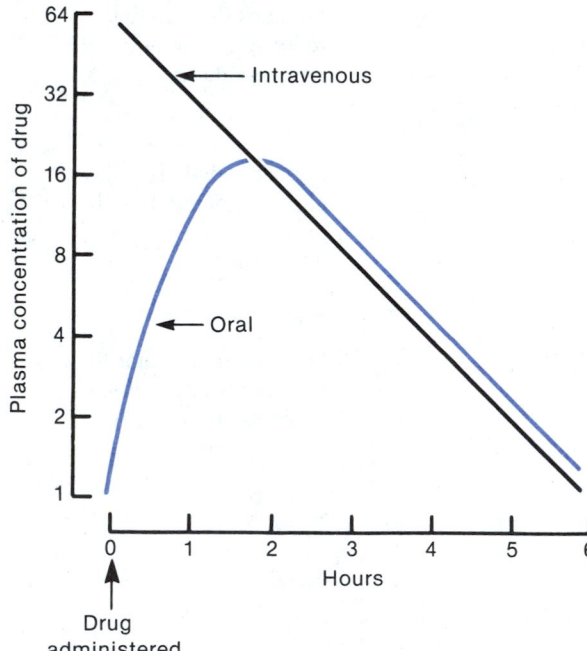

Fig. 32-3 Curve showing therapeutic blood levels.

From Clark, S., and Queener, J.: Pharmacological basis of nursing practice, St. Louis, 1982, The C.V. Mosby Co.

Peak action	Time it takes for a drug to reach its highest effective concentration
Duration of action	Length of time during which the drug is present in a concentration great enough to produce a response
Plateau	Blood serum concentration of a drug that is reached and maintained after repeated fixed doses

The ideal way to achieve a constant therapeutic drug level is continuous intravenous infusions, which eliminate the fluctuating effects of intermittent dosages. If a client receives long-term drug therapy, the physician monitors serum drug levels to prevent toxic effects.

Routes of Administration

The route chosen for administering a drug depends on the drug's properties and desired effect and on the client's physical and mental condition. Table 32-8 summarizes the advantages and disadvantages of various routes of administration. A nurse may be involved in judging the best route for a medication, as in the following hypothetical situation:

The client, Mr. Bush, has progressively worsened physically. His temperature is 39.2° C. Mr. Bush complains of nausea and is unable to tolerate oral fluids. The nurse checks Mr. Bush's order, which reads, "Aspirin 600 mg orally for temperature above 38.5° C." On the basis of the assessment, the nurse believes that Mr. Bush will not be able to tolerate an oral dose of aspirin. By consulting the physician the nurse acquires an order for a rectal suppository instead.

Before administering any medication the nurse should consider which route is best for the client's needs.

Oral Route

The oral route of administration is the easiest and the most commonly used. Orally administered medications are less expensive than intravenous solutions and many topical preparations. Because of their slow absorption, drugs given orally have a slower onset of action and a more prolonged effect than parenteral medications. Clients generally prefer the oral route because of the discomfort of injections. A client who has impaired gastrointestinal function or is unable to swallow, restricted from taking fluids, or unconscious cannot take medications orally.

Parenteral Routes

Parenteral administration involves giving a drug by a route other than the gastrointestinal tract.

INJECTION

One form of parenteral administration is injection of a drug. The following are the four major sites of injection:

1. Subcutaneous—injection into tissues just below the dermis of the skin (hypodermic)
2. Intramuscular—injection into the body of a muscle
3. Intravenous—injection into a vein
4. Intradermal—injection into the dermis just under the epidermis

Often a physician uses additional routes for parenteral injections, including intrathecal or intraspinal (into the spinal canal), intracardiac (into the myocardium), intrapleural (into the pleural space), intra-arterial (into an artery), and intra-articular (into the joint space).

The nurse uses strict sterile technique when preparing medications for parenteral injection. Contamination of medication solutions, syringe needles, or the syringe itself can lead to infection.

TOPICAL ADMINISTRATION

Drugs applied to the skin and mucous membranes principally have local effects. The nurse applies medications to the skin by painting or spreading medication over an area, applying moist dressings, soaking body parts in a solution, or giving medicated baths. Systemic effects can occur if a client's skin is thin, if the drug concentration is high, or if contact with the skin is prolonged. There are relatively new drugs on the market that the nurse applies to the skin to cause systemic effects (for example, Nitro-Bid ointment, a form of nitroglycerin, which dilates coronary arteries).

The nurse also applies drugs to mucous membranes. Because of the vascular nature of most mucous membranes, a medication is absorbed quickly. If the drug concentration is high enough, systemic effects may occur. Drugs given by the buccal and sublingual routes exert systemic actions.

Mucous membranes differ in their sensitivity to medications. The cornea of the eye is particularly sensitive to any chemical. The client may complain of a burning sensation when the nurse administers eye or nose drops. Medications are generally less irritating to vaginal or rectal mucosa.

The nurse uses several methods for applying medications to mucous membranes:

1. Direct application of liquid—eye drops, gargling, swabbing the throat

TABLE 32-8

Factors Influencing Choice of Administration Routes

Route	Advantages	Disadvantages/Contraindications
Oral	Convenient and comfortable to administer; economical; may produce local or systemic effects; rarely causes anxiety	Avoid giving to clients with alterations in gastrointestinal function, e.g., nausea and vomiting, reduced motility (following general anesthesia, inflammation of bowel), and surgical resection of portion of gastrointestinal tract. Certain drugs are destroyed by gastric secretions. Oral administration is contraindicated in clients unable to swallow, e.g., clients with neuromuscular disorders, esophageal strictures, and lesions of the mouth. Oral medications cannot be given when client has gastric suction and are contraindicated in clients before certain tests or surgery. An unconscious or confused client is unable or unwilling to swallow. Oral medications may irritate lining of gastrointestinal tract, discolor teeth, or have an unpleasant taste.
Subcutaneous, intramuscular, intravenous, intradermal	Provides route of administration when oral drugs are contraindicated; more rapid absorption than with topical or oral drugs; intravenous infusion provides drug delivery when client is critically ill or peripheral perfusion is inadequate	There is a risk of introducing infection, the drugs are expensive, and these routes are to be avoided in clients with bleeding tendencies. There is a risk of tissue damage with subcutaneous injections. Intramuscular and intravenous routes are dangerous because of rapid absorption. These routes cause considerable anxiety in many clients, especially children.
Skin	Primarily provides local effect; painless; limited side effects	Extensive applications may be bulky and cause difficulty in maneuvering. Clients with skin abrasions are at risk for rapid drug absorption and systemic effects.
Mucous membranes: buccal, sublingual, eye, ear, nose, vagina, rectum	Therapeutic effects provided by local application to involved sites; aqueous solutions readily absorbed and capable of causing systemic effects; provides route of administration when oral drugs are contraindicated	Mucous membranes are highly sensitive to certain drug concentrations. Insertion of rectal medications often causes the client embarrassment. Client with ruptured eardrum cannot receive irrigations. Rectal suppositories are contraindicated if the client has had rectal surgery or if active rectal bleeding is present.
Inhalation	Provides rapid relief for local respiratory problems; provides easy access for introduction of general anesthetic gases; for seriously weakened or unconscious client, oxygen can still be delivered with appropriate respiratory therapy equipment	Some local agents can cause serious systemic effects. Drugs developed to act on body systems other than the lungs cannot be administered by inhalation.

2. Inserting drug into body cavity—placement of suppository in rectum or vagina, insertion of medicated packing into vagina
3. Instillation of fluid into body cavity—ear drops, nose drops, bladder and rectal instillation (fluid is retained)
4. Irrigation of body cavity—flushing eye, ear, vagina, bladder, or rectum with medicated fluid (fluid is not retained)
5. Spraying—instillation into nose and throat

INHALATION

The deeper passages of the respiratory tract provide a large surface area for drug absorption. The vascular alveolar-capillary network readily absorbs the gases and mists introduced through the airways. Medications introduced into the lung's airways must not interfere with normal gas exchange. Inhaled medications may have local effects; for example, bronchodilators dilate narrowed bronchioles and mucolytic agents liquefy thick mucous secretions. Drugs such as oxygen and general anesthetics create general systemic effects. Some medications given by inhalation are designed to produce local effects but have potentially dangerous systemic side effects; for example, isoproterenol (Isuprel) dilates bronchioles but also produces heart rhythm irregularities. The nurse administers oxygen with the appropriate oxygen delivery equipment (see Chapter 41) and administers locally acting medications with hand-operated inhalers.

Systems of Drug Measurement

The proper administration of a medication depends on the nurse's ability to compute drug dosages accurately and measure medications correctly. A careless mistake in placing a decimal point or adding a zero to a dosage can lead to a fatal error. The physician and client depend on the nurse to check the dosage before administering a drug. The nurse is also responsible for teaching clients the dosages prescribed for them.

Three systems of measurement are used in drug therapy: metric, apothecary, and household. Most nations of the world, including Canada, use the metric system as their standard of measurement. However, the U.S. Congress still has not officially adopted the metric system. Most health professionals in the United States use the metric and apothecary systems. Prescriptions to be self-administered are often written in household measures for clients.

Metric System

As a decimal system, the metric system is the most logically organized of the measurement systems. Metric units can easily be converted and computed through simple multiplication and division. Each basic unit of measurement is organized into units of 10. Multiplying or dividing by 10 forms secondary units. In multiplication, the decimal point moves to the right; in division, the decimal moves to the left. For example:

$$10.0 \text{ mg} \times 10 = 100 \text{ mg}$$
$$10.0 \text{ mg} \div 10 = 1.0 \text{ mg}$$

The basic units of measurement in the metric system are the meter (length), the liter (volume), and the gram (weight). For drug calculations the nurse uses only the volume and weight units. In the metric system small or large letters are used to designate the basic units:

Gram = g or Gm
Liter = l or L

Small letters are abbreviations for other units:

Milligram = mg
Milliliter = ml

A system of Latin prefixes designates subdivision of the basic units: deci- ($\frac{1}{10}$ or 0.1), centi- ($\frac{1}{100}$ or 0.01), and milli- ($\frac{1}{1000}$ or 0.001). Greek prefixes designate multiples of the basic units: deka- (10), hecto- (100), and kilo- (1000). When writing drug dosages in metric units, physicians and nurses use either fractions or multiples of a unit. Fractions are always in decimal form, for example:

500 mg or 0.5 g, *not* ½ g
10 ml or 0.01 L, *not* $\frac{1}{100}$ L

When fractions are used, a zero is always placed in front of the decimal to prevent error.

Apothecary System

The apothecary system of measurement is familiar to most people in the United States and Canada. The standards for measurement can be easily seen in the home: milk is bottled in pints and quarts, a yardstick has inches and feet, and a bathroom scale weighs in pounds.

The basic unit of weight is a grain. In colonial days the gram represented the weight of one grain of wheat. Units of weight derived from the grain are the dram, ounce, and pound. The apothecary unit for volume or fluid measurement is the minim. The minim is the approximate quantity of water that weighs a grain. The fluidram, fluid ounce, pint, quart, and gallon are measures derived from the minim.

In the apothecary system, small letters or symbols are used for measurement units:

Grain = gr
Ounce = oz or ℥
Fluid ounce = f℥
Minim = m
Dram = ℨ

Lower-case Roman numerals designate the quantities of the apothecary units. The Roman numeral follows the unit of measure:

3 grains = gr iii

Physicians often use fractions as well as symbols with apothecary units:

$$2^{1/2} \text{ fluid ounces} = f\bar{\xi} \text{ iiss}$$

$$^{1/2} \text{ fluid ounce} = f\bar{\xi} \, ^{1/2} \text{ or } \bar{\xi} \text{ ss}$$

Household Measurements

The household unit of measurement is also familiar to most people. The problem with household measures is their inaccuracy. Household utensils such as teaspoons and cups often vary in size. Scales to measure pints or quarts are often not well calibrated. Household measures include drops, teaspoons, tablespoons, and cups for volume and pints and quarts for weight. Although pints and quarts are considered household measures, they are also used in the apothecary system.

The advantage of household measurements is their convenience and familiarity for clients. When the accuracy of a drug dosage is not critical, it is safe to use household measures. For example, many over-the-counter drugs, such as laxatives, antacids, and cough syrups, can safely be measured by this method. Table 32-9 gives common equivalents from each of the three measurement units.

Solutions

In clinical practice the nurse uses solutions of various concentrations for injections, irrigations, and infusions. It is helpful for the nurse to understand the terms that describe concentrations of solutions. A solution is a given mass of solid substance dissolved in a known volume of fluid or a given volume of liquid dissolved in a known volume of another fluid. When a solid is dissolved in a fluid, the concentration is in units of mass per units of volume, for example, g/ml, g/L, mg/ml. A concentration of a solution may also be expressed as a percentage. A 10% solution, for example, is 10 g of solid dissolved in 100 ml of solution. A proportion also expresses concentrations. A 1:1000 solution represents a solution containing 1 g of solid in 1000 ml of liquid or 1 ml of liquid mixed with 1000 ml of another liquid.

Converting Measurement Units

A pharmacist does not always dispense a medication in the unit of measure in which it is ordered. Drug companies package and bottle certain standard equivalents. For example, the physician may order 250 mg of a medication that is available only in grams. The nurse is responsible for converting available units of volume and weight to the desired dosages. It is therefore important for the nurse to be aware of approximate equivalents in all of the major measurement systems. In practice, equivalent measurements may not be exactly accurate. For example, 60, 64, 65, and 66⅔ mg are all acceptable equivalents for a grain. The nurse chooses the equivalent that is easiest for computation. For example, if a physician orders 5 grains of a medication but the nurse has only 300 mg tablets available, it is easier to divide 300 mg by 60 mg to calculate grains than it is to divide 300 by 66⅔. Freedom to choose equivalents is convenient, but the nurse should consider the probability of error and keep the number of conversions to a minimum.

CONVERSIONS WITHIN ONE SYSTEM

Converting measurements within one system is relatively easy. In the metric system the nurse simply

---

TABLE 32-9

Equivalents of Measurement

Metric (Volume)	Apothecary	Household
1 ml	15 minims (m)	15 drops (gtt)
15 ml	4 fluidrams (f𝔷)	1 tablespoon (tbsp)
30 ml	1 fluid ounce (𝔷)	2 tablespoons (tbsp)
240 ml	8 fluid ounces (f𝔷)	1 cup (c)
480 ml (approximately 500 ml)	1 pint (pt)	1 pint (pt)
960 ml (approximately 1 L)	1 quart (qt)	1 quart (qt)
3840 ml (approximately 4000 ml)	1 gallon (gal)	1 gallon (gal)

divides or multiplies. To change milligrams to grams the nurse divides by 1000, moving the decimal 3 points to the left.

$$1000 \text{ mg} = 1 \text{ g}$$
$$350 \text{ mg} = 0.35 \text{ g}$$

To convert liters to milliliters the nurse multiplies by 1000 or moves the decimal 3 points to the right.

$$1 \text{ L} = 1000 \text{ ml}$$
$$0.25 \text{ L} = 250 \text{ ml}$$

To convert units of measurement within the apothecary or household system the nurse must consult an equivalent table. For example, when converting fluid ounces to quarts the nurse must first know that 16 ounces is the equivalent of 1 quart. To convert 4 ounces to a quart measurement, for example, the nurse divides 4 by 16 to get the equivalent, ¼ or 0.25 quart.

CONVERSION BETWEEN SYSTEMS

Frequently the nurse must determine the proper dosage of a medication by converting weights or volumes from one system of measurement to another. Commonly apothecary and metric units must be converted to equivalent household measures for a client's use at home. When the time comes to make actual drug calculations, it is easier to work with units in the same measurement system.

Tables of equivalent measurements are available in all health care institutions. The pharmacist is also a good resource.

Before making a conversion the nurse compares the measurement system available with what is ordered. For example, a physician orders morphine gr ⅙ IM. The medication is available only in milligrams. To convert grains to milligrams the nurse must know the equivalents:

$$1 \text{ mg} = \frac{1}{60} \text{ gr}$$
or
$$60 \text{ mg} = 1 \text{ gr}$$

Therefore, by converting gr ⅙ to milligrams, the nurse will have the measurements needed to make the eventual dosage calculation. She divides by 6:

$$60 \text{ mg} \div 6 = \frac{1}{6} \text{ gr}$$
$$10 \text{ mg} = \frac{1}{6} \text{ gr}$$

After calculating that the physician's order for morphine gr ⅙ is the same as 10 mg morphine, the nurse can accurately prepare the medication based on the dosages of morphine available.

DOSAGE CALCULATIONS

There is a simple formula the nurse can use in many different types of dosage calculations. The formula can be applied when preparing solid or liquid forms of medications.

$$\frac{\text{Dose ordered}}{\text{Dose on hand}} \times \text{Amount on hand} = \text{Amount to administer}$$

The *dose ordered* is the amount of pure drug the physician prescribes for a client. The *dose on hand* is the weight or volume of drug available in units supplied by the pharmacy. The dose on hand may be expressed on the drug label as the contents of a tablet or capsule or as the amount of drug dissolved per unit volume of liquid. The *amount on hand* is the basic unit or quantity of the drug that contains the dose on hand. For solid drugs the amount on hand may be one capsule. The amount of liquid on hand may be, for example, a milliliter or liter depending on the capacity of the container. The *amount to administer* is the actual amount of available medication the nurse will administer to the client. The amount to administer is always expressed in the same unit as the amount on hand.

The following example illustrates how to apply the formula. The physician orders the client to receive morphine 10 mg IM. Thus the *dose ordered* is 10 mg. The medication is available only in ampules containing 15 mg per milliliter. Thus the *dose on hand* is 15 mg in an *amount on hand* of 1 ml. The formula is applied as follows:

$$\frac{10 \text{ mg}}{15 \text{ mg}} \times 1 \text{ ml} = \text{Volume of milliliter to administer}$$

To simplify the ¹⁰⁄₁₅ fraction, divide numerator and denominator by 5:

$$\frac{2}{3} \times 1 \text{ ml} = \frac{2}{3} \text{ ml to administer}$$

Syringes are calibrated only in decimals. After converting the fraction ⅔ to 0.66 the nurse can more accurately draw up the correct dosage. Administering 0.7 ml of morphine instead of 0.6 ml would not be likely to cause dangerous side effects. However, with some medications, such as cardiotonics, antihypertensives, or chemotherapeutic agents, even slight inaccuracies can be dangerous.

Another example demonstrates how the formula applies with solid dosage forms. The physician orders 0.125 mg PO* of digoxin. The drug is available in tablets containing 0.25 mg.

$$\frac{0.125 \text{ mg}}{0.250 \text{ mg}} \times 1 \text{ tablet} = \text{Number of tablets to administer}$$

---

*PO is the abbreviation for the Latin phrase *per orum*, by mouth.

The fraction $^{0.125}/_{0.250}$ equals ½ or 0.5. Therefore,

$$0.5 \times 1 \text{ tablet} = 0.5 \text{ or } \frac{1}{2} \text{ tablet to be administered}$$

Many tablets come with scores or indentations across the center of the tablet. A scored tablet is easy to break in half for divided dosages. The nurse should never attempt to estimate the amount of medication in a broken unscored tablet. The potential for giving dangerous doses of medication is high when the nurse must estimate dosage amounts.

Often liquid medications come prepared in volumes greater than 1 ml. In this situation the formula still applies. For example, the medication order is, "Erythromycin suspension 250 mg PO." The pharmacy delivers 100 ml bottles with the labels stating, "5 ml contains 125 mg of erythromycin."

$$\frac{250 \text{ mg}}{125 \text{ mg}} \times 5 \text{ ml} = \text{Volume to administer}$$

The fraction $^{250}/_{125}$ equals 2. Therefore,

$$2 \times 5 \text{ ml} = 10 \text{ ml to administer}$$

In this situation the nurse ignores the total volume of medication available and instead uses the dosage values noted on the label. If the nurse calculated the dosage on the basis of 100 ml available, the following error would occur:

$$\frac{250 \text{ mg}}{125 \text{ mg}} \times 100 \text{ ml} = 200 \text{ ml to administer}$$

On the basis of this calculation the client would receive 20 times the desired dosage.

Pediatric Dosages

Calculating children's drug dosages requires caution. Children are unable to metabolize many drugs as readily as adults. The child's body size also necessitates smaller dosages. In most cases physicians calculate the safe dosage for a child before ordering the medication. However, nurses should be aware of the formulas used to calculate pediatric dosages in order to check dosages that raise suspicion or concern. Most drug references list the normal ranges for pediatric dosages.

BODY SURFACE AREA

The most accurate method of calculating pediatric dosages is based on a child's body surface area. Body surface area is estimated on the basis of the child's weight. Standard nomograms or charts list a child's body surface area by weight and approximate age (Fig. 32-4). The formula is a ratio of the child's body surface area compared with the body surface area of an average adult (1.7 square meters, or 1.7 M²).

$$\text{Child's dose} = \frac{\text{Surface area of child}}{1.7 \text{ M}^2} \times \text{Normal adult dose}$$

For example, what dose of ampicillin does a child weighing 12 kg require if the normal single adult dose for ampicillin is 250 mg? The chart shows that a child weighing 12 kg has a surface area of 0.54 M².

$$\text{Child's dose} = \frac{0.54 \text{ M}^2}{1.7 \text{ M}^2} \times 250 \text{ mg}$$

The M² units can be ignored.

$$\text{Child's dose} = \frac{0.54}{1.7} \times 250 \text{ mg}$$

$$\frac{0.54}{1.7} = 0.3$$

$$\text{Child's dose} = 0.3 \times 250 \text{ mg} = 75 \text{ mg}$$

CLARK'S RULE

A less accurate method for calculating pediatric dosages is Clark's rule. Clark's rule compares a child's body weight with the average weight of an adult (150 lb). The formula is applicable to children of all ages.

$$\text{Child's dose} = \frac{\text{Child's weight in pounds}}{150 \text{ lb}} \times \text{Normal adult dose}$$

For example, what is the correct dose of acetaminophen for a 30-lb child if the normal adult dose is 325 mg?

$$\text{Child's dose} = \frac{30 \text{ lb}}{150 \text{ lb}} \times 325 \text{ mg}$$

$$\frac{30}{150} = \frac{1}{5} = 0.2$$

$$\text{Child's dose} = 0.2 \times 325 \text{ mg} = 65 \text{ mg}$$

Administering Medications

The nurse does not bear sole responsibility for drug administration. The physician and pharmacist play key roles in helping to ensure that the right medication gets to the right client.

Physician's Role

The physician prescribes the client's medications (unless a state's nurse practice act allows nurses to prescribe in specific situations). The physician writes an order on a designated form in the client's medical record, in a physician's order book, or on a legal prescription pad. In an emergency a physician may also order a medication by telephone or by giving the nurse an oral order. The nurse enters and signs all telephone and oral orders, writes the name of the physician ordering the drug, and then has the physician countersign the order when he again becomes available. Most institutions require a physician's sig-

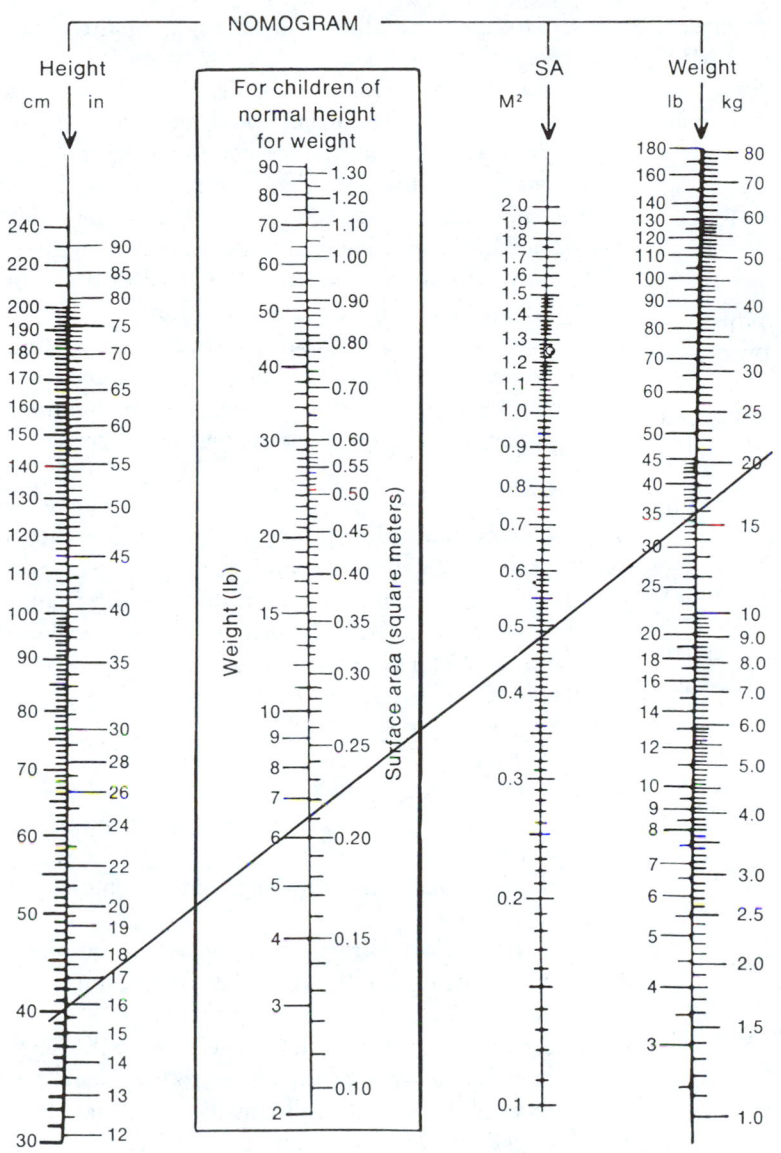

NOMOGRAM

Height

cm   in

For children of
normal height
for weight

SA

M²

Weight

lb   kg

Fig. 32-4 West nomogram for estimation of surface areas in children.

From Whaley, L.F., and Wong, D.L.: Nursing care of infants and children, ed. 2, St. Louis, 1983, The C.V. Mosby Co.

nature within 24 hours after the order is made. Institutional policies vary as to which personnel can take oral or telephone orders. In many institutions nursing students cannot take medication orders. *No medication is to be given without an order.*

Common abbreviations are used when writing orders. The abbreviations indicate dosage frequencies or times, routes of administration, and special information for the nurse to follow in giving the drug.

TYPES OF ORDERS

There are four common types of medication orders, based on the frequency or time intervals for drug administration.

STANDING ORDERS. A standing order is to be carried out until the physician cancels it by another order or until a prescribed number of days elapse. A standing order may have a termination date. Many institutions have policies for the automatic discontinuation of standing orders (for example, for antibiotics and narcotic analgesics). The following are examples of standing orders:

> Tetracycline 500 mg PO q6h*
> Decadron 10 mg qd† × 5 days
> Colace i capsule daily

P.R.N. ORDERS. The physician may order a medication on a p.r.n. basis, or to be given when a client

---

*PO, by mouth; q, every; h, hour.
†qd, every day.

requires it. The nurse uses her judgment in determining the client's need. Often the physician sets maximum intervals for the time of administration. The nurse may decide to lengthen the interval if the client does not need the drug. Examples of p.r.n. orders follow:

Morphine gr ¼ IM q3-4h p.r.n.*
Maalox 30 ml p.r.n.

SINGLE (ONE TIME) ORDERS.

Often a physician will order a medication to be given only once at a specified time. This is common in the case of preoperative medications or medications administered before diagnostic examinations. Examples are:

Atropine 0.4 mg IM on call to OR
Valium 10 mg PO at 0900

STAT ORDERS.

A stat order signifies that a single dose of a medication is to be given immediately and only once. Often stat orders are written in emergency situations when the client's condition changes suddenly. For example,

Give Apresoline 10 mg IM stat

Some conditions change the status of all of a client's medication orders. Surgery automatically cancels all of a client's preoperative medications (see Chapter 47). Since the client's condition changes after surgery, the physician must write new orders. When a client is transferred to another health agency or a different medical service within a hospital, or is discharged, the physician who assumes responsibility for the client orders new medications.

COMPONENTS OF DRUG ORDERS

A medication order is incomplete unless it has seven essential parts:
1. *Client's full name.* This distinguishes the client from other persons with the same last name. Hospitals and other agencies use the client's nameplate to imprint the name and hospital number on order forms.
2. *Date order is written.* The day, month, and year are included. Designating the time an order is written helps to clarify when certain orders are to stop automatically. If an incident occurs involving a medication error (for example, a missed dose), it is easier to document what happened when the order time is available.
3. *Drug name.* Usually the physician orders a generic or trade-name drug. Correct spelling is important in differentiating names with similar spelling.

4. *Dosage.* The amount or strength of the medication is included.
5. *Route of administration.* The physician uses common abbreviations for drug routes. Accuracy is important, since certain drugs are administered by more than one route.
6. *Time and frequency of administration.* The nurse needs to know when to initiate drug therapy. Orders for multiple doses establish a routine schedule for drug administration.
7. *Signature of physician or nurse.* The signature makes the order a legal request. Insurance companies will not reimburse clients for medications unless a signature accompanies the order.

PRESCRIPTIONS

The physician writes prescriptions for clients who are to take medications outside the hospital. The prescription includes more detailed information than a regular order, since the client must understand how to take the medication and when to refill the prescription if necessary. The parts of a prescription include the following:
1. *Superscription.* The client's name, address, age, and date are given for identification purposes. The symbol ℞ ("take thou") is at the top of the form.
2. *Inscription.* This is the drug name, strength, and dose.
3. *Subscription.* Directions are given to the pharmacist as to number of tablets or amount to be dispensed.
4. *Signature.* Information to be written on the label is included, such as directions to the client (for example, take with full glass of water, take between meals), directions for refilling the prescription, and whether the drug name should be on the label.
5. *Personal data.* The physician signs the prescription. If the drug is a controlled substance, the physician includes his or her registration number and address.

Pharmacist's Role

The pharmacist prepares and distributes prescribed drugs. Nurses work with pharmacists employed in health care agencies and retail drugstores. The pharmacist assumes responsibility for filling prescriptions accurately and for being sure prescriptions are valid. If there is any question that a prescription is forged or that the prescribing physician is unlicensed, the pharmacist should not fill the prescription. The pharmacist calls the physician if an ordered dose seems outside the safe therapeutic range.

---

*p.r.n., when necessary.

The pharmacist in a health care agency rarely has to mix compounds or solutions except in the case of intravenous additive solutions. Most drug companies deliver drugs in a form ready for administration. Dispensing the correct drug in the proper dosage and amount with an accurate label is the pharmacist's chief responsibility. The pharmacist is also a resource for information about drug side effects, toxicity, interactions, and incompatibilities.

DISTRIBUTION SYSTEMS

Systems for the storage and distribution of medications vary among health care agencies. Pharmacists provide the drugs, but it is the nurses who distribute medications to clients. Institutions providing nursing care have a designated area for stocking and dispensing drugs. Special medication rooms, portable locked carts, and individual storage units adjacent to clients' rooms are some of the facilities used. Wherever medications are located, nurses keep close watch on the supply, making sure storage areas are locked when unattended.

STOCK SUPPLY. With a stock system medications are available in quantity in stock containers. This system is time consuming and costly, since a nurse must dispense each medication separately for a client.

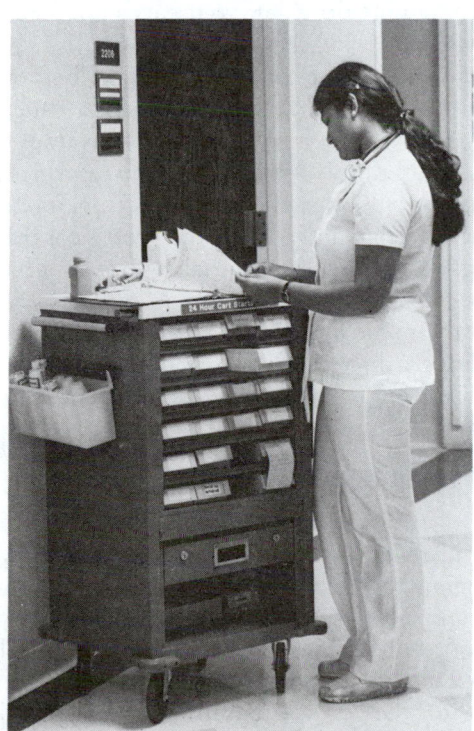

Fig. 32-5 A portable unit dose cart provides a 24-hour supply of prepackaged medications for each client in a nursing division.

INDIVIDUAL CLIENT SUPPLY. A separate supply of medications for each client can be kept in specially labeled drawers or storage bins. Generally the pharmacist dispenses only the amount of medication a client will use for a limited period of time. Nurses distribute a client's medications only from his own supply. This system reduces the time it takes to dispense medications.

UNIT DOSE. The unit dose system is the newest medication distribution system. Portable carts containing a drawer for each client come from the pharmacy with a 24-hour supply of medications. Each tablet or capsule is wrapped in a foil or paper container (Fig. 32-5). At a designated time each day the pharmacist refills the drawers in the cart with a fresh supply of medications. The cart also contains limited amounts of p.r.n. and stock drugs for special situations such as new drug orders or stat orders.

The nurse takes the medication cart around to each client's room. After administering each drug the nurse charts it immediately on the unit dose medication form. Use of the unit dose system reduces the number of medication errors and saves steps in dispensing drugs. When restocking the cart, the pharmacist is more likely to identify missed doses. In some institutions it is the pharmacists who administer medications to clients with the unit dose system.

Nurse's Role

The nurse's role extends beyond simply giving drugs to a client. The nurse has the responsibilities of determining whether a client should receive a drug at a given time, assessing the client's ability to self-administer drugs, providing medications at the proper time, and monitoring the effects of prescribed medications. The nurse uses the nursing process to integrate drug therapy with nursing care.

ASSESSMENT

The nurse assesses the client to determine his need for and potential response to drug therapy. The client's *medical history* reveals indications or contraindications for drug therapy. The client's disorder may put him at risk for adverse effects if he receives certain medications. For example, if the client has a gastric ulcer or bleeding tendency, the nurse should not administer compounds containing aspirin or anticoagulants, which increase the likelihood of bleeding. Long-term health problems such as diabetes, arthritis, or multiple sclerosis, which require medicinal therapies, suggest to the nurse the type of drugs a client is taking. A history of surgical alterations may indicate a client's present use of medications. For example, after a thyroidectomy a client requires hormone replacement.

If the client has a *history of allergies* to medication, the nurse informs other members of the health care team. In a hospital clients wear identification bands that list medications to which they are allergic. The client's medical record also has a label on the front of the chart that lists his allergies. The physician documents medication allergies in the medical progress note.

A *medication history* reveals drugs the client is currently taking or has taken in the recent past. Such medications may be the cause of signs and symptoms observed by the nurse. The nurse questions the client about each drug to determine the name, dosage, frequency of administration, reason for taking, and length of time the client has taken it. The nurse should not assume that every medication prescribed for a client is taken regularly but rather should ask the client whether he follows medication schedules. This will help reveal the client's compliance with medical therapy. The nurse also asks the client whether he takes over-the-counter medications, which clients often forget to mention when asked about medications. Women frequently fail to mention that they take birth control pills. The type of medications a client takes can influence his response to therapy received in a health care setting.

A *diet history* reveals the client's normal eating patterns at home. The nurse can plan a client's dosage schedule more effectively if she knows when the client prefers to eat. It is also helpful to determine if the client regularly snacks between meals.

If the client has *perceptual* or *coordination problems*, the self-administration of medications may be difficult. The nurse must assess the client's ability to take his medications when he returns home. For example, the nurse must be aware of the client's inability to remember dosage times, to pour liquid medications, or to see drug labels well enough to read them. If the client is unable to self-administer drugs, the nurse learns whether family members or friends are available to assist the client.

A client's *knowledge* and *understanding* of medication therapy may influence his willingness or ability to follow a drug regimen. Unless a client understands the purpose of a medication, the importance of regular dosage schedules and proper administration methods, and the possible side effects, he is unlikely to comply with therapy. When assessing the client's knowledge, the nurse asks him to explain what he knows about the medication: What is it for? How does he take it? When does he take it? What side effects if any has he had? Has he ever stopped taking doses? Is there anything he does not understand and would like to know about the drug?

The client's *attitude* about the use of drugs may reveal his level of dependence on a medication. Clients are often reluctant to express their feelings about drugs, particularly if drug dependence is a problem. To assess attitudes, the nurse may have to observe the client's behavior. For example, if the client consistently requests a p.r.n. medication as soon as it can be given or exhibits anxiety before receiving a drug and then suddenly relaxes afterward, drug dependence is a legitimate concern.

The nurse assesses *data about each drug,* including its action, purpose, normal dosages and routes, side effects, and nursing implications for administration and monitoring. Often several resources must be consulted to gather all needed information. Pharmacology textbooks are an excellent source of basic drug information. Professional nursing journals have articles about new drugs and drug classifications. The journals are excellent references for nursing implications. The *Physicians' Desk Reference* (PDR) is accessible in most health care institutions. The PDR provides product information but does not give information related to nursing implications. Inserts or flyers that come packaged with drug products can be useful, especially if a drug has been on the market only for a short time. The nurse is responsible for knowing as much as possible about each medication administered. Many nursing students prepare index cards containing drug data to use as a quick resource when working with clients.

Assessment of the *client's condition* before drug administration will determine whether the client should receive the medication. For example, if a client's heart rate is abnormally slow and irregular, the nurse should consult the physician before giving a medication that acts to slow the heart's contraction. Findings from the assessment also serve as a baseline for later determination of a drug's effects. For example, the nurse auscultates lung sounds before administering a bronchodilator and again after giving the medication to determine if the client's airways become less constricted.

NURSING DIAGNOSIS

The nurse's assessment provides data that can be used to determine actual or potential problems with drug therapy. Alterations in the client's condition may lead the nurse to select a more appropriate route of administration. If the nurse's assessment reveals the client's inability to self-administer drugs, the diagnosis will focus on the nature of the problem and suggest alternative resources. Nursing diagnoses may also reveal behavioral alterations that suggest the client's potential for drug use problems. If the nurse diagnoses a client's knowledge deficit or factors interfering with drug regimen compliance, client edu-

TABLE 32-10

Examples of Nursing Diagnoses With Implications for Drug Therapy

Problem Area	Nursing Diagnoses
Route of administration	Alterations in oral mucosal integrity Alterations in elimination Inability to swallow Alterations in digestion Impaired level of consciousness
Client's ability to self-administer drugs	Impaired sensory perception Alterations in physical mobility
Compliance with therapy	Knowledge deficit concerning drug Anxiety Denial related to disease state
Drug use	Potential dependence on drug use related to chronic pain Predisposition to drug intolerance related to family history

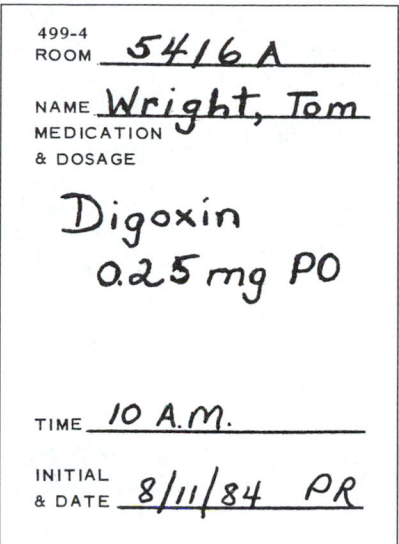

Fig. 32-6   Sample medication ticket.

cation becomes a part of the nursing care plan. Diagnoses help the nurse select the best methods to ensure safe drug administration. Table 32-10 lists examples of nursing diagnoses that may influence drug therapy.

PLANNING

The nurse's goals for drug administration relate to the nurse's responsibilities as well as those of the client. Goals include the following:

1. To administer prescribed drugs in accordance with a client's physical and emotional needs
2. To promote and potentiate the therapeutic effect of prescribed medications
3. To monitor the client's response to medications
4. To maintain the client's safety and comfort
5. To educate clients and family members about drug therapy
6. To prevent the inappropriate use of drugs
7. To prepare clients for self-management of drug therapy

As with any care plan, the nurse's success depends on the creativity and individuality of her actions. For example, clients returning home require adjustments in medication schedules based on their activities of daily living. In the hospital setting the nurse may have to adjust schedules to allow time for diagnostic tests.

The client's participation in the nursing care plan increases the likelihood of achieving safe drug therapy. Clients are less reluctant to receive medications and more likely to use them correctly when they know what to expect.

IMPLEMENTATION

CORRECT TRANSCRIPTION AND COMMUNICATION OF ORDERS. The nurse or a designated unit secretary writes the physician's complete order on the appropriate medication forms, tickets, or Kardex (Figs. 32-6 and 32-7). The transcribed order includes the client's name, the room and bed number, the drug name, the dosage, and the time and route of administration. Each time the nurse prepares a drug dosage, she refers to the medication form or ticket. With the unit dose system only one transcription is necessary, limiting the opportunity for errors. When transcribing orders, the nurse should be sure that names, dosages, and symbols are legible. The nurse rewrites any smudged or illegible transcriptions.

A registered nurse checks all transcribed orders against the original order for accuracy and thoroughness. If an order seems incorrect or inappropriate, the nurse has the responsibility of consulting the physician. The nurse who gives the wrong medication or an incorrect dosage is legally responsible for the error.

ACCURATE DOSAGE CALCULATION AND MEASUREMENT. When measuring liquid medications, the nurse uses standard measuring receptacles. The procedure for drug measurement is systematic to lessen

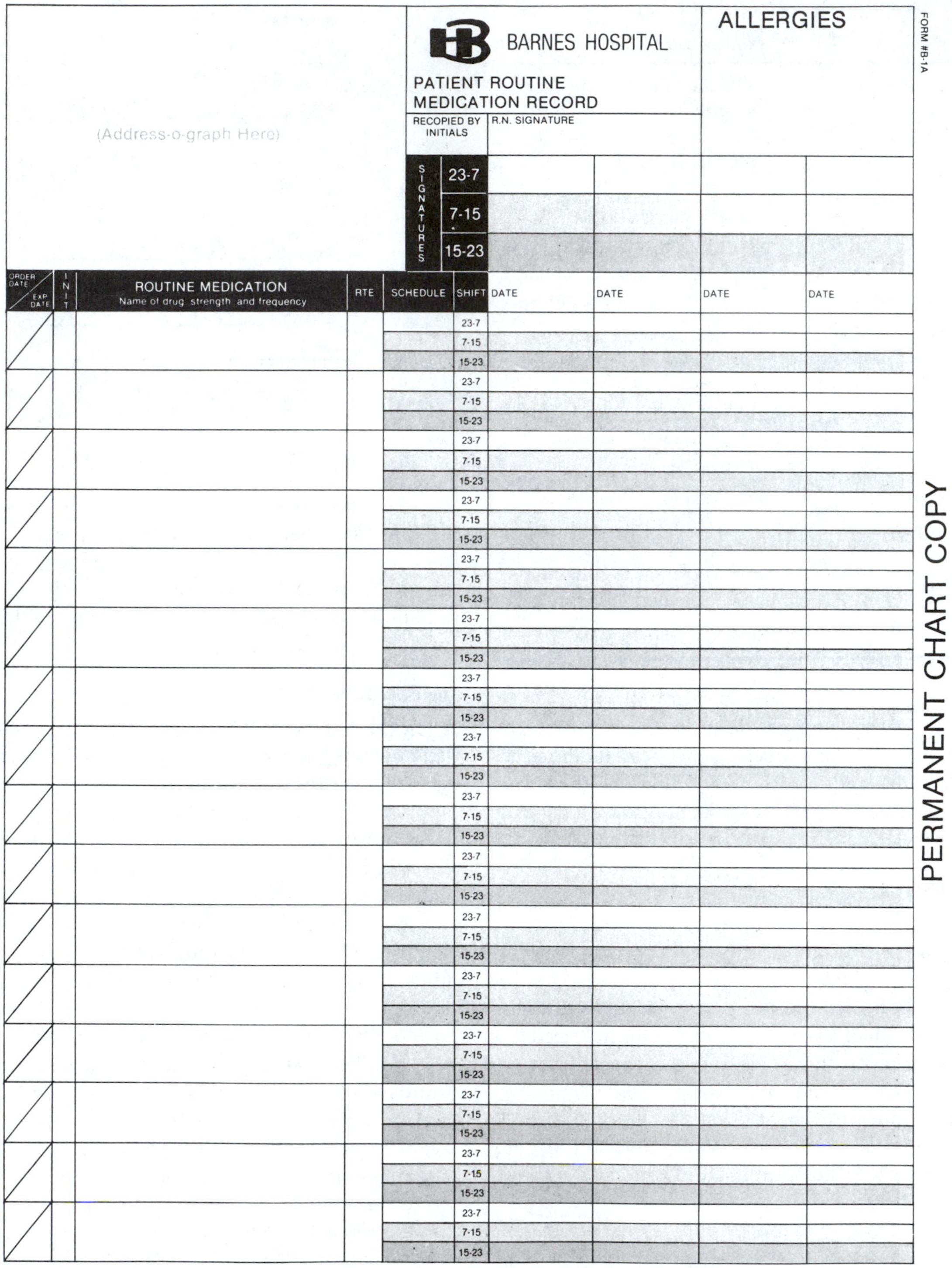

Fig. 32-7 The physician's medication order is transcribed on the medication form or Kardex. Each time the nurse prepares a drug dosage she refers to the medication form. This form is an example of a unit dose sheet, which becomes a permanent part of the medical record. The nurse records all medications administered.

Courtesy Barnes Hospital, St. Louis.

the chance of error. The nurse calculates each dose while preparing the drug. Attention to the process of calculation and avoidance of interference from other nursing activities help minimize mistakes.

CORRECT ADMINISTRATION. To administer a medication safely, the nurse uses aseptic technique and proper procedures in handling and giving medications. Promoting the client's comfort, as by positioning before an injection, increases the efficiency of medication administration. Certain drugs require the nurse to perform additional measures at the time of administration, such as measuring the blood pressure before and after giving an antihypertensive drug or assessing heart rate after giving antiarrhythmic medications.

RECORDING DRUG ADMINISTRATION. After administering a drug the nurse records it immediately in the appropriate record form (Fig. 32-7). *The nurse never charts a medication before administering it.* Recording immediately after administration prevents errors, such as might occur when a nurse gives a medication without knowing that the client had already received the medication from a nurse on the preceding shift, who forgot to record the administration.

The recording of a medication includes the name of the drug, dosage, route, and exact time of administration. Often the medication forms are prepared and the nurse need only record the time. Agency policies may also require that the nurse record the location in which she gives an injection.

If a client refuses a drug or is undergoing tests or procedures that result in a missed dose, the nurse explains in the nurse's notes why the drug was not given. Some agencies require the nurse to circle the prescribed administration time on the medication record (Fig. 32-7).

CLIENT AND FAMILY TEACHING. Unless a client is properly informed about the medications he takes, there is a good chance that he will take the medications incorrectly or not at all. The nurse provides the client with information pertaining to the purpose of medications, their actions, and their effects. Many health care institutions offer easy-to-read leaflets on specific types of drugs. A client must know how to take a drug properly and what the effects will be if he fails to do so. For example, when a client receives a prescription for an antibiotic, he must understand the importance of taking the full prescription. Failure to do this can lead to a worsening of his condition, as well as the development of bacteria resistant to the drug.

Clients who depend on daily injections learn the proper self-administration of drugs through the nurse's demonstrations. The client learns not only how to administer an injection correctly but also how to use aseptic technique. Family members should be taught to give injections in case the client becomes ill or physically unable to handle a syringe. Many audiovisual aids and filmstrips are available to teach diabetics the methods for insulin injections.

Nurses can also provide specially designed equipment for clients with visual alterations. Syringes are available with enlarged calibrated scales for easier reading.

Clients must be made aware of the symptoms of drug side effects or toxicity. For example, clients taking anticoagulants learn to notify the physician immediately when signs of bleeding develop. Family members should be informed of drug side effects, such as changes in behavior, since they are often the first persons to recognize such effects. Clients are better able to cope with problems caused by drugs if they understand how and when to act.

All clients should learn certain basic guidelines for drug safety. These guidelines ensure the proper use and storage of medications in the home setting:
1. Keep each drug in its original labeled container.
2. Be sure the labels are legible.
3. Discard any outdated medications.
4. Discard unused portions of a drug prescribed for a specific illness. Do not save the drug for future illnesses.
5. Dispose of medications in a sink or toilet. Do not place drugs in the trash within reach of children.
6. Do not give a family member a drug prescribed for another individual.
7. Refrigerate medications that require it.
8. Read labels carefully and follow all instructions.

Adequate client preparation will minimize the risk of the client's abusing medications and improve his compliance with prescribed therapies.

MAINTAINING CLIENTS' RIGHTS. In 1973 the American Hospital Association issued a Patient's Bill of Rights (see Chapter 17). This statement acknowledged the rights of health care consumers and addressed the responsibilities of all health care providers. The Patient's Bill of Rights is a comprehensive statement defining rights and responsibilities for a broad area of medical and nursing practice. It helps to clarify the rights of clients in an area of practice such as medication administration.

Because of the potential risks related to medication administration, a client has the following rights:
1. To be informed of drug name, purpose, action, and potential undesired effects

2. To refuse a medication regardless of the consequences

3. To have qualified nurses or physicians assess a drug history, including allergies

4. To be properly advised of the experimental nature of any drug therapy and to give written consent for its use

5. To receive labeled medications safely without discomfort in accordance with the "five rights" of drug administration (see below)

6. To receive appropriate supportive therapy in relation to drug therapy

7. Not to receive unnecessary medications

It is important for the nurse to be aware of clients' rights so she can handle all inquiries by clients and families courteously and professionally. A nurse should not become defensive if a client refuses drug therapy. The nurse must have the necessary knowledge and skill to satisfy the responsibilities of safe and effective drug administration.

EVALUATION

The nurse is responsible for monitoring the client's response to a medication. This is easier if the nurse knows the therapeutic action and common side effects of the medication. When unpredictable reactions occur, the nurse evaluates the client's response in the same manner as after any sudden change in a client's condition. For example, she assesses vital sign changes and observes any physical alterations. The nurse is particularly alert for the occurrence of reactions in a client with multiple drug allergies or with health alterations that increase the client's sensitivity to a drug.

When the nurse's care plan involves teaching the client how to self-administer drugs at home, the nurse must give the client ample time to demonstrate his understanding. The nurse should ask the client to explain when he should take each drug during the day. If the client is to self-administer injections, the nurse should have him do so under supervision. The nurse should ask the client to explain the purpose of each drug and any side effects it may cause. The family should also be involved in the evaluation process, particularly if they are to administer medications.

Medication Delivery

Preparing and administering medications require accuracy on the part of the nurse. The nurse must pay full attention to the task of preparing medications and not attempt to do other tasks simultaneously. The nurse uses five guidelines to ensure safe drug administration—the "five rights" of drug administration:

1. The *right* drug
2. The *right* dose
3. The *right* client
4. The *right* route
5. The *right* time

Right Drug

Before administering any drug the nurse compares the medicine ticket, Kardex, or unit dose recording form with the physician's written orders (Fig. 32-8). If transcriptions are accurate, the nurse then compares the label of the drug container with the form or medicine ticket. The nurse does this three times: (1) before removing the container from the drawer or shelf; (2) as the amount of drug ordered is removed from the container; and (3) before returning the container to storage. With single-dose prepackaged drugs the nurse checks the label with the medicine ticket or form a third time even though there is no permanent container.

Nurses administer only the medications they prepare. A nurse should never administer a drug prepared by another nurse. Should an error occur, the nurse who administers the drug is responsible for its effects.

If a client questions the medication a nurse prepares, it is important not to ignore his concerns. An alert client will know whether a medication is different from those he has received before. For example, the client may ask why he is receiving an injection when he previously received a capsule. In most cases

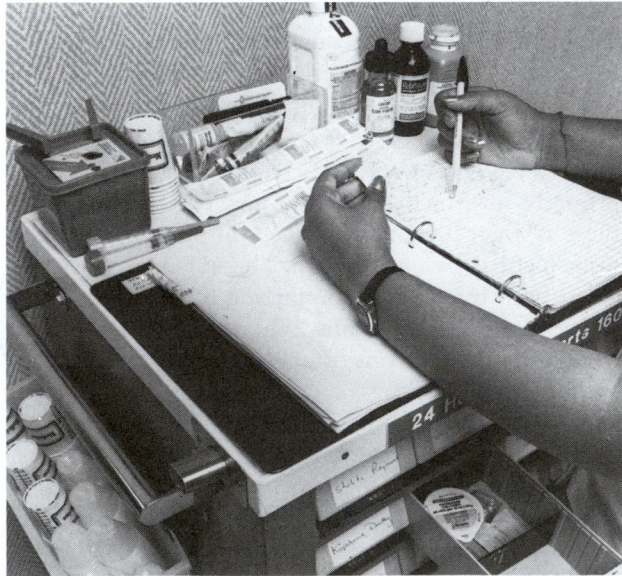

Fig. 32-8 The nurse checks the label of the medication with the transcribed medication order.

the client's medication order has been changed; however, the client's questions might reveal that an error has been made. The nurse should withhold the drug until the preparation can be rechecked against the physician's orders. The client should never be falsely reassured and asked to take a drug if there is any doubt that it is correct.

Clients who self-administer medications should keep the drugs in their original labeled containers. Placing several different pills in single pillboxes is a dangerous habit. A client may easily forget which medication to take when he must select a pill on the basis of appearance only.

To further ensure that the client receives the right drug, the nurse never prepares medications from unmarked containers or containers with illegible labels. If a client refuses a drug, the nurse should never return the medication to the original container or transfer the drug to another container (single-dose prepackaged drugs can be returned to storage areas if unopened).

Right Dose

The unit dose system of drug distribution minimizes errors, since most medications come prepared in proper doses. When a medication must be prepared from a larger than needed volume or strength, or when the physician orders a system of measurement different from what the pharmacist supplies, the chance of error increases. When performing drug calculations or conversions, the nurse should have another qualified nurse check the calculated dosages. Most institutions require that two nurses check all insulin and anticoagulant dosages. The nurse should follow the agency's policies.

After calculating dosages the nurse prepares the medication (see the section on routes of administration). The nurse achieves greater accuracy by using standard measurement devices. For example, many liquid medications come dispensed with a scaled dropper. Graduated cups, syringes, and specially designed spoons can be used to measure medications accurately. In the home setting clients should use kitchen measuring spoons rather than teaspoons and tablespoons, which vary in volume.

When it is necessary to break a scored tablet, the nurse makes sure to break the tablet evenly. A tablet may be cut in half by using a knife edge or by folding a clean paper towel over the tablet and breaking it with the fingers. Any tablets that do not break evenly are discarded. After a tablet is split, the nurse gives the two halves in successive doses.

Often a nurse prepares a tablet by crushing it in a mortar and pestle so the drug can be mixed in the client's food. This is done when a client has difficulty in swallowing and an injection is undesirable. The mortar should always be cleaned out completely before the tablet is crushed. Remnants of previously crushed drugs may increase a drug's concentration or result in the client receiving a portion of an unprescribed drug.

Right Client

An important step in administering drugs safely is being sure the medication is given to the right client. The nurse working in a hospital or extended care setting is frequently responsible for administering drugs to several clients. Often clients have similar last names. It is difficult to remember every client's name and face, especially if a nurse has been off duty for several days. To identify a client correctly, the nurse (1) checks the medicine ticket or form against the client's identification bracelet (Fig. 32-9), and (2) asks the client to state his name.

If an identification bracelet becomes smudged or illegible, the nurse acquires a new one for the client. When asking the client's name, the nurse should not speak the name and assume that the client's response indicates that he is the right person. A client may smile at the nurse even if she happens to say the wrong name, since she is obviously addressing him. Instead, the nurse asks the client to state his full name. This is vital even if the nurse has been caring for the client

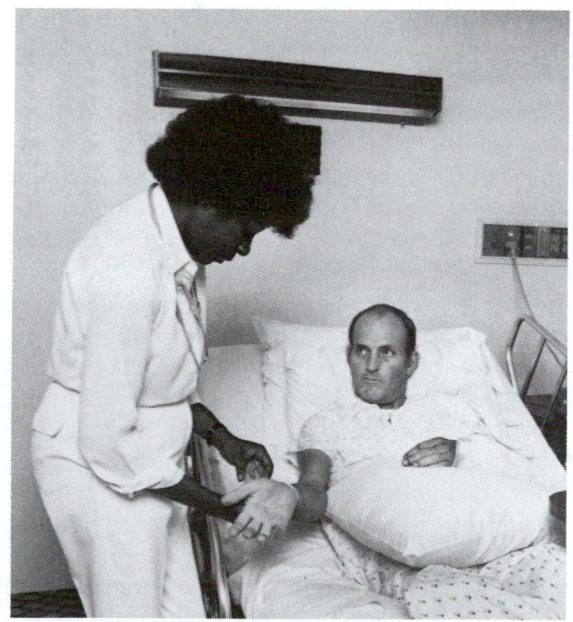

Fig. 32-9 Before administering any medication, the nurse checks the client's identification bracelet to be sure the right client receives the drug.

for several days and recognizes him. To avoid making the client feel uneasy, the nurse simply tells him that the routine for giving a medication requires his identification by name.

Clients who self-administer medications at home should be cautioned never to give a family member one of their medications. A physician should be consulted before one person uses a prescription meant for another, since a drug that is safe for one person can be lethal to another.

Right Route

If a physician's order does not designate a route for medication administration, the nurse consults the physician. Likewise, if the specified route is not the recommended route, the nurse should alert the physician immediately.

When the nurse administers injections (see the section on parenteral routes), certain precautions are necessary to ensure that the medications are given correctly, for example, preventing an intramuscular or subcutaneous injection from directly entering the bloodstream. It is also important to prepare injections only from preparations designed for parenteral use. The injection of a liquid designed for oral use can produce local complications such as a sterile abscess or fatal systemic effects. Drug companies label parenteral drugs for "injectable use only."

Right Time

The nurse must know why a drug is ordered for certain times of the day and whether the time schedule can be altered. For example, two drugs are ordered, one q8h (every 8 hours) and the other t.i.d. (three times a day). Both medications are to be given three times within a 24-hour period. The physician intends the q8h medication to be given around the clock to maintain therapeutic blood levels of the drug. In contrast, the t.i.d. medication is given during the waking hours. Each institution has a recommended time schedule for medications ordered at frequent intervals, for example, q.i.d. medications may be given at 8 AM, noon, 4 PM, and 8 PM; t.i.d. medications may be given at 8 AM, 2 PM, and 8 PM.

Often the physician gives specific instructions about when to administer a medication. A preoperative medication to be given on call means that the nurse is to administer the drug when the operating room notifies the nursing division. A drug ordered p.c. (after meals) is to be given within half an hour after a meal when the client has a full stomach. A stat medication is to be given immediately.

When a nurse is responsible for administering sev-

eral medications, drugs that must act at certain times are given priority. For example, insulin should be administered at a precise interval before a meal. All routinely ordered medications should be given within 30 minutes of the times ordered.

Some medications require the nurse's clinical judgment in determining the proper time for administration. A p.r.n. sleeping medication should be administered when the client is prepared for bed. Many clients prefer to go to sleep earlier than they might normally at home. However, if the nurse is aware that a procedure might interrupt the client's sleep, it is appropriate to withhold the drug until a time when the client can gain full benefit from the medication. A nurse also uses judgment in administering p.r.n. analgesics. When a client's order reads q3-4h, the nurse may give the medication as often as every 3 hours. The nurse assesses the client's level of pain to determine the degree of discomfort. If a client is made to wait until his pain becomes severe, an analgesic is not sufficient. The nurse may need to obtain a stat order from the physician if the client requires a medication before the p.r.n. interval has elapsed.

In the home setting a client may have to take several medications throughout the day. The nurse can help plan medication schedules based on the preferred drug intervals and the client's daily schedule. For example, the schedule for drugs to be given around mealtime can be easily adjusted to the client's preferences. For clients who have difficulty remembering when to take medications, the nurse can make a chart that lists the times when each drug is to be taken.

Avoiding Errors

Most medication errors occur when a nurse fails to follow routine procedures. Unfortunately, many medication errors are never identified. Caution is the rule. Skipping steps in checking orders, calculating dosages, or preparing drugs can prove dangerous. Table 32-11 lists some tips for preventing common administration errors.

When the nurse makes an error, she should acknowledge it immediately. The nurse has the ethical and professional responsibility for reporting the error to the client's physician. Measures to counteract the effects of the error may be necessary, such as administering an antidote when the wrong drug is given, withholding a dose when a medication has been given too soon, or monitoring the drug's effects when an unusually high dosage is given. The nurse is also responsible for completing an incident report that describes the nature of the incident. The report is not an admission of guilt or the basis for punishment and is not a part of the client's legal record. The report

---

TABLE 32-11

How to Prevent Drug Administration Errors

Precaution	Rationale
Read drug labels carefully.	Many products come prepared in similar containers.
Question the administration of multiple tablets or vials for a single dose.	Most doses are one or two tablets or capsules or one single-dose vial. Incorrect interpretation of an order may result in an excessively high dose.
Be aware of drugs with similar names.	Many drug names sound alike, e.g., digoxin and digitoxin, Keflex and Keflin, Orinase and Ornade.
Check the decimal point.	Certain drugs come prepared in quantities that are multiples of one another. For example, Coumadin is available in 2.5 and 25 mg tablets, and Thorazine is available in 30 and 300 mg spansules. An error with a decimal point may not be noticed by the pharmacist.
Question abrupt and excessive increases in dosages.	Most dosage changes are made gradually so the physician can monitor the drug's therapeutic effect and the client's response.
When a new or unfamiliar drug is ordered, consult a resource.	If the physician is also unfamiliar with the drug, there is greater risk of inaccurate dosages being ordered.
Do not administer a drug ordered by a nickname.	Many physicians refer to commonly ordered medications by nicknames. If the nurse or pharmacist is unfamiliar with the name, the wrong drug may be dispensed and administered.
Do not attempt to decipher illegible writing.	When in doubt, ask. Unless the nurse questions an order that is difficult to read, the chance of misinterpreting the order is great.
Know clients with the same last names.	It is common to have two or more clients with the same or similar last names. Special labels on the Kardex or medication book can warn nurses of the potential problem.

provides an objective analysis of what went wrong and is a means for the institution's safety personnel to monitor such occurrences. Without incident reports, nursing supervisory personnel have difficulty identifying errors and solving recurrent problems affecting client care.

Oral Administration

The most desirable way to administer medications is by mouth. Unless the client has impairment of gastrointestinal functioning or is unable to swallow, an oral medication is the safest and easiest to give. Oral medications come in two forms: solid and liquid.

Most tablets and capsules should be swallowed and administered with an adequate amount of fluid. This is a good opportunity for the nurse to increase a client's fluid intake. For clients with nasogastric feeding tubes, tablets can be crushed and capsules opened to mix the medications in a solution for administration through the tube. An enteric-coated tablet should never be crushed or broken for administration because the tablet's contents are irritating to oral and gastric mucosa. A few kinds of tablets must be chewed to create their desired effect. In this case the nurse instructs the client not to swallow the drug whole.

Powdered medications must be mixed with liquids (water or juice) before administration. Several of these drugs (bulk powders) thicken quickly when mixed with liquid. The nurse mixes the drug at the client's bedside so the client can swallow the medication before it thickens. Effervescent powders and tablets should be taken immediately after dissolving. The effervescence helps to improve the unpleasant taste of these preparations and often has therapeutic value for gastrointestinal problems. Administering effervescent tablets in iced liquids also improves the taste.

The client should be warned not to chew or swallow lozenges. The lozenge's therapeutic effect results from a slow absorption through the oral mucosa, not the gastric mucosa. Some liquid preparations such as iron can discolor a client's teeth. The nurse can have the client take these medications through a straw placed well back in the mouth. Some syrups, such as cough syrup, produce local medicating effects on oral mucosa. The nurse instructs a client not to take fluids after swallowing such syrups to avoid washing away the drug.

When administering medication orally, the nurse must protect the client against possible aspiration. Positioning the client in a sitting or side-lying position will prevent the accumulation of liquid or solid medication in the back of the throat. A client who swallows slowly should not be forced to take a large

Administering Oral Medications

EQUIPMENT:
1. Medication cards, Kardex, or record form
2. Medication cart or tray
3. Disposable medication cups
4. Glass of water or juice
5. Drinking straw

STEPS	RATIONALE
1. Gather medication cards or Kardex forms that list all drugs to be given to client at prescribed time.	Cards and forms show which drugs a client receives.
2. Check the accuracy and completeness of each card or form with physician's written medication order, looking at client's name, drug name and dosage, route of administration, and time for administration.	The physician's order is the most reliable resource and the only legal record of drugs the client is to receive. NOTE: Check all orders at least every 24 hours.
3. Recopy any card or portion of the form that is illegible.	Cards that are soiled or illegible can be a source of drug errors.
4. Wash hands.	Removal of microorganisms minimizes their transfer from the nurse's hands to medications and equipment.
5. Arrange medication tray and cups in medicine room or move medication cart to position outside client's room.	Organization of equipment saves time and reduces error.
6. Unlock medicine drawer or cart.	Medications are safeguarded when locked in cabinet or cart.
7. Prepare medications for one client at a time. Keep medication tickets or forms for each client together.	This prevents preparation errors.
8. Select correct drug from stock or unit dose drawer and compare with medication card or form.	Reading the label against the transcribed order reduces error.
9. Calculate the correct dosage.	Calculation will be more accurate when information from drug labels is at hand.
10. If administering tablets or capsules from bottle, pour the required number into the bottle cap and then transfer to medication cup. *Do not touch medicines with your fingers.* Extra tablets or capsules may be returned to bottle.	Aseptic technique maintains cleanliness of drugs.
11. Transfer unit-dose-packaged tablets or capsules to a medication cup. (Do not remove wrapper.) All tablets or capsules given to a client at the same time may be placed in one cup except for those requiring preadministration assessments, such as pulse rate and blood pressure.	Keeping medications that require preadministration assessments separate from others will make it easier for the nurse to withhold those drugs if necessary.
12. To pour liquids, remove bottle cap and place it upside down.	This prevents contamination.
13. Hold bottle with label against palm of hand while pouring.	Spilled liquid will not soil or fade label.
14. Hold medication cup at eye level and fill to desired level. (Scale should be even with fluid level at bottom of meniscus.)	This ensures accuracy of measurement.

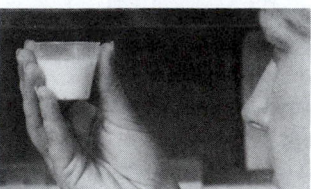

STEPS	*RATIONALE*
15. Discard excess liquid into sink. Wipe lip of bottle with paper towel.	This prevents contamination of bottle's contents and prevents bottle cap from sticking.
16. When preparing a narcotic, check the narcotic record for the previous drug count, remove the necessary volume of drug, record the necessary information on the form, and sign the form.	Controlled substance laws require careful monitoring of dispensed narcotics.
17. Compare the medication card or form with the prepared drug and container.	Reading the label a second time reduces error.
18. Return stock containers or unused unit-dose medications to shelf or drawer and read labels a third time.	This reduces administration error.
19. Place medications and cards together on tray or cart.	Drugs are labeled at all times for identification.
20. Do not leave drugs unattended.	The nurse is responsible for safekeeping of drugs.
21. Take medications to client at correct time.	Medications are administered within a time period of 30 minutes before or 30 minutes after the prescribed time to ensure the intended therapeutic effect.
22. Identify the client by comparing name on card or form with name on the client's identification band. Ask the client to state his name.	Identification bands are made at time of the client's admission and are the most reliable source of identification. Replace any missing identification bands.
23. Perform any necessary preadministration assessment.	Assessment data determine whether medications should be given at that time.
24. Explain the purpose of the medication and its action to the client.	The client's understanding of the purpose of medication will improve compliance with drug therapy.
25. Assist the client to a sitting or side-lying position.	This prevents aspiration during swallowing.
26. Administer drugs properly. Offer the client a choice of water or juice with drugs to be swallowed. The client may wish to hold solid medications in hand or cup before placing in mouth.	Choice of therapy promotes the client's comfort. The client can become familiar with medications by seeing each drug and then will be able to recognize correct drugs.
27. If the client is unable to hold medications, place the medication cup to his lips and gently introduce the drugs into his mouth.	This prevents contamination of medications.
28. If a tablet or capsule falls to the floor, discard it and repeat preparation.	This prevents contamination.
29. Stay with the client until he has completely swallowed each medication. If uncertain whether the client has swallowed the medication, ask him to open his mouth.	The nurse assumes responsibility for ensuring that the client receives the ordered dosage. If left unattended, the client may not take the dose or may save drugs, causing a risk to his health.
30. Wash your hands.	This prevents the spread of microorganisms.
31. Record each drug administered on medication record.	Prompt documentation prevents errors such as repeated doses.
32. Return medication cards to appropriate file for next administration time.	Cards are used as reference for when next dosage is due. Loss of card may lead to administration error.
33. Discard used supplies, replenish stock such as cups and straws, and clean work area.	A clean working space assists other staff in completing duties efficiently.
34. Return within 30 minutes to evaluate the client's response to medications.	By monitoring the client's response, the nurse assesses the drug's therapeutic benefit and can detect the onset of side effects or allergic reactions.

amount of liquid with each swallow. Likewise, a client should swallow only one pill or capsule at a time. If a client begins a coughing spell while taking a medication, the nurse withholds the remaining portion of the drug until the client can breathe easily again.

Procedure 32-1 describes the steps for oral administration of solid and liquid medications.

Administration of Injections

The administration of an injection is an invasive procedure that must be performed using aseptic techniques (Table 32-12). Once a needle pierces the skin, there is the risk of infection. The nurse administers drugs parenterally by one of four routes: subcutaneous, intramuscular, intradermal, and intravenous. Each type of injection requires certain skills to be sure the medication reaches the proper location. The effects of a parenterally administered drug can develop rapidly, depending on the rate of drug absorption. The nurse closely observes the client's response.

TABLE 32-12

Preventing Infection during an Injection

Goal	Actions
Preventing contamination of solution	Draw medication from vial quickly. Do not allow vial to stand open.
Preventing needle contamination	Avoid letting needle touch a contaminated surface: outer edges of ampule or vial, outer surface of needle cap, nurse's hands, countertop, or table surface.
Preventing syringe contamination	Avoid touching length of plunger or inner part of barrel. Keep tip of syringe covered with cap or needle.
Preparing skin	Wash skin soiled with dirt, drainage, or feces with soap and water, and dry. Use friction and a circular motion while cleaning with an antiseptic swab. Swab from center of site and move outward in a 2-inch radius.

Equipment

A variety of syringes and needles are available, each designed to deliver a certain volume of medication to a specific type of tissue. The nurse uses judgment in determining which syringe or needle will be most effective.

SYRINGES

Syringes consist of a cylindrical barrel with a tip designed to fit the hub of a hypodermic needle and a close-fitting plunger (Fig. 32-10). Most hospitals and health care institutions use disposable, single-use plastic syringes. Plastic syringes are inexpensive, and the plunger is easy to manipulate. Glass syringes are more expensive and must be sterilized before each use.

The nurse fills a syringe by aspiration, pulling the plunger outward while the needle tip remains immersed in the prepared solution. During preparation the nurse may handle the outside of the syringe barrel and the handle of the plunger. To maintain sterility the nurse avoids letting any unsterile object touch the tip or inside of the barrel, the shaft of the plunger, or the needle.

Syringes come in a number of sizes, varying in capacity from 1 to 50 ml (Fig. 32-11). It is unusual to use a syringe larger than 5 ml for an injection. A 2 to 3 ml syringe is adequate for intramuscular and subcutaneous injections; a larger volume creates discomfort for the client. The 2.5 or 3 ml hypodermic syringe often comes prepackaged with a needle attached. However, the nurse may change needle sizes. The hypodermic has two scales along the barrel; one is divided into minims and the other into tenths of a milliliter.

An insulin syringe holds 1 ml and is calibrated in units. Most insulin syringes are U-100s, designed for use with U-100 strength insulin. Each milliliter of solution contains 100 units of insulin. At one time there were also U-40 and U-80 syringes for the respective concentrations of insulin.

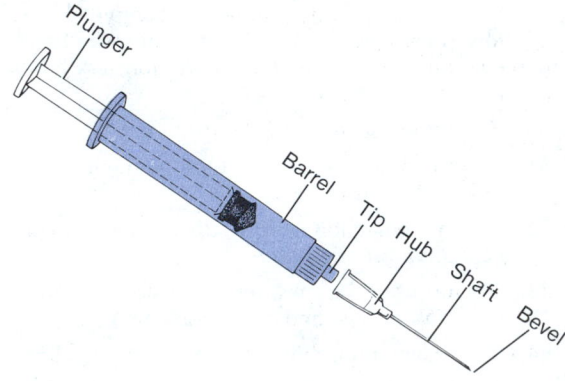

Fig. 32-10 Parts of a syringe and hypodermic needle.

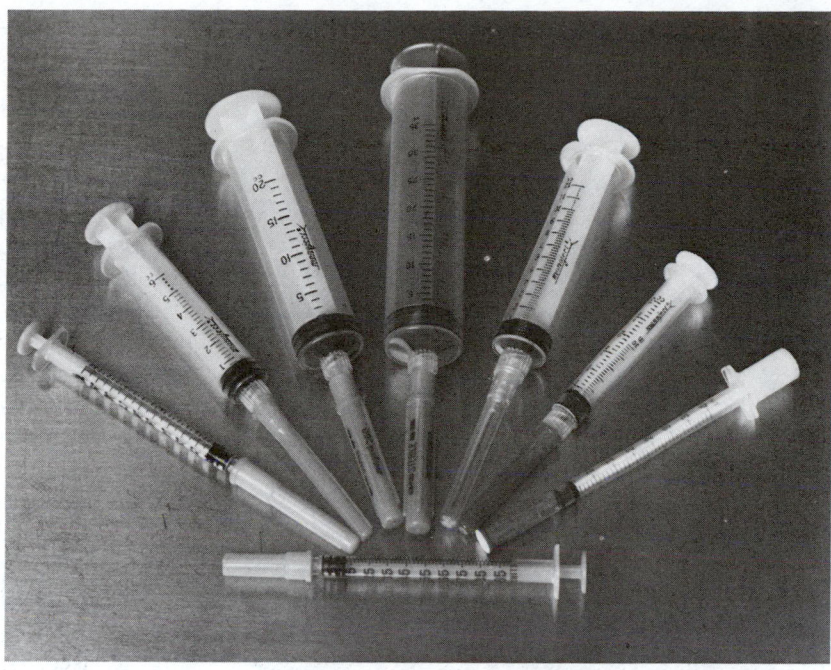

Fig. 32-11 Variety of syringe sizes.

The tuberculin syringe has a long, thin barrel with a preattached thin needle. The syringe is calibrated in sixteenths of a minim and hundredths of a milliliter and has a capacity of 1 ml. The nurse uses a tuberculin syringe to prepare small amounts of potent drugs, such as those used for intradermal skin testing. A tuberculin syringe is also useful in preparing small precise doses for infants or young children.

The nurse uses large hypodermic syringes to administer certain intravenous drugs, add medications to intravenous solutions, and irrigate wounds or drainage tubes.

NEEDLES

Needles come packaged in individual sheaths to allow flexibility in choosing the right needle for a client. Some needles are preattached to standard-sized syringes, for example, insulin and tuberculin syringes. Most needles are made of stainless steel, although several intravenous catheters are plastic. Needles are disposable except for those made from surgical steel, which are attached to glass syringes.

The needle has three parts: the hub, which fits onto the tip of a syringe; the shaft, which connects to the hub; and the bevel or slanted tip (see Fig. 32-10). The nurse may handle the needle hub to ensure a tight fit on the syringe. However, the shaft and bevel must remain sterile at all times.

Each needle has three characteristic features: the slant of the bevel, the length of the shaft, and the needle gauge or diameter. A short bevel is best for intravenous injections, since it does not become easily

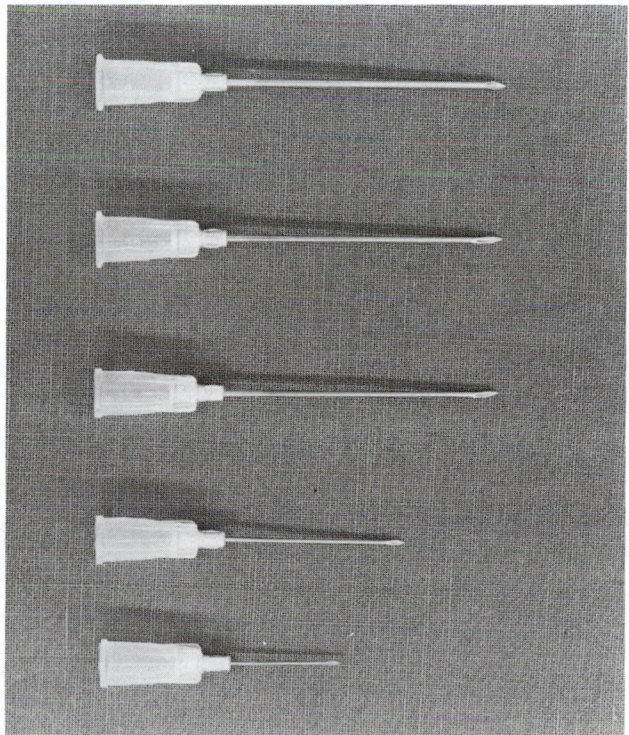

Fig. 32-12 Hypodermic needles arranged in order of gauge. *Top to bottom:* 16 gauge, 19 gauge, 20 gauge, 23 gauge, and 25 gauge.

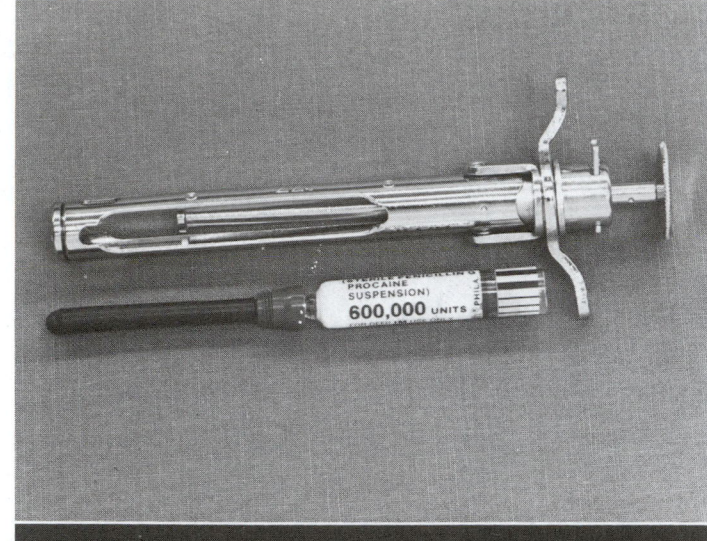

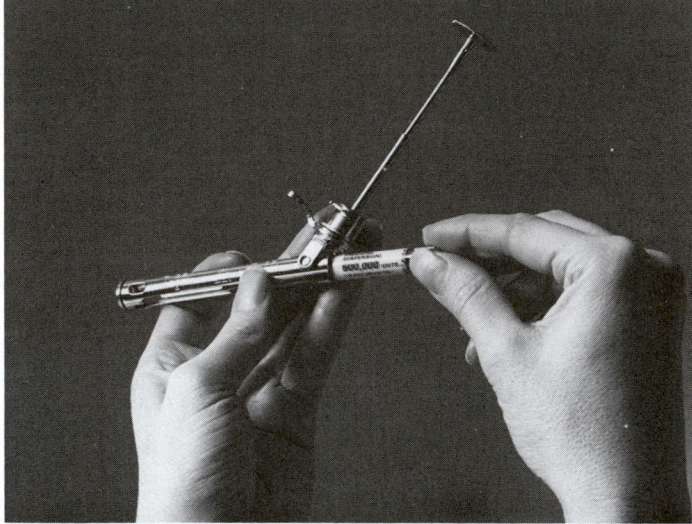

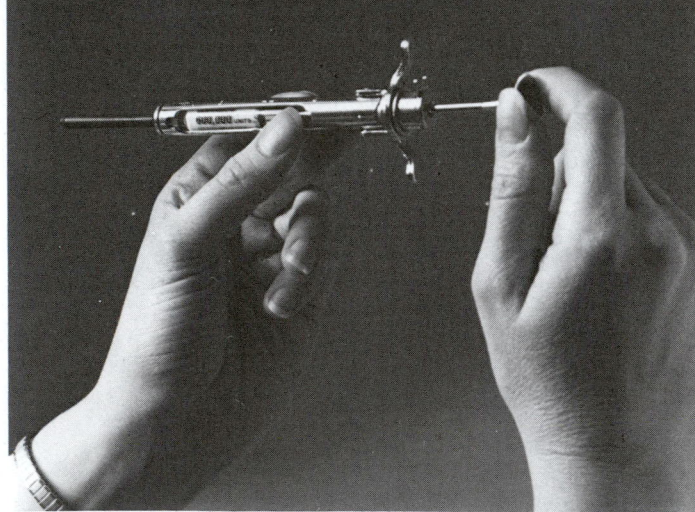

Fig. 32-13 **A,** Tubex metal syringe and prefilled sterile cartridge with needle. **B,** Assembling the Tubex. **C,** The cartridge slides into the syringe barrel and locks at the plunger.

occluded against the inside of a blood vessel wall. Long bevels are sharper, which minimizes the discomfort caused by subcutaneous and intramuscular injections. Needles vary in length from ¼ to 5 inches, although 1½ inches is the maximum length for injections given by nurses. The nurse chooses needle length according to the client's size and weight and the type of tissue into which the medication is to be injected. A child or a slender adult generally requires a shorter needle. The nurse uses a longer needle (usually 1 to 1½ inches) for intramuscular injections and a shorter needle (usually ⅜ to ⅝ inch) for subcutaneous injections.

The smaller the gauge, the larger the needle diameter (Fig. 32-12). The selection of a gauge depends on the viscosity of the fluid to be injected or infused. A 16- or 18-gauge large-diameter needle is ideal for infusing blood products, since the needle causes less trauma to red blood cells. An intramuscular injection usually requires a 20- to 23-gauge needle, depending on the viscosity of the medication. Subcutaneous injections require smaller-diameter needles, for example, a 25-gauge needle, while for an intradermal injection a 26-gauge needle is used.

DISPOSABLE INJECTION UNITS

Disposable, single-dose, prefilled syringes are available for some medications. With these units it is unnecessary for the nurse to prepare doses except perhaps to expel an unneeded portion of the medication.

The Tubex injection system includes a reusable metal syringe that holds prefilled, disposable, sterile cartridge-needle units. The syringe unit opens near the base of the barrel by a hingelike connection (Fig. 32-13). A single medication cartridge slips into the syringe. The nurse locks the cartridge in place and turns the plunger so it screws into the cartridge. The plunger then expels the medication as in a regular syringe. One disadvantage of the system is that clients often complain that the needles are not sharp.

Preparing an Injection from an Ampule

Ampules contain single doses of medication in a liquid form. Ampules are available in several sizes, containing volumes from 1 ml to 10 ml or more (Fig. 32-14). An ampule is made of clear glass with a constricted neck that must be snapped off to allow access to the medication. A colored ring around the neck indicates where the ampule is prescored to be broken easily. The nurse uses a file to scratch the neck of an ampule that is not prescored.

When withdrawing the medication the nurse uses aseptic technique by preventing the needle from touching the ampule's outer surface. Aspiration of

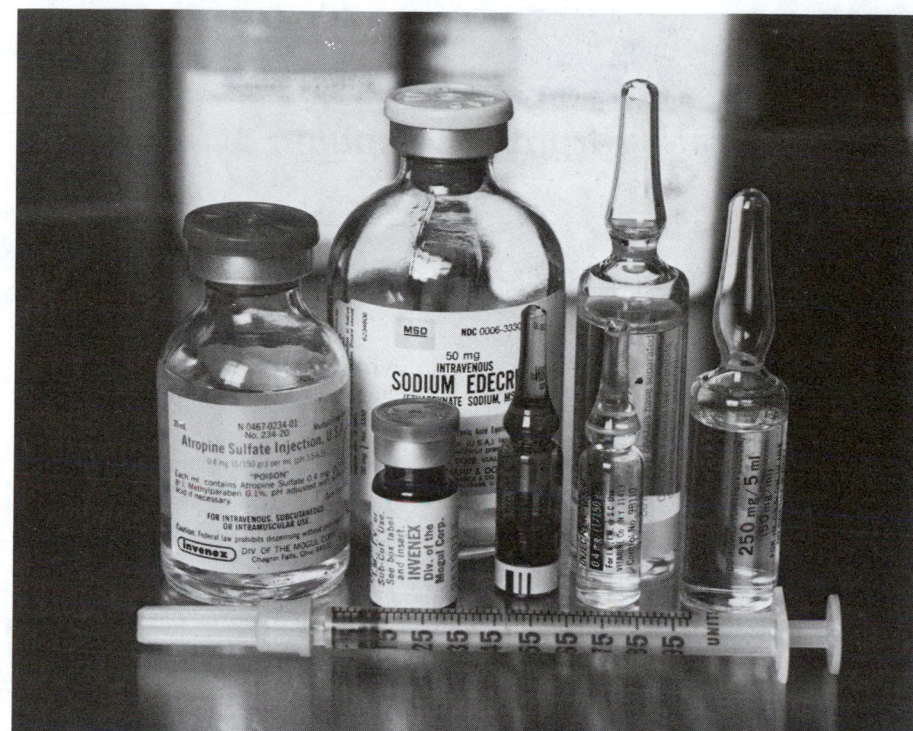

Fig. 32-14 Variety of vials and ampules.

the drug into a syringe occurs easily. Procedure 32-2 describes the techniques of preparing an injectable drug from an ampule.

Preparing an Injection from a Vial

A vial is a single- or multiple-dose glass container with a rubber seal at the top. A metal cap protects the seal until it is ready for use. Vials contain either liquid or dry forms of medications. Drugs that are unstable in solution are packaged in dry form. The vial label specifies the solvent used to dissolve the drug and the amount of solvent needed to prepare a desired drug concentration. Normal saline and sterile distilled water are the solutions commonly used to dissolve drugs.

Unlike the ampule, the vial is a closed system, and air must be injected into it to permit easy withdrawal of the solution. Failure to inject air when withdrawing solution creates a vacuum within the vial that makes withdrawal difficult. Procedure 32-3 summarizes the steps for withdrawing medications from a vial.

To prepare a powdered drug, the nurse draws up the amount of diluent or solvent recommended on the vial's label. The nurse injects the solvent into the vial in the same manner as injecting air into the vial. Most powdered medications dissolve easily, but it may be necessary to withdraw the needle in order to mix the contents thoroughly. Gently shaking or rolling the vial between the hands will dissolve the pow-

dered drug. After mixing multidose vials the nurse makes a label that includes the date of mixing and the concentration of drug per milliliter. Multidose vials may require refrigeration after the contents are reconstituted.

Mixing Medications

If two drugs are compatible, it is possible to mix them together in an injection. A client will appreciate not having to receive more than one injection at a time. Most nursing units have charts that list common compatible drugs. If there is any uncertainty about drug compatibilities, a pharmacist should be consulted.

MIXING MEDICATIONS FROM TWO VIALS

The nurse follows three principles when mixing medications from two vials: (1) not contaminating one medication with another, (2) ensuring that the final dosage is accurate, and (3) maintaining aseptic technique.

When multidose vials are used, the risk of contamination is great. The nurse should draw each dose into a separate syringe and then transfer the contents of one syringe into the other. She takes one of the filled syringes and pulls back on the plunger to aspirate air in excess of the volume to be added. The nurse removes the needle from the syringe, takes the second syringe, and carefully inserts the needle

Preparing an Injectable Medication from an Ampule

STEPS	RATIONALE

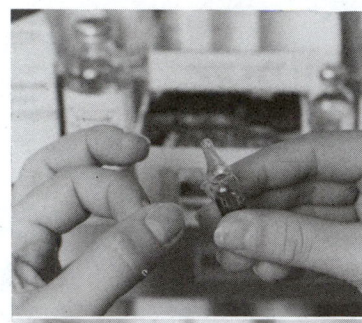
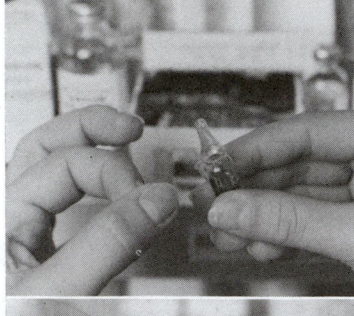
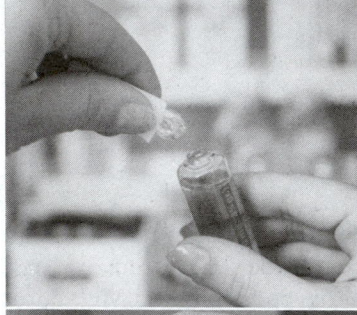
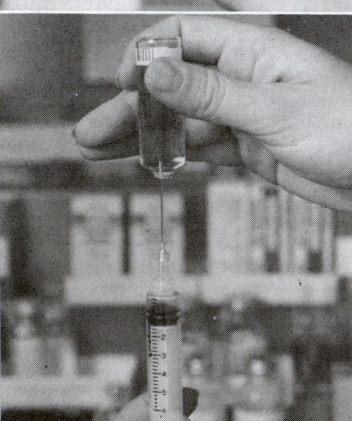
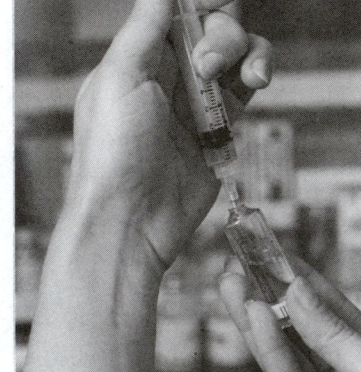

1. Tap the top of the ampule lightly and quickly with a finger.

   This dislodges any fluid that collects above the neck. All of the solution moves into the lower chamber.

2. Place a small gauze pad or dry alcohol swab around the neck of the ampule.

   A pad or swab protects the nurse's fingers from trauma as the glass is broken.

3. Snap the neck of the ampule in a direction away from your hands.

   This prevents shattering the glass toward the nurse's fingers or face.

4. Holding the inverted ampule, insert the needle into the center of the ampule opening. Do not allow the needle tip or shaft to touch the rim of the ampule. NOTE: The ampule may be held upright as long as the needle tip or shaft does not touch ampule's rim.

   The broken rim of the ampule is considered contaminated.

5. Aspirate the medication into the syringe by pulling back on the plunger.

   Withdrawal of the plunger creates a negative pressure within the barrel that pulls fluid into the syringe.

6. Keep the needle tip below the surface of the liquid. Tip the ampule to bring all the fluid within reach of the needle.

   This prevents aspiration of air bubbles.

7. If air bubbles are aspirated, do not expel the air into the ampule.

   Air pressure will force fluid out of the ampule and the medication will be lost.

8. To expel excess air bubbles, remove the needle from the ampule. Hold the syringe with the needle pointing up. Draw back slightly on the plunger, and then push the plunger upward to eject the air. *Do not eject fluid.*

   Withdrawing the plunger too far will pull it from the barrel. Holding the syringe vertically allows fluid to settle in the bottom of the barrel. Pulling back on the plunger allows fluid within the needle to enter the barrel.

9. After withdrawing the required fluid volume, remove the needle from the ampule. Hold the syringe and needle upright and tap the syringe barrel to dislodge air bubbles. Eject the air as described in step 8.

   Air within the barrel displaces medication and causes dosage errors.

10. Cover the needle with its sheath or cap.

    Covering the needle prevents contamination of needles and prevents needle sticks.

PROCEDURE 32-3

Preparing an Injectable Medication from a Vial

STEPS	RATIONALE
1. Remove the metal cap to expose the rubber seal.	The vial comes packaged with the cap to prevent contamination of the seal.
2. With an alcohol swab wipe off the surface of the rubber seal.	This removes dust or grease but does not sterilize surface.
3. Remove needle cap. Pull back on the plunger to draw air into the syringe equivalent to the volume of medication to be aspirated.	To prevent buildup of negative pressure when aspirating medication, air must first be injected into the vial.
4. Insert the tip of the needle, with bevel pointing up, through the center of the rubber seal. Apply pressure to the needle point during insertion.	The center of the seal is thinner and easier to penetrate. Keeping the bevel up and using firm pressure prevents cutting a rubber core from the seal.
5. Inject the air into the vial, holding on to the plunger.	Air must be injected first before aspirating the fluid. The plunger may be forced backward by air pressure within the vial.

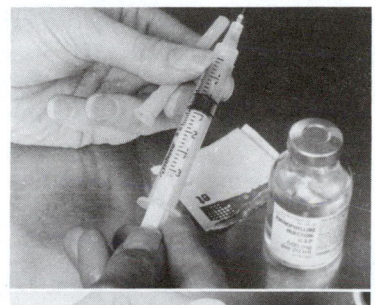
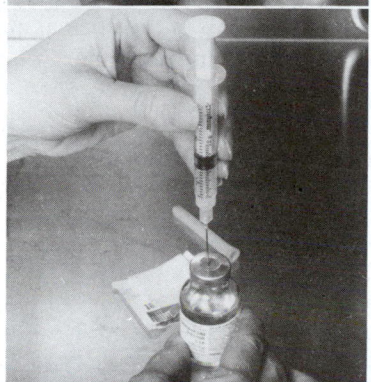

STEPS	RATIONALE
6. Invert the vial while keeping a firm hold on the syringe and a plunger. Hold the vial between thumb and middle finger of the nondominant hand. Grasp the end of the barrel and plunger with thumb and forefinger of the dominant hand.	Inverting the vial allows fluid to settle in the lower half of the container. The position of the hands prevents movement of the plunger and permits easy manipulation of the syringe.
7. Keep tip of needle below fluid level.	This prevents aspiration of air.
8. Allow air pressure to gradually fill the syringe with medication. Pull back slightly on the plunger if necessary.	Positive pressure within the vial forces fluid into the syringe.

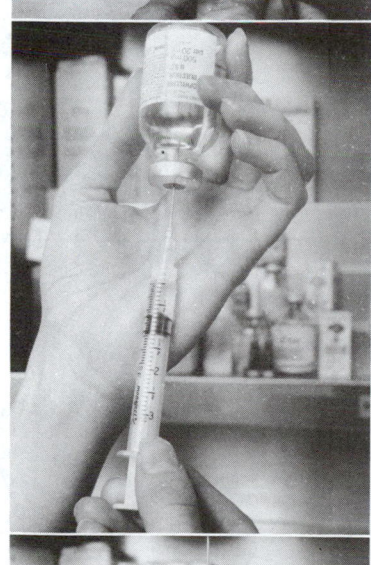

STEPS	RATIONALE
9. Tap the side of the barrel carefully to dislodge any air bubbles. Eject any air remaining at the top of the syringe into the vial.	Forcefully striking the barrel while the needle is inserted in the vial may bend the needle. Accumulation of air displaces medication and causes dosage errors.
10. Once the correct volume is obtained, remove the needle from the vial by pulling back on the barrel.	Pulling the plunger rather than the barrel would cause separation from the barrel and loss of medication.
11. Remove any remaining air from the syringe (see Procedure 32-2, step 9) and cover the needle with its sheath or cap.	This prevents contamination of the needle top.

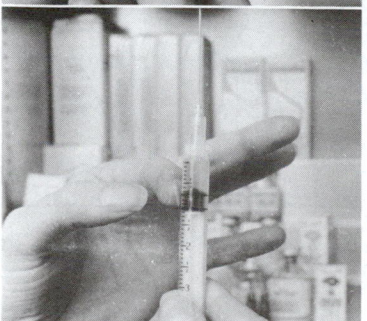

through the tip of the first syringe's barrel. She slowly injects the solution into the barrel, making sure to inject the exact amount of medication desired. She then withdraws the needle and discards the second syringe into an appropriate receptacle. The nurse applies a new needle to the filled syringe, expels any air, and sheaths the needle. She checks the syringe scale to be sure the combined volume of medications is accurate.

If one of the two doses of medication comes from a single-dose vial, it is unnecessary to use two syringes for mixing drugs (Fig. 32-15). The nurse takes a syringe and aspirates the volume of air equivalent to the first medication's dosage (vial A). She injects the air into the vial, making sure the needle does not touch the solution, withdraws the syringe, and then aspirates air equivalent to the second medication's dosage (vial B). Then she fills the syringe with the medication from vial B in the normal manner. At this point medication from vial A has not contaminated vial B. The

nurse applies a new sterile needle to the syringe and inserts it into vial A, being careful not to push the plunger and expel medication into the vial. She carefully withdraws the desired amount of medication from vial A into the syringe. If a vial has excess positive pressure, the plunger may begin to move before the nurse is ready. This can cause an accidental withdrawal of too much medication. After withdrawing the necessary amount of solution the nurse withdraws the needle and sheaths the syringe.

MIXING MEDICATIONS FROM ONE VIAL AND ONE AMPULE

Mixing medications from a vial and an ampule is simple, since it is not necessary to add air in order to withdraw medication from an ampule. The nurse prepares medication from the vial first and then, using the same syringe and needle, withdraws medication from the ampule. This technique prevents contamination of solutions and the needle.

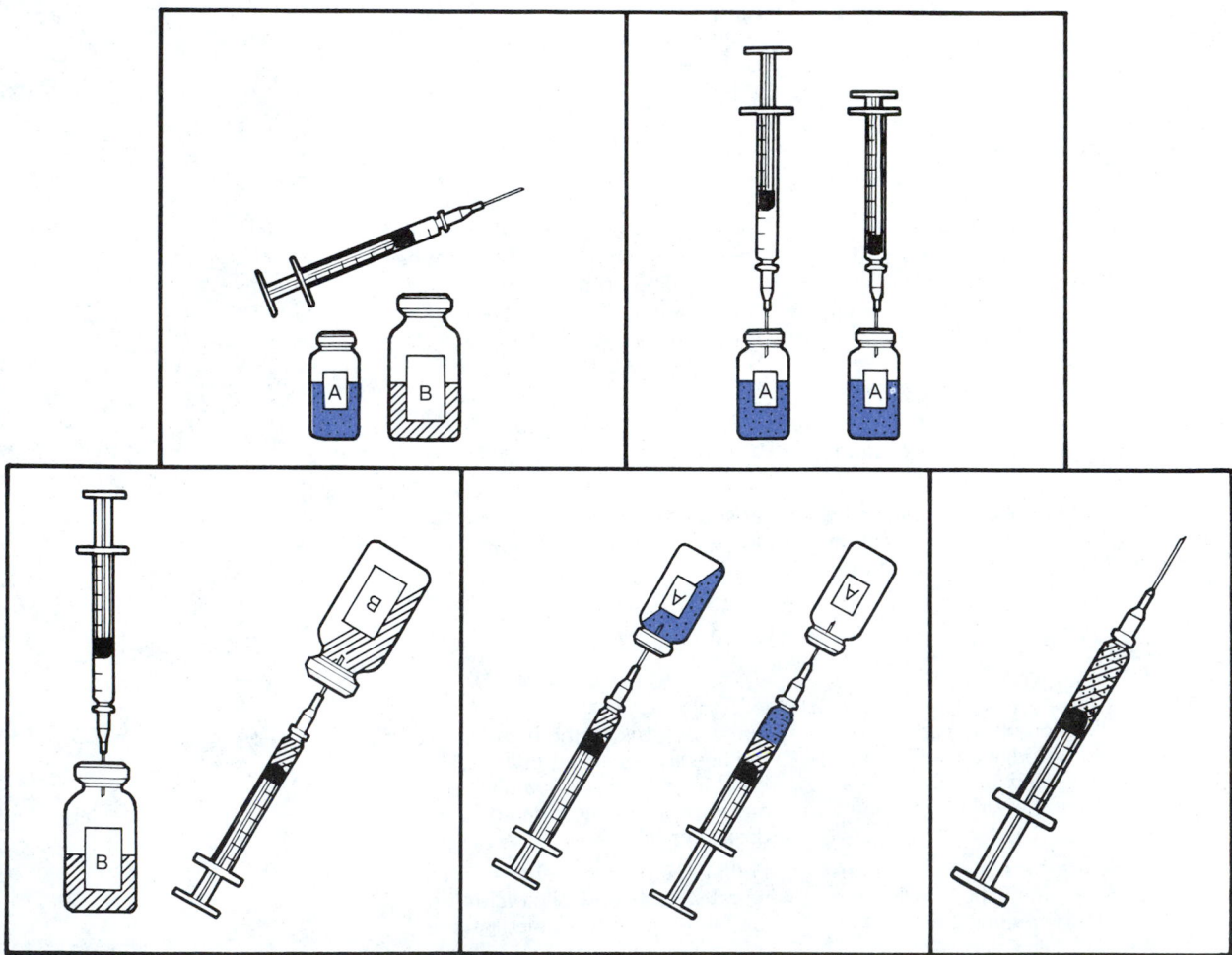

Fig. 32-15 Steps in mixing single and multidose vials.

Administering Injections

Each injection route is unique in regard to the type of tissues into which the medication is injected. The characteristics of the tissues influence the rate of drug absorption and thus the onset of drug action. Before injecting a drug the nurse should know the volume of medication to administer, the characteristics of the medication (for instance, irritating substance, viscosity), and the location of anatomical structures underlying injection sites (for example, major nerves and blood vessels). Procedure 32-4 describes the steps for administering injections.

A nurse's inability to administer injections correctly can have negative consequences. Failure to select an injection site in relation to anatomical landmarks can result in nerve or bone damage during needle insertion. If the nurse fails to aspirate the syringe before injecting a medication, the medication may accidentally be injected directly into an artery or vein. Injecting too large a volume of medication for the site selected causes extreme pain and may result in local tissue damage.

Many clients, particularly children, fear injections. Often a client would rather endure severe pain than be given a "shot." Clients with serious or chronic illness often are subjected to multiple injections daily. The nurse is able to minimize the client's discomfort in several ways:

1. Using a sharp beveled needle in the smallest suitable length and gauge
2. Selecting the proper injection site, using anatomical landmarks
3. Applying ice to the injection sites to create local anesthesia before needle insertion
4. Inserting the needle smoothly and quickly to minimize tissue pulling
5. Holding the syringe steady while the needle remains in tissues
6. Positioning the client as comfortably as possible to reduce muscular tension
7. Diverting the client's attention from the injection by talking with him or asking him to think of something pleasant
8. Massaging the injected area gently for several seconds unless contraindicated

SUBCUTANEOUS INJECTIONS

Subcutaneous injections involve depositing medication into the loose connective tissue under the dermis. Because subcutaneous tissue is not as richly supplied with blood as the muscles, drug absorption is somewhat slower than with intramuscular injections. However, drugs are absorbed completely if the client's circulatory status is normal. Since subcutaneous tissue contains pain receptors, the client may experience some discomfort during an injection.

Subcutaneous injection sites include the outer upper arms, the abdomen from below the costal margins to the iliac crests, the anterior thighs, and the upper back (Fig. 32-16). The injection site chosen should be free of skin lesions, bony prominences, and large underlying muscles or nerves. Clients who self-administer injections usually select the abdomen and upper thighs because of easier accessibility. Only small doses (0.5 to 1 ml) of water-soluble medication should be given by the subcutaneous route. Subcutaneous tissue is sensitive to irritating solutions and large volumes of medication. Collection of medication within the tissues can cause sterile abscesses, which appear as hardened, painful lumps under the skin.

A client's body weight indicates the depth of the subcutaneous layer. Therefore the nurse must choose the needle length and angle of insertion based on the client's weight. Generally a 25-gauge ⅝-inch needle inserted at a 45-degree angle (Fig. 32-17) deposits medication into the subcutaneous tissue of a normal-sized client. A child may require only a ½-inch needle. If the client is obese, the nurse often pinches the tissue and uses a needle long enough to insert through fatty tissue at the base of the skinfold. The preferred needle length is one-half the width of the skinfold. With this method the angle of insertion may be between 45 and 90 degrees. Thin cachectic clients may have insufficient tissue for subcutaneous injections. The upper

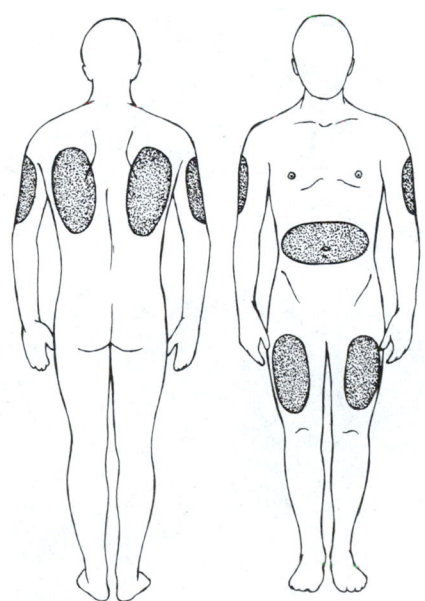

Fig. 32-16 Common sites for subcutaneous injections.

PROCEDURE 32-4

Administering Subcutaneous and Intramuscular Injections

EQUIPMENT:
1. Syringe (size according to volume of drug to be administered)
2. Needle (size varies according to type of tissue and size of client; intramuscular—20- to 23-gauge and ⅝ to 1½ inches in length; subcutaneous—25-gauge and ½ to 1 inch in length
3. Antiseptic swab, e.g., alcohol
4. Medication ampule or vial
5. Medication card or form

STEPS	RATIONALE
1. Assemble equipment and check the medication order as described in Procedure 32-1.	This ensures accuracy of the order.
2. Prepare the medication from the ampule or vial as described in Procedures 32-2 and 32-3.	
3. Provide privacy for the client. Keep a drape over body parts not requiring exposure.	Proper selection of an injection site may require exposure of body parts.
4. Select an appropriate injection site. Palpate the site for masses or tenderness. Avoid areas of scarring, bruising, abrasion, or infection. Palpate muscles to determine firmness and size. NOTE: When administering heparin subcutaneously, use abdominal injection sites.	Injection sites should be free of lesions that might interfere with drug absorption. Sufficient muscle mass is needed to ensure accurate intramuscular injection into the proper tissue. NOTE: An anticoagulant will cause local bleeding and bruising when injected into areas such as the arms and legs, which are involved in muscular activity.
5. Assist the client to a comfortable position.	Relaxation of the muscle receiving an intramuscular medication minimizes discomfort. Promoting the client's comfort helps to reduce his anxiety.
6. Relocate the site using anatomical landmarks.	Accurate injection of a medication requires insertion in the correct anatomical site to avoid injuring underlying nerves, bones, or blood vessels.
7. Cleanse the site with an antiseptic swab. Apply the swab at the center of the site and rotate outward in a circular direction for about 5 cm (2 inches).	The mechanical action of the swab removes secretions containing microorganisms.
8. Hold the swab between the third and fourth fingers of the nondominant hand.	The swab will remain readily accessible when it is time to withdraw the needle.
9. Remove the needle cap from the syringe by pulling the cap straight off.	Preventing the needle from touching the sides of the cap prevents contamination.

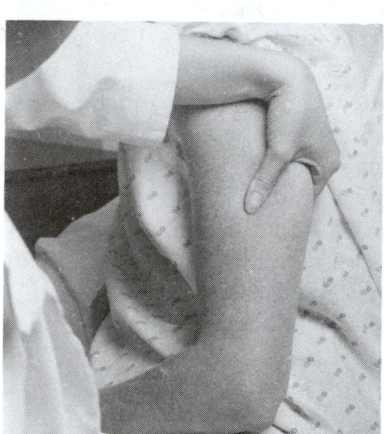

STEPS	RATIONALE	
10. Hold the syringe between the thumb and forefinger of your dominant hand as though the syringe were a dart. (Most nurses hold the syringe palm up for subcutaneous injections and palm down for intramuscular injections because of the different angles of insertion.)	A quick smooth injection requires proper manipulation of the syringe parts.	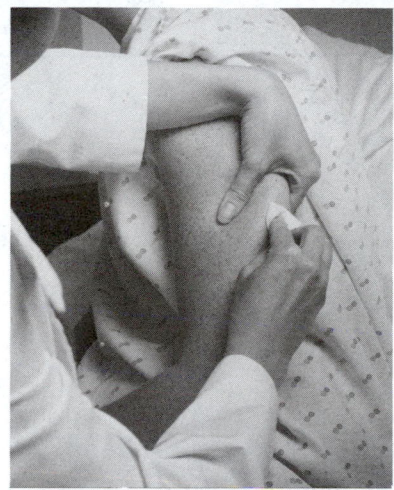
11. Subcutaneous injection:		
a. For the average-sized client, with your nondominant hand spread the skin tightly across the injection site.	The needle penetrates tight skin easier than loose skin.	
b. Inject the needle quickly and firmly at a 45-degree angle.	A quick, firm insertion minimizes the client's anxiety and discomfort.	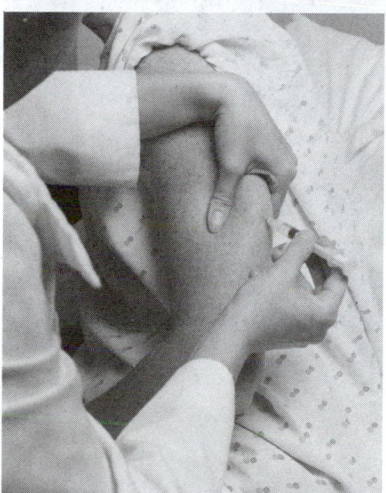
c. For an obese client, pinch the skin at the site and inject the needle below the tissue fold.	Obese clients have a fatty layer of tissue above subcutaneous tissue.	
Intramuscular injection:		
a. Position the nondominant hand at the proper anatomical landmarks and spread the skin tightly. Inject the needle at a 90-degree angle.	This speeds insertion and reduces discomfort.	
b. If the client's muscle mass is small, grasp the body of the muscle and inject the medication.	This ensures that the medication reaches muscle tissue.	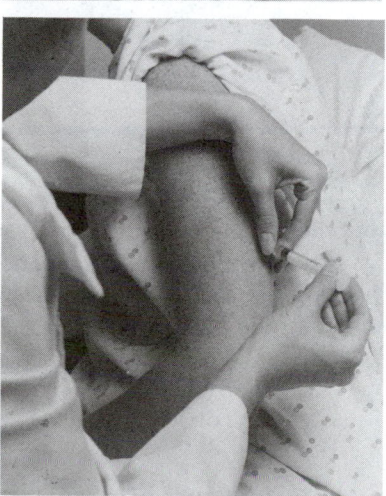
12. Once the needle enters the site, with your nondominant hand grasp the lower end of the syringe barrel. Move your dominant hand to the end of the plunger. Avoid movement of the syringe.	A properly performed injection requires smooth manipulation of syringe parts. Movement of the syringe may displace the needle and cause discomfort.	

PROCEDURE 32-4, *cont'd*

Administering Subcutaneous and Intramuscular Injections

STEPS	RATIONALE
13. Slowly pull back on the plunger to aspirate the medication. If blood appears in the syringe, withdraw the needle, dispose of the syringe, and repeat the medication preparation. If no blood appears, inject the medication slowly. NOTE: Some agencies recommend not aspirating subcutaneous heparin injections.	Aspiration of blood into the syringe indicates intravenous placement of the needle. Subcutaneous and intramuscular medications are not for intravenous use. Slow injection reduces pain and tissue trauma. NOTE: Heparin is an anticoagulant that is typically given in small subcutaneous doses. The drug may cause severe bruising with aspiration. The drug is not harmful if given intravenously.
14. Withdraw the needle quickly while placing the antiseptic swab just above the injection site.	Support of tissues around the injection site minimizes discomfort during needle withdrawal.
15. Massage the site lightly. NOTE: Do not massage a subcutaneous heparin injection site.	Massage stimulates circulation and thus improves drug distribution and absorption. However, it also causes bruising.
16. Recap the needle.	This protects the nurse from accidental injury by a needle stick.
17. Assist the client to a comfortable position.	Assuming a comfortable position gives the client a sense of well-being.
18. Discard needles and syringes into the appropriately labeled receptacles.	Proper disposal prevents injury to clients and hospital personnel.
19. Chart the medication as described in Procedure 32-1.	Timely documentation prevents future drug errors.
20. Return to evaluate the client's response to medication within 15 to 30 minutes.	Parenteral drugs are absorbed into and act more quickly than oral medications. The nurse's observations determine the efficacy of drug action.

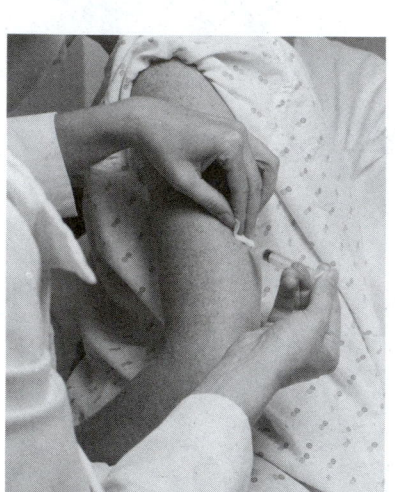

abdomen is the best site for injection when a client has little peripheral subcutaneous tissue.

It is important to rotate injection sites. Repeated administration of medication in the same site will cause tissue sloughing and formation of lesions that impair drug absorption. Diabetics usually have injection site charts on which they record sites of successive injections.

INTRAMUSCULAR INJECTIONS

The intramuscular route provides faster drug absorption than the subcutaneous route because of mus-

cle's greater vascularity. The danger of causing tissue damage is less when medications enter deep muscle, but there is the risk of inadvertently injecting drugs directly into blood vessels. The nurse uses a longer (1- to 1½-inch) and heavier-gauge (23 to 20) needle to pass through subcutaneous tissue and penetrate deep muscle tissue. The angle of insertion for an intramuscular injection is 90 degrees (Fig. 32-17). Muscle is less sensitive to irritating and viscous drugs. A normal, well-developed client can safely tolerate as much as 3 ml of medication without severe muscle discomfort. A larger volume of medication is unlikely

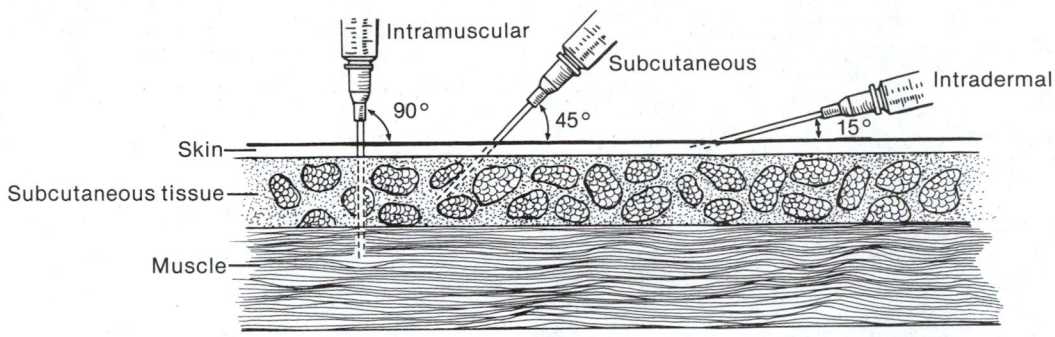

Fig. 32-17 Comparison of the angles of insertion for intramuscular (90 degrees), subcutaneous (45 degrees), and intradermal (15 degrees) injections.

to be absorbed properly. Children, the elderly, and cachectic individuals can tolerate only 2 ml of an intramuscular injection.

The nurse should assess the integrity of a muscle before giving an injection. The muscle should be free of tenderness. Repeated injections in the same muscle will cause considerable discomfort. By asking the client to relax, the nurse can palpate the muscle to rule out the presence of hardened lesions. Normally a muscle feels soft when relaxed and firm when tense.

The nurse can minimize discomfort during an injection by helping the client assume a position that reduces strain on the muscle. For example, the client should sit with the involved arm flexed at the elbow and supported during an injection into the deltoid muscle. For all other injection sites the client should lie down with the body well supported.

SITES. When selecting an intramuscular site, the nurse considers the following: Is the area free of infection or necrosis? Are there local areas of bruising or abrasions? What is the location of underlying bones, nerves, and major blood vessels? What volume of medication is to be administered?

An injection site should be composed of healthy tissue and underlying muscle. The nurse chooses a site only after careful identification of anatomical landmarks such as bony prominences. A large, healthy muscle can withstand larger volumes of medications than a small, emaciated one.

Vastus Lateralis. The vastus lateralis is a preferred injection site for adults and children because of the absence of major nerves and blood vessels and the rapid drug absorption at this site. It is a thick, well-developed muscle on the anterior lateral aspect of the thigh, extending from a handbreadth above the knee to a handbreadth below the greater trochanter of the femur (Fig. 32-18). The middle third of the muscle is the suggested site for injection (see Fig. 32-16). In

width the site extends from the midline of the top of the thigh to the midline of the outer side of the thigh. With young children or cachectic clients it is helpful to grasp the body of the muscle during injection to be sure the drug is deposited in muscle tissue. To help the client relax the muscle, the nurse asks him to lie flat with the knee slightly flexed.

Ventrogluteal. Another preferred site is the ventrogluteal, which involves the gluteus medius and gluteus minimus muscles. These muscles are situated deep and away from major nerves and blood vessels. Thus this site is safe to use in cachectic clients as well as infants and children. Because it is located away from the rectal area, there is less chance of contamination in incontinent clients (a problem when the dorsogluteal site is used).

To locate the ventrogluteal muscle, the nurse places the palm of her right hand over the greater trochanter of the client's right hip (left hand for left hip). She points the thumb toward the client's groin and the fingers toward the client's head, places her index finger over the anterior superior iliac spine, and extends the middle finger back along the iliac crest toward the buttock. The index finger, middle finger, and iliac crest form a V-shaped triangle. The injection site is the center of the triangle (Fig. 32-19).

The client may lie on his side, back, or abdomen as long as the landmarks are easily accessible. Flexing of the knee and hip helps the client relax.

Dorsogluteal. The dorsogluteal site has been a traditional one for intramuscular injections. However, there is considerable risk of striking the underlying sciatic nerve, greater trochanter, and major blood vessels. In many clients the flabby, sagging tissues of the buttocks make it difficult to identify the correct site for needle insertion. Insertion of a needle into the sciatic nerve can cause permanent or partial paralysis of the client's involved leg.

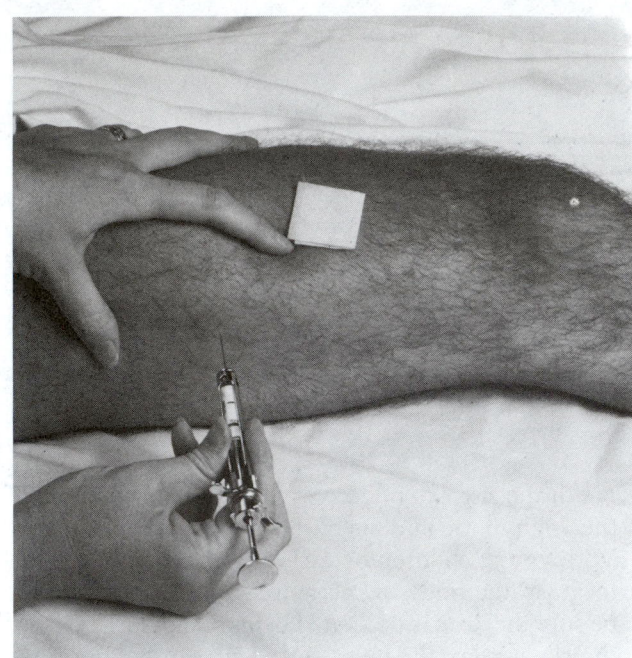

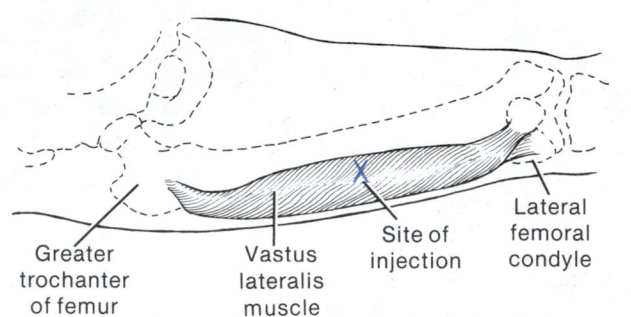

Fig. 32-18 **A,** The injection site into the vastus lateralis muscle is in the middle third of the muscle. **B,** Selected site for intramuscular injection into the vastus lateralis muscle.

When the client is in a prone or side-lying position, the site is located below the iliac crest and above an imaginary diagonal line between the posterosuperior iliac spine and the greater trochanter of the femur. The path of the sciatic nerve is well below this diagonal line (Fig. 32-20). If the nurse has difficulty palpating the greater trochanter, having the client raise his knee and extend his hip will help the nurse locate the bony prominence.

A less accurate method of locating the dorsogluteal muscle is dividing the buttock into quadrants (see Fig. 32-20). The vertical dividing line extends from the gluteal fold up to the iliac crest. The intersecting horizontal line extends from the medial fold to the lateral aspect of the buttock. The injection site is in the upper outer quadrant. This method increases the risk of injury to the sciatic nerve.

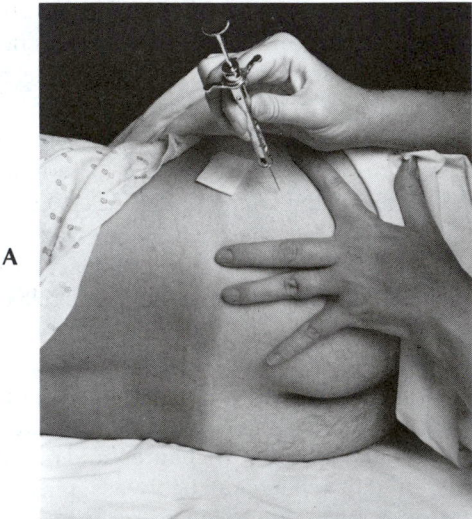

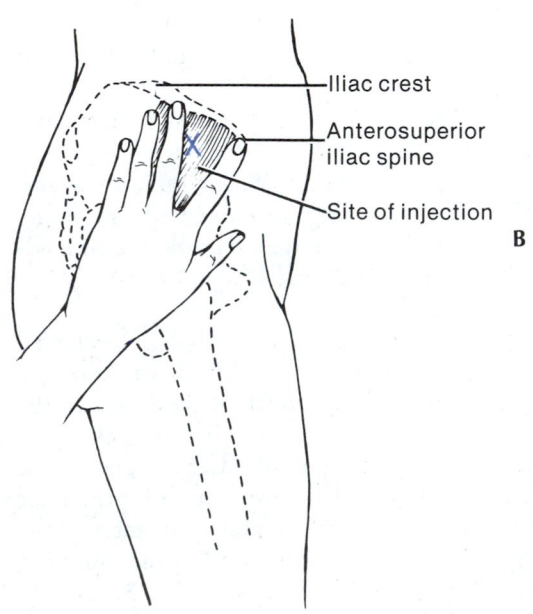

Fig. 32-19 **A,** Injection site into ventrogluteal muscle avoids major nerves and blood vessels. **B,** Ventrogluteal muscle injection site.

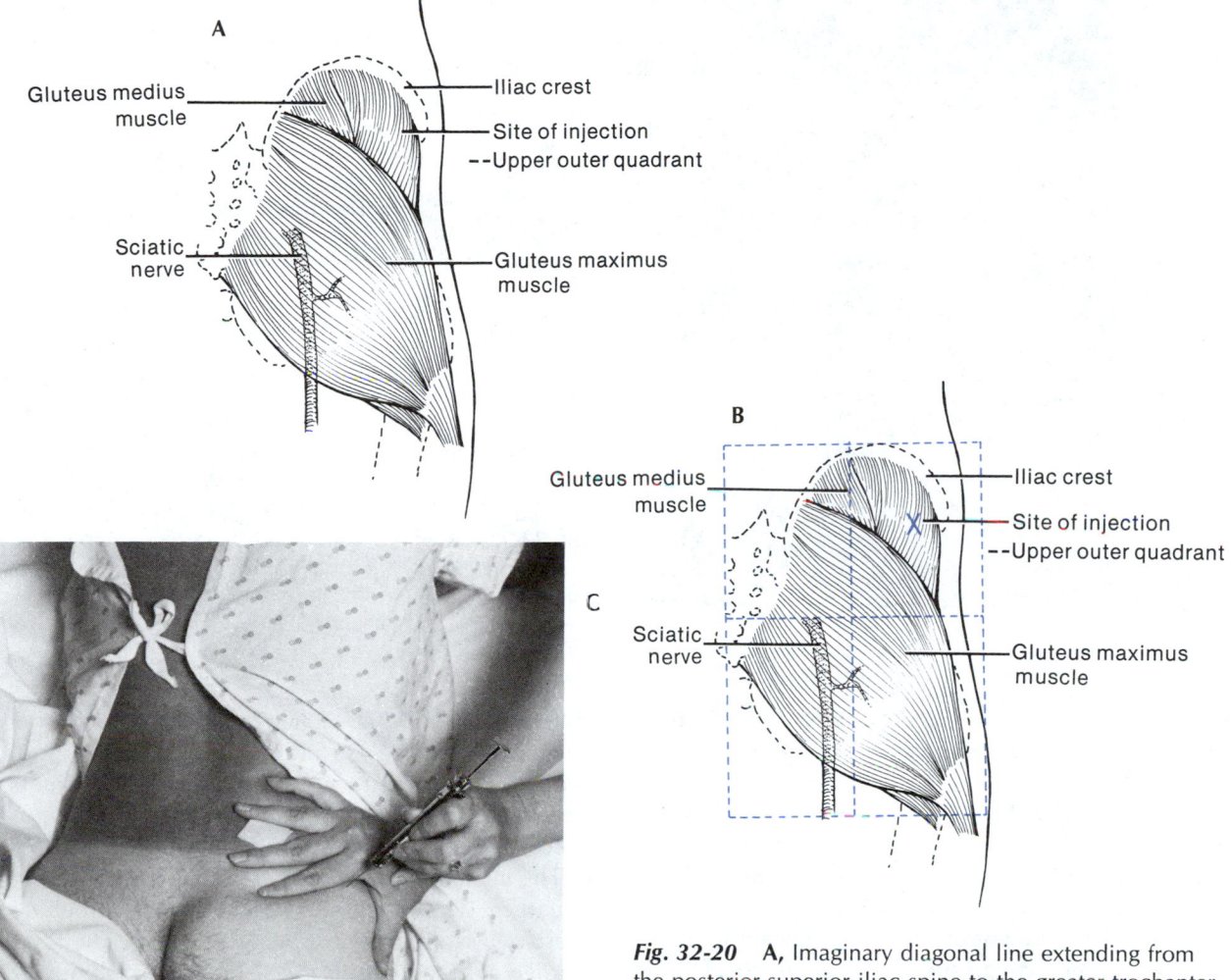

Fig. 32-20 A, Imaginary diagonal line extending from the posterior superior iliac spine to the greater trochanter is the landmark for selecting the dorsogluteal injection site. **B,** The buttocks may be divided into quadrants for selecting the dorsogluteal injection site. **C,** Site of injection into dorsogluteal muscle.

The dorsogluteal site is not recommended for children under 3 years of age. The muscle is developed by walking and is too small in this age group.

Lying prone with the feet turned inward promotes relaxation during injection of the gluteal muscle. Lying on the side with the upper knee and hip flexed and placed in front of the lower leg has the same effect. The dorsogluteal site should never be used while a client stands because this position causes contraction of the muscle.

Before giving an injection in the dorsogluteal muscle the nurse carefully cleanses the skin. The skin surface around the buttock will be contaminated with microorganisms in an incontinent client. If a client's skin is obviously soiled, the nurse washes the area well with soap and water before preparing the skin for the injection.

Deltoid. In many adults and most children the deltoid muscle is not well developed. The radial and ulnar nerves and brachial artery lie within the upper arm along the humerus. The nurse uses the deltoid site to administer small volumes of medication or when other injection sites are inaccessible because of dressings, casts, or other obstructions.

To locate the deltoid muscle the nurse has the client expose the upper arm and shoulder fully. A tight-fitting sleeve should not be rolled up. The nurse has the client relax the arm at the side and flex the elbow (Fig. 32-21, *A*). The client may sit, stand, or lie down. The injection area is a small triangle pointing downward from a line extending along the lower edge of the acromial process. The bottom tip of the triangle is a midpoint of the lateral aspect of the upper arm, in line with the axilla. The injection site is in the center

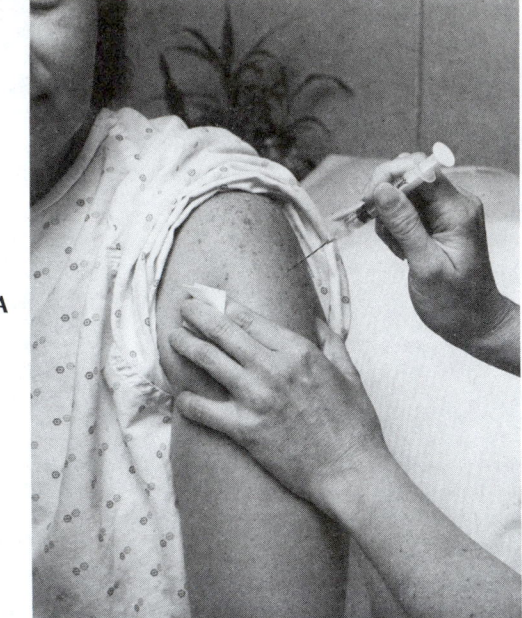

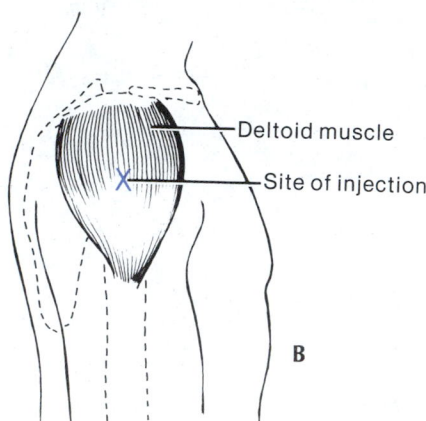

Fig. 32-21 **A,** Site of intramuscular injection into the deltoid muscle. **B,** Site of deltoid muscle injection below acromial process.

of the triangle, approximately 2.5 to 5 cm (1 to 2 inches) below the acromial process (Fig. 32-21, *B*).

AIR LOCK TECHNIQUE. Intramuscular injections administered with the air lock technique are less irritating to subcutaneous tissues. When a small volume of air is injected behind a bolus of medication, the air clears the needle of medication, preventing tracking of the drug through subcutaneous tissues. The air also helps to lock the medication into the muscle for better absorption.

After preparing the proper medication dosage, the nurse draws approximately 0.5 to 1 ml of air into the syringe. Holding the needle upright, the nurse makes a final check of the medication volume. Then the nurse slowly ejects all but 0.2 to 0.3 ml of the air, taking care not to expel any medication. The needle then must be injected downward at a 90-degree angle so that the air rises to the top of the medication toward the plunger (see Fig. 32-17). As the nurse injects the drug into the muscle, the air follows the medication, creating an air lock (Fig. 32-22). If the nurse administers the drug with the needle at an angle less than 90 degrees, the air collects along the barrel of the syringe and enters the muscle too soon. Medication can then easily leak back into subcutaneous tissues.

The air lock technique is also useful for subcutaneous injections when it is necessary for the client to receive all of a dose. Insulin administration is a common example. Injecting 0.2 to 0.3 ml of air through the needle ensures that all medication is expelled through the needle shaft's bore.

Z-TRACK METHOD. When irritating preparations such as iron are given intramuscularly, even an air lock is insufficient to protect the skin and subcutaneous tissues. The Z-track method of injection more successfully seals medication within muscle tissues.

The nurse selects an intramuscular site, preferably in larger, deeper muscles such as the ventrogluteal muscle. It is important to apply a new needle to the syringe after preparing the drug so no solution remains on the outside needle shaft. The nurse draws up 0.2 to 0.3 ml of air to create an air lock. After preparing the site with an antiseptic swab, the nurse pulls the overlying skin and subcutaneous tissues approximately 2.5 to 3.5 cm (1 to 1½ inches) laterally

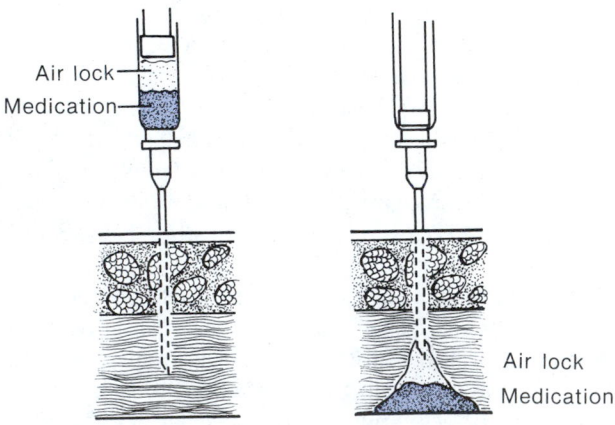

Fig. 32-22 Administering intramuscular injection by the air lock technique prevents tracking of medication through subcutaneous tissues.

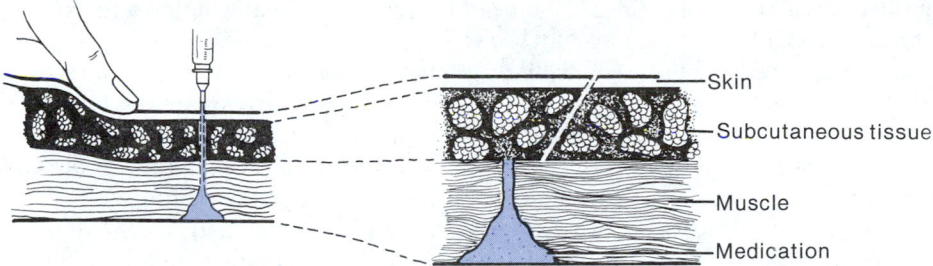

Fig. 32-23 The Z-track method of injection deposits the medication into the muscle without tracking residual medication through sensitive tissues.

to the side. Holding the skin taut with her nondominant hand, the nurse injects the needle deep into the muscle. With practice the nurse learns to hold the syringe and aspirate with one hand. The nurse injects the medication and air slowly if there is no blood return on aspiration. The needle remains inserted for 10 seconds to allow the medication to disperse evenly. The nurse then releases the skin after withdrawing the needle. This leaves a zigzag path that seals the needle track wherever tissue planes slide across each other (Fig. 32-23). The medication cannot escape from the muscle tissue.

INTRADERMAL INJECTIONS

The nurse typically gives intradermal injections for the purpose of skin testing, for example, in tuberculin and allergy tests. Since these medications are potent, they are injected into the dermis where blood supply is reduced and drug absorption occurs slowly. A client may have a severe anaphylactic reaction if the medications enter the client's circulation too rapidly. For clients with a history of numerous allergies the physician often performs skin testing.

Skin testing requires that the nurse be able to clearly see the injection sites for changes in color and tissue integrity. Intradermal sites should be lightly pigmented, free of lesions, and relatively hairless. The inner forearm and upper back are ideal locations.

The nurse uses a tuberculin or small hypodermic syringe for skin testing. A short (¼- to ½-inch), fine-gauge (26 or 27) needle is ideal for injecting medications between the skin layers. After preparing the injection site with an antiseptic swab, the nurse holds the syringe with the bevel of the needle pointing upward (Fig. 32-24, *A*). The needle enters the skin at an angle of 5 to 15 degrees (Fig. 32-24, *B*). As the

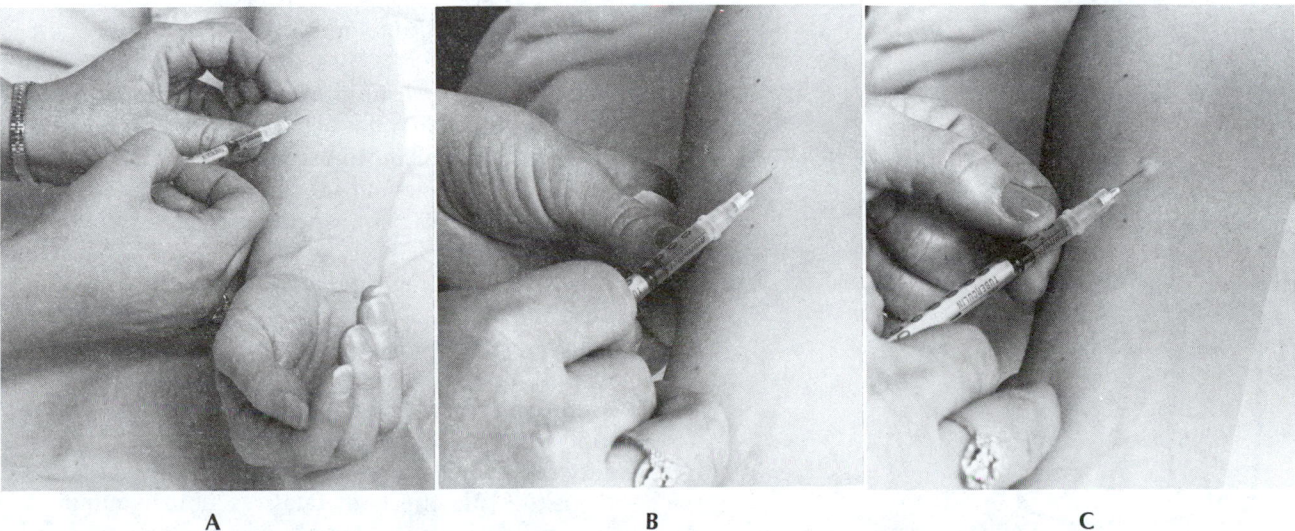

A   B   C

Fig. 32-24 **A** and **B,** For intradermal injections the nurse holds the syringe needle bevel up. **C,** If injected correctly, the medication forms a bleb when deposited in the dermis.

nurse injects the medication, a small wheal resembling a mosquito bite should appear on the skin's surface (Fig. 32-24, C). If a wheal does not appear or if the site bleeds after needle withdrawal, there is a good chance the medication entered subcutaneous tissues. In this case skin test results will not be valid. After the injection the nurse wipes the site lightly but does not massage the area. Brisk massage may disperse the medication into underlying tissues or cause it to escape from the injection site.

Documentation of an intradermal injection includes a description of the precise location and time of administration. The nurse can use a skin pencil to draw a circle around the perimeter of the injection site, which must be "read" within a prescribed time, for example, 48 hours. Because of the drug's toxic nature the nurse observes the client closely for allergic reactions.

INTRAVENOUS ADMINISTRATION

The nurse administers drugs intravenously by three methods (Fig. 32-25):

1. As mixtures within large volumes of intravenous (IV) fluids
2. By injection of a bolus or small volume of medication through an existing intravenous infusion line or heparin lock
3. By "piggyback" infusion of a solution containing the prescribed medication and a small volume of IV fluid through an adjoining or existing IV line

In all three methods the client has either an existing IV infusion line or an IV access site in the form of a heparin lock. In most institutions and settings only physicians are allowed to inject medications directly into a client's vein through venipuncture.

Chapter 42 describes in detail the technique for performing venipuncture and establishing continuous IV fluid infusions. Medication administration is only one reason for supplying IV fluids for a client. IV fluid therapy is used primarily for fluid replacement in clients unable to take oral fluids and as a means of supplying electrolytes and nutrients.

Whichever method of IV drug administration the nurse uses, it is important to observe clients closely for symptoms of adverse reactions to medications. Once a drug enters the bloodstream, the medication begins to act immediately and there is no way to stop its action. Thus the nurse takes special care to avoid errors in dosage calculation and drug preparation. The nurse should double-check the "five rights" of safe drug administration and know the desired action and potential side effects of the medication. If the drug has an antidote, the nurse must have it available during drug administration. When administering potent medications, such as antihypertensives, the nurse assesses vital signs before, during, and after drug infusion.

Administering drugs by the IV route has certain advantages. Often the nurse uses the IV route in emergency situations when a fast-acting drug must be delivered quickly. For example, when a client goes into cardiac arrest, medications are administered intravenously in an attempt to restore heart function. The IV route is also best when it is necessary to establish constant therapeutic blood levels of a drug. For example, if a client is at risk for developing a serious infection, the physician prescribes IV administration of antibiotics to maintain effective concentrations of the drug. Some medications are highly alkaline and irritating to muscle and subcutaneous tissues. These drugs cause less discomfort when given intravenously.

Of the three methods of administering IV medications, mixing drugs in large volumes of fluids is the safest and easiest. Drugs are diluted in large volumes (500 ml or 1000 ml) of compatible IV fluids such as normal saline or lactated Ringer's solution. In most institutions the pharmacist adds medications to the primary container of IV solution to ensure asepsis. Since the drug is not present in a concentrated form, the risk of side effects or fatal reactions is minimal. Vitamins and potassium chloride are two types of drugs commonly added to a client's IV fluids. The danger with continuous infusion is that, if the IV fluid is infused too rapidly, the client may suffer circulatory

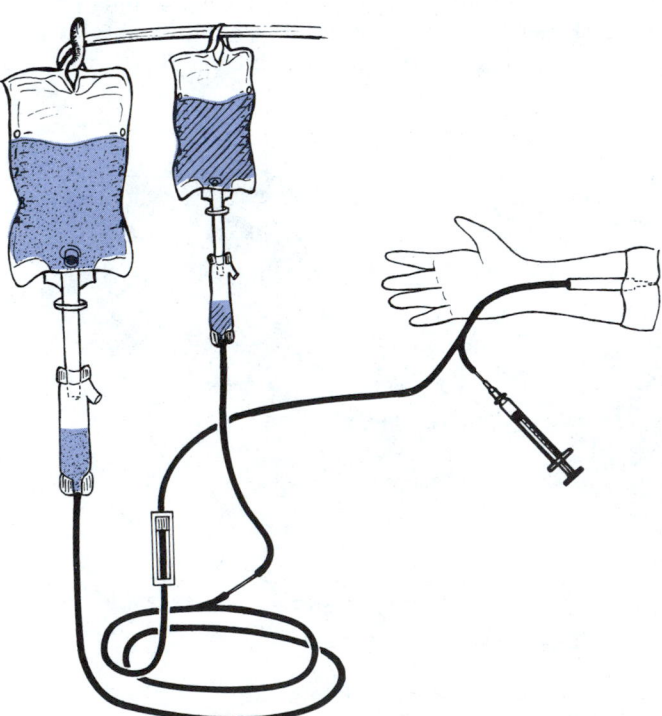

Fig. 32-25 Intravenous medications administered by bolus, piggyback, and large-volume continuous infusion.

PROCEDURE 32-5

Adding Medications to Intravenous Fluid Containers

EQUIPMENT:
1. Prepared medication in a syringe
2. Intravenous fluid container (bag or bottle, 500 or 1000 ml volume)
3. Alcohol or antiseptic swab

STEPS	RATIONALE
BAG	
1. Locate the medication injection port on the infusion bag.	The medication injection port is self-sealing to prevent introduction of microorganisms after repeated use.
2. Wipe off the port with an alcohol or antiseptic swab.	Wiping off the port reduces the risk of introducing microorganisms into the bag during needle insertion.
3. Carefully inject the needle of the syringe through the center of the injection port and inject the medication.	Injection of a needle into the sides of the port may produce a leak and lead to contamination of the fluid.
4. Withdraw the syringe and mix the solution by holding the bag and turning it gently from end to end.	This allows the medication to be distributed evenly throughout the bag of fluid.
5. Rehang the bag and check the infusion rate (see Chapter 42)	This prevents rapid infusion of fluid.
BOTTLE	
1. Locate the medication injection site on the bottle's rubber stopper. The site is usually marked by an "X" or a circle. The air vent and main tubing port are not the injection sites.	Accidental injection through the main tubing port or air vent can alter pressure within the bottle and cause fluid leaks through the air vent.
2. Perform steps 2 through 5 as above.	

fluid overload (see Chapter 42). Procedure 32-5 describes the method of adding medications to large volumes of intravenous fluids.

An IV bolus involves introducing a concentrated dose of medication directly into a client's systemic circulation. Since a bolus requires only a small amount of fluid to deliver the medication, it is an advantage when the amount of fluid the client can take is restricted. The IV bolus is the most dangerous method for administering drugs because there is no time to correct errors. In addition, a bolus may cause direct irritation to the lining of blood vessels. Before administering a bolus the nurse confirms placement of the IV line. This involves obtaining a blood return through the IV catheter or needle. The inability to obtain a blood return suggests that the needle or catheter is in the client's tissues or resting against the vein wall. A drug should never be given intravenously if the insertion site appears puffy or edematous or the IV fluid cannot flow at the proper rate. Accidental injection of a medication into the tissues surrounding a vein can cause pain, necrotic sloughing of tissues, and abscesses, depending on the drug's composition.

A heparin lock is an IV needle with a small "well" covered by a rubber diaphragm (Fig. 32-26). After each medication administration the nurse injects a small volume of diluted heparin into the "well." The presence of heparin in the needle inhibits clot for-

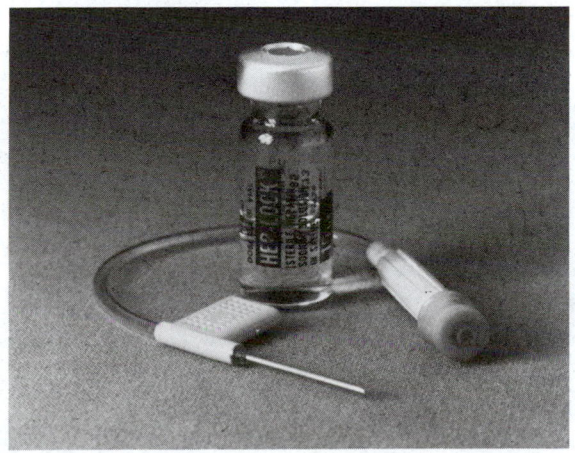

Fig. 32-26 Heparin lock and diaphragm (well).

PROCEDURE 32-6

Administering a Medication by Intravenous Bolus

HEPARIN LOCK

EQUIPMENT:
1. Prepared medication in a syringe with small-gauge (25 or 26) needle
2. Syringe containing 1 ml of 1:1000 heparin solution
3. Alcohol or antiseptic swab
4. Watch with second hand or digital readout

STEPS	RATIONALE
1. Clean the heparin lock's rubber diaphragm with the antiseptic swab.	Cleaning the diaphragm prevents introduction of microorganisms during needle insertion.
2. Insert a 25-gauge needle of the syringe containing prepared drug through the center of the diaphragm.	This prevents damage to the diaphragm and subsequent leakage.
3. Inject the medication bolus slowly over several minutes. (Each medication has a recommended rate for bolus administration. Check package directions.) Use a watch to time the administration.	Rapid injection of an intravenous drug can kill a client.
4. After administering the bolus, withdraw the syringe. Insert the 25-gauge needle of the syringe containing the diluted heparin (heparin flush) solution. Inject the heparin.	This maintains patency of the needle by inhibiting clot formation. Dilution of the heparin solution prevents systemic anticoagulation of the client.
5. Observe the client closely for adverse reaction.	IV medications act rapidly.

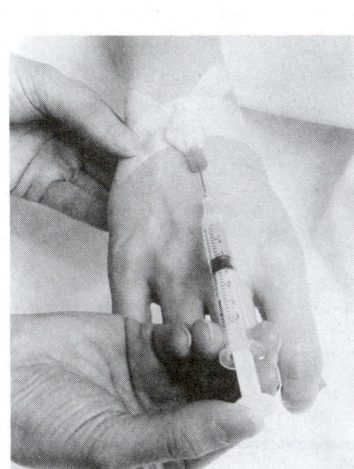

INTRAVENOUS INFUSION LINE

EQUIPMENT:
1. Prepared medication in a syringe with a small-gauge (25 or 26) needle
2. Alcohol or antiseptic swab
3. Intravenous line tubing with injection port
4. Watch with second hand or digital readout

STEPS	RATIONALE
1. Determine if IV fluids are infusing at proper rate (see Chapter 42).	Fluid infusion will deliver the injected medication to the client's vein.
2. Select injection port of tubing closest to needle insertion site.	This allows for easier fluid aspiration to obtain a blood return.
3. Clean off injection port with the antiseptic swab.	Cleaning the injection port prevents introduction of microorganisms during needle insertion.

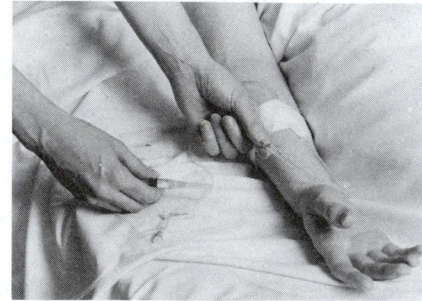

STEPS	RATIONALE	
4. Insert small-gauge needle containing prepared drug through center of port.	This prevents damage to port's diaphragm and subsequent leakage.	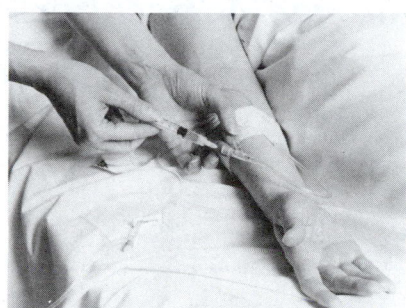
5. Occlude the intravenous line by pinching the tubing just above the injection port. Pull back gently on the syringe's plunger to aspirate for a blood return.	Final check ensures that medication is being delivered into the bloodstream.	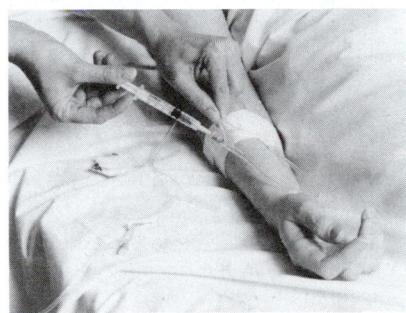
6. After noting a blood return release the tubing and inject the medication slowly over several minutes. (Read directions on drug package.) Use a watch to time the administration.	Release of tubing allows slow infusion of fluids. Rapid injection of an IV drug can prove fatal to a client.	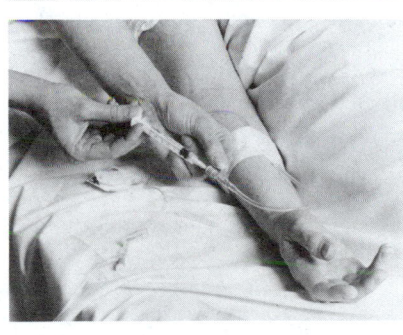
7. After injecting the medication, withdraw the syringe and recheck the fluid infusion rate.	Injection of a bolus may alter the rate of fluid infusion. Rapid fluid infusion can cause circulatory fluid overload.	
8. Observe the client closely for adverse reactions.	IV medications act rapidly.	

mation and thus maintains needle patency despite the absence of a continuous fluid flow. Normally, checking for a blood return in a heparin lock before bolus administration is unnecessary. However, if the needle site becomes puffy or the client complains of discomfort, it is necessary to aspirate the "well" for a blood return. A heparin lock is more comfortable and easier to maintain than an IV fluid line. Procedure 32-6 describes the technique for administering an IV medication bolus.

One way to minimize the risk of rapid dose infusion is to dilute IV medications and infuse the drugs over longer time intervals. The nurse adds the medication to a small amount (50 to 100 ml) of compatible IV fluid. The fluid is contained within a secondary fluid compartment separate from the primary IV fluid bag. The compartment is either a container (for example, Volutrol) that connects directly to the IV line or a small bag or bottle connected to a separate tubing that inserts into the main IV line. The nurse confirms the placement of the IV needle or catheter before beginning infusion of the fluid. Usually intermittent infusions take 30 minutes to be administered (Procedure 32-7).

PROCEDURE 32-7

Administering IV Medications via "Piggyback," through Adjacent or Existing Infusion Lines

INFUSION THROUGH AN ADJACENT LINE

EQUIPMENT:
1. Medication prepared in a 50 or 100 ml infusion bag with an IV infusion tubing set
2. Main IV infusion line
3. 23- or 21-gauge needle
4. Alcohol or antiseptic swab

STEPS	RATIONALE
1. Prepare the secondary infusion line, being sure tubing is completely filled with medication-fluid mixture.	This prevents introduction of air into the primary IV line.
2. Check infusion rate of main IV line (see Chapter 42).	Checking the infusion rate determines the patency of the system. Any obstruction to flow will interfere with medication delivery.
3. Hang the secondary fluid bag at or above the level of the main fluid bag.	The height of the fluid bag regulates the rate of fluid flow to the client.
4. Connect the needle to the end of secondary line tubing. Clean the injection port to the main IV line with an antiseptic swab.	This prevents introduction of microorganisms during needle insertion.
5. Insert the needle of the secondary line through the injection port of main IV line. Regulate the flow rate of the medication solution (usually 30 to 60 minutes).	This provides a direct route for slow intermittent medication infusion. For optimal therapeutic effect, the drug should be infused within 30 to 60 minutes.
6. Observe the client for signs of adverse reactions.	IV medications act rapidly.
7. After medication has infused, turn off flow regulator on secondary IV line. Leave needle, tubing, and secondary bag hanging for future drug administration.	Turning off flow regulator prevents backup of fluid from main line into secondary line. Establishment of secondary line produces route for microorganisms to enter main line. Repeated changes of tubing or needle increase risk of infection transmission.

INFUSION THROUGH A VOLUTROL

EQUIPMENT:
1. Volutrol (plastic graduated container that is part of a main IV line and hangs between the main IV bag or bottle and the infusion tubing)
2. Syringe with prepared medication
3. Alcohol or antiseptic swab

STEPS	RATIONALE
1. Check the infusion rate of the IV line.	This determines patency of the system. Obstruction to flow interferes with medication delivery.
2. Fill the Volutrol with the desired amount of fluid (50 to 100 ml) by opening the clamp between the Volutrol and the main IV bag.	A small volume of fluid dilutes the IV medication and thus reduces the risk of rapid dose infusion.
3. Clean off the injection port on top of the Volutrol.	Cleaning the injection port prevents introduction of microorganisms during needle insertion.
4. Insert the syringe needle into the port and inject the medication. Gently rotate the Volutrol between your hands.	This mixes medication within the Volutrol to ensure equal distribution of the medication.
5. Recheck IV infusion rate (medication should infuse in 30 to 60 minutes).	For optimal therapeutic effect the drug should be infused within 30 to 60 minutes.
6. Observe client for signs of adverse reactions.	IV medications act rapidly.

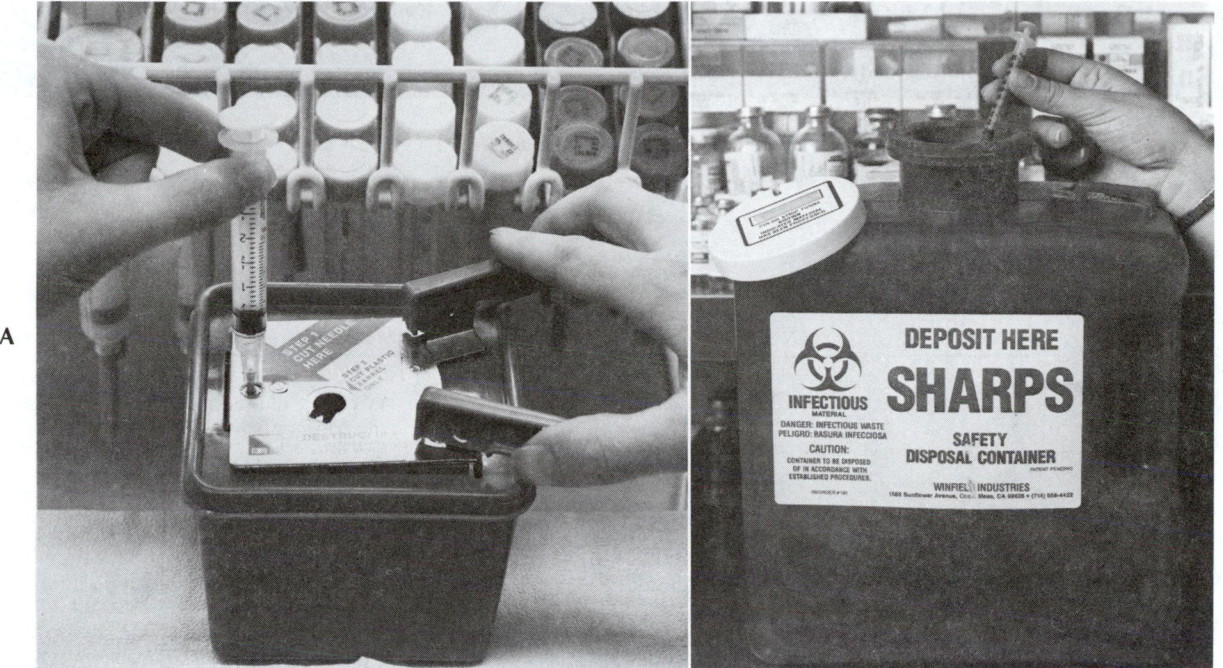

Fig. 32-27 **A,** A needle breaker cuts the needle cleanly off at the hub. The contaminated needle falls into the underlying container without risk of injury to the nurse. **B,** Special containers are available in nursing units for disposal of contaminated syringes.

Disposal of Equipment

After administering injections the nurse must dispose of used equipment properly. A stray needle can injure the client, the nurse, housekeepers, or other health care personnel. The victim of a needle stick with a contaminated needle may need an injection to prevent hepatitis.

The nurse breaks the needle at the hub and discards the needle and syringe into clearly marked appropriate containers. Used needles and syringes should never be placed in wastebaskets, in the nurse's pocket, or on the client's bed or table (Fig. 32-27).

Local Drug Applications

Skin Applications

Since many locally applied medications such as lotions, pastes, and ointments can create both systemic and local effects, the nurse should not apply these medications with a bare hand. The nurse should also avoid direct contact with any skin lesions for which the client is being treated because the chance of cross-contamination is great. If the client has an open wound, the nurse must use sterile technique in applying skin preparations. It is therefore recommended that the nurse use gloves to apply lotions, ointments, or pastes. The client who has disfiguring lesions may feel embarrassed if the nurse appears reluctant to touch an affected area. In this case sterile tongue depressors, cotton-tipped applicators, cotton balls, or gauze sponges can be used to apply skin preparations.

Skin encrustations and dead tissues harbor microorganisms and block the contact of medications with the tissues to be treated. Simply applying new medications over previously applied drugs does little to prevent infection or offer therapeutic benefit. The nurse cleans the skin thoroughly before applying medications by washing the area gently with soap and water, soaking an involved site, or locally debriding tissue.

When applying ointments or pastes, the nurse spreads the medication evenly over the involved surface and covers the area well without applying an overly thick layer. Opaque ointments prevent visualization of underlying skin. Often physicians order that a gauze dressing be applied over the medication to prevent soiling of the client's clothes and wiping away of the drug.

The nurse applies lotions and emollients by patting the medication lightly onto the skin's surface. Rubbing may cause irritation to underlying tissues. In contrast, a liniment is applied by rubbing the medication gently but firmly into the skin.

Administering Eye Drops and Ointment

EQUIPMENT:
1. Medication eyedropper or ointment tube
2. Cotton ball or tissue

EYE DROPS

STEPS	RATIONALE
1. Wash your hands.	Washing hands prevents transfer of microorganisms.
2. Explain the procedure to the client.	This reduces the client's anxiety.
3. Ask the client to lie in the supine position with head slightly hyperextended.	This position provides easy access to eye for medication instillation and minimizes drainage of medication through the tear duct.
4. Hold a cotton ball or clean tissue in the nondominant hand just below the lower eyelid.	Cotton or tissue will absorb any medication that escapes the eye.
5. With tissue resting against the lower lid margin gently retract the lower lid downward with the thumb or finger, pressing against the bony orbit. *Do not press* directly against the eyeball.	This procedure exposes the lower conjunctival sac. Retraction against the bony orbit prevents pressure and trauma to the eyeball.
6. Ask the client to look up toward the ceiling.	This action retracts the sensitive cornea up and away from the conjunctival sac and reduces stimulation of the blink reflex.
7. Hold the eyedropper in the dominant hand approximately 1 to 2 cm (½ to ¾ inch) above the conjunctival sac.	This helps the nurse avoid contact of eyedropper with eye structures, thus reducing risk of injury to eye and transfer of infection to dropper.
8. Drop the prescribed number of medication drops into the conjunctival sac.	The conjunctival sac normally holds 1 to 2 drops. Applying drops to the sac provides for even distribution of medication across the eye.
9. If the client blinks or closes the eye, or if the drops land on outer lid margins, repeat the procedure.	Therapeutic effect of the drug can be obtained only when the drops enter the conjunctival sac.
10. After instilling the drops, ask the client to close the eye gently.	This helps to distribute medication. Squinting or squeezing of the eyelids forces medication from the eyes.
11. When administering drugs that cause systemic effects, protect your finger with clean tissue and apply gentle pressure to the client's nasolacrimal duct for 10 to 15 seconds.	This prevents absorption of medication into the systemic circulation.
12. If there is excess medication on the eyelids, gently wipe it from the inner to the outer canthus. If the client had an eye patch, apply a clean one.	This promotes client comfort and prevents trauma to eye. A clean patch reduces chances of infection.

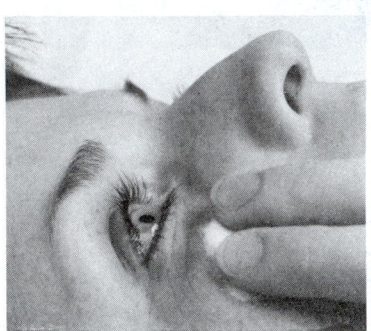

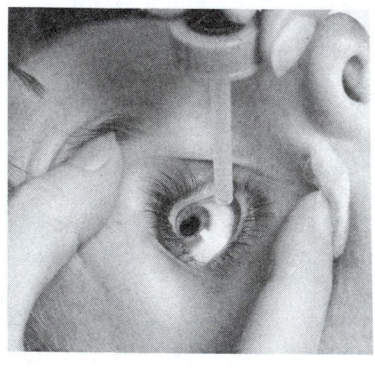

STEPS	RATIONALE

EYE OINTMENT

1. Perform steps 1 through 6 above for eye drops.

2. Apply a thin stream of ointment evenly along the inside edge of the lower eyelid, on the conjunctiva.

   This serves to distribute medication evenly across the eye and lid margin.

3. Have the client close the eye and rub the lid lightly in a circular motion with a cotton ball. NOTE: If the client has blepharitis (infection of eyelash follicles), apply the ointment to both upper and lower lid margins. Be sure the medication is applied around the follicles of both lids.

   This further distributes medication without traumatizing the eye.

Buccal and Sublingual Applications

Medications administered through application to the oral mucous membranes generally exert systemic effects. The buccal and sublingual routes are indicated for drugs that tend to be destroyed by gastric juices or are so rapidly detoxified by the liver that therapeutic blood levels are never attained.

The nurse instructs the client to place a sublingual tablet under his tongue. The client should avoid chewing or swallowing the tablet or taking any fluids. If taken properly, the medication simply dissolves under the tongue. Glyceryl trinitrate (nitroglycerin) is one of the most common sublingually administered drugs.

The client places buccal tablets in the space between the upper molar teeth and gums. Eating, chewing, drinking, or smoking can dislodge the medication and make it ineffective. Drugs given by the buccal and sublingual routes tend to dissolve and be absorbed quickly.

Eye Applications

The eye is the most sensitive organ to which the nurse applies medications. The cornea is richly supplied with sensitive pain fibers. The nurse avoids instilling any form of eye medication directly onto the cornea.

The risk of transmitting infection from one eye to the other is high. The nurse therefore avoids touching the eyelids or other eye structures with the eye dropper or ointment tube. Ophthalmic medications are sterilized and should be used only for the affected eye or eyes. The nurse never allows a person to use another's eye medication.

Crusts or drainage along the eyelid margins and inner canthus harbor microorganisms. The nurse must gently wash away any secretions or crusts before administering medications. Crusts that are dried and difficult to remove can be soaked with a clean, damp washcloth or gauze pad before removing. Procedure 32-8 outlines the steps for administering eye medications.

Ear Instillations

The internal ear structures are very sensitive to temperature extremes. Failure to instill ear drops or irrigating fluid at room temperature may cause vertigo (severe dizziness) or nausea. Although the structures of the outer ear are not sterile, it is wise to use sterile drops and solutions in case the eardrum is ruptured. Entrance of nonsterile solutions into middle ear structures could result in infection. An important rule when instilling ear medications is never to occlude the ear canal with the dropper or irrigating syringe. Forcing medication into an occluded ear canal creates pressure that may injure the eardrum.

The external ear structures of children are different from those of adults. When instilling drops for irrigating the canal (Procedure 32-9), it is necessary to

PROCEDURE 32-9

Instilling Ear Drops and Irrigating the External Ear Canal

INSTILLATION OF DROPS

EQUIPMENT:
1. Medication dropper
2. Cotton-tipped applicator
3. Tissue
4. Cotton ball (optional)

STEPS	RATIONALE
1. Wash your hands.	This reduces transfer of microorganisms.
2. Explain the procedure to the client.	This reduces the client's anxiety.
3. Have the client assume a side-lying position with the ear to be treated uppermost.	This position provides easy access to the ear for instillation of medication. The ear canal is in a position to retain medication.
4. If cerumen occludes the outermost portion of the ear canal, wipe it out gently with a cotton-tipped applicator. *Do not force the wax inward to block or occlude the canal.*	Cerumen may harbor microorganisms. Its presence blocks distribution of medication into the canal. Occlusion of the canal with cerumen interferes with normal sound conduction.
5. Straighten the client's ear canal by pulling the pinna down and back (children) or upward and backward (adults).	Straightening the ear canal provides for direct access to the deeper external ear structures.
6. Instill prescribed drops holding the dropper 1 cm (½ inch) above the ear canal.	Forcing drops into an occluded canal may cause injury to the eardrum.
7. Ask the client to remain in the side-lying position 2 to 3 minutes. Apply gentle pressure to the tragus of the ear with a finger.	This allows complete distribution of the medication. Pressure on the tragus moves the medication inward.
8. At times the physician orders insertion of a portion of a cotton ball into the outermost part of the canal. Do not press the cotton into the canal. Remove the cotton in 15 minutes.	Inserting cotton into the outer canal prevents escape of medication when the client sits or stands.

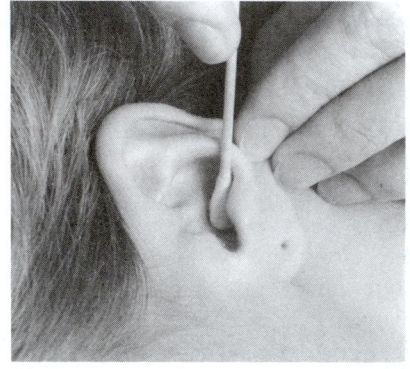

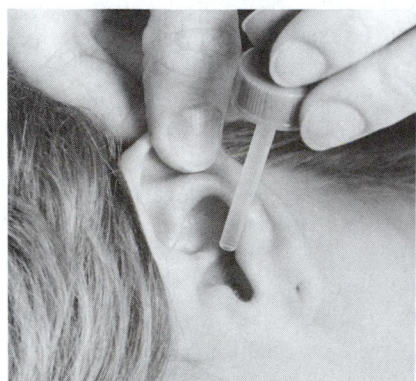
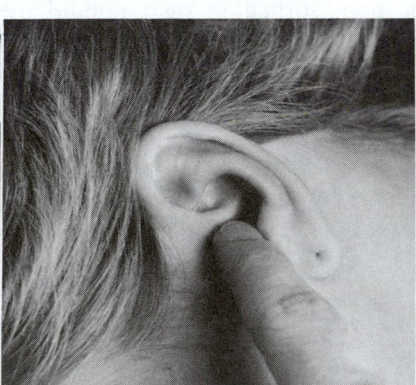
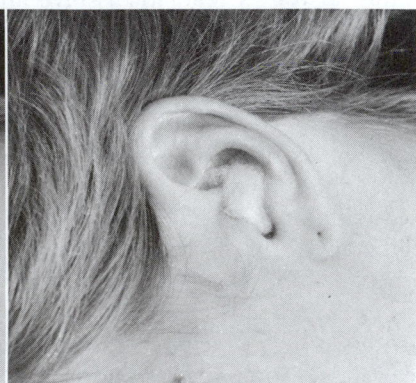

IRRIGATION OF CANAL

EQUIPMENT:
1. Irrigating solution at room temperature
2. Irrigating syringe
3. Kidney-shaped basin
4. Towel

STEPS	RATIONALE
1. Perform steps 1 to 4 above for instilling drops.	
2. Place a towel under the client's head and ask the client to hold the kidney-shaped irrigating basin just under the tragus of the affected ear.	This minimizes leakage of fluid around the neck and facial area for the client's comfort.
3. Have the client tilt his head slightly forward toward the basin.	This allows fluid to drain easily out of the ear into the basin.
4. Straighten the ear canal as in step 3 of drop instillation.	
5. Slowly instill the irrigating solution by holding the tip of the syringe 1 cm (½ inch) above the opening to the ear canal. Allow the fluid to drain out during instillation.	Slow instillation prevents buildup of pressure in the ear canal and ensures contact of the medication with all of the canal surfaces.
6. Dry off the client's ear and allow him to return to a sitting position.	This provides for client comfort.

straighten the ear canal. In infants and young children the nurse straightens the cartilaginous canal by grasping the pinna of the ear and pulling it gently down and backward. In adults the ear canal is longer and composed of underlying bone and is straightened by pulling the auricle upward and backward. Failure to straighten the canal properly may prevent medicinal solutions from reaching the deeper external ear structures.

Nasal Instillations

Clients with nasal sinus alterations may receive drug solutions by spray, drops, or tampons. Decongestants are the drugs most commonly administered as nose drops and sprays. Decongestants have an astringent effect on mucous membranes, helping to relieve symptoms of the common cold by shrinking the swollen membranes. Clients who abuse decongestants may experience a rebound effect: after the initial decongestant action of the dose recedes, the client suffers greater congestion and discomfort than in the original episode.

Nasal drops are effective in treating sinus infections. The nurse must know the proper way of positioning the client to permit the medication to reach the affected sinus. Drugs that create systemic effects may also be given nasally. Hormones of the posterior pituitary gland, such as vasopressin and oxytocin, are available as sprays or as powders to be inhaled.

When administering nasal drops (Procedure 32-10), the nurse makes sure the client is in a comfortable position. Since hyperextending the neck for a time can cause strain on neck muscles, the nurse supports the client's neck muscles when tipping the client's head over the edge of the bed. To instill drops in an infant, the nurse places a small pillow under the shoulders and lets the head tilt backward into her arms. Restraint of an infant's head and arms may be necessary.

Severe nose bleeds often require nasal packing. Nasal tampons are treated with medication containing vasoconstrictors, such as epinephrine, to reduce blood flow. Usually a physician is responsible for placement of nasal tampons.

PROCEDURE 32-10

Instilling Nasal Drops

EQUIPMENT:
1. Clean tissue
2. Prepared medication with dropper
3. Small pillow (optional)

STEPS	RATIONALE
1. Wash your hands.	Washing hands reduces transfer of microorganisms.
2. Explain the procedure to the client.	This reduces the client's anxiety.
3. Instruct the client to blow his nose (unless contraindicated, e.g., risk of intracranial pressure or nose bleeds).	Blowing the nose removes mucus and secretions, which block distribution of medication.
4. Ask the client to assume a supine position. To reach the posterior pharynx and opening of the eustachian tube, tilt the client's head backward. To reach the ethmoid or sphenoid sinuses, tilt the head back over the edge of the bed or place a small pillow under the client's shoulder and tilt his head back. To reach the frontal and maxillary sinuses, tip the head back over the edge of the bed or pillow with the head turned toward the side to be treated.	Proper positioning allows medication to drain into the affected sinus region.
5. Instruct the client to breathe through his mouth.	Mouth breathing reduces the chance of aspirating nasal drops into the trachea and lungs.
6. Hold the dropper 1 cm (½ inch) above the nares and instill the prescribed number of drops toward the midline of the ethmoid bone.	The dropper become contaminated when in contact with mucous membranes. Instilling toward the ethmoid bone facilitates distribution of medication over the nasal mucosa.
7. Have the client remain in a supine position for 5 minutes.	Remaining in the supine position prevents premature loss of medication through the nares.
8. Discard any remaining solution before returning the dropper to the bottle.	This prevents contamination of remaining medication.

It is generally easier to have the client self-administer sprays. In the supine position with head tilted back, the client holds the tip of the spray container just inside the nares. The nurse instructs the client to inhale as the spray enters the nasal passages. For clients who use nasal sprays repeatedly, the nurse checks the nares for signs of irritation.

Vaginal Instillations

Vaginal medications are available as suppositories or creams. Suppositories come individually packaged in foil wrappers. Storage in a refrigerator prevents the solid oval-shaped suppositories from melting. After a suppository is inserted into the vaginal cavity, the client's body temperature causes the suppository to melt and be distributed.

Both suppositories and cream can be administered with an inserter or applicator (Fig. 32-28). A suppository may also be given with a gloved hand. Since the vaginal canal is not sterile, the nurse follows clean technique, using disposable gloves, for suppository or cream insertion.

Often clients prefer administering their own vaginal medications to avoid embarrassment. The client should be given privacy during insertion. After instillation of the drug she may wish to wear a perineal pad to collect excess drainage. Since vaginal medications are frequently given to treat infection, any discharge may be foul smelling. The client should be offered frequent opportunities to maintain perineal hygiene (see Chapter 35).

Procedure 32-11 outlines the methods for vaginal medication administration.

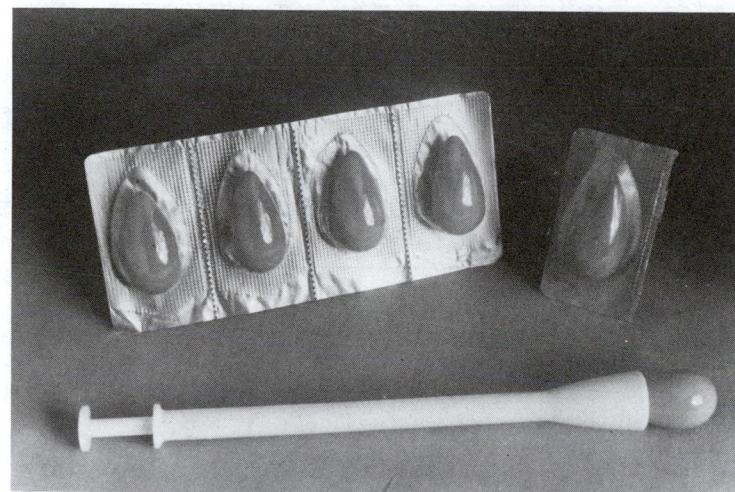

Fig. 32-28 Vaginal suppositories.

PROCEDURE 32-11

Instilling Vaginal Medications

INSERTION OF SUPPOSITORY

EQUIPMENT:
1. Vaginal suppository
2. Clean disposable gloves
3. Lubricating jelly
4. Clean tissues
5. Suppository inserter (optional)
6. Perineal pad (optional)

STEPS	RATIONALE
1. Wash your hands.	Washing hands reduces risk of transferring microorganisms.
2. Explain the procedure to the client.	This reduces the client's anxiety.
3. Have the client lie in the dorsal recumbent position.	This position provides easy access to and good exposure of the vaginal canal. The dependent position of the client allows the suppository to dissolve in the vagina without escaping through the orifice.
4. Keep the abdomen and lower extremities draped.	This minimizes the client's embarrassment.
5. Apply disposable gloves.	Use of gloves prevents transmission of infection between nurse and client.
6. Remove the suppository from the foil wrapper and apply a liberal amount of petrolatum jelly to the smooth or rounded end. Lubricate the gloved index finger of the dominant hand.	This reduces friction against mucosal surfaces during insertion.
7. With the nondominant gloved hand gently retract the labial folds.	This exposes the vaginal orifice.
8. Insert the rounded end of the suppository along the posterior wall of the vaginal canal the length of the index finger (7.5 to 10 cm [3 to 4 inches]).	Proper placement of the suppository ensures equal distribution of medication along the walls of the vaginal cavity.
9. Withdraw the finger and wipe away any remaining lubricant from around the orifice and labia.	This maintains the client's comfort.

Continued.

Instilling Vaginal Medications

INSERTION OF SUPPOSITORY

STEPS	RATIONALE
10. Remove the gloves by pulling them inside out and discard them in an appropriate receptacle.	Removing gloves in this manner prevents spread of microorganisms.
11. Instruct the client to remain on her back for at least 10 minutes.	This position allows medication to melt and be absorbed into the vaginal mucosa.
12. Offer a perineal pad before the client resumes ambulation.	This provides for client comfort.

NOTE: Follow same procedure when using suppository inserter.

INSTILLATION OF CREAM

EQUIPMENT:
1. Vaginal cream
2. Plastic applicator
3. Clean disposable gloves
4. Paper towel

STEPS	RATIONALE
1. Perform steps 1 through 5 of the procedure for suppository insertion.	
2. Fill the cream applicator following package directions.	Dosage is prescribed by volume in applicator.
3. With your nondominant gloved hand gently retract the labial folds.	This exposes the vaginal orifice.
4. With your dominant gloved hand insert the applicator approximately 7.5 cm (3 inches). Push the applicator plunger to deposit the medication.	This allows for equal distribution of medication along the walls of the vaginal cavity.
5. Withdraw the plunger and place it on a paper towel. Wipe off any residual cream from labia or vaginal orifice.	Residual cream on applicator may contain microorganisms.
6. Remove the gloves and turn them inside out. Dispose of them in the appropriate receptacle.	Disposing of gloves in this way reduces transfer of microorganisms.
7. Ask the client to remain flat on her back for at least 10 minutes.	The cream will be distributed and absorbed evenly in the vaginal cavity, rather than being lost through the vaginal orifice.
8. Wash the applicator with soap and warm water and store it for future use.	The vaginal cavity is not sterile. Soap and water will assist in removing bacteria and residual cream.
9. Offer the client a perineal pad when she resumes ambulation.	This provides client comfort.

Rectal Instillations

Rectal suppositories differ in shape from vaginal suppositories, being thinner and bullet shaped (Fig. 32-29). The rounded end prevents anal trauma during the insertion. Rectal suppositories contain medications that exert local effects, such as promoting defecation, or systemic effects, such as reducing nausea. Rectal suppositories are stored in the refrigerator until the time of administration.

During administration it is important to place the suppository past the internal anal sphincter and against the rectal mucosa. Otherwise the suppository may be expelled before it can dissolve and be absorbed into the mucosa. With practice a nurse learns to recognize the sensation of the sphincter relaxing around the finger. The suppository should not be forced into a mass of fecal material. It may be necessary to clear the rectum with a small cleansing

---

PROCEDURE 32-12

Inserting a Rectal Suppository

EQUIPMENT:
1. Rectal suppository
2. Lubricating jelly
3. Clean disposable gloves
4. Tissue

STEPS	RATIONALE
1. Wash your hands.	Washing hands reduces transfer of microorganisms.
2. Explain the procedure to the client.	This reduces the client's anxiety.
3. Ask the client to assume a side-lying (Sims') position with upper leg flexed upward.	This position exposes the anus and helps the client relax the external anal sphincter.
4. Keep the client draped with only the anal area exposed.	Draping the client maintains his privacy and facilitates relaxation.
5. Remove the suppository from its foil wrapper and lubricate the rounded end with jelly. Lubricate the gloved index finger of the dominant hand.	Lubrication reduces friction as the suppository enters the rectal canal.
6. Ask the client to take slow, deep breaths through his mouth and to relax the anal sphincter.	Forcing a suppository through a constricted sphincter causes pain.
7. Retract the client's buttocks with your nondominant hand. With your gloved index finger, insert the suppository gently through the anus, past the internal sphincter, and against the rectal wall: 10 cm (4 inches) in adults, 5 cm (2 inches) in children and infants.	The suppository must be placed against the rectal mucosa for eventual absorption and therapeutic action. 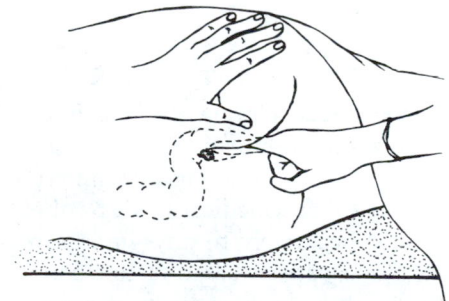
8. Withdraw your finger and wipe off the client's anal area.	This provides client comfort.
9. Discard the gloves by turning them inside out and dispose of them in appropriate receptacle.	Disposing of the gloves in this way reduces transfer of microorganisms.
10. Ask the client to remain flat or on his side for 5 minutes.	This prevents expulsion of the suppository.
11. If the suppository contains a laxative or fecal softener, place the call light in the client's reach so he can obtain assistance to reach a bedpan or toilet.	Being able to call for assistance provides the client with a sense of control over elimination.

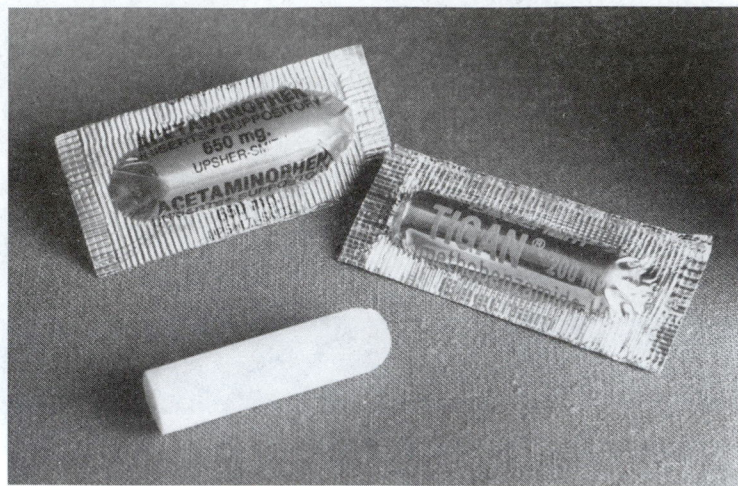

Fig. 32-29   Rectal suppositories.

enema before a suppository can be inserted. Procedure 32-12 outlines steps for a suppository insertion.

Administering Drugs by Inhalation

In most instances only the physician or respiratory therapist administers drugs by inhalation. The nurse, however, plays a key role in administering respiratory gases such as oxygen. Chapter 41 describes in detail the methods for administering inhalants and respiratory gases.

Individualizing Drug Administration

Some clients require special consideration during medication administration. Administering drugs to children and the elderly challenges the nurse's knowledge and skill.

Infants and Children

A child's age and developmental level influence the way he will react to administration of drugs. For example, an infant or toddler usually interprets the nurse's attempt to give medications as a threat. The infant responds negatively to any unpleasant sensation such as that caused by a bad-tasting cough syrup. The toddler, with his new sense of autonomy, may show his independence by refusing to take medicines. An older child is able to understand why he needs medicine. However, if the nurse fails to respect the child's feelings and attitudes, the child may not cooperate with drug therapy.

Taking medications is often accompanied by a sense of fear. When a child receives an injection, he is aware of little except the size of the needle and the knowledge that he is about to feel pain. The antici-

pation usually creates more distress than the needle stick itself.

The nurse must minimize the child's fear of taking medications. A nurse should never use a medication or injection as a way of threatening a child. If receiving a medication is emotionally stressful, the child may learn to mistrust or dislike the nurse. The child should not look on taking a medication as an unpleasant experience but rather as a routine part of the day. The nurse gives a child simple explanations as to why the medicine is needed. The nurse's actions should be gentle and relaxed. In the case of an injection the nurse avoids letting the child see the syringe and needle until just before administration. An injection should be given as rapidly as possible. The nurse does not mislead the child into thinking an injection will not hurt. After giving the injection the nurse comforts and praises the child.

The nurse does not force a child to take medicine. A toddler will likely spit out an orally administered medication. The school-aged child will give a reason for refusing the medicine. Words of praise give toddlers a sense of autonomy in deciding to take medicine. Role playing by giving injections to dolls often helps toddlers and preschoolers express their fears and become less reluctant to receive an injection. School-aged children and adolescents need to discuss their feelings about taking medications. Offering choices increases a child's willingness to cooperate. For example, the nurse may offer the medication as a pill, as a presweetened liquid, or mixed with a pleasant-tasting food.

The parents are important resources when administering medications to children. Parents know their children best and are often more effective in explaining why medicines are needed. A parent can console and support the child. Restraining a child may be necessary during an injection to avoid injuring the child, and a parent may be the best person to do this. However, the nurse should not make the parent the target for the child's anger or resentment. If a parent is reluctant to restrain a child, the nurse must assume the task.

The Elderly

Many elderly clients have some form of disablng or chronic disease. For this reason the elderly population spends more on prescription and over-the-counter drugs than any other age group. The majority of elderly clients self-administer medications at home. An elderly client may take as many as six different medications daily. The section on factors influencing drug actions describes the physiological changes of aging that influence drug absorption, metabolism, and elimination. Equally important are the sensory and cognitive changes an elderly client experiences that make accurate drug administration a difficult task. The nurse's role is largely an educational one in assisting elderly clients with drug therapy. The nurse must consider the client's level of physical, sensory, and cognitive function when teaching a client to purchase and use medications correctly.

The elderly client frequently undergoes changes in vision, hearing, touch, and coordination. An older person has difficulty seeing close objects clearly and often experiences a glare in bright light. Hearing changes make it difficult for the elderly to hear high-pitched sounds. Often several words sound alike to an elderly person. The sensitivity of touch declines, impairing the ability to feel objects in the hands. Conditions such as arthritis and parkinsonism impair coordination and movement so that the elderly person is unable to prepare medications or manipulate a syringe.

The nurse considers the client's sensory limitations when planning teaching sessions and methods for self-administration of drugs. The client with reduced vision should always wear glasses during discussions and when preparing medications. The nurse uses teaching materials with large, boldface type and asks the pharmacist to type drug labels in large print. If the client cannot identify a pill, packaging devices can minimize the need for identification. For example, pill cartridges, similar to those used with oral contraceptives, are now available for other drugs. When giving instructions, the nurse speaks slowly in a low-pitched voice and faces the client. The nurse offers clients opportunities to ask questions or review information to ensure their understanding. If a client is unable to handle drug packages or equipment properly, the nurse asks the client's spouse, child, or close friend to help.

Elderly clients try to retain their independence for as long as possible. Often they deny the fact that they will require medications for the rest of their lives. They may refuse to accept any limitations or to recognize the value of drug therapy. Often elderly clients stop taking drugs prescribed for them as soon as they feel better. A client may self-prescribe over-the-counter drugs or take drugs prescribed for a spouse. An elderly client may believe that two pills are better than one in treating a problem. Elderly clients commonly fail to see the importance of maintaining a regular dosage schedule.

The most common types of drug errors committed by the elderly are (1) omission of dosages, (2) administration of drugs not prescribed or use of incorrect drugs, and (3) use of medications at the improper time or out of sequence.

The nurse provides clients with information pertaining to the importance of safe drug therapy. The client must know the purpose and benefits of each drug prescribed. The nurse reviews the implications of taking drugs incorrectly. Omission of doses usually occurs simply because a client forgets to take the medication. The nurse may devise an egg carton system, in which the carton sections represent times of administration. The nurse teaches the client the type and number of drugs to place in each section. The client then must only keep track of dosage schedules. Some elderly clients have a distorted view of time. Setting an alarm clock to go off at specific times is a helpful reminder for drug administration. The nurse may recommend that the client take drugs at the time of daily events such as bathing or meals. A major problem with this method is that many medications are poorly absorbed when taken with food.

An elderly client should take as few drugs as possible. The nurse must stress the danger of taking multiple over-the-counter drugs, which can interfere with the therapeutic effects of prescribed medications. To monitor drug therapy, clients and family members must be aware of the symptoms of side effects.

Summary

The nurse's responsibilities in administering medications are complex. The nurse must follow legal guidelines that dictate the procedures for prescribing and administering drugs. The nurse must frequently make judgments as to a client's need for drug therapy. It is also the nurse's responsibility to prepare and administer medications safely and effectively.

The nurse must acquire detailed knowledge about a drug as well as the client receiving it. Identifying pertinent nursing diagnoses helps the nurse choose the best methods for drug administration. The preparation of a drug requires a methodical approach. Application of physiological, anatomical, and aseptic principles ensures that the nurse will administer a drug safely. In monitoring a client's response to medications, the nurse applies physical assessment skills and employs knowledge of expected drug effects. The nurse also teaches clients and their families to administer drugs safely.

If a nurse is unwilling to assume the responsibilities related to drug therapy, the results of administering medications can be disastrous. A client's well-being depends on the nurse's intelligent and skillful application of all principles of drug administration.

KEY CONCEPTS

✓ Learning drug classifications improves understanding of nursing implications for administering drugs with similar characteristics.

✓ Nurse practice acts define and set limits on the scope of a nurse's professional functions and responsibilities in giving medications.

✓ Federal drug legislation regulates the production, distribution, prescription, and administration of drugs.

✓ All controlled substances are handled according to strict procedures that account for each drug.

✓ The nurse applies understanding of the physiology of drug action when timing administration, selecting routes, initiating actions to promote drug efficacy, and observing clients' responses to drugs.

✓ Clients with alterations in organs that excrete drugs are at risk for drug toxicity.

✓ The elderly client's body undergoes structural and functional changes that alter drug actions and influence the manner in which nurses provide drug therapy.

✓ An obese client generally requires a larger dose of a drug than an average-sized client.

✓ Children's drug dosages are computed on the basis of body surface area or weight.

✓ Repeated doses of a drug are required to achieve constant therapeutic blood levels.

✓ Drugs given parenterally are absorbed more quickly than drugs administered by other routes.

✓ The metric system is the standard system for drug measurement in most countries of the world.

✓ The least accurate system of drug measurement is the use of household measurements.

✓ Each drug order should include the client's name, the order date, the drug name, dosage, and route and time of administration, and the physician's signature.

✓ A medication history reveals the drugs a client is currently taking as well as the client's compliance with therapy.

✓ A nurse's teaching plan for drug therapy should include guidelines for drug safety.

✓ The "five rights" of drug administration ensure accurate preparation and administration of drug dosages.

✓ Nurses administer only medications they prepare.

✓ Drugs should be charted immediately after administration.

KEY CONCEPTS, *cont'd*

✓ The nurse never administers a drug without accurately identifying a client.

✓ Medications should be given within 30 minutes of the time prescribed.

✓ A nurse uses clinical judgment in determining the best time to administer p.r.n.-ordered medications.

✓ The nurse reports a drug error immediately.

✓ When preparing medications, the nurse checks the drug container label against the medication card or form three times.

✓ The nurse never leaves a prepared medication unattended.

✓ When the nurse prepares and administers an injection, the needle bevel and shaft and the syringe's inner barrel, tips, and plunger must remain sterile.

✓ The nurse rotates injection sites when giving repeated parenteral administrations.

✓ Failure to select injection sites by anatomical landmarks may lead to tissue, bone, or nerve damage.

✓ Air locks prevent tracking of medication through subcutaneous tissues and localize the drug in muscle tissue.

✓ The Z-track method for intramuscular injections protects subcutaneous tissues from irritating parenteral fluids.

✓ When administering medications to children, the nurse should attempt to eliminate their fear or negative feelings associated with taking medications.

✓ The nurse should never force a child to take a medication.

✓ Sensory changes in the elderly client may lead to errors in self-administration of drugs.

READINGS

Allen, M.D.: Drug therapy in the elderly, Am. J. Nurs. 80:1474, 1980.

Bauer, L.A.: Clinical pharmacokinetics, Nurse Pract. 7:42, 1982.

Brandt, P.A., et al.: IM injections in children, Am. J. Nurs. 72:1402, 1972.

Brock, A.: Self-administration of drugs in the elderly: nursing responsibilities, J. Gerontol. Nurs. 6:402, 1980.

Clark, J.B., et al.: Pharmacological basis of nursing practice, St. Louis, 1982, The C.V. Mosby Co.

Davis, N.M., and Cohen, M.R.: Learning from mistakes: 20 tips for avoiding medication errors, Nursing 82 12:65, 1982.

Hayes, J.E.: Normal changes in aging and nursing implications of drug therapy, Nurs. Clin. North Am. 17:253, 1982.

LeSage, J.: Drug therapy in long term care facilities, Nurs. Clin. North Am. 17:331, 1982.

McConnell, E.A.: The subtle art of really good injections, RN 45:24, 1982.

Rettig, F.M., and Southby, J.R.: Using different body positions to reduce discomfort from dorsogluteal injection, Nurs. Res. 31:219, 1982.

Rodman, M.J., and Smith, D.W.: Clinical pharmacology in nursing, ed. 2, Philadelphia, 1979, J.B. Lippincott Co.

Sandroff, R.: Booby-trapped orders, RN 44:26, 1981.

Spencer, R.T., et al.: Clinical pharmacology and nursing management, Philadelphia, 1983, J.B. Lippincott Co.

Tanner, S.: IV bolus leaves no room for error, RN 44:54, 1981.

Thompson, D.A.: Teaching the client about anticoagulants, Am. J. Nurs. 82:278, 1982.

Wong, D.L.: Significance of dead space in syringes, Am. J. Nurs. 82:1237, 1982.

OBJECTIVES

Mastery of content in this chapter will enable the student to:

- Define the terms in the glossary.
- Identify the body's normal defenses against infection.
- Describe the nature of signs of a localized infection.
- Describe the characteristics of each link of the infection chain.
- Identify clients most at risk for acquiring an infection.
- Explain conditions that precipitate the onset of nosocomial infections.
- Describe nursing interventions designed to break each link in the infection chain.
- Correctly perform protective isolation techniques.
- Perform the proper procedure for handwashing.
- Describe the zone of sterility for a sterile gown and sterile field.
- Properly apply a sterile gown, sterile gloves, and a surgical mask.

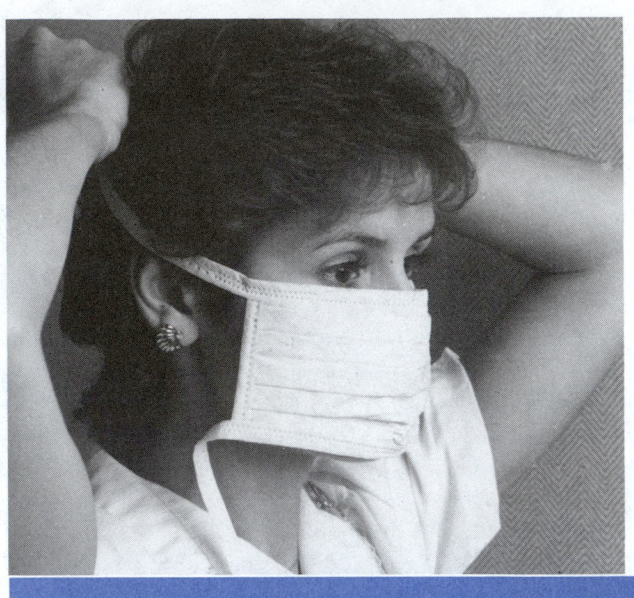

GLOSSARY

antibody Immunoglobulin, essential to the immune system, which is produced by lymphoid tissue in response to bacteria, viruses, or other antigens.

antigen Substance, usually a protein, that causes the formation of an antibody and reacts specifically with that antibody.

antiseptic Tending to inhibit the growth and reproduction of microorganisms.

asepsis Absence of germs or microorganisms.

cannulation Insertion of a flexible tube (cannula) into a body duct or cavity, such as the bladder or a blood vessel.

carrier Animal or person who harbors and spreads a disease-causing organism but who does not become ill.

Centers for Disease Control (CDC) Agency of the U.S. government that provides facilities and services for the investigation, identification, prevention, and control of disease.

colonized Referring to the establishment of a mass of microorganisms, often nonpathogenic, in or on the body.

communicable disease Any disease transmitted from one person or animal to another by direct or indirect contact, or by vectors.

contagious Communicable, as a disease.

cytotoxic Pharmacological compound that inhibits the proliferation of cells within the body.

endogenous Produced within a cell or organism.

epidemiology Study of the occurrence, distribution, and causes of disease.

exogenous Originating outside an organ or part.

expectorate Eject mucus, sputum, or fluids from the trachea and lungs by coughing or spitting.

exudate Fluid, cells, or other substances that have been slowly discharged from cells or blood vessels through small pores or breaks in cell membranes.

fomites Inanimate substances or objects, such as clothing and paper, that absorb and transmit infectious material.

iatrogenic disease Disease caused by a treatment or diagnostic procedure.

immunoglobulin Humoral antibody produced by the body and present in serum and external secretions; it is formed in response to specific antigens.

inflammation Protective response of body tissues to irritation or injury.

invasive Referring to procedures that involve puncture, incision, or insertion of a foreign object, such as a needle or catheter, into the body.

33 Infection Control and Medical Asepsis

leukocytosis Abnormal increase in the number of circulating white blood cells.

lymphocyte One type of leukocyte developing in the bone marrow; responsible for synthesizing antibodies and T cells that attack antigens.

maceration Softening something solid, such as the skin, by soaking.

macrophage Large phagocytic cell of the reticuloendothelial system.

microorganism Any microscopic entity capable of carrying on living processes, such as bacteria, viruses, and fungi.

nosocomial infection Infection acquired during hospitalization or stay in a health care facility.

parasite Organism living in or on another organism and obtaining nourishment from it.

pathogen Any microorganism capable of producing disease.

phagocytosis Process by which certain cells, such as macrophages, engulf and dispose of microorganisms.

purulent Producing or containing pus.

sterile Aseptic.

sterile field Specified area, such as within a tray or on a sterile towel, that is considered free of microorganisms.

virulent Of or pertaining to a very pathogenic or rapidly progressive condition.

A client who enters a health care setting places himself at risk for acquiring an infection. A number of diseases either increase susceptibility to infection or lower immunity to infectious microorganisms. The client may undergo procedures that involve the introduction of foreign objects (for example, needles or catheters) into the body, providing the means for infection to begin. The nurse comes in contact with all types of organisms capable of causing infection. Unless the nurse practices techniques to control or eliminate infection, the client becomes a target for acquiring microorganisms that can cause inflammation and infectious disease.

In the home a client must recognize sources of infection and be able to institute protective measures, such as properly preparing and cooking foods, maintaining personal hygiene, and ensuring a clean environment. The nurse is responsible for teaching clients about the nature of infection, the methods of transmission, the reasons for susceptibility, and methods of control.

The nurse's knowledge of the infectious process, application of infection control principles, and use of common sense help to protect clients from infection. The control of infection is an integral part of every action the nurse performs.

Body's Defenses against Infection

An infection begins with the invasion of the body by pathogens or microorganisms capable of producing disease. Pathogens multiply, causing disease by local cellular injury, release of toxins, or induction of antigen-antibody reactions. The body has normal defenses against infection, but if these fail, the infection can progress to cause serious complications and even death.

Normal Flora

The body normally contains microbial flora that reside on the skin, in the mouth, and in the gastrointestinal tract. A person normally excretes trillions of microbes daily through the intestines. The skin also has a large population of resident flora in concentrations greater than 10,000 microbes per square centimeter of skin. Flora reside on the skin's surface as well as deep within the epithelial skin structures. Another rich source of flora is the saliva and oral mucosa. Normal flora do not cause disease but instead participate in maintaining a person's health.

The flora of the large intestine exist in large numbers without causing injury. These bacterial flora compete with disease-producing microorganisms for food. Flora also secrete antibacterial substances within the intestine's walls. The skin's flora exert a decontaminative action by inhibiting the multiplication of organisms landing on the skin. The mouth and pharynx are also protected by flora that impair the growth of invading microbes. The mass of normal flora maintains a sensitive balance with other microorganisms to prevent the onslaught of infection. Any factor that disrupts this balance places a person at serious risk for acquiring an infectious disease.

Body System Defenses

A number of the body's organ systems have unique defenses against infection (Table 33-1). The skin, respiratory tract, and gastrointestinal tract are easily accessible to microorganisms. Pathogenic organisms can easily adhere to the skin's surface, be inhaled into the lungs, or be ingested with food. Each organ system has defense mechanisms physiologically suited to its structure and function. For example, the lungs cannot completely control the entrance of microorganisms. However, the airways are lined with hairlike projections or cilia, which rhythmically beat to move a blanket of mucus and any adherent organisms up to the pharynx to be swallowed. Any conditions that impair an organ's specialized defenses increase a person's susceptibility to infection.

Inflammation

The body's cellular response to any type of injury such as trauma or infection is inflammation (see Chapter 5). Inflammation is a protective vascular reaction that delivers fluid, blood products, and nutrients to the interstitial tissues in an area of injury. The process neutralizes and eliminates the pathogens or necrotic tissues and establishes a means of repairing body cells and tissues.

Once an infection develops, a series of well-coordinated events comes into play. Acute inflammation is an immediate response to cellular injury. Arterioles supplying the infected area dilate, allowing more blood into the local circulation. The increase in local blood flow causes the characteristic redness of inflammation. The symptom of localized warmth or heat results from a greater volume of blood at the inflammatory site. If the inflamed area is deep within the body, local warmth does not occur, since the maximum body temperature is at the body's core. As the inflammatory process develops, fluid and cells from the bloodstream necessary for healing accumulate to form exudate at the site. When the inflammation is near the skin's surface, the accumulated fluid appears as localized swelling.

Another classic sign of inflammation is pain in the affected part. The swelling of inflamed tissues increases pressure on nerve endings, causing pain. Chemical substances that stimulate nerve endings, such as histamine, are also released. As a result of the physiological changes occurring with inflammation, the involved body part undergoes a loss of function, which may be only temporary. For example, a localized infection of the hand causes the fingers to become swollen, painful, and discolored. The joints may become stiff as a result of swelling, but function of the fingers returns when the inflammation subsides.

In summary, the signs of inflammation are also the signs of a localized infection: redness, localized warmth, swelling, pain or tenderness, and loss of function in the affected body part. When inflammation becomes systemic, other signs and symptoms develop: fever, leukocytosis (increased number of white blood cells), malaise, anorexia, nausea, vomiting, and lymph node enlargement. The specific cause for each symptom is unknown but can be attributed to a generalized impairment in body function.

Fever results from the release of pyrogens at the site of infection or injury. The pyrogens cause the body's thermostat setting to increase, thus causing greater heat production and heat conservation with a rise in body temperature (see Chapter 28). The body's response to systemic inflammation is an increase in the number of white blood cells delivered to the inflamed site. The white blood cells attack the

T A B L E 3 3 - 1

Normal Body System Defense Mechanisms against Infection

System/Organ	Defense Mechanisms	Action	Factors That May Alter Defense
Skin	Intact multilayered surface	Provides mechanical barrier to microorganisms	Cuts, abrasions, puncture wounds, areas of maceration
	Shedding of outer layer of skin cells	Removes organisms that adhere to skin's outer layers	Failure to bathe regularly
Mouth	Intact multilayered mucosa	Provides mechanical barrier to microorganisms	Lacerations, trauma, extracted teeth
	Saliva	Washes away particles containing microorganisms	Poor oral hygiene, dehydration
Respiratory tract	Cilia lining upper airways, coated by a sticky mucus blanket	Trap inhaled microbes and sweep them outward in mucus to be expectorated or swallowed	Smoking, high concentrations of oxygen and carbon dioxide, decreased humidity, cold air
	Macrophages	Engulf and destroy any microorganisms that reach the lung's alveoli	Smoking
Urinary tract	Flushing action of urine flow	Washes away microorganisms on lining of bladder and urethra	Obstruction to normal flow by urinary catheter placement, obstruction from growth or tumor, or delayed micturition
	Intact multilayered epithelium	Provides barrier to microorganisms	Introduction of urinary catheter, continual movement of catheter in urethra
Gastrointestinal tract	Acidity of gastric secretions	Chemically destroys microorganisms incapable of surviving in low pH	Administration of antacids
	Rapid peristalsis in small intestine	Prevents retention of bacterial contents	Delayed motility owing to impaction of fecal contents in large bowel or mechanical obstruction by masses

site of inflammation by releasing enzymes and antimicrobial substances that destroy and remove the foreign material causing inflammation. The increased release of white blood cells from the bone marrow produces a systemic leukocytosis. The flow of lymph accelerates during inflammation. There is a danger that infectious organisms can spread along the course of the lymphatics. Normally, infectious agents travel to the lymph nodes to be phagocytosed or digested by special cells called macrophages. The process commonly results in localized enlargement of lymph nodes.

Immune Response

When a foreign material enters the body's tissues, a response similar to inflammation occurs. Certain foreign materials cause a change in the body's biological makeup so that reactions to subsequent exposures are different from the initial reaction. These altered responses are known as immune responses, and the foreign material is called an antigen. In a normal immune response, the antigen is neutralized, destroyed, or eliminated from the person's body.

Antigens are foreign materials usually composed of

proteins that are not normally found within a person's body. Often antigens exist in complex form as a part of the structure of a bacterium or virus. Once an antigen enters the body, it travels in the blood or lymph and initiates two responses. The cell-mediated response involves the proliferation of lymphocytes, which react specifically with antigens, in the lymph nodes, spleen, thymus gland, and bone marrow. Stimulation of lymphocytes triggers the humoral immune response, which results in the synthesis of immunoglobulins or antibodies that act to destroy antigens.

When the antigen reaches the lymphoid tissue, it reacts with macrophages, which may present the antigen in the proper form to the lymphocytes or change the antigen to make it more susceptible to attack. Antigens react with lymphocytes to cause an increase in the number of lymphocytes and the conversion of certain lymphocytes into antibodies. The immunoglobulin antibodies then circulate widely in the body to provide greater general immunity. Memory lymphocytes prepare the body against future antigenic invasion. Thus, when an antigen of a type to which the body has been exposed enters the body, antibodies form more rapidly than during the first exposure and immunoglobulin levels remain high to attack the antigen.

The formation of immunoglobulins or antibodies is the basis of immunization against disease. The antibodies most commonly found in the blood are in the immunoglobulin G (IgG) class. They are important in providing resistance to infection and can cross the placenta from mother to child, giving the infant passive immunity.

Chain of Infection

The mere presence of a pathogen does not mean that an infection will begin. The development of an infection occurs in a cyclical process that depends on six elements: (1) infectious agent or pathogen, (2) reservoir for pathogen growth, (3) portal of exit from the reservoir, (4) means of transmission, or vehicle, (5) portal of entry to host, and (6) susceptible host (Fig. 33-1). An infection will develop if this chain is uninterrupted. The nurse's efforts to control infection are directed toward breaking the infection chain.

Infectious Agent

Pathogenic organisms include bacteria, viruses, fungi, and yeasts (Table 33-2). The specific characteristics of each organism are beyond the scope of this

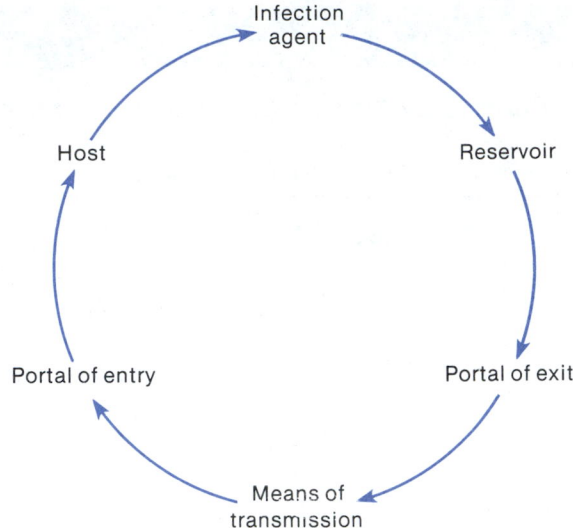

Fig. 33-1 Chain of infection.

text. All organisms require food and the proper environment for growth. A dark, warm, moist habitat, as in the oral cavity, underneath a wound dressing, or within a drainage tube, is ideal.

Pathogens on the hands may be categorized as resident or transient. Resident pathogens are always present in the creases and crevices of the skin. *Staphylococcus aureus* is a resident pathogen found in a large proportion of the population. The resident pathogens are stable in number and attach to skin surfaces by adhesion and absorption. They are not easily removed by washing with soap and water unless considerable friction is used, and they are less susceptible to antiseptics than are transient bacteria.

Transient pathogens are usually picked up by the hands in normal activities of living. For example, when a nurse touches a bedpan or a contaminated dressing, transient bacteria adhere to the skin. The organisms attach loosely to the skin in dirt and grease or under fingernails. Frequent, thorough handwashing removes transient pathogens easily.

The potential for microorganisms to elude the body's defenses and cause disease depends on the number of organisms and their virulence or pathogenicity. Some organisms enclosed in slimy capsules avoid phagocytosis. Other organisms escape destruction by secreting toxins that kill white blood cells. Still other organisms (for example, the tubercle bacillus) have gained resistance to the environment within phagocytes and exist as intracellular parasites.

The nurse's knowledge of microbiology provides the background for understanding how microorganisms survive and proliferate.

TABLE 33-2

Common Pathogens and Some Infections or Diseases They Produce

Organism	Reservoir	Infection or Disease
BACTERIA		
Staphylococcus aureus	Skin, hair, anterior nares	Wound infection, pneumonia, food poisoning, cellulitis
Streptococcus (beta-hemolytic group A)	Oropharynx, skin, peri-anal area	"Strep throat," rheumatic fever, scarlet fever, impetigo
Streptococcus (beta-hemolytic group B)	Adult genitalia	Urinary tract infection, wound infection, endometritis
Escherichia coli	Colon	Enteritis
Neisseria gonorrhoeae	Genitourinary tract, rectum, mouth, eye	Gonorrhea, pelvic inflammatory disease, infectious arthritis, conjunctivitis
Clostridium tetani	Soil, colon	Tetanus
Mycobacterium tuberculosis	Respiratory tract, lymph nodes	Tuberculosis
VIRUSES		
Herpes simplex 1	Lesions of mouth, skin, blood, excretions	Cold sores, aseptic meningitis, sexually transmitted disease
Hepatitis A	Feces, blood, urine	Infectious hepatitis
Hepatitis B	Feces, blood, all body fluids and excretions	Serum hepatitis
YEAST		
Candida albicans	Mouth, skin, colon, genital tract	Thrush, dermatitis
FUNGI		
Aspergillus	Soil, dust	Aspergillosis
Coccidioides immitis	Soil contaminated with spores	Coccidioidomycosis

Reservoir

Microorganisms have many sources or reservoirs for growth. One of the most common is the body itself. A variety of organisms reside on the surface of the skin and within body cavities, fluids, and discharges. The presence of microorganisms does not always cause a person to be ill. *Carriers* are persons or animals who show no symptoms of illness but who have pathogens on or in their bodies that can be transferred to others. For example, a person can be a carrier of tuberculosis without having manifestations of the disease.

Some areas of the body contain larger populations of resident flora than others. These include the skin, respiratory tract, mouth, vagina, colon, and lower urethra. Areas of the body normally considered sterile, without organism growth, are the bloodstream, spinal fluid, peritoneal cavity, urinary tract, muscles, bones, and chambers of the eye. The entrance of a foreign object into a sterile site leads to a high risk for infection.

Animals, plants, insects, and inanimate objects can also be reservoirs for infectious organisms. Shellfish can become contaminated with *Vibrio cholerae*, the bacterium that causes cholera. The tick is a carrier for the microbe that causes Rocky Mountain spotted fever. The deadly bacteria that cause tetanus thrive in the soil.

Food, water, and milk are additional reservoirs for pathogens. *Clostridium botulinus* toxin survives in improperly stored food such as nonrefrigerated milk products to cause botulism. The bacterium *Legionella pneumophila,* which causes Legionnaires' disease, lives in contaminated pooled water.

Environment of Microorganisms

In order to thrive, organisms must exist in a suitable environment. Characteristics of an environment that supports organism growth include the following.

FOOD

Microorganisms require nourishment. Some, such as *Clostridium perfringens,* the microbe that causes gas gangrene, thrive on organic matter. Others, such as *Escherichia coli,* consume undigested foodstuffs in the bowel. Carbon dioxide and inorganic material such as soil provide nourishment for other organisms.

OXYGEN

Aerobic bacteria require free oxygen for their survival and for multiplication sufficient to cause disease. Aerobic organisms tend to cause more infections in humans. Examples of aerobic organisms are *Staphylococcus aureus* and strains of *Streptococcus.*

Anaerobes thrive in environments where little or no free oxygen is available. Infections deep within the pleural cavity, in a joint, or in a deep sinus tract are typically caused by anaerobes. Bacteria that cause tetanus, gas gangrene, and botulism are anaerobes.

WATER

Most organisms require water for their survival. The spirochete that causes syphilis, *Treponema pallidum,* lives only in a moist environment. Some bacteria assume a form resistant to drying. These spore-forming bacteria, such as those that cause anthrax, botulism, and tetanus, can live without water.

TEMPERATURE

Microorganisms can live only in certain temperature ranges. However, some can survive temperature extremes that would be fatal to humans. Some viruses are resistant to boiling water.

pH

The acidity of an environment determines the viability of microorganisms. Most microorganisms prefer an alkaline environment within a pH range of 5 to 8. Bacteria in particular thrive in urine with a high pH. Organisms cannot survive the acid environment of the stomach.

LIGHT

Microorganisms thrive in dark environments such as those under dressings and within body cavities.

Ultraviolet light is effective in killing certain forms of bacteria.

Portal of Exit

Once microorganisms find a site to grow and multiply, they must find a portal of exit if they are to enter another host and cause disease. When the human is the reservoir, microorganisms can exit through a variety of sites.

SKIN AND MUCOUS MEMBRANES

Any break in the integrity of the skin and mucous membranes can lead to an infection. As pathogenic organisms grow and multiply within a wound, they create purulent drainage. For example, *Staphylococcus aureus* creates a characteristic yellow drainage, whereas *Pseudomonas aeruginosa* causes a greenish cast to drainage. The drainage is a potential portal of exit for infection.

RESPIRATORY TRACT

Pathogens residing in the respiratory tract can be released from the body when the person sneezes, coughs, talks, or even breathes. The microorganisms exit via the mouth and nose in normal clients. In clients with artificial airways such as tracheostomy or endotracheal tubes (see Chapter 41), organisms easily exit through these devices.

URINARY TRACT

Normally the urine is sterile. However, in a client who is infected, microorganisms exit during urination or through urinary diversions such as ileostomies and suprapubic drains (see Chapter 39).

GASTROINTESTINAL TRACT

The mouth is one of the more bacterially contaminated sites of the body even though most of the organisms are normal flora. However, organisms that are normal flora in one person can be pathogens in another. Organisms exist when a person expectorates saliva. Kissing can also provide a means of exit from the oral cavity.

Bowel elimination, drainage of bile via surgical wounds or drainage tubes, and the escape of gastric contents during vomiting are additional means of exit from the gastrointestinal tract.

REPRODUCTIVE TRACT

Organisms such as *Neisseria gonorrhoeae* and herpes simplex may exit via the male's urethral meatus or the female's vaginal canal. In the male, urine or semen may be the vehicle of the pathogens. Discharge from the female's vaginal canal may carry pathogens.

TABLE 33-3

Modes of Transmission

Route	Means	Examples of Organisms (Diseases)
Contact	Direct (direct physical transfer between an infected or colonized person and a susceptible host)—turning clients, giving baths, having sexual contact with an infected person	*Staphylococcus, Treponema* (syphilis), herpes simplex virus
	Indirect (personal contact of susceptible host with contaminated inanimate object)—needles, bedpans, intravenous tubing, stethoscopes, instruments and dressings, linen, dishes, and silverware	Measles virus, hepatitis B virus, *Enterococcus*
	Droplet contact (infectious agent coming in contact with conjunctivae, nose, or mouth of susceptible host; droplets travel only up to 3 feet and therefore contact is not airborne)—coughing, sneezing	Influenza virus, *Mycobacterium tuberculosis* (tuberculosis)
Air	Droplet nuclei (residue of evaporated droplets remain suspended in air)—coughing, sneezing, talking	Influenza virus, pneumococcus (pneumonia, meningitis, and other infections)
	Dust (contains infectious agent)	*Aspergillus* (aspergillosis)

Vehicle	Contaminated items
	  Liquids
	    Water
	    Drugs, solutions
	    Blood
	  Food (improperly handled or stored, fresh fruits and vegetables)
		
		Vibrio cholerae (cholera)
		Pseudomonas
		Hepatitis B virus
		Salmonella, Staphylococcus, Enterobacter, and *Klebsiella*

Vectors	Insects
	  Mosquitoes
	  Fleas, ticks, lice
	
	Animals (cows, pigs)
		
		Plasmodium (malaria)
		Rickettsia typhi and *R. prowazekii* (typhus)
		Brucella (brucellosis)

BLOOD

The blood is normally sterile, but in the case of hepatitis or septicemia (presence of bacteria in the circulating blood) it becomes a reservoir for infectious organisms. A break in the skin by needle puncture or a traumatic wound allows pathogens to exit the body in blood.

Modes of Transmission

There are many vehicles for the transmission of microorganisms from the reservoir to the host. Table 33-3 summarizes common modes of transmission. Certain infectious diseases tend to be transmitted more commonly by specific modes. However, the same microorganisms may be transmitted by more than one route. For example, herpes zoster may be spread by the airborne route in droplet nuclei or by direct contact.

Almost any object within the environment (for example, a stethoscope, thermometer, or bandage scissors) can become a means of transmitting infection. All hospital personnel providing direct care, such as nurses, physical therapists, and physicians, and those performing diagnostic and support services, such as laboratory technicians, respiratory therapists, and dietary workers, must be free of infection. Each group of health care workers follows specific procedures for handling equipment and supplies used by clients. For example, respiratory therapists wash their hands before working with each client and dispose of soiled oxygen equipment in a prescribed manner. Recently developed medical devices and procedures provide new avenues for growth and spread of pathogens.

Invasive procedures such as cardiac catheterization and cystoscopy (visualization of the bladder) facilitate the diagnosis of clients' problems but also increase the risk of transmitting infection. Because so many factors can promote the spread of infection to clients, all health care workers must be conscientious in using infection control practices.

Portal of Entry

Organisms can enter a person's body through the same routes they use for exiting. As described previously, factors that reduce the body's defenses enhance the chances of pathogens entering. For example, when a contaminated needle pierces a client's skin, organisms enter the body. Any obstruction to the flow of urine from a urinary catheter allows organisms to travel up the urethra. Mishandling of sterile bandages over an open wound permits pathogens to enter exposed tissues.

Susceptible Host

Whether a person acquires an infection depends on his susceptibility to an infectious agent. Susceptibility is the degree of resistance an individual has to pathogens. Although everyone is constantly in contact with large numbers of microorganisms, an infection will not develop until an individual becomes susceptible to the strength and numbers of those microorganisms. The more virulent an organism, the greater the likelihood of a person's susceptibility.

The integrity of a person's defenses against infection directly influences susceptibility. Factors such as increasing age, poor nutritional status, and stress impair an individual's immunological defenses. The nature of a disease process, hereditary conditions, and the type of medical therapy received may further decrease a person's resistance to infection.

Course of Infection

By understanding components of the infection chain, the nurse can intervene to prevent infections from developing. When the client acquires an infection, the nurse is in an advantageous position to observe early signs and symptoms of infection and to take appropriate actions to prevent its spread. Infections follow a progressive course (Table 33-4). The severity of the client's illness will depend on the extent of the infection, the pathogenicity of the causative microorganisms, and the susceptibility of the host.

If the client's infection is localized to a small wound, antibiotic therapy and proper wound care

TABLE 33-4

Course of Infection

Stage	Description
Incubation period	Interval between entrance of pathogen into the body and appearance of first symptoms; e.g., chickenpox 2-3 weeks, common cold 1-2 days, influenza 1-3 days, mumps 18 days
Prodromal stage of illness	Initial stage of illness manifested by early signs and symptoms, e.g., malaise, low-grade fever, fatigue; client is more capable of spreading disease to others during this stage
Full stage of illness	Client manifests signs and symptoms specific to type of infection; e.g., common cold manifested by sore throat, sinus congestion, rhinitis; mumps manifested by earache, high fever, parotid and salivary gland swelling
Convalescence	Acute symptoms of infection disappear; length of recovery depends on the severity of infection and client's general state of health

will likely control the infection's spread and minimize the client's illness. The client will experience only localized symptoms such as pain, tenderness, and swelling at the wound site. However, a systemic infection such as gram-negative sepsis can prove fatal. Gram-negative bacteria release endotoxin, which is part of the bacterial cell wall. Endotoxins ultimately interfere with the metabolic functions of cells, seriously impairing oxygen delivery to the cells. If the infection progresses and the client fails to respond to therapy, circulatory failure can develop and multiple body systems become involved.

The course of an infection thus influences the level of nursing care provided a client. The nurse is responsible for the proper administration of antibiotics and monitoring the client's response to drug therapy (see Chapter 32). Supportive therapy includes providing adequate nutrition and rest to bolster the client's defenses against the infectious process. The complexity of care further depends on the body systems affected by the infection.

Regardless of whether the client's infection is localized or systemic, the nurse plays a dominant role in minimizing the spread of infection. A simple wound infection can involve the urinary tract if the nurse uses poor technique during perineal hygiene. A client returning from surgery may have a clean wound but develop an infection if the nurse fails to wash her hands after caring for an infected client. Nurses can also acquire infections from clients if their techniques for controlling infection transmission are inadequate.

Asepsis and Nosocomial Infections

A nurse can never be too cautious in efforts to control and prevent the spread of infection. The environment of most health care facilities exposes clients to considerable risk of acquiring infections. The nurse must understand the factors causing infection as well as the principles used to prevent and control the spread of pathogens.

Nosocomial infections are those resulting from the delivery of health services in a health care facility. The acquisition of hepatitis from contact with a contaminated needle and the development of intestinal enteritis after ingesting contaminated food are examples of nosocomial infections. A hospital is one of the most likely places for acquiring an infection. It usually harbors a high population of virulent strains of microorganisms, for example, oxacillin-resistant *Staphylococcus* and toxigenic *Escherichia coli*. The virulent bacteria are usually resistant to antibiotics. Iatrogenic infections are a type of nosocomial infection resulting from a diagnostic or therapeutic procedure. Acquisition of a urinary infection after catheter insertion is an example of an iatrogenic nosocomial infection.

Clients in health care settings are usually vulnerable to infection because they are in high-risk groups. For example, a high percentage of the client population in hospitals is elderly. Most nosocomial infections occur in clients over 60 years of age (Gross et al., 1980). It is estimated that nosocomial infections affect nearly 2 million clients each year in the United States alone (Bennett, 1979). According to Sencer and Axnick (1975), excess hospitalization caused by nosocomial infection costs over 1 billion dollars annually.

Nosocomial infections may be exogenous or endogenous. An exogenous infection arises from microorganisms external to the individual, which do not exist as normal flora, such as *Salmonella*, *Clostridium tetani*, and *Aspergillus*. Endogenous infections can occur when part of the client's flora becomes altered and an overgrowth results; examples are infections caused by enterococci, yeasts, and streptococci. When sufficient numbers of microorganisms normally found in one body cavity or lining are transferred to another body site, an endogenous infection develops. For ex-

ample, transmission of enterococci, normally found in fecal material, from the hands to the skin is a common cause of wound infections. The number of microorganisms needed to cause a nosocomial infection depends on the virulence of the organism, the host's susceptibility, and the body site affected.

A number of factors within a health care setting increase a person's exposure to infectious microorganisms. The number of health care employees having direct contact with clients, the type and number of invasive procedures, the therapy received, and the length of hospitalization all influence the risk of infection. Major sites for nosocomial infection include the urinary tract, surgical or traumatic wounds, the respiratory tract, and the bloodstream (Table 33-5).

The nurse's efforts to minimize the onset and spread of infection are based on the principles of aseptic technique. The term "asepsis" means the absence of germs or pathogens. The two types of aseptic technique the nurse practices are medical and surgical asepsis.

Medical asepsis or clean technique includes the procedures used to reduce the number of microorganisms and prevent their spread from one place or person to another. Since nurses work in environments where pathogens are always present, they carry out precautions to protect themselves, clients, and co-workers from disease-causing microorganisms. Changing a client's linen daily, handwashing, and using clean medication cups are examples of medical asepsis. The principles of medical asepsis are commonly followed in the home. Washing hands before preparing food, using disposable drinking cups in the bathroom, and mopping the kitchen floor are all medical aseptic practices.

Surgical asepsis or sterile technique includes the procedures used to eliminate microorganisms from an area. An object free of microorganisms is termed *sterile*. The process of sterilization destroys all microorganisms and their spores. Sterile technique is practiced by nurses in the operating room, where only sterile instruments are used during a surgical procedure.

Once an object becomes unsterile or unclean, it is *contaminated*. In medical asepsis an area or object is considered contaminated if it contains or is suspected of containing pathogens. For example, a used bedpan, the floor, and a wet piece of gauze are contaminated. In surgical asepsis an area or object is considered contaminated if touched by any object that is not sterile. For example, a tear in a surgical glove exposes the outside of the glove to the skin surface, thus contaminating it.

Special procedures make objects clean or sterile. The process of destroying all pathogenic organisms,

TABLE 33-5

Causes and Sites for Nosocomial Infections

Site	Cause or Source of Infection
Urinary tract	Insertion of urinary catheter; closed drainage system becoming open; catheter and tube becoming disconnected; drainage bag port touching dirty surface; poor specimen collection technique; obstruction or interference with urinary drainage; urine in catheter or drainage tube being allowed to reenter bladder (reflux); poor handwashing technique; repeated catheter irrigations with solutions
Surgical or traumatic wounds	Improper skin preparation (shaving and bathing) before surgery; poor handwashing before dressing changes; failure to cleanse skin surface properly; failure to use aseptic technique during dressing changes; use of contaminated antiseptic solutions
Respiratory tract	Contaminated respiratory therapy equipment; failure to use aseptic technique while suctioning airway; improper disposal of mucous secretions
Bloodstream	Contamination of intravenous (IV) fluids by tubing or needle changes; insertion of drug additives to IV fluid; addition of connecting tubes or stopcocks to IV system; improper care of IV needle insertion site; contaminated needles or catheters; failure to change IV site when inflammation first appears

except spores, is called *disinfection*. The use of boiling water to disinfect a baby's bottle is a common disinfection practice. Disinfectants destroy most pathogens, but many are too strong to be used in or on a living person.

Antiseptics, bacteriostats, and bactericides are solutions or substances that can be applied safely to the skin or a mucosal surface. Frequently the nurse uses such preparations to clean and treat wounds, clean thermometers, or prepare the skin before a needle insertion. Antiseptics inhibit bacterial growth, whereas bacteriostats prevent the growth of bacteria. A bactericide kills bacteria but not necessarily spores. Isopropyl alcohol and iodine-containing solutions, such as povidone-iodine (Betadine) and poloxamer-iodine (Prepodyne), are commonly used antiseptics and bactericides.

The nurse is responsible for providing the client with a safe environment. The effectiveness of aseptic practices depends on the nurse's conscientiousness and consistency in using effective aseptic techniques. It is easy to forget key procedural steps or when hurried to take shortcuts that break aseptic procedures. However, the nurse's failure to be meticulous will place the client at risk for an infection that can seriously impair recovery.

Assessment

The nurse assesses a client's susceptibility to infection and looks for the signs and symptoms of infection in the client. By knowing the factors that increase a client's susceptibility, the nurse is better able to plan preventive therapy that includes aseptic techniques. By recognizing early signs and symptoms of infection, the nurse can alert the physician to the potential need for therapy and initiate supportive nursing measures.

Client Susceptibility

Numerous factors influence the client's susceptibility to infection. The nurse gathers information about each factor through a nursing history.

AGE

Throughout the life span a person's susceptibility to infection changes. At birth an infant has reduced defenses against infection. Born with only the antibodies provided by the mother, the infant has an immature immune system incapable of producing necessary immunoglobulins and white blood cells that attack invading antigens, such as bacteria and viruses. As the child grows, the immune system matures, but the child is still susceptible to organisms that cause the common cold, intestinal infections, and infectious diseases such as mumps, chickenpox, and measles.

The normal young or middle-aged adult has refined defenses against infection. Normal flora, body system defenses, inflammation, and the immune response provide adequate protection against invading microorganisms. Viruses are the most common cause of infectious illness in adults.

With aging an individual's defenses against infection again change. The immune response, particularly cell-mediated immunity, declines. Alterations in the immune system may even be instrumental in triggering the normal aging process. Cells of the immune system, such as lymphocytes, become more diversified with age, and the body undergoes a progressive loss of cellular regulation. When viruses or other antigens and corresponding antibodies lodge in sites such as the kidney and arteries, factors injurious to the tissues are released and deterioration begins. With aging and in autoimmune diseases (alterations of the immune system), cellular changes such as depletion of lymphoid tissues occur. Cancer and adult-onset diabetes mellitus are believed to be diseases of aging that arise from immunodeficiencies. The basic mechanism for the aging process is not understood. However, it is known that with advancing age immunity to infection decreases.

The elderly also undergo alterations in the structure and function of the skin, urinary tract, and lungs. For example, the skin loses its turgor and the epithelium thins. As a result, the skin is more easily abraded or torn. Such alterations increase the elderly client's exposure to pathogens.

NUTRITIONAL STATUS

When a person's protein intake is inadequate as a result of poor diet or debilitating disease, the rate of protein breakdown exceeds that of tissue synthesis (see Chapter 38). This deteriorative process results in a negative nitrogen balance; that is, the output of nitrogen sources such as protein exceeds nitrogen intake. A reduction in the intake of protein and other nutrients such as carbohydrates and fats reduces the body's defenses against infection and impairs wound healing (see Chapter 48).

Clients with illness or disease that increases protein requirements are at further risk. These conditions include traumatic injury, postoperative states, extensive burns, and conditions causing fever.

The nurse assesses the client's dietary habits in terms of the type of foods eaten daily. The client's ability to tolerate the intake of solid foods also influences nutritional status. Clients who have difficulty swallowing, experience alterations in digestion, or are too confused or weak to feed themselves are at risk for inadequate dietary intake.

STRESS

The body responds to emotional or physical stress by what is known as the general adaptation syndrome (see Chapter 5). During the alarm stage the basal metabolic rate increases as the body utilizes available energy stores. Adrenocorticotropic hormone (ACTH)

acts to increase serum glucose levels and decrease unnecessary anti-inflammatory responses through the release of cortisone. If stress continues or becomes intense, the elevated cortisone levels result in decreased resistance to infection. Continued stress leads to a state of exhaustion wherein energy stores are depleted and the body has no resistance to invading organisms. The same conditions that increase clients' nutritional requirements also increase the level of physical stress. After surgery or a traumatic injury the client has a high susceptibility to infection, not only because of trauma to the body but also because of the level of stress endured.

HEREDITY

Certain hereditary conditions impair an individual's response to infection. The client's history of preexisting medical problems should reveal any known hereditary disorders. For example, agammaglobulinemia is an inherited or acquired disorder characterized by the absence of serum immunoglobulins. The client's ability to initiate defenses against infection, as by the release of lymphocytes and formation of antibodies, is virtually absent.

DISEASE PROCESS

Clients with diseases of the immune system are at particular risk for infection. Leukemia, lymphoma, and aplastic anemia are examples of conditions that compromise a host by weakening normal defenses against microbial assault. Clients with these diseases are unable to produce sufficient white blood cells to ward off infection.

Victims of chronic disease such as diabetes mellitus and multiple sclerosis are also more susceptible to infection, because of general debilitation and nutritional impairment. Diseases that impair body system defenses, such as pulmonary emphysema and bronchitis (which impair ciliary action and thicken mucus), cancer (which causes ulceration of previously intact skin and mucous membranes), and peripheral vascular disease (which reduces blood flow to injured tissues), increase susceptibility to infection. Burn clients have a very high susceptibility to infection because of the direct damage of skin surfaces. The greater the depth and extent of the burns, the higher the risk for infection.

MEDICAL THERAPY

Some types of drug and medical therapies compromise a person's immunity to infection. The nurse assesses the client's medication history to determine if the client takes medications at home that increase infection susceptibility. A review of therapies received within the health care setting further reveals any risks to the client. Adrenal corticosteroids are anti-inflammatory drugs, prescribed for a wide variety of conditions, that cause protein breakdown and impair the inflammatory response against bacteria and other pathogens. Cytotoxic or antineoplastic drugs attack cancer cells but cause side effects of bone marrow depression and normal cell toxicity. With bone marrow depression the body is unable to produce lymphocytes and sufficient white blood cells. When normal viable cells become altered by antineoplastic agents, cellular defenses against infection falter.

Cancer clients receiving radiotherapy are also at risk for acquiring infection. The massive doses of radiation, which destroy cancerous cells, can also depress the bone marrow and destroy normal cells.

Clinical Appearance

A client's signs and symptoms of infection will be either local or systemic. Localized infections are most commonly seen in areas of skin or mucous membrane breakdown such as surgical and traumatic wounds, skin ulcers, decubitus ulcers, and mouth lesions. Infections also develop locally in cavities beneath the skin as in an abscess.

To assess an area for localized infection, the nurse first inspects the area for redness and swelling caused by inflammation. There may be drainage from open lesions or wounds. Infected drainage may be yellow, green, or brown, depending on the site of infection. The nurse further asks the client if there is any pain or tenderness around the site. The client may complain of tightness caused by the formation of edema. If the infected area is large enough, the movement of a body part may be restricted. Gentle palpation of an infected area usually results in some degree of tenderness.

A systemic infection causes more generalized symptoms than a local infection. Unlike localized infections, systemic infections usually result in fever. The client complains of fatigue and malaise. Lymph nodes that drain the area of infection often become enlarged, swollen, and tender on palpation. For example, an abscess in the peritoneal cavity may cause enlargement of lymph nodes in the groin. An infection of the upper respiratory tract may cause cervical lymph node enlargement. If an infection is serious and widespread, all major lymph nodes may enlarge. Systemic infections commonly cause a loss of appetite, nausea, and vomiting.

Systemic infections often develop after treatment has failed to control a localized infection. The nurse who cares for a client with a localized infection should be alert for changes in the client's level of activity and responsiveness. As systemic infections develop, the client may become lethargic and complain of a loss of energy. During febrile episodes the client's temperature may become high, leading to episodes of increased heart and respiratory rates. Involvement of major body systems produces specific signs. For example, a pulmonary infection results in a productive cough with purulent sputum. A urinary tract infection may result in cloudy, foul-smelling urine.

The nurse uses knowledge of the client's medical condition to anticipate the development of infection and the extent to which various body systems might become involved.

Nurse's Role in Infection Control

The nurse has two primary responsibilities in controlling infection: (1) preventing the onset and spread of infection and (2) promoting measures for the treatment of infection. To prevent an infection from developing or spreading, the nurse minimizes the numbers and kinds of organisms transmitted to potential infection sites. Eliminating reservoirs of infection, controlling portals of exit and entry, and avoiding actions that transmit microorganisms will prevent bacteria from finding a site to grow. Disinfection and sterilization of supplies and good handwashing are examples of medically aseptic methods the nurse uses to control the spread of microorganisms. A final preventive measure is to strengthen a potential host's defenses against infection. Nutritional support, rest, maintenance of physiological protective mechanisms, and immunization protect a client from invasion by pathogens.

When a client develops an infection, the nurse continues preventive care so health care personnel and other clients do not acquire the infection. Clients with highly communicable diseases require protective aseptic techniques that control the client's environment by forming barriers against bacterial spread.

Treatment of an infectious process includes eliminating the infectious organisms and supporting the client's defenses. The nurse must collect specimens of body fluids or drainage from infected body sites for cultures. When the disease process or causative organism has been identified, the physican prescribes the anti-infective or antibiotic drug most effective for the situation. The nurse administers antibiotics judiciously, watching for allergic reactions, assessing the progress of the client's infection, and administering the drugs by the proper methods.

Systemic infections require measures to prevent the complications of fever (see Chapter 28). Maintaining intake of fluids prevents dehydration resulting from diaphoresis. The client's increased metabolic rate necessitates an adequate nutritional intake. Rest preserves the client's energy for the healing process.

Localized infections often require measures to facilitate removal of infectious organisms. Wet-to-dry dressings (see Chapter 48) are used to remove infected drainage from wound sites. Application of heat compresses promotes blood flow to an infected site and thus the delivery of blood components needed to fight an infection. Drainage tubes are inserted to remove infected drainage from body cavities. The nurse uses medical and surgical aseptic techniques to manage wounds and ensures the correct handling of infected drainage or body fluids.

During the course of any infection the nurse supports the client's body defense mechanisms. For example, if a client is known to have infectious diarrhea, the nurse must maintain skin integrity to prevent breakdown and entrance of microorganisms. Humidified air maintains the function of the lung's protective cilia. Therefore when administering oxygen to a client, the nurse checks to be sure only humidified gas is provided. Routine hygiene measures such as cleansing the oral cavity and bathing further protect the skin and mucous membranes from organism spread.

The needs of a client with an infection can be many. By monitoring the infection's course carefully, the nurse can choose the most appropriate measures to maintain or restore the client's health.

Medical Asepsis

The nurse follows certain principles and procedures in preventing infection and controlling its spread. The nurse uses basic medical aseptic techniques to break the infection chain. When a client acquires an infection, the nurse institutes measures for treating the infection and preventing its spread to others. Infections that are readily transmissible between individuals require the nurse to use protective aseptic techniques. Clients with high susceptibility to infection require special precautions to prevent exposure to pathogens.

General Aseptic Measures

A nurse can never be too careful in using aseptic techniques. In every aspect of client care there are measures that will prevent the development of infection.

CONTROL OR ELIMINATION OF INFECTIOUS AGENTS

The proper cleansing, disinfecting, and sterilization of contaminated objects significantly reduce and often eliminate microorganisms. In large health care centers

a central supply department does most of the disinfecting and sterilizing of reusable supplies. However, the nurse encounters situations during a client's care that require use of these techniques. Many of the principles of cleansing and disinfecting also apply to the home setting.

CLEANSING. Cleanliness inhibits the growth of microorganisms. In the health care setting nurses clean objects to prepare them for disinfection and sterilization. Whenever cleaning equipment soiled by organic material, such as blood, fecal matter, mucus, or pus, it is important to use waterproof gloves, a stiff-bristled brush, and detergent or soap.

These basic steps will ensure that an object is clean:

1. Rinse a contaminated object or article with cold running water to remove organic material. Hot water causes the protein in organic material to coagulate and stick to objects, making removal difficult.
2. After rinsing, wash the object with soap and warm water. Soap or detergent reduces the surface tension of water and emulsifies any dirt or remaining material. Few household detergents, however, have disinfectant properties. Rinse the object thoroughly to remove the emulsified dirt.
3. Use a brush to remove any dirt or material in grooves or seams. Friction dislodges contaminated material for easy removal.
4. Rinse the object in warm water.
5. Dry the object and prepare it for disinfection or sterilization.
6. The brush, gloves, and sink in which the equipment is cleaned should be considered contaminated and should be cleansed.

DISINFECTION AND STERILIZATION. The two primary methods for disinfection and sterilization are physical processes, involving the use of heat or radiation, and chemical processes, in which various solutions or gases are used for disinfection. Both processes act to disrupt the internal functioning of microorganisms by destroying cell proteins. Sterilization and disinfection occur when heat reaches a level sufficient to destroy organisms or when a specific concentration of chemicals has adequate exposure to microorganisms. When the nurse is using heat or radiation, equipment must be packed properly in autoclaves or sterilizing chambers so that organisms receive necessary exposure. Many heat-sensitive products such as rubber, plastic, and paper can be sterilized only by chemical means.

Dry Heat. Dry heat is no longer commonly used in health care agencies, since more effective methods are available. The advantage of dry heat is that some articles to be disinfected cannot be placed in water. Dry heat disinfects but does not destroy all microorganisms. Disinfection occurs when a temperature of 160° C (320° F) is maintained for 2 hours. In the home, articles placed in the oven at 350° F for at least 45 minutes will become disinfected. The density of the article influences the degree of disinfection.

Boiling Water. The least expensive and most practical means for sterilization and disinfection in the home is boiling water. Unfortunately, bacterial spores and some viruses are resistant to boiling. The process is not used in health care agencies. When boiling is used in the home, a minimum of 15 minutes will achieve disinfection.

Steam. There are two methods for using steam in sterilization. Steam or moist heat under pressure is the best means of destroying all microorganisms. As water vapor is subjected to higher pressure, it can achieve a temperature above the boiling point. Such high temperatures kill all pathogens and their spores. An autoclave works on the principle of steam under pressure. The time needed to ensure sterilization depends on the type of equipment, its wrapping, the manner in which it is packed in the autoclave, and the temperature and pressure maintained. Saturated steam at 121° to 123° C (250° to 254° F) at 15 to 17 pounds of pressure per square inch will sterilize items in 15 to 45 minutes.

At one time hospitals relied on this process to flush bedpans and urinals. However, the temperature of free-flowing steam reaches only the boiling point (100° C or 212° F), which is not sufficiently high to kill all pathogens. Nurses should be aware that hoppers or flushers do not sterilize but rather mechanically cleanse.

Radiation. The use of radiation achieves disinfection and sterilization. Nonionizing radiation, such as ultraviolet light, does not penetrate deeply into objects and thus is impractical in a health agency. Ionizing radiation, however, is very effective in sterilizing drugs, foods, and other heat-sensitive items. Because of the complexity and expense of ionizing devices, most are in factories rather than hospitals.

Ethylene Oxide Gas. Ethylene oxide gas destroys spores and microorganisms by altering the cells' metabolic processes. The fumes are released within an autoclave-like chamber at a relatively low temperature of 54.4° to 65.5° C (130° to 150° F) and a humidity of 30% to 60%. Unlike radiation, ethylene oxide gas has excellent penetrating qualities. The danger of the gas is its high toxicity to humans. Ventilation of the sterilizer and aeration of sterilized materials must be strictly controlled.

Chemical Solutions. Chemical disinfectants are frequently used for disinfection of instruments and equipment. Often the nurse soaks surgical instruments in a disinfectant before cleaning and sterilizing them. Glass thermometers may be stored in disinfectant solutions.

Characteristics of an effective chemical disinfectant include the following:
1. Attacks all types of microorganisms
2. Rapid acting
3. Not harmful to body tissues
4. Not inactivated by organic material
5. Works with water
6. Stable in light and heat
7. Will not destroy article being disinfected
8. Retains no odor
9. Inexpensive

Among the effective chemical disinfectants are chlorine, iodine, and alcohol. Chlorine is useful in disinfecting water and for housekeeping purposes. It corrodes metals and should never be mixed with ammonia because of the toxic fumes the combination emits. Although iodine has bactericidal properties, it can stain permeable objects. A solution of detergent and iodine is called an iodophor. Iodophors are frequently used for surgical scrubbing because of their antiseptic properties. Both ethyl (grain) and isopropyl (rubbing) alcohol have antiseptic qualities. In some institutions alcohol is used as a disinfectant. Isopropyl alcohol is the best alcohol for removing fat from the skin. The alcohols have the disadvantages of causing excessive dryness to the skin and damaging plastic material.

CONTROL OR ELIMINATION OF RESERVOIRS

To control or eliminate reservoir sites for infection, the nurse acts to eliminate sources of body fluids, drainage, or solutions that might harbor microorganisms.

When bathing a client, the nurse uses soap and water to remove organisms residing on the skin (see Chapter 35). Any drainage, dried secretions, excess perspiration, and sediment from previously used disinfectant must be washed away.

A dressing or bandage must be changed if it becomes wet and soiled. The dark, moist environment beneath the dressing is an ideal breeding site for microorganisms.

The client's bedside unit, whether at home or in a hospital, should be free of standing water and used bottles of solution. Bedside units should be kept clean and dry, and bottles of solution should be covered or capped. Certain disinfectant solutions will harbor microorganisms if bottles are left open for long periods.

It is important that a surgical wound drains properly (see Chapter 48). The accumulation of serous fluid under the skin can become a reservoir for microorganisms. The nurse looks for swelling of wound sites to detect serous accumulation. If the client has a tube draining the wound, the nurse makes sure it drains freely and remains patent.

Additional reservoirs of infection are suction and drainage bottles and urinary drainage bags. Suction bottles should be emptied and rinsed thoroughly on each shift and changed every 24 hours. Any drainage system (for example, nasogastric tube drainage) should be emptied on each shift unless a physician orders otherwise. Drainage systems should never be raised above the level of the site being drained. For example, when a urinary drainage bag is raised above the level of the bladder while turning or moving a client, microorganisms can easily reenter the bladder via reflux of urine. The drainage tube or catheter should be clamped if it is necessary to raise the bag.

CONTROL OF PORTALS OF EXIT

To control organisms exiting via the respiratory tract, the nurse should avoid talking directly into a client's face or talking, sneezing, or coughing directly over a surgical wound or sterile dressing field (see Chapter 48). The nurse should cover her mouth or nose when sneezing or coughing. The nurse is also responsible for teaching clients how to protect others when they sneeze or cough and for providing clients with disposable wipes or tissues to control spread of microorganisms.

A nurse who has a mild cold and continues to work with clients should wear a mask, especially when changing a dressing or performing a sterile procedure. The nurse should refrain from working with clients who are highly susceptible to infection.

Another way of controlling the exit of microorganisms is the careful handling of exudate such as urine, feces, and emesis. It is wise for the nurse to wear disposable gloves if there is a chance her hands will come in contact with any exudate. The nurse disposes of anything soiled by exudate into appropriate containers. Soiled linen is placed in linen bags. Items moist from body discharges are wrapped in waterproof containers, such as plastic bags, before being discarded. Proper wrapping and disposal protect housekeeping employees from contact with organisms.

CONTROL OF TRANSMISSION

Handwashing is the most important and most basic technique in preventing and controlling the transmission of pathogens. Contaminated hands are a prime cause of cross-infections. For example, a nurse is caring for a client who has excessive pulmonary excretions. The nurse assists the client in expectorating the mucus and disposes of tissues in a bedside container. The client's roommate asks the nurse to open the containers of food on her meal tray. The nurse then leaves the client's room to pour a dose of medication due in 5 minutes. If the nurse fails to wash her hands before each of these actions, organisms from the first client's mucus could easily be transmitted to the roommate's food and to the medication container.

The Centers for Disease Control (CDC) recommends that nurses routinely wash their hands in the following situations:

1. Before and after contact with a client (particularly those with high susceptibility to infection)
2. After touching organic material
3. Before performing invasive procedures, such as administering injections, catheterization, and suctioning
4. Before handling dressings or touching open wounds
5. Before preparing medications
6. After handling contaminated equipment

Before the nurse begins working with clients, a 2-minute handwashing provides good protection. A 30-second handwashing after each routine client contact ensures that transmission of organisms will be minimal. Before a nurse works with sterile equipment, handwashing should last 3 minutes. Whenever the nurse has handled contaminated equipment or organic material, a 1-minute handwashing is recommended.

The nurse instructs clients and visitors on the proper times for handwashing. Teaching handwashing techniques is particularly important if the client's health care is to continue at home. Clients should wash their hands before eating or handling food, after handling contaminated equipment, linen, or organic material, and before and after elimination. Visitors are encouraged to wash their hands before eating or handling food, after coming in contact with infected clients, and after handling contaminated equipment or organic material.

Procedure 33-1 describes handwashing. The principles of handwashing incorporate elements of microbiology, physics, and chemistry. Because skin crevices harbor large numbers of microorganisms, the use of friction is essential to loosen dirt and bacteria. Warm water and soap help to suspend soil and or-

PROCEDURE 33-1

Handwashing

STEPS	RATIONALE
1. Use a sink with warm running water and equipped with soap or disinfectant and paper towels.	Running water facilitates removal of organisms. Paper towels are easy to discard.
2. Push wristwatch and long uniform sleeves up above wrists. Remove jewelry.	This provides complete access to fingers, hands, and wrists. Jewelry may harbor microorganisms.
3. Keep fingernails short and filed.	Dirt and secretions that lodge under the fingernails contain microorganisms. Long fingernails can scratch a client's skin.
4. Inspect the surface of the hands and fingers for any breaks or cuts in the skin and cuticles. Report such lesions when caring for highly susceptible clients.	Open cuts or wounds can harbor high concentrations of microorganisms. Such lesions may serve as portals of exit, increasing a client's exposure to infection, or as portals of entry, increasing the nurse's risk of acquiring an infection.
5. Stand in front of the sink, keeping hands and uniform away from the sink surface. (If hands touch the sink during handwashing, repeat the process.) Use a sink where it is comfortable to reach the faucet.	The inside of the sink is a contaminated area. Reaching over a sink increases the risk of touching the edge, which is contaminated.
6. Turn on the water. Press foot pedals with the foot to regulate flow and temperature. Push knee pedals laterally to control flow and temperature. Turn on hand-operated faucets by covering the faucet with a paper towel.	When the hands come in contact with a faucet, they are considered contaminated. Organisms spread easily from the hands to the faucet.
7. Avoid splashing water against your uniform.	Microorganisms travel and grow in moisture.
8. Regulate flow of water so the temperature is warm.	Warm water is more comfortable. Hot water opens pores of the skin, causing irritation.
9. Wet hands and lower arms thoroughly under running water. Keep the hands and forearms lower than the elbows during washing.	The hands are the most contaminated parts to be washed. Water flows from the least to the most contaminated area.
10. Apply soap to the hands. If bar soap is used, hold it throughout the handwashing period. Soap granules, leaflets, and liquid preparations may be used.	Bar soap should be rinsed before returning it to soap dish. A soap dish that allows water to drain keeps the soap firm. Jellylike soap permits growth of microorganisms.

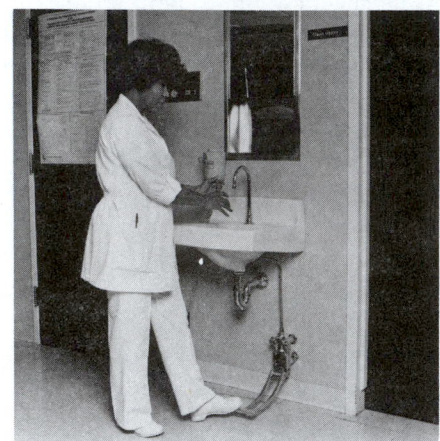

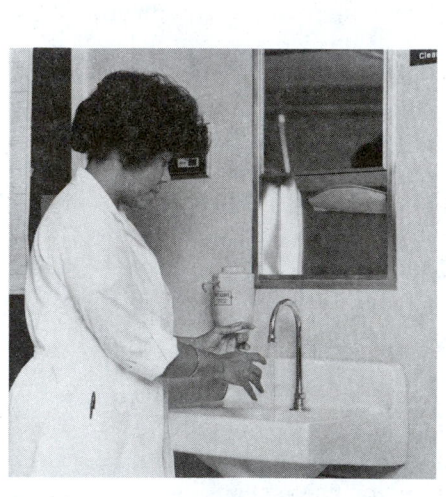

STEPS	RATIONALE	

11. Wash the hands using plenty of lather and friction for 15 to 30 seconds. Interlace the fingers and rub the palms and back of hands with a circular motion.

Soap cleanses by emulsifying fat and oil and lowering surface tension. Friction and rubbing mechanically loosen and remove dirt and transient bacteria. Interlacing fingers and thumbs ensures that all surfaces are cleansed.

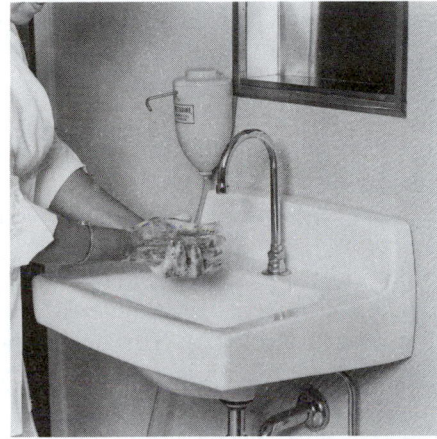

12. If areas underlying fingernails are soiled, clean them with fingernails of the other hand and additional soap or a clean orangewood stick. Do not tear or cut the skin under or around the nail.

Mechanical removal of dirt and sediment under nails reduces microorganisms on hands.

13. Rinse the hands and wrists thoroughly, keeping hands down and elbows up.

Rinsing mechanically washes away dirt and microorganisms.

14. Repeat steps 10 through 12 but extend the actual period of washing for 1-, 2-, and 3-minute handwashings.

The greater the likelihood of the hands being contaminated, the greater the need for thorough handwashing.

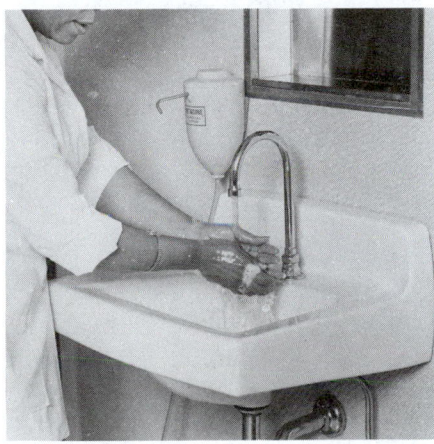

15. Dry the hands thoroughly, wiping from the fingers down to the wrists and forearms.

Dry from the cleanest area (fingertips) to the least clean (wrists) to avoid contamination. Drying hands prevents chapping and roughened skin.

16. Discard paper towel in proper receptacle.

Proper disposal of contaminated objects prevents transfer of microorganisms.

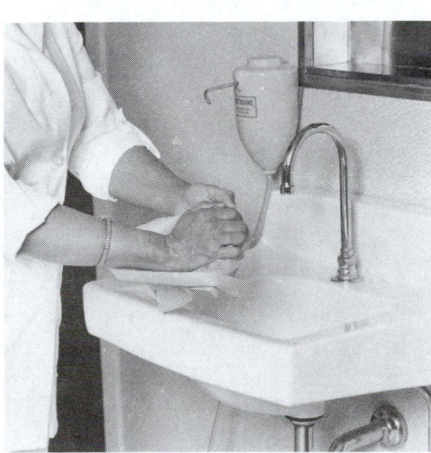

17. Turn off water with foot and knee pedals. To turn off a hand faucet, use a clean, dry paper towel.

A wet towel and wet hands allow the transfer of pathogens by capillary action.

18. Keep hands and cuticles well lubricated with hand lotion or moisturizer.

Dry, chapped skin cracks easily, creating a portal of entry for infection.

ganisms so they can be rinsed away. Regular soap or a mild detergent is best for washing hands. In special care areas such as nurseries, the operating room, or isolation units, soaps with antiseptics or germicides may be required. However, antiseptics can cause dryness and irritation of the skin, creating tiny cracks and cuts that can house microorganisms.

At one time hexachlorophene-containing products were popular for handwashing. However, hexachlorophene was found to cause toxic effects when absorbed through the skin, and in 1972 the Food and Drug Administration removed it from the market. Today hexachlorophene can be obtained only with a prescription.

In addition to handwashing, the nurse takes other actions to reduce microorganism transmission. In the hospital, home, or extended care facility a client should have a personal set of care items. Sharing thermometers, bedpans, urinals, bath basins, and eating utensils can easily lead to transmission of infection. Thermometers, even when individually used, warrant special care. Since the client's own mucus can become a source for microorganism growth, after each use the client's thermometer is washed in soap and water and dried.

Because certain microorganisms travel easily through the air, linens or bedclothes should not be shaken. Dusting with a specially treated or dampened cloth prevents dust particles from entering the air.

To prevent transmission of microorganisms through indirect contact, soiled items and equipment must be kept from touching the nurse's clothing. A common error is to carry dirty linen in the arms against the uniform. Special linen bags should be used, or soiled linen carried with hands held out from the body. Laundry hampers should not be allowed to overflow.

It is important to remember that anything that touches the floor is contaminated. If the nurse accidentally drops a piece of equipment, it should be discarded. When the nurse stoops or bends, the uniform should not touch the floor, and clean or soiled linen should never be put on the floor.

CONTROL OF PORTALS OF ENTRY

Many of the measures that control the exit of microorganisms likewise control the entrance of pathogens. Maintaining the integrity of skin and mucous membranes reduces the chances of microorganisms reaching a host. The client's skin should be kept well lubricated by using hand lotion as appropriate (see Chapter 35). Immobilized and debilitated clients are particularly susceptible to skin breakdown. Clients should not be positioned on tubes or objects that might cause breaks in the skin. Dry, wrinkle-free linen

also reduces the chances of skin breakdown. Frequent oral hygiene prevents drying of mucous membranes. A water-soluble ointment will keep the client's lips well lubricated.

After elimination a woman or girl should clean the rectum and perineum by wiping from the urinary meatus toward the rectum. Cleansing in a direction from the least to the most contaminated area helps reduce genitourinary infections.

Clients, health care personnel, and even housekeepers are at risk for acquiring infections from accidental needle sticks. After administering an injection or inserting an intravenous catheter, the nurse should carefully dispose of contaminated needles (see Chapter 32). A stray needle lying in bed linen or carelessly thrown into a wastebasket is a prime source for pathogens. Hepatitis B or serum hepatitis is the infection most commonly transmitted by contaminated needles. A needle stick should be reported immediately. In most health care agencies the victim of a needle stick completes an injury report and sees a physician for treatment. It may be necessary for the person to receive a series of gamma globulin injections.

Another cause for the entrance of microorganisms into a host is the improper handling and management of catheters and drainage sets. The point of connection between a catheter or drain and tubing should remain closed and intact. As long as such systems are closed, their contents are considered sterile (except for drainage of infectious wounds). When turning, lifting, or moving clients, the nurse should make certain that connecting tubes have enough slack to avoid being pulled apart. At times the nurse obtains specimens from drainage tubes or inserts needles into intravenous tubing ports. The nurse disinfects tubes and ports by wiping them liberally with alcohol or a similar solution before opening the system. Placing squares of sterile gauze around the ends of an opened tube adds further protection against entrance of bacteria.

A final method for reducing the entrance of microorganisms is the technique for cleansing wounds (see Chapter 48). The wound itself is considered to be sterile. To prevent entrance of microorganisms, the nurse should clean outward from a wound site. When applying a disinfectant or cleaning with soap and water, it is important to wipe around the wound edge first and then clean outward. A clean gauze should be used for each revolution around the wound's circumference.

PROTECTION OF THE SUSCEPTIBLE HOST

A client's resistance to infection will improve with adequate nutrition. A well-balanced diet provides the essential proteins, vitamins, carbohydrates, and fats the body uses for building tissue and storing energy. An infection increases the body's need for nutrients. The nurse uses measures to increase a client's appetite and assists in planning meals that contain essential nutrients (see Chapter 38).

Rest is essential to maintain the body's normal reparative processes. The nurse promotes the client's comfort and sleep (see Chapter 36) so that energy stores are replaced daily.

Protection of existing body defense mechanisms is crucial for maintaining a client's resistance to infection. Maintaining skin and mucous membrane integrity and supporting specialized defenses such as the lung's cough reflex and the normal mechanism for urinary excretion (see Table 33-1) protect the client from unnecessary exposure to pathogens.

Immunizations provide a person with additional protection against infectious disease. Children, in particular, require immunization for diseases such as measles and mumps, since their immune systems are immature. Immunization is also important when a person has a history of exposure to certain infectious organisms. For example, if a person receives a traumatic wound from a potentially contaminated object such as a rusty nail, tetanus toxoid stimulates the formation of antibodies against the tetanus bacteria. The nurse's role is to educate clients and their families about the importance of immunization.

PROTECTIVE ASEPSIS

Often clients acquire infectious diseases that can easily be transmitted to other clients, family members, or health care personnel. Communicable diseases, such as measles and tuberculosis, and infections by highly virulent organisms would spread rapidly throughout a health care institution if special precautions were not used for prevention. Clients with low immunity also require special precautions to prevent exposure to organisms normally found in a health care environment.

Protective aseptic techniques or isolation precautions are used to control transmission of pathogens. Environmental barriers such as a private room, a closed door, a mask, or a protective gown and gloves keep pathogens in a confined area. The extent of protection a client requires depends on how transmissible a disease is. Any person caring for the client follows practices either to prevent organisms from leaving the room of the infected client or to prohibit them from entering the room of a highly susceptible client.

In 1983 the CDC issued specific guidelines for isolating the client within a controlled environment (Garner and Simmons, 1983). Two systems are used for implementing protective asepsis. In the disease-specific system, certain practices are followed for each infectious disease. This is the less costly and time-consuming system, since certain diseases require only minimal precautions. The more commonly used system in hospitals is category-specific isolation. Diseases requiring similar isolation precautions, indicated by the manner in which the organisms are transmitted, are grouped in eight categories (Table 33-6). Clients with diseases that can be transmitted by contact and air, such as diphtheria, require strict aseptic practices. The nurse uses all available environmental barriers to provide strict isolation. The client with an infection that spreads only by contact, such as herpes simplex, impetigo, or infection by resistant bacteria, requires *contact isolation*. The nurse uses protective gowns, masks, and gloves only when in contact with infective material. Clients with disease transmissible through the air over short distances (droplet transmission), such as pneumonia, *Haemophilus* influenza in children, bacterial meningitis, and measles, require *respiratory isolation*. In this case the nurse must wear a mask whenever she is in the client's room. Clients with diseases that are spread through fecal material, such as infectious diarrhea, viral hepatitis, and viral meningitis, require *enteric precautions*. The nurse uses gown and gloves to avoid contact with feces. Clients with current active tuberculosis, which may be transmitted by air and through sputum, require *tuberculosis isolation*. Clients with infections transmitted by direct or indirect contact with infected material or drainage from an infected body site require *drainage and secretion precautions*. Abscesses, infected burns, or wound infections may necessitate such precautions. Clients with diseases transmitted by direct or indirect contact with infected blood or body fluids, such as serum hepatitis, acquired immune deficiency syndrome (AIDS), and primary syphilis, require *blood and body fluid precautions*. The nurse wears a gown and gloves only when the risk of coming in contact with infected material is high, such as during blood drawing or dressing changes.

Some institutions practice protective asepsis for clients who are at high risk for acquiring infections. The CDC, however, no longer has a protective or reverse isolation category. Clients with conditions such as leukemia, lymphoma, and burns or who have received organ transplants are protected from acquiring infections from health care personnel and visitors. Anyone caring for the client wears a mask, gloves, and gown to prevent transmission of organisms by air droplet or contact.

Regardless of the type of protective asepsis system, the nurse must follow certain basic principles:

1. The hands should be washed thoroughly before

TABLE 33-6

Category-Specific Isolation

Type of Isolation	Purpose	Example of Disease or Condition	Room	Gown	Gloves	Mask	Precautions
Strict	Prevents transmission of highly contagious or virulent infections spread by air and contact	Chickenpox; diphtheria	Private room with door closed	Required of all persons entering room	Required of all persons entering room	Required of all persons entering room	Discard or bag and label articles contaminated with infective materials. Send reusable articles for disinfection and sterilization.
Contact	Prevents transmission of highly transmissible infections spread by close or direct contact, which do not warrant strict precautions	Acute respiratory infections in infants and young children; impetigo; herpes simplex; infections by multiple resistant bacteria	Private room; clients infected with same organism may share a room	Indicated if soiling or contact is likely	Indicated for persons touching infective material	Indicated for persons coming close to client	Discard or bag and label articles contaminated with infective material. Send reusable items for disinfection and sterilization.
Respiratory	Prevents transmission of infectious diseases over short distances via air droplets	Measles; meningitis; mumps; pneumonia; *Haemophilus influenza* (in children)	Private room; clients infected with same organism may share a room	Not indicated	Not indicated	Indicated for persons who come close to client	Discard or bag and label articles contaminated with infective material. Send reusable items for disinfection and sterilization. Bathroom should not be shared by clients.
Enteric precautions	Prevents infections transmitted by direct or indirect contact with feces	Cholera; diarrhea of an infectious cause; hepatitis A; gastroenteritis caused by highly infectious organism	Private room if client's hygiene is poor (does not wash hands, shares contaminated items); clients with same organism may share a room	Indicated if soiling is likely	Indicated when touching infective material	Not indicated	Discard or bag and label articles contaminated with infective material. Send reusable items for disinfection and sterilization. Bathroom should not be shared by clients.

Category	Description	Disease examples	Private room	Gowns	Gloves	Masks	Articles
Tuberculosis isolation	Special category for clients with pulmonary tuberculosis who have positive results on sputum or chest x-ray examination indicating active disease	Laryngeal tuberculosis	Private room with special ventilation preferred; door closed	Indicated only if needed to prevent gross contamination of clothing	Not indicated	Indicated only if client is coughing and does not reliably cover mouth	Articles are rarely involved in transmission of tuberculosis. Articles should be thoroughly cleansed, disinfected, or discarded.
Drainage/secretion precautions	Prevents infections transmitted by direct or indirect contact with purulent material or drainage from an infected body site	Abscess; burn infection; infected wound; minor infections not included in contact isolation	Private room not indicated	Indicated if soiling or contact with infective material is likely	Indicated for touching infective material	Not indicated	Discard or bag and label articles contaminated with infective material. Send for disinfection or sterilization.
Blood/body fluids precautions	Transmitted by direct or indirect contact with infective blood or body fluids	Acquired immune deficiency syndrome (AIDS); hepatitis B; syphilis	Private room indicated if client's hygiene is poor	Indicated if soiling clothes with blood or body fluids is likely	Indicated for touching blood or body fluids	Not indicated	Discard or bag and label articles contaminated with blood or body fluids. Disinfect and sterilize articles. Avoid needle stick injuries. Dispose of used needles in properly labeled, puncture-resistant container. Clean blood spills promptly with 5.25% solution of sodium hypochlorite diluted 1:10 with water.
Care of severely compromised clients (previously called protective or reverse isolation)	Protects an uninfected client with lowered immunity and resistance from acquiring infectious organisms	Leukemia; lymphoma; aplastic anemia	Private room with door closed	Required of all persons entering room	Required of all persons entering room	Indicated for persons coming in contact with client	For open wounds or burns use sterile gloves.

entering and leaving the room of a client receiving protective asepsis.

2. All contaminated supplies and equipment should be disposed of in a manner that prevents spread of microorganisms to other persons.

3. Knowledge of the disease process and the means of infection transmission should be applied when using protective barriers.

4. Measures should be implemented to protect other people who might be exposed during transport of the client to locations outside the isolation room.

PSYCHOLOGICAL IMPLICATIONS OF ISOLATION. Protective asepsis creates a forced solitude that deprives the client of normal social relationships. The client may need to remain in a private room with limited interpersonal contact for days or weeks. This situation can by psychologically harmful, especially for children.

As a result of the infectious process the client's body image is altered. He may feel unclean, rejected, lonely, or guilty. The aseptic practices the nurse follows further intensify this belief of difference or undesirability. Isolation in a private room limits sensory contact. The client sees few people, and often the isolation precautions require closure of the room door. Unless the nurse acts to minimize the client's feelings of psychological and physical isolation, his emotional state can interfere with recovery.

Before protective aseptic measures are instituted, the client and family must understand the nature of the client's condition, the purposes of protective asepsis, and how to carry out the specific precautions. If they are able to participate in maintaining asepsis, the chances of reducing the spread of infection and lowering the client's risk of complications are great. The client and family should be taught the proper way to wash their hands and don gowns, masks, or gloves. Each procedure should be demonstrated, and the client and family should be given an opportunity for practice. It is also important to explain how infectious organisms can be transmitted so the client understands the difference between contaminated and clean objects. Unless family members know that their clothing becomes contaminated by contact with infected secretions, efforts at controlling infection are wasted.

The nurse also takes measures to improve the client's sensory stimulation during isolation. Reading materials, a radio or television set, a clock, and hobby materials should be available. However, if a book or other inanimate object comes in contact with infected material, it must be disinfected or discarded. An object such as a radio can be wrapped in a protective plastic covering. The room environment should be clean and pleasant looking. The room drapes or shades should be opened and any excess supplies or equipment removed. The nurse plans her activities of care to allow sufficient time with the client receiving protective asepsis. If the nurse rushes through care or shows a lack of interest in the client's needs, the client will feel rejected and even more isolated. The nurse must take the opportunity to listen to the client's concerns or interests. Mealtime is a particularly good opportunity for conversation. Providing comfort measures such as repositioning, a back massage, or a tepid sponge bath increases the client's physical stimulation. If the client's condition permits, the nurse should encourage him to walk and sit up in a chair.

It is important for the nurse to explain to family members the client's risk of depression or loneliness. Visiting family members should be encouraged to avoid expressions or actions that convey revulsion or disgust. The nurse advises family members on ways to provide meaningful stimulation.

PROTECTIVE ENVIRONMENT. A private room reduces the possibility of transmission of infection by separating susceptible clients from those who might be sources of infection and by serving as a reminder for personnel to wash their hands and use medically aseptic precautions. Many kinds of infections do not require isolation in a private room. However, if the client uses poor hygiene or if it would be difficult to separate the client and his personal items from a person sharing the room, a private room is preferable. On the door or wall outside the client's room, the nurse posts a card listing the precautions for the client's isolation category. The card is a handy reference for health care personnel and visitors and alerts anyone who might enter the room accidentally that special precautions must be followed.

The protective environment should contain handwashing, bathing, and toilet facilities. Soap and antiseptic solutions are made available. Personnel and visitors should wash their hands before coming to the client's bedside and again before leaving the room.

When toilet facilities are available, there is no need for portable commodes or special precautions in transporting bedpans, urinals, and emesis basins. Isolation supplies can be stored in an anteroom between the room and hallway or in a special isolation cart in the hallway (Fig. 33-2). The nurse keeps ample supplies of gowns, masks, and gloves in the storage area.

The nurse makes certain that each isolation room contains a special impervious bag for soiled or contaminated linen in addition to a trash container with plastic liners. These receptacles prevent transmission of microorganisms by preventing seepage to and soiling of the outside surface. If a client requires blood

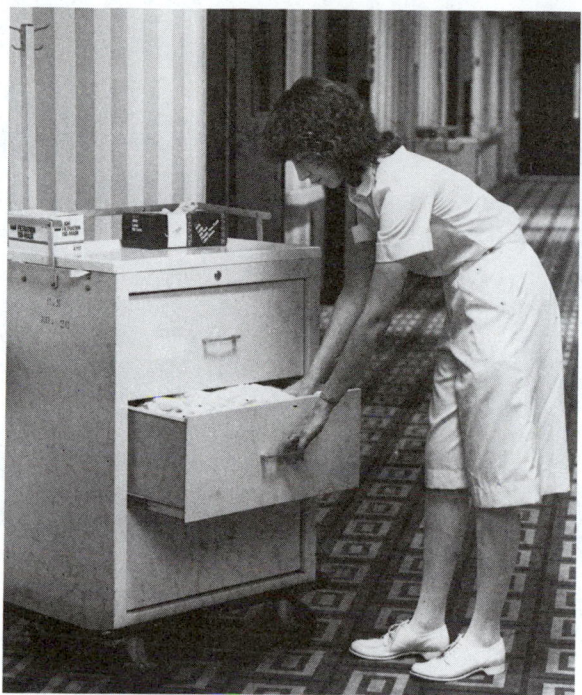

Fig. 33-2 The nurse keeps a supply of gowns, masks, and gloves in a portable isolation unit.

or body fluid precautions, a disposable container should be available in the room to discard used needles and syringes.

The nurse should avoid taking any article or piece of equipment into a client's room that is to be reused outside the isolation area. If such an article becomes contaminated with infected material, it must be discarded or disinfected and sterilized. For this reason many hospitals use disposable dishes for clients receiving protective asepsis. (No special precautions are necessary for china or glass dishes unless they are visibly contaminated with infective material.) A nurse also keeps the client's chart outside at the nurses' station or on the isolation cart. Equipment such as a sphygmomanometer, stethoscope, or other examination devices should be left in the client's room until protective aseptic precautions are no longer required.

GOWNS. The primary reason for gowning is to prevent soiling of clothing during contact with the client. Gowns protect health care personnel and visitors from coming in contact with infected material and also protect clients from organisms on other persons' clothing. Gowns prevent cross-contamination in instances such as changing the linen of a client who has infectious diarrhea or changing dressings for a wound with purulent drainage.

Isolation gowns open at the back and have ties at the neck and waist to keep the gown closed and se-cure. A gown should be long enough to cover all outer garments. Long sleeves with tight-fitting cuffs provide added protection. There is no special technique for donning a clean gown as long as it is fastened securely.

Occasionally the nurse reuses an isolation gown, for example, in the nursery or special isolation unit. If a gown is to be reused, the inside and ties must remain clean. First the waist ties are untied, and then the hands are washed. The neck ties are untied, allowing the gown to fall gently from the shoulders. Care should be taken to remove the hands from the sleeves without touching the outside of the gown. The sleeves should not be allowed to turn inside out. The gown is held inside at the shoulder seams and folded in half with the outside surfaces touching. This keeps the inside surface clean.

To don a previously worn gown, the nurse should grasp it at the top in the inside, with the outside facing away (Fig. 33-3, *A*). The hands are carefully slid into the sleeves (Fig. 33-3, *B*). If the hand cannot move through the cuff, the sleeve should be pulled over the hand with the opposite hand (Fig. 33-3, *C*), which is still covered by the sleeve. A contaminated surface can touch another contaminated surface, but a clean surface must not touch a contaminated one. Once the gown is on, the neck ties should be fastened securely (Fig. 33-3, *D*). If hands become contaminated by touching the gown, they should be washed before the gown is tied. To prevent hand contamination, a colleague should tie the waistbands.

GLOVES. Gloves prevent the transmission of pathogens by direct and indirect contact. The CDC (Williams, 1983) cites three reasons for wearing gloves:

1. Reduces possibility of personnel coming in contact with infectious organisms that infect clients (for example, handling contaminated dressings, suctioning the airway of a client with oral herpes simplex infection, cleaning an incontinent client with hepatitis)
2. Reduces likelihood that personnel will transmit their own endogenous flora to clients
3. Reduces possibility that personnel will become transiently colonized with microorganisms that can be transmitted to other clients (Transient colonization can usually be prevented with handwashing.)

Nurses apply gloves when there is risk of handling infected material. In most cases disposable, single-use gloves are worn. After coming in contact with any infected material, the nurse should change gloves if the client's care is not completed. However, if the nurse's actions will not involve more contact with the client, reapplying gloves is unnecessary.

Family members frequently believe that they can

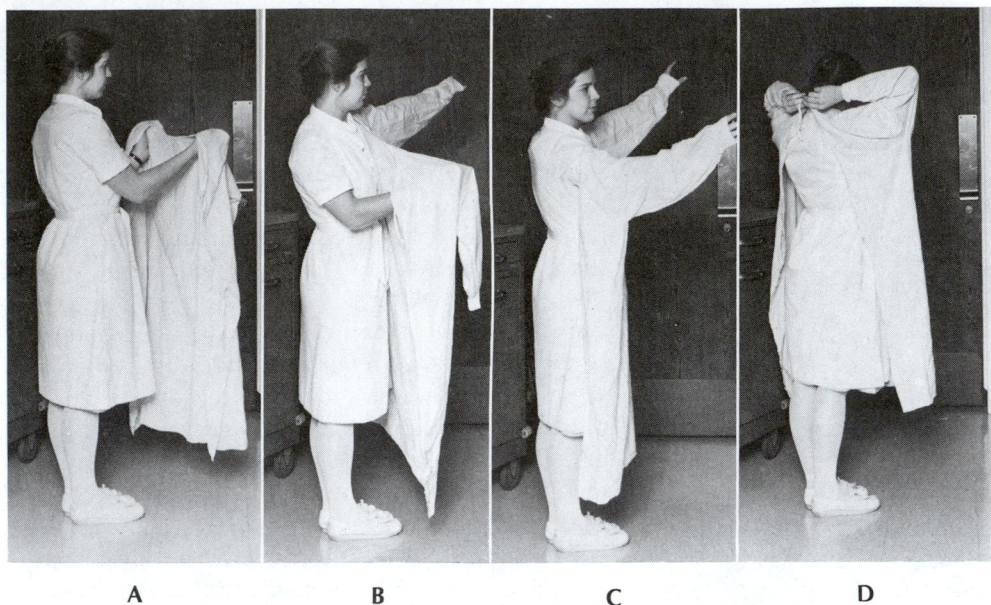

Fig. 33-3 Donning a sterile gown (see text for description).

touch any object once they have applied gloves. The nurse should explain that gloves can also become contaminated after touching infected material or another contaminated object.

MASKS. A mask protects a nurse from inhaling microorganisms from a client's respiratory tract and prevents the transmission of pathogens from the nurse's respiratory tract. The mask protects a wearer from inhaling large-particle aerosols that travel short distances (3 feet) and small-particle droplet nuclei that remain suspended in the air and travel longer distances. At times a client who is susceptible to infection wears a mask to prevent inhalation of pathogens. Clients receiving respiratory precautions who are transported outside their rooms should wear masks during transit to protect other clients and personnel.

According to the CDC, masks may prevent the transmission of infections by direct contact with mucous membranes (Williams, 1983). The presence of a mask discourages the wearer from touching the eyes, nose, or mouth.

A properly applied mask fits snugly over the mouth and nose so pathogens cannot enter or escape through the sides. If a person wears glasses, the top edge of the mask fits below the glasses so they will not cloud over as the person exhales. A mask that has become moist is ineffective and should be discarded. A mask should never be reused. A safe rule is to change a mask every hour. Clients and family members should be warned that a mask can cause a sensation of smothering. If family members become uncomfortable, they should leave the room and discard the mask.

DELIVERING CARE IN AN ISOLATION ROOM. It is important for the nurse to remain aware of medical aseptic technique while working with a client in a protected environment. If the nurse brings any article into the room or exposes an article to infected material and then touches or removes the article, the risk of transmitting infection to other clients or personnel is increased.

During the administration of medications the medication cart or tray remains outside the client's room. The nurse takes the medication into the room in a cup or its individual wrapper. The nurse need not wear a gown if the isolation precautions do not call for it or if direct client contact is avoided. After the client takes the medication, the cup or wrapper should be discarded in the plastic-lined receptacle.

Before administering injections the nurse prepares the syringe in the medication room. Since direct contact is needed during administration, the nurse wears a gown into the client's room except with respiratory infection. In most agencies, disposable needles and syringes are used. Otherwise, reusable syringes, such as a Tubex (see Chapter 32), are disposed of like any other contaminated reusable object. After administering the injection the nurse discards the contaminated needle and syringe into the appropriate container in the client's room. The nurse never discards needles or syringes into the wastebasket. When containers are not available in the client's room, it is proper for the nurse to carry the syringe and needle in a clean paper towel to the medication room for disposal, although this increases the risk of cross-infection. After administering any medication the nurse washes her hands before leaving the client's room and then records the medication.

When hygiene is administered to a client, the gown should not become wet. Carrying a washbasin against the gown or leaning against a wet bedside table soils the gown and provides a direct path for microorganisms to spread to the nurse's uniform. After the gown is removed, anything that comes in contact with the wet uniform, such as fingers or supplies, will be contaminated as well.

The nurse attempts to keep all equipment for assessing vital signs, such as the stethoscope, thermometer, and sphygmomanometer, in the client's room for the duration of protective asepsis. If this is not possible, the nurse uses precautions to prevent cross-contamination. The nurse carries a clean blood pressure cuff into the room and places it on a clean surface such as a paper towel. The client dons a clean short-sleeved gown that covers the arm above the antecubital fossa. The nurse applies the cuff over the thin gown to prevent contact with the client's skin. After measuring the blood pressure, the nurse removes the cuff and returns it to the clean surface before touching the client or any contaminated article. Then the nurse can safely take the cuff out of the room after handwashing.

A stethoscope can also be worn in and out of an isolation room as long as the nurse does not remove the stethoscope and place it on a contaminated surface. After assessing vital signs, the nurse washes the diaphragm or bell with the appropriate disinfectant solution.

If a gown and gloves must be worn while in the client's room, the nurse cannot wear a wristwatch to measure vital signs. The gown's cuffs are to be worn down to the wrist. If the watch fits over the cuff, it will become contaminated. Likewise, if the nurse pushes the cuff up to view the watch, palpates the client's pulse, and then lowers the cuff over the watch, the hand can contaminate the watch. To avoid cross-infection the nurse carries the watch to the client's bedside and places it on a clean paper towel within view. After assessing pulse and respirations the nurse removes the gown and gloves, washes her hands, and picks up the watch by grasping the clean surface of the towel. Once the towel is discarded, the nurse can put on the watch while leaving the client's room.

SPECIMEN COLLECTION. A client with an infectious disease may require numerous laboratory studies. Body fluids and secretions suspected of containing infectious organisms are collected for culture and sensitivity tests. The specimen is placed in a special medium that promotes the growth of organisms. A laboratory technologist then identifies the type of microorganisms growing in the culture. Additional test results indicate the antibiotics to which the organisms are resistant or sensitive. The sensivity reports determine which antibiotics will be used in the client's treatment.

The nurse obtains all culture specimens with sterile equipment. Collecting fresh material from the site of infection, as in the case of wound drainage, ensures that the specimen will not be contaminated by neighboring microbes. All specimen containers should be sealed tightly to prevent spillage and contamination of the outside of the container. Table 33-7 describes the techniques for collecting specimens from the client receiving protective asepsis. In each case a clean container remains outside the client's room or on a clean paper towel in the client's bathroom. After the specimens are transferred to containers, the nurse labels each specimen properly with the client's name, the type of specimen, and the type of protective asepsis. In some institutions nurses place the specimen containers in impervious bags before transporting them to the laboratory.

BAGGING ARTICLES. The nurse uses special bagging procedures for removing contaminated items from the client's environment. Bagging articles prevents accidental exposure of personnel to contaminated articles and prevents contamination of the surrounding environment.

The CDC recommends that a single bag is adequate for discarding or wrapping items if the bag is impervious and sturdy and if the article can be placed in the bag without contaminating the outside of the bag (Williams, 1983). The nurse typically discards reusable equipment such as stethoscopes, forceps, or suction bottles in single bags. The CDC recommends double bagging if it is impossible to prevent contamination of the bag's outer surface.

When trash containers or linen bags become filled, the proper method for disposal is double bagging. To double bag an article such as linen, the nurse puts on a gown to enter the client's room. The nurse places all soiled linen within a single linen bag and then ties the top securely (Fig. 33-4, *A*). A second nurse stands outside the room with a clean bag to receive the linen (Fig. 33-4, *B*). The clean bag may bear a special marking for isolation or be color coded to alert laundry workers to its contents. The nurse outside the room holds the clean bag by folding the top edges back to form a cuff over her hands. As the opening of the bag is separated to receive the contaminated bag, the nurse in the room places her hand inside the clean bag to hold the clean bag open fully so the contaminated bag can easily be dropped into it (Fig. 33-4, *C*). The object is to avoid allowing the contaminated

TABLE 33-7

Specimen Collection Techniques

Specimen Source	Amount Needed*	Collection Device*	Specimen Collection and Transfer
Wound	As much as possible (after cleaning skin to remove flora)	Cotton-tipped swab or syringe	Have clean test tube or culturette tube on clean paper towel. After swabbing center of wound site, grasp collection tube by holding it with paper towel. Carefully insert swab without touching outside of tube. After washing hands and securing tube's top, transfer tube into bag held by nurse outside room.
Blood	10 ml per culture bottle, from two different venipuncture sites	Syringe and culture media bottles	Perform venipuncture at two different sites to decrease likelihood of both specimens being contaminated by skin flora. Have second nurse at client's door holding culture bottles and swabbing off bottletops with alcohol. Change needles after venipuncture. Inject 10 ml of blood into each bottle. Nurse at doorway secures tops of bottles, labels specimens, and sends to laboratory.
Stool	Small amount, approximate size of a walnut	Clean cup with seal top (not necessary to be sterile) and tongue blade	Place cup on clean paper towel in client's bathroom. Using tongue blade, collect needed amount of feces from client's bedpan. Transfer feces to cup without touching cup's outside surface. Wash hands and place seal on cup. Transfer specimen into clean bag held by nurse outside room.
Urine	1-5 ml	Syringe and sterile cup	Place cup or tube on clean towel in client's bathrom. Use syringe to collect specimen if client has a Foley catheter. Have client follow procedure to obtain a clean voided specimen (see Chapter 39) if not catheterized. Transfer urine into sterile container either by injecting urine from syringe or pouring it from used container. Wash hands and secure top of container. Transfer specimen into clean bag held by nurse outside room.

*Agency policies may differ on type of containers and amount of specimen material required.

bag to touch the clean bag's outer edge. The nurse outside the room secures the outer bag and sends the contents to the laundry, making certain that the bag is properly labeled. The outside nurse also hands the nurse inside the room a new bag to collect soiled linen.

Double bagging can be used for any type of article. The agency's policy should be consulted for the proper procedure.

REMOVING PROTECTIVE CLOTHING. The nurse removes used gloves, mask, and gown before leaving the isolation room. The gloves should be removed first because they are more likely to be contaminated.

If the nurse unties a gown with gloves still on, there is a good chance of contaminating hair or a portion of the uniform. When gloves are pulled off, the cuff should be grasped with the other gloved hand and pulled off, turning the glove inside out. With the ungloved hand the nurse tucks the fingers inside the cuff of the remaining glove and pulls it off, turning the glove inside out. The gloves are discarded in a plastic-lined receptable. Masks are usually disposable and made of a specially prepared paper or cotton fiber. The wearer removes the mask and discards it in a plastic-lined receptacle.

Linen gowns should be disposed of in the special

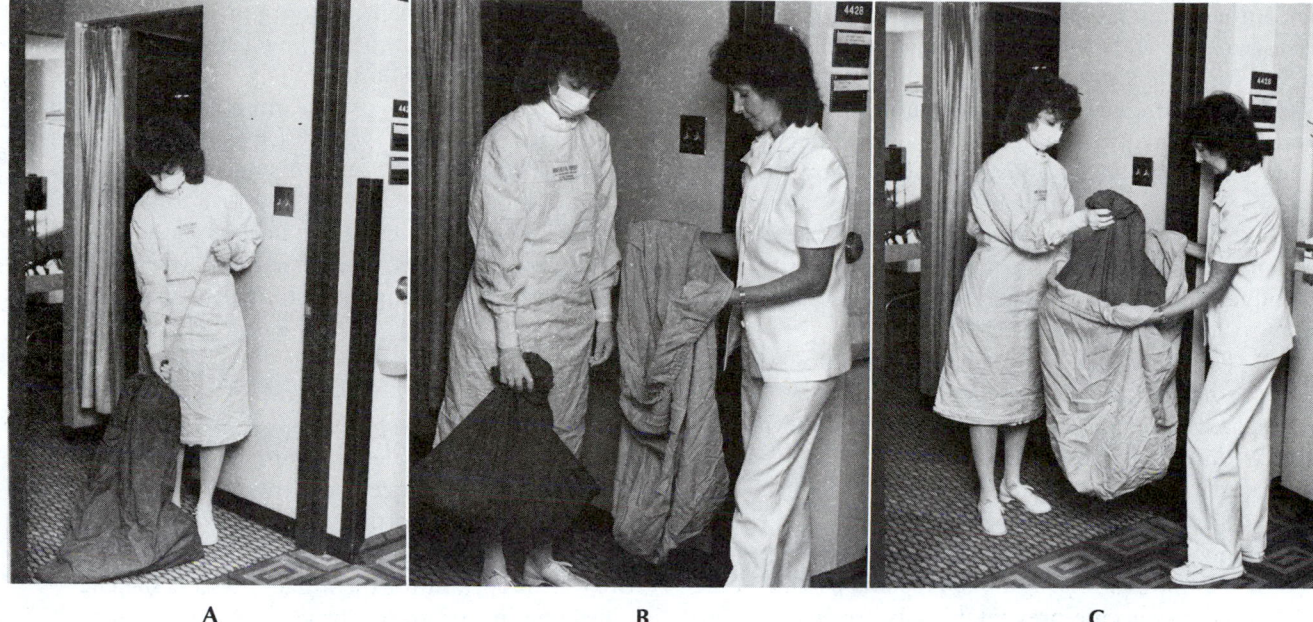

A **B** **C**

Fig. 33-4 **A,** The nurse secures a linen bag. **B,** A nurse standing outside the client's room receives the soiled linen bag. **C,** The nurse drops the contaminated bag into the clean bag.

linen hampers in the client's room. Paper gowns may be discarded in special trash containers. The nurse should never leave a client's room while wearing an isolation gown. When the gown is taken off, it should be turned inside out so hands and clothing do not come in contact with the outside contaminated surface. After the gown is discarded, hands should be washed thoroughly.

TRANSPORTING CLIENTS. Clients infected with virulent organisms should leave their rooms only for essential purposes such as diagnostic procedures or surgery. Before transferring the client to a wheelchair or stretcher, the nurse gives the client a clean gown and an isolation gown to serve as a robe. A client who is infected by an organism transmitted via the respiratory tract must also wear a mask. Personnel transporting the client should also wear masks and gowns as needed.

Unless the client is unable to walk, a wheelchair or stretcher should not be brought into the room. If this is impossible, the nurse must be sure to have the equipment disinfected once the client returns to the room. An extra layer of sheets may be used to cover the stretcher or seat of the wheelchair.

Personnel in diagnostic areas or the operating room should be notified that the client is receiving protective asepsis before arrival. The nurse records the type of isolation on the client's chart and explains to the client how to avoid transmitting infection during transport.

ROLE OF THE INFECTION CONTROL NURSE

Many hospitals employ nurses who are specially trained in the area of infection control. These nurses are responsible for advising hospital personnel on safe aseptic practices and for monitoring infection outbreaks within the hospital. The specific duties of an infection control nurse include the following:

1. Providing staff education on infection control
2. Reviewing infection control policies and procedures
3. Screening clients' laboratory reports for culture results
4. Screening client records for incidence of community-acquired infections
5. Gathering statistics regarding epidemiology of nosocomial infections
6. Notifying public health department of incidence of infections
7. Conferring with support services such as housekeeping and the dietary department
8. Educating clients and their families

An infection control nurse can be a valuable resource for controlling the incidence of nosocomial infections (Nodolny, 1980).

INFECTION CONTROL IN HOSPITAL PERSONNEL

Hospital workers are exposed continually to infectious microorganisms. An employee who becomes ill can expose susceptible clients to any of a number of infectious diseases. For these reasons the CDC has identified the following elements of a personnel health service that will assist in infection control.

1. *Placement evaluation.* A health assessment evaluates an employee's risk for acquiring or transmitting an infectious disease in the place of employment. An immunization history, history of previous infectious disease, and a physical examination determine whether an employee is a carrier of a disease (for example, tuberculosis) or has any condition (for example, immunodeficiency) that increases susceptibility to infection.

2. *Personnel health and safety education.* A hospital's health service should plan frequent in-service programs to acquaint personnel with the policies and procedures for infection control. An infection control nurse can coordinate such an effort. Written policies and guidelines should be provided for all levels of personnel.

3. *Immunization programs.* Hospital personnel are exposed to vaccine-preventable diseases such as rubella and hepatitis B because of contact with clients or the infected material from clients. An immunization program safeguards personnel and protects clients from becoming infected by personnel. It is especially important to immunize employees who work in high-risk areas. For example, nurses working in intensive care units are more susceptible to hepatitis B because they frequently administer blood. Nurses working in obstetric clinics should be immunized against rubella to protect pregnant clients.

4. *Work restrictions and control of job-related illnesses.* When an employee is exposed to an infectious disease, it is up to the health service to determine whether the employee can continue working. The hospital has the responsibility of preventing the spread of infection to clients and employees. It may become necessary to exclude an employee from direct client contact.

5. *Health counseling.* Hospital personnel should know about infection risks. Personnel with certain clinical conditions require health counseling. Female employees who are pregnant or who might become pregnant should know about risks to the fetus from work assignments and measures to reduce these risks.

Surgical Asepsis

Surgical asepsis requires more stringent precautions than medical asepsis. The nurse working with a sterile field or with sterile equipment must understand that the slightest break in technique results in contamination. Surgical asepsis requires the absence of all microorganisms, including pathogens and spores, from an object. The nurse also practices surgical asep-

sis in an effort to keep microorganisms away from an area, for example, when filling a syringe or changing a dressing on a wound.

Although surgical asepsis is commonly practiced in the operating room, labor and delivery area, and major diagnostic areas, the nurse also uses surgical aseptic techniques at the client's bedside, for example, when inserting intravenous or urinary catheters, administering injections, suctioning the tracheobronchial airway, and reapplying sterile dressings.

Assessment

Because surgical asepsis requires exact techniques, the nurse must be able to ensure the client's cooperation. If a client accidentally raises a hand and touches a sterile field during a dressing change, the nurse will have to repeat the entire procedure. Therefore it is important for the nurse to assess the client's understanding of sterile procedure and to identify whether special precautions are necessary to prevent contamination during procedures.

CLIENT KNOWLEDGE

Often clients are reluctant to move or touch objects during a sterile procedure because of fear of interfering or of experiencing pain. Clients rarely understand that sterile equipment cannot be touched by unsterile objects or even what an unsterile object is.

The nurse determines if a client has undergone a sterile procedure in the past. If not, the nurse explains how the procedure is to be performed and what the client can do to avoid contaminating sterile objects:

1. Avoiding sudden movements of body parts covered by sterile drapes
2. Refraining from touching sterile supplies, drapes, or the nurse's sterile gloves and gown
3. Avoiding coughing, sneezing, or talking over a sterile area

PRECAUTIONS

Certain sterile procedures may last a long time. The nurse must assess the client's needs and anticipate any factors that may disrupt a procedure. If a client is in pain, the nurse tries to administer analgesics no more than half an hour before a sterile procedure begins. If the client has an urge to defecate or urinate, measures are taken to care for elimination needs.

Often clients must assume relatively uncomfortable positions during sterile procedures. The nurse assesses the client's ability to assume such positions without distress. For example, a client with respiratory problems may have difficulty lying flat or leaning over. The nurse helps the client assume the most comfortable position that still allows access to a body part.

The client's condition may result in actions or events that cause contamination of a sterile field. For example, the client with a respiratory infection can easily transmit organisms by coughing or breathing. The nurse anticipates such a problem and offers the client a mask during a procedure. For the client with a colostomy or ileostomy, the nurse determines whether the bag is full and either changes or empties it to prevent leakage of contaminating contents.

Principles of Surgical Asepsis

When beginning a surgically aseptic procedure, the nurse follows certain principles to ensure the maintenance of asepsis. If the skin is broken as a result of trauma, disease, or an invasive procedure or if the nurse introduces an object such as a needle or catheter into a body cavity normally free of microorganisms, the nurse uses surgical aseptic principles. Failure to follow each principle conscientiously endangers the client, placing him at risk for an infection. The following principles are important.

1. *A sterile object remains sterile only when touched by another sterile object.* This principle guides the nurse in where to place sterile objects and how to handle them. Sterile touching sterile remains sterile; for example, sterile gloves are worn or sterile forceps are used to handle objects on a sterile field. Sterile touching clean becomes contaminated; for example, if the tip of a syringe or other sterile object touches the surface of a clean disposable glove, the object is contaminated. Sterile touching contaminated becomes contaminated; for example, when the nurse touches a sterile object with an ungloved hand, the object is contaminated. Sterile touching questionable is considered contaminated; for example, when a tear or break in the covering of a sterile object is found, it is discarded regardless of whether the object itself appears untouched.

2. *A sterile object or field out of the range of vision or held below a person's waist is contaminated.* Nurses never turn their backs on a sterile tray or leave it unattended. Contamination can occur accidentally by a dangling piece of clothing, falling hair, or an unknowing client touching a sterile object. If it is necessary to leave a room, the nurse covers a sterile tray with a sterile towel or drape. Any object held below waist level is considered contaminated because it cannot be viewed at all times. Sterile objects should be kept in front with hands as close together as possible.

3. *A sterile object or field becomes contaminated by microorganisms transported to it through the air.* The nurse avoids activities that may create air cur-

rents, such as excessive movements or rearranging linen once a sterile object or field becomes exposed. When sterile packages are being opened, it is important to minimize the number of people walking into the area. Microorganisms also travel by droplet through the air. No one should talk, laugh, sneeze, or cough over a sterile field or when gathering and using sterile equipment. When opening a tray and adding sterile equipment, the nurse should wear a mask. A nurse with a cold or other respiratory ailment should never perform sterile procedures unless she wears a double mask. Microorganisms traveling through the air can fall on sterile items or fields if the nurse reaches over the work area. When opening sterile packages, the nurse holds the item or piece of equipment as close as possible to the sterile field without touching the sterile surface. Minimal movement or rearranging of sterile items also reduces contamination by air transmission.

4. *A sterile object or field becomes contaminated by capillary action when a sterile surface comes in contact with a wet contaminated surface.* Moisture seeps through a sterile package's protective covering, allowing microorganisms to travel to the sterile object. Whenever stored sterile packages become wet, the nurse discards the objects immediately or sends the equipment for resterilization. When working with a sterile field or tray, the nurse may have to pour sterile solutions. Any spill can be a source of contamination unless the object or field rests on a sterile surface that cannot be penetrated by moisture. Urinary catheterization trays contain sterile supplies that rest in a sterile plastic container. In this example sterile solutions spilled within the container will not contaminate the catheter or other objects. In contrast, if a nurse places a piece of sterile gauze in its wrapper on a client's bedside table and the table surface is wet, the gauze is considered contaminated.

5. *Fluid flows in the direction of gravity.* A sterile object becomes contaminated if gravity causes a contaminated liquid to flow over the object's surface. In some institutions the nurse uses forceps to transfer sterile objects to a sterile tray or field. Often the forceps are stored in a container of disinfectant solution. The nurse always holds the tips of wet forceps down. Should the nurse raise the tips up, fluid would flow toward the hands and become contaminated. Then, as the nurse lowered the forceps, the contaminated fluid would travel down to contaminate the tips. The forceps could no longer be used for transferring sterile objects. For this reason many institutions use dry disposable forceps. The same principle applies to the surgical hand scrub. In contrast to basic handwashing, the surgical nurse holds the hands above the elbows during the surgical hand scrub. This allows wa-

ter to flow downward without contaminating the nurse's hands and fingers. The principle of water flow by gravity is also the reason for drying from fingers to elbows with hands held up, after the scrub.

6. *The edges of a sterile field or container are considered to be contaminated.* Frequently a nurse places sterile objects on a sterile towel or drape. Since the edge of the drape touches an unsterile surface, such as a table or bed linen, a 2.5 cm (1-inch) border around the drape is considered contaminated. The edges of sterile containers become exposed to air once they are open and are thus contaminated. After a sterile needle is removed from its protective cap, or after forceps are removed from a container, the objects must not touch the container's edge. The lip of an opened bottle of solution also becomes contaminated once it is exposed to the air. When pouring a sterile liquid, the nurse first pours a small amount of solution and discards it. The solution washes away any microorganisms on the bottle lip. Then the nurse pours a second time to fill a container with the desired amount of solution.

Performing Sterile Procedures

All the equipment that will be needed should be assembled before a procedure. It is important to anticipate what will be required so leaving equipment unattended will not be necessary. A few extra supplies should be available in case objects inadvertently become contaminated. Before the sterile procedure, each step should be explained so the client can cooperate fully. Another nurse should be in attendance during the procedure in case assistance in acquiring supplies is needed.

If an object becomes contaminated during the procedure, the nurse should not hesitate to discard it. An ounce of prevention is worth a pound of cure when performing any sterile procedure.

Surgical Aseptic Technique

When working in areas such as the operating room and delivery room, the nurse follows a series of steps to maintain sterile technique. The nurse first applies a mask and cap, then washes her hands, and finally dons a sterile gown and gloves. If the nurse is working in a general care area, handwashing and donning sterile gloves may be the only procedures followed. Special surgical aseptic techniques are used for preparing sterile equipment such as drapes and sterile supplies.

DONNING AND REMOVING CAPS AND MASKS

For a sterile procedure the nurse first applies a clean cap and surgical mask. Caps are made of paper or cloth. The commonly used disposable paper cap fits over the hair much like a hairnet. All of the nurse's hair must fit under the cap. Loose hair hanging over a sterile area or field results in contamination of all items on the field.

A surgical mask reduces accidental contamination of the nurse's hands and all sterile objects by droplet nuclei. A mask is useless unless it fits snugly around the face and nose. After a mask is worn for several hours, the area over the mouth and nose often becomes moist. Moisture promotes the spread of microorganisms. The nurse in the operating room must apply a second mask over the first, since removing a mask in a surgical area results in immediate contamination of surrounding objects. Procedure 33-2 describes the steps for applying a mask.

Before removing a mask and cap the nurse removes sterile gloves and washes the hands to prevent contamination of the hair, neck, and facial area. After untying the mask the nurse folds it in half with the inner surfaces together and discards it with the cap. Wadding the mask in the hands contaminates the hands.

SURGICAL HANDWASHING

Surgical handwashing requires a greater effort than in medical aseptic practice to remove microorganisms from the hands. In this technique the nurse washes a wider area, from fingertips to elbows. The duration of the scrub is from 5 to 10 minutes depending on institutional policy. The CDC does not recommend an ideal duration for a surgical scrub but does report that 5 minutes appears safe (Williams, 1983). For maximal elimination of bacteria, the nurse removes all jewelry and keeps fingernails short, clean, and free of polish. Brushes are used during scrubbing. Some experts caution that too much brushing removes outer layers of the epidermis, thereby exposing bacterial flora in the deeper skin layers. Antiseptic solutions such as iodophors, chlorhexidine, and hexachlorophene improve the removal of bacteria from the hands and lower arms. Procedure 33-3 describes the steps of the surgical handwashing procedure.

DONNING A STERILE GOWN

The nurse must wear a sterile gown in the operating room and delivery room so sterile objects can be comfortably handled with less risk of contamination. The sterile gown acts as a barrier to decrease shedding of microorganisms from skin surfaces into the air and thus prevents wound contamination. Nurses caring for clients with large open wounds or assisting physicians during major invasive procedures (for example, arterial cannulization) may also wear sterile gowns.

PROCEDURE 33-2

Donning a Surgical Mask

STEPS	RATIONALE
1. Find the top edge of the mask (usually has a thin metal strip along edge).	Pliable metal fits snugly against the bridge of the nose.
2. Hold the mask by the top two strings or loops. Tie the two top ties at the top of the back of your head with the ties above the ears (alternative: slip loops over each ear).	Position of ties at top of head provides tight fit. Ties over ears may cause irritation.

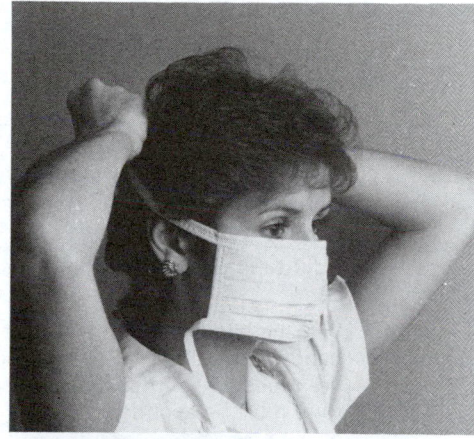

STEPS	RATIONALE
3. Tie the two lower ties snugly around the neck with the mask well under the chin.	This prevents escape of microorganisms through sides of mask as nurse talks or breathes.
4. Gently pinch the upper metal band around the bridge of the nose.	This prevents microorganisms from escaping around nose.

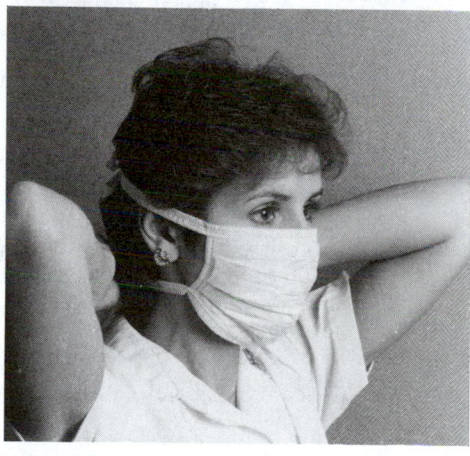

The nurse does not don a sterile gown until after surgical handwashing and after applying a mask and surgical cap. The nurse either picks up the gown from a sterile pack or has a gowned assistant hand her the gown. Only a certain portion of the gown—the area from the anterior waist to but not including the collar and the anterior surface of the sleeves—is considered sterile. The back of the gown, under the arms, the collar, the area below the waist, and the underside of the sleeves are not sterile, since the nurse cannot keep these areas in constant view and ensure their sterility. Procedure 33-4 reviews the steps for applying a gown.

DONNING STERILE GLOVES

Once the nurse completes scrubbing the hands, sterile gloves act as an additional barrier to bacterial transfer. Bacteria can multiply rapidly under gloves and can contaminate a wound or sterile object through a puncture in a glove. Use of antiseptic detergents retards bacterial growth under gloves.

There are two gloving methods: open and closed. Nurses commonly use the open method in the clinical area before changing dressings, inserting catheters, or suctioning a client's airway. Both methods are acceptable in operating rooms, but closed gloving is

PROCEDURE 33-3

Surgical Handwashing

STEPS	RATIONALE
1. Wash hands at a deep sink with foot pedals or knee controls for the dispensing of soap and control of water temperature and flow.	This minimizes risk of hands and lower arms touching dirty surface.
2. Use an appropriate antiseptic detergent such as iodophors and hexachlorophene.	Antiseptics maximally reduce the number of microorganisms on the hands.
3. Have two hand brushes and an orange stick or disposable nail file available.	Brushes are used to enhance the mechanical friction during handwashing. An orange stick facilitates cleansing under fingernails.
4. Remove all jewelry.	Jewelry harbors microorganisms.
5. Apply a face mask, making certain to cover the nose and mouth snugly.	The mask prevents escape of microorganisms into the air, which can contaminate the hands.
6. Adjust the water flow to a lukewarm temperature.	Hot water removes protective oils from the skin and increases the skin's sensitivity to soap.
7. Wet the hands and forearms liberally, keeping the hands above the level of the elbows during the entire procedure. NOTE: Nurse's scrub dress or uniform must be kept dry.	Water runs by gravity from fingertips to elbows. The hands become the cleanest part of the upper extremity. Keeping the hands elevated allows water to flow from least to most contaminated area.
8. Dispense a liberal amount of soap (2 to 5 ml) into the hands and lather hands and arms to 5 cm (2 inches) above the elbows.	Washing a wide area reduces risk of contaminating the overlying gown that the nurse later applies.
9. Clean nails with orange stick or file under running water.	This removes dirt and organic material that harbor large numbers of microorganisms.
10. Rinse hands and arms thoroughly.	Rinsing removes transient bacteria from fingers, hands, and forearms.
11. Lather hands and arms and scrub each hand with a brush for 45 seconds. Using the same brush, scrub each arm to 5 cm (2 inches) above the elbow dividing the arm into thirds: scrub each lower forearm 15 seconds, each upper forearm 15 seconds, and 5 cm above each elbow 15 seconds.	Scrubbing loosens resident bacteria that adhere to skin's surface.
12. Discard brush and rinse hands and arms thoroughly.	After touching skin, brush is considered contaminated. Rinsing removes resident bacteria.
13. Using a second brush, scrub each hand for 30 seconds. Use the same brush to scrub each arm up to the elbow by dividing the arm in half: scrub each lower forearm 15 seconds and each upper forearm 15 seconds.	A second scrubbing ensures thorough cleansing of hands and forearms. The number of resident microorganisms remaining on skin will be minimal.
14. Discard brush and rinse hands and arms thoroughly. Turn off water with foot pedal.	
15. Use a sterile towel to dry one hand thoroughly moving from fingers to elbow. Dry in a rotating motion. NOTE: Nurses wishing to apply sterile gloves for use in a regular clinical area need not use brushes or dry hands with sterile towels. Thorough lathering and friction performed twice according to procedure will ensure clean hands. In this situation the nurse may use clean paper towels for drying.	Dry from cleanest to least clean area. Drying prevents chapping and facilitates donning of gloves.
16. Repeat drying method for other hand, using a different area of the towel or a new sterile towel.	
17. Keep hands higher than elbows and away from the body.	This prevents accidental contamination.
18. Proceed into operating room or labor and delivery area.	

PROCEDURE 33-4

Donning a Sterile Gown

STEPS	RATIONALE	
1. Don a mask and cap. Carry out surgical handscrubbing for at least 5 minutes.	Scrubbing eliminates microorganisms from surface of hands. Mask and cap reduce chances of transmitting organisms to the gown by direct contact and airborne transmission.	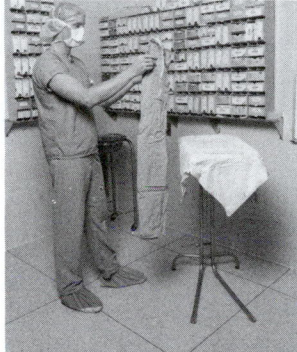
2. Pick up the gown, grasping the inside surface of the gown at the collar.	The hands are not completely sterile. The inside surface of the gown will contact the skin's surface and is thus considered contaminated.	
3. Stand away from the sterile pack and table. Hold the gown at arm's length away from your body and allow the gown to unfold by itself. Be careful not to allow the gown to touch the floor.	Contact of the outer surface of the gown with a dirty or clean surface would result in gown contamination. Shaking of the gown can cause air currents that increase the risk of contamination.	
4. Hold the gown by the inside, open shoulder seams, and insert each hand through the armholes.	The inside surface of the gown is considered contaminated.	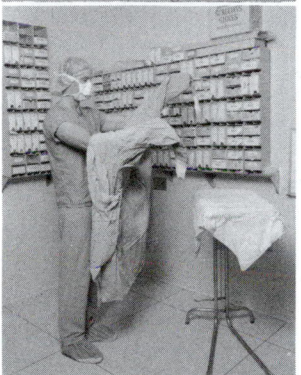
5. Keeping your upper arms in front of you at shoulder height, extend the arms toward the gown cuff. (Do not push the hands through the cuffs if using the closed glove method.)	Extension of the arms straight ahead keeps the sterile surface of the gown in view and reduces the risk of touching the floor or a portion of the body.	
6. Have a circulating nurse (considered unsterile) tie the collar securely from behind and pull the sleeves onto your arms for proper fit and comfort.	Working from behind the gowned person prevents contamination by the circulating nurse.	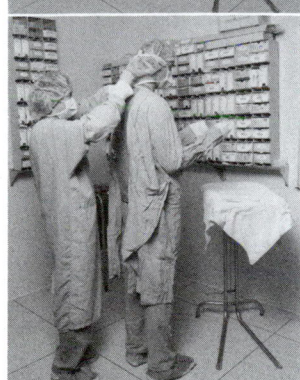
7. If the waist ties or snaps fall in front of the gown, enclose them within a sterile towel and hand the sterile towel to the circulating nurse standing behind you. (Disposable paper gowns have a special tag the circulating nurse may grasp.)	The towel provides a surface the circulating nurse can grasp without contaminating the gown.	
8. Have the circulating nurse tie or snap the waistband securely from behind, making certain the gown is completely closed.	Wrapping the gown securely around the nurse's body reduces air currents and risk of contamination.	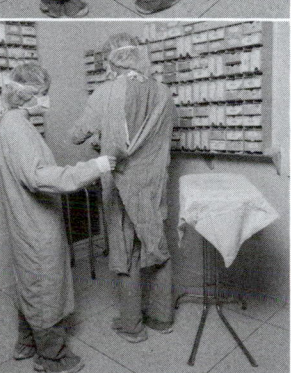

PROCEDURE 33-5

Open Gloving

STEPS	RATIONALE
1. Remove the outer package wrapper by carefully peeling apart the sides.	This prevents inner glove package from accidentally opening and touching contaminated objects.
2. Grasp the inner package and lay it on a clean flat surface just above waist level. Open the package, keeping the gloves on the wrapper's inside surface.	A sterile object held below a person's waist is considered contaminated. The inner surface of the glove package is considered sterile.
3. If gloves are not prepowdered, take the packet of powder and apply lightly to the hands over a sink or wastebasket.	Powder allows gloves to slip on easily. (Some physicians do not use powder for fear of promoting growth of microorganisms.)
4. Identify the right and left glove. Each glove has a cuff approximately 5 cm (2 inches) wide. Glove the dominant hand first.	Proper identification of gloves prevents contamination by improper fit. Gloving of the dominant hand first improves the nurse's dexterity with the procedure.
5. With the thumb and first two fingers of the nondominant hand, grasp the edge of the cuff of the glove for the dominant hand. Touch only the glove's inside surface.	The inner edge of the cuff will lie against the skin and thus is not considered sterile.
6. Carefully pull the glove over the dominant hand, leaving a cuff and being sure the cuff does not roll up the wrist. Be sure the thumb and fingers are in the proper spaces.	If the glove's outer surface touches the hand or wrist, it is contaminated.
7. With the gloved dominant hand, slip the fingers underneath the second glove's cuff.	The cuff protects the gloved fingers. Sterile touching sterile prevents glove contamination.
8. Carefully pull the second glove over the nondominant hand. Do not allow the fingers and thumb of the gloved dominant hand to touch any part of the exposed nondominant hand. Keep the thumb of the dominant hand abducted back.	Contact of gloved hand with exposed hand results in contamination.
9. Once the second glove is on, interlock the hands together. The cuffs usually fall down after application. Be sure to touch only the sterile sides.	This ensures smooth fit over fingers.

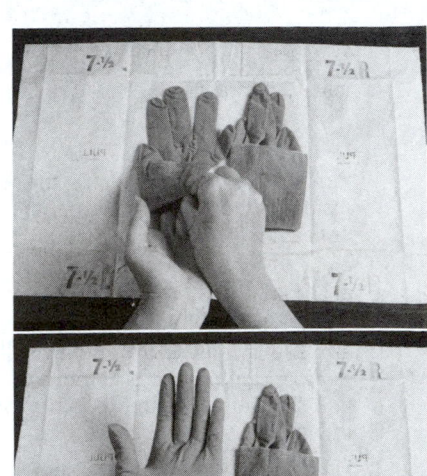
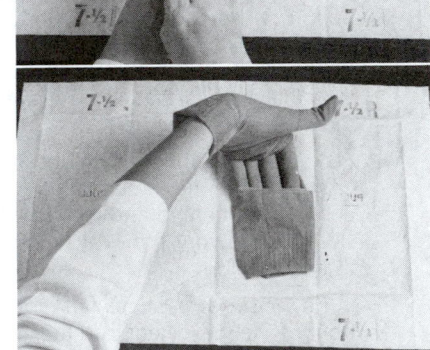
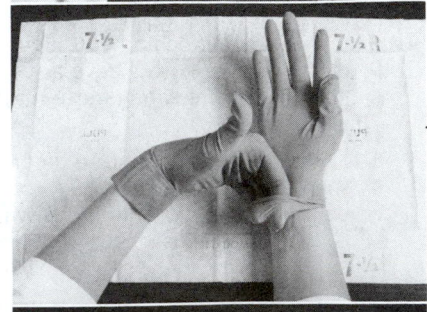
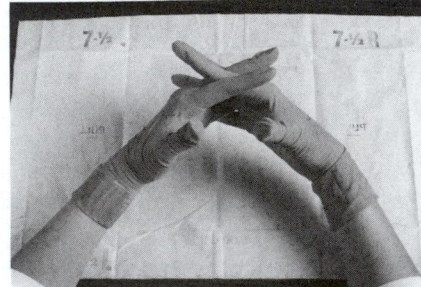

Closed Gloving

STEPS	RATIONALE	
1. Following steps 1 and 2 in the procedure for open gloving, an assistant or circulating nurse prepares the glove package.	Nurse donning gloves wears a sterile gown and cannot prepare gloves without contaminating the gown.	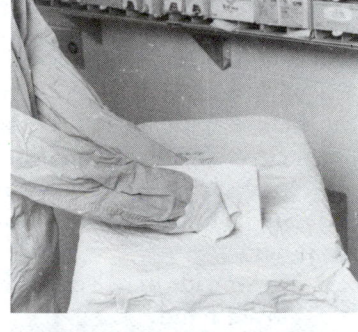
2. Keep scrubbed hands within sleeve of surgical gown at the point of the cuff seams.	This prevents bare hands from contacting sterile exterior of gown.	
3. Grasp the inside of the cuff sleeve covering the nondominant hand. With the same hand pick up the glove for the dominant hand. Place the glove palm side down on the palm of the covered dominant hand, with the glove fingers pointing toward the elbow of the dominant arm.	The gown protects the nurse's fingers. Sterile touching sterile is sterile. Positioning of the glove will allow the nurse to slip it over the gown cuff.	
4. The fingers of the covered dominant hand pinch the underside of the glove's cuff. With the covered nondominant hand, grasp the topside of the glove's cuff for the dominant hand. Pull the glove over the gown cuff and fingers of the dominant hand simultaneously.	Since the fingers do not exit through the gown's cuff, gown and glove contamination is prevented.	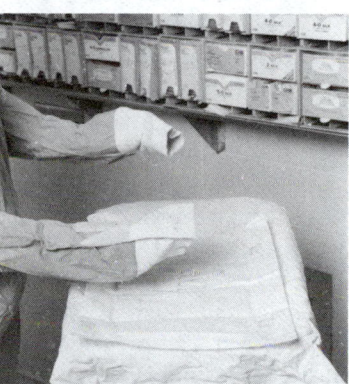
5. Carefully push the fingers into the glove and be sure the glove's cuff covers the gown's cuff.	This ensures proper fit. The glove fits over the gown cuff to provide extra protection against contamination.	
6. With the gloved dominant hand, place the opposite glove palm side down over the palm of the covered nondominant hand with the glove fingers pointing toward the elbow.	Sterile touching sterile is sterile.	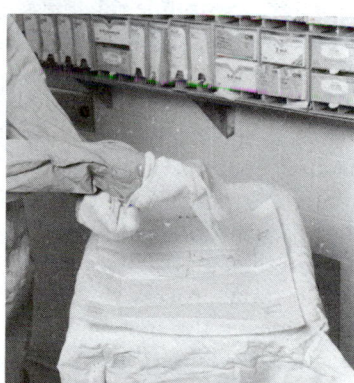
7. Repeat steps 4 and 5 for the nondominant hand.		
8. Interlock the gloved hands.	This ensures smooth fit over the fingers.	

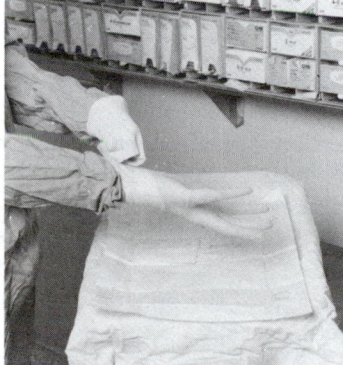 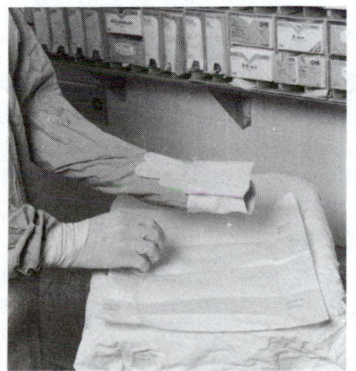 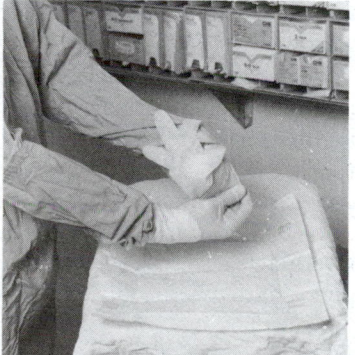

more frequently used for initial gloving and the open method for changing a contaminated glove during the operative procedure. Procedures 33-5 and 33-6 review the steps of each gloving technique.

Sterile gloves come prepackaged with labels indicating the glove size. Each nurse should learn the glove size that is most comfortable and fits best. Common sizes range from small (size 6 to 6½) to large (size 8 to 8½). The glove should not stretch so tightly over the hand that it can easily tear. However, if the glove is too loose, it will be difficult to manipulate or pick up objects and the loose rubber may snag and tear. Before applying a glove the nurse makes certain that the package is dry and intact.

After a sterile procedure the nurse disposes of gloves in the following manner to minimize hand contamination:

1. The outside of one cuff is grasped with the other gloved hand.
2. The glove is peeled off, turned inside out, and discarded in the proper receptacle.
3. The fingers of the bare hand tuck inside the remaining glove's cuff. (The outside of the glove is not touched.)
4. The glove is peeled off, turned inside out, and disposed of in the proper receptacle.

OPENING STERILE PACKAGES

Sterile items such as syringes, gauze dressing, catheters, and irrigation trays are packaged in paper or plastic containers. Some institutions wrap reusable supplies in a double thickness of linen. The wrappers are impervious to microorganisms as long as they are dry and intact. Rooms equipped with clean enclosed storage cabinets are the best place to store sterile items. Sterile supplies are never kept in the same room as dirty equipment.

Sterile supplies have dated labels or chemical tapes that indicate the date when the sterilization period expires (Fig. 33-5). The tapes change color during the sterilization process. Failure of the tapes to change color means the item is not sterile. A sterile supply or piece of equipment should never be used after the expiration date. The item is either discarded or returned to the institution's supply area for resterilization.

Before opening a sterile item the nurse washes the hands thoroughly. The nurse assembles the supplies in the work area such as the bedside or treatment room before opening packages. A bedside table or countertop provides a large, clean working area for opening items. The work area should be above waist level. Sterile supplies should not be opened in a confined space where a dirty object might fall on or strike the supplies.

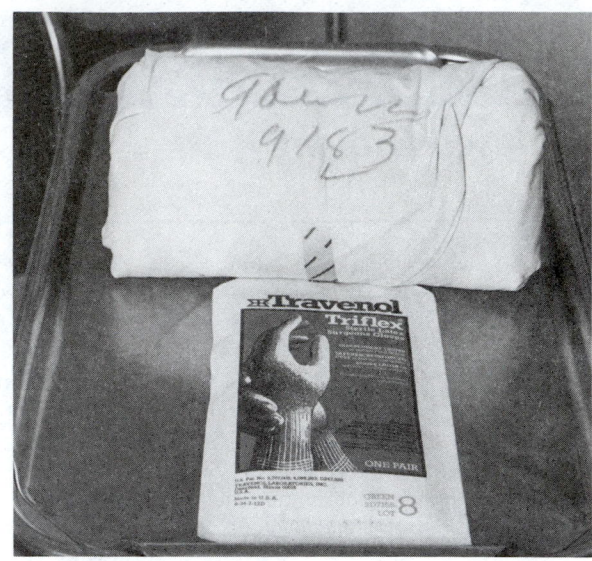

Fig. 33-5 Sterile supplies have dated labels or chemical indicator tapes that show when the sterilization period expires.

Sterile packaged items are wrapped in a way that allows opening without contaminating the contents. Large items must be placed on the work surface. Commercially packaged items are usually designed so the nurse need only tear away or separate the paper or plastic cover. The nurse should always tear the wrapper away from the body and avoid reaching over the sterile contents (Fig. 33-6). One hand can grasp the outside of the wrapper without danger of contamination. While removing wrappers, the nurse avoids touching the inside of the wrapper. Once the inside of the wrapper is contaminated, it can contaminate the sterile item if the wrapper accidentally slips backward over the item.

When opening items packaged in linen, the nurse follows a series of steps to avoid contamination:

1. The nurse removes any tape or seal indicating sterilization date.
2. The nurse grasps the outer surface of the tip of the outermost flap.
3. The nurse opens the flap away from the body, keeping the arm outstretched and away from the sterile field.
4. The nurse grasps the outside surface of the first side flap.
5. The side flap is then opened, allowing it to lie flat on the table surface. The arm is kept to the side and not over the sterile surface.
6. Steps 4 and 5 are repeated for the second side flap.
7. The nurse grasps the outside surface of the last and innermost flap.

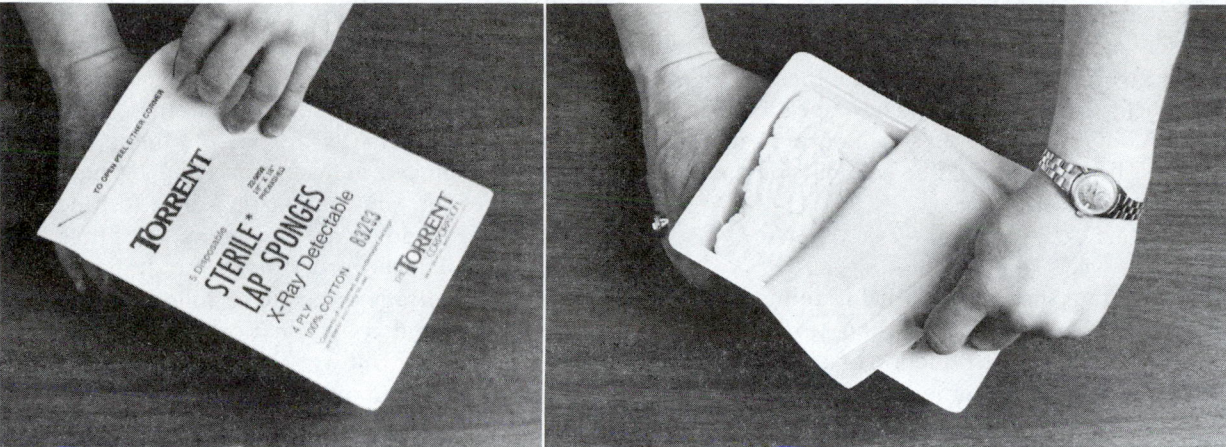

Fig. 33-6 When opening a commercially packaged sterile item, the nurse tears the wrapper away from her body.

8. The nurse stands away from the sterile package and pulls the flap back, allowing it to fall flat on the table.

9. The inner surface of the linen package (except for the 1-inch border around the edges) is sterile. The sterile field can be used to add additional sterile items. The 1-inch border can be grasped to maneuver the field on the table surface.

If the sterile supplies are not to be used immediately, the nurse can close the sterile package. In this case the nurse should touch only the wrapper's outside surface. To close a package the order of unwrapping is reversed and the nurse does not touch the inside contents or reach over the field.

To open small sterile items, the package is held in one hand while the wrapper is pulled away with the other hand. The nurse always holds a portion of the wrapper around the sterile item to avoid touching the item. Often the nurse opens items so they can be handed to a person wearing sterile gloves or transferred to a sterile field.

ADDING STERILE SUPPLIES TO A STERILE FIELD

Occasionally the nurse will add sterile supplies to a sterile field, such as a sterile container or the inside surface of a wrapper. For example, after opening a gauze pack wrapped in linen, the nurse may add sterile instruments to the field. After opening a sterile catheterization kit, the nurse may choose to add a catheter or sterile cotton balls to the kit.

To add supplies the nurse opens the item to be transferred by grasping its outside wrapper in the nondominant hand. After the wrapper is peeled over on the nondominant hand, the item is still sterile and the nurse can safely drop the item onto the sterile field. If the wrapper is long and could fall down on

the sterile field, the nurse takes the dominant hand and carefully holds the wrapper around the wrist of the nondominant hand.

When transferring sterile items, the nurse avoids flipping or throwing objects onto the sterile field. The nurse cannot control where a flipped object lands. An object that comes in contact with the edge of the sterile field must be discarded.

POURING STERILE SOLUTIONS

Often the nurse must pour sterile solutions into sterile containers. For example, before catheterizing a client, a nurse uses a sterile antiseptic solution to prepare the urethral meatus. The nurse pours the solution of choice into a container within the catheterization kit.

A bottle containing a sterile solution is sterile on the inside and contaminated on the outside, including the bottle's neck. The inside of the bottle cap is also sterile. After a cap or lid is opened, it is held in the hand or placed sterile side (inside) up on a clean surface. This means that the inside of the lid can be seen as it rests on the table surface. A bottle cap or lid should never rest sterile side down on a sterile surface because the outer edge of the cap is unsterile and would contaminate the surface. Likewise, placing a sterile cap down on an unsterile surface increases the chances of the inside of the cap becoming contaminated.

The bottle should be held with its label in the palm of the hand. This prevents the possibility of the solution wetting and fading the label. Before pouring the solution into the container the nurse pours a small amount (1 to 2 ml) into a disposable cup or plastic-lined waste receptacle. The discarded solution cleans the lip of the bottle. The edge of the bottle is kept away from the edge or inside of the receiving container. The nurse pours the solution slowly to avoid splashing, which would contaminate the underlying drape or field. The bottle should never be held so high above the container that even slow pouring will cause splashing. The bottle should be held outside the edge of the sterile field.

APPLYING STERILE DRAPES

Draping establishes a sterile field around a treatment site, such as a surgical incision, a venipuncture site, or the site for the introduction of a biopsy needle. The drape provides a larger working surface for placing sterile supplies.

Drapes are available in cloth, paper, and plastic. The ideal drape is waterproof to prevent spread of microorganisms through moisture. Many styles, shapes, and sizes of drapes are available to accommodate the different areas or body parts to be covered. For example, a drape with a hole in the center is used to cover the perineal area before a urinary catheter insertion. A long narrow drape is ideal for covering a body extremity. Sterile treatment sets such as catheter insertion trays, dressing change sets, and diagnostic sets, for example, thoracentesis and lumbar puncture trays, contain sterile drapes.

When applying sterile drapes, the nurse may use gloved or ungloved hands. Gloved hands make the procedure easier, since the nurse is able to touch the entire drape. If gloves are not worn, the nurse may touch only a 1-inch border along the drape's edges. The most important principle to follow in applying drapes is to avoid contamination—by not reaching over a drape, not allowing the drape to touch the nurse's uniform, and not allowing the drape's sterile surface to touch the client.

To apply a drape with ungloved hands, the nurse follows these steps (Fig. 33-7):

1. The nurse grasps the corner of the drape with the dominant hand, taking care that the fingers touch only the 1-inch margin at the corner.
2. The drape is then lifted straight up with one hand and allowed to unfold gently. (The nurse should not shake the drape or allow it to touch the uniform or arm.)
3. With the nondominant hand the adjacent corner of the drape is grasped and held straight.
4. The nurse approaches the area to be draped, being careful not to touch contaminated surfaces.

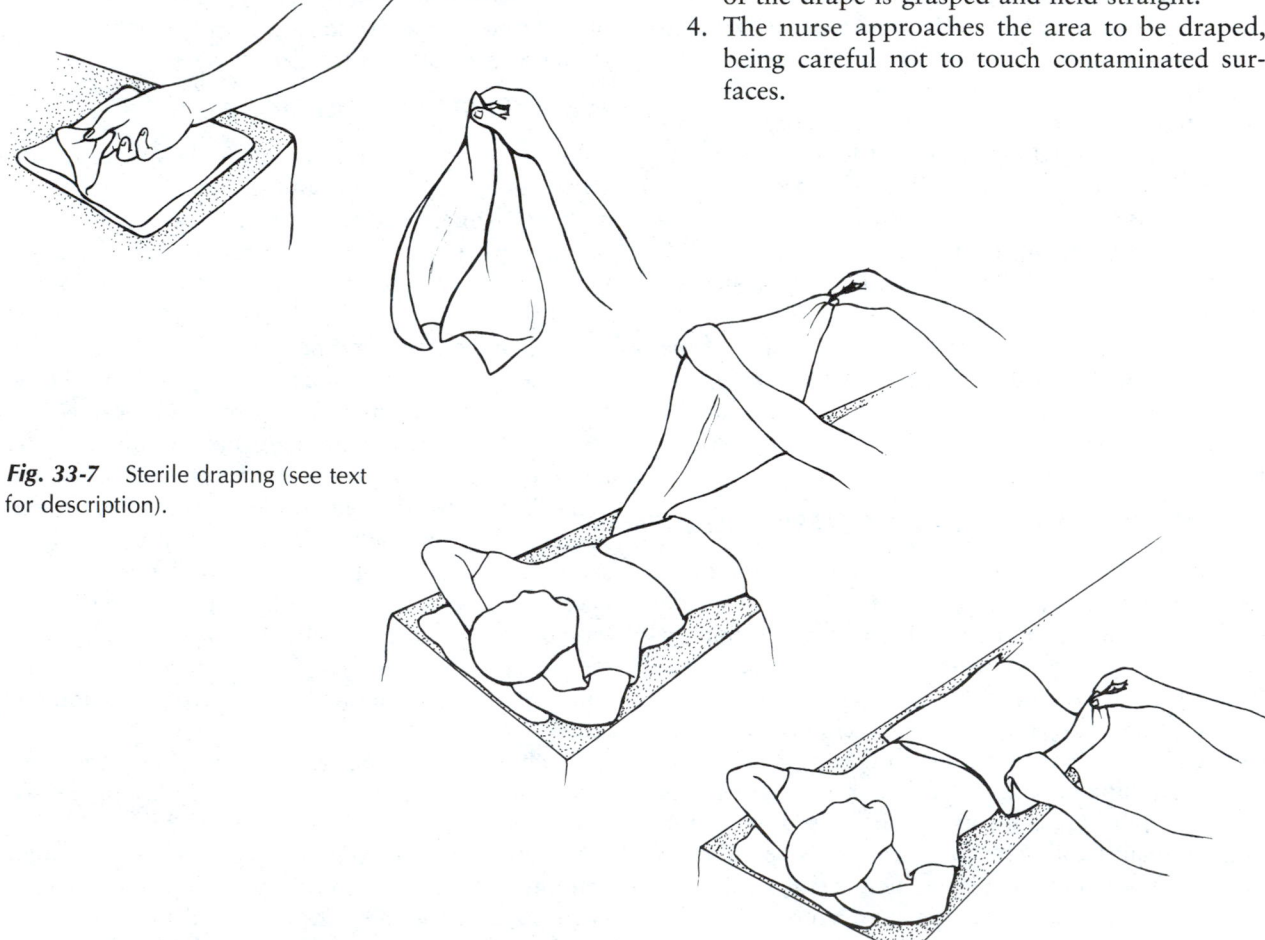

Fig. 33-7 Sterile draping (see text for description).

5. Holding the drape, the nurse positions the bottom half over the area first.
6. The nurse positions the top half last to avoid reaching over the sterile area.
7. The nurse may grasp the 1-inch border around the drape's edges to position it as needed.

When wearing gloves, the nurse protects the fingertips by enclosing them within the drape edges.

Client Education

Often clients must learn to use infection control practices at home. For example, a client may be discharged from the hospital with the task of changing a dressing or administering self-injections. A young mother learns the importance of disinfecting her baby's bottle by boiling. The client with a colostomy learns to handle and dispose of the colostomy bag without exposing family members to potentially infectious microorganisms.

Aseptic technique becomes almost second nature to the nurse practicing it daily. However, the client is less aware of the factors that promote the spread of infection or of the ways to prevent its transmission. The home environment does not always lend itself to the practice of aseptic technique. For example, because of plumbing problems a client may not have access to free-flowing water needed for good handwashing practices. Clients may not be able to afford needed sterile supplies. A nurse must often help a client improvise with the resources available to maintain hygienic techniques. For example, a client may use a laundered washcloth instead of expensive sterile gauze to wash around an open wound.

Once clients are at home, they determine their own compliance with infection control practices. It is the nurse's responsibility to educate clients about the nature of infection and the techniques to employ in preventing or controlling its spread. Useful topics the nurse can discuss in any teaching session include the following:

1. The client's susceptibility to infection
2. The chain of infection with specific reference to means of transmission
3. Basic handwashing practices (when and how)
4. Hygienic practices that minimize organism growth and spread
5. Preventive health care, for example, diet, immunizations, exercise
6. Proper methods for food handling and storage
7. Family members at risk for acquiring infections

Except for the need to administer self-injections, it is more practical for clients to learn clean, medical aseptic techniques than strict sterile techniques. Most physicians do not allow clients to return home with open wounds or conditions that require sterile procedures. Family members who must care for such a client, however, must be actively involved in the nurse's teaching plan. The nurse's efforts must be directed toward teaching clients and family members a common-sense approach for controlling and preventing infection.

Summary

In every aspect of practice the nurse encounters situations that present a risk of an infection developing or being transmitted. Knowledge of the body's normal defenses against infection helps the nurse recognize clients most at risk for acquiring infections. The nature of the infection chain is a useful concept in identifying nursing interventions for infection control.

Nurses use two types of infection control practices, medical and surgical asepsis, to prevent infection transmission. Each set of practices calls for a conscientious and knowledgeable application of infection control principles. The nurse's failure to follow these principles seriously hampers a client's recovery or maintenance of good health.

KEY CONCEPTS

✓ Normal body flora resist infection by releasing antibacterial substances and inhibiting multiplication of pathogenic microorganisms.

✓ The signs of local inflammation and infection are identical.

✓ Immunity to infection is measured by the capacity to produce antibodies in response to exposure to an antigen.

✓ An infection can develop as long as the six elements comprising the infection chain are uninterrupted.

✓ A microorganism's virulence depends on its ability to resist attack by the body's normal defenses.

✓ Microorganisms are transmitted by direct and indirect contact, by airborne spread, and by vectors and contaminated vehicles such as food and liquids.

✓ Increasing age, poor nutrition, stress, inherited conditions, chronic disease, and treatments or conditions that compromise the immune response increase a person's susceptibility to infection.

✓ The major sites for nosocomial infections include the urinary and respiratory tracts, bloodstream, and surgical or traumatic wounds.

✓ Invasive procedures, medical therapies, long hospitalization, and contact with health care personnel increase a hospitalized client's risk for acquiring a nosocomial infection.

✓ Surgical asepsis requires more stringent techniques than medical asepsis and is directed toward eliminating microorganisms on an area or object.

✓ Following aseptic principles is the key to a nurse's success in preventing clients from acquiring infections.

✓ Protective aseptic practices prevent personnel and clients from acquiring infections, as well as preventing the transmission of microorganisms to other persons.

✓ Proper cleansing requires mechanical removal of all organic material from an object or area.

✓ The nurse does not take an article into an isolation room if the article is to be used by another client.

✓ A client receiving protective asepsis is subject to sensory deprivation because of the restricted environment.

✓ Lack of handwashing is the main cause of nosocomial infections.

✓ An infection control nurse monitors the incidence of infections within an institution and provides educational and consultative services to maintain aseptic practices.

✓ If the skin is broken or if the nurse performs an invasive procedure into a body cavity normally free of microorganisms, surgical aseptic practices are enforced.

✓ A sterile object becomes contaminated by direct contact with a clean or contaminated object, by exposure to airborne microorganisms, and by contact with a wet medium containing microorganisms.

REFERENCES

Bennett, J.V.: Incidence and nature of endemic and epidemic nosocomial infections. In Bennett, J.V., and Brachman, P.S., editors: Hospital infection, Boston, 1979, Little, Brown, & Co.

Garner, J.S., and Simmons, B.P.: CDC guidelines for isolation precautions in hospitals, Infect. Control 4(4):249, 1983.

Gross, P.A., et al.: Nosocomial infection: decade-specific risk, Infect. Control 4(3):145, 1983.

Nodolny, M.D.: What does the infection control nurse do? Am. J. Nurs. 80:430, 1980.

Sencer, D.J., and Axnick, H.W.: Utilization of cost/benefit analysis in planning prevention programs, Acta Med. Scand. 576:123, 1975.

Williams, W.W.: CDC guidelines for infection control in hospital personnel, Infect. Control 4(4):325, 1983.

ADDITIONAL READINGS

Axnick, K.J.: Infection control considerations in the care of the immunosuppressed patient, Crit. Care Quarterly 3:79, 1980.

Hargiss, C.O.: The patient's environment: haven or hazard, Nurs. Clin. North Am. 15(4):671, 1980.

Hargiss, C.O., and Larson, E.: Infection control guidelines for prevention of hospital acquired infections, Am. J. Nurs. 81:2175, 1981.

Labet, C.G., and Roderick, M.A.: Infection control in the use of intravascular devices, Crit. Care Quarterly 3(4):67, 1981.

Mallison, G.F.: Decontamination, disinfection, and sterilization, Nurs. Clin. North Am. 15(4):757, 1980.

Marchiondo, K.: The very fine art of collecting culture specimens, Nursing 79 9(4):34, 1979.

Nichols, R.L.: Techniques known to prevent post-operative wound infection, J. Infect. Control 3(1):34, 1982.

Simmons, B.P.: Guidelines for prevention of surgical wound infections, Am. J. Infect. Control 11(4):133, 1983.

Werdegar, D.: Employee health, Nurs. Clin. North Am. 15(4):769, 1980.

7

The basic human needs include those for comfort and security, and the client's ability to meet these needs is often disrupted by health problems. Nursing care therefore assists clients in meeting these needs, which include the needs for physical and psychological safety, effective hygiene, sleep, and relief from pain. Using the nursing process the nurse assesses the client's comfort and safety needs and abilities to meet them, individualizes nursing diagnoses as the basis for care to meet these needs, plans and implements nursing interventions, and evaluates the results of care. Only by focusing on these needs as well as the client's other physiological and psychosocial needs can nursing care holistically assist the client to maximum wellness.

Promoting Comfort and Safety

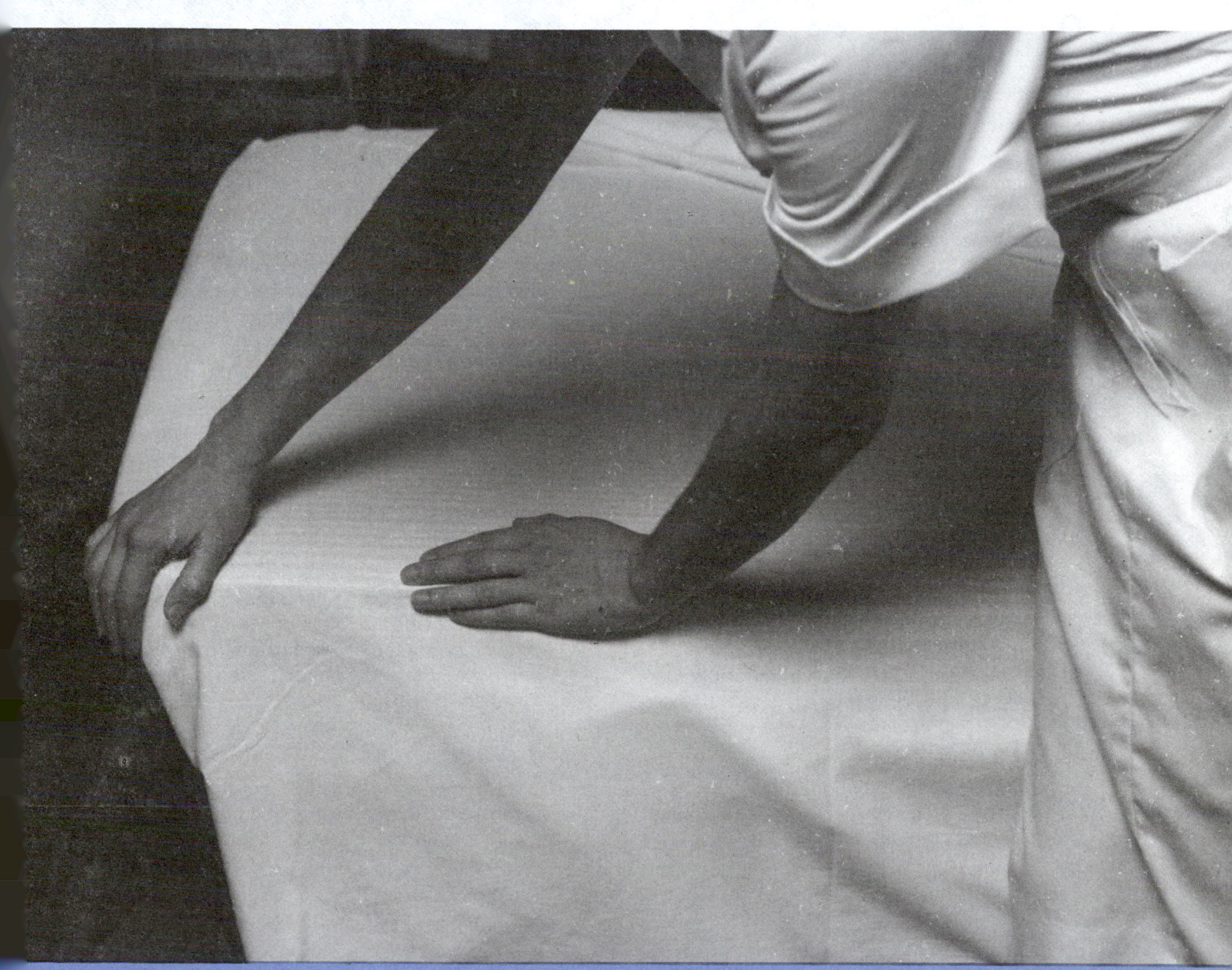

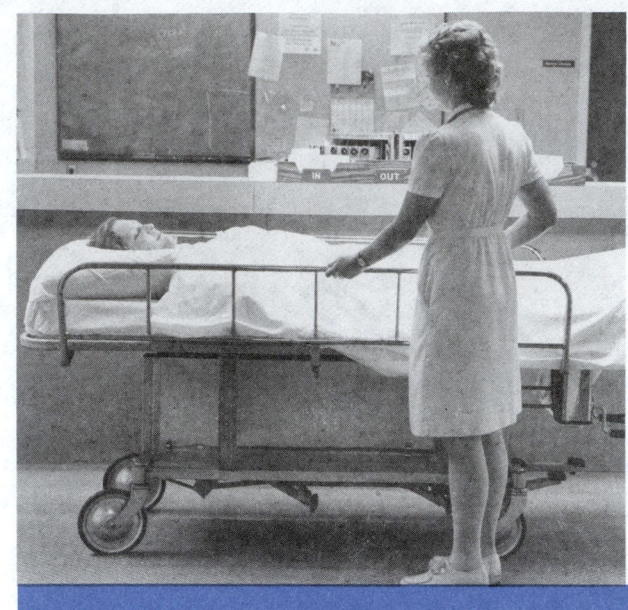

OBJECTIVES

Mastery of content in this chapter will enable the student to:

- Define the terms in the glossary.
- Describe how unmet basic physiological needs of oxygen, fluids, nutrition, and temperature can threaten a client's safety.
- Discuss methods to reduce physical hazards.
- Describe current methods to reduce the transmission of pathogens and parasites.
- Describe present methods of pollution control.
- Discuss the specific risks to safety as they pertain to the client's developmental age.
- Describe the four categories of risks in a health care agency.
- State nursing diagnoses associated with risk to a client's safety.
- Develop a nursing care plan for clients whose safety is threatened.
- Describe nursing interventions specific to the client's age for reducing risk of falls, fires, poisonings, and electrical hazards.
- Describe methods to evaluate interventions designed to maintain or promote a client's safety.

GLOSSARY

air pollution   Contamination of the environmental atmosphere with substances known as pollutants that are not normally found in the air.

carbon monoxide   Colorless, odorless, poisonous gas produced by the combustion of carbon or organic fuels.

decibel   Unit of measure of the intensity of sound.

Food and Drug Administration (FDA)   Federal agency responsible for the enforcement of federal regulations regarding the manufacture and distribution of food, drugs, and cosmetics to ensure protection against the sale of impure or dangerous substances.

food poisoning   Toxic processes resulting from the ingestion of a food contaminated by toxic substances or by bacteria containing toxins.

incident report   Confidential document that describes any client accident while the person is on the premises of a health care agency.

noise pollution   Noise level in an environment when it becomes uncomfortable to its inhabitants.

poison   Any substance that impairs health or destroys life when ingested, inhaled, or absorbed by the body in relatively small amounts.

poison control center   One of a network of facilities that provides information regarding all aspects of poisoning or intoxication, maintains records of their occurrence, and refers clients to treatment centers.

pollutant   A harmful chemical or waste material discharged into the water or atmosphere.

relative humidity   Amount of moisture in the air as compared with the maximum amount that the air could contain at the same temperature.

restraint   Device to aid the immobilization of a client or to immobilize an extremity.

water pollution   Contamination of lakes, rivers, and streams by industrial pollutants.

34 | *Safety*

Nursing care directed toward health maintenance and illness prevention involves promoting the client's safety in the community or within the health care environment, which is just as essential as meeting hygiene and nutrition needs. Protection and safety are basic to survival, and these needs continue throughout the life span.

Potential safety hazards can be obvious, such as a dark, cluttered staircase, or unseen, such as a medication error or toxic fumes from a faulty furnace. The nurse can increase the client's safety by including interventions for a safe environment within the plan of care and with every nursing procedure.

Defined broadly, an environment is all of the many factors, physical and psychosocial, that influence or affect the life and survival of the client. A safe environment in a health care agency is one that is comfortable, maintains the client's privacy, and reduces to a minimum the risks of injury, infection, and untoward effects from treatments or medications. Safety is also evaluated in the client's home, workplace or school, and neighborhood.

A safe health care environment reduces the length of treatment or hospitalization, the frequency of treatment-related accidents, the potential for lawsuits, the number of work-related injuries to personnel, and the overall cost of health services. In addition, a safe health care environment allows the professional and paraprofessional staff to function at its optimal level.

Safety in the home reduces the risk of accidents and illnesses and the subsequent need for health care service. Safety is positively correlated to health promotion: the greater the safety in a home, the greater the level of health promotion in that home.

Environmental Safety

To ensure safety for clients, the nurse must understand what contributes to a safe environment. Threats to safety are tangible and intangible. A safe environment is one in which (1) basic needs are achievable, (2) physical hazards are reduced, (3) transmission of pathogens and parasites is reduced, (4) sanitation is maintained, and (5) pollution is controlled.

Basic Needs

Meeting basic human needs is necessary for achieving safety and security needs (see Chapter 4). Frequently the basic physiological needs, including oxygen, degree of humidity, nutrition, and optimal temperature, influence a person's safety.

OXYGEN

The nurse must be aware of factors in a client's environment that decrease the amount of available oxygen and thus threaten the client. One of the most common environmental hazards affecting available oxygen is an improperly functioning furnace. A furnace that is not operating properly or is not properly vented introduces carbon monoxide into the home, workplace, school, or health care environment. *Carbon monoxide* is a colorless, odorless, poisonous gas produced by the combustion of carbon or organic fuels. Carbon monoxide binds strongly with hemoglobin, preventing the formation of oxyhemoglobin and thus reducing the supply of oxygen delivered to the tissues (see Chapter 41). A client who moves to a new residence or who has an older furnace should be encouraged to have the furnace inspected by the gas company. This inspection is usually performed free of charge or for a nominal fee. Public buildings such as schools, hospitals, and businesses are required by municipal codes to have periodic furnace inspections to reduce the risk of carbon monoxide poisoning. The inspector evaluates furnace installation, function, and exhaust system.

Carbon monoxide poisoning can be caused in other ways, such as the inadvertent inhalation of automobile or truck exhaust fumes in a poorly ventilated area such as a closed garage. The risk of carbon monoxide poisoning increases during blizzard conditions because people stranded in their vehicles in a snowstorm may attempt to keep warm by running the engine. The poisoning can occur if the exhaust system is faulty and leaks into a vehicle with tightly sealed windows. Or the exhaust pipe may be occluded with snow or embedded in a snowbank, thus forcing the toxic exhaust fumes back into the vehicle rather than eliminating them by the exhaust system.

HUMIDITY

The relative humidity of the air in the environment may affect the client's health and safety. *Relative humidity* is the amount of water vapor in the air as compared with the maximum amount of water vapor that the air could contain at the same temperature. The comfort zone for humidity varies from person to person, but most people are comfortable when the humidity is between 60% and 70%.

When the relative humidity is high, the skin's moisture evaporates slowly. Thus during hot, humid weather people feel uncomfortably hot and "sticky." If the relative humidity is low, the skin's moisture evaporates quickly. This is why people feel less hot and uncomfortable when the temperature is 32.2° C (90° F) with a relative humidity of 30% than when the temperature is 32.2° C with a relative humidity of 85%.

Modern air conditioners and forced air furnaces enable people to control the temperature of the home and work environments, but they also remove humidity. As a result, people in these environments may have dry mucous membranes of the nose and throat, increasing their risk of respiratory tract infections. Thus many people have attached humidifiers to their furnaces to raise the humidity of the environment when the furnace is operating.

Increasing the environmental humidity has therapeutic benefits. Children and adults with upper respiratory tract infections usually experience improvement in their symptoms when a humidifier is placed in the room while they sleep. The humidifier increases the relative humidity of the inhaled air, which helps to liquefy secretions and improve breathing.

NUTRITION

Meeting nutritional needs adequately and safely requires environmental controls and knowledge. In the home the client needs a refrigerator and if possible a freezer compartment to keep perishable foods fresh. An adequate water supply is needed to clean fresh produce and dishes. Some provision for garbage collection is necessary to maintain sanitary conditions.

Clients and other food preparers need basic information regarding safety in food handling and preparation. Fresh vegetables and fruits should be washed before storing or use to remove insecticides, dirt, and pathogens. Fresh meat, poultry, and fish that are stored in a refrigerator should be used within 24 to 36 hours unless they are stored in a meat keeper that guarantees freshness for 7 days. The safest approach is to freeze fresh meat immediately and thaw it just before use. Any frozen meat that has thawed partially or entirely should not be refrozen. Large chickens and turkeys should always be defrosted in the refrigerator rather than at room temperature because organisms can quickly grow in poultry. Food products should not be used after their expiration dates. Finally, people who do their own canning of vegetables should take care to perform the canning procedure correctly in order to prevent the growth of botulism-causing organisms and other pathogens. The nurse can assess conditions in the client's home and the client's knowledge of food handling to identify needs for teaching or other interventions in these areas.

TEMPERATURE

The comfort zone for environmental temperature varies among individuals, but the usual comfort range is between 18.3° and 23.9° C (65° and 75° F). Temperature extremes that frequently occur during the winter and summer affect not only comfort and productivity but safety as well.

Exposure to severe cold for prolonged periods causes frostbite and hypothermia. Hypothermia occurs when the core body temperature is 35° C (95° F) or below. The person experiences increased confusion and a declining level of consciousness that can result in coma. Shivering is present in the early stages, and trembling may occur on one side of the body or in one extremity. Ultimately the client's vital signs, pulse, and blood pressure decline, and death ensues.

The elderly are at a higher risk for hypothermia, which is believed to be a result of autonomic nervous system response. Chronic or acute illness increases a person's susceptibility to hypothermia. Similarly, the ingestion of alcohol interferes with the client's temperature regulation and increases the risk for hypothermia.

Exposure to extreme heat can result in heatstroke

or heat exhaustion. In either case the body's electrolyte balance is changed, the core body temperature rises, and brain damage results when the core body temperature reaches 41.1° C (106° F). The client becomes confused, the level of consciousness declines, and coma can result. The chronically ill, the elderly, the young, and the poor are at greatest risk for injury from extreme heat.

Reduction of Physical Hazards

Physical hazards in an environment may threaten a client's safety. These hazards can result in a physical injury, such as a sprained ankle from slipping on an unsecured rug, or a psychological injury, such as occurs when a person finds that his residence has been burglarized. Many physical hazards can be minimized by adequate lighting, reduction in clutter, and security measures.

ENSURING ADEQUATE LIGHTING

Adequate lighting reduces physical hazards by illuminating areas in which the client moves and works. Outside the home lighting brightens walkways from the street to the house, from the garage to the house, and on the stairs up to the front or back door. Inside the house the halls, staircases, and individual rooms need adequate lighting so residents can carry out activities of daily living safely and without eyestrain. Night lights in dark halls, bathrooms, and rooms of children and the elderly help to maintain safety by reducing the risk of falls. A night light in a guest room can help to orient an overnight guest who needs to get up in the middle of the night.

Adequate lighting also helps to protect the home and its inhabitants from crime. Well-lighted garages, walkways, and doorways discourage intruders from entering the premises or hiding in shadows.

DECREASING CLUTTER

Injuries in the home frequently result from objects on the stairs and floor, wet spots on the floor, and clutter on bedside tables, closet shelves, the top of the refrigerator, or bookshelves. The risk of injury from clutter is greatest for the elderly and those with impaired vision.

An ounce of prevention is worth a pound of cure when evaluating a client's environment for clutter. To reduce the risk of injury, all clutter should be removed. Halls and traffic areas should remain free of equipment and furniture. Necessary objects such as clocks, glasses, tissues, or medications should remain on bedside tables within reach of an ill client, but nonessential materials such as books, needlework, or newspapers should be placed elsewhere.

SECURING THE HOME

People need to take precautions to secure their homes from intruders, who constitute a threat to both physical and mental safety. When assessing the client's home for safety, the nurse should evaluate the presence and quality of locks on doors and windows. Adequate exterior lighting can also reduce the risk of home break-ins. Clients, particularly the elderly, should be instructed to keep lights on inside and outside the house while they are away.

For the client who is relocating, it might be helpful to inquire about the crime rate in the proposed location. Statistics about crimes rates can be obtained from the local police department and home insurance companies.

Reduction of Transmission of Pathogens and Parasites

A pathogen is any microorganism capable of producing an illness. A parasite is an organism living in or on another organism and obtaining nourishment from it. Pathogens and parasites can be found in water, food, people, and insects and other animals.

In a health care agency effective and efficient methods are used for the control of pathogen transmission, including techniques of medical and surgical asepsis (see Chapter 33). *Medical asepsis* is the removal or destruction of disease-causing organisms or infected material. *Surgical asepsis* is protection against infection by the use of sterile techniques.

The transmission of pathogens from person to person can be reduced and in some cases prevented by immunizations. *Immunization* is the process by which resistance to an infectious disease is produced or augmented. Immunity is acquired following the oral administration or injection of an antigen, which causes production of an antibody within the body. As a result the body is immune to the effects of the harmful pathogens. The discovery of the immunization process for smallpox led the way for the biomedical advances of immunizations for other communicable diseases. As a result the incidence of many highly communicable diseases has been greatly reduced.

FOOD SANITATION

Improperly processed or contaminated food can cause illness and death by transmission of pathogens and parasites. Commercially processed and packaged foods are subject to Food and Drug Administration (FDA) regulations and usually contain a minimal amount of contaminants. The FDA is a federal agency responsible for the enforcement of federal regulations regarding the manufacture and distribution of food, drugs, and cosmetics to protect consumers against the sale of impure or dangerous substances. The FDA guidelines require commercial food processors to comply with sanitation and preparation standards that decrease the risk of contamination.

The risk of contamination is greatest when food is processed incorrectly. *Food poisoning* is the toxic processes resulting from the ingestion of a food contaminated by toxic substances or by bacteria containing toxins. Kinds of food poisoning include (1) bacterial food poisoning such as botulism, which originates from improper food canning, (2) toadstool poisoning from the mistaken ingestion of toadstools instead of mushrooms, (3) shellfish poisoning from eating contaminated shellfish such as lobster or crab, (4) parasitic infestation from contaminated meat, poultry, or fish, such as *Salmonella* from contaminated poultry, and (5) chemical poisoning from ingesting insecticide sprays on unwashed fruits and vegetables.

INSECT AND RODENT CONTROL

Insects and rodents are carriers of pathogens. The *Anopheles* mosquito is a carrier of malaria, a recurrent disease characterized by chills, fever, anemia, and an enlarged spleen. Hot, humid weather following heavy rain creates swampy areas that result in an increased mosquito population, which in turn increases the human population's risk for malaria. The health departments in some municipalities order the spraying of an insecticide to decrease the mosquito population.

Rodents also transmit pathogens. The rat or mouse can transmit rat-bite fever, which in the United States is caused by the *Streptobacillus moniliformis* organism and in the Far East by the *Spirillum minus* organism. Although both of these organisms are sensitive to penicillin, the best approach to rat-bite fever is prevention, which is achieved by reducing the rodent population.

DISPOSAL OF HUMAN WASTES

The transmission of pathogens and parasites is also controlled by adequate disposal of human waste. The proper construction and repair of sewers and drains are necessary for adequate disposal of human waste. Without a satisfactory sewer and waste system the population is at risk for illnesses that are transmitted by way of human feces. Examples of these diseases are typhoid fever and hepatitis.

Pollution Control

A healthy environment is free of pollution. People commonly think of pollution in terms of air or water pollution, but noise can also be a form of pollution that presents health risks.

Air pollution is the contamination of the environmental atmosphere with substances known as pollutants. A pollutant is a harmful chemical or waste material discharged into the water or atmosphere. In urban regions, industrial wastes and vehicle exhausts are common contributors to air pollution. In the home, school, or workplace, cigarette smoke is the primary cause of air pollution.

Prolonged exposure to air pollution is a safety hazard because it increases the risk for pulmonary disease. The greater the time or severity of exposure, the greater the risk of illness.

Water pollution is the contamination of lakes, rivers, and streams, usually by industrial pollutants. Industries found guilty of polluting the water are often required by the courts to pay for the clean-up.

It is important to keep lakes, rivers, and streams as pollution free as possible because all life depends on water. Water treatment facilities filter harmful contaminants from the water, but there are often flaws within water systems. If water exiting the treatment facility becomes contaminated, the public is notified to boil their water. Flooding frequently causes damage to water treatment stations, requiring boiling of drinking water.

Water purification standards have reduced the spread of waterborne diseases. Before these standards many communities experienced epidemics of cholera, dysentery, and typhoid fever, all of which are caused by waterborne pathogens.

Noise pollution occurs when the noise level in an environment becomes uncomfortable to its inhabitants. Noise levels are measured in units of sound intensity called decibels. Noise level tolerances vary from individual to individual and are influenced by the person's health status. A high noise level over a period of time can produce hearing loss. If the noise level is maintained or the person does not use protective earplugs, complete deafness can result.

The health care agency can also be noise polluted. Even when the noise level is not high enough to affect clients' hearing acuity, it may produce a syndrome called sensory overload. *Sensory overload* is a marked increase in the intensity of auditory and visual stimuli. It disrupts cerebral processing of information and problem solving and increases anxiety, paranoia, hallucinations, depression, and unrealistic feelings (Lindenmuth, Breu, and Malooley, 1980).

Pollution—air, water, and noise—can impair the level of health of all those exposed to the pollutants. A nurse assessing a client's environment may be the first to recognize the potential threat to the client from pollution.

■ ■ ■ ■ ■

Environmental safety is important for the client, family, and health care agency. Healthy, literate, young, and economically stable clients usually need no help in maintaining safety in home and community environments. However, people who are ill, unable to read, poor, or elderly require the nurse's help to achieve a safe environment. To do this the nurse thoroughly assesses the environment in the home or health care agency for threats to the client's safety.

Assessment for Threats to Client Safety

Nurses provide care to clients and their families in their homes or communities, as with community health nursing, or within an institutional setting such as a hospital or an extended care facility. Because level of health is diminished by injury, assessing both the community and health care agency for actual or potential threats to client safety is important.

Community

In the United States and Canada accidents are the leading cause of death in people between 1 and 44 years of age (Table 34-1). Other threats to a client's safety within the community include unmet basic needs, transmission of pathogens and parasites, and pollution.

The threats to safety are influenced by the client's development stage. For example, a toddler is at greater risk for accidental poisoning from an insec-

ticide than is a young adult, and a young adult has a greater risk of injury from an automobile accident than does the toddler. Other risks may be associated with life-style habits, mobility status, sensory impairments, and safety awareness.

RISKS AT DEVELOPMENTAL STAGES

INFANT AND PRESCHOOLER. Home accidents kill, disfigure, and permanently disable thousands of children each year. Children under age 5, at greatest risk for death in home accidents, require adult protection to ensure their safety. Adults are faced with the challenge of protecting their children without stifling their development and creativity. Health education for the parents is not enough to prevent accidents. Action must be taken to remove the dangers. One type of action is mandating safety in products that go into the home, such as the use of flame-retardant materials in children's nightwear and tamper-proof closures on medications.

Two conclusions can be drawn about the underlying causes or precipitating factors in childhood accidents (Roy, 1982). First, accidents involving children are largely preventable, but frequently parents need to be shown the specific dangers by nurses and other health care professionals. Second, as the infant grows, accident potential increases. The newborn's accident potential is influenced by people or external agents, but growth and the acquisition of new motor skills place the active child at risk for injuries (Table 34-2).

SCHOOL-AGE CHILD. When children enter school, their environment expands to include the school and the means of transportation to and from school, whether it is school bus, carpool, or walking.

Through discussions and examples, parents and teachers instruct the child how to cross the street safely. In addition, school-age children are at a greater risk of injury from strangers and therefore it should be continually reinforced that the child does not talk to strangers or accept rides or gifts from strangers.

School-age children are often involved in team and contact sports. They should be taught to play safely. The school sports program should provide protective safety equipment, and teachers and coaches should be sure it is used properly.

ADOLESCENT. As children enter their adolescent years, they begin to develop a sense of identity. This self-identity may lead teenagers into a conflict between their own developing values and those of their parents. In addition, the adoelscent begins to separate emotionally from the family, and the peer group begins to have a stronger influence.

TABLE 34-1

Accidental Death Rates (Per 100,000) in People Ages 1 to 44 in the United States and Canada

Age	United States*	Canada†
1-4	28.2	28.0
5-14	18.0	
5-19		35.0
14-24	60.0	
20-44		45.2
25-44	40.8	

*Data from U.S. Department of Health and Human Services: Health—United States, 1982, Washington, D.C., 1982, U.S. Government Printing Office.
†Data from Statistics Canada, Canada Yearbook, 1980-81, Ottawa, 1981, Minister of Supplies and Services

TABLE 34-2

Motor Development Changes Increasing the Risk of Injury in Infants

Age (months)	Motor Development	Hazard
1	No neck control	If unsupported, infant's head flops forward or backward
2	Presence of grasp reflex; grasps object and holds it for a few moments or longer	Able to grasp electrical cords and other dangerous items on the floor
3	May begin to roll from back to stomach	Risk of falling off beds, changing tables, and counters
4	Increased grasping ability; explores new objects with mouth; increased ability to roll from back to tummy, from side to side, and rocking motion	Able to pick up small objects, which usually go immediately into mouth; increased risk of falling from surfaces
5	Increased ability of locomotion by rocking, rolling, twisting; able to grasp bottle; increased ability to grasp small objects	Able to purposefully move toward objects that may be dangerous; should not be left unattended with bottle because choking on contents may occur; increased risk of choking on small objects
6	Able to creep and propel body on stomach, steering with arms and legs; able to reach out and take objects	Able to move to potential dangers such as electrical outlets and cleansers; able to grab dangerous objects
7	May be crawling	Able to move rapidly from one spot to another
8	May be able to pull to a standing position	Can easily fall unless helped back to a sitting or lying position
9	Begins to crawl up stairs; can stand and move by using pieces of furniture for support (walking may occur anywhere from 9 months on)	Can easily lose balance and fall down the stairs; can easily lose balance with wobbly furniture and be bruised on sharp corners of tables and bookcases
10	Climbs up and down from chairs	Can easily fall from chair (unable to judge distances or own limits)
11	Interested in feeding self	May easily choke unless table foods are cut small
12	May climb out of crib; takes covers off plastic and screw-top containers	Increased risk of falling out of crib or playpen; able to open and possibly taste harmful substances

The struggle toward identity may cause the teenager to experience periods of shyness and fear of people, and anxiety may result. Some adolescents withdraw from close relationships, isolating them from the peer group. Occasionally, psychoactive substances, such as drugs and alcohol, make the world more bearable for the troubled teenager. Unfortunately, substances used for this purpose put the adolescent at a high risk for continued alcohol or drug abuse (Rice and Kibbee, 1983).

Usually substance abuse accompanies other problems. The adolescent abuser is probably in a dysfunctional situation at home, at school, or within the peer group. However, some adolescent substance abusers have stable, healthy families and peer relationships and initially may be successful academically and socially.

Long-term habitual use of drugs or alcohol results in subtle behavioral changes (Table 34-3). Parents and nurses are able to recognize these changes, especially when they reappear over a period of time. The nurse should be aware, however, that medical and emotional problems can produce similar behavioral changes. Moodiness and confusion are typical adolescent behavior patterns (Rice and Kibbee, 1983).

When assessing the adolescent for possible sub-

TABLE 34-3

Changes That May Indicate Substance Abuse

Change	Cause
Bloodshot eyes	Alcohol
Slurred speech	Alcohol, depressants
Restlessness	Alcohol withdrawal, stimulants
Sleepiness	Alcohol, depressants
Erratic appetite	Alcohol, depressants, stimulants
Clumsiness	Alcohol, stimulants, depressants
Urinary frequency	Alcohol
Blackouts	Alcohol
Susceptibility to illness	Alcohol, stimulants, depressants
Dilated pupils	Stimulants

Modified from Rice, M.A., and Kibbee, P.E.: Matern. Child Nurs. **8**:134, 1983.

Physiological Changes Common to the Aging Process That Increase the Risk of Falls

- Decreased circulation in the brain causing dizziness and fainting
- Mechanical obstruction of vertebral arteries to the brain caused by crushed osteoporotic vertebrae
- Decreased auditory acuity
- Decreased night vision, color vision, visual acuity
- Cataracts, glaucoma
- Inner ear problems
- Arteriosclerosis
- Orthostatic hypotension
- Loss of sense of position
- Diminished space perception
- Decreased muscle mass, strength, coordination
- Decreased ability to balance
- Osteoporosis and increased stress on weight-bearing areas resulting in an unsteady gait and susceptibility to fractures
- Decreased muscle activity necessary for adequate venous return
- Decreased capacity of blood vessels
- Slowed nervous system response
- Osteoarthritis and other arthritic conditions

Modified from Witte, N.S.: Am. J. Nurs. **79**:1950, 1979.

stance abuse, the nurse must look for environmental and psychosocial clues. Environmental clues include the presence of drug-oriented magazines, beer and liquor bottles, and drug paraphernalia. Blood spots on clothing or the continual wearing of long-sleeved shirts in hot weather and dark glasses indoors may suggest abuse of drugs. Psychosocial clues include failing grades, change in dress, increased absenteeism from school, increased aggressiveness, changes in interpersonal relationships, isolation, erratic behavior, avoidance of eye contact, bragging about drug abuse, and increased time spent in the bathroom. Chapter 45 describes in more detail the problems related to substance abuse.

ADULT. The threats to an adult client's safety are frequently related to life-style habits. The client who excessively uses alcohol, for example, is at great risk for motor vehicle accidents. The long-term smoker has a greater risk of cardiovascular or pulmonary disease as a result of the inhalation of smoke into the lungs and the effect of nicotine on the circulatory system (vasoconstriction). Likewise, the adult experiencing a high level of stress is more likely to have an accident. Increased stress levels also increase the risk of certain stress-related illnesses such as headaches, gastrointestinal disorders, and infections (see Chapter 5).

ELDERLY. Accidental injury from falls, automobile collisions, and burns was the leading cause of death among the elderly in 1980 (Cooper, 1981). Of all fatal home falls, 82% are experienced by adults over 65 years of age. The elderly are more likely to fall as a result of the physiological changes that occur during the aging process (see box above).

The major causes of falls among the elderly are dizziness, decreased visual acuity, decreased balance, osteoporosis, and proprioceptive problems. For example, on rising from a chair an elderly man may become dizzy and fall. A postmenopausal woman with osteoporosis may place all of her weight on one leg when stepping off a curb and experience a spontaneous ankle break resulting in a fall.

Some of the same physiological changes also increase the elderly client's risk for automobile accidents and burns. The slowed response time of the central nervous system prevents elderly drivers from quickly controlling the automobile in potential accident situations. Sensory impairments decrease the elderly client's ability to identify safety threats.

LIFE-STYLE. A client's life-style can increase safety risks. Clients who drive or operate machinery while under the influence of chemical substances have a greater risk of causing injury to themselves and others. In addition, workers who operate heavy machinery have a greater risk of injury than those who conduct business from a desk in an office.

People who are risk takers or daredevils certainly have an increased risk of injury. Skiers who attempt slopes too advanced for their skill levels are injured more frequently than those who ski within their level of ability. People who skydive, climb mountains, or fly private planes are considered high risks by insurance companies and therefore pay higher premiums for health insurance.

Last, people experiencing great stress or anxiety are more accident prone because they are often too preoccupied with their stressors to notice the source of potential accidents, such as a cluttered stair or a stop sign while driving.

MOBILITY. A client with impaired mobility has many kinds of safety risks. First, immobilization itself can predispose the person to other physiological and emotional hazards, which in turn can further restrict mobility and independence (see Chapter 31). A client with impaired mobility is at risk for injury when entering motor vehicles and buildings that are not equipped for the handicapped. For example, a wheelchair-dependent client may be injured by falling from the chair when reaching for an elevator button that is too high. Handicapped clients are at greater risk for automobile and other kinds of accidents. Injuries incurred in an accident can prevent the person from performing independent tasks and result in greater dependence and depression.

SENSORY IMPAIRMENTS. Clients with visual, hearing, or communication impairments are at greater risk for injury in the community. A visually impaired or hearing-impaired client may not be able to perceive a potential danger that otherwise might be recognized. A client with impaired communication skills may be unable to express needs for assistance by calling the police, fire station, or ambulance dispatcher.

SAFETY AWARENESS. Some clients are unaware of safety precautions such as keeping medicine away from children or reading the expiration date on food products. A complete nursing assessment should help the nurse identify the client's level of knowledge regarding home safety so that deficiencies can be corrected with an individualized nursing care plan.

Health Care Agency

Risks to a client's safety are also present within the health care environment. The basic types of risk to a client's safety are (1) falls, (2) client-inherent accidents, (3) procedure-related accidents, and (4) equipment-related accidents. The nurse learns to recognize factors associated with these four potential problem areas and to take steps to prevent or minimize accidents in the institution.

When an accident occurs in a health care agency, an incident report is filed. An incident report is a confidential document that completely describes any client accident occurring on the premises of a health care agency. It documents how the accident occurred, any reactions by or untoward effects on the client, and what was done for the client. The incident report is for internal use and is filed with the agency's insurance and legal departments. In the event of a lawsuit, the incident report is available to the hospital attorneys (see Chapter 17).

In addition to completing the incident report, the nurse must document the accident in the client's medical record and describe its effects on the client's health status. The nurse does not write "incident report completed" in the medical record because the incident report is for internal use only (Lynn, 1980).

FALLS

Of all clients admitted to a hospital, extended care facility, or nursing home, 2% experience a fall, and 2% of those who fall have a fracture (Lynn, 1980). Falls result from slipping or sliding, knees "buckling under," fainting, or tripping over tubes, equipment, or furniture. A client can fall from the bed, wheelchair, toilet, or commode or while walking. The occurrence of falls increases during the evening and nighttime hours.

The client's age is an important factor in the risk of injury within a health care setting, but age is not the sole risk factor. The client's degree of physical or mental debility, psychomotor status, and use of medications are also important variables (see box at right).

Evening and nighttime falls are common among elderly clients because of a phenomenon known as sundowning, in which elderly institutionalized clients tend to become confused or disoriented at the end of the day (see Chapter 27). Many of these clients have diminished visual acuity and hearing loss. With less light they lose visual cues that help them compensate for their sensory impairments. As a result they become confused and may fall when they try to leave their bed or chair.

CLIENT-INHERENT ACCIDENTS

Client-inherent accidents are accidents other than falls in which the client is the primary factor. Examples of client-inherent accidents are self-inflicted

High-Risk Diagnoses and Conditions Leading to Falls in Hospital Settings

HIGH-RISK DIAGNOSES

- Neurological disorders
  - Parkinson's disease
  - Brain tumor
  - Seizure disorder
  - Cerebrovascular accident
  - Head injury
  - Spinal cord injury
  - Multiple sclerosis
- Debilitating disease
  - Anemia
  - Pulmonary disease
  - Coronary artery disease
  - Cushing's disease
  - Diabetes mellitus
  - Cancers (especially metastatic)

RISK-PRONE CONDITIONS

- Difficulties with gait or locomotion
  - Use of walker, cane, or crutches
  - Prosthesis
  - Dizziness
- Debilitation
  - Nosocomial—bowel preparation, invasive procedures, postoperative status
  - Natural—restrictive pain, diminished caloric intake, prolonged bed rest
- Mental status deterioration
  - Confusion
  - Disorientation
  - Depression
  - Mental retardation
  - Organic brain syndrome
- Central nervous system alterations
  - Tranquilizers
  - Sedatives
  - Substance abuse
  - Anesthesia
- Sensory deficits
  - Blindness
  - Eye patches
  - Hearing loss
  - Hemiplegia
  - Paraplegia
  - Quadriplegia
  - Proprioceptive loss
- Language barrier

Modified from Lynn, F.H.: Am. J. Nurs. **80**:1098, 1980.

cuts, injuries, and burns; ingestion or injection of foreign substances; self-mutilation or setting fires; and pinching fingers in drawers or doors (Lynn, 1980).

The nurse must file a complete and accurate incident report for client-inherent injuries. A thorough report describing the client's physical and behavioral status as well as the incident is necessary for studying risk factors within the agency that require preventive action. This report also can protect the institution and health care professionals from any subsequent lawsuits (see Chapter 17). For example, if an oriented adult client breaks into the medication station and ingests a bottle of aspirin, the agency may not be considered at fault because the medications were properly locked up and the client broke into the area. If, on the other hand, a disoriented, confused client breaks into the medication station and ingests a bottle of aspirin, the agency could be held responsible because a disoriented client should be properly restrained and protected from self-injury.

PROCEDURE-RELATED ACCIDENTS

Procedure-related accidents are those that occur during therapy. They include medication errors, untoward drug effects, improper application of restraints, and accidents during dressing changes and other nursing procedures.

The nurse can prevent many procedure-related accidents. For example, correct administration of medications, using the "five rights" described in Chapter 32, helps to prevent medication errors. In addition, proper administration of intravenous fluids prevents fluid overload or deficit (see Chapter 42). Also, injury from the introduction of pathogens is reduced when surgical asepsis is used for sterile dressing changes (see Chapter 33) or invasive procedures such as insertion of a Foley catheter (see Chapter 39). Finally, correct use of body mechanics and transfer techniques reduces the risk of injuries from transfer procedures (see Chapter 30). Additional interventions for preventing procedure-related injuries are described in the later implementation section of this chapter.

EQUIPMENT-RELATED ACCIDENTS

Equipment-related accidents are those that result from the malfunction, disrepair, or misuse of equipment or from an electrical hazard. Equipment for monitoring or therapy should not be used without instruction. A nurse who is unsure about how to operate a piece of equipment or uncertain whether a piece of equipment is operating properly should ask for assistance. Severe injury can occur if personnel do not ask how to use a piece of equipment properly.

Potential electrical hazards should be assessed both in the client's home and in the health care environ-

---

Checklist for Electrical Hazards

- Ungrounded equipment
- Frayed cords
- Circuits overloaded by too many appliances in one area
- Improperly functioning equipment
- Use of extension cords
- Tangled or cluttered cords
- Use of electrical appliances near sink, bathtub, shower, or damp areas
- Electrical cords or appliances within range of young children
- Noninsulated wiring in basement or crawl-space

Examples of Nursing Diagnoses for Safety Needs

- Risk of falling related to muscle atrophy and weakness from prolonged immobilization
- Risk of falling related to dizziness associated with postural hypotension
- Risk of infant poisoning related to unsecured storage of toxic agents
- Risk of self-medication overdose related to confusion and disorientation
- Risk of suffocation related to improperly vented furnace in home
- Risk of electrocution related to exposed appliance wiring
- Risk of trauma related to cluttered stairway
- Risk of trauma related to driving while intoxicated
- Risk of food poisoning related to lack of knowledge about food storage
- Risk of respiratory illness related to cigarette smoking

---

ment. Using a checklist to identify hazards takes only a few minutes but can reduce the risk of electrical fires, electrocution, or injury from improperly wired equipment (see box above).

Nursing Diagnoses

The nursing diagnosis identifies risks to a client's safety based on the data provided by the nursing assessment. Four categories of nursing diagnoses involve the threats of poisoning, suffocation, trauma, and other variables in the client's internal or external environment. The nursing diagnosis should include specific causative factors so that nursing care can be individualized for the client (box at right).

The variables of age, level of health, presence of stressors, life-style habits, physical or mental impairments, educational level, socioeconomic status, and environmental factors influence the formulation of nursing diagnoses related to a client's safety.

Planning

The care plan for the client's safety has as its primary goal prevention of illness or injury. The secondary goal is reducing developmental and environmental risks to the client's safety. When a client is confused, ill, or helpless, the nurse is the primary professional responsible for maintaining a safe environment and protecting the client from injuries caused by the illness or disability, such as with the confused client who must be restrained to prevent him from climbing over the bed side rails and possibly incurring injury.

Implementation

Nursing interventions are directed toward maintaining the client's safety in the home environment as well as in the health care agency. Because most nursing measures are applicable in both environments, the interventions are presented in two sections: developmental considerations and environmental protections. The first category of interventions includes those specific to each developmental age for reducing risks for that particular age group. Environmental interventions are developed to modify the environment so that present or potential hazards are eliminated or minimized.

DEVELOPMENTAL CONSIDERATIONS

INFANT AND PRESCHOOLER. Infants and preschoolers depend on adults to protect them from injury. Growing children are curious and completely trusting of their environment and do not perceive themselves to be in danger.

Nurses are frequently in a position to educate parents or guardians about reducing risks of injuries for young children. Nurses working in prenatal clinics can easily incorporate safety into the care plan of the childbearing family. Community health nurses can assess the home environment and show parents how to promote safety in their homes. The pediatric nurse

TABLE 34-4

Nursing Interventions to Promote Safety of Infants and Preschoolers

Intervention	Rationale
Use large soft toys with plastic eyes, nose, or mouth.	The small parts can be dislodged by baby and accidental aspiration can occur.
If a playpen with mesh sides is used, do not leave one side down.	The baby's head can become wedged between the playpen pad and the lowered mesh side, and asphyxiation can occur.
Never leave the sides of the crib down or turn away from a baby on a changing table.	The child can suddenly roll and fall from the crib or changing table.
Hold baby at feeding time; do not prop the bottle.	This increases bonding and reduces the risk of choking.
If formula is used, be sure to read the instructions. Most formulas must be diluted with water.	Using undiluted formula can cause fluid and electrolyte imbalances in the newborn.
Discontinue the use of the pumpkin seat at 3 months or earlier if the infant is very mobile.	At 3 months an active infant may be able to propel himself out of the pumpkin seat and fall.
Baby proof the house for small objects, sharp objects, and toxic and poisonous substances.	Babies explore their world with their hands and mouth, and small objects can result in choking. Toxic and poisonous substances require prompt action (see later section on poison).
Cover electrical outlets with protective covers (see Fig. 34-1).	Electrical wall outlets are at babies' eye level and stimulate their curiosity. A crawling baby will frequently attempt to play with electrical wall plates regardless of the number of toys available.
Use guardrails at the top and bottom of stairs and at the doorway of rooms considered off limits to a crawling or walking toddler.	This prevents the child from falling down the stairs.
Never leave baby unattended in pumpkin seat, walker, stroller, or high chair.	An active child can easily slide out of these devices and fall.
Never leave a baby or child unattended in a bath or wading pool.	Accidental drowning may occur.
Never attach a pacifier to a child with a string around the neck.	The string may become easily tangled, and strangulation can result.
Restrain a child in the back seat of an automobile. Children under 4 should be in an approved car seat (see Fig. 34-2). Older children should be restrained with a seat belt.	In the event of a sudden stop or an auto accident, an unrestrained child is bounced against hard, sharp surfaces of the vehicle's interior and injuries result.
Plastic bags such as those for storing fruit or dry cleaning should be removed from the home.	If the child places these over the head, the air supply decreases and the child suffocates.
Install strong dead-bolt locks on doors well beyond the toddler's reach, even when the child is standing on a chair.	This prevents the child from leaving the home without the parents' knowledge, which reduces the danger of the child getting lost, freezing to death, or being abducted.
Use the words "no" and "don't" to convey that an object or action increases the child's risk of injury, such as playing with matches (see Fig. 34-3).	Improperly using these words renders them meaningless to the child.
Teach the child to swim at an early age, but always provide supervision.	The child will be able to enjoy the water safely. A child who knows how to swim can still get in difficulty in the water and needs supervision.

Continued.

TABLE 34-4, cont'd

Nursing Interventions to Promote Safety of Infants and Preschoolers

Intervention	Rationale
Teach the child how to cross the street and how to walk in parking lots.	This provides the child with self-protection against dangers from automobiles.
Teach the child not to talk to or accept anything from a stranger and to notify parents if approached by a stranger.	This reduces the risk of injury or abduction by a stranger. Reporting the stranger's presence helps law enforcement personnel investigate and remove a threat.
Do not allow the child to run with a sucker or popsicle in the mouth.	The child may fall and the stick from the sucker or popsicle can cause injury.
Impress on the child not to eat anything found on the street or in the grass.	The substance may be poisonous and can cause severe illness.
Use back burners on stoves and get into the habit of turning pot handles toward the wall.	This reduces the risk of the child pulling down a pot of hot liquid and being burned.
Remove doors from unused refrigerators and freezers, and instruct the child not to hide in these items.	The door may latch and on older models cannot be released from the inside; as a result asphyxiation can occur.

can teach both the child and the parent or guardian about safety. Other nursing interventions that should be incorporated into the plan of care for safety of a child are listed in Table 34-4 and illustrated in Figs. 34-1 to 34-3.

SCHOOL-AGE CHILD. School-age children increasingly explore their environment. They have friends outside their immediate neighborhood, they may walk to school, and they become more active in school, church, and community activities. All of these activities help the child to develop social skill and independence, but they also increase the risk of injury. The school-age child begins to align some activities with those of the adult, learning from parents, teachers, and often television heroes. This patterning of behavior and activities is not necessarily a threat to the child, except when the child imitates an adult behavior that presents safety risks, such as operating an electric saw. Some nursing interventions help to guide the parent to provide for the safety of the school-age child (Table 34-5).

ADOLESCENT. When children approach their adolescent years, much of their time is spent away from home and with their peer group. Risks to the adolescent's safety therefore involve many factors outside the home environment. Adults serve as role models for adolescents and through example and education can help the adolescents minimize risks to their safety. While seeking independence and identity, adolescents

are also trying to assume adult activities and roles. In so doing, they need help in understanding the responsibilities that go along with these new activities. The box on p. 918 lists measures by which nurses and parents can help the adolescent prevent accidents.

ADULT. Risks to young and middle adults frequently result from life-style factors, such as child rearing, high stress states, inadequate nutrition, and excessive alcohol intake. Adults need to be taught that their safety is in fact threatened, and as a result their life-style needs to be modified.

Stress management centers and health promotion activities have been incorporated into many community service programs as well as hospitals. In addition, neighborhood centers, community clinics, and

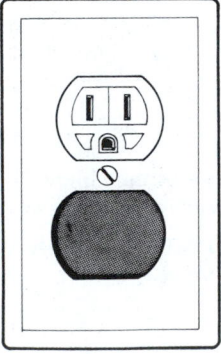

Fig. 34-1 Safety covers for electrical outlets.

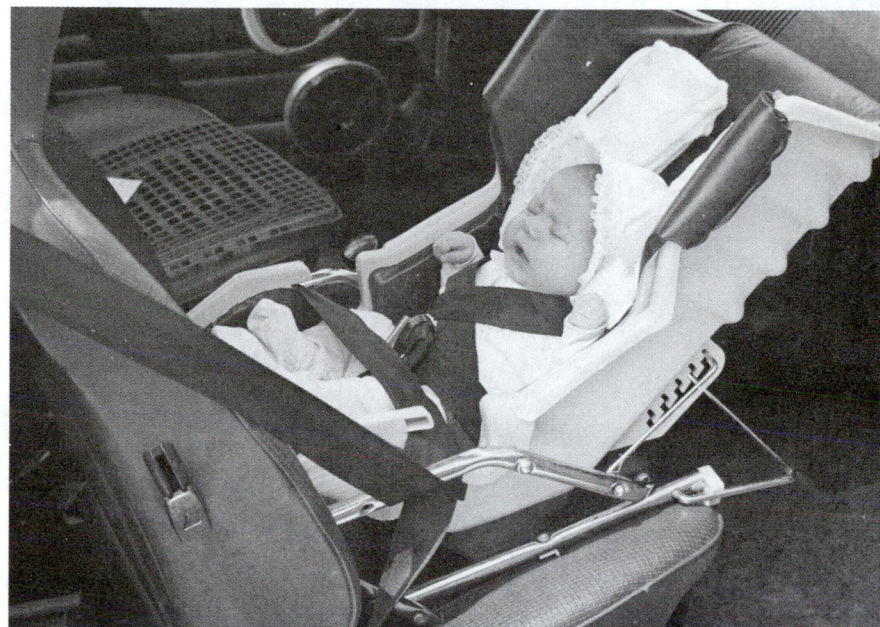

Fig. 34-2 Infant car seat.

From Whaley, L.F., and Wong, D.L.: Nursing care of infants and children, ed. 2, St. Louis, 1983, The C.V. Mosby Co.

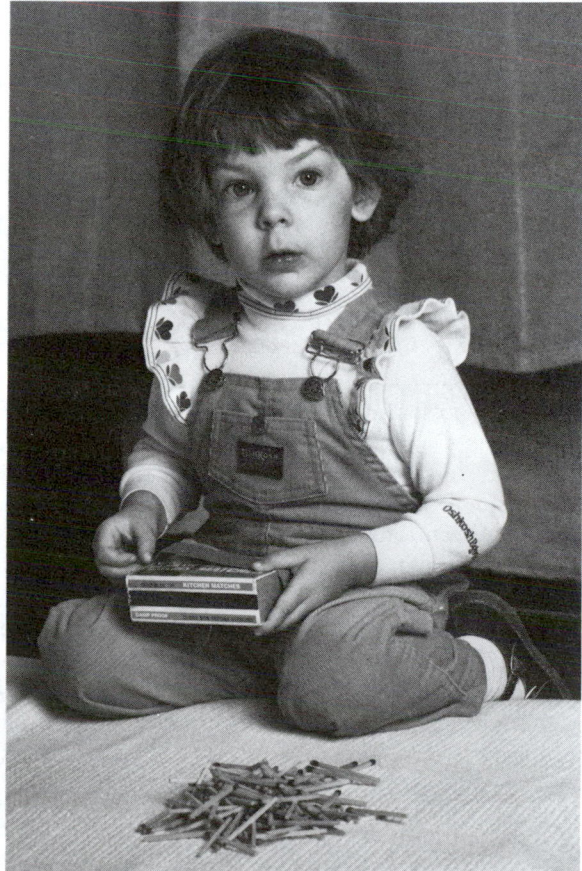

Fig. 34-3 Playing with matches.

TABLE 34-5

Nursing Interventions to Promote Safety of the School-Age Child*

Intervention	Rationale
Teach the child the safe use of equipment for play and work activities.	The child needs to learn that some equipment is for play and other for work and that improper use can result in injury.
Teach the child how to ride a bicycle safely and the responsibilities that go with bicycling.	If bicycling is prohibited on sidewalks, the child must learn to obey traffic signals and ride with traffic patterns.
Teach the child, when roller skating, to wear protective helmets and knee and elbow pads.	When children roller skate, they fall; protective devices reduce the risk of serious injury.
Never allow the child to operate appliances while alone in the house.	If an electrical mishap were to occur, there would not be anyone available to help the child.
If a parent chooses to have firearms in the house, teach the parent to keep them unloaded, locked up, and out of reach.	This prevents injury from accidental discharge or improper use.

*In addition to those in Table 34-4 that are appropriate for the school-age child.

Measures for Adolescents to Prevent Accidents

- Enroll teenagers in a driver's education course and make practice drives with them in good and bad weather. Teach them how to handle a motor vehicle in a skid.
- Teach them to wear seat belts while driving or as passengers.
- Instruct them not to drive after using a psychoactive substance or enter an automobile when the driver has been using such substances.
- Form a contract with teenagers that, if they drink at a party, they call home for a ride with no questions asked.
- Help them develop safe eating, sleeping, and relaxation habits.
- Inform them of the dangers of psychoactive substances.
- Recognize changes in adolescents' behavior and mood.
- Listen to them.
- Do not try to be a buddy; remain a parent.

Steps the Elderly Can Take to Prevent Automobile Accidents

- See your physician if you suspect you have a hearing problem.
- Leave your car window partially open to let you hear warning signals.
- Set the air conditioner or heater and the radio low so that their noise does not mask outside sounds.
- Place mirrors on both sides of the car, and use them and a wide rear-view mirror when you change lanes or pass other vehicles.
- Stop frequently to stretch your muscles and rest your eyes.
- Schedule regular eye examinations to check for vision changes or health problems that may affect your vision.
- Follow the physician's recommendations, if any, about limiting when and where you drive.
- Before driving, give yourself time to adjust to new lenses, especially bifocals or trifocals.
- Wear good quality sunglasses (usually gray or green) to reduce glare. Wear them only in the daytime.
- Keep windshield and all windows clean inside and out. Replace worn wiper blades. Keep headlights, tail lights, and turn signals clean to maintain maximum lighting.
- If you take medication, know its long- and short-term effects on your driving ability.
- Do not smoke while driving at night. Smoking impairs vision.
- Do not drive when you have been drinking.
- Enroll in a driver training course through your state motor vehicle department.

From Cooper, B.A.: Geriatr. Nurs. **2:**287, 1981.

---

outpatient clinics are equipped to assist the adult in modifying life-style habits that present risks to health, such as smoking, overeating, lack of exercise, and alcoholism. Chapters 2 and 5 detail the appropriate nursing interventions.

ELDERLY. As noted earlier, most injuries to the elderly involve falls, auto accidents, and burns (Cooper, 1981). The advancing age and the concurrent physiological changes in vision, hearing, mobility, circulation, and the ability to make quick judgments all predispose the elderly to falls (see Chapter 27). In addition, many of the medications given to the elderly make falls more likely (Cooper, 1981). Nursing interventions designed to reduce the risk of falls compensate for the physiological changes of aging (Table 34-6).

Automobile accidents are more likely to occur with the elderly because of three specific physiological changes. Changes in visual acuity and depth perception prevent the client from quickly observing situations in which an accident is likely to occur. Because their visual changes have occurred gradually, many elderly drivers do not realize that their vision is limited. Second, decreased hearing acuity alters the elderly client's ability to hear emergency vehicle sirens or car and truck horns. Last, because of decreased nervous system response, the elderly are unable to react as quickly as they once could to avoid an accident. Interventions directed toward preventing automobile accidents are designed to compensate for these changes (see box above).

Pedestrian accidents among the elderly can also be reduced by persuading the elderly to take five precautions: (1) wear reflectorized garments when walking at night, (2) stand on the sidewalk, not in the street, when waiting to cross a street, (3) always cross at corners, not in the middle of the block, particularly if the street is a major one, (4) whenever possible, cross with the traffic light, not against it, and (5) look left, right, and left again before entering the street or crosswalk.

TABLE 34-6

Measures to Prevent Falls by the Elderly

Measure	Rationale
STAIRS	
Install treads with a uniform depth of 9 inches and 9-inch risers (vertical face of the steps).	If stairs are of uniform size, the elderly need not continually adjust their vision.
Install uniform-textured or plain-colored surfaces on each tread, and mark the edge of the tread with a contrasting color.	Uniform textures or color help to decrease vertigo. Marking the edge of the tread provides the client with an obvious visual clue to the end of the stair.
Ensure proper lighting of each tread. Block sun or light-bulb glare with translucent shades or screen, or use lower wattage bulbs.	An elderly client's vision is unable to accommodate quickly to changes in lighting.
Ensure adequate head room so users need not duck to negotiate stairs.	Sudden changes in a client's head position may result in dizziness.
Remove protruding objects from staircase walls.	Decreased peripheral vision may prevent the client from seeing the object.
Maintain outdoor walkways and stairs in good condition, free of holes, cracks, and splinters.	Decreased visual acuity can prevent the elderly from seeing any structural defect.
HANDRAILS	
Install smooth but slip-resistant handrail at least 2 inches from the wall.	The 2-inch distance allows the client to grasp the handrail firmly for support.
Secure handrail firmly so that user's weight is supported, especially at the bottom and top of the stairway.	The elderly have the greatest risk of falling at the top and bottom of stairs because their center of gravity is being shifted and their balance is unstable.
Install grab rails in the bathroom near the toilet or tub.	This enables the elderly to have support while rising from a sitting to standing position.
FLOOR COVERINGS	
Secure all carpeting, mats, and tile; place nonskid backing under small rugs.	A sudden slip may cause dizziness and inability of an elderly person to regain balance.

Burns and scalds are also more apt to occur with the elderly who are at greater risk for several reasons. They may forget and leave hot water running or become confused when turning the dials on a stove. Impaired visual acuity and sense of smell increase the danger that the elderly may not detect smoke or gas fumes (Cooper, 1981). The nursing measures developed for preventing burns are designed to minimize the risk from impaired vision and hearing (see box at left on p. 920).

■ ■ ■ ■ ■

Nursing interventions designed to reduce the developmental risks to a client's safety need to be specific to the appropriate age level. For example, teaching a 15-month-old how to climb stairs holding the handrail is an appropriate intervention to promote safety, whereas this teaching would be ineffective at

a much earlier age. The nursing care plan developed for a client's safety should be individualized to the client's age, mobility status, level of orientation, environment, level of health, and personal goals.

ENVIRONMENTAL CONSIDERATIONS

Potential accidents in the client's environment include falls and client-inherent, procedure-related, or equipment-related accidents. The most common types of injuries are falls, fires, poisonings, and electrical injuries. Based on the assessment and diagnosis of these risks, the nurse designs interventions to reduce risks and promote the client's safety in these areas.

FALLS. Modifications in the client's home or health care environment can easily reduce the risk of falls. Falls can occur when a heavy or debilitated client in bed or a wheelchair or on a toilet or commode is not

Steps the Elderly Can Take to Prevent Burns

- Do not smoke in bed or when sleepy.
- When cooking, do not wear loose-fitting clothing (bathrobes, night gowns, pajamas).
- Set thermostats for water heater or faucets so that the water does not become too hot.
- Install a portable hand fire extinguisher in the kitchen.
- Keep access to outside door(s) unobstructed.
- Identify emergency exits in public buildings.
- If you consider entering a boarding or foster home, check to see that it has smoke detectors, a sprinkler system, and fire extinguishers.
- Wear clothing that is nonflammable or treated with a permanent flame-retardant finish. Fabrics of animal hair, wool, or silk are less flammable.
- Use several electrical outlets to avoid overloading.

From Cooper, B.A.: Geriatr. Nurs. **2**:287, 1981.

Safeguards to Reduce the Risk of Falls

- Place bedside tables and over-bed tables close to the client.
- Encourage the client to rise from the bed or chair slowly to prevent dizziness resulting from postural hypotension.
- Remove clutter from bedside tables, hallways, bathrooms, and grooming areas.
- Mount grab bars around toilets and showers, and instruct the client how to use them (see Fig. 34-4).
- Advise that rugs and carpets be securely attached to floors and stairs.
- Advise that bath mats and nonskid strips be attached to bathtubs and floor of shower stalls.
- Advise that electrical cords be secured against baseboards so the client cannot easily trip over them.
- See that the nurse's call bell is within easy reach of the hospitalized client, who should be instructed as to where emergency call bells are located in bathrooms.
- See that wheelchairs remain locked when transporting a client from bed to wheelchair or back to bed (see Fig. 34-5).
- Check that the side rails are up and the safety straps secured around the client who is on a stretcher (see Fig. 34-6).

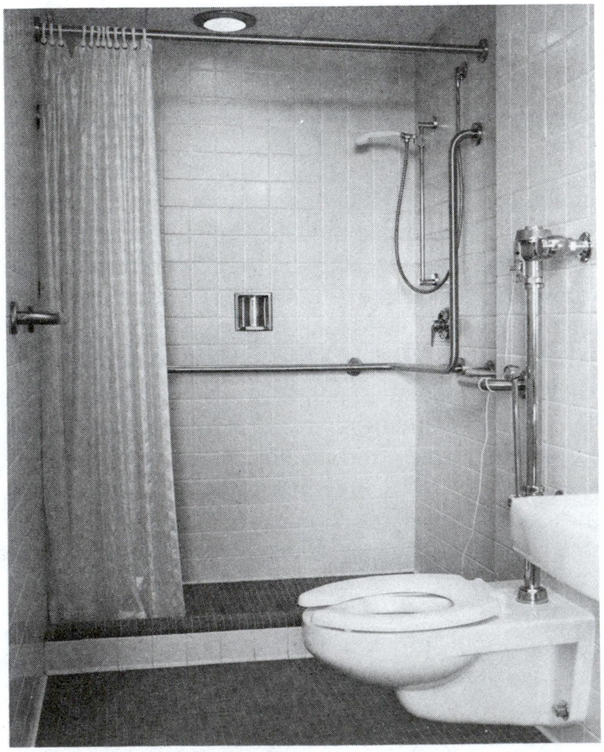

Fig. 34-4 Safety bars around toilets and showers.

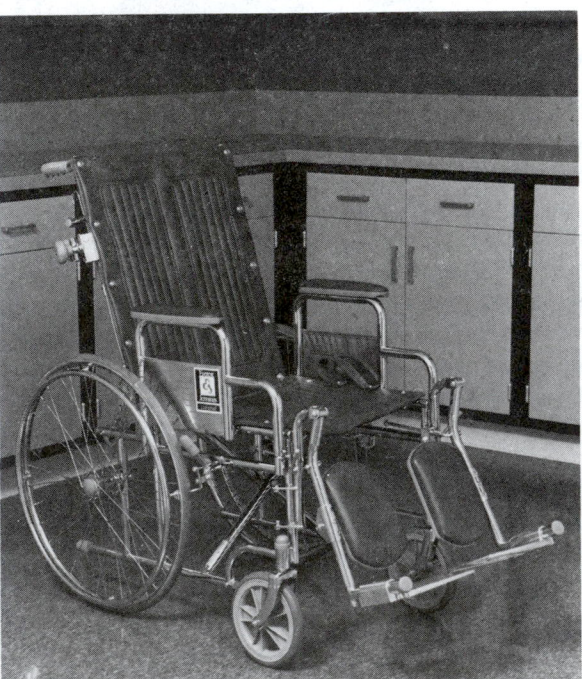

Fig. 34-5 Safety lock on wheelchair.

properly secured or supported. Excess furniture and equipment increase clutter and the risk of falling. The nurse should be sure that a weakened client, walking with the support of nurses or family, wears rubber-soled shoes or slippers to prevent a fall from slipping or sliding along the floor.

Clients and others need to be instructed how to inspect the tips of canes, walkers, and crutches to be sure the rubber tip is intact. The rubber tip increases friction, and without it the walker or other adaptive device could easily slide along a waxed surface, causing the person to fall (see Chapter 30).

With clients in the home or hospital setting, certain safeguards can be implemented or taught to the family to minimize the risk of falls (see box at left and Figs. 34-4 to 34-6). In addition, confused, disoriented, very young, or very old clients may require the use of restraints and side rails to protect them from falling out of bed.

Restraints. A restraint is any one of numerous devices used to immobilize a client or an extremity. The use of restraints involves a psychological adjustment for the client and family, and the nurse should assist them in adapting to this necessary change. Restraints are most effective when used consistently. A restraint applied too tightly causes skin irritation, and if applied too loosely does not serve the purpose of restricting the client's movement to promote safety.

The use of restraints is a nursing procedure, and as with other procedures, the nurse must follow specific guidelines (Table 34-7 and Fig. 34-8). The overall objectives for restraints are:

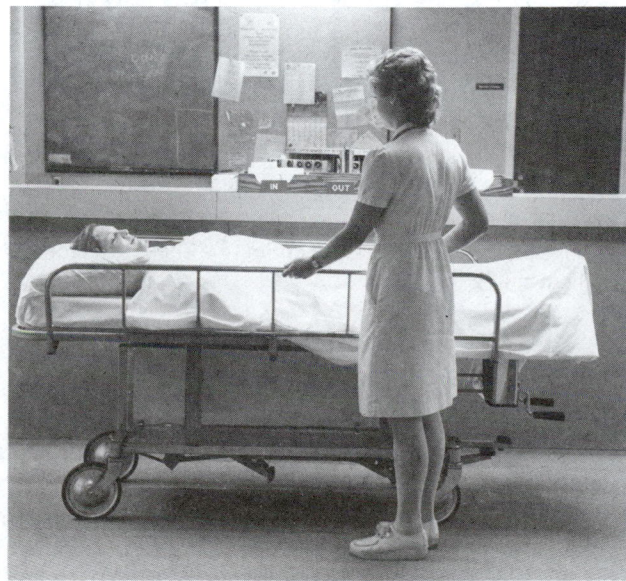

Fig. 34-6 Side rails in the up position on a stretcher.

TABLE 34-7

Guidelines for the Use of Restraints

Guideline	Rationale
The restraint should be selected to reduce the client's movement only as much as necessary.	Overrestraining a client so activities are unduly restricted can exacerbate the hazards of immobility.
If a restraint is necessary, the nurse should carefully explain to the client and family the type of restraint and why the restraint is needed.	Restraint can increase confusion or hostility in both the client and family. Explanation of the restraint can reduce or even prevent some of these negative perceptions.
Restraint should not exacerbate the client's health problem.	Restraints that are too tight can impair circulation to the distal extremities.
Restraint should not interfere with treatment.	Restraints placed over intravenous sites can impede the flow of fluid into the client's circulation. Restraints attached to fractured or dislocated extremities can impair healing.
Bony prominences should be padded before applying a restraint.	Padding reduces the risk of injury to the skin from pressure.
Restraints should be changed whenever they become soiled or damp.	Soiled or damp restraints increase the risk of skin breakdown.
Restraints should be secured in such a manner that they cannot be undone by the client.	When a client is able to undo restraints, the whole purpose of the restraint is negated.
Any restraint applied to a client in bed should be attached to the bed frame (see Fig. 34-7), not the side rails.	Release of the side rails while the restraint remains attached can result in injury to the client's musculoskeletal system.
Restraints should be removed every 4 hours. The client should not be left unattended.	This provides an opportunity to assess skin integrity and to provide skin care, often by massaging the areas on which the restraints were applied. A previously restrained client who is left unattended can cause self-injury or can injure others.

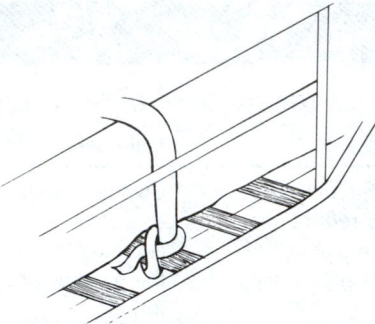

Fig. 34-7 Attachment of restraint ties to the bed frame.

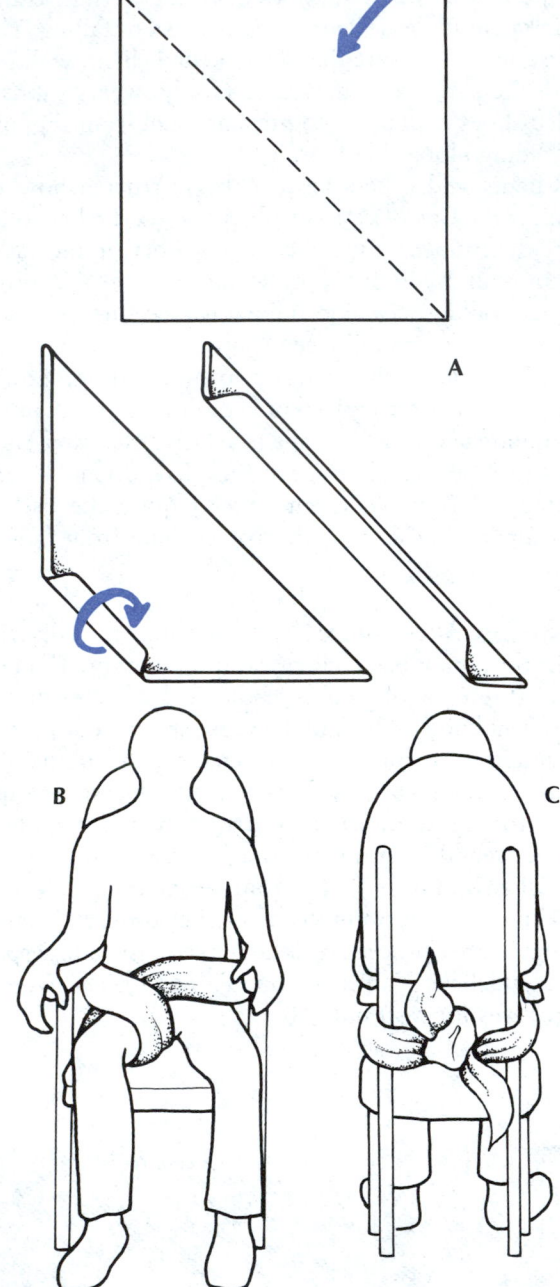

Fig. 34-8 **A,** Modified restraint, folding bed sheet along the bias. **B,** Sheet is continuously folded along bias until a long strip is achieved. **C,** Securing the sheet restraint on a client sitting in a chair.

1. To reduce the risk of the client falling out of bed or from chair or wheelchair
2. To prevent interruption of therapy such as traction, intravenous infusions, nasogastric tube feeding, or Foley catheter
3. To prevent the confused or combative client from removing life support equipment
4. To reduce the risk of injury to others by the client

When used correctly, restraints benefit the client. The decision to use restraints can be made by the nurse or the physician. Some agencies have specific guidelines regarding which health professional should order restraints. For legal purposes it is important that the nurse be familiar with agency policy and procedures for the appropriate use of restraints. Situations arise in which the nurse must make an independent judgment and apply restraints. When this occurs, it is important that the nurse document the assessment of the client's activity and behavior, the conclusions about the client's status, the nursing action, and the fact that the action was explained to both the client and family. In addition, the nurse should note specifically the type of restraint selected and where the restraints were applied.

The nursing assessment helps the nurse in determining the type of restraint to use. The nurse first determines the client's need and identifies the purpose of the restraint. Second, the nurse selects a restraint to match the client's need. For example, if a client is at risk for falling out of the chair, a jacket restraint is needed rather than restraint of only one arm, which would be appropriate for maintaining an intravenous infusion.

Basically four types of restraints are available for use with clients in both the community and institutional settings: jacket restraints, mitten restraints, clove hitch restraints, or elbow restraints.

The *jacket restraint* is a vestlike garment that usually overlaps in the back of the client with ties that

the nurse attaches to the bed frame or under the mattress (see Chapter 30). When jacket restraint is used to restrain a client seated in a chair, the ties are fastened under the arms of the chair.

When a jacket restraint is unavailable, the nurse can create a modified restraint by folding a bed sheet on the bias (Fig. 34-8, *A*). The sheet is then rolled

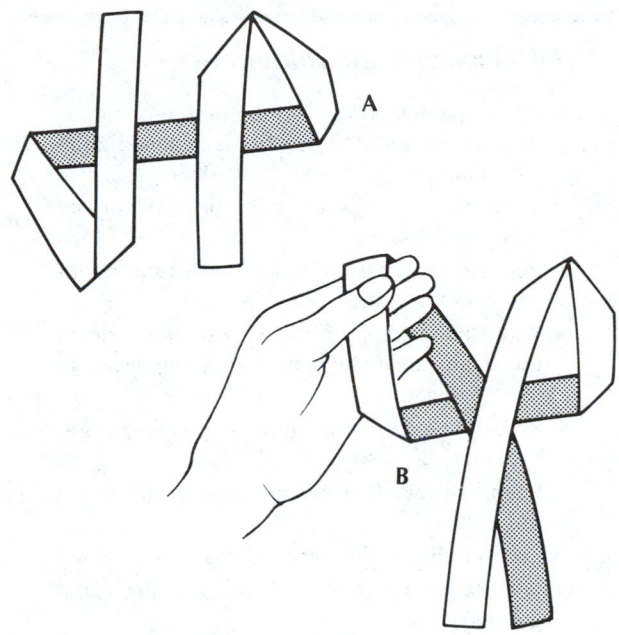

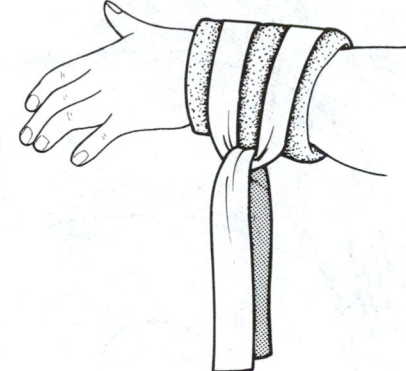

Fig. 34-10 Applying the clove hitch restraint directly over a padded extremity.

Fig. 34-9 **A,** To make a clove hitch restraint, the nurse first makes a figure eight with a strip of cloth. **B,** Picking up the loops of the clove hitch.

along the bias fold to achieve a long strip (Fig. 34-8, *B*). The nurse secures the restraint around one thigh and across the chest of the client. The ends of the restraint are passed underneath the arms of the chair and tied in the back of the chair (Fig. 34-8, *C*). The ties must be secured underneath the chair's armrest to prevent the client from standing up and sliding the entire restraint over the top of the chair and thus being released from the restraint.

A sheet folded on the bias is also useful to restrain a client in bed. The nurse places the sheet across the client's chest and attaches each end to the bed frame. Although this restraint is certainly not as comfortable as the jacket restraint, it is effective in maintaining a disoriented or combative client in bed until a jacket restraint can be obtained. In such a case the restraint reduces the risk of the client falling or injuring another person.

Mitten restraints are used to prevent clients from dislodging equipment, such as intravenous lines, Foley catheters, cardiac monitors, or dressings, or from scratching themselves. These restraints are designed with a thumbless mitten to which ties are attached. The ties are then secured to the bed frame or the arm of a chair.

Other types of restraints are used to restrain one or all extremities. Limb restraints are commercially available. These consist of a soft sheepskin pad that comes in direct contact with the client's skin and is attached to the bed frame with ties.

The *clove hitch restraint* for limb restraint is made from a strip of cloth that does not tighten if the client pulls against it. The clove hitch itself is made in two steps. The nurse first makes a figure eight with the strip of cloth (Fig. 34-9, *A*) and then picks up the loops (Fig. 34-9, *B*). The nurse should first place gauze or padding around the extremity to be restrained and then place the loops of the clove hitch directly over the padded surface (Fig. 34-10).

Under no circumstances should the nurse restrain an extremity with a slip knot. This type of crude restraint is a threat to the client's circulation and skin integrity. If the client were to pull against a slip-knot restraint, the restraint would become tighter, decreasing the blood supply and oxygen delivery to the distal extremity.

An *elbow restraint* is frequently used with children. The objective of this type of restraint is to prevent the child from bending the elbow. Thus the youngster can neither tamper with intravenous infusions and surgical dressings nor scratch. The elbow restraint is a piece of fabric with slots in which tongue blades are placed so the elbow joint remains rigid (Fig. 34-11).

The client with whom restraints are used may become more confused and combative because of the restraint. The nurse schedules additional time with the restrained client to offer reassurance and in controlled situations release from the restraints for a period of time. Restraints are beneficial, but if used incorrectly they can reduce the client's overall level of physical and mental health.

Side Rails. Chapter 30 discusses side rails as a device for increasing the client's mobility and stability in bed or when moving from bed to chair. Side rails are also of benefit in preventing the client from falling out of bed. The side rail is attached to the side of the bed and can be raised or lowered.

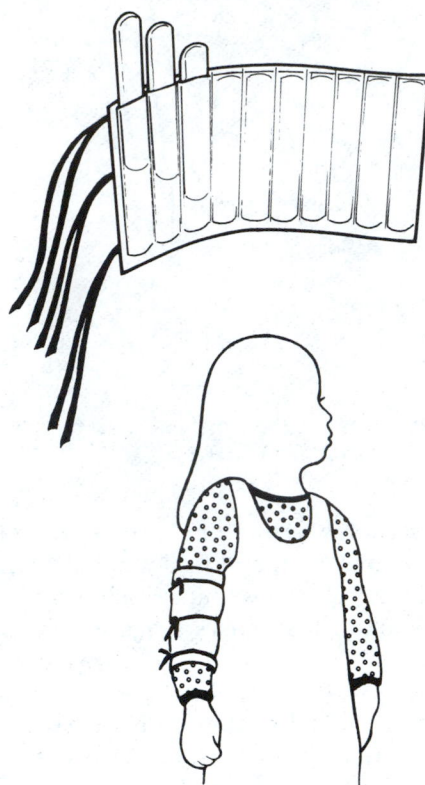

Fig. 34-11 Elbow restraint.

Side rails are effective in protecting an unconscious client from falling out of bed. However, the use of side rails alone for a disoriented client may cause only more confusion and further injury. Frequently a confused client who is determined to get out of bed attempts to climb over the side rail or climbs out at the foot of the bed. Either attempt usually results in a fall. Therefore for the confused client a jacket restraint is often used with the side rails elevated. It is particularly important to remember this with the elderly client who may experience the sundowning phenomenon discussed earlier.

FIRES. Both the home and the hospital environment are always at risk of fires. Accidental home fires typically result from smoking in bed, careless extinguishing of cigarette butts in trash cans, grease fires, or electrical fires resulting from faulty wiring or appliances. Institutional fires typically result from a client smoking in bed or from an electrical or anesthetic-related fire.

The interventions described here are directed toward fires occurring in health care agencies, but the same principles apply for fires in the home. First, it is important to have a plan of action in the event a fire occurs (see boxed material).

If a nurse observes a fire, its exact location should

> ## *Fire Prevention Guidelines*
>
> - Know the telephone number for reporting a fire, and be sure the number is attached to all telephones.
> - Know the agency's or unit's fire drill or fire evacuation routine.
> - Post accurate, easy-to-follow routes for the location of fire exits.
> - Know the location of fire extinguishers, how to use them, and which type of extinguisher to use for specific fires (see Table 34-8).
> - Report a fire before attempting to extinguish it, regardless of its size.
> - Keep hallways free of unnecessary equipment or furniture.
> - Keep fire hoses clear at all times.
> - Periodically check the efficiency of fire extinguishers.
> - Post signs on the outside of elevators warning people to take the stairs in the event of a fire.

be reported immediately. If there is no immediate threat to clients, after reporting the fire the nurse may attempt to extinguish it. Most fire departments want to be notified of the fire before the person attempts to extinguish it so they can be on the scene as quickly as possible.

If a fire occurs in a health care agency, the nurse has two major goals: to protect clients from injury and to contain the fire.

Clients who are close to the fire, regardless of its size, are at risk of injury and should be moved to another area. If a client requires oxygen but not life support, the nurse first discontinues the oxygen. Oxygen is not itself flammable, but it is combustible and can fuel an existing fire. If the client is on life support, the nurse may need to maintain the client's respiratory status manually with an Ambu bag (see Chapter 41) until the client is moved away from the threat of fire. Ambulatory clients can be directed to walk by themselves to a safe area, and in some cases ambulatory clients may be able to assist in moving clients in wheelchairs.

Bedridden clients are generally moved from the scene of a fire by a stretcher, their bed, or a wheelchair. If none of these methods is appropriate, the clients must be carried from the area. In hospital or institutional fires all personnel are mobilized to evacuate clients. If a client must be carried, the nurse should be careful not to overextend physical limits for lifting, since injury to the nurse can result in fur-

TABLE 34-8

Types of Fire Extinguishers and Their Uses

Type	Class of Fire	How to Use	Precautions
Carbon dioxide (CO$_2$)	Grease, electrical	Direct CO$_2$ into the flame, thus cutting off the fire's oxygen supply.	
Soda and acid (water extinguisher)	Paper and rubbish, wood	Turn canister upside down, thereby mixing the soda and acid. CO$_2$ is then produced, releasing the water extinguisher under pressure. To stop the flow, turn canister right side up.	Ineffective against grease and electrical fires because it causes grease to spatter, thereby spreading the fire, and water conducts electricity
Dry chemical	Rubbish, electrical	Pull a pin or press a level on the extinguisher, blanketing the fire with foam, and thus cutting off the fire's oxygen supply.	Ineffective against grease because it causes grease to spatter and thus spreads the fire
Water pump	Rubbish, wood	Pump the handle while pointing the nozzle toward the fire.	Ineffective against grease and electrical fires because the grease can spatter, spreading fire, and because water conducts electricity
Antifreeze or water	Rubbish, wood, grease, anesthetics	Pull pin and handle of extinguisher, and direct extinguisher toward fire.	Ineffective against electrical fires because water conducts electricity

ther injury to the client. If fire department personnel are on the scene, they can help evacuate the clients.

Once a fire has been reported and it has been determined that there is no danger to clients or the clients have been removed from danger, nurses and other personnel must take measures to contain or put out the fire. One means of containing a fire is to reduce its oxygen source by closing doors and windows and turning off oxygen. Electrical equipment should also be turned off. The nurse should know how to use a fire extinguisher. The three basic types of fires for which extinguishers are used are paper and rubbish (type A), grease and anesthesia (type B), and electrical (type C). The appropriate extinguisher must be used for each type (Table 34-8). The wrong extinguisher will not put out the fire and may even worsen the situation, especially with electrical and grease fires.

POISONING. Accidental poisonings are a greater risk for the toddler, the preschooler, and the young school-age child. The nurse can help parents take preventive measures to reduce the risk of accidental poi-

soning by placing poison labels on hazardous substances (Fig. 34-12). In the adolescent and young or middle adult poisonings are usually caused by insect or snake bites. Drug poisonings with this age group are commonly related to suicide attempts or result from drug experimentation. The elderly client is also

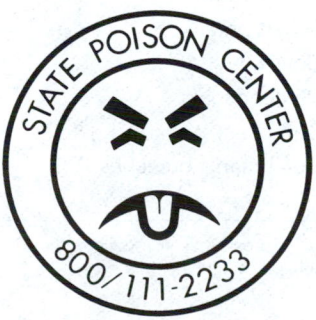

Fig. 34-12 "Mr. Yuk" label.
From Billings, D.M., and Stokes, L.G.: Medical surgical nursing: common health problems of adults and children across the life span, St. Louis, 1982, The C.V. Mosby Co.

Poisonous Plants

These plants contain a wide variety of poisons, and symptoms may vary from a mild stomach ache, skin rash, and swelling of the mouth and throat to involvement of the heart, kidneys, or other organs. The poison center can give you more specific information on these plants or others that may be poisonous and are not on this list. Many plants do not cause toxicity unless ingested in very large amounts.

- Acorn (oak)
- Akee fruit
- Anemone
- Angel trumpet tree
- Apricot (kernels, leaves)
- Arrowhead
- Autumn crocus
- Avocado (leaves)
- Azalea
- Baneberry
- Belladonna
- Betel nut palm
- Bird of paradise
- Bittersweet
- Black locust
- Bleeding heart
- Buckeye
- Buttercup
- Caladium
- Calla lily
- Castor bean
- Century plant
- Cherries (pits)
- Chinaberry
- Choke cherry
- Christmas rose
- Climbing nightshade
- Cowbane
- Daffodil
- Daphne
- Deadly nightshade
- Delphinium
- Desert potato
- Devil's ivy
- Dieffenbachia
- Dumbcane
- Dutchman's breeches

- Elderberry
- Elephant ear
- English ivy
- Euonymus
- Fava bean
- Flags (iris)
- Four o'clock
- Foxglove
- Goldenchain
- Holly berries
- Horsetail reed
- Hyacinth
- Hydrangea
- Indian turnip
- Inkberry
- Iris
- Jack-in-the-pulpit
- Japanese yew
- Jasmine
- Jequirty bean
- Jerusalem cherry
- Jimson weed seeds
- Jonquil
- Lantana
- Larkspur
- Lingustrum
- Lily of the valley
- Lobelia
- Locoweed
- Lucky nut
- Marsh marigold
- Mayapple
- Mistletoe berries
- Monkshood
- Moonseed
- Morning glory
- Mother-in-law plant

- Mountain laurel
- Mulberries (green)
- Narcissus
- Nightshade
- Oleander
- Peach (seeds)
- Pencil tree
- Peony
- Periwinkle
- Peyote
- Philodendron
- Pigeonberry
- Poison hemlock
- Poison ivy
- Pokeweed/pokeberries
- Potato (all green parts)
- Primrose
- Privet
- Ranunculus
- Rhododendron
- Rhubarb leaves
- Rosary pea
- Snow drop
- Sorrel
- Star of Bethlehem
- Swiss cheese plant
- Thornapple
- Threadleaf
- Tobacco
- Tomato (all green parts)
- Tulip bulb
- Virginia creeper
- Water hemlock
- Wisteria
- Yellow jessamine
- Yew berries

Modified from St. Louis Regional Poison Center Network: Poisonous plants, St. Louis, 1983, Cardinal Glennon Memorial Hospital for Children.

Poisonous Household Chemicals

- Alcoholic beverages
- Ammonia
- Antifreeze
- Ant syrup or paste
- Automotive products
- Bathroom bowl cleaner
- Bleach
- Boric acid
- Camphophenique
- Charcoal lighter
- Cleaning fluid
- Clinitest tablets
- Cologne
- Copper and brass cleaners
- Corn and wart remover
- Detergents
- Dishwasher detergents
- Disinfectants
- Drain cleaners
- Epoxy glue kit

- Furniture polish
- Garden sprays
- Gasoline
- Gun cleaners
- Hair dyes
- Insecticides
- Iodine
- Iron medications
- Kerosene
- Lighter fluid
- Model cement
- Muriatic acid
- Mushrooms
- Nail polish
- Nail polish remover
- Oven cleaner
- Paint
- Paint remover
- Paint thinner
- Perfume

- Permanent wave solutions
- Pesticides
- Pine oil
- Plants
- Prescription and nonprescription medicines
- Rat poisons
- Rubbing alcohol
- Shaving lotion
- Silver polish
- Snail bait
- Spot removers
- Strychnine
- Sulfuric acid
- Super glue
- Turpentine
- Veterinary products
- Weed killers
- Window wash solvent

From St. Louis Regional Poison Center Network: Poisonous household chemicals, St. Louis, 1983, Cardinal Glennon Memorial Hospital for Children.

at risk for poisoning because diminished eyesight may cause an accidental ingestion of a toxic substance. The impaired memory of some elderly clients may also result in accidental overdosage of prescribed medications.

A poison is any substance that impairs health or destroys life when ingested, inhaled, or absorbed by the body. In the home the two major sources of poisons are plants (see boxed material on p. 926) and household cleaners (boxed material above). However, insect bites or the accidental ingestion of drugs or cosmetics may also result in poisoning.

For some types of poisons specific antidotes or treatments are available, but for other types there is no treatment. The capacity of body tissue to recover from the poison determines the reversibility of the effect. Poisons can impair the respiratory, circulatory, central nervous, hepatic, gastrointestinal, and renal systems of the body.

Experts recommend that in a suspected case of poisoning the nurse or family member should call a poison control center. A poison control center is a facility that provides information regarding all aspects of intoxication, treatment, and referrals. The nurse should teach parents that calling such a center for informa-

tion before attempting home remedies can save their child's life. People may mistakenly induce vomiting for corrosive or petroleum-based substances, thus potentially worsening the victim's condition.

Procedure 34-1 lists accepted interventions for accidental poisonings that the nurse may teach to a parent or guardian. In addition, the parent may be instructed to give milk to neutralize an acid substance or lemon juice or vinegar to neutralize an alkaline substance.

ELECTRICAL HAZARDS. Much of the equipment used in health care settings is electrical. Most hospital beds and examining tables have electric motors so a client's position can be changed easily and quickly. Any piece of electrical equipment used in a health care agency must be well maintained in a safe condition to prevent electrical hazards.

The electrical plug of grounded equipment has three prongs (Fig. 34-13). The rounded, longer prong is the ground. Theoretically the grounding prong carries any stray electrical current back to the ground, hence its name. The other two prongs carry the power to the piece of electrical equipment (Cooper, 1983). Electricity follows a path of least resistance, and with

PROCEDURE 34-1

Intervening in Accidental Poisonings

STEPS	RATIONALE
1. Identify the type and amount of the substance ingested.	This information will help to determine the correct type and amount of antidote needed for the victim.
2. Call the poison control center before attempting any intervention.	Poison control centers have all the information needed to treat the poisoned client or to offer referral to treatment centers.
3. If instructed to induce vomiting: administer 1 tablespoon (15 ml) of syrup of ipecac followed by a glass of water; repeat once if vomiting does not occur in 15 to 20 minutes. Do not administer if child is under 1 year of age.	Households should keep syrup of ipecac in an easily accessible place. Ipecac causes vomiting and emptying of the stomach, rather than gagging or retching.
If ipecac is unavailable:	
a. Administer one or two glasses of warm water followed by tickling the back of the throat.	This induces vomiting but may not ensure complete emptying of stomach contents.
b. Administer 1 tablespoon of salt or 1 to 2 teaspoons of mustard in a glass of warm water.	This induces vomiting but may not ensure complete emptying of stomach contents.
4. If requested to do so, save vomitus and deliver to poison control center.	Laboratory analysis can determine what further treatment is necessary.
5. Place the victim with the head turned to the side.	This reduces the risk of aspiration.
6. Vomiting is *never* induced for the following substances: lye, household cleansers, grease or petroleum products, furniture polish.	Vomiting can increase the area of internal burns (in the case of lye) and the risk of aspiration.
7. Vomiting is *never* induced in an unconscious victim.	Vomiting increases the risk of aspiration.
8. If instructed by the poison control center to bring the person to the emergency room, call an ambulance.	Ambulance personnel will be able to provide emergency measures if needed. In addition, the parent or guardian may be too upset to drive safely.

electrical short circuits or other accidents the path of least resistance may not be the intended circuit but may be through a person in contact with the equipment. If the grounding prong is intact and operational, it will act as a path of least resistance and divert all stray current into the ground.

Improperly grounded or malfunctioning electrical equipment increases the risk of electrical injury and

fire. Many electrical injuries or fires from electrical sources can be prevented if nurses and others observe for hazards. The use of a prevention checklist when assessing the client's environment can reduce injuries in both the health care agency and the home (see box on p. 929).

Evaluation

The nursing care plan directed toward the promotion of the client's safety is evaluated on the basis of reduced potential for injury and the absence of actual injury. The nursing plan and the interventions are designed to reduce injuries from actual or potential developmental or environmental risks. The nurse continually assesses risks in both areas to identify any new or continuing hazards. If such a risk is identified or if the client does experience injury, the nurse must modify the nursing care plan to develop interventions for these safety needs.

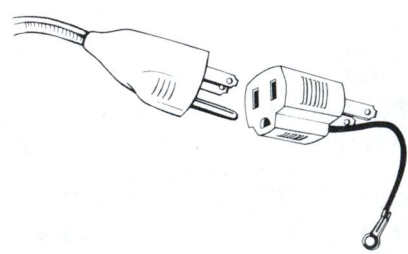

Fig. 34-13 Three-pronged ground plug with adapter.

Prevention of Electrical Hazards

- Use only grounded equipment.
- Check electrical equipment for frayed cords or visible signs of damage before use.
- Avoid overloading outlets.
- If extension cords must be used, make sure they are taped to the ground with *electrical tape* to prevent others from tripping over the cord and pulling out the plug.
- Never pull a plug using the cord. Pull a plug by gripping it firmly and pulling it straight out of the wall socket.
- Send equipment that has been dropped to the biomedical department before reuse.
- Report any shocks experienced while using equipment.
- Believe a client who reports a tingling sensation or shocks from the equipment, and have the equipment evaluated for stray current. If possible, unplug equipment until evaluation takes place.
- If you do not understand how to operate a piece of equipment, ask for assistance.

Modified from Cooper, K.C.: Focus **10**:17, 1983.

Summary

A safe environment is essential to maintaining and restoring a client's health. Nurses working in a structured health care setting or in a community-based agency are the client's first line of defense against falls, environmental hazards, medication errors, poisoning, and other injuries.

The client's risk for injury increases with declining health status, decreases in mobility, and reduced functioning of special senses. In addition, clients at opposite ends of the life span, the very young and the elderly, have greater risks to their safety.

The nursing process is used to reduce the risk of injury through specific nursing interventions and client education. The nurse promotes a safe environment by removing threats to safety and by teaching clients and their families about hazards in their homes.

KEY CONCEPTS

✓ Protection and safety are basic to survival throughout the life span.

✓ A safe environment in a health care agency is one that is comfortable, maintains the client's privacy, and reduces the risks of injury, infection, and untoward effects from treatment or medications.

✓ A safe health care environment reduces the length of treatment or hospitalization, the frequency of treatment-related accidents, the potential for lawsuits, the number of work-related injuries to personnel, and the overall cost of health service.

✓ Safety in the home reduces the risk of accidents, illnesses, and the need for health care services.

✓ In the community a safe environment is one in which basic needs are achievable, physical hazards are reduced, transmission of pathogens and parasites is reduced, pollution is controlled, and sanitation is maintained.

✓ Factors that reduce the amount of available atmospheric oxygen include an improperly functioning furnace and high carbon monoxide levels from automobile exhaust and cigarette smoke.

✓ Excessive relative humidity causes the skin's moisture to evaporate slowly, whereas low relative humidity causes the skin's moisture to evaporate quickly and the skin to become excessively dry.

✓ Controlled increases in environmental humidity can liquefy respiratory tract secretions and reduce the risk of respiratory tract infections.

✓ Prolonged exposure to extremely hot or cold environmental temperatures can reduce the client's level of health or even cause death.

✓ Air pollution, water pollution, and noise pollution in the work or community environment are health risks.

✓ Reduction of physical hazards in a client's environment includes providing adequate lighting, decreasing clutter, and securing the home.

✓ Pathogens and parasites can be found in water, food, people, and insects and other animals.

✓ The transmission of pathogens and parasites is reduced through medical and surgical asepsis, immunization, food sanitation, insect and rodent control, and disposal of human wastes.

✓ Every developmental stage involves specific risks the nurse should assess.

✓ Children under 5 years of age are at greatest risk for home accidents that may result in severe injury and death.

✓ The school-age child is at risk for injury at home, at school, and traveling to and from school.

✓ Adolescents are at risk of abusing drugs and alcohol.

✓ Threats to an adult's safety are frequently associated with life-style habits.

✓ Risks of injury for the elderly are directly related to the physiological changes of the aging process.

✓ Risks to client safety within a health care agency include falls and client-inherent, procedure-related, and equipment-related accidents.

KEY CONCEPTS, cont'd

✓ Nursing interventions for promoting a client's safety are individualized for the client's developmental stage, life-style, and environment.

✓ Nursing interventions are developed to modify the client's environment for protection from falls, fires, poisonings, and electrical hazards.

✓ The nursing care plan to promote safety is continually evaluated to identify new or continued risks to the client.

REFERENCES

Cooper, K.L.: Electrical safety: the electrically sensitive ICU patient, Focus 10:17, 1983.

Cooper, S.: Common concern—accidents and older adults, Geriatr. Nurs. 2:287, 1981.

Davidson, M., and Grant, E.: Accidental hypothermia: a community hospital perspective, Postgrad. Med. 70:42, 1981.

Lindenmuth, J.E., Breu, C.S., and Malooley, J.A.: Sensory overload, Am. J. Nurs. 80:1456, 1981.

Lynn, F.H.: Incidents—need they be accidents, Am. J. Nurs. 80:1098, 1980.

Maslow, A.H.: Toward a psychology of being, ed. 2, New York, 1968, Van Nostrand Reinhold Co., Inc.

Rice, M.A., and Kibbee, P.E.: Review: identifying the adolescent substance abuser, Matern. Child Nurs. J. 8:139, 1983.

ADDITIONAL READINGS

Baptiste, M.S., and Feck, G.: Preventing tap water burns, Am. J. Public Health 70:727, 1980.

Ferguson, D., and Beck, C.: H.A.L.F.—a tool to assess elder abuse within the family, Geriatr. Nurs. 4:30, 1983.

Ford, A.H.: Use of automobile restraining devices for infants, Nurs. Res. 29:281, 1980.

Hayne, W.E.: Retirement cypen tower: a design for retirement living, Aging 4:18, 1983.

Meth, I.M.: Electrical safety in the hospital, Am. J. Nurs. 80:1344, 1980.

Riffle, K.L.: Falls: kinds, causes and prevention, Geriatr. Nurs. 3:165, 1982.

Rivara, F.P., and Berger, C.R.: Consumer product hazards: setting priorities for research and regulatory action, Am. J. Public Health 70:701, 1980.

Roy, G.: Home accidents—can they be prevented? Nurs. Times Community Outlook, August 11, 1982, p. 212.

Roy, G.: Home accidents: developmental risks, Nurs. Times Community Outlook, August 11, 1982, p. 217.

Witte, N.S.: Why the elderly fall, Am. J. Nurs. 75:1950, 1979.

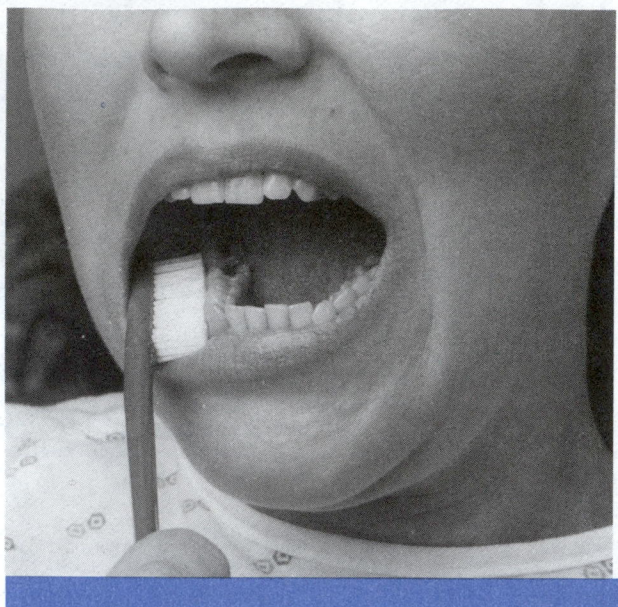

OBJECTIVES

Mastery of content in this chapter will enable the student to:

- Define the terms in the glossary.
- List the factors that influence a client's personal hygiene.
- Develop a nursing care plan based on the client's personal preferences and hygiene practices.
- Identify common skin problems and related nursing interventions.
- Discuss conditions that may put a client at risk for impaired skin integrity.
- Describe the types of bathing techniques used depending on the physical condition of the client.
- Discuss the basic guidelines the nurse should follow when giving any type of bath.
- Successfully peform a complete bed bath and backrub.
- List the steps involved in bathing an infant.
- List common foot and nail problems and their related nursing interventions.
- List five nursing goals in providing oral hygiene.
- Describe two major types of oral problems, their causes, and related nursing interventions.
- Successfully assist or provide a client with daily oral care.
- Discuss the care involved in providing oral hygiene for an unconscious client.
- List common hair and scalp problems and their related nursing interventions.
- Describe the procedures of inserting and removing contact lenses and artificial eyes.
- Successfully make an occupied, an unoccupied, and a surgical hospital bed.

GLOSSARY

AM care   Routine hygiene care performed before breakfast or early in the morning.

apocrine gland   One of the large, deep exocrine glands located in the axillary, anal, genital, and mammary areas of the body; secretes sweat having a strong odor.

bath blanket   Thin, lightweight cotton blanket used to cover the client during the bath; it absorbs the water and provides warmth.

callus   Common, usually painless thickening of the epidermis at locations of external pressure or friction.

cerumen   Waxy substance secreted in the ear.

complete bed bath   Bath in which the entire body of a client is washed in bed.

corn   Horny mass of condensed epithelial cells overlying a bony prominence (usually on a toe).

dandruff   Excessive amount of scaly material composed of dead epithelium shed from the scalp.

dental caries (cavity)   Abnormal destructive condition in a tooth caused by a complex interaction of food, especially starches and sugars, with bacteria that form dental plaque.

drawsheet   Sheet, smaller in size than a bottom or top sheet, that is placed over the middle of the bottom sheet to keep the mattress and bottom linens dry; can also be used to turn and move clients in bed.

eccrine gland   One of the two types of sweat glands; eccrine glands are present throughout the

35 | *Hygiene*

body and promote cooling by evaporation of their secretions.

erythema Redness or inflammation of the skin or mucous membranes that is a result of dilation and congestion of superficial capillaries; sunburn is an example.

gingiva Gum of the mouth; a mucous membrane with supporting fibrous tissue that overlies the crowns of unerupted teeth and encircles the necks of those that have erupted.

halitosis Offensive breath resulting from poor oral hygiene, dental or oral infection, ingestion of certain foods, or systemic disease.

keratosis Any skin condition in which there are overgrowth and thickening of the cornified epithelium; types are actinic and seborrheic.

oral hygiene Condition or practice of maintaining the tissues and structures of the mouth.

paronychia Infection of the fold of skin at the margin of a nail.

partial bed bath Bath in which body parts that might cause the client discomfort if left unbathed, that is, face, hands, axillary areas, back, and perineum, are washed in bed.

perineal care Cleansing procedure prescribed for cleaning the genital and anal areas as part of the daily bath or after various obstetrical and gynecological procedures.

periodontal disease (pyorrhea) Disease of the tissues around the tooth, such as an inflammation of the periodontal membrane or ligament.

plantar wart Painful lesion on the sole of the foot, primarily at pressure points, caused by the common wart virus.

PM care Routine hygiene care performed before bedtime.

pruritus Symptom of itching, an uncomfortable sensation leading to the urge to scratch, which may result in secondary infections.

sebum Normal secretion of the sebaceous glands of the skin; when combined with sweat, forms a moist, oily, acidic film that protects the skin from drying.

Trendelenburg position Position in which the body and legs are on an inclined plane with the head lowermost.

Maintenance of physical hygiene is necessary for an individual's comfort, safety, and sense of well-being. Hygiene practices include measures that maintain personal cleanliness and good grooming. Normally a well person is capable of meeting his own hygiene needs. However, an ill person may require the nurse's assistance to carry out routine hygiene practices. The nurse has the responsibilities of determining a client's ability to perform self-care and providing hygiene care according to the client's needs and preferred practices. The nurse must also determine whether a client's hygiene practices are adequate and if the client is aware of specific hygiene needs. As a client's physical condition changes, so do hygiene needs.

While providing routine hygienic care, the nurse has the opportunity to perform assessments of the client's physical and emotional state. The nurse can assess the integument and identify any alterations or the potential for integumentary changes. Since hygienic care often requires intimate contact with the client, the nurse is able to use communication skills to promote the therapeutic relationship and to learn about the client's emotional needs. Providing hygiene also gives the nurse an excellent opportunity to offer emotional support and teach clients about health promotion practices. By incorporating nursing therapies into daily hygiene care, the nurse can more efficiently meet the client's total needs. For example, while bathing a surgical client the nurse can inspect the condition of a dressing or wound, discuss the activity limitations resulting from surgery, and assist the client with lower extremity exercises.

A client's hygiene practices are influenced by the individual's beliefs, values, habits, and health status. The nurse must consider these, as well as the client's specific physical limitations, when planning hygiene care. Every client is likely to perform hygiene measures differently. For example, some people are accustomed to bathing in the evening rather than in the morning or to shampooing their hair once a week instead of daily. Such preferences do not significantly affect health and can usually be incorporated into the nurse's plan of care. The important goals are preserving as much of the client's independence as possible, providing a setting conducive to the client's privacy, and ensuring that hygiene measures are performed often enough to promote the client's physical well-being.

Factors Influencing Hygiene Practice

An ill person who enters the health care system must adjust to the role of client, which may mean giving up some or all independence. Even a client with moderate physical limitations soon realizes that he is dependent on the nursing staff for assistance with or provision of his hygiene care. The feeling of dependence represents a loss of control for the client and may increase feelings of discomfort resulting from the psychological stress. It is imperative that the nurse understand the client's perspective and consider factors that influence the client's hygiene practices.

Body Image

The client's general appearance indicates the importance hygiene holds for him. If the client is meticulously groomed, the nurse must consider all details of grooming when planning care and must consult the client before making decisions about how hygienic care should be provided. In contrast, the client who appears unkempt or uninterested in hygiene requires education about the importance of hygiene. The nurse must not convey feelings of disapproval or revulsion when caring for a client whose hygiene is obviously poor.

When the client's body image changes as a result of surgery or a physical ailment, the nurse must make an extra effort to promote hygiene. For example, a young woman who has undergone a thyroidectomy may be concerned about the appearance of the scar in her neck. In addition to helping the client maintain good grooming practices, the nurse can discuss ways to cover the scar with ties or scarves until it becomes fainter.

Socioeconomic Status

A person's economic resources influence the type and extent of hygienic practices used. The nurse should determine if the client can afford necessary hygiene supplies such as deodorant, shampoo, toothpaste, and cosmetics.

Knowledge

Knowledge about the importance of hygiene and its implications for well-being influences a person's hygiene practices. However, knowledge alone is not enough; the person must also be motivated to maintain self-care. Often learning about his illness or condition will encourage the client to improve his hygiene. For example, when a diabetic client is made aware of the effect of diabetes on the circulation to the feet, he is more likely to learn the proper techniques for foot care.

Cultural Variables

A client's cultural beliefs, personal values, and familial practices influence hygienic care. Persons from diverse cultural backgrounds follow different self-care practices. In North America, for example, many people take daily showers or tub baths. In the Far East cleanliness is viewed as essential to a person's well-being. In European countries, however, it is not unusual to bathe completely only once a week. When a nurse works with a client whose hygiene practices are different from her own, she should not be judgmental or force a change in the client's practices unless hygiene is inadequate for the client's physiological needs.

Familial habits also influence hygiene practices. Members of a large family that has only one bathtub may be accustomed to bathing only once or twice a week. If a mother routinely brushes her teeth after each meal, her children are likely to do the same. A father who does not use shaving cologne or antiperspirant will be unlikely to encourage his son to do so. As children grow and become influenced by peers, hygiene habits can change. A teenage girl will become concerned with her hairstyle and makeup when a young man becomes interested in her.

Personal Preferences

When planning a client's hygiene care the nurse must be aware of the times of day at which the client prefers to bathe, shampoo his hair, shave, or brush his teeth. Likewise, the nurse should consider the hygiene products the client prefers, such as type of soap, toothpaste, or shaving cream. Each client will also have preferences regarding how hygiene is performed. For example, one man may prefer to shave before his bath, whereas another shaves after taking a shower. Respecting client's preferences helps the nurse develop a more individualized plan of care.

Types of Hygiene Care

The nurse provides a variety of hygiene measures throughout the course of a day. The client's own preferences and habits influence how the nurse organizes her care so hygiene can be provided. The nurse can often schedule other care measures around the times hygiene is planned. The following paragraphs describe the types of hygienic care commonly performed at certain times of day.

Early Morning Care

Nursing personnel on the night shift are responsible for providing basic hygiene to clients getting ready for breakfast or scheduled for early morning surgery or diagnostic tests. Such "AM care" includes offering a bedpan or urinal if the client is not ambulatory, washing the client's hands and face, and assisting with oral care.

Morning or After Breakfast Care

After breakfast the nurse performs or assists the client with necessary hygiene measures. These include offering the bedpan or urinal if the client is not ambulatory; assisting the client with oral care; shaving the male client; assisting with or providing a complete bed bath, shower, or tub bath; giving a back massage; changing the client's gown or pajamas; shampooing, brushing, or combing the client's hair; and changing the bed linens and straightening the client's bedside unit and room.

Afternoon Care

A hospitalized client frequently undergoes many exhausting tests or procedures in the morning. In rehabilitation centers clients may participate in various therapy programs during the morning hours. After lunch the nurse may provide additional hygienic care such as washing the hands and face, assisting with oral care, and fluffing pillows or straightening bed linen. These simple measures give the client a refreshed feeling before family members and other visitors arrive.

Evening or Hour of Sleep Care

Just before bedtime the nurse offers personal hygiene care that helps the client relax so he can fall asleep more easily. Such "PM care" may include changing soiled bed linens, gowns, or pajamas; assisting the client in washing the face and hands; providing oral hygiene; giving a back massage; and offering the bedpan or urinal if the client is not ambulatory.

Care of the Skin

The skin is an active organ with the functions of protection, secretion, excretion, temperature regulation, and sensation (Table 35-1). The skin has three primary layers: epidermis, dermis, and subcutaneous. The epidermis is composed of several thin layers of cells undergoing different stages of maturation. The innermost layer of the epidermis generates new cells

---

TABLE 35-1

Function of the Skin and Implications for Care

Function	Description	Implications for Care
Protection	The epidermis is a relatively impermeable layer that prevents entrance of microorganisms. Although microorganisms reside on the skin surface and in hair follicles, the relative dryness of the skin's surface inhibits bacterial growth. Sebum removes bacteria from hair follicles. The acidic pH of the skin further retards bacterial growth.	Weakening of the epidermis occurs by scraping or stripping its surface as by use of dry razors, tape removal, or improper turning or positioning techniques. Excessive dryness causes cracks and breaks in the skin and mucosa that allow bacteria to enter. Emollients soften skin and prevent moisture loss, soaking of the skin improves moisture retention, and hydration of the mucosa prevents dryness. However, constant exposure of the skin to moisture causes maceration or softening, which promotes bacterial growth. Bed linen and clothing should be kept dry. Misuse of soap, detergents, cosmetics, deodorant, and depilatories can cause chemical irritation. Alkaline soaps neutralize the protective acid condition of the skin. Cleansing of the skin removes excess oil, sweat, dead skin cells, and dirt that can promote bacterial growth.
Sensation	The skin contains sensory organs for touch, pain, heat, cold, and pressure.	Friction should be used judiciously to avoid causing discomfort during bathing. Smoothing linen removes sources of mechanical irritation. Removing rings prevents the nurse from accidentally injuring the client's skin.
Temperature regulation	Body temperature is controlled by radiation, evaporation, conduction, and convection.	Factors that interfere with heat loss can alter a person's temperature control. Wet bed linen or gowns interfere with convection and conduction. Excess blankets or bed coverings can interfere with heat loss through radiation and conduction. Coverings can promote heat conservation.
Excretion and secretion	Sweat acts to promote heat loss by evaporation. Sebum lubricates skin and hair.	Perspiration and oil can harbor microorganism growth. Bathing removes excess body secretions, although excessive bathing can cause drying of skin.

that migrate slowly toward the epidermal surface. These cells replace the dead cells that are continuously shed from the skin's outer surface. The epidermis also contains melanocytes, special cells that produce the melanin or dark pigment of the skin. Darker-skinned races have more active melanocytes, which produce more melanin.

The dermis is a thicker skin layer containing bundles of collagen and elastic fibers to support the epidermis. Nerve fibers, blood vessels, sweat glands, sebaceous glands, and hair follicles course through the dermal layer. Sebaceous glands secrete sebum, an oily, odorous fluid, into the hair follicles. Sebum lubricates the skin and hair to keep them supple and pliant. There are two types of sweat glands: eccrine and apocrine. The eccrine glands are distributed throughout the skin but are more abundant in the forehead, palms, and soles. Sweat excreted from the eccrine glands assists in temperature control through evaporation. The apocrine glands can be found in the axillary and genital areas. The bacterial decomposition of sweat from these glands is responsible for body odor. In the ears ceruminous glands secrete cerumen into the external ear canal. This heavy, oily substance traps foreign material entering the ear.

Although the oral mucosa contains the dermal layer, it does not have sebaceous or sweat glands, hair follicles, or ceruminous glands. Instead, salivary glands secrete saliva through ducts at the base of the mouth. Saliva aids in the mechanical cleansing and hydration of the external mucosa. The skin is generally tough and pliable, but mucous membranes are much more sensitive. Therefore extra caution is necessary when cleansing the oral cavity.

The subcutaneous tissue layer contains blood vessels, nerves, lymph, and loose connective tissue filled with fat cells. The fatty tissue serves as a heat insulator of the body. Subcutaneous tissue also provides support for upper skin layers. Very little subcutaneous tissue can be found underlying the oral mucosa.

The skin and mucosa exchange oxygen, nutrients, and fluid with underlying blood vessels, synthesize new cells, and eliminate dead nonfunctioning cells. The cells of the integument require adequate nutrition and hydration to resist injury and disease. Adequate circulation is essential to maintain cell life. When a person's physical condition changes, the skin often reflects this by alterations in color, thickness, texture, turgor, temperature, and hydration (see Chapter 29). As long as the skin remains intact and healthy, its physiological function remains optimal.

Assessment

As the nurse prepares to assist the client with personal hygiene needs, it is important to remember that assessment is ongoing. The nurse does not assess all body parts before giving a bath or shampooing the client's hair. However, the nurse must determine whether the client can tolerate hygiene procedures, which can often be exhausting. For example, if a client is short of breath or complains of fatigue, the nurse either limits hygiene measures or provides total care without the client's assistance.

Most assessment occurs as the nurse ministers to the client's hygienic needs. For example, while bathing a client's back the nurse may look for skin rashes, decubitus ulcers (see Chapter 31), or pressure sites. Hygiene care gives the nurse the opportunity to make assessment findings for a wide variety of health care problems and thus helps the nurse set priorities for the client's care plan.

PHYSICAL ASSESSMENT OF THE SKIN

Assisting a client with his personal hygiene affords the nurse opportunities for assessing all external body surfaces. Using the skills of inspection and palpation (see Chapter 29) the nurse looks for alterations in the integument, determines the client's need for hygiene, and notes changes of the integument in response to nursing and medical therapies.

The nurse determines the condition of the skin by observing its color, texture, thickness, turgor, temperature, and hydration. Chapter 29 describes in detail the techniques for assessing each of these characteristics. The nurse gives special attention to the characteristics most influenced by hygiene measures. Are there areas of dry skin as a result of too frequent baths, excessive use of soap, or use of harsh alkaline soaps? Have areas of skin maceration formed as a result of improper drying? Are there callused areas on the feet or hands that might benefit from soaking and the application of lotion?

While inspecting the skin the nurse notes the presence and condition of any lesions. Chapter 29 describes the various types of skin lesions. Certain types have implications with regard to hygiene measures (Table 35-2). When the nurse observes any skin problems, it is helpful to explain proper skin care to the client. For example, a rash on the client's skin is often indicative of an allergic reaction. The nurse can teach the client about the proper use of medications prescribed for the rash and caution the client against use of over-the-counter drugs that may prove useless or even worsen the rash. Likewise, the nurse may educate the client about avoiding use of irritants, such as harsh soaps or cosmetics, that can aggravate the skin rash condition.

TABLE 35-2

Common Skin Problems

Problem	Characteristics	Implications	Interventions
Dry skin	Flaky, rough texture on exposed areas such as hands, arms, legs, or face	Skin may become infected if the epidermal layer is allowed to crack.	Bathe less frequently. Rinse body of all soap well, since residue left on skin can cause irritation and breakdown. Add moisture to air through use of humidifier. Increase fluid intake when skin is dry. Use moisturizing lotion to aid in healing process. The lotion forms a protective barrier and helps maintain fluid within the skin. Use creams to clean skin that is dry or allergic to soaps and detergents.
Acne	Inflammatory, papulopustular skin eruption, usually involving bacterial breakdown of sebum; appears on face, neck, shoulders, and back	Infected material within pustule can spread if area is squeezed or picked. Permanent scarring can result.	Wash hair and skin thoroughly each day with hot water and soap to remove oil. Cosmetics should be used sparingly, since oily cosmetics or creams accumulate in pores and tend to make the condition worse. Dietary restrictions may need to be implemented. Foods found to aggravate the condition should be eliminated from diet. Exposure to ultraviolet rays, either from sunshine or a heat lamp, may help control acne. Caution should be used to prevent burning of skin. Use prescribed topical antibiotics for severe forms of acne.
Hirsutism	Excessive growth of body and facial hair, especially in women	Hirsutism may cause a negative body image by giving a female a male appearance.	The following may be used to remove unwanted hair: depilatories (can cause infection, rashes, or dermatitis); shaving (safest method); electrolysis (permanently removes hair by destroying hair follicles); tweezing (lasts only temporarily); bleaching of hair (lasts only temporarily).

TABLE 35-2, cont'd

Common Skin Problems

Problem	Characteristics	Implications	Interventions
Skin rashes	Skin eruption that may result from over exposure to sun or moisture or from an allergic reaction; may be flat or raised, localized or systemic, pruritic or nonpruritic	If the skin is continually scratched, inflammation and infection may occur. Rashes can also cause discomfort.	Wash area thoroughly and apply antiseptic spray or lotion to prevent further itching and aid in healing process. Warm soaks may relieve inflammation.
Contact dermatitis	Inflammation of skin characterized by abrupt onset with erythema, pruritus, pain, and appearance of scaly oozing lesions; seen on face, neck, hands, forearms, and genitalia	Dermatitis is often difficult to eliminate because the person is usually in continual contact with a substance causing the skin reaction. The substance may be hard to identify.	The condition usually disappears when exposure to causative agents (e.g., cleansers and soaps) is avoided.
Abrasion	Scraping or rubbing away of epidermis; may result in localized bleeding and later weeping of serous fluid	Infection occurs easily owing to loss of protective skin layer.	Nurses should be careful not to scratch clients with jewelry or fingernails. Wash abrasions with mild soap and water. Use of a dressing or bandage could increase risk of infection owing to retained moisture.

DEVELOPMENTAL CHANGES

A client's age influences the normal condition of the skin and the type of hygiene measures required. The neonate's skin is relatively immature with the epidermis and dermis loosely bound together. The skin is extremely thin. Since any friction against the skin layers can cause bruising, the nurse must handle the neonate carefully during bathing. A break in the neonate's skin can easily lead to infection.

In a toddler the skin layers are more tightly bound together. The child thus has a greater resistance to infection and skin irritation. However, because of the child's more active play and the absence of established hygiene habits, greater attention is needed from parents and care givers to provide thorough hygiene.

During adolescence the growth and maturation of the integument are increased. In girls estrogen secretion causes the skin to become soft, smooth, and thicker in texture with increased vascularity. In boys male hormones produce an increased thickness of the skin with some darkening in color. Sebaceous glands become more active, predisposing adolescents to acne. Eccrine and apocrine sweat glands become fully functional during puberty. Adolescents usually begin to use antiperspirants. More frequent bathing and shampooing also become necessary to reduce body odors. Sweating is usually more pronounced in boys. The growth of body hair increases during adolescence as a result of hormonal changes. The body hair has a characteristic pattern of distribution, which the nurse can assess (see Chapter 29). Pubic and axillary hair develops in both sexes. Beard and mustache hair grows in boys as a result of testicular androgens. Some girls and women have increased androgen levels causing hirsutism, or growth of facial hair.

The condition of an adult's skin depends on the person's hygiene practices and exposure to environmental irritants. Normally the skin is elastic, well hydrated, firm, and smooth. With age the skin loses its resiliency and moisture. Sebaceous and sweat glands become less active. Thus many older adults do not need antiperspirants. The epithelium thins, and elastic collagen fibers shrink. Therefore the elderly client's skin is very fragile. Activities such as moving up in bed, sitting on a bedpan, or turning from side to side can cause bruising and even breaks in the skin. Removal of tape from an elderly client's skin can result in loss of an entire skin layer if caution is not used. Typically the elderly person's skin is dry and wrinkled. Excessive exposure to the sun can aggravate the wrinkling and drying. Daily bathing may cause the skin to become excessively dry.

RISKS FOR SKIN IMPAIRMENT

The nurse should look for certain conditions when assessing a client's risk for impaired skin integrity.

IMMOBILIZATION. A client who is unable to move freely as a result of illness or some external restraint is at risk for skin breakdown. The dependent body parts are exposed to pressure from underlying surfaces. A mattress, a body cast, or even a wrinkled layer of linen exerts pressure against skin surfaces, reducing circulation to affected body parts. Chapter 31 describes how impairment of circulation to dependent body parts can result in decubitus ulcer formation. The nurse should be aware of clients who require assistance to turn and change position. Localized redness and tenderness are early signs of pressure on dependent body parts.

REDUCED SENSATION. Many clients are unable to sense an injury to the skin's surface. Clients with paralysis, circulatory insufficiency, or local nerve damage do not receive normal transmission of nerve impulses when excessive heat or cold, pressure, friction, or chemical irritants are applied to the skin. The nurse can easily assess the status of a client's sensory nerve function by checking for pain, tactile, or temperature sensation (see Chapter 29). The nurse attempts to protect the client's skin from exposure to irritants. For example, diabetes causes a loss of sensation in the extremities. The nurse must carefully check the temperature of bath water before allowing a diabetic client to bathe.

NUTRITIONAL ALTERATIONS. Adequate nutrients are essential for maintaining the normal integrity of integumentary structures. Clients with limited caloric and protein intake have impaired tissue synthesis. The skin becomes thinner, less elastic, and smoother and there is a loss of subcutaneous tissue. Poor digestion and absorption of nutrients (as caused by inflammatory conditions of the bowel or bowel surgery), excessive protein metabolism (as caused by fever,

burns, surgery, or extensive wound healing), and excessive loss of protein (as caused by blood loss, wound exudate, or burns) place clients at risk for nutritional imbalances. Any hospitalized client who is not permitted to eat is a candidate for nutritional problems.

Intravenous fluids such as dextrose in water do not contain the calories needed to prevent protein breakdown. For example, a liter of dextrose in water contains fewer than 200 calories. For a client to receive a normal daily intake of 2000 to 2500 calories it would be necessary to infuse over 10 liters of intravenous fluid.

SECRETIONS AND EXCRETIONS ON THE SKIN. Moisture on the skin's surface is a medium for bacterial growth and can cause softening of epidermal cells. Perspiration, urine, watery fecal material, and wound drainage can accumulate on the skin's surface, resulting in skin breakdown and infection. The nurse gives particular attention to body areas, such as under the woman's breasts, the perineal area, or under the arms, where moisture may collect and skin surfaces may rub against each other and cause friction.

VASCULAR INSUFFICIENCY. In peripheral vascular disease either the arterial blood supply to tissues is inadequate or venous return is impaired, causing circulatory stasis in dependent extremities. Inadequate blood flow to the skin results in ischemia and breakdown. Clients with this disease have a high risk of infection because delivery of nutrients and white blood cells to injured tissues is inadequate.

EXTERNAL DEVICES. Often a client has some type of external device applied to or around the skin that has the potential for exerting pressure or friction against the skin's surface. A cast, cloth restraint, bandage, dressing, or orthopedic brace can rub against the skin and cause breakdown. The nurse assesses all skin surfaces exposed to any external device.

Nursing Diagnosis

The nurse's assessment findings reveal whether the client has actual or potential alterations in skin integrity (Table 35-3). If the client has the potential for skin breakdown, the nurse plans preventive measures. The factors contributing to the problem determine the nurse's interventions. For example, the diagnosis of potential alterations in skin integrity related to insufficient dietary intake requires the nurse not only to maintain meticulous hygiene but also to provide the client with necessary nutritional support.

If the client has actual skin breakdown, the nurse

TABLE 35-3

Examples of Nursing Diagnoses Related to Skin Integrity

Problem	Causes
Potential alterations in skin integrity	Related to: Physical immobility Inadequate nutritional intake Fecal incontinence Wound drainage Leg cast application Reduced sensation
Altered skin integrity	Related to: Pressure sores (decubiti) Dry, cracked skin Open wound Vascular insufficiency Burns

must provide care that promotes healing of injured skin surfaces and prevents infection. The nurse also eliminates factors that may lead to further tissue injury.

Planning

Providing skin care has many purposes other than maintaining a client's cleanliness. A bath or shower helps the client relax, stimulates circulation to the skin, provides exercise through range of joint motion during bathing, improves self-image, and stimulates the rate and depth of respirations. The interaction between nurse and client during bathing and skin care gives the nurse an opportunity to develop a meaningful relationship with the client.

Planning should focus not only on the types or methods of skin care the nurse will deliver but also on the variety of nursing care measures the nurse can perform as a client bathes. Teaching, providing emotional support, and values clarification are just some of the types of interaction the nurse can include during hygiene.

Considering the client's hygiene preferences before planning care is also important. One client may prefer only a partial bath in the morning, and another may enjoy showering just before bed. The type of hygiene the client desires or requires will determine the supplies and equipment the nurse must prepare.

The client's condition influences the plan for delivering hygiene. A seriously ill client usually needs a daily bath because body secretions accumulate and the client is able to do little to maintain cleanliness. An elderly client at home may require a visit from the nurse to assist with a tub bath. If the client is normally inactive during the day and his skin tends to be dry, the nurse may need to visit only twice a week.

Timing is also important in planning hygiene care. Being interrupted in the middle of a bath to go to an x-ray examination can frustrate and embarrass a client. The nurse should plan hygiene care around tests and procedures she knows the client must undergo.

Implementation

BATHING A CLIENT

Bathing a client may primarily serve the purpose of cleanliness or may have specific therapeutic benefits, depending on the type of bath administered (Table 35-4). A physician's order is necessary for baths designed for specific therapeutic purposes, such as sitz baths and soaks.

The extent of a client's bath and the methods used for bathing depend on the client's physical capabilities and the degree of hygiene required. A *complete bed bath* is for clients who are totally dependent on the nurse because of illness and who require total hygienic care. Procedure 35-1 details the steps for giving a complete bed bath.

A *partial bed bath*, as the name implies, consists of bathing only body parts that would cause discomfort if left unbathed. Typically, dependent clients in need of only partial hygiene or self-sufficient bedridden clients who are unable to reach all body parts receive a partial bed bath. The nurse assists in bathing the face, hands, axillary areas, perineum, and back.

The *tub bath* or *shower* can be used to give a more thorough bath than a bed bath (Procedure 35-2). In a tub or shower, washing and rinsing of all body parts are easier. Safety is of primary concern because the surface of a tub or shower stall is slippery. An ambulatory client may require only minimal assistance from the nurse. The more dependent client may need assistance to lower himself into a tub or may sit in a chair underneath the shower.

Tepid sponging is used when a client's temperature reaches a serious elevation. The procedure can be soothing but can also be uncomfortable, depending on the client's skin temperature. Tepid water is used to avoid the chilling effect of cold water applications. Since cooling occurs slowly, temperature fluctuations are avoided. Procedure 35-3 details the steps involved in tepid sponging.

Text continued on p. 949.

PROCEDURE 35-1

Giving a Bed Bath

EQUIPMENT:

1. Two bath towels, one for the face and one for the body
2. Two washcloths
3. Washbasin with water temperature adjusted for the client's comfort (43° to 46° C [110° to 115° F])
4. Soap and soap dish
5. Bath blanket to cover the client during the bath
6. Clean gown or pair of pajamas
7. Additional bed linens if required
8. Hygienic aids: powder, deodorant, skin lotion, antiperspirant
9. Bedpan or urinal
10. Linen hamper or laundry bag

STEPS	RATIONALE
1. Review the client's chart for orders or specific precautions concerning movement and positioning.	Reviewing the chart ensures client and nurse safety, as well as proper use of body mechanics for the nurse and client during the procedure.
2. Explain the bathing procedure, assess the client's physical ability to assist with the bath, and determine the client's preferences for hygiene practices.	Explanations promote the client's cooperation and participation. Involvement of the client in planning the bath promotes the client's independence and results in a plan consistent with his hygiene habits.
3. Assemble the equipment and arrange it for convenience on the bedside and overbed stand. Remove all unnecessary equipment such as call light or water pitcher.	Planning and assembling the equipment permits a smooth flow of the procedure. This contributes to the efficiency of the procedure and provides client comfort.
4. Adjust the room temperature and ventilation. Make sure all doors and windows are closed to prevent drafts.	A warm room prevents rapid loss of body heat during bathing.
5. Provide privacy by drawing the curtain or closing the door.	Ensuring the client's mental comfort is as important as ensuring his physical comfort.
6. Offer the bedpan or urinal.	Client will feel more comfortable after voiding, and interruption of the bath may be avoided.
7. Wash your hands.	This prevents transmission of microorganisms.
8. Lower the side rail and assist the client to a comfortable position, maintaining body alignment.	The client's comfort is maintained throughout the procedure.
9. Bring the client toward the side closest to you. Place the bed in the high position.	When the nurse does not have to reach across the bed, strain on back muscles is minimized.
10. Loosen the top covers at the foot of the bed. Fold and remove the top sheet from underneath. If possible, have the client hold the bath blanket while you withdraw the top sheet. If the client is unable to hold the blanket, hold the bath blanket with one hand while removing the top sheet with the other.	Removal of top linens prevents their becoming soiled or moist during bath. The bath blanket provides warmth and privacy.

STEPS	RATIONALE

11. If the top sheet is to be reused, fold it for replacement. If not, dispose of the sheet in the laundry bag, taking care not to allow linen to come in contact with your uniform.

Proper disposal prevents transmission of microorganisms.

12. Remove the client's gown or pajamas. If an extremity is injured, begin removal from the *uninjured* side. If the client has an intravenous (IV) tube, remove the gown from the arm *without* the IV first, then lower the IV container and slide the gown over the IV tubing and over the IV container. Rehang the IV container and check the flow rate.

Removal of the gown allows full exposure of body parts during bathing. Undressing the unaffected side first allows easier manipulation of the gown over the body part with reduced range of motion.

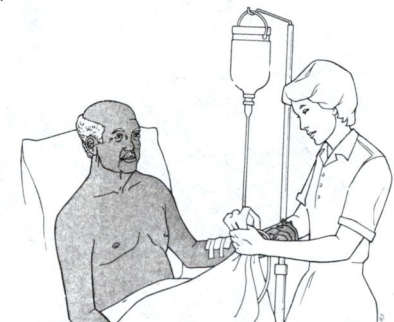

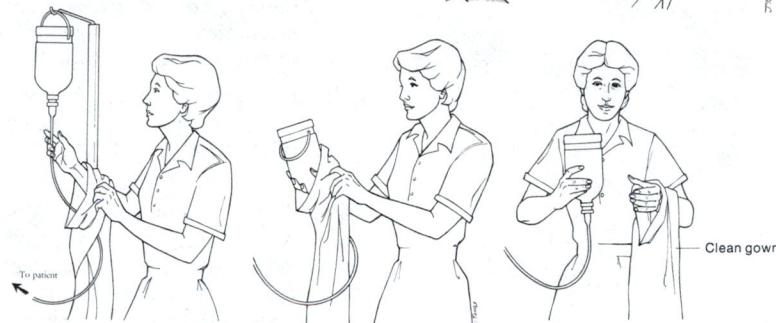

13. Pull the side rails up. Fill the washbasin two-thirds full with water between 43° and 46° C (110° and 115° F). Keep the water and room temperatures warm.

The side rails maintain the client's safety as the nurse leaves the bedside. Warm water promotes comfort and prevents unnecessary chilling.

14. If allowed, remove the pillow and raise the head of the bed 30 degrees. Place a bath towel under the client's head. (Some clients, e.g., those with breathing difficulties, require a pillow or the head of the bed elevated at all times.)

Pillow removal makes it easier to wash the client's ears and neck. Placement of a bath towel under the head prevents bed linen from becoming wet.

15. Make a mitt with the washcloth.

A mitt retains the water and heat better than a loosely held washcloth, keeps cold edges from rubbing against the client, and prevents splashing.

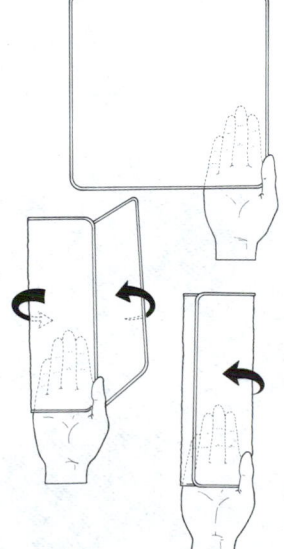
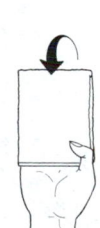

16. Place a face towel over the client's chest.

This prevents soiling of the bath blanket.

Continued.

Giving a Bed Bath

STEPS	RATIONALE

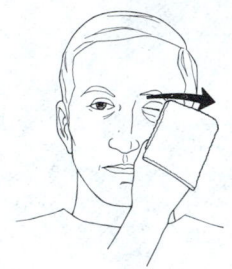

17. Wash the client's eyes without soap, using a different section of the mitt for each eye. Move the mitt from the inner toward the outer canthus. Do not apply direct pressure to the eyes. Encrustations on eyelids may require soaking before removal. Dry the eyes thoroughly.

Soap irritates the eyes. Use of separate sections of the mitt prevents spread of microorganisms. Bathing from the inner to the outer canthus prevents secretions from entering the nasolacrimal ducts. Pressure over the eyes can cause internal injury.

18. Ask the client if he prefers soap used on his face. Wash, rinse, and dry well the forehead, cheeks, nose, neck, and ears. (Men may wish to shave either at this point or after the bath.)

Soap tends to dry the face more quickly, since it is exposed to air more than other parts of the body.

19. Expose the arm farther from you and place the bath towel lengthwise under it.

By bathing the farther side first, the nurse avoids having to reach over a clean area. The towel protects the bed from becoming wet.

20. Bathe the arm with soap and water using long, firm strokes from distal to proximal areas. Raise and support the arm above the head (if possible) while washing the axilla thoroughly.

Soap lowers surface tension and facilitates removal of debris and bacteria when friction is applied during washing. Long, firm strokes stimulate circulation. Movement of the arm above the head exposes the axilla for thorough cleansing and facilitates normal range of motion.

21. Rinse and dry the arm and underarm well. If the client uses deodorant or talcum powder, apply it.

Excess moisture can cause skin maceration or softening.

22. Fold the towel in half and place the basin on it so the client's hand can be immersed in the water.

23. Allow the client's hand to soak for a few minutes before washing the hand and fingernails in the basin. Clean and trim the nails if necessary. Remove the basin and dry the hand well.

Soaking the hands softens the cuticle and loosens debris beneath the nails; soaking helps the client feel his hands are really clean. Drying the hands well removes moisture from between the fingers.

Repeat steps 20 to 23 for the opposite arm.

24. Cover the client's chest with the bath towel and fold the bath blanket down to the client's umbilicus.

This prevents unnecessary exposure of body parts.

25. With one hand lift the edge of the towel away from the chest. With the mitted hand, bathe the chest using long, firm strokes. Take special care to wash skinfolds under the female client's breasts. It may be necessary to lift the breast upward while

The towel maintains warmth and privacy. Firm strokes stimulate circulation and help prevent chilling. Secretions and dirt collect in skinfolds.

STEPS	RATIONALE

bathing underneath it. Keep the client's chest covered between the wash and rinse periods.

26. Place the bath towel lengthwise over the abdomen. Fold the blanket down to the pubic region.

This prevents unnecessary exposure of body parts.

27. With one hand lift the bath towel. With the mitted hand bathe the abdomen, giving special attention to bathing the umbilicus and abdominal folds. Stroke from side to side. Keep the abdomen covered between washing and rinsing. Dry well.

Moisture and sediment that collect in skinfolds predispose the client to skin maceration and irritation.

28. Expose the far leg by folding the bath blanket over toward the midline. Drape the perineum.

This prevents unnecessary exposure.

29. Bend the client's leg at the knee by positioning your arm under the leg. While grasping the client's heel elevate the leg from the mattress slightly and slide the bath towel lengthwise under the leg.

The towel protects the bed linen from wetness. Support of the joint and extremity during lifting prevents strain on musculoskeletal structures.

30. Place the basin on a towel on the bed and secure its position near the foot to be washed.

31. With one hand supporting the leg, raise the leg and slide the basin under the lifted foot. Make sure the foot is firmly placed on the bottom of the basin. Let the foot soak while you wash the leg.

Position the foot to avoid pressure from the edge of the basin on the calf. Soaking softens calluses and rough skin.

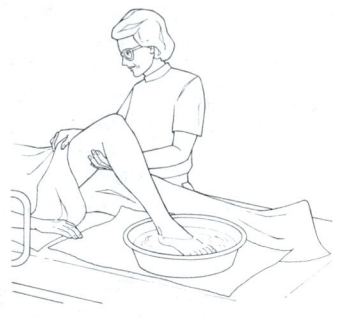

32. Use long, smooth, firm strokes, washing from ankle to knee and from knee to thigh. Dry well.

This promotes venous return.

33. Cleanse the foot, making sure to bathe between the toes. Clean and clip the nails as needed. Dry well. If the skin is dry, apply lotion.

Secretions and moisture may be present in the skinfolds between the toes. Lotion helps to retain moisture and soften skin.

Repeat steps 28 to 33 for the other foot.

34. Cover the client with the bath blanket and change the bath water. Remember to raise the side rails for the client's safety.

A drop in water temperature during the bath can cause chilling. Clean water reduces microorganism transmission.

35. Help the client to a prone or side-lying position to wash the back and buttocks. Place a towel lengthwise along the client's side.

Continued.

Giving a Bed Bath

STEPS	RATIONALE
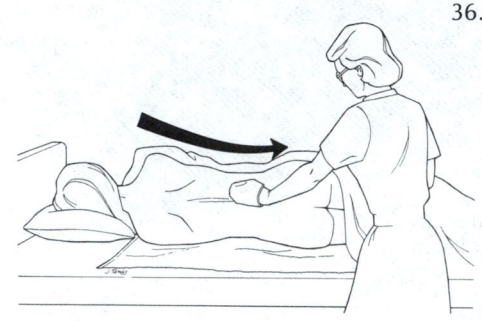 36. Cover the client by sliding the bath blanket down from shoulder to thighs and tuck securely under the thighs.	The bath blanket maintains warmth and prevents unnecessary exposure.
37. Wash, rinse, and dry the back from neck to buttocks using long, firm strokes. Pay special attention to folds of the buttocks and anus.	Skinfolds near the buttocks and anus may contain fecal secretions that harbor microorganisms.
38. Change the water and washcloth.	This prevents transfer of microorganisms from the anal area to the genitalia.
39. Assist the client to a supine or side-lying position. Cover the chest and upper extremities with a towel and the lower extremities with the bath blanket. Expose only the genitalia. (If the client can assist, covering the entire body with the bath blanket may be preferable.) Wash, rinse, and dry the perineum (see Procedures 35-4 and 35-5), giving special attention to skinfolds.	
40. Apply body lotion or oil to moisturize the skin, if desired.	Moisturizing prevents dry chapped skin.
41. Assist the client in dressing.	
42. Comb the client's hair; women may want to apply makeup.	
43. Make the client's bed (see Procedure 35-12).	
44. Clean and replace the bathing equipment. Replace the call light and personal possessions and leave the room as comfortable as possible.	A clean environment promotes the client's comfort. Keeping the call light and articles of care within reach promotes the client's safety.
45. Wash your hands.	Washing prevents microorganism transmission.
46. Report and record on the client's chart any significant findings or abnormal data such as reddened skin areas or joint or muscle pain on movement. Record the level of assistance required by the client.	Timely documentation maintains accuracy of the client's record.

PROCEDURE 35-2

Assisting a Client with a Tub Bath or Shower

STEPS	RATIONALE
1. Schedule use of the bathtub or shower if the client does not have a private bathroom.	This prevents unnecessary waiting that can fatigue the client.
2. Check the tub or shower to determine if it needs cleaning. Use cleaning techniques according to agency policy. Place a rubber mat on the tub or shower bottom. Place a disposable bath mat or towel on the floor in front of the tub or shower.	Cleaning prevents transmission of infection. Mats prevent slipping and falling.
3. Collect the following equipment and place it within easy reach of the tub or shower: washcloth, two bath towels, soap, gown or pajamas, and hygienic aids and toiletries requested by the client.	Placing items close at hand prevents possible falls when the client reaches for equipment.
4. Assist the client to the bathroom if necessary. Have the client wear a robe and slippers en route to the bathroom.	Assistance prevents accidental falls. Robe and slippers prevent chilling.
5. Demonstrate to the client how to use the call signal for assistance.	Bathrooms are equipped with signaling devices in case the client feels faint or weak and needs immediate assistance.
6. Place an "occupied" sign on the bathroom door.	This maintains the client's privacy.
7. Fill the bathtub halfway with warm water (41° C [105.8° F]). Ask the client to test the water, and adjust the water temperature if it is too warm. Explain which faucet controls the hot water. If the client is taking a shower, turn the shower on and adjust the water temperature before the client enters the shower stall.	Adjusting the temperature prevents accidental burns.
8. Instruct the client to use safety bars when getting in and out of the tub or shower.	Safety bars prevent slipping or falls.
9. Instruct the client not to remain in the tub longer than 20 minutes. Check on the client every 5 minutes.	Prolonged exposure to warm water may cause vasodilation and pooling of blood, leading to lightheadedness or dizziness.
10. Return to the bathroom when the client signals and knock before entering.	
11. For a client who is unsteady, drain the tub of water before the client attempts to get out of it.	This prevents accidental falls.
12. Assist the client out of the tub as necessary and help with drying.	Moisture may cause softening of skin and promote spread of infection.
13. Assist the client as needed in donning a clean gown or pajamas, slippers, and robe.	Clothing maintains warmth to prevent chilling.
14. Assist the client to his room and help him assume a comfortable position in bed or a chair.	This maintains the relaxation gained from bathing.
15. Clean the tub or shower according to agency policy. Remove soiled linen and place it in the dirty linen bag. Discard any disposable equipment in the proper receptable. Place an "unoccupied" sign on the bathroom door. Return supplies to the storage area.	Cleaning prevents transmission of microorganisms through soiled linen and moisture.
16. Wash your hands.	Washing prevents transmission of microorganisms.
17. Record and report the client's response to the bath or shower and the condition of the client's skin.	Timely recording provides accurate documentation.

PROCEDURE 35-3

Tepid Sponging

EQUIPMENT:

1. Bath basin
2. Tepid water (32° C [90° F])
3. Bath thermometer
4. Washcloths
5. Waterproof pads
6. Bath blanket
7. Ethyl alcohol (optional)
8. Thermometer

STEPS	RATIONALE
1. Explain to the client that the purpose of tepid sponging is to cool the body slowly. Describe in brief the steps of the procedure.	The procedure can be uncomfortable because of cool water application. Anxiety over the procedure can increase the body temperature.
2. Measure the client's temperature and pulse.	Measurements provide a baseline to measure the effects of sponging.
3. Place waterproof pads under the client and remove the gown.	Pads prevent soiling of the bed linen. Removing the gown provides access to all skin surfaces.
4. Keep the bath blanket over body parts not being sponged. Close the windows and door to prevent drafts in the room.	The bath blanket prevents chilling.
5. Check the water temperature. Add equal parts ethyl alcohol and water (optional).	Alcohol evaporates at low body temperature to increase heat loss.
6. Immerse washcloths in water and apply wet cloths under each axilla and over the groin.	The axilla and groin are areas containing large superficial blood vessels. The application of sponges promotes cooler temperature of the body's core by conduction.
7. Gently sponge an extremity for 5 minutes. Note the client's response. The opposite extremity may be covered by a cool washcloth.	This prevents a sudden temperature fall and minimizes the risk of developing chills.
8. Dry the extremity and reassess the client's pulse and body temperature. Observe the client's response to therapy.	The client's response to therapy is monitored to prevent a sudden temperature change.
9. Continue sponging the other extremities, back, and buttocks for 3 to 5 minutes each. Reassess the temperature and pulse every 15 minutes.	
10. Change the water and reapply sponges to the axilla and groin as needed.	The water temperature rises as a result of exposure to the client's warm body surface.
11. When the body temperature falls to slightly above normal, discontinue the procedure.	This prevents a temperature drift to a subnormal level.
12. Dry the extremities and body parts thoroughly. Cover the client with a light bath blanket or sheet.	Drying and covering the client prevent chilling. An excessively heavy covering may increase body temperature.
13. Dispose of equipment and change the bed linen if soiled.	This controls the transmission of infection.
14. Measure the client's body temperature.	The temperature indicates the response to therapy.
15. Record the time the procedure was started and terminated, vital sign changes, and the client's response.	Recording communicates the care provided in an accurate and timely fashion.

TABLE 35-4

Types of Therapeutic Baths

Type of Bath	Purpose
Hot water tub bath	Immersion in hot water helps relieve muscle soreness and spasm. However, there is a danger of causing burns. Water temperature should be 45°-46° C (113°-114.8° F).
Warm water tub bath	Bathing in warm water relieves muscle tension. Water temperature should be 43° C (109.4° F).
Cool water bath	Bathing in cool water can relieve tension or lower body temperature. Precautions must be taken to avoid chilling. Water temperature should be tepid (32° C [90° F]) rather than cold. This type of bath is especially effective in reducing the body temperature of a small child with a fever.
Soak	Local application of water or medicated solution can remove dead tissue or soften crusted secretions. Aseptic technique is necessary when cleaning open or abraded areas of the skin. Soaks are also useful in reducing pain and swelling of inflamed or irritated skin surfaces.
Sitz bath	A sitz bath cleanses and reduces inflammation of the perineal and anal areas of a client who has undergone rectal surgery or childbirth or who has local rectal irritation from hemorrhoids or fissures. Water temperature depends on the client's condition but should be 43°-45° C (109.4°-113° F).

Whatever type of bath the client receives, the nurse should follow these guidelines:

1. Provide privacy. Close the door or pull room curtains around the bathing area. While bathing the client expose only the areas being bathed.
2. Maintain safety. Keep side rails up while you are away from the client's bedside. (This is particularly important for dependent or unconscious clients.) Place the call light in the client's reach if you must leave the room temporarily.
3. Maintain warmth. The room should be kept warm, since the client is partially uncovered and may easily be chilled. Control drafts and keep windows closed.
4. Promote the client's independence as much as possible during bathing activities. Offer assistance as needed.

PERINEAL CARE

Usually perineal care is part of the complete bed bath. Clients most in need of meticulous perineal care are those at greatest risk for acquiring an infection, for example, clients who have indwelling urinary catheters, are recovering from rectal or genital surgery, or have undergone childbirth. A client who is able to perform self-care should be allowed to do so. Many nurses are embarrassed about providing perineal care, particularly to clients of the opposite sex. Male nurses often seek out a female team member to provide hygiene to female clients, and vice versa. Embarrassment should not cause the nurse to overlook the client's hygiene needs. A professional, dignified attitude can reduce embarrassment and put the client at ease.

If a client performs self-care, various problems such as vaginal or urethral discharge, skin irritation, and unpleasant odors may go unnoticed. The nurse must be alert for complaints of burning during urination or localized soreness or pain in the perineum. The nurse also inspects bed linen for signs of discharge. Clients most at risk for skin breakdown in the perineal area are those with urinary or fecal incontinence, rectal and perineal surgical dressings, and indwelling urinary catheters.

Procedures 35-4 and 35-5 detail the steps involved in providing perineal care for female and male clients. An essential part of the nurse's care is to instruct clients on the importance of perineal hygiene in preventing infection. Catheter care is usually performed as part of perineal care. Chapter 39 describes the procedure for catheter care.

BACKRUB

A backrub usually follows the client's bath. It promotes relaxation, relieves muscular tension, and stimulates circulation to the skin. The nurse can also provide a backrub in the evening to help a client relax and fall asleep. During the backrub the nurse can assess the condition of the client's skin.

An effective backrub takes 3 to 5 minutes to complete. The nurse should inquire if the client would like a backrub, since some clients dislike the close physical contact a backrub requires. The nurse should also consult the client's record before offering a backrub, which is contraindicated when the client has frac-

PROCEDURE 35-4

Female Perineal Care

EQUIPMENT:

1. Washbasin
2. Soap dish with soap
3. Disposable or cloth washcloths (two or three)
4. Bath towel
5. Bath blanket
6. Waterproof pad or bedpan
7. Toilet tissue
8. Disposable gloves
9. Disposable bag

STEPS	RATIONALE
1. Explain the procedure and its purpose to the client.	Explanation helps minimize anxiety during a procedure that is often embarrassing to nurse and client.
2. Pull the curtain around the client's bed or close the room door. Assemble the supplies at the bedside.	The client's privacy is maintained.
3. Raise the bed to a comfortable working position.	This facilitates good body mechanics and the nurse's safety.
4. Lower the side rail. Assist the client to a dorsal recumbent position.	This position provides easy access to the female genitalia.
5. Position the waterproof pad under the client's buttocks or place the bedpan under the client.	This prevents bedclothes from becoming wet.
6. Drape the client by placing the bath blanket with one corner between the client's legs, a corner pointing toward each side of the bed, and a corner at the client's chest. Wrap the bath blanket around the client's far leg by bringing a side corner around the leg and tucking it under the hip. Drape the near leg in the same way.	Draping prevents unnecessary exposure of body parts and maintains the client's warmth and comfort during the procedure.
7. Raise the side rail. Fill the washbasin with water that is approximately 41° to 43° C (105° to 109.4° F).	The rail maintains the client's safety from an accidental fall. A proper water temperature prevents burns to the perineum.
8. Place the washbasin and toilet tissue on the overbed table. Place the disposable or regular washcloths in the washbasin.	
9. Lower the side rail and help the client flex her knees and spread her legs (a client with knee or hip disease may keep her legs straight).	This position provides full exposure of the female genitalia.
10. Put on disposable gloves. Fold the lower corner of the bath blanket up between the client's legs onto her abdomen.	Use of gloves minimizes the transmission of microorganisms. Keeping the client draped until the procedure begins minimizes anxiety.
11. Using your nondominant hand, retract the labia from the thigh and with your dominant hand wash carefully in the skin folds.	Skinfolds may contain body secretions that harbor infection and cause body odor. Wiping from the perineum to the rectum reduces the chance of transmitting fecal organisms to the urinary meatus.

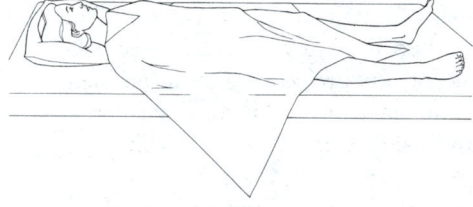

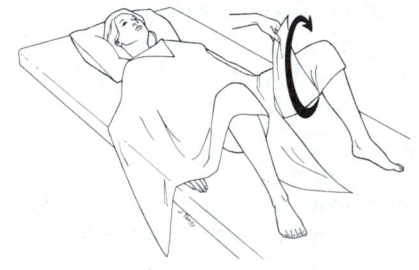

STEPS	RATIONALE

Wipe from the perineum toward the rectum. Repeat on the opposite side using a separate section of the washcloth. Rinse and dry the area thoroughly.

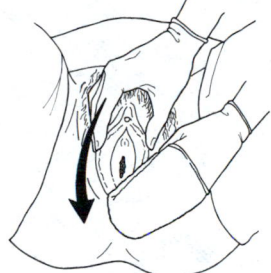

12. Separate the labia with your nondominant hand. With the other hand wash downward from the pubic area toward the rectum in one smooth stroke. Use a separate section of washcloth for each stroke. Pay particular attention to areas around the labia minora, clitoris, and vaginal orifice.

This cleansing method reduces the chance of transmitting microorganisms to the urinary meatus.

13. If the client is on a bedpan, pour warm water over the perineal area.

Rinsing removes soap and microorganisms more effectively than wiping.

14. Dry the perineal area thoroughly.

Retained moisture harbors microorganisms.

15. Fold the center corner of the bath blanket back between the client's legs over the perineum. Help the client off the bedpan, lower her legs, and assist her to a side-lying position.

The bath blanket prevents unnecessary exposure of body parts. The side-lying position provides easy visualization of anal area.

16. Clean the anal area by wiping off excess fecal material with toilet tissue. Wash the area by wiping from vagina toward anus with one stroke. Discard the washcloth. Repeat with a clean cloth until the skin is clear of fecal material.

Cleaning prevents the transmission of microorganisms.

17. Rinse the area well and dry with a towel.

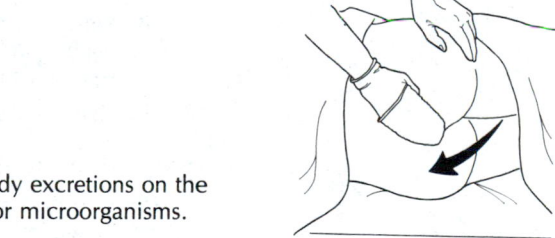

18. Remove the disposable gloves and dispose of them in the proper receptacle.

Moisture and body excretions on the gloves can harbor microorganisms.

19. Assist the client to a comfortable position and cover her with a sheet.

Making the client comfortable minimizes the emotional stress of the procedure.

20. Remove the blanket and dispose of all soiled bed linen. Return unused equipment to the storage area.

21. Raise the side rail and lower the bed to the proper height. Return the client's room to its condition before the procedure.

The side rail protects the client from a fall. A clean environment promotes the client's comfort.

22. Wash your hands.

Washing prevents the transmission of microorganisms.

23. Record and report any observations (i.e., amount and character of discharge, condition of genitalia).

Timely recording ensures accurate documentation of care.

PROCEDURE 35-5

Male Perineal Care

STEPS	RATIONALE
1. Collect the same equipment as in Procedure 35-4. Follow steps 1 through 8 of Procedure 35-4.	
2. Lower the side rail and don disposable gloves.	Gloves prevent exposure of the nurse's hands to microorganisms.
3. Raise the bottom corner of the bath blanket above the client's perineum. Gently raise the penis and place the bath towel underneath.	The towel prevents moisture from collecting in the inguinal area.
4. Gently grasp the shaft of the penis. If the client is uncircumcised, retract the foreskin.	Secretions capable of harboring microorganisms collect underneath the foreskin.
5. Wash the tip of the penis at the urethral meatus first. Using a circular motion, clean from the meatus outward. Discard the washcloth and repeat until the penis is clean. Rinse and dry gently.	Cleansing moves from the area of least contamination to the most contaminated area, preventing entrance of microorganisms into the urethra.
6. Return the foreskin to its natural position.	Tightening of the foreskin around the shaft of the penis can cause localized edema and discomfort.
7. Wash the shaft of the penis with gentle but firm downward strokes. Pay special attention to the underlying surface of the penis.	Vigorous massage of the penis can lead to an erection, which can cause embarrassment for the client and nurse.
8. Rinse and dry the penis thoroughly. Instruct the client to spread his legs apart slightly.	Spreading the legs provides easy access to scrotal tissues.
9. Gently cleanse the scrotum. Lift it carefully and wash underlying skinfolds. Rinse and dry.	Pressure on scrotal tissues can be very painful to the client.
10. Fold the bath blanket back over the client's perineum and assist the client in turning to a side-lying position.	The bath blanket maintains the client's comfort and minimizes anxiety during the procedure. The side-lying position provides access to the anal area.
11. Follow steps 16 through 23 of Procedure 35-4.	

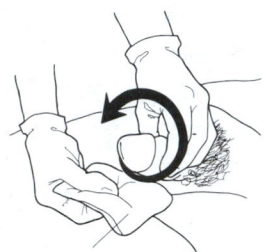

Disposable washcloth

PROCEDURE 35-6

Administering a Backrub

EQUIPMENT:

1. Bath blanket
2. Bath towel
3. Lotion (cream, alcohol, or powder)

STEPS	*RATIONALE*
1. Explain the procedure and the desired position to the client.	Explanation helps relieve anxiety about the procedure.
2. Adjust the bed to a high, comfortable position.	This reduces strain on the nurse's back.
3. Help the client assume either a prone position or a side-lying position with the back toward the nurse. Close the curtain around the bed.	The positions make it easier to apply necessary pressure to the back muscles.
4. Expose the client's back, shoulders, upper arms, and buttocks. Cover the rest of the body with the bath blanket. Lay a towel alongside the client's back.	Body parts are not exposed unnecessarily.
5. Wash your hands in warm water. Warm the lotion either in your hands or by placing the container under warm water.	Cold causes muscle tension.
6. Explain to the client that the lotion may feel cold and wet.	Warning the client reduces the startle response.
7. Apply lotion to the sacral area and stroke upward from the buttocks to the shoulders, over the upper arms, and back to the buttocks, using a continuous, firm stroke. Follow muscle groups. Do not let your hands leave the client's skin. Continue for at least 3 minutes.	Continuous contact is soothing and stimulates circulation to the tissues. 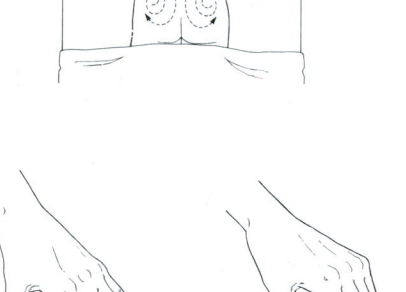
8. Knead the skin by grasping tissue between your thumb and fingers. Knead upward along one side of the spine from the buttocks to the shoulders and nape of the neck. Knead or stroke down. Repeat along the other side of the back.	Kneading increases circulation to muscles. Continuous motion is soothing and relieves muscle tension. 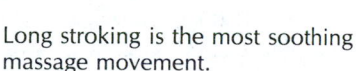
9. End the massage with long stroking movements and tell the client you are ending it.	Long stroking is the most soothing massage movement.
10. Wipe excess lubricant from the client's back with a bath towel. Retie the gown or assist with pajamas. Help the client to a comfortable position.	Excess lotion can be an irritant. A comfortable position enhances the backrub's effects.
11. Dispose of the soiled towel and wash your hands.	These hygiene measures promote infection control.
12. Record the client's response and the condition of the skin.	

tured ribs, burns, or open wounds. Clients with a history of cardiac arrhythmias may experience irregularities in heart rate, possibly as a result of circulatory changes. Procedure 35-6 reviews the steps for administering a backrub.

BATHING AN INFANT

An infant can be bathed in much the same way as an adult, either by a sponge bath or in a small tub. However, there are special precautions the nurse should take. Because an infant's temperature control mechanisms are still immature, prolonged exposure of body parts may cause rapid cooling. When giving a sponge bath the nurse keeps the infant covered as much as possible. When giving a tub bath the nurse should work quickly and be sure the water temperature is warm enough to prevent chilling. Henningson, Nyström, and Tunnell (1981) note that bathing a newborn by immersion causes less heat loss and less crying. The infant's thin sensitive skin requires gentle handling and avoidance of soaps or toiletry items that might irritate the skin. Care of the umbilical cord is a special consideration for the newborn. The neonate must have sponge baths until the umbilical cord falls off and the skin heals. Immersion of the umbilicus in a tub of water before the skin heals can result in a serious infection. The nurse also gives special care to infants who have been circumcised. A small amount of bleeding normally occurs from the penis. The physician applies a sterile gauze dressing impregnated with petrolatum jelly around the circumcised area. The nurse may periodically clean the penis with moistened cotton balls until the dressing can be removed permanently (Whaley and Wong, 1983).

In hospitals where there is rooming-in of the infant and mother, the infant's bath is an excellent opportunity to involve the parents in the child's care. The parents can examine the infant's body parts and learn about normal variations in skin characteristics. A parent may worry about minor birth injuries unless the nurse explains how they occur and when they will disappear.

SPONGE BATH. A sponge bath is given to newborns until the umbilicus heals. Washing a newborn immediately after birth is unnecessary except to cleanse blood from the face and head. The vernix caseosa, a grayish white, cheeselike substance covering the infant's skin, can temporarily provide insulation and prevent infection. The vernix caseosa dries and disappears within 24 to 48 hours.

Supplies for the bath include a shirt, a diaper (disposable or plain cloth), safety pins, a soft washcloth, cotton balls, a towel, and facial tissue. Plain water is best for the infant's bath to prevent irritating the skin

and sensitive mucous membranes. A mild soap can be used for soiled areas such as around the anus. Oils should not be used, since they clog pores and are a medium for bacterial growth. Powders should also be avoided, both because the infant may inhale the particles and because powder has a tendency to cake with moisture and cause irritation. Optional supplies include alcohol for cleansing the umbilical cord, petrolatum jelly to prevent diaper rash, and lotion to provide pleasurable tactile stimulation for the infant during massage of the skin.

The nurse prepares a basin with water at 38° to 40.5° C (100° to 105° F) so it feels comfortably warm when tested on the inside surface of the nurse's forearm. To prevent cooling, the nurse washes the infant's face, eyes, ears, and scalp before removing his shirt and diaper. The towel may also be kept over the infant for warming. The nurse cleans the infant's eyes and ears with clean, moistened cotton balls or a washcloth. The eyes are gently wiped from the inner to the outer canthus, using a clean cotton ball with each stroke or turning the cloth so only a clean part touches the eyes. While washing the face the nurse inspects the nares for crusted secretions. Cotton-tipped swabs should not be used to clean the nares or ears because an infant may move suddenly, causing the swab to break and damage the eardrum or mucous membranes. A rolled wisp of dampened cotton or the twisted end of the washcloth works well for cleaning the external ear canal and pinna. The infant's scalp can be cleaned by wiping off any secretions with a washcloth. However, if shampooing is necessary, the nurse secures the baby's head with one hand and positions it over the bath basin. A mild soap is best for shampooing. The nurse rinses the scalp by pouring water from a small cup or container over the infant's head into the basin. Thorough drying is necessary to prevent evaporative heat loss.

The nurse then undresses the infant for the remainder of the bath. The towel is again used to drape areas not being washed. Keeping the infant covered may be difficult, since infants often kick and twist. Because of the infant's sensitive skin, little rubbing should be done when cleansing. However, the nurse gives special attention to the folds in the neck and axillae and creases at joints. For example, neck creases often collect regurgitated food, which may cause a rash. The umbilical cord should be cleansed with mild soap and water and dried thoroughly. Alcohol may be applied to the umbilicus to help dry it and to reduce chances of infection. Then the nurse dresses the infant in a shirt.

The nurse bathes the infant's buttocks and genitalia last. For a girl it is important to retract the labia fully in order to remove the vernix caseosa. If the vernix caseosa is thick and adherent, the nurse may choose to remove it gradually during successive diaper changes to avoid causing unnecessary irritation during one bath. The vulva is cleaned from front to back to prevent spread of microorganisms from the anal area to the urethra. This technique for preventing urinary infection should be explained to the parents.

In male infants the nurse washes carefully around the penis and scrotum. Noncircumcised infants should not have the foreskin retracted, since it is often too tight. Later, after the foreskin loosens, the nurse should teach the parents how to retract the foreskin, cleanse the area, and return the foreskin to its position. No special care is required around a circumcised penis. The nurse usually cleans off any blood with a clean cotton ball or washcloth. The original petrolatum jelly dressing remains in place for only a day.

The nurse bathes the buttocks last. Fecal material can be removed with facial tissue. Using mild soap helps ensure thorough cleansing of the anal area. After thorough drying, the application of a thin layer of petrolatum jelly helps retain skin moisture and prevents diaper rash.

After the bath the nurse applies a clean diaper, which should fit snugly around the thighs and abdomen to prevent leakage of urine. If the child is circumcised, the diaper should fit loosely to prevent friction against the penis. The diaper should always be below the umbilical site until it is completely healed. The nurse fastens the diaper with the back overlapping the front to permit full flexion of the hips.

TUB BATH. Infants can be given a tub bath after the umbilicus has healed (within 1 to 2 weeks). Supplies for the tub bath are the same as those for a sponge bath. Supplies should be within easy reach. The face, neck, ears, eyes, and scalp are washed before the infant is undressed and immersed in the tub. The nurse lowers the infant slowly into the tub to avoid startling him. The child must always be held firmly with one hand. A child is never left unattended in the bathinette. Often infants enjoy the sensation of being immersed in water, and older infants may enjoy playing during the bath. Body creases are much easier to clean and rinse in a tub bath. After the bath the nurse wraps the infant completely in a towel and gently pats him dry, paying special attention to body creases. Application of body lotion to dry, cracked areas of the skin is soothing and provides important tactile stimulation.

Evaluation

The nurse evaluates skin care after bathing on the basis of the following expected outcomes:

1. The skin is clean, dry, elastic, well hydrated, and without areas of local inflammation.
2. There are no new skin lesions, such as abrasions, pressure sores, or excoriations.
3. Existing lesions are clean, without drainage, and smaller with each bath.

The general benefits of bathing are evaluated on the basis of these criteria:

1. The client expresses a sense of comfort and relaxation.
2. Joints are capable of moving freely through a full range of motion.
3. The client makes positive statements regarding his sense of well-being.

Care of the Feet and Nails

The feet and nails often require special attention to prevent infection, odors, and injury to tissues. Many people are unaware of foot or nail problems until pain or discomfort occurs. Problems result from abuse or poor care of the feet and hands such as biting nails or trimming them improperly, exposure to harsh chemicals such as ammonia or chlorine, and wearing ill-fitting shoes.

The feet are important to a person's physical and emotional health. Foot pain can often lead a person to change his walking gait, causing strain on different muscle groups. Many people must walk or stand comfortably to perform their jobs effectively. Poor job performance can lead to emotional stress. Thus any disorder of the feet or nails can cause a variety of problems.

The nails are epithelial tissues that grow from the root of the nail bed, located in the skin at the nail groove. A normal healthy nail is transparent, smooth, and convex, with a pink nail bed and translucent white tip. Disease can cause changes in the shape and curvature of the nail (see Chapter 29). Inflammatory lesions of the nail bed cause the formation of thickened, horny nails, which can separate from the nail bed.

Assessment

PHYSICAL ASSESSMENT

Assessment of the feet involves a thorough examination of all skin surfaces. The nurse inspects for presence of lesions and notes whether there are areas of dryness, inflammation, or cracking. The areas between the toes should be carefully checked. The heels, soles, and sides of the feet are prone to irritation from ill-fitting shoes. Table 35-5 reviews common types of foot problems.

TABLE 35-5

Common Foot and Nail Problems

Condition	Characteristics	Implications	Interventions
Callus	Thickened portion of epidermis, consisting of a mass of horny, keratotic cells; usually flat, painless, and found on undersurface of foot or on palm of hand; caused by local friction or pressure	Condition may cause discomfort when wearing tight-fitting shoes.	Advise the client to wear gloves when using tools or objects that may create friction on palmar surfaces. Encourage the client to wear comfortable shoes. Soak callus in warm water and Epsom salts to soften cell layers. Use a pumice stone to remove callus after it softens. Applications of creams or lotions can reduce reformation.
Corns	Keratosis caused by friction and pressure from shoes; seen mainly on toes, over a bony prominence; usually cone shaped, round, and raised	Conical shape compresses underlying dermis, making it thin and tender. Pain is aggravated when tight-fitting shoes are worn. Tissue can become attached to bone if allowed to grow. Client may suffer alteration in gait owing to pain.	Surgical removal may be necessary depending on severity of pain and size of corn. Avoid use of oval corn pads, which increase pressure on toes and reduce circulation.
Plantar warts	Fungating lesion that appears on sole of foot; caused by papilloma virus	Warts may be contagious. They are painful and make walking difficult.	Treatment ordered by physician may include applications of salicylic acid, electrodesiccation (burning with an electrical spark), or freezing with solid carbon dioxide.
Athlete's foot (tinea pedis)	Fungal infection of the foot; scaliness and cracking of skin between toes and on soles of feet; small blisters containing fluid may appear; apparently induced by wearing of constricting footwear, e.g., sneakers	Athlete's foot can spread to other body parts, especially the hands. It is contagious and frequently recurs.	Feet should be well ventilated. Drying feet well after bathing and applying powder help prevent infection. Wearing of clean socks or stockings reduces incidence. Physician may order application of griseofulvin, miconazole, or tolnaftate.
Ingrown nails	Toe or fingernail growing inward into soft tissue around nail; often results from improper nail trimming	Ingrown nails can cause localized pain when pressure is applied.	Treatment is frequent hot soaks in antiseptic solution and removal of portion of nail that has grown into the skin. Instruct the client on proper nail trimming techniques.
Ram's horn nails	Unusually long curved nails	Attempt by nurse to cut nails may result in damage to nail bed with risk of infection.	Refer the client to a podiatrist.
Paronychia	Inflammation of tissue surrounding nail after a hangnail or other injury; occurs in people who frequently have their hands in water; common in diabetic clients	Area can become infected.	Treatment is hot compresses or soaks and local application of antibiotic ointments. Paronychia can be prevented by careful manicuring.
Foot odors	Result of excess perspiration promoting microorganism growth		Frequent washing, use of foot deodorants and powders, and wearing clean footwear will prevent or reduce this problem.

It is also important to assess the client's gait. Painful disorders of the feet can cause limping or an unnatural gait. The nurse asks if the client has discomfort of the feet and what factors aggravate the pain. Foot problems may result from bone or muscular alterations rather than skin disorders.

Clients with peripheral vascular disease, such as those with diabetes, should be assessed for adequacy of circulation to the feet. Chapter 29 describes the signs of arterial and venous insufficiency. Palpation of the dorsalis pedis and posterior tibial pulses indicates whether adequate blood flow is reaching peripheral tissues. Edema and changes in skin color, texture, and temperature can indicate that the client is in need of special hygienic care.

The nurse inspects the color, shape, texture, and thickness of the nails. Skin around the nail beds and cuticles should be smooth and without inflammation. The nurse should ask female clients if they frequently polish their nails and use polish remover, since chemicals in these products can cause excessive nail dryness.

DEVELOPMENTAL FACTORS

Foot care for the elderly deserves special attention from the nurse. Many older people cannot care for their feet properly because of poor vision, hand tremors, obesity, or the inability to bend over. Unless foot and nail problems are resolved, an elderly person can easily become disabled and lose his independence.

The nurse's assessment considers common problems of the aged. They often have dry feet because of a decrease in sebaceous gland secretion, dehydration of epidermal cells, and poor condition of footwear. Fissures that result in itching commonly develop. Fungal infections commonly occur under toenails, causing dirty yellow streaks or total discoloration. The nails also become opaque, scaly, and hypertrophied.

If an elderly client has chronic foot problems, the nurse should assess the type of home remedies used. Many over-the-counter preparations, such as those to treat corns, can damage normal skin layers. Burns or ulcerations resulting from these products increase the risk of infection.

FOOTWEAR

The types of footwear worn can predispose clients to foot and nail problems. Children or young adults who frequently fail to wear socks may have excess perspiration that promotes fungal growth. Tight or ill-fitting shoes or socks may cause certain skin lesions and interfere with circulation in the feet. Many elderly women wear garters or knee-high nylons that constrict circulation in the legs. The nurse also assesses

---

Examples of Nursing Diagnoses Related to Problems of the Feet and Nails

Problem	Causes
Altered skin integritiy	Related to: Corns Fissures Athlete's foot
Impaired tissue perfusion	Related to: Arterial insufficiency Poor venous return
Pain	Related to: Callus formation Ingrown toenails
Impaired mobility	Related to: Pain from corns Pain from ingrown nails Pain from "ram's horn" nails

---

whether clients wear clean footwear, since repeated use of soiled footwear can lead to infection. Shoes should fit snugly, not tightly, and provide support for the arch of the foot. When the person stands, there should be at least a ¾-inch space between the great toe and the widest part of the shoe.

Nursing Diagnosis

Diagnoses related to problems of the feet and nails are given in Table 35-6.

Planning

The nurse may provide foot and nail care during the client's bed bath or at a separate time in the day according to the client's preference. Many community health nurses visit clients at home solely to provide foot and nail care.

The nurse's goals of care include the following:
1. Maintaining integrity of skin surfaces
2. Promoting the client's comfort and sense of cleanliness
3. Maintaining proper function of the feet

Implementation

Foot and nail care involves soaking to soften cuticles and layers of horny cells, thorough cleansing,

PROCEDURE 35-7

Nail and Foot Care

EQUIPMENT:

1. Washbasin
2. Bath towel, face towel
3. Washcloth
4. Emesis basin
5. Nail clippers, orange stick
6. Emery board or nail file
7. Lotion
8. Disposable bath mats
9. Paper towels

STEPS	RATIONALE
1. Explain the procedure to the client.	Explanation promotes the client's participation in care procedures.
2. Arrange the equipment on the overbed table. Pull the curtain around the bed or close the room door.	Easy access to equipment prevents delays. Maintaining the client's privacy reduces anxiety.
3. Assist the client to a bedside chair if possible. Place the disposable bath mat on the floor under the client's feet. Place the call light within the client's reach.	A chair makes it easier to immerse the feet in the basin.
4. Fill the washbasin with water at 109° to 110° F (43° to 44° C).	Warm water softens the nails, reduces inflammation of the skin, and promotes circulation.
5. Place the basin on the bath mat and help the client place his feet in the basin.	
6. Adjust the overbed table to a low position and place it over the client's lap.	Easy access prevents accidental spills.
7. Fill the emesis basin with water at 109° to 110° F (43° to 44° C) and place the basin on the paper towels on the overbed table.	Warm water softens the nails and thickened epidermal cells.
8. Instruct the client to place his fingers in the emesis basin and place his arms in a comfortable position.	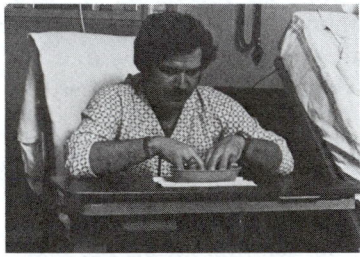
9. Allow the client's feet and fingernails to soak for 10 to 20 minutes. Rewarm the water in 10 minutes.	
10. Clean gently under the fingernails with the orange stick. Remove the emesis basin and dry the fingers thoroughly.	The orange stick can be used to remove debris under the nails that harbors microorganisms. Thorough drying impedes fungal growth and prevents maceration of tissues.
11. With the nail clippers, clip the fingernails straight across and even with the tops of the fingers. Shape the nails with an emery board or nail file.	Cutting straight across prevents splitting of nail margins and formation of sharp nail spikes that can irritate lateral nail margins. Filing prevents cutting the nail too close to the nail bed.
12. Push the cuticle back gently with the orange stick.	This reduces the incidence of inflamed cuticles.
13. Move the overbed table away from the client.	
14. Put on disposable gloves and scrub callused areas of the feet with the washcloth.	Gloves prevent transmission of fungal infections to the nurse. Friction removes dead skin layers.

STEPS	RATIONALE
15. Clean gently under the nails with the orange stick. Remove the feet from the basin and dry them thoroughly.	Removal of debris and excess moisture reduces the chances of infection.
16. Clean and trim the toenails using procedures in steps 11 and 12.	
17. Apply lotion to the feet and then assist the client back to bed and into a comfortable position.	Lotion lubricates dry skin by helping to retain moisture.
18. Make sure the call light is within reach. Raise the side rail.	The call light and side rail provide for the client's safety.
19. Clean and return equipment and supplies to the proper place. Dispose of soiled linen. Wash your hands.	This controls the transmission of microorganisms.
20. Record and report the procedure and any pertinent observations (i.e., breaks in skin or areas of inflammation).	Accurate documentation is timely and descriptive.

drying, and proper trimming of nails. The nurse may provide the care in bed for an immobilized client or have the client sit in a chair for easier access and more thorough cleansing. Procedure 35-7 describes the steps for foot and nail care. It is important for the nurse to take time during the procedure to teach the client the proper techniques for cleaning and nail trimming. By allowing the client to perform a part of foot and nail care, the nurse can stress principles related to preventing infection and injury to tissues and promoting good circulation.

A diabetic client or one with peripheral vascular disease is at risk for foot and nail problems because of impaired circulation. Any minor break or irritation in the skin has the potential for developing into a serious infection. A diabetic foot ulcer may lead to gangrene unless the client follows meticulous hygiene techniques. The nurse takes additional precautions when caring for these clients' feet and nails:

1. Do not cut the client's corns or calluses or use commercial removers, which contain ingredients that may be irritating. A physician or podiatrist should be consulted if corns or calluses appear.
2. File the client's toenails; do not use scissors or clippers, which are likely to slip and cut the surrounding tissue.
3. Do not use over-the-counter preparations to treat athlete's foot or ingrown toenails because the ingredients may cause infection. The physician or podiatrist should be consulted when these conditions appear.

4. Teach the client to avoid wearing elastic stockings or constricting garters and not to cross the legs. Both impair circulation to the lower extremities.
5. Wash the client's feet at least daily.
6. Keep the client's feet dry and warm.
7. Explain to the client that going barefoot should be avoided, since injury or infection might result.
8. Make sure the client's shoes fit well. The soles should be flexible and nonslipping.
9. Advise the client to wear clean socks or hose each day.

Evaluation

Following nail and foot care, the nurse evaluates the interventions on the basis of the following expected outcomes:

1. The skin around nails is intact and well lubricated.
2. Nails are short and straight without split edges.
3. Localized pain or tenderness around nails or on the surface of the foot is absent or reduced.
4. The client is able to walk comfortably in shoes.

Oral Hygiene

The teeth are hard, bonelike structures that extend from the jawbones. The major part of a tooth is the dentin, an ivory-like substance that is harder than bone. Dentin surrounds the tooth's pulp cavity. A layer of enamel, visible in the oral cavity, covers the upper portion of the tooth, called the crown. The periodontal membrane, just below the gum margins, surrounds the tooth root and holds it firmly in place. A tooth receives its blood, lymph, and nerve supply from the base of the tooth socket within the jaw. Healthy teeth appear white, smooth, shiny, and properly aligned.

Oral hygiene helps maintain the healthy state of the mouth, teeth, gums, and lips. Brushing cleans the teeth of food particles, plaque, and bacteria, massages the gums, and relieves discomfort resulting from unpleasant odors and tastes. Flossing further helps to remove plaque and tartar between teeth to reduce gum inflammation and infection. Complete oral hygiene gives a sense of well-being and thus can stimulate appetite.

The nurse's responsibilities in oral hygiene are maintenance and prevention. The nurse can help clients maintain good oral hygiene by teaching them correct techniques or by actually performing hygiene for weakened or disabled clients. Often the nurse must make referrals to a dentist for problems requiring special care. Educating clients about common gum and tooth disorders and methods of prevention can motivate them to follow good oral hygiene practices.

Assessment

PHYSICAL ASSESSMENT

Chapter 29 describes in detail the assessment of the lips, teeth, buccal mucosa, gums, palate, and tongue. The nurse inspects all areas carefully for color, hydration, texture, and presence of lesions. Clients who do not follow regular oral hygiene practices may have receding gum tissue, inflamed gums, discolored teeth (particularly along gum margins), dental caries, missing teeth, and halitosis. Localized pain is a common symptom of gum disease and certain tooth disorders. Whenever palpating lesions in the mouth, the nurse must wear gloves and wash hands thoroughly before and after the examination. Infections of the mouth may involve organisms such as *Treponema pallidum*, *Neisseria gonorrhoeae*, *Mycobacterium tuberculosis*, and herpesvirus hominis.

DEVELOPMENTAL CHANGES

Throughout life physiological changes occur in the mouth structures (Table 35-7). In addition, as a person matures, social factors influence oral hygiene practices. The nurse considers the client's developmental level when determining the types of hygiene problems to expect.

TABLE 35-7

Physiological Development of the Mouth

Developmental Level	Changes
Infant	The deciduous teeth begin to erupt at about 5 months of age. Solid food can be taken in the mouth at about 5-6 months of age with chewing beginning by 6-8 months.
18 months–6 years	The 20 deciduous teeth are present. By the age of 6, "baby" teeth begin to fall out and are replaced by the permanent teeth. By age 2, child can begin to brush teeth and learn hygiene practices of parents. Dental caries may become a problem if dental hygiene is neglected.
6-12 years	Deciduous teeth are replaced by permanent teeth. All permanent teeth are present by age 12 except second and third molars. Diet is similar to adult's. Definite food preferences become apparent. Dental caries and irregularity in the spacing of teeth are significant health problems.
12-18 years	All permanent teeth are present. Dental hygiene practices tend to improve because of increased awareness of body image.
18-40 years	Third molars appear. If good oral hygiene and nutrition practices are not kept up at this time, problems can result in later years.
40-65 years	Loss of teeth, usually a result of periodontal disease, is common. Most people over age 55 have lost some or all of their teeth because of poor oral care.
65 years and over	Aging teeth become brittle, drier, and darker in color. Teeth become uneven, jagged, and fractured after years of crushing and grinding. Gums lose vascularity. Gum recession occurs from loss of tissue elasticity, causing dentures to fit poorly. Eating habits often change, and malnutrition may be a problem.

HYGIENE PREFERENCES

The nurse must determine the client's oral hygiene practices in order to identify errors in technique, deficiencies in types of practices, and the client's knowledge level about dental care. Some helpful questions include the following:

1. How often does the client brush his teeth?
2. What type of toothpaste or dentifrice does he use?
3. Does the client have dentures? When and how does he clean them?
4. Does the client use mouthwash or lemon-glycerin preparations?
5. Does the client floss? If so, how often?
6. When was the client's last dental visit?
7. How often does the client visit a dentist?

Asking the client to demonstrate brushing and flossing techniques will be useful in developing a teaching plan.

RISK FACTORS FOR ORAL HYGIENE PROBLEMS

Certain clients have more difficulty maintaining oral hygiene than others. The seriously ill client depends on the nurse to attend to all hygiene needs. A combative client may resist the nurse's oral care measures. Clients who are confused, depressed, or paralyzed also require special attention from the nurse.

Certain clients who undergo physiological alterations also require more aggressive oral hygiene measures. The client who is dehydrated or unable to eat or drink is likely to have dry mucous membranes and thick secretions on the tongue and gums. Clients with nasogastric tubes and mouth breathers require more attention to maintaining hydration of oral structures. In clients receiving chemotherapeutic drugs, ulcerations and inflammation of the mouth develop because of the drugs' effects on cell growth. Such clients undergo considerable discomfort and are at risk for infection. Leukemic clients have severe swelling of the gums and are prone to bleeding. Frequent meticulous hygiene is the only way to maintain the integrity of their oral mucosa. Other clients requiring aggressive mouth care include those who have undergone oral surgery, have had trauma to the mouth, or have endotracheal tubes or oral airways in place.

Common Oral Problems

Before performing an assessment of oral structures it is important to be familiar with the common oral problems. Each problem presents recognizable signs and symptoms and influences not only for the type of hygiene but also the type of teaching the nurse must provide.

The two major types of oral problem are dental caries (cavities) and periodontal disease (pyorrhea). *Dental caries* is the most common oral problem of younger people. The development of cavities is a pathological process that involves the eventual destruction of the tooth enamel through decalcification. Decalcification is a result of an accumulation of mucin, carbohydrates, and lactic acid bacilli in the saliva normally found in the mouth, which forms a coating on the teeth called *plaque*. Plaque is transparent and colorless and adheres to the teeth, particularly near the base of the crown at the gum margins. The plaque prevents normal acid dilution and neutralization and thus prevents the dissolution of bacteria in the oral cavity. The acid eventually destroys the tooth enamel and in severe cases the pulp or inner spongy tissue of the tooth. A cavity first begins as a chalky white discoloration of the tooth. As the cavity advances, the tooth takes on a brown or black discoloration.

To prevent tooth decay the client may have to change his eating habits by reducing intake of carbohydrates, especially sweet snacks between meals. Candy, soft drinks, ice cream, or jellies should be limited. If the client does eat sweets, it is important to brush within 30 minutes to reduce the action of plaque. Rinsing the mouth thoroughly with water or eating an acid-containing fruit such as an apple also helps reduce plaque. Using fluoridated water or a fluoride rinse can also reduce dental caries. Brushing after each meal and before bedtime and daily flossing are basic measures for prevention of dental caries.

For people over 35 years of age, the most common oral problem is *periodontal disease* or pyorrhea. Periodontal disease is a long-term process involving infection and destruction of the supporting structures of the teeth: the gingivae (gums), cementum, ligaments, and alveolar bone. Periodontal disease progresses in four stages: (1) gingivitis or inflammation of the gums, (2) periodontitis, (3) acute necrotizing ulcerative gingivitis, and (4) destruction of the tooth-supporting structure (Levine, 1973). Symptoms of periodontal disease include bleeding gums, swollen inflamed tissues, receding gumlines with the formation of gaps or pockets between the teeth and gums, and the eventual loss of teeth. If proper oral health care is not maintained, dead bacteria, called tartar, can collect at the gumline. The tartar attacks the gums and fibers attached to the teeth, resulting in lost teeth. The best preventive measures are regular flossing and brushing.

Other oral problems include *stomatitis*, an inflammatory condition of the mouth resulting from contact with irritants such as tobacco or from vitamin deficiency, infection by bacteria, viruses, or fungi, or use of chemotherapeutic drugs; *glossitis*, an inflammation of the tongue resulting from infectious disease or injury from a burn, bite, or other injury; and *gingivitis*, an inflammation of the gums usually resulting from poor oral hygiene or occurring as a sign of leukemia, vitamin deficiency, or diabetes mellitus.

Halitosis (bad breath) is a common problem of the oral cavity. It may be the result of poor oral hygiene, ingestion of certain foods, or an infection or disease process. Proper oral hygiene can eliminate the odors unless the cause is a systemic condition such as liver disease or diabetes.

The nurse frequently encounters *cheilosis* in clients. The disorder involves cracking of the lips, especially at the angle of the mouth. Riboflavin deficiency, mouth breathing, and excess salivation may cause cheilosis. Lubrication of the lips helps retain moisture, and antifungal or antibacterial ointments discourage microorganism growth.

A final problem the nurse should be able to recognize is *oral malignancy*. Malignancies appear as lumps or ulcers in or around the mouth. The most common site is at the base of the tongue. Early detection of oral cancers is vital to the success of treatment. Any sore in the mouth that does not heal should be brought to the attention of a dentist.

Nursing Diagnosis

The nurse's assessment may reveal actual or potential alterations in the integrity of mouth structures. Likewise, pertinent nursing diagnoses may reflect problems or complications resulting from alterations of the oral cavity (Table 35-8).

Planning

Developing a care plan for maintaining oral hygiene involves consideration of the client's personal preferences, the physical and emotional status, and physical capabilities. The nurse must establish a good relationship with the client to assist with oral hygiene practices. Some clients are very sensitive about the condition of their mouths and are reluctant to let someone else care for them. In many cases clients are also unaware that they are at risk for serious dental and periodontal disease and thus require extensive education.

The nurse's goal in providing oral hygiene include the following:

1. Maintaining an intact, well-hydrated oral mucosa
2. Preventing infection and dental caries
3. Developing client's understanding of the importance of oral hygiene
4. Promoting client's self-esteem and comfort
5. Developing client's skills in performing oral hygiene measures

Implementation

Good oral hygiene involves cleanliness, comfort, and moisturizing of mouth structures. Proper prophylactic care will prevent oral disease and tooth destruction. Unfortunately, clients in hospitals or long-term care facilities often do not receive the aggressive care they need. Simple swabbing of the mouth is ineffective in removing food debris. The lemon-glycerin swab used in many institutions creates more problems than benefits. Glycerin has an astringent effect, drying and shrinking gums and mucous membranes. The lemon, if used extensively, exhausts the salivary reflex through overstimulation and can erode teeth enamel (MacMillan, 1981). Since swabbing fails to clean teeth adequately, plaque accumulates around the base of the teeth. The glycerin provides nourishment for

---

TABLE 35-8

Examples of Nursing Diagnoses Related to Alterations of the Oral Cavity

Problem	Causes
Altered mucous membrane integrity	Related to: Dehydration Restriction of fluid and food intake Ineffective hygiene Medication
Potential alterations in oral mucosa	Related to: Endotracheal intubation Ill-fitting dentures Comatose state
Pain of oral cavity	Related to: Loose teeth Gingivitis Glossitis
Altered nutritional intake	Related to: Ill-fitting dentures Gingivitis Absence of teeth
Body image disturbance	Related to: Absence of teeth Dental caries Halitosis

bacteria. Mouthwash has value only in providing a pleasant aftertaste. Used over a long period of time mouthwash dries the mucosa.

Brushing, flossing, and irrigation are necessary for proper cleansing. Clients will also benefit from a proper diet that excludes foods promoting plaque formation and tooth decay and promotes healthy mucosa and periodontal structures. A well-balanced diet ensures the integrity of tissues. Eating fibrous foods such as fresh fruits and vegetables helps to cleanse the teeth of plaque. The acidic quality of fruits also helps eliminate bacteria that form on teeth from simple carbohydrates.

BRUSHING

Thorough brushing of the teeth at least four times a day (after meals and at bedtime) is basic to an effective oral hygiene program. A toothbrush should have a straight handle and a brush small enough to reach all areas of the mouth. Elderly clients with reduced dexterity and grip may require an enlarged toothbrush handle that provides an easier grip. This can be accomplished by piercing a soft rubber ball and pushing the brush handle through or by gluing a short piece of plastic tubing around the handle. An even, rounded brushing surface with soft, multitufted, nylon bristles is best. Rounded, soft bristles stimulate the gums without causing abrasion and bleeding. All tooth surfaces—inner, outer, and chewing—should be brushed thoroughly (Fig. 35-1). Dentists recommend holding the toothbrush at a 45-degree angle to the gumline in order to reach all tooth surfaces. Electric toothbrushes may be used, but the nurse must check for any electrical hazards. Toothettes, pieces of foam rubber attached to a stick, are useful for clients who have sensitive gums or who have had oral surgery. Brushing the tongue reduces the number of bacteria in the mouth, although many people cannot tolerate this without gagging. A fluoride toothpaste should be used. Most products are pleasant tasting.

When teaching clients about mouth care the nurse reminds them not to share toothbrushes at home and not to drink directly from a bottle of mouthwash. Cross-contamination occurs easily. The use of disclosure tablets or drops to stain the plaque that collects at the gumline can be useful for showing clients how effectively they brush.

The amount of assistance needed by the client in brushing the teeth may vary. Many clients are able to perform their own oral care and should be encouraged to do so. The nurse observes the client to be sure proper techniques are used. Other clients need total assistance with hygiene. Procedure 35-8 reviews steps for assisting partially dependent clients with mouth care.

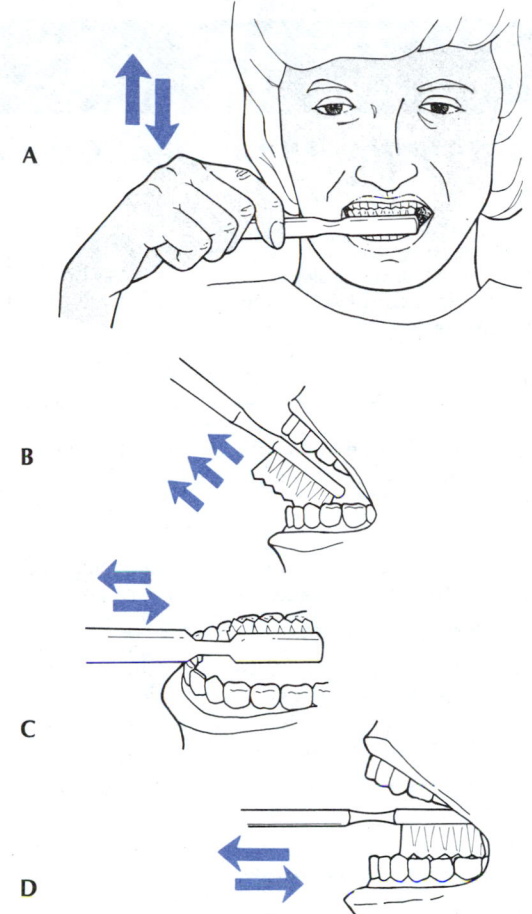

Fig. 35-1 **A,** Position the brush horizontally and brush up and down with short strokes. **B,** Position the brush at a 45-degree angle against the inside of the front teeth. Brush from gum to crown of the teeth with short strokes. Reposition the brush until all of the front teeth have been brushed. **C,** Hold the brush horizontally against the inner surfaces of the teeth and brush up and down. **D,** Position the brush on the biting surfaces of the teeth and brush back and forth.

Modified from Sorrentino, S.A.: Mosby's textbook for nursing assistants, St. Louis, 1984, The C.V. Mosby Co.

The unconscious client requires the nurse's special attention. Providing mouth care for this individual requires consideration of three factors: (1) the client is unable to eat or drink; (2) the client frequently breathes through an open mouth; and (3) the client often is attached to some type of oxygen equipment. All of these factors cause drying of the mucosa and the formation of crusts on the tongue and mucous membranes. Since the unconscious client cannot often swallow, salivary secretions accumulate in the mouth. The secretions frequently contain gram-negative bacteria that can cause pneumonia if aspirated. Proper care keeps the mouth moist and eliminates secretions that can lead to infection.

PROCEDURE 35-8

Assisting the Dependent Client with Brushing Teeth

EQUIPMENT

1. Toothbrush
2. Toothpaste or dentifrice
3. Water glass with cool water
4. Mouthwash
5. Straw
6. Emesis basin
7. Face towel and paper towels

STEPS	RATIONALE
1. Explain the procedure to the client and inquire about preferences regarding hygiene aids.	Certain clients may feel uncomfortable about having a nurse care for their basic hygiene needs. Participation by the client promotes his relaxation during the procedure.
2. Place the paper towels on the overbed table and arrange other equipment within easy reach.	The towel collects spills from the emesis basin.
3. Pull the curtain or close the room door.	This provides privacy.
4. Raise the bed to a comfortable working position. Raise the head of the bed to a position in which the client is comfortable. Move the client or help the client move to a position near you.	Raising the bed prevents muscle strain as the nurse attends to the client's needs. The semi-Fowler's position prevents the client from aspirating or choking.
5. Lower the side rail and place the towel on the client's chest.	This prevents soiling of bed linen.
6. Position the overbed table within easy reach and adjust the height as needed.	Easy accessibility of supplies ensures a smooth procedure.
7. Apply toothpaste to the toothbrush and hold the toothbrush over the emesis basin. Pour a small amount of water over the end of the brush.	Moisture aids in the distribution of toothpaste over tooth surfaces.
8. Brush the inner and outer surfaces of the upper and lower teeth by brushing from the gum to the crown of each tooth. Apply the brush at a 45-degree angle to the gumline and use short strokes. Brush one tooth at a time. Clean the biting surfaces of the teeth by holding the brush parallel with the teeth and brushing gently back and forth. Brush the sides of the teeth by moving the bristles back and forth.	This angle allows the bristles to clean under the gumline where most plaque and tartar accumulate. A back-and-forth motion dislodges food particles caught between teeth and along chewing surfaces.
9. Hold the brush at a 45-degree angle and lightly brush over the surface and sides of the tongue. Avoid initiating the gag reflex.	Microorganisms grow abundantly on the tongue's surface. Gagging causes discomfort and may result in aspiration of toothpaste.
10. Allow the client to rinse the mouth thoroughly by taking several sips of water, swishing it across all tooth surfaces, and spitting it into the emesis basin.	Irrigation removes food particles.
11. Allow the client to gargle or rinse the mouth with mouthwash.	Mouthwash leaves a pleasant taste in the mouth.
12. Assist the client to a comfortable position, remove the bedside table, raise the side rail, and lower the bed to its original position.	This provides the client's comfort and safety.
13. Wipe off the overbed table, discard soiled linen and paper towels in the appropriate container, and return equipment to the proper place.	This controls the transmission of microorganisms.
14. Wash your hands.	Washing prevents the transmission of microorganisms.
15. Record and report the procedure, noting the condition of the oral cavity.	Recording documents the response of the client to hygiene measures.

PROCEDURE 35-9

Mouth Care for the Unconscious Client

EQUIPMENT:
1. Mouthwash or antiseptic solution
2. Toothettes or tongue blade wrapped in single layer of gauze
3. Padded tongue blade
4. Face towel
5. Emesis basin
6. Paper towels
7. Water glass with cool water
8. Petrolatum jelly

STEPS	RATIONALE
1. Explain the procedure to the client.	Although unconscious, the client may retain the ability to hear explanations.
2. Wash your hands.	Washing prevents transmission of microorganisms.
3. Place the paper towels on the overbed table and arrange equipment for ease in providing care.	
4. Pull the curtain around the bed or close the door to the room.	This provides privacy.
5. Raise the bed to its highest horizontal level. Lower the side rail.	Use of good body mechanics prevents injury to nurse and client.
6. Position the client on the side near you. Make sure the client's head is turned toward the mattress.	Proper positioning of the head protects the client from aspirating secretions.
7. Place the towel under the client's face and the emesis basin under the client's chin.	This prevents soiling of bed linen.
8. Carefully separate the upper and lower teeth with the padded tongue blade.	This prevents the client from biting down on the nurse's fingers and provides access to the oral cavity.
9. Clean the mouth using the toothettes or tongue blade moistened with mouthwash or water. Suction as needed during cleansing. Clean the chewing and inner surfaces first. Swab the roof of the mouth and inside cheeks and lips. Swab the tongue but avoid causing the gag reflex. Moisten a clean applicator with water and swab the client's mouth to rinse. Repeat as needed.	Swabbing stimulates the gums and helps remove large food particles when brushing is impossible. Water or mouthwash provides a lubricant for dry mucosa. Rinsing helps remove secretions and food particles.

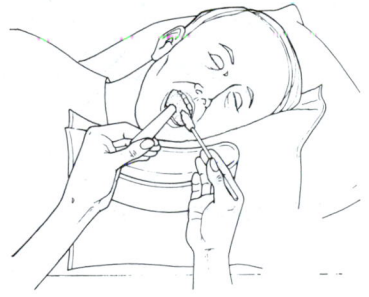

10. Apply petrolatum jelly to the lips.	Petrolatum jelly prevents the lips from drying and cracking.
11. Explain to the client that you have completed the procedure.	
12. Reposition the client comfortably, raise the side rail, and return the bed to its original position.	This maintains the client's comfort and safety.
13. Clean equipment and return it to its proper place. Place the soiled linen in the "dirty" utility room.	Proper disposal of soiled equipment prevents the spread of infection.
14. Wash your hands.	Washing prevents the transmission of microorganisms.
15. Record and report the procedure and pertinent observations (e.g., presence of bleeding gums, dry mucosa, or crusts on tongue).	Accurate documentation should be timely and descriptive.

While providing hygiene to an unconscious client, the nurse must protect the client from choking and aspirating. Positioning the client on one side with the head turned well toward the dependent side allows excess fluid to drain from the mouth instead of collecting in the back of the pharynx. The safest technique is to have two nurses provide the care: one to do the actual cleaning and the other to remove secretions with suction equipment. The client's mouth must remain open during mouth care to give the nurse access to all oral structures. A padded tongue blade is useful for keeping the mouth open and the teeth separated without causing trauma to sensitive mucous membranes. The nurse should never use her fingers to hold the mouth open, since the client may bite down accidentally. A human bite is highly contaminated and can lead to a serious infection. The nurse should never use the tongue blade to force the mouth open because of the danger of breaking teeth.

It may be necessary to perform mouth care at least every 2 hours for an unconscious client to maintain the condition of oral mucosa. The nurse should remember that the client may be able to hear although he cannot speak. The nurse explains to the client how mouth care is to be provided and the sensations the client will feel and tells the client when the procedure

---

PROCEDURE 35-10

Flossing Teeth

EQUIPMENT:

1. Dental floss (waxed or unwaxed)
2. Glass with water
3. Emesis basin

STEPS	RATIONALE
1. Use 12 to 18 inches of floss wrapped around the index or middle fingers of both hands to hold taut a section ½ to 1 inch long.	Taut floss is easier to place between the teeth. 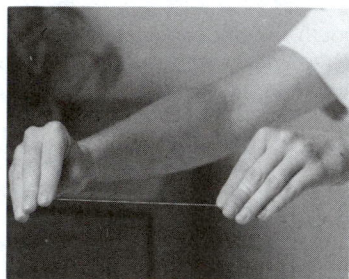
2. To clean lower teeth hold the floss so the forefingers of both hands are on top of the strand. Gently place the floss on either side of a tooth and pull ends forward into a curve.	Curving floss around a tooth ensures removal of all food particles.
3. Carefully move floss up and down in a seesaw motion between the tooth surfaces. Be sure the floss slides under the gumline and up toward biting surfaces. Repeat the seesaw motion two or three times. Be sure to clean the outer surface of the back molar.	Movement helps remove plaque and tartar from tooth enamel. Thicker layers of plaque and tartar form at and below the gumline.
4. To clean upper teeth hold the floss over the thumb of one hand and the forefinger of the other. Move the floss as on the upper teeth. Repeat until the teeth on both sides are clean.	The thumb helps to retract and support the cheek.
5. As the floss becomes frayed, move to another part of the floss by unwinding the part that is around the fingers.	Frayed floss becomes caught between teeth and can be torn off and lodge between the teeth. This can lead to gum inflammation and infection.
6. Allow the client to rinse his mouth.	Rinsing removes plaque and tartar from the oral cavity.

is completed. Procedure 35-9 details the steps involved in providing mouth care for the unconscious client.

FLOSSING

Dental flossing is necessary for effective removal of plaque and tartar between teeth. Brushing alone cannot do the job. If toothpaste is applied to the teeth before flossing, the fluoride can come in direct contact with tooth surfaces, aiding in cavity prevention. Flossing once a day is sufficient.

The nurse uses approximately 40 to 46 cm (16 to 18 inches) of lightly waxed or unwaxed floss. Unwaxed floss tends to be thinner and more absorbent, and it slides easily between teeth. Since it is important to clean all teeth surfaces thoroughly, the nurse should not rush to complete flossing (Procedure 35-10). If the client is able, the nurse should encourage him to floss several teeth so she can observe his technique. Placing a mirror in front of the client will help the nurse demonstrate the proper methods for holding the floss and cleaning between the teeth.

FLUORIDE USE

In many communities the water supply now contains fluoride. Even though fluoride has not been proved to eliminate tooth decay, it is known to prevent dental caries (Whaley and Wong, 1984). People who do not have fluoridated water available can obtain fluoride in the form of mouthwash, toothpaste, or supplements. Most toothpastes on the market today contain fluoride and can help prevent tooth decay. Fluoride supplements can be given to children beginning at the age of 2 weeks. Supplements are available without a prescription and can be taken with water, juice, or milk. The family dentist should be consulted concerning the amount of fluoride to be given.

Excessive fluoridation can result in a discoloration of tooth enamel. Clients should be advised to watch for this condition. Parents should keep fluoride supplements out of the reach of children.

DENTURE CARE

Often the nurse must clean dentures for clients who are unable to do so themselves. Dentures should be cleaned as frequently as natural teeth to prevent gingival irritation and infection. The nurse should remember that dentures are the client's personal property and should be handled with care, since they can easily be broken. Replacing lost or broken dentures can be expensive. A disposable plastic denture cup with the client's name and room number should be kept in the client's bedside drawer. The nurse should caution clients against wrapping dentures in facial or

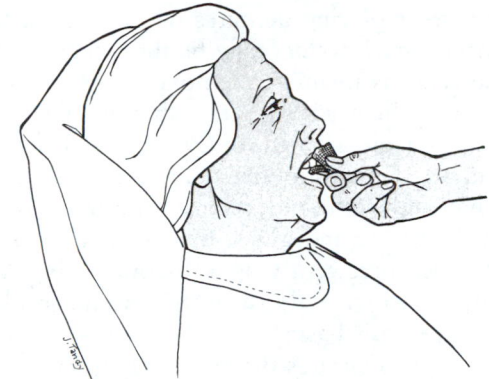

Fig. 35-2 Remove the upper denture by grasping it with the thumb and index finger of one hand. Use a piece of gauze to grasp the slippery denture and to prevent the spread of microorganisms.

From Sorrentino, S.A.: Mosby's textbook for nursing assistants, St. Louis, 1984, the C.V. Mosby Co.

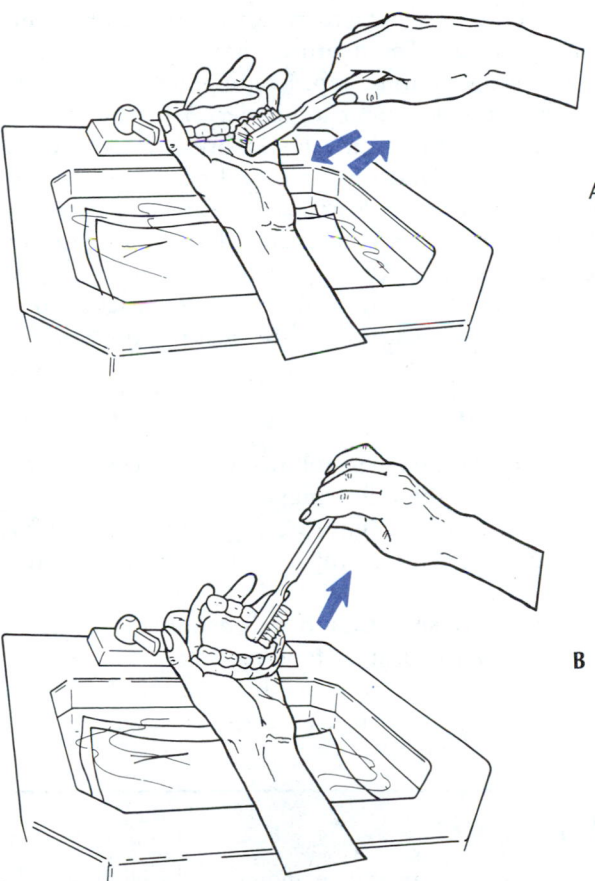

Fig. 35-3 **A,** The outer surfaces of the upper denture are brushed with back and forth motions. The denture is held over the sink, which is half filled with water and lined with a towel. **B,** Position the brush vertically to clean the inner surfaces of the denture. Use upward strokes.

From Sorrentino, S.A.: Mosby's textbook for nursing assistants, St. Louis, 1984, The C.V. Mosby Co.

toilet tissue or placing dentures on meal trays, since the dentures may accidentally be thrown away.

If the client is unable to remove his dentures, the nurse grasps them with the thumb and index finger wrapped in a piece of gauze (Fig. 35-2). The gauze prevents accidental slipping while the dentures are being handled. Often dentures form a tight seal against the palate and gums. It may be necessary to move the dentures gently up and down to break the seal. After removing the dentures the nurse places them in an emesis basin.

To clean the dentures the nurse may use an emesis basin or sink half filled with clean tap water. A washcloth placed in the bottom of the sink helps prevent damage to the dentures during brushing (Fig. 35-3). The nurse uses a toothbrush and dentifrice to brush each denture on the inner and outer surfaces of the teeth, the biting surfaces, and the denture plate. Cleansing prevents food and bacteria from collecting under the dentures. Rinsing the dentures with warm water ensures complete removal of dentifrice and food particles. The dentures may be stored in cool water in the denture cup. Keeping the dentures well moistened makes insertion easier. Before reinserting the dentures the client should brush his gums and tongue gently and rinse the oral cavity thoroughly. When the client needs assistance to reinsert dentures, the nurse should ask the client which denture he prefers to insert first. Usually clients prefer inserting the bulkier upper denture first. The nurse presses the dentures firmly in place to secure their position.

Evaluation

Expected outcomes following complete oral hygiene include the following:
1. Oral mucosa, gums, and tongue are well hydrated, without inflammation or areas of tenderness.
2. Lips are smooth and well hydrated.
3. Teeth are clear of food particles.
4. The client is able to demonstrate the proper techniques for brushing and flossing.

Hair Care

A person's appearance and general feeling of well-being often depend on the way the person's hair looks and feels. Illness or disability may prevent a client from maintaining daily hair care. An immobilized client's hair soon becomes tangled if not brushed or combed routinely. Dressings of the face or neck may leave sticky adhesive, blood, or antiseptic solutions on the hair. Clients who take chemotherapeutic drugs often lose much of their hair. The nurse should remember that proper hair care is very important to the client's body image. Brushing, combing, and shampooing are basic hygiene measures.

Hair grows from follicles in the dermis. The tiny blood vessels supplying each follicle give the hair its nourishment. Each hair has a shaft extending from the follicle. The shaft is normally shiny and pliant and is not excessively oily, dry, or brittle.

Hair growth, distribution, and pattern can be indicators of a person's general health status (see Chapter 29). Hormonal changes, emotional and physical stress, aging, infection, and certain diseases can affect characteristics of the hair. The hair shaft is an inert structure; any changes in its color or condition occur as a result of hormonal activity and nutrient supply to the hair follicle. Therefore "turning gray" does not occur overnight but is a slow process in response to the metabolic changes affecting hair growth.

Assessment

PHYSICAL ASSESSMENT

While assisting with hair care the nurse assesses the condition of the client's hair and scalp. Normally the hair is clean, shiny, and untangled and the scalp is clear. The nurse notes the overall distribution of hair, which varies from thick to thin. Evenness of hair growth can be influenced by several factors. Baldness in men is usually a genetic condition. However, the loss of hair (alopecia) can also be the result of chemotherapy. The nurse assesses the degree of oiliness in hair. Adolescents frequently have excessively oily hair. People with dry hair, which results from aging and protein deficiency, require less frequent shampooing. The texture of hair varies from soft to coarse. An infant has very soft hair, whereas a person who has had a permanent wave often has coarse hair.

The nurse also carefully inspects the scalp for abnormalities such as lesions, areas of inflammation or tenderness, and presence of infection or infestation (lice or ticks). The presence of scalp problems influences the type of hair care the nurse provides.

HAIR CARE PRACTICES

The nurse can usually determine whether a person follows good hair care practices. Dull, tangled, dirty hair indicates improper care. However, before judging the client's appearance the nurse should consider whether unkempt hair is the result of a lack of interest, depression, or inability to care for the hair.

The nurse should determine the client's preferred hairstyle. If a young girl normally wears pigtails or an elderly woman fixes her hair in a bun, the nurse should attempt to arrange their hair in the same fashion. Asking the client to assist or teach the nurse how to style the hair correctly gives the client a greater sense of independence.

Clients also generally prefer use of certain hair care products. For example, many dark-skinned persons apply oil to their hair when it is dry. Some clients use a brush to groom their hair while others use a comb. Frequency of shampooing varies according to individual preference. The nurse also learns the time of day when clients prefer to care for their hair.

COMMON HAIR AND SCALP PROBLEMS

The nurse may encounter several types of problems in persons who do not practice routine hair care. Table 35-9 lists common problems and related nurs-

ing interventions. When such problems are identified, the nurse assumes responsibility for discussing with clients the importance of maintaining cleanliness and good grooming. If left unattended many of these problems can spread to affect other members of the client's family.

Implementation
BRUSHING AND COMBING

Frequent brushing helps keep hair clean and distributes oil evenly along hair shafts. Combing merely prevents hair from becoming tangled. Short-tooth combs are adequate for short hair, but large-tooth combs are preferred for curly hair. Combs with sharp,

---

TABLE 35-9

Hair and Scalp Problems

Problem	Characteristics	Implications	Interventions
Dandruff	Scaling of the scalp accompanied by itching; in severe cases, dandruff on eyebrows	Dandruff causes a person embarrassment. If dandruff enters the eyes, conjunctivitis may develop.	Shampoo regularly with a medicated shampoo. In severe cases a physician's advice may be needed.
Ticks	Small gray-brown parasites that burrow into the skin and suck blood	Ticks transmit several diseases to people. The most common are Rocky Montain spotted fever and tularemia.	Do not pull ticks from skin because the sucking apparatus remains and may become infected. Placing a drop of oil or ether on the tick or covering it with petrolatum jelly eases removal. Oil suffocates the tick.
Pediculosis (lice)	Tiny grayish white parasitic insects that infest mammals		
Pediculosis capitis (head lice)	Found on the scalp attached to hair strands; eggs look like oval particles, similar to dandruff; bites or pustules may be observed behind ears and at hairline	Head lice are difficult to remove and may spread to furniture and other people if not treated.	Shampoo with Kwell soap and repeat 12-24 hours later.
Pediculosis corporis (body lice)	Tends to cling to clothing so may not be easily seen; body lice suck blood and lay eggs on the clothing or furniture	The client itches constantly. Scratches seen on skin may become infected. Hemorrhagic spots may appear on the skin where lice are sucking blood.	Client should bathe or shower thoroughly. After skin is dried, Kwell lotion should be applied. After 12-24 hours another bath or shower should be taken. Bag any infested clothing or linen until laundered.
Pediculosis pubis (crab lice)	Found in pubic hair; crab lice are grayish white with red legs	Lice may spread through bed linen, clothing, or furniture or between persons via sexual contact.	Shave hair off affected area. Cleanse as for body lice. If lice were sexually transmitted, partner must be notified.

irregular teeth may scratch the scalp. The client able to care for himself should be encouraged to maintain routine hair care. However, clients with limited mobility and poor coordination and those who are confused or seriously weakened by their illness require the nurse's help.

Clients in a hospital or extended care facility appreciate the opportunity to have their hair brushed and combed before they are seen by others. For example, the nurse should offer to brush the client's hair before a physician's visit, a diagnostic test, or the arrival of family members.

An acutely ill client may prefer not to have his hair groomed. This can lead to problems, especially if the client's hair is long. Long hair easily becomes matted and tangled. Unless the hair is brushed frequently, the nurse will have to spend many hours combing out tangles, which can be a painful procedure.

To brush hair properly the nurse parts the hair into two sections and then separates each section into two more sections. Parting allows for ease in brushing smaller sections of hair. The nurse brushes from the scalp toward the hair ends. If tangles are present, the nurse uses the fingers to separate a small lock of hair, grasps it firmly near the scalp, and combs the loose end of the lock. Anchoring the tangled hair prevents painful pulling of the scalp during combing. If hair is excessively tangled, the nurse should comb out only a few sections at a time. Moistening hair with water or alcohol often frees tangles for easier combing. The nurse never cuts the client's hair without written consent.

If a client is likely to be confined to bed for several days, the nurse may ask the client's permission to braid the hair. This promotes the client's comfort by reducing the need for grooming. Making two braids, one on each side of the head, is usually more comfortable than one large braid, which the client would have to lie on.

SHAMPOOING

Frequency of shampooing depends on a person's daily routines. Some people wash their hair every day, while others shampoo only once a week or less frequently. The nurse should remind hospitalized clients that staying in bed, excess perspiration, or treatments that leave blood or solutions in the hair may require more frequent shampooing. For clients in the home setting the nurse's greatest challenge may be to find ways the client can shampoo the hair without injury. For example, a client with a long leg cast may need to wash his hair at a sink until it is safe to shower or until the cast is removed and tub baths can be resumed.

If the client is able to take his own shower or bath, the hair can usually be shampooed without difficulty. A shower chair may be used for the client who is ambulatory but becomes tired or faint. Handheld shower nozzles allow clients to wash their hair during a tub bath or shower. For safety purposes the nurse should be sure all shampoo and hair care items are within the client's reach.

Clients who are allowed to sit in a chair can usually be shampooed in front of a sink. The individual should be positioned facing away from the sink, with the head and neck hyperextended over the sink's edge. A folded towel placed under the neck on the edge of the sink provides added comfort. If the client is forced to sit at the bedside, it is possible to shampoo the hair as the client leans forward over a washbasin.

If a client is unable to sit but can be moved, the nurse may transfer the client to a stretcher and transport him to a sink or shower equipped with a handheld nozzle. This procedure is commonly used for quadriplegic clients in rehabilitation centers. The nurse must be sure the stretcher wheels are locked during this procedure. The nurse places a towel or small pillow under the client's head and neck, allowing the head to hang slightly over the stretcher's edge. This position allows water to flow away from the head and neck. Caution is needed with clients who have suffered neck injuries, since hyperextension of the neck could cause further injury.

If the client is unable to sit in a chair or be transferred to a stretcher, shampooing must be done with the client in bed. Many institutions require a physician's order for the procedure because positioning the client in the necessary manner or allowing moisture to come in contact with wounds or incisions may be undesirable. Procedure 35-11 details the steps involved in shampooing the client's hair in bed.

SHAVING

Shaving of facial hair can be done after the bath or shampoo. Women may prefer to shave their legs or axillae during the bath. When assisting a client, the nurse should take care to avoid cutting the client with razor blades. Clients prone to bleeding, such as those receiving anticoagulant medications (heparin or coumadin) or high doses of aspirin and those with bleeding disorders (hemophilia or leukemia), may prefer to use an electric razor. Before using an electric razor it is important to check for any electrical hazards.

When a razor blade is used for shaving, the skin must be softened to prevent pulling, scraping, or cuts. For example, placing a warm washcloth over the male client's face for a few seconds, followed by the application of shaving cream or a lathering of mild soap,

PROCEDURE 35-11

Shampooing Hair in Bed

EQUIPMENT:

1. Two bath towels
2. Face towel or washcloth
3. Shampoo (hair conditioner and cream rinse optional)
4. Water pitcher
5. Plastic trough
6. Washbasin
7. Bath blanket
8. Waterproof pad
9. Clean comb and brush
10. Hair dryer

STEPS	RATIONALE
1. Explain to the client what you are going to do.	The client may be apprehensive about positioning or the risk of water entering the eyes.
2. Arrange equipment in a convenient place.	
3. Place a waterproof pad under the client's shoulders, neck, and head. Position the client with head and shoulders at the top edge of the bed. Place a plastic trough under the client's head and a washbasin at the end of the trough.	This prevents soiling of bed linen. The trough allows water to drain away from the client's face into the washbasin. 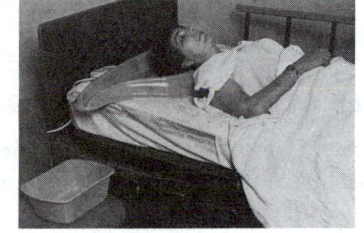
4. Place a rolled towel under the client's neck and a bath towel across the client's shoulders.	Towels prevent water from draining down the back of the neck.
5. Brush and comb the client's hair.	Removing tangles results in more thorough cleansing.
6. Obtain water at 110° F (43° to 44° C).	Proper water temperature prevents burns to the scalp.
7. Ask the client to hold a face towel or washcloth over the eyes.	This prevents soapsuds or water from entering the eyes.
8. With the water pitcher slowly pour water over the hair until it is completely wet. Apply a small amount of shampoo.	Water aids in distribution of shampoo suds over the hair.
9. Work up a lather with both hands. Start at the hairline and work toward the back of the neck. Lift the head slightly with one hand to wash the back of the head. Massage the scalp by applying pressure with your fingertips.	Massage increases scalp circulation.
10. Rinse the hair with water. Make sure water drains into the basin properly. Repeat rinsing until the hair is free of soap.	Retained soap leaves a dull finish on the hair. Soap may cause scalp irritation.
11. Repeat steps 8 through 10.	
12. Apply conditioner if requested and rinse the hair thoroughly.	Conditioner prevents excess drying. Cream rinse makes combing and brushing easier after drying.
13. Wrap the client's head in a bath towel. Dry the client's face with the cloth used to protect his eyes.	
14. Dry the client's hair and scalp. Use the second towel if the first becomes saturated.	In clients who are ill, retained moisture may cause cooling and chills.
15. Comb the hair to remove tangles and dry hair as quickly as possible.	Drying the hair prevents chilling.
16. Assist the client to a comfortable position.	
17. Return equipment to its proper place. Discard any disposable equipment and place soiled linen in the "dirty" utility room. Wash your hands.	This maintains cleanliness of the client's immediate environment and controls transmission of infection.
18. Record and report any observations (i.e., lesions, dry flaky scalp, localized areas of inflammation).	Accurate documentation should be timely and descriptive of the client's response and pertinent observations.

will effectively soften the skin. If the client is unable to shave his own face, the nurse may perform the shave. To avoid causing discomfort or razor cuts the nurse gently pulls the skin taut and uses short, firm razor strokes in the direction the hair grows. Short downward strokes work best to remove hair over the upper lip. Often a client can explain the best way to move the razor.

MUSTACHE AND BEARD CARE

Male clients with mustaches or beards require daily grooming. Keeping these areas clean is important, since food particles can easily collect in the hair. If the client is unable to care for himself, the nurse should trim, comb, or wash the beard or mustache when needed or at the client's request. The nurse never shaves off a mustache or beard without the client's consent.

Care of the Eyes, Ears, and Nose

Special attention is given to the cleansing of the eyes, ears, and nose during the client's bath. However, clients may also have special problems requiring cleansing of these organs throughout the day. Care centers on the prevention of infection and the maintenance of normal organ function.

Eyes

The eyes are one of the most important organs. The partial or total loss of vision is devastating, not only because it leads to dependence on others, but also because the person's ability to view the world is lost. Normally no special care is required for the eyes, since they are continually cleansed by tears and the eyelids and lashes prevent entrance of foreign particles. A person needs only to remove any dried secretions that have collected on the inner canthus or the eyelashes. Unconscious clients are at risk for eye injury because the blink reflex may be absent. In these clients excessive drainage frequently collects along eyelid margins. Special attention is also needed for clients who have had eye surgery or who have conjunctivitis or external eye irritation resulting from increased discharge or drainage. The nurse often has the responsibility of assisting clients in the care of eyeglasses, contact lenses, or artificial eyes.

ASSESSMENT

The nurse carefully inspects all external eye structures (see Chapter 29). Normally the conjunctivae are clear and without inflammation. The eyelid margins are in close approximation with the eyeball, and the lashes are turned outward. The lid margins are normally without inflammation, drainage, or the presence of lesions. The client's eyebrows should be symmetrical. Flaking of skin around the eyebrows may indicate dandruff.

IMPLEMENTATION

BASIC CARE. Cleansing of the eyes simply involves washing with a clean washcloth moistened in water. The use of soap may cause burning and irritation. The nurse wipes from the inner to the outer canthus. A separate section of the washcloth is used each time to prevent spread of infection. If a client has dried secretions that are not removed easily with wiping, the nurse may place a damp cloth or cotton ball on the lid margins to loosen the secretions. Direct pressure should never be applied over the eyeball, since this may cause serious injury.

The unconscious client may require more frequent eye care. Secretions may collect along the lid margins and inner canthus when the blink reflex is absent or when the eye does not close totally. It may be necessary to place an eye patch over the involved eye(s) to prevent corneal drying and irritation. Lubricating eye drops may be administered according to the physician's orders.

SPECIAL CARE. Eyeglasses or contact lenses are prescribed to correct visual acuity problems. Eyeglasses may be worn to see at a distance, throughout the day, or only for reading. Contact lenses are worn continuously during the day, and newer types of lenses can be worn while sleeping.

EYEGLASSES. Glasses are made of hardened glass or plastic that is impact resistant to prevent shattering. Nevertheless, because of the cost of glasses, the nurse must exercise care when cleaning glasses and should protect them from breakage or other damage when not worn. Glasses should be put in their case and in a drawer of the bedside table when not in use.

Warm water is sufficient for cleaning glass lenses. A soft tissue is best for drying to prevent scratching of the lens. Plastic lenses in particular are scratched easily, and special cleansing solutions and drying tissues are available for plastic lenses.

CONTACT LENSES. A contact lens is a small, round, sometimes colored disk that fits over the cornea of the eye. Table 35-10 gives the advantages and disadvantages of the three common types of contact lenses. Two major disadvantages of any contact lenses are that (1) if lost they are difficult to find (unless colored) and (2) if scratched they are irritating to the cornea and require replacement.

TABLE 35-10

Types of Contact Lenses

Type	Advantages	Disadvantages
Hard	Provides excellent vision, easy to care for, durable, low cost	Can cause corneal injury after prolonged use, cannot be worn through the night
Soft	More comfortable than hard lenses, can be worn for longer periods	Vision less acute, possible growth of bacteria on lens surface, easier to break than hard lens
Gas permeable	Provides excellent vision, easy to care for, durable, can be worn continuously for several days	Possible growth of bacteria on lens surface

Many people wear contacts for cosmetic reasons. They are also useful for correcting certain types of astigmatisms, which occur when the curvature of the cornea is uneven. Contact lenses are safer than eyeglasses for sports activities or active jobs.

Contact lenses usually are not worn continuously, although the new gas-permeable lenses can be worn for up to 6 months at a time. Continuous wearing of lenses can irritate the eyes and cause serious corneal abrasions. They should be removed when sleeping or sunbathing. If a client cannot remove his own lenses, the nurse should assist him.

Before a lens can be removed, it must be positioned directly over the cornea. If it is not, gentle pressure against the eyelid will position the lens properly. To remove a hard lens the nurse first gently retracts the upper and lower eyelids with the thumb and index finger. Retraction against the bony orbit prevents pressure from being applied directly on the eyeball. With the lid margins at the edge of the contact lens the nurse presses the lower lid against the lower edge of the lens. This pressure causes the upper edge of the lens to tip forward so it can easily be grasped and removed. A small storage container with separate cups labeled *R* for right eye and *L* for left eye holds the lenses until needed.

To remove a soft lens the nurse instructs the client to look forward. Using the thumb the nurse retracts the lower lid and with the index finger slides the lens down to the inferior aspect of the eye. Pinching the lens slightly between the thumb and index finger causes the lens to double up. Air enters underneath the lens to release the suction, allowing easy removal of the lens.

While a client is seriously ill, reinserting contact lenses is generally unnecessary. However, once the client becomes more active in his care and needs the lenses to see properly, the nurse should assist with lens reinsertion. The most important thing to check when inserting a contact lens is that it goes into the correct eye. Each lens is ground to fit an individual eye. Before insertion the lenses should be cleaned in a sterile, nonirritating solution. Application of a sterile wetting solution allows the lens to glide easily over the cornea. Clients should be discouraged from using saliva or tap water as wetting solutions, since they can cause infection. To insert the lens the nurse asks the client to lie supine or to sit with the head tilted backward. The nurse places the lens, inside up, on the tip of the index finger. After retracting the upper and lower eyelids apart the nurse places the lens directly over the cornea as the client looks straight ahead.

ARTIFICIAL EYES. Clients with artificial eyes have had an enucleation of an entire eyeball as a result of tumor growth, severe infection, or eye trauma. Some artificial eyes are permanently implanted. Others should be removed daily for cleansing. Clients with artificial eyes usually prefer to care for their own eyes rather than having a nurse assist them. The nurse should respect the client's wishes and help by obtaining necessary equipment. If the client is unconscious, incapable of using his arms, or unable to move his head or neck, the nurse must assist with removal of the eye.

To remove an artificial eye the nurse retracts the lower eyelid and exerts slight pressure just below the eye. This action causes the artificial eye to rise from the socket because the suction holding the eye in place has been broken. The nurse may also use a small, rubber-bulb syringe or medicine dropper bulb to create a suction effect. The suction created by placing the bulb tip directly over the eye and squeezing lifts the artificial eye from the socket.

The artificial eye is usually made of glass or plastic. Warm normal saline will clean the prosthesis effectively. The nurse should also clean the edges of the eye socket and surrounding tissues with saline or clean tap water. Any signs of infection should be reported immediately, since bacteria can spread to the neighboring eye, underlying sinuses, or underlying brain tissue. To reinsert the eye the nurse retracts the lower lid and gently slips the eye into the socket, fitting it neatly under the upper eyelid.

Ears

Disturbances in the sense of hearing are frustrating and anxiety provoking for most people. A person with normal hearing also becomes frustrated when the hearing-impaired individual cannot understand what is being said. Hygiene of the ears has implications for hearing acuity only when wax or foreign substances collect in the external ear canal and interfere with sound conduction. The nurse should be sensitive to any behavioral cues that might indicate a hearing impairment (see Chapter 44). When caring for a client with a hearing aid, the nurse must use communication techniques that promote hearing of the spoken word. Enunciating clearly, standing close to the client's unaffected or more functional ear, speaking slowly, and using a normal tone of voice enhance communication.

ASSESSMENT

Assessment of the external ear structures includes inspection of the auricle, external ear canal, and tympanic membrane (see Chapter 29). While performing hygiene measures the nurse is most concerned with noting the presence of accumulated cerumen or drainage in the ear canal or local inflammation.

IMPLEMENTATION

The nurse makes sure that cleansing of the ears occurs as part of the complete bed bath (see Procedure 35-1). The clean end of a moistened washcloth, rotated gently into the ear canal, works best for cleaning. When cerumen is visible, gentle downward retraction at the entrance of the ear canal may cause the wax to loosen and slip out. The nurse instructs clients never to use bobby pins or toothpicks to remove ear wax. The use of such objects can cause trauma to the ear canal and rupture of the tympanic membrane. Use of cotton-tipped applicators should also be avoided, since they can cause wax to become impacted within the canal.

HEARING AIDS. Chapter 44 discusses the need for and use of hearing aids. The nurse must remember to clean the earpieces daily with mild soap and water. Cleansing prevents the buildup of wax and other debris that could interfere with sound amplification. The batteries should be checked to maintain the hearing aid's proper working order.

Nose

The nose provides for the sense of smell but also controls the temperature and humidity of inhaled air and prevents entrance of foreign particles into the respiratory system. The accumulation of crusted secretions within the nares can impair olfactory sensation and breathing. Irritation of nasal mucosa can cause swelling, leading to obstruction of the nares. Typically hygiene care of the nose is simple, but clients with nasogastric, enteral feeding, or endotracheal tubes that enter the nose may require special attention.

ASSESSMENT

The nurse inspects the nares for signs of inflammation, discharge, lesions, edema, and deformity (see Chapter 29). The nasal mucosa is normally pink, clear, and without discharge. For clients with any form of tubing exiting the nose, the nurse should look at the nares surfaces that come in contact with the tubing. Friction from tubing can cause tissue sloughing, localized tenderness, inflammation, and even bleeding.

IMPLEMENTATION

The client can usually remove secretions from the nose by gently blowing into a soft tissue. This may be all the daily hygiene that is needed. The nurse cautions the client against harsh blowing that creates pressure capable of injuring the eardrum, nasal mucosa, and even sensitive eye structures. Bleeding from the nares is a key sign of harsh blowing.

If the client is unable to remove nasal secretions, the nurse assists by using a wet washcloth or a cotton-tipped applicator moistened in water or saline. The applicator should never be inserted beyond the length of the cotton tip. Excessive nasal secretions can also be removed by suctioning. Nasal suctioning is contraindicated in clients who have had brain surgery.

When clients have tubes inserted through the nose, the nurse should change the tape anchoring the tube at least once a day. When tape becomes moist from nasal secretions, the skin and mucosa can easily become macerated. The up and down movement of tubing causes tissue sloughing. The nurse should know how to tape tubing correctly to minimize tension or friction on the nares (see Chapter 41). When sloughing occurs, it may be necessary to remove the tube and insert one through the other naris. The nurse should always clean the nares thoroughly around the tubing because secretions accumulate.

Client's Room Environment

Attempting to make clients' rooms as comfortable as their home environments is one of the nurse's priorities. Clients with severe illness may be restricted to bed for many days. Likewise clients immobilized by traction apparatus, casts, or monitoring equipment do not always enjoy the luxury of leaving their rooms as they wish. Clients who are hospitalized in semiprivate rooms must share their environment with another person. Chronically disabled persons living in nursing homes or skilled care facilities are often confined to their rooms for long periods. The client's room environment should be comfortable, safe, and large enough to allow the client and visitors to move about freely. The nurse is able to control such factors as room temperature, ventilation, noise, and odors to create a more comfortable environment. Keeping the room neat and orderly also contributes to the client's sense of well-being.

Maintaining Comfort

Providing a comfortable environment depends on the client's age, severity of illness, and level of normal daily activity. Depending on the client's age and physical condition, the room temperature should be maintained between 20° and 23° C (68° and 74° F). Infants, the elderly, and the acutely ill may need a warmer room temperature. However, certain critically ill clients benefit from cooler room temperatures to lower the body's metabolic demands. A client who is physically active will usually be more comfortable in a cool room.

A good ventilation system keeps stale air and odors from lingering in the room. Since drafts may occur as the air moves about the room, however, the nurse must protect the acutely ill, infants, and the elderly by ensuring that they are adequately dressed and covered with a lightweight blanket. Clients who complain of excess drafts, despite the nurse's interventions, may need to be moved to a different room.

Good ventilation also reduces lingering odors caused by draining wounds, vomitus, bowel movements, and the failure to empty bedpans and urinals promptly. Body, breath, or smoking odors may also be offensive to some people. Room deodorizers can be helpful in eliminating many unpleasant odors. Nurses should always empty and rinse bedpans or urinals promptly after use. Thorough hygiene measures are the best way to control body or breath odors. Hospitalized clients can generally choose to stay in a room where smoking is not permitted. The nurse should monitor visitors who attempt to smoke in client's rooms and explain that smoke can be irritating to the client's breathing. Many health care institutions prohibit smoking in nursing care areas.

Ill clients seem to be more sensitive to the noises commonly heard within a hospital environment: the clanging of metal equipment, wheelchairs or stretchers moving down halls, or loud talking and laughter at the nurse's station. Until the client is familiar with the hospital noise, the nurse should try to control the noise level by handling equipment properly, making sure equipment is in proper working order, and controlling voice volume. The nurse also explains the source of any unfamiliar noises.

Proper lighting is necessary for the safety and comfort of the client and health care workers. A brightly lit room is usually stimulating. When clients attempt to fall asleep, the nurse should try to reduce lighting levels. Room lighting can be adjusted by closing or opening drapes, regulating overbed and floor lights, and closing or opening room doors.

Controlling stimuli within the room environment helps to promote the client's feeling of security. A comfortable environment enhances the client's ability to gain needed rest and sleep so all energy can be directed to recovery.

Room Equipment

A typical hospital room contains certain basic pieces of furniture: overbed table, bedside stand, chairs, lamp, and bed. Clients confined to bed at home usually have similar room furnishings. The overbed table rolls on wheels and can be adjusted to various heights over the bed or a chair. Usually two storage areas are under the tabletop. The table provides ideal working space for the nurse performing procedures and also serves as a surface to place meal trays, toiletry items, and objects frequently used by the client. The bedside stand is used to store the client's personal possessions as well as hygiene equipment such as the bath basin, extra towels, or an emesis basin. The telephone, water pitcher, and drinking cup are commonly found on a bedside table.

Most hospital rooms contain two types of chairs: an armless straight-backed chair and an upholstered lounge chair with arms. The lounge chair is used by the client and visitors and is usually placed at the foot of the bed or alongside it. Straight-backed chairs are convenient when temporarily transferring the clients from the bed, as during bedmaking. A straight-backed chair is also more maneuverable than the larger lounge chair. Nurses frequently place clean linen on the chair or hang linen bags over the chair back.

Each room usually has an overbed light in addition to a floor or table lamp. Movable lights that extend over the bed from the wall should be positioned for easy reach but moved aside when not in use to prevent clients or staff from bumping their heads. Gooseneck or special examination lights are portable standing lights used to provide extra illumination during bed-side procedures.

Other equipment usually found in a client's room includes a call light to signal the nurse when assistance is needed, a television set or radio, a blood pressure gauge mounted to the wall, oxygen and vacuum wall outlets, and personal care items supplied either by the hospital or by the client.

BEDS

When a person becomes seriously ill, many days may pass before he can escape the confines of his bed. Because a bed is the piece of equipment used most by a client, it should be designed for comfort, safety, and adaptability for changing positions.

The typical hospital bed consists of a firm mattress on a metal frame that can be raised and lowered horizontally. The frame is divided into three sections so the operator can raise and lower the head and foot of the bed, in addition to inclining the entire bed with the headboard up or down. Table 35-11 lists common bed positions. Most beds are powered by electrical motors, but some beds are run manually or by hydraulic power.

The position of a bed is usually changed by electrical controls on the side of the bed, at the foot of the bed, or in a bedside cable. Clients can thus raise or lower sections of the bed without expending much energy. It is important for nurses to instruct clients on the proper use of controls and to caution them against raising the bed to a position that might cause harm. A hospital bed is usually 65 to 70 cm (26 to 28 inches) above the floor at its lowest level. In the home most beds are 50 to 55 cm (20 to 22 inches) high. The greater height of a hospital bed prevents undue musculoskeletal strain on the nurse and the client. It is unnecessary for the nurse to reach across or bend down while caring for clients, and clients can move from the bed to a chair with minimal stress on their hips and knees.

Beds contain safety features such as locks on the wheels or casters. The wheels should be locked whenever the bed is stationary to prevent accidental movement during performance of a procedure (such as transferring the client from the bed to a stretcher). Side rails protect clients from accidental falls. The headboard can be removed from most beds, which is important in emergency situations when the medical team must have easy access to the client's head during cardiopulmonary resuscitation (see Chapter 41).

Most beds have firm, water-repellent mattresses. Special foam, sponge, rubber, water, and alternating air pressure mattresses can be placed on top of the mattress. These devices are useful in reducing pressure sores during prolonged immobilization (see Chapter 31). There are also special types of beds available for clients with severe mobility restrictions, such as the CircOlectric and Stryker beds. A detailed discussion of the use of these beds can be found in Chapter 31.

TABLE 35-11

Common Bed Positions

Position	Description	Uses
Fowler's	Head of bed raised to an angle of 45 degrees or more; semi-sitting position	Preferred while client eats; used during nasogastric tube insertion and nasotracheal suction; promotes lung expansion
Semi-Fowler's	Head of bed raised approximately 30 degrees; incline less than Fowler's position	Promotes lung expansion
Trendelenburg (see Fig. 35-4)	Entire bedframe tilted downward with head of bed down	For postural drainage; facilitates venous return in clients with poor peripheral perfusion
Reverse Trendelenburg	Entire bedframe tilted downward with foot of bed down	Used infrequently; promotes gastric emptying and prevents esophageal reflux

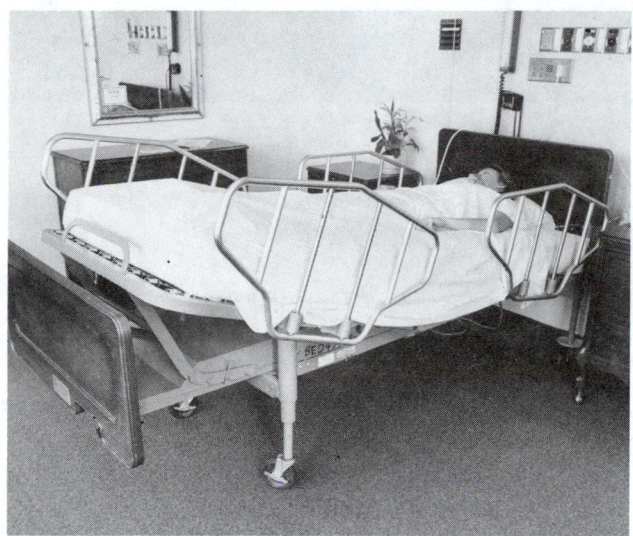

Fig. 35-4 The Trendelenburg position.

BEDMAKING. Making a bed is an important responsibility of the nurse. Clients spend much of their time in bed, eating, bathing, using bedpans or urinals, and undergoing numerous therapeutic procedures. It is essential for the nurse to keep the bed as clean and comfortable as possible. This requires frequent inspections to be sure linen is clean, dry, and wrinkle free.

The nurse usually makes a bed in the morning after the client's bath or as the client is bathing and showering. Another convenient time for bedmaking is when the client is out of the room for tests or procedures. Throughout the day the nurse straightens linen that becomes loose or wrinkled. The bed linen should also be checked for food particles after meals and for wetness or soiling. Any linen that becomes wet or soiled should be changed.

When changing the bed linen the nurse follows basic principles of asepsis by keeping soiled linen away from the uniform. It is best to place soiled linen in special linen bags before discarding in the linen hamper. The nurse never fans linen, since air currents can spread microorganisms throughout a room. The nurse also never places dirty linen on the floor as the chances for transmitting infection are great. If clean linen touches the floor, it is immediately discarded.

During bedmaking it is essential for the nurse to use proper body mechanics. The bed should always be raised to its highest position before changing linen so the nurse does not have to bend or stretch over the mattress. When making an occupied bed the nurse should also use the principles of body mechanics while turning and repositioning the client (see Chapter 30).

The client's privacy, comfort, and safety are all important when making a bed. When preparing an occupied bed the nurse keeps the client covered at all times and closes room curtains or dividers so the client can turn without fear of exposing body parts. Using side rails, keeping call lights within the client's reach, and maintaining the proper bed position help promote a client's comfort and safety. After making a bed the nurse always returns it to the lowest horizontal position to prevent accidental falls.

Whenever possible the nurse should make the bed while it is unoccupied. Having the client get out of bed is a way of promoting ambulation. If the client is confined to bed, the nurse organizes bedmaking activities to conserve time and energy. For example, the nurse collects all needed supplies at one time, moves furniture such as the overbed table away from the bed, places linen within easy reach on a chair or bedside table, and makes as much of one side of the bed as possible before going to the other side.

Procedure 35-12 details the steps involved in making an occupied bed. When making an unoccupied bed the nurse follows the same basic principles for bedmaking. However, the nurse loosens the bed linen on both sides, removes all soiled linen simultaneously, and places the clean base and top linen on one side before going to the other side. The surgical, recovery, or postoperative bed is a modified version of the unoccupied bed. This type of bed is usually indicated for clients who are brought to the room on a stretcher. The nurse prepares the top linen in a special manner so the client can easily be transferred to the bed and covered promptly with the top sheet. Fan-folding the top sheet lengthwise along one side of the bed prevents the linen from being wrinkled as the client is transferred to the bed. If a client is returning from surgery, the nurse always makes a complete linen change. Once a client is discharged, all bed linen is sent to the laundry, the mattress and bed are cleaned by housekeeping personnel, and new bed linen is applied.

Linens. The nurse collects linens in order of their use. This makes it easier for the nurse to make the bed without having to stop and search for specific linen pieces. It is important to collect not only bed linens but also the client's personal linens such as bath towels and washcloths. The nurse should avoid bringing excess linen to the client's room, since it can easily become contaminated. Linen should be collected in the following order: linen bag for soiled linen, mattress pad (optional), bottom sheet (flat or fitted), cotton or plastic-backed drawsheet, top sheet (flat), blanket, bedspread, pillowcase(s), bath towel(s), hand towel, washcloth(s), hospital gown, and blanket.

PROCEDURE 35-12

Making an Occupied Bed

EQUIPMENT:

1. Linen bag
2. Mattress pad
3. Bottom sheet (flat or fitted)
4. Top sheet (flat)
5. Drawsheet
6. Blanket
7. Bedspread
8. Pillow case(s)
9. Bedside chair for placing linen in order of use.

STEPS	RATIONALE
1. Review the client's chart for orders or specific precautions for movement and positioning.	Reviewing the chart ensures client and nurse safety, as well as proper use of body mechanics for the nurse and client during the procedure.
2. Explain the procedure to the client and assess the client's physical capability to move.	Explanation promotes the client's cooperation during bedmaking.
3. Assemble the equipment and arrange it for convenience on the bedside chair. Remove all unnecessary equipment, i.e., the bedside table.	Planning and assembling the equipment provides for a smooth flow of the procedure and ensures the client's comfort. Placing linen on a clean surface minimizes the spread of infection.
4. Provide privacy by drawing the curtain or closing the door.	Ensuring the client's mental comfort is as important as ensuring his physical comfort.
5. Wash your hands.	Washing prevents transmission of microorganisms.
6. Lower the side rail on your side of the bed. Remove the call light.	Lowering the side rail provides easy access to bed and linen.
7. Adjust the bed height to a comfortable working position. Position the client supine or as flat as possible (unless the client is short of breath).	Raising the bed minimizes strain on the nurse's back and muscles. The client's position maintains his comfort throughout the procedure.
8. Loosen the top sheet at the foot of the bed.	Loosening linen makes it easier to remove.
9. Remove the bedspread and blanket separately and place them in the linen bag if they are not to be reused. If they are to be reused, fold them in the following manner: Bring top and bottom edges together. Fold the side farther from your working side over onto the nearer side. Bring the top and bottom edges together again. Place the folded linen over the back of the chair.	This folding method facilitates replacement and prevents wrinkling.
10. Cover the client with the bath blanket in the following manner: Unfold the bath blanket over the top sheet. Ask the client to hold the bath blanket. If the client is unable to assist in this manner, tuck the top of the bath blanket	The bath blanket provides warmth and privacy during linen removal.

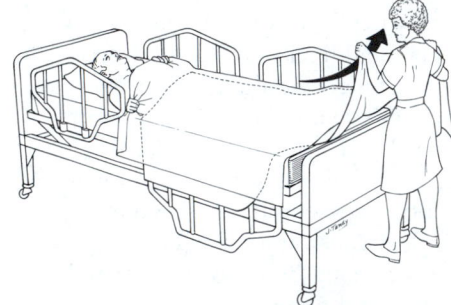
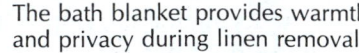

STEPS	*RATIONALE*

under the client's shoulder. Grasp the top sheet under the bath blanket at the client's shoulders and bring the sheet down to the foot of the bed. Remove the sheet and discard it in the linen bag.

11. With assistance from another nurse slide the mattress toward the head of the bed.

If the mattress slides toward the foot of the bed when the head of the bed is raised, it is difficult to tuck the linen and is uncomfortable for the client.

12. Position the client on his side on the far side of the bed, facing away from you. Adjust the pillow under the client's head.

Moving the client provides space for placement of clean linen.

13. Loosen bottom linens, moving from the head to the foot of the bed. Fan fold the bottom linens toward the client, first the drawsheet and then the bottom sheet. Tuck the edges of the linen just under the client's buttocks, back, and shoulders. Do not fan fold the mattress pad if it is to be reused.

This method provides maximum work space for placing clean linen.

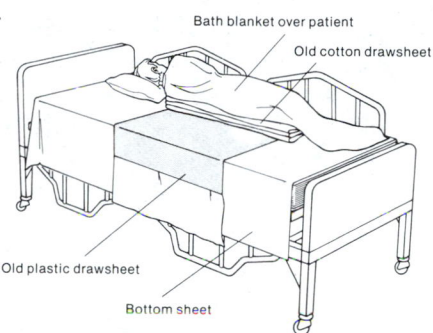

Bath blanket over patient
Old cotton drawsheet
Old plastic drawsheet
Bottom sheet

14. Apply clean linen to the exposed half of the bed.
   a. Place a clean mattress pad on the bed by unfolding it lengthwise with the center crease in the middle of the bed. Fan fold the top layer toward the client and smooth the bottom layer over the mattress. (If the pad is to be reused, simply smooth out the wrinkles.)

Applying linen over the bed in successive layers minimizes the energy needed during bedmaking.

   b. Unfold the bottom sheet lengthwise so the center crease is situated lengthwise along the center of the bed. Fan fold the sheet's top layer toward the center of the bed alongside the client. Smooth the bottom layer of the sheet over the mattress and bring the edge toward the side at which you are standing. Allow it to hang about 25 cm (10 inches) over the mattress edge. The lower hem of the bottom sheet should lie seam down, even with the bottom edge of the mattress.

Proper positioning of linen on one side ensures that adequate linen will be available to cover the opposite side of the bed. Keeping the seam edges down eliminates a source of irritation to the client's skin.

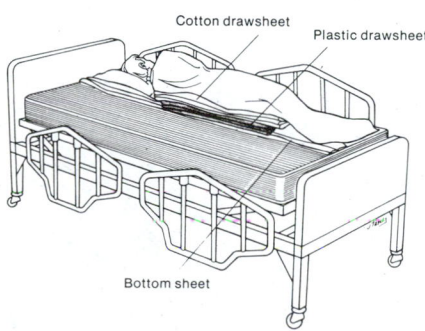

Cotton drawsheet
Plastic drawsheet
Bottom sheet

Continued.

Making an Occupied Bed

STEPS	RATIONALE

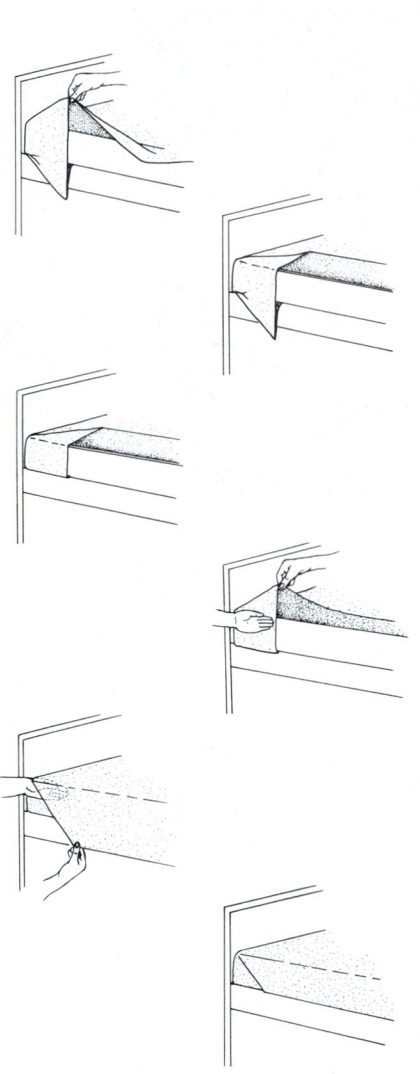

15. Miter the bottom sheet at the head of the bed.

A mitered corner is not loosened easily.

   a. Face the head of the bed diagonally. Place your hand under the top corner of the mattress near the mattress edge and lift.

   b. Tuck the top edge of the bottom sheet smoothly under the mattress so the edges of the sheet above and below the mattress would meet if brought together.

   c. Face the side of the bed and pick up the top edge of the sheet approximately 45 cm (18 inches) from the top of the mattress.

   d. Lift the sheet and lay it on top of the mattress to form a triangular fold, with the lower base of the triangle even with the mattress edge.

   e. Tuck the lower edge of the sheet, which is hanging free below the mattress, under the mattress. Tuck with palms down.

Tucking sheets palms down prevents fingernails from catching on bedsprings.

   f. Hold the sheet covering the side edge of the mattress in place with one hand. With the other hand pick up the top of the triangular linen fold and bring it down over the side of the mattress. Tuck this portion of the sheet under the mattress.

   g. Tuck the remaining portion of the sheet under the mattress, keeping linen smooth.

Folds of linen are a source of irritation against the client's skin.

16. Open the drawsheet so it folds in half. Lay the center fold along the middle of the bed lengthwise.

This ensures that enough linen is available to cover the opposite side of the bed.

17. Position the drawsheet so it will lie under the client's buttocks and torso. Fan fold the top layer toward the client with the edge alongside the client's back. Smooth the bottom layer out over the mattress and tuck the excess edge under the mattress (keep the palms down).

The drawsheet is used to lift and reposition the client. Placement under the torso distributes most of the client's body weight over the sheet.

STEPS	RATIONALE
18. Raise the side rail on the working side and go to the other side of the bed. Lower the side rail.	This maintains the client's safety during turning.
19. Assist the client to roll slowly onto his other side, over the folds of linen.	This exposes the opposite side of the bed for removal of soiled linen and placement of clean linen.
20. Loosen the edges of the soiled linen from underneath the mattress.	
21. Remove soiled linen by folding it into a bundle with the soiled side turned in. Discard it in the linen bag.	This reduces transmission of microorganisms.
22. Spread clean fan-folded linen smoothly over the edge of the mattress from the head to the foot of the bed.	
23. Assist the client in rolling back into the supine position. Reposition the pillow.	Client comfort is maintained.
24. Miter the top corner of the botton sheet (see step 15). When tucking the corner, be sure the sheet is taut.	A taut sheet eliminates wrinkles and folds that can irritate the client's skin.
25. Facing the side of the bed grasp the remaining edge of the bottom sheet. Lean back and pull to tuck the excess linen tightly under mattress. Proceed from the head to the foot of the bed. (Avoid lifting the mattress to ensure a tight fit.)	
26. Smooth the drawsheet over the bottom sheet. Grasp the edge of the sheet with palms down, lean back, and tuck the sheet tightly under the mattress. Tuck from the middle to the top and then to the bottom.	
27. Place the top sheet over the client with the center fold lengthwise down the middle of bed. Open the sheet from head to foot and unfold it over the client.	This ensures equal distribution of the sheet over the bed.
28. Ask client to hold the clean top sheet, or tuck the sheet around the client's shoulders. Remove the bath blanket and discard it into the linen bag.	The sheet prevents exposure of body parts. Having the client hold the sheet encourages client participation.
29. Place the blanket on the bed, unfolding it so the crease runs lengthwise along the middle of	The blanket should be placed to cover the client completely and provide adequate warmth.

Continued.

Making an Occupied Bed

STEPS	RATIONALE
the bed. Unfold the blanket so it covers the client. The top edge should be even with the edge of the top sheet and 6 to 8 inches from the top mattress edge.	
30. Make a cuff by turning the top hem of the bedspread under the top hem of the sheet.	This provides a neat appearance to the bed linen.
31. At the foot of the bed lift the mattress corner slightly with one arm and tuck the top linens under the mattress. The top sheet, blanket, and bedspread are tucked under together. Be sure linens are loose enough to allow movement of the client's feet.	Pressure sores can develop on the toes and heels from the client's feet rubbing between tight-fitting bed-sheets.
32. Make a modified mitered corner from the top sheet and blanket: Pick up the edge of the blanket and top sheet approximately 45 cm (18 inches) from the foot of the mattress. Lift the blanket and top sheet to form a triangular fold and lay it on the bed. With one hand hold the linen already tucked under the mattress. With the other hand tuck the loose edge hanging down under the side of the mattress. Pick up the triangular fold and bring it down over the mattress, holding the linen in place on the side of the mattress. Do not tuck.	A modified mitered corner secures the top linen but keeps an even edge of the blanket and top sheet draped over the mattress.
33. Raise the side rail. Make the other side of the bed repeating step 32.	The side rail prevents the client from accidentally falling from the bed.
34. Change the pillowcase: Remove the soiled pillowcase and discard it into linen bag with one hand. Grasp a clean pillowcase at the center of the closed end. Gather the case, turning it inside out over the hand holding it. With the same hand pick up the middle of one end of the pillow. Pull the pillowcase down over the pillow with the other hand.	This method makes it easy to slide the case smoothly over the pillow.
35. Supporting the client's head, place the pillow under the head.	Support prevents a hyperextension of the neck.
36. Place the call light within the client's reach and return the bed to a comfortable position.	This provides comfort and safety.

STEPS	RATIONALE
37. Open the room curtains. Rearrange the furniture. Place personal items within easy reach on the overbed table or bedside stand.	A neat environment promotes a sense of well-being.
38. Discard dirty linen in the linen hamper.	This prevents transmission of microorganisms.
39. Wash your hands.	

Linens are pressed and folded in a manner to prevent the spread of microorganisms and to make bedmaking easier. Bed linens have a center crease that the nurse places in the center of the bed from the head to the foot. The linens unfold easily to the sides, with creases often fitting over the mattress edge.

When removing soiled linen the nurse rolls up the linen with the side on which the client was lying rolled inside. Soiled linen should never come in contact with the nurse's uniform (Fig. 35-5).

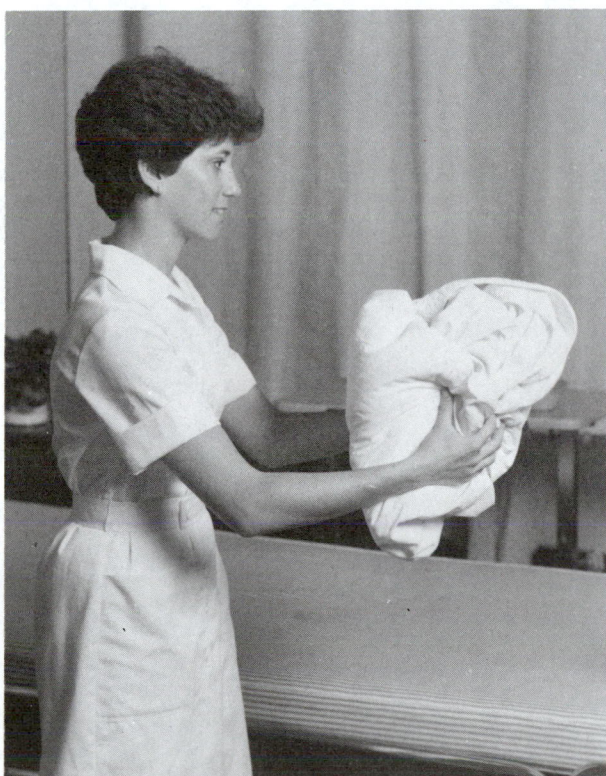

Fig. 35-5 The nurse carries dirty linens away from her body to avoid contaminating her uniform.

A complete linen change is not always necessary. The nurse may reuse the mattress pad, drawsheet, blanket, and bedspread for the same client if they are not wet or soiled. All linen should be removed from the client's room at the time of discharge.

Summary

Hygiene measures cover a variety of basic physical needs that clients are often unable to meet themselves. The nurse may spend a good part of a working day assisting clients with bathing, oral care, hair and nail grooming, and bedmaking in an attempt to provide them with a clean, safe, comfortable environment. The nurse's responsibility includes assessing a client's physical condition, personal hygiene habits, and body image to provide individualized hygienic care. Promoting a client's independence and participation in health care is one goal the nurse can often achieve while assisting with hygiene practices.

A nurse should be resourceful when delivering hygiene measures. Because hygienic care involves close, prolonged contact with clients, there is time for therapeutic communication, client teaching, and providing emotional support. Likewise, whenever the client needs assistance with bathing or other hygiene measures, the nurse has an excellent opportunity to conduct portions of a physical examination.

Basic hygiene measures may appear to require little skill, but actually the nurse must use considerable judgment and planning to anticipate certain clients' hygiene needs. Debilitated and seriously ill clients create significant challenges to the nurse. Unless the nurse provides extensive hygiene measures for these clients, they will likely develop serious health alterations.

KEY CONCEPTS, cont'd

✓ The nurse assumes responsibility for providing a client's daily hygiene needs if the client is unable to care for himself adequately.

✓ Hygiene is a personal matter, and the nurse must consider all factors influencing a client's hygiene as she prepares the care plan.

✓ Providing hygienic care gives the nurse the opportunity to assess all external body surfaces, as well as the client's emotional state.

✓ Assisting the client with or providing daily hygiene needs allows the nurse to use her teaching and communication skills to develop a meaningful relationship with the client.

✓ The client's personal preferences must always be considered as the nurse plans the client's daily hygiene care.

✓ The nurse must be careful to maintain the client's privacy and comfort when providing the client's daily care.

✓ The evaluation of hygiene care is based on the client's expression of a sense of comfort, relaxation, and well-being.

REFERENCES

Henningson, A., Nyström, B., and Tunnell, R.: Bathing or washing babies after birth? Lancet **2**:1401, 1981.

Levine, P.: Safeguarding your patients against periodontal disease, RN **36**:38, 1973.

Macmillan, K.: New goals for oral hygiene, Can. Nurse 77(3):40, 1981.

Whaley, L.F., and Wong, D.L.: Nursing care of infants and children, ed. 2, St. Louis, 1983, The C.V. Mosby Co.

ADDITIONAL READINGS

Davis, M.: Getting to the root of the problem: hair grooming techniques for black patients, Nursing 77 7:60, 1977.

Dyer, E., et al.: Dental health in adults, Am. J. Nurs. **76**:1156, 1976.

Ebersole, P., and Hess, P.: Toward healthy aging: human needs and nursing response, ed. 2, St. Louis, 1984, The C.V. Mosby Co.

Gannon, E.P., and Kadezabek, E.: Giving your patients meticulous mouth care, Nursing 80 **10**:14, 1980.

Maurer, J.: Providing optimal oral health, Nurs. Clin. North Am. **12**:4, 1977.

Michelson, D.: How to give a good back rub, Am. J. Nurs. **78**:1197, 1978.

Roach, L.B.: Assessing skin changes: the subtle and the obvious, Nursing 74 4:64, 1974.

Schweiger, J.L., Lang, J.W., and Schweiger, J.W.: Oral assessment: how to do it, Am. J. Nurs. **80**:654, 1980.

Sorrentino, S.: Mosby's textbook for nursing assistants, St. Louis, 1984, The C.V. Mosby Co.

Sykes, J.: Black skin problems, Am. J. Nurs. **79**:1092, 1979.

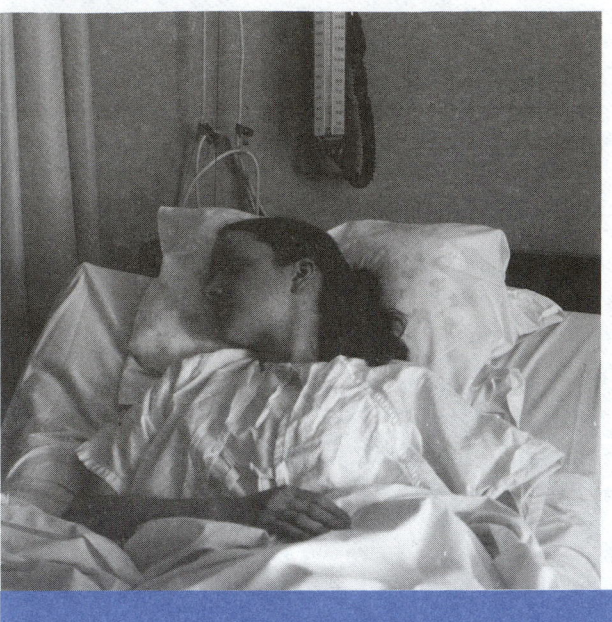

OBJECTIVES

Mastery of content in this chapter will enable the student to:

- Define the terms in the glossary.
- Describe the differences and similarities between rest and sleep.
- Describe circadian rhythms and their influence on biological function.
- Identify areas of the central nervous system responsible for controlling the sleep cycle.
- Describe the characteristics of each stage of the sleep cycle.
- Discuss the nature of dreams.
- Compare and contrast the sleep requirements of clients at different age levels.
- Describe three functions of sleep.
- Identify factors that normally promote and disrupt sleep.
- Discuss characteristics of common sleep disorders.
- Identify nursing interventions designed to promote a normal sleep cycle for an adult and child.

GLOSSARY

apnea Cessation of air flow through the nose and mouth.

biological clock Cyclical nature of body functions; functions controlled from within the body are synchronized with environmental factors; same meaning as biorhythm.

cataplexy Condition characterized by sudden muscular weakness and loss of muscle tone.

central sleep apnea Sleep disorder characterized by the absence of attempts to breathe; person is momentarily unable to move respiratory muscles or maintain airflow through the nose and mouth.

circadian rhythm Repetition of certain physiological phenomena within a 24-hour cycle.

enuresis Involuntary passage of urine; incontinence.

hypersomnia–sleep apnea Condition in which a person sleeps for an excessively long time; sleep disorder involving daytime sleepiness and disordered breathing patterns during sleep; many clients experience forms of sleep apnea resulting in sleep deprivation.

infradian rhythm Repetition of certain physiological phenomena within a cycle exceeding 24 hours.

insomnia Condition characterized by chronic inability to sleep or remain asleep through the night.

narcolepsy Syndrome involving sudden sleep attacks that a person cannot inhibit; uncontrollable desire to sleep may occur several times during a day.

nocturia Urination at night; can be a symptom of renal disease or may occur in persons who drink excessive amounts of fluids before bedtime.

nocturnal enuresis Incontinence of urine during the night.

nonREM or NREM sleep Abbreviation for non-rapid eye movement, which occurs during the first four stages of normal sleep.

obstructive sleep apnea Temporary cessation of airflow (apnea) but with continuation of chest and abdominal movements; occurs while a person is sleeping.

parainsomnias Group of sleep disorders, including somnambulism, night terrors, and nocturnal enuresis.

reflux Abnormal backward flow of fluid, as in the case of gastric contents reentering the esophagus.

REM sleep Abbreviation for rapid eye movement, occurring during stage of sleep in which dreaming and rapid eye movements are prominent; important for mental restoration.

36 | *Sleep*

reticular activating system Group of specialized nerve cells located in the brainstem, upper spinal cord, and cerebral cortex.

sedative Medication that produces a calming effect by decreasing functional activity, diminishing irritability, and allaying excitement.

somnolence Condition characterized by constant sleepiness or drowsiness.

tranquilizer Medication that calms agitated or anxious persons without causing loss of consciousness.

ultradian rhythm Repetition of certain physiological phenomena within a cycle lasting less than 24 hours.

Basic to the quality of life are the needs for rest and sleep. Physical and emotional health depends on the ability to fulfill these essential human needs. Without rest and sleep the ability to concentrate and make judgments lessens, irritability increases, and ability to participate in daily activities is reduced. The nurse works with clients who often have preexisting sleep disturbances as well as clients who develop sleep problems as a result of specific health alterations. A sleep disturbance may cause a client to seek health care or it may be a problem to which the client has adjusted reasonably well. When a person becomes ill, rest and sleep are important for normal recovery. During illness, a client often requires more sleep and rest than normal. However, the nature and implications of an illness may prevent the client from gaining adequate rest and sleep. The environment of a hospital or long-term care facility and the activities of health care personnel may also make it difficult for the client to sleep, as in the following hypothetical situation.

Carol, a 28-year-old woman, is hospitalized for acute inflammation of the gallbladder. Pain has caused additional symptoms of nausea and vomiting. She has two young children at home, and her husband is out of town on business. Carol is concerned that it will be difficult for her parents to watch over the children. The nurses are ordered to monitor Carol's condition by checking vital signs every 4 hours. An intravenous (IV) line is inserted into Carol's left arm, adding to her discomfort. Her anxiety seems to grow as the pain worsens. Carol continually watches the slow drip of the IV. Whenever she lies flat on her back the pain increases, but this is her normal sleeping position. Despite having received an analgesic late in the preceding evening, Carol reports in the morning that she was unable to sleep.

Nurses work with clients like Carol every day. To help a client gain needed rest and sleep a nurse must understand the nature of sleep, the factors influencing it, and the client's sleep habits. Each client requires an individualized approach. The nurse's interventions can be effective for both short-term and long-term sleep disturbances.

Differentiating Sleep and Rest

A person at rest feels mentally relaxed, free from anxiety, and physically calm. Rest does not imply inactivity, although we often think of it as settling down in a comfortable chair or lying in bed. A person may become rested by reading a book, taking a long walk, or playing a game of backgammon. Rest is a reduction in bodily work that leaves the person feeling refreshed, rejuvenated, and ready to resume the activities of the day.

Sleep is a state of rest that occurs for sustained periods. The reduced consciousness during sleep provides time for the repair and recovery of body systems. A sleeping person has reduced interaction with the environment. Sleep restores a person's energy and feeling of well-being.

The nurse must constantly be aware of a client's need for rest. Without proper rest an individual becomes tired, irritable, and less capable of making sound decisions. The stress of inadequate rest can result in illness or worsen existing illness. In all health care settings nurses may care for clients whose illnesses were caused by the inability to engage in restful forms of activity. The nurse plays an important role in helping clients learn the importance of rest and ways to promote it.

Promoting Rest

A number of factors determine a person's ability to gain adequate rest. In a home setting the nurse helps the client develop behaviors conducive to rest and relaxation. In a health care setting, such as a hospital, the nurses must be able to promote rest in an environment that often produces stress. Unfamiliar noises, loss of privacy, frequent examinations and procedures, and a variety of health care personnel are all challenges to the client's achievement of rest.

FREEDOM FROM WORRY

The client must have a sense that there is nothing requiring concern or worry. A feeling of control is essential to sufficient rest. Allowing a client to make decisions about his own care creates a sense of control. Promoting client participation in care helps to relieve the client's concerns. The client who remains active feels a greater sense of self-worth. The nurse's ability to perform care competently and smoothly helps to eliminate some of the uncertainties the client may have about his well-being. Thorough client education provides the client with the information needed to manage personal health problems. By encouraging the client's questions or expressions of concern, the nurse alleviates the client's worries and helps him gain a sense of security.

In the home setting a person learns to put aside daily concerns long enough to rest the mind and body. For example, after a stressful day in the office, a person can gain rest from a competitive game of tennis or racquetball. A homemaker may escape the worries of daily chores by taking time out to read a book or watch a favorite soap opera. It is often difficult for a person to practice restful activities after becoming accustomed to a fast-paced way of life. The nurse can help by learning about the activities the client enjoys and then helping the client find time for them each day.

PHYSICAL COMFORT

By promoting the client's comfort, the nurse improves the client's ability to gain needed rest (see Chapter 35). The nurse must eliminate any sources of irritation that interfere with the client's ability to relax. At home, basic comfort measures such as a warm bath, a backrub, or the application of a heating pad may be enough to eliminate painful stimuli so the client can rest.

SUFFICIENT SLEEP

Without sufficient sleep a client will not feel rested throughout the day. Even though a client may be able to practice restful behaviors, physical and mental fatigue will develop if sleep is disturbed or inadequate. The nurse can promote proper sleep only by understanding the physiology of sleep and the conditions that promote and hinder sleep.

Physiology of Sleep

In recent years there have been many studies of people as they sleep. Information gained from recording of brain activity, heart rate, muscular activity, and other body functions reveals that sleep is a cyclical phenomenon.

Circadian Rhythms

Each person's life is a series of rhythms that influence and regulate physiological function and behavioral responses. The most familiar rhythm is the 24-hour, day-night cycle known as the diurnal or circadian rhythm. Another rhythm is the woman's menstrual cycle, an infradian (longer than 24 hours) rhythm. The stage of sleep known as REM (rapid eye movement) is an ultradian (less than 24 hours) rhythm lasting from 10 to 60 minutes. Circadian rhythms are particularly influential in controlling the pattern of major biological functions. The fluctuation and predictability of body temperature, heart rate, blood pressure, hormone and electrolyte secretions, and sensory acuity depend on the 24-hour circadian cycle.

Ordinarily we perceive the sleep-wake cycle as simple. We wake in the morning, stay active during the day and evening hours, fall asleep at night, dream, and again awaken. Thus it seems that sleep is governed by light and darkness. Indeed, light and temperature are the most potent regulators of circadian rhythm, including sleep-wake cycles. However, many stimuli can influence a circadian rhythm—for example, social and occupational habits. Each person has an individualized biological clock that synchronizes the sleep cycle. Some people are able to fall asleep at 8 PM, while others go to bed at midnight or early in the morning.

Biological cycles have an obvious influence on human lives. Some people prefer to work early in the morning, while others perform best in the afternoon. Research using psychological and physiological tests has shown that people perform differently at different hours of the day. Also, the symptoms of diseases, such as the pain of glaucoma and the respiratory difficulties of asthma, are more severe at certain hours. Most people try to synchronize activity with the demands of society and the schedule of modern life. However, the body does not adjust instantly to change. For example, a person who normally sleeps during the night but who must begin to work in the evenings will not adjust physiologically for several weeks. Alterations in the sleep-wake cycle, such as sleeping during the day and remaining awake at night, can signal serious illness.

The biological rhythm of sleep frequently becomes synchronized with other body functions. Changes in body temperature, for example, correlate with sleep patterns. Normally, body temperature peaks in the afternoon, decreases gradually, and then drops sharply after a person falls asleep (see Chapter 28). When a person's sleep-wake cycle becomes disrupted—for example, by rotating job shifts or frequent environmental disturbances—other physiological functions change as well. The integrity of a client's sleep-wake cycle can influence the client's overall state of health.

Two specialized areas of the brainstem control the cyclical nature of sleep: (1) the reticular activating system (RAS) in the brainstem, spinal cord, and cerebral cortex, and (2) the bulbar synchronizing region (BSR) in the medulla (Fig. 36-1). The two systems work together, intermittently activating and suppressing the brain's higher centers. The RAS receives sensory input in the form of visual, auditory, pain, and tactile stimuli. These stimuli maintain a person's alertness and wakefulness. Activity in the higher centers of the cerebral cortex (for example, thought processes and emotions) also stimulates the RAS. Researchers

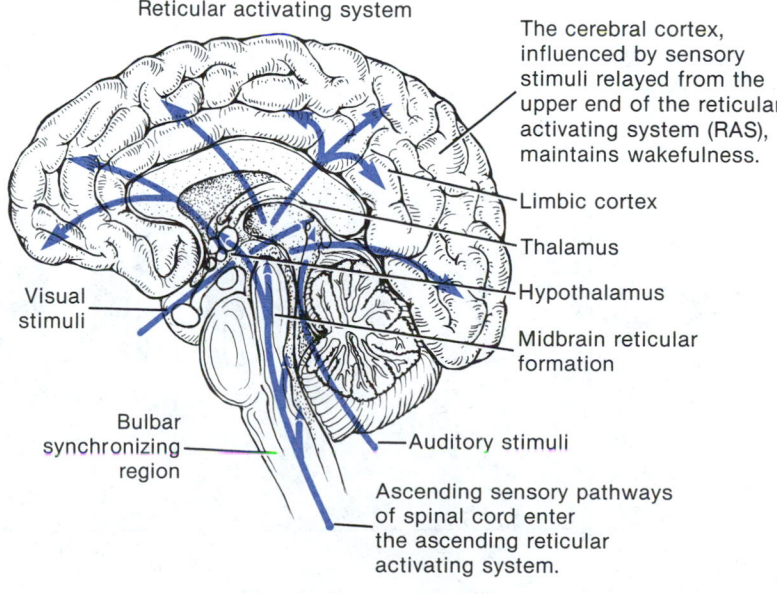

Fig. 36-1 The reticular activating system (RAS) and the bulbar synchronizing region (BSR) control sensory input, intermittently activating and suppressing the brain's higher centers to control sleep and wakefulness.

Reticular activating system

The cerebral cortex, influenced by sensory stimuli relayed from the upper end of the reticular activating system (RAS), maintains wakefulness.

Limbic cortex

Thalamus

Hypothalamus

Midbrain reticular formation

Auditory stimuli

Ascending sensory pathways of spinal cord enter the ascending reticular activating system.

Bulbar synchronizing region

Visual stimuli

know less about the BSR. However, it is known that activity of the BSR increases with the onset of sleep. As a person attempts to fall asleep, he closes his eyes and assumes a relaxed position. Stimuli to the RAS diminish. If the room is dark and quiet, activation of the RAS further declines. At some point the BSR takes over, causing the person to fall asleep. Normally it is not until early in the morning, with the glimmer of sunrise or the ringing of an alarm clock, that the RAS again becomes stimulated and the person awakes.

Sleep Cycle

Sleep is a rhythm within the circadian rhythm. In an adult the routine sleep pattern begins with a pre-sleep period during which the person is aware only of a gradually developing drowsiness. Normally the presleep period lasts from 10 to 30 minutes, but in some people it may last an hour or more.

An adult falling asleep initially passes through a sleep cycle in which there are four stages of nonREM or NREM sleep, lasting approximately 90 minutes, and then a 5-minute burst of REM. A typical night consists of four to six such cycles. As the period of sleep progresses, stages III and IV shorten and the period of REM lengthens. REM sleep may last as long as 30 to 60 minutes during the last sleep cycle.

NONREM STAGE I. Stage I is the lightest level of sleep, lasting only a few minutes. The person is easily aroused by noise, touch, or other sensory stimuli. When awakened, the person feels as though he had been daydreaming. The heart rate, temperature, respiration, and basal metabolic rate begin to decrease. The person may be awakened by muscle jerks or the sensation of falling as a result of muscle relaxation.

NONREM STAGE II. If undisturbed the person quickly enters stage II. The sleeper becomes more relaxed and is less aware of surroundings but may still be awakened quite easily. Stage II lasts 10 to 20 minutes. Body functions continue to slow.

NONREM STAGE III. In stage III, the initial stage of deep sleep, the sleeper is difficult to arouse and rarely moves. Occasional sensory stimuli usually will not disturb the sleeper. The slowing of body processes continues. Stage III lasts approximately 15 to 30 minutes.

NONREM STAGE IV. Stage IV is the deepest stage of sleep. It is extremely difficult to arouse most sleepers in this stage, which is believed to be responsible for restoring and resting the body. Persons deprived of stage IV sleep experience feelings of depression, general malaise, apathy, and lethargy. In stage IV the heart and respiratory rates are significantly lower than during waking hours. The stage lasts approximately 15 to 30 minutes. Sleepwalking and enuresis may occur.

REM SLEEP. REM sleep resembles the sleep pattern of stage I, with electrical brainwaves reflecting a more wakeful and active state. However, the individual in REM sleep is the most difficult to arouse. Dreaming is prominent during this period, although it occurs during all sleep stages. The process of mental restoration depends on dreaming. There is an increase in autonomic activity. The sleeper's heart rate, respirations, blood pressure, and basal metabolic rate increase and fluctuate. Breathing can become so irregular that the person may become temporarily apneic. The oxygen saturation in arterial blood falls during REM sleep, which may be the reason for nocturnal anginal attacks. There are also bursts of eye movements during REM sleep and depression of head, neck, and skeletal muscle tone as well as deep tendon reflexes. Men often have penile erections. Gastric secretions increase. The REM stage serves to discharge

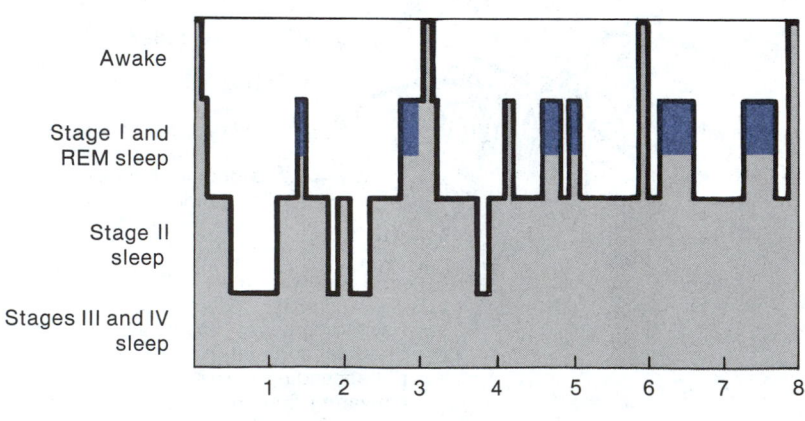

Fig. 36-2 Normal sleep pattern of a young adult.

a person's drive centers (for example, learning and libido) and aids in metabolism in the central nervous system. Deprivation of REM sleep causes irritability and anxiety. The length of the REM stage increases with each successive sleep cycle. The average duration is 20 minutes.

The cyclical pattern of sleep progresses from stage I through IV, followed by a reversal from stages IV to II, ending with a period of REM sleep (Fig. 36-2). A person may fluctuate for short intervals between stages II, III, and IV before entering the REM stage. The amount of time spent in each stage varies throughout the night. The number of sleep cycles depends on the total amount of time spent sleeping.

Functions of Sleep

Sleep has a protective and restorative function for all organisms. During nonREM sleep a person's biological functions slow. A healthy adult's normal heart rate throughout the day averages 70 to 80 beats per minute, unless the individual is in excellent physical condition. However, during sleep the heart rate falls to 60 beats per minute or less. This means the heart beats 10 to 20 fewer times in each minute during sleep or 60 to 120 fewer times in each hour. Clearly, then, restful sleep is beneficial in preserving cardiac function.

During nonREM sleep the body repairs and renews epithelial and specialized cells, such as brain tissue. Stage IV sleep may be responsible for triggering production of growth hormone for bone growth, protein synthesis, and tissue repair. This is especially true in children, who experience more stage IV sleep.

The body conserves energy during sleep. The skeletal muscles relax progressively during sleep, and the absence of muscular contraction preserves chemical energy for more vital cellular processes. The lowering of the basal metabolic rate further conserves the body's energy supply.

REM sleep appears to be a cycle of brain activity important for learning, memory, and behavioral adaptation. The brain filters stored information related to the day's activities. The person who is asleep may be able to solve problems and gain new insights. Dreaming allows a person to clarify emotions and prepare the mind for events of the next day. The benefits of sleep become more obvious when a person suffers sleep deprivation; people deprived of REM sleep are anxious and irritable.

Dream Theories

Dreams may occur during both nonREM and REM sleep. The dreams of REM sleep are more vivid and elaborate. REM dreams progress in content throughout the night from dreams about current events to emotional dreams of childhood or the past. Personality can influence the quality of dreams; for example, a creative person usually has creative dreams and a depressed person usually dreams of helplessness.

Most persons dream about immediate concerns such as an argument with a spouse, plans for a wedding, or worries over unpaid bills. Sometimes a person is unaware of fears that are represented in bizarre dreams. Psychologists attempt to analyze the symbolic nature of dreams. For example, an apple may represent a forbidden object, the sense of hurrying or rushing to an unknown destination may represent an unresolved conflict, or a lion may symbolize rage. A person's ability to describe a dream and interpret its significance may help resolve personal concerns or fears.

The dreams accompanying REM sleep are believed to have great functional importance; however, there are varying views as to the precise function of REM sleep. Sigmund Freud was the first to describe dreams as a hidden realm of mental activity. Freud believed that dreams were a product of a person's unconscious wishes or desires and served to release psychological tensions. Thus the occurrence and nature of dreams are the basis for psychotherapy. Since dreams were believed to be the result of complicated forms of mental activity, the psychotherapist's chore was to help bring dream content to a person's awareness and explore the dream's real significance.

Another theory suggests that dreams serve to erase certain fantasies or nonsensical memories. Most dreams are forgotten. In fact, during REM sleep, consolidation of short-term memory is impaired. To remember a dream a person must consciously think about the dream on awakening. People who recall dreams vividly usually awake just after a period of REM sleep. Some theorists therefore believe that people dream in order to forget. They discourage clients from attempting to remember dreams so that undesirable thought patterns are effectively forgotten.

Other theorists believe that dreams serve to consolidate memories for emotional and mental equilibrium.

Sleep Requirements

The amount of sleep an individual needs gradually decreases from infancy to old age (Fig. 36-3). There is, in fact, no specific number of hours of sleep needed to ensure adequate rest. One person may function well with 4 hours of sleep while another requires 12 hours. Each person has his own biological clock for determining sleeping intervals.

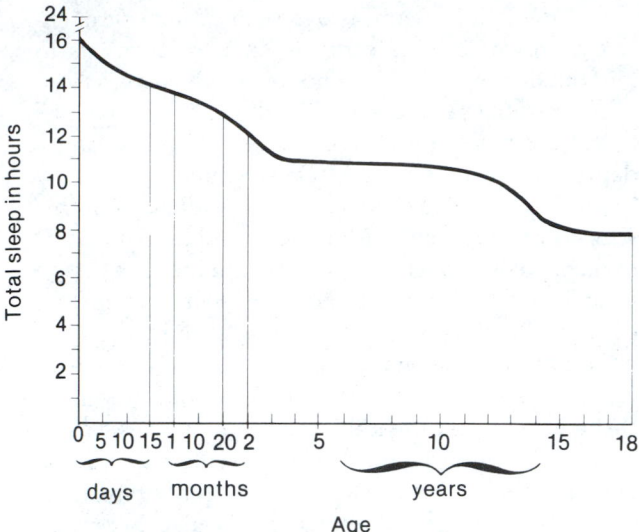

Fig. 36-3 Age changes in total amounts of daily sleep and percentage of REM sleep.

From Whaley, L.F., and Wong, D.L.: Nursing care of infants and children, ed. 2, St. Louis, 1983, The C.V. Mosby Co.

Neonates

A neonate sleeps approximately 16 hours daily; however, this may range from 10 to 23 hours. The child enters the world in a state of wakefulness, with eyes open wide and sucking behavior vigorous. After about an hour the newborn becomes quiet and less responsive to internal and external stimuli. A period of sleep lasting up to 4 hours follows. The child will then awaken again and often become overly responsive to stimuli. Hunger, pain, cold, or other stimuli frequently elicit crying. For the first week the neonate sleeps almost constantly to recover from the birth process. Approximately 50% of the sleep of a newborn is REM sleep, which stimulates the higher brain centers. This is essential for development, since the neonate is not awake long enough for significant external stimulation.

Infants

In contrast to neonates, infants usually develop a nocturnal pattern of sleep by age 3 months. The infant may take several naps during the day but usually sleeps an average of 10 to 12 hours a night. The infant commonly awakens early in the morning, although it is not unusual for an infant to awaken during the night. If awakening during the night continues, the problem may be with diet because hunger frequently awakens the child. Large infants sleep longer than smaller ones because of their greater stomach capacity. Infants between 1 month and 1 year of age sleep an average of 14 hours a day. REM sleep predominates in the infant's sleep cycle.

Toddlers

By the age of 2 years children sleep through the night and take one or two daily naps. At 3 years the second nap is usually eliminated. The percentage of REM sleep begins to fall because the toddler has access to a variety of meaningful external stimuli. As the brain matures there is less need for internal stimulation. One problem frequently faced by the parents of a toddler is the child's unwillingness to go to bed at night. This usually is an expression of the child's need for autonomy. The child prefers to stay awake and spend time with parents and siblings to satisfy the need to explore and be curious.

Preschoolers

The preschooler's primary problem in acquiring necessary sleep is difficulty in relaxing or quieting down after a long active day. Many preschoolers also have problems with bedtime fears, waking during the night, or nightmares. Parents are most successful in getting preschoolers to bed by establishing a consistent bedtime ritual. Children should not be allowed to become manipulative by sleeping with parents or by staying up past a reasonable hour. When nightmares occur, the parent should comfort the child in the child's own bed. The total daily sleep needs for a preschooler average 10 to 11 hours.

School-Age Children

The amount of sleep needed during the school years is highly individualized because of children's varying states of activity and level of health. The school-age child usually does not require a nap. Throughout the school years a child is in need of 10 to 12 hours of sleep. The 6- or 7-year-old child can usually be persuaded to go to bed by encouraging quiet activities beforehand. The older child becomes resistant out of a need to be independent. Many older children seek a later bedtime as a symbol of dominance over younger children. Parents are usually successful in getting the older child to bed by using a firm, consistent approach.

Adolescents

An adolescent usually spends an active day that is both mentally and physically exhausting. Often the desire to spend time with peers prevents adolescents from realizing their need for sleep. Once bedtime approaches, however, the adolescent offers little resistance to sleep. An adolescent averages 8 to 9 hours of sleep nightly.

Adults

The average daily amount of sleep varies considerably among adults. The majority of adults in the 20- to 50-year-old age group average 6 to 8½ hours of sleep. However, 5% to 10% of this age group sleep more than 9 hours, and 2% to 5% sleep less than 6 hours without difficulty. Approximately 20% of the time is spent in REM sleep, 50% to 60% in a light stage I or II sleep, and 20% in the deeper stage III or IV sleep. One of the more inconsistent sleep habits among adults is the time they go to sleep. Most healthy adults do not require regular naps.

Older Adults

Older adults require fewer hours of sleep than any other age group. Most elderly persons sleep 6 to 7 hours daily during intervals distributed throughout the day. Frequent naps lasting 15 minutes to an hour are common. Napping is a normal pattern that increases with age and should not be interfered with. Long periods of sleep during the day, however, are not natural and indicate boredom, oversedation from the previous night or from drugs, or physical illness. The quality of sleep deteriorates with advancing age. An elderly adult needs more time to fall asleep. Women tend to go to bed earlier than men. Sleep becomes fragmented with frequent long periods of wakefulness during the night. Interruptions in sleep often occur because of nocturnal micturition, leg cramps, nightmares, worry, or bereavement. The percentage of stage IV sleep declines, and generally the elderly are more easily aroused.

Factors Affecting Sleep

Sleep is not always easy to attain. There are diverse causes for disturbances in sleep. Factors that promote sleep in one person may hinder sleep in another. Also, a single factor may not be the consistent cause for a person's inability to sleep. Both physiological and psychological factors may alter the quality and quantity of sleep.

Sleep Patterns

The length of time a person sleeps as well as the time sleep begins will influence succeeding attempts to fall asleep. For example, when a person awakens earlier than usual, there is a resetting of the circadian rhythm. The next night the person will be able to fall asleep earlier than the previous night. If a person follows the natural sleep rhythm and sleeps an extra hour, the rhythm will be delayed an hour the first night, 2 hours the second night, and so on (Hauri, 1982). A person who experiences temporary sleep deprivation as a result of an active social evening, lengthened work schedule, or late-night television watching usually feels sleepy the next day. Sleep deprivation may result in difficulty performing tasks and remaining attentive. Chronic lack of sleep is much more serious than temporary sleep deprivation and can cause serious alterations in a person's ability to perform daily functions.

Illness

A number of illnesses have the potential for disturbing sleep. Any condition characterized by pain will interfere with the person's ability to fall asleep. Pain stimuli accompanied by muscular tension prevent an individual from achieving full relaxation. Conditions characterized by recurrent pain may also cause a person to awaken during the night.

Hypertension often causes early morning awakening and tiredness. Anxiety may be influential in the hypertensive client's sleep problem. Hypothyroidism decreases stage IV sleep, while hyperthyroidism lengthens the presleep period. Since gastric secretions increase during REM sleep, a person with gastric or duodenal ulcers may experience a worsening of symptoms.

Respiratory disease commonly interferes with sleep. Clients with emphysema, chronic bronchitis, and pulmonary edema experience severe shortness of breath and frequently cannot sleep without two or three pillows to elevate their heads. Asthma, bronchitis, and allergic rhinitis alter the rhythm of a person's breathing and disturb sleep. A person with a common cold has nasal congestion, sinus drainage, and an inflamed throat, all of which impair breathing and the ability to relax.

Nocturia, or urination during the night, disrupts sleep and the sleep cycle. This condition is most common in elderly people with reduced bladder tone. Men with prostatic enlargement also experience nocturia.

The elderly often experience "restless leg syndrome," which occurs during the presleep stage. The person experiences recurrent, rhythmical movements of the feet and legs. An itching sensation is felt deep in the muscles. Relief comes only from moving the legs, which prevents the person from relaxing long enough to fall asleep. The restless leg syndrome is a benign condition. In contrast, a person who has severe leg cramps during the night may have arterial insufficiency.

Medications

Certain drugs and their side effects may interfere with sleep patterns. Drugs such as antihypertensives and diuretics can interfere with sleep because of side effects such as nocturia. Tranquilizers, antidepressants, barbiturates, and stimulants suppress REM sleep. Few of these drugs actually promote normal sleep. Common sleeping pills are effective only for approximately a week. Thereafter a rebound effect occurs, with the person having more difficulty initiating and maintaining sleep than before taking medication. A person also often feels groggy the day after taking a sedative. When sedatives are withdrawn, the amount of REM sleep increases. Dreaming and nightmares may be especially vivid.

Alcohol and Stimulants

The excessive intake of alcohol may interfere with sleep in the same fashion as sedative drugs. Alcohol often speeds the onset of sleep but disrupts REM sleep. After alcohol becomes metabolized during the night, the person may awaken and have difficulty returning to sleep because of an interrupted sleep cycle. The hangover following alcohol consumption may be the result of REM deprivation. A recovering alcoholic may experience sleep disturbances for a year or more after giving up drinking.

Stimulants such as caffeine and nicotine can also disturb sleep. A single cup of hot chocolate or coffee or a glass of cola may keep a person awake for hours. Caffeine may also cause the sleeper to awaken during the night. Heavy smokers do not sleep as well as nonsmokers, but nicotine is not as powerful a stimulant as caffeine.

Life-Style

The routine a person follows during the course of a day may influence sleep patterns. An individual working a rotating shift—for example, 2 weeks of days followed by a week of nights—has difficulty adjusting to the altered sleep schedule. The body's internal clock might be set for the person to fall asleep at 11 PM but the work schedule forces him to go to sleep at 9 AM instead. The individual often can sleep only 3 or 4 hours, since the body's clock perceives that it is time to be awake and active. Only after several weeks of working a nightshift does a person's biological clock adjust. Alterations in routine that are capable of disrupting sleeping patterns include per-

forming unaccustomed heavy work and changing the evening mealtime. A person usually needs a cooling down period before going to sleep. Active exercise 2 hours before bedtime promotes sleep, but the same exercise immediately before bedtime may cause a person to lie awake for hours.

Psychological Stress

Preoccupation with personal problems or situational crises can disrupt sleep. Stress causes a person to be tense and often leads to frustration when sleep does not come. The stress that disrupts a person's sleep may result from an event as serious as a death in the family or as insignificant as hearing a sound from outside.

Stress may cause a person to try too hard to fall asleep, awaken frequently during the sleep cycle, or oversleep after initial difficulties falling asleep. As a result of continued stress, poor sleep habits develop. For example, a person who tries too hard to fall asleep becomes preoccupied with the process and then is unable to sleep. Often, rather than getting out of bed and engaging in quiet activities that direct attention away from the inability to sleep, the person stays in bed and becomes angry and frustrated.

A person's emotional health also influences the ability to sleep. Clients with depression often waken several times during the night or early in the morning. The elderly client who has experienced the loss of physical abilities, friends, spouse, or personal belongings may experience anxiety that prevents adequate sleep.

Environment

The environment in which a person sleeps has a significant influence on ability to fall asleep and remain asleep. For example, some people require silence to fall asleep, whereas others need a certain amount of background noise, such as soft music. Good ventilation is essential to promote restful sleep. The size, firmness, and position of the bed can promote or inhibit sleep. If a person normally sleeps with another individual, sleeping alone can cause wakefulness. Changes in the environment, such as different lighting levels or intermittent and unexpected noises, also disrupt sleep.

In a health care environment such as a hospital, it is difficult to reproduce the conditions in which a client normally sleeps. Nurses entering rooms late at night, the sound from a roommate's television, and conversations of nurses in the hallway are examples of stimuli that can interfere with a client's sleep patterns.

The intensive care unit (ICU) setting is one location where clients frequently experience sleep deprivation. Environmental stimuli in the ICU are continuous and varied. Physicians and nurses make frequent observations of the client's condition, discuss orders at the bedside, and perform numerous procedures. Monitoring devices and life support equipment give off continuous noise. Intravenous catheters, monitoring wires, and drainage tubing are sources of physical stimulation for the client. Clients constantly subjected to stimuli ultimately undergo mental changes as a result of sleep deprivation.

Exercise and Fatigue

A person who is moderately fatigued usually achieves restful sleep. This is especially true if the fatigue is the result of enjoyable work or exercise. Exercising 2 hours before bedtime allows the body to cool down and maintains a state of fatigue that promotes relaxation. However, excess fatigue resulting from exhausting or stressful work can make falling asleep difficult.

Caloric Intake

Weight loss or gain influences a person's sleep pattern. When a person gains weight, sleep periods become longer with fewer interruptions. Weight loss can cause short and fragmented sleep. Certain sleep disorders may be the result of the semistarvation diets popular in our weight-conscious society.

Hormonal Changes

Changes in hormone levels influence sleep. During menopause women commonly have disrupted sleep patterns, although this may partially be attributable to anxiety. Hypothyroidism decreases stage IV sleep, whereas hyperthyroidism lengthens the presleep period and causes short sleep stage intervals.

Common Types of Sleep Disturbances

A significant percentage (12% to 15%) of persons in industrialized nations have serious sleep disorders (Walseben, 1982). This figure does not include the common disorder of insomnia, or difficulty initiating and maintaining sleep. The more serious disorders include somnambulism (sleepwalking), night terrors, nocturnal enuresis (urinating during sleep), narcolepsy (falling asleep suddenly during the day), sleep apnea (cessation of breathing during sleep), and hypersomnia (excess daytime sleep).

The most effective way to diagnose sleep disorders is by a nocturnal polysomnogram. Three electrodes connect a client to a polygraph to measure three parameters during sleep: electrical brainwaves, extraocular eye movements, and muscle movements of the chin. Additional electrodes may monitor heart rate, respiratory effort, and leg movements. An ear oximeter may be used to measure oxygen saturation of the client's blood.

Insomnia

Insomnia is a symptom of clients with chronic difficulty falling asleep (initial insomnia), difficulty remaining asleep (intermittent insomnia), or inability to go back to sleep after awakening (terminal insomnia). The insomniac complains of insufficient quantity and quality of sleep. Frequently, however, the client gets more sleep than is realized. Insomnia may signal an underlying physical or psychological disorder.

Insomnia is most commonly associated with poor sleep habits. If the condition continues, the fear of not being able to sleep can be enough to cause wakefulness. During the day a person with chronic insomnia may feel sleepy, fatigued, depressed, and anxious.

Insomnia is not merely a temporary inability to fall asleep but may become a condition that continues for years. Treatment is usually symptomatic, including improved sleep hygiene measures, biofeedback, and relaxation techniques. The exact cause of insomnia is unknown. In drug-dependence insomnia the client is unable to fall asleep because of excessive use of hypnotic medications. Such a client benefits from a gradual withdrawal of hypnotics.

Parainsomnias

Parainsomnias are a group of disorders associated with sleep stages or partial arousals. Typically there is an abrupt onset of autonomic and motor activity while the person is still asleep. Somnambulism, nocturnal enuresis, and night terrors are parainsomnias. The disorders are rarely seen in persons over the age of 20.

Somnambulism, or sleepwalking, occurs most commonly during stage III or IV of nonREM sleep. During sleepwalking, a person is unaware of his surroundings and slow to react. The chances of injury from a fall are great. When awakened the person is unable to remember sleepwalking but instead thinks he has been asleep. A sleepwalker has a normal percentage of REM sleep. The nurse encountering a sleepwalker should not startle him. The nurse gently lays a hand on the person's shoulder, awakens him, leads him back to bed, and explains what has occurred. Children with somnambulism generally have fewer incidents of sleepwalking as they grow older.

Nocturnal enuresis begins during stage IV of nonREM sleep. The person urinates when passing from stage IV to a lighter stage II sleep, before REM sleep. The condition's cause is unknown, although it seems to be hereditary in many cases. Enuresis occurs more often in boys than in girls and in lower socioeconomic groups. Bedwetting occurs less frequently in homes where cleanliness is prized, a toilet is nearby, fluid intake is restricted before bedtime, a parent makes a special effort with toilet training, or a child is taken from bed to empty his bladder at night. Treatment primarily involves teaching parents to deal with the child's problem fairly and consistently. Imipramine (Tofranil) is an antidepressant medication that has been effective in treating bedwetters. The drug produces an anticholinergic effect that reduces bladder contraction and urethral sphincter relaxation.

Night terrors are a disorder occurring during stage III sleep. A child suddenly sits up and gets out of bed, screams and shakes, and appears very frightened. A parent's fear may be equal to the child's, since it is difficult to calm the child. The disorder tends to affect toddlers and preschool-age children and is rare in children over the age of 6.

Narcolepsy

Narcolepsy is a disorder characterized by sudden sleep that a person cannot inhibit. During the day the person may suddenly feel an overwhelming wave of sleepiness and fall asleep. The cause is unknown, although a central nervous system disorder is believed to be involved. Narcolepsy begins in adolescence or young adulthood and continues throughout life. Sleep studies show the occurrence of REM sleep during a person's waking period, resulting in the sleep attack. The attacks may occur several times in a day. Accompanying the sleep attack is a momentary loss of muscle tone (cataplexy), which may also occur after the person is asleep. Often individuals experience visual and auditory hallucinations at the onset of sleep.

The greatest problem with narcolepsy is that persons fall asleep at inappropriate times. Unless a person understands the disorder, a sleep attack can easily be mistaken for laziness, lack of interest in activities, or drunkenness. Treatment with stimulants such as amphetamines or methylphenidate (Ritalin) has shown some success. Any factors that increase a narcoleptic's drowsiness—for example, liquor, exhausting activities, or certain medications—should be avoided.

Sleep Apneas

Sleep apneas are a form of disordered breathing. These conditions are believed to have a significant effect on disease entities, such as heart disease and chronic obstructive pulmonary disease, because they cause reduced oxygen saturation in the blood during sleep. Sleep apneas may be a major factor in client mortality occurring during sleep.

Apnea is the cessation of airflow through the nose and mouth for at least 10 seconds (Block, 1980). *Obstructive apnea* is caused by pharyngeal obstruction in the upper airway. Although airflow has ceased, a person with obstructive apnea still attempts to breathe and abdominal and chest movements persist. *Central apnea,* the cessation of all attempts of breathing, may be caused by defects in the brain's respiratory center. *Hypopnea* is a reduction in the amplitude of ventilation. Airflow in the nose and mouth and movement of the chest and abdomen are decreased.

A combination of sleep-disordered breathing patterns is common in a large percentage of the population. It is only those who suffer symptoms as a result of the disorders who are a cause for concern. Men are more frequently affected by sleep apneas. Repeated episodes may cause cardiac arrhythmias, pulmonary hypertension, and anginal attacks when oxygen saturation falls. The most frequent time of naturally occurring death is 6 AM, and some researchers believe that sleep apneas are a precipitating factor.

Hypersomnia–sleep apnea is a syndrome involving daytime sleepiness and disordered breathing patterns during sleep. Sleep is disturbed during the night, with snoring, restlessness, and periodic episodes of apnea. The disorder affects both men and women, particularly those who are overweight and have airway deformities (such as a short neck, thick tongue, or de-

---

Components of a Sleep History

- Description of client's sleeping problem
- Nature of sleep disturbance
- Severity of sleep problem
- Daytime symptoms
- Normal sleep pattern
- Medical history
- Current life events
- Emotional and mental status
- Bedtime rituals and environment
- Report from bed partner
- Sleep log
- Behaviors of sleep deprivation

viated nasal septum). Such clients sometimes fall asleep during an examination. As a result of sleep deprivation, these clients often experience mental and emotional changes such as jealousy, suspicion of others, anxiety, and depression.

In a recently developed treatment for sleep apnea, a surgeon removes a portion of tissue from the posterior pharynx to enlarge the airway. Since the clients are often overweight, a weight reduction program may be helpful. A tracheotomy (see Chapter 41) to bypass the upper airway is also effective; however, it is disfiguring. Clients treated with tracheotomies have special tubes positioned in the trachea through a neck incision that permits them to plug the external opening during the day so they can breathe more normally.

Assessment

In an effort to promote a normal restful sleep for a client, the nurse should assess a client's sleep history (see boxed material). The choice of sleep therapies will depend on the factors and conditions that typically promote the client's sleep.

Description of Sleeping Problem

The client should be asked to describe the sleep problem. Open-ended questions such as, "Now, you've said you're having trouble sleeping?" encourage the client to describe the nature of any difficulties. As the client relates the problem, the nurse begins to focus on specific concerns.

Nature of Sleep Disturbance

The nature of the sleep disturbance may help to indicate the source of the problem. The client should be asked if he has trouble getting to sleep or staying asleep, if he wakes up too early, or if there is a combination of problems. Often the client can recall specific situations or circumstances that led to the disturbance. Questions such as, "Can you remember anything that occurred before you went to bed that kept you from falling asleep?" or "When you awakened, was there a reason for it?" help to clarify the problem. Sometimes, however, clients are unable to recall situations that consistently seemed to cause the sleep disturbance.

Children frequently are able to relate fears or worries that inhibit their ability to fall asleep. If a child frequently awakens in the middle of a bad dream, the parent can identify the problem but perhaps does not understand the meaning of the dream. Parents can also describe the typical behavior patterns that foster or impair a child's sleep. For example, excessive stim-ulation from active play, having several friends home to visit, or undergoing numerous tests in a hospital may predictably impair the child's sleep.

Severity of the Problem

Questions such as the following can help the nurse determine the severity of the problem. How long has the client noticed a sleep disturbance? How many nights a week does the client have difficulty sleeping? How long does it take to fall asleep? How frequently does the client awaken? How long does it take the client to fall asleep again after awakening?

The severity of the problem will be reflected in the client's overall condition. For example, a chronic sleep disturbance will influence a client's ability to perform daily activities. If the problem is recent, the client may be better able to recall factors leading to the disturbance.

Parents are usually the best source of information about a child's sleeping problem. They can tell the nurse how long the problem has existed, how it has progressed, and the child's response to the disturbance. The nurse can then assess the severity of the condition based on information about the frequency of episodes of night terrors, bad dreams, enuresis, or difficulty falling asleep at night.

Daytime Symptoms

It is important to learn if the client's sleep problem interferes with daily functioning. Does the client feel tired, irritable, or have difficulty concentrating? Is it necessary for the client to nap during the day? Has the client noticed a problem in meeting work responsibilities or maintaining interpersonal relationships since the sleep disturbance began?

During the history the nurse observes the client's behaviors. If the client moves slowly and without energy or appears apathetic and unenthusiastic, inadequate sleep may be the problem. Failure to remain alert and failure to concentrate during questioning are other relevant observations.

Young children often display symptoms of sleep problems during play or in school. A child may easily become irritable or angry. Some children fall asleep in school at inappropriate times. A nurse can often sense a young child's overall lack of energy and enthusiasm during play or during interactions with other children.

Normal Sleep Patterns

The client or the parent should be asked to describe the normal sleep pattern that existed before the sleep disturbance. Questions might concern the typical hour the person went to sleep, the average length of sleep, and the number of times the person awakened during the night. The client's problem may be drastically different from his "normal" pattern or may prove to be relatively minor.

Medical History

The nurse should determine if the client has any preexisting health problems that might interfere with sleep. Does the client have a history of psychiatric problems? Has the client had hypothyroidism or hyperthyroidism? A medication history, including a description of over-the-counter drugs, may reveal the source of a sleep problem.

Current Life Events

It is important to learn if the client has recently experienced any stressful events. Change of job or marital status, financial difficulties, loss of a loved one, and the uncertainty of a medical diagnosis are examples of changes sufficient to disrupt the ability to sleep. The client should be asked whether any such stressor seemed to precipitate the sleep alteration.

Emotional and Mental Status

The client's description of his personality and feelings about himself may reveal emotional factors contributing to sleep disturbances. Is the client usually content, anxious, excitable, or prone to worry or loneliness? The client's emotions before going to bed will determine the likelihood of mental preoccupations disturbing sleep.

Bedtime Rituals and Environment

Determining the client's bedtime rituals is very helpful. What does the client do before retiring? Does the client drink a glass of milk, watch television, eat a snack, or exercise? From this information the nurse can determine habits that are important to maintain, as well as factors that may disturb the client's sleep.

The client should be asked to describe bedroom conditions. Is the bedroom dark, or are there any sources of light? Is the door to the room usually open or closed? Does the client listen to the radio or watch television in the bedroom? On what type of bed and mattress does the client sleep? Does any type of noise prevent the client from falling asleep? The nurse can attempt to reproduce the client's bedtime environment in a hospital or extended care facility to promote sleep.

The nurse should pay special attention to a child's bedtime rituals. The parents can report whether it is necessary, for example, to read the child a bedtime story, rock the child to sleep, or engage in quiet play. The child's sleeping environment is also important. Many children fear the dark or are unable to fall asleep without the presence of a parent.

Bed Partner

Information from a client's bed partner may help to reveal the nature of certain sleep disorders. A bed partner, for example, can identify the pattern of awakening. Partners of clients with sleep apneas often complain that their sleep is disturbed by the client's snoring and restless movement. Often a partner must sleep in a different bed or room. The nurse should ask the client's bed partner whether the client has pauses or interruptions of breathing or snoring during sleep. Some partners mention becoming fearful when the client apparently stops breathing and then struggles before airflow returns. The partner may also be the best source to describe the frequency of narcoleptic attacks in a client.

Sleep Log

After recording a history of the client's sleeping pattern, the nurse may desire additional information from the client if the cause of the sleep problem is unclear. The nurse should not rely only on the client's casual description of the problem, since the client may emphasize the worst sleeping nights and thus distort the picture of the problem. A sleep log requires the client to keep a written record of activities performed 2 to 3 hours before bedtime, the hour the client decides to retire, the hour the client tries to go to sleep, the estimated hour he falls asleep, the frequency of middle-of-the-night awakenings, and the time of awakening in the morning. A client in a hospital cannot provide a sleep log. However, the log can be useful for assessing clients seen in a community or home setting.

Behaviors of Sleep Deprivation

The nurse must look for behaviors reflecting sleep deprivation in clients unaware of their sleep problems. Clients with sleep deprivation initially exhibit irritability, slurred speech, and disorientation. This condition is similar to a drunken state. As sleep deprivation continues, psychotic behavior such as delusions and feelings of paranoia may develop. For example, the client may report seeing strange objects or colors in the room or hearing strange noises. The client may react fearfully whenever someone enters the room.

Clients with chronic sleep problems usually exhibit the milder symptoms of sleep deprivation. In some clients acute symptoms develop as a result of events occurring during prolonged hospitalization. Clients hospitalized in intensive care units for an extended period may show the "ICU syndrome" of sleep deprivation. The constant environmental stimuli within an ICU, such as strange noises from equipment, frequent monitoring by nurses, and ever-present light, confuse clients. A client's mental status deteriorates when it is impossible to tell the difference between night and day. The repeated stimuli, coupled with the client's poor physical status, lead to sleep deprivation.

Nursing Diagnosis

On the basis of assessment findings the nurse can describe the nature of the client's sleep problem and the contributing factors. For example, the diagnosis of inability to fall asleep is appropriate only for clients who have unusually long presleep periods. The contributing factors may be numerous, but the nurse should attempt to identify the most important factor. A nursing diagnosis of an inability to fall asleep related to symptoms of physical illness is the basis for planning therapies that minimize the client's symptoms. If the contributing factor for a hospitalized client is a change in sleep rituals, the nurse should plan to initiate rituals similar to those the client uses at home.

The client's problem may be diagnosed as difficulty throughout the sleep cycle. Thus the diagnosis of alterations in sleep pattern reflects the complexity of the client's sleep disorder. Again, the contributing factors identified from the assessment will determine the nursing therapy.

Certain sleep disorders may cause changes or create risks for the client. The nursing diagnosis, then, should focus on the nature of the problem, as well as on the contributing factors. For example, risk of injury related to somnambulism should direct the nurse's attention to providing a safe environment. Safety measures should become the nurse's first priority before attempting to find therapies that may reduce the incidence of somnambulism. Table 36-1 lists examples of nursing diagnoses related to sleep disorders.

TABLE 36-1

Examples of Nursing Diagnoses Related to Sleep Disturbances

Problem	Causes
Inability to fall asleep, difficulty remaining asleep, or premature awakening	Related to: Changes in sleep rituals Alterations in life-style Changes in sleeping environment Drug or alcohol ingestion Symptoms of physical illness Emotional or mental unrest
Alterations in sleep pattern	Same as above
Risk of injury	Related to: Somnambulism Narcolepsy
Alterations in behavior	Related to: Sleep deprivation Hypersomnia—sleep apnea syndrome
Loss of self-esteem	Related to: Nocturnal enuresis Narcolepsy

Planning

Planning sleep therapy requires incorporating factors that normally promote sleep with a sleep pattern the client defines as normal. In a hospital or other health care facility, one of the nurse's greatest challenges is planning treatments, procedures, and routines so they do not interfere with a client's rest. The nurse has the greatest control over interruptions that disrupt a hospitalized client's sleep patterns.

The success of sleep therapy also depends on an individualized approach corresponding to the client's life-style and the nature of the sleep disorder. Extensive planning will be wasted if the client does not participate in the planning. For example, using measures to promote sleep at a time when the client prefers to be awake is not in the client's best interest.

The goals of the nurse's care should be:

1. To promote a sleep-rest pattern conducive to the client's needs and preferences
2. To minimize symptoms of sleep deprivation
3. To improve the client's and family members' understanding of factors that promote or disrupt sleep and rest

Implementation

In an acute care setting sleep is sometimes given less importance than therapies or procedures. However, unless clients obtain necessary rest and sleep, their physical condition can deteriorate. In the home setting the ability to acquire sleep depends largely on the client's willingness and ability to use sleep therapies. The nurse's creativity is important in helping clients integrate sleep therapies with their daily routines.

The main types of sleep therapy include environmental controls, promotion of bedtime rituals, prevention of physiological disturbances, promotion of comfort, maintenance of psychological well-being, and establishment of consistent periods of sleep and rest. The client's age can also influence the type of therapies that are most effective.

Controlling the Environment

The environmental conditions most conducive to improving a client's sleep must be individualized. However, certain interventions are generally applicable to various age groups.

NEWBORNS AND INFANTS

The room temperature should be maintained at a comfortable level, 18° to 21° C (65° to 70° F) during the day and 15.5° to 18° C (60° to 65° F) at night. The crib is positioned away from open windows and drafts. The infant is covered with a warm blanket.

A safe environment should be provided. To reduce the chance of suffocation, pillows or the ends of loose blankets should not be placed in the crib. A loose-fitting plastic mattress cover should not be used, since an infant might pull it over the face and cause suffocation. Infants are positioned in bed in a way that prevents suffocation or aspiration of stomach contents. An infant should be placed on his side until he is capable of turning his head from side to side.

Infants prefer sleeping in a softly lit room. Light should not shine directly on the infant's eyes. A small table lamp should be lit so the infant is not left in total darkness.

CHILDREN AND ADULTS

The room temperature should be comfortable for the client. Elderly clients often require extra blankets or covers on a bed. Some clients choose to sleep wearing socks or with a hot-water bottle near their feet.

Some clients prefer to sleep in total darkness, whereas others like a source of soft light. If street lights shine through windows or if the client sleeps during the day, room-darkening shades or blinds are useful. A small amount of light provides easier identification of the environment and reduces confusion.

Clients usually sleep better on a firm mattress. Bedboards can be applied underneath mattresses to add support.

Sources of distracting noise should be eliminated, and bedrooms should be kept as quiet as possible. In a hospital, nurses should minimize discussion outside of clients' rooms. Clients should be asked if they prefer to have the room door closed or open. It may be necessary to ask hospital roommates to turn down the volume on their television or radio. Clients may be accustomed to sleeping with a familiar inside noise, such as the steady hum of a fan or appliance.

Promoting Bedtime Rituals

Bedtime rituals or routines relax the client in preparation for sleep. In the case of children, going to bed should never be used as a punishment.

NEWBORNS AND INFANTS

Newborns and infants sleep through so much of the day that a specific ritual is hardly necessary. However, quieting activities, such as holding the infant snugly in a blanket, singing or talking softly, and gentle rocking, will help infants fall asleep.

TODDLERS AND PRESCHOOLERS

A bedtime ritual should be used consistently for a young child to avoid the child's attempt to delay sleeping. The child may be too excited and full of energy to want to go to bed. Reading the child a story, allowing him to sit in the care giver's lap while listening to music, and listening to a child say his prayers are examples of routines that can become associated with preparing for bed.

SCHOOL-AGE CHILDREN

Quiet activities before bedtime, such as coloring, reading, or listening to music, may still be necessary for school-age children.

ADULTS

When preparing for bed an adult should avoid excessive mental stimulation. Reading a light novel, watching a relaxing television program, or listening to music is helpful. Clients should not attempt to finish office work or resolve family conflicts or financial problems before bedtime.

The nurse may help the client relax by offering bedtime nourishment such as a glass of milk or a small snack. Milk products contain L-tryptophan, which may have a sedative effect.

Clients should avoid using the bedroom to work

or watch television. The bedroom should be associated with sleep.

In a hospital or health care facility part of the bedtime ritual is assuring clients of their safety and well-being. Side rails are kept up for clients who are prone to confusion and falls. A call light should be placed within the client's reach so the client may obtain assistance when needed.

Clients should be encouraged to void before retiring so they are not kept awake by a full bladder.

Relaxation exercises are useful in giving a client control over insomnia. Learning guided imagery or progressive relaxation techniques (see Chapter 37) frees the client from becoming preoccupied with worries or concerns.

Preventing Physiological Disturbances

If the client has a preexisting disease, the nurse should consider ways of controlling symptoms that can interrupt or prevent sleep. For example, a client with respiratory abnormalities should sleep with two pillows or in a semisitting position to ease the effort to breathe. The client may benefit from taking prescribed bronchodilators before sleep to prevent development of airway obstruction. A client with a hiatus hernia also needs special care. After meals the client may experience a burning sensation as a result of gastric reflux. To prevent sleep disturbances the client should eat a small meal several hours before bedtime and sleep in a semisitting position.

The ingestion of alcohol or stimulants such as caffeine before bedtime can cause physiological alterations affecting the client's sleep cycle. Caffeine impairs the ability to fall asleep and can cause cardiac arrhythmias. The client can often feel the irregularity or rapid beat of the heart and is unable to relax.

Promoting Comfort

A person must feel comfortable in order to relax and fall asleep. Even a minor irritant may cause wakefulness.

NEWBORNS AND INFANTS

The diapers should be changed before putting the newborn or infant to bed. Soft cotton nightclothes keep an infant warm and comfortable.

CHILDREN AND ADULTS

A sleep disorder may result from a painful illness. The nurse should encourage the administration of analgesics at least ½ hour before bedtime. Application of dry or moist heat to a painful area (see Chapter 48) may help reduce inflammation or muscle tension

and promote relaxation. Proper positioning also can be useful in eliminating stress on painful body parts. Measures designed to alleviate pain have the potential for promoting restful sleep (see Chapter 37). The nurse or a family member can provide a gentle backrub to ease muscle tension and aches.

Pajamas or nightgowns should be loose fitting to allow freedom of movement. In a health care setting the client should be given a clean gown before bedtime. Linen should be dry and wrinkle free. Any tubes or objects lying under the client should be removed.

Providing for personal hygiene improves a client's sense of comfort. A warm bath or shower before bedtime can be relaxing. Clients restricted to bed should be offered the opportunity to wash the face and hands. Toothbrushing and care of dentures also help to prepare the client for sleep.

A client experiencing sleep problems at home may have difficulty remaining in bed if a bed partner snores or is restless. It may be necessary for the client to sleep in another room until a satisfactory sleep pattern returns.

Maintaining Psychological Well-Being

The inability to sleep causes psychological stress. A number of sleep disorders may threaten a person's sense of well-being.

CHILDREN

Children often have bedtime fears, awaken during the night, or have nightmares. The fears are usually normal for the child's age, for example, fear of the dark, strange noises, intruders, or monsters. After a nightmare, the parents should talk to the child about fears to provide a cooling-down period. The child is comforted but left in his own bed. The child's fears should not be used as an excuse to delay bedtime.

A child with enuresis needs encouragement and patience. The nurse should include the child in any discussion of treatment with the parents. Enuresis should not be considered an act of misbehavior. Parents should not scold, shame, threaten, or punish the child, but rather should be supportive and minimize feelings of guilt and shame. The child must be given the support to help himself and remain confident that his problem can be controlled.

ADULTS

Clients with sleep deprivation can easily become irritable and anxious. The nurse must take time to discuss the influence of these behaviors on their work habits and interpersonal relationships. Including family members in discussions of sleep disorders will enable them to be supportive.

A client who has difficulty falling asleep may find it helpful to get up and pursue a relaxing activity rather than staying in bed and thinking about sleep. Reading, sewing, and knitting are examples of relaxing activities.

In a health care setting a nurse on the nightshift should take time to sit and talk with clients who are unable to sleep. This will help the nurse determine the factors that are keeping the client awake. Explaining procedures or answering questions may give the client the peace of mind he needs to fall asleep.

Establishing Periods of Sleep and Rest

A client needs to depend on established routines for sleep and for restful activities such as exercise. Clients should be encouraged to go to bed and arise at approximately the same times every day. Scheduling regulates the client's biological clock.

In a hospital or extended care setting it is difficult to provide clients with the time needed to rest and sleep. The nurse can help by scheduling treatments, procedures, and routines for times when clients are awake. For example, if a client's physical condition has been stable, the nurse should avoid awakening

---

Instructions for Promoting Good Sleep Habits

TECHNIQUES TO FOLLOW

- Attempt to go to sleep and awaken at the same times each day.
- Control sources of unnecessary noise and light.
- Follow established sleep rituals.
- Exercise at least 1 to 2 hours before going to sleep.
- Keep bedroom at a comfortable temperature and well ventilated.
- Have a comfortable mattress.
- Use relaxation techniques, particularly when the day has been stressful.
- Eat a light snack or drink a glass of milk before bedtime.

HABITS TO AVOID

- Avoid ingestion of alcohol and stimulants before bedtime.
- Do not take work to bed.
- Avoid watching television in bed.
- Avoid repeated use of hypnotics.
- Avoid exhausting exercise just before bedtime.

---

the client to check vital signs. Unless maintaining a drug's therapeutic blood level is essential, medications should be given during waking hours. The nurse should work with the radiology department and other support services to plan therapies at intervals that allow clients time for rest.

When the client's condition demands more frequent monitoring, the nurse can schedule activities to allow extended rest periods. For example, if a client needs frequent dressing changes, is receiving intravenous therapy, and has drainage tubes from several sites, the nurse should not make a separate trip into the room to check each individual problem. Instead the nurse should use a single visit to change the dressing, regulate the intravenous system, and empty the drainage tubes.

Good-quality sleep may depend on proper exercise. Exercise requires physical work but can free the client's mind from day-to-day worries and concerns. Clients should exercise several hours before bedtime to produce a feeling of fatigue that fosters sleep. Walking, bicycling, and swimming are good forms of exercise.

It is common for elderly people to nap for short intervals throughout the day. However, younger clients should avoid taking daytime naps as a way of passing time. Napping can lead to disruption of sleep at night.

Medications and Pharmaceutically Active Substances

Several hypnotic drugs are considered safe in promoting sleep: flurazepam (Dalmane), chlordiazepoxide (Librium), chloral hydrate, methaqualone (Quaalude), and diazepam (Valium). These hypnotics cause least disruption to the sleep cycle. Nurses should caution clients against taking hypnotics with alcoholic beverages. Clients should also avoid activities requiring motor coordination while under the influence of hypnotics.

L-Tryptophan, a substance that is believed to promote sleep, has not yet been approved as a drug by the Food and Drug Administration. L-Tryptophan occurs naturally in foods such as milk, cheese, and meats. It seems to increase sleeping time and reduce the time it takes to fall asleep. Eight glasses of milk equal 1 g of L-tryptophan. However, the amount of L-tryptophan in a typical dinner accompanied by a glass of milk may be enough to promote sleep.

Client Teaching

It is important for clients to develop good sleep habits in the home environment. The nurse instructs clients or the parents of children with sleeping problems about the techniques that promote sleep and the conditions that interfere with sleep (see boxed material).

The client will be more likely to follow the nurse's suggestions if the nurse has gathered information about the client's home setting as a basis for the suggestions. For example, a recommendation that the client try controlling environmental noise has little use if the client lives near a busy airport. A recommendation for relaxing activities should include activities the client enjoys.

The client should also be taught how disease states can interfere with sleep. For example, the client with a hiatus hernia should learn to avoid eating large meals before bedtime in order to prevent irritating esophageal reflux that would keep him awake. A client must also understand the proper way to take hypnotics to avoid side effects or drug-dependence insomnia.

Evaluation

The nurse should evaluate the effectiveness of sleep therapies on the basis of the expected outcomes of care. Evaluation of efforts to promote a more normal sleep and rest pattern should be based on the following criteria:

1. The client's ability to fall asleep within 20 to 30 minutes
2. A reduction in episodes of awakening from sleep
3. A return to sleep within minutes after awakening
4. An increase in the duration of sleep to the length of time desired by the client
5. The client's ability to recall episodes of dreaming

Efforts to minimize symptoms of sleep deprivation are evaluated on the basis of the following:

1. The client's subjective report of how he feels after sleeping
2. Absence of previous behaviors indicating anxiety or depression
3. The client's ability to fulfill work-related responsibilities successfully

Efforts to improve a client's or family member's understanding of sleep therapies are evaluated on the basis of the following:

1. Use of therapies in the home setting
2. The ability of the client and family to describe factors that promote or disrupt sleep

An important factor in evaluating the outcomes of sleep therapies is the recognition that each client has a different need for sleep and rest. Clients in relatively good health do not require as much sleep as those whose physical condition is poor.

Summary

During a 24-hour period each person needs sleep to protect and restore body functions. Normally the sleep-wake cycle follows a 24-hour rhythm that is coordinated with other physiological functions such as body temperature and hormonal regulation. Sleep is a rhythm within a rhythm. After falling asleep, a person passes through a series of stages that allows the body to rest and recuperate.

A person's age dictates the amount of sleep he normally needs. Older people require less sleep. The sleeping habits of the client's age group can influence the nurse's choice of sleep therapy.

Numerous factors have the potential for promoting or disrupting sleep. In an attempt to establish a normal sleeping pattern for the client, the nurse should use factors that foster relaxation and sleep and eliminate those that disrupt sleep. The nurse must thoroughly assess a client's sleeping pattern to plan an individualized and effective approach to sleep therapy.

KEY CONCEPTS

✓ Sleep is a sustained unbroken period of rest during which a person experiences a reduced level of consciousness.

✓ The sleep cycle is a circadian rhythm that affects the fluctuation of body temperature, heart rate, blood pressure, and hormone and electrolyte secretions.

✓ Although light and temperature are the main regulators of the sleep cycle, social and occupational habits can also influence a person's sleep pattern.

✓ Activation and suppression of the brain's higher centers by the reticular activating system (RAS) and the bulbar synchronizing region (BSR) are responsible for controlling the sleep cycle.

✓ During a typical night's sleep a person passes through four to six sleep cycles, each of which is comprised of five sleep stages.

✓ The amount of sleep a person normally needs decreases from infancy to old age.

✓ Newborns and infants have a higher percentage of REM sleep than older age groups because they have a greater need for the mental stimulation of REM sleep.

✓ A common psychological stressor that interferes with a child's ability to sleep is fear of the unknown.

✓ As children grow and begin to seek autonomy or independence, it is important for parents to enforce consistent sleep rituals.

✓ The elderly commonly have difficulty falling asleep and experience frequent interruptions in their sleep patterns.

✓ During sleep many physiological functions slow down, the body conserves energy, and brain activity promotes memory and learning.

✓ Symptoms of various disease processes may disrupt sleep.

✓ Long-term use of sleeping pills may eventually lead to difficulty in initiating and maintaining sleep.

✓ The hectic pace of a person's life-style, emotional and psychological stress, and alcohol ingestion all disrupt the sleep pattern.

✓ An environment conducive to sleep is a darkened room with reduced noise, a comfortable bed, and good ventilation.

✓ The most common type of sleep disorder is insomnia, which is characterized by the inability to fall asleep or remain asleep during the night.

✓ Assessment of a client's sleep history involves an analysis of the client's normal sleep pattern, the nature of the sleep disturbance, and the identification of factors that impair the client's sleep.

✓ Diagnosing a client's sleep problem depends on identifying factors that impair sleep.

✓ In using environmental controls to promote sleep, the nurse should consider the client's home environment.

✓ A bedtime ritual of relaxing activities prepares a person physically and mentally for sleep.

✓ Pain control is essential to promote a client's ability to sleep.

✓ One of the most important nursing interventions for promoting sleep is establishing periods for sleep and rest.

✓ L-Tryptophan, a natural component of milk products and meat, and hypnotic drugs may stimulate sleep.

REFERENCES

Block, A.J.: Respiratory disorders during sleep. I. Heart Lung 9:1011, 1980.

Hauri, P.: Current concepts: the sleep disorders, ed. 2, Kalamazoo, Mich., 1982, The Upjohn Co.

Walseben, J.: Sleep disorders, Am. J. Nurs. 82:936, 1982.

ADDITIONAL READINGS

Ebersole, P., and Hess, P.: Toward healthy aging: human needs and nursing response, St. Louis, 1981, The C.V. Mosby Co.

Fass, G.: Sleep, drugs, and dreams, Am. J. Nurs. 71:2316, 1971.

Fernsebner, B.: Sleep deprivation in patients, AORN J. 37:35, 1983.

Fosnot, H.: When the patterns of sleep go askew, Patient Care 14:122, 1980.

Hartmann E.: The sleeping pill, London, 1978, Yale University Press.

Hayter, J.: The rhythm of sleep, Am. J. Nurs. 80:457, 1980.

Helton, M.C., et al.: The correlation between sleep deprivation and the intensive care unit syndrome, Heart Lung 9:464, 1980.

Kales, A., et al.: Psychophysiological and biochemical changes following use and withdrawal of hypnotics. In Kales, A., editor: Sleep: physiology and pathology, Philadelphia, 1969, J.B. Lippincott Co.

Luce, G.G.: Biological rhythms in human and animal physiology, New York, 1971, Dover Publications, Inc.

Melnechuk, T.: The dream machine, Psychology Today 17:22, 1983.

Narrow, B.W.: Rest is. . . , Am. J. Nurs. 67:1646, 1967.

Schirmer, M.S.: When sleep won't come, J. Gerontol. Nurs. 9:16, 1983.

Whaley, L.F., and Wong, D.L.: Nursing care of infants and children, ed. 2, St. Louis, 1983, The C.V. Mosby Co.

Williams, D.H.: Sleep and disease, Am. J. Nurs. 71:2321, 1971.

Zelechowski, G.P.: Helping your patient sleep: planning instead of pills, Nursing 77 7:63, 1977.

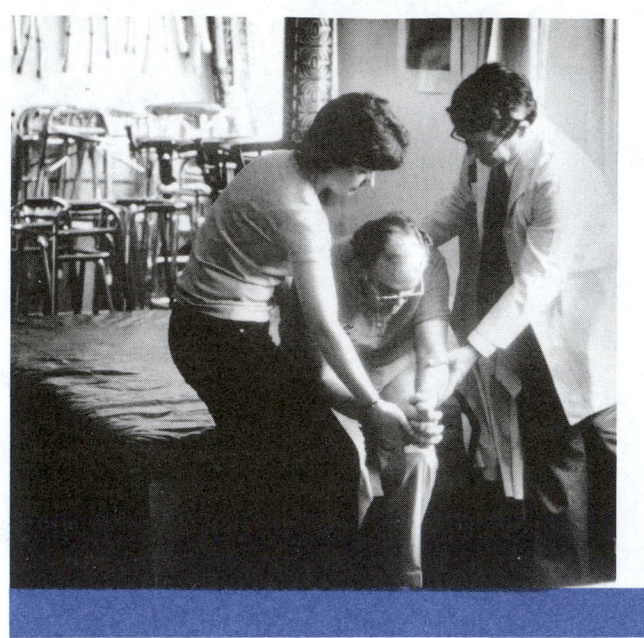

OBJECTIVES

Mastery of content in this chapter will enable the student to:

- Define the terms in the glossary.
- Discuss common misconceptions about pain.
- Identify the three components of the pain experience.
- Compare and contrast the characteristics of acute and chronic pain.
- Perform an assessment of a client experiencing pain.
- Identify the physiological and psychological mechanisms for pain relief measures.
- Institute pain relief measures.

GLOSSARY

addiction Compulsive, uncontrollable, physical and psychological dependence on a substance or habit, for example, a narcotic, to the point that withdrawal causes severe emotional, mental, and physiological reactions.

afferent Proceeding toward a center, as with nerves, arteries, and veins.

analgesic Relieving pain; a drug that relieves pain.

chordotomy Surgical resection of the anterolateral nerve tracts in the spinal cord for pain relief.

colic Sharp visceral pain resulting from obstruction or smooth muscle spasm of a hollow organ, such as a ureter or the intestines.

concomitant symptom Symptom that accompanies a primary symptom.

efferent Directed away from a center, as with nerves, arteries, and veins.

endorphin Naturally occurring neuropeptide that is composed of amino acids and is secreted within the central nervous system to reduce pain.

exacerbation Increase in the seriousness of a disease or disorder as marked by greater intensity in the signs or symptoms.

narcotic Drug substance, derived from opium or produced synthetically, that alters perception of pain and that with repeated use may result in physical and psychological dependence.

pain Subjective, unpleasant sensation caused by noxious stimulation of sensory nerve endings.

remission Partial or complete disappearance of the clinical and subjective characteristics of a chronic or malignant disease; remission may be spontaneous or the result of therapy.

rhizotomy Surgical resection of the dorsal root of a spinal nerve for pain relief.

threshold Point at which a person first perceives a painful stimulus as being painful.

tolerance Point at which a person is not willing to accept pain of greater severity or duration.

transcutaneous electrical nerve stimulation (TENS) Technique in which battery-powered device blocks pain impulses from reaching the spinal cord by delivering weak electrical impulses directly to the skin's surface.

37 | Pain

Every person has experienced some type or degree of pain. Pain that results from a stubbed toe, cut finger, or decayed tooth is self-limiting, predictable, and tolerated well by most individuals. Pain that arises from a terminal illness, an unknown or undiagnosed source, or a serious injury is indeterminate in length, unpredictable in its course, and less well tolerated.

A client often values above all else the nurse's ability to bring relief from his suffering. However, the nurse caring for the client cannot see or feel the pain that is being treated. No two persons experience pain in the same way, and no two painful events create identical responses or feelings in a person. For many individuals in pain total relief never comes, and the nurse can only use interventions that minimize the pain.

Nurses work with clients during various activities throughout the day. Familiarity with a client's ongoing needs gives the nurse a unique opportunity to help promote his comfort. The nurse has a responsibility to discover what the experience of pain is like for a client and then to initiate measures that either provide relief or help the client learn to cope with discomfort.

Nature of Pain

Pain is a subjective and highly individualized experience, and the interpretation and meaning of pain involve various psychosocial and cultural factors. The person experiencing pain is the only authority about his pain. According to McCaffery (1980), "Pain is whatever the experiencing person says it is, existing whenever he says it does." Pain cannot be objectively measured, such as with a roentgenogram or blood test. Although certain types of pain create predictable signs and symptoms, often the only way a nurse can assess pain is by relying on the client's words and behavior. Only the client can reveal whether pain is present and what the experience is like. To help a client gain pain relief, the nurse must believe that the pain exists.

Pain is a protective physiological mechanism. With a sprained ankle, a person avoids bearing full weight on the foot to prevent further injury. Pain is a warning that tissue damage has occurred. The client who is unable to feel sensations, such as one who has a spinal cord tumor or a peripheral nerve disorder, will be unaware of pain-inducing injuries.

Pain is a leading cause of disability and one of the most common reasons for seeking health care. As the average life span increases, more people have chronic disease in which pain is a common symptom. In addition, medical advances have resulted in diagnostic and therapeutic measures that are often uncomfortable. Pain is one of the most common problems faced by nurses in their practice, yet it is also a source of frustration and is frequently one of the most misunderstood problems the nurse confronts.

Prejudices and Misconceptions

The following hypothetical situation illustrates one of the common misconceptions health care workers and nurses can have about a client's pain:

Ms. Truman has been hospitalized four times in the last 2 years with severe back pain. Multiple tests have failed to reveal the source of Ms. Truman's discomfort. She takes several pain medications at home, but she reports that none provides relief. In the hospital Ms. Truman always requests a pain shot a half hour before the scheduled administration time.

The nurses are frustrated in caring for Ms. Truman. They are unconvinced that she needs the routine pain medications. There are times when she does not seem to be in pain, yet she begins to complain when a nurse comes to her bedside. Much of the nurses' frustration stems from knowing that a client down the hall who has a severe leg fracture does not call for help half as often as Ms. Truman.

Too often health care personnel assume that they can determine whether pain really exists and to what extent. When there is a lack of objective evidence pointing to the source of pain, nurses find it hard to believe that the client is uncomfortable. Frequently nurses needlessly avoid administering analgesics for fear of fostering drug dependence. Another misconception is that the amount of tissue damage in an injury can accurately predict pain intensity.

Such myths and misconceptions about pain limit the nurse's ability to assess a client's pain. Unfortunately, all people are influenced by prejudices that originate in their culture, education, and experience. Typically a mother tells her child with a cut finger, "Now, don't cry, it will go away." Such statements create expectations as to how the child should experience pain and will expect others to react to pain.

Nurses often hold biases toward certain types of clients experiencing pain. Clients with minor illnesses such as a hernia or hemorrhoids are frequently viewed skeptically if they claim to feel intense pain. Strong biases are often held against alcoholics or drug abusers, yet these clients are as subject to pain as anyone else. The nurse should not project personal values onto the client experiencing pain. Too often the obese, the elderly, and members of certain ethnic groups are made to feel that they deserve the pain they have. Personal prejudices are not conducive to effective and efficient relief of a client's pain.

Most nurses feel more comfortable in dealing with concrete problems that are predictable and that respond to specific therapies. For example, the administration of an antihypertensive drug will lower a dangerously high blood pressure and reduce the client's risk of more serious complications. Pain is not as simple to manage. Too often nurses infer there is less pain than the client is really experiencing. Nurses may assume a fatalistic attitude toward pain relief. In many cases total pain relief never comes and the nurse faces failure. Many nurses even avoid acknowledging a client's pain because of their own fear and denial

of it. In order to help a client gain comfort or relief, the nurse must view the experience through the client's eyes. Acknowledging personal prejudices or misconceptions will also help the nurse address the client's problem more professionally. The nurse who becomes an active, knowledgeable observer of a client in pain will be able to achieve a more objective analysis of the pain experience. The client makes the diagnosis that pain is present, and the nurse works to apply techniques and skills that ultimately give the client relief.

Components of the Pain Experience

The pain experience consists of a three-stage process: reception, perception, and reaction. An understanding of each stage will assist the nurse in recognizing the factors that can cause pain, the symptoms that accomany pain, and the actions of various therapies.

Reception

Reception is the neurophysiological component of the pain experience. Special receptors receive painful stimuli and transmit the impulses via afferent peripheral nerves to the spinal cord. After the impulses cross over to the opposite side of the spinal cord, they ascend via the spinal cord to higher centers of the central nervous system. Fig. 37-1 illustrates the normal pain reception pathway via the spinothalamic tract.

Special pain receptors are found in skin, muscle, bone, mucous membranes, and tendons. There are very few pain receptors in the visceral organs themselves. Therefore, the pain of a broken bone can be severe, but a tumor of the lung rarely causes a client pain.

Two types of nerve fibers conduct painful stimuli: C fibers are very small and conduct impulses slowly, and A fibers are larger and conduct impulses rapidly. The A fibers send impulses that localize the source of pain, whereas C fibers relay impulses of a more diffuse nature. For example, after stepping on a nail, a person initially feels a sharp localized pain, which is the result of A fiber transmission. Within a few seconds the pain becomes more diffuse and widespread until the whole foot aches because of C fiber innervation.

Numerous physical factors are stimuli for pain. Thermal stimuli result from contact of the skin with hot or cold substances. Pressure, friction, tension, and stretching are mechanical stimuli. Chemical stimuli originate from substances within the body, such as gastric enzymes and histamines, or from substances outside the body. Table 37-1 summarizes physical

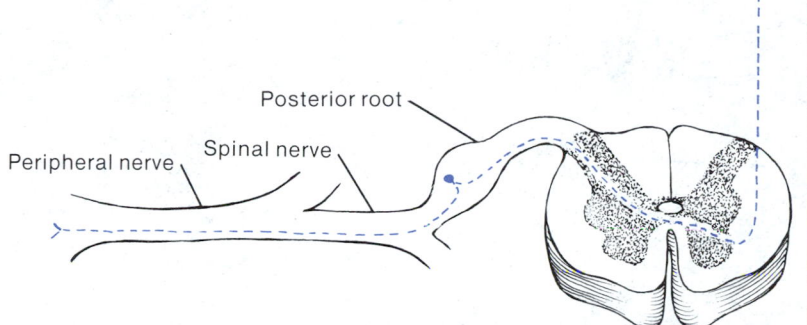

Fig. 37-1 Pain reception pathway.

Peripheral nerve Spinal nerve Posterior root Spinal cord (spinothalamic tract)

alterations that elicit pain-producing stimuli. The nurse's knowledge of physical factors that elicit pain can aid in the selection of appropriate pain relief therapies.

Impulses travel quickly to bring information to the higher brain centers. However, there is also a protective reflex response that occurs with pain reception (Fig. 37-2). A fibers send sensory impulses to the spinal cord, where they synapse with spinal motor neurons. The motor impulses travel via a reflex arc along efferent nerve fibers back to a peripheral muscle near the site of pain stimulation. Contraction of the muscle leads to a protective withdrawal from the source of pain. For example, when a person accidentally touches a hot iron, a burning sensation is felt but the hand also reflexively withdraws from the iron's surface. When superficial fibers in the skin are stimulated, a person moves away from the pain source. If internal tissues such as muscle or mucous membranes become stimulated, tightening and guarding of muscles occur.

For pain reception to occur the person must have an intact peripheral nervous system and spinal cord. Common factors that can disrupt pain reception in-

TABLE 37-1

Physical Sources of Pain

Source	Type of Stimulus	Pathophysiological Processes
Trauma	Mechanical, chemical	Tissue damage, inflammation, direct irritation of nerve endings
Ischemia	Chemical	Decreased blood flow to body part (i.e., blocked coronary artery)
Alteration in body fluids	Mechanical	Edema distending body tissues
Duct distention	Mechanical	Overstretching of duct's narrow lumen (i.e., passage of kidney stone through ureter)
Perforated visceral organ	Chemical	Chemical irritation of secretions on sensitive nerve endings (i.e., ruptured appendix or duodenal ulcer)
Space-occupying lesion (tumor)	Mechanical	Irritation of peripheral nerves by growth of lesion within a confined space
Burn (heat or extreme cold)	Thermal	Inflammation or loss of superficial layers of epidermis causing increased sensitivity of nerve endings.

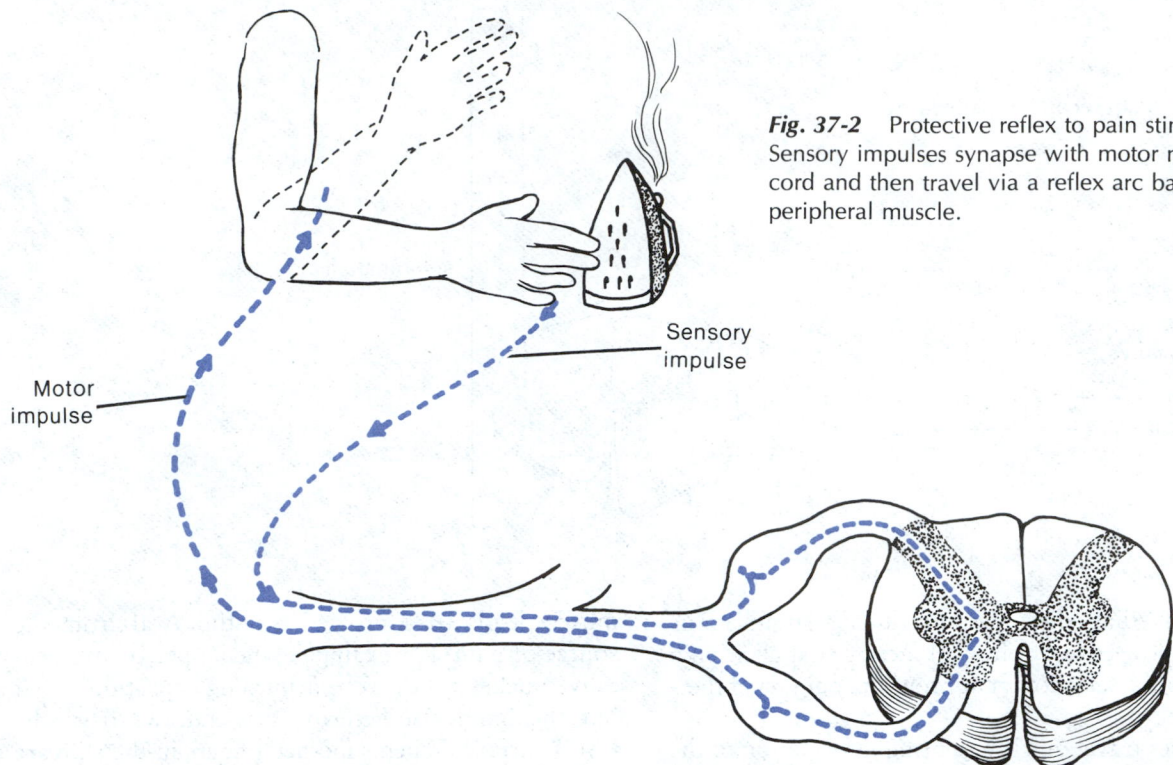

Fig. 37-2 Protective reflex to pain stimulus. Sensory impulses synapse with motor neurons in cord and then travel via a reflex arc back to a peripheral muscle.

Motor impulse

Sensory impulse

clude trauma, drugs, tumor growth, and metabolic disorders.

Perception

Perception involves the interpretation of the pain experience, beginning when a client first becomes aware of pain. Both physiological and psychological factors are involved in the client's pain perception.

PHYSIOLOGICAL FACTORS

Pain impulses traveling up the spinothalamic tract activate the reticular formation within the brainstem and the limbic system, which lies near the thalamus and hypothalamus. In addition, the impulses continue to travel to higher centers in the cerebral cortex. The interaction of reticular, limbic, and cortical centers provides perceptual information about the location, severity, and character of the pain stimulus. Activation of the reticular formation brings the pain experience to a person's conscious awareness. Reticular and limbic system activation creates a motivational drive to take some action as a result of the painful stimulus. The cerebral cortex controls higher levels of perceptual function, allowing a person to interpret the multitude of psychological factors comprising the pain experience.

Since perception requires a functional central nervous system, any factor that lowers consciousness lowers pain perception. Analgesics, anesthetics, and cerebral and spinal cord disease decrease a person's pain perception. In contrast, conditions that heighten a person's awareness or sensitivity to stimuli increase pain perception. Sensory restriction and sleep deprivation are common factors that increase the perception of pain. Clients frequently experience more pain during the night than during the day because the number of other incoming sensory stimuli decreases during the night.

Sleep deprivation lowers a person's adaptive capacity to all forms of stimuli, thus intensifying pain perception. The client who has undergone a rigorous schedule of diagnostic examinations that have interfered with normal sleep may react strongly even to the application of a blood pressure cuff.

GATE CONTROL THEORY. Literature on pain frequently refers to the Melzack-Wall (1965) gate control theory of pain perception. Although it continues to be a source of disagreement among neurophysiologists, it provides a simple model of pain perception. According to this theory the transmission of potentially painful impulses can be altered or blocked by a gating mechanism. The gate control theory assumes that peripheral pain fibers synapse in the gray matter of the dorsal horns of the spinal cord. The synapses are theorized to be gates that when closed block impulses from reaching the brain and when open allow

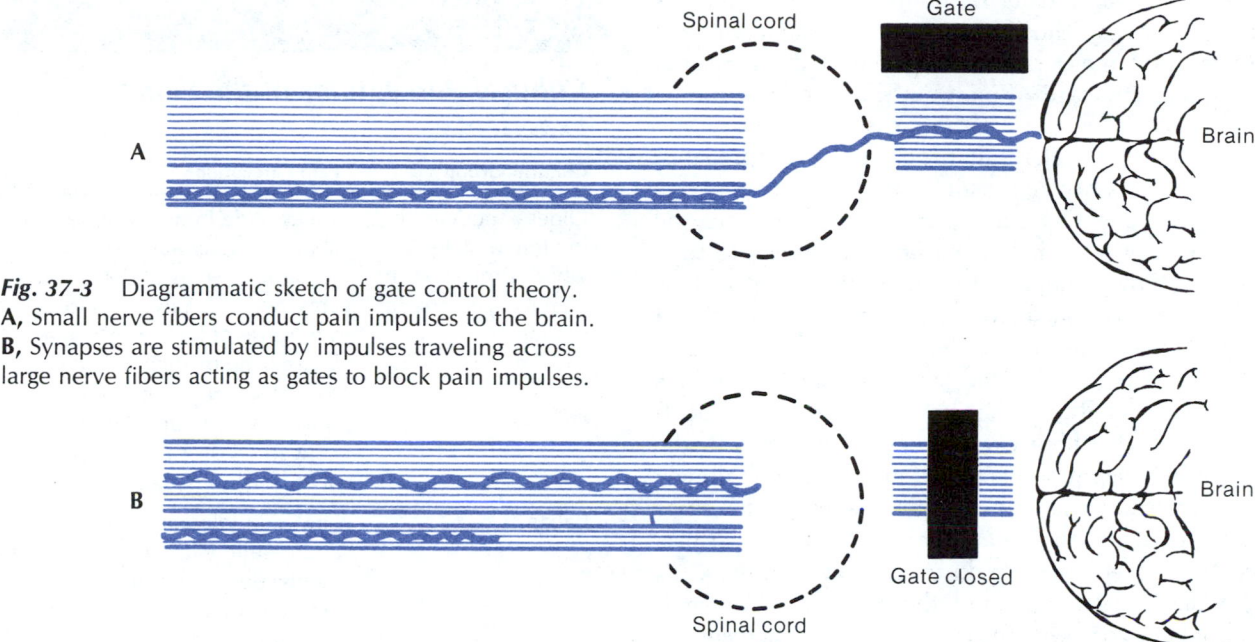

Fig. 37-3 Diagrammatic sketch of gate control theory. **A,** Small nerve fibers conduct pain impulses to the brain. **B,** Synapses are stimulated by impulses traveling across large nerve fibers acting as gates to block pain impulses.

impulses to ascend. Larger nerve fibers stimulated by heat, cold, and touch convey impulses through the same synapses as those through which pain impulses travel. Whether the gates open or close depends on whether competing messages from the larger nerve fibers stimulate the gates (Fig. 37-3). A bombardment of large-fiber sensory impulses such as those from the pressure of a backrub or the heat of a warm compress will close the synaptic gates to pain stimuli. It is now believed that gating mechanisms may also exist in the brainstem. The transmission of pain impulses from the spinal cord to the cerebral cortex can be inhibited or facilitated, thus altering pain perception. Although the gate control theory is still being developed, it offers nurses a conceptual basis for various pain relief measures.

ENDORPHINS. The discovery of endorphins offers further insight into pain perception. Endorphins are the body's natural supply of opiate-like substances. The hypothalamus, thalamus, pons, and limbic system are some of the sites that contain opiate receptors. It is believed that endorphins transmit, modify, and inhibit painful stimuli. People who have less pain than others from a similar injury generally have higher endorphin levels. Certain pain relief measures such as transcutaneous electrical nerve stimulation and acupuncture are believed to cause the release of endorphins. The effects of placebos may also be related to endorphin levels. Endorphins may also influence the psychological component of pain perception. Endorphin levels are higher in a person who feels euphoric or happy than in a depressed individual. Endorphins

may also reduce anxiety, since it has been found that opiate antagonists increase anxiety in healthy people. Greater understanding of how endorphins are formed and released will provide more insight into the mechanisms of pain relief.

PSYCHOLOGICAL FACTORS

For many years researchers believed that all people had the same capacity for perceiving pain. However, theories regarding a uniform pain threshold (the point at which a person first perceives a stimulus as painful) and a correlation between tissue damage and pain intensity have been abandoned and are not useful ways to understand pain. A person's pain threshold is a part of the sensory component of pain and is related primarily to physiological factors; however, psychosocial influences can affect the willingness of a person to perceive or label even mild sensory stimuli as painful.

Not all individuals perceive pain in the same manner. The higher centers of the central nervous system work collectively to perceive the onset of pain, determine its nature, and identify the significance or meaning of the pain. Perception is largely influenced by the cerebral cortex, the center for all thought processes. As a result, the pain experience is the product of a person's past experiences with pain, values, cultural expectations, and emotions, as well as the physical pain stimulus itself.

Each person learns from past painful experiences in an individual way. Previous experience does not necessarily mean a person will accept pain more easily in the future. If a person has had frequent episodes of pain without relief or bouts of severe pain, his perceptions are those of apprehension or even fear. In contrast, if a person has had repeated experiences with the same type of pain but the pain has successfully been relieved, it becomes easier to interpret the pain sensation. As a result, the client is better prepared to take necessary actions in relieving the pain.

When a client has had no experience with pain, the first perception of pain can impair his ability to cope with it. For example, after abdominal surgery it is common for a client to experience severe incisional pain for several days. Unless the client is aware of this, he may perceive the onset of pain as a serious complication. Rather than participate actively in postoperative breathing exercises (see Chapter 48), the client may lie immobile in bed and breathe shallowly in fear that something has gone wrong. The nurse should attempt to prepare the client with a clear perception of what he can do to minimize the pain.

Values about pain and the manner in which it should be expressed are also a part of pain perception. If the client views pain as a personal weakness or a deserved punishment, he may refrain from expressing any discomfort. If the client perceives pain as unwarranted or as a threat to his comfort and existence, the individual is less hesitant to express pain. If a person values the support of significant others, he is likely to perceive the need to express pain more openly.

People learn cultural expectations regarding the meaning and significance of pain. Children learn that certain behavioral responses are either rewarded or punished. For example, a child who cries because of a fall or injury may be held and comforted, ignored, or even reprimanded. Adults have acquired firmly established perceptions about pain and the reactions to it (see next section). Table 37-2 summarizes common pain perceptions of specific ethnic populations studied by Zborowski (1952). Although culture has a dominant influence on pain expectancy and acceptance, such information should never be generalized to all members of a cultural group. It is too easy to stereotype how a person might react to pain, thus prohibiting a nurse's objective assessment. In addition, cultural perceptions have likely changed over the decades since this study in 1952. However, this information can give the nurse an idea of the importance of recognizing a client's cultural orientation to pain.

A person's emotions play an influential role in pain perception. If an individual feels happy and contented and is actively involved in activities, there is little time to attend to sources of minor or even moderate discomfort. However, once a person becomes depressed, lonely, angry, or bored, there is more time to concentrate on pain and the perceptions are heightened.

TABLE 37-2

Cultural Perceptions of the Pain Experience

Cultural Group	Pain Perception
Older American (born in United States, white, Protestant, no identity with ethnic group)	Takes pride in not complaining about pain; avoids crying or screaming, signs of defeat; in presence of family, tries to retain sense of humor; may delay seeking medical advice; if pain is severe, withdraws and isolates self; future oriented—concerned over pain but confident it will be treated
Italian	Low pain tolerance; may cry and gesture with body movements; does not complain to family but likes them around as a distraction; wants palliative relief immediately; present oriented—concerned primarily with the pain sensation and not the reason for the pain
Jewish	Low pain tolerance; gives dramatic accounts of pain; cries and moans to bring family around for sympathy; does not want to be alone; future oriented—concerned with cause of pain; seeks curative measures

Modified from Zborowski, M.: J. Soc. Issues **8**:16, 1952.

Anxiety has frequently been shown to increase a person's perception of pain. An emotionally healthy person is usually able to tolerate mild to moderate pain, and often even severe pain, more effectively than one whose emotions are less stable.

Reaction

Reaction to pain includes both physiological and behavioral responses in any combination. Even though there are overt physiological signs indicating the presence of pain, a person may behave as though the pain did not exist.

PHYSIOLOGICAL RESPONSES

As pain impulses ascend the spinal cord toward the brainstem and thalamus, the autonomic nervous system becomes stimulated as part of the stress response.

TABLE 37-3

Physiological Responses to Pain

Response	Cause or Effect
SYMPATHETIC STIMULATION*	
Dilation of bronchial tubes and increased respiratory rate	Provides greater O_2 intake
Increased heart rate	Provides greater O_2 transport
Peripheral vasoconstriction (pallor, elevation in blood pressure)	Elevates blood pressure with shift of blood supply from periphery and viscera to skeletal muscles and brain
Increased blood glucose	Provides additional energy
Diaphoresis	Controls body temperature during stress
Increased muscle tension	Prepares muscles for action
Dilation of pupils	Affords better vision
Decreased gastric motility	Frees energy for more immediate activity
PARASYMPATHETIC STIMULATION†	
Pallor	Blood supply shift away from periphery
Muscle tension	Result of fatigue
Decreased heart rate and blood pressure	Vagal stimulation
Rapid, irregular breathing	Body defenses begin to fail under prolonged stress of pain
Nausea and vomiting	Return of gastric function
Weakness or exhaustion	From expenditure of physical energy

*Pain of low to moderate intensity and superficial pain.
†Severe or deep pain.

Pain of low to moderate intensity and superficial pain elicit the "flight-or-fight" reaction of the general adaptation syndrome (see Chapter 5). Stimulation of the sympathetic branch of the autonomic nervous system results in the physiological responses summarized in Table 37-3. If the pain is unrelenting, severe, or deep, typically originating from involvement of the visceral organs (such as with a myocardial infarction and colic from gallbladder or renal stones), the par-

asympathetic nervous system goes into action. Sustained physiological responses to pain could cause serious harm to an individual. Except in cases of severe traumatic pain, which may send a person into shock, most individuals reach a level of adaptation in which physical signs return to normal. Thus a client in pain will not always exhibit physical signs throughout the period of discomfort.

BEHAVIORAL RESPONSES

Behavioral responses to pain can be quite varied. A person's tolerance to pain refers to the point at which the individual is unwilling to accept pain of a greater severity or duration. How well a person tolerates pain and the nature of his reaction depend on attitudes, motivational factors, values, and cultural expectations.

People learn to express their reactions by observing others. The experiences and attitudes of a person's family are important factors in determining how that person will react to a painful experience. For example, if a child's parents dread a visit to the dentist, it is likely the child will acquire the same apprehension. Because pain is often equated with disease or illness, the reactions of a given cultural or social group are often the result of their attitudes toward sickness and health.

Pain is a threat to a person's physical and psychological well-being. A client may be reluctant to express pain, considering it a sign of personal weakness. Often clients believe that being a "good patient" means to refrain from expressing pain to avoid inconveniencing the people around them. Another reason clients may not express pain is that maintaining self-control is important in their culture. The client with high pain tolerance is able to endure periods of severe pain without assistance. Often a nurse must coerce such a client to accept pain-relieving measures so his activity or nutritional intake is not seriously curtailed. To maintain a positive self-image, this client minimizes his responses to pain. Fatigue lessens the extent to which the client reacts to painful stimuli, and the client may simply run out of energy and fall asleep even though the pain still exists.

In contrast, a client with low pain tolerance may seek relief before the pain occurs. For example, a client may request an aspirin in anticipation of a headache. The client's ability to tolerate pain significantly influences the nurse's perceptions of how serious the discomfort is. Often the nurse is more than willing to attend to the client whose pain tolerance is high. Yet it is unfair to discount or ignore the needs of the client who is unable to tolerate even minor pain.

Typical body movements and facial expressions that indicate pain include clenched teeth, holding the

TABLE 37-4

Types of Pain

Type	Definition	Characteristics	Examples
Superficial or cutaneous	Pain resulting from stimulation of the skin	Short duration, localized; usually a sharp sensation	Needle stick; small cut or laceration
Deep visceral	Pain resulting from stimulation of internal organs	Diffuse, may radiate in several directions; duration varies but usually lasts longer than superficial pain; pain may be sharp, dull, or unique to organ involved	Crushing sensation (e.g., angina pectoris); burning sensation (e.g., gastric ulcer)
Referred	Common phenomenon in visceral pain, since many of the organs themselves have no pain receptors; however, sensory neurons from the affected organ enter the same spinal cord segment as neurons from areas where the pain is felt; the brain perceives pain in unaffected areas	Pain is felt in a part of the body separate from the source of pain and may assume any characteristic	A myocardial infarction may cause referred pain to the jaw, left arm, and left shoulder; kidney stones may refer pain to the groin area
Radiating	A sensation of pain extending from the initial site of injury to another body part	Pain feels as though it travels down or along a body part; may be intermittent or constant	Low back pain from a ruptured intravertebral disc accompanied by pain radiating down the leg from sciatic nerve irritation
Phantom limb	Abnormal sensation or feeling as though an amputated body part still remains; may be psychogenic or the result of stimuli from nerves located above amputation site	Pain continues long after stump heals; burning, sharp pain is common immediately after amputation; the amputated part may feel as though it is elevated above the bed while the client is lying down	Amputated limb

painful part, bent posture, facial grimacing, and tensing of abdominal muscles. A client may respond more expressively by crying or moaning. Often the client is attempting to express discomfort through frequent requests to the nurse. The nurse soon learns to recognize different patterns of behavior that reflect pain. However, the lack of pain expression does not necessarily mean that the client is not experiencing pain. Unless a client openly reacts to pain, it is extremely difficult for the nurse to determine the nature and extent of the discomfort. A major role of the nurse is helping the client communicate his pain response more effectively. Knowledge of the disease or illness helps the nurse anticipate the type of pain the client will endure. For example, a ruptured intravertebral disc in a lower lumbar vertebra typically causes severe low back pain in addition to pain that radiates or extends down the leg. The pain of menstrual cramping is characterized by lower abdominal and low back discomfort. Table 37-4 summarizes some common types of pain.

■ ■ ■ ■ ■

Pain is a complex series of physical and psychological responses. The receptive, perceptive, and reactive components of the pain experience interact to produce the various reactions of a person in pain (Fig. 37-4). The nurse's aim in providing pain relief is to control or eliminate any one of the three components. Knowledge of the factors influencing each component provides the nurse with a means of finding creative pain relief measures.

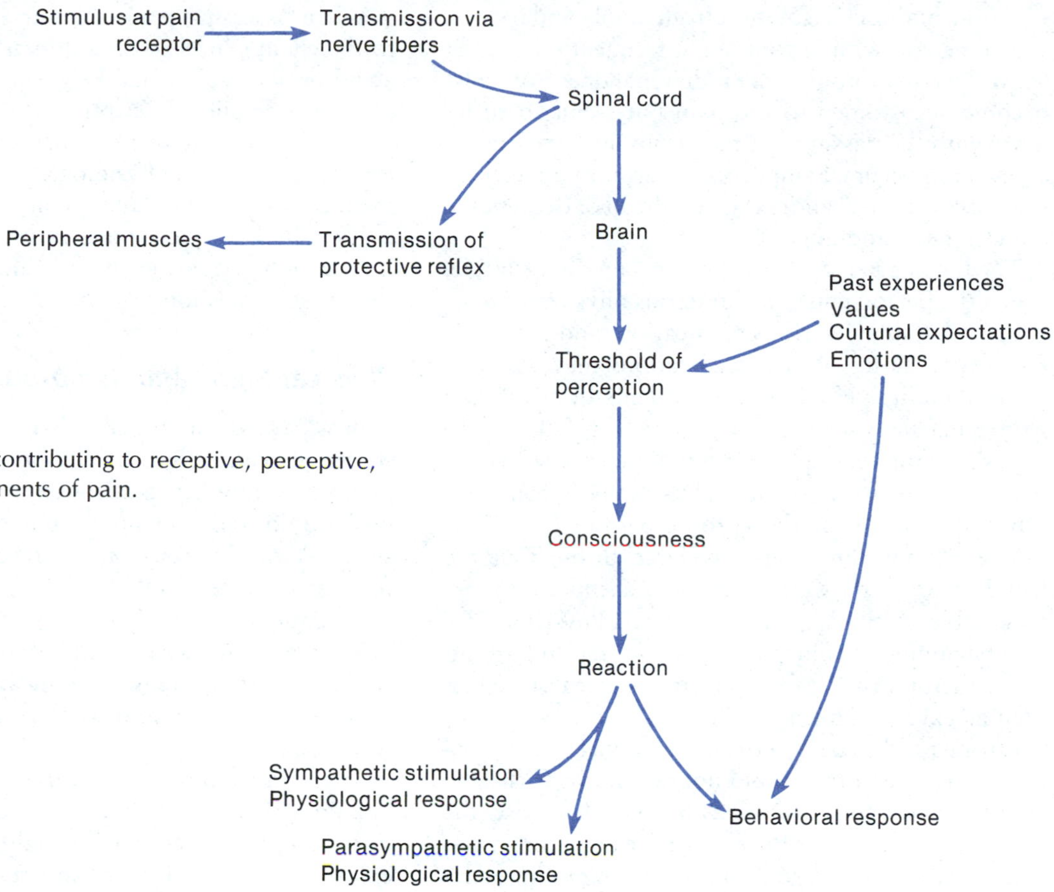

Fig. 37-4 Factors contributing to receptive, perceptive, and reactive components of pain.

Acute and Chronic Pain

The pain experience varies according to the length of time it lasts. Whether pain is acute or chronic influences an individual's behavior and manner of coping with the pain experience. The ability of a client to be receptive to the nurse's care depends on whether pain is of short or long duration.

Acute pain is of brief duration, and the end is expected. The onset is immediate, and the pain may subside with or without treatment. The pain is a new experience, often frightening, and typically individuals show overt behavioral responses.

The client in acute pain has expectations that complete relief will come soon. Conflict may arise between nurse and client if the nurse is unable to provide quick pain relief. Since acute pain is self-limiting, the nurse may fall into the trap of thinking the client will soon get over the discomfort. The nurse with such an attitude may be less inclined to pursue a variety of pain relief measures.

Acute pain is a potentially serious threat to a client's recovery and thus should be one of the nurse's priorities of care. For example, acute postoperative pain hampers the client's ability to become active and increases the risks of complications from immobility (see Chapter 47). A client cannot progress physically or psychologically as long as acute pain persists, for it causes the client to focus all of his interest on pain relief. The nurse's efforts at teaching and motivating the client toward self-care will be fruitless unless pain is eliminated or controlled. Once pain is relieved, the client and health care team can direct full attention toward activities that promote recovery rather than remedies to relieve pain and its consequences.

Chronic pain lasts a prolonged period of time, and many persons never gain complete relief. It may begin as acute pain or as gradually increasing discomfort. The client with chronic pain often experiences periods of remissions (partial or complete disappearance of symptoms) and exacerbations (increase in severity of signs or symptoms). The unpredictability of chronic pain causes frustration in the client, frequently leading to psychological depression. The pain becomes part of every aspect of the individual's life. Chronic pain is a major cause of psychological and physical disability leading to problems such as loss of job, divorce, inability to perform simple daily activities, sexual dysfunction, and social isolation from family and friends.

The person with chronic pain frequently does not show overt symptoms. The individual does not really become accustomed to the pain but seems to suffer more with the passing of time as physical and mental exhaustion occurs. Symptoms of chronic pain include fatigue, insomnia, anorexia, weight loss, depression, hopelessness, and anger.

The life of a person with chronic pain can be tragic. Often the person consults numerous physicians in order to accumulate various medications and therapies. However, taking several medications may result in many undesirable side effects. Clients desperate for pain relief may seize on any hope and fall prey to quackery, for example, special liniments, diets, or pain-relief devices. Alcohol abuse may become another alternative for the chronic pain sufferer. Fortunately, pain clinics are available throughout the United States and Canada to help clients find more acceptable methods of pain control. Physicians are also beginning to understand pain better and are offering therapies other than pharmacological remedies, such as exercise and biofeedback.

Caring for the client with chronic pain is an unusual challenge. The nurse should not become as frustrated as the client when relief measures fail. Likewise, the nurse should not offer the client false hope for a cure. The nurse's primary goal may be to minimize or reduce the client's perception of pain. Providing physical therapy to strengthen weakened muscles, offering a pleasing and attractive meal, and encouraging the expression of feelings are some activities that will help decrease the client's preoccupation with pain. Later sections discuss other types of intervention.

Assessment of the Client's Pain

The key to assessing pain is knowing not to ignore the client. The nurse should believe what the client says and explore the pain experience thoroughly with him. Pain is a real experience, and nurses cannot allow personal biases to prejudice the assessment of pain. Viewing the pain from the client's perspective will enable the nurse to gain a more accurate assessment.

Even though it is difficult to assess pain objectively because it has so many subjective elements, pain has certain basic characteristics that the nurse can measure objectively. The client's pain history offers a wealth of information about the typical course of an episode of pain. The nurse also learns what factors commonly aggravate or relieve the client's discomfort. Awareness of the influence pain has on the client's normal life-style allows the nurse to identify practical approaches for pain relief.

When assessing pain, the nurse must be sensitive to the client's level of discomfort. If a client's pain is acute or severe, it is unlikely that he will be able to provide a detailed description of the pain experience. During an episode of acute pain the nurse primarily assesses the client's physiological responses as well as the location, severity, and quality of the pain. A thorough pain assessment takes time and should be conducted only when the client is alert and attentive to the nurse's questions.

Physical Signs and Symptoms

Basic to assessing a client's pain response is measurement of the signs of autonomic nervous system involvement. When a client expresses discomfort or his behavior reflects pain, the nurse should assess vital signs. With the early onset of pain the heart rate, respiratory rate, and blood pressure increase. The nurse compares vital sign values with the client's baseline measurements recorded before the onset of pain. A change in vital signs is significant. There is no prescribed level or extent of change that signifies a pain response.

The nurse should not confuse signs and symptoms of pain with other behavioral or pathological changes. For example, a client who is highly anxious will also exhibit an elevated heart and respiratory rate; one who is seriously dehydrated has an increased pulse because of volume depletion. The nurse takes into account all of the client's signs and symptoms before determining that pain is the cause.

It is helpful to determine which clients are at greater risk for having pain. The client's health status indicates whether pain is an anticipated symptom. The postoperative client, the person with incurable cancer, and the victim of serious trauma are just three examples of clients who will probably experience severe pain.

If a client's pain continues unrelieved, the nurse looks for signs of physical exhaustion. Decreasing vital sign values indicate parasympathetic nerve response. The client becomes less responsive to stimuli within the environment. The nurse should measure vital signs more frequently if the client's condition deteriorates.

Client's Subjective Report

Some characteristics of pain can be detailed only by the client. The nurse assesses the location, severity, and quality of the pain with techniques designed to minimize the subjectivity of the client's descriptions.

LOCATION

The first step in assessing pain involves asking the client to identify its location. Generally, superficial pain is easier to locate than deep or visceral pain. Pain may be localized, diffuse, referred, or radiating. To localize the pain, the nurse asks the client to trace the area from the most severe point outward. This may be difficult to do if pain is diffuse, involving large segments of the body. The nurse should be patient as the client attempts to localize the pain and be sure of the final location chosen. The determination of the location of pain will affect the methods of diagnosis and treatment. It would be unfortunate for the client to have an x-ray study made of the abdomen, only to learn that the pain was actually in the chest.

Knowing the underlying disease or illness assists the nurse in locating the pain. Pancreatitis, for example, causes widespread abdominal pain, whereas an inflamed gallbladder causes localized right-sided subcostal pain radiating to the right shoulder. The nurse may not always be aware of the client's diagnosis; however, knowing where certain types of pain typically originate helps the nurse to understand the client's description and provides guidelines for further assessment.

When describing pain location, the nurse should use anatomical landmarks and descriptive terminology. The statement, "The pain is localized in the upper right quadrant of the abdomen" is more specific than "The client states the pain is located in his abdomen." The following is an example of a nurse's note describing a client's pain:

The client has a sharp, "knifelike" pain on the radial side of his right wrist. The pain radiates along the right thumb and to the palmar surface of the hand. The pain began immediately when the client attempted to stop a fall from a ladder with his right hand. The pain has increased in severity since the fall, approximately 1 hour ago. The client describes the pain as "the worst I've ever had." There are redness, bruising, and swelling of the right wrist and thumb. The pain is aggravated by flexion and rotation of the wrist. The client applied an ice pack to the wrist with little relief.

When speaking with children, the nurse uses words they can understand (such as "tummy") as they locate the pain. Parents can often be helpful in assisting their children to describe pain.

SEVERITY

Perhaps the most subjective characteristic of pain is its severity or intensity. Certain types of pain are obviously more severe than others. For example, the pain of a ruptured appendix is more severe than that of a mild sunburn. The client's perceptions greatly influence the reported severity of pain.

Numerical

0	1	2	3	4	5	6	7	8	9	10

No pain   Severe pain

Descriptive

No pain	Mild pain	Moderate pain	Severe pain	Unbearable pain

Visual analog

No pain   Unbearable pain

Client designates a point on the scale that corresponds to his perception of the pain's severity at the time of assessment.

Fig. 37-5 Sample descriptive pain scales.

Descriptive scales are one of the most objective means of measuring pain severity (Fig. 37-5). A numerical scale consists of a line divided by numbered points, which indicate various pain intensities. A descriptive scale follows the same principle except that the points are described by increasing levels of severity. A visual analog scale does not have labeled subdivisions. Only the ends of the scale are labeled, giving the client total freedom in identifying the severity of pain. A pain scale should be designed so that it is easy for the nurse to administer and is not time consuming for the client to complete. If the client can easily understand the scale, his description of pain severity should be more accurate.

Descriptive scales are useful not only in determining the severity of pain but also in assessing changes in the client's condition. The nurse can use the scales after therapy or when symptoms become aggravated to judge whether pain has decreased or increased in severity. The pain scales are therefore useful in evaluation as well as assessment.

The nurse should not use pain scales to compare one client with another. Although the scales lend relative objectivity to measurement, the severity of pain is too subjective to permit comparisons between individuals.

A less objective means of assessing pain severity involves having the client describe pain as mild, moderate, severe, or unbearable. The problem with such questioning is the meaning these terms actually have for the client and the nurse. The nurse gains clearer understanding of the client's pain by using a graded assessment scale.

QUALITY

Another subjective characteristic of pain is its quality. Because there is no common or specific pain vocabulary in general usage, the words a client may choose to describe pain can apply to any number of things. Frequently, a client describes pain as "crushing," "throbbing," "sharp," "dull," or "burning."

When assessing the quality of a client's pain, the nurse should not provide descriptions for the client. For example, the nurse should not ask, "Is your pain throbbing?" The client may simply find it convenient to answer yes, even though the pain feels quite different. To gain a more accurate description, the nurse uses direct or open-ended questions (see Chapter 15) so the client is free to choose his own descriptions. The nurse might say, "Tell me what your pain feels like," or "Describe your pain for me." Only when the client is unable to describe pain should the nurse offer to list various descriptive terms.

There is some consistency in the way people describe certain types of pain. The pain associated with a myocardial infarction is often described as crushing or viselike, whereas the pain of a surgical incision is often described as sharp and stabbing in quality. When the client's descriptions fit the pattern forming in the nurse's assessment, a clearer analysis can be made of the nature and type of pain.

Client's Pain History

Each pain experience follows a certain course. After repeated episodes the client can generally describe the history of the pain experience. If the assessment reveals a predictable pattern of symptoms and events, it will become easier for the nurse to develop an effective treatment plan.

TIME AND DURATION

The nurse asks questions to determine the pattern of onset, periodicity, and duration of pain. When did the client's pain begin? Does it occur at the same time each day? How long does it last with each occurrence? When did the client last notice the pain? How frequently does it recur?

Episodes of sudden excruciating pain call for different nursing measures than a steady, unrelenting, dull discomfort. An understanding of the time cycle of a client's pain helps the nurse anticipate when to intervene. Certain types of pain are characterized by specific patterns of onset and duration. For example, labor pains become progressively more severe, more frequent, and of longer duration.

PRECIPITATING EVENTS AND AGGRAVATING FACTORS

It can be helpful to know if specific events or conditions precipitate pain. Likewise, the nurse must learn what factors aggravate or increase the severity of the client's pain. The client should be asked what he was doing when he first noticed the pain. Can he connect pain with any body function or activity? A change in body position is often a precipitating or aggravating event. Table 37-5 summarizes precipitating and aggravating factors commonly associated with specific sources of pain.

Once the nurse identifies precipitating or aggravating factors, it is easier to plan interventions to avoid exacerbating the pain. For example, if the client notices more pain between meals when his stomach is empty, the nurse can provide frequent small serv-

---

TABLE 37-5

Examples of Precipitating and Aggravating Factors Related to Specific Sources of Pain

Source of Pain	Precipitating/Aggravating Factors
Angina pectoris (insufficient blood flow through coronary arteries)	Physical exertion; emotional stress; exposure to cold temperature; eating large meal
Ruptured intravertebral disc	Bending over or stretching; lifting objects
Gastric ulcer	Tension; going to work; coffee or liquor ingestion
Urinary tract infection	Micturition (urinating)
Gallbladder inflammation	Eating foods high in fat content
Appendicitis	Sudden jarring or vibration of bed while lying down
Pharyngitis (sore throat)	Swallowing; talking
Peripheral vascular disease (insufficient blood flow to extremities)	Exercise (walking or running)
External otitis (inflammation of outer ear canal)	Rubbing or scratching ear canal; excessive drying of skin
Pleuritis	Inhaling deeply and coughing

ings of food. If bending over worsens the client's back pain, the nurse instructs him to bend his knees when picking up objects from the floor.

RELIEVING FACTORS

It is important to learn whether the client has discovered an effective method for relieving the pain. Position change, a heating pad, an ice bag, eating, rest, and analgesics are among the ways the client may relieve pain. What works best for the client will often work best for the nurse. The client gains a sense of comfort from knowing the nurse is willing to try his relief measures. If the client takes analgesics, the nurse should find out the type of medication, the dosage, and the frequency. If the client uses heat or cold applications, the nurse makes sure it is done in a way that avoids injury to the skin (see Chapter 48). While assessing relieving factors, the nurse may also ask the client if only a physician has been consulted for pain, or if the services of other practitioners (such as chiropractors, naturopaths, yoga instructors, or acupuncturists) have been sought. The client with chronic pain is more likely to have tried alternative health care modes.

CONCOMITANT SYMPTOMS

Acute pain is often accompanied by sudden changes in vital signs, as described earlier. It is imperative, however, not to overlook the possibility that some other underlying disorder is responsible for vital sign changes. The concomitant symptoms may become as much a priority as the pain itself. The nurse may have to treat pain, a fall in blood pressure, and an irregular heart beat all at once.

Pain frequently triggers other symptoms such as nausea, dizziness, and restlessness. Some types of pain have predictable concomitant symptoms; superficial pain is often accompanied by local areas of heat, redness, and swelling, and the pain of blocked arterial blood flow to an extremity results in color changes such as cyanosis and diminished or absent arterial pulses.

PAST EXPERIENCES

When the client describes the problem of his pain, it is valuable for the nurse to know the client's previous experiences. A pain history can reveal whether the discomfort is a long-term, chronic problem. If the client has experienced acute episodes in the past, he should be asked what can he recall of the events. The nurse can plan therapies to prevent the recurrence of unpleasant pain experiences. For example, if the client has previously undergone surgery and experienced severe pain afterward, the nurse can help the client anticipate and understand postoperative pain. By

teaching the ways of relieving pain through non-pharmacological measures, the nurse can help the client cope better with the next surgical experience.

Effects of Pain on the Client

Pain is a stressful event that has the potential for altering the client's life-style and psychological well-being. The nurse attempts to learn the extent to which pain has altered the client's life. The nurse's assessment of the effects of pain will offer guidelines to assist the client in adjusting to change.

INFLUENCE ON ACTIVITIES OF DAILY LIVING

Clients who live with pain daily experience changes in their ability to participate in routine activities. An assessment of these changes reveals to the nurse the extent of the client's disability and the adjustments that will be necessary to help the client participate in self-care.

The nurse asks the client if pain interferes with sleep. Does he have difficulty falling asleep? Are sleeping pills or other medications needed to induce sleep? Does the pain awaken him during the night? The client may have become an insomniac as a result of the pain. The nurse attempts to introduce principles of good sleep hygiene (see Chapter 36) and initiates pain relief measures to promote a more normal sleep pattern.

Depending on the location of pain the client may have difficulty performing normal hygiene measures. Can the client dress independently? Is the client able to shampoo his hair? Does the pain restrict mobility to the point that the client is no longer able to bathe in a bathtub? A client with severe arthritis, for example, may find it painful to grasp eating utensils. The nurse can determine from the assessment the client's need for self-help devices such as Velcro strips to replace buttons on clothing, enlarged utensil handles to facilitate grasping, or safety bars to protect the client while bathing. The nurse also considers the need for family members or friends to assist the client with basic hygiene measures.

Pain can seriously impair a client's ability to maintain normal sexual relations. Conditions such as arthritis, degenerative diseases of the hip, and chronic back pain make it difficult for a person to assume the usual positions during sexual intercourse. When assessing the extent to which pain has affected sexual activity, the nurse determines the frequency of sexual relations before and after the onset of pain. It is also helpful to learn if a client is physically unable to participate or if the desire for sexual intercourse has been lost.

The ability of a person to engage in normal work

activities can be seriously threatened by pain. The more physical activity required in a job, the greater the risk of discomfort when the pain is associated with musculoskeletal and certain visceral alterations. Pain related to emotional stress will likely be increased in the individual whose job involves tension-laden decision making. The nurse assesses the type of work the client does, as well as his ability to function in a regular job. The daily chores of the homemaker are assessed in the same manner as a full-time job outside the home. The nurse determines if it is necessary for the client to stop all activity occasionally because of the pain. Often the nurse can help the client to select ways of minimizing or controlling the pain so he can remain productive in a regular job.

It is also important to include an assessment of how pain affects the client's normal social activities. The pain may be so debilitating that the client becomes too exhausted to socialize. If the pain threatens the client's self-concept, he may no longer feel comfortable interacting with friends. The nurse identifies the client's normal social activities, the extent to which the activities have been disrupted, and whether the client wishes to participate.

PSYCHOSOCIAL EFFECTS

A client's perception of pain, molded by psychological and social variables, is a significant part of the pain experience. The nurse cannot fully understand the client's pain without knowing his values, past experiences, and emotional responses to pain. A client's perceptions of body image, role within the family, level of family acceptance, and the threat of pain disrupting personal goals must all be considered in assessment.

The best time to assess psychosocial factors is when the client is not suffering severe pain. The client spends a considerable amount of energy during an episode of severe pain and at such times will be less willing to respond to questions that explore his true feelings and emotions. The nurse should select a time when the client acknowledges relief. The client should know that the nurse's goal is a full understanding of his perceptions of pain. Conveying a sense of caring to the client may be the most important thing a professional nurse does.

Client's Coping Resources

The experience of having pain can be a lonely one. The pain may be severe enough to cause partial or total disability. Clients often find a variety of ways to cope with the physical and psychological effects of pain. The nurse's pain assessment includes the identification of the client's coping resources. These resources can be incorporated into the nurse's plan of care to provide support to the client and to afford a degree of pain relief.

Coping resources are more than just methods or techniques that relieve pain. A client may depend on the emotional support of a spouse, children, other family members, or friends. Although the client will still experience pain, the presence of a loved one can minimize the associated loneliness and fear. A client's religious beliefs can also provide a source of comfort. Reading scriptures or saying a prayer in quiet gives many individuals an inner strength to cope more effectively with their discomfort. Being actively involved in household chores or activities at work can be another mechanism for coping with pain.

The nurse asks the client what factors help in accepting or adjusting to the pain experience. Having the client describe what he typically does during an episode of pain may reveal the presence or absence of coping resources.

Nonverbal Responses to Pain

Throughout the assessment the nurse should closely observe the client's nonverbal behaviors. Subtle facial expressions or body movements often reveal more about the character of pain than precise questioning. Does the client grimace or begin to toss or turn at regular intervals? Does the amount of body movement increase as the assessment progresses? Does the client react more uncomfortably as he assumes different positions?

Nonverbal cues may be the only indicators of pain for clients who are unable to describe their discomfort. The infant, the unconscious client, the disoriented or confused person, the aphasic, and the client who speaks a foreign language are unable to clearly explain the character or meaning of pain.

Certain types of nonverbal expressions characterize sources of pain. The client with chest pain often grabs or holds the chest. A child or adult with severe abdominal pain often assumes a fetal position. A client experiencing a severe headache may squint or rub the temples.

The client's nonverbal expression of pain may support or contradict data previously collected by the nurse. If a young woman in labor reports that her labor pains are occurring more frequently and if she begins to massage her abdomen with greater regularity, the client's report is confirmed. If a client complains of severe abdominal pain but continues to grasp his chest, a more detailed assessment may be necessary.

Nursing Diagnosis

The nurse often has a wealth of data to use in determining the extent of the client's problem. However, once the final analysis has been made, the nurse is specific in diagnosing the client's pain. Some typical diagnoses that focus on the nature of the client's pain are "alteration in comfort related to incisional pain," "alteration in comfort related to chronic back pain," and "alteration in comfort related to recurrent chest pain."

Focusing on the specific nature of the pain helps the nurse identify the types of interventions most useful for a specific source of pain. Teaching a client back exercises will help to alleviate low back pain but will do little for the pain of an abdominal incision. Splinting an incision and frequent repositioning of the client will effectively lessen the pain from an incision but will not alleviate a client's chest pain.

The nursing diagnosis may also serve to summarize the effects of pain on a client. Assessment of the influence pain has on a client's life-style might result in such diagnoses as "impaired mobility related to right hip pain," "alterations in self-care related to bilateral hand pain," and "alterations in self-image related to chronic pain."

In these examples the diagnoses provide the nurse with guidelines for intervening in problems created by pain. The nurse may provide other therapies beyond those aimed toward pain relief. For example, the client who is unable to perform self-care measures because of the disabling effects of pain may benefit from pain relief therapies, but the nurse will also provide the client with alternative methods for performing self-care. Suggestions for rearranging bathing facilities, teaching the client dressing techniques, or providing utensils the client can more easily manipulate are ways of improving a client's ability to perform self-care without directly relieving the client's pain. The nurse's assessment will indicate the extent to which the effects of the client's pain can be minimized.

The nursing diagnosis may also focus on a component of the pain experience—perception. Increased pain perception is related to environmental isolation, anxiety, fatigue, and fear. When the client's pain perception is heightened, the nurse directs care toward reducing pain perception or minimizing pain reception and reaction. For example, a bedridden client's fatigue from the pain of a fractured leg can cause the pain to be perceived as severe. In addition, the client is more aware of other sources of discomfort. The nurse will attempt to preserve and increase the client's level of energy so the client has the ability to attend to stimuli other than the pain. In addition, the nurse will eliminate sources of discomfort while the client lies in bed so pain reception is minimal.

When diagnosing the client's pain, the nurse should consider all factors contributing to the pain experience. A diagnosis should be descriptive of a specific problem and useful in directing the nurse toward appropriate interventions. Table 37-6 lists examples of nursing diagnoses for several types of pain. The characteristics of each type of pain have implications for the nurse in identifying treatment measures.

Plan of Care

Whatever the related source of the client's pain, the nurse's goals are to (1) promote a sense of comfort and well-being; (2) maintain existing physical, emotional, and mental functioning; and (3) improve the client's understanding of the pain experience.

Together the nurse and client set realistic expectations for the type and degree of pain relief desired. A therapy that works for one client will not work for all. It is important for the client to understand that complete pain relief cannot always be guaranteed, but that it will be attempted. A knowledgeable and honest analysis of the client's problem gives the client confidence in the nurse's ability to provide pain relief.

Before implementing any pain relief measures the nurse includes two important elements in the care plan: ensuring that a therapeutic relationship is established with the client and educating the client about pain. Both elements are critical to the success of any intervention.

Therapeutic Relationship

The client in pain is highly vulnerable and is at the mercy of anyone who may attempt halfheartedly to "make him feel better." The client is not always convinced that someone is concerned with his welfare. The client in pain needs someone to trust. If the nurse is unable to establish a therapeutic relationship with the client, any resultant mistrust can heighten the client's awareness of pain. Unless the client has a means to express his concerns or fears about pain, the reaction to the pain experience may become inappropriate. Often a client will become angry, orally abuse the nurse, or complain about the nurse's care when his needs for pain relief are ignored.

The nurse can best help by seeing the client as a total person and conveying a sense of caring. Giving careful attention to the client's concerns during the assessment is one way of building the client's confi-

TABLE 37-6

Examples of Pain Diagnoses

Diagnosis	Pain Sources	Type of Pain	Subjective Characteristics	Historical Factors	Effects on Client
Alteration in comfort related to low back pain	Injury to back: ruptured intravertebral disc	Deep, localized, radiating	Sharp, localized pain in lumbosacral area; sharp radiating pain along sciatic nerve (compression on sciatic nerve); numbness and tingling of leg (compression of spinal cord)	Aggravated by bending or twisting at trunk, lifting heavy objects, sitting, climbing stairs, and coughing; pain minimized by using proper body mechanics during ambulation and sitting, lying supine on a flat firm mattress, applying heat to lumbosacral area, and strengthening back muscles	May interfere with client's ability to perform work depending on amount of physical activity required; often cause of chronic pain, resulting in depression, fatigue, insomnia
Alteration in comfort related to anginal chest pain	Narrowing of coronary arteries, reducing efficiency of oxygen delivery to myocardium when heart's demands for oxygen increases	Deep, visceral	Crushing, stabbing sensation to chest, left shoulder, and frequently left arm	Attack precipitated by exercise or increased physical activity, emotional stress, exposure to cold environment, or after eating heavy meal; relieved by immediately stopping all physical activity, assuming a comfortable position in a quiet, nonstressful environment, avoiding cold temperatures	Depending on severity of angina client may be unable to perform any type of physical activity (walking, climbing stairs, performing household chores); social activities affected since client is often unable to walk distances; client often fearful of having "heart attack"
Alteration in comfort related to terminal cancer	Invasion of cancerous tumor to the bone, pelvic, and abdominal structures	Deep, visceral; may be referred or radiating depending on extent of tumor involvement	Often throbbing, burning, knifelike, and excruciating; pain usually continuous with only partial relief and ranges from severe to moderate; localized or diffuse depending on extent of tumor	Pain progressively increasing in intensity; location of tumor influences aggravating factors (e.g., bone pain increased by movement, abdominal pain influenced by eating, deep breathing, and movement); pain relieved by altering perceptions (e.g., distraction, maintaining independence, and relaxation techniques); concomitant symptoms associated with area of involvement (e.g., abdominal tumors cause nausea, vomiting, altered bowel habits)	Constant pain; client depressed, hopeless, often angry; chronic use of analgesics can distort perceptions and alter level of consciousness; only concerned about present and forgets future goals; often isolates self from others if pain does not lessen in severity

TABLE 37-6, cont'd

Examples of Pain Diagnoses

Diagnosis	Pain Sources	Type of Pain	Subjective Characteristics	Historical Factors	Effects on Client
Alteration in comfort related to sunburn	Overexposure of skin to sun's rays	Superficial	Burning or irritating sensation; pain felt only in exposed areas	Pain usually most severe in first 24 hours after exposure; duration depends on extent of burn; skin overly sensitive to tactile stimuli and exposure to heat; relieved by tepid sponging and topically applied sprays and creams containing anesthetics	Has minimal effect on activities of daily living; bathing in a hot shower or tub can increase pain intensity
Alteration in comfort related to rheumatoid arthritis	Inflammation of synovial membrane lining joints; joint becomes stiff, tender, and often immobile	Cutaneous or deep, depending on joints affected	Localized tenderness commonly in joints of the hands, knees, elbows, shoulders, and hips; pain can be severe and immobilizing	Aggravated by movement of affected joint, anxiety, stress, and fatigue; prolonged inactivity worsens joint stiffness and pain; relieved by rest, muscle strengthening exercises, and locally applied heat; other associated symptoms include swelling and localized warmth; range of joint motion may be reduced	Activities of daily living can be seriously impaired; when hands are involved, client may have difficulty grasping or manipulating objects; involvement of weight-bearing joints (e.g., knees) limits mobility; with advanced disease permanent physical deformity develops; involvement of knees and hips makes sexual intercourse difficult

dence in the nurse. Promptness in attending to the client's needs further establishes a strong therapeutic relationship. Clients can easily sense when the nurse does not genuinely care about them. Making judgments about the validity of the client's pain, bartering pain relief in return for "good" client behavior, and controlling sources of pain relief are behaviors that will destroy the client's trust in the nurse.

A successful nurse-client relationship depends in part on the nurse's ability to respect the client's response to pain. Many nurses value firm self-control. However, a client may need to cry, moan, or even become angry. Whatever the client's response, he should not feel ashamed or fearful that the nurse will not be accepting.

Ideally, the relationship between nurse and client is a collaborative one. The nurse is willing to recognize that the client knows something the nurse does not about his pain and its relief. If the client suffers chronic pain, it is essential that he assume responsibility for the therapy.

Education

A client is better prepared to handle almost any situation when he understands it. The experience of pain is no exception. Teaching a client about the pain experience reduces anxiety and helps the client achieve a sense of control. For example, a client may be entering a clinic or hospital the first time for the purpose of undergoing diagnostic tests. If the client knows there are to be tests but does not understand them, he begins to fantasize about the experience. The client's fears are enhanced if friends have had unpleasant experiences in similar circumstances. Fear increases the client's perception of painful stimuli. Teaching the client about pain and its relief will eliminate the fantasies and allow the client to focus on activities that help control the pain. Preparing a client for a painful experience eliminates any sudden surprises that make the client feel victimized.

Pain is predictable after surgery, during invasive procedures, and during certain illnesses. The nurse discusses with the client the occurrence of the pain, its onset and duration, the location and quality, causative factors, and steps the client and nurse can take for pain relief. The more the client knows, the better he can prepare for the painful experience. It has been demonstrated repeatedly that clients who are prepared preoperatively for postoperative pain (see Chapter 47) recover more quickly than those who receive no teaching.

A clinic nurse might explain about a blood specimen collection to a client in this way:

Mr. Tillis, you will have three blood specimens drawn, but it only takes one needle stick to get the blood we need. First, you will have a thin rubber tubing, which is called a tourniquet, tied around your upper arm. This helps to keep your veins filled. Then I will wipe off your arm with some alcohol that might feel cool. You will feel a sharp burning sensation as the needle enters the skin. Once it is in, the burning will be much less. As I collect your blood, your arm may begin to feel numb or tingling, but that's normal as long as the tourniquet is on. It only takes about a minute to get the blood, and then I will take off the tourniquet and remove the needle.

Ideally the nurse teaches the client early about any impending painful experiences. This allows the client an opportunity to consider the situation, ask questions, and make decisions. However, for some clients early forewarning of pain can be a problem. The highly anxious or fearful client is often irrational and unable to learn from the nurse's explanations. Such clients tend to fantasize horrible events if they receive information too early about painful procedures. If a client seems unlikely to benefit from advance preparation, it is best to explain invasive procedures a short time before they occur. It is not always easy to know whether a client can accept an impending unpleasant experience. If a client is typically anxious or if previous teaching has not relieved anxiety, the nurse must use judgment in knowing when to tell the client.

Relevant play is a type of teaching that works well with children. Play reduces the anxiety that might otherwise be created if the nurse tries to explain complicated procedures. For example, if a child is to have a laceration of the arm sutured, it helps to let the child put sutures into a doll's arm. Almost any procedure or situation can be acted out through the use of dolls or other appropriate toys.

Guidelines for Individualizing Pain Therapy

In planning pain relief measures it is important for the nurse to choose therapies suited to the client's unique pain experience. McCaffery (1979) suggests nine useful guidelines for individualizing pain therapy:

1. *Use different types of pain relief measures.* Using more than one therapy has an additive effect in reducing pain. In addition, the character of a client's pain may change throughout the day, requiring several different therapies. Combining physical and psychological approaches, for example, analgesics and relaxation, controls all components of the pain experience.

2. *Provide pain relief measures before pain becomes severe.* An ounce of prevention is worth a pound of cure. It is easier to prevent severe pain than to relieve it once it exists. Giving an analgesic half an hour before a client must walk or perform an activity is an example of controlling pain early.

3. *Use measures the client believes are effective.* The client is the expert on his own pain. The client may have ideas about what measures to use and when to use them that will make pain therapy successful. Even if the client's remedies are unscientific, such as rubbing hand lotion on a swollen finger, they should be included as long as they are not harmful to the client.

4. *Consider the client's ability or willingness to participate in pain relief measures.* Some clients cannot actively assist with pain therapy because of fatigue, sedation, or altered levels of consciousness. However, there are variations of pain relief measures that require little effort, such as performing relaxation exercises in bed or listening to music as a distraction. The nurse will not relieve pain by forcing an unwilling client to participate in therapy. The depressed client with chronic pain has little motivation to participate in his own care.

5. *Choose pain relief measures on the basis of the client's behavior reflecting the severity of pain.* It would be poor judgment to administer a potent narcotic if a client has only mild pain. The nurse carefully assesses what the client says and how he behaves before choosing pain therapy. Some clients acquire relief from severe pain after using only mild analgesics. Only the client can determine the potency of an effective therapy.

6. *If a therapy is ineffective at first, encourage the client to try it again before abandoning it.* Often the client's anxiety or doubt prevents a therapy from relieving the pain. Some approaches, such as distraction, require practice. Some measures that seem ineffective may merely require adjustment in order to become effective. For example, the dosage of an analgesic may be increased if a client's severe pain is initially unrelieved. The nurse should exhibit patience and understanding in helping the client learn to use measures that do not afford immediate relief.

7. *Keep an open mind about what may relieve pain.* New ways are frequently found to control pain. There is still much to be learned about the pain experience. Rejecting a client's nonconventional therapies will lead to mistrust. It is, however, the nurse's responsibility to monitor therapies to ensure the client's safety and well-being.

8. *Keep trying.* The nurse can easily become frustrated when efforts at pain relief fail. It is important not to abandon the client when the pain persists. The client in severe chronic pain who is ignored may choose suicide as an alternative. If the nurse fails to provide the client comfort, she should reassess the situation and consider whether alternative therapies are needed.

9. *Protect the client.* A pain therapy should not cause more distress than the pain itself. The nurse always observes the client's response to therapy. Any pain relief measure may cause side effects, such as fatigue, anxiety, or additional pain. The nurse's aim is to relieve pain without disabling the client mentally, emotionally, or physically.

Implementation for Pain Relief

The nurse can independently implement a variety of pain relief measures that can complement therapies prescribed by a physician. If there is ever any doubt about using a nursing therapy, the nurse must consult the client's physician. Generally, the least invasive or safest therapy should be tried first.

Nursing Measures

The nurse institutes different kinds of pain relief measures to alter different components of the pain experience. Nursing therapies may prevent pain reception, lessen pain perception by cutaneous stimulation and increasing sensory input, or modify the client's reaction to pain.

PREVENTING PAIN RECEPTION

One of the most basic nursing responsibilities is protecting the client from harm. The nurse can directly intervene in providing comfort for a client by removing painful stimuli from the environment. Smoothing wrinkles from a bed, removing tubes on which the client is lying, loosening a constricting bandage, and changing a wet dressing are examples of removing painful stimuli.

The nurse must consider the types of stimuli that may cause pain. To prevent exposure to chemical stimuli the nurse protects the client's skin from caustic substances. For example, after a client has a diarrheal stool, the nurse washes irritating intestinal secretions from the skin. Hydrogen peroxide is typically diluted to half strength to avoid burning the mucosa during oral hygiene. Lifting rather than pulling a client up in bed and positioning the client anatomically are ways of avoiding the mechanical stimuli of stretching or pulling body parts. To prevent exposure to thermal stimuli that might injure tissues, the nurse carefully checks the temperature of bath water, heating pads, and cold and hot compresses.

Often it takes only a simple consideration of the client's comfort and a little extra time to avoid pain-producing situations. The nurse learns that raising the head of the bed makes sitting on a bedpan more comfortable for the client. Giving the arthritic client a chair with an elevated seat prevents knee discomfort as the client rises to a standing position.

Knowledge of factors that precipitate or aggravate an episode of pain helps the nurse prevent discomfort. The client with coronary artery disease is taught to avoid stressful exercise and eating large meals. Learning proper lifting techniques helps a client avoid back pain while on the job. A client with glaucoma is taught to visit a physician regularly and take prescribed medications to avert an acute attack resulting in eye pain.

The nurse also intervenes to reduce the extent to which pain receptors are stimulated. Covering an open wound with bandages reduces irritation to sensitive nerve endings. Turning a client stops transmission of impulses from pressure sites on bony prominences. Applying local anesthetics to the skin blocks the reception of painful stimuli.

LESSENING PAIN PERCEPTION

CUTANEOUS STIMULATION. Application of the gate control therapy through nursing care measures prevents pain impulses from reaching the client's conscious awareness. Cutaneous stimulation can activate the large-diameter sensory nerve fibers in the skin and alleviate pain by preventing painful stimuli from reaching higher centers of the brain. A massage, backrub, warm bath, and the application of heat and cold (see Chapter 48) and liniment are simple ways to reduce pain perception. The touch of the hands or the soothing sensation of a cool compress creates impulses that close the synaptic gates to pain transmission. Closure of the gate may not be complete, and the client may still feel some pain. However, cutaneous stimulation methods can reduce the severity of pain. As a side benefit, the proper use of cutaneous stimulation helps the client relax muscle tension that otherwise might increase pain. When using these methods, the nurse helps the client assume a comfortable position, eliminates sources of environmental noise, and explains the purpose of the therapy. A client or the family can often learn to use cutaneous stimulation measures in the home.

The nurse avoids using cutaneous stimulation when the skin is overly sensitive to stimuli, as with burns, bruising, skin rashes, inflammation, and underlying bone fractures.

INCREASING SENSORY INPUT. Researchers have proposed that the reticular formation in the brainstem inhibits painful stimuli if the person receives sufficient or excessive sensory input. With meaningful sensory stimuli a client can in effect ignore or become unaware of the pain. A person who is bored, lonely, or in isolation and has only his pain to think about is more susceptible to perceiving pain. Techniques that increase sensory input tend to work best when the pain is mild to moderate.

Distraction is a technique with which the client focuses his attention on stimuli other than the pain sensation. Activities such as listening to music, watching television, knitting, carrying on a conversation, or playing with a pet are effective in reducing a person's pain perception. Distraction tends to lower the client's awareness of the pain and often increases pain tolerance. Once distraction stops, however, the client's pain again becomes the center of attention. The nurse's assessment often reveals activities the client participates in at home that act as distractions. Many of these activities can also be used in a hospital or long-term care facility.

It is helpful for the nurse to explain the use and benefits of distraction to the client's family. Out of concern, the family often gives too much attention to a client's pain. Asking questions about the pain or offering to help the client perform basic activities of daily living can cause the client to become pain conscious. The family can easily participate in planning distractions that afford the client comfort.

MODIFYING PAIN REACTION

Modifying anxiety associated with pain not only directly relieves pain but also potentiates the effects of other pain relief measures. For example, a client gains an added benefit from a backrub if he is able to relax and feel that the pain will subside. Anxiety may be useful, however, when a client anticipates a painful experience. A moderate level of anxiety helps the client prepare to take action, such as using relaxation techniques and guided imagery, so he can cope with the impending pain.

When anxiety is severe or if it occurs while pain is present, the perceived intensity of pain often increases. The client's attention becomes focused on the pain experience. When anxiety aggravates the client's discomfort, the nurse should let the client know he is not alone. Explaining the reason for the client's pain and the effects of certain therapies will improve the client's understanding and reduce anxiety. The nurse can also help the client express anxiety by listening, discussing the client's feelings about pain, and accepting the client's emotions.

A nurse can also relieve anxiety and potentiate the effects of other therapies by using a positive approach in administering therapy. For example, while giving an analgesic or a treatment, simply saying, "I believe this will help you," provides relief for many clients. The nurse does not give false reassurance but instead conveys a sense of confidence that the therapy will work.

Relaxation is mental and physical freedom from tension or stress. The ability to relax physically promotes mental relaxation as well. Relaxation techniques provide clients with a sense of self-control when pain occurs. These techniques reverse the physical and emotional stress that occurs with pain. Clients who use relaxation techniques successfully experience slowing of heart and respiratory rates, reduction in blood pressure, and lessening of muscle tension. The nurse obtains a physician's order for relaxation therapy if there is any question of the legality of the nurse's action or if the client's physical condition is unstable.

A client can learn a variety of relaxation techniques, including meditation, yoga, Zen, guided imagery, and progressive relaxation exercises. Guided imagery and progressive relaxation can easily be incorporated into a client's pain therapy.

For relaxation techniques to be effective, the client's full participation and cooperation are necessary. The nurse explains the techniques in detail to help the client form realistic goals for pain relief. Considerable practice is generally needed to achieve consistent pain reduction. The nurse describes common sensations the client may experience, such as a decrease in temperature, a feeling of heaviness, or numbness of a body part. The sensory changes are the feedback to which the client attends as he progresses through the exercises. The nurse acts as a coach, guiding the client slowly through the steps of the exercise. The nurse should never attempt to teach relaxation techniques while the client is in acute discomfort because inability to concentrate will make the exercise ineffective.

The client may use guided imagery and relaxation exercises together or separately. In either case the nurse arranges for the environment to be as quiet as possible. Reducing light by closing curtains or turning off room lights decreases irritating stimuli. Every effort is made to minimize distractions. The client sits in a comfortable chair or lies in bed with all body parts well supported to enhance relaxation. A light sheet or blanket to maintain the client's temperature often helps the client feel more comfortable.

In guided imagery the client creates an image in his mind, concentrates on that image, and gradually becomes less aware of pain. The nurse coaches the client in forming the image and helping him concentrate on the sensory experience. Initially the nurse asks the client to think of a pleasant scene or experience that enables him to use all the senses. The client describes the image and the nurse records it so it can be used during later exercises. The nurse uses only specific information given by the client. The nurse guiding the client through the imagery does not make changes in the client's image. For example, if the client typically imagines a scene in which he is relaxing on a cool bed of grass, the nurse does not unexpectedly add the description of a small dog entering the scene. If the client is fearful of dogs, the nurse's description may create tension and anxiety. The following is an example of a portion of a guided imagery exercise:

Imagine yourself lying on a cool bed of grass with the sounds of rushing water from a nearby stream. It's a warm, balmy day. You turn to see a patch of blue wildflowers in bloom and can smell their fragrance.

Guided imagery works best when the client is able to use all of the senses. The nurse sits close enough to the client to be heard but is not intrusive. A calm, soft voice helps the client focus more completely on the suggested image. As the client relaxes, he becomes engrossed in the image and it is unnecessary for the nurse to speak continuously. If the client shows signs of agitation, restlessness, or discomfort, the nurse should stop the exercise and begin later when the client is more at ease.

Progressive relaxation exercises begin by having the client assume the most comfortable position possible. Some clients are less easily distracted if their eyes are closed, whereas others attempt to focus on a particular spot in the room. Soft background sound provided by a radio or tape masks outside noise and helps the client relax and concentrate.

The relaxation exercise involves a combination of controlled breathing exercises and a series of contractions and relaxations of muscle groups. The client begins by breathing slowly and diaphragmatically, allowing the abdomen to rise slowly and the chest to expand fully. The nurse coaches the client in breathing slowly and gradually relaxing his entire body. While the client establishes a regular breathing pattern, the nurse begins to coach the client to pay attention to any tense muscle groups. The nurse directs the client to locate the area of muscular tension, think about how it feels, tense the muscles fully, and then completely relax them. This creates the sensation of removing all discomfort and stress. Gradually the client can relax the muscles without first tensing them. Once the client achieves full relaxation, pain perception is lowered and anxiety toward the pain experience becomes minimal. The following is an example of how a nurse coaches a client:

Let's begin by finding as comfortable a position as possible. Arms at your side . . . legs uncrossed. . . . Move until you feel at ease. . . . Take a deep breath. Feel your stomach and chest slowly rise. . . . Relax. . . . Now breathe out slowly . . . slowly . . . and relax. Breathe in slowly again . . . and let it out. Your body is beginning to relax. . . . Think relax. . . . Feel the parts of your body. . . . Notice any tension in your muscles. . . . Continue to breathe slowly . . . and relax. Concentrate on any tension in your hands. . . . Notice how it feels. . . . Now make a fist. A tight fist! As you begin to exhale, relax your fist. . . . Good! Notice how your hand feels. . . . Think relax. . . . Your hand may feel warm or cool . . . heavy or light. . . . Just relax more . . . and more. Now focus on your forearms. . . . Notice any tension. . . . Relax your arms. . . . Feel your body relaxing. . . . Let the feelings of relaxation spread from your fingers and hands through the muscles of your arms.

As with guided imagery, if the client becomes agitated or uncomfortable, the nurse stops the exercise. If the client seems to have difficulty relaxing only part of his body, the nurse can slow the progression of the exercise and concentrate on the tensed body part. The client must also know from the beginning that he may stop the exercise at any time. With practice the client can learn to perform relaxation exercises independently.

Relaxation techniques are particularly effective for chronic pain, labor pains, and relief of procedure-related pain. The techniques are less effective for episodes of acute or severe pain.

Medical Measures

Numerous medical measures used alone or in combination with other therapies provide temporary or permanent pain relief. The nurse's methods for controlling pain complement those of the physician. The nurse has the responsibility of understanding the mechanisms of action of medical therapies in order to monitor their administration.

ADMINISTERING ANALGESICS

Pharmacological agents act at different levels of the nervous system to create pain relief. A given drug may act at the peripheral receptor level, at the level of the spinal cord, or at higher levels in the brainstem and cerebral cortex. Nonnarcotic analgesics such as acetylsalicylic acid (aspirin) and acetaminophen (Tylenol) act primarily on peripheral receptors to diminish reception of painful stimuli. Narcotic analgesics such as morphine, meperidine (Demerol), and codeine act on higher centers of the brain to modify the perception of and reaction to pain. Morphine is a derivative of opium and has three characteristic analgesic effects: (1) raising the pain threshold and thereby reducing a person's pain perception; (2) reducing anxiety and fear, which are components of the reaction to pain; and (3) inducing sleep even in the presence of severe pain. The danger of morphine and other narcotic analgesics is the potential for depression of vital nervous system functions. Opiates cause respiratory depression by depressing the respiratory center within the brainstem.

Although nonnarcotic analgesics are safer because they have fewer side effects, they are effective only in relieving mild pain. If the client is experiencing moderate to severe pain as in the case of a traumatic injury, surgery, cancer, or severe inflammation, narcotic analgesics are more effective. The one limitation of opiates is the minimal relief provided for isolated, sharp pain such as anginal chest pain. Table 37-7 compares the level of analgesia produced by selected pharmacological agents. The following are the characteristics of an ideal analgesic:

1. Having rapid onset
2. Effective over a prolonged time
3. Effective for all ages
4. Used orally and parenterally
5. Free of severe side effects
6. Nonaddicting
7. Inexpensive

The proper use of analgesics requires careful assessment, application of pharmacological principles (see Chapter 32), and common sense. A person's response to an analgesic is highly individualized. A relatively mild nonnarcotic may prove as effective as a potent narcotic for some clients, or an orally administered analgesic may bring the same relief as an injectable form of analgesic. It is the nurse's responsibility to follow a few basic principles:

TABLE 37-7

Comparison of Narcotic Analgesics

Level of Pain	Drug	Equivalent Analgesic Dose (mg)	Time for Peak Effect (minutes)	Duration of Effect (hours)
Severe	Morphine	10	30-90	Up to 7
	Dihydromorphinone (Dilaudid)	1.5	30-90	4-5
	Oxymorphone (Numorphan)	1-1.5	30-90	36
	Methadone (Dolophine)	7.5-10	60-120	3-6
Moderate to severe	Anileridine (Leritine)	25-30	30-60	2-3
	Butorphanol (Stadol)	1.5-3.5	30	3-4
	Meperidine (Demerol)	75-100	30-60	2-4
	Pentazocine (Talwin)	40-60	30-60	2-3
Mild to moderate	Codeine	120	60-90	4-6
	Propoxyphene (Darvon)	180-240	60	4-6

1. Know the client's previous response to analgesics.
2. Select the proper medication.
3. Know the accurate dosage.
4. Assess the right time and interval for administration.

It is helpful to know whether the client has previously gained relief from analgesics. The client can usually tell the nurse whether a medication proved effective. If possible it should be noted whether a nonnarcotic was as successful as a narcotic. Previous dosages and routes of administration should be assessed. A client who has remained comfortable receiving an oral dose of codeine every 6 hours will look skeptically at the nurse who enters the room with a syringe. If a client has not recently received any form of analgesic, the nurse must obtain a history of allergies.

Selecting the proper medication can often be difficult. Frequently a physician will order several analgesics from which to choose. Generally a more potent medication is ordered for episodes of severe pain, whereas a milder analgesic is prescribed for less acute pain. For pain that is mild to moderate, it is safer to start with a nonnarcotic or a milder form of narcotic. Nonnarcotics can also be alternated with narcotics. Pain may be aggravated as a result of physical distress and fatigue and require a more potent medication. Later in the day when the pain has subsided, a nonnarcotic may be adequate.

Too often nurses and physicians undertreat acute pain, particularly when administering narcotics. Many nurses fear they will cause the client to become drug dependent or that the dosage will cause respiratory depression. Clients vary considerably in their ability to absorb and metabolize drugs. A helpful rule to follow is that severe pain requires a greater amount of analgesic to relieve it, and doses at the upper end of the normal prescribed ranges are usually safe. If a well-meaning nurse administers a low dose that proves ineffective, the client may be forced to suffer a prolonged time until a drug can again be given.

The nurse has the primary role in determining the time and interval for analgesic administration. Narcotic analgesics are usually ordered on a p.r.n. (as needed) basis. For example, the medication order is oral codeine 30 mg every 3 to 4 hours p.r.n. If a client receives a dose at 7 AM, the nurse may not administer the drug again until 10 AM at the earliest. However, the client may not require the drug until late afternoon. The nurse must learn the normal duration of action for analgesics. The nurse must also anticipate the client's pain. Using a preventive approach requires that the nurse assess the client's discomfort frequently and recognize the nonverbal expression of pain. If any pain-producing procedure is scheduled, such as walking, sitting up, or a dressing change, the nurse should give an analgesic before the activity. The drug should be administered so that its peak effect is reached during the client's most active time.

LOCAL ANESTHETICS. Physicians often use local anesthesia to eliminate pain while suturing a wound, manipulating a painful body part, delivering an infant, and performing certain types of surgery. Local anesthesia eliminates the risks of general anesthesia, which involves loss of consciousness and depression of vital functions.

The administration of a local anesthetic produces a loss of sensation by inhibiting nerve conduction. Local anesthetics can be applied topically on skin and mucous membranes or injected into an area to anesthetize a part of the body. Local anesthetics block the function of sensory, motor, and autonomic neurons supplying the affected area. Thus, when the client temporarily loses sensation of a body part, motor and autonomic function is also lost. Smaller sensory nerve fibers are more sensitive to local anesthetics than large motor fibers. As a result, the client loses sensation before losing motor function, and conversely, motor activity returns before sensation.

Local anesthetics have the potential for creating side effects depending on their level of absorption into the circulation. Topical application to the skin is the safest method of administration, since the skin is relatively avascular. Itching and burning of the skin or even a localized rash may occur. Topical application to vascular mucous membranes increases a client's susceptibility to systemic effects. The physician uses the lowest possible concentration of anesthetic to avoid serious reactions.

Injection of local anesthetics increases the risk of systemic side effects, depending on the amount of anesthetic used and the area injected. The physician should take the precaution of aspirating, or pulling back the syringe plunger, before injecting the medication. If blood enters the syringe, the physician pulls the needle back to avoid injecting the anesthetic directly into the bloodstream. When aspiration produces no blood, it is safe to inject the anesthetic.

Table 37-8 and Fig. 37-6 summarize the types of local anesthesia by injection. Each produces a different level of anesthesia as a result of the amount of anesthetic used and the location of the spinal nerve affected.

The nurse assists the physician during the use of local anesthesia by providing emotional support to the client, watching for systemic side effects, and protecting the client from injury. Many clients are apprehensive about whether an anesthetic will prevent

TABLE 37-8

Local Anesthesia Techniques

Type	Area Injured	Area Anesthetized	Indications for Use
Infiltration	Superficially under skin or mucous membranes	Small peripheral nerves to area infiltrated	Small incisions of the skin; insertion of sutures to close cuts or wounds; minor dental repairs
Nerve block	Area surrounding large peripheral nerve at point above bifurcation of nerve	Wider area than with infiltration; numbs entire body part (e.g., hand, upper gums, foot)	Major dental repairs; manipulation or reduction of extremity fractures; minor hand and foot surgery
Epidural	In lumbosacral region of spinal cord; anesthetic injected around major nerve roots exiting from base of spinal cord at site outside dura mater	Lower trunk and extremities	Delivery of newborn; major surgery to lower trunk and extremities (e.g., hemorrhoidectomy, appendectomy, vascular repair)
Spinal	Anesthetic injected around major nerve root within subarachnoid space of spinal cord	Lower trunk and extremities	Major surgery to lower trunk and extremities; clients who would be at risk with general anesthesia

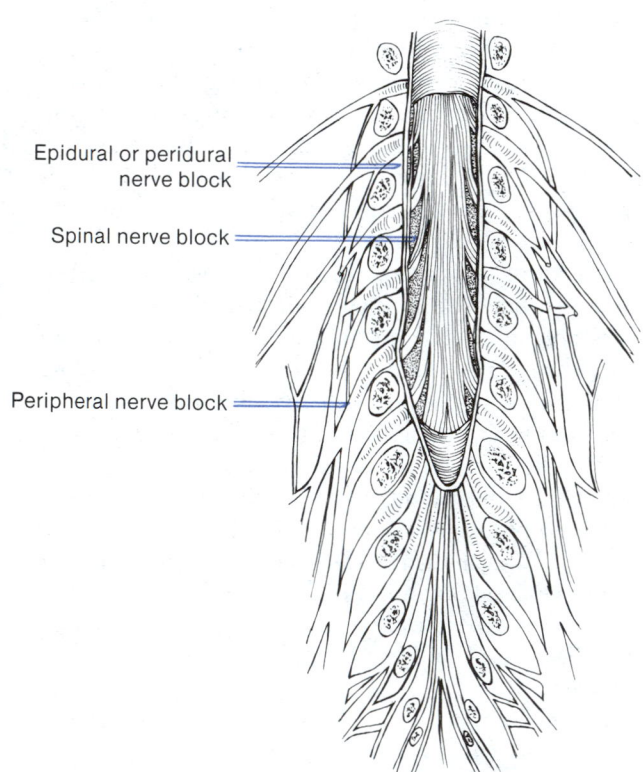

Epidural or peridural nerve block

Spinal nerve block

Peripheral nerve block

Fig. 37-6 Injection sites for peripheral, spinal, and epidural nerve blocks.

pain. The nurse explains how the local anesthetic will be applied and the sensations the client will experience. The initial injection of an anesthetic can be painful if the physician does not first numb the injection site. The nurse prepares the client for such discomfort.

It is common for clients to fear paralysis, since epidural and spinal injections come close to the spinal cord. The nurse explains where the needles are inserted and warns clients that they will temporarily lose motor and autonomic function (for example, bowel and bladder function).

Before the client receives an anesthetic, the nurse determines the client's history of allergies. To monitor systemic effects of local anesthetics, the nurse assesses the blood pressure and pulse. Spinal anesthesia may also cause variations in respiratory rate.

After administration of a local anesthetic the nurse protects the client from injury until full sensory and motor function returns. Pain is a normal protective mechanism. Until a local anesthetic is absorbed and metabolized, the client must be careful in using an anesthetized body part. For example, after an injection into a joint, the nurse warns the client to avoid using the joint until function returns. For clients with topical anesthesia the nurse avoids applying heat or cold to numb areas. Likewise, the nurse assists in positioning a client after spinal anesthesia, since the client will be unaware of wrinkles in the sheets or other sources of irritation. After spinal anesthesia the client is restricted to bed until sensory and motor function returns. The nurse assists the client during the first attempt at getting out of bed.

PLACEBOS. Often a nurse's reassuring words will seem to bring about pain relief even though there are no direct physiological or chemical effects on a client. A placebo is a dosage form that contains no pharmacologically active ingredient but may relieve pain. Commonly used placebos are normal saline, sterile water, and sugar. The pharmacy can prepare placebos in the form of capsules or tablets to make them look the same as medications.

Considerable argument exists over how placebos relieve pain. Some researchers believe that placebos increase endorphin levels. Others believe that the placebo creates a psychological sense of pain relief, lowering a person's pain perception. Whatever the mode of action, when the placebo is administered correctly, the client is convinced that it will provide pain relief. The client's conviction that a placebo is a legitimate form of therapy may be the necessary factor in relieving pain.

The nurse acquires a physician's order before administering a placebo. The placebo is not to be used as a form of punishment or as a test to prove whether the client is really in pain. The nurse may choose to give the placebo by telling the client it is a medication or by explaining to the client its purpose and desired effect.

The nurse can enhance the chances of a placebo working by explaining that the intent of the placebo is to relieve pain. It is also helpful to provide a quiet, comfortable environment that enables the client to relax. Trust in the nurse relieves any doubt the client might have about the therapy's benefit. The nurse administers the placebo as though it were an actual pain medication, assesses the client's pain carefully, and evaluates the placebo's effects.

SURGICAL MEASURES

When a client's pain persists despite medical attempts to relieve it, and when it is clear that the pain is physiologically rather than psychologically caused, surgical correction may provide relief. Surgical interventions are designed to block or interfere with the ability of pain impulses to travel up the spinal cord.

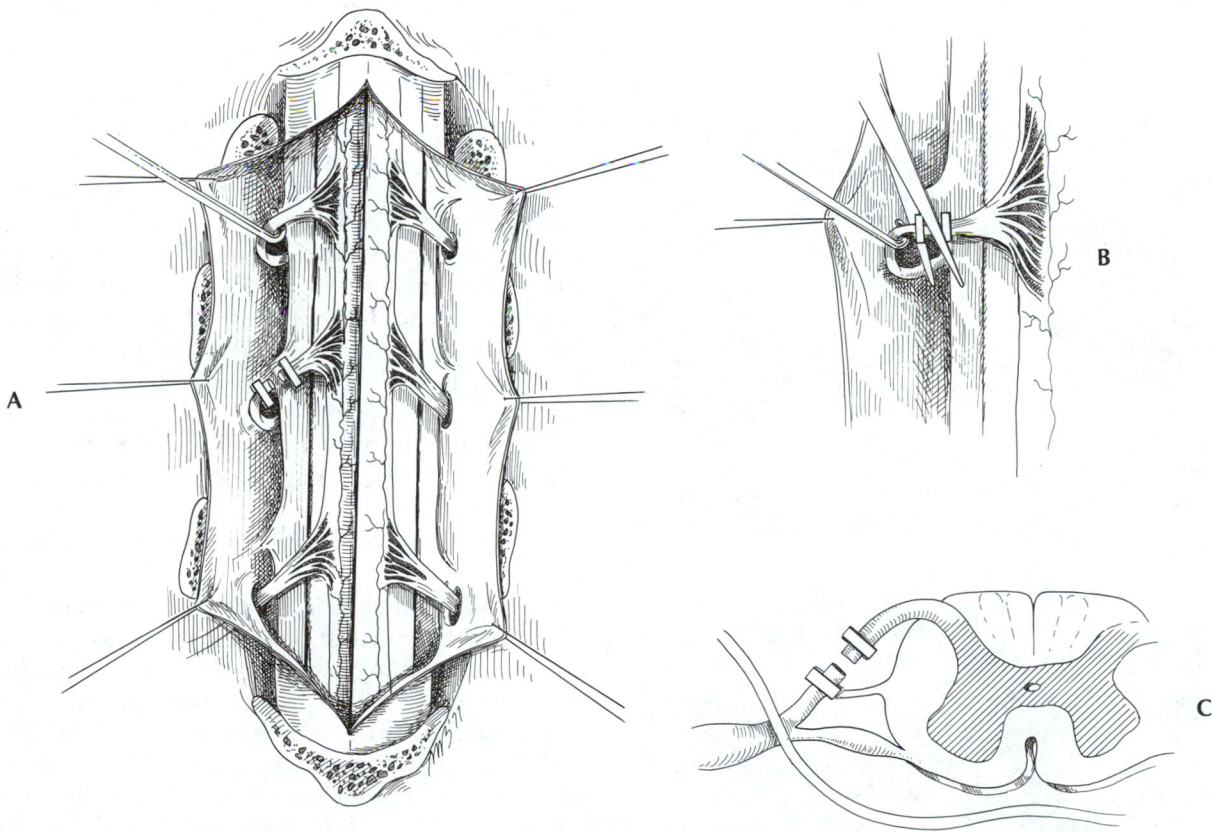

Fig. 37-7 Posterior rhizotomy after laminectomy. **A,** Spinal cord and roots exposed. **B,** Posterior root identified. **C,** Cross section of spinal cord and posterior root.

From Conway-Rutkowski, B.L.: Carini and Owens' neurological and neurosurgical nursing, ed. 8, St. Louis, 1982, The C.V. Mosby Co.

SURGICAL RESECTION OF NERVE PATHWAYS. A posterior *rhizotomy* involves the surgical resection of the dorsal roots of a spinal nerve (Fig. 37-7). The resection occurs intradurally in the posterior root just outside the posterior horn cells of the spinal cord. It is effective for relieving both localized acute pain in the area supplied by the nerve root and deep visceral pain. In treating deep visceral pain the physician must be certain to resect enough posterior roots at various spinal segment levels. Although the sensation of pain is destroyed, the client retains full motor function.

A *chordotomy* is a more extensive surgical procedure involving resection of the thoracic or cervical spinal cord at various levels. The procedure is successful in treating intractable or unrelieved pain. The higher the focus of pain, the higher the site selected for a chordotomy. For example, pain in the thorax, upper extremities, and shoulders requires a high cervical chordotomy. The risks of the procedure are great, since permanent paralysis may result from edema of the cord or accidental resection of motor nerves. After the procedure the client has a permanent loss of both pain and temperature sensation in the affected areas. If the surgery is uncomplicated, the client retains the sense of touch and position.

BLOCKING IMPULSE TRANSMISSION. Within the last 15 years, new electrical stimulation devices have helped in pain relief. The *dorsal column stimulator* is a battery-powered device that blocks pain impulses from reaching the spinal cord. A small electrode is surgically implanted near a sensory nerve believed to be transmitting the pain impulses. The client wears a battery-powered transmitter that sends electrical signals to block pain stimuli. When pain is felt, the client turns on the transmitter, which creates a mild buzzing or tingling sensation. The buzzing may last as long as pain relief occurs. The transmitter stimulates large sensory fibers entering the spinal cord and inhibits small pain fibers.

Transcutaneous electrical nerve stimulation (TENS) is a technique that follows the same principle as dorsal column stimulation. However, with TENS the electrodes are placed externally on the skin's surface (Fig. 37-8). Usually the client places the electrode directly over the site of pain. For example, for incisional pain, an electrode is placed next to the incision. The TENS device has a battery pack that can be regulated to increase the amplitude of the electrical stimulation. The client learns to use the amplitude setting that feels most comfortable and is most effective in pain relief.

ACUPUNCTURE

Acupuncture is not a surgical procedure, but it is an invasive procedure involving the insertion of long slender needles into body tissues. First practiced in the Orient, the treatment is now being used by some Western physicians. The most fascinating aspect of acupuncture analgesia is the distribution of acupuncture sites for the insertion of needles. For example, during a thyroid operation special needles are inserted at a point in the client's forearm above the wrist. Insertion of acupuncture needles at a given site produces an effect at a distant part of the body, which has no known direct anatomical relationship to the insertion site.

No one is sure exactly how acupuncture works. Once the needles are inserted, the tissues must be continuously stimulated. Sometimes the acupuncturist connects an electrical current between two needles. Rotating or twirling the needles with the hand also stimulates tissues. The needles must be placed not only at key meridians or points (Fig. 37-9), but also at the correct depth into the tissues. Eastern theory suggests that acupuncture corrects the disharmony between the life forces of yin and yang. When the balance of yin and yang is disturbed, disease and pain occur. Some physicians believe that acupuncture may be effective as a form of self-hypnosis. Most Western physicians believe that acupuncture works as a form

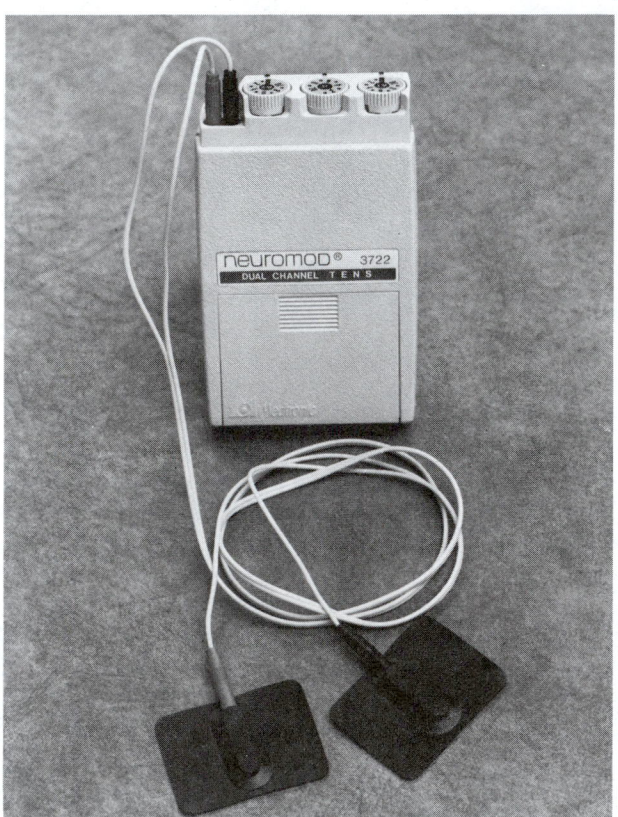

Fig. 37-8 Transcutaneous electrical nerve stimulator.

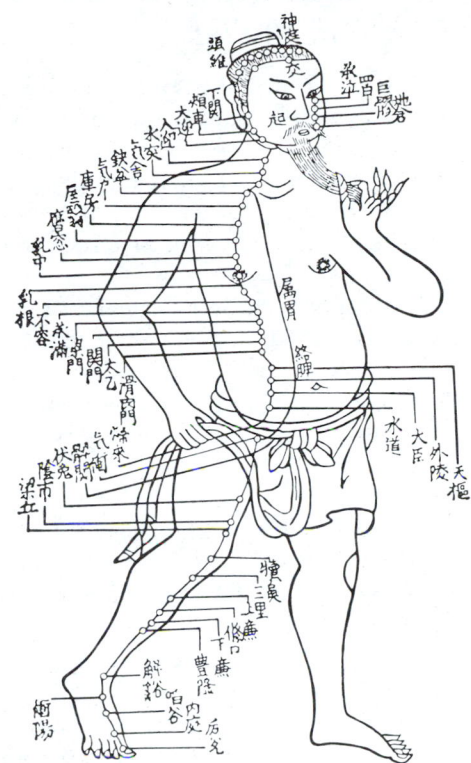

Fig. 37-9 Acupuncture meridians.

From Weisenberg, M.: Pain: clinical and experimental perspectives, St. Louis, 1975, The C.V. Mosby Co.

of counterirritation, closing the gating mechanism for pain impulse transmission.

Intractable Pain of Cancer

For clients with cancer the fear of pain is a common emotion. Clients and families associate pain with a diagnosis of cancer at any stage. A significant number of cancer clients experience pain that is chronic or intractable (not easily relieved).

Suffering from prolonged pain is a demoralizing experience. The client often assumes a dependent role in the family because his ability to care for his own needs is limited. Coping with chronic pain is made more difficult by fatigue and mental depletion. The anxiety resulting from the pain experience can be lessened by the nurse's support and understanding.

When therapy to control the spread of cancer fails, analgesic medications may be the only way of alleviating the cancer client's suffering. The administration of analgesics in the treatment of cancer-related pain requires the application of principles different from those used to treat acute pain. When a client with cancer first experiences pain, it is best to begin with a higher medication dosage than will be needed

for relief. The physician slowly decreases the dosage to the amount needed, thus providing the client with immediate pain relief. Too often physicians, nurses, and cancer clients themselves fear drug dependence. However, studies show that drug dependence is low among clients with cancer-related pain. Administering the right drug and the required dosage at the proper interval alleviates the fear of pain, protects the client from drug-seeking behavior, and reduces the incidence of tolerance and dependence. For clients with cancer the aim of drug therapy is to anticipate and prevent pain rather than treat it. It is therefore necessary to administer required doses on a regular basis. Prescribing analgesics on a p.r.n. basis for cancer clients is ineffective and causes more suffering. The cancer client must take an analgesic regularly, even when the pain, nausea, and other symptoms subside.

Methadone is a popular form of therapy for cancer clients. Its advantages include (1) a high oral potency, (2) long duration of action, (3) a cumulative effect that maintains a steady analgesic level to prevent pain, and (4) a relative lack of interference with a client's mood (Maxwell, 1980). Once a client's methadone dosage becomes regulated, only two daily doses may be required.

Opiate cocktails are also effective in achieving a pain-free state for the client with terminal cancer. Brompton's mixture, Val-Steck elixir, and modified Brompton's mixtures have the advantage of keeping a client alert and oriented so meaningful interpersonal relationships can be continued. Brompton's mixture includes a combination of drugs: morphine or methadone (narcotic analgesic), cocaine or an amphetamine (central nervous system stimulant that reduces sedation and respiratory depression caused by the narcotic), a phenothiazine (antipsychotic and antiemetic), and ethyl alcohol. The mixture often contains a fruit-flavored syrup to improve its taste. Brompton's mixture is easier to take than repeated injections. The client learns to adjust the dosage to ensure adequate pain relief. Taken regularly, the cocktail prevents the occurrence of pain. There is argument that Brompton's mixture is not as effective as morphine alone. However, the limited sedative effect of the cocktail offers an advantage to the client.

A currently popular measure for treatment of severe intractable cancer pain is morphine administered by continuous intravenous (IV) drip. Continuous drip provides more uniform and better pain control because lower doses of the drug are used and thus there are fewer side effects. Although a client receives a continuous infusion of morphine, the total daily dose may be less than with regular conventional intramuscular injections. Candidates for continuous drip therapy include clients with severe pain for which oral and intermittent parenteral narcotics provide minimal relief, clients with severe vomiting who are unable to take medications orally, clients with clotting disorders who cannot tolerate injections without bruising, and clients unable to swallow orally administered medications.

The physician orders the desired dosage and infusion rate of morphine, which is mixed in a crystalloid solution such as 5% dextrose in water (D5W) or lactated Ringer's solution. The morphine is delivered by way of an infusion control pump through microdrip intravenous tubing. The infusion pump ensures a safe, accurate, and steady rate of infusion.

The prescribed dosage of morpine depends on the severity of the client's pain, tolerance to the medication, and previous history of drug use. Doses may range from 4 mg per hour, with 100 mg morphine added to 500 ml IV fluid, to higher doses with 200 mg morphine added to 500 ml IV fluid. The higher the concentration of morphine, the smaller the amount of fluid the client receives. Each agency or institution has its own guidelines for morphine dosage and infusion rates.

While the client receives morphine by continuous drip, the nurse must closely monitor the client's vital signs. To prevent overdosage and central nervous system depression, the nurse records a baseline blood pressure and respiratory rate before the infusion begins. Once the infusion starts, the nurse monitors vital signs as often as every 15 to 30 minutes for the first few hours until the client gains pain relief at a constant dosage. If blood pressure or respirations decrease, the infusion rate is reduced according to physician's order or agency policy. If the client continues to show signs of severe respiratory depression, the physician will order the infusion discontinued. The narcotic antagonist naloxone (Narcan) should be available to the nurse to reverse the respiratory depression.

The use of irradiation may also be a successful means of providing the cancer client with pain relief. Radiotherapy reduces the size of the tumor, thus minimizing pain from pressure on nerve roots. Clients with bone lesions gain considerable relief from radiation.

The nurse uses all available pain relief measures for the client with cancer. The nurse-client relationship can be a positive factor in helping the client adapt to chronic pain. The client must feel that those responsible for managing the pain are competent and dependable.

Evaluating Pain Relief

The client is the principal resource for evaluating the efficacy of pain relief measures. The nurse must continually determine whether the character of the client's pain has changed and whether individual therapies are effective. Using descriptive pain scales after therapy provides a relatively objective interpretation of a treatment's effect.

If the nurse determines that a client continues to experience discomfort after therapy, it may be necessary to try additional therapies. For example, if an analgesic provides only partial relief, the nurse may add relaxation exercises or guided imagery exercises to control the client's pain.

The nurse also evaluates the client's perceptions of the effectiveness of therapy. The client may be able to help decide the best times to attempt a given treatment. For example, the client is the best judge of whether a given therapy works when anxiety and irritability are absent or when the pain is most severe.

The nurse also determines the client's tolerance to therapy, as well as the overall relief obtained. For example, if a nurse administers an analgesic, the occurrence of side effects from the medication must be assessed in addition to the client's reported pain relief. Similarly, after turning a client the nurse should return to determine if the client is tolerating the new position and if the pain has subsided. If a therapy aggravates the client's discomfort, the nurse stops it immediately and seeks an alternative pain relief measure.

The nurse and client should not become frustrated if a given therapy does not act quickly. Time and patience are necessary to maximize the chances of a therapy working. The nurse considers what factors may be influencing the client's perceptions or reactions to pain. For example, guided imagery may be ineffective if during the exercise the client is irritated by constant interruptions or noises from the environment. A backrub may prove ineffective if the client has just learned the results of diagnostic tests and has had no opportunity to express his concerns. The nurse evaluates the entire pain experience to determine what therapies are most effective and when they should be administered.

In order to achieve pain relief, the client and the nurse must work together. The nurse becomes familiar with the client's behaviors and expressions of pain. The client learns to trust the nurse and not to be fearful of expressing discomfort. The nurse must be willing to acknowledge that a particular therapy is not working and that new treatment is required.

Summary

The experience of pain is different for each person. The meaning pain conveys, the threat to comfort, and the potential implications of serious illness make the experience highly subjective but very real. Pain is a problem faced in every health care setting. The nurse is most effective in providing comfort to a client by understanding the nature of pain and the client's perceptions, eliminating personal prejudices about pain, and working closely with the client to find the best pain relief measures.

KEY CONCEPTS

✓ Pain is largely a subjective experience.

✓ Pain is a protective mechanism that warns a person of tissue injury.

✓ A nurse's misconceptions about pain often result in doubt as to the degree of the client's suffering and unwillingness to provide relief.

✓ Knowledge of the three components of the pain experience—reception, perception, and reaction—provides the nurse with guidelines for determining pain relief measures.

✓ Reception of painful stimuli requires an intact peripheral nervous system and spinal cord.

✓ Stimulation of synaptic gates is theorized to have the potential for blocking pain impulses and thus decreasing a client's pain perception.

✓ A number of therapies that provide pain relief may act by causing an increase in endorphin levels.

✓ The nature of a person's past experience with pain will affect his ability and willingness to cope with future discomfort.

✓ A client's cultural background influences the meaning and significance of pain and thus affects the person's behavior during pain.

✓ Acute pain causes stimulation of the sympathetic branch of the autonomic nervous system.

✓ A client's pain tolerance influences the nurse's perceptions of the seriousness of the discomfort.

✓ The difference between acute and chronic pain involves the duration of discomfort, physical signs and symptoms, and the client's perceptions regarding pain relief.

✓ The nurse does not attempt to assess the pain history while the client is experiencing severe discomfort.

✓ Pain scales lend objectivity to the measurement of pain severity and serve as tools to evaluate efficacy of pain therapies.

✓ Clients who live with daily pain experience changes in their routine living activities.

✓ Nursing diagnoses focus on the nature of the pain, the effect of pain on a client, or a component of the pain experience.

✓ Central to a nurse's plan for pain relief is developing a therapeutic relationship with the client and educating the client about pain.

✓ The nurse individualizes pain therapy by collaborating closely with the client, using assessment findings, trying a variety of therapies, and maintaining the client's well-being.

✓ Eliminating sources of painful stimuli is a basic nursing measure for promoting a client's comfort.

✓ Progressive relaxation exercises and guided imagery promote a sense of relaxation and lessen the client's awareness of pain.

✓ The proper administration of analgesics requires the nurse to know the client's response to the drugs, select the proper medication, and administer an accurate dose in a timely manner.

✓ Using a regular schedule for analgesic administration helps to prevent pain.

✓ The administration of a local anesthetic causes temporary loss of sensation, motor function, and possibly autonomic function.

✓ The nurse's primary role in caring for a client who receives local anesthesia is protecting the client from injury.

✓ Surgical measures for pain relief alter the ability of pain impulses to travel up the spinal cord.

✓ The client with intractable cancer-related pain requires dosages of analgesics that give immediate relief so that drug-seeking behaviors leading to drug dependence are avoided.

✓ The aim of therapy for cancer clients is to anticipate and prevent pain rather than treat it.

✓ Evaluation of the client's pain therapy requires a consideration of the changing character of pain, response to therapy, and the client's perceptions of a therapy's effectiveness.

REFERENCES

Maxwell, M.B.: How to use methadone for the cancer patient's pain, Am. J. Nurs. **80**:1606, 1980.

McCaffery, M.: Understanding your patient's pain, Nursing 80 **10**:26, 1980.

McCaffery, M.: Nursing management of the patient with pain, ed. 2, Philadelphia, 1979, J.B. Lippincott Co.

Melzack, R., and Wall, P.D.: Pain mechanisms: a new theory, Science **150**:978, 1965.

Zborowski, M.: Cultural components in responses to pain, J. Soc. Issues **8**:16, 1952.

ADDITIONAL READINGS

Anderson, J.L.: Nursing management of the cancer patient in pain: a review of the literature, Cancer Nurs. **5**:33, 1982.

Bagley, C.S., et al.: Pain management: a pilot project, Cancer Nurs. **5**:191, 1982.

Beyerman, K.: Flawed perceptions about pain, Am. J. Nurs. **82**:302, 1982.

Boyer, M.W.: Continuous drip morphine, Am. J. Nurs. **82**:603, 1982.

Cummings, D.: Stopping chronic pain before it starts, Nursing 81 **11**:60, 1981.

Donovan, M.I.: Relaxation with guided imagery: a useful technique, Cancer Nurs. **3**:27, 1980.

Levin, R.F.: Choice of injection site, locus of control, and the perception of momentary pain, Image **14**:26, 1982.

McCaffery, M.: Patients shouldn't have to suffer: how to relieve pain with injectable narcotics, Nursing 80 **10**:34, 1980.

McCaffery, M.: Relieve your patients' pain fast and effectively with oral analgesics, Nursing 80 **10**:58, 1980.

Melzack, R.: How acupuncture can block pain. In Weisenberg, M., editor: Pain: clinical and experimental perspectives, St. Louis, 1975, The C.V. Mosby Co.

Storlie, F.: Pointers for assessing pain, Nursing 78 **8**:37, 1978.

Wells, N.: The effect of muscle relaxation on postoperative muscle tension and pain, Nurs. Res. **31**:236, 1982.

West, B.A.: Understanding endorphins: our natural pain relief system, Nursing 81 **11**:50, 1981.

8

The six chapters in Unit 8 consider fundamental physiological needs: nutrition, urinary elimination, bowel elimination, oxygenation, fluid and electrolyte balance, and acid-base balance. The nurse in any setting may encounter clients whose health problems disrupt their ability to meet these needs, or the health problem may be the unmet need itself. Through an understanding of the physiological processes in body systems in which these needs arise, the nurse applies the nursing process to assist the client in meeting physiological needs in both health and illness.

Caring for Clients with Physiological Needs

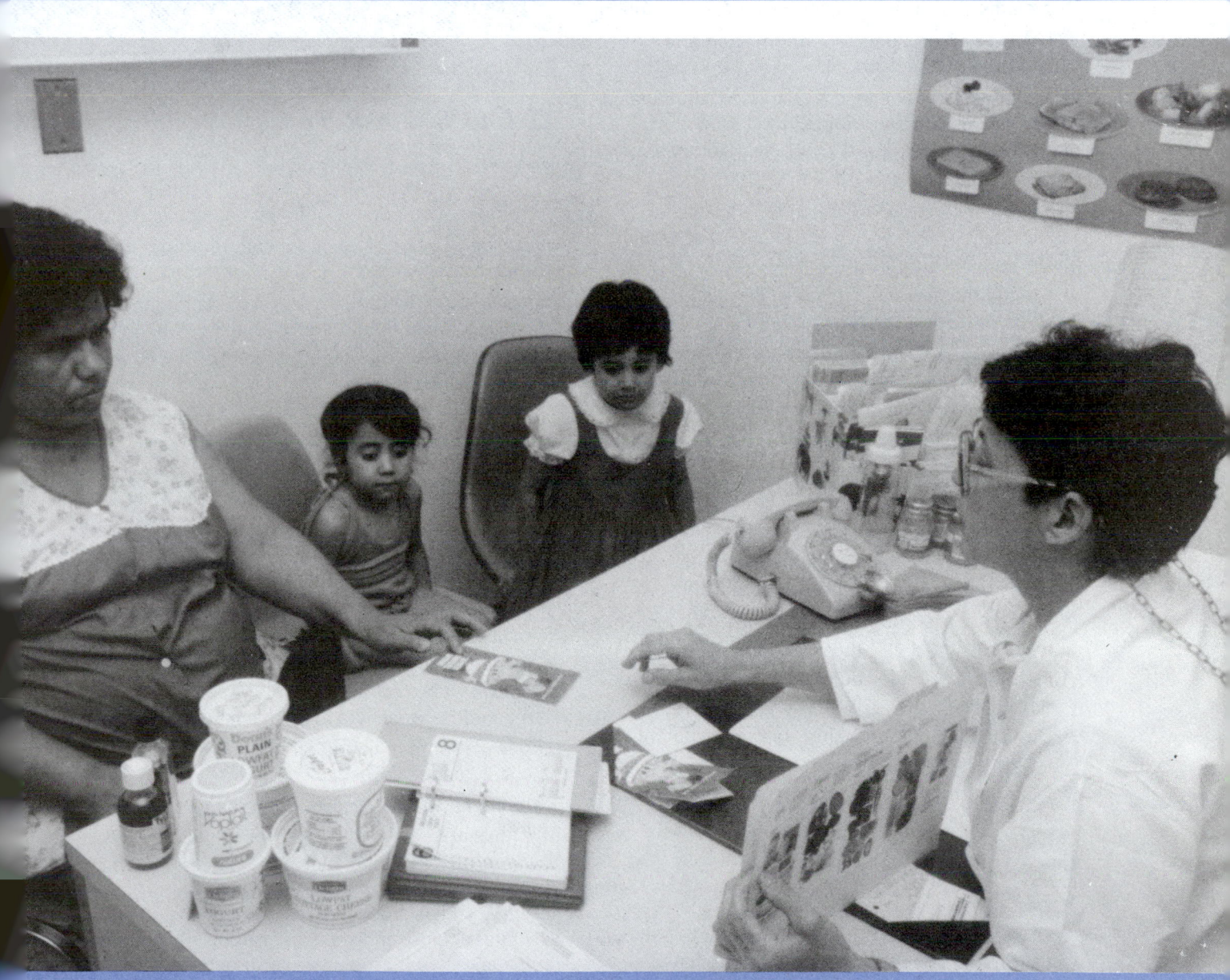

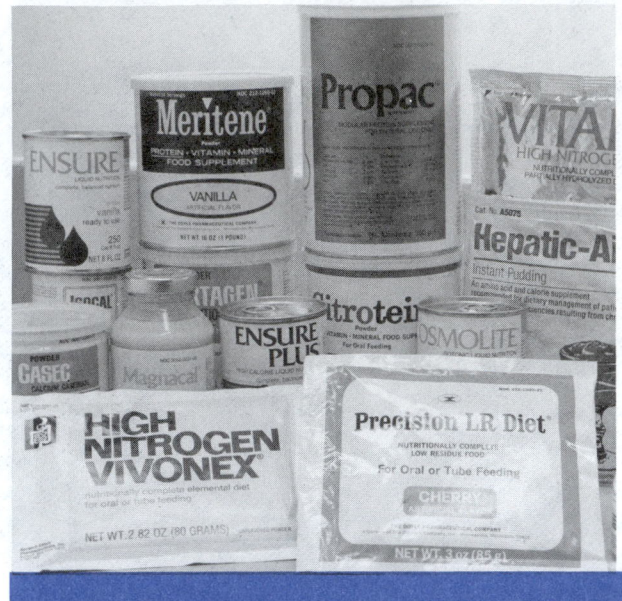

OBJECTIVES

Mastery of content in this chapter will enable the student to:

- Define the terms in the glossary.
- List the six categories of nutrients and explain why each is necessary for nutrition.
- Explain how energy is measured and the importance of a balance between energy intake in foods and energy output.
- Describe the role of water in digestion and absorption.
- Differentiate between complete and incomplete proteins and discuss their importance in nutrition.
- List the end products of carbohydrate, protein, and lipid metabolism.
- Explain the significance of saturated, unsaturated, and polyunsaturated lipids in nutrition.
- List the water- and fat-soluble vitamins and their major functions and sources.
- Differentiate between macrominerals and microminerals and discuss the significance of important minerals in nutrition.
- Identify the areas in the gastrointestinal tract where nutrients are absorbed.
- Describe the basic four food groups, and discuss their value in planning meals for good nutrition.
- Explain recommended daily allowances (RDAs).
- List seven dietary guidelines for health promotion.
- Describe variations in dietary needs based on age.
- Discuss the major areas of nutritional assessment.
- Discuss the differences between the nutritional needs of the sick and those of the healthy.
- Name some of the factors that influence a client's dietary patterns and nutritional status.
- Identify three major nutritional problems and describe clients at risk for these problems.
- Describe the different kinds of diet commonly used in health care facilities.
- Explain principles to follow when feeding clients and the nurse's responsibility in assisting them with eating.
- Describe enteral feeding methods.
- Describe total parenteral nutrition (TPN).
- Discuss the importance of diet counseling in evaluation and client teaching before discharge.

GLOSSARY

anabolism Constructive metabolism characterized by conversion of simple substances into more complex compounds of living matter.

anorexia Lack or loss of appetite resulting in the inability to eat.

antioxidant Agent that inhibits oxidation and thus prevents deterioration through oxidation.

ariboflavinosis Condition caused by dietary deficiency of vitamin B_2.

atherosclerosis Common arterial disorder characterized by yellowish plaques of cholesterol, lipids, and cellular debris in the inner layers of the walls of the large and medium-sized arteries.

basal metabolism rate (BMR) Amount of energy used in a unit of time by a fasting, resting subject to maintain vital functions.

beriberi Disease of the peripheral nerves caused by a deficiency of or an inability to assimilate thiamin.

cachexia General ill health and malnutrition marked by weakness and emaciation.

caries Abnormal condition of the teeth or bones characterized by decay.

carpopedal spasm Spasm of the hands, thumbs, feet, or toes that sometimes accompanies tetany.

catabolism Complex metabolic process in which energy is liberated for use in work, energy storage, or heat production by oxidation of carbohydrates, lipids, and proteins; carbon dioxide and water, as well as energy, are produced.

38 *Nutrition*

catalyst   Substance that influences the rate of a chemical reaction without being permanently altered by the process.

collagen   Substance that combines to form the white, glistening, inelastic fibers of tendons, ligaments, and fasciae.

compliance   Fulfillment by the client of the care giver's prescribed course of treatment.

cretinism   Condition characterized by severe congenital hypothyroidism.

eclampsia   Gravest form of toxemia of pregnancy, characterized by grand mal convulsions, coma, hypertension, proteinuria, and edema.

emaciation   Excessive leanness caused by disease or malnutrition.

enzyme   Protein produced by living cells that catalyzes chemical reactions in organic matter.

gluconeogenesis   Formation of glucose or glycogen from substances that are not carbohydrate, such as protein or lipid.

glycerol   Alcohol that is a component of lipids and that is soluble in ethyl alcohol and water.

glycogen   Polysaccharide that is the major carbohydrate stored in animal cells.

glycolysis   Series of enzymatically catalyzed reactions within cells by which glucose and other sugars are broken down to yield lactic acid or pyruvic acid, releasing energy in the form of adenosine triphosphate.

hemosiderosis   Abnormal deposition of iron in a variety of tissues.

hepatomegaly   Abnormal enlargement of the liver.

hypermetabolism   Increased metabolism, producing above normal body heat.

hyperosmolarity   Increased osmotic concentration of a solution.

intrinsic factor   Substance that is secreted by the gastric mucosa and is essential for the intestinal absorption of vitamin B_{12}.

ketoacidosis   Acidosis accompanied by an accumulation of ketones in the body, resulting from faulty carbohydrate metabolism.

legume   Fruit or pod of beans, peas, and lentils.

levodopa   Drug used in the treatment of parkinsonism.

malnutrition   Any nutritional disorder such as unbalanced, insufficient, or excessive diet or impaired absorption, assimilation, or utilization of food.

megadose   Dose greatly in excess of that usually prescribed.

metabolism   Aggregate of all chemical processes that take place in living organisms, resulting in growth, generation of energy, elimination of wastes, and other functions concerned with the distribution of nutrients in the blood after digestion.

oliguria Diminished capacity to form and pass urine, preventing efficient excretion of the end products of metabolism.

organic foods Foods grown in soils that have been treated only with organic matter (manure or compost).

osmolarity Osmotic pressure of a solution.

osmotic diuresis Increased urinary secretion that follows increased blood volume resulting from increased osmolarity of blood; fluid is pulled from cells, leading to cellular dehydration.

osteoporosis Disorder characterized by abnormal rarefaction of bone.

oxidation Any process in which the oxygen content of a compound is increased.

paresthesia Abnormal sensation such as burning or tingling.

pellagra Disorder resulting from a deficiency of niacin or tryptophan.

peristalsis Coordinated, rhythmical, serial contractions of smooth muscle that force food through the digestive tract.

pH Scale representing the relative acidity or alkalinity of a solution.

prostaglandin One of several potent, hormone-like, unsaturated fatty acids that act in exceedingly low concentrations on target organs.

recommended daily allowances (RDAs) Suggested or recommended amounts of various nutrients used in planning diets.

reduction Process in which oxygen is removed from a substance.

satiety Satisfied feeling of being full.

splenomegaly Abnormal enlargement of the spleen.

stria Streak or linear scar that results from rapid development of tension in the skin.

tryptophan Essential amino acid, precursor of serotonin and niacin.

villi Tiny projections, barely visible to the unassisted eye, clustered over the entire mucosa of the small intestine.

The science of nutrition is relatively young, although nutritional support has always been a factor in the care of the sick. Because most other forms of treatment were lacking, early client care relied heavily on the preparation and administration of food to maintain the body's strength to fight disease. Information about foods that appealed to sick people and were likely to be retained by diseased bodies was shared and became an important part of early medical lore.

Most nursing schools before World War II provided instruction in nutrition and diet therapy, laboratory courses in food preparation, and clinical experience in the preparation and serving of therapeutic diets.

The war brought a tremendous increase in knowledge about disease and injury and changed the attitudes of people toward hospitalization. People began to regard hospitals as facilities for the restoration of health rather than shelters for the terminally ill. As hospital use increased, nurses were given more responsibilities. As a result of this and a postwar shortage of nurses, numerous ancillary services were developed to assist in client care. Because of nurses' greater involvement in other aspects of client care, they delegated many functions to the growing number of technicians and aides. Dietitians were increasing in number. They had responsibility for planning and preparing all hospital meals, including therapeutic diets. They also assumed responsibility for the dietary teaching of clients. Nurses' aides prepared clients for meals, and dietary aides served the meals. Consequently, nurses' involvement in diet therapy was reduced to recording dietary intake in the nurse's notes.

Dietitians, left with almost complete responsibility for this aspect of client care, rarely received more than token support from other members of the health team. Hospital clients were often discharged before their dietary instruction had been completed. In clinics, ambulatory care centers, and physicians' offices, dietary instruction often consisted of mimeographed diets, presented without explanation or encouragement to comply. Since the dietary aspects of care were not emphasized, clients did not feel bound to accept radical departures from their usual food intake. As nursing schools tried to incorporate all the new medical knowledge into the curriculum, other aspects of the curriculum were allotted less time and emphasis. Nutrition and diet therapy often became integrated into medical-surgical nursing courses and in many instances consisted only of reading assignments. In schools where courses in nutrition and diet therapy were retained, these courses were taught by nonnursing faculty and the content was seldom reinforced when the students gave nursing care in the clinical areas.

Today there is renewed interest in a holistic approach to client care. With many effective treatment modalities available, clients are frequently involved in the decision of which one will be prescribed for them. People in general are becoming more interested in foods and how certain nutrients affect their health and well-being. Claims abound for natural foods, organically grown foods, and diets to cure all ills, often without any scientific basis. Nonetheless, responsible research is uncovering relationships between food intake and certain diseases. More is being learned about the essential nutrients, particularly vitamins and minerals. Nurses are renewing their interest in nutrition for their own benefit as well as their clients'. Nutritionists in private practice provide counseling to the public. Primary nurses in hospitals and nurse practitioners in the community are responsible for all aspects of client care, including nutritional support and education.

The increasing interest in health promotion and prevention of disease has also led to a greater role of nutrition in health care. Nurses are in an excellent position to assess nutritional status, observe nutritional intake, evaluate response to therapy, and support the dietary teaching and regimen prescribed for the client.

At the present time, interest in nutrition is high. Diet therapy is recognized as an important adjunct to treatment and remains the only treatment for some conditions. Nutritional interest has spread beyond medicine to the public domain as people seek reliable information. Scientific research continues to provide answers, and nutrition experts are establishing guidelines for good nutrition and issuing warnings related to diet and disease.

Human bodies need food for fuel in order to carry on life processes. Research has established many nutrients that are essential to health. Newer studies indicate that what a person eats may have a profound effect not only on health but also on behavior, intellect, emotions, and sleep habits.

Principles of Nutrition

The body requires food to (1) provide energy for organ function, body movement, and work, (2) maintain body temperature, and (3) provide raw materials for enzyme function, growth, replacement of cells, and repair.

Metabolism refers to all the biochemical reactions that take place within the body. Metabolism consists of anabolic reactions that build substances and body tissue and catabolic reactions that break down substances. These reactions require energy. Food is ingested, digested, and absorbed in order to produce this energy. Energy is measured in calories.

People's energy requirements vary and are influenced by many factors. The energy requirement of an awake person at rest is called the basal metabolism rate (BMR). The BMR is the energy need at a person's lowest level of cellular function. Such things as age, body size, body temperature, activity, environmental temperature, growth, sex, nutritional state, emotional state, and food intake affect individual energy requirements beyond the BMR.

When energy requirements are completely met by calorie intake in food, people maintain their activity level without weight change. When the number of calories ingested exceeds the energy needs, the person gains weight. When the number of calories ingested fails to meet energy requirements, the person will burn body fat for energy and will lose weight. Energy requirements vary from day to day, reflecting changes in the factors that influence them. For example, illness frequently increases energy requirements through increased body temperature, hypermetabolism, and stress.

Nutrients are foods that contain the elements necessary for body function. Six categories of nutrients are needed: water, carbohydrates, proteins, lipids, vitamins, and minerals. These categories are discussed separately in the following sections. Energy needs are met by the metabolism of carbohydrates, proteins, and lipids. Water too is needed because nutrients must be in solution for absorption and transportation. Although vitamins and minerals do not provide energy, they are involved in the reactions that produce energy.

Foods are sometimes described according to the density of their nutrients. Nutrient density is the proportion of essential nutrients to the number of calories. Foods with the most nutrients in proportion to their total calories are said to have high density. Foods with low nutrient density are also called "empty calories" because they provide an energy source but lack essential nutrients. Alcohol and refined sugar are examples of low-density nutrients or empty calories.

Water

Of the six nutrients, water is the most important because the function of cells depends on a fluid environment. Water comprises 60% to 70% of total body weight. A lean person's body contains more water than an obese person's body. Infants have the greatest percentage of total body weight as water, and elderly people have the least. The proportion of water in total body weight decreases with age. Infants and elderly people are most vulnerable to water deprivation or water loss. Yet no one, when deprived of water, can survive for more than a few hours in a desert or a few days in the most protective environment.

We meet the fluid needs of our bodies by drinking liquids, by the large fluid component of the solid foods we eat, and to a lesser degree by the water produced when food is oxidized. In a healthy person the fluid intake from all sources equals the fluid output from all sources over a 3-day period. The ill person usually has increased fluid needs because of increased body temperature or a hypermetabolic state. Diseases also affect fluid output through reduced kidney output or increased fluid losses of urine, perspiration, and other body secretions. Fluid may be trapped in a body compartment (edema) and not be available for the body to use.

Thirst is the protective symptom that alerts the conscious person to the need for fluids. Thirst is a less reliable guide to the need for fluids in the older or confused client. Infants experience thirst, although they may not be able to communicate this need.

Water is essential to energy production even though it does not provide calories. Cells cannot function without it. Nutrients must be in solution to be absorbed into the bloodstream and transported to body cells.

Carbohydrates

Carbohydrates are composed of carbon, hydrogen, and oxygen. The ratio of hydrogen to oxygen is the same as in water: two hydrogen ions for every oxygen ion. Carbohydrates are obtained primarily from plant foods; the only important source of animal carbohydrate is the lactose in milk (milk sugar). The carbohydrate content of the diet tends to be greater for families with limited resources for food expenditure and less for more affluent families. Carbohydrates may contribute as much as 90% of the total caloric intake in other parts of the world where grains, such as rice and corn, are a major ingredient of every meal.

Carbohydrates are classified according to their sugar units or saccharides. A monosaccharide is a simple sugar that cannot be broken down into any more basic sugar unit. Examples of monosaccharides are glucose (dextrose), galactose, and fructose; these monosaccharides have the same chemical composition but different arrangements of molecules.

A carbohydrate with two sugar units is a disaccharide. When two monosaccharides unite, they form a disaccharide and water. During digestion the reverse occurs: a disaccharide takes up water and is split into two simple sugars. Sucrose, lactose, and maltose are disaccharides.

Polysaccharides are composed of many sugar units. They are insoluble in water and digested with varying degrees of completeness. Glycogen is a polysaccharide; it is the form in which the body stores carbohydrate. Glycogen is synthesized from glucose in the liver and muscles and is also stored in the liver and muscles.

Plants store carbohydrate as starch. Starch is made up of granules enclosed by cellulose walls. When starch is cooked, the granules swell and burst their cellulose wall. Raw starch foods are more difficult to digest than the same foods after cooking, since the freeing of the granules from the cellulose permits greater contact with digestive enzymes and more complete digestion.

The digestion of starch consists of several steps. Starch is first broken down into dextrins, then into maltose, and finally into glucose. Dextrin, an intermediate product of starch digestion, is also produced commercially and is used to increase the digestibility of foods, such as baby foods and cereals. Small amounts of dextrin are produced when bread is toasted or flour is browned.

Some polysaccharides cannot be digested because humans do not have enzymes capable of breaking them down. Nevertheless, these polysaccharides have a role in human nutrition, since they add fiber to the diet. Fiber is receiving increasing attention as a dietary factor in disease prevention and treatment. Examples of fiber are agar and pectin, which are used to form gels and as thickening agents, carrageenan (Irish moss), which is used to increase the smoothness of ice creams and sauces, and lignin, a woody substance added to breads.

The metabolism of 1 g of carbohydrate produces 4 calories. Carbohydrate metabolism may produce three different results: catabolism into energy, carbon dioxide, and water; anabolism into glycogen for storage; and conversion into fat (adipose tissue) for storage. Carbohydrates contribute to the total caloric requirements, but there are no specific required daily allowances for carbohydrates. Carbohydrates are the body's preferred energy source and are needed for the metabolism of lipids and for protein sparing (replacing protein in meeting energy needs). In order to keep the body in acid-base balance, at least 50 to 100 g of carbohydrate is needed daily. Recent guidelines and nutritional plans advocate an increase in the percentage of total daily calories provided by carbohydrates to 60% or more. This increase should be derived from natural sugars and polysaccharides.

Proteins

Proteins are composed of hydrogen, oxygen, carbon, and nitrogen. Most proteins also contain sulfur and phosphorus. Because of their high molecular weight and tendency to form colloidal solutions, proteins do not readily pass through body membranes. Amino acids are the most important components of proteins; they are essential for synthesis of body tissue in growth, maintenance, and repair. Protein can also be used as a source of energy.

Protein foods tend to be expensive, and their contribution to total caloric intake is usually higher in affluent families and developed countries. Protein intake is of particular importance during periods of rapid growth and after disease and injury.

Proteins are classified as simple, conjugated, or derived. Simple proteins are hydrolyzed into amino acids or their derivatives. Albumin and globulin are simple proteins. The combination of a simple protein with a nonprotein substance will produce a conjugated protein. Examples of conjugated protein are mucoprotein, which is formed by the combination of a carbohydrate group and a simple protein, and lipoprotein, formed by a combination of a lipid and a simple protein. Derived proteins are formed during the hydrolysis of protein. For example, peptides and proteoses occur during stages in the digestion of protein.

Another method of classifying protein is based on its nutritional value. This classification identifies proteins as either complete or incomplete. A complete protein is one that contains all the essential amino acids in sufficient quantity to support growth and maintain nitrogen balance. Complete proteins are also referred to as high–biological value proteins. Examples of complete or high–biological value proteins are meat, fish, poultry, milk, and eggs.

An incomplete protein either does not contain all the essential amino acids or does not have them in sufficient quantity to support growth and maintain nitrogen balance. Examples of incomplete proteins are cereals, legumes, and vegetables. The combination of one incomplete protein with another incomplete protein (which contains the missing amino acids or increases the amount of amino acids) in the same dish or meal will supply the essential amino acids to support growth and maintain nitrogen balance. Incomplete proteins that combine to act as complete proteins are called complementary proteins. Grains and legumes are complementary proteins. Incomplete proteins can also be made complete by the supplementation of synthetic amino acids. The addition of synthetic lysine to wheat is an example of amino acid supplementation.

Amino acids are classified as essential or nonessential:

ESSENTIAL	NONESSENTIAL
Histidine	Alanine
Isoleucine	Arginine
Leucine	Asparagine
Lysine	Aspartic acid
Methionine	Citrulline
Phenylalanine	Cysteine
Threonine	Cystine
Tryptophan	Glutamic acid
Valine	Glycine
	Hydroxyglutamic acid
	Hydroxyproline*
	Norleucine*
	Proline
	Serine
	Thyroxine*
	Tyrosine

Since the body cannot synthesize essential amino acids, it is essential that they be provided by the diet. Nonessential amino acids need not be present in the diet because the body can manufacture them from the breakdown of other amino acids.

Protein is the body's only source of nitrogen, and 16% of protein is nitrogen. Nitrogen balance is an important concept. The body is in nitrogen balance when the intake and output of nitrogen are equal. When the intake of nitrogen exceeds the output, the body is in positive nitrogen balance, as in growth, normal pregnancy, and wound healing. The nitrogen retained by the body is used for building, repair, or replacement of body tissues.

Negative nitrogen balance occurs when the body is losing more nitrogen than it is taking in. The increased nitrogen loss is the result of body tissue de-

struction. Negative nitrogen balance is associated with infection, fever, starvation, injury, and prolonged immobilization.

Protein can be used to provide energy, but because of protein's essential role in growth, maintenance, and repair, it is important that protein be spared to carry out its own unique functions. Protein sparing refers to the provision of sufficient carbohydrate in the diet to meet the energy needs of the body in order to spare protein for its role in nitrogen balance and tissue building.

Protein is metabolized to yield amino acids, nitrogen, and 4 kcal (17 joules) per gram. Amino acids are anabolized into tissues, hormones, and enzymes. Amino acids can also be converted to fat and stored as adipose tissue or catabolized into energy, carbon dioxide, and water.

The required daily allowance for protein ranges from 2.2 g/kg body weight for infants under 6 months of age to 56 g for males over the age of 15 years (see Table 38-8). Pregnant women require an additional 30 g and lactating women an additional 20 g above their usual daily need of 44 to 46 g.

Nutrition experts believe that the intake of protein in America is generally greater than required. Protein foods are expensive to buy and to produce in terms of the economic use of land and fodder. In addition, meats, whole milk, cheese, and eggs are not pure protein; they also contain significant amounts of saturated fatty acids and cholesterol. Nutritional guidelines recommend the reduction of saturated fats and cholesterol.

Lipids

Lipid is a comprehensive term applied to compounds that are insoluble in water but soluble in organic solvents, such as ethanol, ether, benzene, and acetone. Lipids include fats that are solid at room temperature and oils that are liquid at room temperature. Lipids are composed of carbon, hydrogen, and oxygen, but the proportion of each element differs from that of carbohydrate.

Lipids are classified as simple, compound, or derived. Simple lipids, such as monoglycerides, diglycerides, and triglycerides, are esters of glycerol and fatty acids. A monoglyceride contains one fatty acid, a diglyceride contains two fatty acids, and a triglyceride contains three fatty acids. Compound lipids are simple lipids combined with a nonlipid substance, such as carbohydrate in glycolipids, phosphorus in phospholipids, and protein in lipoproteins. Derived lipids, such as cholesterol, steroid hormones, and the fat-soluble vitamins, are produced during the breakdown of simple or compound lipids.

---

*Whether these are true amino acids is questionable.

Approximately 98% of the lipid in foods and 90% of the lipid in the human body is in the form of triglycerides. Triglycerides are termed simple when the three fatty acids that comprise them are the same. A mixed triglyceride is composed of two or three different fatty acids. High blood levels of triglycerides have been linked to atherosclerosis.

Health care workers are also interested in the relationship between dietary intake of fatty acids and blood cholesterol levels. Increased blood cholesterol levels are associated with atherosclerosis and resulting cerebrovascular accidents (stroke) and coronary occlusion.

A saturated fatty acid contains as much hydrogen as it can hold. An unsaturated fatty acid can take up another hydrogen atom, and a polyunsaturated fatty acid can take up many more hydrogen atoms. Unsaturated and polyunsaturated fatty acids are oils. They have a low melting point and are liquid at room temperature. Hydrogenation is a process by which these oils are made more solid by the addition of hydrogen. The addition of hydrogen also makes them more saturated. Ingestion of saturated fatty acids appears to increase blood cholesterol levels. Ingestion of unsaturated fatty acids has a minimal effect on blood cholesterol, and polyunsaturated fatty acids appear to lower blood cholesterol levels.

Fatty acids are usually not purely saturated, unsaturated, or polyunsaturated. Most animal fats have high proportions of saturated fatty acids; most vegetable fats have higher amounts of unsaturated and polyunsaturated fatty acids (see boxed material).

Linoleic acid is the only essential fatty acid. Since the body is unable to synthesize linoleic acid, it is dependent on an adequate dietary intake. Linoleic acid is a polyunsaturated fatty acid found in safflower, soybean, corn, cottonseed, and peanut oils.

Fat is the body's form of stored energy. The glycerol portion of lipids can be converted to glucose by gluconeogenesis. All body cells except the red blood cells and the central nervous system cells can oxidize fatty acids for energy. After a period of starvation, even the central nervous system can adapt to the use of amino acids and ketones as energy sources.

The metabolism of 1 g of lipid yields 9 kcal (38 joules), more than twice the energy provided by carbohydrates or proteins. Lipids account for 35% to 45% of the American diet, with the percentage usually increasing with affluence. Nutritional guidelines recommend a reduction of lipid intake to 30% of the total caloric intake, with some authorities suggesting even lower intakes.

RDA is not listed for lipids. Lipids contribute to energy production and are the vehicles for required fat-soluble vitamins.

Spectrum of Polyunsaturation of Oils

Percent

Percent	Oil
100	
95	
90	
85	
80	
75	Safflower oil
70	
65	
60	Soybean oil
55	Corn oil
50	Cottonseed oil
45	
40	
35	
30	Peanut oil
25	
20	Olive oil
15	
10	Lard, palm oil
5	
	Butterfat, cocoa butter, palm kernel, coconut oil
0	

From Bodinski, L.: The nurse's guide to diet therapy, New York, 1982, John Wiley & Sons, Inc.

Vitamins

Vitamins are organic substances, present in minute amounts in foods, that are essential to normal metabolism. The body is unable to synthesize vitamins in the required amounts and depends on dietary intake. Research is constantly improving the understanding of the role of vitamins in human physiology. New vitamins have been identified and recommended allowances established or revised.

Although they are contained in many foods, vitamins are affected by processing, storage, and preparation. Vitamin content is usually highest in fresh foods that are used quickly after minimal exposure to heat, air, or water. Vitamins are classified as water soluble and fat soluble.

WATER-SOLUBLE VITAMINS

The water-soluble vitamins are vitamin C and vitamin B complex, which consists of eight different vitamins. Water-soluble vitamins cannot be stored in the body and must be provided in the daily food intake. It was once assumed that, because water-soluble vitamins are not stored in the body, hypervitaminosis of these vitamins does not occur. However,

TABLE 38-1

Water-Soluble Vitamins

Vitamin	Functions	Results of Deficiency	Results of Excess	Sources	RDA Range*
C (ascorbic acid)	Production of collagen, integrity of capillary walls, formation of red blood cells, metabolism of amino acids, reduction of iron salts, protection of other vitamins from oxidation	Scurvy, poor wound healing, bleeding gums, loose teeth, bruising	Kidney stones, scurvy on withdrawal, urinary tract infection	Citrus fruits, potatoes, cabbage, tomatoes, broccoli, strawberries, cantaloupe, green peppers	35-60 mg/day
VITAMIN B COMPLEX					
B₁ (thiamin)	Component of enzymes, carbohydrate oxidation	Beriberi (rare), polyneuritis, mental confusion, muscular weakness, ataxia, tachycardia, cardiac enlargement	None known	Pork, fish, eggs, poultry, dried beans, whole grains, wheat germ, oatmeal, bread, pasta	0.3-1.5 mg/day
B₂ (riboflavin)	Metabolism of nutrients, essential for growth	Ariboflavinosis: cracks at mouth corners, scaly desquamation of skin around mouth, eye irritation, glossitis, photophobia	Ulcer, elevated blood glucose level, increased uric acid levels in blood	Milk, whole grains, green vegetables, liver	0.4-1.7 mg/day
Niacin	Essential for protein utilization, glycolysis, fat synthesis, tissue repair	Pellagra: weakness, anorexia, lassitude, indigestion; severe pellagra: dermatitis, diarrhea, dementia	Ulcer, liver dysfunction, elevated blood glucose level, increased blood uric acid levels	Meats, dairy products, whole grains, cereals, tuna	6-19 mg/day

*See Table 38-8 for detailed recommendations.
†From Estimated safe and adequate daily dietary intakes, Committee on Dietary Allowances, Food and Nutrition Board, National Academy of Sciences–National Research Council, Washington, D.C., 1980.

TABLE 38-1, cont'd

Water-Soluble Vitamins

Vitamin	Functions	Results of Deficiency	Results of Excess	Sources	RDA Range*
B_6 (complex of pyridoxine, pyridoxal, pyridoxamine)	Metabolism of nutrients, synthesis of nonessential amino acids, conversion of tryptophan to niacin, proper function of blood and central nervous system cells	Gastrointestinal upsets, irritability, weakness, nervousness, convulsions	Reverses antiparkinson effects of levodopa; megadoses: peripheral nerve damage, loss of sensation, numbness, awkward gait	Whole grains, liver, fish, poultry, green beans, nuts, meats, potatoes	0.3-2.2 mg/day
Folacin, folic acid	Metabolism of some amino acids, maturation of red blood cells	Macrocytic anemia	None known; potentially harmful because body is able to store folacin	Liver, green leafy vegetables, meat, fish, poultry, whole grains	30-400 μg/day
B_{12} (cobalamin)	Manufacture of enzymes essential to the metabolism of nutrients, nucleic acid, and folic acid; proper function of the cells of the bone marrow, gastrointestinal tract, and nervous system	Absence of the intrinsic factor in gastric juice prevents absorption of vitamin B_{12} and results in pernicious anemia	None known	Milk, eggs, cheese, meat, fish, poultry, foods of animal origin (plant foods contain no vitamin B_{12})	0.5-3 μg/day
Pantothenic acid	Metabolism of nutrients, synthesis of cholesterol and steroid hormones, activity of adrenal cortex	None known	Increased need for thiamin	Meats, whole grain cereals, legumes	2-7 mg/day†
Biotin	Synthesis of fatty acids, utilization of glucose, metabolism of protein, utilization of vitamin B_{12} and folic acid	Produced by the ingestion of large amounts of raw egg whites that contain a protein substance, avidin, which binds biotin to itself	None known	Liver, kidneys, dark green vegetables, egg yolk, green beans	35-200 μg/day†

recent studies of people who took megadoses of vitamin C and vitamin B_6 indicate that toxicity can occur. Vitamins are chemicals used as catalysts in biochemical reactions. When there is enough of any specific vitamin to meet the catalytic demands, the rest of the vitamin supply acts as a free chemical and may be toxic to the body. Table 38-1 lists the characteristics of water-soluble vitamins.

FAT-SOLUBLE VITAMINS

The fat-soluble vitamins—A, D, E, and K—can be stored in the body, and therefore daily intake is not needed. However, with the exception of vitamin D, these vitamins should be provided by dietary intake. Toxicity to some fat-soluble vitamins has been recognized for years. Toxicity is usually the result of megadoses of synthetic vitamins, but it has also been reported in people whose diet includes a large intake of fish liver.

Processing, storage, and preparation of foods have less effect on fat-soluble vitamin content, and many foods are fortified by the addition of vitamin A and D. The characteristics of the fat-soluble vitamins are listed in Table 38-2.

Minerals

Minerals are inorganic elements that are essential to the body because of their role as catalysts in biochemical reactions. Minerals are classified as macrominerals when the daily requirement is 100 mg or more and microminerals when less than 100 mg is needed daily. Because the required amount of microminerals is usually very small or a trace, microminerals are also referred to as trace elements. The characteristics of macrominerals are summarized in Table 38-3. Those of microminerals are summarized in Table 38-4.

TABLE 38-2

Fat-Soluble Vitamins

Vitamin	Functions	Effects of Deficiency	Effects of Excess	Sources	RDA Range*
A (retinol, retinal, and retinoic acid)	Growth and maintenance of epithelial tissue, maintenance of visual acuity in dim light	Night blindness, rough scaly skin, dry mucous membranes, decreased resistance to infection, faulty tooth and bone development	Nausea, vomiting, abdominal pain, and growth failure in children; weight loss in adults; megadoses: hair loss, bone swelling and tenderness, joint pain, hepatomegaly, splenomegaly	Whole milk, whole milk products, eggs, green leafy vegetables, yellow fruits and vegetables	400-1000 μg/day as retinol equivalents
D (cholecalciferol, ergosterol)	Absorption and utilization of calcium in bone and tooth development	Rickets and delayed dentition in children, osteomalacia in adults	Megadoses: loss of appetite, vomiting, diarrhea, fatigue, growth failure, drowsiness, kidney stones	Sunlight, fortified milk, fortified margarines, fish liver oils	5-10 μg/day
E (tocopherol)	Protection of vitamins A and C and polyunsaturated fatty acids from oxidation, synthesis of heme	Increased hemolysis of red blood cells and macrocytic anemia in premature infants	Interference with the utilization of vitamins A and K, prolonged prothrombin time, intestinal irritability	Vegetable oils, green leafy vegetables, milk, eggs, meats, cereals	3-10 mg/day as alpha-tocopherol equivalents
K	Essential to prothrombin formation and blood clotting	Hemorrhagic disease of the newborn, prolonged clotting time in adults	Hyperbilirubinemia in infants, vomiting in adults	Green leafy vegetables	10-140 μg/day†

*See Table 38-8 for more detailed recommendations.
†From Estimated safe and adequate daily dietary intakes, Committee on Dietary Allowances, Food and Nutrition Board, National Academy of Sciences–National Research Council, Washington, D.C., 1980.

TABLE 38-3

Macrominerals

Mineral	Functions	Effects of Deficiency	Effects of Excess	Sources	RDA Range*
Calcium	Formation of teeth and bones, contraction of muscle fibers, transmission of nerve impulses, activation of enzymes, permeability of cell membranes, coagulation of blood, cardiac function	Tingling of fingers and around mouth, muscle cramps, carpopedal spasm, tetany, convulsions	Relaxed skeletal muscles, deep bone pain, kidney stones, pathological fractures	Milk, milk products	360-1200 mg/day
Chloride	Regulation of osmotic pressure, component of gastric juice, activation of amylase in saliva, regulation of acid-base balance	Alkalosis	Acidosis	Salt added to food in preparation, preservation, processing, and seasoning	275-5100 mg/day†
Magnesium	Supports function of B vitamins; utilization of calcium, potassium, and protein; maintenance of electrical activity in nerves and muscles	Neuromuscular irritability, disorientation, confusion, leg cramps, hallucinations, tachycardia, convulsions, hypertension	Lethargy, respiratory dysfunction, coma, death	Whole grains, fish, nuts, legumes, green vegetables	50-400 mg/day
Phosphorus	Formation of bone and teeth, activation of B vitamins, transfer of energy within cells, promotion of normal muscle and nerve activity, metabolism of carbohydrate, regulation of acid-base balance, transmission of hereditary traits	Hemolytic anemia, defective white blood cell function, delayed clotting, bone pain, pathological fractures	None known	Pork, beef, dried peas and beans	240-1200 mg/day
Potassium	Maintenance of osmotic pressure within cells, participation in intercellular enzyme reactions, conversion of glucose to glycogen, transmission of nerve impulses, contraction of muscle fibers, transmission of electrical impulses in heart	Fatigue, muscle weakness, ileus, paresthesia, weak irregular pulse, increased sensitivity to digitalis, heart block	Anxiety, irritability, hyperactivity of gastrointestinal tract, arrhythmias	Apricots, oranges and orange juice, bananas, tomatoes and tomato juice, potatoes	350-5625 mg/day

Continued.

*See Table 38-8 for more detailed recommendations.
†From Estimated safe and adequate daily dietary intakes, Committee on Dietary Allowances, Food and Nutrition Board, National Academy of Sciences—National Research Council, Washington, D.C., 1980.

TABLE 38-3, cont'd

Macrominerals

Mineral	Functions	Effects of Deficiency	Effects of Excess	Sources	RDA Range*
Sodium	Maintenance of osmotic balance, maintenance of blood volume, participation in intracellular chemical reactions, regulation of acid-base balance	Apprehension, increased gastrointestinal motility, personality change, postural hypotension, cold clammy skin	Thirst, rough red dry tongue, flushed skin, restlessness, agitation, oliguria	Salt, salted foods, ham, preserved meats, milk, meat, eggs, carrots, beets, celery	115-3300 mg/day†
Sulfur	Activation of many oxidation-reduction reactions, participation in detoxification of harmful compounds	None known	None known	Cheese, eggs, poultry, fish	None established

TABLE 38-4

Microminerals

Mineral	Functions	Effects of Deficiency	Effects of Excess	Sources	RDA Range*
Chromium	Proper glucose metabolism, efficient use of insulin, activation of several enzymes	None known	None known	Whole grains, animal protein (except fish and cheese)	0.01-0.2 mg/day†
Cobalt	Component of vitamin B_{12}	None known	None known	Organ meats	Not established
Copper	Essential to hemoglobin formation, cofactor in synthesis of phospholipids, formation and activity of some enzymes, synthesis of prostaglandin	Abnormal blood cell development in infants, bone demineralization	Headache, dizziness, heartburn, weakness, nausea, vomiting, diarrhea, Wilson's disease	Liver, kidney, shellfish, nuts, raisins	0.5-3 mg/day†
Fluoride	Formation of teeth, prevention of dental caries	Poor dental health	Mottling, pitting, and discoloration of tooth enamel	Fluoridated water, seafood, toothpaste, mouthwash gels	0.1-4 mg/day†

*See Table 38-8 for more detailed recommendations.
†From Estimated safe and adequate daily dietary intakes, Committee on Dietary Allowance, Food and Nutrition Board, National Academy of Sciences–National Research Council, Washington, D.C., 1980.

TABLE 38-4, cont'd

Microminerals

Mineral	Functions	Effects of Deficiency	Effects of Excess	Sources	RDA Range*
Iodine	Basic component of thyroid hormones	Cretinism in infants, simple goiter in children and adults	Toxic goiter	Iodized salt, seafood, food additives, dough oxidizers, dairy disinfectants, coloring agents	40-150 µg/day
Iron	Essential to the formation of hemoglobin, synthesis of vitamins, purines, and antibodies	Anemia, fatigue, weakness, lethargy	Hemosiderosis, acute iron poisoning from accidental ingestion in infants and children: cramps, abdominal pain, nausea, vomiting, black stools	Liver, lean meats, whole grains, enriched breads and cereals	10-18 mg/day; pregnant women need 30-60 mg/day of supplemental iron
Manganese	Essential to bone formation, reproduction, and central nervous system function; metabolism of carbohydrate; synthesis of protein	None known	None known	Whole grains, nuts, fruits, vegetables	0.5-5 mg/day†
Molybdenum	Involved in bone formation, growth, and metabolism	None known	Interferes with copper metabolism	Beef liver, whole grains, legumes, organ meats	0.03-0.5 mg/day†
Selenium	Prevents red blood cell destruction, acts as an antioxidant	None known	Dental caries in children	Meats, seafoods, grain content varies with selenium level in soil	0.01-1.2 mg/day†
Zinc	Connective tissue integrity, involvement in immune response, formation of enzymes	Impaired wound healing, decreased sensations of taste and smell	None known	Oysters, liver, meats, poultry, legumes, nuts	3-15 mg/day

In addition to the microminerals in Table 38-4, arsenic, nickel, silicon, tin, vanadium, and possibly cadmium are known to play as yet unidentified roles in human nutrition. The field of minerals is currently a major area of nutrition research.

Digestion

The only nutrients the body can use in their ingested form are monosaccharides, water, vitamins, some minerals, and alcohol. All other foods must be broken down into simpler form for absorption.

Digestion consists of mechanical breakdown by chewing, churning, mixing with fluid, and chemical reactions by which food is reduced to its simplest form. The flow of digestive juice is under hormonal control. Enzymes are an essential component of the chemistry of digestion. They are proteinlike substances that act as catalysts to speed up biochemical reactions. As catalysts, enzymes are not part of the end product of the reaction. Most enzymes have one specific function, although some enzymes are able to enter into several closely related reactions. Enzyme activity is regulated by the pH of the intestinal contents. Each enzyme functions best at a specific pH and will be inactivated by major variations from that level. The secretions of the gastrointestinal tract have vastly different pH levels; saliva is relatively neutral, gastric juice is highly acid, and the secretions of the small intestine are alkaline.

The mechanical, chemical, and hormonal activities of digestion are interdependent. Enzyme activity is dependent on the mechanical breakdown of food to increase its surface area for chemical action. Hormones regulate the flow of digestive secretions needed for enzyme supply, and digestion may also be slowed down or speeded up by strong emotional states. The secretion of digestive juice and motility of the gastrointestinal tract are regulated by physical, chemical, and hormonal factors, and they are intricately bound to psychological, emotional, and nervous system alterations.

Digestion begins in the mouth where food is mechanically broken down by chewing. The food is mixed with saliva, which contains ptyalin (salivary amylase), an enzyme that acts on cooked starch to begin its conversion to maltose. The longer food is chewed, the more starch digestion occurs in the mouth. Proteins and fats are broken down physically but remain unchanged chemically because there are no enzymes in the mouth to act on them. Chewing reduces food particles to a size suitable for swallowing, and saliva provides lubrication to further ease swallowing.

Swallowed food enters the esophagus and is moved along by peristaltic waves. At the cardiac sphincter, the upper opening of the stomach, the presence of the food mass causes the sphincter to relax and allow the food to enter the stomach.

The stomach acts as a reservoir for food. Food remains in the stomach for varying periods depending on the type of meal, gastric motility, and psychological influences. In general, carbohydrate meals spend the least amount of time in the stomach, lipid meals the longest, and protein meals an intermediate period. Large food intake decreases gastric motility and increases the length of time food remains in the stomach. Food remains in the stomach for an average period of 3 hours, with a range of 1 to 7 hours.

The activity of ptyalin continues in the stomach until the presence of hydrochloric acid decreases the pH sufficiently to inactivate it. The stomach churns the food mass, mixing it with gastric secretions and causing further breakdown in the size of the food particles. The acid environment favors the action of pepsin. Pepsin is an enzyme that splits proteins into proteoses and peptones. Lipase, an enzyme that functions best in an alkaline medium, is able to act on emulsified fats such as butter, egg yolk, milk, and cream at near-neutral pH levels. Lipase splits emulsified fats into fatty acids and glycerol.

Food leaves the stomach at the pyloric sphincter as an acid, liquefied mass called chyme. Chyme flows into the duodenum and is quickly mixed with bile, intestinal juices, and pancreatic secretions. Bile emulsifies fat to permit enzyme action, and it holds fatty acids in solution.

Intestinal secretions contain seven enzymes: lipase for fat digestion, aminopolypeptidase and dipeptidase for protein digestion, and amylase, sucrase, lactase, and maltase for carbohydrate digestion.

Pancreatic juice contains five enzymes: amylase, which digests starch; lipase, which breaks down emulsified fats; and trypsin, chymotrypsin, and carboxypolypeptide, which enter into reactions with proteins.

Peristalsis continues in the small intestine, mixing the secretions with the chyme. The mixture becomes increasingly alkaline, inhibiting the action of the gastric enzymes and promoting the action of the duodenal secretions. The major portion of digestion occurs in the small intestine, producing glucose, fructose, and galactose from carbohydrates; amino acids from proteins; and fatty acids and glycerol from lipids.

Absorption

The small intestine is also the site of absorption of simple nutrients. The small intestine is lined with numerous villi that project into the lumen and greatly

TABLE 38-5

Sites of Absorption of Nutrients

Upper Duodenum	Lower Duodenum	Upper Jejenum	Lower Jejenum	Ileum
	←———— Glucose ————→		←——— Sucrose ———→	
	←———— Amino acids ————→		←——— Lactose ———→	
	←——— Fats ———→		←——— Maltose ———→	
Cholesterol	←—— Lumen of the small intestine ——————————————→			
←———————— Iron ————————————→				
←———————— Calcium ————————————→				
		Vitamin D*		Vitamin D*
←———————— Vitamin A ————————→				
Vitamin E		Vitamin B$_6$		
Vitamin K				
Folic acid				
Riboflavin				
Thiamin	Minerals	Ascorbic acid		Vitamin B$_{12}$

Modified from Bodinski, L.: The nurse's guide to diet therapy, New York, 1982, John Wiley & Sons, Inc.
*Site of absorption controversial.

increase the surface area available for absorption. Table 38-5 illustrates the areas of absorption of specific nutrients. Table 38-6 depicts the means and route of absorption of major nutrients.

The intestinal contents continue to move by peristaltic action into the large intestine. Water is the only nutrient that is absorbed from the large intestine. Other nutrients remaining in the intestinal contents when they reach the large intestine are lost to the body and will be excreted as waste products. When intestinal motility is increased, as in diarrhea, the body loses nutrients that move through the small intestine too quickly for complete absorption.

METABOLISM

Nutrients absorbed in the intestines, including water, are transported through the circulatory system to body tissues. Through metabolism, nutrients are converted by chemical changes into a number of substances the body requires. Carbohydrates, protein, and fat undergo metabolism to produce chemical energy and to maintain a dynamic balance of tissue buildup and breakdown. In order to carry out the body's work the chemical energy produced by metabolism is converted to other types of energy by different tissues. Muscle contracture involves mechanical energy, the nervous system involves electrical energy, the mechanisms of heat production involve thermal energy, and so on, and these forms of energy all originate in metabolism. The interrelationships of protein, carbohydrate, and fat metabolism are depicted in Fig. 38-1.

The two basic types of metabolism are anabolism and catabolism. Anabolism is the production of more complex chemical substances by synthesis of nutrients. Catabolism is the breakdown of chemical substances into simpler substances. Although catabolism produces some energy, both processes require energy, which must be provided from either food or stored energy sources.

STORAGE

Some but not all of the nutrients required by the body are stored in body tissues. The body's major form of stored energy is fat stored in the adipose tissue, which has an almost unlimited capacity. Glycogen is stored in small reserves in liver and muscle tissue, and protein is stored in muscle mass. When the body's energy requirements exceed the energy supplied by ingested nutrients, stored energy is used; conversely, unused energy is stored, principally in fat.

Fat-soluble vitamins are also stored in limited reserves and are released to meet the body's needs when not provided sufficiently by dietary intake. Water-soluble vitamins are not stored and therefore must be provided by daily dietary intake.

TABLE 38-6

Intestinal Absorption of Some Major Nutrients

Nutrient	Form	Means of Absorption	Control Agent or Required Cofactor	Route
Carbohydrate	Monosaccharides (glucose and galactose)	Competitive Selective Active transport via sodium pump	— — Sodium	Blood
Protein	Amino acids	Selective	—	Blood
	Some dipeptides	Carrier transport systems	Pyridoxine (pyridoxal phosphate)	Blood
	Whole protein (rare)	Pinocytosis	—	Blood
Fat	Fatty acids	Fatty acid–bile complex (micelles)	Bile	Lymph
	Glycerides (mono-, di-)		—	Lymph
	Few triglycerides (neutral fat)	Pinocytosis	—	Lymph
Vitamins	B$_{12}$	Carrier transport	Intrinsic factor (IF)	Blood
	A	Bile complex	Bile	Blood
	K	Bile complex	Bile	From large intestine to blood
Minerals	Sodium	Active transport via sodium pump	—	Blood
	Calcium	Active transport	Vitamin D	Blood
	Iron	Active transport	Ferritin mechanism	Blood (as transferritin)
Water	Water	Osmosis	—	Blood, lymph, interstitial fluid

From Williams, S.R.: Nutrition and diet therapy, ed. 4, St. Louis, 1984, The C.V. Mosby Co.

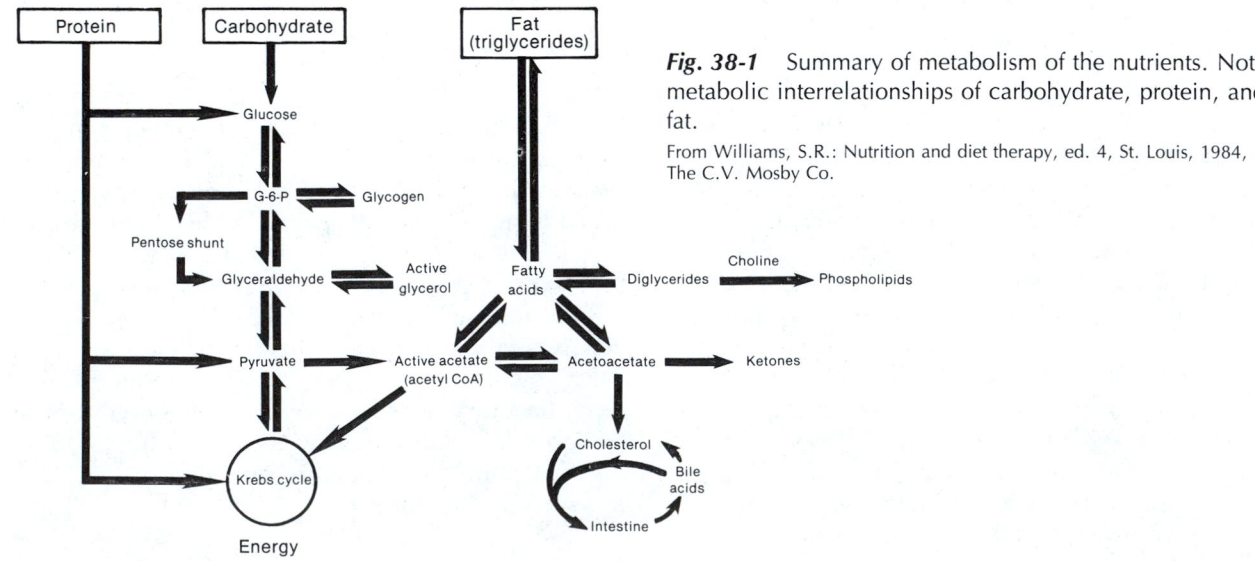

Fig. 38-1 Summary of metabolism of the nutrients. Note metabolic interrelationships of carbohydrate, protein, and fat.

From Williams, S.R.: Nutrition and diet therapy, ed. 4, St. Louis, 1984, The C.V. Mosby Co.

Elimination

The intestinal contents move through the various segments of the large intestine by peristalsis. As the material moves toward the rectum, water is absorbed into the mucosa. The longer the material stays in the large intestine, the more water is absorbed and the firmer the remaining solid material becomes.

The end products of digestion include cellulose and similar fibrous substances that the body is unable to digest, sloughed cells from the intestinal walls, mucus, digestive secretions, water, and microorganisms.

TABLE 38-7

Daily Dietary Guide—the Basic Four Food Groups

Food Group	Main Nutrients	Daily Amounts*
Milk		
Milk, cheese, ice cream, or other products made with whole or skimmed milk	Calcium, protein, riboflavin	Children under 9: 2-3 cups Children 9-12: 3 or more cups Teenagers: 4 or more cups Adults: 2 or more cups Pregnant women: 3 or more cups Nursing mothers: 4 or more cups (1 cup = 8 ounces fluid milk or designated milk equivalent†)
Meats		
Beef, veal, lamb, pork, poultry, fish, eggs	Protein, iron, thiamin	2 or more servings Count as 1 serving: 2-3 ounces of lean, boneless, cooked meat, poultry, or fish 2 eggs
Alternates: dry beans, dry peas, nuts, peanut butter	Niacin, riboflavin	1 cup cooked dry beans or peas 4 tbsp peanut butter
Vegetables and fruits		4 or more servings Count as 1 serving: ½ cup of vegetable or fruit or a portion such as 1 medium apple, banana, orange, potato, or ½ a medium grapefruit, melon Include
	Vitamin A	A dark-green or deep-yellow vegetable or fruit rich in vitamin A at least every other day
	Vitamin C (ascorbic acid)	A citrus fruit or other fruit or vegetable rich in vitamin C daily
	Smaller amounts of other vitamins and minerals	Other vegetables and fruits including potatoes
Bread and cereals	Thiamin, niacin, riboflavin, iron, protein	4 or more servings of whole grain, enriched or restored Count as 1 serving: 1 slice of bread 1 ounce (1 cup) ready to eat cereal, flake or puff varieties ½-¾ cup cooked cereal ½-¾ cup cooked pastes (macaroni, spaghetti, noodles) Crackers: 5 saltines, 2 squares graham crackers, etc.

From Williams, S.: Nutrition and diet therapy, ed. 4, St. Louis, 1984, The C.V. Mosby Co.
*Use additional amounts of these foods or added butter, margarine, oils, sugars, etc., as desired or needed.
†Milk equivalents: 1 ounce cheddar cheese, 3 servings cottage cheese, 1 cup fluid skimmed milk, 1 cup buttermilk, ½ cup dry skimmed milk powder, 1 cup ice milk, 1⅔ cups ice cream, ½ cup evaporated milk.

Foundations of an Adequate Diet

Basic Four Food Groups

The identification of nutrients essential to life and the establishment of recommendations of the approximate amounts of these nutrients needed by the body led to the search for a formula for an adequate diet. One of the earliest recommendations for healthful food intake was to ingest a well-balanced diet. It was theorized that, because almost every living thing depends on intake of similar amounts of the same chemicals for health, selecting foods from a wide variety of different animal, vegetable, and fish products would ensure the required amounts of needed nutrients.

The well-balanced diet, although a sound concept, was too nonspecific for sound meal planning. The seven basic food groups, later revised to four basic groups, was developed as a guide to meal planning.

The basic food group guide lists the number of servings from each of the four groups needed to meet daily requirements of essential nutrients. Recommended intakes vary with age, and the guide includes serving size (Table 38-7).

The basic four food group plan in the recommended amounts provides approximately 1200 kcal. Additional foods to round out meals and meet energy requirements can be selected from unenriched cereals and flours and products made from them, sugars, and butter, margarine, and other fats.

Recommended Dietary Allowances

The Committee on Dietary Allowances of the Food and Nutrition Board of the National Academy of Sciences has published a list of recommended dietary allowances (RDAs) since 1943. The RDAs are the level of intake of essential nutrients considered, in the judgment of the committee on the basis of scientific

TABLE 38-8

Food and Nutrition Board, National Academy of Sciences–National Research Council,

	Age (years)	Weight (kg)	Weight (lb)	Height (cm)	Height (in)	Protein (g)	Fat-Soluble Vitamins Vitamin A (μgRE)[b]	Vitamin D (μg)[c]	Vitamin E (mgα-TE)[d]	Vitamin C (mg)
Infants	0.0-0.5	6	13	60	24	kg × 2.2	420	10	3	35
	0.5-1.0	9	20	71	28	kg × 2.0	400	10	4	35
Children	1-3	13	29	90	35	23	400	10	5	45
	4-6	20	44	112	44	30	500	10	6	45
	7-10	28	62	132	52	34	700	10	7	45
Males	11-14	45	99	157	62	45	1,000	10	8	50
	15-18	66	145	176	69	56	1,000	10	10	60
	19-22	70	154	177	70	56	1,000	7.5	10	60
	23-50	70	154	178	70	56	1,000	5	10	60
	51 +	70	154	178	70	56	1,000	5	10	60
Females	11-14	46	101	157	62	46	800	10	8	50
	15-18	55	120	163	64	46	800	10	8	60
	19-22	55	120	163	64	44	800	7.5	8	60
	23-50	55	120	163	64	44	800	5	8	60
	51 +	55	120	163	64	44	800	5	8	60
Pregnant						+30	+200	+5	+2	+20
Lactating						+20	+400	+5	+3	+40

From Recommended dietary allowances, ed. 9, Washington, D.C., 1980, National Academy of Sciences, by permission of the Academy.
[a]The allowances are intended to provide for individual variations among most normal persons as they live in the United States under usual environmental stresses. Diets should be based on a variety of common foods to provide other nutrients for which human requirements have been less well defined. See text for detailed discussions of allowances and of nutrients not tabulated.
[b]Retinol equivalents. 1 retinol equivalent = 1 microgram of retinol or 6 micrograms of β-carotene. See text for calculation of vitamin A activity of diets as retinol equivalents.
[c]As cholecalciferol; 10 micrograms of cholecalciferol = 400 International Units of vitamin D.
[d]α Tocopherol equivalents; 1 milligram of d-α-tocopherol = 1 α-TE. See text for variation in allowances and calculation of vitamin E activity of the diet as α-tocopherol equivalents.

knowledge, to be adequate to meet the nutritional needs of practically all healthy people. The RDAs were originally designed as a guide for planning and securing food supplies for national defense during World War II. Now they are revised every 5 years to incorporate changes and new knowledge based on research. The RDAs are designed for population groups, not for individuals, and they exceed the requirements for most healthy individuals. The nutrients in the RDAs should be supplied by a wide variety of foods. The 1980 RDAs include an estimated safe and adequate intake of some minerals for which RDAs are not established. These estimates were used in the preparation of Tables 38-1 through 38-4. RDAs for 1980 appear in Table 38-8.

In 1941 the Food and Drug Administration established minimum daily requirements, standards that represented minimum intake for each nutrient. These standards were replaced in 1968 by the U.S. recommended daily allowances (U.S. RDAs), which are used only in food labeling. Unless a food has added nutrients or the manufacturer makes nutritional claims for it, nutritional labeling is voluntary. In most cases the single value used is the highest amount listed in the RDA (excluding recommendations for infants or pregnant or lactating women). In labeling, amounts present are expressed as a percentage of the U.S. RDAs. The U.S. RDA for iron is 18 mg, for example, and if a serving of oatmeal contains 0.72 mg of iron, the container would be labeled to indicate that one serving contains 4% of the U.S. RDA for iron.

The Canadian recommended daily nutrient intakes—published by the Committee for Revision of the Canadian Dietary Standard, Bureau of Nutritional Sciences, Health and Welfare—are similar to those of the United States. The Canadian standards for 1982, which include the same nutrients, list 20 age categories compared to 17 in the U.S. tables (Table 38-9.)

Recommended Daily Dietary Allowances,[a] Revised 1980

Water-Soluble Vitamins						Minerals					
Thiamine (mg)	Riboflavin (mg)	Niacin (mg NE)[e]	Vitamin B$_6$ (mg)	Folacin[f] (µg)	Vitamin B$_{12}$ (µg)	Calcium (mg)	Phosphorous (mg)	Magnesium (mg)	Iron (mg)	Zinc (mg)	Iodine (µg)
0.3	0.4	6	0.3	30	0.5[g]	360	240	50	10	3	40
0.5	0.6	8	0.6	45	1.5	540	360	70	15	5	50
0.7	0.8	9	0.9	100	2.0	800	800	150	15	10	70
0.9	1.0	11	1.3	200	2.5	800	800	200	10	10	90
1.2	1.4	16	1.6	300	3.0	800	800	250	10	10	120
1.4	1.6	18	1.8	400	3.0	1,200	1,200	350	18	15	150
1.4	1.7	18	2.0	400	3.0	1,200	1,200	400	18	15	150
1.5	1.7	19	2.2	400	3.0	800	800	350	10	15	150
1.4	1.6	18	2.2	400	3.0	800	800	350	10	15	150
1.2	1.4	16	2.2	400	3.0	800	800	350	10	15	150
1.1	1.3	15	1.8	400	3.0	1,200	1,200	300	18	15	150
1.1	1.3	14	2.0	400	3.0	1,200	1,200	300	18	15	150
1.1	1.3	14	2.0	400	3.0	800	800	300	18	15	150
1.0	1.2	13	2.0	400	3.0	800	800	300	18	15	150
1.0	1.2	13	2.0	400	3.0	800	800	300	10	15	150
+0.4	+0.3	+2	+0.6	+400	+1.0	+400	+400	+150	[h]	+5	+25
+0.5	+0.5	+5	+0.5	+100	+1.0	+400	+400	+150	[h]	+10	+50

[e]1 NE (niacin equivalent) is equal to 1 milligram of niacin, or 60 milligrams of dietary tryptophan.

[f]Folacin allowances refer to dietary sources as determined by *Lactobacillus casei* assay after treatment with enzymes (conjugases) to make polyglutamyl forms of the vitamin available to the test organism.

[g]The recommended dietary allowances for vitamin B$_{12}$ in infants are based on the average concentration of the vitamin in human milk. The allowances after weaning are based on energy intake (as recommended by the American Academy of Pediatrics) and consideration of other factors, such as intestinal absorption; see text.

[h]The increased requirement during pregnancy cannot be met by the iron content of habitual American diets or by the existing iron stores of many women; therefore the use of 30 to 60 milligrams of supplemental iron is recommended. Iron needs during lactation are not substantially different from those of nonpregnant women, but continued supplementation of the mother for 2 to 3 months after parturition is advisable to replenish stores depleted by pregnancy.

TABLE 38-9

Recommended Nutrient Intakes for Canadians: Average Energy Requirements and

Age	Sex	Average Height (cm)[c]	Average weight (kg)[c]	Requirements[a,b]					
				kcal/kg[c,d]	MJ/kg[d]	kcal/day[e]	MJ/day[f]	kcal/cm[g]	MJ/cm[f]
MONTHS									
0-2	Both	55	4.5	120-100	0.50-0.42	500	3.0	9	0.04
3-5	Both	63	7.0	100-95	0.42-0.40	700	2.8	11	0.05
6-8	Both	69	8.5	95-97	0.40-0.41	800	3.4	11.5	0.05
9-11	Both	73	9.5	97-99	0.41	950	3.8	12.5	0.05
YEARS									
1	Both	82	11	101	0.42	1100	4.8	13.5	0.06
2-3	Both	95	14	94	0.39	1300	5.6	13.5	0.06
4-6	Both	107	18	100	0.42	1800	7.6	17	0.07
7-9	M	126	25	88	0.37	2200	9.2	17.5	0.07
	F	125	25	76	0.32	1900	8.0	15	0.06
10-12	M	141	34	73	0.30	2500	10.4	17.5	0.07
	F	143	36	61	0.25	2200	9.2	15.5	0.06
13-15	M	159	50	57	0.24	2800	12.0	17.5	0.07
	F	157	48	46	0.19	2200	9.2	14	0.06
16-18	M	172	62	51	0.21	3200	13.2	18.5	0.08
	F	160	53	40	0.17	2100	8.8	13	0.05
19-24	M	175	71	42	0.18	3000	12.4		
	F	160	58	36	0.15	2100	8.8		
25-49	M	172	74	36	0.15	2700	11.2		
	F	160	59	32	0.13	1900	8.0		
50-74	M	170	73	31	0.13	2300	9.6		
	F	158	63	29	0.12	1800	7.6		
75+	M	168	69	29	0.12	2000	8.4		
	F	155	64	23	0.10	1500	6.0		
Pregnancy (additional)[h]									
First trimester									
Second trimester									
Third trimester									
Lactation (additional)[h]									

From Bureau of Nutritional Sciences, Department of National Health and Welfare, Ottawa, Canada, 1982.
[a]Recommended nutrient intakes for Canadians, 1982—Committee for the revision of the Dietary Standard for Canada, Bureau of Nutritional Sciences, Department of National Health and Welfare. Recommended intakes of energy and of certain nutrients are not listed in this table because of the nature of the variables upon which they are based. The figures for energy are estimates of average requirements for expected patterns of activity. For nutrients not shown, the following amounts are recommended: thiamin, 0.4 mg/100 kcal (0.48 mg/5000 kJ); riboflavin, 0.5 mg/1000 kcal (0.6 mg/5000 kJ); niacin, 6.6 NE/1000 kcal (7.9 NE/5000 kJ); vitamin B_6, 15 μg, as pyridoxine, per gram of protein intake; phosphorus, same as calcium. Recommended intakes during periods of growth are taken as appropriate for individual representative of the midpoint in each age group. All recommended intakes are designed to cover individual variations in essentially all of a healthy population subsisting upon a variety of common foods available in Canada. It is emphasized that these are examples of the application of the RNI to particular classes of individuals and/or particular situations.
[b]Requirements can be expected to vary within a range of ±30%.
[c]Figures rounded to the closest whole number when ≥10 and to the closest 0.5 when <10.
[d]First and last figures are averages of the beginning and at the end of the 3-month period.
[e]Figures rounded to the nearest 50 when <1000 and to the nearest 100 when ≥1000.
[f]Figures include 2 decimals if value is <1 and 1 decimal if ≥1.

Summary Examples of Recommended Nutrient Intakes

Protein (g/day)[i]	Fat-Soluble Vitamins			Water-Soluble Vitamins			Minerals				
	Vit A (RE/day)[j]	Vit D (µg/day)[k]	Vit E (mg/day)[l]	Vit C (mg/day)	Folacin (µg/day)[m]	Vit B_{12} (µg/day)	Ca (mg/day)	Mg (mg/day)	Fe (mg/day)	I (µg/day)	Zn (mg/day)
11[n]	400	10	3	20	50	0.3	350	30	0.4[o]	25	2[p]
14[n]	400	10	3	20	50	0.3	350	40	5	35	3
16[n]	400	10	3	20	50	0.3	400	45	7	40	3
18	400	10	3	20	55	0.3	400	50	7	45	3
18	400	10	3	20	65	0.3	500	55	6	55	4
20	400	5	4	20	80	0.4	500	65	6	65	4
25	500	5	5	25	90	0.5	600	90	6	85	5
31	700	2.5	7	35	125	0.8	700	110	7	110	6
29	700	2.5	6	30	125	0.8	700	110	7	95	7
38	800	2.5	8	40	170	1.0	900	150	10	125	6
39	800	2.5	7	40	170	1.0	1000	160	10	110	7
49	900	2.5	9	50	160	1.5	1100	220	12	160	9
43	800	2.5	7	45	160	1.5	800	190	13	160	8
54	1000	2.5	10	55	190	1.9	900	240	10	160	9
47	800	2.5	7	45	160	1.9	700	220	14	160	8
57	1000	2.5	10	60	210	2.0	800	240	8	160	9
41	800	2.5	7	45	165	2.0	700	190	14	160	8
57	1000	2.5	9	60	210	2.0	800	240	8	160	9
41	800	2.5	6	45	165	2.0	700	190	14[q]	160	8
57	1000	2.5	7	60	210	2.0	800	240	8	160	9
41	800	2.5	6	45	165	2.0	800	190	7	160	8
57	1000	2.5	6	60	210	2.0	800	240	8	160	9
41	800	2.5	5	45	165	2.0	800	190	7	160	8
15	100	2.5	2	0	305	1.0	500	15	6	25	0
20	100	2.5	2	20	305	1.0	500	20	6	25	1
25	100	2.5	2	20	305	1.0	500	25	6	25	2
20	400	2.5	3	30	120	0.5	500	80	0	50	6

[g]Figures rounded to the nearest 0.5.
[h]Pregnancy: Add 100 kcal during the first trimester and 300 for the second and third trimesters. Lactation: Add 450 kcal/day.
[i]The primary units are grams per kilogram of body weight. The figures shown here are only examples.
[j]One retinol equivalent (RE) corresponds to the biological activity of 1 µg of retinol, 6 µg of β-carotene or 12 µg of other carotenes.
[k]Expressed as cholecalciferol or ergocalciferol.
[l]Expressed as d-α-tocopherol equivalents, relative to which β-and-γ-tocopherol and α-tocotrienol have activities of 0.5, 0.1 and 0.3 respectively.
[m]Expressed as total folate.
[n]Assumption that the protein is from breast milk or is of the same biological value as that of breast milk and that between 3 and 9 months adjustment for the quality of the protein is made.
[o]For the infant it is assumed that breast milk is the source of iron up to 2 months of age.
[p]Based on the assumption that breast milk is the source of zinc up to 2 months of age.
[q]After the menopause the recommended intake is 7 mg/day.

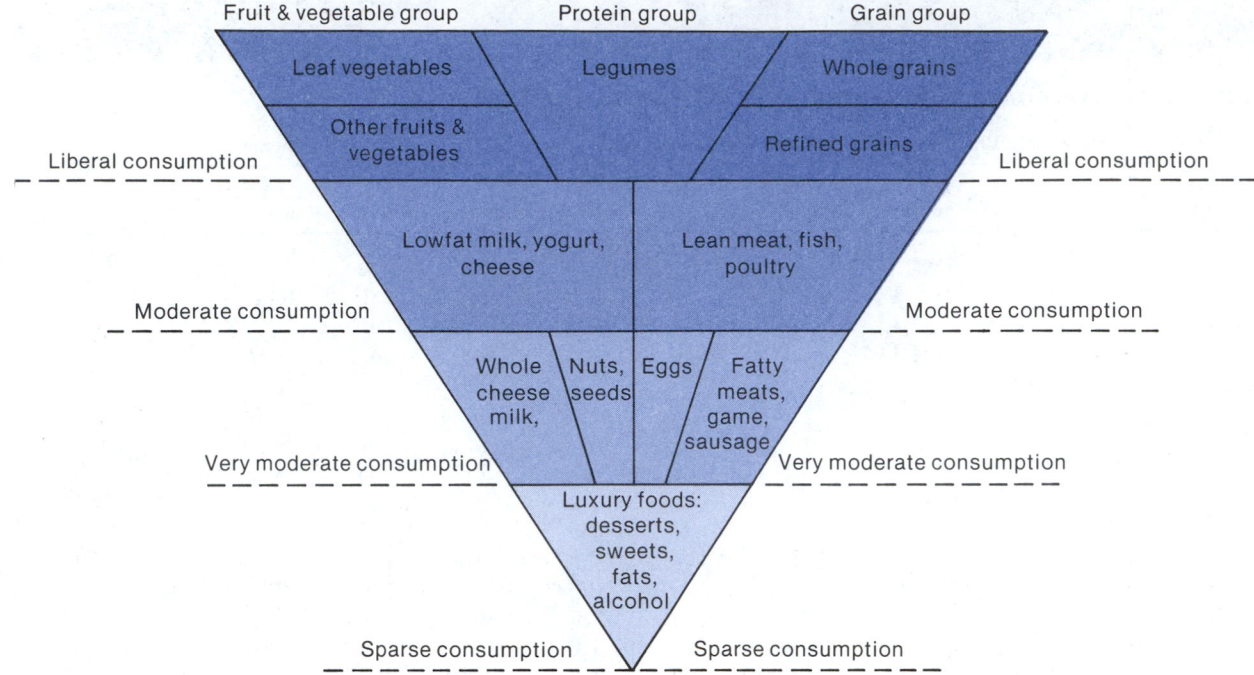

Fig. 38-2 A suggested food guide.
From Pennington, J.: J. Nutr. Education **13**:53, 1981.

Other Dietary Guidelines

In 1977 the Senate Select Committee on Nutrition and Human Needs formulated guidelines for Americans, designed to help them avoid some of the nutrition-related problems identified by research studies. These guidelines, directed at the problems of obesity, excessive intake of fats, cholesterol, sugar, salt, and inadequate intake of fiber, relate to heart disease, cancer, gastrointestinal disorders, diabetes mellitus, and other health problems. The seven recommendations are to:

1. Avoid overweight by controlling caloric intake and increasing exercise
2. Increase intake of complex carbohydrates and naturally occurring sugars from 28% to 48% of the energy intake
3. Reduce intake of refined sugars from 45% to 10% of total caloric intake
4. Reduce fat intake from 40% to 30% of energy intake
5. Reduce saturated fat intake to 10% and receive the rest of fat intake from 10% each of unsaturated and polyunsaturated fats
6. Reduce cholesterol to approximately 300 mg per day
7. Reduce salt intake to 5 g (2+ teaspoonfuls)

The U.S. Department of Agriculture and the Department of Health and Human Services issued dietary guidelines for Americans in 1980. These guidelines are more general and recommend approximately the same changes, although they do not specify amounts of intake. They also include a recommendation related to alcohol intake, which was not included in the earlier Senate committee guidelines. The seven recommendations advise Americans to:

1. Eat a variety of foods
2. Maintain ideal body weight
3. Include adequate starch and fiber in the diet
4. Avoid too much sugar
5. Avoid too much fat, saturated fat, and cholesterol
6. Avoid too much sodium
7. Consume alcohol in moderation if at all

Opponents of the guidelines believe that the 1977 guidelines were too radical and that recommendations should not be formulated for an entire population but should be based on individual evaluation.

A recent food guide (Pennington, 1981) attempts to incorporate limitation of problem nutrients, available food supplies, and health promotion into the basic recommendations. This plan consists of four food groups and four levels of consumption. The four food groups are group I: vegetables and fruit; group II: grains; group III: vegetable, dairy, and meat sources of protein; and group IV: luxury foods such as desserts, sweets, fats, and alcohol.

The four levels of consumption are level I: liberal; level II: moderate; level III: very moderate; and level

TABLE 38-10

Portion Sizes and Suggested Servings Per Day from the Inverse Pyramid Food Guide

Food Group	Example of Portion Sizes	Suggested Servings Per Day	
		Teens and Adults	Children
Vegetables and fruits	¼-1 c raw, ½ c cooked leafy greens ¼-½ c dried fruit ½ c fruit or vegetable juice ¼ c other fruits and vegetables	6 or more with at least 1 from leafy greens	4 or more with at least 1 from leafy greens
Grains and grain products	1 slice bread, 1 waffle, 1 tortilla ½ c cooked cereal ½ c rice, noodles, grits ¾-1 c ready to eat cereal	6 or more with at least 3 from whole grains	4 or more with at least 2 from whole grains
Protein foods*	1 c milk, yogurt 1 oz cheese, meat, fish, poultry 1 egg ½ c cooked legumes 2 tbsp peanut butter 2 oz seeds, nuts	6 to 15 with at least 2 from dairy foods and at least 4 from others	6 to 15 with at least 3 from dairy foods and at least 3 from others

Luxury foods	Desserts
	  ½ c pudding, ice cream
	  2 cookies
	  Small slice cake
	Fats
	  1 tbsp butter, oil
	Sweets
	  1 tbsp sugar, honey
		Children, Teens, and Adults
		Desserts
		  1 or less
		Fats
		  4 or less
		Sweets
		  4 or less	

	Alcohol 1 oz liquor 4 oz wine 12 oz beer	**Adults Only** Alcohol—1 or less	

From Pennington, J.: J. Nutr. Education **13**:54, 1981.
*Small portion sizes are specified in order to encourage a wide variety.

IV: sparse. Food groups I and II should be taken at the first level of consumption. Food group III contains foods to be taken at three different levels. Legumes in group III are to be consumed liberally or at level I and skim and low-fat milk dairy products, lean meat, and poultry at level II or moderate intake. Luncheon meats, whole milk dairy products, sausage, nuts, seeds, peanuts, eggs, and fatty meats or game should be consumed at level III or very moderately. Sparse consumption of foods in the luxury group IV is recommended. Fig. 38-2 shows the food guide as a reverse pyramid. Table 38-10 lists the recommended intake and serving sizes.

Alternative Food Patterns

Long before recommended allowances and guidelines were issued, many people followed special patterns of food intake based on religion, cultural background, ethics, health beliefs, personal preference, or concern for the efficient use of land to produce food. Such special diets are not necessarily more or less nutritional than diets based on the basic four food groups or other nutritional guidelines, since good nutrition depends on a balanced intake of all required nutrients. Two common dietary patterns are vegetarian diets and "natural" or "health food" diets.

VEGETARIAN DIETS

Vegetarianism is the consumption of a diet consisting predominantly of plant foods. Vegetarians may be ovolactovegetarians, who avoid meat, fish, and poultry but include eggs and milk in their diet, or lactovegetarians, who include milk in the diet but avoid eggs. Vegans, or pure vegetarians, consume only plant foods, avoiding meat, poultry, fish, seafood, eggs, and dairy products. A semivegetarian may eat seafood or poultry or both in addition to plant foods.

Vegetarian diets are of concern because some of the foods that are excluded from the diet are important sources of essential nutrients. Animal foods, for example, are the only source of vitamin B_{12}. Protein is apt to be insufficient in the vegan diet, especially for growing children and pregnant women. Plant foods contain amino acids but not in sufficient quantity or variety. The use of complementary proteins usually solves this problem in the well-planned vegan diet. Combining grains with legumes or legumes with seeds supplies all the essential amino acids in adequate amounts.

Calcium deficiency is a possible problem when milk is excluded from the diet. Soybean milk fortified with calcium, leafy green vegetables, and tofu (soybean curd) that has been precipitated by the addition of calcium can protect against deficiency. In the absence of red meat intake, iron deficiency is a possibility unless the diet is rich in whole grains, green leafy vegetables, and vitamin C to enhance iron absorption.

NATURAL OR HEALTH FOOD DIETS

Some people adhere to diets that include only foods produced without chemical fertilizers or organically grown. The label "organically grown" does not always ensure that a food is free from chemicals or that it is superior to other foods. The use of chemical fertilizers often improves foods by increasing the nutrient content of the soil in which they are grown. Chemicals used in processing and preservation of foodstuffs make some foods available when they are normally out of season, as well as protecting against insect and bacterial invasion.

"Health foods" are foods for which specific health promotion claims are made. These claims are usually unfounded, and often these foods are significantly more expensive (see later section on food fads).

Natural foods and health foods are not harmful if they are part of a well-balanced diet; the major danger is that the higher cost of these special foods may limit expenditures for essential nutrients.

Developmental Variables in Nutrition

Infants

Infancy is a period characterized by rapid growth and high energy requirements. The average birth weight of an American baby is 3.2 to 3.4 kg (7 to 7½ pounds). The infant usually doubles birth weight

at 4 to 5 months and triples it at 1 year of age. An energy intake of approximately 117 kcal/kg body weight is needed in the first half of infancy and 108 kcal/kg in the second half.

A full-term newborn infant is able to digest and absorb simple carbohydrates, proteins, and a moderate amount of fat. Amylase, the starch-splitting enzyme, is not present at birth. Because a large proportion of the infant's total body weight is water, fluid requirements are high.

BREAST-FED INFANTS

Breast milk is the ideal food for infants. The current recommendation is that breast milk be the major source of nutrients in the first 6 months of life. Breast-feeding reduces the incidence of infantile allergy by avoiding the early introduction of antigens often present in infant formulas and foods. As the infant grows, the gastrointestinal tract provides a more secure barrier against antigenic proteins.

In addition to supplying the essential nutrients, breast milk also provides protective maternal antibodies and promotes bonding. The lipid content of breast milk is more readily absorbed than the lipid content of other infant foods. Breast milk provides more of the essential fatty acid linoleic acid than other foods. There is some indication that breast-feeding may prevent infant obesity and protect against hypercholesterolemia in later life. At the end of the nursing period, breast milk has a higher fat content that is thought to provide satiety and stop the infant from sucking. The higher cholesterol level of breast milk in comparison with other infant formulas is thought by some authorities to foster the development of more efficient cholesterol metabolism.

Breast-fed infants need a source of vitamin C, fluoride, vitamin D, and iron. Diluted orange juice can be introduced at 1 to 2 months of age, with the amount of diluent gradually decreased until the infant is receiving full-strength juice. Vitamin C can be supplied as a supplement for the infant with a family history of allergy. Fluoride should be given as a supplement in areas where the water supply is not fluoridated or if the infant does not drink enough fluoridated water to meet the needs for this mineral. Vitamin D is also given as a vitamin supplement. After 4 months, when the fetal store of red blood cells is exhausted, the infant needs a dietary source of iron. Premature infants, who lacked the opportunity to store iron, need iron earlier and appear to absorb it better than full-term infants.

BOTTLE-FED INFANTS

Bottle-fed infants are usually given 5% to 10% glucose 4 hours after birth. This practice is questioned by those who advocate reduced intake of refined sugar, believing that early introduction to sugar fosters a desire for sweet foods. The infant who handles the glucose feeding well progresses to diluted formula and then to full-strength formula. Infant formulas, designed to duplicate human milk as closely as possible, can also be fortified with vitamins and minerals. Many formulas are available premixed and bottled for individual feedings.

Neither undiluted whole milk nor skim milk should be used as a basis for infant formulas. Whole milk has excessive protein and requires dilution, and skim milk lacks linoleic acid. Although whole milk may be given when the bottle-fed infant is 4 to 6 months of age, skim milk should not be given to infants. Bottle-fed babies need a fluoride supplement if the water supply is not fluoridated. They also should be given diluted orange juice or a vitamin C supplement at 1 to 2 months of age.

Bottle-fed infants need the opportunity for non-nutritive sucking and should be given boiled water or allowed to suck nonsweetened pacifiers. Bottle-fed babies should not be expected to finish the bottle at every feeding as long as weight gain and growth proceed normally. Feedings should not be used as a method of keeping the infant from fussing.

INTRODUCTION TO SOLID FOOD

The ability to swallow voluntarily is not fully developed until 10 to 12 weeks of age. Before that time swallowing must be stimulated by sucking. The amount of saliva needed to ease the swallowing of solid food is not secreted until about 3 months of age. The extrusion reflex (pushing food out of the mouth with the tongue) lasts until the infant is 4 months old. Taste sensation is not present until 3 to 4 months of age. Consequently, spoon feeding is not developmentally sound until 4 to 6 months of age.

Enriched rice cereal, the first solid food for both breast-fed and bottle-fed infants, may be introduced at 4 to 6 months of age. Other grain cereals will follow later. Cereals provide iron, calcium, phosphorus, thiamin, riboflavin, and niacin. Meat is an alternative first food for breast-fed babies. Some pediatricians prefer it because of its iron and protein content. Vegetables are usually given at 7 months, fruits at 8 months, and meat and cottage cheese at 9 months. Earlier introduction of meat for the bottle-fed infant results in excessive protein intake.

Infants should be introduced to new foods in small servings, one new food at a time, to permit recognition of allergies. They should be exposed to a wide variety of foods to ensure intake of essential nutrients. The texture of solid food progresses from strained to mashed to minced to chopped to cut table foods. When the teeth begin to emerge, the infant will enjoy toast, zwieback, and crackers.

Toddlers and Preschoolers

The growth rate slows during the toddler period (1 to 3 years of age). The toddler needs fewer calories but an increased amount of protein in relation to body weight. Toddlers, struggling for autonomy, are more interested in their environment and increasing motor skills than in food.

The toddler needs two servings (16 ounces) daily from the milk group to supply protein, calcium, riboflavin, and vitamins A and B_{12}. Fortified milk provides vitamin D and additional vitamin A. Whole milk should be used until the toddler reaches 2 years of age because of the linoleic acid in the milk fat. Fortified soybean milk can be used in vegan diets. One half of the toddler's protein intake should consist of high–biological value proteins. Toddlers who consume more than 24 ounces of milk daily in preference to other foods may develop a milk anemia. Lean red meats, as a part of the 1 to 3 ounces of meat group foods, are a good source of iron. Whole grains and enriched cereals and breads also contribute iron to the toddler's diet.

The toddler should receive four servings daily from the fruit and vegetable group. One serving daily should be a good source of vitamin C. Green leafy vegetables and deep yellow fruits and vegetables should be served frequently. Toddlers often prefer bite-sized raw vegetables rather than cooked vegetables. Raw carrots should not be given, since the toddler could choke on them. Individual salad vegetables should be served separately because toddlers usually dislike mixtures.

The toddler's four servings from the bread and cereal group should include whole grain or enriched breads, cereals, and pastas. Infant cereals may continue to be used because of their higher iron content. Sugar-coated cereals and the use of sugar on cereals should be avoided. Toddlers often prefer cereal in dry form as a finger-fed snack. In addition to the basic four food groups, the toddler should have 1 to 2 teaspoons of margarine or butter for its vitamin A content.

Good nutritional habits should be started early, with fruit desserts, custards, puddings, and ice cream emphasized instead of cake, pies, and cookies.

During the preschool years, from ages 3 to 6, children gain an average of 2 kg (4½ pounds) of body weight and 5 to 8 cm (2 to 3 inches) in height a year. At the end of the preschool period the child's weight is double that at 1 year of age and height is 1½ times that at 1 year. The average 6-year-old weighs 19 kg (42 pounds) and stands 105 cm (42 inches) high. Growth slows during the preschool period, but energy requirements are increased.

Daily protein needs are increased to 40 g, half of which should be provided by proteins of high biological value. Calcium and iron intake remains important. Fruits and vegetables as finger food snacks should be encouraged to provide vitamins A and C, which are frequently low in the preschooler's diet. Interest in food continues to be overshadowed by interest in the enlarging environment and motor skills. Several small meals may be preferable to the traditional three. Families who eat their largest meal in the evening should provide a different meal schedule for the preschooler, who may be too tired to eat at the end of a busy day.

Preschoolers need 16 ounces of milk daily, 1 to 3 ounces from the meat group, four servings from the fruit and vegetable group (including a daily source of vitamin C and frequent servings of leafy green and deep yellow vegetables and fruits), four servings of whole grain or enriched foods from the bread and cereal group, and 1 to 2 teaspoons of margarine or butter.

School-Age Children

School-age children, 6 to 12 years old, are growing at a slower and more steady rate. There is a gradual decline in energy requirements per unit of body weight. The school-age child gains 3 to 5 kg (6½ to 11 pounds) in weight and 6 cm (2½ inches) in height a year until puberty.

The appetites of school-age children are greater than those of younger children, and food intake is more varied. Recommended intake includes two servings from the milk group, 2 to 3 ounces of meat group foods, three to four servings from the fruit and vegetable group (with a daily source of vitamin C and a source of vitamin A every other day), three to four servings from whole grain and enriched breads and cereals, and 1 to 2 teaspoons of margarine or butter.

Despite better appetites and more varied food intake, the diets of school-aged children should be carefully assessed for adequate protein intake and vitamin A and C content. Milk intake usually exceeds the recommendations, but failure to eat a proper breakfast and unsupervised intake at school may result in improper or inadequate food intake.

Adolescents

During adolescence, physiological age is a better guide to nutritional needs than chronological age. Adolescence begins with the growth spurt of puberty that marks the end of childhood and ends with the completion of physical growth. Caloric needs are greatly increased to meet the increased metabolic demands. Girls need approximately 2000 to 2500 kcal a day; boys need 2500 to 3000 kcal a day. Protein

needs increase to a daily requirement of 50 to 60 g. Calcium is essential for the rapid bone growth of adolescence, and girls need a continuous source of iron to replace menstrual losses. Iodine is required to support increased thyroid activity, and B complex vitamins support the heightened metabolic activity.

Adolescents' requirements from the basic four groups include three or more servings from the milk group; two or more servings from the meat group; four or more servings from the vegetable-fruit group (with a daily source of vitamin C and a source of vitamin A every other day); two to six or more servings from the bread and cereal group, with emphasis on whole grains; and 1 to 2 tablespoons of margarine or butter.

The adolescent's diet is influenced by many factors other than nutritional needs. Adolescents are concerned about their body images and adapting their self-images to rapid physical changes. Striving for independence may lead to rejection of the family's nutritional standards, as well as other family values. Heightened interest in nutrition may stem from an interest in sports or achieving a fashionable figure. Fad diets are a constant threat to an adequate intake.

Nutritional deficiencies may occur in adolescent girls as a result of dieting and the use of oral contraceptives. The nutrients involved are folic acid, vitamin B_6, vitamin C, thiamin, riboflavin, and iron. The adolescent boy's diet may be inadequate in total calories, protein, iron, folic acid, B vitamins, and iodine.

Pregnant teenage girls must meet their own nutritional needs, as well as the additional demands of pregnancy. Pregnancy occurring within 4 years after the menarche (which usually occurs at 10½ to 13 years in America) places both mother and fetus at risk because of anatomical and physiological immaturity. There is an increased incidence of eclampsia in pregnant adolescents. In addition, the fetus has an increased risk of low birth weight, malformation, and mortality.

Research into teenage pregnancies will provide more definitive dietary recommendations. At present, nutritional requirements for the pregnant teenager are the sum of the recommended daily allowances for pregnancy and those appropriate for the expectant mother's age, the same procedure followed for the mature pregnant woman.

The caloric intake of the pregnant adolescent should permit an 11 to 13 kg (24- to 30-pound) total weight gain, usually achieved by increasing the caloric intake by 300 kcal daily. Protein requirements are 1.7 g/kg body weight for girls under 15 years and 1.5 g for those 15 years and older. Six daily servings from the milk group are recommended to satisfy protein and calcium needs.

Most teenage girls do not want to gain weight. Counseling related to the nutritional needs of pregnancy may be very difficult, and suggestions based on the teenager's usual diet meet with more success than rigid directions. The diet of a pregnant adolescent is most apt to be deficient in calcium, iron, vitamin A, and vitamin C.

Young and Middle Adults

The demands for most nutrients are reduced as the growth period ends. Mature adults need nutrients for energy, maintenance, and repair. Energy needs usually decline as life becomes more sedentary. Life-styles are changing, and many adults are assuming responsibility for food selection for themselves and others for the first time. Obesity may become a problem because of decreased physical exercise, increased dining out, or the ability to afford more luxury foods.

Adult women who use oral contraceptives need extra folic acid, vitamin C, riboflavin, vitamin B_6, and vitamin B_{12}. Those who use intrauterine devices need additional vitamin C and iron to compensate for increased menstrual flow.

Young and middle-aged adults are subject to the same recommendations from the basic four food groups: two or more servings from the milk group, four or more servings from the vegetable-fruit group (with the recommendation for a daily source of vitamin C and three to four weekly servings of sources of vitamin A continuing), four or more servings from the whole grain or enriched bread and cereal group, and 1 to 2 tablespoons of margarine or butter.

PREGNANCY

Poor nutrition during pregnancy can lead to the birth of an infant with a low birth weight and decreased chances of survival. Generally, the fetus' needs are met at the expense of the mother's needs. However, if nutrient sources are not available, both mother and fetus will suffer. The nutritional status of the mother at the time of conception is important in terms of nutritional reserves and basic eating habits. Often significant aspects of fetal growth and development occur before pregnancy is even suspected, which makes good nutrition especially important for women in their childbearing years.

The energy requirements of pregnancy are related to body weight and activity. A gain of 1 to 2 kg (2⅕ to 4⅖ pounds) a week should occur in the first trimester, with a 0.4 kg (1 pound) gain per week during the second and third trimesters. A total weight gain of 10 to 15 kg (22 to 28 pounds) is recommended.

Caloric intake should be sufficient to meet energy needs and to spare protein for anabolism. A 14% to 15% increase over prepregnancy caloric requirements (or an increase of 300 kcal a day) is usually sufficient. Inadequate weight gain is not desirable even in the mother who is markedly obese. Weight gain above 15 kg (33 pounds) is not desirable either. Weight is carefully monitored during pregnancy. In the event of undesirable gains or losses the food intake should be evaluated. Pregnant women should be cautioned against fasting as a method of weight control, since fasting leads to ketoacidosis, which can be dangerous to the fetus.

Food intake in the first trimester should consist of balanced portions of essential nutrients with emphasis on quality of intake. Protein intake throughout pregnancy is increased by 30 g or a 65% to 68% increase over prepregnancy requirements. High-risk mothers are advised to double their normal protein intake. In pregnancy, protein is needed for the development of the fetus, uterus, mammary glands, placenta, and amnionic fluid and for increased blood production and protein reserves. High–biological value protein should supply two thirds of the protein intake.

Calcium intake should be increased by 0.4 g (50%), an intake of 1.2 g per day. Calcium is needed for fetal tooth and bone development and blood clotting. Calcium intake is especially critical in the third trimester when fetal bones are mineralized.

Pregnant women need more iron than can be supplied by even the most ideal diet; mineral supplementation is required. Iron needs are increased by 30 to 60 mg a day. Iron is needed to correct preexisting deficiencies and to provide for increased maternal blood volume, for fetal blood storage (a 3- to 4-month supply is stored in the fetal liver), and for blood loss during delivery.

Iodine needs are increased by 25 mg (15% to 17%) because of increased activity of the thyroid gland.

Because vitamin A is needed for cell development, epithelial tissue maintenance, and tooth and bone development, requirements are increased by 200 retinol equivalents (20% to 25%).

Thiamin requirements are increased by 0.4 mg (40%); riboflavin by 0.3 mg (20% to 25%); niacin by 0.2 mg (15% to 17%); vitamin B_6 by 0.6 mg (30%); folic acid by 400 μg (100%); and vitamin B_{12} by 1 μg (100%). The B vitamins are needed for enzyme production necessitated by increased metabolic activity. Folic acid intake is particularly important for its role in DNA synthesis and the maturation of red blood cells. Inadequate intake of folic acid may lead to megaloblastic anemia, a type of anemia seen in women who have had many pregnancies.

Vitamin C requirements are increased by 20 mg (30%) in order to provide the intercellular cement in connective and vascular tissue and to enhance the absorption of iron. Vitamin D needs are increased by 5 μg (100%), since this vitamin promotes the absorption of calcium and phosphorus, necessary for fetal tooth and bone development.

In terms of the basic four food groups, the pregnant woman should have four or more servings from the milk group; four or more servings from the meat group; five to seven servings from the vegetable-fruit group (including a citrus fruit and a potato daily, and leafy green or dark yellow vegetables and fruits three to four times a week); two to four or more servings from the enriched or whole grain bread and cereal group; and at least 1 to 2 tablespoons of margarine or butter daily.

Pregnant women should increase their fluid intake by drinking 6 to 8 glasses of water daily. They should avoid saccharine, alcohol, excessive caffeine, and all drugs not specifically ordered by their obstetricians.

Vegans can satisfy their protein requirement by the use of complementary plant proteins. They will need iron, calcium, and vitamin B_{12} supplementation because of the absence of animal protein and should be encouraged to add milk to their diets during pregnancy.

LACTATION

Lactation necessitates further increases in nutritional support above those required for pregnancy. The production of breast milk requires 400 kcal a day; the caloric content of breast milk increases these demands by 20 kcal per ounce. The lactating woman needs 300 kcal a day in addition to her pregnancy requirement or 500 kcal above her prepregnancy requirement.

Protein requirements are reduced to 20 g per day, 10 g less than during pregnancy. The need for calcium, which is now required as a component of breast milk, remains the same as during pregnancy. Although the lactating woman requires less protein, folacin, and iron as compared to the pregnancy requirements, there is an increased need for vitamin A, niacin, riboflavin, iodine, and zinc over pregnancy needs. The need for vitamins C, D, E, B_6, B_{12}, and thiamin and for the minerals calcium, phosphorus, and magnesium are the same for the pregnant and the lactating woman, but the lactating woman requires more fluid intake.

The lactating woman's selections from the basic four food groups should be a continuation of her pregnancy diet with the following additions. The increased calories should be provided by leafy green vegetables, citrus fruits, whole grains, milk, meats, and poultry to provide vitamins A and C, niacin, riboflavin, and zinc. She should continue to drink a quart of milk daily or its equivalent from the milk group. Fluid intake should total at least 3 quarts a day.

The lactating woman does not need to restrict her intake of spicy foods, since these foods have been shown to be nonirritating to the infant's gastrointestinal tract. Caffeine, alcohol, and drugs are excreted in breast milk and should be used only under a physician's supervision.

Older Adults

Adults 65 years and older have decreased needs for niacin, thiamin, and riboflavin, B vitamins associated with energy production. Decreased activity of the thyroid gland reduces the need for iodine. Present knowledge does not indicate an increased need for any nutrient.

There are numerous factors that influence the nutritional status of the older adult. Income is probably the most important. Adults with fixed incomes often limit their food expenditures when other financial obligations increase. Health is another important influence; the older adult may be on a therapeutic diet or have difficulty eating because of physical symptoms, lack of teeth, or dentures. Food shopping and preparation may be difficult because of physical disability or lack of transportation. Living alone decreases the interest and pleasure of preparing and eating meals.

There is a normal decline in taste acuity with age. The taste buds that recognize sweet and salt are the first to deteriorate, leaving bitter and sour as the dominant taste sensations. Dentures also increase bitter and sour taste sensations. There is a normal decline in gastric secretions that results in less efficient digestion.

The basic four food group selections for older adults are the same as for younger adults, although there may need to be some changes in the way foods are prepared or the types of foods selected. Diets of older adults are typically low in protein foods and high in breads, cakes, and cereals. Meats may be avoided because of cost or because they are difficult to chew. Cheese, eggs, and peanut butter are good protein substitutes. Milk continues to be an important food, particularly for the older woman who needs adequate calcium to protect against osteoporosis. Whole grain cereals and breads should be encouraged. Cream soups and meat-based vegetable soups will nourish the older adult with chewing problems. The diet of the older adult should be low in fat and high in fiber and iron and should include good sources of calcium and vitamin B_{12}. Meals on Wheels and group eating at senior citizens' centers improve the older adult's nutritional intake, as well as morale.

Nutrition and the Nursing Process

Nurses are in an excellent position to recognize signs of poor nutrition and to take steps to initiate change. Close daily contact with the hospitalized client enables nurses to make observations of the client's physical status, food intake, and response to therapy. Nurses should inform the physician of observations that indicate nutritional problems and should incorporate approaches to solving the problem in their care plans. They should investigate the reasons for reduced food intake and provide alternative types of food or methods of intake. An equally important nursing responsibility is awareness of indications that intravenous feedings can be replaced by oral feedings or that a nasogastric tube is no longer needed. Clients may receive intravenous feedings or inadequate liquid diets longer than necessary when nurses do not take the initiative in suggesting changes. The nurse who reads the laboratory test results and understands their implications can bring the results to the physician's attention.

Nurses in ambulatory care centers and physicians' offices can check current weight measurements against previous values and alert the physician to major deviations. Nurses can also interview clients before they see the physician and stress the importance of sharing relevant information and concerns.

Nurse practitioners and community health nurses can use their physical assessment and interviewing skills to identify nutritional problems and provide sound counseling or appropriate referral.

Nurses in all settings should be alert to clients at risk because of nutritional problems. Both overweight and underweight clients are at risk because a deviation of 20% from ideal body weight is considered a high risk factor. Both gross increases and decreases in body weight may reduce protein reserve.

Any client with a condition that interferes with the ability to ingest, digest, or absorb adequate nutrients should be considered at risk. Congenital anomalies and surgical revisions of the gastrointestinal tract interfere with the normal function of the tract. Clients maintained exclusively by intravenously administered glucose or saline for more than 10 days are at risk for nutritional deficiencies.

Increased demand for nutrients to meet heightened metabolic needs is a factor in the care of infants, pregnant women, and clients with burns, fever, cancer, and infections. Increased loss of body fluids because of draining wounds, hemorrhage, vomiting, or diarrhea places clients at risk. Infants and the elderly are especially vulnerable to fluid loss.

In the assessment step of the nursing process, the nurse gathers data to make a diagnosis of the client's nutritional problem or the potential for nutritional complications. Once the nutritional needs of the client are identified, the nurse is involved in activities designed to meet those needs.

Assessment of Nutritional Status

Nurses committed to health maintenance and promotion will make nutritional assessment part of every nurse-client relationship. Because food and fluid are basic biological needs of all human beings, a nutritional assessment is an essential part of an overall nursing assessment. In addition, nutritional assessment is particularly important for clients potentially at risk for nutritional problems related to illness, hospitalization, life-style habits, and other factors. A complete nutritional assessment includes observation, a nursing history focusing on diet, anthropometric measurements, diagnostic tests, and consideration of factors that influence the client's dietary patterns (see Chapter 29).

Observation

As in other kinds of nursing assessment, the nurse observes the client for signs of actual or potential nutritional needs. Because improper nutrition affects all body systems, clues to malnutrition may be observed during physical assessment (see Chapter 30). When the general physical assessment of body systems is complete, the nurse can recheck pertinent areas to evaluate the client's nutritional status. The clinical signs of nutritional status (Table 38-11) provide guidelines for observation during the physical assessment.

Nursing History

In addition to the general nursing history (see Chapter 8), the nurse can obtain a more specific diet history to assess the client's actual or potential nutritional needs. The diet history focuses on the client's habitual intake of food and liquids, as well as information about preferences, allergies, problems, and other relevant areas. Fig. 38-3 provides an example of a diet history.

In addition, a detailed record can be kept of the client's food intake over a 3-day period, including a weekend day. This record allows the nurse to calculate the client's nutritional intake and to compare this with recommended daily allowances in order to determine whether the client's usual dietary habits are providing all nutrients in required amounts.

In the nursing history the nurse also gathers infor-

TABLE 38-11

Clinical Signs of Nutritional Status

Body Area	Signs of Good Nutrition	Signs of Poor Nutrition
General appearance	Alert, responsive	Listless, apathetic, cachectic
Weight	Normal for height, age, body build	Overweight or underweight (special concern for underweight)
Posture	Erect, arms and legs straight	Sagging shoulders, sunken chest, humped back
Muscles	Well developed, firm, good tone, some fat under skin	Flaccid, poor tone, undeveloped, tender, "wasted" appearance, cannot walk properly
Nervous control	Good attention span, not irritable or restless, normal reflexes, psychological stability	Inattentive, irritable, confused, burning and tingling of hands and feet (paresthesia), loss of position and vibratory sense, weakness and tenderness of muscles (may result in inability to walk), decrease or loss of ankle and knee reflexes
Gastrointestinal function	Good appetite and digestion, normal regular elimination, no palpable organs or masses	Anorexia, indigestion, constipation or diarrhea, liver or spleen enlargement
Cardiovascular function	Normal heart rate and rhythm, no murmurs, normal blood pressure for age	Rapid heart rate (above 100 beats per minute tachycardia), enlarged heart, abnormal rhythm, elevated blood pressure
General vitality	Endurance, energetic, sleeps well, vigorous	Easily fatigued, no energy, falls asleep easily, looks tired, apathetic
Hair	Shiny, lustrous, firm, not easily plucked, healthy scalp	Stringy, dull, brittle, dry, thin, and sparse, depigmented, can be easily plucked
Skin (general)	Smooth, slightly moist, good color	Rough, dry, scaly, pale, pigmented, irritated, bruises, petechiae
Face and neck	Skin color uniform, smooth, pink, healthy appearance, not swollen	Greasy, discolored, scaly, swollen, skin dark over cheeks and under eyes, lumpiness or flakiness of skin around nose and mouth
Lips	Smooth, good color, moist, not chapped or swollen	Dry, scaly, swollen, redness and swelling (cheilosis), or angular lesions at corners of the mouth or fissures or scars (stomatitis)
Mouth, oral membranes	Reddish pink mucous membranes in oral cavity	Swollen, boggy oral mucous membranes
Gums	Good pink color, healthy, red, no swelling or bleeding	Spongy, bleed easily, marginal redness, inflamed, gums receding
Tongue	Good pink color or deep reddish in appearance, not swollen or smooth, surface papillae present, no lesion	Swelling, scarlet and raw, magenta color, beefy (glossitis), hyperemic and hypertrophic papillae, atrophic papillae
Teeth	No cavities, no pain, bright, straight, no crowding, well-shaped jaw, clean, no discoloration	Unfilled caries, absent teeth, worn surfaces, mottled (fluorosis), malpositioned

From Williams, S.R.: Nutritional guidance in prenatal care. In Worthington-Roberts, B.S., Vermeersch, J.A., and Williams, S.R.: Nutrition in pregnancy and lactation, ed. 2, St. Louis, 1981, The C.V. Mosby Co.

TABLE 38-11, cont'd

Clinical Signs of Nutritional Status

Body Area	Signs of Good Nutrition	Signs of Poor Nutrition
Eyes	Bright, clear, shiny, no sores at corner of eyelids, membranes moist and healthy pink color, no prominent blood vessels or mound of tissue or sclera, no fatigue circles beneath	Eye membranes pale (pale conjunctivas), redness of membrane (conjunctival injection), dryness, signs of infection, Bitot's spots, redness and fissuring of eyelid corners (angular palpebritis), dryness of eye membrane (conjunctival xerosis), dull appearance of cornea (corneal xerosis), soft cornea (keratomalacia)
Neck (glands)	No enlargement	Thyroid enlarged
Nails	Firm, pink	Spoon shape (koilonychia), brittle, ridged
Legs, feet	No tenderness, weakness, or swelling; good color	Edema, tender calf, tingling, weakness
Skeleton	No malformations	Bowlegs, knock-knees, chest deformity at diaphragm, beaded ribs, prominent scapulas

mation about the client's activity level in order to determine the energy need and compare it with the client's food intake.

Anthropometry

Anthropometry is a system of measurement of the size and makeup of the body and specific body parts. Anthropometric measurements that aid in the recognition of nutritional problems include weight, height, mid–upper arm circumference, and measurement of triceps skinfold. Unless contraindicated by the client's physical condition, height and weight measurements should be obtained on hospital admission. When height or weight cannot be measured, the client should be asked about usual measurements and any recent variations. The client's present height and weight can be compared both to the usual measurements and to standards for normal height-weight relationships (see Table 29-5 in Chapter 29). General observations about weight variations can also be made on the basis of overall appearance. Loose skinfolds, temporal hollowing, sunken eyes, and wasted muscles are common clues to weight loss. Purple striae indicate recent weight gain.

The triceps skinfold measurement (measured by special calipers and the value compared to a table of norms) provides information about the amount of subcutaneous fat. Comparing the upper arm circumference to the norm provides information about skeletal muscle mass (Table 38-12).

Diagnostic Tests

Laboratory values useful in nutritional assessment include the complete blood count, serum albumin level, transferrin level, and urinary concentrations of sodium, potassium, urea nitrogen, and creatinine. A low red blood cell count and depressed hemoglobin value indicate anemia. The hemoglobin and hematocrit values reflect the state of hydration. Serum levels of albumin and transferrin are useful in the identification of protein-calorie malnutrition (PCM). Reduced levels of albumin and transferrin in adults also indicate a visceral protein deficit. Transferrin is an iron-carrying protein, normally found in the blood, that is rapidly depleted in acute illnesses. Protein is also lost rapidly in catabolic states.

Urine specimens collected every 24 or 48 hours are helpful in assessing nutritional status. Urinary levels of sodium and potassium are useful indicators of renal function and response to intravenous electrolyte therapy. The urea nitrogen level is related to the use of exogenous protein and to nitrogen balance. Creatinine, another by-product of protein metabolism, is used in conjunction with height as an indicator of changes in lean tissue mass.

TABLE 38-12

Standards for Anthropometric Measures

	Male	Female
Arm circumference (cm)	29.3	28.5
Triceps skinfold (mm)	12.5	16.5
Arm muscle circumference (cm)	25.3	23.2

Data from Jelliffe, D.B.: The assessment of the nutritional status of the community, Geneva, 1966, World Health Organization.

Name _____ Date _____

Age _____ Hospital number _____

Family composition _____

Present weight _____ Usual weight _____

Height _____ Recent changes in weight _____

Number of meals per day _____ Number of snacks per day _____

Meals prepared by _____

Food preferences	Food allergies	Food aversions	Nonfavored but acceptable foods

Fig. 38-3 Diet history.

From Bodinski, L.H.: The nurse's guide to diet therapy, New York, 1982, John Wiley & Sons, Inc.

List any foods that cause indigestion.

List any foods that cause diarrhea.

List any foods that cause flatulence (gas).

Any difficulty chewing or swallowing?

Dentures?

Usual bowel movements.

History of dietary problems.

History of diseases, surgical procedures, or weight problems.

Physical activity.

Appetite _____ Recent changes in appetite _____

Breakfast at _____ AM With _____

Usual breakfast   Serving size

_____   _____
_____   _____
_____   _____
_____   _____
_____   _____

Occasional breakfasts _____

Weekends _____ Holidays _____ Special _____

Eats lunch/dinner at _____ PM With _____

At home _____ At work _____

Usual lunch/dinner   Serving size

_____   _____
_____   _____
_____   _____
_____   _____
_____   _____

Occasional lunches/dinners _____

Weekend _____ Holiday _____ Special _____

Eats supper/dinner at _____ PM With _____

Usual supper/dinner   Serving size

_____   _____
_____   _____
_____   _____
_____   _____
_____   _____

Occasional supper/dinner _____

Weekends _____ Holidays _____ Special _____

Snacks   Time   Serving size

_____   _____   _____
_____   _____   _____
_____   _____   _____
_____   _____   _____

Factors Influencing Dietary Patterns

A final area for the nurse to assess is a set of factors that influence the client's dietary pattern and thus nutritional status. These factors include the client's health status, cultural background, religion, socioeconomic status, personal preference, psychological factors, use of alcohol or drugs, and misinformation or beliefs about food values.

HEALTH STATUS

A good appetite is generally accepted as a sign of health, while anorexia is an almost universal symptom of disease. Anorexia also occurs as a side effect of drug therapy and as a response to treatment. Yet medical personnel tend to be unconcerned about anorexia and believe that a client's appetite will return when the condition is corrected. It is important, however, to recognize that nutritional support is an essential part of recovery.

CULTURE AND RELIGION

The influence of religion and culture on a client's attitude toward food is often overlooked. Health care workers often attribute a client's refusal to eat or to comply with a dietary regimen to anorexia or lack of understanding. Thus they may ignore the symptom or, if they believe lack of understanding is the problem, may increase nutritional education. Interpreters are brought in when language appears to be a barrier to understanding. Yet nurses should also inquire whether religious or cultural food habits might be the basis for refusal of hospital food or a special diet. If this is the case, they can investigate and revise food offerings.

It is not possible to be familiar with all the dietary practices of all religions and cultures, but nurses should be familiar with the food practices of the predominant religions and cultures in their area of practice. If they ask questions about individual practices, clients are usually happy to explain their practices and grateful for the interest and concern expressed.

Cultural patterns should be considered in planning therapeutic diets; ethnic dishes should be included whenever appropriate. Nurses need to familiarize themselves with the ingredients in ethnic foods to recognize their contribution to the diet.

Many clients of various ethnic backgrounds have adopted an American diet, others retain their cultural influence in food selection, and still others choose foods from both. Older clients are more apt to cling to ethnic food habits. Illness often causes regression and a desire for childhood comforts, which might include ethnic foods. Whatever the situation, it is worthwhile to consider religion or culture as possible reasons for food refusal or dietary noncompliance.

SOCIOECONOMIC STATUS

The amount of family income that is available for buying food varies. Food expenses are not a fixed amount as are rent and mortgage payments. When money is tight, therefore, many people spend less on food. On the other hand, food can be a status symbol, and buying luxury foods may boost self-esteem.

It is generally assumed that people with higher incomes purchase more proteins and fats and fewer complex carbohydrates, while people with lower incomes do the opposite. This is not always true because some people with an interest in nutrition are convinced of the soundness of dietary guidelines and plan their meals accordingly. Some people with limited income also follow dietary guidelines and purchase adequate amounts of protein foods despite a limited budget.

In addition to food purchases, a family must consider food preparation. When no one is at home to prepare meals, more convenience foods must be used. When someone has the time to convert inexpensive foods into appealing meals, more of the food budget can be used to ensure that all necessary nutrients are included.

The impact of advertising and the lack of knowledge about the contents of processed foods also influence food purchases. It cannot be assumed that the person with enough money will purchase foods containing the essential nutrients.

PERSONAL PREFERENCE

Individual food likes and dislikes are perhaps the strongest influence on food intake. A given food preference may have a tie to the past; the reason for the preference may no longer be remembered although the food remains a favorite. Food aversions can also be traced to the past, but unpleasant circumstances are more apt to be remembered. Certain foods, usually those associated with childhood, make people feel safe and protected and are often desired during periods of stress. Foods associated with childhood memories are apt to be favorites with an adult who had a happy childhood and rejected by a person with less pleasant memories. Children tend to adopt the food preferences of their parents, and these preferences may persist throughout life. Luxury foods may be popular because they indicate a person's ability to serve the "best." Some people derive status from buying wholesome foods, since this underscores their knowledge of nutrition and awareness of current research findings.

Clients who follow a therapeutic diet need help to understand the reasons for the diet. The client's food preferences should be considered in planning the diet. When a client does not like a particular food on the diet, a substitute should be found, since every effort should be made to increase the palatability of the diet. The nurse interviews the client before evaluating adherence to the dietary regimen. The nurse should demonstrate a willingness to explore possible adaptations when a client fails to comply with dietary instructions.

PSYCHOLOGICAL FACTORS

Closely related to matters of personal preference are psychological factors, which also influence clients' dietary patterns. Food is a basic human need for all people, but eating patterns vary widely among individuals as a result of differences in education, family influences, values, attitudes, behavioral patterns, and other factors. One person may be highly motivated to eat balanced meals every day, for example, whereas another may be less interested in nutrition and may eat whatever is most convenient most of the time. Perceptions about diet also vary: one person may perceive that vitamins are important and daily supplements necessary, whereas another may believe that vitamin needs are satisfied by eating an occasional fresh fruit or vegetable. The nurse assesses such psychological factors in planning and implementing dietary teaching or counseling.

Another psychological factor is the symbolic value of food. For some people, milk symbolizes maternal security, whereas to others it may symbolize helplessness; therefore some clients may drink a great deal of milk whereas others reject it because of symbolic associations. Similarly, to some clients meat symbolizes strength and masculinity and vegetables and fruits symbolize femininity, significantly affecting dietary patterns.

ALCOHOL AND DRUGS. The client's ingestion of alcohol and use of prescription, over-the-counter, or illegal drugs may also affect nutritional status either directly or indirectly by influencing dietary patterns.

The excessive ingestion of alcohol contributes to nutritional deficiencies in several ways. Money used to buy alcoholic beverages might otherwise have been spent on more nutritional foods. Alcohol may replace part of the diet, thus reducing the intake of nutrients from other foods. Alcohol can also depress the appetite. Furthermore, excessive ingestion of alcohol can affect gastrointestinal organs, reducing the efficiency of digestion and absorption of nutrients. A vicious circle develops in which the malnourished body is less able to cope with the toxic effects of alcohol, thus increasing the effects of alcohol on nutrition.

The effects of drugs on nutrition vary widely, de-

TABLE 39-13

Examples of Food Fads and Myths

Food	Common Misinformation	Nutritional Facts
Honey	Thought healthier than sugar, a curative for coughs or colds, better than sugar for digestion	No special curative powers, no significant differences in digestion
Yogurt	Thought to ensure good health, more nutritious than milk	Essentially equivalent to milk in nutritional qualities
Citrus fruits	Thought to cause "acid indigestion"	Stomach acid production unaffected by citrus fruits
Cabbage, onions	Thought to taint breast milk	Lactation requires specific nutrients, and breast milk is not tainted by any food
Gelatin	Thought in large amounts to build strong nails	Not necessary for nail formation, which depends on general nutrition, nail care, and other factors
Oysters, raw egg, rare lean beef	Thought to increase fertility or sexual potency	No food alone affects sexual potency
Raw milk	Thought more nutritious than pasteurized milk	Pasteurized milk may contain slightly less vitamin C but also includes vitamin D; raw milk carries a greater risk of contamination

pending on the type and actions of the drug. Drugs that depress the appetite, including nonprescription drugs sold to dieters, can lower the intake of essential nutrients. Other drugs can deplete stores of nutrients or lessen their absorption in the intestines. The nurse should therefore take note of any drugs in the nursing and medical histories in order to minimize or counteract their effects on the client's nutritional status.

MISINFORMATION AND FOOD FADS. For many people dietary patterns are influenced by misinformation or myths about the values of certain foods. A food fad is a shared perception that a particular food is especially healthy, can cure an illness, can increase sexual potency, should be avoided because of negative health effects, and so on. Some food myths are rooted in cultural background, some arise because of the popular interest in "natural" foods, some involve peer pressure, and some persist because of the desire to exert greater control over health status through diet. Although it is true that good nutritional practices improve health, many food fads and myths have no scientific basis. Often the foods do not have the properties claimed by those believing in the fad or myth. If such beliefs have the potential to disrupt a client's dietary pattern, the nurse may use teaching or counseling techniques to ensure that the client's diet provides adequate nutrition. Because people's food beliefs are often closely related to their philosophy of life or other life-style factors, the nurse must be careful not to seem condescending or put the client on the defensive when discussing food values and correcting misinformation. This is particularly true when the client is from a culture different from the nurse's.

Table 38-13 presents a few examples of food fads and myths and the truth about these foods.

Nursing Diagnosis

On the basis of assessment data, the nurse determines a nursing diagnosis for the client's nutritional status. These diagnoses fall into three general types: actual or potential nutritional deficits related to lack of or insufficiency in the diet of one or more nutrients; nutritional problems related to eating habits, including obesity, anorexia nervosa, and bulimia; and potential nutritional problems related to illness in postoperative clients, clients with cancer who are receiving radiotherapy, and immobilized clients. The later section on planning and intervention discusses general nursing actions related to nutritional problems, and the following sections on specific diagnoses include specific treatments in addition to the general nursing interventions for hospitalized clients.

Nutritional Deficits

Clients who are otherwise healthy and who are not experiencing the specific nutritional problems of obesity, anorexia, or bulimia may have actual or potential nutritional deficits related to poor diet. A deficit may occur with any one or more of the nutrients necessary for high-level wellness. Specific diagnoses are related to the actual deficiency of the particular nutrient, as discussed earlier in relation to carbohydrates, proteins, lipids, vitamins, and minerals. For example, a diagnosis for a specific nutritional deficit might be anemia and fatigue related to insufficient dietary intake of iron.

The nursing diagnosis may also involve a general nutritional deficiency rather than a known deficit of one or more specific nutrients—for example, potential risks to the fetus related to maternal dietary deficiencies in protein, vitamins, and minerals.

Both specific and generalized nutritional deficits can be diagnosed on the basis of clinical observations, dietary history, and diagnostic tests.

OBESITY

Overnutrition is a major health problem in the United States today. Obesity is a condition in which there is a 20% increase above ideal body weight. Obesity cuts across all socioeconomic levels and is a risk factor in most of the leading causes of death. Although some cultures consider overweight attractive or a status symbol, most people strive for a slender figure. Excessive weight causes psychological problems, inconvenience, and unhappiness in addition to its impact on health.

There are countless programs for weight loss. The most popular promise rapid weight loss with a minimum of food deprivation. The sheer number of these diet plans indicates their lack of effectiveness. Most people consider diets a temporary measure; they "go on a diet" to lose a specified number of pounds, and when the poundage is lost they "go off the diet" and return to their former eating habits.

To lose weight, a person must burn some of the body's store of fat. When insufficient calories are ingested to meet the daily energy needs, the body is forced to burn its reserve stores for energy. A person may lose weight either by reducing food intake or increasing energy needs through increased activity. The best plan for weight loss combines reduced food intake with increased exercise. Exercise provides distraction from the thoughts of food, firms tissues as weight is lost, and may decrease appetite. The best diet plan is the adoption of a well-balanced diet for life. The basic four food groups in the recommended serving sizes supply approximately 1200 kcal a day and provide a safe basis for weight reduction. Once the ideal body weight is reached, the intake can be adjusted upward to maintain this weight. This prevents the common problem with most diets: the tendency to regain weight after the dieting stops. Following the guidelines and reducing intake of fats and refined sugars should also result in weight loss. The elimination of part of the saturated fat intake by reducing butter intake and removing fats from meat and the elimination of sugar in beverages or on cereals can considerably reduce calories over a period of time. One tablespoon of butter contains 108 kcal, and 1 teaspoon of sugar contains 32 kcal.

The safest and most effective treatment for obesity is the combination of reduced food intake and increased energy expenditure. The use of drugs to suppress appetite or surgical procedures to bypass digestion or absorption has attendant dangers and does not require commitment on the part of the dieter.

ANOREXIA NERVOSA

Anorexia nervosa is a biopsychosocial disorder in which self-imposed starvation is used to establish identity and control. There may be a metabolic and possibly a hereditary predisposition to the condition. Usually a problem in family dynamics is present. Early feeding patterns and attitudes toward food have also been implicated. The desirability of a slender figure in today's society is considered a potent factor.

The client with anorexia nervosa is usually an adolescent girl. This condition is characterized by denial on the part of the client: denial of being underweight despite emaciation and progressive weight loss; denial of hunger despite prolonged food deprivation; and denial of fatigue despite frantic activity.

The extreme undernutrition leads to secondary endocrine disorders such as amenorrhea and delayed sexual development. In addition to food refusal, the client may go on food binges followed by self-induced vomiting or cathartic purges. The treatment of anorexia nervosa is a combination of psychotherapy, behavior modification, and dietary therapy.

BULIMIA

Bulimia or the binge-purge syndrome is a recently identified nutritional condition. Bulimia occurs in half of the clients with anorexia nervosa, but not all bulimic clients have anorexia nervosa. The syndrome appears to develop in the presence of an abnormal craving for food accompanied by the desire to remain slender. The client gorges on food to satisfy the craving and then induces vomiting to prevent the digestion of food. The client may also use laxatives or enemas to increase gastric motility so nutrients are not absorbed. The practice of secretly vomiting after eating usually starts with occasional binges and gradually becomes a daily activity and the preferred way of controlling weight.

Frequent vomiting, laxative abuse, and overuse of enemas lead to electrolyte imbalances (hypokalemia being the most serious), esophageal lesions, dental caries, endocrine disturbances, and metabolic changes.

Treatment modalities include dietary education, hospitalization, psychotherapy, drug therapy with phenytoin (Dilantin), group therapy, and behavioral modification. The incidence of bulimia is growing, and more definitive information is needed.

Clients at Risk for Nutritional Problems
POSTOPERATIVE CLIENTS

The surgical experience necessitates interference with food intake. Preoperative preparation usually involves at least an 8-hour period of fasting. Clients rarely receive an appreciable amount of nutrients on the day of surgery, and resumption of food intake in the postoperative period varies with the individual client, the surgical procedure, the presence of complications, and the surgeon's protocol.

Unless the surgical procedure dictates an alternative feeding method, clients who have had mouth and throat surgery must chew and swallow food in the presence of excision sites, sutures, or otherwise manipulated tissue. The ingestion of food causes discomfort, and clients are usually reluctant to eat or drink. Fluids are usually offered first. The use of a straw may be helpful in some cases, such as dental surgery, but is specifically contraindicated in others, such as cleft palate repairs. Soft foods are sometimes easier to swallow than liquids. Hot fluids, tart juices, and fiber should be avoided after throat and mouth surgery. Milk, yogurt, sherbet, ice cream, ginger ale, and diluted fruit juices are usually allowed. It is important to encourage intake and swallowing, and any food that is appropriate to the prescribed diet should be given in the early postoperative period. Once dysphagia subsides, concern for the nutrient content of the intake can be resumed.

When surgery is performed on the stomach and intestines, an alternative method of food intake is usually prescribed to allow the suture line to heal and edema to subside. Nasogastric suction may also be used to prevent gastric and intestinal secretions from irritating the resected areas. When oral intake is restricted for a short period, fluids are usually given intravenously. Long periods of restriction indicate the need for enteral feedings introduced distal to the operative site or for total parenteral nutrition. Gastric surgery may limit the amount of food that can be ingested at any one time. Intestinal surgery may interfere with absorption of nutrients, depending on the length of intestine involved and the location (see Table 38-5).

The diversion of intestinal wastes through the creation of artificial openings in the abdomen (ileostomy, colostomy) affects fluid loss and electrolyte balance. Clients with ileostomies also lose some of their ability to absorb vitamin B_{12}. Clients with ileostomies and colostomies have dietary concerns related to the consistency of the ostomy waste and control of odor.

CANCER AND RADIOTHERAPY

Cancer is a complex variety of disorders with diverse causes. Malignant cells compete with normal cells for nutrients, increasing the metabolic needs of the client. Clients with cancer typically complain of anorexia and taste distortions.

Nutritional support and the correction of nutritional deficits can enable clients to benefit from therapies previously denied them because of their cachectic state. Optimal nutrition improves cancer survival rates as well as the quality of life.

Although radiotherapy destroys the rapidly dividing neoplastic cells, it also destroys normal cells. Clients in good nutritional states can tolerate larger doses of radiation. Radiotherapy usually causes anorexia, nausea, and vomiting. The area of the body irradiated also determines the type of reactions. Irradiation of the head and neck can lead to taste and smell distortions, decreased salivation, and dysphagia. Irradiation of the abdomen and pelvis can result in malabsorption and diarrhea. Most clients find that radiotherapy causes profound fatigue.

Clients receiving radiotherapy should try to eat well before treatments. After anorexia subsides, breakfast is an important meal. Since meats are often rejected because of taste distortions, milk and eggs become important protein sources. Cold foods are often preferred. Commercial preparations are available that provide essential nutrients in a concentrated, palatable liquid form. Tube feedings or total parenteral nutrition can also be used for clients with obstinate anorexia.

IMMOBILIZED CLIENTS

Extended immobilization can result in deossification and osteoporosis of bones and in hypercalcemia. Hypercalcemia predisposes clients to kidney and bladder stones; it is a particular problem in children and adolescents because of their rapid bone growth.

Early ambulation is the best way to prevent problems associated with immobilization. When ambulation is not possible, adequate quantities of high–biological value protein help prevent skin breakdown and infections, and high phosphorus intake in the early weeks of immobilization reduces blood calcium levels. Generous fluid intake also protects against kidney stones. Range of motion exercises for noninvolved joints provide some activity.

Nutrition Planning and Intervention for Hospitalized Clients

Maintaining a proper nutritional status is a better nursing intervention than correcting deficits. The recognition of clients who are at risk for nutritional problems should result in a care plan that will prevent nutritional problems or minimize them if they do occur. The nurse should be as concerned with the client's nutritional state as with every other aspect of care. Nutritional education and counseling are important for the client on a regular diet to prevent disease and promote health. The better clients on a therapeutic diet understand the rationale for the diet, the more likely they are to comply with it.

Stimulating Appetite

Hospitalized clients usually have poor appetites despite the efforts of hospital dietitians to increase the appeal of meals. Nurses can help by displaying an interest in the client's intake, by understanding the influences that reduce appetite, and by a willingness to do everything possible to improve intake. One of the most disruptive influences on a client's intake is diagnostic testing. Blood and x-ray tests frequently require that the client be in a fasting state. Therefore breakfast is withheld and food often is not available when the client is permitted to eat. With present-day food packaging and microwave ovens it should be possible to serve a hot meal promptly when tests are complete.

To overcome the scheduling problem, a different meal pattern is used in some hospitals. A continental breakfast is served at the usual breakfast time, brunch is served at 11 AM, dinner at 4 PM, and an easily digested but substantial snack at bedtime. The client scheduled for tests is less hungry in the morning because of the previous evening snack, and usually the testing is over in time for brunch. Mealtimes differ from those of the unit staff, permitting more personnel to be available to prepare clients for meals, assist and encourage clients to eat, socialize with clients while they eat, and evaluate and record their intake.

Stress is another important influence on hospitalized clients' food intake. Clients are worried about their condition, their families, their jobs, and all the unknown aspects of hospitalization. The nurse should listen to clients' concerns, provide reassurance when appropriate, and carefully explain all unfamiliar procedures.

Nurses are also responsible for providing an environment conducive to eating. The client's room should be free of reminders of treatments completed or yet to come, and the environment should be free of odors. Mouth care should be provided when necessary to remove unpleasant tastes, and the client should be positioned comfortably for maximum independence. The client should be given advance notice of mealtime to permit anticipation of the meal. When a client refuses a particular item on the tray, every effort should be made to replace it with a suitable substitute.

Diet Therapist

After a meal the client's intake is evaluated and charted on the basis of the four food groups. Nurses should recognize that they share responsibility with the dietitian for food intake and should work cooperatively with the diet therapist. Sharing information about a client's concerns and response to diet therapy will benefit the nurse, the diet therapist, and the client. The client's education about the therapeutic diet should be a shared responsibility. The dietitian is the expert in diet therapy, but the nurse can relate the dietary modification to the client's condition and explain how the diet contributes to the overall plan of care.

Special Diets

Nurses should be familiar with the special diets used in client care so they can select appropriate between-meal liquids and snacks, monitor food brought in by visitors, and offer acceptable substitute foods (Fig. 38-4).

A regular hospital diet contains approximately 2500 kcal and consists of appropriate servings from the basic four food groups. A regular diet is about 15% protein, 50% carbohydrate, and 35% lipid, which is similar to the usual American diet. In some hospitals the regular diet has been changed to reflect the dietary guidelines by decreasing lipids and increasing complex carbohydrates. There are no particular food restrictions on the regular diet, but foods that are difficult to digest and fried foods are usually kept to a minimum.

A *light diet* is composed of foods that are easily digested and quickly emptied from the stomach. Rich, heavy foods such as fatty foods, pastries, concentrated sweets, and fibrous fruits and vegetables are eliminated from the light diet. Foods are usually prepared simply.

The major modification in the *soft diet* is texture. The soft diet usually contains sufficient calories in the same percentages of protein, carbohydrate, and lipid as in the regular diet. The soft diet is designed to include foods that are easily chewed and digested. Harsh, fibrous foods, rich foods, and strongly flavored foods are omitted.

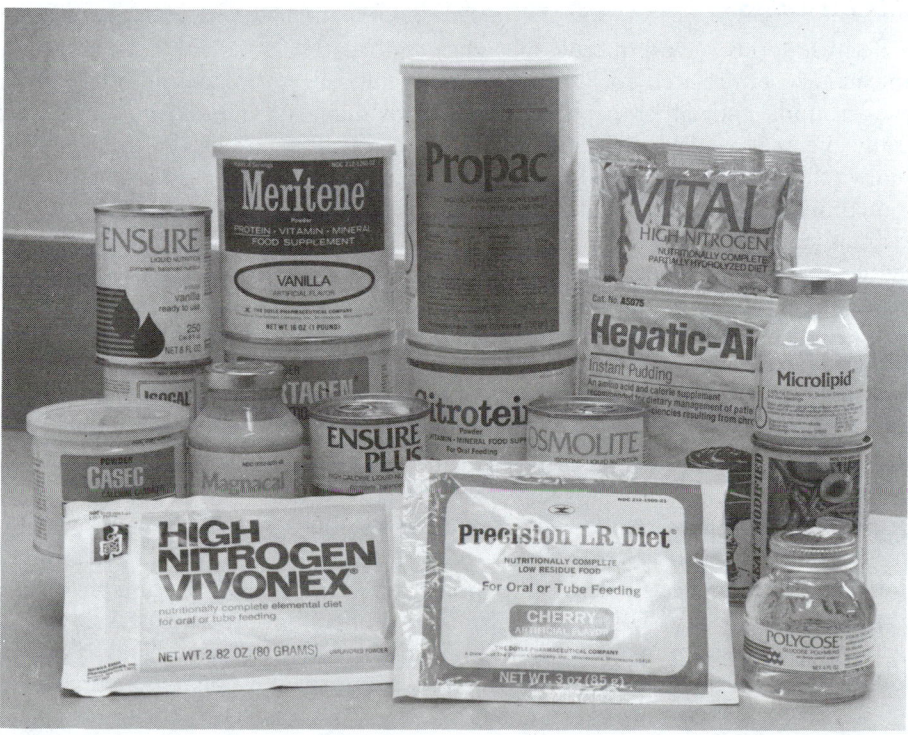

Fig. 38-4 Various diet supplements.

Liquid diets may be clear liquid (transparent fluids) or include full liquids (foods that are liquid at room or body temperature). A clear liquid diet does not provide sufficient calories and usually is given for only 1 to 2 days. Clear liquids, which do not provide lipid, contain only about 480 kcal of carbohydrate and 40 kcal of protein. Caloric and protein intake can be increased by the inclusion of egg white and gelatin to clear liquid diets. Although full liquid diets provide adequate calories, they usually are low in iron and lack fiber.

A *bland diet* is designed to eliminate any food that is chemically, mechanically, or thermally irritating. Stimulating liquids and spicy foods are eliminated, and foods are served warm or cool rather than hot or cold.

A *low-residue diet* is designed to reduce the contents of the intestinal tract. This diet limits fiber and other foods that leave a high level of residue in the intestines. Milk and milk products leave a high intestinal residue and are limited to 8 ounces a day in a low-residue diet. Clear fluids, meats, fats, and eggs are permitted. Cheese, fried foods, and highly seasoned foods are avoided. Only refined cereals and white bread are permitted, and all vegetables except peeled white potato are excluded. Although fruits are not permitted, fruit juices are allowed. A low-residue diet usually provides insufficient calcium, iron, and vitamins. It is not designed to be used for more than 3 or 4 days.

PSYCHOSOCIAL EFFECTS OF SPECIAL DIETS

Because foods have symbolic meanings for clients and are closely related to life-style, habits, cultural background, and other aspects of the individual, many clients have difficulty adjusting to special diets. Many clients had previously considered mealtime something to look forward to, a pleasurable period distinct from routines or an interlude from work activities. The special diet, especially a bland diet, makes eating a dull affair. In addition, eating with others may have been a primary form of social interaction for the client, but now the client eats alone in a hospital room or at home and cannot eat the same foods as other family members. In such situations the nurse and other health care professionals should recognize the actual or potential psychosocial factors and make plans to counteract negative effects. For example, the nurse can find substitutes for dietary foods to match the client's preference or can make meals more appealing with spices or condiments. Family members or others can also be involved, both to maintain the social value of mealtimes and to provide support

when practical by joining in the client's diet. Counseling techniques may be employed to help family members support the client through conversation and other means. A little imagination can go a long way to make a restricted diet more satisfactory.

Assisting Clients with Feeding

Before attempting to feed a client, every nurse should be spoon-fed a meal that includes soup in order to understand this experience. Being fed deprives clients of the independence they gained over their food intake as toddlers. At best, being fed is an unpleasant experience. Nurses can improve client feeding by carefully protecting clients' dignity and actively involving them in the process. Any material used to protect a client's clothing should be referred to as a napkin, not a bib. The nurse should allow the client time to empty the mouth after every spoonful, attempting to match the speed of feeding to the client's readiness and asking frequently if it is too fast or slow. The nurse should also allow clients to direct the order in which they wish to eat food items, and conversation about topics other than food should be an integral part of the process. The nurse who has several clients to feed should use ingenuity to prevent an assembly line approach that is devastating to the client's self-esteem.

HANDICAPPED CLIENTS

Clients with disabilities that interfere with independent food intake should be allowed to do as much as possible for themselves. The nurse should prepare the tray, cutting food into bite-sized pieces, buttering bread, and pouring liquids (Fig. 38-5). Special eating utensils should be used if they will contribute to the client's independence. Some disabled clients may become tired from their efforts to feed themselves. The nurse should ascertain whether the client who stops eating is still hungry and needs assistance to finish the meal. The results of self-feeding should be evaluated on the basis of food intake and not neatness. The client's success should be recognized and commended. The nurse who finds a way to aid the disabled client to eat more independently should share this information by incorporating it in the care plan.

TUBE FEEDING

Clients may be fed by the oral, enteral, or parenteral route. The oral route is the most desirable. Clients who are unable to take in, chew, or swallow food but who are able to digest and absorb it may be given tube feedings. Feeding tubes can be placed in the esophagus, stomach, or upper small intestine. The

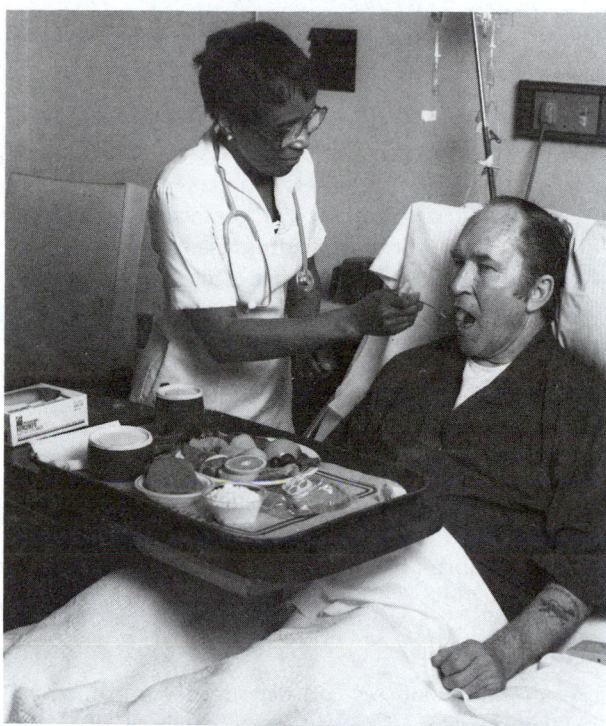

Fig. 38-5 When assisting a client to eat, the nurse should make sure the food is cut into bite-sized pieces.

tube may be inserted through the nose or mouth or surgically implanted. Tube feedings may be given intermittently (bolus feedings) or by slow constant drip. Bolus feedings more closely resemble the normal feeding pattern and permit the client more freedom. Continuous drip feedings are delivered through a small-caliber feeding tube and flow by gravity, or they are controlled by a pump. The slow constant feeding increases absorption and reduces diarrhea.

The solutions used for tube feedings must be nutritionally adequate, tolerated by the client, and appropriate to the area of the gastrointestinal tract to which they are delivered. Tube feedings that are placed directly in the stomach are usually finely chopped or pureed to resemble food after it has been chewed, mixed with saliva, and swallowed. Tube feedings introduced directly into the small intestine must contain nutrients in their simplest form, ready to be absorbed. Tube feedings can be prepared in a home or hospital kitchen. Regular meals can be liquefied in a blender for gastric feedings. The wide variety of commercial products available have become popular for tube feedings. They are easy to prepare and offer standard nutritional content. The commercial preparations differ in osmolarity, digestibility, caloric density, lactose content, viscosity, and lipid content. Ensure is an example of a commercial food for

clients who can digest protein and fat. Like similar products from other manufacturers, it provides 1 kcal/ml. Flexical is an example of a food for tube feeding that is ready to be absorbed. It (and similar products) provides 1 kcal/ml. A high-density product for tube feeding is available for clients with fluid restrictions. It is concentrated and provides 2 kcal/ml.

Clients may be maintained indefinitely on tube feedings, which can provide all the essential nutrients except fiber. Although cramping and diarrhea are commonly associated with tube feedings, these symptoms usually subside when the flow rate or the concentration of the solution is reduced.

TOTAL PARENTERAL NUTRITION

When clients are unable to handle nutrient intake via the enteral route, they may be given parenteral nutrition. All the essential nutrients are available in intravenous solutions. However, in order to meet the client's total nutritional needs parenterally, it is necessary to use concentrated glucose solutions in order to avoid fluid overload. Concentrated solutions would also damage peripheral blood vessels. Total parenteral nutrition (TPN) is accomplished by introducing a fine catheter into a vein (usually the subclavian or cephalic) and guiding the catheter tip into the superior vena cava or right atrium of the heart. The proximal end of the catheter is anchored in place, connected to intravenous tubing and covered by an occlusive dressing. Placing the tip of the catheter in a large central vein or in the right atrium provides rapid dilution for the hyperosmolar solution. TPN solutions can be individually formulated to meet the client's needs. Basic solutions consist of hypertonic glucose, hypertonic or isotonic amino acid solution, and all the vitamins and minerals for which requirements are known. Special solutions are available that are low in protein, specific electrolytes, or fluid content or high in specific electrolytes or minerals. Lipid needs are usually met by insertion into a peripheral vein, since lipids are not mixed with TPN solutions. Fat emulsions can be "piggybacked" to the TPN catheter under special precautions. The major concern with TPN is the risk of infection. Dressing changes, bottle changes, and tubing changes are all performed under sterile conditions.

The flow rate of the solution, which is another critical aspect of care, is usually controlled by an infusion pump. The flow rate must be carefully monitored, since deviations from the prescribed rate are dangerous. If the infusion falls behind schedule, a new rate must be calculated. Increasing the flow rate to catch up can result in circulatory overload, hyperglycemia, and osmotic diuresis.

Diet Therapy in Disease Management

Good nutrition is important in both health and illness, but the specific dietary intake pattern that results in good nutrition must often be modified for clients with particular diseases. Diet modifications are necessary to correspond with the body's ability to metabolize certain nutrients, to correct nutritional deficiencies related to the disease, and to eliminate certain foods from the diet that may be harmful to persons with the disease.

In all cases the nurse works with the physician and diet therapist in planning and implementing specific diet therapies for clients with disease. The following sections are intended as examples of diet modifications for specified diseases, not as guidelines for diet planning.

GASTROINTESTINAL DISEASES

The treatment of *ulcerative colitis* may include a liquid diet in the acute stage, a low-residue diet during recovery, and thereafter a bland diet high in protein, calories, vitamins, and minerals and low in fat. Vitamins and iron supplements are generally required because absorption is decreased.

The treatment of *diarrhea* may include a diet high in vitamins to counteract decreased absorption, low in residue, and high in calories if the client is emaciated.

The treatment of *malabsorption syndrome,* including sprue and celiac disease, includes a gluten-free diet. Gluten is present in wheat, rye, and oats.

The treatment of *acute enteritis* generally involves fasting initially, followed by a liquid diet, and thereafter a bland diet.

Acute gastritis is generally treated by a liquid diet initially, with a gradual transition to a low-residue diet and thereafter a bland diet. The treatment for *chronic gastritis* involves eliminating from the diet the foods or liquids that cause inflammation and thereafter permitting only easily digested foods.

The treatment of *diverticulitis* in which perforation has not occurred includes a liquid diet or low-residue diet until the infection subsides, after which a high-fiber diet is generally prescribed.

Diet therapy for *peptic ulcer* traditionally involves a diet that is bland and leaves a low residue, that omits very sweet, sour, or spicy foods, that does not permit serving foods at very hot or cold temperatures, and that is high in protein and fat to neutralize and inhibit acidity. The size and frequency of food servings are also gradually changed from initial small hourly feedings to a bland convalescent diet at normal mealtimes.

CARDIOVASCULAR DISEASES

The general goals of dietary treatment of cardiovascular diseases include preventing stomach distention to avoid pressure against the heart, reducing the client's weight if needed, and lowering blood lipids to lessen the risk of atherosclerosis.

The treatment of *myocardial infarction* includes a liquid diet for several days, progressing to a low-fat, low-sodium, high-carbohydrate, soft diet during recovery, followed by a diet moderately low in fat and protein and high in carbohydrates.

The exact role of cholesterol and saturated fat intake in *atherosclerosis* remains debatable, but dietary therapy for treatment and prevention generally includes maintaining a recommended weight and a diet low in saturated fats and cholesterol.

The treatment of *hypertension* includes weight reduction to normal if the client is overweight and a diet low in sodium and moderately low in fats.

DIABETES

Adult-onset diabetes can usually be controlled by diet therapy alone; juvenile-onset diabetes requires both insulin and dietary restrictions. In both cases the diet is individualized according to the client's age, build, weight, and activity level. Fats are moderately controlled, and complex carbohydrates make up a higher percentage of the diet than simple carbohydrates. Foods for dietary planning are classified in six exchange groups, in which each item has about the same value as other foods in the same group. Meals are planned around balanced numbers of food exchanges.

URINARY TRACT DISEASES

The dietary treatment of *acute glomerulonephritis* depends on individual tolerances but may begin with a limited liquid diet for a few days, gradually returning to a normal diet limited in protein. The diet for *chronic glomerulonephritis* is generally high in carbohydrates and fat, with protein amounts equal to normal plus the amount lost in urine.

The treatment of *uremia* may begin with a diet of fruit juices only or beverages containing carbohydrates and fats. A diet of essential amino acid protein and carbohydrates follows.

Dietary treatment for *renal stones* depends on the type of stones. For calcium phosphate stones the diet is low in calcium and high in acid ash. For uric acid stones the diet is low in purines. For calcium oxalate stones the diet avoids all foods high in calcium and oxalates.

Evaluation

The value of the nurse's activities in meeting the client's nutritional needs is unknown until they are evaluated. Nutritional assessment must be ongoing to evaluate the results of nursing interventions. Care plans must be constantly updated to avoid continuing ineffective actions and to strengthen support of effective interventions. Adequate time should be allowed to test a nursing approach to a problem. Behavior change in a client is as valid an indicator of success as weight gain or laboratory results.

Nurses should establish outcomes for nursing actions and be alert for signs that goals are being met. Whenever possible the client should be an active participant in the planning and evaluation of care.

Client and Family Counseling

Clients discharged from a hospital with a diet prescription often need dietary counseling to plan meals that meet specific diet requirements or general nutrition needs. Similarly, in other health care settings clients with nutrition deficits or specific problems such as overweight may require assistance in menu planning and compliance with recommended diet therapies. The nurse's counseling role often includes the family and community resources as well.

Meal planning must take into account the family's budget and differences in the preferences of family members. Specific foods are chosen on the basis of the dietary prescriptions or standard dietary guidelines such as the basic four food groups. But meals should also provide a variety of foods and contrasting colors and consistencies. For families on limited budgets, substitutes can be used. For example, beans or cheese dishes can often replace meat in a meal, and evaporated or dry skim milk can be used for many cooking purposes. The method of preparation may also be modified when it is necessary to minimize certain substances; for example, baking rather than frying reduces fat intake, and lemon juice or spices can be used to replace salt in a low-sodium diet.

Planning menus a week in advance has several benefits. In addition to helping ensure good nutrition or compliance with a specific diet, such planning based on three balanced meals a day helps family members avoid impulse eating of less nutritional foods. Fruit and other nutritional items can be included in the plan for between-meal snacks. Careful advance planning can also help the family stay within the allotted budget because planned food buying is generally more economical than last-minute shopping, which may include more expensive processed and packaged foods. Often a simple tip can be of value in meal planning, such as the advice to avoid grocery shopping when hungry, which can lead to spontaneous purchases of more expensive or less nutritional foods not included in meal plans.

Finally, the nurse can assist the client with referral to community resources for assistance with dietary problems. Assistance in obtaining food is provided by several government programs such as food commodities, food stamps, and school lunch programs. Private organizations such as Meals on Wheels programs also provide assistance. Volunteer health agencies, such as the American Heart Association and the American Diabetes Association, provide nutrition consultation, diet counseling, and educational materials. Other community groups also offer planned menus and other nutritional guidelines.

Summary

The nurse has the responsibility to work cooperatively with other members of the health team to meet the nutritional needs of clients.

Nurses must understand the functions of the basic nutrients and how they are metabolized to produce energy. An understanding of the guidelines for the selection of an adequate diet is essential so that nurses can teach clients about diet and answer questions related to diet. Nurses should also be alert to current research findings and their impact on dietary recommendations. They should be familiar with alternative food patterns followed by some clients and have a knowledge of the influence of age on dietary needs.

Nurses must be able to assess the nutritional status of clients. They must also recognize that many divergent factors influence a client's food intake and that these factors must be considered in attempting to modify food intake.

Nurses must be able to identify clients at risk for nutritional problems and be aware of common nutritional conditions. They should be aware of the importance of their interaction with others in the area of food intake, be familiar with common hospital diets, and be able to assist clients at mealtime.

Finally, nurses must evaluate their activities in the area of nutritional support in order to revise those that prove ineffective and continue those that are effective.

KEY CONCEPTS

✓ The nutrients needed by the body to carry out vital functions are water, carbohydrates, proteins, lipids, vitamins, and minerals.

✓ Water, vitamins, and minerals do not provide calories. Water is needed for cellular function and absorption. Vitamins and minerals act as catalysts in metabolic processes. Some minerals are essential in the formation of body cells.

✓ Body weight is maintained when food intake equals energy output. Increased food intake or reduced energy output will result in weight gain. Decreased food intake or increased energy output will result in weight loss.

✓ Carbohydrates are anabolized into glycogen and adipose tissue or catabolized into energy.

✓ Proteins are anabolized into tissues, hormones, or enzymes or catabolized into energy.

✓ Lipids may be anabolized into adipose tissue or catabolized into energy.

✓ Proteins are essential for growth, maintenance, and repair. They are the only nutrients that contain nitrogen. Nitrogen balance exists when the body's intake and output of nitrogen are equal.

✓ The essential amino acids and the essential fatty acids must be supplied by dietary intake because the body is unable to synthesize them from other ingested substances.

✓ Polyunsaturated fatty acids are believed to lower serum cholesterol levels and protect against atherosclerosis.

✓ Water-soluble vitamins cannot be stored in the body and must be provided daily. Fat-soluble vitamins can be stored in the body, and a less frequent intake will meet body needs.

✓ Digestion is the mechanical and chemical process by which food is broken down into its simplest form for absorption. Digestion and absorption occur mainly in the small intestine.

✓ Recommended daily allowances (RDAs), another basis for diet selection, were formulated for population groups, not individuals.

✓ Guidelines for dietary change advocate reduced intake of fat, saturated fat, salt, refined sugar, and cholesterol and increased intake of complex carbohydrates and fiber.

✓ Vegetarian diets can be made adequate with the use of appropriate plant foods and supplementation with vitamin B_{12}.

✓ Age affects the requirements for essential nutrients. Periods of rapid growth increase the need for protein, vitamins, and minerals.

✓ The many factors that influence dietary patterns must be considered in a client's nutritional plan of care.

✓ Because improper nutrition can affect all body systems, nutritional assessment includes a review of the total physical assessment.

✓ Obesity is a major health problem for which there are many proposed treatments.

✓ Anorexia nervosa and bulimia are becoming more commonly recognized as health problems in adolescent girls.

KEY CONCEPTS, cont'd

✓ Nurses can improve food intake of clients by thoughtful attention to the preparation of both client and environment before meals are served.

✓ Disabled clients should be supported in their efforts to eat as independently as possible.

✓ Proper feeding techniques can protect the dependent client from loss of dignity and self-esteem.

✓ Special hospital diets alter the composition, texture, digestibility, and residue of foods to suit client's particular needs.

✓ Tube feedings can be used for clients who are unable to ingest food but are able to digest and absorb foods.

✓ Total parenteral nutrition (TPN) supplies essential nutrients in appropriate amounts to support life through the introduction of a concentrated nutrient solution into a large central vein or the right atrium of the heart.

✓ Evaluation of the outcomes of nursing intervention in the area of nutritional support is essential to revise, update, or continue nursing activities.

REFERENCE

Pennington, J.: Considerations for a new food guide, J. Nutr. Education 13:2, 1981.

ADDITIONAL READINGS

Bodinski, L.: A nurse's guide to diet therapy, New York, 1982, John Wiley & Sons, Inc.

Buergel, N.: Monitoring nutritional status in the clinical setting, Nurs. Clin. North Am. 14:2, 1979.

Butterworth, C.: The skeleton in the hospital closet, Nutr. Today 9:4, 1974.

Butterworth, C., and Blackburn, G.: Hospital malnutrition and how to assess the nutritional status of the patient, Nurs. Digest 4:6, 1976.

Caly, J.: Assessing adults' nutrition, Am. J. Nurs. 77:10, 1977.

Ciseaux, A.: A view from the mirror, Am. J. Nurs. 80:8, 1980.

Claggett, M.: Anorexia nervosa: a behavioral approach, Am. J. Nurs. 80:8, 1980.

Copeland, E., Van Elys, J., and Shils, M.: Nutrition and cancer, 1978, American Cancer Society.

Department of Agriculture and Department of Health and Human Services: Nutrition and your health: dietary guidelines for Americans, Washington, D.C., 1980, U.S. Government Printing Office.

Dwyer, J.: Vegetarianism, Contemp. Nutr. 4:6, 1979.

Goodhart, R., and Shils, M., editors: Modern nutrition in health and disease, ed. 6, Philadelphia, 1980, Lea & Febiger.

Greenburg, J.: Why your hospitalized patient won't eat, Consultant 19:9, 1979.

Howard, R., and Herbold, N.: Nutrition in clinical care, ed. 2, New York, 1982, McGraw-Hill Book Co.

Hui, Y.: Human nutrition and diet therapy, Belmont, Calif., 1983, Wadsworth Publishing Co.

Keithley, J.: Proper nutritional assessment can prevent hospital malnutrition, Nursing 79 9:2, 1979.

Krause, M., and Mahan, L.: Food, nutrition, and diet therapy, Philadelphia, 1979, W.B. Saunders Co.

Lucas, A.: Anorexia nervosa, Contemp. Nutr. 3:8, 1978.

Lucas, A.: Bulimia and vomiting syndrome, Contemp. Nutr. 6:4, 1981.

Massachusetts General Hospital Dietary Department: Diet manual, Boston, 1976, Little, Brown & Co.

McDaniel, J.: Diet therapy in the nursing school curriculum, J. Am. Diet. Assoc. 70:3, 1977.

Mertz, W.: Trace elements, Contemp. Nutr. 3:2, 1978.

Mosby's medical and nursing dictionary, St. Louis, 1983, The C.V. Mosby Co.

Richardson, T.: Anorexia nervosa: an overview, Am. J. Nurs. 80:8, 1980.

Robinson, C., and Weigley, E.: Basic nutrition and diet therapy, New York, 1984, Macmillan, Inc.

Rose, J.: Nutritional problems in radiotherapy patients, Am. J. Nurs. 78:6, 1978.

Rose, J., editor: Nutrition and killer diseases, Park Ridge, N.J., 1982, Noyes Publications.

Rudman, D., and Williams, P.: Megavitamins: use and misuse, N. Engl. J. Med. 309:8, 1983.

Schaumburg, H., et al.: Sensory neuropathy from pyridoxine abuse: a new megavitamin syndrome, N. Engl. J. Med. 309:8, 1983.

Senate Select Committee on Human Needs: Dietary goals for the United States, Washington, D.C., 1977, U.S. Government Printing Office.

Shapcott, D.: Essential trace mineral deficiencies and cardiovascular disease. In Rose, J., editor: Nutrition and killer diseases, Park Ridge, N.J., 1982, Noyes Publications.

Suitor, C., and Hunter, M.: Nutrition: principles and application in health promotion, Philadelphia, 1980, J.B. Lippincott Co.

Thiele, V.F.: Clinical nutrition, ed. 2, St. Louis, 1980, The C.V. Mosby Co.

Williams, S.R.: Nutrition and diet therapy, ed. 4, St. Louis, 1984, The C.V. Mosby Co.

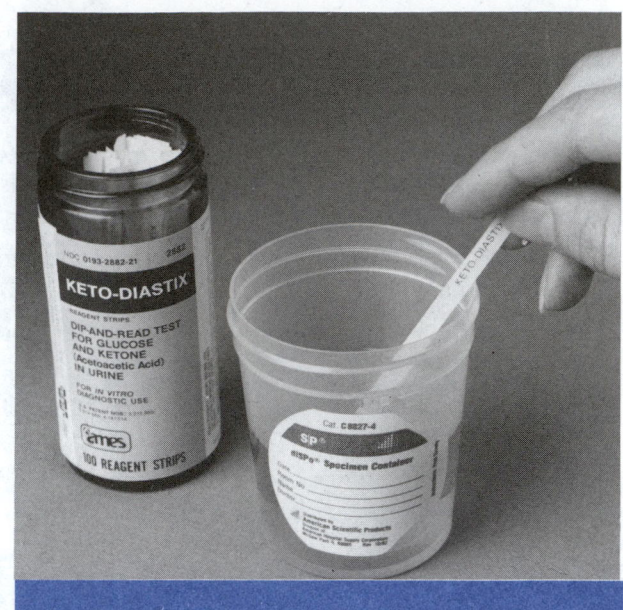

OBJECTIVES

Mastery of content in this chapter will enable the student to:

- Define the terms in the glossary.
- Explain the function of each organ in the urinary system.
- Describe the process of urination.
- Identify factors that commonly influence urinary elimination.
- Compare and contrast common alterations in urinary elimination.
- Explain how urethral catheterization predisposes a client to a urinary tract infection.
- Describe physical assessment techniques used to assess urinary elimination.
- Obtain a nursing history for a client with urinary elimination problems.
- Obtain a clean-voided urine specimen.
- Describe characteristics of normal and abnormal urine.
- Describe the nursing implications of common diagnostic tests of the urinary system.
- Describe nursing measures that stimulate the micturition reflex.
- Insert a urinary catheter.
- Apply a condom catheter.
- Instruct a client on Credé's bladder compression and pelvic floor muscle exercises.

GLOSSARY

anuria Cessation of urine production.

bacteriuria Presence of bacteria in the urine.

Credé's method Manual compression of the bladder externally to promote expulsion of urine.

cystitis Inflammation of the urinary bladder, characterized by pain, urgency, and frequency of urination.

diuresis Increased formation and excretion of urine.

dysuria Painful urination resulting from bacterial infection of the bladder and obstructive conditions of the urethra.

glomerulus Cluster or collection of capillary vessels within the kidney involved in the initial formation of urine.

glycosuria Abnormal presence of glucose in the urine.

hematuria Abnormal presence of blood in the urine.

ketonuria Presence in the urine of excessive amounts of ketone bodies by products of fat metabolism such as occurs in diabetes mellitus.

meatus Opening through any part of the body, for example, the urethral meatus.

micturition Urination; act of passing or expelling urine voluntarily through the urethra.

nephron Structural and functional unit of the kidney containing a renal glomerulus and tubule.

39 *Urinary Elimination*

neurogenic bladder   Dysfunctional urinary bladder resulting from impaired neurological innervation.

neuropathy   Abnormal condition characterized by inflammation and degeneration of peripheral nerves.

polyuria   Excretion of an abnormally large volume of urine.

renal   Of or pertaining to the kidney.

residual urine   Volume of urine remaining in the bladder after a normal voiding; the bladder normally is almost completely empty after micturition.

ureterostomy   Diversion of urine away from a diseased or defective bladder through an artificial opening in the skin.

urgency   Sensation of the need to void soon.

urinary frequency   Symptom involving increased voiding.

urinary incontinence   Inability to control urination.

The ability to maintain control of urination is a basic function most people take for granted. As with bowel elimination, any alteration in urinary elimination may result in considerable embarrassment. A client forced to depend on a catheter for urinary drainage feels self-conscious and dependent on care givers. A client who wets his clothing because of poor urination control feels a sense of uncleanliness and revulsion.

Clients with urinary elimination problems require understanding and sensitivity to their needs. Elimination alterations may cause serious changes in a client's body image and pose other health problems. With elderly clients in particular the nurse must be aware of the reasons for their problems and find acceptable solutions.

Physiology of Urinary Elimination

Urinary elimination depends on the function of four organs: kidneys, ureters, bladder, and urethra. The kidneys remove wastes from the blood and form urine. The ureters transport urine from the kidneys to the bladder. The bladder holds urine until the urge to urinate develops. The urethra is the final passageway through which urine leaves the body. All organs of the urinary system must be intact and functional for the successful removal of urinary wastes (Fig. 39-1).

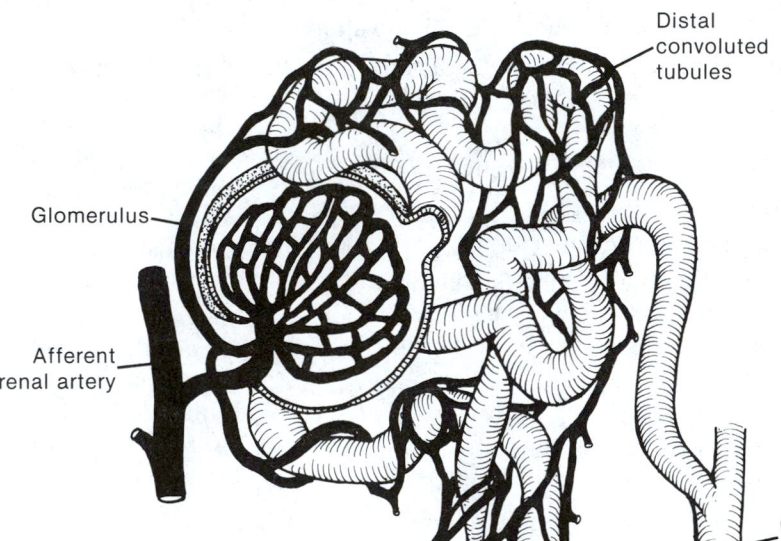

Fig. 39-1   Organs of the urinary system.

Diaphragm
Adrenal gland
Right kidney
Ureters
Orifices of ureters
Urethra
Adrenal gland
Left kidney
Bladder
Trigone

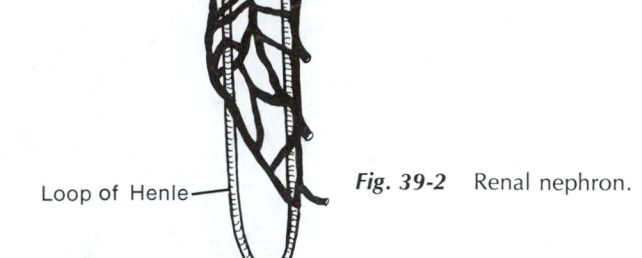

Fig. 39-2   Renal nephron.

Distal convoluted tubules
Glomerulus
Afferent renal artery
Collecting duct
Loop of Henle

Kidneys

The kidneys are reddish brown, bean-shaped organs that lie on either side of the vertebral column behind the abdominal peritoneum and against the deep muscles of the back. The kidneys rest at a level with the twelfth thoracic and third lumbar vertebrae. Normally the left kidney is 1.5 to 2 cm ($^6/_{10}$ to $^8/_{10}$ inch) higher than the right.

The kidneys contain specialized cells called nephrons, which remove waste products from the blood and regulate water and electrolyte concentrations in body fluids (Fig. 39-2). Blood reaches the nephrons by way of the renal artery, which branches into smaller arteries, eventually giving rise to the afferent arterioles that supply the nephrons. A cluster of blood vessels leading from the afferent arteriole forms the glomerulus, which is the initial site of urine formation. The glomerular capillaries are relatively porous and permit the filtration of water and substances such as glucose, amino acids, urea, uric acid, creatinine, creatine, and major electrolytes. Protein is the one substance that does not normally filter through the glomerulus. Therefore the appearance of protein in the urine is a sign of glomerular injury. The hydrostatic pressure of blood within the capillaries acts as the force for blood filtration through the glomerulus. The filtration pressure remains relatively constant because of the kidneys' ability to adapt to changes in systemic arterial blood pressure. Normally 180 liters of blood filter through the nephrons of each kidney daily. This is about 21% of the cardiac output. The kidneys' normal glomerular filtration rate is 125 ml per minute.

Not all of the glomerular filtrate is excreted as urine. Once the filtrate leaves the glomerulus, it passes through a system of tubules where certain substances such as glucose, amino acids, uric acid, sodium and potassium ions, and water are selectively reabsorbed back into the plasma. Other substances such as hydrogen ions, potassium ions, and ammonia are secreted back into the tubules. Approximately 99% of the filtrate is reabsorbed into the plasma, with the remaining 1% comprising urine. The normal range of urine production for an adult is 0.6 to 1.6 liters a day. Various factors, such as fluid intake and body temperature, may affect urine production. An output of 50 ml of urine per hour is generally normal, and an output of less than 30 ml per hour may indicate kidney failure. The normal composition of urine is 95% water and 5% solutes. These solutes include electrolytes (sodium, potassium, chloride, phosphate, magnesium, and bicarbonate) and organic solutes (such as urea, uric acid, creatinine, and ammonia).

Ureters

Urine leaves the kidney tubules and enters collecting ducts that transport it to the renal pelvis. A ureter joins each kidney pelvis to provide the initial exit route for urinary wastes. The ureters are long tubular structures, 25 cm (10 inches) long and 1.25 cm (½ inch) in diameter in the adult. They extend downward behind the peritoneum to join at the floor of the bladder in the pelvic cavity. Urine draining from the ureters to the bladder is sterile.

Three layers of tissue form the wall of the ureter. The inner layer is a mucous membrane continuous with the lining of the renal tubules and urinary bladder. The mucous lining is an excellent medium for the growth and spread of microorganisms. The middle layer consists of smooth muscle fibers. This muscular layer helps transport urine through the ureters by peristaltic waves that are stimulated by the presence of urine in the renal pelvis. An outer layer of fibrous connective tissue provides support to the ureters.

Peristaltic waves cause the urine to enter the bladder in spurts rather than in a steady flow. To prevent the reflux of urine from the bladder back into the ureters, a small flaplike fold of mucous membrane acts as a valve and covers the juncture of the ureters with the bladder.

An obstruction within the ureters, such as a kidney stone (renal calculus), results in strong peristaltic waves that attempt to move the obstruction into the bladder. Simultaneously a reflex sympathetic response causes constriction of the renal arterioles so that urine production in the kidney on the affected side declines.

Bladder

The urinary bladder is a hollow, distensible, muscular organ that serves as a reservoir for urine and the organ of excretion. When empty the bladder lies in the pelvic cavity behind the symphysis pubis. In the male the bladder lies against the rectum posteriorly, and in the female it rests against the anterior wall of the uterus and vagina.

The bladder's shape changes as it becomes filled with urine. Normally it holds approximately 600 ml of urine. When the bladder is full, the superior surface expands upward into a dome and pushes above the symphysis pubis. A greatly distended bladder may reach the level of the umbilicus. In a pregnant woman the fetus pushes against the bladder, causing a feeling of fullness and reducing the bladder's capacity.

At the base of the bladder is a triangular area, the trigone. An opening exists at each of the trigone's three angles: two at the base of the trigone for the ureters and one at the apex for the urethra.

The wall of the bladder consists of four layers: the inner mucous coat, which is continuous with the ureters and urethra, a submucous coat of connective tissue, a muscular coat, and an outer serous coat. The muscular layer consists of bundles of muscle fibers that form the detrusor muscle. Parasympathetic nerve fibers supply the detrusor muscle for function during urination. At the base of the bladder is the internal urethral sphincter, composed of a ringlike band of muscle. The sphincter prevents the escape of urine from the bladder and is under involuntary control by the autonomic nervous system.

Urethra

Urine travels from the bladder through the tube-shaped urethra and passes to the outside of the body through the urethral meatus. A mucous membrane lines the urethra, and urethral glands secrete mucus into the urethral canal. Thick layers of smooth muscle surround the urethra.

In women the urethra is approximately 4 cm (1½ inches) long. The external urethral sphincter, located about halfway down the urethra, permits voluntary control of urine flow. The short length of the urethra in women and girls provides an easy access for bacterial microorganisms. In men the urethra, which functions as a urinary canal and a passageway for cells and secretions from reproductive organs, is 20 cm (8 inches) long. The male urethra has three sections: the *prostatic urethra,* which passes from the bladder's base through the prostate gland, the *membranous urethra,* which is surrounded by the external urethral sphincter, and the *penile urethra.*

Act of Urination

Urination, micturition, and voiding are all terms for the process by which urine is expelled from the urinary bladder. The bladder normally holds as much as 600 ml of urine. However, the desire to urinate can be sensed when the bladder contains only a small amount of urine (150 to 200 ml in an adult, 50 to 100 ml in a child). As the volume of urine increases, the bladder walls stretch, sending sensory impulses to the micturition center in the sacral spinal cord. Parasympathetic impulses from the micturition center stimulate the detrusor muscle to contract rhythmically. The internal urethral sphincter also relaxes so urine may enter the urethra, although voiding does not yet occur. As the bladder contracts, nerve impulses travel up the spinal cord to the midbrain and cerebral cortex. A person is thus conscious of the need to urinate. If the person chooses not to void, the external urinary sphincter remains contracted and the micturition reflex is inhibited. However, when a person is ready to void, the external sphincter relaxes, the micturition reflex stimulates the detrusor muscle to contract, and urination occurs. Damage to the spinal cord above the sacral region causes loss of voluntary control of urination, but the micturition reflex pathway may remain intact, allowing urination to occur reflexively. This condition is called an *automatic bladder.*

Factors Influencing Urination

Numerous factors influence the volume of urine entering the bladder and the ability to urinate.

Growth and Development

Infants and young children are unable to concentrate urine and reabsorb water effectively. Their urine thus appears light yellow or watery. In relation to their small body size, infants and children excrete large volumes of urine. For example, a 6-month-old child who weighs between 10 and 16 pounds excretes 400 to 500 ml of urine daily. The child weighs about 10% of an adult's weight but excretes 33% as much urine.

A child is unable to control micturition voluntarily until the age of 18 to 24 months. It is usually more difficult for children to control urination than defecation. A child must be able to recognize the feeling of bladder fullness, to hold urine for 1 to 2 hours, and to communicate the sense of urgency to a parent. As in the case of toilet training for defecation, the young child needs a parent's understanding, patience, and consistency. A child may not gain full control of micturition until the age of 4 or 5. Boys are generally slower than girls. Daytime control of micturition is easier to accomplish than nighttime control and occurs earlier in the child's development, usually by 2 years of age.

The adult normally voids 1600 ml of urine daily. The kidney is able to concentrate urine effectively, producing a normal amber-colored urine. Normally a person does not void excessively during the night because of a reduction of renal blood flow during rest and because of the kidney's ability to concentrate urine.

The process of aging impairs micturition. Problems of mobility sometimes make it difficult for the elderly to reach a toilet in time. Elderly people may be too weak to rise from a toilet seat without assistance. Chronic neurological disease, such as parkinsonism or cerebrovascular accident (stroke), impairs the sense of balance and makes it difficult for men to stand while voiding. If an elderly person loses control of thought processes, the ability to control micturition is unpredictable. The person may lose the ability to sense a full bladder or be unable to recall the procedure for voiding.

Changes in kidney and bladder function also occur with aging. The kidney's ability to concentrate urine declines. Thus the elderly often experience nocturia, excessive urination at night. The bladder loses its muscle tone and capacity to hold urine, resulting in increased frequency of urination. Because the bladder cannot contract as effectively, an elderly person often retains urine in the bladder after voiding. Residual urine increases the risk for bacterial growth.

Sociocultural Factors

A person's social habits are the result of familial and cultural influences. The habits of micturition are no exception. North Americans expect toilet facilities to be private. Many Europeans, in contrast, accept less private communal toilet facilities as a way of life. There are also gender differences in toilet behavior. Men share public urinals and women use enclosed cubicles.

Toileting habits begin when children attempt to mimic parents' behaviors. Social expectations influence the time when it is proper to urinate. For example, schoolchildren are expected to wait until recess to urinate or to raise their hands for permission to use the toilet.

The nurse's approach to a client's elimination needs must consider the client's cultural and social habits. If a client prefers privacy, the nurse makes every attempt to prevent interruptions as the client voids. A client who is less sensitive to the need for privacy should be treated with understanding and acceptance.

Psychological Factors

Anxiety and emotional stress do not change the characteristics of urine, although they may affect the character of feces. However, a client who is highly anxious may feel a greater sense of urgency and experience increased frequency of urination. An anxious person may have the urge to void even after voiding only a few minutes earlier.

Anxiety may also prevent a person from being able to urinate completely. Emotional tension makes it difficult to relax abdominal and perineal muscles. If a person is unable to relax the external urethral sphincter completely, voiding may be incomplete and urine will be retained in the bladder.

Personal Habits

Some people follow complex routines before defecation. Usually fewer rituals precede urination. Privacy is the most essential condition for most people. Taking time to urinate allows a person to relax fully so that urine retention does not occur. During urination some individuals need distractions to promote relaxation, such as reading or singing.

Muscle Tone

Weakness of abdominal and pelvic floor muscles impairs bladder contraction and control of the external urethral sphincter. Poor control of micturition can result from muscle wasting caused by prolonged immobility, stretching of muscles during childbirth, menopausal muscle atrophy, and damage to muscles from trauma.

Continuous drainage of urine through an indwelling catheter causes loss of bladder tone. The bladder remains relatively empty and thus is never stretched to its capacity. When a muscle fails to be stretched regularly, atrophy develops. When a catheter is removed, the client may have difficulty regaining urinary control.

Fluid Intake

The kidneys maintain a sensitive balance between the retention and excretion of fluids. If fluids and the concentration of electrolytes and solutes are in equilibrium, an increase in fluid intake causes an increase in urine production. Ingested fluids increase the body's circulating plasma and thus increase the volume of glomerular filtrate and urine excreted.

The ingestion of certain fluids has a direct influence on urine production and excretion. Alcohol inhibits the release of antidiuretic hormone (ADH) and thus promotes urine formation. Coffee, tea, cocoa, and cola drinks that contain caffeine increase diuresis and the frequency of micturition. Foods that contain a high fluid content, such as fruits and vegetables, may also increase urine production.

Disease Conditions

Several disease conditions affect the ability to micturate. Any lesion of peripheral nerves leading to the bladder causes loss of bladder tone, reduced sensation of bladder fullness, and difficulty in controlling urination. For example, diabetes mellitus and multiple sclerosis cause neuropathies that alter bladder function.

Diseases that slow or hinder physical activity interfere with the person's ability to void. Rheumatoid arthritis, degenerative joint disease, and parkinsonism are examples of conditions that make it difficult to reach and use toilet facilities. A client with rheumatoid arthritis often cannot sit on or rise from a toilet without an elevated seat.

Renal and bladder disease obviously affects micturition. Acute renal disease, such as glomerulonephritis, reduces the volume of urine produced. Chronic renal disease initially causes the kidney to release large volumes of poorly concentrated urine. Irritation or inflammation of the bladder caused by infection or obstruction results in incomplete bladder emptying during micturition. Benign prostatic hypertrophy or enlargement of the prostate gland, a common condition in older men, results in obstruction to urine outflow and impairment of bladder tone.

Febrile conditions influence urine production. The client who becomes diaphoretic loses a large amount of fluids through insensible water loss, which causes a decrease in urine production. However, the increased body metabolism associated with fever increases the accumulation of body wastes. Although urine volume may be reduced, the urine is highly concentrated.

Surgical Procedures

The stress of surgery initially triggers the general adaptation syndrome (see Chapter 5). The posterior pituitary gland releases an increased amount of ADH, which increases water reabsorption and reduces urine output. The surgical client is often in an altered state of fluid balance before surgery, which aggravates the reduction in urine output. The stress response also reduces the level of aldosterone, resulting in reduction in urine output in an effort to increase circulatory fluid volume.

Anesthetic agents and narcotic analgesics slow the glomerular filtration rate, reducing urine output. These pharmacological agents also interfere with sensory and motor impulses traveling between the bladder, spinal cord, and brain. Clients recovering from anesthesia and deep analgesia are often unable to sense bladder fullness and are unable to initiate or inhibit micturition. Spinal anesthetics, in particular, create the risk of urinary retention because of the inability to sense the need to void.

Surgery involving lower abdominal and pelvic structures can impair urination because of local trauma to surrounding tissues. The edema and inflammation associated with the healing process (see Chapter 5) may obstruct the flow of urine from the bladder or urethra, interfere with relaxation of pelvic and sphincter muscles, or cause discomfort during voiding. After surgery involving the bladder and urethra, clients routinely need urinary catheters. The surgical formation of a ureterostomy (urinary diversion) either temporarily or permanently bypasses the bladder and urethra as the exit routes for urine. The client with a ureterostomy has a stoma on the abdomen for the purpose of draining urine.

Medications

Various medications influence the volume of urine excreted or change the characteristics of urine. Diuretics prevent the reabsorption of water and certain electrolytes in the kidney tubules, resulting in increased urine output. Because of the high proportion of water in the urine a client taking diuretics has light-colored urine. Certain medications change the color of urine. Table 39-1 lists some common medications and their effects on urine.

Diagnostic Examinations

Examinations of the urinary system can influence micturition. Certain procedures such as an intravenous pyelogram or urogram require that the client not take fluids orally before the test. A restriction in fluid intake commonly lowers urine output. Diagnostic examinations (for example, cystoscopy) that involve direct visualization of urinary structures may cause localized edema of the urethral passageway and spasm of the bladder sphincter. The client often has urinary retention following such a procedure and may pass red- or pink-tinged urine because of bleeding resulting from trauma to the urethral or bladder mucosa.

Alterations in Urinary Elimination

The most common urinary problems encountered by the nurse involve disturbances in the act of mic-

TABLE 39-1

Drugs That Discolor Urine

Drug	Color of Urine
Amitriptyline (Elavil)	Blue-green
Cascara	Yellow to red
Danthron (Modane, Dorbane)	Pink to red
Phenytoin (Dilantin)	Pink to red to red-brown
Indomethacin (Indocin)	Green
Methyldopa (Aldomet)	Red
Phenazopyridine (Pyridium)	Orange to red
Phenothiazines (Thorazine, Mellaril)	Pink to red to red-brown
Riboflavin (vitamin B$_2$)	Yellow
Rifampin (Rifadin)	Bright orange-red
Warfarin sodium (Coumadin)	Orange

turition. These disturbances result from impaired bladder function, obstruction to urine outflow, or inability to voluntarily control micturition. Some clients may have permanent or temporary changes in the normal pathway of urinary excretion. The ureterostomy client has special problems, since urine drains to the outside through an artificial opening (stoma) on the abdominal wall.

Urinary Retention

Urinary retention is the inability of the bladder to empty fully. Urine accumulates in the bladder, stretching its walls and causing feelings of pressure, discomfort, tenderness over the symphysis pubis, restlessness, and diaphoresis. A key sign is the absence of urine output over several hours and the development of a distended bladder. The client under the influence of anesthetics or analgesics may feel only pressure, but the alert client will experience severe pain as the bladder distends beyond its normal capacity. In severe urinary retention the bladder may hold as much as 2000 to 3000 ml of urine.

As retention progresses, *retention with outflow* may develop. Pressure in the bladder builds to a point that the external urethral sphincter is unable to hold back urine. The sphincter temporarily opens to allow a small volume of urine (25 to 60 ml) to escape. As urine exits, the bladder pressure falls enough to allow the sphincter to regain control and close. Thus a vicious circle develops. The client voids small amounts of urine two or three times an hour with no real relief of distention or discomfort.

Retention occurs as a result of urethral obstruction, alterations in motor and sensory innervation of the bladder, and emotional anxiety (Table 39-2). Low fluid intake may also cause distention, although it is a less common cause. Gradual urine production fills the bladder slowly and prevents activation of the stretch receptors. After distending beyond a certain point the bladder becomes unable to contract.

Lower Urinary Tract Infections

Urinary tract infections are the most common type of hospital-acquired (nosocomial) infections in the United States, accounting for nearly half of such infections. The formation of bacteria in the urine (bacteriuria) is a serious problem that may lead to the spread of organisms into the bloodstream and kidneys.

Microorganisms can enter the urinary tract through

TABLE 39-2

Causes of Urinary Elimination Disorders

Disorder	Physiological Alteration	Causes
Urinary retention	Obstruction of urine flow	Prostate gland enlargement, fecal impaction, pregnancy in third trimester, urethral stricture or edema following childbirth, urethral edema following surgery or diagnostic examination
	Alterations in motor and sensory innervation	Spinal cord and peripheral nerve trauma, degeneration of peripheral nerves (e.g., diabetic neuropathy)
	Inability to relax sphincters	Emotional anxiety, muscle tension
Lower urinary tract infection	Obstruction to urine flow	Kinked or blocked urethral catheter, urinary retention
	Introduction of media for bacterial spread	Poor perineal hygiene, frequent sexual intercourse, improperly handled diagnostic instruments, improperly sterilized instruments, contaminated urine receptacles
Urinary incontinence	Incompetent or weakened sphincter	Multiple childbirths, surgery of pelvic organs, removal of prostate
	Loss of voluntary control of voiding	Mental confusion, sedation or analgesia, spinal cord injury, bladder spasm, bladder atrophy

the urethral meatus or through the bloodstream. The ascending route through the urethra is more common. Bacteria inhabit the perineum, the periurethral meatus, the distal urethra, and the vagina in women. Organisms thus enter the urethral meatus easily and travel up along the inner mucosal lining to the bladder. Women are more susceptible to infection because of the proximity of the anus to the urethral meatus and because of the female's short urethra. In the male, prostatic secretions contain an antibacterial substance that reduces the occurrence of urinary tract infection.

In a healthy person with good bladder function, organisms are flushed out spontaneously during voiding. However, bladder distention reduces blood flow to the mucosal and submucosal layers. Tissues become more susceptible to bacterial invasion. Residual urine in the bladder is an ideal site for microorganism growth. The pH and chemical makeup of urine also affect the spread of organisms. Bacteria grow more readily in an acid environment and in high concentrations of urea.

The most common cause of infection is urinary tract instrumentation. For example, the introduction of a catheter or diagnostic instrument through the urethra provides a direct route for microorganisms. With an indwelling bladder catheter, bacteria ascend along the outside of the catheter on the urethral wall or travel up the catheter's lumen. The catheter interferes with the normal voiding mechanism that acts as a defense against organisms entering the urethra. Local irritation to the urethra or bladder further predisposes tissues to bacterial invasion.

Urinary tract infections acquired in health institutions also result from contaminated hands of personnel, irrigation fluids, catheter lubricants, urinals, bedpans, and rectal thermometers.

Poor perineal hygiene is a common cause of urinary tract infection in females. Inadequate handwashing, failure to wipe from front to back after voiding or defecating, and frequent sexual intercourse predispose females to urinary tract infection. In some young girls cystitis develops as a result of exposure to ingredients in bubble baths. Any interference with the free flow of urine predisposes clients to infection. A kinked or obstructed catheter and any condition resulting in urinary retention can cause infection of the bladder.

Clients with urinary tract infections experience pain or burning during urination (dysuria) as urine flows past inflamed tissues. Fever, chills, nausea and vomiting, and malaise develop as the infection worsens. An irritated bladder causes a frequent and urgent sensation of the need to void. Irritation to bladder and urethral mucosa results in blood-tinged urine (hematuria). The urine appears concentrated and cloudy because of the presence of bacteria. If infection spreads to the kidneys, flank pain, tenderness, and chills are common symptoms.

Urinary Incontinence

Urinary incontinence is the loss of control over micturition. The condition may be temporary or permanent and can be caused by urinary infections, physiological changes of aging, mental confusion, weakened pelvic muscles, spinal cord injury, loss of bladder tone, or the effects of sedatives or analgesics.

The client is no longer able to control the external urethral sphincter. Complete incontinence is total uncontrollable emptying of the bladder. When a client loses only a portion of urine from the bladder, or dribbles, the condition is partial incontinence. Incontinence is not the same as urinary retention overflow. With incontinence the bladder does not normally reach full capacity or become distended.

There are two main types of incontinence: stress incontinence and urge incontinence. In *stress incontinence* an increase in intra-abdominal pressure from activities such as coughing, vomiting, lifting, or laughing interferes with the weakened urethral sphincter and forces expulsion of urine. The condition is most common in women with displacement of the bladder following hysterectomy or multiple childbirths. Men who have had surgical removal of the prostate gland may also experience stress incontinence.

Urge incontinence occurs when a person develops a sudden urge to urinate and is unable to reach toilet facilities in time. Urge incontinence may be precipitated by any number of factors. Bladder infections, bladder spasms, and neuromuscular dysfunction are common causes.

Incontinence should not be associated only with the elderly and senile. It may develop in people of every age, although it is more common in adults. Incontinence causes a person to feel like a social outcast. Clothing becomes wet with urine, and the accompanying odor adds to the embarrassment. Clients with this problem often avoid social activities for fear of an episode occurring.

The elderly do have special problems with incontinence because of their physical limitations and the environment in which they live. An elderly person with restricted mobility has a greater chance of being incontinent because of inability to reach toilet facilities in time. Low-set chairs and beds raised well above the floor may be obstacles for the elderly who must get up to reach a toilet. An elderly client who has difficulty undoing buttons or manipulating zippers faces another obstacle in using toilet facilities. The elderly client often lacks the energy to walk very far at one time, and if there is only one toilet in the home, the distance may be too far for the client with urge incontinence.

Continued episodes of incontinence create the potential for skin breakdown. The acidic character of urine is irritating to the skin. The immobilized client who has frequent incontinence is especially at risk for decubitus ulcers (see Chapter 31).

Enuresis

Enuresis is repeated involuntary urination in children who have reached the age when voluntary bladder control is possible. Episodes occur more commonly at night (nocturnal enuresis), usually during deep sleep (see Chapter 36). Enuresis may occur during the day (diurnal enuresis) when the child is engaged in play and is unaware of a full bladder. Some children are enuretic during a temper tantrum or dispute with a sibling. Such an accident may be an attention-seeking behavior.

Primary enuresis means that the child has never had a long dry or symptom-free period. *Secondary* or *acquired enuresis* occurs after a dry period of at least a year. The combined incidence of both types of enuresis is 5% to 17% in otherwise normal children between 3 and 15 years of age (Whaley and Wong, 1983).

Several theories have been developed about the cause of enuresis. The condition has been shown to be associated with hereditary factors. Parents, siblings, and close relatives of enuretic children often have histories of the problem. These people have had difficulty inhibiting the micturition reflex. Delayed development, sibling rivalry, emotional trauma during toilet training, food allergies, and behavior problems are additional possible causes of enuresis. Behavior problems, however, are more likely to be the result than the cause of enuresis.

Ureterostomies

With surgery it is possible to divert the drainage of urine from a diseased or dysfunctional bladder. A

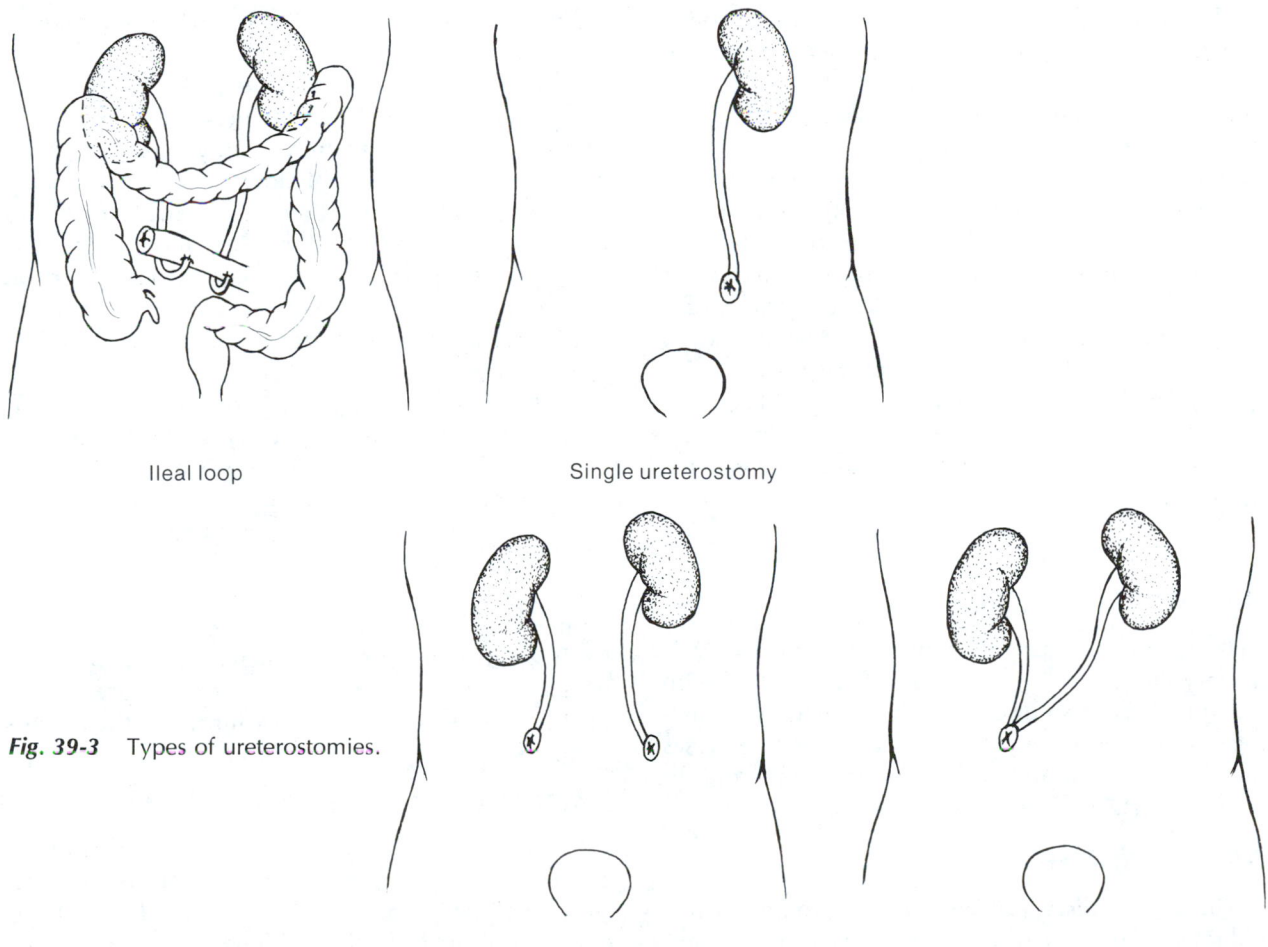

Ileal loop

Single ureterostomy

Double ureterostomy

Transureterostomy

Fig. **39-3** Types of ureterostomies.

ureterostomy or urinary diversion is any one of several surgical procedures that create stomas on the outer abdominal wall for urine drainage. Typically the client with a ureterostomy has had the bladder removed surgically because of a malignant growth, or had birth defects, or has undergone spinal cord injury. A ureterostomy is the treatment of choice for problems related to chronic incontinence.

Fig. 39-3 illustrates several types of ureterostomies. The ileal loop or conduit involves separating a loop of intestinal ileum with its blood supply intact. The surgeon implants the ureters into the ileum, which serves as an outlet for urine drainage. The ileum is not a reservoir or bladder. The remaining ileum is reconnected to the rest of the digestive tract. The disadvantage of this procedure is that, if urine outflow becomes obstructed, the ileal conduit absorbs fluids and electrolytes and can cause metabolic alterations.

A ureterostomy involves bringing the end of one or both ureters to the abdominal surface. To avoid the need for two collecting devices, a transureterostomy connects the ureters and brings one out through the abdominal wall.

The client with a ureterostomy must wear a stomal pouch continuously because there is no sphincter control for regulation of urine flow. Because of continuous urinary drainage a major challenge in the care of the client with a ureterostomy is maintenance of skin integrity. Any obstruction within a ureterostomy may lead to serious fluid and electrolyte alterations.

A ureterostomy poses the same threats to a client's body image as a colostomy. The client must wear an artificial device to collect urine, and he must learn the skills to manage it. This requires physical and social rehabilitation. The client with a ureterostomy can wear normal clothing, engage in any physical activity, travel, and have sexual relations. It is not necessary for the client with an ostomy to adopt an isolated life-style.

Assessment

To identify the presence and nature of a client's urinary elimination problem and gather data for an individualized plan of care, the nurse obtains a nursing history, performs a physical assessment, assesses the client's urine, and reviews information from diagnostic tests and examinations.

Nursing History

The nursing history reviews the status of the client's kidney and urinary tract function, as well as conditions that may alter urination.

PATTERN OF URINATION

The nurse questions the client as to the approximate number of times voiding occurs each day. Frequency varies significantly among individuals. The common times for urination are on awakening from sleep, following meals, and before bedtime. If the client voids frequently during the night, this pattern may indicate renal disease. Information about the client's pattern of urination is necessary to establish a baseline of comparison for the client's urination pattern during the nurse's care. *Polyuria* is excessive urination; *oliguria* is the voiding of scant amounts of urine. If the client is suffering from any diagnosed illness, the nurse also determines if the urination pattern has recently changed.

PAST ILLNESSES OR SURGERY

Through the nursing history the nurse determines whether the client has had a history of elimination problems such as urinary tract infections, prostatic hypertrophy, or neurogenic bladder. A history of urinary alterations increases the client's risk for recurrent problems. Chronic diseases such as diabetes and multiple sclerosis, which impair bladder function, require the nurse to use preventive measures in the plan of care.

Surgical trauma to perineal or pelvic areas creates the potential for elimination problems. The nurse carefully assesses clients returning from surgery who have difficulty voiding. Bladder distention or retention overflow indicates that the client is unable to control micturition fully. If the client has had previous surgery for the purpose of creating a urinary diversion or ostomy, the nurse assesses its location and reviews the client's usual methods for management, including the following:

1. The type of appliances or pouch
2. The type of skin barriers or applications
3. The methods used to reduce or prevent skin irritation
4. The frequency of appliance changes
5. The type of nighttime drainage system

If the client is at home, the nurse determines if management methods promote urine outflow and effectively prevent complications such as skin irritation or urinary infection. In the hospital or long-term care facility, the nurse attempts to integrate the client's methods into the routine of care.

SYMPTOMS OF URINARY ALTERATIONS

Certain symptoms specific to urinary alterations may occur in more than one type of disorder. During an assessment the nurse asks the client if any of the symptoms listed in Table 39-3 have been experienced. The nurse also assesses if the client is aware of any conditions or factors that precipitate or aggravate the symptoms.

MEDICATIONS

The nurse reviews the client's medication history to determine if the use of any drugs may be influencing the client's elimination pattern or the character of the urine. The history should include use of over-the-counter medications.

ENVIRONMENTAL BARRIERS

For the elderly client or the client with mobility problems the nurse should assess conditions in the environment that may make urination difficult. If the client has limited knee or hip mobility or has weakened lower extremity muscles, are there elevated toilet seats, grab bars, or toilet seat arms available? What is the distance between the client's bed and the bathroom? Would a portable commode be useful in preventing accidents of incontinence?

Clients with visual alterations may have difficulty reaching toilet facilities. The bathroom or bedroom should have a night light. If the client has difficulty with hand coordination, the nurse should assess the client's types of clothing and the client's ease in using clothing fasteners.

Physical Assessment

During the initial inspection it is important for the nurse to assess skin integrity. Often problems with urinary elimination are associated with fluid and electrolyte disturbances. The nurse assesses the skin's hydration status by noting texture and turgor. Assessment of the oral mucosa also reveals whether the client's hydration is adequate. Chapter 42 describes additional assessment data for detecting fluid and electrolyte imbalance.

To assess urinary function the nurse examines the kidneys, bladder, and urethral meatus. Chapter 29 describes in detail the techniques of assessment.

KIDNEYS

The location of the kidneys makes it difficult for the nurse to assess their integrity. The only way to assess the position, shape, and size of the kidneys is by deep palpation of the abdomen. Much practice is required for the nurse to become adept at kidney palpation.

If the kidneys become infected or inflamed, flank pain typically develops. The nurse can assess for tenderness early in the course of the disease by percussing the costovertebral angle (the angle formed by the spine and twelfth rib). The client may sit or stand, and the nurse uses either direct or indirect percussion

TABLE 39-3

Common Symptoms of Urinary Alterations

Symptom	Causes
Urgency	Full bladder, inflammation or irritation to bladder mucosa, incompetent urethral sphincter
Dysuria	Cystitis, trauma or inflammation of urethra
Difficulty starting stream	Prostate enlargement, anxiety, urethral edema
Polyuria	Increased fluid intake, diuretics, diabetes insipidus (deficiency of ADH), acute glomerulonephritis, ingestion of fluids containing alcohol or caffeine
Oliguria	Dehydration, renal failure

over the costovertebral angle. Inflammation of the kidney results in pain during percussion.

BLADDER

Normally the bladder rests below the symphysis pubis and cannot be examined by the nurse. When distended, the bladder rises above the symphysis pubis at the midline of the abdomen and just below the umbilicus. During the physical assessment the nurse may note a swelling or convex curvature of the lower abdomen. This observation is easier to make in clients of low or average body weight.

When distention is not visible, the nurse lightly palpates the lower abdomen. The bladder normally feels smooth and rounded. As the nurse applies light pressure to the bladder, the client may feel tenderness or even pain, depending on the degree of bladder fullness. Palpation may also cause the urge to urinate.

Percussion of the bladder provides minimal assessment data except for distinguishing the bladder from other abdominal organs or abnormalities. A full distended bladder produces a dull percussion note.

URETHRAL MEATUS

The female client assumes a dorsal recumbent position to provide full exposure of the genitalia. The nurse uses the nondominant hand to retract the labial folds in order to visualize the urethral meatus. Normally the meatus is pink and appears as a small slitlike opening below the clitoris and above the vaginal orifice. There is normally no discharge from the meatus. Any drainage may indicate presence of infection. The nurse notes the color and consistency of any drainage. A clear watery drainage is likely to be urine.

Women with vaginal infections are susceptible to urinary tract infections, since the vaginal discharge may travel easily to the urethral meatus. Elderly women commonly have vaginitis as a result of hormonal deficiencies. The nurse inspects the vaginal orifice carefully and describes the character of any drainage. Infection is indicated by reddened, inflamed vaginal mucosa.

The male's urethral meatus is normally a small opening at the tip of the penis. A *hypospadias* is a congenitally formed opening of the urethra on the undersurface of the penis. The nurse inspects the meatus for the presence of discharge and inflammation. It may be necessary to retract the foreskin in uncircumcised males in order to visualize the meatus clearly.

Assessment of Urine

The assessment of urine involves measuring the client's fluid intake and urine output and observing the characteristics of the client's urine.

INTAKE AND OUTPUT

The nurse assesses the client's average daily fluid intake. Clients in the home setting can report their fluid intake in units of cups, cans, and glasses rather than milliliters. If a more precise measurement of fluid intake is needed, the nurse may ask the client to show a commonly used glass or cup on which the intake estimate is based.

In a health care setting the nurse measures all of a client's fluid intake when the physician orders intake and output measurement (see Chapter 42). The nurse includes all sources of fluid intake, such as fluids taken during meals and with medications, intravenous infusions, and nasogastric tube feedings.

Because it is often difficult for the client to estimate volumes of urine voided, the nurse must obtain measurements rather than depend on the client's estimate in the nursing history. A change in urine volume is a significant indicator of fluid imbalance or kidney disease. While caring for the client, the nurse assesses volume by measuring the urinary output with each voiding. Plastic receptacles are available that fit under toilet seats to collect urine. The nurse also measures urine from bedpans or male urinals. If the client has a catheter, the drainage bag collects all urine for measurement. Special urimeters attach to the catheter drainage tubing and are a convenient means of measuring urine volume on an hourly or more frequent

basis. A urimeter is a plastic cylinder that holds from 100 to 200 ml of urine. After measuring urine from a urimeter the nurse can drain the cylinder into the urinary drainage bag or into a receptacle for disposal.

CHARACTERISTICS OF URINE

The nurse inspects the client's urine for color, clarity, and odor.

COLOR. Normal urine ranges in color from a pale, straw color to amber, depending on its concentration. Urine is usually more concentrated when a person awakens in the morning. As the person drinks more fluids, the urine becomes less concentrated.

Bleeding from the kidneys or ureters causes urine to become dark red; bleeding from the bladder or urethra causes a bright red urine. Various medications also change the urine's color (see Table 39-1). Certain foods may change the urine color to red, including beets, rhubarb, and blackberries. Special dyes used in intravenous diagnostic studies eventually become excreted by the kidneys and discolor the urine. Dark amber urine may be the result of high concentrations of bilirubin caused by jaundice of the liver. Whenever the client's urine changes to an abnormal color, the nurse reports it to the physician.

CLARITY. Normal urine appears transparent at the time of voiding. Urine that stands several minutes in a container becomes cloudy. Freshly voided urine in clients with renal disease may appear cloudy because of the protein concentration. Urine also appears thick and cloudy as a result of the presence of bacteria.

ODOR. A person's urine has a characteristic aromatic odor. The more concentrated the urine, the stronger the odor. Presence of bacteria in the urine causes an ammonia odor; this is common in clients who are repeatedly incontinent.

Urine Testing

The nurse is frequently responsible for collecting urine specimens for laboratory testing. The type of test determines the method of urine collection. A urinalysis, involving measurement of the common constituents of urine, requires only a specimen obtained with normal voiding. A urine specimen for culture and sensitivity must be sterile in order to get an accurate measurement of bacterial growth in the urine. A 24-hour urine collection requires a client to collect all urine during a specific 24-hour period. A double-voided specimen, which is used to test urinary glucose, requires the client to void twice in succession, discarding the first specimen.

SPECIMEN COLLECTION

URINALYSIS SAMPLE. A simple urinalysis does not require a sterile urine specimen. The client may void into a clean urine cup, a urinal, or a bedpan. The client must void before defecating so feces do not contaminate the specimen. If a woman is having a menstrual period, the nurse makes note of this on the specimen requisition in case red blood cells appear in the urine. The nurse transfers the urine to the proper container and sends it to the laboratory. All specimens are labeled with the client's name, the date, and the time of collection.

CLEAN-VOIDED OR MIDSTREAM SPECIMEN. To obtain a specimen relatively free of the microorganisms growing in the lower urethra, the nurse instructs the client on the method for obtaining a clean-voided specimen. Both female and male clients receive a clean washcloth with soap or a disinfectant towel to wash the urethral meatus. The woman should wipe from the meatus toward the rectum or from the least contaminated to the most contaminated area. The man cleans the meatus in a circular motion moving from the meatus up the glans penis. The nurse cautions the client against wiping repeatedly with the contaminated cloth.

The client receives a sterile urine cup in which to void. The nurse instructs the client to allow the first part of the urine stream to go discarded. The initial stream cleans or flushes the urethral orifice and meatus of any resident bacteria. During the midstream or middle portion of voiding, the nurse or client collects the specimen. It is easier for the client to obtain the specimen while using toilet facilities rather than sitting on a bedpan. Immediately after obtaining the specimen the nurse places a sterile top securely over the container and labels it with the client's name, the date, and the time of collection. Urine specimens must reach the laboratory within 1 hour of collection or else be refrigerated to 4° C. Urine that stands in a container at room temperature fosters bacterial growth.

STERILE SPECIMEN. Another method for collecting a sterile urine specimen for culture is by catheterizing a client (see Procedure 39-2) or by obtaining the specimen from an indwelling catheter already in place. Urine specimens should not be collected for culture from urine drainage bags unless it is the first urine drained into a new sterile bag. Bacteria grow rapidly in drainage bags and would give a false measurement of bacteria in bladder urine.

When catheterizing a client, the nurse collects the specimen as soon as urine flows from the catheter's end. After filling the sample container the nurse either withdraws the catheter (if the catheterization is performed only for a sample) or connects the indwelling catheter to a drainage tube.

If a client already has an indwelling catheter, the nurse uses a sterile syringe to withdraw the urine specimen. A 3 ml syringe with a small-gauge needle (23- or 25-gauge) is best. A large-gauge needle is more likely to leave a permanent hole through which urine may leak from the system. It is safe to insert a needle directly into the end of a self-sealing rubber catheter. Silastic, plastic, or silicone catheters are not self-sealing. Some urine drainage tubes have special ports to withdraw specimens. The nurse wipes the catheter or port with a disinfectant swab. Inserting the needle at a 30-degree angle ensures entrance into the catheter lumen. To ensure that urine will be in the tubing or catheter, the nurse may clamp the tubing just below the site chosen for specimen withdrawal. This allows fresh sterile urine to collect in the tube. The nurse must be careful not to raise the tubing, which returns urine to the bladder.

After obtaining the specimen the nurse transfers the urine into a sterile container using sterile aseptic technique. The laboratory requisition should indicate how the specimen was collected (by catheterization or needle aspiration).

TWENTY-FOUR-HOUR URINE SPECIMENS. Some tests of renal function and urine composition, such as the measurement of levels of adrenocortical steroids and hormones and creatinine clearance tests, require a 24-hour collection of urine. The 24-hour collection period begins after the client urinates. The nurse indicates the starting time on the gallon urine jar or bottle and on the laboratory requisition. The nurse discards the first sample. The client then collects all urine voided in the 24-hour period. Any missed specimens will make the test results inaccurate. The nurse should remind the client to void before defecating so that urine is not contaminated by feces. The 24-hour collection jar usually either contains a preservative or requires refrigeration. The laboratory should be consulted for instructions. The client should void the last specimen as close as possible to the end of the 24-hour period.

DOUBLE-VOIDED SPECIMEN. For accurate measurement of glucose and ketones in the urine the specimen must be "fresh." Stagnant urine that has been in the client's bladder for several hours does not reveal the amount of glucose and ketones in the urine at the time of testing. Ideally the client voids 30 to 45 minutes before the time a test specimen is required. The nurse discards the first specimen and then has the client drink at least 8 ounces of water or another preferred liquid. The client then voids a second or double-voided specimen for testing. The second specimen accurately reflects the urine that was recently filtered by the kidney.

URINE COLLECTION IN CHILDREN. Specimen collection from infants and children is often difficult. Adolescents and school-age children are usually able to cooperate, although they may be easily embarrassed. Preschool children and toddlers have difficulty voiding on request. Offering a young child fluids 30 minutes before requesting a specimen may help. The nurse must use terms for urination that the child can understand, such as "pee-pee" or "tinkle." A young child may be reluctant to void in unfamiliar receptacles. A potty chair or bedpan placed under the toilet is usually effective. The nurse must use special collection devices for infants or toddlers who are not toilet trained. Clear, plastic, single-use bags with self-adhering material can be attached over the child's urethral meatus.

The nurse prepares an infant by first washing the genitalia, perineum, and surrounding skin with soap and water or an antiseptic. Thorough drying is necessary, since the bag's adhesive does not stick to a moist, powdered, or oily surface. The nurse attaches the bag from back to front, first to the perineum and then toward the symphysis pubis. In girls the perineum should be stretched tightly to ensure that the bag has a leak-proof fit. In boys the scrotum and penis fit inside the collection bag. A diaper is placed over the bag. The nurse checks the bag frequently and removes it as soon as urine is available. An active child can easily loosen the bag and cause a leak. For a clean-voided specimen the nurse uses a sterile collection bag.

COMMON URINE TESTS

Four of the common urine tests are urinalysis, specific gravity measurement, urine culture, and a test for glucose and ketones.

URINALYSIS. The laboratory performs the urinalysis on a routine or clean-voided specimen or on a specimen obtained from a catheter. Table 39-4 lists the normal values for a urinalysis. The urinalysis is a

TABLE 39-4

Routine Urinalysis Values

Measurement	Normal Value	Interpretation
pH	4.6 to 8.0	Helps to indicate acid-base balance; urine that stands for several hours becomes alkaline from bacterial invasion
Protein	Up to 8 mg/100 ml	Normally not present in urine; seen in renal disease because damage to glomerular membrane allows protein to enter urine
Glucose	Not normally present	Diabetic clients have glucose in urine as a result of inability of tubules to reabsorb high glucose concentrations (over 180 mg/100 ml); ingestion of high concentrations of glucose may cause some to appear in urine of healthy persons
Ketones	Not normally present	Poorly controlled diabetic clients experience a breakdown of fatty acids; the end product of fatty acid metabolism is ketones; clients suffering dehydration, starvation, or excessive aspirin ingestion also have ketonuria
Blood	Up to two red blood cells	Damage to glomerulus or tubules may cause blood cells to enter urine; trauma or disease of lower urinary tract also causes hematuria
Specific gravity	1.01 to 1.025	Measures concentration of particles in the urine; a high specific gravity reflects concentrated urine; a low specific gravity reflects a diluted urine; dehydration, reduced renal blood flow, and an increase in ADH secretion elevate specific gravity; overhydration and inadequate ADH secretion reduce specific gravity

helpful screening test for renal disease, metabolic disorders, lower urinary tract alterations, and fluid imbalances. For a quick screening the nurse can perform certain portions of the urinalysis with special reagent strips or tablets (see Procedure 39-1). The reagent tablets work in much the same way, with the nurse dropping urine onto the tablet and watching for a color change.

SPECIFIC GRAVITY. To measure specific gravity the nurse uses a urinometer and cylinder (Fig. 39-4). The urinometer has a specific gravity scale at the top and a weighted mercury bulb at the bottom. The nurse pours a urine specimen into a clean, dry cylinder. Next the nurse suspends the weighted urinometer into the cylinder of urine. The concentration of dissolved substances in the urine determines the depth at which the urinometer will float. The point the level of urine reaches on the scale is the specific gravity measurement.

URINE CULTURE. A urine culture simply requires the nurse to obtain a sterile sample of urine. It takes approximately 72 hours before the laboratory can report significant findings of bacterial growth. If bacteria are present, an additional test for sensitivity determines which antibiotics are effective and which are ineffective against the bacteria.

GLUCOSE AND KETONES. An accurate measurement of glucose and ketones always requires a double-voided specimen. A Keto-Diastix or Multistix reagent strip easily detects glucose and ketone. The strips contain chemicals that change color when exposed to urine constituents such as glucose and ketone. Procedure 39-1 reviews the steps in measuring glucose with a reagent strip.

Reagent tablets also measure glucose and ketone concentrations in urine. The Clinitest tablet method requires a test tube, a medicine dropper, and a reagent tablet. The nurse drops 10 drops of water into the tube followed by 5 drops of well-mixed urine. After a Clinitest tablet is dropped into the tube, the tablet causes the urine to boil. The resultant color change indicates the glucose concentration in the urine. To measure ketone the nurse drops a single drop of urine onto an Acetest tablet. If acetone is present, varying shades of lavender appear. Within a specified time the nurse compares the tablet's color with a color chart. The Keto-Diastix and Clinitest tablet tests can easily be performed by clients in the home.

Diagnostic Examinations

There are two approaches for visualizing urinary structures: direct and indirect. It is possible to perform some examinations without the client being hospitalized.

The nursing implications for urinary diagnostic examinations are similar to those for gastrointestinal examinations (Table 39-5). The nurse is responsible for:

1. Explaining the procedure to the client
2. Restricting solid food intake as ordered
3. Administering cathartics as needed
4. Maintaining fluid intake as ordered
5. Administering pretest medications
6. Positioning the client
7. Providing support to the client during the procedure
8. Observing for postprocedural complications

INDIRECT VISUALIZATION

To view the entire urinary system the physician orders indirect visualization examinations. The client receives an intravenous injection of either a contrast dye or radioisotope. Normally the injected medium takes only a few minutes to circulate and be excreted into the urinary system. Since the kidneys and ureters lie behind the intestines, it is necessary with tests such as the intravenous pyelogram (IVP) to give the client a bowel preparation. Cathartics are usually sufficient to promote adequate emptying of the bowel. The client's dietary intake before the examination is restricted. Renal scanning uses radioactive isotopes to outline urinary structures. The isotope can be detected without the need of a bowel preparation.

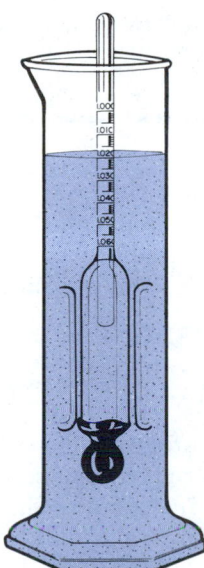

Fig. 39-4 Measurement of urine specific gravity using a urinometer.

PROCEDURE 39-1

Measurement of Glucose and Ketone Concentration in the Urine Using a Keto-Diastix

EQUIPMENT:
1. Double-voided urine specimen
2. Keto-Diastix reagent strip
3. Color-coded test chart
4. Wristwatch with second hand or digital readout

STEPS	RATIONALE
1. Acquire a double-voided urine specimen from the client.	A double-voided specimen ensures that the glucose concentration is an accurate measure of glucose in bladder urine.
2. Immerse the end of the strip impregnated with the chemical reagent into the urine specimen.	Immersion exposes the reagent to urine constituents.
3. Remove the strip immediately.	Immediate removal prevents dilution of reagents.
4. Hold the strip horizontally and start counting for 30 seconds.	Horizontal position prevents mixing of chemical reagents.
5. Read the color of the ketone reading at 15 seconds by comparing the strip's color to the color chart on the Keto-Diastix bottle.	In 15 seconds the reagent will indicate presence of ketones from negative to 3+ (large).
6. Read the color of the glucose reading at 15 additional seconds by comparing the strip's color to the color chart.	In 30 seconds the reagent indicates the presence of glucose from negative to 4+ (2%).
7. Dispose of the reagent strip in a trash receptacle.	Disposal prevents transmission of microorganisms.
8. Record results of the glucose and acetone test in the client's medical record.	Timely documentation permits early treatment intervention.

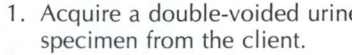

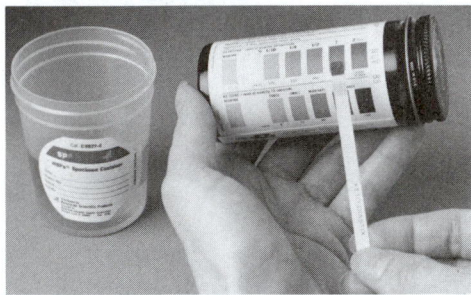

The intravenous pyelogram requires that x-ray studies be taken at specific intervals over a 30- to 60-minute period as the dye concentrates. The client may also be asked to void during the procedure in order to measure bladder emptying. A renal scan measures radioactive concentrations while the client assumes a supine, prone, or sitting position. Since a very low dosage of radioisotope is used, no precautions against radioactive exposure are needed.

The indirect urinary examinations are relatively painless except for the intravenous injection of dye or isotope. The client may feel a sense of dizziness or warmth during the dye injection. The nurse does not routinely administer a sedative before the test unless the physician views the client as highly anxious. The intravenous dye used in this procedure contains iodine and thus has the potential for creating serious allergic reactions. The nurse routinely assesses the client's history of allergies before the examination.

DIRECT VISUALIZATION

To view the interior of the bladder and urethra the physician performs a cystoscopy. The cystoscope looks much like a urinary catheter although it is not as flexible. The instrument consists of an outer plastic or rubber sheath, an obturator that keeps the scope rigid during insertion through the urethra, a telescope for viewing the bladder and urethra, and a channel for inserting catheters or special surgical instruments.

The procedure is painful during instrument inser-

TABLE 39-5

Diagnostic Examinations of Urinary Structures

Test Name	Purpose	Nursing Implications		
		Before Test	During Test	After Test
Intravenous pyelogram (IVP)	The IVP allows indirect visualization of kidneys, renal pelvis, ureters, and bladder following injection of an intravenous radiopaque dye. The physician observes for presence of renal artery blockage, urinary tumors, vascular abnormalities, and evidence of trauma.	1. Client signs informed consent for the procedure. 2. Assess client for history of iodine allergy. 3. Client receives a cathartic on evening before the test. 4. Client takes nothing by mouth after midnight. 5. Explain that flushing of the face is normal during dye injection and that client may feel dizzy or warm. 6. Explain that physician starts an intravenous infusion for dye injection. 7. Explain that procedure involves x-ray studies taken at several intervals, with client instructed to void near end of procedure.	1. Assess intravenous site for signs of infiltration of dye into tissues (swelling, redness, pain). 2. Observe for signs of allergic reaction to dye, e.g., respiratory distress, fall in blood pressure. 3. Remind client of normal sensations caused by dye injection.	1. Client may receive normal diet after examination. 2. Encourage fluid intake to minimize dehydration effect from fasting.
Renal scan	This test allows indirect visualization of urinary tract following intravenous injection of a radioisotope. Physician observes for renal artery blockage and primary renal disease indicated by delay in isotope excretion. Test is indicated for clients unable to receive IVP drugs.	1. Client signs an informed consent. 2. Explain that radioisotope is injected intravenously through an existing IV line or needle. 3. Explain that client will feel no discomfort, but that it is necessary to lie still. 4. Explain that there is no risk of radioactive exposure.	1. Assist client to change positions during procedure. 2. Explain that machine measuring uptake of isotope is similar to a Geiger counter.	1. Instruct client to resume normal activities.

Continued.

TABLE 39-5, cont'd

Diagnostic Examinations of Urinary Structures

Test Name	Purpose	Nursing Implications		
		Before Test	**During Test**	**After Test**
Cystoscopy	This allows direct visualization of urethra and bladder through the transurethral insertion of a cystoscope into bladder. Physician directly views urethral canal, bladder, and prostate in males. During procedure urine specimens and tissue specimens can be collected. Ureteral catheters may also be inserted.	1. Client signs an informed consent. 2. Client receives cathartics on evening before the test. 3. *Local anesthetics:* Encourage oral fluids. 4. *General anesthetics:* Client takes nothing by mouth after midnight. 5. Explain that insertion of cystoscope is similar to urethral catheter insertion. 6. Explain importance of lying still during procedure. 7. Explain that an intravenous line will be started to administer fluids during procedure. 8. Administer sedative and/or analgesic.	1. Assist client to assume a lithotomy position. 2. Prepare perineal area with antiseptic solution. 3. Explain (if client is awake) that insertion of cystoscope causes urge to void. 4. Remind client to lie still.	1. Instruct client to remain in bed as ordered. 2. Assess for signs of urinary retention. 3. Observe characteristics of urine, noting blood or cloudy urine. 4. Encourage increased fluid intake. 5. Observe for fever, dysuria, drop in blood pressure.

tion. Unless the client lies still, there is risk of serious tissue injury, such as bladder perforation. The client may have the test under general anesthesia or receive sedatives and analgesics just before the examination. Since the examination requires insertion of a foreign object into a sterile cavity, the client receives large amounts of fluids (intravenously or orally) before and during the procedure to maintain a continuous urine flow and to flush out any bacteria.

When performing a cystoscopy with general anesthesia, the physician orders the client to fast after midnight the evening before the examination. General anesthetics have the potential for causing nausea and vomiting. The client does not receive a bowel preparation.

The physician performs the cystoscopy in a hospital cystoscopy room or in an office. The nurse helps the client assume a lithotomy position, which facilitates instrument passage. Special cystoscopy tables minimize the stress and fatigue clients may experience from maintaining one position for a prolonged time.

The nurse drapes the client to minimize embarrassment. If the client is awake during the procedure, the physician or nurse explains each step. After the examination the nurse observes the client for signs and symptoms of bleeding or infection resulting from instrument trauma.

Nursing Diagnosis

The nurse's assessment of the client's urinary function may indicate an actual or potential elimination problem or an associated problem resulting from urinary elimination alterations (Table 39-6). Specifying the contributing factors for each diagnosis allows the nurse to select individualized nursing interventions. For example, measures that relieve urinary retention will not minimize urinary tract infection.

Associated problems require interventions that often have no direct effect on urinary elimination. For example, skin breakdown associated with repeated

TABLE 39-6

Examples of Nursing Diagnoses Related to Urinary Elimination Problems

Problem	Causes
Alterations in urination	Related to: Urinary retention Urinary tract infection Incontinence Enuresis Ureterostomy
Potential or actual skin breakdown	Related to exposure to urine
Alterations in comfort	Related to: Dysuria Urinary retention
Body image alterations	Related to: Incontinence Ureterostomy Enuresis
Risk of urinary tract infection	Related to: Catheterization Cystoscopic examinations Poor hygiene habits
Risk of altered fluid and electrolyte balance	Related to impaired ureterostomy drainage

urinary incontinence requires measures that do not influence micturition. As with bowel elimination problems (see Chapter 40), unless the nurse intervenes the associated problems are likely to continue. Problems involved with urinary elimination alterations are often interrelated and complex.

Interventions designed to relieve or prevent urinary elimination alterations may cause certain associated problems. The client who is catheterized for urinary retention acquires a risk for developing urinary tract infections. Therefore the nurse must also identify problems that may potentially develop as a result of therapy.

Planning

The nurse plans therapeutic interventions for clients with urinary elimination problems, and preventive interventions may be required for clients with potential urinary problems. The nurse plans therapies according to the severity of risks to the client. For example, the risk of infection or fluid and electrolyte

imbalance may temporarily outweigh the priorities given to maintaining skin integrity or comfort.

The client with actual or potential alterations in urinary elimination learns to recognize the signs of change and to prevent the development of serious problems. Alterations in urinary elimination pose more risk to a client's overall state of health than common bowel elimination problems.

Planning the client's care also involves an understanding of the individual's need to control body function. Alterations in urinary elimination can be embarrassing, uncomfortable, and often frustrating. The nurse and client work together to establish ways of maintaining client involvement in nursing care. For example, some clients can learn to perform self-catheterization and other independent measures.

In an effort to promote normal urinary elimination, the goals of the nursing care plan include:

1. Promotion of the client's understanding of urinary elimination
2. Promotion of normal micturition
3. Promotion of complete bladder emptying
4. Prevention of infection
5. Maintenance of skin integrity
6. Promotion of comfort
7. Return of bladder function

Implementation

The nurse's success depends in part on the client's understanding of normal urinary elimination. The client should know the basic mechanism for urine production and voiding. Likewise, if the client is unaware of the normal sterility of the urinary tract, the nurse will be less successful in helping the client establish good hygiene practices. The client should also learn the significance of symptoms of urinary alterations so early preventive health care can be initiated.

Client education is best promoted as the nurse provides care for the client's needs. For example, if the nurse is attempting to increase the client's fluid intake, a good time to discuss the benefits is while giving fluids with medications or meals. The nurse may be more successful in teaching the client about perineal hygiene during a bath or while giving catheter care. Much of the information the nurse offers is practical in nature. The nurse can easily include family members in informal discussions with the client.

Promoting Normal Micturition

Many nursing measures have been designed to promote normal voiding in clients at risk for urination difficulties and in clients with established urination problems. The nurse can initiate many of the measures independently.

STIMULATING MICTURITION REFLEX

The client's ability to void depends on feeling the urge to urinate and on being able to control the urethral sphincter. One factor that commonly interferes with micturition is the client's inability to relax. The nurse can help foster relaxation and stimulate the reflex to void by helping clients assume the normal position for voiding. Females are better able to void by assuming a squatting position. This position promotes contraction of the pelvic and intra-abdominal muscles that assist in sphincter control and bladder contraction. If the client is unable to use toilet facilities, the nurse positions the client in a squatting position on a bedpan (see Chapter 40) or bedside commode. The male client voids more easily in the standing position. At times it may be necessary for one or more nurses to assist the male client to stand. If the male client cannot reach toilet facilities, he may stand at the bedside and void into a urinal, a metal or plastic receptacle for urine (Fig. 39-5).

Other measures that promote a client's relaxation and ability to initiate micturition include the use of sensory stimuli. The sound of running water helps many clients void through the power of suggestion. Stroking the inner aspect of the client's thigh may stimulate sensory nerves and promote the micturition reflex. Placing the client's hand in a pan of warm water often promotes voiding. It is easier for a person to relax and void when sitting on a bedpan that has been warmed. The nurse can also pour warm water over the client's perineum and create the sensation to urinate. If the client's urine output is to be measured,

the nurse must first measure the volume of water to be poured over the perineal area.

MAINTAINING ELIMINATION HABITS

Many clients follow set routines to promote normal voiding. In a hospital or long-term care facility the nurse's routines may conflict with those of the client. Integrating the client's habits into the plan of nursing care fosters a more normal voiding pattern.

The client usually requires time to void. Asking a client to void quickly so he can be transported to x-ray testing, or requesting a urine specimen as soon as possible, does not contribute to normal voiding habits. The client should be given at least 30 minutes to provide a specimen. The nurse learns the times when a client normally voids, such as on awakening or before meals, and offers the opportunity to use toilet facilities at those times. Also important in timing is the need to respond to the client's urge to urinate. Delay in assisting the client to the bathroom may interfere with normal micturition.

Privacy is essential for normal voiding. If the client cannot reach the bathroom, the nurse makes sure the bedside area is enclosed by a curtain. In the home the debilitated client may prefer using a bedside commode enclosed behind a partition or room divider. Some clients are embarrassed by the sound of voiding. Running water or flushing the toilet masks the sound effectively. Often young children are unable to void in the presence of persons other than their parents.

If the client typically uses special measures to void, the nurse should encourage their continued use at home and, when possible, in the institution. The client may be able to relax and void more easily while reading or listening to music. A drink of coffee or a sip of beer may also promote urination.

MAINTAINING ADEQUATE FLUID INTAKE

A simple method of promoting normal micturition is maintaining a good fluid intake. A client with normal renal function who does not have heart disease or alterations requiring fluid restriction should drink 2000 to 2500 ml of fluid daily. Fluids promote normal urine formation and thus improve the flow of urine through the urinary system. When fluid intake is increased, the excreted urine flushes out any solutes or particles that may collect in the urinary system. For example, urinary flow removes bacteria from near the urethra and thus reduces the chances of infection in the lower urinary tract. Since a client is unlikely to be willing to drink 2500 ml of water daily, the nurse should offer fluids the client prefers. In a home setting it may be helpful to set a schedule for drinking fluids, for example, with meals, with medications, or after

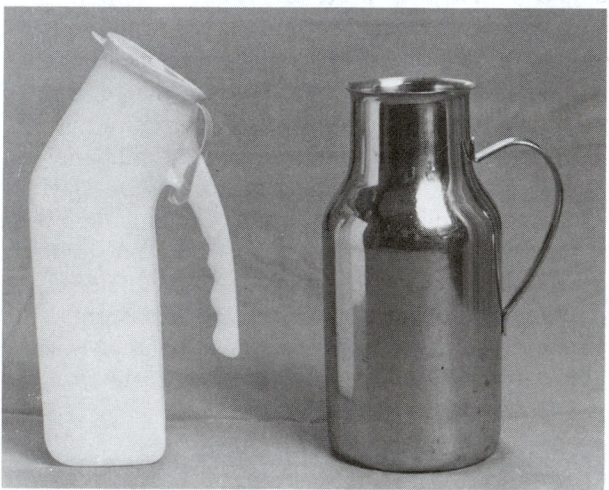

Fig. 39-5 Types of male urinals.

exercise. To prevent nocturia, fluids should not be taken just before bedtime.

Promoting Complete Bladder Emptying

Clients with urinary retention and incontinence are frequently unable to empty the bladder fully. Measures that promote micturition may help, but additional techniques are useful to foster bladder emptying.

STRENGTHENING PELVIC FLOOR MUSCLES

Clients who have difficulty starting and stopping the urine stream may benefit from exercises to strengthen pelvic muscles. The client may practice the exercises anytime or anywhere, for example, while sitting or standing, during work, or while watching television.

The client first learns to feel the pelvic muscles. The nurse instructs the client to try to stop the flow of urine during urination and then to restart it. The client does this with each voiding. This maneuver helps the client feel the anterior muscles of the pelvic floor.

Second, while in a sitting or standing position, the client tries to tighten the muscles around the anus without tensing leg, buttock, or abdominal muscles. This maneuver allows the client to identify the posterior muscles of the pelvic floor.

The client exercises by tightening the posterior muscles and then slowly contracting the anterior muscles while counting to four. Then the client relaxes the muscles completely. The exercise should be repeated at least four times an hour while the client is awake; this exercise schedule should be continued for 2 to 3 months.

Sit-ups also aid in bladder control by strengthening the abdominal muscles. Of course, many clients are unable to perform repeated numbers of sit-ups. Starting with a few at a time and gradually increasing the number of repetitions will improve pelvic muscle strength.

MANUAL BLADDER COMPRESSION

By manually compressing the walls of the bladder a person can improve bladder emptying. Credé's method helps stimulate micturition, as well as manually expelling urine when bladder tone is reduced. The client places both hands flat on the abdomen below the umbilicus and above the symphysis pubis with the fingers pointed down toward the bladder's dome. The client compresses the hands downward against the bladder's walls while simultaneously tightening the perineum, contracting the abdominal wall, and holding the breath. When urine is in the bladder, Credé's compression causes the sensation of bladder fullness. The maneuver also promotes bladder emptying by relaxing the urethral sphincter.

DRUG THERAPY

Drug therapy alone or in conjunction with other therapies can be useful for treating problems of incontinence and retention. Commonly used medications include those that increase bladder emptying and decrease bladder hyperactivity (for example, urge incontinence).

The bladder is innervated by the parasympathetic nervous system. When urine is present in the bladder, stress or urge incontinence may occur as a result of hyperactivity of the bladder muscle that suddenly increases intravesicular pressure. The uncontrolled bladder contractions may be caused by local irritants to the bladder such as stones or infection. Drugs that depress the neurotransmitter acetylcholine, which stimulates the bladder, reduce incontinence caused by bladder irritation. Examples of these anticholinergic drugs include propantheline (Pro-Banthine) and methantheline (Banthine). The anticholinergics can cause cardiac arrythmias and should be used with caution in clients with heart disease.

When the bladder empties, the detrusor muscle contracts in response to parasympathetic stimulation. Incomplete bladder emptying results from impaired innervation or weakness of the detrusor muscle. The client experiences retention and overflow incontinence. Therapy with cholinergic drugs is aimed at increasing contraction of the bladder and improving emptying. Bethanechol (Urecholine) stimulates parasympathetic nerves to increase bladder wall contraction and relax the sphincter. Bethanechol can be given by subcutaneous or oral routes. The nurse should administer the first dose 3 to 4 hours after the last voiding to be sure the bladder contains urine. To gain the peak effect of the drug, the nurse administers it shortly before micturition is attempted (15 to 30 minutes subcutaneously, 30 to 60 minutes orally). The effect of the drug can be augmented by using Credé's method or other measures for stimulating micturition.

CATHETERIZATION

Catheterization of the bladder involves the introduction of a rubber or plastic tube through the urethra and into the bladder. The catheter provides for a continuous flow of urine in clients unable to control micturition or in clients with obstructions to urine outflow. Because bladder catheterization carries the risk of the development of urinary tract infection, it is preferable to rely on other measures to promote bladder emptying.

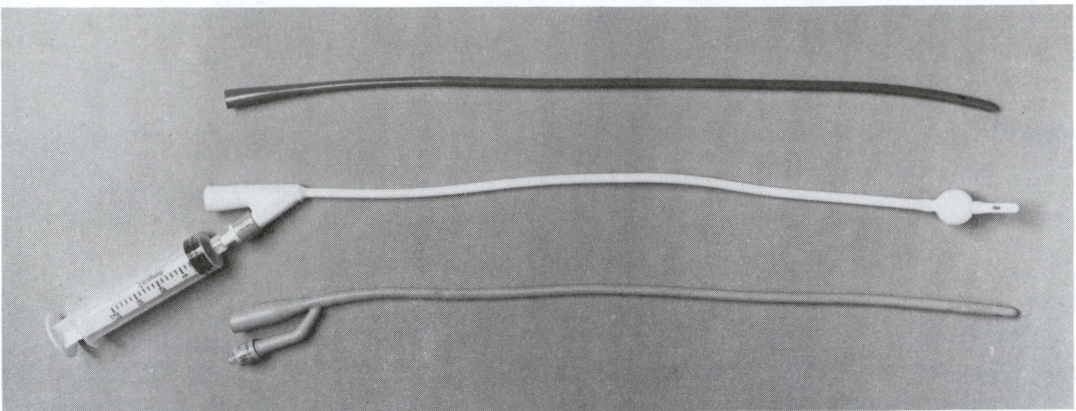

Fig. 39-6 Straight and indwelling catheters. *Top,* straight catheter; *middle,* indwelling catheter with inflated balloon; *bottom,* indwelling double-lumen catheter.

TYPES OF CATHETERIZATION. Intermittent and indwelling catheterization are the two forms of catheter insertion. With the *intermittent* technique a straight single-use catheter is introduced for a period long enough to drain the bladder (5 to 10 minutes). When the bladder is empty, the nurse immediately withdraws the catheter. Intermittent catheterization can be repeated as necessary. An *indwelling* or Foley catheter remains in place for an extended period until a client is able to void completely and voluntarily. It may be necessary to change indwelling catheters periodically.

The straight single-use catheter (Fig. 39-6) has a single lumen with a small opening approximately 1.3 cm (½ inch) from the tip. Urine drains from the tip, through the lumen, to a receptacle. An indwelling Foley catheter has a small inflatable balloon that encircles the catheter just below the tip. When inflated, the balloon rests against the bladder outlet to anchor the catheter in place. The indwelling catheter also has as many as two or three separate lumens within the body of the catheter. One lumen drains urine through the catheter to a collecting tube. A second lumen carries sterile water to and from the balloon when it is inflated or deflated. A third (optional) lumen may be used to instill fluids or medications into the bladder. It is easy to determine the number of lumens by the number of drainage and injection ports at the catheter's end.

Bladder catheters come in a variety of diameters to accommodate the size of a client's urethral canal. The French system indicates the catheter gauge. The larger the gauge number, the larger the catheter. Children usually require a size #8 or #10 French. Women require a #14 to #16 size, while men need a #16 to #20 French gauge catheter. The use of an overly large catheter can cause trauma to the urethral tissue. If a catheter is too small, blood clots or urine sediment may obstruct urine outflow.

INDICATIONS FOR USE. Catheterization may be indicated for a variety of reasons. When the need for catheterization is short term and minimizing infection is a priority, the intermittent method is best. Indwelling catheterization is used when long-term bladder emptying is necessary.

Intermittent catheterization is indicated in the following situations:

1. For immediate relief of bladder distention
   a. Clients unable to void 8 to 12 hours following surgery
   b. Clients with acute retention following trauma to the urethra
   c. Clients unable to void as a result of the effects of sedatives or analgesics
2. For long-term management of clients with incompetent bladders
   a. Spinal cord injuries
   b. Progressive neuromuscular degeneration
3. To obtain a sterile urine specimen
4. To assess for the presence of residual urine after voiding

Intermittent catheterization with good aseptic technique is associated with a lower incidence of infection than indwelling catheterization. However, if a client's condition requires frequent intermittent catheterization, an indwelling catheter may be preferable.

Indwelling catheterization is indicated in these situations:

1. When there is an obstruction to urine outflow
   a. Prostate enlargement
   b. Urethral stricture

Text continued on p. 1114.

PROCEDURE 39-2

Female Urinary Catheterization: Indwelling and Straight

EQUIPMENT:

1. Sterile catheterization tray
   a. Sterile gloves
   b. Sterile drapes, one fenestrated
   c. Lubricant
   d. Antiseptic cleansing solution
   e. Cotton balls or gauze sponges
   f. Forceps
   g. Straight or indwelling catheter
   h. Prefilled syringe with solution to inflate balloon for indwelling catheter
   i. Receptacle or basin (usually the bottom of tray)
   j. Specimen container

2. Flashlight or gooseneck lamp
3. Sterile drainage tubing and collection bag
4. Tape, rubber band, and safety pin
5. Bath blanket
6. Waterproof pad
7. Trash bag
8. Basin with warm water and soap
9. Bath towel

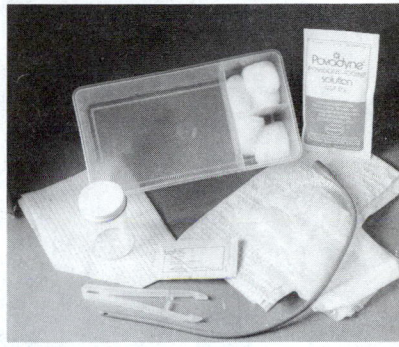

STEPS	*RATIONALE*
1. Explain the procedure to the client.	Explanation minimizes the client's anxiety and promotes cooperation.
2. Stand on the left side of the bed if you are right handed and on the right side if left handed. Clear the bedside table and arrange equipment.	Successful catheter insertion requires the nurse to assume a comfortable position with all equipment easily accessible.
3. Close the cubicle or room curtains.	Privacy reduces the client's embarrassment and aids in relaxation during the procedure.
4. Place the waterproof pad under the client.	The pad prevents soiling of bed linen.
5. Assist the client to a dorsal recumbent position (supine with knees flexed). Ask the client to relax the thighs so as to externally rotate them.	This position provides good access to perineal structures.
6. Drape the client with the bath blanket. Place the blanket diamond fashion over the client; one corner at the client's neck, one corner over each foot, and the last corner over the perineum.	Unnecessary exposure of body parts is avoided and the client's comfort is maintained.
7. Wash the perineal area with soap and water as needed, and dry.	The presence of microorganisms near the urethral meatus is reduced.
8. Wash your hands.	Transmission of bacteria from nurse's hands is prevented.
9. If inserting an indwelling catheter, open the drainage system. Place the drainage bag over the edge of the bottom bed frame. Bring the drainage tube up between side rail and mattress.	Once the catheter is inserted, the nurse will immediately connect the drainage system. Easy access prevents possible contamination. The system is positioned to promote gravity drainage.
10. Position the lamp to illuminate the perineal area. (When using a flashlight, have another nurse hold it.)	This permits accurate identification and good visualization of urethral meatus.
11. Open the catheterization kit according to directions, keeping the bottom of the container sterile.	Transmission of microorganisms from table or work area to sterile supplies is prevented.
12. Don sterile gloves (see Chapter 33).	
13. Pick up the solid sterile drape by one corner and allow it to unfold. Be sure the drape does not touch a contaminated surface (see Chapter 33).	Sterility of drape to be used as work surface is maintained.
14. Allow the top edge of the drape to form a cuff over both of your hands. Place the drape down on the bed between the client's thighs. Slip the cuffed	The outer surface of the drape covering the hands remains sterile. Sterile drape against sterile gloves is sterile.

Continued.

Female Urinary Catheterization: Indwelling and Straight

STEPS	RATIONALE
edge just under the client's buttocks, taking care not to touch a contaminated surface with your gloves.	
15. Pick up the fenestrated sterile drape and allow it to unfold as in step 12. Apply the drape over the client's perineum exposing the labia and being sure not to touch a contaminated surface.	The fenestrated drape provides a clean work area near the catheter insertion site.
16. Place the sterile tray and its contents on the sterile drape between the client's thighs.	Easy access to supplies during catheter insertion is provided.
17. Open the packet containing the antiseptic cleansing solution and pour the contents over the sterile cotton balls or gauze. (Be sure not to pour solution in the receptacle that is to receive urine).	All equipment is prepared before handling the catheter to maintain aseptic technique during the procedure.
18. Open urine specimen container, keeping the top sterile.	
19. Apply the lubricant to the bottom 2.5 to 5 cm (1 to 2 inches) of the catheter tip.	Lubricant allows easy insertion of the catheter tip through the urethral meatus.
20. With your nondominant hand carefully retract the labia to fully expose the urethral meatus. Maintain the position of your nondominant hand throughout the remainder of the procedure.	Full visualization of the meatus is provided. Full retraction prevents contamination of the meatus during cleansing. Closure of the labia during cleansing requires that procedure be repeated.
21. With your dominant hand pick up a cotton ball with the forceps and clean the perineal area, wiping front to back from the clitoris toward the anus. Use a new clean cotton ball for each wipe: along near labial fold, directly over meatus, and along far labial fold.	Cleansing reduces the number of microorganisms at the urethral meatus. Use of a single cotton ball for each wipe prevents transfer of microorganisms. Preparation moves from the area of least contamination to that of most contamination. The dominant hand remains sterile.
22. With your dominant hand pick up the catheter approximately 7.5 to 10 cm (3 to 4 inches) from the tip. Place the end of catheter in the urine tray receptacle.	Collection of urine prevents soiling of the client's bed linen and allows accurate measurement of urinary output. Holding the catheter near the tip allows easier manipulation during insertion into the meatus.
23. Ask the client to bear down gently to void and slowly insert the catheter through the meatus.	Relaxation of the external sphincter aids in insertion of the catheter.
24. Advance the catheter approximately 5 to 7.5 cm (2 to 3 inches) in an adult, 2.5 cm (1 inch) in a child, or until urine flows out the catheter's end. When urine appears, advance the catheter another 1.2 cm (½ inch).	The female urethra is short. Appearance of urine indicates that the catheter tip is in the bladder or lower urethra. Further advancement of the catheter ensures bladder placement.
25. Release the labia and hold the catheter securely with your nondominant hand.	Bladder or sphincter contraction may cause accidental expulsion of catheter.
26. Collect urine specimen as needed: Fill specimen cup or jar to desired level (20 to 30 ml) by holding the end of the catheter in your dominant hand over the cup. With your dominant hand pinch the catheter to stop urine flow temporarily. Release the catheter to allow remaining urine in the bladder to drain into the collection tray. Cover the specimen cup and set it aside for labeling.	
27. Allow the bladder to empty fully (unless institution policy restricts the maximal volume of urine to drain with each catheterization).	Retained urine may serve as reservoir for growth of microorganisms. (Caution is taken to avoid hypotension resulting from sudden release of pressure against the pelvic floor blood vessels under the bladder.)

PROCEDURE 39-2, cont'd

Female Urinary Catheterization: Indwelling and Straight

STEPS	RATIONALE
28. With a straight single-use catheter, withdraw the catheter slowly but smoothly until removed.	Discomfort to the client is minimized.
29. With indwelling catheter: a. While holding catheter with thumb and little finger of nondominant hand at meatus, take the end of the catheter and place it between the first two fingers of the nondominant hand.	The catheter should be anchored while the syringe is manipulated.
b. With the free dominant hand attach the syringe to the injection port at the end of the catheter.	The port connects to the lumen leading to the inflatable balloon.
c. Slowly inject the total amount of solution. If the client complains of sudden pain, aspirate back solution and advance the catheter farther.	Balloon within bladder is inflated. If balloon is malpositioned in urethra, pain will occur during inflation.
d. After inflating the balloon fully, release the catheter with the nondominant hand and pull gently to feel resistance.	Inflation of the balloon anchors the catheter tip in place above the bladder outlet.
30. Attach the end of catheter to the collecting tube of the drainage system.	A closed system for urine drainage is established.
31. Tape the catheter to the client's inner thigh with a strip of nonallergenic tape. Allow for slack so that movement of the thigh does not create tension on the catheter.	Anchoring of the catheter minimizes trauma to the urethra and meatus during the client's movement. Nonallergenic tape prevents skin breakdown.
32. Be sure there are no obstructions or kinks in the tubing. Place the excess coil of tubing on bed and fasten it to the bottom bedsheet with a clip from the drainage set or with a rubber band and safety pin.	Patent tubing allows free drainage of urine by gravity and prevents backflow of urine into the bladder.
33. Remove gloves and dispose of equipment, drapes, and urine in proper receptacles.	Transmission of microorganisms is prevented.
34. Assist the client to a comfortable position. Wash and dry the perineal area as needed.	The client's comfort and security are maintained.
35. Instruct the client on ways to position herself in bed with the catheter: side lying—facing drainage system with catheter and tubing on bed unobstructed; supine—catheter and tubing draped over thigh; side lying—facing away from system, catheter and tubing extend between legs.	Urine should drain freely without obstruction. Placing the catheter under extremities can result in obstruction as a result of compression of tubing from the client's weight. When the client is on one side facing away from the system, the catheter should not be placed over the upper thigh; this forces urine to drain uphill.
36. Caution the client against pulling on the catheter.	

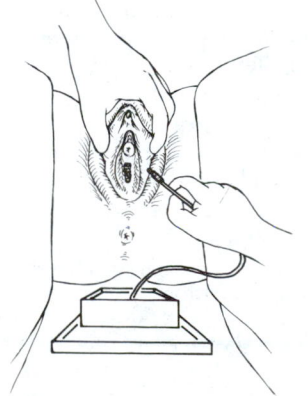

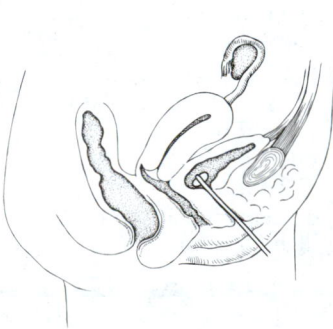

PROCEDURE 39-3

Male Urinary Catheterization: Indwelling and Straight

EQUIPMENT:
Same equipment listed for procedure of female catheterization (flashlight or gooseneck lamp is not required).

STEPS	RATIONALE
1. Explain the procedure to the client.	Explanation minimizes the client's anxiety and promotes cooperation.
2. Follow steps 2 through 4 for the female catheterization procedure.	
3. Assist the client to assume a supine position with the thighs slightly abducted.	Supine position prevents tensing of abdominal and pelvic muscles.
4. Drape the client's upper trunk with a bath blanket and cover the lower extremities with the bedsheets, exposing only the genitalia.	Unnecessary exposure of body parts is prevented and the client's comfort is maintained.
5. Wash the perineum with soap and water as needed. In uncircumcised males be sure to retract the foreskin to cleanse the urethral meatus.	Presence of microorganisms near the urethral meatus is reduced.
6. Follow steps 8, 9, 11, and 12 of the female catheterization procedure.	
7. Apply sterile drapes: Pick up the solid sterile drape by the corner and allow it to unfold. Be sure the drape does not touch a contaminated surface (see Chapter 33). Apply the drape over the client's thighs just below the penis. Pick up the fenestrated sterile drape, allow it to unfold, and drape it over the penis with the fenestrated slit resting over the penis.	Sterility of the drape as work surface is maintained.
8. Place the sterile tray and its contents on the drape alongside the client's thigh or on top of the thighs.	Easy access to supplies during catheter insertion is provided.
9. Prepare cotton balls or gauze with antiseptic solution. Open the urine specimen container, keeping the top sterile.	
10. Apply the lubricant to the bottom 12.5 to 17.5 cm (5 to 7 inches) of the catheter tip.	Lubricant allows easy insertion of the catheter tip through the urethral meatus.
11. With your nondominant hand retract the foreskin of the uncircumcised male. Grasp the penis at the shaft just below the glans. Retract the urethral meatus between the thumb and forefinger. Maintain the nondominant hand in this position throughout the procedure.	A firm grasp minimizes the chance of an erection occurring (if an erection develops, discontinue procedure). Accidental release of the foreskin or dropping of the penis during cleansing requires the process to be repeated.
12. With the dominant hand pick up a cotton ball with the forceps and clean penis. Move it in a circular motion from the meatus down to the base of the glans. Repeat cleansing two more times using a clean cotton ball each time.	Preparation reduces the number of microorganisms at the meatus and moves from the area of least contamination to most contamination. The dominant hand remains sterile.
13. Pick up the catheter with the gloved dominant hand approximately 5 to 7.5 cm (2 to 3 inches) from catheter tip. Hold the end of the catheter loosely coiled in the palm of the dominant hand (optional: may grasp catheter with forceps).	Holding the catheter near the tip allows easier manipulation during insertion into the meatus and prevents the distal end from striking the contaminated surface.
14. Lift the penis to a position perpendicular to the client's body and apply light traction.	This position straightens the urethral canal to ease catheter insertion.

Male Urinary Catheterization: Indwelling and Straight

STEPS	RATIONALE

15. Ask the client to bear down as if to void and slowly insert the catheter through the meatus.

Relaxation of external sphincter aids in insertion of the catheter.

16. Advance the catheter 17.5 to 20 cm (7 to 8 inches) in an adult and 5 to 7.5 cm (2 to 3 inches) in a young child, or until urine flows out the catheter's end. If resistance is felt, withdraw the catheter; do not force it through the urethra. When urine appears, advance the catheter another 1.2 cm (½ inch).

The adult male urethra is long. Appearance of urine indicates the catheter tip is in the bladder or urethra. Resistance to catheter passage may be caused by urethral strictures or an enlarged prostate. Further advancement of catheter ensures proper placement.

17. Lower the penis and hold the catheter securely in the nondominant hand. Place the end of the catheter in the urine tray receptacle.

The catheter may be accidentally expelled by the bladder or urethral contraction. Collection of urine prevents soiling and provides output measurement.

18. Collect the urine specimen according to step 26 in the female catheterization procedure.

19. Allow the bladder to empty fully (unless institution policy restricts the maximal volume of urine to drain with each catheterization).

Retained urine serves as a reservoir for the growth of microorganisms. (Precaution prevents hypotension resulting from the sudden release of pressure against the pelvic floor blood vessels under the bladder.)

20. With straight single-use catheters withdraw slowly but smoothly until removed. Replace foreskin over glans.

21. With indwelling catheters inflate the balloon and check for proper anchoring as in step 29 of the female catheterization procedure.

22. Attach the end of the catheter to the collecting tube of the drainage system.

Closed system for urine drainage is established.

23. Tape the catheter to the client's inner thigh or lower abdomen (with penis directed toward the client's chest) with a strip of nonallergenic tape. Provide slack so movement does not create tension on the catheter.

Anchoring of the catheter minimizes trauma to the urethra and meatus. Taping to the abdomen minimizes irritation at the angle of the penis and scrotum. Nonallergenic tape prevents skin breakdown.

24. Be sure there are no obstructions or kinks in the tubing. Place the excess coil of tubing on the bed and fasten it to bottom bedsheet with a clip to drainage set or with a rubber band and safety pin.

Patent tubing allows free drainage of urine by gravity and prevents backflow of urine into bladder.

25. Remove gloves and dispose of all equipment.

Transmission of microorganisms is prevented.

26. Assist the client to a comfortable position and wash and dry perineal areas as needed.

Client's comfort is promoted.

27. Instruct the client on proper positioning technique and the importance of not pulling on the catheter (see steps 35 and 36 for female catheterization).

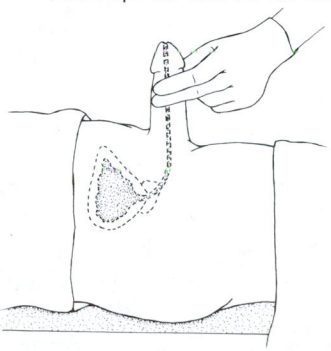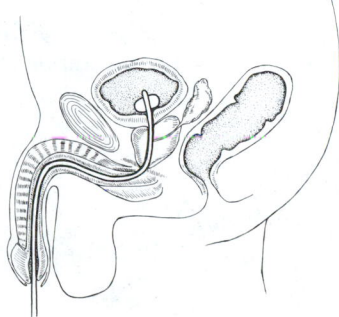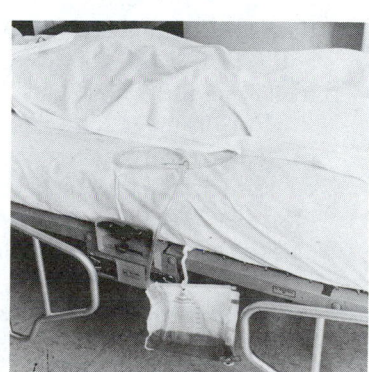

2. For clients undergoing surgical repair of the urethra and surrounding structures (transurethral resection)
3. To prevent urethral obstruction from blood clots
   a. Bladder tumors
   b. Surgical repair of urethra
4. To provide a means of recording output measurements in critically ill or comatose clients
5. To prevent skin breakdown in comatose clients who are incontinent or severely disoriented
6. To provide continuous or intermittent bladder irrigations

CATHETER INSERTION. Urethral catheterization requires a physician's order. The nurse must use strict aseptic technique. Before beginning the procedure the nurse describes the steps of catheterization to the client in detail, since the procedure will be easier to perform if the client cooperates. The nurse should organize all equipment to prevent interruptions during the procedure and to avoid a break in sterile technique.

The steps for inserting an indwelling and a single-use straight catheter are the same. The difference lies in the procedure taken to inflate the indwelling catheter balloon and secure the catheter in place. While inserting an indwelling catheter the nurse has the opportunity to collect needed specimens. Procedures 39-2 and 39-3 list steps for performing female and male urethral catheterization.

CLOSED DRAINAGE SYSTEMS. After inserting an indwelling catheter it is necessary to maintain a closed urinary drainage system to minimize the risk of infection. Urinary drainage bags are plastic and capable of holding approximately 1000 to 1500 ml of urine. The bag should hang on the bed frame without touching the floor when the bed is in its lowest position (Fig. 39-7). A drainage bag should not be placed over the bed's side rails. The bag also fits on the frames of most wheelchairs. When the client ambulates, the nurse or client carries the bag below the client's waist. *The nurse should never raise a drainage bag and tubing above the level of the client's bladder.* Urine in the bag and tubing can become a medium for bacteria, and infection is likely to develop if urine is returned to the bladder.

Most drainage bags contain an antireflux valve to prevent urine from reentering the drainage tubing and contaminating the client's bladder. A spigot at the base of the bag provides a means for the nurse to empty the bag of urine. The spigot should always be clamped, except during emptying, and tucked into the protective pouch at the bag's side.

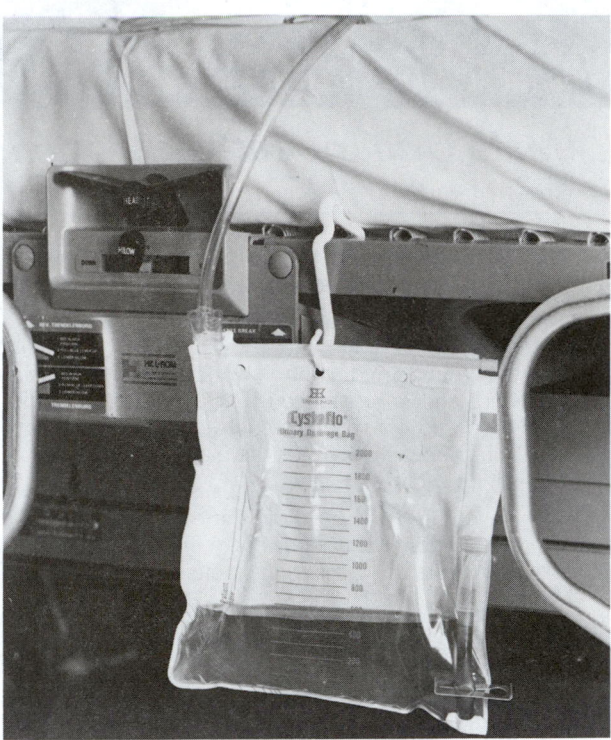

Fig. 39-7 The urine drainage bag hangs on the bed frame below the level of the client's head.

Some urinary drainage bags have special urimeters between the collection tubing and bag. The urimeter is a clear graduated cylinder that measures small volumes (100 to 200 ml) of urine. The urimeter is useful for clients requiring frequent urine output measurements, since it eliminates the need to empty the drainage bag each time a measurement is due. The nurse simply notes the volume of urine in the urimeter and then opens the valve that allows urine from the urimeter to enter the drainage bag. When urine from the drainage bag is measured, it is best to use a separate graduated receptacle for measurement accuracy. Scales on the bags offer only approximate volumes.

To keep the drainage system patent the nurse: (1) checks for kinks or bends in the tubing; (2) avoids positioning the client on the drainage tubing; and (3) observes for clots or sediment that may occlude the collecting tubing.

REMOVAL OF INDWELLING CATHETER. There are two important principles to follow when removing an indwelling catheter: (1) promote normal bladder function and (2) prevent trauma to the urethra. Bladder dysfunction in the form of loss of muscle tone is a common problem following prolonged catheterization. One method that serves to reduce the loss of bladder tone is bladder reconditioning. The procedure requires a physician's order and is initiated at least 10 hours before catheter removal (Williamson, 1982). The nurse clamps the indwelling catheter to allow urine to accumulate in the bladder. The volume of urine stretches the bladder's walls to stimulate muscle tone. Three hours later the nurse unclamps the catheter and allows urine to drain for 5 minutes, simulating voiding. The process is repeated two more times. After the conditioning procedure the nurse removes the catheter. Clients who receive bladder conditioning are able to feel the urge to void sooner than those clients who have no conditioning. Once a client voids, the effects of conditioning promote more complete bladder emptying and thus reduce the amount of residual urine remaining in the bladder.

To remove a catheter the nurse requires a clean towel, a trash receptacle, and a sterile syringe the same size as the volume of solution within the catheter's inflated balloon. The end of each catheter contains a label that denotes the volume of solution (5 to 30 ml) within a balloon.

The nurse positions the client in the same position assumed during catheterization. After removing the tape anchoring the catheter, the nurse places the towel between the female's thighs or over the male's thighs. The nurse inserts the syringe into the injection port. Most ports are self-sealing and require only the tip of the syringe to be inserted. A syringe needle is usually not necessary. The nurse slowly withdraws all of the solution to deflate the balloon totally. If a portion of the solution remains, the partially inflated balloon will cause trauma to the urethral canal as the catheter is removed. Following deflation the nurse explains that the client will feel a burning sensation as the catheter is withdrawn. The nurse then pulls the catheter out smoothly and slowly.

It is normal for the client to experience dysuria, especially if the catheter has been in place several days or weeks. The catheter causes inflammation of the urethral canal. Until the bladder regains full tone, the client may also have frequency of urination.

The nurse notes when the client first voids after catheter removal. If over 8 hours elapses before the client voids, it may become necessary to catheterize the client again. If the volume of urine voided is small, residual urine may be in the bladder.

ALTERNATIVES TO CATHETERIZATION

To avoid the risks associated with catheters inserted through the urethra there are two alternatives for urinary drainage. *Suprapubic* catheterization involves placing a catheter directly into the bladder through an abdominal incision. This method is useful in clients with chronic incontinence or loss of bladder control. Suprapubic catheterization reduces the risk of infec-

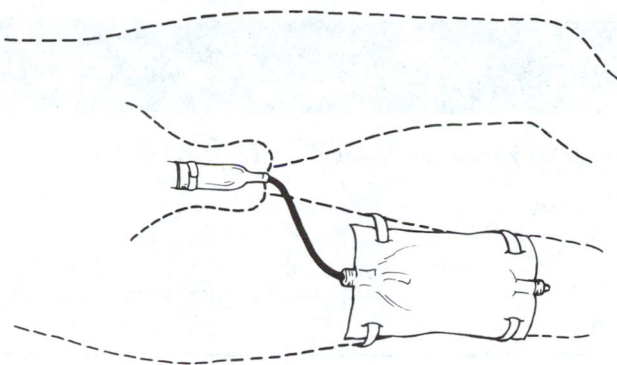

Fig. 39-8 Condom catheter with leg drainage bag.

tion ascending along the urethra to the bladder. There are also less urethral irritation and obstruction of urethral and prostatic glands in the male. Extra care must be given to the abdominal wound to prevent infection and skin irritation. Bladder infection may still develop in the client with a suprapubic catheter. Spread of the infection to the kidneys may necessitate removal of the catheter.

The external application of a urinary drainage device is a convenient and safe method to drain urine in male clients. The *condom* catheter is suitable for incontinent or comatose clients who still have complete and spontaneous bladder emptying. The condom is a soft, pliable, rubber sheath that slips over the male's penis. A strip of self-adhesive tape fits around the top of the condom to secure it in place (Fig. 39-8). Care must be taken not to tighten the band tightly, or blood supply to the penis will be impaired. The end of the condom fits into a plastic drainage tubing. A drainage bag can be attached to the side of the client's bed or strapped to the client's leg. The condom catheter poses little risk of infection unless the client is uncooperative or confused. Infections with condom catheters usually result from trauma to the urethral meatus or buildup of pressure in the outflow tubing. Procedure 39-4 reviews application of the condom catheter.

A condom catheter may remain in place 1 to 2 days. With each catheter change the nurse cleans the urethral meatus and penis thoroughly and looks for signs of skin irritation. Twisting of the condom near the drainage tube can cause irritation and obstruct urine outflow. The nurse checks the tubing frequently for patency.

Prevention of Infection

One of the most important considerations for a client with urinary alterations is the need to prevent

PROCEDURE 39-4

Applying a Condom Catheter

EQUIPMENT:

1. Rubber condom sheath
2. Strip of elastic or Velcro adhesive
3. Urinary collection bag with drainage tubing
4. Basin with warm water and soap
5. Towel and washcloth
6. Bath blanket

STEPS	RATIONALE
1. Explain the procedure to the client.	Explanation of the procedure reduces the client's anxiety and improves cooperation.
2. Assist client to a supine position. Place the bath blanket over the upper trunk and cover the lower extremities with bedsheets so only the genitalia are exposed.	A supine position promotes comfort, and draping prevents unnecessary exposure of body parts.
3. Cleanse the genitalia with soap and water, and dry thoroughly.	Secretions that may irritate the client's skin are removed. The rubber sheath rolls onto dry skin more easily.
4. Prepare the urinary drainage bag by attaching it to the bed frame. Bring the drainage tubing up through the side rails onto the bed.	Easy access to equipment during connection of the condom catheter is provided.
5. Grasp the penis firmly along the shaft with your nondominant hand. With your dominant hand hold the condom sheath at the tip of the penis and smoothly roll the sheath up onto the penile shaft.	A firm grasp reduces chances of an erection occurring. The condom should fit smoothly to prevent sites of constriction.
6. Be sure the tip of the penis is 2.5 to 5 cm (1 to 2 inches) above the end of the condom catheter.	This position allows free passage of urine into the collecting tubing during voiding.
7. Encircle the penile shaft with the strip of Velcro or adhesive. Be sure the strip touches only the condom sheath. Apply snugly but not tightly.	The adhesive strip anchors the condom in place. Snug fit prevents constriction of blood flow.
8. Connect the drainage tubing to the end of the condom catheter.	Connection of the drainage system prevents soiling of bed linen and provides for collection of all voided urine.
9. Place the excess coil of tubing on the bed and secure to the bottom bedsheet.	Patent tubing promotes free drainage of urine.

infection. Several nursing measures that decrease the risk of infection are discussed in the following sections.

PERINEAL HYGIENE

The client at risk for a urinary tract infection should consistently receive scrupulous perineal cleansing. Chapter 35 describes the techniques for providing hygiene to clients.

For clients with catheters, hygiene measures are necessary at least twice a day and after each bowel movement. Any secretions or encrustations at the catheter insertion site must be completely removed. In some institutions iodophor solutions such as povidone-iodine (Betadine) are used for cleansing and

iodophor ointments are applied at the urethral meatus. The client should refrain from applying powders or lotions, which favor growth of microorganisms.

CATHETER MANAGEMENT

Infection can develop in a catheterized client in a number of ways. Maintaining a closed urinary drainage system is important in infection control. Any break in the system can lead to introduction of microorganisms (Fig. 39-9). In addition, the nurse monitors the patency of the system to prevent pooling of urine within drainage tubing. Urine in the drainage bag is an excellent medium for microorganism growth. Bacteria can travel up drainage tubing to grow in pools of urine. If this urine flows back into

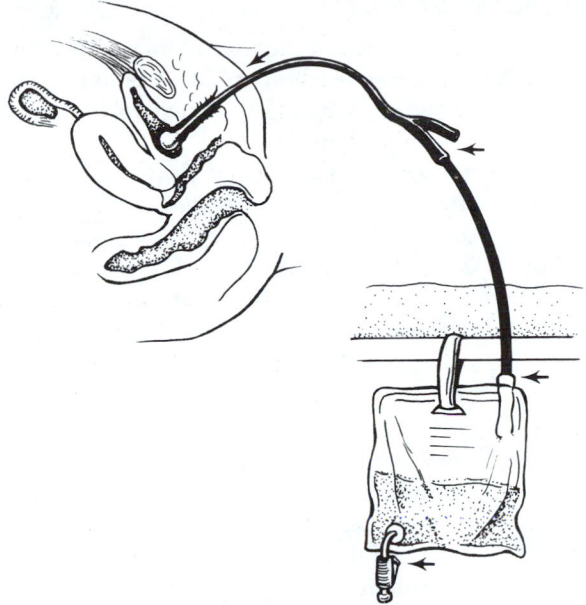

Fig. 39-9 Potential sites for introduction of infectious organisms into a urinary drainage system.

> ### *Tips for Preventing Infection in Catheterized Clients*
>
> - Do not allow the spigot on the drainage bag to touch a contaminated surface.
> - Do not open the drainage system at connection points to obtain specimens or measure urine.
> - If the drainage tubing becomes disconnected, do not touch the ends of the catheter or tubing. Wipe the ends of the tube with antiseptic solution before reconnecting.
> - Prevent pooling of urine and reflux of urine into the bladder.
>   - Avoid raising the drainage bag above the level of the client's bladder.
>   - If it becomes necessary to raise the bag during transfer of the client to a bed or stretcher, clamp the tubing.
>   - Avoid making large loops in the tubing.
>   - Before the client exercises or ambulates, drain all urine from the tubing into the bag.
> - Avoid prolonged clamping or kinking of the tubing (except during conditioning).
> - Empty the drainage bag at least every 8 hours.

the client's bladder, an infection will likely develop. The boxed material gives suggestions for ways to prevent infections in catheterized clients.

HANDWASHING

Good handwashing practices are basic to infection control. Handwashing is necessary before the nurse handles a catheter or the drainage system. When the nurse goes from a client with a catheter to one without, handwashing can prevent cross-contamination. The nurse also cautions clients against handling a catheter with unclean hands.

ACIDIFYING URINE

An acid urine tends to inhibit growth of microorganisms. The intake of foods such as meats, eggs, whole-grain breads, cranberries, prunes, and plums increases urine acidity. The foods metabolize into acid end products that eventually enter the urine. Cranberry juice increases urine acidity, whereas fruit juices such as orange or grapefruit juice produce an alkaline urine. There is evidence that high doses of ascorbic acid lower the urine pH.

Maintenance of Skin Integrity

The normal acidity of urine causes it to be irritating to the skin. When urine becomes alkaline, encrustations or precipitate collects on the skin, fostering breakdown. Continuous exposure to urine of the perineal area or the skin surrounding an ostomy leads to gradual maceration and excoriation. Washing with mild soap and warm water is the best way to remove urine from the skin. Body lotion keeps the skin moisturized and provides a barrier to the urine. Clients who wet their clothing should receive a clean set of clothes after each voiding. Allowing a client with chronic incontinence or a child with enuresis to lie in wet clothes or on a soiled bed pad is unacceptable.

When the skin becomes irritated or inflamed, the physician may prescribe a cream or spray containing steroids to reduce inflammation of tissues. Kenalog is a popular form of cortisone spray. If fungal growth develops, the antifungal medication nystatin (Mycostatin), available in cream or powder form, is effective.

The client with an ostomy has a special hygiene problem because urine drains from the ostomy site continuously. Frequently the drainage pouch or appliance becomes moist and slips from the skin. Continual oozing of urine around the stoma causes skin breakdown. Skin barriers, similar to those used with colostomies and ileostomies (see Chapter 40) provide a layer of protection between the client's skin and the ostomy pouch. When urine leaks, it frequently covers the outer skin barrier. It is also helpful for the client with an ostomy to select an appliance that fits snugly against the skin's surface around the stoma.

Heatlamp treatments are useful for severe skin excoriations (see Chapter 48). Short-term exposure of the skin to heat improves blood supply to the area and promotes drying. The nurse checks the client frequently to prevent the development of a skin burn.

Promotion of Comfort

Clients with urinary alterations become uncomfortable as a result of the symptoms of urinary problems. The frequent or unpredictable voiding associated with enuresis and incontinence, dysuria resulting from bladder infections, and the painful distention from urinary retention are all sources of discomfort.

The incontinent client gains comfort from having clean, dry clothing. When stress incontinence is the problem, a protective pad or sanitary belt offers protection against soiling. Wet clothing adheres to the skin and can cause rubbing and irritation.

Dysuria may be relieved by the administration of urinary analgesics that act on the urethral and bladder mucosa. Phenazopyridine is helpful in relieving dysuria, burning, and itching associated with urinary tract infections. The drug comes combined with sulfonamide antibiotics in preparations such as Azo Gantanol and Azo Gantrisin. The sulfonamide provides additional antibacterial action. Clients taking medications with phenazopyridine should be informed that their urine may appear orange in color. They must drink large amounts of fluids to prevent toxicity from the sulfonamides and to maintain optimal flow through the urinary system.

If the client has local discomfort from an inflamed urethra, a warm sitz bath may provide pain relief (see Chapter 48). The warm water soothes inflamed tissues near the urethral meatus by improving blood supply. The client is often relaxed after a sitz bath so voiding occurs easily.

The pain of distention cannot be relieved unless the client is able to empty the bladder. Methods for stimulating micturition, for example, the sound of running water, Credé's method, or catheterization, may be the only sources of pain relief.

Establishing Return of Bladder Function

Clients with incontinence often are able to learn a routine that reverses or controls the incontinent episodes. The nurse and client work together to develop a bladder training program that promotes physical and psychological well-being. Some measures useful in treating incontinence are also beneficial to an enuretic child. The training program can begin only when the physician determines that the client is ready.

BLADDER TRAINING

For a client with incontinence to gain reliable bladder control, there must be remaining bladder function. The client must be alert enough to follow the established training program.

The nurse's first step is to assess the client's current voiding pattern. Comparing this data with information regarding the client's usual voiding pattern provides a baseline for developing the plan of care. The client requires the nurse's understanding and support. Anger, apathy, social isolation, and depression are common with incontinence, and a bladder training program can give the client renewed self-esteem and the ability to assume a more normal life-style.

The following measures will help the incontinent client gain control over urination:

1. Learning exercises to strengthen the pelvic floor
2. Voiding after meals, at bedtime, and when the urge to urinate occurs
3. Using methods to relax to ensure complete bladder emptying
4. Never ignoring the urge to void
5. Taking fluids approximately 30 minutes before planned voiding
6. Limiting fluids after supper to no more than 150 to 200 ml (5 to 7 ounces)
7. Taking prescribed diuretic medications or fluids that increase diuresis (such as tea or coffee) early in the morning
8. Following a weight control program if obesity is a problem

These guidelines help the client to establish a routine for voiding and to control factors that might increase the number of incontinent episodes.

Evaluation

To evaluate the plan of care the nurse sets expected outcomes that measure whether interventions in promoting normal urinary elimination were effective. The optimal outcome is the client's ability to urinate voluntarily without dysuria, urgency, or frequency. The urine should be an amber color, clear, without abnormal constituents, and within the normal range of pH and specific gravity.

The nurse can also evaluate specific interventions designed to promote normal urinary function and prevent the complications associated with urinary alterations.

Nursing care to promote normal micturition is evaluated on the basis of the following:

1. The client's ability to void an amount equal to fluid intake (ideally 2000 ml intake/2000 ml output)

2. The client's ability to void without the use of medications, bladder compression, or catheterization

Measures to promote complete bladder emptying are evaluated on the following bases:

1. The absence of bladder distention
2. A residual urine volume, as determined by straight catheterization, of less than 25 ml
3. A patent, free-flowing drainage system

Interventions designed to prevent urinary tract infection are evaluated using these criteria:

1. A urine culture that is negative for bacteria
2. The absence of dysuria, burning, itching at the urethral meatus, urgency, or frequency

Maintenance of skin integrity is evaluated on the basis of the following:

1. A dry perineal area that is without inflammation or excoriation
2. Skin around a ureterostomy client's stoma that is dry and without inflammation or excoriation

The following criteria are used to evaluate interventions designed to promote client comfort:

1. The client's ability to void without dysuria
2. The absence of bladder distention
3. The incontinent client's expression of a feeling of well-being

An effective bladder training program is evaluated on the basis of these criteria:

1. A reduction in the number of incontinent episodes
2. The client's ability to void when the urge to urinate occurs

Summary

Normal urinary function provides a means for the excretion of body wastes. The kidneys also play a vital role in regulating fluid and electrolyte balance. The nurse's knowledge of urinary tract structure and function provides a basis for selecting nursing therapies appropriate for a client's alterations.

Using the nursing process to organize care for actual or potential urinary problems, the nurse collects data related to the client's voiding pattern, exposure to risks for urinary tract alteration, and physical condition. The laboratory analysis of urine specimens and diagnostic review of urinary structures provide further information for the nurse's data base. Nursing diagnoses are the basis for the plan of care.

Nursing interventions promote normal urination and provide support to clients unable to maintain continence. Because of the urinary tract's vulnerability to infection, one of the nurse's primary concerns is infection control. The client with urinary alterations may also suffer considerable embarrassment, social isolation, and depression. Whether the client's alteration is only temporary (as with catheterization) or long term (as with ureterostomy), the nurse must maintain the client's privacy and dignity at all times.

KEY CONCEPTS

✓ The mucous lining of the urethra, bladder, and ureters provides an excellent medium for microorganism growth.

✓ The act of micturition or voiding is influenced by voluntary control from higher brain centers, as well as involuntary control from the spinal cord.

✓ Problems of mobility and changes in kidney and bladder function cause the aged to be at risk for urinary elimination alterations.

✓ In a healthy adult an increase in fluid volume results in increased urine output.

✓ A normal pattern of urination involves voiding after awakening from sleep, after meals, after a large intake of fluids, and before bedtime.

✓ Symptoms common to urinary disturbances include urgency, dysuria, polyuria, oliguria, and difficulty in starting the urinary stream.

✓ In the home setting the nurse's assessment of the client's elimination function should include a review of environmental barriers that might make it difficult for the client to reach toilet facilities.

✓ Certain foods, medications, dyes used in diagnostic examinations, and serum bilirubin levels can influence urine color.

✓ When collected properly, a clean-voided urine specimen does not contain bacteria picked up from the urethral meatus.

✓ A urine specimen should never be obtained from a catheter drainage bag.

✓ Accurate measurement of glucose concentration in urine requires a double-voided specimen.

✓ A client can better understand the importance of perineal hygiene by knowing that the urinary tract is normally sterile.

✓ Methods of promoting the micturition reflex assist clients in sensing the urge to urinate and controlling urethral sphincter relaxation.

✓ Provision for privacy helps promote normal voiding.

✓ An increased fluid intake results in urine formation that flushes particles and solutes from the urinary system.

✓ Exercises that strengthen muscles of the pelvic floor increase a client's urethral sphincter control.

✓ The greatest risk of urinary catheterization is urinary tract infection.

✓ An indwelling urinary catheter remains in the bladder for an extended period, making the risk of infection greater than with intermittent catheterization.

✓ A urinary drainage system should always remain closed.

✓ A catheter drainage system should be positioned to allow free drainage of urine by gravity.

✓ Backflow of urine from a catheter system into the bladder may cause infection.

✓ An indwelling catheter should never be removed before the balloon is deflated fully.

✓ Condom catheters are applied snugly but not so tightly as to constrict blood flow.

✓ Since urine drains almost continuously from a ureterostomy, there is a risk of skin breakdown around a stoma site.

REFERENCES

Whaley, L.F., and Wong, D.L.: Nursing care of infants and children, ed. 2, St. Louis, 1983, The C.V. Mosby Co.

Williamson, M.L.: Reducing post-catheterization bladder dysfunction in reconditioning, Nurs. Res. **31**:28, 1982.

ADDITIONAL READINGS

Bates, P.: A troubleshooter's guide to indwelling catheters, RN **44**:63, 1981.

Bielski, M.: Preventing infection in the catheterized patient, Nurs. Clin. North Am. **15**:703, 1980.

Brink, C.: Assessing the problem, Geriatric Nurs. **1**:241, 1980.

Demmerle, B., and Bantol, M.A.: Nursing care of the incontinent person, Geriatric Nurs. **1**:246, 1980.

Finkbeiner, A.E.: Helpful drugs, Geriatric Nurs. **1**:270, 1980.

Jeter, K.F.: Urinary ostomies, a guidebook for patients, ed. 2, 1978, United Ostomy Association, Inc.

Mandelstam, D.: Strengthening pelvic floor muscles, Geriatric Nurs. **1**:251, 1980.

Murray, B.S., et al.: The patient has an ileal conduit, Am. J. Nurs. **71**:1560, 1971.

Pagana, K.D., and Pagana, T.J.: Diagnostic testing and nursing implications, St. Louis, 1982, The C.V. Mosby Co.

Taylor, J.W., and Ballenger, S.: Neurological dysfunctions and nursing interventions, New York, 1980, McGraw-Hill, Inc.

Thomas, B.: Problem solving: urinary incontinence in the elderly, J. Gerontol. Nurs. **6**:533, 1980.

Underwood, M.A.: Urinary tract infections, Crit. Care Q. **3**:63, 1980.

Wells, T.: Promoting urine control in older adults, Geriatric Nurs. **1**:236, 1980.

Wells, T., and Brink, C.: Helpful equipment, Geriatric Nurs. **1**:264, 1980.

OBJECTIVES

Mastery of content in this chapter will enable the student to:

- Define the terms in the glossary.
- Discuss the role of the gastrointestinal organs in digestion and elimination.
- Describe four functions of the large intestine.
- Explain the physiology of normal defecation.
- List and discuss psychological and physiological factors that influence the elimination process.
- Compare and contrast common physiological alterations in elimination.
- Assess a client's elimination pattern.
- Perform a guaiac test for occult blood.
- List nursing diagnoses related to alterations in elimination.
- Describe nursing implications for common diagnostic examinations of the gastrointestinal tract.
- Administer an enema.
- List nursing measures aimed at promoting normal elimination.

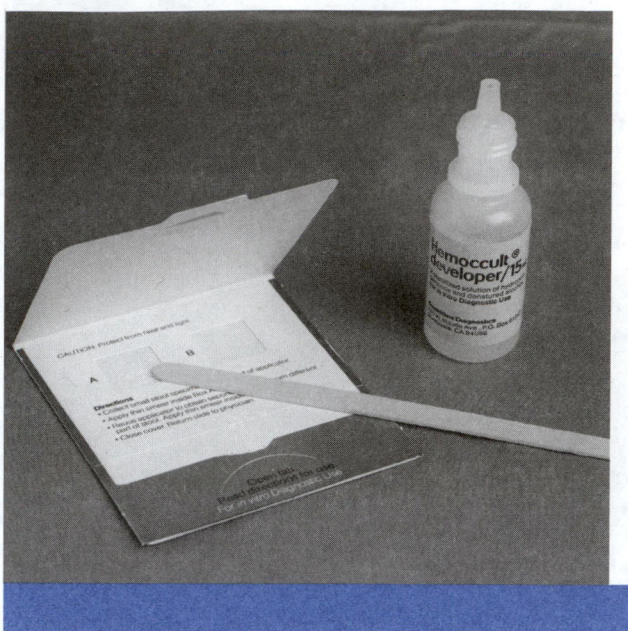

GLOSSARY

biopsy Removal of a small piece of living tissue from an organ or other part of the body for microscopic examination.

bolus Round mass of chewed food ready to be swallowed.

cathartic Drug that acts to promote bowel evacuation.

chyme Viscous, semifluid contents of the stomach present during digestion of a meal, which eventually pass into the intestines.

colitis Inflammatory condition of the large intestine.

colon Portion of the large intestine from the cecum to the rectum.

constipation Condition characterized by difficulty in passing stool or an infrequent passage of hard stool.

contrast medium Radiopaque substance injected into the body to improve visualization of internal structures that are otherwise difficult to see on x-ray examination.

defecation Passage of feces from the digestive tract through the rectum.

diarrhea Increase in the number of stools and the passage of liquid, unformed feces.

diverticula Pouchlike herniations through the muscular wall of a tubular organ; may be present in the stomach, small intestine, or, most commonly, the colon.

endoscopy Visualization of the interior of body organs and cavities with an endoscope.

enema Procedure involving introduction of a solution into the rectum for cleansing or therapeutic purposes.

excoriation Injury to the skin's surface caused by abrasion.

feces Waste or excrement from the gastrointestinal tract.

flatulence Condition characterized by the accumulation of gas within the lumen of the intestines.

guaiac test Test of feces for the presence of occult (hidden) blood.

haustral contraction Type of peristaltic contraction that occurs in the large intestine; produces a large sac in the colon's wall to increase surface area for nutrient absorption.

hemorrhoids Permanent dilation and engorgement of veins within the lining of the rectum.

laxative Drug that acts to promote bowel evacuation.

masticate To chew or tear food with the teeth while it becomes mixed with saliva.

melena Abnormal black, sticky stool containing digested blood; indicative of gastrointestinal bleeding.

40 | *Bowel Elimination*

ostomate   Person with an ostomy.

ostomy   Surgical procedure in which an opening is made into the abdominal wall to allow the passage of intestinal contents from the bowel (colostomy) or urine from the bladder (urostomy).

regurgitation   Return of swallowed food into the mouth.

stoma   Artifically created opening between a body cavity and the body's surface, for example, a colostomy, formed from a portion of the colon pulled through the abdominal wall.

tarry   Sticky quality of feces containing blood.

The regular elimination of fecal waste products is essential for normal body functioning. Disturbances in elimination influence the gastrointestinal and other body systems. Normal bowel function requires a balance of physiological, psychological, social, and cultural factors. A client's developmental needs also affect the pattern of bowel elimination. Because normal bowel function depends on the balance of several factors, each individual has a unique pattern of elimination.

Clients often require assistance from the nurse to maintain normal elimination habits. Illness may impair a client's ability to follow a good bowel management program. For example, certain conditions impair a client's ability to eat regularly or maintain a necessary fluid intake. A client may also be restricted physically from being able to use normal toilet facilities. The home environment may present obstacles for the client with altered mobility, requiring changes in bathroom fixtures.

Disturbances in elimination can cause embarrassment and discomfort for clients. Clients often view the need to use a bedpan or to receive assistance with perineal hygiene after defecation as offensive. The nurse should show a respect for the client's privacy and emotional needs when delivering care. Measures designed to promote normal elimination should also minimize discomfort for clients. The nurse's competence in managing a client's elimination problems rests on a clear understanding of normal elimination and the factors that may create alterations.

Normal Elimination Process

The gastrointestinal tract consists of a series of hollow mucous membrane–lined, muscular organs whose primary purpose is to absorb fluid and nutrients (Fig. 40-1). The volume of fluids absorbed by the gastrointestinal tract is high, making fluid balance a key function of the elimination process. In addition to ingested fluids and foods, the gastrointestinal tract receives a large volume of secretions from organs such as the gallbladder and pancreas (Table 40-1). Any disorder that seriously impairs the normal absorption or secretion of gastrointestinal fluids will cause fluid imbalance.

To facilitate the absorption and transport of solid nutrients, the gastrointestinal tract mechanically and chemically breaks down nutrients into a suitable size and form. All of the digestive organs work together to ensure that the mass or bolus of food reaches the areas of nutrient absorption safely and effectively. The teeth masticate (chew) food, breaking it down to a suitable size for swallowing. Salivary secretions contain enzymes that initiate the digestion of certain food elements. The saliva dilutes and softens the bolus of food in the mouth for easier swallowing.

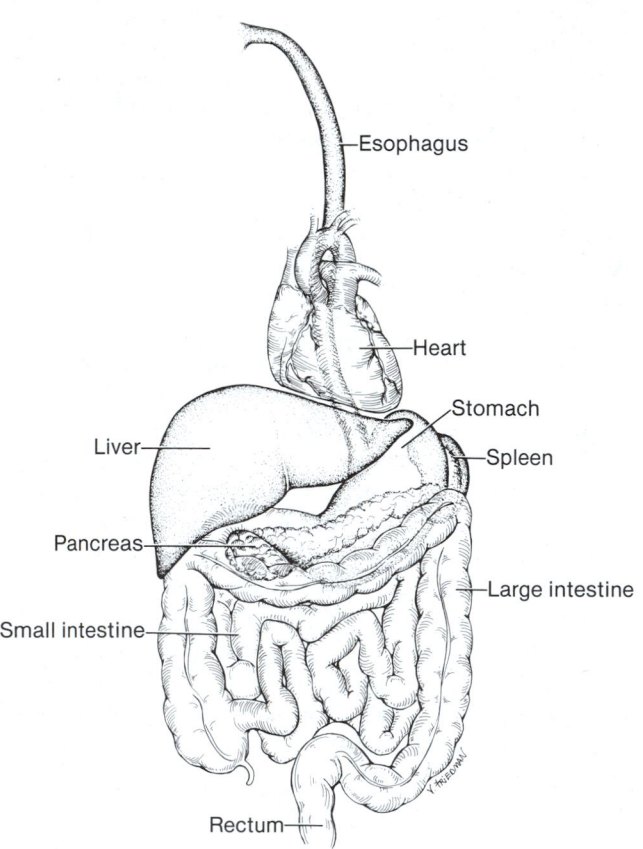

Fig. 40-1 Organs of the gastrointestinal system.

Esophagus

As food enters the upper esophagus, it passes through the upper esophageal sphincter. The sphincter is a circular muscle that prevents air from entering the esophagus and food from refluxing or moving backward into the throat. The bolus of food travels approximately 45 cm (18 inches) down the esophagus. Food is pushed along by slow peristaltic waves, which are produced by alternating contractions of underlying smooth muscle. As a portion of the esophagus contracts behind the food bolus, the circular muscle in front of the bolus relaxes. A peristaltic wave propels food toward the next wave, similar to the way a wave in the ocean pushes a raft ashore. Peristalsis moves gastrointestinal contents throughout the length of the gastrointestinal tract.

In 15 seconds the bolus of food moves down the esophagus and reaches the lower esophageal sphincter. There is no identifiable muscular sphincter between the esophagus and the stomach. There is, however, a pressure difference existing at the lower end of the esophagus. The lower esophageal pressure is 10 to 40 mm Hg, while the pressure within the stomach is 5 to 10 mm Hg. The pressure gradient normally prevents the reflux of stomach contents back into the esophagus. Numerous factors can influence the lower esophageal sphincter pressure. Antacids increase pressure at the sphincter to minimize reflux. Ingestion of fatty foods and nicotine from smoking lower the pressure and increase risk of reflux.

Stomach

In the stomach food is temporarily stored and mechanically broken down for eventual digestion and absorption. The stomach secretes hydrochloric acid (HCl), mucus, the enzyme pepsin, and intrinsic factor.

TABLE 40-1

Gastrointestinal Tract Fluid Balance

	Ingested and Secreted (ml)	Absorbed (ml)
Food and drink	1500	
Saliva	1500	
Gastric juice	3000	
Pancreatic juice	2000	
Bile	500	
Small intestine		5850
Colon		2500
Feces		150
TOTAL	8500	8500

The concentration of HCl influences stomach acidity and the body's systemic acid-base balance (see Chapter 43). For every HCl molecule secreted into the stomach, a bicarbonate (HCO_3) molecule enters the blood plasma. HCl aids in the mixing and breakdown of food elements within the stomach. Mucus protects the stomach mucosa from acidity and enzyme activity. Aspirin and alcohol are known to cause damage to the stomach's mucous lining. Pepsin serves to digest proteins, although a minimal amount of digestion occurs in the stomach. Intrinsic factor is the essential component needed for vitamin B_{12} absorption in the intestine. Lack of intrinsic factor results in pernicious anemia.

Before food leaves the stomach, it has been changed into a semifluid state called chyme. Food converted into chyme is more easily digested and absorbed than solid food. Clients who have portions of their stomach removed or who have rapid stomach emptying (as with colitis) have serious digestive problems because food is not broken down into chyme. Food enters the small intestine before being adequately broken down to a semifluid form. Absorption is less efficient, and nutritional alterations can develop.

Small Intestine

In the course of normal digestion, chyme leaves the stomach and enters the small intestine. The small intestine is approximately 600 cm (20 to 21 feet) long and contains three anatomical divisions: duodenum, jejunum, and ileum. The chyme mixes with digestive enzymes (such as bile and amylase) while traveling through the small intestine. Segmentation (alternating contraction and relaxation of intestinal smooth muscle) churns the chyme, further breaking down food elements for digestion (Fig. 40-2). As the chyme

mixes, the forward peristaltic movement temporarily ceases to permit nutrient absorption. The chyme travels slowly down the small intestine to allow time for nutrient absorption.

Most nutrients are absorbed in the small intestine as are electrolytes, including sodium, chloride, potassium, magnesium, bicarbonate, and calcium. Enzymes from the pancreas (such as amylase) and bile from the gallbladder are released into the duodenum. The intestine breaks down fats, proteins, and carbohydrates into their basic elements. Nutrients are almost entirely absorbed by the duodenum and jejunum. The ileum absorbs certain vitamins, iron, and bile salts. If the function of the small intestine is impaired, the digestive process is greatly altered. For example, inflammation, surgical resection, or obstruction can disrupt peristalsis, reduce the area of absorption, or block the passage of chyme. As a result, electrolyte and nutrient deficiencies develop.

Large Intestine

The remaining chyme that is unabsorbed enters the large intestine (colon) through the ileocecal valve. The valve is a circular muscle layer that prevents colon contents from regurgitating or returning to the small intestine. The large intestine is the primary organ of bowel elimination. Although chyme enters the colon in a watery state, the volume of water lessens as the chyme moves along the length of the colon.

The large intestine extends 1.5 m (5 feet) from the cecum to the anal canal (Fig. 40-3). Throughout its length the colon is made up of muscular tissue. An internal layer of circular muscle is surrounded by longitudinal fibers. The muscular quality of the colon allows it to eliminate large quantities of waste.

The colon has four interrelated functions: absorption, protection, secretion, and elimination. A large volume of water and a significant amount of sodium and chloride are absorbed by the colon daily. As food passes through the large intestine, haustral contractions occur. Haustral contractions are similar to the segmental contractions of the small intestine but last longer, up to 5 minutes. The contractions produce large sacs in the colon's wall, providing a large surface area for absorption to occur.

As much as 2.5 liters of water may be absorbed by the colon in 24 hours. On the average 55 milliequivalents (mEq) of sodium and 23 mEq of chloride are absorbed daily. The amount of water absorbed from the chyme depends on the speed at which the colonic contents move. The chyme is normally concentrated into a soft, formed mass. If the speed of peristaltic contractions is abnormally accelerated, there is less time for the water to be absorbed and the stool will

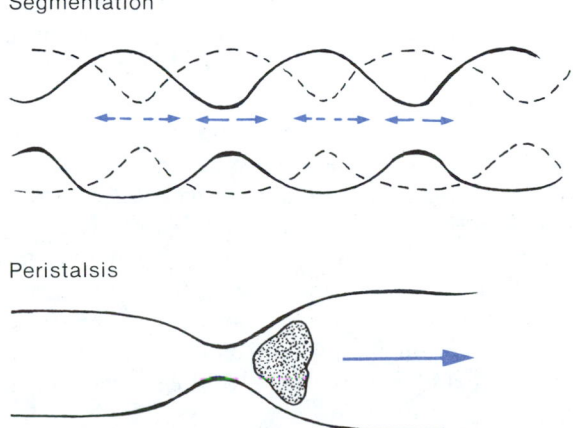

Segmentation

Peristalsis

Fig. 40-2 Segmental and peristaltic waves.

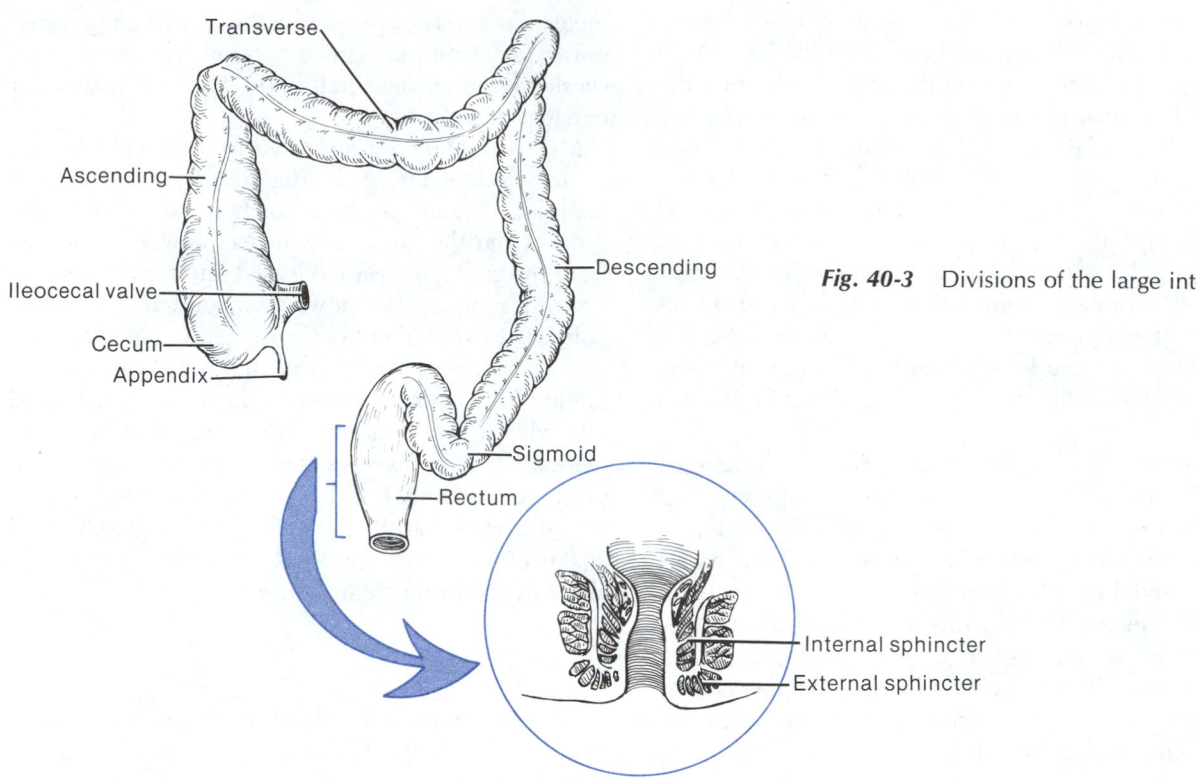

Fig. 40-3 Divisions of the large intestine.

be watery. If peristaltic contractions slow down, a hard mass of stool forms, resulting in constipation.

The colon protects itself by releasing a supply of mucus. The mucus lubricates the contents of the colon, preventing trauma to its lining. Lubrication is especially important near the distal end of the colon where contents become drier and harder.

The secretory function of the colon aids in electrolyte balance. Bicarbonate is secreted in exchange for chloride. Approximately 4 to 9 mEq of potassium is released each day by the large intestine. Serious alterations in colon function can contribute to electrolyte imbalance.

The final function of the colon is elimination. The colon removes waste products of digestion in addition to gas. The gas is the result of air swallowing and bacterial action on nonabsorbable carbohydrates. Fermentation of the carbohydrates produces a variety of forms of intestinal gas. The gas can act as a stimulant to peristalsis.

Slow peristaltic contractions move contents through the colon. Intestinal contents serve as the main stimulus for contraction. Waste products and gas exert pressure against the walls of the colon. As a result, the muscle layer stretches, stimulating the reflex that initiates contraction.

Mass peristaltic movements push the undigested food toward the rectum. These movements are unlike the frequent peristaltic waves found in the small in-

testine in that they typically occur only three or four times daily. Large segments of the colon contract as a result of two reflex responses—gastrocolic and duodenocolic—which occur when the stomach or duodenum is filled with food. Filling of the stomach or duodenum initiates nerve impulses that stimulate the colon's muscular walls. Mass peristalsis is strongest during the hour after mealtime. This is helpful for the nurse to know in planning and implementing elimination measures for a client.

Rectum

Once waste products reach the sigmoid portion of the colon, they are called feces. The sigmoid stores feces until just before defecation, or the act of having a bowel movement. The rectum, which is approximately 10 to 15 cm (4 to 6 inches) in length, is the final division of the gastrointestinal tract. Normally it remains empty of feces until defecation begins. It contains vertical and transverse folds of tissue believed to play a role in retaining feces. Each vertical fold contains an artery and veins. If the veins become repeatedly distended from pressure during the straining of defecation, permanent dilations called hemorrhoids form. The presence of hemorrhoids can make defecation painful.

When the fecal mass or gas moves into the rectum to distend its walls, the act of defecation begins. The process involves both involuntary and voluntary control. The internal sphincter is a smooth muscle innervated by the autonomic nervous system. As the rectum distends, sensory nerves are stimulated and carry impulses via sacral nerves that cause the internal sphincter to relax, allowing more feces to enter the rectum. At the same time impulses travel to the brain to create awareness of the need to defecate.

As the internal sphincter relaxes, so does the external sphincter, a voluntary striated muscle. The person who is toilet trained can voluntarily control the external sphincter. If the time for defecation is not right, constriction of the levator ani muscle closes the anus and defecation is delayed. At the time of defecation, the external sphincter relaxes. Pressure can be exerted to expel feces through an increase in intra-abdominal pressure or a Valsalva maneuver. A Valsalva maneuver is the voluntary contraction of the abdominal muscles during forced expiration with a closed glottis (holding one's breath). Relaxation of the levator ani muscle allows the feces to be expelled. If the act of defecation is voluntarily stopped, feces remain in the rectum until the defecation reflex is restimulated.

The act of defecation can be promoted by flexion of the thigh muscles and taking a sitting position. Flexion of the thigh places additional pressure on the abdomen. Defecating in a normal sitting position increases downward pressure on the rectum.

Factors Affecting Elimination

Many factors promote or impair elimination (Table 40-2). Knowledge of these factors allows the nurse to anticipate the measures required to maintain a normal elimination pattern. An understanding of how specific factors alter normal elimination provides guidelines for reversing their effects.

Psychological Factors

The function of virtually all body systems can be impaired by prolonged emotional stress (see Chapter 5). The function of the gastrointestinal tract is easily affected by stress. If an individual becomes anxious, afraid, or angry, the stress response initiates impulses from the parasympathetic division of the autonomic nervous system. The overall response allows the body to restore defenses. The digestive process is accelerated and peristalsis is increased to provide nutrients needed for defense. Side effects of increased peristalsis are diarrhea and gaseous distention.

A number of diseases of the gastrointestinal tract are believed to be aggravated by stress. For example,

TABLE 40-2

Factors Affecting Elimination

Factors Promoting Elimination	Factors Impairing Elimination
Stress-free environment	Emotional stress (anxiety or depression)
Ability to follow personal bowel habits, privacy	Failure to heed the defecation reflex, lack of time or privacy
High-fiber diet	High-carbohydrate and high-fat diet
Normal fluid intake (fruit juices, warm liquids)	Reduced fluid intake
Exercise	Immobility or inactivity
Ability to assume a squatting position	Inability to squat because of immobility, advanced age, musculoskeletal deformities, pain, or advanced pregnancy; pain during defecation
Properly administered laxatives and cathartics	Use of narcotic analgesics, antibiotics, or general anesthetics and overuse of cathartics

ulcerative colitis, a chronic inflammation and ulceration of the colon, worsens when a client suffers psychological stress. The client with colitis commonly exhibits behavior indicative of emotional tension. For many years the cause of ulcerative colitis and other gastrointestinal disorders such as Crohn's disease and gastric ulcers was believed to be largely psychosomatic. It is now known that the primary cause of these disorders is physiological but that emotional stress exacerbates the symptoms and the course.

A factor that may contribute to a child's emotional stress and interfere with gastrointestinal function is the method of toilet training. Bowel training should not begin until a child is at an age (usually 2 to 3 years) when the nervous and muscular systems have developed the ability to control elimination. A child must be able to recognize the urge to defecate, be able to communicate this sensation to a parent, and be able to delay defecation. The child's motivation to please the parent by defecating at the proper time is also important. Forcing a child to sit on a potty chair for long intervals or spanking the child for having accidents will make toilet training a stressful process. The battle between a frustrated parent and a reluctant toddler may cause the child to rebel by retaining feces, which may lead to chronic constipation. The child needs a parent's understanding and patience. Positive reinforcement through the use of training pants, providing the child with a potty chair, and encouraging imitation by having the child watch a parent in the bathroom will prove beneficial.

It is important for the nurse to realize that psychological stress may be a key factor in an elimination problem. The nurse learns to question whether an emotional trauma is linked to a gastrointestinal alteration. Persons with chronic disease may have adapted with a variety of coping strategies. Clients' behaviors will yield important clues regarding their emotional state.

Personal Elimination Habits

An individual's personal elimination habits influence bowel function. The act of defecation is a private matter. Most people benefit from being able to use their own toilet facilities at a time during the day that is most effective and convenient for them. A busy work schedule is one factor that may disrupt a person's normal habits and result in alterations such as constipation. A person should learn the time of day that is best for establishing regular elimination patterns (for example, after meals or on awakening).

Hospitalized clients rarely can maintain privacy during defecation. The client must often share bathroom facilities with a roommate whose hygienic habits may be quite different. The nature of the client's illness often limits physical activity, thus necessitating use of a bedpan or bedside commode. The sights, sounds, and odors associated with sharing toilet facilities or using bedpans are often humiliating to the client. Embarrassment prompts clients to ignore the urge to defecate. Failure to heed the normal defecation reflex begins a vicious circle of discomfort. If alterations such as constipation develop, therapies may be needed, making the problem even more significant and anxiety producing.

The client requires the nurse's understanding and support. If the nurse becomes easily embarrassed or nervous when the client requires assistance with elimination, the client will sense the nurse's reaction. When a client has an "accident," the nurse should not show disapproval or revulsion. The nurse must be able to discuss the individual's elimination problems and needs openly. Gaining knowledge of the client's personal elimination habits is necessary in developing a plan of care. The measures the client uses at home to maintain bowel function should be followed in the health care setting, if possible.

Diet

The character of a person's dietary intake significantly affects the process of elimination. Certain foods promote normal peristaltic movement. Thus, breast-fed infants have a softer, more liquid stool than infants who are bottle fed. A food that promotes normal elimination in one individual may cause diarrhea or constipation in another.

The presence of fiber, the undigestible residue in the diet, provides the bulk in fecal material. For this reason many people use the words "bulk" and "fiber" interchangeably when discussing the content of certain foods. Bulk-forming foods generally stretch the bowel walls, creating peristalsis and initiating the defecation reflex. (An infant's immature bowel cannot usually tolerate fiber-containing foods until several months of age.) By stimulating peristalsis, the bulk foods pass quickly through the intestines, keeping the stool soft. Certain foods, such as the following, contain a higher amount of fiber than others:

1. Raw fruits (apples, oranges)
2. Cooked fruits (prunes, apricots)
3. Greens (spinach, kale, cabbage)
4. Raw vegetables (celery, zucchini)
5. Whole grains (cereal, breads)

Ingestion of a high-fiber diet improves the likelihood of a normal elimination pattern if all other factors are normal. Gas-producing foods such as onions, cauliflower, and beans also stimulate peristalsis. The gas that is formed distends intestinal walls, increasing colon motility.

Certain foods, such as milk and milk products, are difficult or impossible for some people to digest. The person who is unable to digest milk successfully has a lactose intolerance. Lactose, a simple form of sugar found in milk, is normally broken down by the enzyme lactase. The inability to digest lactose results from the individual's failure to produce lactase. Intolerance to specific foods may result in diarrhea, gaseous distention, and cramping.

Fluid Intake

The gastrointestinal tract has a major role in controlling fluid balance. If a fluid deficiency develops as a result of an alteration in another body system, more fluid is absorbed from the intestine in compensation. Deficiencies in intake or disturbances causing loss of fluid (such as vomiting) directly affect the character of the fecal mass. Fluid liquefies intestinal contents, easing their passage through the colon. A reduction in fluid intake slows the passage of food through the intestines. As peristalsis slows, there is an increased absorption of fluid and a hardening of the feces. Normally, an adult should drink six to eight glasses or

1400 to 2000 ml of fluid daily. Hot beverages and fruit juices are especially effective in promoting softening of stool and increasing peristalsis.

Exercise

Physical activity promotes peristalsis, whereas immobilization depresses colonic motility. Early ambulation after illness therefore is encouraged to ensure the maintenance of normal elimination.

Maintaining the tone of the skeletal muscles used during defecation is important. Weakened abdominal and pelvic floor muscles impair the ability to increase intra-abdominal pressure and to control the external sphincter. Muscle tone may be weakened or lost as a result of long-term illness or of neurological disease that impairs nerve transmission.

Position during Defecation

Squatting is the normal position assumed during defecation. Modern toilets are designed to facilitate this posture, allowing the person to lean forward, exert intra-abdominal pressure, and contract the thigh muscles. However, an elderly client or a client with joint disease such as arthritis may be unable to rise from a low toilet seat. Attachments that raise the level of the seat enable the client to get off the toilet without assistance. Clients who use such attachments, as well as short people, may require a footstool on which to place their feet in order to achieve proper hip flexion.

For the client immobilized in bed, the act of defecation is often difficult. In a supine position it is impossible to contract the muscles used during defecation. Assisting the client to a more normal sitting position on a bedpan enhances the ability to defecate.

Age

Developmental changes that affect the function of elimination occur throughout life. The infant has a small stomach capacity and less secretion of digestive enzymes. Certain foods such as complex starches are tolerated poorly. Food passes quickly through an infant's intestinal tract because of rapid peristalsis. The infant is unable to control defecation because of a lack of neuromuscular development.

During the adolescent growth spurt there is rapid growth of the large intestine. The secretion of hydrochloric acid increases, particularly in males. Adolescents typically eat more during this growth period.

The elderly frequently experience changes in the gastrointestinal system that can impair digestion and elimination. Many elderly people lose their teeth and

thus the ability to chew food thoroughly. Morsels of food enter the digestive tract only partially chewed and cannot be digested, since the amount of digestive enzymes in saliva and the volume of gastric acids fall with aging. The inability to digest fat-containing foods reflects a loss of the enzyme lipase.

With age, peristaltic action declines and esophageal emptying is slowed. Sluggish emptying of the esophagus can cause discomfort in the epigastric section of the abdomen. The absorptive properties of the intestinal mucosa change, causing protein, vitamin, and mineral deficiencies. The elderly also lose muscle tone in the internal sphincter of the large intestine. Although the integrity of the external sphincter may remain intact, the elderly client may have difficulty controlling bowel evacuation. Because of slowing of nerve impulses, some elderly clients are less aware of the need to defecate.

Pain

Normally the act of defecation is painless. However, a number of conditions, including hemorrhoids, rectal surgery, and abdominal surgery, may result in significant discomfort during defecation. In these instances the client often suppresses the urge to defecate in an effort to avoid pain. Constipation is a common problem for clients with pain during defecation.

Pregnancy

As a woman's pregnancy advances and the size of the fetus increases, pressure is exerted on the rectum. A temporary obstruction created by the fetus impairs the free passage of feces. Constipation is a common problem during the last trimester of pregnancy. A pregnant woman's frequent straining during defecation may result in the formation of permanent hemorrhoids.

Surgery and Anesthesia

The use of general anesthetic agents during surgery causes the temporary cessation of peristalsis (see Chapter 47). Inhaled anesthetic agents block parasympathetic impulses to the intestinal musculature. The anesthetic's action results in slowing or cessation of peristaltic waves. The client who receives local or regional anesthesia is less at risk for elimination alterations, since bowel activity is affected minimally or not at all.

Any surgery that involves the direct manipulation of the bowel temporarily stops peristalsis. This condition, called paralytic ileus, usually lasts approximately 24 to 48 hours. If the client remains inactive or is unable to eat after surgery, return of normal bowel function may be further delayed.

Medications

Medications are available for promoting defecation. Laxatives and cathartics are drugs that soften the stool and promote peristalsis. When used judiciously, laxatives and cathartics safely maintain normal elimination patterns. Problems arise when cathartics are taken for prolonged periods. Cathartics are more potent than laxatives in stimulating motility. Chronic use of cathartics causes the large intestine to lose muscle tone and become less responsive to stimulation. It can also cause serious diarrhea that may lead to dehydration and electrolyte depletion.

Several medications have side effects that may impair elimination. Narcotic analgesics depress peristalsis in the gastrointestinal tract. Opiates commonly cause constipation. Anticholinergic drugs, such as atropine, glycopyrrolate (Robinul), and methantheline (Banthine), inhibit gastric acid secretion and depress gastrointestinal motility. Although useful in treating hyperactive bowel disorders, anticholinergics can cause constipation in a client with normal bowel function. Many antibiotics produce diarrhea as a result of irritation and inflammation of the gastrointestinal mucosa. If the diarrhea and associated abdominal cramping become severe, the client may need to change medications.

Diagnostic Tests

Diagnostic examinations involving visualization of gastrointestinal structures often require that portions of the bowel be empty or clear of contents. A client is not allowed to eat or drink after midnight of the day preceding such examinations as a barium enema, endoscopy of the lower gastrointestinal tract, or an upper gastrointestinal (UGI) series. In the case of a barium enema or endoscopy, the client usually receives cathartics and an enema. Emptying the bowel of its contents interferes with elimination until the client is able to resume eating normally.

Barium examination procedures pose an additional problem. Barium hardens if allowed to stay in the gastrointestinal tract. This can lead to constipation or bowel impaction. A client should receive a cathartic to promote elimination of barium. Failure to evacuate all barium may require that the client receive an enema.

Common Bowel Elimination Problems

The nurse may encounter many clients who have or are at risk for developing elimination problems. Problems result from physiological changes in the gastrointestinal tract, surgical alteration of intestinal structures, or disorders that impair defecation.

Constipation

Constipation is the passage of hard, dry stools that typically require much straining during defecation. For various reasons intestinal motility slows, causing prolonged exposure of the fecal mass to the intestinal walls. Most of the fecal water content is absorbed, leaving little to soften and lubricate the stool. Often passage of a dry stool creates rectal pain.

Constipation is not solely defined according to the frequency of defecation. A person who has soft-formed stools only two or three times a week is not constipated. However, if normal elimination is delayed for a prolonged time, the chance of becoming constipated is high, since the feces remain in the colon longer than usual.

The causes of constipation are numerous. It often results from irregular bowel habits. For example, an aggressive businessperson who cannot miss a meeting and a person forced to stand in a long line for groceries are at risk for constipation if they repeatedly ignore the defecation reflex. Other contributing factors include an inadequate fluid intake, lack of exercise, and a low-fiber diet. Foods likely to cause constipation include lean meats, cheese, eggs, and pasta. The client restricted to bed or immobilized because of injury or disease is especially at risk for constipation. During the third trimester of pregnancy the growing fetus compresses the rectum. The pregnant woman can counteract this problem somewhat by eating high-fiber foods and increasing fluid intake.

Another common cause of constipation is the habitual use of laxatives. Individuals who rely on laxatives for regular bowel movements develop a physical dependence on the medication. Laxatives promote complete emptying of the colon, and a period of time is then necessary to refill the colon with bulk. However, the client may become anxious to have another bowel movement and take repeated doses of laxatives. Through lack of use the colon's normal reflexes eventually diminish in strength. The colon loses its muscle tone and becomes responsive only to the stimulating effect of laxatives or enemas.

For many clients constipation is a significant hazard to health. Straining during defecation presents an obvious problem to the client who has had recent abdominal or rectal surgery. The effort to pass a stool can cause stress on the suture line, and sutures may actually rupture, reopening the wound. In addition, clients with a history of cardiovascular disease or diseases causing elevated intraocular pressure (glaucoma) and intracranial pressure should use measures to prevent constipation and should avoid using the Valsalva maneuver. Straining during defecation is usually accompanied by holding the breath, and, as a result, the intrathoracic pressure and the heart rate drop. This sudden change in heart rate can be easily withstood by a person with a healthy heart, but the client with any degree of cardiac instability should avoid a Valsalva maneuver. Exhaling through the mouth during straining helps prevent a Valsalva maneuver from occurring.

Impaction

Fecal impaction results from unrelieved constipation. It is a collection of hardened feces, wedged in the rectum, that cannot be expelled. In cases of severe impaction the mass may extend up into the sigmoid colon. Clients who are debilitated, confused, or unconscious are most at risk for impaction. These individuals are too weak or unaware of the need to defecate. Frequent repetition of practices that promote constipation can also cause impaction, as can failure to pass barium contrast medium after a gastrointestinal examination.

An obvious sign of impaction is the inability to pass a stool for several days despite a repeated urge to defecate. The client with a history of constipation is most at risk. When a continuous oozing of diarrheal stool suddenly develops in such a client, impaction should be suspected. The liquid portion of feces located higher in the colon seeps around the edges of the impacted mass. Loss of appetite (anorexia), abdominal distention and cramping, and rectal pain may accompany the condition. The nurse who suspects an impaction can gently perform a digital examination of the rectum and palpate the impacted mass. Some institutions require a physician's order for a nurse to perform a rectal examination because of the risk of causing vagal stimulation that slows a client's heart rate.

Diarrhea

Diarrhea is an increase in the number of stools and the passage of liquid, unformed feces. It is a symptom of disorders affecting digestion, absorption, and secretion in the gastrointestinal tract. Intestinal contents pass through the small intestine and colon too quickly to allow the usual absorption of fluid. Irritation

within the colon may be an added factor that results in an increased mucus secretion. As a result, feces become watery. It is often difficult to assess diarrhea in infants because of their wide variation in bowel habits. An infant who is bottle fed may have one firm stool every second day, while a breast-fed baby may pass five to eight small, soft stools daily. It is important for the mother or nurse to note (1) any sudden increase in number of stools, (2) any reduction in fecal consistency with an increase in fluid content, and (3) a tendency for feces to be greenish.

The excessive loss of colonic fluid can result in

TABLE 40-3

Conditions That Cause Diarrhea

Condition	Physiological Effects
Emotional stress (anxiety)	Increased intestinal motility
Intestinal infection (streptococcal or staphylococcal enteritis)	Inflammation of intestinal mucosa, increased mucus secretion in colon
Food allergies	Reduced digestion of food elements
Food intolerance (greasy foods, coffee, alcohol, spicy foods)	Increased intestinal motility, increased mucus secretion in colon.
Medications	
Iron	Irritation of intestinal mucosa
Antibiotics	Suprainfection allowing overgrowth of normal flora, inflammation and irritation of mucosa
Laxatives	Increased intestinal motility
Colon disease (colitis, Crohn's disease)	Inflammation and ulceration of intestinal walls, reduced absorption of fluids, increased intestinal motility
Surgical alterations	
Gastrectomy	Loss of reservoir function of stomach, food dumped into duodenum too quickly for proper absorption
Colon resection	Reduced size of colon, reduced amount of absorptive surface

serious fluid and electrolyte imbalance. Infants and the elderly are particularly susceptible (see Chapter 42). Diarrhea was once the chief cause of death in infancy. Since repeated passage of diarrheal stools also exposes the skin of the perineum and buttocks to irritating intestinal contents, meticulous skin care is needed to prevent skin breakdown. The client may experience abdominal cramping, nausea, and vomiting, depending on the severity of the diarrhea.

Many conditions cause diarrhea (Table 40-3). The aim of treatment is first to remove all precipitating conditions and then to slow peristalsis. Any source of irritation to the intestinal mucosa must be eliminated. The client may need to refrain from eating or drinking if the diarrhea is severe and aggravated by oral intake. Often the client's nausea results in a loss of appetite. Fluids may need to be given intravenously to maintain necessary hydration. The nurse must carefully measure intake and output to determine overall fluid balance.

Incontinence

Fecal incontinence is the inability to control the passage of feces and gas from the anus. Any physiological or psychological condition that impairs function of the anal sphincter may lead to incontinence. Common physiological causes are those that alter sacral nerve transmission to the sphincter muscle, such as spinal cord trauma and multiple sclerosis. Tumors or growths of the sphincter tissue can also cause incontinence. Mental disorders such as schizophrenia, severe depression, and dementia may prevent the client from being aware of the need to defecate.

Incontinence can be devastating to the client's body image. In many situations the client is mentally alert but physically unable to avoid defecation. The embarrassment of soiling one's clothes can lead to social isolation. The client must depend on the nurse for a very basic need. Clients with mental or sensory alterations often are unaware that they have passed a stool. The nurse must express understanding and support of the client even though the repeated need to clean an incontinent client can become frustrating.

Like diarrhea, incontinence predisposes the client to skin breakdown. The nurse must check frequently to be sure the client's anal and perineal regions are clean and dry.

Flatulence

As gas accumulates in the lumen of the intestines, the bowel wall stretches and distends. This condition, known as flatulence, is a common cause of abdominal fullness, pain, and cramping. Normally intestinal gas escapes through the mouth (belching) or the anus (passing of flatus). However, if there is a reduction in intestinal motility resulting from factors such as opiates, general anesthetics, abdominal surgery, or immobilization, the client's flatulence may become severe enough to cause abdominal distention with shortness of breath. The accumulation of gas forces the diaphragm upward and reduces lung expansion.

A person normally produces several hundred milliliters of intestinal gas daily. Swallowed air makes up over 75% of intestinal gas in the form of nitrogen and oxygen. Bacterial decomposition of food in the colon releases the gas methane. Carbon dioxide is a product of fermentation in the bowel as intestinal acids become neutralized. Any factor that potentiates gas formation will increase intestinal flatulence. For example, certain foods (such as onions, beans, and cauliflower) contain nonabsorbable carbohydrates. In some individuals these foods remain within the colon to be broken down by bacteria into methane. A person with flatulence will benefit from avoiding foods that increase gas production.

Hemorrhoids

Hemorrhoids are dilated, engorged veins in the lining of the rectum. They are classified as either external or internal depending on their location on the outer anal surface or within the inner rectal wall. External hemorrhoids are clearly visible as protrusions of skin. If the underlying vein is thrombosed or hardened, there may be a purplish discoloration. Internal hemorrhoids have an outer mucous membrane. Increased venous pressure resulting from straining at defecation, pregnancy, congestive heart failure, and chronic liver disease is a causative factor in hemorrhoids.

Hemorrhoids are friable tissues that bleed easily when stretched. Passage of a hard stool commonly precipitates bleeding. The hemorrhoids become inflamed and tender, and clients may complain of itching and burning. Since pain worsens during defecation, the client may ignore the urge to defecate, resulting in constipation.

Ostomies

Certain diseases create conditions that prevent the normal passage of feces through the rectum. This necessitates the temporary or permanent formation of an artificial opening (stoma) in the abdominal wall. Surgical openings are formed in the ileum (ileostomy) or colon (colostomy). Ends of the intestines are then brought through the opening to create the stoma (Fig. 40-4). A person with an ostomy covers the stoma with a plastic pouch or bag to collect all fecal material that is passed.

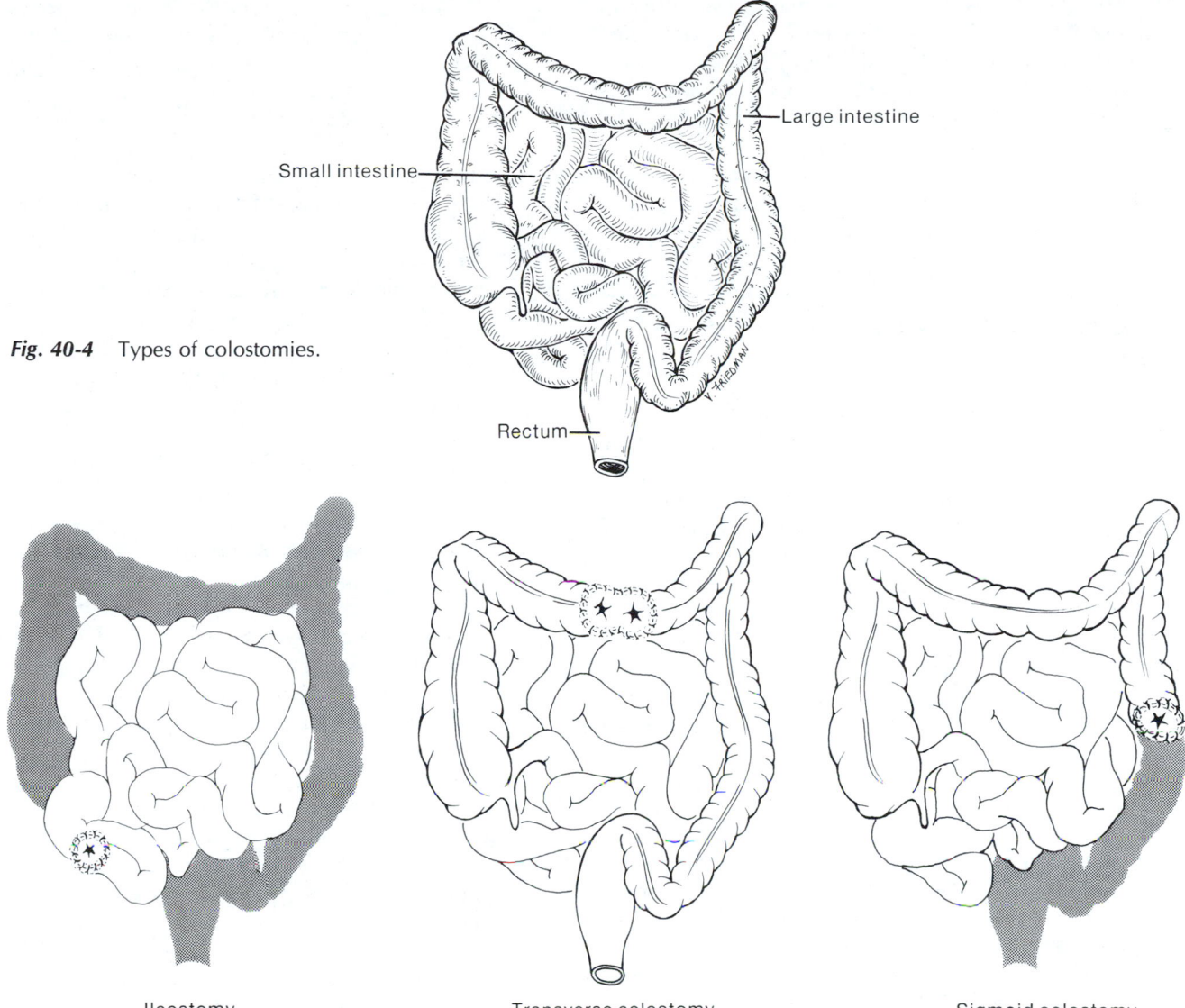

Fig. 40-4 Types of colostomies.

Ileostomy   Transverse colostomy   Sigmoid colostomy

The location of the ostomy determines the consistency of stool that is passed. An ileostomy bypasses the entire large intestine. As a result, stools are frequent and liquid. The same fecal characteristics hold true for a colostomy of the ascending colon. A colostomy of the transverse colon generally results in a more solid, formed stool. The sigmoid colostomy emits stool almost identical to that normally passed through the rectum.

Ostomies that emit frequent liquid stools create a management challenge. A bag or pouch must be worn at all times. A regular schedule of defecation cannot be achieved, since usually there is a continuous oozing of stool. The bag must be emptied, washed, and replaced throughout the day. Skin care is vital to prevent exposure to fecal irritants.

A colostomy in the transverse or sigmoid colon is simpler to manage. The client may continue to wear a pouch at all times even though bowel movements may occur only once or twice daily. Dietary regulation allows some clients to eat selected foods at prescribed intervals so that bowel movements occur at a convenient time. Therefore the client may not need to wear a pouch. Routine irrigations of the ostomy, similar to administration of an enema, allow the person to empty the bowel regularly and eliminate the need for a pouch.

The client with an ostomy experiences serious body image changes, particularly if the ostomy is permanent. Clients often perceive the construction of an artificial opening in the abdominal wall for the passage of feces as a form of mutilation. Even though clothing conceals the ostomy, the client feels different and unusual. Many clients have difficulty maintaining or initiating normal sexual relations with a partner. An important factor in the client's reactions is the character of fecal excretions and the ability to control them. Foul-smelling odors, spillage, or leakage of liquid stools and inability to regulate bowel movements give the client a sense of powerlessness and loss of self-esteem.

General Assessment of Bowel Function

To assess a client's elimination pattern and determine the presence of any abnormalities, the nurse should collect the following data:

1. Nursing history of the client's normal and present elimination pattern, with identification of measures used by the client to maintain elimination
2. Physical assessment of the abdomen
3. Inspection of fecal characteristics
4. Review of pertinent diagnostic test results

If the nurse identifies the presence of any abnormalities, assessment can focus on the specific nature of the problem.

Nursing History

The nursing history provides a review of the client's normal bowel pattern and habits. What a client describes as "normal" may be very different from the factors and conditions that tend to promote normal elimination. Identifying normal and abnormal patterns and habits allows the nurse to determine the nature of the client's problems, as well as methods most conducive to alleviating any problems. Much of the content in the nursing history can be organized around the factors that affect elimination. The nurse then applies this knowledge through a series of questions to determine the presence and extent of any gastrointestinal alterations. A typical nursing history of a client's elimination status includes the following:

1. *Determination of the individual's normal elimination pattern.* Frequency and time of day are included.
2. *Identification of any routines the client follows to promote normal elimination.* Examples are drinking hot liquids, using a laxative, eating specific foods, or taking time to defecate during a certain part of the day.
3. *Description of any recent change in elimination pattern.* This information is perhaps most significant, since elimination patterns are var-

iable and the client is the best resource to detect change. The nurse asks the client what he believes the change is associated with and how long he has noticed it.

4. *Client's description of normal characteristics of his stool.* The nurse determines if the client's stool is normally watery or formed, soft or hard, and the typical color. The client also describes a normal stool's shape.
5. *Diet history.* It is helpful to identify the client's normal dietary preferences for a day. The nurse asks the client to give examples of foods typically eaten for each daily meal. It is especially significant to determine if mealtime is usually irregular or if a given meal is infrequent.
6. *Description of daily fluid intake.* This includes the type and amount of fluid. The client may have to estimate the amount using common household measurements.
7. *History of exercise.* The nurse asks the client to describe the type and amount of exercise performed daily. Simply asking the client if he exercises is a poorly designed question because it leaves the judgment solely to the client. For example, a client who walks back and forth in his office may perceive this as adequate exercise. Therefore, the nurse should ask for a specific description of exercise patterns.
8. *Assessment of the use of artificial aids at home.* The nurse should determine if the client requires the use of enemas, laxatives, or special foods before having a bowel movement. If so, the nurse asks how often the client uses an artificial aid.
9. *History of surgery or illnesses affecting the gastrointestinal tract.* This information can often help explain the client's symptoms. In addition, it provides the nurse with an idea of the potential for maintaining or restoring a normal elimination pattern.
10. *Presence of artificial orifices.* If the client has a colostomy or ileostomy, the nurse should ask the client to describe the methods used to maintain the ostomy's normal function.
11. *Medication history.* It is essential to know if the client is taking any medications (such as laxatives, antacids, iron supplements, and analgesics) that might alter defecation or fecal characteristics.
12. *Emotional state.* The client's emotions can significantly alter the frequency of defecation. During assessment, observation of the client's affect, tone of voice, and mannerisms can reveal significant behaviors indicating emotional stress.

Physical Assessment of Gastrointestinal Function

The nurse determines the status of gastrointestinal function through physical assessment of the abdomen and rectum. Chapter 29 describes in detail the techniques for assessing the abdomen and rectum.

ABDOMINAL ASSESSMENT

The nurse describes all findings in relation to the abdominal landmarks. Dividing the abdomen into quadrants or nine equal sections permits a more systematic review of findings.

The nurse should inspect the contour, shape, symmetry, and skin color of the abdomen. Inspection should also include observation of masses, scars, venous patterns, artificial orifices, or lesions. While viewing the abdomen's shape, the nurse looks for distention or protuberance. Intestinal gas, tumors, or fluid in the abdominal cavity may cause distention. Inspecting the abdomen of an obese client is often difficult because what appears to be a distended abdomen may actually be simply an excess of fatty tissue. A distended abdomen feels tight and the skin appears taut as if stretched. The client with distention will describe a feeling of fullness.

Daily measurement of the abdomen's girth will reveal whether distention is increasing. The nurse measures girth or circumference by placing a tape measure around the client's abdomen at the level of the umbilicus. It is important to measure the girth at the same point each time.

The nurse should perform auscultation of the abdomen next because if palpation comes first the frequency of bowel sounds may be changed. The nurse should use the diaphragm of the stethoscope to assess bowel sounds in each of the quadrants or sections. While auscultating, the nurse should note the character and frequency of bowel sounds. Normally air and fluid move through the intestines, creating soft gurgling or bubbling sounds. Bowel sounds do not occur regularly; normally 5 to 20 seconds is needed to hear the first sound. Loud growling sounds or borborygmi indicate increased gastric motility. The nurse records bowel sounds as normal or audible, absent, hyperactive, or hypoactive. If a client has a gastrointestinal drainage tube connected to suction, the suction should be turned off during auscultation to allow the nurse to hear bowel sounds clearly.

During palpation and percussion of the abdomen, it is important for the client to relax. Tensing of abdominal muscles interferes with the nurse's ability to palpate underlying organs or masses. Conversing with a client often creates a distraction that helps the client relax. The nurse should palpate with a light, gentle touch. Palpation of a tender or sensitive area elicits a guarding or voluntary tightening of abdominal muscles. If the nurse locates an unusual mass, deep palpation may be necessary for further examination. However, the nurse should not apply deep palpation unless trained thoroughly in the skill.

Percussion allows the nurse to detect the presence of lesions, fluid, or gas within the abdomen. Familiarity with the five percussion notes (see Chapter 29) also permits a clear identification of underlying abdominal structures. The presence of gas or flatulence will create a tympanic note. Masses, tumors, and fluid are dull to percussion.

RECTAL ASSESSMENT

The nurse should first inspect the area surrounding the anus for the presence of lesions, discolorations, inflammation, and hemorrhoids. Any abnormalities should be carefully recorded. To examine the rectum the nurse must use gentle palpation. After donning a clean disposable glove, the nurse lubricates the index finger with petrolatum jelly. The nurse then asks the client to bear down and, as the client does so, the nurse passes the index finger through the relaxed anal sphincter toward the client's umbilicus. The sphincter usually constricts around the nurse's finger. The nurse should methodically palpate all sides of the rectal wall for nodules or irregularities in texture. The rectal mucosa is normally smooth and soft. Pushing the index finger forcefully against the rectal wall or extending the finger too far may cause discomfort for the client. Vigorous stimulation should be avoided to prevent triggering a vagal nerve reflex that can lower the client's heart rate.

The findings of an abdominal assessment may give clues as to the nature of gastrointestinal alterations. For example, abdominal distention coupled with auscultation of hyperactive bowel sounds suggests gaseous formation, presence of obstruction, or inflammation of the bowel. The nurse's assessment will then focus on other factors or conditions to help clarify the nature of the client's problem.

FECAL CHARACTERISTICS

Further assessment of a client's elimination status is made through inspection of fecal characteristics. Table 40-4 lists the essential characteristics to look for in normal feces. A number of factors can influence each characteristic. The key for the nurse to remember in reviewing characteristics is whether there have been recent changes. The client will likely be the most knowledgeable about whether changes have occurred. The nurse should consider any change significant and report it in the nursing history.

The normal brown color of feces is produced by the presence of bile pigments. In the infant the yellow

TABLE 40-4

Fecal Characteristics

Characteristic	Normal	Abnormal	Cause
Color	Infant: yellow; adult: brown	White or clay	Absence of bile
		Black or tarry	Iron ingestion or upper gastrointestinal (GI) bleeding
		Red	Lower GI bleeding
		Pale with fat	Malabsorption of fat
Odor	Pungent; affected by food type	Noxious change	Blood in feces or infection
Consistency	Soft, formed	Liquid	Diarrhea, reduced absorption
		Hard	Constipation
Frequency	Varies: infant four to six times daily (breast fed) or one to three times daily (bottle fed); adult daily or two to three times a week	Infant more than six times daily or less than once every 1 to 2 days; adult more than three times a day or less than once a week	Hypomotility or hypermotility
Amount	150 g per day		
Shape	Resembles diameter of rectum	Narrow, pencil-shaped	Obstruction, rapid peristalsis
Constituents	Undigested food, dead bacteria, fat, bile pigment, cells lining intestinal mucosa, water	Blood, pus, foreign bodies, mucus, worms	Internal bleeding, infection, swallowed objects, irritation, inflammation

color is caused by the rapid rate of peristalsis. As the child's intestinal motility slows, the stool takes on characteristics of the adult's feces. Lack of bile production or any obstruction to its flow results in a white or clay-colored stool, which is typical of the client with biliary tract obstruction caused by the formation of stones. Black stools may indicate two conditions: the continued ingestion of iron supplements or the presence of upper gastrointestinal bleeding as with a slow bleeding gastric ulcer. Bleeding can be singled out if, in addition to the black color, the stool has a tarlike or sticky consistency. Melena is blood in the feces. Bright red blood in the stool indicates lower gastrointestinal tract bleeding. This may simply be the result of hemorrhoids, but it could also indicate a more serious problem such as gastrointestinal hemorrhage. Any bright red bleeding should be reported to the physician immediately if the nurse fails to find the presence of hemorrhoids. In malabsorption syndromes the undigested fat mixes with the feces, resulting in a pale-colored stool.

Normally the stool is soft and consistent in form. The quality and quantity of a client's fluid and diet intake will directly affect the stool consistency. The

speed of peristalsis also determines if stool has a high liquid content or if it is well formed.

Feces possess a strong pungent odor with which most people obviously are familiar. Various foods can create changes in odor that may be noticed only by the client. However, the experienced nurse is familiar with changes resulting from the presence of blood or infection in the intestinal tract.

The frequency of bowel movements is highly individualized and depends on the client's age, diet, and personal habits and the presence of gastrointestinal abnormalities. For these reasons the nurse must determine the client's normal elimination pattern. Although two or three times a week is normal for some adults, the client who is accustomed to daily bowel movements will be anxious if infrequent bowel movements develop. More than three stools a day in an adult suggests an abnormal increase in motility. The infant is especially susceptible to dehydration if frequent watery stools develop.

The amount of fecal material passed is difficult to measure. The nurse's only means of measurement is by observing the stool. Usually the client is the best source of information. If the client notices an increase or decrease in the amount of stool, this should be reported to the nurse.

The shape of a normal stool is equivalent to the diameter of the client's rectum. This characteristic is again best measured by the client. However, the nurse should be alert to any narrowing of stool size. Feces that are forced past an internal obstruction in the sigmoid colon or rectum may be expelled in a thin, pencil-shaped form. Rapid intestinal motility may also cause pencil-shaped stool.

The presence of any unusual fecal constituents should also be recorded. Any foreign objects swallowed should normally be passed in the stool. Worms may be visible to the unassisted eye. Although intestinal worms are more commonly found in other parts of the world, they are not uncommon in North America. Inflammatory and infectious conditions of the bowel can cause evacuation of pus and mucus.

Laboratory and Diagnostic Tests

Laboratory and diagnostic examinations yield useful information concerning the nature of elimination problems. Laboratory analysis of fecal contents can detect the presence of pathological conditions such as tumors, hemorrhage, and infection. Diagnostic studies allow the physician to visualize all segments of the gastrointestinal tract. Certain diagnostic tests such as endoscopy permit direct visualization of structures. Tests such as the barium enema or an upper gastrointestinal (UGI) series require ingestion of a contrast medium that outlines structures on x-ray examination.

FECAL SPECIMENS

The nurse is directly responsible for ensuring that all specimens are accurately obtained, properly labeled in appropriate containers, and transported to the laboratory on time. Institutions provide special containers for fecal specimens. Certain tests require that the specimens be placed in chemical preservatives. To ensure that the correct container is used, the nurse refers to the institution's policy and procedures or the laboratory manual.

Medical aseptic technique should be implemented during the collection of any stool specimen (see Chapter 33). Certain bacteria can easily be acquired by a person who handles a specimen improperly. Handwashing is necessary for anyone who might come in contact with the specimen. Often the client is capable of obtaining the specimen if properly instructed. Explain to the client that feces cannot be mixed with urine or water. For this reason the client must defecate into a clean, dry bedpan or special container that can be placed under the toilet seat. After defecation, the

toilet paper is discarded into the toilet or a disposable bag.

Tests for occult (microscopic) presence of blood in the stool and stool cultures require only a small sample of fecal material. The nurse collects approximately an inch of formed stool or 15 to 30 ml of liquid diarrheal stool. To avoid contact with feces while transferring solid specimens to a container, the nurse should use a wooden tongue depressor. The nurse must pour the liquid specimens carefully into the proper container. Tests for measuring the output of fecal fat require a 3- to 5-day collection of stool. In such a test all fecal material must be saved throughout the test period.

After obtaining a specimen the nurse should tightly seal the container and complete the appropriate laboratory requisition forms. The nurse then records all specimen collections in the client's medical record. It is important to avoid any delays in sending specimens to the laboratory. Some tests require the stool to be warm, and thus it must be delivered immediately. When stool specimens are allowed to stand at room temperature, bacteriological changes that alter test results can occur.

GUAIAC TEST.
A common fecal laboratory test that the nurse performs is the guaiac test. It measures the presence of microscopic amounts of blood in the feces. Normally individuals lose small amounts of blood daily in the feces from minor abrasions of the nasopharyngeal and oral surfaces. Quantities of blood greater than 50 ml arising from the upper gastrointestinal tract can be seen as melena. Guaiac tests help to reveal the presence of blood undetectable by visual examination.

Clients who are receiving anticoagulants or have a bleeding disorder or a gastrointestinal disorder known to cause bleeding should be guaiac tested. Intestinal tumors, inflammation of the bowel, and ulcerations are examples of alterations that may cause gastrointestinal bleeding. The most common guaiac tests are the Hemoccult slides and the Hematest tablets. Both are easy to perform (Procedure 40-1).

DIAGNOSTIC EXAMINATIONS

A client may have a diagnostic examination on an outpatient or inpatient basis. Hospitals and clinics have facilities that enable the client to come for examinations without being hospitalized. Visualization of gastrointestinal structures may be by a direct or an indirect approach.

The nursing implications for gastrointestinal diagnostic examinations involve the following:
1. Explanation of the procedure
2. Restriction of dietary intake as ordered

PROCEDURE 40-1

Measuring Occult Blood

HEMOCCULT TEST

EQUIPMENT:

1. Cardboard Hemoccult slide
2. Wooden applicator
3. Hemoccult developing solution
4. Disposable gloves

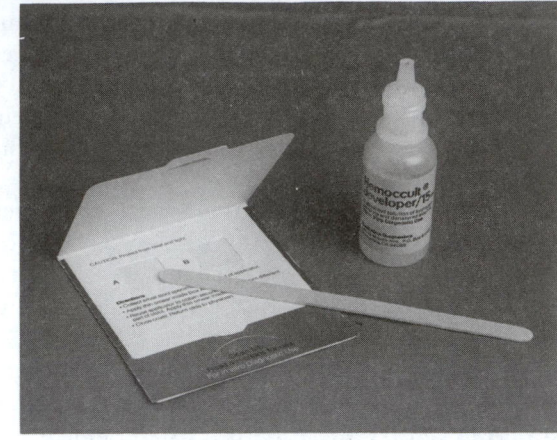

STEPS	RATIONALE
1. Explain the procedure to the client.	The client's understanding of the test's purpose facilitates cooperation with the procedure and relieves anxiety.
2. Instruct the client to defecate in a clean dry bedpan or collecting device attached to the toilet. Warn the client against combining urine with stool.	Contents of the urine may contaminate the fecal specimen.
3. Don clean disposable gloves.	Gloving reduces transmission of microorganisms from the fecal specimen to the nurse's hands.
4. With the tip of the wooden applicator obtain a small portion of feces.	A small specimen is sufficient for measuring blood content.
5. Smear the specimen thinly inside the first box of the cardboard slide.	The paper inside the box is guaiac paper, sensitive to fecal blood content. A thick accumulation of specimen is not necessary for guaiac measurement.
6. Obtain a second specimen from a different portion of the stool and apply it thinly to the slide's second box.	Findings of occult blood are more conclusive for gastrointestinal bleeding when the entire specimen is found to contain blood.
7. Close the slide cover and turn the slide over to the reverse side. Open the cardboard flap and apply 2 drops of Hemoccult developing solution on the guaiac paper.	The developing solution penetrates the underlying fecal specimen. The presence of blood is indicated by a change in color of the guaiac paper.
8. Read the results of the test after 30 to 60 seconds.	A bluish discoloration indicates presence of occult blood in the stool (guaiac positive). If there is no change in the guaiac paper's color, the test is negative for blood (guaiac negative).
9. Dispose of the test slide in a proper receptacle. Remove gloves by pulling them inside out. Wash hands thoroughly.	Aseptic practices prevent transmission of microorganisms.
10. Record results of the test in the client's record.	All specimen test results are documented in the client's chart.

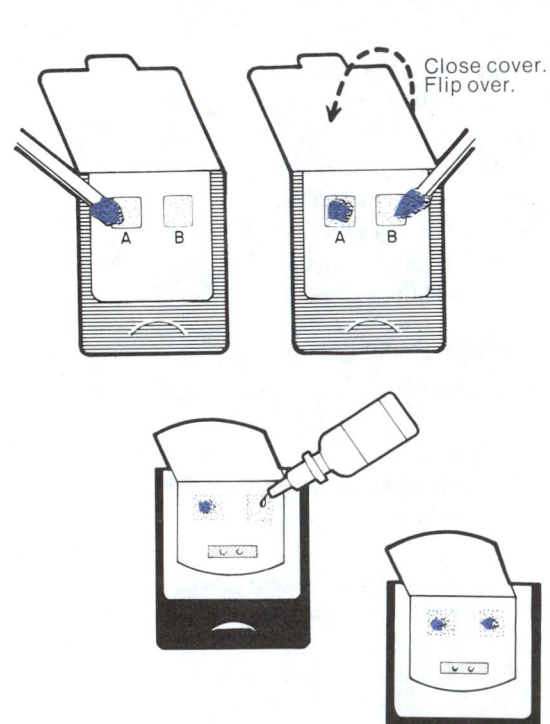

Close cover. Flip over.

HEMATEST TABLETS

EQUIPMENT:
1. Hematest tablets
2. Guaiac paper
3. Sink with running water
4. Wooden applicator
5. Disposable gloves

STEPS	RATIONALE
1. Follow steps 1 through 4 of the Hemoccult procedure.	
2. Place a small amount of fecal specimen on the guaiac paper.	Guaiac paper is sensitive in detecting fecal blood content.
3. Place a Hematest tablet on top of the stool specimen.	The tablet contains a solid form of developing solution.
4. Apply 2 to 3 drops of tap water on the tablet, allowing the water to flow onto the guaiac paper.	Tap water dissolves the Hematest tablet and thus dispenses the developing solution over the specimen and guaiac paper.
5. Observe the color of the guaiac paper.	Bluish discoloration is guaiac positive. No color change is guaiac negative.
6. Follow steps 9 and 10 of the Hemoccult test.	

3. Administration of bowel preparation
4. Administration of pretest medications
5. Positioning of the client
6. Providing support to the client during the procedure
7. Observation for postprocedural complications

DIRECT VISUALIZATION. Special instruments introduced either through the mouth (upper gastrointestinal viewing) or the rectum (lower gastrointestinal viewing) allow the physician to inspect the integrity of mucosa, blood vessels, and specific organ parts. A fiberoptic endoscope is an optical instrument consisting of a lens viewer, a long flexible tube, and a light source at the end. The tube looks much like a catheter with several hollow internal channels that allow the physician to view structures at the tip of the tube and to insert special instruments for biopsy of tissues. The tube is flexible to minimize trauma and discomfort to the client as it is introduced through a body orifice.

Proctoscopes and sigmoidoscopes are rigid tube-shaped instruments with an attached light source. The proctoscope looks much like a speculum with a light. These instruments are less flexible than fiberoptic scopes and more capable of causing the client discomfort. The physician uses a proctoscope to visualize the rectum and distal colon and a sigmoidoscope to visualize the sigmoid colon.

The client about to undergo any of these procedures is generally highly anxious unless the nurse explains the procedure thoroughly. It is embarrassing and distressing to have a tube inserted into the rectum or through the mouth. The client remains awake during the procedures, although the physician usually orders a sedative to be given. Unless the client cooperates fully, it is impossible to insert the instruments safely and effectively. The nurse should explain the purpose of each test and warn the client of any sensations that might be felt as the instruments are inserted (Table 40-5). The nurse should allow the client to express any fears and ask questions before the test.

Starting at midnight the day before most gastrointestinal examinations, the client refrains from eating or drinking. The absence of contents in the stomach or duodenum prevents the chance of the client vomiting during the procedure. The physician may allow the client to have a light liquid breakfast before examination of rectal or colonic structures. The client usually receives enemas and laxatives on the evening

TABLE 40-5

Diagnostic Examinations of Gastrointestinal Structures

Test Name	Purpose	Before Test	Nursing Implications during Test	After Test
Upper gastrointestinal (GI) endoscopy or gastroscopy	This test allows visualization of esophagus, stomach, and duodenum. The physician inspects for tumors, vascular changes, mucosal inflammation, ulcers, hernias, and obstructions. A gastroscope enables the physician to remove tissue specimens for biopsy, remove abnormal tissue growth (polyps), and coagulate sources of bleeding	1. The client signs an informed consent for the procedure. 2. The client takes nothing by mouth after midnight the night before the test. 3. Remove the client's dentures. 4. Explain that the client may feel fullness in the throat and sense of gagging during the test. 5. Explain that the client will be unable to speak as the endoscope enters the esophagus. 6. Position the client in left Sims' or left lateral position. 7. Administer sedative and anticholinergic.	1. Describe steps of procedure to client. 2. Place tissue specimens in a properly labeled container that is sealed tightly. 3. Have emergency equipment available in case of respiratory complications.	1. Since client's throat is anesthetized, the nurse instructs the client to avoid eating or drinking until the gag reflex returns (2-4 hours). 2. Explain that hoarseness and the sensation of a sore throat are normal for several days. Cool fluids and gargling relieve soreness. 3. Observe for bleeding, fever, abdominal pain, difficulty swallowing, and difficulty breathing.
Sigmoidoscopy	This test allows visualization of anus, rectum, and sigmoid colon.	1. The client signs an informed consent for procedure. 2. The client receives an enema the night before and morning of procedure. 3. Laxatives are optional. 4. Light breakfast may be allowed. 5. Explain that the client will feel discomfort and the urge to defecate as the instruments are inserted. 6. During the examination the physician uses air to distend the bowel for better visualization. Explain that the client will feel "gas pains."	1. Keep the client draped and observe for any respiratory distress (especially in clients with lung disease who cannot tolerate a head-down position). 2. Provide the physician with long cotton swabs for removing mucus. 3. Place tissue specimens in a properly labeled container and seal tightly.	1. Observe for rectal bleeding, rectal or abdominal pain, and fever. 2. Caution the client to observe for any blood in stools and to report bleeding to a physician.
Proctoscopy	This test allows visualization of anus and rectum. Both examinations enable physician to collect tissue specimens and coagulate sources of bleeding.			

T A B L E 40 - 5 , cont'd

Diagnostic Examinations of Gastrointestinal Structures

Test Name	Purpose	Before Test	Nursing Implications during Test	After Test
		7. Position the client in a knee-chest position face down. Sims' position on left side is acceptable. 8. Drape the client to avoid unnecessary exposure and minimize embarrassment.		
Upper gastrointestinal study (UGI)	X-ray study of ingested contrast medium allows the physician to visualize lower esophagus, stomach, and duodenum. The physician notes the presence of ulcerations, inflammation, and tumors and anatomical malposition of the organs. The patency of organs and the pyloric valve are also observed.	1. The client signs informed consent. 2. The client takes nothing by mouth after midnight the night before. 3. Explain that the test may take several hours and requires frequent position changes. Explain that discomfort is minimal except for lying on a hard examination table. 5. Explain that barium has a chalky taste. (Some preparations contain artificial flavoring.)	1. The test is performed in the radiology department. A technician explains steps of the procedure.	1. The client may resume eating after the examination is completed. 2. It is important for the client to expel the barium to avoid bowel impaction. Instruct the client to increase fluid intake (at least 2 liters of fluid after the examination). The physician may order mild laxative or enema. Stools are light in color until barium is expelled.
Small bowel follow-through (continuation of UGI)	This allows physician to examine the small intestine. Flow of barium through the intestine may suggest motility problems.			
Barium enema	This allows indirect visualization of the colon to reveal the presence and location of tumors, polyps, and diverticula. The physician also can detect positional abnormalities.	1. The client signs informed consent. 2. Bowel preparation varies among physicians. The client may receive any combination of the following the evening before the examination: a. Clear liquids for lunch and supper	1. Client expels barium after first set of x-ray films (30 minutes). A repeat film is then taken to check for barium retention.	1. The client may resume eating after the examination is completed. 2. Instruct the client to increase intake of oral fluids to promote barium evacuation and to counteract dehydrating effects of cathartics.

Continued.

TABLE 40-5, cont'd

Diagnostic Examinations of Gastrointestinal Structures

Test Name	Purpose	Before Test	Nursing Implications during Test	After Test
Barium enema, cont'd		b. One glass of water 8 to 10 hours before the study c. Stimulant cathartics d. An enema 3. On the day of examination the client receives additional cathartic by suppository. 4. Explain to the client the purpose of extensive bowel preparation. 5. Explain to the client that a lengthy procedure may cause fatigue. 6. Observe results of all enemas and cathartics to ensure that the bowel is empty before the study. 7. Explain that the client may feel cramping and fullness once the barium is instilled. 8. Explain that the client will be instructed to change positions frequently: supine, prone, and side lying.		3. Instruct the client to observe stools for presence of barium. The physician may order a mild cathartic. 4. Offer the hospitalized client a warm bath for comfort.

and morning before lower gastrointestinal examinations. It is important for the large intestine and rectum to be empty for the physician to visualize structures clearly.

Before the examination the client usually receives a sedative such as diazepam (Valium). For upper gastrointestinal visualization the client also receives an anticholinergic medication such as atropine to reduce oral secretions. Before inserting a fiberoptic endoscope through the mouth, the physician applies a local anesthetic spray to the posterior pharynx to minimize discomfort and the client's gag reflex.

Examinations are conducted in special endoscopy rooms or in treatment rooms in the nursing divisions. The nurse assists the client to take a position on the examination table that facilitates passage of the instruments (Table 40-5). Clients weakened by illness may require extra pillows to help maintain the proper position. The nurse should drape the client to minimize any embarrassment. Throughout the procedure the nurse and physician explain the steps taken (for example, passage of the instrument, suctioning of collected fluid, or biopsy of tissue). After the examination is completed, the nurse assists the client to a comfortable position and transports him either to his room or to a holding area for observation. The nurse observes the client for signs of complications such as pain, bleeding, and difficulty swallowing or breathing. These signs are indicative of trauma or perforation of some portion of the gastrointestinal tract by the examination instrument. If the client is discharged, the nurse instructs him to report any signs of complications.

INDIRECT VISUALIZATION. When direct visualization is impossible (as with deeper gastrointestinal structures), the physician relies on indirect x-ray examination. The client either ingests a contrast medium or has the medium administered in the form of an enema. One of the most common media is barium, a white, chalky, radiopaque substance that the client drinks like a milkshake. It is used in upper gastrointestinal (UGI) studies and barium enemas. Contrast media usually contain a flavoring agent for better palatability.

For any x-ray contrast examination of the gastrointestinal tract, the client is instructed not to eat or drink after midnight the night before the examination. Food and fluid in the gastrointestinal tract will prevent contrast media from accurately outlining gastrointestinal structures. What may look like a tumor could be a mass of undigested food. For studies such as a barium enema, the client requires bowel preparation with cathartics and enemas.

The nurse explains what happens during the procedure. The clients may experience unusual sensations during the examination (such as the chalky taste of barium or abdominal cramping and gas pains during a barium enema). The procedures are relatively painless but can be time consuming. The nurse explains that several x-ray films are taken to visualize structures as the contrast medium moves through the gastrointestinal tract. The client assumes several positions to promote barium flow by gravity. During barium enemas a difficult task for the client is retaining the volume of barium (500 to 1500 ml) until all x-ray films are taken.

The client does not receive a sedative before x-ray studies. A radiologist and a technician are available to explain the procedure to the client. After completion of the examination the nurse's primary concern is that the client expels all of the barium. Retained barium absorbs fecal water and causes a hardened intestinal impaction. The client should drink large amounts (1 to 2 liters) of fluids and the nurse observes the color of stools. Barium creates a light or white stool color. If the client is unable to expel all of the barium, a mild cathartic or enema may be necessary.

Nursing Diagnosis

The nurse's assessment of the client's bowel function reveals data that may indicate an actual or potential elimination problem or a problem resulting from elimination alterations (Table 40-6). The contributing factors enable the nurse to select interventions directed at the specific cause of the elimination problem. For example, the nurse's interventions for altered elimination related to constipation will be different than those aimed at the contributing factor of diarrhea. Associated problems such as body image changes or skin breakdown require interventions unrelated to the impairment of bowel function. However, in some instances the nurse must direct as much attention to the elimination problem as to the associated problem. For example, the nurse can use meticulous skin care and apply ointments to reduce the skin's exposure to fecal irritants. However, unless the client's diarrhea is resolved, the nurse's efforts at preventing skin breakdown may fail.

The nurse's ability to identify the correct diagnosis depends not only on the thoroughness of assessment but also on recognition of factors that can impair

TABLE 40-6

Examples of Nursing Diagnoses Related to Bowel Elimination Problems

Problem	Causes
Alterations in elimination	Related to: Constipation Impaction Diarrhea Incontinence Flatulence
Alterations in defecation	Related to: Rectal pain Incontinence Immobility
Body image alterations	Related to: Ostomy Fecal incontinence Diarrhea
Potential or actual skin breakdown	Related to exposure to liquid feces
Insufficient nutritional intake	Related to loss of appetite from flatulence or impaction
Fluid and electrolyte imbalance	Related to diarrhea

elimination. It is the nurse's responsibility to determine the client's risk and institute measures to ensure maintenance of normal bowel function.

Planning

One of the nurse's primary goals is to help the client maintain or regain a normal elimination pattern. Education is important so clients can understand their own normal elimination patterns and the relatively easy ways of promoting normal elimination. The nurse's plan should include frequent discussion periods to help family members and clients understand the factors that influence elimination.

Each person's defecation pattern is unique. Foods or activities that cause constipation in one person may cause diarrhea in another. For this reason the nurse and client must collaborate closely to plan interventions that will likely be effective. For example, if a client is to be hospitalized for several days, the dietary department can provide the client with a daily serving of prunes. If the client's illness restricts dietary intake, it is the nurse's responsibility to identify alternative measures for preventing elimination problems. Likewise, the client at home may not be able to afford the high-fiber foods most effective in producing soft-formed stools. The nurse must consider the client's needs in the plan of care and use the client's food preferences in recommending less expensive high-fiber foods.

In an effort to promote normal bowel elimination the nurse's plan should focus on the following:
1. The client's understanding of normal elimination
2. Proper fluid and food intake
3. Regular exercise
4. Regular bowel habits
5. Normal defecation
6. Comfort
7. Skin integrity
8. Positive body image

Implementation

The success of the nurse's interventions depends on improving the client's and family members' understanding of bowel elimination. The client or a family member can easily acquire the knowledge needed to prevent elimination problems. In the home, hospital, or long-term care facility, clients capable of learning can be taught effective bowel habits. The more the client understands about normal elimination, the more able he is to inform the nurse about the nature of any problems.

The nurse should teach the client and family about proper foods in the diet, adequate fluid intake, and the type of fluids that stimulate or slow peristalsis. The client also needs to learn the importance of establishing regular bowel routines, maintaining regular exercise, and taking appropriate measures when elimination problems develop. When complications develop from elimination problems, the nurse can teach the client and family members how to give proper skin care, administer enemas, and monitor the effects of medications.

Maintenance of Proper Fluid and Food Intake

In choosing the proper diet for promoting normal elimination, the nurse should consider the frequency of defecation, characteristics of feces, and types of foods that either impair or promote defecation in the client. The client with frequent constipation or impaction requires an increased intake of high-fiber foods and more fluids such as fruit juices and warm liquids. However, the client should realize that diet therapy provides only long-term relief of elimination problems and may not give immediate relief from problems such as constipation.

When diarrhea is a problem, the nurse can recommend foods of low fiber content and discourage the intake of foods that typically cause gastric upset or abdominal cramping. The client with diarrhea is susceptible to potassium loss from the excessive loss of gastrointestinal contents. However, although foods such as fruit and vegetables are high in potassium, they also have high fiber content that can worsen diarrhea. Less irritating foods with high potassium content include baked chicken, seafood, pork, veal, molasses, and evaporated and dry nonfat instant milk. Potassium supplements may be ordered by the physician, but they are extremely irritating to gastric mucosa.

Illnesses causing diarrhea can be debilitating. If the client is unable to tolerate foods or liquids orally, intravenous therapy will be necessary. Potassium supplements are usually added to intravenous fluids. The client returns to a normal diet slowly, often beginning with a diet consisting only of fluids. Excessively hot or cold fluids stimulate peristalsis, causing abdominal cramping and further diarrhea. As the client's tolerance to liquids improves, the physician orders the addition of solid foods to the diet.

Clients with colostomies usually benefit from low-fiber diets that reduce the amount of feces evacuated. If the client remains on a low-fiber diet, vitamin supplements may be necessary. The following are common low-fiber foods:

1. Coffee in small amounts, tea
2. Enriched bread, plain rolls
3. Noodles, rice, puffed rice, rice flakes
4. Cottage cheese, cream cheese
5. Plain cake, ice cream, pudding
6. Eggs cooked any way except fried
7. Strained fruit juices
8. Tender lean meats, fish, poultry
9. Butter, margarine

The nurse should warn ostomates against eating high-fiber foods such as corn-on-the-cob, popcorn, celery, or nuts, all of which may accumulate and block passage to the stoma.

Clients with flatulence or ostomies that emit foul odors should avoid eating gas-forming foods. In addition to beans, cabbage, onions, and cauliflower, beer is a common cause of intestinal gas production. The client should become familiar with the foods that cause gaseous distention for him.

Promotion of Regular Exercise

A daily exercise program often helps prevent elimination problems. The exercise need not be strenuous. Walking, riding a stationary bicycle, or taking a relaxing swim is enough to stimulate normal peristalsis. Clients who are sedentary at work, such as typists, keypunch operators, computer technicians, and secretaries, are most in need of regular exercise routines.

For a client temporarily immobilized by illness or surgery, the nurse should attempt to begin ambulation as soon as possible. If the client's condition permits, the nurse will assist a postoperative client to walk to a chair on the evening of the day of surgery. The postsurgical client should walk farther each day.

Some clients have difficulty passing stool because of a weakening of abdominal and pelvic floor muscles. The nurse may instruct the client to practice simple exercises:

1. While lying supine, tighten the abdominal muscles as though you were pushing them to the floor. Hold the muscles tight to a count of three and then relax. Repeat the exercise five to 10 times as tolerated.
2. Flex and contract the thigh muscles by raising the knees one at a time slowly toward the chest. Repeat the exercise for each leg at least five times and increase the frequency as tolerated.

These exercises are especially helpful for bedridden clients who are forced to use a bedpan.

Promotion of Regular Bowel Habits

One of the most important habits a nurse can teach a client regarding bowel habits is to take time for defecation. Ignoring the urge to defecate and not tak-ing time to defecate completely are common causes of constipation. To establish regular bowel habits, a client must know when the urge to defecate normally occurs. Ignoring the urge or rushing will prevent the client from determining this.

The nurse advises the client to begin establishing a routine during a time when defecation is most likely to occur, usually an hour after meals. If a client attempts to defecate during the time when mass colonic peristalsis occurs, the chances of being successful are great. If a client is restricted to bed or requires assistance in ambulating, the nurse should offer a bedpan or help the client reach the bathroom when the urge to defecate develops. The nurse must be prompt in assisting the client before the urge disappears.

Many clients have already established rituals for defecation. In a hospital or long-term care facility, the nurse should make certain that treatment routines do not interfere with the client's schedule. It is also important to provide privacy during defecation. When a client forced to use a bedpan shares a room with another person, the nurse should curtain off the client's area so the client can relax, knowing that interruptions will not occur. Bathroom doors should be closed, although the nurse may stand close by in case the client needs assistance.

Promotion of Normal Defecation

Although good dietary habits and regular exercise are the major ways of promoting normal defecation, there are other specific interventions that stimulate the defecation reflex, affect the character of fecal contents to produce normal stools, or enhance intestinal peristalsis. The goal of all these interventions is to help the client evacuate bowel contents normally without discomfort. Interventions designed to promote normal defecation include assisting the client to defecate in a squatting position, positioning the client properly on a bedpan, administering cathartics and antidiarrheal agents, and giving enemas.

SQUATTING POSITION

The nurse may need to assist clients who have difficulty squatting because of muscular weakness and mobility problems. Regular toilets are too low for clients unable to lower themselves to a squatting position because of orthopedic repair of hip and knee joints, arthritis, degenerative joint disease, or diseases causing muscular wasting of thigh muscles. The nurse can advise clients to purchase special elevated toilet seats for the home. With such a seat the client uses less effort to sit or stand. In orthopedic and rehabilitation units in a health care center, toilet seats are elevated.

POSITIONING ON BEDPAN

A client restricted to bed must use a bedpan for defecation. Women use bedpans to pass both urine and feces, while men use bedpans only for defecation. Sitting on a bedpan can be extremely uncomfortable. The nurse should help the client assume a position similar to the natural squatting position.

Two types of bedpans are available (Fig. 40-5). The regular bedpan, made of metal or hard plastic, has a curved smooth upper end and a sharp-edged lower end. The pan is approximately 5 cm (2 inches) deep. A fracture pan, designed for clients with body or leg casts, has a shallow upper end approximately 1.3 cm (½ inch) deep that slips easily under a client. The upper end of either pan fits under the client's buttocks toward the sacrum, with the lower end just under the upper thighs. The nurse must be sure the pan is placed high enough so feces enter the pan. A metal bedpan is very cold and should be warmed before the client is positioned. The nurse places the pan under warm running water for a few seconds and quickly dries it. The warmth helps the client relax the anal sphincter.

The most important element for the nurse to consider in positioning the client is preventing muscle strain and discomfort. A client should never be placed on a bedpan with the bed flat unless activity restrictions demand it. If the bed is flat, the client will be forced to hyperextend the back to lift the hips onto the pan. Raising the client to a 90-degree angle can also make positioning difficult. In a sitting position the client must rise straight up, using the strength of the arms as the pan is positioned. Most clients are too weak to accomplish this maneuver, and clients who have had abdominal surgery are hesitant to exert strain on suture lines. Furthermore, the nurse is unable to lift the client in such a position without risk of injury.

Fig. 40-6 demonstrates proper and improper techniques for positioning clients on bedpans. The best method is to be sure the client is positioned high in the bed. The nurse raises the client's head approximately 30 degrees. This position prevents hyperextension of the back and provides support to the upper torso as the client raises the hips by bending the knees and lifting the hips upward. The nurse places a hand under the client's sacrum to help in lifting, while slipping the pan under the client. It is not necessary to expose the client's body while placing the bedpan. The bedsheet is lifted just enough to slip the pan under the client. Clients who have overhead trapeze frames connected to their beds can easily lift themselves by grasping the trapeze bar.

If the client is unable to lift the hips or if the nurse judges it is unsafe to allow the client to exert such effort, the client can roll onto the pan. The nurse lowers the head of the bed to a flat position and asks the client to roll over onto one side. The nurse places the bedpan firmly against the client's buttocks and down into the mattress. The client then rolls back onto the pan. After positioning the pan correctly, the nurse raises the client's head 30 degrees. A rolled towel or small pillow placed under the lumbar curve of the back provides comfort. A light application of powder on the back and buttocks prevents the client's skin from sticking to the pan. Raising the knee gatch of the bed or having the client bend the knees assists the client in assuming a squatting position. The knee gatch should never be raised if it is contraindicated (as in clients with vascular stasis, orthopedic repair

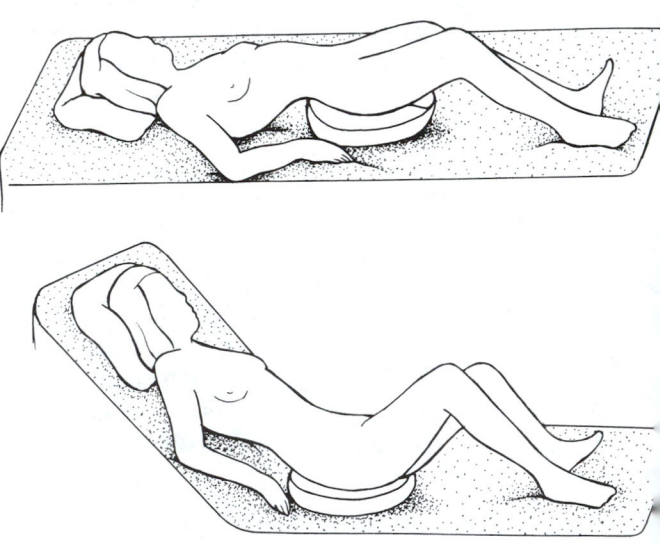

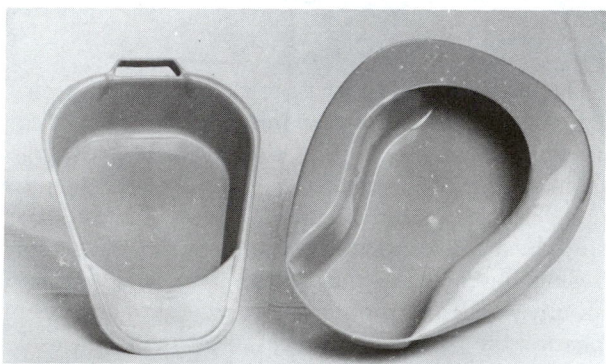

Fig. 40-5 Types of bedpans: fracture bedpan (on left) and regular bedpan.

Fig. 40-6 Positioning on a bedpan. *Top,* Improper technique for positioning client. *Bottom,* Proper technique, avoiding back strain.

of hips and knees, or vascular surgery involving the lower extremities).

The nurse should maintain the privacy of a client sitting on a bedpan. The call light and a supply of toilet paper should be within easy reach. When the client finishes, the nurse responds to the call signal immediately and removes the pan. The client may require the nurse's assistance with wiping. To remove the pan the nurse asks the client to roll off to the side or raise the hips. The nurse holds the pan steady to avoid spilling its contents. The nurse should avoid pulling or shoving the pan from under the client's hips, since this can pull the client's skin and cause tissue injury. The nurse should assist the client in cleansing the anal and perineal area after defecation and should offer the client a washcloth to wipe the hands. If an unpleasant odor remains in the room, the nurse can use a deodorizing spray.

The nurse should immediately empty the bedpan's contents either into the client's toilet or in a special receptacle in the utility room. A spray faucet attached to most toilets allows the nurse to rinse the client's bedpan thoroughly. The client uses the same bedpan each time.

It is important for the nurse to offer the bedpan frequently to a client. The client may accidentally soil bedclothes if forced to wait for a bedpan. Many clients try to avoid using a bedpan because it is embarrassing and uncomfortable. Such clients may attempt to get to the bathroom even though their conditions prohibit ambulation. The nurse must warn these clients about the risk of falls or accidents.

CATHARTICS AND LAXATIVES

Often a client is unable to defecate normally because of pain, constipation, or impaction. Cathartics and laxatives have the short-term action of promoting emptying of the bowel. They are also used in bowel evacuation for clients undergoing gastrointestinal examination and abdominal surgery. Although the terms "cathartic" and "laxative" are often used interchangeably, cathartics have a stronger effect on the intestines.

Cathartics and laxatives are available in oral and suppository dosage forms (see Chapter 32). Although the oral route is more commonly used, cathartics that come prepared as suppositories are more effective because of their stimulant effect on the rectal mucosa. Cathartic suppositories such as bisacodyl (Dulcolax) may act within 30 minutes. The nurse should administer the suppository shortly before the client's usual time to defecate or immediately after a meal.

The nurse teaches clients about the potential harmful effects of repeated use of laxatives. Laxatives are readily available in drugstores and groceries. The client should understand that laxatives and cathartics are not meant for long-term maintenance of bowel function.

Five types of cathartics are available: stimulant cathartics, saline (osmotic) agents, wetting (softening) agents, bulk-forming agents, and lubricants. The drug classes are based on the method by which the agent promotes defecation.

Stimulant cathartics cause local irritation to the intestinal mucosa and inhibit reabsorption of water in the large intestine. Intestinal irritation increases intestinal motility. The rapid movement of feces causes retention of water in the stool. The drugs can cause formation of a soft to fluid stool in 6 to 12 hours. Clients tend to abuse stimulants more than other cathartics. Overuse leads to loss of intestinal tone.

Commonly used stimulant cathartics include castor oil, cascara, phenolphthalein (Ex-Lax or Feen-A-Mint), and bisacodyl (Dulcolax). Nurses should warn mothers who breast feed that cascara is excreted in the milk. Phenolphthalein comes in a chewable gum or candy form and thus should be kept away from children, since it can be toxic in large doses.

Saline or osmotic agents contain a salt preparation that is not absorbed by the intestines. The cathartic exerts an osmotic effect, drawing water into the fecal mass. The osmotic action increases the bulk of the intestinal contents and enhances lubrication. Magnesium hydroxide (milk of magnesia) and sodium phosphate (Phospho-Soda) are examples of saline cathartics. Clients with impaired kidney function should avoid using these drugs because they cannot excrete the excess salt.

Wetting agents or stool softeners are detergents that lower the surface tension of feces, allowing penetration by water and fat. These drugs also inhibit absorption of water by the intestines. The fecal mass becomes large and soft. Commonly used wetting agents are dioctyl sodium sulfosuccinate (Colace) and dioctyl calcium sulfosuccinate (Surfak). A wetting agent is most effective when the goal is to prevent the client from straining during defecation.

Bulk-forming cathartics have the effect their name implies. The drugs consist of cellulose and polysaccharides that absorb water and increase solid intestinal bulk. The fecal bulk stretches the intestinal walls, stimulating peristalsis. Bulk laxatives are the least irritating and safest of all cathartics. When mixed with water, they can solidify if not swallowed quickly. Clients should be encouraged to take bulk cathartics with plenty of fluids to prevent hardening of the drug and intestinal obstruction. Bulk-forming laxatives can also relieve a mild watery diarrhea by absorbing water to produce a soft-formed stool. Common bulk-forming cathartics are methylcellulose (Hydrolose) and psyllium hydrocolloid (Metamucil).

Lubricants soften the fecal mass, thus easing the strain of defecation. Clients with painful hemorrhoids particularly benefit from a lubricant. The only lubricant laxative available is mineral oil. Regular use of mineral oil interferes with absorption of the fat-soluble vitamins A, D, E, and K. The drug can also cause a dangerous form of pneumonia if aspirated.

ANTIDIARRHEAL AGENTS

For clients with diarrhea the frequent passage of liquid stools becomes a problem. The most effective antidiarrheal agents are opiates such as codeine phosphate, paregoric, diphenoxylate (Lomotil), and bismuth subsalicylate (Pepto-Bismol). Antidiarrheal agents decrease intestinal muscle tone to slow the passage of feces. Opiates inhibit peristaltic waves that move feces forward, but they also increase the segmental contractions that mix intestinal contents. As a result more water is absorbed by the intestinal walls. Antidiarrheal agents should be used with caution, since opiates are habit forming. The effective antidiarrheal dose is lower than the dose that can cause analgesia or feelings of euphoria.

ENEMAS

An enema is the instillation of a solution into the rectum and sigmoid colon. The primary reason for enema administration is to promote defecation by stimulating peristalsis. The volume of fluid instilled breaks up the fecal mass, stretches the rectal wall, and initiates the defecation reflex. Enemas are also given as a vehicle for medications that exert a local effect on rectal mucosa.

The most common use for an enema is the temporary relief of constipation. Other indications include the following:

1. Removal of feces resulting from impaction
2. Emptying of the bowel in preparation for x-ray examination, endoscopic visualization, surgical procedure, or delivery of a baby
3. Evacuation of feces to institute a program for bowel training

Clients should be discouraged from relying on enemas to maintain bowel regularity. Enemas do not treat the cause of constipation. As with laxative abuse, frequent use of enemas destroys normal defecation reflexes. A client with recurrent constipation should consult a physician.

TYPES OF ENEMAS. There are several types of enemas. *Cleansing enemas* promote the complete evacuation of feces from the colon. They act by stimulating peristalsis through the infusion of a large

TABLE 40-7

Suggested Maximum Volumes for Saline and Tap Water Enemas

Age Group	Volume (ml)
Infant	150-250
Toddler	250-350
School-age child	300-500
Adolescent	500-750
Adult	750-1000

volume of solution (Table 40-7) or through local irritation of the colon's mucosa. Cleansing enemas include tap water, normal saline, hypertonic saline, and soapsuds solution. Each solution exerts a different osmotic effect (see Chapter 42), influencing the movement of fluids between the colon and interstitial spaces beyond the intestinal wall. Infants and children can tolerate only normal saline because of their predisposition to fluid imbalance.

Tap water is hypotonic and exerts a lower osmotic pressure than fluid in the interstitial spaces. After infusion into the colon, tap water escapes from the bowel lumen into the interstitial spaces. The net movement of water is low; the infused volume stimulates defecation before significant amounts of water leave the bowel. Tap water enemas should not be repeated because water toxicity or circulatory overload can develop if significant amounts of water are absorbed.

Physiological normal saline is the safest solution to use because it is isotonic; that is, it exerts the same osmotic pressure as fluids in the interstitial spaces surrounding the bowel. The volume of infused saline stimulates peristalsis. Administering saline enemas does not create the danger of excess fluid absorption. If prepared saline is not available at home, 500 ml (1 pint) of tap water mixed with 1 teaspoon of table salt is an appropriate substitute.

Hypertonic solutions infused into the bowel exert osmotic pressure that pulls fluids out of the interstitial spaces. The colon fills with fluid, and the resultant distention promotes defecation. Clients unable to tolerate large volumes of fluid benefit most from this type of enema. A hypertonic solution of 120 to 180 ml (4 to 6 ounces) is usually effective. The commercially prepared Fleet Enema is the most commonly used hypertonic enema.

Soapsuds may be added to tap water or saline to create the additional effect of intestinal irritation. Only pure castile soap is safe to use. Harsh soaps or

PROCEDURE 40-2

Administering an Enema

ADMINISTRATION VIA RECTAL TUBE WITH CONTAINER

EQUIPMENT:

1. Enema container
2. Ordered volume of solution warmed to 40.5° to 43° C (105° to 109° F) (with soap, salt, or other additives)
3. Rectal tube with rounded tip
4. Tubing to connect rectal tube to container
5. Regulating clamp on tubing
6. Bath thermometer to measure solution's temperature
7. Lubricating jelly
8. Waterproof pad
9. Bath blanket
10. Toilet paper
11. Bedpan or commode
12. Washcloth and towel
13. Disposable gloves

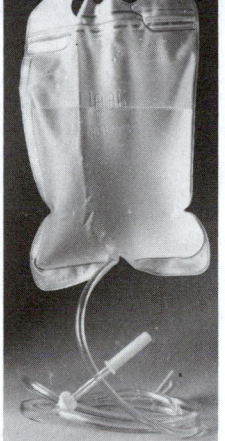

STEPS	RATIONALE
1. Explain the procedure to the client.	This reduces the client's anxiety and promotes cooperation during the procedure.
2. Close room or cubicle curtains.	This provides client privacy.
3. Assist the client into the left side-lying (Sims') position with the right knee flexed. Children may also be placed in the dorsal recumbent position. (Position clients with poor sphincter control on the bedpan.)	Sims' position allows enema solution to flow downward by gravity along the natural curve of the sigmoid colon and rectum, thus improving retention of the solution. (Clients with poor sphincter control cannot retain all of the enema solution.)
4. Place the waterproof pad under the client's hips and buttocks.	This prevents soiling of bed linen.
5. Drape the client's trunk and lower extremities with the bath blanket, leaving only the anal area exposed.	Draping prevents unnecessary exposure of body parts and reduces the client's embarrassment.
6. Assemble the enema container, connecting tubing, clamp, and rectal tube. The size of the rectal tube should be #10 to #12 French for an infant or child and #22 to #26 French for an adult.	Rectal tubing should be small enough to fit the diameter of the client's rectum and large enough to prevent leakage of solution from around the tube.
7. Close the regulating clamp.	Closure prevents initial loss of solution as it is added to the container.
8. Add warmed solution to the container (see Table 40-7 for appropriate volumes). Warm tap water as it flows from the faucet. Place a saline container in a basin of hot water before adding saline to enema container. Check temperature of solution with bath thermometer or by pouring a small amount of solution over the inner wrist.	Hot water can burn intestinal mucosa. Cold water can cause abdominal cramping and is difficult to retain.
9. Raise the container, release the clamp, and allow the solution to flow long enough to fill tubing.	This removes air from the tubing.
10. Reclamp tubing.	Clamping prevents further loss of solution.
11. Place the bedpan near the bedside unit.	The bedpan is easily accessible if the client is unable to retain enema.
12. Don disposable gloves.	Gloving prevents transmission of organisms from feces.
13. Lubricate 3 to 4 inches of the tip of the rectal tube with lubricating jelly.	Lubricant allows smooth insertion of the rectal tube without risk of irritation or trauma to the mucosa.

Continued.

PROCEDURE 40-2, cont'd

Administering an Enema

STEPS	RATIONALE
14. Gently separate the buttocks and locate the rectum. Instruct the client to relax by breathing out slowly through the mouth.	Breathing out promotes relaxation of the external anal sphincter.
15. Insert the tip of the rectal tube slowly by pointing the tip in the direction of the client's umbilicus. Length of insertion varies: 7.5 to 10 cm (3 to 4 inches) for an adult; 5 to 7.5 cm (2 to 3 inches) for a child; 2.5 to 4 cm (1 to 1½ inches) for an infant. Withdraw tube immediately if it meets with obstruction.	Careful insertion prevents trauma to the rectal mucosa from accidental lodging of the tube against the rectal wall. Insertion beyond the proper limit can cause bowel perforation.
16. Hold tubing constantly until the end of fluid instillation.	Bowel contraction can cause expulsion of a rectal tube.
17. Open the regulating clamp and allow solution to enter slowly with the container at the client's hip level.	Rapid infusion can stimulate evacuation prematurely before sufficient volume of solution is infused.
18. Raise height of enema container slowly to the appropriate level above the anus (30 to 45 cm or 12 to 18 inches). Infusion time varies with volume of solution administered (e.g., 1 liter in 10 minutes).	This allows for continuous slow infusion of solution. Raising the container too high causes rapid infusion and possible painful distention of the colon.
19. Lower the container or clamp tubing if the client complains of cramping or if fluid escapes around the rectal tube.	Temporary cessation of infusion prevents cramping. Cramping may prevent the client from retaining all fluid.
20. Clamp the tubing after all solution is infused.	Clamping prevents entrance of air into the rectum.
21. Place layers of toilet tissue around the tube at the anus and gently withdraw the rectal tube.	This provides for client's comfort and cleanliness.
22. Explain to the client that the feeling of distention is normal. Ask the client to retain the solution as long as possible while lying quietly in bed. (For an infant or young child gently hold the buttocks together for a few minutes.)	Solution distends the bowel. The length of retention varies with type of enema and the client's ability to contract the anal sphincter. Longer retention promotes more effective stimulation of peristalsis and defecation. (Infants and young children have poor sphincter control.)
23. Discard enema container and tubing in proper receptacle or rinse out thoroughly with warm soap and water if container is to be reused.	This controls transmission and growth of microorganisms.
24. Remove gloves by pulling them inside out and discard in trash can.	This prevents microorganism transmission.
25. Assist the client to the bathroom or help position the client on bedpan.	The normal squatting position promotes defecation.
26. Observe character of feces and solution (caution the client against flushing toilet before inspection).	When enemas are ordered "until clear," it is essential to observe the contents of solution passed.
27. Assist the client as needed to wash the anal area with warm soap and water.	Fecal contents can irritate the skin. Hygiene promotes the client's comfort.
28. Wash your hands and record the results of the enema.	Prompt recording improves documentation of treatment results.

detergents can cause serious bowel inflammation. The recommended ratio of soap to solution is 5 ml (1 teaspoon) of castile soap to 1000 ml of warm water or saline.

Oil retention enemas act by lubricating the rectum and colon. The feces absorb the oil and become softer and easier to pass. To enhance the action of the oil, the client retains the enema for several hours if possible.

Carminative enemas provide relief from gaseous

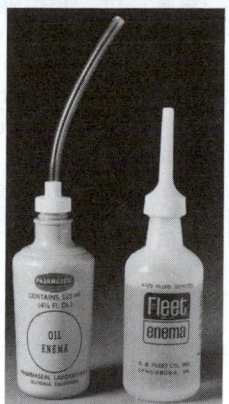

ADMINISTRATION VIA PREPACKAGED DISPOSABLE CONTAINER

EQUIPMENT:

1. Prepackaged bottle with rectal tip
2. Disposable gloves
3. Lubricating jelly
4. Waterproof pad
5. Bath blanket
6. Toilet paper
7. Bedpan or commode
8. Washcloth and towel

STEPS	RATIONALE
1. Follow steps 1 through 5 of previous procedure.	
2. Place the bedpan near the bedside unit.	The bedpan is easily accessible if the client is unable to retain the enema.
3. Don disposable gloves.	Gloving prevents transmission of organisms from feces.
4. Remove the plastic cap from the rectal tip. The tip is already lubricated, but more jelly can be applied as needed.	Lubrication provides for smooth insertion of rectal tube without causing rectal irritation or trauma.
5. Gently separate the buttocks and locate the rectum. Instruct the client to relax by breathing out slowly through the mouth	Breathing out promotes relaxation of the external anal sphincter.
6. Insert the tip of the bottle gently into the rectum. Advance the tip 7.5 to 10 cm (3 to 4 inches) in the adult. (Children and infants usually do not receive prepackaged hypertonic enemas.)	Gentle insertion prevents trauma to the rectal mucosa.
7. Squeeze the bottle until all of the solution has entered the rectum and colon. (Most bottles contain approximately 250 ml of solution.)	Hypertonic solutions require only small volumes to stimulate defecation.
8. Follow steps 21 through 28 of the previous procedure.	

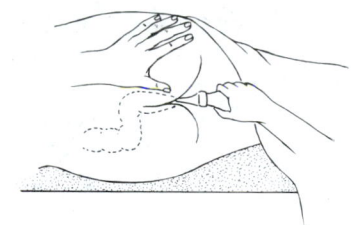

distention. Their administration improves the client's ability to pass flatus. An example of a carminative enema is MGW solution, which contains 30 ml of magnesium, 60 ml of glycerin, and 90 ml of water. Some physicians order more unusual solutions such as milk and molasses.

Medicated enemas contain pharmacological therapeutic agents. An example is polystyrene sodium sulfonate (Kayexalate), used to treat clients with dangerously high serum potassium levels. This preparation contains a resin that exchanges sodium ions for potassium ions in the large intestine. Another medicated enema is neomycin solution, an antibiotic used to reduce bacteria in the colon before bowel surgery.

ENEMA ADMINISTRATION. The nurse administers enemas in commercially packaged disposable units or with reusable equipment prepared before use. Sterile technique is unnecessary, since the colon normally contains bacteria. However, the nurse does need to wear gloves to prevent the transmission of fecal microorganisms.

The nurse should explain the procedure to the client, including the position to assume, precautions to take to avoid discomfort, and the length of time necessary to retain the solution before defecation. If the client is to receive the enema at home, the nurse explains the procedure to a family member.

Often the physician orders "enemas till clear." This means that the enema is repeated until the client passes fluid that is clear and contains no fecal material. It may be necessary to give as many as three enemas (check agency policy), but the nurse should caution the client against using more than three. Excess enema administration seriously depletes fluids and electrolytes. If the client's enema fails to return a clear solution after three administrations, the physician should be notified.

When an enema is administered to a child, it is helpful to have a parent assist with the procedure. The child should understand each step of the procedure and be able to see the equipment beforehand.

Administering an enema to a client unable to contract the external sphincter can pose difficulties. The nurse administers the enema with the client positioned on the bedpan. Administering the enema with the client sitting on the toilet is unsafe because the curved rectal tubing can abrade the rectal wall.

Procedure 40-2 outlines the steps for enema adminstration.

OSTOMY IRRIGATION

To establish a pattern of regular defecation, clients with sigmoid colostomies should irrigate their colostomy routinely (daily or every other day). The irrigation procedure is identical to that of giving an enema; however, the shape of the stoma requires the use of a special cone-tipped irrigating tube (Fig. 40-7). Clients typically use warm tap water to cleanse the bowel. Emptying the bowel at a scheduled time prevents stomal discharges between irrigations. The client gains greater freedom without the need to wear a stomal pouch continuously.

Most clients prefer sitting on the toilet during the

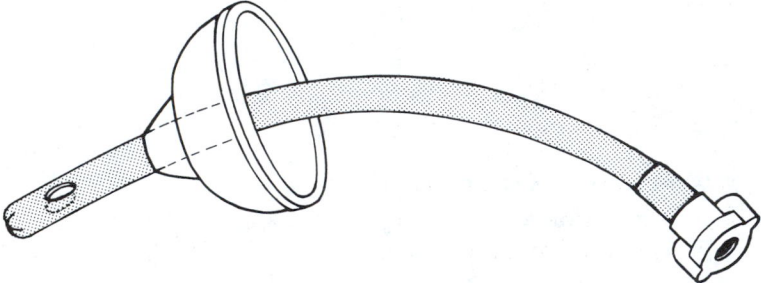

Fig. 40-7   Cone tip for administration of stomal irrigations.

irrigation. Since the stoma has no sphincter, the irrigating solution begins to drain when the cone is removed. The client wears a long plastic irrigating sheath or bag that extends from the stoma down into the toilet. The irrigating solution drains from the stoma into the toilet without soiling the client's skin. It may take up to an hour for feces and solution to be totally expelled. After the greatest portion has passed, the client may choose to close the bottom of the irrigating sheath and wear it as a bag until drainage stops. This allows the client to resume normal activity more quickly.

DIGITAL REMOVAL OF STOOL

For clients with an impaction, the fecal mass may be too large to be passed voluntarily. If enemas fail to promote defecation, the nurse must break up the fecal mass with her fingers and remove it in sections. The procedure can be very uncomfortable for the client. Excessive rectal manipulation may cause irritation to the mucosa, bleeding, and stimulation of the vagus nerve. Vagal nerve stimulation results in a reflex slowing of the heart rate. Because of the procedure's potential complications, in many institutions only physicians are allowed to remove impactions digitally. If the nurse performs the procedure, a physician's order is necessary. Procedure 40-3 lists steps for the digital removal of stool.

BOWEL TRAINING

The client with incontinence is unable to maintain bowel control. A bowel training program can help some clients achieve normal defecation, especially those who still have some neuromuscular control of abdominal muscles and the anal sphincter. The training program involves setting up a daily routine for elimination. By attempting to defecate at the same time each day and using measures that promote defecation, the client gains control of bowel reflexes. The program requires time, patience, and consistency on the part of the nurse and the client. The physician determines the client's physical readiness and ability to benefit from bowel training. A successful program includes the following elements:

1. Assessing the client's normal elimination pattern and recording times when the client is incontinent
2. Choosing a time in the client's pattern to initiate defecation control measures
3. Administering stool softeners orally every day or a cathartic suppository at least half an hour before the selected defecation time
4. Offering the client a hot drink or fruit juice (or whatever fluids normally stimulate peristalsis for the client) before the defecation time

Removing Stool Digitally

STEPS	RATIONALE
1. Explain the procedure to the client, noting that manipulation of the rectum can cause discomfort.	Explanation reduces the client's anxiety. The client's cooperation is necessary to minimize the risk of injury.
2. Assist the client to a side-lying position with knees flexed.	This position provides access to the rectum.
3. Drape the client's trunk and lower extremities with a bath blanket.	Draping prevents unnecessary exposure of body parts.
4. Place a waterproof pad under the client's buttocks.	This prevents soiling of bed linen.
5. Place a bedpan next to client.	The bedpan is the receptacle for the stool.
6. Don disposable gloves.	Gloving prevents transmission of microorganisms.
7. Lubricate the glove's index finger with lubricating jelly.	Lubrication permits smooth insertion of the finger into the rectum.
8. Insert the index finger into the rectum and advance the finger slowly along the rectal wall toward the client's umbilicus.	This allows nurse to reach impacted stool high in the rectum.
9. Gently loosen the fecal mass by massaging around it. Work the finger into the hardened mass.	Loosening the mass allows nurse to penetrate it with less discomfort to the client.
10. Work the stool downward toward the end of the rectum. Remove small sections of feces at a time.	This prevents the need to force the finger up into the rectum and minimizes trauma to the mucosa.
11. Periodically assess the client's heart rate and look for signs of fatigue. Stop the procedure if the client's heart rate drops or the rhythm changes.	Vagal stimulation slows the heart rate. The procedure may exhaust the client.
12. Continue to clear the rectum of feces and allow the client to rest at intervals.	Rest improves the client's tolerance of the procedure.
13. After disimpaction provide a washcloth and towel to wash the buttocks and anal area.	Washing promotes the client's sense of comfort and cleanliness.
14. Remove the bedpan and dispose of the feces. Remove the gloves by turning them inside out and discard in proper receptacle.	This prevents transmission of microorganisms.
15. Assist the client to the toilet or a clean bedpan.	Disimpaction may stimulate the defecation reflex.
16. Wash your hands and record the results of disimpaction. Describe the fecal characteristics. (The procedure may be followed by enemas or cathartics.)	Prompt recording improves the accuracy of documentation.

5. Assisting the client to the toilet at the designated time (A training program is less effective if the client uses a bedpan.)
6. Providing the client with privacy and setting a time limit for defecation (15 to 20 minutes)
7. Instructing the client to lean forward at the hips while sitting on the toilet, to apply manual pressure with the hands over the abdomen, and to bear down but not strain in order to stimulate colon emptying
8. Not criticizing the client or conveying a sense of frustration if the client is unable to defecate
9. Providing regular meals with adequate fluids and fiber
10. Maintaining normal exercise within the client's physical ability

The client will require positive reinforcement and encouragement. It often takes several days before a training program is successful.

Promotion of Comfort

Many clients experience discomfort as a result of alterations in elimination. The client with hemorrhoids experiences pain whenever the hemorrhoidal tissues are directly irritated. Flatulence can also create discomfort, particularly if abdominal distention develops. The nurse's interventions for promoting comfort ultimately promote normal elimination as well.

The primary goal for the client with hemorrhoids is to have soft-formed stools. Proper diet, fluids, and regular exercise improve the likelihood of stools being soft. If the client becomes constipated, passage of hard stools will cause bleeding and irritation of hemorrhoidal tissues.

Local application of heat provides temporary relief to swollen hemorrhoids. A sitz bath is the most effective means of heat application (see Chapter 48).

Often hemorrhoids become so enlarged that they cover the rectum. To prevent trauma to tissues the nurse must use caution when inserting rectal thermometers, suppositories, or rectal tubes. A generous application of lubricating jelly will reduce friction when inserting an object past a hemorrhoid. Often the client is better able to insert an object safely into the rectum. The nurse should never attempt to force an object into the rectum without full view of the anus. When hemorrhoids cause chronic pain, surgical removal is the treatment of choice.

To relieve the discomfort of flatulence the nurse should use measures that either reduce formation of flatus or promote its escape. Air swallowing increases the formation of flatus. The client can reduce the amount of air swallowed by not drinking carbonated beverages, not using straws for drinking, and not chewing gum or hard candies. When flatulence becomes severe as a result of reduced peristalsis, a nasogastric tube is often used (see Chapter 47). For example, after major abdominal surgery a nasogastric tube is inserted to empty gastric contents until normal peristalsis returns.

When flatulence results in abdominal cramping, ambulation promotes the passage of flatus. Having the client walk down the hall may be enough to stimulate peristalsis and relieve gaseous accumulation in the bowel.

When conservative measures fail, flatulence can be relieved by insertion of a rectal tube. The client assumes a side-lying position while the nurse inserts the tube in the same manner as for an enema administration (see Procedure 40-2). Since fluid is not instilled into the bowel, the nurse can advance the tube deeper to reach areas where flatus has accumulated (15 cm or 6 inches in an adult, 5 to 10 cm or 2 to 4 inches in a child).

After inserting the tube the nurse instructs the client to lie quietly in bed. To prevent the tube from being dislodged, the nurse may tape it to one of the client's buttocks. A gauze dressing or waterproof pad placed around the open end of the rectal tube will catch any liquid fecal material.

Continual use of rectal tubes can cause irritation and eventual excoriation of the anus and rectal mucosa. A rectal tube should not remain in place longer than 30 minutes. The physician will determine the frequency with which the tube can be inserted. If flatulence persists, the nurse should notify the physician.

Maintenance of Skin Integrity

The client with diarrhea or fecal incontinence has a predisposition to skin breakdown when fecal contents remain on the skin. The same problem exists for the client with a colostomy that drains liquid stool. Liquid stool is usually acidic and contains digestive enzymes. Prolonged contact with the skin will result in inflammation and excoriation. Irritation from repeated wiping with toilet tissue aggravates skin breakdown. Bathing the skin after soiling is helpful but may result in more breakdown unless the skin is thoroughly dried.

The nurse should instruct the client on cleansing the anal area with mild soap and water after each passage of stool. When caring for a debilitated, incontinent client who is unable to ask for assistance, the nurse should check frequently for occurrence of defecation. The anal areas can be protected with an application of petrolatum jelly, zinc oxide, or other ointment. Ointments hold moisture in the skin, preventing drying and cracking. Yeast infections of the skin can develop easily, since the organisms thrive in feces. Several antifungal agents, available in powder form, are effective against yeast. Baby powder or cornstarch should not be applied to the skin. They have no medicinal properties, and they frequently cake on the skin and become difficult to remove.

The client with an ostomy has the continuous challenge of maintaining skin integrity. Stool from ileostomies and colostomies of the ascending and transverse colon usually contains digestive enzymes. To protect the skin, an ostomate wears a special skin barrier made of karaya or a gelatinous amalgam, substances that assume the contour of the underlying skin (Fig. 40-8). There is no need for adhesives, since the barriers adhere to the skin surface. A hole in the center of the barrier permits protusion of the stoma. The pouch or bag that collects feces is attached directly to the skin barrier (Fig. 40-9). The barriers last several days, eliminating the need for frequent removal and reapplication of the pouch. As long as the pouch and skin barrier remain intact, the client's skin will remain dry.

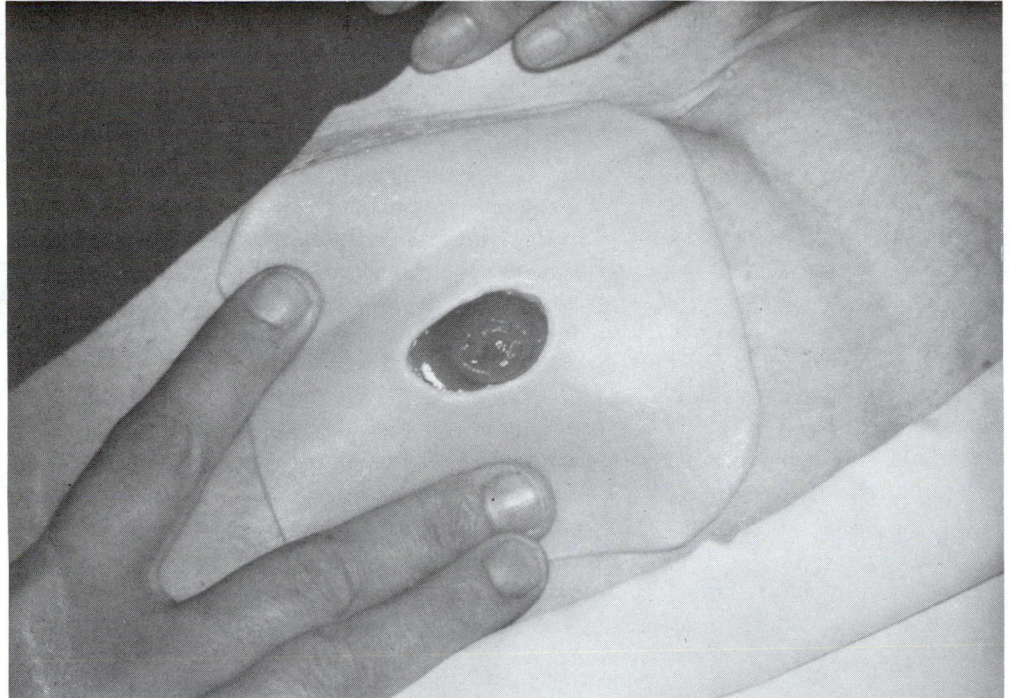

Fig. 40-8 HolliHesive applied to skin. No skin is exposed. A pouch will be applied as a separate step.
From Managing the ostomy patient, Chicago, 1980, Hollister Inc.

Evaluation

The effectiveness of the nurse's therapies depends on success in meeting the expected outcomes of care. The ultimate goal is the client's normal defecation of soft-formed stools. Short-term interventions are used to achieve this goal. Therapies designed to promote a proper diet and fluid intake are evaluated on the following basis:

1. The client's or family member's ability to develop a meal plan and prepare meals consisting of high- or low-fiber foods (depending on tendency to have constipation or diarrhea)
2. The client's success in drinking 2000 to 3000 ml of fluid daily (except clients whose elimination problems result from fluid restrictions)

Nursing therapies designed to promote normal defecation are evaluated on the basis of these criteria:

1. The client's ability to maintain bowel control without the use of medications or enemas
2. The client's participation in a regular exercise program
3. The client's ability to pass stools without straining

Because of the various effects of elimination disorders, the nurse's therapies should also focus on min-

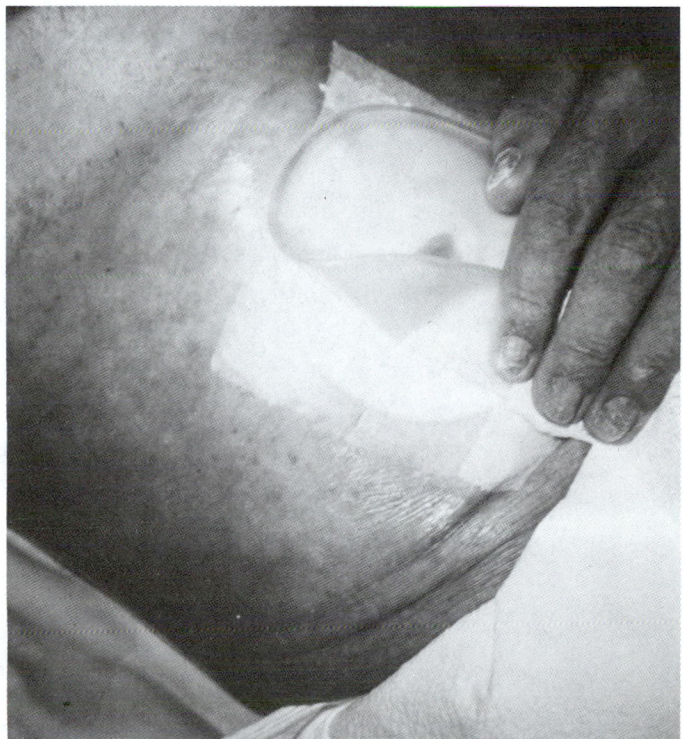

Fig. 40-9 Pouching system. Darting of Stomahesive and pouch will allow edges to move with the client's movements, especially respirations.
From Broadwell, D.C., and Jackson, B.S.: Principles of ostomy care, St. Louis, 1982, The C.V. Mosby Co.

imizing complications. Therapies designed to promote comfort when the client has hemorrhoids or flatulence are evaluated on these bases:

1. The client's ability to defecate without discomfort
2. The absence of bleeding from or inflammation of hemorrhoidal tissues
3. The absence of abdominal cramping and distention

Evaluation of therapies designed to maintain the skin integrity of clients with diarrhea, incontinence, or an ostomy includes the following criteria:

1. The client's perianal area remaining dry without signs of inflammation or excoriation
2. The skin around a stoma site remaining dry without signs of inflammation or excoriation

Summary

The normal elimination of fecal wastes requires maintenance of gastrointestinal function. The nurse's therapies either promote or minimize the factors that influence peristalsis and the absorption and secretion of intestinal contents.

Each client has a different pattern of defecation. The client can become preoccupied with being unable to pass a normal stool. Nursing care begins with educating clients about simple daily activities or habits that promote defecation.

Clients become dependent on the nurse when they lose the ability to control body functions. Measures designed to promote normal defecation can be embarrassing and uncomfortable. The nurse's approach requires sensitivity and understanding of the client's needs.

KEY CONCEPTS

✓ A primary function of the elimination process is fluid balance.

✓ The mechanical breakdown of food elements, gastrointestinal motility, and the selective absorption and secretion of substances by the large intestine influence the character of feces.

✓ Mass peristalsis in the large intestine is strongest an hour after mealtime.

✓ Emotional and physical stress increases peristalsis.

✓ Bowel training cannot be effective until a child's nervous and muscular systems have matured.

✓ Disruption of normal elimination habits places a person at risk for constipation.

✓ Food high in fiber content and an increased fluid intake keep feces soft.

✓ Analgesics and anesthetics slow peristalsis.

✓ Regular use of laxatives can lead to constipation.

✓ Straining during defecation slows the heart rate.

✓ The greatest danger from diarrhea is development of fluid and electrolyte imbalance.

✓ The location of an ostomy influences the consistency of the stool.

✓ Assessment of a person's elimination pattern should focus on bowel habits, an analysis of factors that normally influence defecation, and a review of recent changes in elimination.

✓ The client is the best source of information about changes in fecal characteristics.

✓ A guaiac test is recommended for clients who are receiving anticoagulants or who have a bleeding disorder or gastrointestinal disorder that causes bleeding.

KEY CONCEPTS, *cont'd*

✓ Indirect and direct visualization of the lower gastrointestinal tract requires cleansing of the bowel before the procedure.

✓ The nurse should consider the frequency of defecation, fecal characteristics, and the effect of certain foods on gastrointestinal function when selecting a diet that promotes normal elimination.

✓ Proper positioning on a bedpan allows the client to assume a position similar to squatting without experiencing muscle strain.

✓ Cathartics or laxatives should be administered shortly before the usual time a client defecates.

✓ The safest form of laxative is a bulk-forming cathartic.

✓ Proper administration of an enema is the slow instillation of a warm solution in the proper volume.

✓ Irrigation of an ostomy follows the same principles as an enema administration except a special irrigating tube is needed and the client cannot control passage of feces.

✓ Dangers during the digital removal of stool include traumatizing the rectal mucosa and promoting vagal stimulation.

✓ Skin breakdown can occur after repeated exposure to liquid stool.

✓ Ostomates should wear skin barriers to protect underlying skin from breakdown.

READINGS

Aman, R.A.: Treating the patient, not the constipation, Am. J. Nurs. 80:1634, 1980.

American Cancer Society: Care of your sigmoid colostomy, New York, 1979, The Society.

Battle, E.H., and Hanna, C.E.: Evaluation of a dietary regimen for chronic constipation: report of a pilot study, J. Gerontol. Nurs. 6:527, 1980.

Guyton, A.C.: Human physiology and mechanisms of disease, ed. 3, Philadelphia, 1982, W.B. Saunders Co.

Mahoney, J.M.: What you should know about ostomies, Nursing 78 8:74, 1978.

Pagana, K.D., and Pagana, T.J.: Diagnostic testing and nursing implications, St. Louis, 1982, The C.V. Mosby Co.

Whaley, L.F., and Wong, D.L.: Nursing care of infants and children, ed. 2, St. Louis, 1983, The C.V. Mosby Co.

Winkelstein, C., and Lyons, A.S.: Insight into the emotional aspects of ileostomies and colostomies (reprint), New York, 1971, Medical Insight.

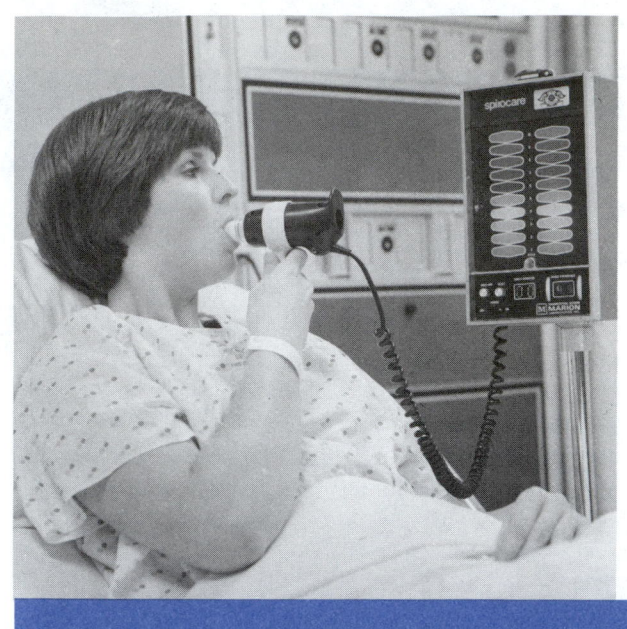

OBJECTIVES

Mastery of content in this chapter will enable the student to:

- Define the terms in the glossary.
- Describe the gross structure and function of the respiratory system.
- Identify the processes involved in ventilation, perfusion, and the exchange of respiratory gases.
- Describe the neural and chemical regulation of respiration.
- Explain how a client's level of health, age, lifestyle, and environment can affect tissue oxygenation.
- Identify the causes and effects of hyperventilation, hypoventilation, and hypoxemia.
- Perform a nursing assessment of the respiratory system.
- Develop nursing diagnoses for altered oxygenation.
- Describe nursing interventions to maintain or promote lung expansion, promote mobilization of pulmonary secretions, maintain a patent airway, promote oxygenation, and restore cardiopulmonary function.
- Develop evaluation criteria for the nursing care plan for the client with altered oxygenation.

GLOSSARY

abdominal-diaphragmatic breathing   Respiration in which the abdomen moves out while the diaphragm descends on inspiration.

alveolar hyperventilation   Respiratory rate in excess of that required to maintain normal carbon dioxide levels in the body tissues.

alveolar hypoventilation   Respiratory rate insufficient to prevent carbon dioxide retention.

atelectasis   Collapse of alveoli, preventing the normal respiratory exchange of oxygen and carbon dioxide.

bronchoscopy   Visual examination of the tracheal and bronchial tree using the standard rigid, tubular metal bronchoscope or the narrower, flexible fiberoptic bronchoscope.

carbon monoxide poisoning   Toxic condition in which carbon monoxide gas has been inhaled and absorbed in the lungs, displacing oxygen from hemoglobin and decreasing the capacity of the blood to carry oxygen.

cardiac arrest   Sudden cessation of cardiac output and effective circulation.

cardiopulmonary resuscitation   Basic emergency procedures for life support consisting of artificial respiration and manual external cardiac massage.

chest percussion   Striking of the chest wall with a cupped hand to promote mobilization and drainage of pulmonary secretions.

chest physiotherapy   Group of therapies used to mobilize secretions.

41 | *Oxygenation*

coccidioidomycosis Infectious fungal disease caused by the inhalation of windborne spores of the bacterium *Coccidioides immitis*.

cough Sudden, audible expulsion of air from the lungs.

diffusion Movement of molecules from an area of high concentration to an area of lower concentration.

erythrocyte Red blood cell.

flail chest Condition caused by multiple rib fractures, resulting in instability in part of the chest wall and paradoxical breathing, with the lung underlying the injured area contracting on inspiration and expanding on expiration.

hemoptysis Coughing up of blood from the respiratory tract.

hemothorax Accumulation of blood and fluid in the pleural cavity between the parietal and visceral pleurae.

hypovolemia Decreased circulatory blood volume resulting from extracellular fluid losses.

hypoxia Inadequate cellular oxygenation that may result from a deficiency in the delivery or use of oxygen at the cellular level.

incentive spirometry Method of encouraging voluntary deep breathing by providing visual feedback to clients of the inspiratory volume they have achieved.

intermittent positive-pressure breathing Method of achieving lung hyperinflation by applying positive pressure to the airways.

nebulization Process of adding moisture to inspired air by the addition of water droplets.

orthopnea Abnormal condition in which the client must sit, stand, or use multiple pillows when lying down in order to breathe.

oxygen therapy Administration of oxygen by any route to a client to prevent or relieve hypoxia.

pectus excavatum Depression of the sternum.

pneumothorax Collection of air or gas in the pleural space.

polycythemia Abnormal increase in the number of erythrocytes in the blood.

postural drainage Use of positioning along with percussion and vibration to drain secretions from specific segments of the lungs and bronchi into the trachea.

pulmonary function tests Procedures for determining the capacity of the lungs to exchange oxygen and carbon dioxide efficiently.

pursed-lip breathing Deep inspiration and prolonged expiration through pursed lips.

thoracentesis Surgical perforation of the chest wall and pleural space with a needle for the aspiration of fluid or a specimen for diagnostic or therapeutic purposes.

ventilation Respiratory process by which gases are moved into and out of the lungs.

vibration Fine, shaking pressure applied to the chest wall only during exhalation.

Oxygen is a basic human need and is required for life. The nurse frequently encounters clients who are unable to meet their oxygen needs independently. To assist clients to meet their oxygen needs the nurse needs to understand respiratory physiology.

Respiratory physiology involves the oxygenation of the body through the mechanisms of ventilation, perfusion, and transport of respiratory gases. In addition, neural and chemical regulators control fluctuations in respiratory rate and depth to meet tissue oxygen demands.

The individual's level of health, age, life-style, and environment also affect the ability to meet tissue oxygen needs. When a client is unable to meet his oxygen requirements, hyperventilation, hypoventilation, or hypoxemia may result.

This chapter discusses respiratory physiology, factors affecting oxygenation, hyperventilation, hypoventilation, hypoxia, and the care of the client who is unable to meet oxygen needs. Through the nursing process the nurse assesses and diagnoses oxygenation needs and plans and implements nursing interventions to meet those needs.

Respiratory Physiology

The majority of cells in the human body obtain most of their energy from chemical reactions involving oxygen, and cells must also eliminate carbon dioxide (Vander, Sherman, and Luciano, 1980). For this exchange of respiratory gases to occur, the organs, nerves, and muscles of respiration must be intact. In addition, the central nervous system must be able to regulate the cycle of inspiration and expiration.

Structure and Function

Respiration can be altered by conditions or disease processes that occur in various regions of the pulmonary system, resulting in changes in both structure and function. The airways, pulmonary circulation, lungs, and respiratory muscles are essential to the three major purposes of the respiratory system: ventilation, perfusion, and the exchange of respiratory gases.

The primary functions of the lungs are to transfer oxygen from the atmosphere into the alveoli and to transfer carbon dioxide from the alveoli to the atmosphere as a waste product. In addition, the lungs filter toxic materials from the circulation, metabolize some compounds, such as angiotensin I, bradykinin, and prostaglandins, and serve as a reservoir for blood (West, 1979). Each lung lies in a pleural space that surrounds the lung except at the medial attachment. This medial attachment is the hilus, which contains the mainstem bronchi and pulmonary vessels (Bushnell, 1981). Actually the pleural space is a potential space, the thickness of which is only a thin film of liquid lying between the outer layer of the lung (visceral pleura) and the inner cell layer of the chest cavity (parietal pleura). The purpose of this film is to permit an easy gliding movement of the lung along the chest wall; however, a great deal of force would be required to pull the pleura away from the chest wall (Wade, 1977). The vessels of the pulmonary circulation are also contained within the lung, as described in the later section on perfusion.

The alveoli are tiny air sacs at the terminal end of the lower airway (Fig. 41-1). The alveolar wall is composed of the alveolar membrane, a network of capillaries and interstitial fluid that contains collagen fibers (Bushnell, 1981). The exchange of respiratory gases, oxygen (O_2) and carbon dioxide (CO_2), takes place in the alveoli. A unique characteristic of these tiny air sacs is their ability to expand during inspiration, greatly increasing the surface area over which the exchange of gases can occur.

Ventilation

Ventilation, perfusion, and the exchange of respiratory gases are the three processes that provide blood oxygenation. Ventilation is the process by which gases are moved into and out of the lungs. Adequate ventilation requires proper coordination of the muscular and elastic properties of the lung and thorax and intact innervation. The major inspiratory muscle is the diaphragm, which is innervated by the phrenic nerve. The phrenic nerve exits the spinal cord at the fourth vertebra. The diaphragm descends on inspiration, thereby increasing lung volume. Disruption of the spinal cord at the fourth cervical level can sever the phrenic cervical nerve and impair the function of the diaphragm. The cervical vertebrae are quite commonly injured in diving and automobile accidents. These clients may be dependent on a ventilator for the remainder of their lives because the diaphragm does not descend for inspiration.

The other inspiratory muscle groups elevate the chest cage and expand its anterior-posterior diameter, which also increases lung volume. For adequate ventilation to occur, the lungs must be able to accomplish the work of breathing and to move respiratory gases into and out of the lungs.

WORK OF BREATHING

The work of breathing is the total amount of effort required to expand and contract the lungs. It is determined by the degree of compliance of the lung tissue, the resistance of the airway, the presence of active expiration, and the use of the accessory muscles of respiration (Groër and Shekleton, 1983).

Compliance is the intrinsic ability of the lungs and thorax to expand in response to an increase in intra-alveolar pressure (Groër and Shekleton, 1983). Simply stated, compliance is the ability of the lungs to expand for inspiration. Compliance is decreased in certain diseases, such as pulmonary edema, interstitial fibrosis, or pleural fibrosis. In addition, congenital or traumatic structural abnormalities, such as kyphosis or fractured ribs, decrease lung compliance.

Airway resistance is the pressure difference between the alveoli and the mouth in relation to the rate of flow of the inspired gas. Airway resistance can be increased by an airway obstruction, such as the presence of a foreign body, small airway disease, asthma, or tracheal edema. When airway resistance is increased, the amount of air traveling through the anatomical airways is decreased.

Active expiration is the active use of muscle groups to contract the lungs. Expiration is normally a passive process that depends on the elastic recoil properties of the lungs and that requires little or no muscle work. The elastic recoil is produced by elastic fibers in the lung tissue and by the surface tension in the fluid film lining the alveoli (Bushnell, 1981). In addition, passive recoil of the chest wall and abdominal musculature further enhances expiration. Active expiration can also be altered by certain disease processes.

The accessory muscles of respiration, the sterno-cleidomastoid muscle groups, can be used to increase lung volume during inspiration. Clients with chronic

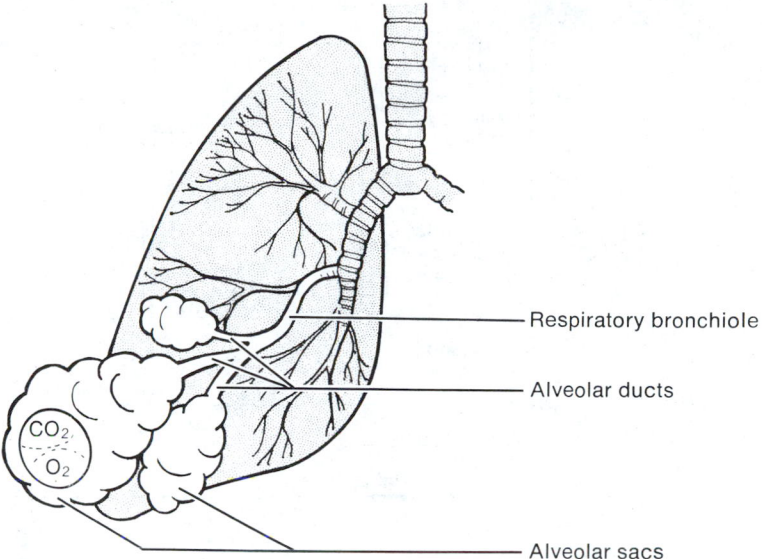

Fig. 41-1 Alveoli at the terminal end of the lower airway.

From Groër, M.W., and Shekleton, M.E.: Basic pathophysiology: a conceptual approach, ed. 2, St. Louis, 1983, The C.V. Mosby Co.

obstructive pulmonary disease, especially emphysema, frequently use these muscle groups to increase lung volume. During assessment the nurse may observe the client's clavicles being elevated in the inspiratory phase of respiration.

Decreased compliance, increased airway resistance, active expiration, or use of the accessory muscles increases the work of breathing, resulting in an increased energy expenditure by the body. To meet this expenditure the body increases its metabolic rate, and consequently the need for oxygen is increased. This sequence can set up a vicious circle for a client with impaired ventilation and can cause further deterioration in the respiratory status.

VOLUMES

The normal volumes within the lung are measured through pulmonary function testing. Some of these measurements can be determined with a spirometer, which measures the volume of air entering or leaving the lungs (Fig. 41-2). Variations in lung volumes may be associated with health states such as pregnancy, exercise, obesity, or obstructive and restrictive pathological conditions of the lung. Factors such as the presence of surfactant, compliance, and paralysis of respiratory muscles can affect normal pressures and volumes within the lungs as well.

PRESSURE

Gases are moved into and out of the lungs through a process involving pressures (Fig. 41-3). Intrapleural pressure is negative to (less than) atmospheric pres-

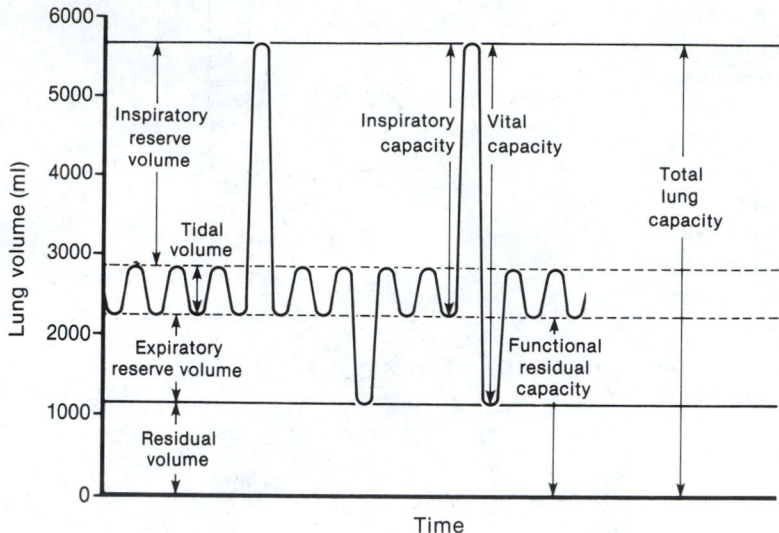

Fig. 41-2 Normal lung volume measured by spirometry.

From Perry, A.G., and Potter, P.A., editors: Shock: comprehensive nursing management, St. Louis, 1983, The C.V. Mosby Co.

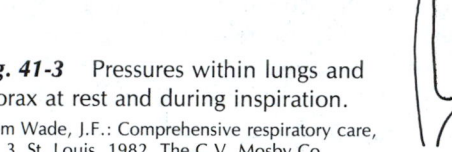

Fig. 41-3 Pressures within lungs and thorax at rest and during inspiration.

From Wade, J.F.: Comprehensive respiratory care, ed. 3, St. Louis, 1982, The C.V. Mosby Co.

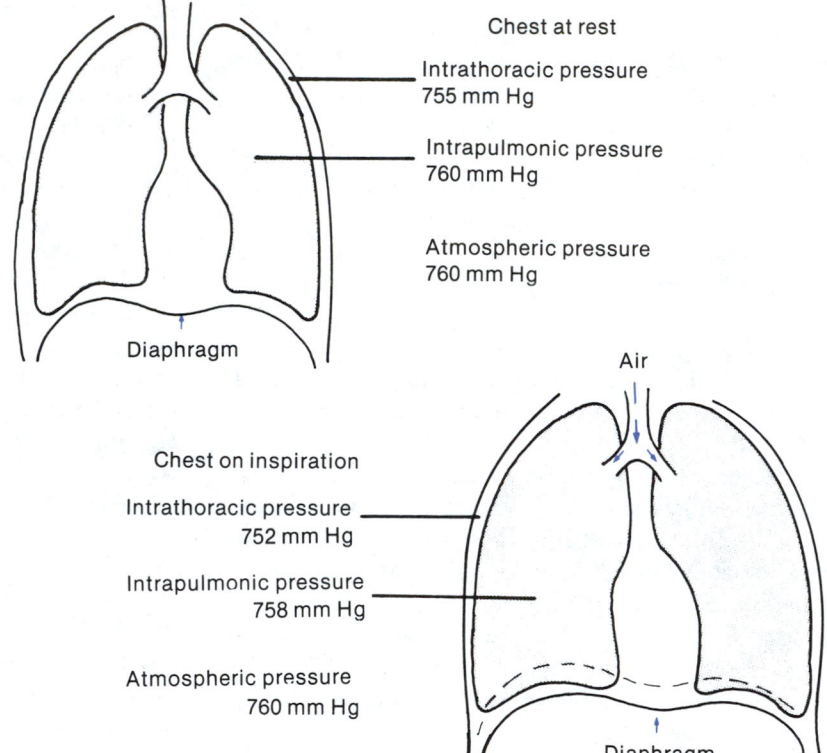

Chest at rest

Intrathoracic pressure
755 mm Hg

Intrapulmonic pressure
760 mm Hg

Atmospheric pressure
760 mm Hg

Chest on inspiration

Intrathoracic pressure
752 mm Hg

Intrapulmonic pressure
758 mm Hg

Atmospheric pressure
760 mm Hg

sure, which is 760 mm Hg at sea level. For air to flow into the lungs, the intrapleural pressure must become negative, setting up a pressure gradient between the atmosphere and the alveoli, which causes a suctioning of air into the lungs. In addition, intra-alveolar pressures become slightly negative with respect to atmospheric pressure, increasing airflow into the air sacs. Once atmospheric air is introduced into the intrapleural space, the negative pull is abolished, resulting in contraction of the lung (Fig. 41-3).

Perfusion

The primary function of the pulmonary circulation is to move blood to and from the blood-gas barrier so gas exchange can occur. The pulmonary circulation also serves as a reservoir for blood so the lung can increase its blood volume without large increases in the pulmonary artery or venous pressures. Finally, this circulatory system filters blood so small thrombi are removed before they reach the brain or other vital organs (West, 1979).

PULMONARY CIRCULATION

The pulmonary circulation begins at the pulmonary artery, which receives mixed venous blood from the right ventricle. The blood flow through this system depends on the pumping ability of the right ventricle, which has an output of approximately 5 to 6 liters per minute. The flow continues from the pulmonary artery through the pulmonary arterioles, pulmonary capillaries, pulmonary venules, and pulmonary veins; it finally returns oxygenated blood to the left atrium.

DISTRIBUTION

The pressures within the pulmonary circulatory system are low in comparison to those in the systemic circulatory system. The pulmonary systolic arterial pressure is between 20 and 30 mm Hg, the pulmonary diastolic pressure is less than 12 mm Hg, and the mean pulmonary pressure is less than 20 mm Hg (Daily and Schroeder, 1981). With low pressure and low resistance the walls of the pulmonary vessels are thinner than those in the systemic circulation and contain a smaller amount of smooth muscle. The lung accepts the total cardiac output from the right ventricle and, except in cases of alveolar hypoxia, is not required to direct blood flow from one region to another.

Exchange of Respiratory Gases

Respiratory gases are exchanged in the alveoli and body tissues. Oxygen is transferred from the lungs to the blood, and carbon dioxide is transferred from the blood to the lungs to be exhaled as a waste product. At the tissue level, oxygen is transferred from the blood to the tissues, and carbon dioxide is transferred from the tissues to the blood to return to the lungs and be exhaled. This transfer depends on the process of diffusion.

DIFFUSION

Diffusion is the movement of molecules from an area of high concentration to an area of lower concentration. The diffusion of respiratory gases can be affected by the thickness of the membrane across which the gases diffuse and by the surface area of the membrane.

An increased thickness of the membrane decreases the rate of diffusion because respiratory gases take longer to diffuse across a thicker membrane. In clients with pulmonary edema, pulmonary infiltrate, or a pulmonary effusion, the thickness of the respiratory membrane is increased. As a result, diffusion is slowed and the delivery of oxygen to the tissues may be impaired.

The surface area of the membrane can be altered as a result of a chronic disease process (such as emphysema), an acute disease process (such as a pneumothorax), or a surgical process (such as a lobectomy). The surface area is decreased when fewer alveoli are functioning.

OXYGEN TRANSPORT

The oxygen transport system consists of the lungs and cardiovascular system. Adequacy of oxygen delivery depends on the amount of oxygen entering the lungs (ventilation), the blood flow to the lungs and to the tissues (perfusion), the adequacy of diffusion, and the capacity of the blood to carry oxygen. The blood's capacity to carry oxygen is influenced by the amount of dissolved oxygen in the plasma, the amount of hemoglobin, and the affinity of hemoglobin for oxygen.

Only a relatively small amount of the required oxygen, approximately 3%, is dissolved in the plasma. Most of the oxygen is transported by hemoglobin. The hemoglobin molecule serves as the carrier for both oxygen and carbon dioxide. The hemoglobin molecule combines with oxygen to form oxyhemoglobin. The maximal amount of oxygen that can be combined with hemoglobin is called the oxygen capacity. Each gram of hemoglobin can combine with 1.39 ml of oxygen (West, 1979). When the total hemoglobin is multiplied by this figure, the product is the total oxygen-carrying capacity of hemoglobin. The oxyhemoglobin molecule is easily reversible, allowing hemoglobin and oxygen to dissociate and freeing oxygen to enter the tissues.

CARBON DIOXIDE TRANSPORT

The transport of respiratory gases includes the movement of carbon dioxide. The fate of carbon dioxide in the blood is summarized in the following outline*:

1. In plasma
   a. Dissolved
   b. Formation of carbamino compounds with plasma protein
   c. Hydration, H^+ buffered, HCO_3^- in plasma
2. In red blood cells
   a. Dissolved
   b. Formation of carbamino compounds
   c. Hydration, H^+ buffered, 70% of HCO_3^- diffuses into plasma
   d. Cl^- shifts into cells; mOsm/L in cells increases

Carbon dioxide diffuses into red blood cells and is rapidly hydrated into carbonic acid as a result of the

*From Ganong, W.F.: Review of medical physiology, ed. 11, Los Altos, Calif., 1983, Lange Medical Publications.

presence of carbonic anhydrase. The carbonic acid then dissociates into hydrogen (H^+) and bicarbonate (HCO_3^-) ions. The hydrogen ion is buffered by hemoglobin, and the HCO_3^- diffuses into the plasma (Ganong, 1983) (see also Chapter 43). In addition, some of the carbon dioxide in the red blood cells reacts with amino acid groups, forming carbamino compounds. This reaction can occur rapidly without the presence of an enzyme. Reduced hemoglobin (deoxyhemoglobin) can combine with carbon dioxide more easily than oxyhemoglobin, and therefore the majority of carbon dioxide is transported by venous blood.

Regulation of Respiration

The main purpose of respiratory regulation is to supply sufficient oxygen to the blood to meet varying demands, such as exercise, infection, or pregnancy. In addition, respiratory regulation promotes exhalation of metabolically produced carbon dioxide, which is a determinant of acid-base status. The adequacy of respiratory regulation is measured by arterial blood gases (see Chapter 43).

There are two types of respiratory regulators: neural regulators and chemical regulators. Neural regulation includes the central nervous system control of respiratory rate and depth. Chemical regulation involves the influence of chemicals, such as carbon dioxide and hydrogen ions, on the rate and depth of respiration.

NEURAL REGULATION

Synchronized inspiration and expiration can be regulated through either voluntary or automatic control. The center for voluntary control is located in the cerebral cortex and delivers impulses to the respiratory motor neurons by way of the spinal cord (Ganong, 1983). An individual voluntarily controls respiration to accommodate various activities, such as speaking, eating, and swimming. The medulla oblongata contains the center for the automatic control of respiration, which occurs continuously through sleeping and most waking activities. This neural regulation maintains the appropriate rhythm and depth of respiration, in addition to the balance in length between inspiration and expiration.

CHEMICAL REGULATION

The respiratory chemoreceptors are located in the medulla and in the aortic carotid bodies. Changes in the blood's carbon dioxide, oxygen, and hydrogen ion content are identified by these chemoreceptors. They then stimulate the neural regulators to adjust the rate or depth of ventilation to maintain the arterial pressure of carbon dioxide ($Paco_2$) at a constant level, to alter the effects of excess hydrogen ion concentration, and to raise the arterial pressure of oxygen (Pao_2) (Ganong, 1983). For example, after jogging the person's respiratory rate remains increased to permit the lungs to excrete the excess carbon dioxide that results from the increased metabolic activity of the cells during exercise. Rapid respiration following an exercise period allows the body to correct metabolic imbalances.

The chemoreceptors also assist in the regulation of respiration in certain illnesses. For example, the respiratory rate of the febrile client is elevated because the febrile state increases metabolic activities, resulting in greater oxygen demand and more carbon dioxide production. To adapt to the increased oxygen need the chemoreceptors stimulate the respiratory center in the medulla oblongata to increase the rate and depth of respiration. More oxygen is inspired, and the excess carbon dioxide is expired. This is a short-term adaptive mechanism that cannot continue over a long period without the client experiencing respiratory distress or acid-base imbalance (see Chapter 43).

Factors Affecting Oxygenation

The adequacy of ventilation, perfusion, and the transport of respiratory gases from the lungs to the tissues is influenced by four major factors: the client's (1) level of health, (2) age, (3) life-style, and (4) environmental exposures.

Level of Health

Any condition that affects the functioning of the respiratory system directly affects the client's ability to meet the body's oxygen demands. The general classifications of respiratory disorders include hyperventilation, hypoventilation, hypoxia, and hypercapnia. These disorders are described in detail later in the chapter.

Other disease processes also affect oxygenation. These include alterations that affect the oxygen-carrying capacity of the blood, such as the anemias; alterations in the ability of the myocardial pump to perfuse the ventilated regions of the lung and to deliver oxygenated blood to the tissues; and increases in the body's metabolic demands. The increased demand may be increased normally, such as during pregnancy, or may result from an abnormal process, such as fever and infection. Alterations that affect chest wall movement or the central nervous system also affect oxygenation.

DECREASED OXYGEN-CARRYING CAPACITY

As noted earlier, hemoglobin carries 97% of the diffused oxygen to the tissues. Thus any process that decreases or alters hemoglobin decreases the oxygen-carrying capacity of the blood. Anemia and inhalation of toxic substances are two disorders that decrease the carrying capacity.

Anemia is characterized by a decrease in hemoglobin in the blood to levels below normal. Anemia reflects one or more of three basic processes: decreased hemoglobin production, increased red cell destruction, or blood loss. Assessment findings in clients with anemia include fatigue, decreased activity tolerance, increased breathlessness, pallor, and increased heart rate. Severe anemia in the elderly can precipitate cardiac failure.

Carbon monoxide is the most common toxic inhalant decreasing the oxygen-carrying capacity of the blood. Carbon monoxide gas that has been inhaled and absorbed in the lungs displaces oxygen from hemoglobin and decreases the capacity of the blood to carry oxygen. The bond of the carbon monoxide molecule with the hemoglobin molecule is approximately 20 times stronger than the bond between hemoglobin and oxygen. Because of the strength of the bond, carbon monoxide is not easily dissociated from hemoglobin.

Assessment findings for clients with carbon monoxide poisoning depend on the percentage of hemoglobin saturated with carbon monoxide. An outstanding clinical feature is the absence of cyanosis. The skin of carbon monoxide victims can appear normal or cherry red. When 10% or less of the hemoglobin is saturated with carbon dioxide, there are usually no symptoms. If 10% to 20% of the hemoglobin is saturated, the client complains of a headache, which is the result of cerebral vasodilation. A 20% to 30% saturation causes chest pain as a result of myocardial hypoxia. When 30% to 40% of the hemoglobin is saturated, the client experiences a severe headache, chest pain, weakness, nausea, and vomiting. As the amount of hemoglobin saturated with carbon monoxide increases, the client's heart rate and respiratory rate increase. When the hemoglobin is more than 50% saturated, Cheyne-Stokes respiration, coma, and death may result (Luce, Tyler, and Pierson, 1984).

Treatment of carbon monoxide poisoning includes the administration of high concentrations of oxygen. The objective of treatment is to displace the carbon monoxide from the hemoglobin. This displacement occurs in direct proportion to the arterial concentration of oxygen. As arterial oxygenation increases, carbon monoxide is more rapidly displaced from the blood.

DECREASED INSPIRED OXYGEN CONCENTRATIONS

Whenever the concentration of inspired oxygen declines, the oxygen-carrying capacity of the blood is decreased. Decreases in inspired oxygen concentration (FIO_2) can be caused by an upper or lower airway obstruction, decreased environmental oxygen (as occurs at high altitudes), or decreased inspiration as the result of an incorrect oxygen concentration setting on respiratory therapy equipment.

An airway obstruction is a barrier that limits the amount of inspired oxygen delivered to the alveoli. As a result the amount of oxygen available for diffusion into the blood is decreased.

High altitudes lower the inspiratory oxygen concentration because the atmospheric oxygen is at a lower concentration. People who reside at high altitudes adapt to the lowered atmospheric oxygen by increasing hemoglobin production.

An incorrect oxygen flow rate setting on oxygen therapy equipment can cause decreases in the inspired oxygen concentration. To avoid such problems the nurse should determine that the oxygen therapy is at the correct rate, by the correct route, for the correct client. Oxygen should be treated as a drug, and the "five rights" of drug administration should be followed (see Chapter 32).

DECREASED CARDIAC OUTPUT

Decreases in cardiac output reduce the perfusion of the ventilated regions of the lung. As a result, there is a decrease in the amount of oxygen circulating to the peripheral tissues. Common factors that decrease cardiac output are hypovolemia and left-sided heart failure.

HYPOVOLEMIA. Hypovolemia is a reduced circulating blood volume resulting from extracellular fluid losses. If the loss is significant, the amount of fluid available for circulation is diminished. The body attempts to adapt to hypovolemia by increasing the heart rate and peripheral vasoconstriction in an effort to raise cardiac output.

LEFT-SIDED HEART FAILURE. Left-sided heart failure is an abnormal cardiac condition characterized by impaired function of the left side of the heart and by elevated pressure and congestion in the pulmonary veins and capillaries. If the failure of the left ventricle is significant, the amount of blood ejected from the left ventricle drops greatly. As a result, the cardiac output also falls.

The delivery of oxygen-rich hemoglobin to the tissues depends on the cardiac output. Decreases in cardiac output can cause tissue hypoxia, which may result in lower activity tolerance, breathlessness, dizziness, and confusion.

INCREASED METABOLIC RATE

Increases in the metabolic activity of the body result in an increased oxygen demand. If the body is unable to meet this demand, the level of oxygenation declines. An increased metabolic rate is a normal response of the body to pregnancy, wound healing, and exercise, because the body in these situations is building tissue, that is, the fetus, new tissue to replace damaged tissue, or increased muscle mass, respectively. Most people are able to meet the greater need for oxygen and do not display any signs of an oxygen deficit.

The increased metabolism of the body during fever or infection is an adaptive response. The body is attempting to meet the increased need for energy. If the infection or febrile state persists, the metabolic rate remains high and the body begins to break down protein stores without adequate replacement of protein. Because the oxygen demand continues as a result of decreased muscle mass and muscle wasting, the client may not be able to carry out the work of breathing and may eventually display signs and symptoms of hypoxemia.

CONDITIONS AFFECTING CHEST WALL MOVEMENT

Any factor or condition that reduces chest wall movement can result in decreased ventilation. If the diaphragm cannot fully descend with breathing, the volume of inspired air decreases and less oxygen is delivered to the alveoli and subsequently to the tissues.

PREGNANCY. As the fetus grows within the pregnant woman, the greater size of the uterus pushes the stomach upward against the diaphragm. During the last trimester of pregnancy the inspiratory capacity of the pregnant woman declines. Thus she may experience some shortness of breath on exertion and may be easily fatigued. However, this condition is temporary. After the pregnancy the diaphragm can again descend fully and the lung volumes return to normal.

OBESITY. Obese clients often have a heavy lower thorax and abdomen, which severely reduces lung volumes, particularly in the recumbent and supine positions. In some obese clients an obesity-hypoventilation syndrome develops in which oxygenation is decreased and carbon dioxide is retained, resulting in daytime sleepiness. The body tries to compensate for the decreased oxygenation by increasing red blood cell production. This results in polycythemia, an abnormally increased number of red blood cells.

The obese client is also susceptible to pneumonia following an upper respiratory tract infection because the lungs cannot be fully expanded and pulmonary secretions are not mobilized in the lower lobes. The postoperative or immobilized obese client is at high risk for hypostatic bronchopneumonia. Pulmonary hygiene measures should always be included in the nursing care plan in an attempt to reduce the risks of hypostatic bronchopneumonia.

MUSCULOSKELETAL ABNORMALITIES

Musculoskeletal impairments in the thoracic region reduce oxygenation. Such impairments may result from abnormal structural configurations, trauma, muscular diseases, or diseases of the central nervous system.

ABNORMAL STRUCTURAL CONFIGURATIONS. Abnormal structural configurations affecting oxygenation include those that affect the rib cage, such as pectus excavatum, and those that affect the vertebral column. Pectus excavatum is a depression of the sternum that interferes with complete lung expansion. Kyphosis is an abnormal condition of the vertebral column characterized by increased convexity of the thoracic spine as viewed from the side. This abnormality produces a structural barrier to lung expansion, and the angle of curvature can progress with time, resulting in severe hypoventilation and hypoxemia.

TRAUMA. Trauma to the chest wall may also impede inspiration. The person with multiple rib fractures develops a flail chest, a condition in which the fractures cause instability in part of the chest wall and paradoxical breathing, with the lung underlying the inspired area contracting on inspiration and bulging on expiration. If uncorrected this asynchronous chest wall movement can result in hypoxia.

Incisional trauma to the chest wall or upper abdomen may also decrease chest wall movement and oxygenation. The client may breathe shallowly in an attempt to minimize chest wall movement in order to avoid pain, thereby increasing the risk for hypostatic bronchopneumonia. Certain analgesics may also decrease the client's respiratory rate. Therefore, with clients who have had surgery of the chest or upper abdomen, the nurse must correctly use analgesics along with the techniques of coughing and deep breathing. To minimize the pain associated with deep breathing and coughing the nurse may administer the analgesic 20 to 30 minutes before the procedure. The risks of pain and hypostatic bronchopneumonia are reduced by having the client turn, cough, and deep breathe at the time of the analgesic's peak effect (see Chapter 47).

MUSCLE DISEASES. Muscle diseases such as muscular dystrophy ultimately affect the oxygenation of tissues. If muscular disease decreases the client's ability to expand and contract the chest, ventilation is impaired and atelectasis can occur. Frequently the cause of death in these clients is pneumonia and severe hypoxemia.

NERVOUS SYSTEM DISEASES. Myasthenia gravis, Guillain-Barré syndrome, and poliomyelitis are nervous system diseases that can affect respiratory functioning. Myasthenia gravis interferes with the normal transmission of impulses from the nerves to the muscles. The disease involves the whole body, including the muscles of respiration.

Guillain-Barré syndrome and poliomyelitis cause inflammation and paralysis of muscle groups. Guillain-Barré syndrome usually results in an ascending type of paralysis, which can be reversed, leaving the client with little or no residual paralysis. If the paralysis ascends to the thoracic region, the respiratory muscles become paralyzed. Poliomyelitis may lead to generalized or localized paralysis. As with Guillain-Barré syndrome the paralysis may be reversed, but poliomyelitis usually leaves more residual paralysis.

CENTRAL NERVOUS SYSTEM ALTERATIONS. Diseases or trauma involving the central nervous system, specifically the medulla oblongata and spinal cord, may result in impaired respiration. When the medulla oblongata is affected, neural regulation of respiration is damaged and abnormal breathing patterns may develop. Damage to the spinal cord can affect respiration in two ways. If the phrenic nerve is damaged, the diaphragm may not descend, thus reducing inspiratory lung volumes and causing hypoxemia. Spinal cord trauma below the fifth cervical vertebra usually leaves the phrenic nerve intact but damages nerves that innervate the intercostal muscles, resulting in an inability of the chest to expand in the anterior-posterior diameter. These clients are at risk for atelectasis and subsequent pneumonia.

INFLUENCES OF CHRONIC DISEASE

The level of oxygenation can be decreased as a direct consequence of chronic disease, as with cardiopulmonary disease, or as a secondary effect, as with anemia in a client with osteoarthritis.

Chronic illness may also affect oxygenation as an indirect result of depression. A depressed client may not be interested in preparing meals or eating. When the dietary intake declines, the production of hemoglobin is diminished, and the oxygen-carrying capacity of the blood declines.

Age

The developmental stage of the client and the normal aging process can affect the level of tissue oxygenation.

PREMATURE INFANT

A premature infant is at risk for hyaline membrane disease, which is thought to be caused by a surfactant deficiency. The surfactant-synthesizing ability of the lungs develops during later stages of fetal development and therefore may be lacking in premature infants (Groër and Shekleton, 1983).

INFANT AND TODDLER

The infant and toddler are at risk for upper respiratory tract infections as a result of frequent exposure to other children. In addition, during the teething process some infants develop nasal congestion, which encourages bacterial growth and increases the potential for a respiratory tract infection.

Upper respiratory tract infections are usually not dangerous, and the infant or toddler recovers with little difficulty. However, in children of this age group airway obstructions can develop as a result of respiratory tract infections. The two most common airway diseases are bronchiolitis and acute epiglottitis. Both of these are acute conditions with rapid onset, and the child shows symptoms of hypoxia. Fortunately, most infants and toddlers respond rapidly to treatment with antibiotics.

SCHOOL-AGE CHILD AND ADOLESCENT

School-age children and adolescents are exposed to respiratory infections and respiratory risk factors such as smoking. The healthy child usually does not experience any adverse pulmonary effects from respiratory infections. The person who starts smoking in adolescence and continues to smoke through adulthood into middle age, however, has an increased risk for cardiopulmonary disease.

OLDER ADULT

The respiratory system undergoes changes throughout the aging process. The connective tissue and bronchial tree undergo structural changes as the lungs lose some of their elasticity. The alveoli are often enlarged and the bronchial ducts are dilated (Groër and Shekleton, 1983).

Both ventilation and the transfer of respiratory gases decline with age. The normal arterial oxygen concentration also declines. Osteoporotic changes of the thoracic cage and kyphosis of the vertebrae occur normally with aging. With these changes the lungs are unable to expand fully, leading to lower oxygenation levels.

The normal changes in the lungs during the aging process increase the elderly adult's susceptibility to severe complications of infections, stress, and cardiac problems. Minor pulmonary infections can set off a series of responses leading eventually to cardiopulmonary dysfunction.

Life-Style

A person's life-style may directly or indirectly affect the body's ability to meet oxygen requirements. Life-style factors that influence respiratory functioning include nutrition, exercise, cigarette smoking, substance abuse, and stress.

NUTRITION

Nutritional intake can affect respiratory function in three ways. First, severe obesity can decrease lung expansion because of the pressure of the abdomen against the diaphragm. The decline in lung expansion may be very evident when the obese person attempts to lie flat. In fact, such a client may be unable to tolerate the supine position because of "air hunger" and may need support from several pillows to sleep. Second, the malnourished client may experience respiratory muscle wasting that increases the work of breathing. The client may have a low activity tolerance demonstrated by dyspnea on exertion. The muscle weakness may also decrease the ability to cough productively, putting the client at risk for the accumulation of pulmonary secretions. Finally, both obese and malnourished clients are at risk for anemia, which decreases the blood's oxygen-carrying capacity.

EXERCISE

Any type of exercise increases the body's metabolic activity and thus the body's oxygen demands. During exercise the respiratory rate and depth of respirations increase, enabling the person to inhale more oxygen and expire excess carbon dioxide.

A physical exercise program benefits the client in several ways (see Chapter 31). People who exercise regularly have a lower pulse rate and blood pressure, an increased blood flow, and greater oxygen extraction by working muscles. Fully conditioned people can increase their oxygen consumption by 10% to 20% because of the increased cardiac output. Regular exercise also benefits the client psychologically by providing the ability to perform activities of daily living and increasing the person's sense of well-being (Luce, Tyler, and Pierson, 1984).

CIGARETTE SMOKING

Cigarette smoking is associated with a number of diseases, including lung cancer. The risk of lung cancer is 60 times greater for a person who smokes two packs of cigarettes a day than for someone who has never smoked. The mortality for persons with lung cancer is approximately 90%, and the illness is frequently diagnosed only when it has reached an advanced stage (Groër and Shekleton, 1983).

Cigarette smoking may lead to cardiovascular disease. The inhaled nicotine causes vasoconstriction of peripheral and coronary blood vessels. Thus cigarette smoking can worsen peripheral vascular and coronary artery diseases.

Smoking is also associated with recurrent respiratory tract infections, especially emphysema and chronic bronchitis. Smoking itself damages the ciliary clearance mechanism within the lungs and paralyzes the cilia. As a result, the cilia are unable to clear mucus from the airways; accumulation of mucus leads to the development of chronic bronchitis.

SUBSTANCE ABUSE

Excessive use of alcohol or drugs can impair tissue oxygenation in two ways. First, the person who chronically abuses substances frequently has a poor nutritional intake. With the resultant decrease in iron-rich foods, hemoglobin production declines. Second, excessive use of large quantities of alcohol and certain drugs can depress the respiratory center in the central nervous system. The rate and depth of inspiration are reduced, decreasing the amount of oxygen inhaled. Thus less oxygen is available for delivery to the tissues. Chapter 45 discusses more fully the physiological problems associated with substance abuse.

ANXIETY

A continuous state of severe anxiety increases the body's oxygen demand. The body responds to anxiety and other stresses by an increased rate and depth of respiration. Most people can adapt to this increased oxygen need, but some, particularly those with chronic illnesses or acute life-threatening illnesses such as a myocardial infarction, cannot tolerate the oxygen demands associated with anxiety. These clients may require pharmacological interventions to reduce their anxiety. For example, a client may have a myocardial infarction because of an occlusion of a coronary artery, which blocks the blood supply and oxygen to a region of the myocardium and causes ischemia. The body's response to any anxiety in this client competes with the injured myocardium for available oxygen. To help protect the myocardium from further damage, the nurse intervenes to reduce the client's anxiety.

Environment

The environment in which a client lives and works can also influence the level of oxygenation. The incidence of pulmonary disease is higher in smoggy urban areas than in rural areas. In addition, children or family members of smokers have a greater risk for respiratory tract infections or chronic illnesses because they passively inhale smoke.

A client's workplace similarly may increase the risk for pulmonary disease. Occupational pollutants include asbestos, talcum powder, dust, and airborne fibers. Farm workers in dry regions of the southwestern United States are at risk for coccidioidomycosis, a fungal disease caused by the inhalation of spores of the windborne bacterium *Coccidioides immitis*.

Finally, the altitude of the work or home environment can affect oxygenation. In high altitudes the atmospheric oxygen pressure is lower, resulting in a lower percentage of inspired oxygen and decreased concentration of arterial oxygen. The body adapts to high altitudes by increasing the heart rate, the respiratory rate, and erythrocyte production. After living at a high altitude for a time people usually become acclimated and can tolerate exercise without any adverse consequences.

■ ■ ■ ■ ■

Knowledge of factors that can affect normal respiratory functioning helps the nurse anticipate actual or potential respiratory alterations. For example, if the nurse anticipates anemia in a client with a chronic disease, the nurse may assess the client's activity tolerance and increase the dietary intake of iron-rich foods, which will assist the body in its production of hemoglobin.

Similarly, a nurse who works in a high-altitude region may design a more gradual progressive exercise program for a person with chronic pulmonary disease than would be used in a low-altitude area, or may instruct clients with cardiopulmonary disease to use supplemental oxygen during exercise.

Alterations in Respiratory Functioning

Alterations in respiratory function are caused by illnesses and conditions that affect ventilation or oxygen transport. The three primary alterations are hyperventilation, hypoventilation, and hypoxia.

Hyperventilation

The term "hyperventilation" is often used to refer to alveolar hyperventilation. Alveolar hyperventilation is a state of ventilation in excess of that required to maintain normal carbon dioxide levels in the body tissues (Groër and Shekleton, 1983). The carbon dioxide level in arterial blood falls because carbon dioxide is expired in larger than normal amounts. Because less carbon dioxide is available to combine with water to form carbonic acid, respiratory alkalosis can occur (see Chapter 43).

Hyperventilation can be induced by anxiety or severe stress. Anxiety attacks can lead to hyperventilation to the point of unconsciousness. Hyperventilation can also be induced by injuries to or infections of the respiratory center in the medulla.

Fever can result in hyperventilation as a result of compensatory mechanisms within the body. For each degree Fahrenheit increase in body temperature, there is a 7% increase in the metabolic rate (Groër and Shekleton, 1983). Higher metabolic rates increase carbon dioxide production, and rising carbon dioxide levels in the blood lead to increased respiration in clients without chronic obstructive pulmonary disease.

Hyperventilation may also be chemically induced. Salicylate poisoning causes excessive stimulation of the respiratory center because of the body's attempt to compensate for carbon dioxide excess. Amphetamines also increase ventilation, primarily by raising the body's metabolic rate.

Last, hyperventilation can occur as the body tries to compensate for metabolic acidosis. Ventilation increases in order to reduce the amount of carbon dioxide available to form carbonic acid (see Chapter 43).

Alveolar hyperventilation can produce many signs and symptoms that can be identified by assessment

---

Signs and Symptoms of Alveolar Hyperventilation

- Shortness of breath
- Chest pain
- Dizziness
- Light-headedness
- Decreased concentration
- Paresthesia
- Numbness (extremities, circumoral)
- Tinnitus
- Blurred vision
- Disorientation

(see box on p. 1169). Blood flow to the major organs is diminished as a result of the vasoconstrictor effect of low carbon dioxide and reduced cardiac output. The hemoglobin does not release oxygen to tissues as readily, and tissue hypoxia results. The client may experience the subjective symptoms of shortness of breath and chest pain. In addition, because the brain is extremely sensitive to hypoxia, dizziness, light-headedness, inability to concentrate, tinnitus, blurred vision, and disorientation can develop. As the symptoms worsen, the client may become more agitated and the respiratory rate may further increase.

The objectives of therapy for hyperventilation are to treat the underlying cause and to help the client retain more carbon dioxide. Treatment of the underlying cause may include correcting an acid-base imbalance, reducing a fever, or calming the client. The client can retain carbon dioxide by breathing into a paper bag, thus rebreathing expired carbon dioxide.

Hypoventilation

Alveolar hypoventilation is a respiratory rate insufficient to prevent carbon dioxide retention. Hypoventilation results in hypercapnia, elevated carbon dioxide levels in the blood, and hypoxemia. Because too much carbon dioxide is available, carbonic acid is increased and respiratory acidosis occurs (see Chapter 43).

Hypoventilation is caused by a pathophysiological mechanism. The central nervous system may be affected, as with a drug overdose or trauma to the brainstem, or the lungs themselves may be affected. Severe atelectasis can produce hypoventilation. Atelectasis is a collapse of the alveoli that prevents the normal respiratory exchange of oxygen and carbon dioxide. If enough alveoli collapse, less of the lung is capable of being ventilated and hypoventilation occurs.

The inappropriate administration of oxygen can also result in hypoventilation. Clients with chronic obstructive pulmonary disease have adapted to a higher than normal carbon dioxide level, and their only stimulus to breathe is the hypoxic drive. The administration of high concentrations of oxygen, greater than 24% to 28%, will obliterate the hypoxic drive. Thus the elimination of the stimulus to breathe depresses or in some cases suppresses respiratory function and hypoventilation occurs.

The client with hypoventilation may have many signs and symptoms that are revealed through physical assessment (see the boxed material). Dizziness, headache, and confusion are caused by the vasodilator effect of carbon dioxide in the brain. A throbbing occipital headache may occur and be most intense on awakening in the morning. Behavioral

> ### Signs and Symptoms of Alveolar Hypoventilation
>
> - Dizziness
> - Headache (may be occipital only on awakening)
> - Lethargy
> - Disorientation
> - Decreased cooperation
> - Cardiac arrhythmias
> - Electrolyte imbalances
> - Convulsions
> - Coma
> - Cardiac arrest

changes may include lethargy, disorientation, and lack of cooperation. In addition, these clients may have cardiac arrhythmias and electrolyte imbalances.

If hypoventilation is not treated, the client's status can rapidly decline, and convulsions, unconsciousness, and death can result.

The goals of treatment for hypoventilation are first to restore or maintain optimal ventilatory function, second to improve tissue oxygenation, and third to restore or maintain acid-base balance (Groër and Shekleton, 1983).

Hypoxia

Hypoxia is a state of inadequate cellular oxygenation that results from a deficiency in the delivery or the use of oxygen at the cellular level (Groër and Shekleton, 1983). Hypoxia can be caused by (1) a decreased hemoglobin level and lowered oxygen-carrying capacity of the blood; (2) a diminished concentration of inspired oxygen as may occur at high altitudes; (3) inability of the tissues to extract oxygen from the blood as with cyanide poisoning; (4) decreased diffusion of oxygen from the alveoli to the blood as with pneumonia; and (5) poor tissue perfusion as with shock.

The clinical signs and symptoms of hypoxia include apprehension, inability to concentrate, declining level of consciousness, dizziness, and behavioral changes (see the box opposite). The hypoxic client is unable to lie down and appears fatigued and agitated. Changes in vital signs include an increased pulse rate and increased rate and depth of respiration. However, as the hypoxia worsens, the respiratory rate may decline as a result of fatigue. During the early stages of hypoxia the blood pressure is elevated unless the hy-

Signs and Symptoms of Hypoxia

- Apprehension, anxiety
- Decreased ability to concentrate
- Decreased level of consciousness
- Increased fatigue
- Dizziness
- Behavioral changes
- Increased pulse rate
- Increased rate and depth of respiration
- Elevated blood pressure
- Cardiac arrhythmias
- Pallor
- Cyanosis
- Clubbing
- Dyspnea

poxia is caused by shock. Cyanosis, a blue discoloration of the skin and mucous membranes caused by the presence of desaturated hemoglobin in capillaries, is a late sign of hypoxia. Cyanosis observed in the tongue and soft palate, where blood flow is high, indicates hypoxemia. Cyanosis elsewhere, as in the fingers, may merely reflect stagnant blood flow (Luce, Tyler, and Pierson, 1984). Cyanosis is apparent when 5 g of hemoglobin per 100 ml of blood has been reduced to deoxyhemoglobin and has reached the superficial capillaries (Groër and Shekleton, 1983). The presence or absence of cyanosis, however, is not an absolute indicator of oxygenation status.

Dyspnea is another clinical sign of hypoxia. Dyspnea is shortness of breath or a difficulty in breathing. Pathological dyspnea must be differentiated from physiological dyspnea, which is the not unpleasant shortness of breath experienced by healthy people after exercise or excitement. Pathological breathlessness is a distressing sensation of not being able to catch one's breath (Groër and Shekleton, 1983).

Hypoxia is a life-threatening condition. Left untreated, it can produce cardiac arrhythmias that may result in death. Hypoxia is treated by the administration of oxygen, or by treatment of the underlying cause, such as shock or pneumonia.

Assessment

The nursing assessment of a client's respiratory functioning includes a nursing history, physical examination, and collection of laboratory data and specimens.

Nursing History

The nursing history described here focuses on the client's ability to meet oxygen needs. The complete nursing history is described in Chapter 7. The nursing history for respiratory function includes cough, shortness of breath, wheezing, pain, environmental exposures, frequency of respiratory tract infections, pulmonary risk factors, and medications.

COUGH

Cough is a sudden, audible expulsion of air from the lungs. The person breathes in, the glottis is partially closed, and the accessory muscles of expiration contract to expel the air forcibly from respiratory passages. Coughing is a protective reflex to clear the trachea, bronchi, and lungs of irritants and secretions. In addition, the cough reflex prevents the aspiration of foreign bodies into the lungs.

The presence of a cough is difficult to evaluate. Almost everyone sometimes experiences periods of coughing. Furthermore, clients with a chronic cough tend to deny, underestimate, or minimize their coughing, often because they are so accustomed to coughing that they are truly unaware of how frequently it occurs. A family member or significant other may provide more objective information about the client's frequency of coughing.

Once the nurse determines that the client has a cough, the cough must be identified as productive or nonproductive and its frequency must be assessed. A *productive cough* is one that results in sputum. Sputum is material coughed up from the lungs that may be expectorated through the mouth. It contains mucus, cellular debris, and microorganisms, and it may contain pus or blood. If a client is producing sputum, the nurse must obtain information regarding its color, consistency, odor, and the presence of blood (see the box on p. 1172). The nurse should also inquire if the sputum is produced at all times, just on rising from bed, or only when the client has a cold. If the sputum is discolored, the nurse should inquire if the sputum clears with coughing. Occasionally yellow sputum produced in the early morning may clear with the second or third cough. The nurse inquires whether the amount of sputum has recently increased or decreased. The client should try to produce some sputum so the nurse can inspect it for color, consistency, and odor.

Coughing is classified as to the time when the client most frequently coughs. Clients with chronic sinusitis may cough only in the early morning or immediately after rising from a sleeping position. This coughing clears the airway of mucus resulting from sinus drainage. Clients with chronic bronchitis generally produce sputum all day, although greater amounts are pro-

---

Range of Sputum Characteristics

COLOR
- Clear
- White
- Yellow
- Green
- Brown
- Red
- Streaked with blood

CONSISTENCY
- Frothy
- Watery
- Tenacious, thick

ODOR
- None
- Foul

BLOOD
- All the time
- Occasionally
- Early morning

---

duced after rising from a semirecumbent or flat position. This is the result of the dependent accumulation of sputum in the airways associated with reduced mobility (see Chapter 31).

Finally, the nurse should ask if the client has ever noticed streaks or flecks of blood in the sputum. Hemoptysis, the coughing up of blood from the respiratory tract, often occurs with minor upper respiratory tract infections or bronchitis. Bright red sputum may indicate *Aspergillus* infection, lung abscess, tuberculosis, bronchogenic carcinoma, or congestive heart failure. When a client reports bloody or blood-tinged sputum, diagnostic tests, such as examination of sputum specimens, chest x-ray examinations, bronchoscopy, or other x-ray studies, should be performed to determine the cause.

DYSPNEA

Dyspnea, or shortness of breath, can be a subjective finding (the client states that he feels short of breath) or an objective finding (exaggerated respiratory effort, use of the accessory muscles of respiration, flaring of the nares, and an extreme increase in the rate and depth of respirations) (Groër and Shekleton, 1983). Dyspnea is not always a direct reflection of the state of tissue oxygenation but may be a symptom of a discrepancy between the need for respiration and the body's ability to meet that need. The perception and occurrence of dyspnea depend on the client's state of mind, the concentrations of carbon dioxide and oxygen in the blood, and the adequacy of ventilation, perfusion, and transport of respiratory gases (Groër and Shekleton, 1983).

The nursing history of dyspnea includes the circumstances of its occurrence, such as with exertion, stress, or respiratory tract infection. The nurse also determines whether the client's perception of dyspnea affects the ability to lie flat. The client with true dyspnea is unable to lie flat. Orthopnea is an abnormal condition in which the person must sit, stand, or use multiple pillows when lying down in order to breathe. The presence of orthopnea is usually quantified, such as two- or three-pillow orthopnea. This means that the client perceives shortness of breath unless he uses two or three pillows for sleeping.

WHEEZING

Wheezing is a form of rhonchus and is characterized by a high-pitched musical quality. It is caused by the high-velocity movement of air through a narrowed airway. Wheezing may be associated with asthma and acute bronchitis. Clients who have periods of wheezing can usually describe when they wheeze and if the wheeze is present on inspiration or expiration.

The nurse should also obtain information about any precipitating factors such as the presence of a respiratory infection, allergens, exercise, or stress. Likewise, the nurse should determine what methods the client uses to relieve the wheezing, such as rest or sitting upright. If the client uses a medication for relief, the nurse should determine what medication is used.

PAIN

Pain associated with respiration must be evaluated with regard to location, duration, radiation, and effect on respiration. Pleuritic chest pain is peripheral in location and may radiate to the scapular regions. It is worsened by inspiratory maneuvers, such as coughing, yawning, or sighing. Clients often describe pleuritic pain as knifelike. It lasts from a minute to hours and is always associated with inspiration.

Musculoskeletal pain may be present following exercise, rib trauma, or prolonged coughing episodes. This type of pain is also aggravated by inspiratory movements and may easily be confused with pleuritic chest pain (Smith, 1982).

ENVIRONMENTAL EXPOSURE

Environmental exposure to many inhaled substances is closely linked with respiratory disease. The nurse should investigate potential exposures in the client's home and workplace.

The most common environmental exposure involves cigarette smoking. The nurse should determine whether a client who is a nonsmoker is passively exposed to smoke. Passive smoke exposure occurs when the client breathes air containing the smoke from another person's cigarette.

An employment history should be obtained to assess potential exposure to substances such as asbestos, dust, fibers, or toxic fumes. Exposure to other substances may occur during travel. Schistosomiasis can be acquired during travel to Asia, Africa, the Caribbean, and South America. Coccidioidomycosis can be acquired in southwestern desert regions of the United States. Histoplasmosis may result from exposure in chicken farms and great river valleys, such as the Ohio and Mississippi valleys (Smith, 1982).

RESPIRATORY INFECTIONS

In the nursing history the nurse obtains information about the frequency and duration of respiratory tract infections. Although everyone occasionally experiences a cold, with some people the common cold frequently results in bronchitis or pneumonia. The nurse also asks about any known exposure to tuberculosis and inquires about the results of any tuberculin skin test the client has had.

RISK FACTORS

The nurse must also investigate familial and environmental risk factors. A family history of cancer, particularly lung cancer, or cardiovascular diseases should be noted. If the client's family has such a history, it is necessary to document which blood relatives have had the disease and their present level of health or their age at time of death.

Other family risk factors include the presence of infectious diseases, particularly tuberculosis. The nurse should determine who in the client's household has been infected and the status of their treatment.

Last, a complete employment history is necessary to identify exposure to substances such as asbestos, coal, or dust. These data are particularly important with middle-aged and elderly adults who may have worked in places that were not regulated to protect the workers from carcinogens.

MEDICATIONS

The last component of the nursing history should be medications the client is using. These include prescribed, over-the-counter, and illicit drugs and substances. Such medications may have adverse effects in themselves or by interaction with other drugs. A person using a prescribed bronchodilator drug, for example, may decide that using an over-the-counter inhalant as well will be beneficial. This product may react with the prescribed medication by potentiating or decreasing its effect.

Illicit drugs, particularly parenterally administered narcotics, are often diluted with talcum powder. Injections of these drugs can cause pulmonary disorders as a result of the irritant effect of talcum powder on the lung tissues.

■ ■ ■ ■ ■

The nursing health history of the respiratory system provides the nurse with a data base for the subsequent physical examination. As with the total nursing history, this history helps to identify factors that may affect the client's present and future level of health.

Physical Examination

The physical examination performed to assess the client's level of tissue oxygenation includes evaluation of the entire cardiopulmonary system. The skills of assessment, inspection, palpation, and percussion are used. The examination described here focuses on the client's respiratory status more specifically than the general physical assessment described in Chapter 29.

INSPECTION

Using inspection techniques the nurse observes the client's skin color, general appearance, level of consciousness, breathing patterns, and chest wall movement.

Breathing patterns include respiratory rate, depth, and rhythm (Table 41-1). Breathing patterns can be altered by exercise, obesity, and an increased metabolic rate. Certain breathing patterns may indicate a change in the client's level of tissue oxygenation or a change in the acid-base balance.

Chest wall movements are observed to determine if the chest expands symmetrically or if abnormal paradoxical breathing is present. Abnormal chest wall movements can occur with a disease process or as a result of chest wall trauma (Table 41-2).

PALPATION

Palpation of the chest provides assessment data in several areas. Palpation documents the type and amount of thoracic excursion, elicits any areas of tenderness on light and deep palpation, and can identify the presence of tactile fremitus and rales. With palpation the nurse can locate the cardiac point of maximal impulse (PMI). Palpation also allows the nurse to feel for any abnormal masses or lumps in the axilla and breast tissue (see Chapter 29).

PERCUSSION

With percussion the nurse can detect the presence of fluid in the lung fields. Fluid in the lungs is an abnormal finding that occurs with pulmonary infiltrations, pneumonia, or atelectasis. When fluid is present, the sound produced by percussion is dullness (Chapter 29).

TABLE 41-1

Assessment of Breathing Patterns

Pattern	Causes
Eupnea—normal respiratory rate; an adult range of 12-22 breaths/minute; normal tidal volume is 5-7 ml/kg body weight*	
Tachypnea—increased respiratory rate above the client's normal rate; characterized by quick shallow respirations	Exercise, pregnancy, fever, pulmonary diseases, anxiety, neurological conditions, airway obstruction
Bradypnea—decreased respiratory rate below the client's normal rate	Drug overdose, central nervous system dysfunction, airway obstruction
Kussmaul respiration—abnormally deep, very rapid sighing type of respiration; tidal volume is increased as well as rate	Diabetic ketoacidosis
Ataxic respirations—uncoordinated respiratory patterns; no coordinated rate or depth of respiration	Central nervous system disorders
Cheyne-Stokes respiration—breathing pattern characterized by alternating periods of apnea and deep rapid breathing; cycle begins with slow, shallow breaths that gradually increase to abnormal depth and rate; respiration gradually subsides as breathing slows and becomes shallow	Congestive heart failure, bronchopneumonia, drug overdose, sleep, central nervous system damage

*Data from Luce, J.M., Tyler, M.L., and Pierson, D.J.: Intensive respiratory care, Philadelphia, 1984, W.B. Saunders Co.

If the nurse identifies areas of dullness on percussion, nursing interventions should be directed toward mobilizing pulmonary secretions and maintaining a patent airway. Fluid in the lungs provides a medium for bacterial growth and increases the risk of infection.

Dullness on percussion may also indicate a pleural effusion, which is the presence of fluid in the pleural space. Pleural effusions may result from an infectious process, such as tuberculosis, or from a neoplasm in the lung. The fluid is removed by thoracentesis. Fol-

TABLE 41-2

Assessment of Abnormal Chest Wall Movement

Abnormality	Cause
Retraction—visible sinking in soft tissues of chest between and around firmer tissue of cartilaginous and bony ribs; retractions have a specific beginning point and worsen and there is a need for increased inspiratory effort; retractions may be observed at intercostal space, intraclavicular space, trachea, and substernally*	Any condition that causes increased inspiratory effort (e.g., airway obstruction, asthma, tracheobronchitis)
Paradoxical breathing—asynchronous breathing; chest contracts during inspiration and expands during expiration	Flail chest

*Infants can experience sternal and substernal retractions with only slight inspiratory effort because of their chest pliability.

lowing removal and resolution of the effusion, the lung expands and the client's dyspnea declines.

AUSCULTATION

Auscultation is used to identify abnormal lung sounds (see Chapter 29). Adventitious sounds occur with collapse of a lung region, the presence of fluid in the lung field, or airway obstruction. Auscultation is also used to evaluate the response of the client to nursing interventions for improving respiratory status.

■ ■ ■ ■ ■

Physical examination enables the nurse to document abnormalities described in the nursing history as well as to identify abnormalities not included in the nursing history. In addition, repeated physical examination provides objective criteria for evaluating nursing care. The use of diagnostic tests to gather further information completes the assessment data base.

Diagnostic Tests

Many different diagnostic tests can be performed to obtain data for the respiratory assessment. Diagnostic tests can determine the adequacy of ventilation and oxygenation, allow the inspection of structures of the respiratory system, and determine the presence of abnormal cells or infection in the respiratory tract.

TESTS TO MEASURE ADEQUACY OF VENTILATION AND OXYGENATION

PULMONARY FUNCTION TESTS. Pulmonary function tests are procedures for determining the ability of the lungs to exchange oxygen and carbon dioxide efficiently. Basic ventilation studies are performed with a spirometer and recording device as the client breathes through a mouthpiece into a connecting tube. Measurements include tidal volume, inspiratory reserve volume, residual volume, and force expiration volume (see Fig. 41-2).

Pulmonary function tests are usually performed in a pulmonary function laboratory. The nurse prepares the client by explaining the procedure. A nose clip is used to prevent air from being inhaled or exhaled through the nose. The client is instructed to breathe through a mouthpiece attached to a spirometer for measuring lung volume. The client is asked at appropriate times in the test to inhale or exhale as much air as possible. The nurse seeks the client's cooperation to ensure accurate results.

Preparing the client by providing information about the procedure decreases anxiety and encourages cooperative participation. Usually no other preparation is needed, although it may be beneficial if the client does not eat a large meal immediately before the test. A large meal may diminish the client's ability to inhale deeply, and the results of the test may be inaccurate.

ARTERIAL BLOOD GASES. Arterial blood gas measurement is performed in conjunction with pulmonary function tests to determine the hydrogen ion concentration, partial pressure of carbon dioxide and oxygen concentration, and oxyhemoglobin saturation. Arterial blood gas tests provide information about the diffusion of gas across the alveolar capillary membrane and the adequacy of tissue oxygenation (see Chapter 43).

COMPLETE BLOOD COUNT. The complete blood count is a determination of the number of red and white blood cells per cubic millimeter of blood. The nurse obtains a venous blood sample by using the venipuncture technique (see Chapter 42).

The complete blood count includes the measurement of hemoglobin. Hemoglobin is the complex protein-iron compound in the blood that carries oxygen to the cells from the lungs and carbon dioxide from the cells to the lungs. Each erythrocyte, or red blood cell (RBC), contains 200 to 300 molecules of hemoglobin. Each molecule of hemoglobin contains several molecules of heme, and each molecule of heme can carry one molecule of oxygen.

The normal values for a complete blood count vary with age and sex. The newborn's hemoglobin level is quite high, from 14 to 20 g/100 ml of blood. This value declines during the first year of life to 11 to 14 g/100 ml. From age 1 year through puberty, the normal hemoglobin value ranges between 11 and 13 g/100 ml of blood. The normal value for adult men is 14 to 18 g/100 ml, and for adult women the normal value is 12 to 16 g/100 ml. The older adult is more likely to have deficiencies in hemoglobin as a result of the presence of chronic illness, decreased appetite, and nutritional deficiencies.

TESTS TO VISUALIZE STRUCTURES OF THE RESPIRATORY SYSTEM

CHEST X-RAY EXAMINATION. A chest x-ray examination consists of a roentgenogram of the thorax that allows the physician and nurse to observe the lung fields for fluid (such as occurs with pneumonia), for masses (as with lung cancer), for fractures (as with rib and clavicular fractures), and for the presence of other abnormal processes (such as tuberculosis).

A chest x-ray examination is a painless procedure, requiring only that the client hold his breath during inspiration. An expiratory film is taken occasionally.

BRONCHOSCOPY. Bronchoscopy is the visual examination of the trachea and bronchial tree. The standard rigid, tubular metal bronchoscope or the narrower, flexible fiberoptic bronchoscope may be used. Bronchoscopy is performed to obtain biopsy and fluid or sputum samples for examination. The procedure can also be used to remove mucus plugs or foreign bodies that have become lodged in the airways.

The client is maintained in a fasting state before bronchoscopy. As with many invasive procedures, there is a risk that the client may gag and vomit. Maintaining the client in a fasting state reduces the risk of vomiting and aspiration of stomach contents.

The nurse also administers proper medications before the procedure. A sedative is usually administered, and atropine may be used occasionally to reduce oral secretions. The nurse continues to observe the client after the procedure for signs and symptoms of respiratory distress or hypoxia.

LUNG SCAN. The most common lung scan is the computed tomogram (CT scan). CT scanning combines x-ray and computer technology. X-ray beams pass through a section or plane of the thorax from different angles, and the computer calculates tissue absorption and displays a printout and scan picture of the tissues showing the densities of various intrathoracic structures. A CT scan can identify abnormal masses by size and location. The CT scan cannot identify tissue type, which requires a biopsy.

CT scans are noninvasive and painless. The client usually requires no preprocedure preparation. Occasionally a contrast medium may be injected during the procedure to assist with the visualization of structures. If a contrast medium is ordered, venipuncture is used to gain access to the client's circulatory system.

TESTS TO DETERMINE THE PRESENCE OF ABNORMAL CELLS OR INFECTION IN THE RESPIRATORY TRACT

THROAT CULTURES. A throat culture sample is obtained by swabbing the oropharynx and tonsillar regions with a culture swab (see Chapter 33). The purpose of the throat culture is to determine the presence of pathogenic microorganisms and the antibiotics to which they are most sensitive.

When obtaining a throat culture sample, the nurse inserts the swab into the pharyngeal region and passes it along reddened areas and areas of exudate. Some clients have an active gag reflex, making it difficult to obtain the specimen. The gag reflex may be less active if the client is sitting straight and leaning slightly forward. In addition, the client may be able to control the gagging if informed that the procedure will take only a few seconds.

SPUTUM SPECIMENS. Sputum specimens are obtained to identify a specific microorganism and its drug sensitivities. This type of specimen is referred to as "sputum for culture and sensitivity." A sputum specimen may also be obtained to identify the presence of the tubercle bacillus (TB). This sputum specimen is called "sputum for acid-fast bacillus" (AFB). The AFB specimen is obtained serially in the early morning, usually for 3 consecutive days. Finally, sputum specimens are obtained to identify the presence of abnormal cells. This is called a "sputum for cytology" and involves a serial collection of three early morning sputum specimens. Cytological sputum examination is performed to identify any cancers in the lung by cell type.

If a client is unable to cough or produce sputum, the nurse may have to suction the airway to obtain the specimen. The nurse attaches a sputum trap to the suction catheter (Fig. 41-4), which traps mucus during suctioning. In this procedure the nurse must avoid suctioning large amounts of sterile saline into the sputum trap. Sterile saline dilutes the sputum and can make analysis difficult or impossible.

When sputum specimens are obtained, the nurse should record the color, consistency, amount, and

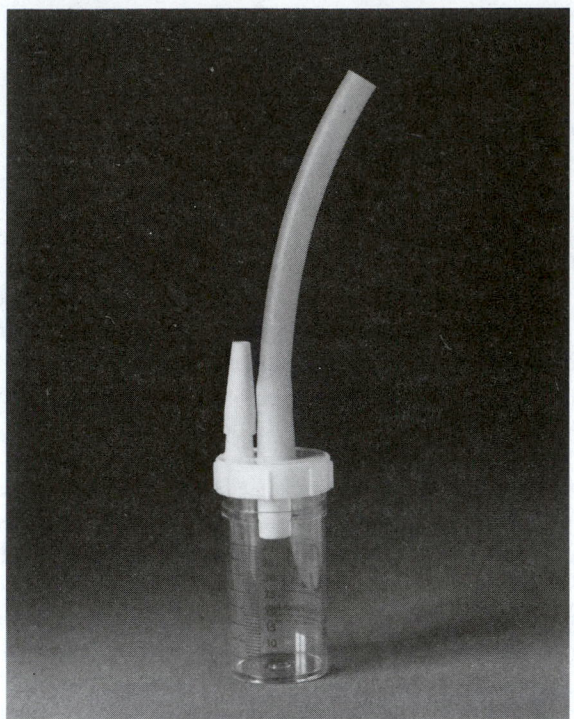

Fig. 41-4 Sputum trap for collecting sputum specimens during suctioning. The rubber tubing is connected to the suction catheter. Once the specimen has been collected, the rubber tubing is removed from the suction catheter and placed over the air vent on the sputum trap. This reduces the spread of bacteria from the sputum.

odor of the sputum and that the specimen was sent to a specific laboratory for analysis on a specific date and time.

THORACENTESIS. Thoracentesis is the surgical perforation of the chest wall and pleural space with a needle to aspirate fluid for diagnostic or therapeutic purposes or to remove a specimen for biopsy. The procedure is performed with aseptic technique, using a local anesthetic. The client usually sits upright with the anterior thorax supported by pillows or an over-the-bed table (Fig. 41-5).

Whether this procedure is painful depends on the client's tolerance to pain (see Chapter 37). The nurse can reduce the client's anxiety by making sure that the procedure has been thoroughly explained and that the client knows what to expect. The client must understand the importance of holding his breath as requested and of not coughing during the procedure. Sudden movements of the thorax may result in the lung being punctured by the thoracentesis needle. The client is also instructed to notify the physician before coughing or sneezing so the needle can be withdrawn.

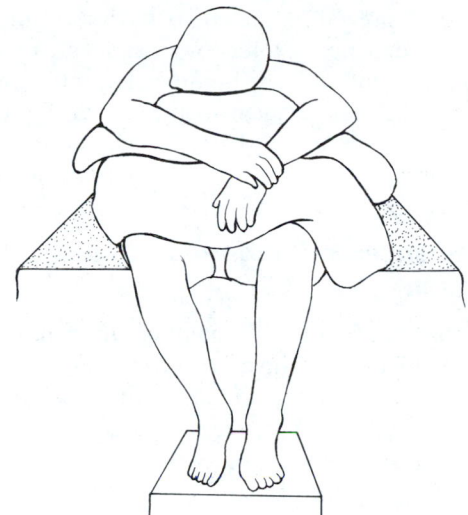

Fig. 41-5 Position of client for thoracentesis.

Nursing Diagnosis

There are four major categories of nursing diagnoses for clients with an altered level of oxygenation: (1) ineffective airway clearance, (2) impaired gas exchange, (3) ineffective breathing patterns, and (4) altered cardiac output. Within each category are multiple nursing diagnoses for a client with an actual or potential respiratory dysfunction (Table 41-3). The specific diagnoses presented here are only examples of nursing diagnoses in each category.

Ineffective Airway Clearance

A client's inability to clear the airway effectively may result from airway secretions, airway obstruction, ineffective cough, immobilization, or unconsciousness. The nursing assessment may include one or more of five findings. The client may have noisy respirations that are audible to the ear or auscultation. Sputum may be present with or without a cough. A nonproductive cough may indicate the client's inability to mobilize pulmonary secretions as a result of fatigue, pain, immobility, or poor coughing efforts. The presence of dyspnea or changes in the respiratory rate or depth can indicate ineffective airway clearance. Occasionally, the body is able to adapt to partial occlusions in the airway by increasing the rate of respirations. Last, cyanosis may result from the client's inability to maintain a patent airway.

Impaired Gas Exchange

Impaired gas exchange may be caused by the same factors as ineffective airway clearance. In addition,

TABLE 41-3

Examples of Nursing Diagnoses for Actual or Potential Respiratory Dysfunction

Problem	Causes
Ineffective airway clearance	Related to: Impaired cough reflex Impaired pulmonary secretions Incisional pain Immobility Decreased level of consciousness
Impaired gas exchange	Related to: Decreased lung expansion Decreased level of consciousness Presence of pulmonary secretions Acid-base imbalance Inadequate oxygen intake
Ineffective breathing patterns	Related to: Chest wall abnormality Immobility Use of analgesics Neuromuscular damage Airway obstruction
Altered cardiac output	Related to: Acid-base disturbances Electrolyte imbalance Reduced extracellular volume

this nursing diagnosis may be associated with structural deficits such as a flail chest, which affects lung expansion, or with an acid-base abnormality (see Chapter 43). The signs and symptoms of impaired gas exchange may include those of hyperventilation, hypoventilation, or hypoxia.

Ineffective Breathing Patterns

Ineffective breathing patterns can be caused by neuromuscular impairment, pain, musculoskeletal impairment, anxiety, decreased energy, fatigue, or the use of analgesics. Characteristic findings include dyspnea, tachypnea, fremitus, abnormal arterial blood gas levels, cyanosis, cough, nasal flaring, change in depth of respiration, pursed-lip breathing, prolonged expiration, increased anterior-posterior diameter of the chest, use of accessory muscles, and altered excursion of the chest wall.

Altered Cardiac Output

Alterations in cardiac output are caused by factors that decrease extracellular blood volume or by electrolyte or acid-base imbalances that affect myocardial contractility and, ultimately, cardiac output. Characteristic findings include changes in blood pressure, fatigue, jugular vein distention, color changes of the skin and mucous membranes, oliguria, decreased peripheral pulses, cold clammy skin, rales, dyspnea, orthopnea, and restlessness. Additional signs and symptoms include changes in mental status, shortness of breath, syncope, vertigo, edema, coughing frothy sputum, abnormal heart sounds, and weakness. The number and severity of symptoms are directly related to the extent of decline in cardiac output. Not all clients have all of these signs and symptoms.

Planning

Clients with impaired respiration require a nursing care plan directed toward meeting the actual or potential oxygenation needs of the client. The plan is based on one or more of the following goals:
1. Maintenance and promotion of lung expansion
2. Mobilization of pulmonary secretions
3. Maintenance of a patent airway
4. Maintenance or promotion of tissue oxygenation
5. Restoration of cardiopulmonary function

The client's overall level of health, age, life-style, and environmental risks all affect the level of tissue oxygenation. Clients with severe impairments in oxygenation frequently require nursing interventions directed toward all five goals.

Implementation

Nursing interventions for promoting and maintaining adequate oxygenation include independent nursing actions, such as positioning, coughing techniques, and preventive health behaviors, and independent or dependent interventions, such as oxygen therapy, lung inflation techniques, hydration, medications, and in some agencies the use of chest physiotherapy. These are the basic categories of nursing interventions, the goals of which are listed above.

Maintenance or Promotion of Lung Expansion

Nursing interventions to maintain or promote lung expansion include noninvasive techniques such as positioning and breathing exercises. Lung expansion is also promoted by procedures using equipment such as incentive spirometers, blow bottles, and intermittent positive-pressure breathing machines. Lung expansion can also be achieved by invasive procedures such as insertion of a chest tube.

POSITIONING

In the healthy, completely mobile person, adequate ventilation and oxygenation are maintained by frequent changes of position during the activities of daily living. However, when a person's mobility is restricted as a result of illness or injury, he is at risk for respiratory impairment. The most common types of impairments are stasis of pulmonary secretions and decreased chest wall expansion (see Chapter 31).

Frequent changes of position of the partially or completely immobilized client are simple and cost-effective methods for reducing the risks of pulmonary complications. Postoperative clients whose incisional pain limits chest wall expansion require frequent changes of position. Because chest wall expansion is limited, these clients are at risk for pooling of respiratory secretions and subsequent hypostatic bronchopneumonia. The care plan for the immediate postoperative period should include changing a client's position at least every 2 hours, and, unless contraindicated, the ambulation schedule should gradually increase the amount of time the client spends out of bed. These two interventions in the postoperative nursing care plan promote full lung expansion and help reduce the risk of postoperative pulmonary complications (see Chapter 47).

BREATHING EXERCISES

Breathing exercises include various techniques to improve ventilation and oxygenation. The three basic techniques are deep breathing and coughing exercises, pursed-lip breathing, and abdominal-diaphragmatic breathing. The first, deep breathing and coughing exercise, is routinely used with postoperative clients. The procedure for deep breathing and coughing is detailed in Chapter 47.

Pursed-lip breathing involves a deep inspiration and a prolonged expiration through pursed lips. Originally this breathing exercise was thought to decrease airway collapse by increasing intraluminal airway pressure near the mouth. However, recent research indicates that this technique benefits clients primarily by slowing the ventilatory rate, thereby increasing tidal volume and decreasing dead space ventilation. Alveolar ventilation remains the same, but the work of breathing decreases (Luce, Tyler, and Pierson, 1984).

Pursed-lip breathing exercises are useful in promoting adequate oxygenation and ventilation in anxious clients, as well as those with chronic obstructive pulmonary diseases. The client is instructed to take a deep breath and to exhale slowly through pursed lips while counting to four silently. Since this exercise affects exhalation, the client should be encouraged to increase the exhalation time. The client is usually able to perfect this technique by increasing the count during exhalation from four to eight. This exercise is best performed with the client sitting upright.

Abdominal-diaphragmatic breathing requires the client to relax the intercostal and accessory respiratory muscles while taking deep inspirations and watching the abdomen move outward as the diaphragm descends. During expiration the client slowly and forcefully contracts the abdominal muscles and observes the abdomen for inward movement as the diaphragm ascends. These exercises are initially taught with the client in the supine position and then are practiced while sitting and standing. Frequently the exercise is used along with the pursed-lip breathing technique. The pulmonary results of this exercise pattern include decreased air trapping and reduced work of breathing (Luce, Tyler, and Pierson, 1984). This exercise is also useful for clients with pulmonary disease and for postoperative clients or women in labor to promote relaxation and provide pain control.

INCENTIVE SPIROMETRY

Incentive spirometry is a method of encouraging voluntary deep breathing by providing visual feedback to clients concerning their inspiratory volume. Incentive spirometry is used to prevent or treat atelectasis and is particularly useful for postoperative clients (Luce, Tyler, and Pierson, 1984). The two general types of incentive spirometers are flow-oriented and volume-oriented spirometers.

Flow-oriented incentive spirometers consist of one or more plastic chambers that house freely movable, colored balls. The client is instructed to inhale briskly to elevate the balls and to keep them floating as long as possible. Clients need to be instructed that the goal is to keep the balls elevated for as long as possible in

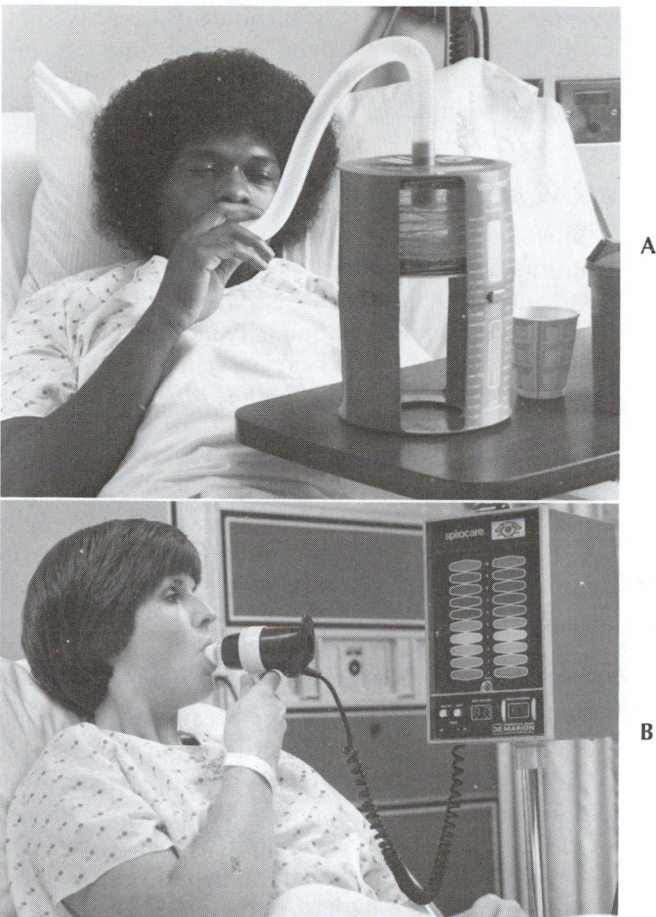

Fig. 41-6 Volume-oriented incentive spirometry. **A,** Bellows visible to client. **B,** Achievement light indicator.

order to ensure a maximal sustained inhalation. The goal is *not* to snap the balls to the top of the chamber with a rapid, very brief, low-volume breath. Even if a very slow inspiration does not elevate the balls, this pattern may achieve greater lung expansion (Luce, Tyler, and Pierson, 1984). The advantage of flow-oriented inspiratory spirometry is its low cost, but it does not determine the volume of inspiration.

Volume-oriented incentive spirometry devices have a bellows that is raised to a predetermined volume by an inhaled breath (Fig. 41-6, *A*). An achievement light or counter is used instead in some devices (Fig. 41-6, *B*). Some devices are constructed so the light will not turn on unless the bellows is held at a minimal desired volume for a specified period to enhance lung expansion. The advantage of volume-oriented incentive spirometry is that a known volume of inspiration can be maintained.

Incentive spirometry encourages clients to breathe to their normal inspiratory capacity. When this method is used with a postoperative client, it is helpful to know his preoperative inspiratory capacity. Because of postoperative pain, a postoperative inspiratory capacity one half to three fourths of the preoperative volume is acceptable (Luce, Tyler, and Pierson, 1984).

BLOW BOTTLES

Blow bottles are devices in which fluid is moved from one container to another by air pressure. The disadvantage of blow bottles is that they provide feedback only about exhalation. Hyperinflation of the lungs and the presumed benefit occur *only if a deep breath is taken before blowing into the bottle*.

A client who is not properly instructed in using the blow bottle may use frequent small breaths and the Valsalva maneuver to move the liquid. Therefore the nurse should teach the client to inhale deeply and then seal the lips tightly around the mouthpiece and exhale. Unless deep inhalation is achieved, expansion of lung alveoli does not occur.

INTERMITTENT POSITIVE-PRESSURE BREATHING

Intermittent positive-pressure breathing (IPPB) devices assist lung hyperinflation by applying positive pressure to the airways. Hyperinflation depends on the amount of pressure applied and on the compliance of the chest wall. Clients with low compliance require higher IPPB pressures to achieve hyperinflation. Following the inspiration phase of the cycle, the machine automatically shuts off and passive exhalation occurs. The client's next inspiratory cycle triggers the machine to deliver the preset pressure.

CLINICAL INDICATIONS. Clients with respiratory muscle weakness, chest wall deformity, or thoracic or abdominal incisions are unable to take large inspiratory breaths voluntarily. These clients benefit from IPPB or incentive spirometry. Aerosol medications such as bronchodilators or mucolytics can also be administered with the IPPB treatment. In addition, IPPB treatments promote clearing of bronchial secretions and are also used preoperatively to promote lung expansion and to prepare the client for postoperative maneuvers.

CONTRAINDICATIONS. IPPB should not be used with semicomatose, restless, or confused clients. Because these clients are unable to cooperate fully, they are likely to swallow large volumes of air, leading to esophageal and gastric distention and often vomiting.

COMPLICATIONS. As with any procedure, there are potential complications with IPPB treatment. Nosocomial tracheobronchitis and pneumonia have been observed in some clients receiving IPPB therapy. The source of contamination in these cases was found to be the nebulizer, which adds humidification or medication to the inhaled gas (Luce, Tyler, and Pierson, 1984).

A second complication is barotrauma, a physical injury resulting from increased inhalation pressure. Barotrauma may occur with any procedure that distends the lung, but its incidence can be reduced if the pressure generated by the IPPB machine does not produce large lung volumes.

A third complication is respiratory alkalosis (see Chapter 43). This may occur if the IPPB machine is set to deliver rapid inspiration that is inappropriate for the client's normal breathing pattern.

NURSING MANAGEMENT. Some institutions have a specialized respiratory therapy team to administer IPPB treatments. However, the nurse should not assume that this treatment is solely the responsibility of respiratory therapists.

The nurse has the opportunity to observe the client during IPPB treatment. In some agencies and particularly in the home, the nurse is responsible for assisting the client with IPPB therapy (Procedure 41-1).

CHEST TUBES

A chest tube is a catheter inserted through the thorax to remove fluid or air and thus promote lung reexpansion. Chest tubes are used after chest surgery and for pneumothorax or hemothorax.

A *pneumothorax* is the collection of air or other gas in the pleural space. The gas causes the lung to collapse because it exerts a counterpressure against the lung, which is then unable to expand. A pneumothorax may occur spontaneously, result from an open chest wound or the rupture of an emphysematous vesicle on the surface of the lung, or follow a severe bout of coughing or an invasive procedure, such as a thoracentesis or insertion of a subclavian intravenous line.

A client with a pneumothorax usually feels pain as the atmospheric air irritates the parietal pleura. The pain may be sharp and pleuritic. Dyspnea is common and worsens as the size of the pneumothorax increases.

Hemothorax is an accumulation of blood and fluid in the pleural cavity between the parietal and visceral pleurae, usually as the result of trauma. The hemothorax produces a counterpressure and prevents the lung from full expansion. A hemothorax can also be caused by rupture of small blood vessels from inflammatory processes, such as pneumonia or tuberculosis. In addition to pain and dyspnea, signs and symptoms of shock can develop if the blood loss is severe.

PROCEDURE 41-1

Assisting Clients with IPPB Therapy

STEPS	RATIONALE
1. Explain the procedure to the client and have him practice using the mouthpiece before the procedure.	Explaining the procedure reduces procedure-related anxiety, and practice assists the client in becoming accustomed to an airtight seal that he must create with his lips for the IPPB machine to work correctly.
2. Place the client in a high Fowler's position.	A high Fowler's position promotes optimal lung expansion.
3. Encourage the client to relax during the inspiratory cycle.	Relaxation during the inspiratory cycle promotes optimal lung expansion.
4. Encourage the client to exhale normally.	Exhalation is usually twice as long as inspiration. The IPPB machine is preset to click on with the client's normal beginning inspiratory maneuvers.
5. If the client is breathing through his nose and is not able to breathe entirely through his mouth, a nose clip may be needed.	Nose clips produce an airtight seal needed for the IPPB system to function effectively.
6. Observe the client's chest wall movements. If the movements are asymmetrical or if chest pain occurs, stop the procedure and assess the client's respiratory system.	Early identification of barotrauma may be indicated by asymmetrical chest wall movement or chest pain.
7. Observe any sputum production after treatment.	Discolored sputum indicates a pulmonary infection. If discolored sputum is a new finding, it should be reported.
8. Change oxygen tubes and nebulizer every 24 hours.	The risk of nosocomial infection is reduced when oxygen tubes and nebulizer are changed every 24 hours.
9. Record the time and duration of the IPPB treatment, as well as the client's response.	Recording the time, duration, and response to therapy documents that the client did receive IPPB therapy.

Mobilization of Pulmonary Secretions

The ability of a client to mobilize pulmonary secretions may make the difference between a short, smooth postoperative recovery period and a long period involving complications with greater difficulty in achieving a maximal level of health. The nursing interventions that promote mobilization of pulmonary secretions include hydration, humidification, nebulization, and chest physiotherapy.

HYDRATION

Maintenance of an adequate systemic hydration is essential for keeping mucociliary clearance within normal limits. In clients with adequate hydration, pulmonary secretions are thin, white, watery, and easily removed with minimal coughing. Excessive coughing required to clear thick, tenacious secretions is fatiguing and leaves the client with little energy to do anything else (Feldman, 1982). Unless contraindicated, most clinicians recommend a fluid intake of 1500 to 2000 ml per day (Luce, Tyler, and Pierson, 1984). The adequacy of hydration can be determined by the color and consistency of secretions.

HUMIDIFICATION

Humidification is the process of adding water to a gas mixture. Temperature is the most important factor affecting how much water vapor a gas can hold. The actual percentage of water in the gas in relation to the gas's total capacity for water is the relative humidity. Air or oxygen with a high relative humidity keeps the airways moist and loosens and mobilizes pulmonary secretions.

Humidification is necessary for clients receiving oxygen therapy. Oxygen delivered to the upper airways, as with a nasal catheter, nasal cannula, or face mask, is humidified by bubbling the gas through water (Fig. 41-7). Heating of these humidifiers is impractical because condensed moisture fills the narrow oxygen delivery tubing. Therefore the relative humidity of gas delivered to the upper airways is only 30% (Luce, Tyler, and Pierson, 1984).

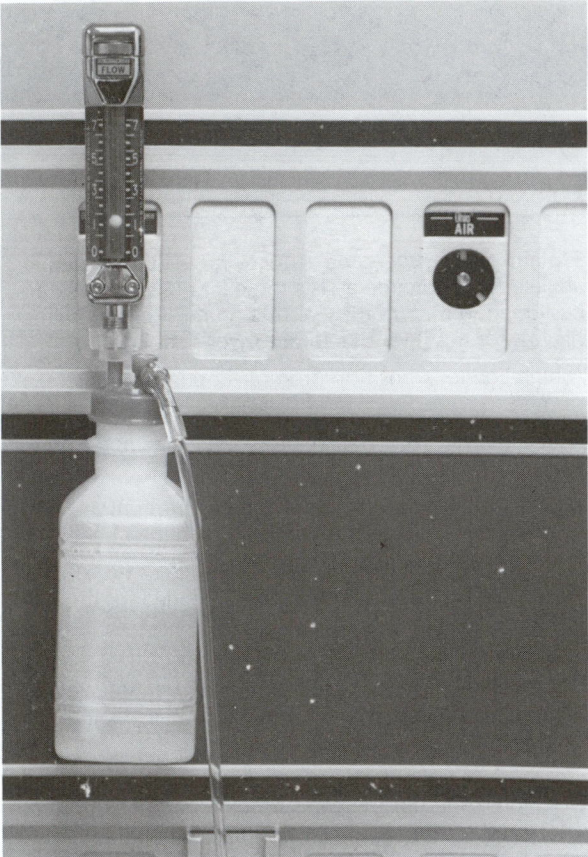

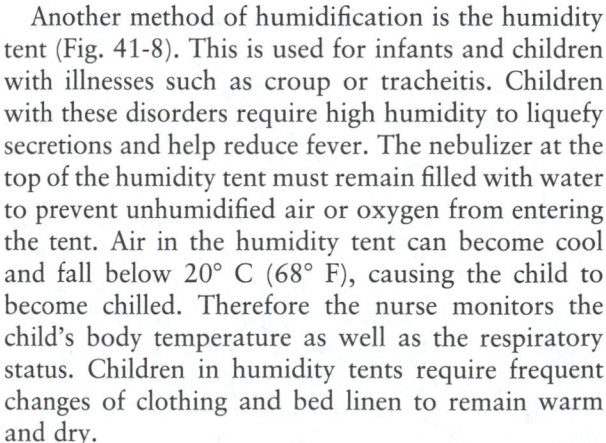

Fig. 41-7 Humidification of oxygen by bubbling the gas through water.

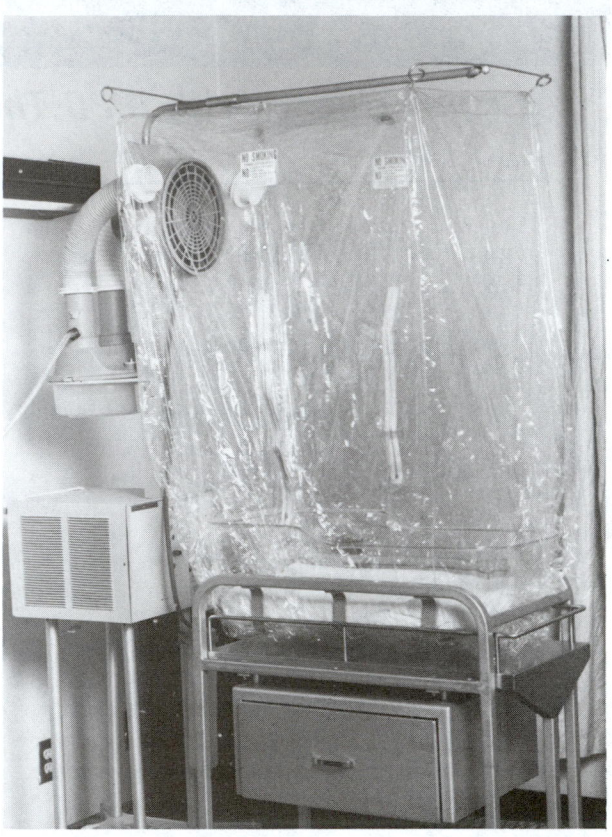

Fig. 41-8 Humidification by a humidity tent: an infant Croupette.

Another method of humidification is the humidity tent (Fig. 41-8). This is used for infants and children with illnesses such as croup or tracheitis. Children with these disorders require high humidity to liquefy secretions and help reduce fever. The nebulizer at the top of the humidity tent must remain filled with water to prevent unhumidified air or oxygen from entering the tent. Air in the humidity tent can become cool and fall below 20° C (68° F), causing the child to become chilled. Therefore the nurse monitors the child's body temperature as well as the respiratory status. Children in humidity tents require frequent changes of clothing and bed linen to remain warm and dry.

NEBULIZATION

Nebulization is a process of adding moisture or medications to inspired air by mixing particles of varying sizes with the air. A nebulizer uses the aerosol principle to suspend a maximal number of water drops or particles of the desired size in inspired air. The goal of nebulization is to improve the clearance of pulmonary secretions by altering the tracheobronchial mucosa. Therefore, nebulization is often used for administration of bronchodilators or mucolytic agents.

The two major types of nebulizers are the jet-aerosol nebulizer and the ultrasonic nebulizer. A jet-aerosol nebulizer uses gas under pressure, and the ultrasonic nebulizer uses high-frequency vibrations to break up the water or medication into fine drops or particles. The drops or particles, when inspired with the air or administered oxygen, are then deposited throughout the tracheobronchial tree.

CHEST PHYSIOTHERAPY

Chest physiotherapy (CPT) is a group of therapies used in combination to mobilize pulmonary secretions. These therapies include postural drainage, chest percussion, and vibration. Chest physiotherapy should be accompanied by productive coughing or suctioning if the client's ability to cough is inadequate.

Chest percussion involves striking the chest wall over the area being drained. The hand is positioned

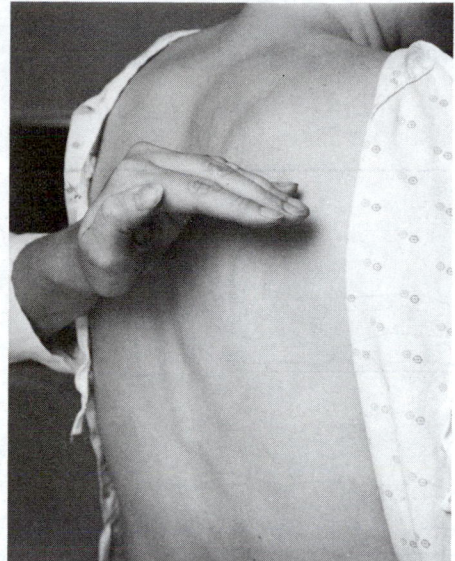

Fig. 41-9 Hand position for chest wall percussion during chest physiotherapy.

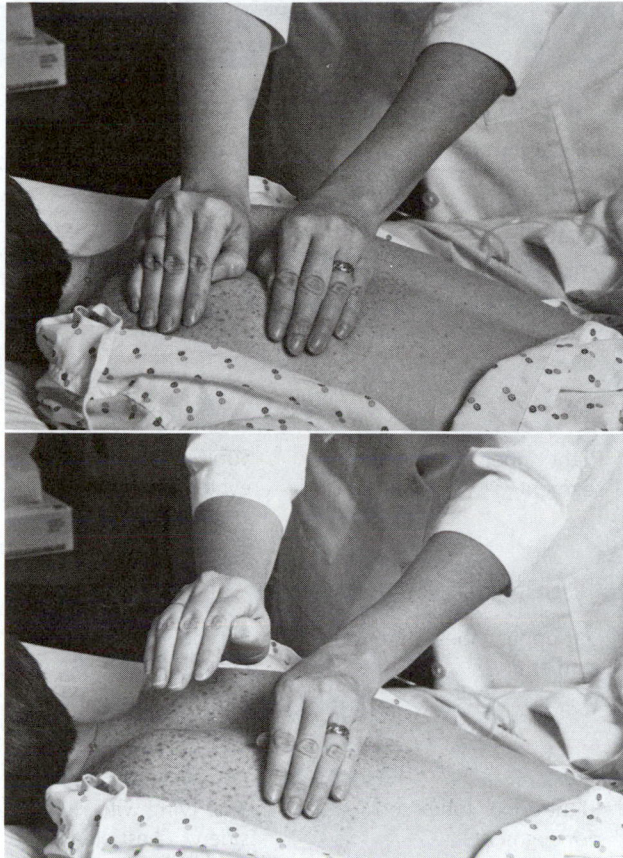

Fig. 41-10 Chest wall percussion, alternating hand motion against the client's chest wall.

so the fingers and thumb touch and the hand is cupped (Fig. 41-9). Percussion on the surface of the chest wall sends waves of varying amplitude and frequency through the chest. The force of these waves can change the consistency of the sputum or dislodge it from airway walls (Luce, Tyler, and Pierson, 1984). Chest percussion is performed by alternating hand motion against the client's chest wall (Fig. 41-10).

Percussion is contraindicated in clients with bleeding disorders, osteoporosis, or fractured ribs. Caution should be taken to percuss the lung fields and not the scapular regions, or trauma may occur to the skin and underlying musculoskeletal structures.

Vibration is a fine, shaking pressure applied to the chest wall only during exhalation (Luce, Tyler, and Pierson, 1984). Vibration increases the exhalation of trapped air and may shake mucus loose and induce a cough.

Postural drainage is the use of positioning techniques that draw secretions from specific segments of the lungs and bronchi into the trachea. Coughing or suctioning normally removes the secretions from the trachea. The procedure for postural drainage can include most lung segments (Table 41-4). Because not all clients require postural drainage of all lung segments, the nurse bases the procedure on the clinical assessment findings. For example, clients with left lower lobe atelectasis may require postural drainage of only the affected region, whereas a child with cystic fibrosis may require postural drainage of all lung segments.

Frequently postural drainage is accompanied by chest percussion and vibration. The decision to use percussion and vibration is based on the client's clinical status.

Not all clients can tolerate the various positions used with postural drainage. Lung hemorrhage, increased intracranial pressure, and uncontrolled hypoxia are some contraindications to placing the client in a Trendelenburg position. The nurse continually evaluates the client's response to position changes and discontinues positions that worsen dyspnea significantly or that cause other symptoms.

■ ■ ■ ■ ■

The evaluation of chest physiotherapy, nebulization, humidification, and hydration is based on the mobilization and removal of secretions from the respiratory tract. With clients unable to clear secretions, the nurse must implement nursing measures to maintain a patent airway.

TABLE 41-4

Various Positions for Postural Drainage

Lung Segment	Position of Client	
ADULT		
Bilateral Apical segments	High Fowler's Sitting on side of bed (see Fig. 41-5)	
Right upper lobe—anterior segment	Supine with head elevated	
Left upper lobe—anterior segment	Supine with head elevated	
Right upper lobe—posterior segment	Side lying with right side of chest elevated on pillow	
Left upper lobe—posterior segment	Side lying with left side of chest elevated on pillows	
Right middle lobe	Three-fourths supine position with dependent lung in Trendelenburg position	
Right middle lobe—posterior segment	Prone with thorax and abdomen elevated	

TABLE 41-4, cont'd

Various Positions for Postural Drainage

Lung Segment	Position of Client	
Both lower lobes—anterior segments	Supine in Trendelenburg position	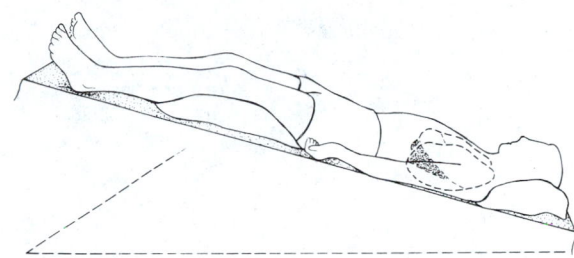
Left lower lobe—lateral segment	Right side lying in Trendelenburg position	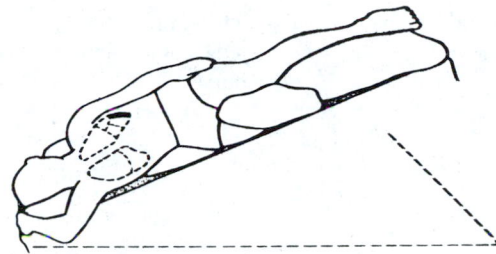
Right lower lobe—lateral segment	Left side lying in Trendelenburg position	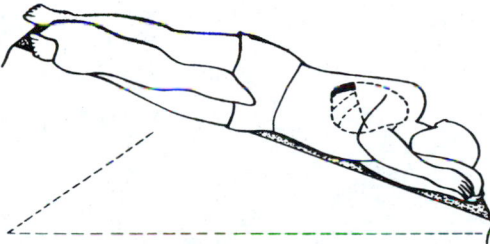
Right lower lobe—posterior segment	Prone with right side of chest elevated in Trendelenburg position	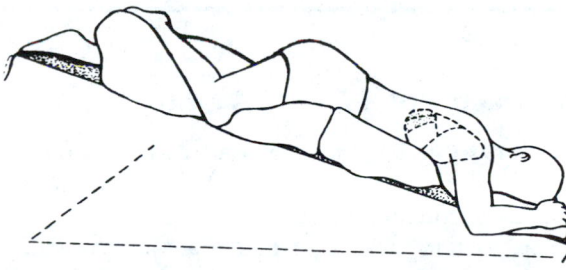
Both lower lobes—posterior segments	Prone in Trendelenburg position	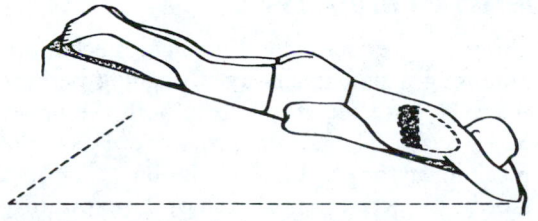

T A B L E 41 - 4 , cont'd

Various Positions for Postural Drainage

Lung Segment	Position of Client	
CHILD		
Bilateral—apical segments	Sitting on nurse's lap, leaning slightly forward flexed over pillow	
Bilateral—middle anterior segments	Sitting on nurse's lap, leaning against nurse	
Bilateral lobes—anterior segments	Lying supine on nurse's lap, back supported with pillow	

Maintenance of a Patent Airway

The airway is patent when the trachea, bronchi, and large airways are free from obstructions caused by mucus or foreign objects. Three types of interventions are used to maintain a patent airway: coughing techniques, suctioning, and artificial airway.

COUGHING TECHNIQUES

Coughing is an effective and efficient mechanism for maintaining a patent airway. Coughing permits the client to remove secretions from both the upper and lower airways. The normal series of events in the cough mechanisms are (1) deep inhalation, (2) closure of the glottis, (3) active contraction of the expiratory muscles, and (4) glottis opening. Deep inhalation increases lung volume and airway diameter. Thus air can pass to partially obstructing mucus plugs or other foreign matter. The contraction of the expiratory muscles against the closed glottis allows a high intrathoracic pressure to develop. As a result, when the glottis is opened, air is expelled in a large flow at a high speed, providing momentum for mucus to move to the upper airway. After the cough the mucus can be expectorated or swallowed (Traver, 1982).

Various coughing techniques can be taught to different clients. Chapter 47 details the technique of deep breathing and coughing. Other cough techniques are cascade, huff, and quad coughing.

With the *cascade cough* the client takes a deep breath and coughs several times while exhaling until he feels that there is no air left in his lungs. Thus the client coughs at progressively lowered lung volumes.

This technique is effective in promoting airway clearance and a patent airway in clients with large volumes of sputum.

With the *huff cough* the client, while exhaling, opens the glottis by saying the word "huff." The huff cough is effective in stimulating a natural cough reflex. This cough is generally effective only for clearing central airways, but with practice the client inhales more air and may be able to progress to the cascade cough.

The *quad cough* technique is used for clients without abdominal muscle control, such as those with spinal cord injuries. The client or nurse pushes inward and upward on the abdominal muscles toward the diaphragm while the client breathes with maximal expiratory effort, causing the cough (Luce, Tyler, and Pierson, 1984).

The efficacy of any cough is evaluated by sputum expectoration, the client's report of swallowed sputum, or the clearing of adventitious sounds on auscultation. Clients with chronic pulmonary diseases, upper respiratory tract infections, and lower respiratory tract infections should be encouraged to cough at least every 2 hours when awake. Clients with a copious amount of sputum should be encouraged to cough every hour while awake and every 2 to 3 hours while asleep until the acute phase of mucus production has ended.

SUCTIONING TECHNIQUES

When a client is unable to clear respiratory tract secretions with coughing techniques, the nurse must use a suctioning technique to clear the airways. The three primary suctioning techniques are oropharyngeal and nasopharyngeal suctioning, orotracheal and nasotracheal suctioning, and suctioning of an artificial airway.

These three techniques are based on common principles. Because the oropharynx and trachea are considered sterile, sterile technique is required for suctioning. The mouth is considered clean, and therefore the suctioning of oral secretions should be performed after suctioning of the oropharynx and trachea. Each type of suctioning requires the use of a beaded-tip catheter with a ring of holes along the side of the catheter at the distal end.

OROPHARYNGEAL AND NASOPHARYNGEAL SUCTIONING.
The oropharynx extends behind the mouth from the soft palate above the level of the hyoid bone and contains the tonsils. The nasopharynx is located behind the nose and extends to the level of the soft palate. Oropharyngeal or nasopharyngeal suctioning is used when the client is able to cough effectively but is unable to clear secretions by expec-

torating or swallowing. The suction procedure (Procedure 41-2) is used after the client has coughed. As the amount of pulmonary secretions is reduced and the client is less fatigued, he may be able to expectorate or swallow the mucus so this type of suctioning is no longer required.

OROTRACHEAL AND NASOTRACHEAL SUCTIONING.
Orotracheal or nasotracheal suctioning is necessary when the client with pulmonary secretions is unable to cough and does not have an artificial airway present. The catheter is passed through the mouth or nose into the trachea. The nose is the preferred route because stimulation of the gag reflex is minimal. The procedure is similar to nasopharyngeal suctioning, but the catheter tip is moved farther into the client to suction the trachea. The entire procedure from catheter passage to its removal cannot take more than 15 seconds because oxygen does not reach the lungs during suctioning. Unless the client is in respiratory distress, he should be allowed to rest between passes of the catheter. If the client is using supplemental oxygen, the oxygen cannulae or mask should be replaced during rest periods.

ARTIFICIAL AIRWAY

An artificial airway is an oral airway or an endotracheal, nasotracheal, or tracheostomy tube. Indications for an artificial airway include decreased level of consciousness, airway obstruction, mechanical ventilation, and removal of tracheal secretions.

ORAL AIRWAY.
The oral airway, the simplest type of artificial airway, is used to prevent obstruction of the trachea by displacement of the tongue into the oropharynx in the unconscious client (Fig. 41-11). The oral airway extends from the teeth to the oro-

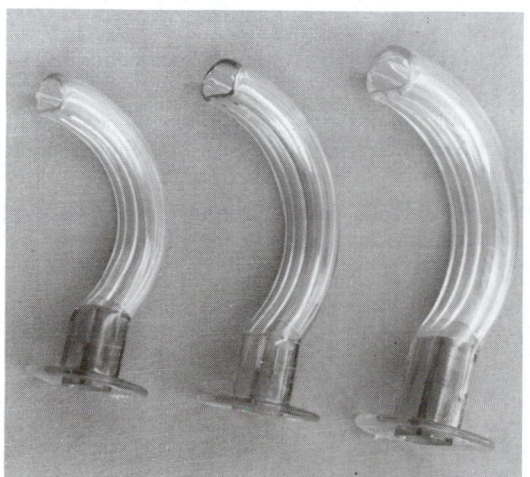

Fig. 41-11   Artificial oral airways.

PROCEDURE 41-2

Oropharyngeal and Nasopharyngeal Suctioning

EQUIPMENT:
1. Portable or wall suction unit with connecting tubing with Y connector if needed
2. Sterile catheter
3. Sterile water or normal saline
4. Sterile gloves
5. Drape or towel to protect linen and client's bedclothes

STEPS	RATIONALE
1. Prepare equipment at the bedside.	Preparation of equipment allows smooth performance of the procedure without interruption.
2. Explain to the client how the procedure will help to clear the airway and relieve some of the breathing problems. Explain that coughing, sneezing, or gagging is normal.	Explanation of the procedure relieves the client's anxiety about the procedure.
3. Properly position the client. a. Place a conscious client with a functional gag reflex for oral suctioning in the semi-Fowler's position with head turned to one side. Place such a client for nasal suctioning in the semi-Fowler's position with neck hyperextended.	The gag reflex helps prevent aspiration of gastrointestinal contents. Positioning of the head to one side or hyperextending the neck promotes smooth insertion of the catheter into the oropharynx or nasopharynx, respectively.
b. Place an unconscious client in the lateral position facing the nurse.	The lateral position prevents the client's tongue from obstructing the client's airway, promotes drainage of pulmonary secretions, and prevents aspiration of gastrointestinal contents.
4. Place a towel on the pillow or under the client's chin.	Soiling of the bed linen or the client's bed clothes from secretions is prevented. Secretions on the towel can be discarded, thus reducing spread of bacteria.
5. Select the proper suction pressure for the client and the type of suction unit. For wall suction units this is 110 to 150 mm Hg in adults, 95 to 110 mm Hg in children, or 50 to 95 mm Hg in infants.	Proper suction pressure provides safe negative pressure according to the client's age. Excessive negative pressure can precipitate a pneumothorax.
6. Pour sterile water or saline into sterile container.	Sterile solution is needed to lubricate the catheter to decrease friction and promote smooth passage of the catheter.
7. Apply a sterile glove to your dominant hand.	The sterile glove maintains asepsis as catheter is passed into client's mouth or nose.
8. Using gloved hand, attach catheter to suction machine.	Sterility is maintained.
9. Approximate the distance between the client's ear lobe and tip of the nose and place the thumb and forefinger of gloved hand at that point.	This distance ensures that the suction catheter remains in the pharyngeal region. Insertion of the catheter past this point places the catheter into the trachea.
10. Moisten the catheter tip with sterile solution. Apply suction with catheter tip in the solution.	Moistening the catheter tip reduces friction and eases insertion of catheter. Applying suction while the catheter is in the sterile solution ensures that suction equipment is functioning before catheter is inserted.

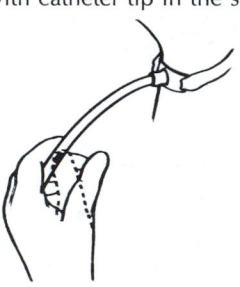

STEPS	*RATIONALE*
11. Suction.	
a. For oropharyngeal suctioning, gently insert the catheter into one side of the mouth, and glide the catheter to the oropharynx. Do not apply suction during insertion.	Stimulation of the gag reflex is reduced.
b. For nasopharyngeal suctioning, gently insert catheter into one nostril. Guide the catheter medially along the floor of the nasal cavity. Do not force the catheter. If one nostril is not patent, try the other. Do not apply suction during insertion.	The catheter avoids the nasal turbinates and enters more easily into nasopharynx. The risk of trauma to the oral and nasal mucosa during catheter insertion is reduced.
12. Apply suction by occluding suction port with your thumb. Gently rotate the catheter as you withdraw it. The entire procedure should not take longer than 15 seconds.	Occlusion of suction port activates suction pressure. Suctioning is intermittently done as the catheter is withdrawn. Rotation removes secretions from all surfaces of the airway and prevents trauma from suction pressure on one area of the airway. Suctioning also removes air. The client's oxygen supply could be severely reduced if the procedure lasts longer than 15 seconds.
13. Flush the catheter with sterile solution by placing it in the solution and applying suction.	Flushing the catheter with sterile solution removes secretions from the catheter and lubricates the catheter for the next suctioning.
14. If the client is not in respiratory distress, allow him to rest for 20 to 30 seconds before reinserting the catheter.	Time between suctionings provides the client with the opportunity to increase his oxygen intake.
15. If the client is able, ask him to deep breathe and cough between suctions.	Deep breathing and coughing promote mobilization of secretions to the upper airway where they can be removed with the catheter. If the client is able to cough productively, further suctioning may not be needed if his airways are clear on auscultation.
If resuctioning is needed, repeat steps 11 through 13.	
16. Suction secretions in mouth or under tongue after suctioning the oropharynx or nasopharynx.	Sterile asepsis is maintained. The mouth should be suctioned only after the sterile areas are thoroughly suctioned.
17. Discard catheter by wrapping it around gloved hand and pulling glove off around catheter.	The spread of bacteria from suction catheter is reduced.
18. Prepare equipment for next suctioning.	Ready access to suction equipment is provided, especially if the client is experiencing respiratory distress.
19. Record the amount, consistency, color, and odor of secretions and the client's response to the procedure.	Recording this information documents that the procedure was completed and the client's status during and after the procedure.

pharynx, maintaining the tongue in the normal anatomical position. The correct size airway must be used. If the airway is too small, the tongue is not held in the anterior portion of the mouth. If the airway is too large, it may force the tongue toward the epiglottis and obstruct the airway.

The artificial oral airway is inserted by turning the curve of the airway toward the client's cheek and placing it over the tongue into the oropharynx. When the airway is in the oropharynx, the nurse turns it so the opening points downward. The correctly placed airway moves the tongue forward away from the oropharynx. The flange, the flat portion of the airway, should rest against the client's teeth.

If the nurse attempts to insert the oral airway with a curve toward the tongue, the client's natural airway can be further obstructed. Inserting the airway incorrectly merely forces the tongue back into the oropharynx.

The oral airway is commonly used for postoperative clients under general anesthesia. The client generally dislodges the airway by coughing it out on regaining consciousness.

The oral airway also promotes orotracheal suctioning in the unconscious client. The suction catheter can be passed through the center of the airway or along its side to gain access to the trachea.

TRACHEAL AIRWAY. Artificial tracheal airways include endotracheal, nasotracheal, and tracheal tubes. These tubes allow easy access to the client's trachea for deep tracheal suctioning. The removal of tracheal secretions must be aseptic, atraumatic, and effective.

Asepsis involves using a freshly opened sterile suction catheter that is handled with a sterile glove. Secretion removal should be as atraumatic as possible. To avoid trauma, suction should never be applied during insertion of the catheter, but only during its withdrawal. The catheter is rotated and suction is applied intermittently during withdrawal.

Effective suctioning removes secretions from the right and left mainstem bronchi. Unless the catheter is unusually long, this procedure is almost impossible to accomplish with a nasotracheal tube (Wade, 1982). To suction each bronchus, the nurse turns the client's head away from the direction of the bronchus to be suctioned. Thus, before the left bronchus is suctioned, the client's head is turned to the right.

■ ■ ■ ■ ■

The frequency of suctioning is determined by continued client assessment. If secretions are identified by inspection or auscultation techniques, suctioning is required. Sputum is not produced continuously or every 1 or 2 hours but occurs as a response to a pathological condition. Therefore there is no rationale for routine suctioning of all clients every 1 to 2 hours.

Maintenance and Promotion of Oxygenation

Promotion of lung expansion, mobilization of secretions, and maintenance of a patent airway all assist the client in meeting oxygenation needs. However, some clients also require oxygen therapy in order to keep the level of tissue oxygenation within a healthy range. Oxygen therapy involves the administration of oxygen by any route to a client to prevent or relieve hypoxia.

GOALS OF OXYGEN THERAPY

The goal of oxygen therapy is to prevent or relieve hypoxia. Any client with impaired tissue oxygenation can benefit from controlled oxygen administration. Oxygen is not a substitute for other forms of treatment, however, and should be used only when indicated. Oxygen should be treated as a drug; it is expensive and has dangerous side effects. As with any drug, the dosage or concentration of oxygen should be continuously monitored. The nurse should routinely check the physician's orders to verify that the client is receiving the prescribed oxygen concentration.

SAFETY PRECAUTIONS WITH OXYGEN THERAPY

Oxygen is a highly combustible gas. Although it will not spontaneously burn or cause an explosion, it can easily cause a fire to ignite in a client's room if it comes into contact with a spark, as from a cigarette. Oxygen in high concentrations has a great combustion potential and fuels fires readily.

The nurse should promote the client's safety by using the following measures. First, "no smoking" signs should be placed on the client's room door and over the head of his bed. The client, his visitors and roommates, and all personnel should be informed that smoking is not permitted in areas where oxygen is in use. The nurse should determine that all electrical equipment in the room is functioning correctly and is properly grounded (see Chapter 34). An electrical spark in the presence of oxygen can result in a severe fire. Finally, the nurse should know the hospital's fire procedures and the location of the closest fire extinguisher.

SUPPLY OF OXYGEN. Oxygen is supplied to the client's bedside either by oxygen tanks or through a permanent pipe system. Oxygen tanks are transported on wide-based carriers that allow the tank to be placed upright at the client's bedside. Regulators are used with oxygen tanks to control the amount of oxygen delivered to the client. One common type is an upright flowmeter with a flow-adjustment valve at the top. A second type is a cylinder indicator with a flow-adjustment handle.

In the hospital or home, oxygen tanks are delivered with the regulator already in place. In the hospital, connecting the regulator is usually the responsibility of the respiratory therapy department. Private oxygen vendors are generally responsible for connecting the oxygen tank to the oxygen regulator for home use.

METHODS OF OXYGEN DELIVERY

Oxygen can be delivered to the client by nasal cannula, nasal catheter, face mask, or mechanical ventilator.

NASAL CANNULA. A nasal cannula is a simple, comfortable device for delivering oxygen to the client (Fig. 41-12 and Procedure 41-3). The two cannulae, about 1.5 cm (½ inch) long, protrude from the center of a disposable tube and are inserted into the nostrils. Oxygen is delivered via the cannulae with a flow rate up to 5 to 6 liters per minute. Higher flow rates dry airway mucosa and do not further increase inspired oxygen concentrations (Luce, Tyler, and Pierson, 1984). The nurse must know what flow rate produces a given percentage of inspired oxygen concentration (FIO_2) (Table 41-5).

NASAL CATHETER. Nasal catheters are used less frequently than nasal cannulae, but they are not obsolete. The procedure involves inserting an oxygen cath-

TABLE 41-5

Correlation of Oxygen Flow Rate with Inspired Oxygen Concentration

Flow (liters/minute)	Concentration (FIO_2)
1	24%
2	28%
4-6	35%-40%

eter into the nose to the nasopharynx (Procedure 41-4). Because securing the catheter can cause pressure on the nostril, the catheter must be changed at least every 8 hours and inserted into the other nostril. For this reason the nasal catheter is often a less desirable method because the client may experience pain when the catheter is passed into the nasopharynx and because trauma can occur to the nasal mucosa.

The relationship of oxygen flow rate in liters per minute and inspired oxygen concentration is the same as for the nasal cannula.

OXYGEN MASKS. An oxygen mask is a device used to administer oxygen. It is shaped to fit snugly over the mouth and nose and is secured in place with a strap. There are two primary types of oxygen masks: high- and low-concentration.

A plastic face mask with a reservoir bag (Fig. 41-13) and a Venturi mask (Fig. 41-14) are capable of delivering higher concentrations of oxygen. The plastic face mask with a reservoir bag can deliver 70% oxygen with a flow rate of 10 liters per minute. This

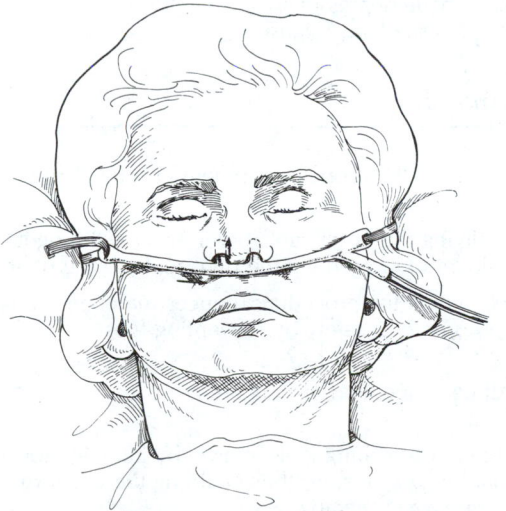
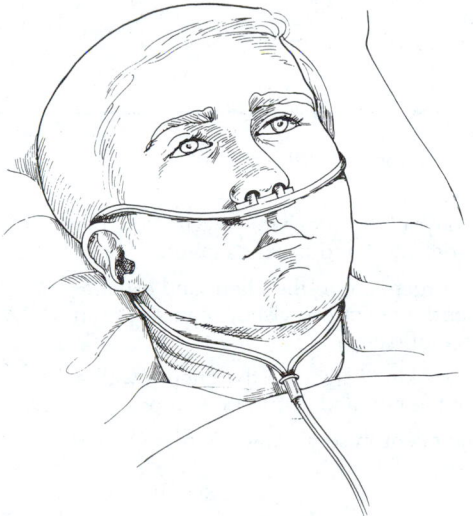

Fig. 41-12 Two types of nasal cannula.
From Wade, J.F.: Comprehensive respiratory care, ed. 3, St. Louis, 1982, The C.V. Mosby Co.

PROCEDURE 41-3

Applying a Nasal Cannula

STEPS	RATIONALE
1. Attach the nasal cannula to a humidified oxygen source adjusted to the prescribed flow rate.	The proper rate prevents drying of mucous membranes and secretions.
2. Place the prongs into the client's nose and adjust the band to the client's comfort.	The chance of the client removing the cannula because of discomfort is reduced.
3. Check the cannula every 8 hours.	Patency of cannula and oxygen flow are ensured.
4. Keep the humidification jar filled at all times.	Inhalation of dehumidified oxygen is prevented.
5. Assess the client's nares and external nose for skin breakdown every 6 to 8 hours.	Prolonged use of nasal oxygen can increase the risk of skin breakdown in the client's nares and external nose.
6. Check the oxygen flow rate and the physician's orders every 8 hours.	Delivery of the prescribed oxygen flow rate is ensured.

PROCEDURE 41-4

Inserting a Nasal Catheter

EQUIPMENT:
1. Appropriate size nasal catheter: small diameter (#8 or #10 French) for children; larger diameter (#10 to #14 French) for adults
2. Oxygen tubing
3. Humidifier
4. Oxygen source with flowmeter
5. Lubricating jelly (must be water soluble)
6. Nonallergenic tape
7. Flashlight or penlight
8. Tongue depressor
9. "No smoking" signs

STEPS	RATIONALE
1. Prepare the equipment at the bedside.	Preparing the proper equipment ensures completion of the procedure without interruption.
2. Verify the physician's order for oxygen flow rate, method of delivery, and nasal catheter.	Verifying the physician's order ensures the right amount of oxygen via the right route to the right client.
3. Explain the procedure to the client and explain why neither the client nor visitors can smoke in the presence of oxygen.	Explaining the procedure reduces the client's anxiety and promotes safety by preventing fires.
4. Place "no smoking" signs on the client's wall at the head of the bed and outside the door.	All personnel and visitors are notified.
5. Position the client in semi-Fowler's or high Fowler's position.	Work of breathing is decreased by allowing for maximal lung expansion, thus enabling the client to benefit from oxygen therapy.
6. Attach catheter to oxygen tubing. Attach oxygen tubing to humidifier.	Oxygen therapy must be humidified to prevent consolidation of pulmonary secretions.

STEPS	RATIONALE
7. Measure the proper length of the nasal catheter to be inserted: measure the distance from the client's nose to his earlobe. Mark the point with a piece of tape.	This measurement approximates the distance to the oropharynx.

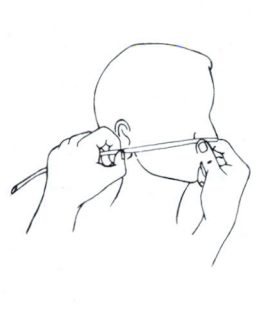 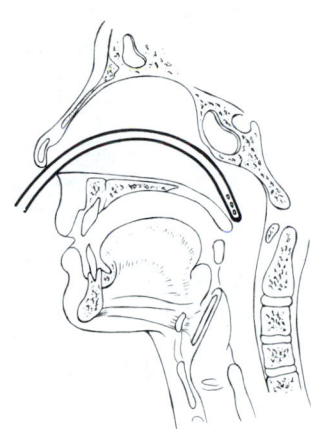 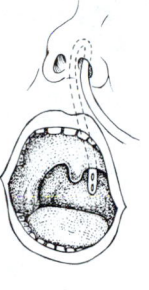 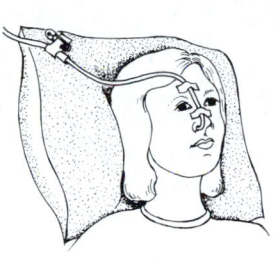

STEPS	RATIONALE
8. Lubricate the tip of the catheter with *water-soluble* jelly.	Smooth insertion of catheter is promoted by reducing friction. A lipid-base lubrication should never be used, since if aspirated it can cause severe lung irritation and pneumonia.
9. Set the flow rate to 2 to 3 liters per minute before inserting the catheter.	Plugging of the catheter by secretions during insertion is prevented.
10. Gently place the catheter into one nostril. Glide the catheter medially along the floor of the nasal cavity. Stop at the premarked point.	Smooth passage of the catheter past nasal turbinates and into the oropharynx is promoted.
11. Inspect the oral cavity using a tongue depressor and flashlight. The tip of the catheter should be visible on either side of the uvula.	Inspecting the oral cavity verifies that the catheter is in the oropharynx.
12. Withdraw the catheter tip so it is no longer visible.	The amount of oxygen swallowed by the client is reduced by withdrawing the catheter tip until it cannot be seen.
13. Secure the catheter to the client's nose.	Displacement of the oxygen catheter is prevented.
14. Readjust the flow rate to the prescribed setting.	Readjusting the flow rate ensures that the prescribed amount of oxygen is delivered to the client.
15. Secure connecting tubing to the client's gown, allowing for slack in the tube.	The client is allowed to move without displacing the catheter.
16. Assess the client's respiratory status following the procedure.	Assessment of the client's status provides data about how the client tolerated the procedure and therapy.
17. Record the procedure in the client's record.	Recording this information documents when the procedure was begun, the oxygen flow rate, the route of administration, and the client's response.

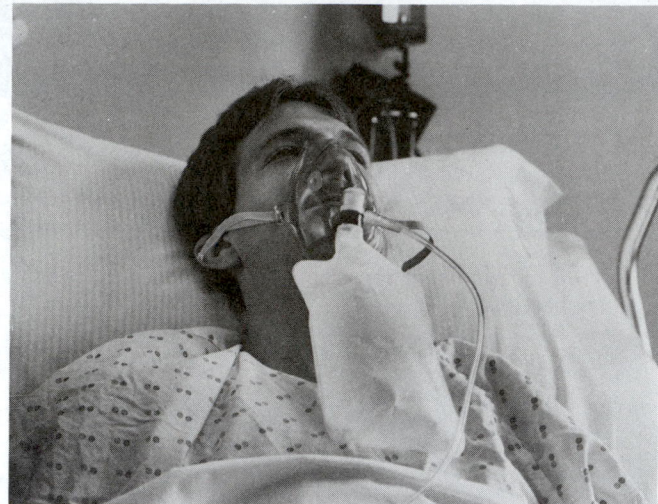

Fig. 41-13 Plastic face mask with reservoir bag.

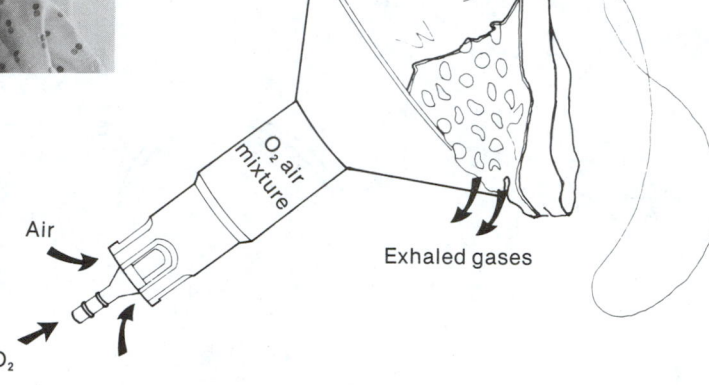

Fig. 41-14 Venturi mask.
From Wade, J.F.: Comprehensive respiratory care, ed. 3, 1982, St. Louis, The C.V. Mosby Co.

oxygen mask maintains a continuous high-concentration oxygen supply in the reservoir bag. The nurse should frequently inspect the bag to make sure it is inflated. If the bag is deflated, the client may be breathing large amounts of the exhaled carbon dioxide.

The Venturi mask can be used to deliver oxygen concentrations of 24%, 28%, 35%, and 40% with oxygen flow rates of 4, 6, 8, and 10 liters per minute, respectively (Wade, 1982).

The simple face mask (Fig. 41-15) is used for short-term oxygen therapy. It fits loosely and delivers oxygen concentrations varying from 30% to 60%. The mask is contraindicated for clients with carbon dioxide retention.

Restoration of Cardiopulmonary Functioning

If a client's hypoxia is severe and prolonged, cardiac arrest may result. A cardiac arrest is a sudden cessation of cardiac output and circulation. When a cardiac arrest occurs, oxygen is not delivered to the tissues, carbon dioxide is not transported from the tissues, tissue metabolism becomes anaerobic, and metabolic and respiratory acidoses occur. Tissue damage, including permanent heart and brain damage, occurs within 5 minutes.

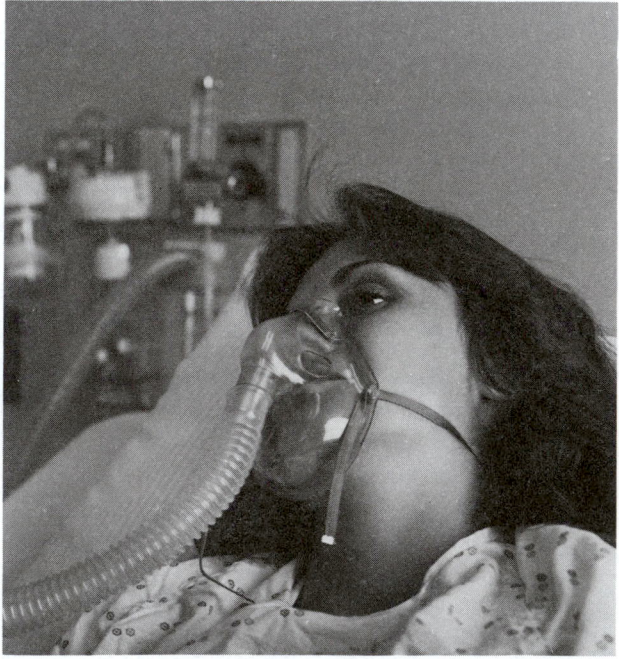

Fig. 41-15 Simple face mask.

Cardiopulmonary Resuscitation (Two Nurses)

STEPS	RATIONALE
1. If immediately available, obtain an Ambu bag with a face mask and oxygen connecting tube.	This equipment produces consistent lung volumes with each artificial respiration.
2. Place the client on a hard surface, such as the floor, or use a backboard.	External compression of the heart is facilitated. The heart is compressed between the sternum and the hard surface.
3. Maintain an open airway by hyperextending the neck. Place one hand behind the victim's neck and the other hand on the forehead. Lift the neck and apply pressure on the forehead. Do not hyperextend the neck if a spinal cord injury is suspected. If the victim is a child, tilt the head backward only slightly.	Airway obstruction from the tongue is relieved.

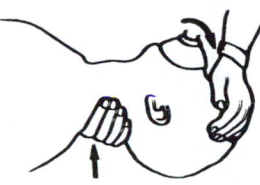 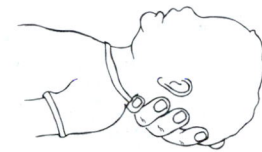

4. Begin artificial respiration.	
a. For mouth-to-mouth resuscitation of an adult, pinch the victim's nose and occlude his mouth with yours. For a child, place your mouth over the child's nose and mouth.	An airtight seal is formed and air is prevented from escaping from the nose.

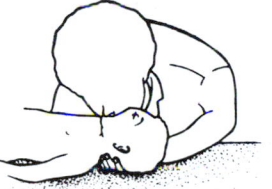

b. For Ambu bag resuscitation, use the proper size face mask and apply it over the victim's mouth and nose.	An airtight seal is formed as the bag is compressed and oxygen enters the client.

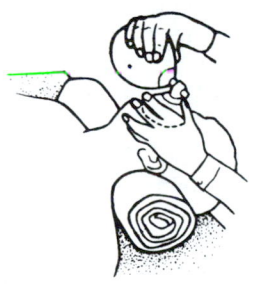

5. Administer artificial respiration.	
a. For mouth-to-mouth resuscitation of an adult, blow four quick breaths into the victim's mouth. Each breath should have increasing volume and strength. The victim is allowed to exhale passively. Then administer one breath every 5 seconds.	Hyperoxygenation is promoted and assists in maintaining blood oxygen levels.
b. For mouth-to-mouth resuscitation of a child, administer short puffs from cheeks once every 3 seconds.	Overinflation of the child's lungs with adult volumes is prevented.
c. For artificial respiration with an Ambu bag in an adult, compress the bag fully for four breaths. Repeat every 5 seconds.	Hyperoxygenation is promoted and assists in maintaining blood oxygen levels.
d. For Ambu bag resuscitation in a child, perform quick, small compressions of the bag every 3 seconds.	Overinflation of the child's lungs is prevented.

Continued.

Cardiopulmonary Resuscitation (Two Nurses)

STEPS	RATIONALE
6. Observe for rise and fall of the chest wall with each respiration. If lungs do not inflate, reposition the head and neck and check for visible airway obstruction, such as vomitus.	Observing chest wall movement ensures that artificial respirations are entering the lungs.
7. Suction any secretions from the airway. If suction is unavailable, turn the victim's head to one side.	Suctioning prevents airway obstruction. Turning the client's head to one side allows gravity to drain secretions.
8. Assess for presence of the carotid pulse. Absence or a questionable pulse indicates the need for external cardiac compression.	The presence and quality of the client's pulse are ensured.
9. Begin external cardiac compression.	
Adult:	
a. Locate the xiphoid process below the sternum. Place the heel of one hand 4 to 5 cm (1½ to 2 inches) above the xiphoid process, and place heel of other hand over the first hand.	Compressions directly over the xiphoid process can lacerate the victim's liver.
b. Keep the hands parallel and the fingers away from victim's chest. Fingers may be interlocked. Keep elbows extended.	Compression occurs only on the sternum. The pressure necessary for external compression is created by the nurse's upper arm muscle strength.
c. Compress the chest 4 to 5 cm (2 to 2½ inches) once every second. Count one, one thousand, two, one thousand, etc.	Sixty compressions a minute should be delivered to ensure adequate cardiac output.
d. Ventilate the lungs after each fifth compression.	Adequate ventilation is promoted during CPR.
Small children and infants:	
e. Compress sternum 1 to 2 cm (½ to 1 inch) with both thumbs while supporting the back, or use the fingertips of the index and middle fingers of one hand.	Damage to external structures from excessive pressure is prevented.

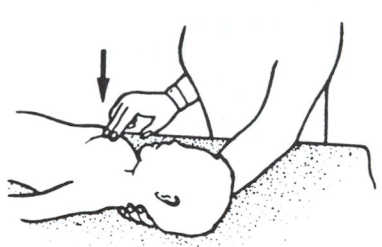 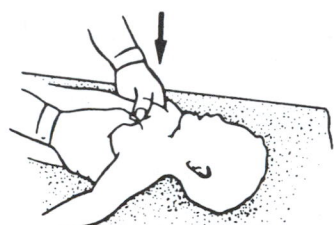

STEPS	RATIONALE
f. Deliver 80 to 100 compressions per minute.	The more rapid heart rate of infants and children is simulated.
g. Ventilate lungs every 3 seconds.	Adequate ventilation is promoted during CPR.
10. Palpate for carotid pulse with each external chest compression.	Assessment of pulse validates that an adequate stroke volume is achieved with each compression.
11. If the carotid pulse is not palpable, compressions are not strong enough. Continue CPR until relieved or until victim regains spontaneous pulse and respirations.	Artificial cardiopulmonary function is maintained.

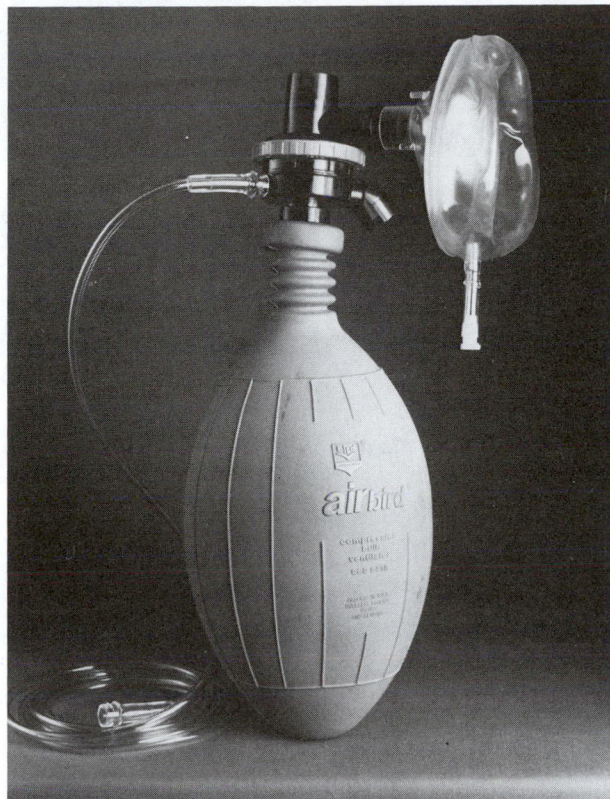

Fig. 41-16 Ambu bag with face mask and oxygen-connecting tubing.

CARDIOPULMONARY RESUSCITATION

Cardiac arrest is characterized by an absence of pulse and respiration and by dilated pupils. If the nurse determines that the client has experienced cardiac arrest, cardiopulmonary resuscitation (CPR) must be initiated. CPR is a basic emergency procedure for life support, consisting of artificial respiration and manual external cardiac massage (Procedure 41-5). CPR has three main goals, called the ABCs of cardiopulmonary resuscitation: to establish an *a*irway, initiate *b*reathing, and maintain *c*irculation.

Evaluation

All nursing interventions are evaluated by comparing the client's response to nursing therapies to the goals of the nursing care plan. Each of the five goals and five categories of interventions has objective evaluation criteria. These criteria are examples of evaluation criteria for clients with altered oxygenation; other evaluation criteria are based on the specific nursing diagnoses and goals of care.

Evaluation of maintenance or promotion of lung expansion is based on:

1. Symmetrical lung expansion on inspection and palpation
2. Increased lung expansion as demonstrated by incentive spirometry
3. Decreased dyspneic respiratory movements
4. Ability to lie flat
5. Presence of breath sounds in all fields on auscultation
6. Absence of abnormal movements such as retractions or movements of accessory muscles

The criteria for successful mobilization of pulmonary secretions are:

1. Productive cough
2. Removal of secretions with suction
3. White, watery sputum
4. Chest clear on auscultation

Maintenance of a patent airway is evaluated on the basis of:

1. Improved coughing ability of client
2. Productive cough
3. Absence of retractions or abnormal chest wall motion

Maintenance or promotion of tissue oxygenation has the following criteria:

1. Absence of signs of hypoxemia
2. Absence of cyanosis
3. Decreased dyspnea
4. Return of vital signs to baseline
5. Normal arterial blood gas results

The evaluation of restoration of cardiopulmonary function is based on:

1. Return of spontaneous pulse and respiration
2. Return of consciousness

As always, if the client does not show improvement in respiratory status, the nurse must reassess the client and reevaluate the care plan to determine the need for new interventions to restore the client's level of oxygenation. Therefore the evaluation process occurs throughout the client's nursing care.

Summary

Clients with impaired oxygenation require planned nursing care that focuses on returning the client to a maximal level of wellness. Many nursing interventions can be used to promote lung expansion, to mobilize secretions, to maintain a patent airway, to promote oxygenation, or to restore cardiopulmonary functioning.

Nursing interventions are individualized to the client's level of health, age, life-style, and needs. Many nursing skills are used to help the client achieve a maximal level of oxygenation.

KEY CONCEPTS

✓ Metabolic activities of the cells require oxygen.

✓ The primary function of the lung is to transfer oxygen from the atmosphere into the alveoli and to transfer carbon dioxide out of the body as a waste product.

✓ Ventilation is the process of providing adequate oxygenation from the alveoli to the blood.

✓ Breathing requires the body to generate energy to expand the lungs; this is called the work of breathing.

✓ Compliance, or the ability of the lungs to expand and contract, depends on the function of musculoskeletal and neurological systems and on other physiological factors.

✓ Inspiration is an active process, and expiration is a passive process.

✓ The process of moving air in and out of the lungs is achieved with lung pressures and lung volumes.

✓ Adequate oxygenation requires the heart to perfuse the ventilated regions of the lung.

✓ Respiratory gases are primarily transported by hemoglobin.

✓ Respiration is controlled by the central nervous system and by chemicals within the blood.

✓ The client's level of tissue oxygenation is affected by the level of health, age, lifestyle habits, and environment.

✓ Decreased hemoglobin levels alter the client's ability to transport oxygen.

✓ An increased metabolic rate increases the tissue oxygen demand.

✓ Impaired chest wall movement reduces the level of tissue oxygenation.

✓ The normal aging process decreases the elasticity of the lungs.

✓ Hyperventilation is a respiratory rate greater than that required to maintain normal levels of carbon dioxide.

✓ Hypoventilation causes carbon dioxide retention.

✓ Hypoxia occurs if the amount of oxygen delivered to the tissues is too low.

✓ The nursing history includes information about the client's cough, dyspnea, wheezing, pain, environmental exposures, respiratory infection, risk factors, and use of medications.

✓ The nurse uses all assessment techniques when evaluating a client's level of oxygenation.

✓ Diagnostic and laboratory tests may be needed to complete the data base for a client with decreased oxygenation.

✓ The nursing process is used to restore or maintain the client's maximal level of wellness.

✓ Improper positioning can decrease ventilation and oxygenation.

✓ Breathing exercises improve ventilation and oxygenation.

✓ Incentive spirometry increases inhalation volumes.

KEY CONCEPTS, cont'd

✓ Hydration and humidification help to liquefy and mobilize pulmonary secretions.

✓ Nebulization delivers small drops of water or particles of medication to the airways.

✓ Chest physiotherapy includes postural drainage, percussion, and vibration to mobilize pulmonary secretions.

✓ Coughing and suctioning techniques are used to maintain a patent airway.

✓ Oxygen therapy is used to improve levels of tissue oxygenation.

✓ Oxygen therapy is delivered by nasal cannula, nasal catheter, or oxygen mask.

✓ Cardiac arrest requires the use of cardiopulmonary resuscitation.

REFERENCES

Bushnell, S.S.: Respiratory intensive care nursing, ed. 2, Boston, 1981, Little, Brown & Co.

Daily, E.K., and Schroeder, J.S.: Techniques in bedside hemodynamic monitoring, ed. 3, St. Louis, 1985, The C.V. Mosby Co.

Feldman, J.: Chronic obstructive pulmonary disease. In Traver, G.A.: Respiratory nursing: the science and the art, New York, 1982, John Wiley & Sons, Inc.

Ganong, W.F.: Review of medical physiology, ed. 13, Los Altos, Calif., 1983, Lange Medical Publications.

Groër, M.W., and Shekleton, M.S.: Basic pathophysiology: a conceptual approach, ed. 2, St. Louis, 1983, The C.V. Mosby Co.

Luce, J.M., Tyler, M.L., and Pierson, D.J.: Intensive respiratory care, Philadelphia, 1984, W.B. Saunders Co.

Perry, A.G., and Potter, P.A., editors: Shock: comprehensive nursing management, St. Louis, 1983, The C.V. Mosby Co.

Smith, S.J.: Clinical assessment of the pulmonary patient. In Traver, G.A.: Respiratory nursing: the science and the art, New York, 1982, John Wiley & Sons, Inc.

Traver, G.A.: Respiratory nursing: the science and the art, New York, 1982, John Wiley & Sons, Inc.

Vander, A.J., Sherman, J.H., and Luciano, D.S.: Human physiology: the mechanism of body function, ed. 3, New York, 1980, McGraw-Hill Book Co.

Wade, J.F.: Respiratory nursing care, ed. 3, St. Louis, 1982, The C.V. Mosby Co.

West, J.B.: Respiratory physiology, the essentials, ed. 2, Baltimore, 1979, The Williams & Wilkins Co.

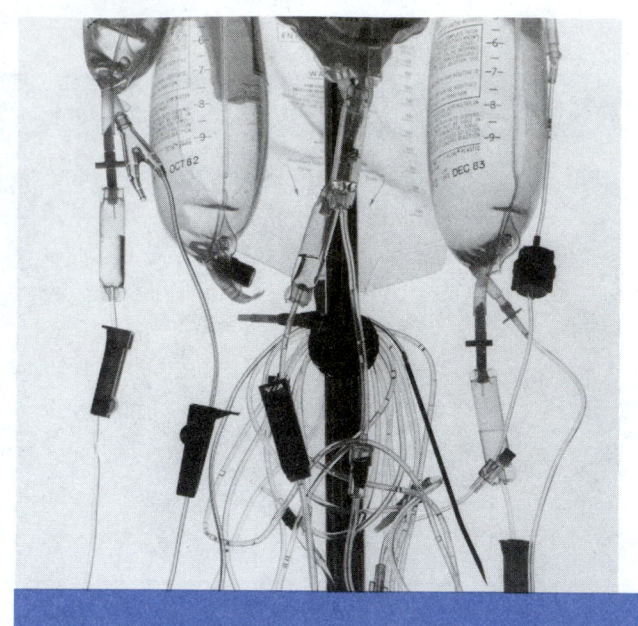

OBJECTIVES

Mastery of content in this chapter will enable the student to:

- Define the terms in the glossary.
- Describe the distribution and composition of body fluids.
- Describe the mechanisms by which body fluids move and are regulated.
- Describe the regulation and imbalances of sodium, potassium, calcium, magnesium, chloride, bicarbonate, and phosphate.
- Describe the volume disturbances of dehydration and overhydration.
- Discuss the variables that affect fluid and electrolyte balance.
- Compile a nursing history and complete a physical examination for fluid and electrolyte balances.
- Measure and record fluid intake and output.
- Describe laboratory studies associated with fluid and electrolyte imbalances.
- State nursing diagnoses associated with fluid and electrolyte imbalances.
- Describe a nursing care plan for clients with fluid and electrolyte disturbances.
- Describe fluids used for oral replacement of fluid losses.
- Discuss the objectives of intravenous therapy.
- Describe different types of intravenous solutions.
- Describe the procedure for initiating and maintaining an intravenous line.
- Demonstrate how to calculate intravenous flow rate and how to use an infusion pump.
- Demonstrate how to change intravenous solutions, tubing, and dressing and how to discontinue an infusion.
- Discuss the complications of intravenous therapy.
- Describe different blood groups and types of transfusion reactions.
- Discuss the procedure for administering a blood transfusion and nursing actions for a transfusion reaction.
- State the goals of total parenteral nutrition.
- List the components of total parenteral nutrition solutions.
- Describe the procedure for initiating and maintaining total parenteral nutrition.
- Discuss how to prevent infections and identify complications of total parenteral nutrition.

GLOSSARY

active transport Movement of materials across the cell membrane by means of chemical activity that allows the cell to admit larger molecules than would otherwise be possible.

aldosterone Mineral corticoid, produced by the adrenal cortex, that regulates sodium and potassium balance.

anions Negatively charged electrolytes.

42 Fluid and Electrolyte Balance

antidiuretic hormone (ADH)   Hormone that decreases the production of urine by increasing reabsorption of water by the kidney tubules.

cations   Positively charged electrolytes.

dehydration   Extracellular water loss that is beyond the normal regulatory system's ability to repair.

electrolyte   Element or compound that, when melted or dissolved in water or other solvent, dissociates into ions and can carry an electric current.

extracellular fluid   Portion of the body fluid comprised of the interstitial fluid and blood plasma.

hemolysis   Breakdown of red blood cells and release of hemoglobin as may result by administration of hypotonic intravenous solutions that cause progressive swelling and rupture of the erythrocytes.

hemosiderin   Iron-rich pigment that is the product of red blood cell hemolysis.

hydrostatic pressure   Pressure exerted by a liquid.

hypervolemia   Increase in the amount of fluid in the circulating blood volume.

interstitial fluid   Fluid that fills the spaces between most of the cells of the body and provides a substantial portion of the liquid environment of the body.

intracellular fluid   Liquid within the cell membrane.

milliequivalent per liter   Number of grams of a specific electrolyte dissolved in 1 liter of plasma.

osmosis   Movement of a pure solvent through a semipermeable membrane from a solution with a lower solute concentration to one with a higher solute concentration.

osmotic pressure   Drawing power for water, which depends on the number of molecules in the solution.

overhydration   Excess of water in the extracellular fluid.

plasma   Watery, colorless, fluid portion of the lymph and blood.

sodium pump   Physiological mechanism that transports sodium ions across cellular membranes against an opposing concentration gradient.

urine specific gravity   Measurement of the degree of concentration of the urine.

urinometer   Device for determining the specific gravity of urine.

venipuncture   Technique in which a vein is punctured transcutaneously by a sharp rigid stylet (such as a butterfly needle), a cannula (such as an angiocatheter that contains a flexible plastic catheter), or a needle attached to a syringe.

F luid and electrolyte balance within the body is necessary to maintain health and function in all body systems. The balance is maintained by the intake and output of water and electrolytes and their distribution in the body. Imbalances may result from many factors and are associated with many illnesses, and therefore nursing care for many different kinds of clients includes assessment and correction of imbalances or maintenance of balance. The nurse who bottle feeds an infant or helps a handicapped or visually impaired elderly client to eat is implementing nursing activities to maintain the client's fluid and electrolyte status.

A healthy, mobile, well-oriented adult is usually capable of maintaining normal fluid balance, even when minor fluid losses occur, as with gastroenteritis. This person is able to maintain fluid balance because of the body's adaptive mechanisms and thirst response. However, the infant, the severely ill adult, the disoriented or immobile client, and the elderly are frequently unable to respond independently to the thirst mechanism, and after a period of time the body's adaptive capacities are no longer capable of maintaining fluid or electrolyte balance.

A person's body composition is over half fluid, which is referred to as total body water (TBW). The percentage of TBW ranges between 60% and 80% (Metheny and Snively, 1983). The variables that account for the differences in TBW include age, sex, and body fat. The newborn's TBW is 80% of kilogram weight. In general, the younger the person, the higher the percentage of TBW. If the adult male's TBW is 70 kg, it constitutes 60% of his kilogram weight. The percentage is slightly less in women. The TBW of the obese adult is approximately 40% to 50%, less than that of the emaciated adult, whose TBW is 70% to 75% (Groër, 1981).

This chapter describes the distribution and composition of body water, how body water moves from one compartment to another, and the factors that regulate fluid balance, as well as specific electrolyte and volume disturbances. Through the nursing process the nurse cares for clients with fluid imbalances and maintains intravenous and blood infusions and total parenteral nutrition.

Distribution of Body Fluids

Body fluids are distributed in two distinct compartments, one containing extracellular fluids and the other intracellular fluids (Table 42-1).

Extracellular fluids are the portion of the body fluids comprising the interstitial fluid and blood plasma. Interstitial fluid fills the spaces between most of the cells of the body and provides a substantial portion of the liquid environment of the body. About 16% of the body weight (or 11.2 liters) consists of interstitial fluids. Plasma, the watery, colorless, fluid portion of the lymph and the blood in which the leukocytes, erythrocytes, and platelets are suspended, comprises 4% (or 2.8 liters).

Intracellular fluids are liquids within cell membranes throughout most of the body, containing dissolved solutes essential to fluid and electrolyte balance and metabolism. Many of the materials in the intracellular fluid compartment are the same as those located in the extracellular fluid space. However, the proportion of the substances is different. For example, there is a greater proportion of potassium in intracellular fluids than in the extracellular fluid compartment. The intracellular and extracellular distributions of major ions are described in a later section.

Composition of Body Fluids

The fluids that circulate throughout the body in the extracellular and intracellular fluid spaces are composed of electrolytes, minerals, and cells.

An *electrolyte* is an element or compound that, when melted or dissolved in water or another solvent, dissociates into ions and is able to carry an electric current. Positively charged electrolytes are *cations*. Students may find it helpful to associate the "t" in cation (which has a positive charge) with a plus (+) sign. Negatively charged electrolytes are called *anions*. The concentrations of electrolytes differ in extracellular and intracellular fluids.

TABLE 42-1

Body Fluid Distribution

Compartment	Percent of Total Body Weight	Fluid Volume (liters)
Extracellular fluid		
Interstitial fluid	16	11.2
Plasma	4	2.8
Intracellular fluid	80	42.0

Electrolytes are commonly measured in milliequivalents per liter (mEq/L). This value represents the number of grams of the specific electrolyte (solute) dissolved in 1 liter of plasma (solution). The only electrolyte concentrations that are not recorded in milliequivalents per liter are calcium, bicarbonate, and phosphate.

Minerals, which are ingested as compounds, are usually referred to by the name of a metal, nonmetal, radical, or phosphate rather than by the name of the compound of which they are a part. Minerals play a vital role in regulating many body functions. They are constituents of all body tissues and fluids, and they are important in maintaining physiological processes. Minerals also act as catalysts in nerve response, muscle contraction, and the metabolism of nutrients in foods. In addition, they regulate electrolyte balance and hormone production, and they strengthen skeletal structures.

Cells, which are also located in body fluids, are the functional fundamental units of all living tissue. Examples of cells within body fluids are the red blood cell (RBC) and the white blood cell (WBC).

Body fluids composed of electrolytes, minerals, and cells comprise a major portion of the total body weight. For body fluids to remain in appropriate intracellular or extracellular compartments, their movement must follow specific patterns.

Movement of Body Fluids

Fluids within the body are not static. Fluids and electrolytes shift from compartment to compartment to meet a variety of metabolic needs such as tissue oxygenation; response to illness, for example, acid-base disturbances (see Chapter 43); or response to drug therapies, for example, diuretics. Body fluid and electrolyte movement is effected through diffusion, osmosis, active transport, or fluid pressures. In addition, the movement of fluid components is dependent on cellular permeability.

Diffusion

Diffusion is a process in which solid, particulate matter in a fluid moves from an area of higher concentration to an area of lower concentration, resulting in an even distribution of the particles in the fluid. Substances that are diffusing therefore move down their concentration gradients or, more simply, in a downhill direction (Groër, 1981). Fluids and electrolytes also diffuse across cellular membranes. For a substance to cross the membrane the membrane must be permeable to that substance.

Osmosis

Osmosis is the movement of a pure solvent, such as water, through a semipermeable membrane from a solution that has a lower solute concentration to one that has a higher solute concentration. The membrane is permeable to the solvent but it is impermeable to the solute, the particulate matter. The rate of osmosis depends on four factors: (1) the concentrations of the solutes in the solutions, (2) the temperature of the solutions, (3) the electrical charges of the solutes, and (4) the differences between the osmotic pressures exerted by the solutions.

The concentration of a solution is measured in osmols. An osmol is the amount of a substance in solution in the form of molecules, ions, or both that has the same osmotic pressure as one mole of an ideal nonelectrolyte. The osmotic pressure of a solution is expressed as osmolarity, which is expressed in osmols or milliosmols per kilogram of the solution.

If the concentration of the solute is greater on one side of the permeable membrane, the rate of osmosis is quicker and there is a more rapid transfer of solvent across the membrane. This continues until an equilibrium is reached.

Active Transport

Active transport is the movement of materials across the cell membrane by means of chemical activity that allows the cell to admit larger molecules than it would otherwise be able to admit. Unlike diffusion and osmosis, active transport requires metabolic activity and energy expenditure.

Enhancing active transport are carrier molecules, such as insulin, within a cell that bind themselves to incoming molecules. For example, insulin binds itself to glucose and serves as a transport vehicle to permit entry of glucose into the cell. Active transport is the mechanism by which the cell absorbs glucose and other substances to carry out metabolic activities.

The criteria for active transport include movement against a concentration gradient, saturation motion, and metabolic work by the cell. Active transport can be inhibited by cooling the cell, starving the cell as by withholding glucose, and poisoning the cell (Groër, 1981).

Fluid Pressures

The pressures exerted by different types of fluids also direct the movement of fluid between the extracellular and intracellular fluid compartments. The two basic pressures exerted on fluids are osmotic and hydrostatic pressures.

Osmotic pressure refers to the drawing power for water and depends on the number of molecules in the solution (Metheny and Snively, 1983). Osmotic pressure is exerted through a semipermeable membrane and is dependent on the activity of the solutes that are separated by the membrane. A solution that has the same osmotic pressure or osmolarity as blood plasma is called isotonic. The intravenous administration of an isotonic solution prevents the shifting of fluid and electrolytes from the intracellular compartments. Two of the substances that affect osmotic pressure are albumin and mannitol. Albumin is a serum protein naturally produced by the body; it exerts colloid osmotic pressure, which assists in maintaining fluids in their proper fluid compartments. Mannitol, a hypertonic saturated sugar solution given therapeutically, alters osmotic pressure and causes osmotic diuresis.

A hypotonic solution that has a lesser concentration of solutes may be administered to a client to help maintain fluid and electrolyte balance. For example, half normal saline (½ NS) may be ordered for clients recovering from ketoacidosis. This hypotonic solution is ordered in combination with other electrolyte solutions.

Hydrostatic pressure is the pressure exerted by a liquid. Blood and fluid entering the capillaries do so at a certain pressure. Basically the hydrostatic pressure of this fluid is caused by gravity, and some capillary beds have a higher pressure because of their location, such as those in the feet. Like osmotic pressures, hydrostatic pressures assist in maintaining body fluids in their appropriate compartments.

■ ■ ■ ■ ■

Body fluids have the capacity to move from one fluid compartment to another. The shift in fluids usually results from an adaptive regulatory mechanism that the body institutes to maintain fluid and electrolyte balance.

Regulation of Body Fluids

Body fluids are regulated by three processes: fluid intake, fluid output, and hormonal controls.

Fluid Intake

Fluid intake is regulated primarily through the thirst mechanism. When thirsty, a person takes in some fluid. The thirst control center is located within the hypothalamus in the brain. The major physiological stimuli to the thirst center are increased plasma osmolarity and decreased blood volume. In addition, psychological factors and the sensation of a "dry throat" create the sensation of thirst (Groër, 1981) (Fig. 42-1).

Receptor cells called osmoreceptors continually monitor the osmotic pressure. When too much fluid is lost, the osmoreceptors detect the loss and activate the thirst center. As a result the person feels thirsty and seeks water.

Water is also acquired from food intake, such as fruits, vegetables, and meats, and from the oxidation of food substances during digestion. As discussed in Chapter 38, water is one of the end products of the metabolism of carbohydrates, proteins, and fats. For each 100 calories of food metabolized, about 14 ml is acquired (Guyton, 1982).

The adult male (70 kg) requires an average daily fluid intake of 2600 ml. Of this amount approximately 1300 ml is from fluid intake, 1000 ml from foods, and 300 ml from metabolism (Metheny and

Fig. 42-1 Stimuli affecting the thirst mechanism.
Modified from Groër, M.W.: Physiology and pathophysiology of the body fluids, St. Louis, 1981, The C.V. Mosby Co.

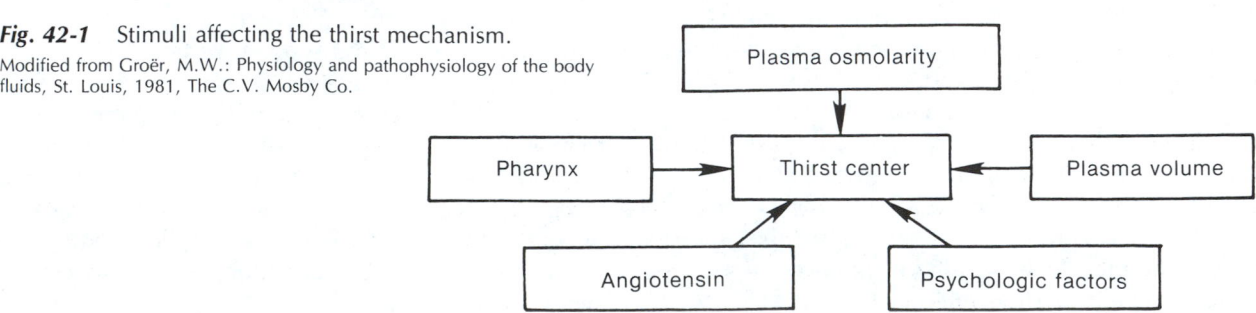

Snively, 1983). Fluid intake requires an alert state. Infants, clients with neurological or psychological impairments, and some of the elderly are unable to perceive or respond to their thirst mechanism; as a result they are at risk for developing dehydration.

Fluid Output

Fluid output occurs through four organs of water loss: the kidneys, the skin, the lungs, and the gastrointestinal tract.

The *kidneys* are the major regulatory organs of fluid balance. They receive about 170 liters of plasma to filter each day and produce 1.5 liters (1500 ml) of urine to be excreted. The amount of urine produced by the kidneys can be influenced by two hormones, antidiuretic hormone (ADH) and aldosterone. These two hormones affect water and sodium excretion and can be stimulated by changes in blood volume. The regulatory effects of these hormones on the kidneys and total fluid balance are described in the following section.

Water loss from the *skin* is regulated primarily by the sympathetic nervous system, which activates the body's sweat glands. Stimulation of the sweat glands can occur as the result of muscular exercise, elevated environmental temperature, and increased metabolic activity as is the case with a fever.

Water loss from the skin can be either a sensible or an insensible loss. Insensible water loss is continuous and is not perceived by the person. The average insensible water loss is 15 to 20 ml/kg/24 hours (Groër, 1981). Sensible water loss occurs through excessive perspiration and is perceived by the person. The amount of sensible perspiration is directly related to the amount of exercise, environmental temperature, and metabolic activity. As these three factors increase, so do the amount of sweat produced and the amount of water lost through the skin. Sensible water loss can range up to 5000 ml depending on exercise and external and body temperatures (Groër, 1981).

The *lungs* expire approximately 400 ml of water daily. This insensible loss may increase in response to changes in respiratory rate and depth, as is the case with increased exercise or the presence of a fever. In addition, devices for the administration of oxygen can increase insensible water loss from the lungs.

The average fluid loss from the *gastrointestinal tract* is about 100 ml/24 hours. Obviously vomiting or diarrhea increases fluid loss.

The nurse who is assessing clients' hydration status must also account for all fluid losses (Table 42-2). As fluid loss increases, the nurse needs to adjust the plan of care to increase fluid intake either orally or parenterally in order to maintain fluid balance. In addition, the nurse must be aware of the hormonal controls on fluid and electrolyte balance.

Hormones

The two major hormones affecting fluid and electrolyte balance are ADH and aldosterone. *ADH* decreases the production of urine by increasing the reabsorption of water by the kidney tubules. During transient periods of fluid volume deficit, as with vomiting and diarrhea or hemorrhage, the amount of this hormone in the blood increases. As a result the water reabsorbed by the kidney tubules increases and is returned to the circulating blood volume. Urinary output declines in response to the action of the hormone.

The stimulus for ADH secretion is an increase in blood osmolarity, which indicates a state of water deficit. The hormone itself is released by the posterior pituitary gland.

Aldosterone is the other major hormone affecting water and electrolyte balance. Aldosterone is a mineral corticoid, produced by the adrenal cortex, that regulates sodium and potassium balance. The presence of aldosterone causes the kidney tubules to excrete potassium and reabsorb sodium, and as a result water is also reabsorbed and returned to the blood volume. Fluid deficits such as those produced by hemorrhage or gastrointestinal losses can stimulate the secretion of aldosterone into the blood.

A third class of hormones, *glucocorticoids,* also affects water and electrolyte balance. While normal glucocorticoid hormone secretion does not result in major fluid imbalances, excesses of the hormone in the circulation alter fluid and electrolyte balance. For example, a client with a disease such as Cushing's syndrome retains sodium and water because of the action of excess glucocorticoids. Likewise, a client

TABLE 42-2

Average Daily Fluid Output in a 70 Kg Adult

Organ or System	Amount (ml)
Kidneys	1500
Skin	
Insensible loss	600-900
Sensible loss	0-5000
Lungs	400
Gastrointestinal tract	100
TOTAL*	2600-2900

*Excludes sensible loss.

who is receiving steroid medications, such as cortisone or prednisone, retains sodium and water.

The regulatory mechanisms for fluid and electrolyte balance are short-term methods of maintaining fluid balance during transient states such as exercise, viral illness, vomiting, or diarrhea. However, when these conditions are prolonged, the body's regulatory mechanisms are insufficient, and fluid and electrolyte imbalances can occur.

Electrolyte Regulation and Imbalances

Electrolytes are present in both the intracellular and extracellular fluids. An electrolyte can be a cation (a positively charged electrolyte) or an anion (a negatively charged electrolyte).

Cations

Major cations within the body fluids include sodium (Na^+), potassium (K^+), calcium (Ca^{++}), and magnesium (Mg^{++}). Cations may be interchanged when one cation exits the cell and is replaced by another cation entering the cell. This replacement phenomenon occurs because cells tend to maintain electrical neutrality. Therefore one positively charged ion must be exchanged with another positively charged ion.

SODIUM

Sodium is the most abundant cation in the extracellular fluid. Sodium ions are involved in the process of maintaining water balance, the transmission of nerve impulses, and the contraction of muscles. The normal extracellular concentration of sodium is 136 to 144 mEq/L.

An important physiological principle in fluid and electrolyte balance is that where sodium goes, water goes. If the kidneys retain sodium, water is retained. Conversely, if the kidneys excrete sodium, water is also excreted. The action of many drugs, such as diuretics, is based on this principle.

SODIUM REGULATION. Sodium is regulated by salt intake, aldosterone, and urinary output. The major source of sodium is dietary, such as table salt, processed meats, snack foods, and canned vegetables. In healthy individuals without diminished cardiovascular or renal function, excretion of urine sodium can be increased to maintain the serum sodium level within normal limits.

When sodium intake decreases or a person loses body fluids, as with burns or trauma, the body attempts to conserve sodium through the hormone aldosterone. As noted earlier, aldosterone is a mineralocorticoid hormone, produced by the adrenal cortex, that increases sodium retention and potassium excretion. Aldosterone exerts its action on the kidney tubules to reabsorb sodium, thus returning sodium to the extracellular fluid. When sodium is retained, water is also retained.

HYPONATREMIA. Hyponatremia is a less than normal concentration of sodium in the blood, which can occur when there is a net sodium loss or net water excess (Table 42-3). Usually hyponatremia includes a decrease in the osmolarity of plasma and extracellular fluid, as occurs with diabetes (Groër, 1981).

When there is a sodium loss, the body initially adapts by reducing water excretion in an attempt to maintain serum osmolarity at near-normal levels. As the sodium loss continues, the body continues to preserve the blood and interstitial (tissue) volume. As a result the sodium in the extracellular fluid becomes more dilute. Hyponatremia caused by sodium loss can result in vascular collapse and shock. When there is a pure sodium deficit, there is a distinct loss of extracellular fluid volume, a condition different from hyponatremia resulting from water excess.

Hyponatremia can develop when there are large excesses of extracellular fluid volume, which is also called water excess. With water excess there are dilutional effects on all of the blood components. This is referred to as dilutional hyponatremia and is characterized by an increase in the client's weight; edema; low hemoglobin, hematocrit, and serum albumin values; normal or excessive urine volume; and frequently a normal urine specific gravity.

HYPERNATREMIA. Hypernatremia is a greater than normal concentration of sodium in the extracellular fluid, which can be caused by excessive water loss or an overall sodium excess (Table 42-4.) When hypernatremia occurs, the body attempts to conserve as much water as possible through renal reabsorption. As a result the urine output of the client is decreased and the specific gravity may be elevated. Whether the cause of hypernatremia is water deficit or sodium excess, there is an increase in the interstitial osmotic pressure, and as a result fluid shifts from the cells into the extracellular fluid. This fluid shift causes the cells to shrink and interrupts most of the physiological cellular processes.

Closely aligned to the regulation of sodium balance and imbalance is the electrolyte potassium. Frequently when sodium is retained, potassium is excreted, as is the case when aldosterone is secreted.

TABLE 42-3

Hyponatremia

Net Sodium Loss*	Net Water Excess*	Signs and Symptoms
Kidney disease	Syndrome of inappropriate ADH secretion (SIADH)	*Physical examination:* apprehension, anxiety, personality change, postural hypotension, postural dizziness, abdominal cramping, nausea and vomiting, diarrhea, tachycardia, convulsions and coma, cold, clammy skin
Addison's disease	Increase of water over solute intake, when renal mechanisms are not functioning properly	
Gastrointestinal losses		
Increased sweating		
Diuretics	Hyperaldosteronism	*Laboratory findings:* serum sodium < 136mEq/L, urine specific gravity < 1.010
Interruption of Na^+,K^+ pump with decreased cell K^+ and decreased serum Na^+	Diabetic ketoacidosis	
	Oliguria caused by renal failure	
Use of diuretics combined with low sodium diet	Psychogenic polydipsia	
Metabolic acidosis		

*Data from Groër, M.W.: Physiology and pathophysiology of the body fluids, St. Louis, 1981, The C.V. Mosby Co.

TABLE 42-4

Hypernatremia

Net Water Deficit*	Net Sodium Excess*	Signs and Symptoms
Water deprivation	Ingestion of large amounts of concentrated salt solutions	*Physical examination:* thirst, dry flushed skin, dry tongue and mucous membranes, pyrexia, agitation, convulsions, restlessness, excitability, oliguria or anuria
Urea diuresis		
Greatly increased insensible water loss	Iatrogenic administration of hypertonic saline solution parenterally	
Disorders in which thirst is either absent or not perceived		*Laboratory findings:* serum sodium > 144 mEq/L, urine specific gravity > 1.030 (if water loss is not caused by renal dysfunction)
Nephrogenic diabetes insipidus		

*Data from Groër, M.W.: Physiology and pathophysiology of the body fluids, St. Louis, 1981, The C.V. Mosby Co.

POTASSIUM

Potassium is the predominant intracellular cation that regulates neuromuscular excitability and muscle contraction. The sources of potassium are primarily dietary and include whole grains, meat, legumes, fruits, and vegetables. Potassium is needed for glycogen formation, protein synthesis, and correction of acid-base imbalances.

Potassium assists in the regulation of acid-base balance because the potassium ion (K^+) is in competition with the hydrogen ion (H^+) for exchange for sodium ions in renal tubular excretion (Metheny, 1981). Therefore, in an acidotic state, a potassium ion is conserved and an hydrogen ion is excreted. The opposite occurs in alkalosis (see Chapter 43).

POTASSIUM REGULATION. Potassium is regulated primarily by the kidneys. In the presence of increased aldosterone secretion, more potassium is excreted through the urine and the serum potassium level can fall. The second mechanism of potassium regulation is the exchange with the sodium ion in the kidney tubule. When sodium is retained, potassium is excreted.

The normal range for serum potassium is 3.5 to 5.5 mEq/L. The major alterations of potassium balance are hypokalemia and hyperkalemia.

HYPOKALEMIA. Hypokalemia is a condition in which an inadequate amount of potassium is circulating in the extracellular fluid. When severe, hypo-

TABLE 42-5

Hypokalemia

Causes	Signs and Symptoms
Use of potassium-wasting diuretics	*Physical examination:* weakness and fatigue, muscle fatigue, decreased muscle tone, intestinal distention, decreased bowel sounds, weak, irregular pulse, heart block (severe hypokalemia), paresthesia
Diarrhea, vomiting, or other gastrointestinal losses	
Alkalosis	*Laboratory findings:* serum potassium < 4 mEq/L,* ECG abnormalities: low voltage, flattening of T waves, depressed ST segments, ECG changes likely when potassium is < 3.0 mEq/L*
Cushing's syndrome or adrenal hormone–producing tumors	
Renal disease	
Extreme diaphoresis	
Excessive use of potassium-free intravenous solutions	

*Data from Metheny, N.M., and Snively, W.D., Jr.: Nurse's handbook of fluid balance, ed. 4, Philadelphia, 1983, J.B. Lippincott Co.

TABLE 42-6

Hyperkalemia

Causes	Signs and Symptoms
Renal failure	*Physical examination:* anxiety, irritability, cardiac irregularities, hypotension, paresthesia, weakness
Hypertonic dehydration	
Massive cellular damage such as burns and trauma	*Laboratory findings:* serum potassium > 5 mEq/L,* ECG findings: bradycardia—serum potassium > 7 mEq/L, heart block—serum potassium > 9 mEq/L
Iatrogenic administration of large amounts of potassium intravenously	
Hypoadrenalism (Addison's disease)	
Acidosis	
Rapid infusion of stored blood	
Potassium-retaining diuretics	

*Levels > 8.5 mEq/L are frequently fatal as a result of cardiac arrest (Metheny and Snively, 1983).

kalemia can affect cardiac conduction and function. Because the normal amount of potassium is so small, there is little tolerance for fluctuations in serum potassium levels.

Hypokalemia can result from several conditions (Table 42-5.) In addition, hypokalemia is often observed in clients recovering from burns, crush injuries, or massive trauma. Initially the extracellular fluid becomes hyperkalemic because of the release of potassium from the damaged cells, but if renal function is normal, the excess potassium is excreted by the kidneys (Groër, 1981).

The symptoms associated with hypokalemia depend on its onset and the client's ability to adapt. Common symptoms include muscle weakness, confusion, lethargy, and cardiac conduction disturbances. In addition, decreased gastric motility can result in a paralytic ileus, anorexia, and polyuria.

HYPERKALEMIA. Hyperkalemia is a greater than normal amount of potassium in the blood. Severe hyperkalemia produces marked cardiac conduction abnormalities.

The primary cause of hyperkalemia is renal failure, but other illness also result in increased potassium (Table 42-6). Any decrease in renal function dimin-

---

TABLE 42-7

Hypocalcemia

Causes	Signs and Symptoms
Rapid administration of blood transfusions that contain citrate	*Physical examination:* numbness and tingling of fingers and circumoral region, hyperactive reflexes, positive Trousseau's sign, positive Chvostek's sign, tetany, muscle cramps, pathological fractures (chronic hypocalcemia)
Hypoalbuminemia	
Parathyroid disease	
Vitamin D deficiency	*Laboratory findings:* serum calcium < 4.5 mEq/L or 10 mg/100 ml, ECG changes—prolonged Q-T interval
Neoplastic diseases	
Pancreatitis	
Rapid administration of citrated blood	

---

ishes the amount of potassium the kidney can excrete. As mentioned previously, soon after burns and trauma the client is hyperkalemic.

The primary symptom of hyperkalemia is irregular electrocardiographic configurations. In addition, there are muscle weakness, paresthesias, and smooth muscle irritability.

CALCIUM

Calcium is the fifth most abundant element in the body. The body requires calcium for cellular membrane integrity and structure, adequate cardiac conduction, blood coagulation, and bone growth and formation. Calcium is present in three forms in the body fluids: (1) ionized (4.5 mg/100 ml), (2) nondiffusible, which is calcium complexed to protein anions (5 mg/100 ml), and (3) calcium salts such as calcium citrate and calcium phosphate (1 mg/100 ml). Calcium in the body fluid is a small percentage of the total body calcium. The major portion of calcium is in bones and teeth.

CALCIUM REGULATION. Calcium in the extracellular fluid is regulated primarily through actions of the parathyroid and thyroid glands. Parathyroid hormone (PTH) controls the balance among bone calcium, gastrointestinal absorption of calcium, and kidney excretion of calcium. Thyrocalcitonin from the thyroid gland also has a minor role in determining serum calcium levels by inhibiting bone resorption of calcium. The two alterations associated with calcium balance are hypocalcemia and hypercalcemia.

HYPOCALCEMIA. Hypocalcemia is present when the serum calcium concentration falls below 8.5 mg/100 ml, which also reflects a drop in ionized calcium to

less than 4 mg/100 ml (Groër, 1981). Hypocalcemia can result from several illnesses, some of which directly affect the thyroid and parathyroid glands (Table 42-7).

The signs and symptoms of hypocalcemia are directly correlated to the physiological role of serum calcium. Because calcium contributes to neuromuscular excitability, hypocalcemia results in muscle cramping, muscle spasms, paresthesia, and tetany. Tetany is continuous muscle contraction, which may be observed as a muscle spasm such as the carpopedal spasm. In addition, hypocalcemia affects the excitability of the cardiac muscle and, if uncorrected, can result in heart failure. The gastrointestinal effects of hypocalcemia are cramping and diarrhea.

HYPERCALCEMIA. Hypercalcemia exists when the total serum concentration of calcium rises to a value greater than 12 mg/100 ml, which reflects an increase of ionized calcium above 5 mg/100 ml. Frequently hypercalcemia is a symptom of an underlying disease resulting in excessive bone resorption with release of calcium (Table 42-8).

The symptoms commonly associated with hypercalcemia are also related to the physiological action of calcium. Initially, there is decreased neuromuscular irritability, resulting in fatigue, muscle pain, and weakness. In addition, personality changes such as irritability, increased sleepiness, and confusion are common. Gastrointestinal disturbances include anorexia, abdominal pain, nausea, and vomiting.

MAGNESIUM

Magnesium is the second most important cation of the intracellular fluids in the body and is essential for enzyme activities, neurochemical activities, and mus-

TABLE 42-8

Hypercalcemia

Causes	Signs and Symptoms*
Hyperparathyroidism Metastic tumors of bone Paget's disease Osteoporosis Prolonged immobilization	*Physical examination:* decreased muscle tone, anorexia, nausea and vomiting, weakness and lethargy, low back pain (retrorenal region from kidney stones), decreased level of consciousness, cardiac arrest *Laboratory findings:* serum calcium > 5.8 mEq/L or 10 mg/100 ml; roentgenographic examination shows generalized osteoporosis, widespread bone cavitation, radiopaque urinary stones; elevated BUN caused by fluid volume deficit or renal damage

*Data from Metheny, N.M., and Snively, W.D., Jr.: Nurse's handbook of fluid balance, ed. 4, Philadelphia, 1983, J.B. Lippincott Co.

TABLE 42-9

Hypomagnesemia

Causes*	Signs and Symptoms

Inadequate intake
  Malnutrition
  Alcoholism
Inadequate absorption
  Diarrhea, vomiting, nasogastric drainage, fistulas
  Excessive dietary calcium—competes with magnesium for transport sites
  Diseases of the small intestine
  Hypoparathyroidism
Excessive loss
  Thiazide diuretics
  Aldosterone excess
  Polyuria
	Physical examination: muscular tremors, hyperactive deep tendon reflexes, confusion and disorientation, hallucinations, convulsions, tachycardia, hypertension
	
	Laboratory findings: serum magnesium level < 1.4 mEq/L

*Data from Groër, M.W.: Physiology and pathophysiology of the body fluids, St. Louis, 1981, The C.V. Mosby Co.

cular excitability. Plasma concentrations of magnesium range from 1.5 to 2.5 mEq/L.

MAGNESIUM REGULATION. Magnesium is indirectly regulated through renal excretion and some actions of parathyroid hormone. Altered magnesium levels, hypomagnesemia and hypermagnesemia, are often associated with serious disease and produce symptoms that reflect altered neuromuscular function (Groër, 1981).

HYPOMAGNESEMIA. Hypomagnesemia is present when the serum concentration level drops below 1.5 mEq/L. The multiple causes of hypomagnesemia (Table 42-9) produce symptoms very similar to hypocalcemia. Assessment findings may include muscle cramps, tetany, weakness, tremors, nausea, vomiting, behavioral changes, and changes in central nervous system and cardiovascular functioning.

HYPERMAGNESEMIA. Hypermagnesemia occurs when the serum concentration of magnesium rises above 2.5 mEq/L. Hypermagnesemia has three primary causes: renal failure, excessive doses of parenterally administered magnesium, and hyperparathyroidism. The clinical symptoms of hypermagnesemia include cardiac arrhythmias, depressed deep tendon reflexes, and depressed respiration.

■ ■ ■ ■ ■

The major cations—sodium, potassium, calcium, and magnesium—are located in the extracellular as well as intracellular fluid. Their actions affect neurochemical and neuromuscular transmissions, which in turn influence muscular function, cardiac rhythm and contractility, mood and behavior, and gastrointestinal functioning.

Anions

There are three major anions of body fluids. These negatively charged electrolytes are chloride, bicarbonate, and phosphate ions. Each has specific functions, regulatory mechanisms, and symptoms that indicate deficiencies or excesses.

CHLORIDE

Chloride is the major anion in the extracellular and intracellular fluid. The major role of the chloride ion is to balance cations within the extracellular fluid. If a negatively charged ion leaves the extracellular fluid and enters the intracellular fluid, a chloride ion will be exchanged and enter the extracellular fluid. The ion exchange maintains electrical neutrality of the cell.

CHLORIDE REGULATION. Chloride is regulated via the kidneys. The amount of chloride excreted is related to dietary intake. The person with normal kidneys who has a high chloride intake will excrete an elevated amount of urine chloride. Normal serum chloride levels range from 95 to 105 mEq/L.

HYPOCHLOREMIA. Hypochloremia occurs when the serum chloride level falls below 95 mEq/L. There are three common causes of hypochloremia. Vomiting or prolonged and excessive nasogastric or fistula drainage can result in hypochloremia. A newborn can quickly develop hypochloremia as a result of diarrhea. Certain diuretics also result in increased chloride excretion.

When serum chloride levels fall, the body attempts to adapt by increased reabsorption of the bicarbonate ion, affecting acid-base balance, and metabolic alkalosis results (see Chapter 43.)

HYPERCHLOREMIA. Hyperchloremia occurs when the serum chloride level rises above 105 mEq/L and usually occurs when the serum bicarbonate value falls.

Hypochloremia and hyperchloremia rarely occur as single disease processes but commonly are associated with acid-base imbalance (see Chapter 43). As a result there is no single set of symptoms associated with these two alterations.

BICARBONATE

Bicarbonate (HCO_3^-) is the major chemical base buffer within the body. The bicarbonate ion is found in the extracellular and intracellular fluid. The regulation of bicarbonate is primarily through the kidneys. When the body needs to retain more base, the kidneys reabsorb greater quantities of bicarbonate and return it to the extracellular fluid. Normal bicarbonate levels range between 22 and 26 mEq/L. The bicarbonate ion is an essential component of the carbonic acid–bicarbonate buffering system essential to acid-base balance (see Chapter 43).

PHOSPHATE

Phosphate (PO_4^-) is a buffer anion that is present both intracellularly and extracellularly. Phosphate together with calcium contributes to the development and maintenance of bones and teeth. In addition, phosphate promotes normal neuromuscular action, participates in carbohydrate metabolism, and assists in acid-base regulation.

Serum phosphate concentration is regulated by parathyroid hormone and by activated vitamin D (Groër, 1981). Phosphate is normally absorbed through the gastrointestinal tract in a range of 3 to 12 mg/100 ml. Calcium and phosphate are inversely proportional. If one rises, the other falls.

■ ■ ■ ■ ■

All body electrolytes need to remain within normal limits for cellular metabolism to be maintained. The body is able to adapt to transient changes in some electrolytes, but this is only a short-term process. Eventually the cause of the electrolyte balance must be corrected. Electrolyte imbalances usually do not occur without some change in fluid volume.

Volume Disturbances

The two basic types of volume disturbance are fluid volume deficits and fluid volume excesses. Fluid volume deficit, or dehydration, is a state of water loss that is beyond the normal regulatory system's ability to repair (Groër, 1981). Fluid volume excess, or overhydration, is an excess in the extracellular fluid.

Dehydration

As described earlier, water balance is maintained by fluid intake, fluid output, and hormonal regulation. When fluid output exceeds intake, dehydration occurs. Likewise, decreased antidiuretic hormone secretion or aldosterone secretion can result in dehydration.

TABLE 42-10

Isotonic Dehydration

Causes	Signs and Symptoms
Losses from the gastrointestinal system, such as diarrhea, vomiting, or drainage from fistulas or tubes	*Physical examination:* initial hypotension, tachycardia, cardiac arrhythmias, dry skin, poor skin turgor, dry mucous membranes, pallor, lethargy, weakness, oliguria
Third-space fluid shifts	*Laboratory findings:* urine specific gravity >1.025
Loss of plasma or whole blood, as with burns or hemorrhage	
Excessive perspiration	

Dehydration is an excessive loss of water from the body tissues. Dehydration is accompanied by a disturbance in the balance of essential electrolytes: sodium, potassium, and chloride. When a water loss occurs, the various regulatory mechanisms within the body attempt to maintain cardiovascular function and perfusion to the vital organs. In addition, the hormonal controls assist in the conservation of the remaining body water.

One result of these mechanisms is an activation of the sympathetic nervous system and vasoconstriction of the arterioles to maintain blood pressure and perfusion of the heart, lungs, and brain. In addition, the renal blood flow and glomerular filtration rate decrease, and urine output falls in order to maintain fluid in the extracellular fluid.

Clinically, dehydration can be observed in three forms: isotonic, hypernatremic, and hyponatremic.

Isotonic dehydration is a loss of fluid from the extracellular space, but there is no important effect on the solutes within the plasma itself. The causes of isotonic dehydration are numerous (Table 42-10). When there is a loss of extracellular fluid, the major response of the body is activation of the sympathetic nervous system. The degree of sympathetic response is proportionate to the degree of extracellular fluid deficit. For example, after 24-hour gastrointestinal flu, the person may be pale, and the urine output is somewhat decreased. However, this response of the sympathetic nervous system is minimal compared to that in a person in shock. In shock, activation of the sympathetic nervous system reduces blood pressure, causes vasoconstriction, increases heart rate, and maintains blood supply to the vital organs and the kidney.

Hypernatremic dehydration signifies a loss of fluid accompanied by sodium excess. It is not characterized by the cardiovascular signs and ultimate circulatory collapse of isotonic dehydration. Rather it results from the loss of excess water from the extracellular fluid, which becomes hyperosmolar, causing cellular dehydration with relative maintenance of the extracellular fluid volume. Hypernatremic dehydration (serum Na^+ 150 mEq/L) is associated with increased insensible water loss (Table 42-11).

Normally with increased insensible water loss, as occurs with hyperventilation, the body responds with thirst and increased water intake and a decrease in urinary output. Clients who are elderly, young, immobile, confused, or neurologically impaired may be unable to perceive or respond to their increased thirst.

Hyponatremic dehydration is observed less frequently than the other two forms and results from a loss of sodium from the extracellular fluid in excess of water loss. Hyponatremic dehydration is frequently associated with chronic illness and malnutrition. When accompanying a chronic process, hyponatremic dehydration usually develops without symptoms. Clients with renal disease are susceptible to this type of dehydration.

The nurse must understand how these three forms of dehydration differ in regard to pure volume loss, volume loss with sodium retention, and volume and sodium loss. Each form is associated with different assessment findings.

Overhydration

Overhydration is a clinical state characterized by an excess of water in the extracellular fluid. Overhydration is not a disease in itself but rather a symptom of disease such as liver, renal, or cardiovascular disease. Overhydration can be caused iatrogenically by the administration of large amounts of isotonic saline solution, or it may occur because of shifts of interstitial fluid into the plasma. It can also follow humoral alterations. Clinically, overhydration is characterized by water intoxication.

Water intoxication is a condition in which the total body water volume is increased because of excessive

TABLE 42-11	

Hypernatremic Dehydration

Causes	Signs and Symptoms
Diabetes insipidus	Weight loss, poor skin turgor, thirst, muscle tremors, hypotension, tachycardia, fever, nuchal rigidity
Interruption of the neurologically driven thirst mechanisms	
Diabetes mellitus (occasionally)	
Head trauma, tumors, or CNS lesions	
Infantile gastroenteritis	

water ingestion or excessive antidiuretic hormone secretion. The overall effect is dilution of the extracellular fluid volume with osmosis of water into the cells and expansion of intracellular fluid (Groër, 1981). This condition is easily confused with hyponatremic dehydration because hyponatremia is present. However, in water intoxication the hyponatremia results from water excess rather than sodium loss.

When clients are overhydrated, the excess fluid can be stored in interstitial spaces, and the nurse observes edema in the dependent body regions. However, during water intoxication there are increases in the extracellular or circulating blood volume as well as in the cells. As a result, signs and symptoms of water intoxication are present in all body systems.

The clinical assessments of fluid and electrolyte imbalances are described in detail in the later assessment section.

EXTRACELLULAR FLUID EXCESS

Extracellular fluid excess occurs when sodium and water are retained in the circulating blood volume. It may be referred to as isotonic excess or circulatory overload. Isotonic excess indicates that the retention of sodium and water has been within isotonic proportions, and the circulating blood volume is increased. Clinical signs of extracellular fluid excess are hypervolemia and edema.

Hypervolemia is an increase in the amount of fluid in the circulating blood volume. To compensate for the increase, the client's urinary output may increase in relation to fluid intake. There may be an increase in blood pressure; however, if the client's kidneys are able to excrete the excess sodium and water, this rise in blood pressure is transient. If the kidneys are unable to excrete the excess volume, neck vein distention, liver enlargement, increased venous pressure, and signs of pulmonary edema may be present.

Edema is the abnormal accumulation of fluid in interstitial spaces of tissues—in the pericardial sac,

intrapleural space, peritoneal cavity, or joint capsules. The nurse must be able to recognize and assess edema (see Chapter 29). When edema is present, the client's body weight increases. Edema is a symptom of many different conditions:

1. Increased venous pressure
2. Increased blood volume with decreased cardiac output
3. Fluid overload
4. Sodium retention
5. Increased aldosterone
6. Increased steroid production or administration
7. Liver disease
8. Loss of serum proteins
9. Malnutrition
10. Allergic reaction
11. Neoplastic disease
12. Blocked lymphatic drainage

Variables Affecting Fluid and Electrolyte Balance

A client's fluid and electrolyte status is not static, nor is it a single physiological entity. Many variables can change the distribution of body fluid and electrolytes. In some instances, as with the normal changes during pregnancy and exercise, the fluid and electrolyte imbalance is a normal and expected response. However, certain disease conditions, such as nausea and vomiting, have a more severe consequence, particularly with infants and the elderly.

In the nursing assessment the nurse identifies altered fluid states. To assess clients effectively, the nurse considers the variables that influence fluid status, how normal balance changes, and whether the change is a normal anticipated change or a consequence of a pathological process. The major factors that can affect fluid and electrolyte status include the client's age, body size, environmental temperature, life-style, and level of health.

Age

The age of the client affects the distribution of body fluids and electrolytes. The major differences are observed in infants, the elderly, and pregnant clients.

INFANTS

The infant's proportion of total body water is greater than that of the school-aged child, adolescent, or adult. However, although infants have a greater proportion of body water, they are not protected from fluid loss, such as that which occurs with diarrhea. In fact, infants are at greater risk for dehydration because their body water loss is proportionately greater per kilogram of body weight.

CHILDREN

In childhood illnesses the regulatory and compensatory responses to imbalances are less stable and tend to operate within a more narrow range with less tolerance for large changes in balance. Children frequently respond to illness with a fever of higher temperature or longer duration than that of adults. Fever in childhood can profoundly affect water and electrolyte balance (Groër, 1981).

ADOLESCENTS

In adolescence rapid and major changes occur in both anatomy and physiology. The increased growth rate increases metabolic processes and, as a result, the amount of water produced as an end product of metabolism. Changes in fluid balance are greater in adolescent girls because of hormonal changes associated with the menstrual cycle.

PREGNANT WOMEN

The pregnant woman experiences several changes in fluid and electrolyte balance. At about the fifteenth week of pregnancy, aldosterone secretion and excretion begin to rise, and in some cases the elevation can be 10 times normal (Metheny and Snively, 1983). Some physicians believe that this is a cause of fluid retention.

As the fetus and uterus grow, reaching their preterm size, they begin to exert pressure on the inferior vena cava. This pressure, along with the pressure of vascular congestion of the pelvis, further increases venal caval pressure. As a result there is increased filtration of fluid from the vascular bed to the tissues, and hydrostatic edema results (Metheny and Snively, 1983). However, when the woman lies down, pressure on the vena cava is relieved, and after a period of time the edema disappears.

At the end of pregnancy, before delivery of the infant, the average woman's body has 6.5 liters of extra fluid. Of this amount, 3.5 liters is from the fetus, placenta, and amniotic fluid. The additional 3 liters results from increases in the mother's blood volume, her breast size, and the mass of the uterus (Metheny and Snively, 1983).

The increase of 40% to 45% in circulating blood volume, which is reached about 2 to 6 weeks before delivery, includes increases in both serum plasma and red blood cells. Following delivery, the excess circulating blood volume declines rapidly, returning to near-normal ranges by the end of the first postpartum week (Metheny and Snively, 1983).

OLDER ADULTS

The elderly client's risk of fluid and electrolyte imbalance may be closely associated with decreased renal function and a consequent lack of urine concentration. The elderly may also have chronic illness, such as diabetes mellitus, cardiovascular disorders, or cancer, which can also impair fluid balance. In addition, the total amount of body water decreases with age. For example, water comprises approximately 60% of the total body weight in young men and 52% in elderly men; 52% in young women, and 46% in elderly women (Metheny and Snively, 1983).

■ ■ ■ ■ ■

Fluid and electrolyte changes normally occur with developmental changes. However, when an illness is also present, the client may be unable to adapt adequately to these changes. Therefore the nurse needs to include the fluid changes associated with aging and development in the nursing assessment.

Body Size

Body size has an effect on the total body water. Since fat contains no water, the obese client has proportionately less body water. Women have more fat deposits, such as in their breasts and hips, than men. As a result, the total body water in women is less than in men of the same age.

Environmental Temperature

Fluid and electrolyte imbalances are associated with extremes in environmental temperature and relative humidity. The overall body response to environmental temperatures exceeding 28° to 30° C (82.4° to 86° F) is to increase sensible water loss by sweating. The sweating cools the peripheral blood and helps to reduce body temperature.

The healthy adult can sweat about 1 liter per hour for 2 hours, losing about 5% of body weight without straining the cooling mechanism. However, once a body weight loss of 7% is exceeded, the cooling mechanism declines to conserve body water (Metheny and Snively, 1983).

The relative humidity of the environmental temperature also affects body water loss and body temperature regulation. The evaporation of sweat decreases at 60% humidity and ceases at 75% (Burch, Knochil, and Murphy, 1979).

The body responds with fluid changes in four ways to excessive environmental temperature. First, there is increase in peripheral vasodilation, which allows more blood to come to the surface for cooling. Second, sweating increases body fluid loss, which results in loss of sodium and chloride ions. Third, there is an increased cardiac output and pulse rate. Last, increased aldosterone secretion occurs, resulting in sodium retention and potassium excretion by the kidneys (Metheny and Snively, 1983). Each of these can affect overall fluid and electrolyte balance, and the nurse needs to include assessment of the client's environment to determine actual or potential alterations in fluid and electrolyte balance.

Life-Style

Life-style can have an indirect effect on fluid and electrolyte balance. The habits that can affect fluid balance include diet, stress, and exercise.

DIET

Dietary intake of fluids, salt, potassium, calcium, and necessary carbohydrates, fats, and proteins helps to maintain normal fluid and electrolyte status. When nutritional intake is inadequate, the body tries to preserve its protein stores by breaking down glycogen and fat stores. However, once those resources are depleted, the body begins to destroy protein sources. Serum protein levels drop below normal, and hypoalbuminemia results. In hypoalbuminemia the serum colloid osmotic pressure is decreased and fluid shifts from the circulating blood volume and enters the interstitial fluid spaces, resulting in edema.

STRESS

The impact of stress on fluid and electrolyte balance can be understood in terms of the general adaptation syndrome (see Chapter 5). Stress causes an increase in aldosterone and glucocorticoids, leading to sodium and water retention. In addition, increased antidiuretic hormone secretion decreases urine output. The overall effect of the stress response on fluids is to increase fluid volume. As a result cardiac output, blood pressure, and perfusion to the major organs are increased.

EXERCISE

Exercise results in the increase of sensible water loss through sweat. The client who exercises can respond to the thirst mechanism and help to maintain fluid and electrolyte balance by increasing fluid intake. Athletes undergoing sustained vigorous exercise need to have their fluid loss replaced by a liquid that contains electrolytes. One such substance is Gatorade, which contains glucose, sodium, chloride, and potassium.

Level of Health

Generally, the better the client's health, the easier it will be to tolerate fluid and electrolyte changes.

SURGERY

Surgical procedures result in changes in fluid balance because of the body's stress response to surgical trauma during the second to fifth days after surgery. The more extensive the surgery, the greater the response of the body. Postoperative fluid imbalances result from the increased secretion of aldosterone, glucocorticoids, and antidiuretic hormone. The aldosterone and glucocortocoid increases result in sodium and chloride retention and potassium excretion. The increased antidiuretic hormone results in a decreased urinary output. These three hormonal increases, along with the activity of the sympathetic nervous system, help to maintain the client's circulating blood volume and blood pressure during the postsurgical period.

After the immediate postoperative period, the hormone secretion returns to normal levels, and the excess sodium and water are excreted from the body. Postoperative fluid and electrolyte changes are normal and should be anticipated in surgical clients.

BURNS

In clients with severe second- or third-degree burns, body fluids are lost. The greater the body surface burned, the greater the fluid loss. The burned client loses body fluids by one of five routes. First, plasma leaves the intravascular space and becomes trapped as edema; this is also called the plasma–to–interstitial fluid shift. Along with the shifting of fluid, serum proteins are lost from the extracellular fluids. Second, plasma and interstitial fluids are lost as burn exudate. This is a visible fluid loss on the burned surface and is common with second-degree burns. Third, water vapor and heat are lost because burned skin can no longer serve as a barrier against such losses. This water vapor and heat loss increases in proportion to the amount of skin burned. Fourth, blood leaks from damaged capillaries, contributing to an already decreased extracellular fluid volume. Last, sodium and water shift into the cells, again depleting extracellular fluid volume (Metheny and Snively, 1983).

CARDIOVASCULAR DISORDERS

The failing heart has a diminished cardiac output. As a result, perfusion to the kidneys is decreased and urinary output drops. The client retains sodium and water, and edema, circulatory overload, and pulmonary edema may result.

The fluid and electrolyte imbalances associated with heart failure can be controlled for a time with diuretics, cardiotonic drugs, and fluid and sodium restrictions. The overall goal of this treatment is to reduce the work of the left ventricle by relieving the excess extracellular fluid volume.

RENAL DISORDERS

Failing kidneys obviously alter fluid and electrolyte balance. There is an abnormal buildup of sodium, chloride, and potassium, along with an excess of toxic extracellular fluid. The fluid becomes toxic because the kidneys are unable to filter and excrete the waste products of cellular metabolism.

The severity of fluid and electrolyte imbalance is proportional to the degree of renal failure. Occasionally, acute renal failure, induced by shock or a decrease in extracellular fluid, may be reversible. Although chronic renal failure is progressive, the client may be treated successfully with dietary control of protein and salt intake, diuretics, and fluid restrictions.

CANCER

The types of fluid and electrolyte imbalances observed in a cancer client depend on the type and progression of the cancer. All of the electrolyte imbalances discussed earlier can be present in the client with cancer. In addition, cancer clients can develop third-space fluid accumulations that increase total body water, while there is actually a decrease in extracellular fluid volume (Metheny and Snively, 1983).

■ ■ ■ ■ ■

In addition to these categories of illness, fluid and electrolyte imbalances also occur with gastrointestinal disturbances and disease of the endocrine system. The changes described are predictable, and therefore the nurse should anticipate fluid and electrolyte imbalances in postoperative or cancer clients.

In addition to these specific illnesses, the client's overall level of health influences fluid and electrolyte status. Clients with chronic illness and concomitant depression of the immune system and decreases in nutritional intake are at a greater risk for fluid and

electrolyte imbalance than the healthier person who has gastroenteritis for 24 to 36 hours. In all cases the nurse must assess the actual or potential risk factors for fluid and electrolyte balances.

Assessing Fluid and Electrolyte Balance

With the assessment of fluid and electrolyte balance the nurse identifies fluid volume overload and deficits. In addition, this assessment helps the nurse to determine the effectiveness of therapy. For example, if a diuretic is prescribed for a client with congestive heart failure, the nurse assessing the client after the therapy expects to note a decreased weight, increased 24-hour urine output, and decrease or absence of dependent edema. The nurse also assesses fluid and electrolyte balance to detect adverse reactions to therapy. For example, if intravenous fluids are ordered for a client with progressive renal failure, the nurse expects on the third day to find that the client's 24-hour fluid intake exceeds renal output by four to one, that the client's weight is increased, and that dependent edema and abnormal lung sounds are present. Finally, fluid and electrolyte assessment helps the nurse anticipate needs for nursing care. For example, a client with edema who is placed on diuretic therapy should have a care plan to anticipate needs such as an increased use of the bathroom, bedpan, or urinal or instruction for a salt-restricted diet.

The assessment of fluid and electrolyte balance includes four areas: nursing history, physical examination, measuring and recording intake and output, and laboratory studies.

Nursing History

To collect data regarding a person's fluid and electrolyte status the nurse must understand fluid regulation, electrolyte imbalances, and volume disturbances. In addition, the nurse needs to know why and how some diseases, treatments, drug therapies, and diet changes will alter fluid balance.

Clients with cardiovascular and renal diseases, severe burns or trauma, and endocrine disorders are at high risk for fluid and electrolyte disturbances. In addition, prolonged gastrointestinal upsets, particularly in the very young and the very old, can result in fluid or electrolyte imbalance.

Certain treatments such as intravenous therapy and total parenteral nutrition alter the fluid balance. Prescribed drugs also increase the client's risk for fluid and electrolyte disturbances. For example, diuretics usually increase the client's risk for sodium loss, which results in hypotonic dehydration. Conversely, the administration of steroid preparations results in sodium retention and can cause a fluid overload in some clients.

The nurse also collects the nursing history to identify potential or actual risk factors that increase the client's chances of fluid and electrolyte imbalances (see boxed material). Eventually all types of chronic diseases have the potential to cause fluid or electrolyte imbalances. Because the progression of these diseases is usually slow, imbalances can be controlled. When nurses care for clients with chronic illnesses, however, often their disease process is no longer stabilized and fluid and electrolyte imbalances are present.

Head injuries can result in cerebral edema. Occasionally this creates pressure on the pituitary gland, and as a result antidiuretic hormone secretion is changed. Two alterations can occur. Diabetes insipidus occurs when too little antidiuretic hormone is secreted and the client excretes large volumes of dilute urine with a low specific gravity. The second alteration is the syndrome of inappropriate secretion of antidiuretic hormone (SIADH), in which there is continued secretion of antidiuretic hormone, which is

seen clinically as water intoxication (Kubo and Grant, 1978). There are six indicators of SIADH*:

1. Hyponatremia with hypo-osmolarity of serum and extracellular fluids
2. Continued renal excretion of sodium
3. No other signs of volume depletion
4. Urine osmolarity above normal range
5. Normal renal function
6. Normal adrenal function

In addition, the client's physical assessment and laboratory findings are consistent with fluid volume overload.

Burns can result in the loss of plasma through the burned skin surface. Thus there is a loss of both fluid and electrolytes.

Drug therapies increase the client's risk for fluid and electrolyte disturbances. Although diuretics cause excretion of water, they can be potassium sparing such as spironolactone (Aldactone), or potassium wasting such as furosemide (Lasix).

Gastroenteritis and nasogastric suctioning result in the loss of potassium and chloride ions. Hydrogen ions are also lost, causing a disturbance in acid-base balance (see Chapter 43).

Fistulas can also result in a loss of potassium. As a result these clients are at risk for hypokalemia. As with clients with gastrointestinal disorders, the loss of potassium increases the risk for acid-base disturbances (see Chapter 43).

If they are not delivered at the correct rate, parenteral fluids (intravenous fluids or total parenteral nutrition) increase the risk of fluid and electrolyte imbalance. A later section describes the procedure the nurse follows in administering parenteral fluids. The nursing history helps the nurse develop a plan of care to anticipate and prevent fluid and electrolyte imbalances.

Physical Examination

The physical examination for fluid and electrolyte disturbances requires the nurse to use the four basic assessment techniques: inspection, palpation, percussion, and auscultation.

Because fluid and electrolyte disturbances can affect all the client's systems, the nurse must systematically identify any abnormalities and determine if the cause is related to fluid volume deficit or overload or if levels of specific electrolytes are elevated or decreased. A head-to-toe assessment pattern is useful for organizing the physical assessment (Table 42-12). In addition, daily weighing indicates the depletion or reten-

---

*From Lane, G., and Pierce, A.G.: When persistence pays off, Nursing 82 **12**:44, 1982.

Risk Factors for Fluid and Electrolyte Imbalances

- Chronic diseases
  - Cancer
  - Cardiovascular disease, such as congestive heart failure
  - Endocrine disease, such as Cushing's disease and diabetes mellitus
  - Malnutrition
  - Pulmonary disease, such as cor pulmonale
  - Renal disease, such as progressive renal failure
- Trauma
  - Crush injuries
  - Head injuries
- Burns
- Drug therapy
  - Diuretics
  - Steroids
  - Spironolactone (Aldactone) or other aldosterone inhibitor agents
- Gastroenteritis
- Nasogastric suctioning
- Fistulas
- Intravenous therapy
- Total parenteral nutrition

TABLE 42-12

Physical and Behavioral Nursing Assessment for Fluid and Electrolyte Status

	Assessment	Imbalance	Frequency
Weight	2%-5% loss	Mild dehydration	On admission
	6%-9% loss	Moderate dehydration	and daily
	10%-14% loss	Severe dehydration	
	20% loss	Death	
	2% gain	Mild volume overload	
	5% gain	Moderate volume overload	
	8% gain	Severe volume overload	
Head (HEENT)			
Fontanels (infant)	Inspection:		Every hour
	Depressed	Fluid volume deficit	
	Bulging	Fluid volume overload	
Eyes	Inspection:		Every 4 hours
	Sunken		
	Dry conjunctivae	} Fluid volume deficit	
	Decreased or absence of tearing		
	Inspection:		Every 4 hours
	Periorbital edema	Fluid volume overload	
	Blurred vision		
	Papilledema		
Ears	None		
Bridge of nose	Palpation: pinched skin remains raised	Fluid volume deficit	Every 2 hours
Throat and mouth	Inspection:		
	Sticky dry mucous membranes		
	Dry cracked lips	} Fluid volume deficit	Every 4 hours
	Decreased saliva		
	Increased viscosity of saliva	Hyponatremia	
	Longitudinal furrows on tongue	Hyponatremia	} Every 2 hours
	Palpation: Chvostek's sign	Hypocalcemia, hypomagnese-mia	
Cardiovascular System	Inspection:		Every hour
	Flat neck veins	Fluid volume deficit	
	Distended neck veins	Fluid volume overload	
	Palpation:		
	Increased pulse rate		
	Decreased pulse rate	} Fluid volume deficit	
	Weak pulse		
	Decreased capillary filling		
	Bounding pulse rate	Fluid volume overload	
	Auscultation:		
	Blood pressure low with or without orthostatic changes	Fluid volume deficit	
	Third heart sound	Fluid volume excess	
	ECG: cardiac arrhythmias	Hypokalemia	

TABLE 42-12, cont'd

Physical and Behavioral Nursing Assessment for Fluid and Electrolyte Status

	Assessment	Imbalance	Frequency
Respiratory System	Inspection:		Every hour
	Increased rate	Fluid volume overload or deficit	
	Dyspnea	Fluid volume overload	
	Auscultation:		
	Rales	Fluid volume overload	
	Rhonchi		
Gastrointestinal System	Inspection:		Every 2 hours
	Sunken abdomen		
	Vomiting	Fluid volume deficit	
	Diarrhea		
	Abdominal cramps		
	Palpation: poor skin turgor	Fluid volume deficit	
	Auscultation: hyperperistalsis with diarrhea or hypoperistalsis	Fluid volume deficit	
Renal System	Inspection:		Every 2 hours
	Oliguria or anuria	Fluid volume deficit or fluid volume overload	
	Diuresis (if kidneys normal)	Fluid volume overload	
	Specific gravity increased	Fluid volume deficit	
Neuromuscular System	Inspection:		Every hour
	Muscle cramps, tetany	Hypocalcemia	
	Irritability, lethargy, coma	Fluid volume deficit	
	Disorientation	Fluid volume overload	
	Palpation:		
	Hypotonicity	Fluid volume deficit and hyponatremia	
	Hypertonicity	Hypernatremia	
	Percussion:		
	Deep tendon reflexes decreased or absent	Hypercalcemia, hypermagnesemia	
	Increased or hyperactive	Hypocalcemia, hypomagnesemia	
Skin			Every 1-2 hours
Body temperature	Increased	Hypernatremia	
	Decreased	Fluid volume deficit	
Body surface	Inspection:		
	Velvety sheen	Hypernatremia	
	Dry, scaly skin	Fluid volume deficit	
	Palpation:		
	Poor skin turgor	Fluid volume deficit	
	Cold, clammy	Hyponatremia	
	Warm, normal, "doughy" quality	Hypernatremia	
Extremities or dependent body parts: sacrum, back, legs	Inspection:	Fluid volume deficit or fluid volume overload	
	Slow venous filling		
	Palpation: edema (1+ to 4+)	Fluid volume overload or slow venous return (e.g., pregnancy)	

Data from Groër, M.W.: Physiology and pathophysiology of the body fluids, St. Louis, 1981, The C.V. Mosby Co.; Keithley, J.K., and Frauline, K.E.: Nursing 82 **12**:44, 1982; and Metheny, N.M.: Natl. Intravenous Ther. Assoc. **4**:38, 1981.

Barnes Hospital **B-8**
DAILY INTAKE AND OUTPUT RECORD

17-4 Rev. 2/83

FROM 0700 / / TO 0700 / /   Addressograph Plate

INTAKE	OUTPUT

		ORDERS: (CIRCLE)	SOURCE KEY:	SOURCE KEY:
Coffee mug	- 180cc		V = VOIDED	VOM. = VOMITUS
Ice tea container to clear line (without ice)	- 250cc	NPO	C = CATHETER	LIQ. S. = LIQUID STOOL
Ice cream container (melted)	- 30cc	WATER	INC = INCONTINENT	HV. = HEMOVAC
Sherbet container (melted)	- 50cc	CLEAR FLUIDS		L.T. = LEVIN TUBE
Juice container	- 120cc	FULL FLUIDS		T.T. = T. TUBE
Milk carton	- 240cc			OTHER
Paper cup (1/4 from brim)	- 240cc	AMT. DESIRED		
Soup bowl (broth)	- 180cc	CC		
Gelatin container (melted)	- 100cc			

RATE   GTTS/MIN.   CC/HR.

	PARENTERAL			ORAL		URINE		OTHER	
TIME	SOLUTION IN BOTTLE		AMT. (CC) ABSORBED	KIND	AMT. (CC)	SOURCE	AMT. (CC)	SOURCE	AMT. (CC)
	KIND	AMT. (CC)							
0700 0800									
0800 0900									
0900 1000									
1000 1100									
1100 1200									
1200 1300									
1300 1400									
1400 1500									
8 HR. TOT.			8 HR. TOT.		8 HR. TOT.		8 HR. TOT.		
1500 1600									
1600 1700									
1700 1800									
1800 1900									
1900 2000									
2000 2100									
2100 2200									
2200 2300									
8 HR. TOT.			8 HR. TOT.		8 HR. TOT.		8 HR. TOT.		
2300 2400									
2400 0100									
0100 0200									
0200 0300									
0300 0400									
0400 0500									
0500 0600									
0600 0700									
8 HR. TOT.			8 HR. TOT.		8 HR. TOT.		8 HR. TOT.		
24 HR. TOT.			24HR. TOT.		24 HR. TOT.		24 HR. TOT.		

Fig. 42-2 Eight-hour fluid intake and output record.
Courtesy Barnes Hospital, St. Louis.

B-17

BARNES HOSPITAL
24 HOUR
INTAKE AND OUTPUT SUMMARY
(Retain in Patient's Record)

STAMP ADDRESSOGRAPH PLATE HERE

DATE	SHIFT	INTAKE		OUTPUT		
		ORAL and/or TUBE FEEDING	IV (Incl. Blood and Plasma)	URINE	GASTRIC	OTHER (specify)
	07000 1500					
	1500 2300					
	2300 0700					
	TOTAL					
	07000 1500					
	1500 2300					
	2300 0700					
	TOTAL					
	07000 1500					
	1500 2300					
	2300 0700					
	TOTAL					
	07000 1500					
	1500 2300					
	2300 0700					
	TOTAL					
	07000 1500					
	1500 2300					
	2300 0700					
	TOTAL					
	07000 1500					
	1500 2300					
	2300 0700					
	TOTAL					
	07000 1500					
	1500 2300					
	2300 0700					
	TOTAL					

156-0 Rev. 10/83

Fig. 42-3 Twenty-four-hour intake and output record.
Courtesy Barnes Hospital, St. Louis.

tion of fluid. A weight gain or loss of 1 kg (2⅕ pounds) corresponds to 1 liter (1 quart) of fluid retention or loss.

Measuring and Recording Intake and Output

Measuring and recording all liquid intake and output during a 24-hour period helps to complete the assessment data base for fluid and electrolyte balance. The nurse is responsible for collecting and recording these data. Intake includes all liquids taken orally, by feeding tube, and parenterally. Liquid output includes urine, diarrhea, vomitus, gastric suction, and drainage from postsurgical tubes, such as chest tubes or Penrose drains. Frequently the recording of such data is referred to as the client's I & O.

Generally, intake and output are routinely measured for clients after surgery and clients whose condition is unstable, who have fever, whose fluids are restricted, or who are receiving diuretic or intravenous therapy. The nurse neither needs nor should wait for a physician's order to begin intake and output measurements. Clients with chronic cardiopulmonary or renal illnesses and those whose health status has declined also receive such measurements.

Obviously oral intake includes all liquids, including gelatin and ice cream taken by mouth. Liquid intake also includes fluids administered through nasogastric or jejunostomy feeding tubes and liquids administered as intravenous fluids as well as blood or its components.

Ambulatory clients' urinary output is recorded after each trip to the bathroom. These clients are instructed to save their urine in a container for the nurse to record the amount, or clients may be instructed to measure and record their own output. When a client has an indwelling Foley catheter, drainage tube, or suction, that output is recorded at the end of each nursing shift or more frequently (possibly every 2 hours) as the client's condition requires.

In the hospital setting 8-hour intake and output records are attached to the client's bedside chart or room door (Fig. 42-2). The 24-hour totals are included on the 24-hour record in the client's chart (Fig. 42-3). These 24-hour totals are usually recorded at midnight or 6 AM, depending on the hospital's policy.

Taking intake and output measurements is a procedure that requires help from the client and family and instructions from the nurse (Procedure 42-1).

The recording of fluids administered parenterally (intravenous fluid solutions and blood components) is discussed in a later section. Fluids given as enteral tube feeding via nasogastric tubes, gastrostomy tubes, or jejunostomy tubes are considered oral intake and should be recorded as such.

Occasionally clients receive a specific amount of a liquid medication every 1 to 2 hours. For example, antacids are commonly ordered in 30 ml doses every hour for clients who have or who are at risk for gastrointestinal bleeding. Over a 24-hour period this hourly antacid can amount to a significant intake and should always be recorded on the client's intake record.

The amounts of fluid intake and output are essential for obtaining an accurate data base. In addition, this information helps to maintain an ongoing evaluation of the client's hydration status and to prevent severe imbalances.

PROCEDURE 42-1

Placing a Client on Intake and Output Measurements

STEPS	RATIONALE
1. Explain to the client why intake and output measurements are important.	Ambulatory clients in particular need to be actively involved. If they have coffee or juice in the hospital cafeteria, for example, they can record their intake.
2. Provide the client with a copy of the hospital's metric conversions.	This provides the client with an easy and accurate conversion method for recording intake.
3. Instruct the client not to empty the urinal, Foley drainage bag, bedpan, or commode but to ask the nurse to empty the container and record the amount.	This maintains accurate record of output.
4. Ask the client who is using the toilet to record each episode of urination and whether the amount was small, moderate, or large.	Toward the end of a postoperative or postpartum period the frequency of voiding is recorded with approximation of the amount voided.

Laboratory Studies

Laboratory tests are performed to obtain further objective data about a client's fluid and electrolyte status, as well as the overall functioning of the renal system. These tests include serum electrolytes, complete blood count, blood urea nitrogen, and urine specific gravity.

SERUM ELECTROLYTES

Serum electrolytes are measured to determine the hydration status, the electrolyte concentration of the blood plasma, and acid-base balance. The electrolytes frequently measured include sodium, potassium, chloride, and bicarbonate ions. How often these electrolytes are measured depends on the severity of the client's illness. For example, the critically ill client with burns, trauma, or postoperative complications and the client whose diabetes mellitus is out of control may have electrolytes measured every hour. On the other hand, a postoperative client who is stable may have electrolytes measured twice a day during the first and second days after surgery and then, if levels remain within normal limits, just once before discharge.

COMPLETE BLOOD COUNT

The complete blood count (CBC) is a determination of the number and type of red and white blood cells per cubic millimeter of blood. Changes in the CBC occur in response to dehydration or overhydration. In dehydration, hemoconcentration takes place, and thus the red or white blood cell count is falsely elevated because the proportion of blood cells to plasma rises. The opposite occurs during overhydration, when there is an excessive amount of extracellular fluid and the proportion of serum to cellular components rises, resulting in hemodilution. Therefore, along with overhydration, there can be a false lowering of CBC values.

BLOOD UREA NITROGEN

The blood urea nitrogen (BUN) test shows the amount of nitrogen substances present in the blood as urea. It is a rough indicator of kidney function. Like the CBC, the BUN responds to changes in hydration. When a client is dehydrated and the extracellular fluid is hemoconcentrated, the BUN is falsely elevated. Likewise, if hemodilution occurs, as is the case with overhydration, the BUN is falsely lowered. Normal BUN values are 10 to 25 mg/100 ml.

URINE SPECIFIC GRAVITY

The urine specific gravity test measures the degree of concentration of the urine. The specific gravity can be measured at the bedside using an urinometer. Normally the urine specific gravity ranges between 1.010 and 1.020. During dehydration the urine becomes more concentrated, and the specific gravity is higher than normal. When overhydration occurs, the urine is more dilute and the specific gravity falls below normal (see Chapter 39).

Nursing Diagnosis

The nursing diagnoses associated with fluid and electrolyte disturbances fall into three broad categories: fluid volume deficit, fluid volume overload, and electrolyte disturbances (Table 42-13).

A fluid volume deficit, or dehydration, is a less than normal amount of extracellular fluid, and the deficit may be accompanied by specific electrolyte disturbances. There are many causes of dehydration, ranging from decreased oral intake to severe trauma or burns. If these are unrecognized and untreated, the dehydrated client may die. The causes and symptoms of dehydration are described in earlier sections.

Fluid volume overload, or overhydration, is the result of excessive extracellular fluid. The excess can occur from a disease process, such as renal failure, or from a treatment, such as rapid administration of parenteral fluids. Fluid volume excess may also be accompanied by electrolyte disturbances. When clients have impaired cardiovascular function, fluid volume excesses can be life threatening because the heart is unable to pump the increased amount of extracellular fluid out of the left ventricle and congestive heart failure occurs. The causes and clinical symptoms of overhydration are detailed in earlier sections.

Electrolyte disturbances can result from a fluid imbalance, a disease process, or treatment. Occasionally, specific electrolyte disturbances manifest their own symptoms, such as tetany resulting from hypocalcemia, but more commonly electrolyte disturbances occur together. For example, hypernatremia is accompanied by hypokalemia.

Planning

When caring for a client with altered fluid and electrolyte status, the nurse develops a plan of care with goals that are individualized to the client's needs. The goals are (1) to correct the imbalance itself, (2) to correct the cause of the disturbance, (3) to maintain fluid and electrolyte balance, and (4) to prevent complications that might result from therapies needed to restore fluid and electrolyte balance.

To correct fluid or electrolyte disturbances, the nurse can increase the client's oral fluid intake, restrict fluid or sodium intake, or administer fluids parenterally.

TABLE 42-13

Examples of Nursing Diagnoses for Fluid and Electrolyte Imbalances

Problem	Cause
FLUID VOLUME DEFICIT	
Isotonic dehydration	Related to loss of plasma associated with burn
Hypernatremic dehydration	Related to CNS lesion
Hyponatremic dehydration	Related to chronic malnutrition
FLUID VOLUME OVERLOAD	
Overhydration and edema	Related to sodium retention
Overhydration and water intoxification	Related to excessive water ingestion
ELECTROLYTE IMBALANCES	
Hyponatremia	Related to use of diuretics
Hypernatremia	Related to excessive insensible water loss
Hypokalemia	Related to gastrointestinal losses with diarrhea
Hyperkalemia	Related to renal failure
Hypocalcemia	Related to rapid blood transfusion containing citrate
Hypercalcemia	Related to osteoporosis
Hypomagnesemia	Related to malnutrition associated with alcoholism
Hypermagnesemia	Related to hyperparathyroidism
Hypochloremia	Related to prolonged vomiting
Hyperchloremia	Related to acid-base disturbances

Implementation

Fluid and electrolyte imbalances require the use of nursing interventions directed toward the following:
1. Correcting fluid volume deficit
2. Decreasing fluid volume overload
3. Correcting electrolyte disturbances
4. Maintaining fluid and electrolyte balance
5. Preventing complications from the therapeutic measures used to restore fluid and electrolyte balance

When a client's volume is depleted, fluids and electrolytes can be replaced orally, with intravenous administration of fluids and blood components, or through total parenteral nutrition if the fluid deficit is caused by malnutrition. For clients with fluid volume excess the nurse implements measures to reduce fluids, such as fluid intake restrictions, reduced sodium intake, and administration of diuretics.

When implementing specific measures to increase or reduce fluid, two nursing interventions are necessary: daily weighing and intake and output measurements.

Daily Weighing

All clients with fluid and electrolyte disturbances should be weighed daily. Otherwise, a client can gain 2.7 to 3.6 kg (6 to 8 pounds) before edema is observed (Folk-Lightly, 1984). Weight should be determined at the same time each day, and the same scale should be used. It is also important that the client wear the same clothes or, if a bed scale is used, that the same number of sheets be used on the scale with each daily weighing.

Intake and Output Measurement

In addition to providing assessment data, intake and output records provide current information about the client's fluid balance. Intake and output measurements can indicate if excess fluid volume is being excreted in the urine. Likewise, they can show if the excretion of fluids through the kidneys has diminished.

It is important to measure, not estimate, intake and output. Both the client and family should be aware that *all* the client's intake and output must be measured.

Oral Replacement of Fluids

Unless contraindicated, oral replacement of fluids and electrolytes is appropriate as long as the client is not vomiting, is not experiencing a profound fluid loss, or does not have a mechanical obstruction in the gastrointestinal tract. Clients who are unable to tolerate solid foods may still be able to ingest fluids.

Oral fluid replacement is easily implemented in the home, as well as the hospital. Mild illness such as viral diarrhea, respiratory tract infections, and fevers may cause fluid and electrolyte disturbances. In ad-

TABLE 42-14

Oral Fluids

Solution	Calories (Kcal/30 ml)	HCO₃⁻ (mEq/L)	Na⁺ (mEq/L)	Ca⁺⁺ (mEq/L)	K⁺ (mEq/L)	Mg⁺⁺ (mEq/L)	Cl⁻ (mEq/L)	Predominant Carbohydrate
Water								
Pedialyte (oral electrolyte solution)	6.0		30.0	4.0	20.0	4.0	30.0	Dextrose
Lytren (oral electrolyte solution)	9.0 (isotonic)		30.0	4.0	25.0	4.0	25.0	Glucose
5% glucose in water	6.0							Glucose
10% glucose in water	12.0							Glucose
Pepsi-Cola	13.2	7.3	6.5		0.8			Sucrose
Coca-Cola	14.4	13.4	0.4		12.0			Sucrose
Ginger ale	10.0	3.6	3.5					Sucrose
Gatorade	5.5		23.0		3.0		17.0	Glucose, sucrose
Lemon-lime soda	9.6		7.5	0.3	0.2			
Broth, beef (canned)	6.0		55.0					
Tea, unsweetened	0.25				Trace			

From Groër, M.W.: Physiology and pathophysiology of the body fluids, St. Louis, 1981, The C.V. Mosby Co.

dition, clients recovering from anesthesia or gastrointestinal surgery usually first receive clear liquids and then advance to a regular diet if they tolerate the liquids.

Fluids need not be replaced by mouth. They can also be replaced internally through nasogastric, gastrostomy, or jejunostomy feeding tubes.

When replacing fluids by mouth in a client with fluid deficit, it is wise to choose fluids with adequate calories and electrolyte content (Table 42-14). If fluids are replaced through a feeding tube, the client's physician usually prescribes the nutritional supplement to be used (see Chapter 38).

Restriction of Fluids

Clients who retain fluids and have a fluid volume overload require restricted fluid intake. Such clients include those with renal failure, congestive heart failure, cor pulmonale, or syndrome of inappropriate antidiuretic hormone secretion.

Fluid restriction is often difficult for clients, particularly if they are taking medications that dry the oral mucous membranes. The nurse should explain to the client and family why fluids are being restricted. In addition, the client needs to know how much fluid is permitted orally and should understand that ice chips, gelatin, and ice cream are considered fluid.

Given this information, the client should be asked to help decide the amount of fluid with each meal, between meals, before bed, and with medications. Frequently clients on fluid restriction can swallow a number of pills with as little as 1 ounce (30 ml) of liquid.

A good rule of thumb for fluid restrictions is to allow half the allotted total oral fluids between 8 AM and 4 PM, the period when clients usually are more active and receive two meals and most of their oral medications. Then an additional two fifths of the allotted total fluid is permitted between 4 PM and 11 PM. This permits fluids with meals and evening visitors. Between the hours of 11 PM and 8 AM the remainder of the total fluid allotment is permitted. Since the client is usually asleep during this period, fluid needs are decreased.

The nurse should also make sure that clients receive

the type of fluids they like best (unless contraindicated). For example, if a client can have only 200 ml of fluid with breakfast and hates orange juice but likes tomato juice, the nurse should be sure that the diet kitchen has this information.

Parenteral Replacement of Fluids

Fluids may be replaced through infusion directly into the blood rather than intake through the digestive system. Parenteral replacement includes intravenous fluid and electrolyte therapy, blood replacement, and total parenteral nutrition.

INTRAVENOUS FLUID AND ELECTROLYTE THERAPY

The overall goal of intravenous fluid administration is to correct or prevent fluid and electrolyte disturbances in clients who are or may become acutely ill. For example, a client with third-degree burns over 40% of the body is critically ill and has severe fluid and electrolyte imbalances. Fluid therapy must be continuously regulated in burn clients because of the continual changes in their fluid and electrolyte balance. A client who is allowed to ingest nothing by mouth for 2 days after an appendectomy receives intravenous fluid replacement to prevent fluid and electrolyte imbalances; the infusion is discontinued on the client's resumption of normal intake.

When intravenous fluid administration is required, the nurse must know the correct solution, the equipment needed, and how to initiate an infusion, regulate the fluid infusion rate, maintain the system, identify and correct problems, and discontinue the infusion.

TYPES OF SOLUTIONS.

Many prepared electrolyte solutions are available for use. Electrolyte solutions fall into three general categories: isotonic, hypotonic, and hypertonic. A solution is *isotonic* if the total electrolyte content approximates 310 mEq/L. A *hypotonic* solution is one in which the total electrolyte content is below 250 mEq/L. A *hypertonic* solution has a total electrolyte content of 375 mEq/L or greater (Metheny and Snively, 1983).

In general, isotonic fluids are used for extracellular volume replacement, as for fluid deficit following prolonged vomiting. The decision to use a hypotonic or hypertonic solution is based on the client's specific electrolyte imbalance.

Certain additives are frequently instilled into intravenous solutions, most commonly vitamins and potassium chloride (KCl). The physician's order includes required additives, for example:

Bottle #1: 1000 ml—D5W with 20 mEq KCl and 1 ampule of multivitamins

Clients with normal kidneys who are receiving nothing by mouth should have potassium added to their intravenous solutions. If the physician's order for such a client does not include potassium, the nurse should double-check the order. Kidneys routinely excrete potassium, and if there is no potassium intake either orally or parenterally, hypokalemia can quickly develop.

The nurse collects and, if necessary, prepares the solution using the "five rights" of medication administration described in Chapter 32.

EQUIPMENT.

The correct selection and preparation of equipment assist in the safe and quick placement of an intravenous line. Because fluids are to be instilled into the client's bloodstream, sterile technique is necessary, and therefore the nurse must have all needed equipment organized and at the client's bedside (Fig. 42-4). The nurse who has to leave the bedside to obtain another piece of equipment must then start the procedure over again. The standard equipment needed includes the following:

1. The correct solution in an intravenous solution container
2. Intravenous tubing to deliver the prescribed rate
3. Proper needle for venipuncture (Fig. 42-5)
4. Alcohol and povidone-iodine (Betadine) cleansing swabs
5. Tourniquet
6. Arm board, if needed
7. 2 × 2 gauze sponge with Betadine ointment
8. Tape that is cut and ready to use

The arm board is used for two purposes: to reduce movement of the extremity with the intravenous infusion in place and to maintain the extremity in a flat position. Arm boards may be used when inserting an intravenous line on the dorsal surface of the hand.

Other intravenous equipment that may be used includes various solution containers, tubing of various types, and volume control devices. An injectable antibiotic such as ampicillin may be added to a small intravenous solution bag containing 50 ml and "piggybacked" into the main intravenous line to be administered over a 30- to 40-minute period (see Chapter 32). The type and amount of solution depend on the medication to be added and the client's physiological status. For example, when ampicillin is administered parenterally, it must be infused within 1 hour after the drug was prepared; otherwise the medication loses its potency. Different tubing types are used to administer a medication. A drug that is to be given rapidly needs to be infused with macrodrip tubing. In addition, clients may require intravenous extension tubing to increase their mobility or to facilitate changes in position. Volume control devices are

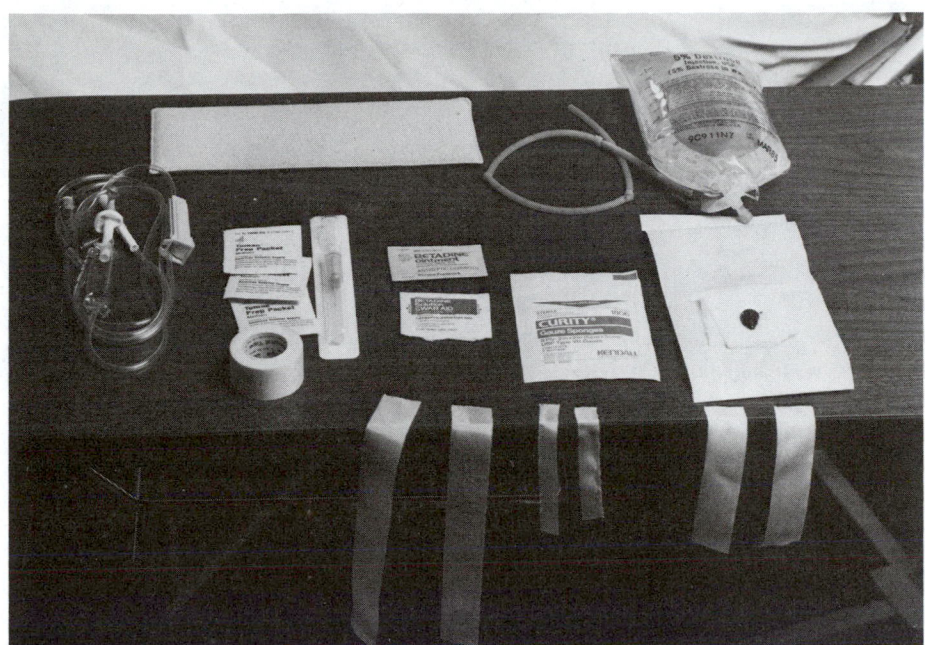

Fig. 42-4 Equipment needed for starting an intravenous infusion.

used with children, with clients with renal or cardiac failure, or with critically ill clients to prevent sudden uncontrolled rapid infusion of large volumes. (Additional information on volume control devices is presented in the section on regulating the infusion rate.)

INITIATING THE INTRAVENOUS LINE. After the equipment is collected at the bedside, the nurse prepares to place the intravenous line by assessing the client for the venipuncture site. A venipuncture is a technique in which a vein is punctured transcutaneously by a sharp rigid stylet (for example, a butterfly needle or cannula such as an angiocatheter that contains a flexible plastic catheter) or by a needle attached to a syringe. The general purposes of a venipuncture are to collect a blood specimen, to instill a medication, to start an intravenous infusion, or to inject a radiopaque substance for radiological examination of a body part or system. The procedure described here is for venipuncture for intravenous infusion.

The nurse assessing the client for potential venipuncture sites should consider conditions, cautions, and contraindications that exclude certain sites. Because very young and elderly clients have fragile veins, the nurse should avoid sites that are easily moved or bumped such as the dorsal surface of the hand. It is often difficult to insert an intravenous line in clients who have had numerous venipunctures because their veins may be sclerosed with scar tissue. An obese client presents problems for venipuncture because of the difficulty in locating superficial veins. The thin

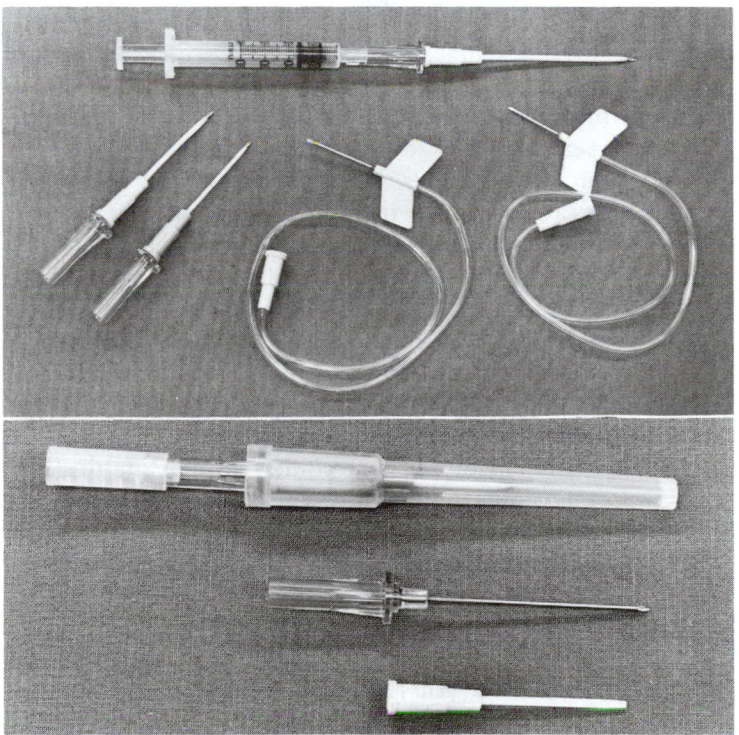

Fig. 42-5 **A,** *Beginning at top and moving clockwise:* angiocatheter attached to syringe, two angiocatheters of different gauges, two butterfly needles of different gauges. **B,** Components of an angiocatheter. *Top to bottom:* angiocatheter in its sterile container, metal stylet to pierce the skin, plastic catheter to remain in the vein.

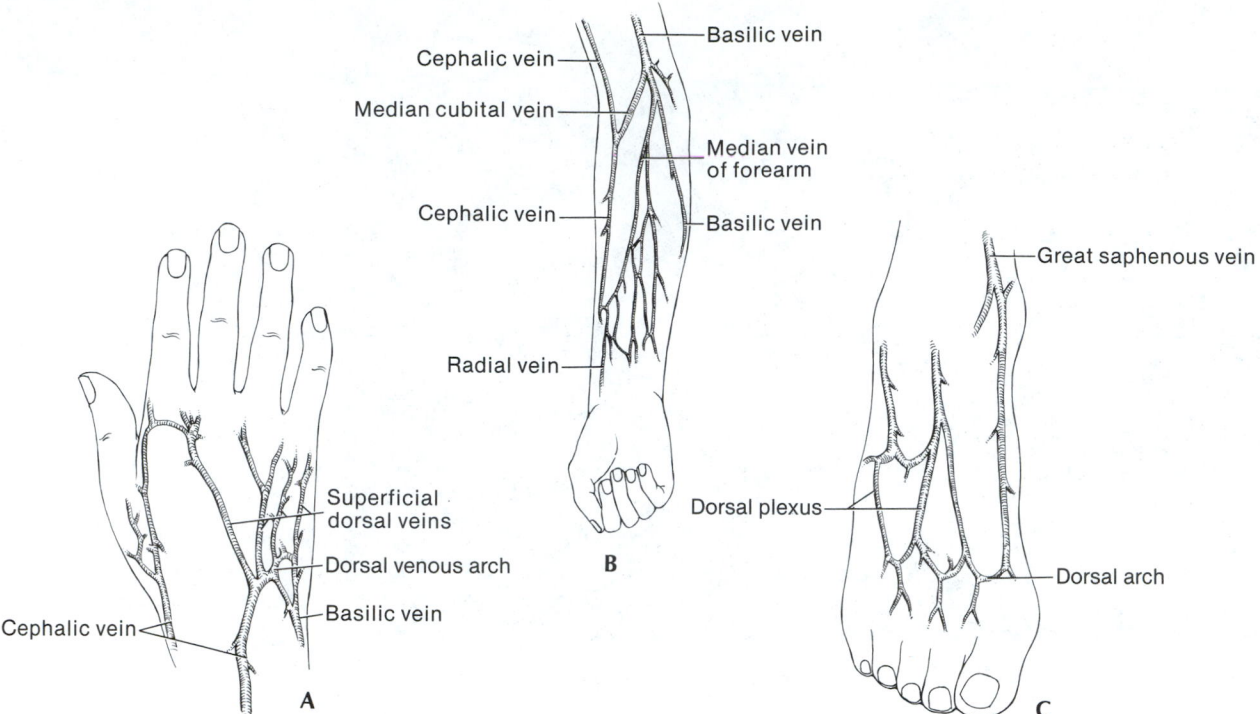

Fig. 42-6 Common intravenous sites. **A,** Inner arm. **B,** Dorsal surface of the hand. **C,** Dorsal surface of the foot.

and emaciated client's veins are also difficult to puncture. Although they may be visible, they are quite fragile, and as a result the nurse may puncture through the entire vein instead of placing the needle or catheter within the vein. When a client is severely dehydrated or has decreased extracellular fluid, as with shock, the veins may collapse. The collapse results from decreased circulating blood volume. When a client's veins collapse, venipuncture becomes extremely difficult, but it is also a lifesaving measure. For these difficult clients venipuncture should be performed by someone with requisite expertise.

Venipuncture is contraindicated in a site that has signs of infection, infiltration, or thrombosis. An infected site is red, tender, swollen, and possibly warm to the touch. Exudate may be present. An infected site is not used because of the danger of introducing bacteria from the skin surface into the bloodstream. Common intravenous puncture sites include the hand and the arm (Fig. 42-6, *A* and *B*). However, the superficial veins of the foot can be used if the client is nonambulatory (Fig. 42-6, *C*).

After completing the assessment for sites for venipuncture, the nurse carefully explains the procedure to the client. The nurse should explain why the infusion was ordered, specifically what will happen, and what is expected of the client.

The venipuncture and intravenous infusion procedure includes multiple steps. Procedure 42-2 describes the steps for using an angiocatheter, but the procedure is the same with a butterfly needle.

Large catheters placed into a central vein such as the subclavian vein are used to monitor a client's central venous pressure (CVP) and to deliver large volumes of fluids and total parenteral nutrition. Although these catheters are inserted by physicians, nurses are responsible for maintaining them.

REGULATING THE INFUSION FLOW RATE. After the intravenous infusion is secured and the intravenous line is patent, the nurse has the responsibility of regulating the rate of infusion according to physician's orders (Procedure 42-3). An infusion rate that is too slow can lead to further cardiovascular and circulatory collapse in a client who is dehydrated, in shock, or critically ill. A too rapid infusion rate can result in fluid overload, which is particularly dangerous in certain cardiovascular, kidney, and neurological disorders. The nurse calculates the infusion rate to prevent too slow or too rapid administration.

INFUSION PUMPS. Recently infusion pumps have been developed to regulate the flow of intravenous fluids. An *infusion pump* is designed to deliver a measured amount of fluid over a period of time. Intravenous infusion pumps monitor intravenous fluids

PROCEDURE 42-2

Venipuncture with an Angiocatheter

EQUIPMENT:

1. Correct solution
2. Infusion set
3. Intravenous tubing to deliver prescribed rate
4. Angiocatheter
5. Alcohol and Betadine cleansing swabs
6. Tourniquet
7. Arm board
8. 2 × 2 gauze and Betadine ointment
9. Tape that is cut and ready to use
10. Towel to place under the client's hand
11. Intravenous pole

STEPS	RATIONALE
1. Gather all the equipment needed and bring it to the client's bedside (see Figs. 42-4 and 42-5).	This maintains organization and avoids having to leave the client to get more equipment. More than one of each piece of equipment is recommended in case a piece of sterile equipment becomes contaminated.
2. Organize the equipment on a clutter-free bedside stand or over-the-bed table.	This reduces the risk of contamination and accidents.
3. Open sterile packages using aseptic technique (see Chapter 33).	This prevents contamination of sterile objects.
4. Check the solution, using the "five rights." Make sure any prescribed additives, such as potassium and vitamins, have been added.	IV solutions are medications and should be double-checked at this point to reduce the risk of error
NOTE: When using a bottled intravenous solution, remove the metal cap and metal and rubber disks beneath the cap.	This permits entry of infusion tubing into the solution.
5. Have infusion set opened, maintaining sterility of both ends.	This prevents bacteria from entering the infusion equipment and thus the client's bloodstream.
6. Place the roller clamp about 2 to 4 cm (1 to 2 inches) below the drip chamber.	Close proximity of the roller clamp to the drip chamber allows more accurate regulation of the flow rate.
7. Move the roller clamp up to the *off* position.	This prevents accidental spillage of intravenous fluid on the client, the nurse, the bed, or the floor.
8. Insert the infusion set into the fluid bag.	
a. Remove the protective cover from the intravenous bag without touching the opening.	This maintains sterility of the solution.

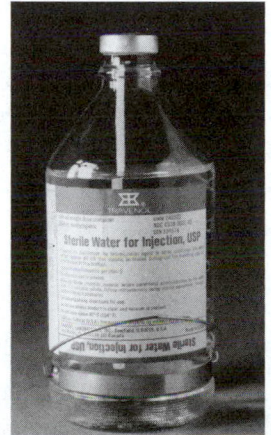

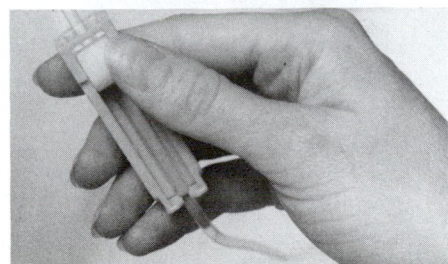

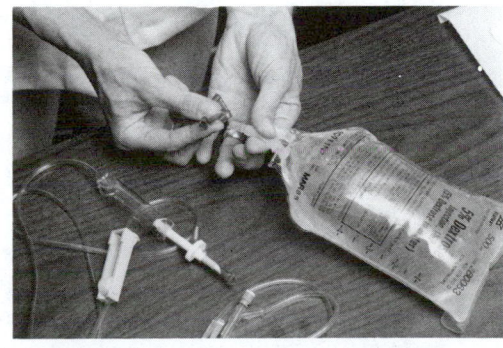

Continued.

PROCEDURE 42-2, cont'd

Venipuncture with an Angiocatheter

STEPS	RATIONALE

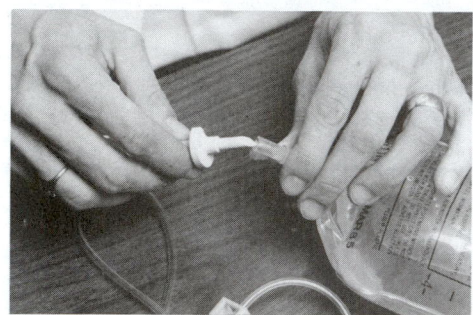

b. Remove the protector cap from the insertion spike, not touching the spike, and insert the spike into the opening of the intravenous bag.

This prevents contamination of solution from a contaminated insertion spike.

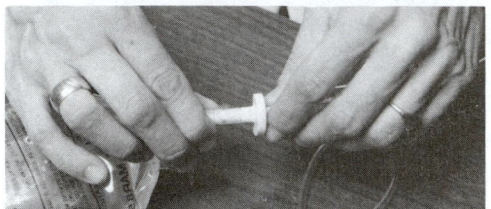

c. Be sure the insertion spike is completely inserted into the opening of the intravenous bag.

This permits the insertion spike to puncture the membrane at the end of the intravenous bag opening, thereby allowing fluid to flow from the bag into the tubing.

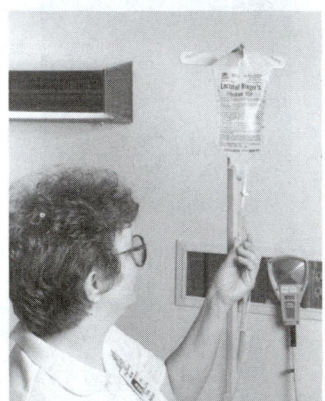

9. Fill infusion tubing.

   a. Compress the drip chamber and release.

This creates a suction effect, and fluid enters the drip chamber.

   b. Remove the needle protector and release the roller clamp to allow fluid to travel from the drip chamber through the needle adapter. Return the roller clamp to the *off* position.

This removes air from the tubing and permits it to fill with solution.

   c. Check tubing for air bubbles. If air bubbles are present, remove them by allowing more fluid to flow through the tubing. Collect excess solution in a basin and discard.

Large air bubbles can act as emboli.

   d. Replace the needle protector.

This maintains sterility of the system.

10. Prepare for venipuncture; select appropriate IV needle.

11. Select a distal site of the vein to be used.

If sclerosing or damage to the vein occurs, a proximal site of the same vein is still usable.

12. If a large amount of body hair is present at the insertion site, shave it off.

Shaving off excess body hair reduces risk of contamination from bacteria that may be present on the hair. The removal of excess body hair also makes removal of adhesive tape less painful.

13. If possible, place the extremity in a dependent position.

This permits venous dilation and visibility of the vein.

STEPS	RATIONALE
14. Place a tourniquet 10 to 12 cm (5 to 6 inches) above the insertion site. The tourniquet should obstruct venous, not arterial, flow.	Diminished arterial flow prevents venous filling. Check for pressure of the distal pulse.
NOTE: Do not tie the tourniquet in a knot; use a loop tie.	This permits quick release of the tourniquet with one hand.
15. Select a well-dilated vein. The client may have to make a fist.	Muscle contraction increases venous distention.
NOTE: Be sure the needle adapter end of the infusion set is nearby and on a sterile gauze or towel.	This permits smooth, quick connection of the infusion to the intravenous needle.

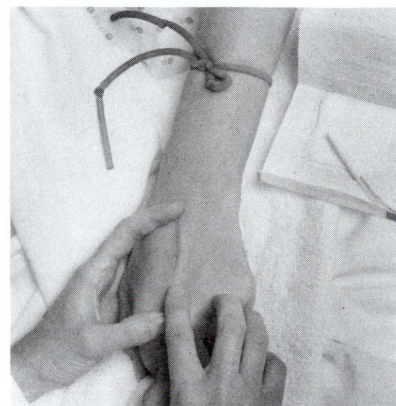

STEPS	RATIONALE
16. Cleanse the insertion site with Betadine solution, followed by alcohol.	Betadine is a topical anti-infective; alcohol is a topical antiseptic. Together these agents reduce skin surface bacteria.

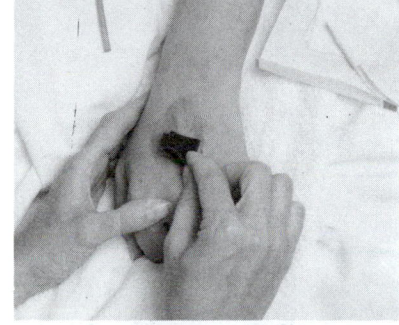

STEPS	RATIONALE
17. Venipuncture with a butterfly needle. Place the needle at a 30-degree angle with the bevel up about 1 cm (½ inch) distal to the actual site of venipuncture. The angiocatheter is inserted bevel up at a 30-degree angle distal to the actual site of venipuncture.	This allows the nurse to place the needle parallel with the vein. Thus, when the vein is punctured, the risk of puncturing both sides of the vein is reduced.

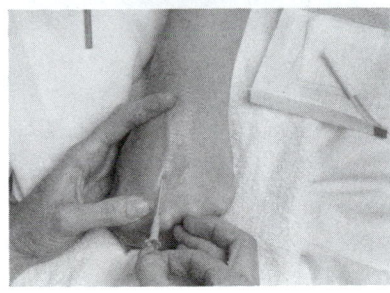

STEPS	RATIONALE
18. Look for a blood return through the tubing of a butterfly needle or an angiocatheter, indicating that the needle has entered the vein. Remove the needle from the angiocatheter, leaving the catheter in place.	Increased venous pressure from the tourniquet increases the backflow of blood into the catheter or tubing. The small flexible catheter remains to permit the entry of intravenous fluids.

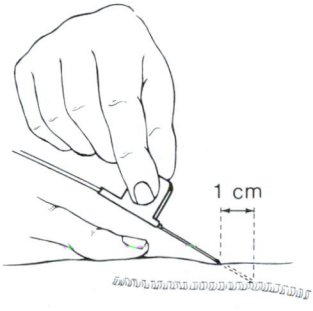

1 cm

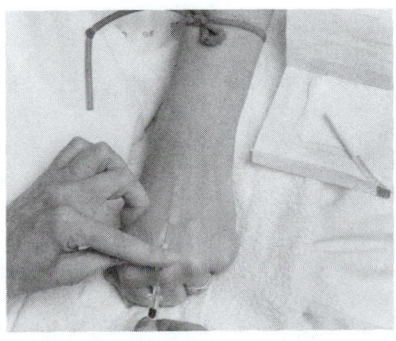

Continued.

PROCEDURE 42-2, cont'd

Venipuncture with an Angiocatheter

STEPS	RATIONALE
19. Connect the needle adapter of the infusion set to the hub of the angiocatheter. To maintain sterility, do not touch the point of entry of either the needle adapter or the hub of the angiocatheter.	Prompt connection of infusion set maintains patency of the vein.
20. Stabilizing the catheter with one hand, release the tourniquet.	This permits venous flow and prevents clotting of the vein and obstruction of the flow of intravenous solution.
21. Place Betadine ointment at the point of catheter insertion.	Betadine ointment is a topical antiseptic-germicide that reduces bacteria on the skin and as a result decreases the risk of local or systemic infection.
22. Secure the intravenous catheter.	This prevents accidental removal of the catheter from the vein.
a. Place a narrow piece (½ inch) of tape under the catheter, and cross the tape over the catheter.	
b. Place a second piece of narrow tape directly across the catheter.	
c. Place a third piece of narrow tape under the intravenous insertion needle adapter, and cross the tape over the infusion tubing. Place a 2 × 2 gauze over the catheter and secure it with a 1-inch piece of tape.	This prevents accidental disconnection of intravenous infusion.
d. Secure the infusion tubing to the dressing with a piece of 1-inch tape.	This further stabilizes the connection of the infusion to the catheter.
23. Note the date and time of placement of the intravenous line. The intravenous tubing dressing should be changed daily, following steps 21 and 22.	This reduces the presence of bacteria in the infusion tubing and on the skin surface.
24. Record the type of fluid, the insertion site, and the type of catheter or needle used at the time the infusion was begun.	This documents in the client's record what was done.

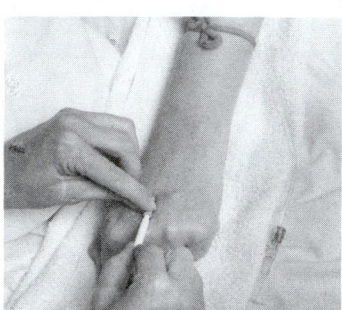

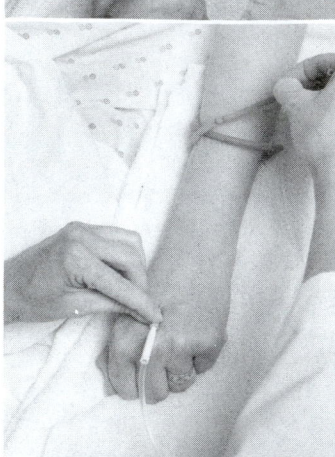

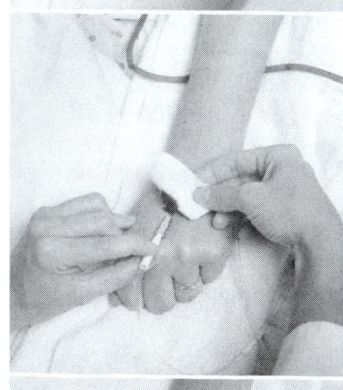

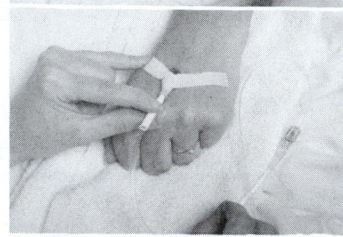
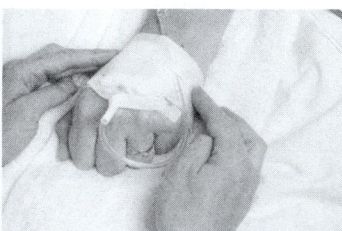

Regulating Intravenous Flow Rates

STEPS	RATIONALE
1. Read the physician's orders and follow the "five rights" to be sure you have the correct solution and proper additives.	IV fluids are medications; following the "five rights" decreases the chance of medication error.
2. Intravenous fluids are usually ordered for a 24-hour period, indicating how long each liter of fluid should run. For example, IV orders for a client are:	The amount of fluid required for a client depends on size, age, illness and amount and type of fluid loss. The amounts are usually calculated over a 24-hour period.

Bottle #1: 1000 ml D5W c̄ 20 mEq KCl

    8 AM–4 PM

Bottle #2: 1000 ml D5W c̄ 20 mEq KCl

    4 PM–12 mn

Bottle #3: 1000 ml D5W c̄ 20 mEq KCl

    12 mn–8 AM

Total 24-hour IV intake: 3000 ml

| 3. To determine the hourly rate, divide volume by hours: | This provides an even infusion of fluid over the 24 hours. |

$$\frac{3000 \text{ ml}}{24} = 125 \text{ ml/hr}$$

| 4. Intravenous fluid orders for a 24-hour period may also be written as: | Fluid needs vary; the rate must be given over the time ordered. |

Bottle #1: 1000 ml D5W c̄ 20 mEq KCl

    8 AM–4 PM

Bottle #2: 1000 D5W c̄ 20 mEq KCl

    4 PM–12 mn

Bottle #3: 500 D5W

    12 mn–8 AM

The hourly rate would be:

$$\frac{2000}{16} = 125 \text{ ml from 8 AM to 12 mn}$$

$$\frac{500}{8} = 63 \text{ ml from 12 mn to 8 AM}$$

| 5. Once the hourly rate has been determined, the minute rate is calculated based on drop factor of the infusion set. A minidrip or microdrip infusion set has a drop factor of 60 drops (gtt) per milliliter. A regular drip or macrodrip infusion set has a drop factor of 15 gtt/ml. | This allows the nurse to calculate hourly flow rate based on this formula:

$$\frac{\text{Total volume} \times \text{Drop factor}}{\text{Infusion time in minutes}}$$ |

Continued.

Regulating Intravenous Flow Rates

STEPS	RATIONALE

6. Using the formula, calculate minute flow rates:

   Bottle #1: 1000 ml c̄ 20 mEq KCl

   Microdrip:

   $$\frac{125 \text{ ml} \times 60 \text{ gtt/ml}}{60 \text{ minutes}} = \frac{7500 \text{ gtt}}{60 \text{ minutes}} = 125 \text{ gtt/minute}$$

   Volume is divided by time.

   Macrodrip:

   $$\frac{125 \text{ ml} \times 15 \text{ gtt/ml}}{60 \text{ minutes}} = 31\text{-}32 \text{ gtt/minute}$$

7. Time the flow rate by counting the drops in the drip chamber for 1 minute by watch, then adjust the roller clamp to increase or decrease speed of the infusion. Check this rate hourly.

   This determines if fluids are being administered too slowly or too fast.

8. Place adhesive tape on the intravenous bag next to the volume markings. This figure is based on 125 ml in an 8-hour period.

   Time taping an intravenous bag gives the nurse a visual cue as to whether the fluids are being administered over the correct period of time.

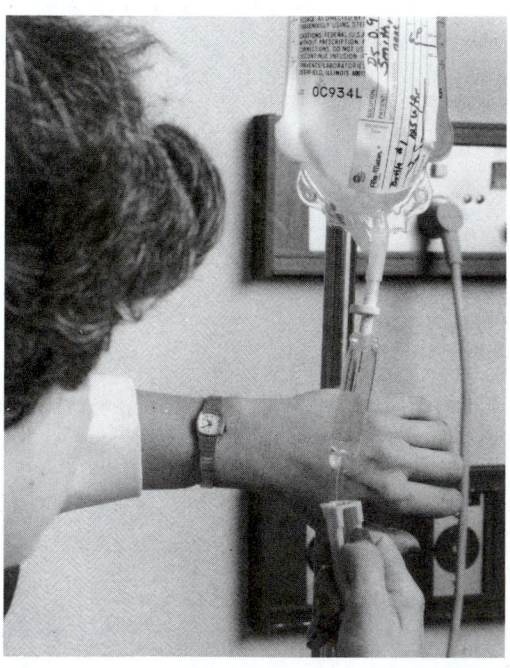
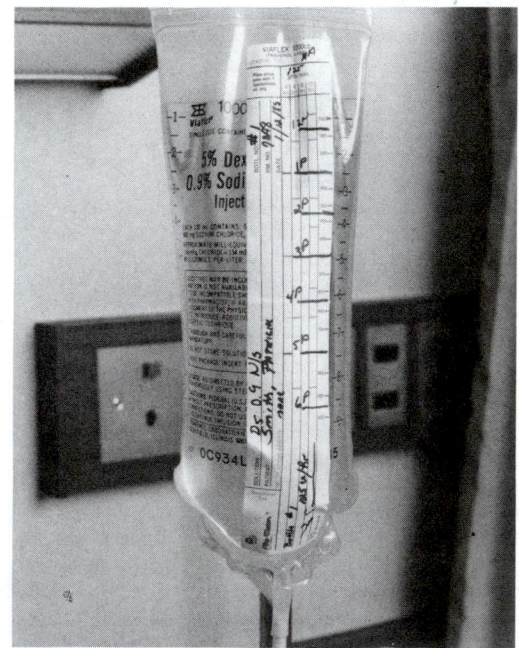

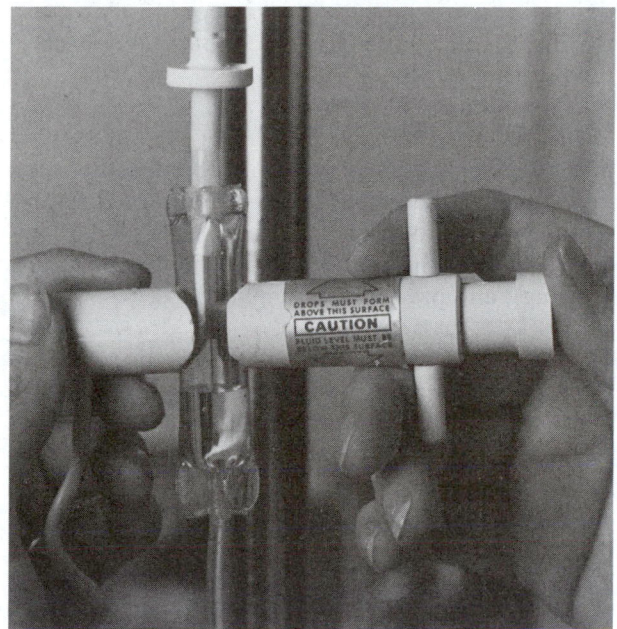

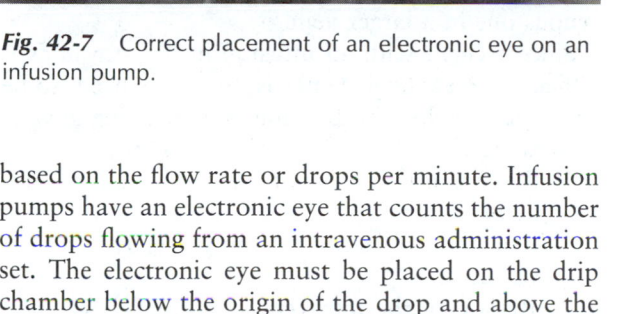

Fig. 42-7 Correct placement of an electronic eye on an infusion pump.

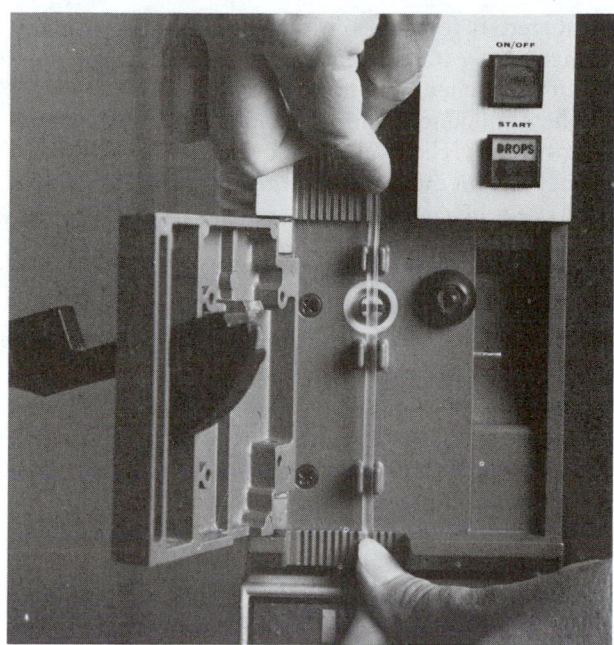

Fig. 42-8 Placement of intravenous tubing in an infusion pump.

based on the flow rate or drops per minute. Infusion pumps have an electronic eye that counts the number of drops flowing from an intravenous administration set. The electronic eye must be placed on the drip chamber below the origin of the drop and above the fluid level in the chamber (Fig. 42-7).

The intravenous infusion tubing is placed within the ridges of the control box in the direction of flow; that is, the portion of the tubing nearest the intravenous bag is at the top and the portion of tubing nearest the client is at the bottom. The required drops per minute are selected, the door to the control chamber is shut, the power button is turned on, and the start button is pressed (Fig. 42-8).

The infusion pump's electronic eye monitors the drip rate; if the required number of drips per minute is not achieved, an alarm will sound. The alarm can be sounded if the intravenous bag is empty, the infusion tubing is kinked, or the vein is clotted. If the alarm sounds, the nurse investigates and corrects the cause of the drip rate problem.

Influences on Flow Rate. Intravenous flow rates can be affected by patency of the intravenous needle or catheter, infiltration, a knot or kink in the intravenous tubing, the height of the intravenous solution, and the position of the client's extremity.

Patency of the intravenous needle or catheter means that there are no clots at the tip of the needle or the catheter and that the catheter or needle tip is not

against the vein wall. The nurse can assess patency by lowering the intravenous bag below the level of the intravenous insertion site and observing for a blood return. If there is no blood return and fluid does not flow easily from the drip chamber when the roller clamp is opened, a clot may be present at the catheter tip.

An *infiltration* may be present when the intravenous insertion site is cool, clammy, swollen, and in some cases painful. An infiltration occurs when the intravenous needle or catheter has become dislodged from the vein and is in the subcutaneous space. When an infiltration is present, the intravenous line must be discontinued and a new line inserted.

A *knot* or *kink* in the tubing can decrease the rate of flow. Occasionally the tubing is kinked underneath the intravenous dressing, which requires the nurse to open the dressing to locate the problem. Frequently the rate of flow will resume once the tubing is straight. The client may also occlude the intravenous tubing by lying or sitting on it.

The *height* of the intravenous bag can affect flow rates. Raising the bag may increase the rate of flow because of the effect of gravity.

The *extremity* position can decrease flow rates, particularly with intravenous sites at the wrist. Occasionally the use of an arm board to keep the wrist flat helps. Sometimes it is more comfortable for the client to have an infusion started in a new location rather than dealing with a site that causes problems.

However, before discontinuing the infusion that is hampered by an extremity position, the nurse must be sure the client has other accessible veins.

These influences on intravenous flow rates can occur with any client at any time. When caring for a client with an intravenous infusion, the nurse should assess the intravenous site and the infusion rate at least every hour.

Prevention of Sudden Increases in Infusion Volume.

Children, the elderly, clients with severe head trauma, and clients susceptible to volume overload need to be protected from sudden increases in infusion volumes. Sudden increases can occur accidentally. For example, a restless client may with a sudden movement loosen the roller clamp and increase the flow rate, or the flow rate may be accidentally increased if the client ambulates. A sudden increase in intravenous volume can kill the client or make him critically ill. Volume control devices, such as a Volutrol or buret, can prevent a sudden increase in intravenous volume (Fig. 42-9).

The volume control device is placed between the intravenous bag and the insertion spike of the infusion set. Most control devices can hold 150 ml. Nurses usually put 2 hours' worth of fluid in the buret. Therefore, if the client is to have only 30 ml per hour, the nurse places 60 ml in the volume control device. If the nurse does not return to the client in exactly 1 hour, the intravenous line does not run dry. In ad-

dition, if there is an accidental increase in flow rate, the client receives at most only 2 hours' allotment of fluid instead of 500 or 1000 ml.

MAINTAINING THE SYSTEM.

After the intravenous line is in place and the flow rate is regulated, the nurse must maintain the system. This includes regulating the flow rate, providing for client needs such as hygiene, changing the intravenous solutions, tubing, and dressings, and preventing complications.

Providing for Client Needs.

The nurse provides for client needs by comfort and hygiene measures, assistance with meals, and assistance with ambulation. Intravenous catheters and medications, especially those with potassium added, can cause discomfort and a burning sensation. Clients need to be reassured that occasional discomfort is normal. Sometimes the discomfort is relieved by repositioning the extremity, but occasionally it is necessary to start a new intravenous line in a larger vein.

Since a client with an infusion in the arm finds it difficult to meet hygiene needs, the nurse needs to be available to help with bathing and changing gowns. Gowns are changed by following six steps:

1. Removing the sleeve of the gown from the uninvolved arm
2. Removing the sleeve of the gown from the involved arm
3. Removing the intravenous bottle or bag from its stand and passing it and the tubing through the sleeve
4. Placing the intravenous bottle or bag and tubing through the sleeve of the clean gown
5. Placing the involved arm through the gown sleeve
6. Placing the uninvolved arm through the gown sleeve

This method allows the client maximum arm mobility and takes very little time. Except during emergencies a hospital gown should never be cut off in order to put a fresh gown on a client with an infusion in his arm.

The client with an arm or a hand infusion is able to walk unless other conditions contraindicate ambulation. A walking intravenous pole, which is a standard intravenous pole with wheels, is needed. The nurse helps the client out of bed and places the intravenous pole next to the involved arm. The client is instructed to hold onto the pole with the involved hand and to push the pole while walking. The nurse should assess the intravenous equipment to make sure that the intravenous bag is at the proper height, that there is no tension on the tubing, and that the flow rate is correct. The nurse should instruct the client to

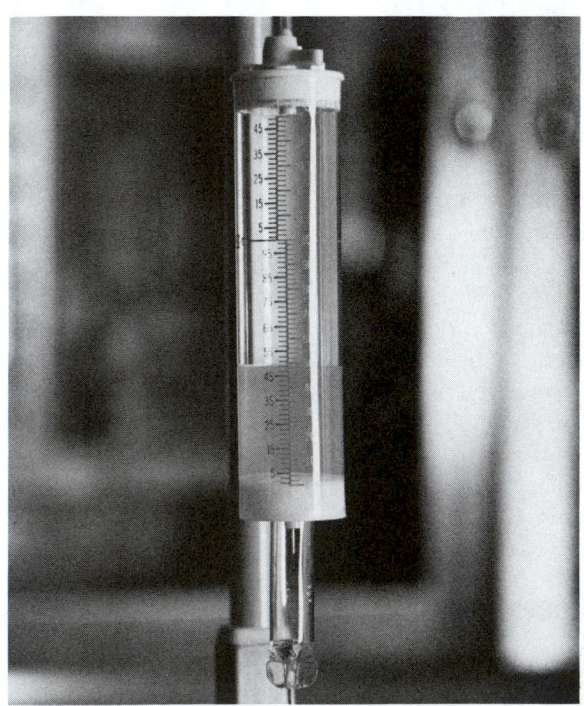

Fig. 42-9 Volume control device.

PROCEDURE 42-4

Changing Intravenous Solutions

STEPS	RATIONALE
1. Have the next intravenous solution prepared at least 1 hour before it is needed. If the solution is prepared in the pharmacy, be sure it has been delivered to the floor. Check that the solution is correct and properly labeled.	This prevents finding an empty intravenous bag without having a replacement bag. Checking prevents medication error.
2. Prepare to change the solution when it remains in the neck of the bottle or bag.	This prevents air from entering the intravenous tubing and the vein from clotting from lack of intravenous flow.
3. Be sure the drip chamber is half full.	This provides intravenous fluid to the vein while the bag is being changed.
4. Prepare new solution for hanging:	This permits a quick, smooth, and organized change from the old solution to the new solution.
a. Plastic bag—remove protective cover from entry site.	
b. Glass bottle—remove metal cap, metal disk, and rubber disk.	
5. Move the roller clamp to reduce the flow rate.	This prevents solution remaining in the drip chamber from emptying.
6. Remove the old solution from the intravenous pole.	This brings the work to the nurse's eye level.
7. Quickly remove the spike from the old intravenous solution, and without touching the tip, spike the new intravenous solution bottle.	This reduces the risk of the solution in the drip chamber (step 3) running dry and maintains sterility.
8. Hang the new bag or bottle of solution.	This allows gravity to assist with delivery of intravenous fluid.
9. Check for air in the intravenous tubing.	This reduces the risk of an embolus.
10. Make sure the drip chamber contains solution.	This reduces the risk of air entering intravenous tubing.
11. Regulate the flow rate to the prescribed rate.	This maintains measures to restore fluid balance.
12. Record the amount and type of fluid infused and the amount and type of the new fluid.	This provides documentation that solution has infused and a new solution has been started.

report any blood in the intravenous tubing, a stoppage in the flow, or increased discomfort.

Changing Intravenous Solutions. Since clients receiving intravenous therapy to restore a fluid volume deficit may require frequent changing of intravenous solutions, the nurse should allow adequate time for this.

Occasionally clients have an infusion to deliver intravenous medication every 4, 6, or 8 hours. In this case an hourly infusion flow of about 10 to 15 ml per hour is used to keep the vein open (KVO) and usually a microdrip infusion set is used. Generally these clients do not use an entire intravenous solution bag. However, they need to have a new solution bag or bottle at least once in every 24 hours because the sterility of the solution cannot be guaranteed for longer than 24 hours. Whenever an intravenous solution container is changed, the nurse uses sterile technique and follows an organized procedure (Procedure 42-4).

Changing the Infusion Tubing. Technically, intravenous tubing can remain sterile for 48 hours. However, most institutions recommend that new sterile tubing be used every 24 hours. The hospital or agency policy manual contains specific guidelines as to when intravenous tubing is to be changed (Procedure 42-5). The procedure is much simpler and more efficient if the nurse changes the infusion tubing when preparing to hang a new intravenous bag or bottle. To prevent the entry of bacteria into the client's bloodstream, sterility must be maintained.

Changing Infusion Tubing

STEPS	RATIONALE
1. Prepare new intravenous solution.	Changing the infusion tubing with a new intravenous solution bag is an easier and safer method.
2. Open the infusion set and move the roller clamp to the *off* position.	This prevents spillage of intravenous solution after the bag or bottle is spiked.
3. Place the insertion spike into the intravenous solution opening.	This permits flow of fluid from the solution to the tubing.
4. Hang the intravenous solution on a pole.	This frees both of the nurse's hands.
5. Compress and release the drip chamber.	This allows the drip chamber to fill with solution.
6. Open the roller clamp, remove the protective cap from the needle adapter, and flush the tubing with solution.	This removes air from the tubing and replaces it with fluid.
7. Replace the protective cap.	This maintains sterility of the needle adapter.
8. Place new intravenous tubing, with the protective cap off, on a sterile 2 × 2 gauze near the client's intravenous site.	This provides smooth, quick insertion of the new intravenous tubing and solution.
9. Remove the top and gauze on the intravenous site dressing one piece at a time. Do not remove the tape securing the intravenous catheter or needle.	This reduces the chance of accidental intravenous catheter or needle removal.
10. Turn the roller clamp to the *off* position on the old tubing.	This prevents spillage of fluid as the tubing is removed from needle hub.
11. Stabilize the hub of the intravenous catheter or needle, and gently pull out the old intravenous tubing. Maintain stability of the hub, and insert the needle adapter of the new tubing into the hub.	This prevents accidental displacement of the intravenous catheter or needle.
12. Open the roller clamp.	This permits new intravenous solution to enter the intravenous catheter or needle.
13. Apply the new dressing (see Procedure 42-6).	This reduces the risk of bacterial infection from the skin.
14. Regulate the intravenous drip according to physician's orders.	This maintains fluid and electrolyte balance.
15. Record the changing of tubing and solution on the client's record.	This provides documentation that measures to maintain sterility were carried out.

Changing the Intravenous Dressing. The dressing over the intravenous insertion site is changed daily to enable the nurse to inspect the site for possible signs of infection or early signs of infiltration (Procedure 42-6). In addition, daily dressing changes reduce the risk of infection at the site. The procedure is sterile and requires the nurse to follow the principles of asepsis (see Chapter 33).

COMPLICATIONS OF INTRAVENOUS THERAPY.

The major complications of intravenous therapy are infiltration, phlebitis, fluid overload, and bleeding.

Infiltration. An infiltration occurs when intravenous fluids enter the subcutaneous space surrounding the venipuncture site. This is manifested as swelling and pallor around the venipuncture site. The swelling results from increased tissue fluid. If enough fluid accumulates, pitting edema forms. The pallor is caused by decreased circulation to the region. In addition, the fluid may be flowing through the intravenous line at a decreased rate or may have stopped flowing. Pain may also be present with an infiltration. Pain usually results from the edema and increases proportionately as the infiltration worsens.

PROCEDURE 42-6

Changing an Intravenous Dressing

STEPS	RATIONALE
1. Remove the old tape and gauze one piece at a time, leaving the tape that secures the intravenous needle or catheter in place.	This prevents accidental displacement of the catheter or needle.
2. Gently remove the tape securing the needle or catheter. Stabilize the needle or catheter with one hand.	This exposes the venipuncture site. Stabilization prevents accidental displacement of the catheter or needle.
3. Cleanse the insertion site with povidone-iodine (Betadine) solution followed by alcohol.	Betadine is a topical anti-infective; alcohol is a topical antiseptic. Together these agents reduce skin surface bacteria.
4. Cleanse with a circular motion, gradually moving away from the venipuncture site.	This prevents cross-contamination from skin bacteria near the venipuncture site.
5. Place Betadine ointment on the venipuncture site.	Betadine ointment is a topical antiseptic germicide that reduces bacteria on the skin and therefore reduces the risk of local or systemic infection.

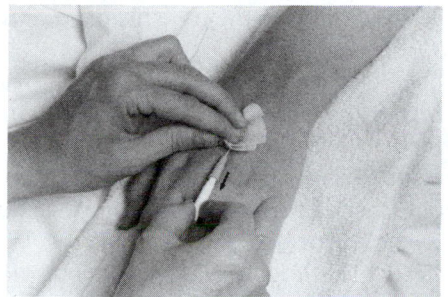

Follow steps 22 and 23 of Procedure 42-2.

6. Record the day and time of change in the nurse's notes.	This documents when the dressing change occurred and who carried out the procedure.

When infiltration occurs, the infusion must be discontinued and, if necessary, reinserted into another extremity. Nursing measures to reduce the discomfort caused by the infiltration are elevation of the extremity, which promotes venous drainage and helps decrease the edema, and wrapping the extremity in a warm towel for 20 minutes, which increases circulation and reduces the pain and edema.

Phlebitis. Phlebitis is an inflammation of the vein caused by the intravenous catheter or by the chemical irritation of additives and medications given intravenously. The signs and symptoms of phlebitis include pain, increased skin temperature over the vein, and in some instances a red line that travels along the path of the vein. When phlebitis is present, the intravenous line must be discontinued and a new intravenous line inserted in another vein. Warm, moist heat on the site of phlebitis can offer some relief to the client.

Phlebitis is potentially dangerous because blood clots (thrombophlebitis) can occur and in some cases may result in emboli.

Fluid Overload. Fluid overload occurs when the client has received too rapid administration of intravenous solutions. The assessment findings are similar to those of fluid volume overload, described earlier. The nurse, on identifying fluid volume overload, should *slow* the rate of infusion, notify the physician, and be prepared to administer diuretics. Prompt action is necessary to prevent worsening of the client's condition or even death.

Bleeding. Bleeding can occur around the venipuncture site while the infusion is taking place. Bleeding is common in clients who have received heparin or who have a bleeding disorder. If bleeding occurs around the venipuncture site and the catheter is within the vein, a dressing may be applied over the site to control the bleeding. Bleeding from a vein is usually a slow, continuous seepage. Clients do not bleed to death from this slight continuous bleeding around the venipuncture.

DISCONTINUING INTRAVENOUS INFUSIONS. Discontinuing an infusion is necessary after the prescribed amount of fluids has been infused, when an infiltration occurs, if phlebitis is present, or if the infusion catheter or needle develops a clot at its tip. The nurse discontinuing an infusion first removes the tape and dressing in the same manner as for the daily infusion dressing changes. Next the nurse moves the roller clamp to the *off* position to prevent spillage of intravenous fluid on the bed, client, nurse, or floor. The nurse places a gauze or alcohol pad over the venipuncture site and, using the other hand, withdraws the catheter or needle by pulling straight back away from the puncture site (see figure with Procedure 42-6). The nurse applies pressure to the site for 1 to 2 minutes to control bleeding and prevent hematoma formation. Clients who have received heparin require longer pressure because of the action of heparin on blood clotting mechanisms. If needed, the nurse applies a sterile dressing over the venipuncture site; a Band-Aid may be sufficient. The nurse records the amount of fluid infused and the time of the discontinuation.

BLOOD REPLACEMENT

Blood replacement or transfusion is the intravenous administration of whole blood or a component such as plasma, packed red blood cells, or platelets. The objectives for blood transfusions are as follows:

1. To increase circulating blood volume following surgery, trauma, or hemorrhage
2. To increase the number of red blood cells and to maintain hemoglobin levels in clients with severe chronic anemia
3. To provide plasma clotting factors to help control bleeding in clients with hemophilia

BLOOD GROUPS AND TYPES. The most important blood grouping for transfusion purposes is the ABO system, which includes four main groups: A, B, O, and AB. Individuals with type A blood naturally produce anti-B antibodies in their plasma. Similarly, type B individuals naturally produce anti-A antibodies in their plasma. A type O individual naturally produces both antibodies, which is why a person with type O blood is considered a universal donor. An AB type individual produces neither antibody, which is why type AB individuals can be universal recipients. If blood that is mismatched with the client's blood is transfused, a transfusion reaction occurs. The transfusion reaction is an antigen-antibody reaction and can range from a mild response, such as itching, rash, or chilling, to severe anaphylactic shock.

Another consideration when matching for blood transfusions is the Rh factor. The *Rh factor* is an antigenic substance present in the erythrocytes of most people. A person having the factor is Rh positive, and a person lacking the factor is Rh negative. If the blood administered to an Rh-positive person is Rh negative, *hemolysis,* or red blood cell destruction, and anemia will occur. If an Rh-negative mother gives birth to an Rh-positive baby, the infant may be exposed to antibodies to the mother's Rh-negative factor, and red blood cell destruction and erythroblastosis fetalis result.

BLOOD TRANSFUSIONS. The administration of blood or blood components is a nursing procedure. The nurse is responsible for a pretransfusion assessment, assessment during the transfusion, and the regulation of the transfusion.

Pretransfusion Assessment. If the client has an intravenous line in place, the nurse should assess the venipuncture site for signs of infection or infiltration. The nurse should also determine that the intravenous venipuncture was performed with a size 18- or 19-gauge angiocatheter. The large catheter promotes flow because the molecules of blood and its components are larger than the molecules of intravenous fluids. In addition, a large catheter prevents hemolysis. The nurse should determine that the intravenous catheter

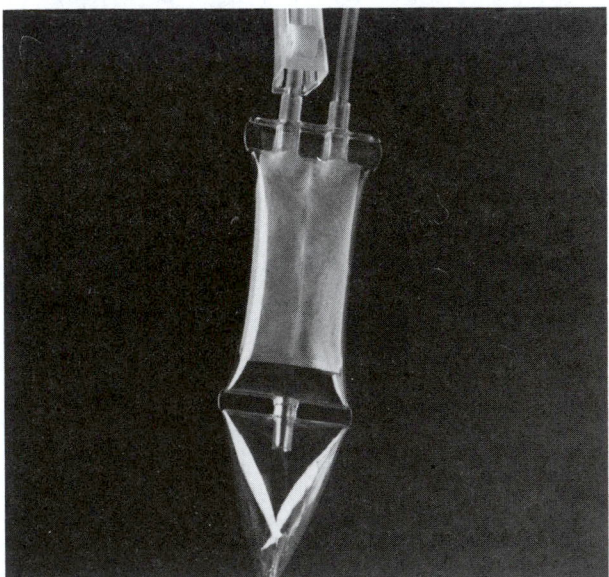

Fig. 42-10 In-line filter infusion tubing for the administration of blood.

PROCEDURE 42-7

Administering a Blood Transfusion

STEPS	RATIONALE
1. Explain the procedure to the client. Determine if there has been any prior transfusion and note reactions, if any.	Clients who have had blood transfusion in the past may have greater fear of transfusion.
2. Ask the client to report to the nurse any of the following symptoms immediately: chills, headache, itching, rash.	These can be signs of a transfusion reaction. Prompt reporting and discontinuation of transfusion can help to minimize a reaction.
3. Be sure client has signed any necessary consent forms.	Some agencies require clients to sign consent forms before receiving any blood component transfusions.
4. Establish intravenous line with large-gauge (#18 or #19) catheter. Refer to Procedure 42-2 for venipuncture technique.	Large-gauge catheters permit infusion of whole blood and prevent hemolysis.
5. Use infusion tubing that has an in-line filter. Tubing should also be a Y-type administration set.	The filter removes any debris and tiny clots from the blood. Using a Y-type set permits (1) administration of additional products or volume expanders easily and (2) an immediate infusion of 0.9% sodium chloride solution after completion of the infusion.

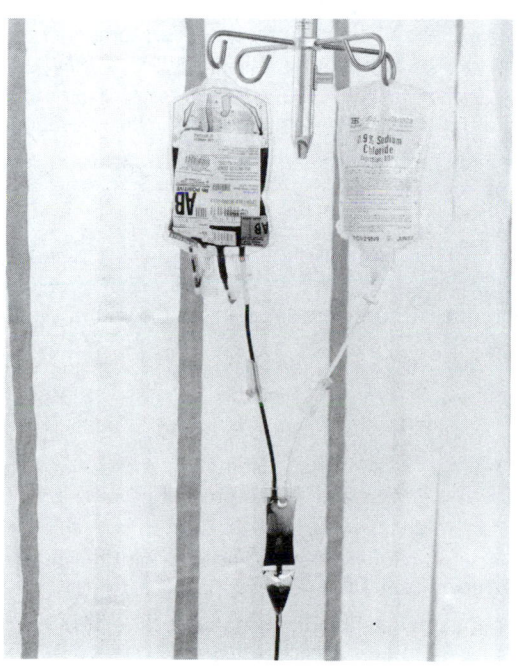

6. Hang a solution container of 0.9% normal saline to be administered following blood infusion.	This prevents hemolysis of red blood cells.
7. Follow agency protocol in obtaining blood products from the blood bank. Request blood when you are ready to use it.	Whole blood or packed red blood cells must remain in a cold (1° to 6° C) environment.
8. With another registered nurse, correctly identify blood product and client.	One nurse reads out loud while the other nurse listens and double-checks the information.
a. Check the compatibility tag attached to the blood bag and the information on the bag itself.	This verifies that the ABO group, Rh type, and unit number match.
b. For whole blood, check ABO group and Rh type, which is on client's chart.	This verifies that they match those on the compatibility tag and blood bag.

Continued.

PROCEDURE 42-7, cont'd

Administering a Blood Transfusion

STEPS	RATIONALE
c. Double-check the blood product with the physician's order.	This verifies correct blood component.
d. Check expiration date on the bag.	After 21 days, blood has only 70% to 80% of the original number of cells and 23 mEq/L of potassium.*
e. Inspect the blood for clots.	An anticoagulant, citrate-phosphate-dextrose (CPD), is added to blood and permits preserved blood to be stored for 21 days. A newer anticoagulant, citrate-phosphate-dextrose-adenine (CPD-A), allows storage for 35 days.* If clots are present, return blood to the blood bank.
f. Ask the client's name, and check armband.	This verifies correct client. Do not administer blood to a client without an arm band. The identification name and number on the wristband must be identical to those on the blood compatibility tag.
9. Monitor vital signs.	
a. Take the client's baseline vital signs before administering the transfusion.	This verifies the client's pretransfusion temperature, pulse, blood pressure, and respirations.
b. Take vital signs every 5 minutes for the first 15 minutes of the transfusion.	This documents any change in vital sign status that could indicate early warning of a transfusion reaction.
c. Observe client for flushing, itching, dyspnea, hives, or rash.	This may indicate an early sign of a transfusion reaction.
10. Begin transfusion	
a. Prime the infusion line with 0.9% normal saline.	This prevents hemolysis.
b. Begin transfusion slowly by first filling the in-line filter.	If the filter is not filled, the transfusion will not infuse properly.
c. Adjust the rate to 2 ml per minute for the first 15 minutes, and remain with client. If you suspect a reaction, *stop* the transfusion and notify the blood bank and the physician.	
11. Maintain the prescribed infusion rate using infusion pumps, if necessary.	Infusion pumps maintain the prescribed rate.
12. Continually observe for adverse reactions.	Adverse reactions can occur at any point during the transfusion (see Table 42-15).
13. Record the administration of the blood or blood product.	This documents the administration of the blood component.

*Data from Metheny, N.M., and Snively, W.D., Jr.: Nurse's handbook of fluid balance, ed. 4, Philadelphia, 1983, J.B. Lippincott Co.

is patent and functioning properly. The nurse should have the proper in-line filter and tubing for blood transfusions (Fig. 42-10). The nurse should prime the tubing with 0.9% normal saline to prevent hemolysis of red blood cells. Other solutions such as D5W (dextrose 5%) cause the red blood cells to swell and rupture because of the hypotonicity of the solution compared with whole blood or packed red blood cells.

The pretransfusion assessment also includes obtaining information from the client. The nurse asks whether the client knows the reason for the blood transfusion and whether the client has ever had a transfusion or a transfusion reaction. A client who has had a transfusion reaction is usually at no greater risk for a reaction with a subsequent transfusion. However, the individual may experience anxiety about the transfusion, necessitating nursing intervention.

The pretransfusion assessment must include a baseline measurement of vital signs. It is important to record these values before administration of any blood products because a change in vital signs can indicate a transfusion reaction.

Procedure 42-7 describes the administration of a blood transfusion. When clients have a severe blood loss such as with a hemorrhage, they may receive rapid transfusions through a central venous pressure catheter. In such a case a blood warming device is necessary because the tip of the central venous pressure catheter lies in the superior vena cava, above the right atrium. Rapid administration of cold blood can result in cardiac arrhythmias (Querin and Stahl, 1983).

Assessment during Transfusion. During the infusion of blood the client is at risk for a reaction, particularly during the first 15 minutes. Therefore the nurse should remain with the client and assess color and vital signs. The various kinds of transfusion reactions are described in a subsequent section.

Regulation of Transfusion. The rate of a transfusion is usually specified in the physician's orders. Ideally a unit of whole blood or packed red blood cells is transfused in 2 hours. However, a client with a low fluid tolerance can have a transfusion over a 4-hour period (Querin and Stahl, 1983).

TRANSFUSION REACTIONS. A transfusion reaction is a systemic response by the body to the administration of blood incompatible with that of the recipient. The causes include red cell incompatibility or allergic sensitivity to the leukocytes, the platelets, or the plasma protein components of the transfused blood or to the potassium or citrate preservative in the blood. Blood transfusion can also result in the transmission of disease.

Types of Reactions. Several types of reactions can result from blood transfusions. General adverse reactions (Table 42-15) range from immediate onset of fever, chills, and skin rash to hypotension, shock, and a delayed reaction that may not occur until several days or weeks after the transfusion.

A second category of reactions includes diseases transmitted by blood donors who are asymptomatic. Common diseases that can be transmitted through transfusions are malaria, hepatitis, and acquired immune deficiency syndrome (AIDS). Since all units of blood collected must undergo serological testing, the risk of acquiring syphilis from blood transfusions is almost nonexistent.

Preventing Reactions. Correct administration of blood and blood products reduces the risk of transfusion reactions. The nurse, although not actually a participant in the blood labeling process, is responsible for determining that the blood delivered to the nursing unit corresponds to the client's blood type as listed in the medical record. Two nurses should check the blood against the client's identification number, blood group, and complete client name. If there is even a minor discrepancy, the blood should not be given and the blood bank laboratory should be notified. It is possible that two clients with the same name are in the hospital. For example, in Unit 4 South there is a Mrs. Sandra Johnson, while in 12 East there is a Mrs. Sandra L. Johnson. If the nurse in 12 East is to administer a unit of blood, the name on the unit should be "Sandra L. Johnson" and the identification number should match Sandra L. Johnson's identification number.

Risks. In addition to allergic reactions and the transmission of illnesses, certain risks are associated with blood transfusions. These include hyperkalemia, hypocalcemia, and circulatory overload.

Stored blood may cause *hyperkalemia*. Blood that is 1 day old has a plasma potassium content of approximately 7 mEq/L, and blood stored for 21 days has a plasma potassium content of 23 mEq/L (Metheny and Snively, 1983). The increase in potassium is related to the destruction of red blood cells. At the end of 21 days about 20% to 30% of the cells are destroyed. Because the major intracellular cation is potassium, potassium enters the plasma as cells are destroyed. A client who receives several units of blood should have the potassium level measured frequently. If it is elevated, the client should be given an ion exchange resin such as polystyrene sulfate (Kayexelate).

In some clients the infusion of blood can result in *hypocalcemia* because of the action of the citrated blood as it combines with the client's ionized calcium (Metheny and Snively, 1983). The two preservatives often added to blood, citrate-phosphate-dextrose and citrate-phosphate-dextrose-adenine, both contain more citrate than is needed to combine with calcium in the blood collected for the transfusion. Therefore, when the transfused blood is infused into the client's bloodstream, the preservative combines with the ionized calcium, and tetany can result. The risk for hypocalcemia increases with the number of blood transfusions the client receives.

Iron overload can occur in clients who receive frequent transfusions. One milliliter of blood contains 1 mg of iron (Mountcastle, 1979). The clinical term for iron overload is hemosiderosis. Hemosiderosis is an abnormal deposition of iron in a variety of tissues, usually in the form of hemosiderin, an iron-rich pigment that is a product of red blood cell hemolysis. Clients at risk for hemosiderosis are those with illnesses that involve chronic, extensive destruction of

TABLE 42-15

Adverse Reactions to Blood Transfusions

Type	Cause	Onset	Signs or Symptoms	Nursing Actions
Febrile nonhemolytic (most common reaction; usually occurs in previous transfusion recipients or multiparous clients)	Antigen-antibody reaction to white blood cells or platelets contained in blood product	Immediately or within 6 hours after transfusion	Fever (with or without chills), headache, nausea and vomiting, nonproductive cough, hypotension, chest pain, dyspnea	1. Stop transfusion. 2. Keep vein open. 3. Notify physician and blood bank. 4. Take vital signs p.r.n.
Allergic urticarial (generally innocuous)	Allergic reaction to plasma-soluble antigen contained in blood product	Anytime during transfusion or within 1 hour after transfusion	Skin rash	1. Slow transfusion to keep-vein-open rate. 2. Notify physician and blood bank. 3. Take vital signs p.r.n.
Delayed hemolytic (more common than acute hemolytic; frequently missed; occurs in previous transfusion recipients or multiparous clients)	Incompatibility of RBC antigens other than ABO group	Days to weeks after transfusion	Decreasing hemoglobin level, possible persistent low-grade fever	1. Notify physician and blood bank.
Acute hemolytic (potentially life threatening)	ABO group incompatibility	Usually during first 5 to 15 minutes, but may occur any time during transfusion	*Mild form:* fever, chills, back pain, hypotension, nausea, vomiting, flushing, hematuria, oliguria *Severe form (in addition to above):* dyspnea, chest pain, anuria, shock, disseminated intravascular coagulation	1. Stop transfusion. 2. Keep vein open. 3. Notify physician and blood bank. 4. Take vital signs p.r.n. Assess for signs and symptoms of shock. 5. Monitor intake and output; check for decreased urinary output. 6. Start resuscitative measures p.r.n.
Anaphylactic (extremely rare; potentially life threatening)	Idiosyncratic reaction in patients with immunoglobulin A (IgA) deficiency, sensitized to IgA through previous transfusion or pregnancy	Immediately (after transfusion of only few milliliters of blood)	Severe respiratory and cardiovascular collapse (with dyspnea and tachypnea, tachycardia, hypotension, and cyanosis), severe gastrointestinal disturbances (with nausea, vomiting, diarrhea, and cramping)	1. Stop transfusion. 2. Keep vein open. 3. Notify physician and blood bank. 4. Take vital signs every 15 minutes (or p.r.n.) 5. Start resuscitative measures p.r.n.

From Querin, J.J., and Stahl, L.D.: Nursing 83 **13**:34, 1983.

red blood cells, such as anemias, thalassemia major, or splenic dysfunction.

Circulatory overload is a risk when a client is receiving massive whole blood or packed red blood cell transfusions for massive hemorrhagic shock or when a client with normal blood volume receives blood. Clients particularly at risk for circulatory overload are the elderly and those with cardiopulmonary diseases.

Nursing Actions during Blood Reactions. A client who is having a transfusion reaction needs prompt and correct nursing actions. Frequently reactions occur when a physician is not immediately available. The overall goal for a client having a blood reaction is to maintain life. Blood reactions are life threatening, but the following basic nursing measures can maintain the client's physiological stability (see also Table 42-15):

1. If a blood reaction is suspected, the nurse *stops* the transfusion immediately.
2. The nurse keeps the intravenous line open by "piggybacking" 0.9% normal saline into the intravenous line (see Chapter 32). The nurse should not turn off the blood and turn on the 0.9% normal saline on the Y-tubing infusion set. This will merely infuse the blood in the tubing into the client. Even a small amount of mismatched blood can cause a major reaction.
3. The nurse notifies the physician or asks someone to do so.
4. The nurse remains with the client, observing signs and symptoms and monitoring vital signs.
5. The nurse prepares to administer emergency medications such as antihistamines, vasopressors, fluids, and steroids.
6. The nurse prepares to perform cardiopulmonary resuscitation.
7. The nurse completes any necessary paperwork.

Although anaphylactic transfusion reactions are relatively rare, they can occur with any client. Correctly administering blood and blood products prevents blood reactions that would be caused by giving the client the wrong blood. When a client is having a transfusion reaction, prompt nursing actions can decrease the severity of the response.

Total Parenteral Nutrition

Total parenteral nutrition (TPN) is the administration of a nutritionally adequate hypertonic solution consisting of glucose, protein hydrolysates, minerals, and vitamins through an indwelling central catheter, usually placed into the jugular or subclavian vein and threaded to the tip of the superior vena cava. The solution used for TPN is quite hypertonic, and therefore a large-gauge catheter, #14 or #16, is recommended.

TPN has been used increasingly over the last 5 years. The use of the nutritional solution decreases muscle and protein wasting in the presence of a severe illness. In some cases TPN has meant the difference between life and death.

Objectives of Total Parenteral Nutrition

The objectives of TPN are as follows:

1. To maintain a positive nitrogen balance in clients whose illnesses prevent them from absorbing sufficient amounts of nutrients (see the boxed material)
2. To increase the delivery of essential amino acids and vitamins for protein synthesis to repair body tissues, as in the severely traumatized client
3. To allow the gastrointestinal tract to heal, as in the client with ulcerative colitis
4. To deliver nutrients to clients with severe psychological illness that affects their nutrition, such as anorexia nervosa

Solutions for Total Parenteral Nutrition

Typically a TPN solution for an adult supplies 1000 calories per liter (Metheny and Snively, 1983). The solution contains 25% dextrose and 4% amino acids. In addition, a fat emulsion, interlipid, may be infused through a Y-type administration set to provide more calories.

Common Conditions Requiring Total Parenteral Nutrition

- Gastrointestinal problems
  - Short bowel syndrome
  - Bowel obstruction
  - Fistulas
  - Pancreatitis
  - Inflammatory bowel disease, such as ulcerative colitis
- Severe burns or trauma
- Malignant disease, particularly when the client is responding to chemotherapy
- Anorexia nervosa
- Preparation of malnourished clients for surgery

Because potassium is needed to transport glucose and amino acids across the cell membrane, approximately 40 mEq of potassium per 1000 calories is added to the solution. In addition, magnesium, calcium, sodium, phosphates, and water-soluble vitamins are added. Depending on the client's overall nutritional status, fat-soluble vitamins are added weekly (Metheny and Snively, 1983).

Prepared solutions can safely be stored at 4° C in the dark for 48 hours (Metheny and Snively, 1983). However, most agencies have the pharmacy prepare the solutions on a daily basis for delivery when needed.

Initiating Total Parenteral Nutrition

Total parenteral nutrition requires a large-gauge intracatheter threaded into a central vein such as the jugular or subclavian. Nurses do not insert such catheters but assist in the procedure.

The procedure is a sterile one and requires the following equipment:
1. Sterile drapes
2. Sterile gloves
3. Sterile Betadine swabs
4. Alcohol
5. Topical anesthetic (lidocaine)
6. Betadine ointment
7. Sterile 4 × 4 and 2 × 2 gauze pads
8. Tape
9. Parenteral solution
10. Parenteral infusion tubing
11. Intracatheter needle
12. Sutures
13. In-line filter
14. Infusion pump

The nurse explains the procedure to the client and obtains consent. The client is taught to perform the Valsalva maneuver, bearing down with mouth closed and holding the breath. This maneuver during the insertion procedure is necessary to increase venous filling of the vein and reduce the risk of an air embolism. Once the client has learned the technique satisfactorily, the catheter can be inserted.

The client is placed in the Trendelenburg position to dilate the central veins in the neck and shoulder. The physician drapes the venipuncture site with sterile barriers and cleanses the site with Betadine swabs followed by alcohol wipes. Lidocaine is injected to provide local anesthesia. The physician punctures the vein and looks for a nonpulsatile blood return. A pulsating blood return indicates that an artery, not the vein, was punctured. When the physician begins to thread the intracatheter through the needle, the nurse instructs the client to do the Valsalva maneuver.

After placement of the catheter the needle is removed and an intravenous infusion is connected to the hub of the catheter. The physician sutures the catheter in place and covers the site with a sterile dressing. A chest x-ray film is obtained to identify any intrathoracic complications.

Beginning the Infusion

Before beginning the infusion the nurse compares the physician's order with the solution prepared by the pharmacy. The nurse connects the TPN infusion tubing to a filter and places the insertion spike in the solution. The tubing is primed with the solution and hung at the bedside. The nurse attaches the tubing to the infusion pump. The nurse removes the dressing and turns off the previous solution. The client is instructed to perform the Valsalva maneuver, the old solution is quickly disconnected, and the new infusion is connected and begun. Munro-Black (1984) recommends using a Kelly clamp to hold the catheter hub to provide better leverage and prevent contamination of the hub. The catheter hub and infusion tubing with top are secured. Finally, the site is covered with a sterile dressing (Munro-Black, 1984).

Infusion Flow Rate

Clients initially receive low doses of TPN solution, such as 1 or 2 liters per 24 hours, gradually increasing to 4 to 5 liters per 24 hours. The solution should be delivered over a 24-hour period; the rate is included in the physician's orders.

Too rapid administration of this hypertonic infusion can result in osmotic diuresis, dehydration, and death. Infusion pumps help to regulate the flow. If an infusion falls behind schedule, the nurse should not attempt to catch up because a hyperosmotic reaction could result (Metheny and Snively, 1983).

Caring for the Client Receiving Total Parenteral Nutrition

Nursing care for the client receiving TPN is based on four major nursing goals: preventing infection, maintaining the TPN system, preventing complications, and promoting the client's well-being (Munro-Black, 1984).

PREVENTING INFECTION

To prevent infection the infusion tubing should be changed every 24 hours. It is best to change the tubing with the first new bottle to be administered each day. The procedure is the same as that for changing infusion tubing (see Procedure 42-5) except that an in-

PROCEDURE 42-8

Changing a Total Parenteral Nutrition Dressing

EQUIPMENT:
1. One pair sterile gloves
2. One sterile barrier
3. Three sterile Betadine swabs
4. Three sterile alcohol swabs
5. Betadine ointment
6. One 2 × 2 gauze pad
7. One 4 × 4 gauze pad
8. Tape
9. Sterile cotton-tipped catheter

STEPS	RATIONALE
1. Collect the equipment.	This prevents the nurse from needing to leave the bedside to collect more supplies.
2. Remove the old dressing slowly, one layer at a time. Touch only the outside or corners of the dressing.	Careful removal prevents accidental dislodging of the catheter and contamination of the puncture site.
3. Assess the venipuncture site for infection and the catheter for knots or kinks.	This prevents systemic contamination that would occur by administering fluid through a contaminated site and maintains catheter patency.
4. Spread the sterile barrier and place the supplies with sterile technique on the field (see Chapter 33). Open and don sterile gloves (see Chapter 33).	This maintains sterility of the field.
5. Clean the site with alcohol swabs beginning at catheter site and moving outward. Repeat two more times. Follow this procedure using Betadine swabs.	This removes bacteria from the venipuncture site; circular motion moving outward prevents cross-contamination with other skin bacteria.
6. Using sterile cotton-tipped applicator, apply Betadine ointment directly over the catheter exit site.	This reduces the risk of bacterial infection.
7. Cover the site with 2 × 2 and 4 × 4 gauze pads, and cover it completely with tape.	Airtight dressing reduces entry of airborne bacteria.
8. Date and initial the dressing.	This identifies to nursing and medical personnel when the dressing change occurred.
9. Record the dressing change in the client's chart.	This provides documentation of the procedure.

line filter is added to trap bacteria. The filter of choice is a 0.22 μm filter because it blocks all bacteria including *Pseudomonas* (Maxwell and Klienan, 1980).

According to the recommendations of the Centers for Disease Control, the venipuncture dressing should be changed every 48 hours. Some experts have found that the less the dressing is manipulated, the lower the infection rate (Munro-Black, 1984) and that if the dressing remains clean, dry, and intact, it does not need to be changed more frequently than every 48 hours (Procedure 42-8).

Clients receiving TPN should have their vital signs measured and their urine checked for sugar and acetone every 4 to 6 hours. The nurse should be alert for changes and report any to the physician.

Medications or blood should not be administered through the TPN line because this increases the risk of bacterial contamination. In a life-or-death situation the TPN line may be the only intravenous line available and will need to be used for emergency treatment.

Maintaining the Total Parenteral Nutrition System

The infusion flow should be assessed every hour by the nurse. All clients receiving TPN should be connected to an infusion pump. The nurse should also evaluate the catheter and infusion line for patency.

PREVENTING COMPLICATIONS

After the catheter is inserted, a chest x-ray film is obtained to document correct placement of the catheter in the superior vena cava, proximal to the right atrium (Munro-Black, 1984). In addition, the film can show the presence of a pneumothorax, which may occur if the needle punctures the pleura during insertion. The assessment findings consistent with a pneumothorax include chest pain, dyspnea, and coughing; the rapidity of onset and the degree of symptoms depend on the severity of the pneumothorax.

A second complication is the development of an air

embolus during insertion of the catheter or changing of the tubing. This can be prevented by having the client do the Valsalva maneuver and placing the client in the Trendelenburg position.

The last major category of complications, which can occur because of the hyperosmolar solution that is being administered, concerns the client's metabolic system. *Hyperglycemia* is caused by a high concentration of dextrose in the TPN solution. Client risk factors for hyperglycemia include increased secretion of adrenal hormones, increased age, and renal disease (Metheny and Snively, 1983). Hyperglycemia, which can cause dehydration, nausea, headache, and weakness, can also occur in the client receiving TPN when the rate of infusion is too rapid. The risk of hyperglycemia can be reduced by administering the solution at the prescribed rate. If the solution falls behind schedule, the nurse should not increase the rate of flow unless ordered by the physician. Checking the urine for glucose and acetone every 4 to 6 hours can identify signs of glucose intolerance. Clients receiving TPN may be given insulin injections to increase the body's ability to metabolize the increased glucose. Once the TPN has been discontinued, the insulin injections are discontinued.

Hypoglycemia can occur if the infusion rate is too slow or TPN is abruptly discontinued. The high glucose concentration of the TPN solution has stimulated the client's pancreas to secrete more insulin. In addition, the client may also be receiving supplemental insulin injections. If the TPN infusion is too slow or abruptly discontinued, there is too little blood glucose and too much insulin, and hypoglycemia occurs. Symptoms of hypoglycemia include occipital headaches, cold clammy skin, dizziness, tachycardia, and tingling of the extremities and circumoral regions (Metheny and Snively, 1983). Hypoglycemia can be prevented by maintaining an accurate infusion rate and a gradual reduction of the TPN solution. The gradual reduction allows the pancreas time to adapt to the decreased glucose load. If the TPN solution must be discontinued abruptly, a solution of 5% dextrose in quarter-strength normal saline, with appropriate potassium chloride added, should be administered at the previous parenteral nutrition rate until the pancreatic insulin rate decreases in about 12 to 24 hours (Grant, 1980).

Fluid overload causes an increase in extracellular fluid volume. If severe, fluid overload can result in pulmonary edema and congestive heart failure. Signs and symptoms of fluid overload include shortness of breath, tachycardia, weak pulse, hypertension or hypotension, confusion, decreased urine output, rales, or pitting edema. Fluid overload can be prevented by maintaining an accurate rate of infusion and monitoring the client's central venous pressure. If signs of fluid overload occur, the nurse *slows* the infusion rate, notifies the physician, and remains with the client, continually assessing the individual's status.

The major metabolic complications of TPN can be prevented by continually implementing seven nursing interventions (Table 42-16). These interventions are designed for early identification and treatment of these complications.

TABLE 42-16

Interventions for Preventing Metabolic Complications of TPN

Intervention	Rationale
Weigh client daily.	Documents that the client is maintaining or gaining weight and has a proper fluid balance
Record intake and output.	Provides data base for ongoing fluid balance assessment
If client is allowed oral intake, maintain calorie count of foods eaten.	Provides data needed to calculate TPN caloric requirement
Obtain urine to measure glucose and acetone every 4 to 6 hours.	Determines if client is excreting glucose in the urine and whether an insulin supplement is needed
Obtain blood samples for measurement of iron, transferrin, and white blood cells.	Evaluates cellular nutritional status
Continually assess the client's fluid and electrolyte status.	Prevents circulatory overload or dehydration
Maintain infusion rate as ordered. Do not speed up or slow down infusion unless instructed by the physician or a severe complication occurs.	Prevents hyperglycemia, osmotic diuresis, hypoglycemia, and fluid overload

PROMOTING THE CLIENT'S WELL-BEING

Teaching the client about the procedure and what measures the nurse will be taking to maintain the system will decrease anxiety. If the nurse is unable to answer all the client's questions, the physician or another nurse should be asked to talk with the client.

If the client cannot have anything by mouth, the nurse should provide mouth care every hour. The client who is independent can be taught how to care for a dry mouth. It may also be helpful to move the client to a private room so the client does not see other people eating, and the nurse should not talk about meals.

The nurse should encourage the client who can tolerate activity to walk frequently. This helps the client meet psychosocial needs while increasing muscle mass and activity tolerance.

Evaluation

The evaluation of nursing care for clients with altered fluid and electrolyte status is based on the individualized nursing care plan. First, the nurse determines if the imbalance itself has been corrected. Second, the nurse uses the evaluation component to resolve the cause of the fluid or electrolyte disturbance. Third, the nurse uses her assessment findings to determine that the client is able to maintain his own fluid and electrolyte balance. Last, the nurse determines whether complications have resulted from therapies, such as intravenous therapy or total parenteral nutrition, that were needed to correct fluid and electrolyte imbalances.

Summary

Clients with altered fluid and electrolyte status require nursing care plans designed to assist in restoring normal fluid volume and electrolyte concentrations. The nurse restores fluid balance through oral fluid replacement or fluid restrictions. In addition, electrolytes can be administered orally or parenterally. Other measures are used to treat underlying illness that may cause fluid and electrolyte imbalances.

If a client's fluid imbalance has occurred because of malnutrition, the use of total parenteral nutrition will help correct the deficits. The replacement of nutrients permits body fluids to return to their normal compartments and prevents further loss of electrolytes and fluids.

When providing care to clients with altered fluid or electrolyte states, the nurse uses all components of the nursing process to maintain and restore fluid balance. In so doing, the nurse continually monitors for changes in the client's status.

KEY CONCEPTS

✓ Body fluids are distributed in extracellular and intracellular fluid compartments.

✓ Body fluids are composed of electrolytes, minerals, and cells.

✓ Body fluids move from compartment to compartment by diffusion, osmosis, or active transport.

✓ The movement of body fluids depends on membrane permeability.

✓ Two fluid pressures, osmotic and hydrostatic, influence the movement of body fluids.

✓ Body fluids are regulated through fluid intake, output, and hormonal regulation.

✓ Three hormones affect fluid and electrolyte balance: antidiuretic hormone, aldosterone, and glucocorticoids.

✓ Major electrolyte cations in the body fluids are sodium, potassium, calcium, and magnesium.

✓ Major electrolyte anions include chloride, bicarbonate, and phosphate.

✓ Volume disturbances include fluid volume deficits and excesses.

✓ The three types of fluid volume deficit are isotonic, hypernatremic, and hyponatremic dehydration.

✓ Two syndromes associated with fluid volume excess are edema and water intoxication.

✓ Fluid and electrolyte balance is affected by acute and chronic illness, developmental factors, increases in environmental temperature and humidity, and life-style habits including diet, stress, and exercise.

✓ Assessment for fluid and electrolyte alterations includes the nursing history, physical and behavioral assessment, measurements of intake and output, daily weighing, specific laboratory data such as complete blood counts and measurement of serum electrolytes, blood urea nitrogen, and specific gravity.

✓ Fluid deficits can be corrected by parenteral administration of fluid.

✓ Parenteral administration of fluid requires a venipuncture procedure with a butterfly needle, angiocatheter, intracatheter, or needle and syringe.

✓ The infusion flow rate is determined by the physician's order.

✓ An infusion flow rate can be influenced by patency of the needle and infiltration, patency of the catheter, height of the intravenous bag, and position of the extremity.

✓ The nurse maintains the intravenous system by changing solutions as needed, the infusion tubing, and the dressing.

✓ Complications of intravenous therapy include infiltration, phlebitis, fluid overload, and bleeding.

✓ Blood transfusions replace fluid volume lost because of hemorrhage, anemia, or coagulation disorders.

✓ Incorrectly matched blood can result in a transfusion reaction.

✓ Before administering a blood transfusion the nurse must assess the client and obtain baseline vital sign measurements.

KEY CONCEPTS, cont'd

✓ During the transfusion the nurse remains with the client for the first 15 minutes and frequently assesses the vital signs.

✓ Administration of blood or blood products requires that the nurse follow a specific procedure to identify transfusion reactions quickly.

✓ In addition to transfusion reactions, the risks of transfusion include hyperkalemia, hypocalcemia, and circulatory overload.

✓ Clients having blood transfusion reactions need prompt, correct nursing actions.

✓ Total parenteral nutrition is the administration of a nutritionally adequate hypertonic solution to maintain positive nitrogen balance.

✓ Total parenteral nutrition requires the nurse to assist in placement of the intravenous line, regulate the infusion to prevent infection, prevent complications, and maintain client comfort.

REFERENCES

Burch, G., Knochil, J., and Murphy, R.: Stay on guard against heat syndromes, Patient Care 13:1, 1979.

Folk-Lightly, M.: Solving the puzzles of patients' fluid imbalances, Nursing 84 14:34, 1984.

Grant, J.: Handbook of total parenteral nutrition, Philadelphia, 1980, W.B. Saunders Co.

Groër, M.W.: Physiology and pathophysiology of the body fluids, St. Louis, 1981, The C.V. Mosby Co.

Guyton, A.C.: Textbook of medical physiology, ed. 6, Philadelphia, 1982, W.B. Saunders Co.

Keithley, J.K., and Frauline, K.E.: What's behind that IV line, Nursing 82 12:33, 1982.

Kubo, W.M., and Grant, M.M.: The syndrome of inappropriate secretion of antidiuretic hormone, Heart Lung 7:465, 1978.

Lane, G., and Pierce, A.G.: When persistence pays off, Nursing 82 12:44, 1982.

Maxwell, M., and Klienan, C., editors: Clinical disorders of fluid and electrolyte metabolism, ed. 3, New York, 1980, McGraw-Hill Book Co.

Metheny, N.M.: Overview of fluid and electrolyte imbalances, Natl. IV Ther. Assoc. 4:38, 1981.

Metheny, N.M., and Snively, W.D., Jr.: Nurse's handbook of fluid balance, ed. 4, Philadelphia, 1983, J.B. Lippincott Co.

Mountcastle, V.C.: Medical physiology, ed. 14, St. Louis, 1979, The C.V. Mosby Co.

Munro-Black, J.: The ABC's of total parenteral nutrition, Nursing 84 14:50, 1984.

Querin, J.J., and Stahl, L.D.: Twelve simple sensible steps for successful blood transfusion, Nursing 83 13:34, 1983.

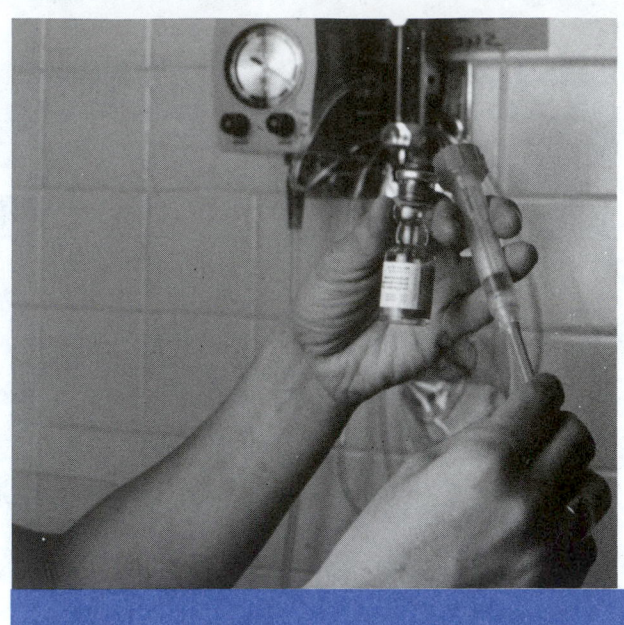

OBJECTIVES

Mastery of content in this chapter will enable the student to:

- Define the terms in the glossary.
- Discuss the chemical, biological, and physiological buffers in the body.
- List and discuss factors that affect acid-base balance.
- Describe the four major types of acid-base imbalance.
- List and discuss the clinical assessments associated with the four major types of acid-base imbalance.
- Discuss the nursing care of clients with acid-base imbalances.
- Evaluate the nursing care plan of a client with an acid-base imbalance.

GLOSSARY

acidemia Increased concentration of hydrogen ions in the blood, causing a reduced pH.

alkalemia Decreased concentration of hydrogen ions in the blood, causing an elevated pH.

arterial blood gases Oxygen and carbon dioxide concentrations, pH, and oxygen saturation of the hemoglobin in arterial blood; also refers to the laboratory tests that measure these levels.

buffer Substance or group of substances that can absorb or release hydrogen ions to correct an acid-base imbalance.

compensation Action by the body's chemical, biological, or physiological buffering systems to correct an acid-base imbalance.

metabolic acidosis Abnormal condition of high hydrogen ion concentration in the extracellular fluid caused by either a primary increase in hydrogen ions or a decrease in bicarbonate.

metabolic alkalosis Abnormal condition characterized by the significant loss of acid from the body or by increased levels of bicarbonate.

plasma proteins Albumin, fibrinogen, prothrombin, and the gamma globulins, which constitute about 6% to 7% of the blood plasma in the body.

respiratory acidosis Abnormal condition characteried by increased arterial carbon dioxide concentration, excess carbonic acid, and increased hydrogen ion concentration.

respiratory alkalosis Abnormal condition characterized by decreased arterial carbon dioxide concentration and decreased hydrogen ion concentration.

43 Acid-Base Balance

For metabolism and other cellular processes to occur, body fluids must be alkaline. Metabolic processes produce acids, however, and therefore physiological processes are necessary for maintaining a relatively stable balance between alkalinity and acidity—the acid-base balance.

Acid-base balance exists when the net rate at which the body produces acids or bases equals the rate at which acids and bases are excreted. The acid-base balance results in a stable concentration of hydrogen ions (H^+) in body fluids.

The concentration of hydrogen ions in a body fluid is expressed as the pH value. The pH is a scale for measuring the acidity or alkalinity of a fluid, such as extracellular fluid. The numerical value of the pH is inversely proportionate to the number of hydrogen ions in the solution. A value of 7.0 is neutral. A value below 7.0 is an acid solution and has a lower level of hydrogen ions, while a value greater than 7.0 is an alkaline solution with a higher level of ions. Normal pH values for extracellular fluids range from 7.36 to 7.44.

A client's state of acid-base balance or imbalance is determined by arterial blood gas tests. Arterial blood gas tests measure the pH, oxygen and carbon dioxide concentrations, and oxygen saturation of hemoglobin in an arterial blood sample. Acid-base balance is necessary for many physiological processes, and imbalances resulting from many causes can threaten a client's health by altering respiration, metabolism, central nervous system function, and other processes.

The nurse must be aware of how to assess a client's acid-base balance and how to interpret the results of arterial blood gas tests. The nurse can then use the nursing process to help correct any acid-base disturbance.

Acid-Base Regulation

The human body has regulatory mechanisms for maintaining the acid-base balance and for adapting to short-term changes in hydrogen ion concentration. Such changes occur, for example, during physical exercise, moderate anxiety states, and minor gastrointestinal upsets. The body can make adjustments for transient changes in pH. This correction is called compensation. However, with more severe changes, such as severe trauma, uncontrolled diabetes mellitus, or shock, the body is unable to correct the pH and the acid-base balance is uncompensated. In such cases prompt medical intervention is required.

There are three general types of acid-base regulators within the body: chemical, biological, and physiological buffering systems. A buffer is a substance or a group of substances that can absorb or release hydrogen ions to correct an acid-base imbalance.

Chemical Regulation
CHEMICAL BUFFERS

The largest chemical buffer in the extracellular fluid is the carbonic and bicarbonate buffer system. This system can be expressed as the following equation:

$$CO_2 + H_2O \leftrightharpoons H^+ + HCO_3^-$$

carbon dioxide   water   carbonic acid   hydrogen   bicarbonate

The carbonic acid–bicarbonate buffer system is the first buffering system to react to change in the pH of extracellular fluid. The excretion of carbon dioxide that results from metabolism is controlled primarily by the lungs. The excretion of hydrogen and bicarbonate ions is controlled by the kidneys. The reaction of these two groups of substances buffers a strong acid or base to maintain a relatively constant pH.

The carbonic acid–bicarbonate buffering system is the only strictly chemical buffering reaction that combines excess ions of either charge. This system can either accept or donate hydrogen ions to correct an acid state (acidosis) or strongly alkaline state (alkalosis) (Lee, Stroot, and Schaper, 1975).

The carbonic acid–bicarbonate buffer responds immediately to acid-base imbalance. It is an adaptive system, and its effect is relatively brief.

PROTEIN BUFFERS

A second chemical buffering system involves the plasma proteins. Plasma proteins are albumin, fibrinogen, prothrombin, and the gamma globulins, which constitute about 6% to 7% of the blood plasma. These proteins have the capacity to bind with or release hydrogen ions to correct acidosis or alkalosis. However, their capacity to maintain acid-base balance of the extracellular fluid is limited, and they cannot correct long-term imbalances.

Biological Regulation

Biological buffering occurs when hydrogen ions are absorbed or released by the body cells. The hydrogen ion has a positive charge and must be exchanged with another positively charged ion, frequently potassium (K^+). In conditions with excessive acid, a hydrogen ion enters the cell and a potassium ion leaves the cell and enters the extracellular fluid. The extracellular fluid is thus less acidic because fewer hydrogen ions are present. As a result of this exchange, however, people with acidosis are also hyperkalemic. Once the acidosis is corrected, the potassium reenters the cells and potassium levels return to normal.

Biological buffering occurs after the process of chemical buffering and takes 2 to 4 hours. A second type of biological buffer is the hemoglobin-oxyhemoglobin system. When blood is oxygenated, chloride travels from the hemoglobin to the plasma. As chloride leaves the cell, bicarbonate enters. This process is part of the chloride shift and is a reciprocal exchange between these anions (Lee, Stroot, and Schaper, 1975).

Physiological Regulation

LUNGS

The two physiological buffers in the body are the lungs and the kidneys. The lungs can provide a rapid adaptation to an acid-base imbalance; in fact, the lungs can act to return the pH to normal before the action of the biological buffers.

Ordinarily, hydrogen ions and carbon dioxide provide the stimulus for respiration. When the concentration of hydrogen ions is altered, the lungs react to correct the imbalance by alternating the rate and depth of respiration. In alkalosis, the rate of respiration is reduced and the person retains carbon dioxide. The carbon dioxide combines with water in the blood to form carbonic acid, which helps to correct the alkaline excess. If an acid excess is present, the respiratory rate is increased and the lungs excrete greater amounts of carbon dioxide (Lee, Stroot, and Schaper, 1975).

KIDNEYS

The kidneys can take from a few hours to several days to regulate acid-base abnormalities. The kidneys use three mechanisms to regulate the hydrogen ion concentration. First, they can reabsorb bicarbonate in cases of acid excess and excrete it in cases of acid deficit. Second, the kidneys use a phosphate ion ($PO_4^{\equiv}$) to carry hydrogen ions (H^+) by excreting phosphoric acid (H_3PO_4) and forming an acid base. Last, the kidneys can convert ammonia (NH_3) to ammonium (NH_4) by attaching a hydrogen ion to ammonia.

Factors Influencing Acid-Base Balance

Three major factors may influence a client's risk for an acid-base imbalance: level of health, age, and life-style.

Level of Health

Clients with chronic disease such as pulmonary disease, diabetes mellitus, or anemia are at greater risk for acidosis or alkalosis because of altered respiration or metabolism. Clients with acute febrile conditions and those who take medications such as steroids or diuretics are also at risk for acid-base imbalances because of metabolic alterations.

The body is constantly undergoing metabolic activities. To maintain adequate metabolism, the kidneys and the lungs maintain a 20:1 ratio between bicarbonate and carbonic acid (Fig. 43-1). When the bicarbonate concentration of the blood rises or the carbonic acid concentration falls, the proportion of

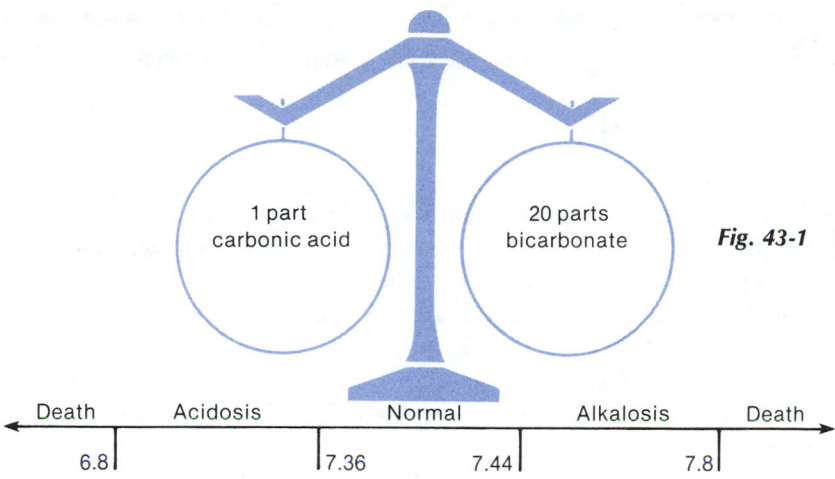

Fig. 43-1 Carbonic acid/bicarbonate ratio and pH.

bicarbonate increases and the pH is greater than 7.44, reflecting a decrease in hydrogen ion concentration and alkalosis. When the bicarbonate concentration of the blood falls or carbonic acid concentration increases, the proportion of bicarbonate is decreased and the pH drops below 7.36, reflecting a decrease in hydrogen ion concentration and acidosis (Groër and Shekleton, 1983). Cellular metabolism cannot tolerate excessively prolonged high or low hydrogen ion concentrations. A pH less than 6.8 or greater than 7.8 usually results in death.

During illness the body's metabolic activities are altered. As a consequence, the bicarbonate/carbonic ratio is less stable and alkalosis or acidosis can occur quickly. Continual nursing assessment can quickly identify symptoms associated with acidosis or alkalosis.

Age

The very young and the very old are most susceptible to acid-base imbalances, in part because of the fluid balance and metabolic activities in these age groups (see Chapter 42). In addition, the aging process changes lung function. Whenever there is a change in fluid balance, metabolic rate, or respiratory functioning, the client is at risk for an acid-base imbalance.

Life-Style

Certain extremes in life-style can result in acid-base imbalances.

FAD DIETING

Acidosis can develop in people who experiment with fad diets. Such diets frequently cause early rapid weight loss, which represents loss of body water. This water loss can predispose the client to dehydration, or extracellular fluid loss (see Chapter 42). In addition, some fad diets encourage near-starvation, altering the metabolic processes and resulting in acid-base imbalance. Not all fad diets are dangerous, but clients attempting rapid weight loss with these diets are at risk for acidosis.

ANXIETY

Anxiety can cause some people to hyperventilate. This may be so severe that respiratory alkalosis develops. These clients frequently need counseling and supportive measures to control their anxiety.

ALCOHOLISM

Chronic alcoholism can increase the client's risk of acidosis because alcoholism is frequently associated with malnutrition. The alcoholic's caloric intake may come primarily from beer, wine, or whiskey, which have little or no nutritional value.

DRUGS

The use of prescription or nonprescription drugs can increase the risk of acid-base imbalance. Diuretics or steroids can cause an acid-base imbalance, particularly if the client uses the drugs inappropriately.

Drugs that are commonly abused can also cause acid-base imbalances. An imbalance may result from depressed ventilation, as with depressant drugs, or hyperventilation, as with amphetamines.

Types of Acid-Base Imbalance

There are four primary types of acid-base imbalance: respiratory acidosis, respiratory alkalosis, metabolic acidosis, and metabolic alkalosis.

Causes of Respiratory Acidosis

- Pneumonia
- Respiratory failure
- Atelectasis
- Drug overdose
- Paralysis of respiratory muscles (Guillain-Barré syndrome, poliomyelitis, myasthenia gravis)
- Traumatic injuries to the thorax (flail chest)
- Obesity
- Airway obstruction
- Head injuries
- Cerebrovascular accident (stroke)
- Drowning
- Cystic fibrosis

Causes of Respiratory Alkalosis

- Anxiety
- Fear
- Anemia
- Hypermetabolic states
- Disorders of the central nervous system (head injuries, infections)
- Drugs (aspirin overdose)
- Asthma
- Pneumonia
- Inappropriate mechanical ventilator settings

Causes of Metabolic Acidosis

- Starvation
- Dehydration
- Diabetic ketoacidosis
- Renal failure
- Shock
- Diarrhea
- Drugs (methanol, ethanol, formic acid, paraldehyde, aspirin)
- Renal tubular acidosis

Causes of Metabolic Alkalosis

- Excessive vomiting
- Prolonged gastric suctioning
- Electrolyte disturbance
- Cushing's disease
- Drugs (steroids, sodium bicarbonate, diuretics)
- Hyperaldosteronism

Respiratory Acidosis

Respiratory acidosis is an abnormal condition characterized by an increased arterial carbon dioxide concentration ($Paco_2$), excess carbonic acid (H_2CO_3), and an increased hydrogen ion concentration (decreased pH). Respiratory acidosis is caused by any condition that depresses ventilation or by hypoventilation (see box above). Decreased ventilation may originate in the respiratory system, as with respiratory failure, or outside the respiratory system, as with a drug overdose.

In clients experiencing respiratory acidosis the cerebrospinal fluid and brain cells become acidic, causing neurological changes. Hypoxemia occurs because of the respiratory depression, resulting in further neurological impairments (see Chapter 41). Electrolyte changes may accompany the acidosis.

Respiratory Alkalosis

Respiratory alkalosis is an abnormal condition characterized by decreased $Paco_2$ and decreased hydrogen ion concentration (increased pH). Respiratory alkalosis results from excessive exhalation of CO_2, or hyperventilation (see top box at right). Like respiratory acidosis, respiratory alkalosis can originate outside the respiratory system, as with anxiety, or within the respiratory system, as with asthma.

Metabolic Acidosis

Metabolic acidosis is an abnormal condition that results from a rise in hydrogen ion concentration (decreased pH) in the extracellular fluid, caused by either a primary increase in hydrogen ion or a decrease in bicarbonate (Groër, 1981). There are many causes of metabolic acidosis (see middle box above). The two types of metabolic acidosis, normochloremic and hyperchloremic, are classified according to the client's plasma chloride concentration.

Metabolic Alkalosis

Metabolic alkalosis is an abnormal condition characterized by the significant loss of acid from the body or by increased levels of bicarbonate. The most common cause is vomiting. Normally the stomach content is high in acid. With prolonged vomiting the acid contents are expelled and the client experiences an acid loss. In addition, metabolic alkalosis may result when a client with a gastric acidity disturbance ingests large amounts of sodium bicarbonate. Other causes are listed in the bottom box at left.

Assessment

The nursing assessment of acid-base disturbances is complex, and frequently it is difficult to discriminate clearly among different types of imbalance. The nursing assessment for clients with actual or potential acid-base disturbances includes a nursing history, a physical examination, and laboratory data. The following sections discuss these assessment areas for each of the four types of imbalance.

Arterial blood gas tests are used to determine the client's acid-base status. The procedure for obtaining the specimen of arterial blood is detailed in the later nursing intervention section (Procedure 43-1). Assessment includes interpreting the results of arterial blood gas testing (see box above).

Respiratory Acidosis

The nursing history for a client with actual or potential respiratory acidosis should identify the presence of any acute or chronic pulmonary disease. The nurse determines whether the client is using any chemical, such as drugs or alcohol, that causes respiratory depression. The nurse should ask the client or the family about any recent head or chest trauma that is not obvious on initial inspection. The nurse should also inquire whether the client has had any recent cold or flulike symptoms. The Guillain-Barré syndrome frequently occurs following a period of such symptoms.

A variety of findings on physical examination may result in clients with respiratory acidosis. The signs and symptoms observed are a response of the body to the acidosis and depend on the client's overall health and age and the cause of respiratory acidosis. See the box above for common clinical symptoms associated with respiratory alkalosis.

Laboratory tests are required for confirmation of any acid-base imbalance. To analyze the results of the arterial blood gas test, the nurse should follow a step-by-step approach. First the pH value is considered. A value below 7.36 indicates that the blood is in a state of acidemia.

The $Paco_2$ value is considered. If the client does not have chronic obstructive pulmonary disease (COPD), and the $Paco_2$ is elevated, the origin of the acid-base imbalance is respiratory. If the pH is below 7.36, respiratory acidosis is present. The client with COPD has adapted to an elevated $Paco_2$, and with compensation his pH remains within a normal range. However, if the client is no longer compensating, the pH begins to fall, indicating acidemia. In addition, the $Paco_2$ may be elevated beyond the compensation.

The Pao_2 value is considered to determine whether the client in respiratory acidosis is also hypoxemic. Hypoxemia should be suspected when the Pao_2 falls below 80 mm Hg. However, the client with COPD usually has a lower than normal Pao_2 owing to the disease process.

The percentage of oxygen saturation is determined. Hemoglobin remains 80% saturated with a Pao_2 of 55 mm Hg.

Finally, the bicarbonate (HCO_3) value is considered. If early uncompensated respiratory acidosis is present, the bicarbonate concentration is within the normal range. If the kidneys are trying to compensate for the acidosis, they retain bicarbonate. Therefore an elevated bicarbonate reading can indicate that the kidneys are functioning as physiological buffers.

The laboratory assessment of acid-base imbalance should include serial blood gas tests to identify any trend of improvement or decline. Clients with acid-base imbalances have arterial blood samples taken repeatedly to evaluate the acid-base balance.

Serum electrolyte determinations are also obtained repeatedly. In respiratory acidosis the serum potassium level is elevated, resulting in hyperkalemia, because of the biological buffering capacity of the cells. Because acidemia is present, the cells attempt to act as a buffer by absorbing hydrogen ions from the extracellular fluid. Hydrogen ions are positively charged and must be exchanged with another intracellular positively charged ion. Therefore, as hydrogen ions are absorbed into the cell, potassium ions are excreted and the potassium level is elevated in extracellular fluid.

Respiratory Alkalosis

The nursing history of the client with suspected respiratory alkalosis identifies the presence of respiratory diseases, any hypermetabolic states, and repeated episodes of acute anxiety. The nurse must also determine whether drug overdose has occurred. Initially a salicylate overdose produces hyperventilation because the lungs are attempting to act as physiological buffers against the ingestion of acetylsalicylic acid.

If the client is on a mechanical ventilator, the nurse should suspect inappropriate ventilator settings and should check the settings against the physician's orders. The nurse should consider as well the possibility of hyperventilation induced by the central nervous system, such as occurs with some head injuries or meningitis.

The nurse's findings in the physical examination of clients with respiratory alkalosis also differ among

---

Common Clinical Symptoms of Respiratory Alkalosis

PHYSICAL EXAMINATION
Central Nervous System

- Anxious appearance
- Irritability
- Tingling of the extremities
- Fainting
- Dizziness

Cardiopulmonary System

- Tachypnea
- Cardiac arrhythmias

Musculoskeletal System

- Tetany
- Muscle weakness

LABORATORY DATA

- pH 7.44 or greater
- $Paco_2$ less than 36 mm Hg
- Pao_2 normal
- O_2 saturation normal
- HCO_3 normal
- K^+ below 3.5 mEq/L

---

clients. The signs and symptoms observed are the body's response to acid-base imbalances (see the box above).

The analysis of laboratory data confirms the presence of respiratory alkalosis. The pH is above 7.44, indicating that the blood is alkalemic. The $Paco_2$ is below normal, showing that the cause of the alkalemia is respiratory. Clients without lung disease should have normal Pao_2 and oxygen saturation recordings. If the client has lung disease, the initial Pao_2 and oxygen saturation findings are within normal ranges but are subject to decline, particularly during an acute asthmatic attack. The bicarbonate level is within normal range during the early stages of respiratory alkalosis. When the kidneys begin to act as physiological buffers, however, they excrete bicarbonate and the serum bicarbonate level falls as the kidneys attempt to correct the acid-base imbalance.

Serum electrolyte tests frequently reveal hypokalemia, which results as the cells act as biological buffers. In an alkalotic state the cells attempt to add more hydrogen ions to the extracellular fluid to restore the pH to normal range. When the cells release hydrogen ions, they absorb potassium ions and serum potassium levels fall.

Metabolic Acidosis

The nursing history of a client with potential or actual metabolic acidosis should include identification of any endocrine imbalances such as diabetes mellitus. The nurse should also obtain information about any dieting practices, such as a fad diet or inappropriate use of diuretics. Any familial history of renal disease is important. Information about substance abuse or ingestion of large quantities of aspirin should also be obtained.

With the physical examination the nurse identifies signs and symptoms representing the body's response to the acid-base imbalance. The most pronounced clinical sign with metabolic acidosis is the compensatory respiratory effort of Kussmaul respirations. Kussmaul respirations usually occur in the client with diabetic ketoacidosis and indicate the client's attempt to exhale excessive carbon dioxide (see Chapter 41). Other assessment findings may be related to potas-

sium excess and the body's response to acidosis (see box at left).

Laboratory tests reveal a pH less than 7.36, reflecting acidemia. The $Paco_2$ is below the normal range; in clients with COPD the $Paco_2$ is less than their baseline value. The drop in $Paco_2$ demonstrates the ability of the lungs to compensate for the metabolic acidosis by exhaling carbon dioxide. The other respiratory parameters, Pao_2 and oxygen saturation, generally remain within normal ranges or the client's baseline ranges. The bicarbonate concentration is low because the body stores of this ion are depleted in response to the acidotic pH.

The serum electrolyte analysis reveals an elevated potassium level, for the same reason as in respiratory acidosis. The potassium level rises in response to cells functioning as biological buffers.

Metabolic Alkalosis

The nursing history for the client with metabolic alkalosis should identify the presence of endocrine disorders such as Cushing's disease or hyperaldosteronism. The nurse should determine whether the client is using prescription or nonprescription medications such as steroids or diuretics. The nurse should also obtain information about any recent episodes of vomiting.

The physical examination to detect and identify the signs and symptoms of metabolic alkalosis is usually more difficult than with other acid-base imbalances because metabolic alkalosis frequently occurs in response to another disease process. Nonetheless, some common signs and symptoms are associated with metabolic alkalosis (see box on p. 1260).

Laboratory tests include a pH greater than 7.44, indicating a blood alkalemia. The $Paco_2$ level may be normal if the lungs are not compensating. If the lungs are compensating, the $Paco_2$ is elevated to retain some carbon dioxide, which is combined with water to form carbonic acid. The bicarbonate level is elevated because of the body's inability to excrete excess amounts.

Serum electrolyte tests reveal hypokalemia, which occurs as a result of the biological buffer mechanisms, in the same way as for respiratory alkalosis.

■ ■ ■ ■ ■

The medical diagnosis of an acid-base imbalance is based on the findings of the arterial blood gas analysis. However, the nursing history and physical examination enable the nurse to identify clients at risk for acid-base imbalances. Ongoing physical examination can also identify subtle changes in the client's physiological function, particularly with respect to

Common Clinical Symptoms of Metabolic Alkalosis

PHYSICAL EXAMINATION
Central Nervous System

- Headache
- Irritability
- Lethargy
- Decreases in level of consciousness

Cardiopulmonary System

- Atrial tachycardia
- Slow, shallow respirations with periods of apnea
- Bradycardia

Gastrointestinal System

- Nausea
- Vomiting

Musculoskeletal System

- Numbness and tingling of extremities
- Hypertonicity of muscles
- Tetany

LABORATORY DATA

- pH greater than 7.44
- $PaCO_2$ normal or greater than 44 mm Hg if lungs are compensating
- PaO_2 normal
- O_2 saturation normal
- HCO_3^- above 26 mEq/L
- K^+ less than 3.5 mEq/L

TABLE 43-1

Examples of Nursing Diagnoses Associated with Acid-Base Imbalances

Problem	Causes
RESPIRATORY ACIDOSIS	
Impaired ventilation	Related to: Airway obstruction Decreased lung expansion Central nervous system depression Decreased exchange of respiratory gases
RESPIRATORY ALKALOSIS	
Hyperventilation	Related to: Anxiety Airway obstruction Hypermetabolic condition Iatrogenic causes
METABOLIC ACIDOSIS	
Excessive metabolic acids	Related to: Starvation Dehydration Endocrine imbalance Drug ingestion
METABOLIC ALKALOSIS	
Decreased metabolic acids	Related to: Endocrine imbalance Prolonged gastric losses Drug ingestion

the central nervous system. Thus the nurse can identify clinical symptoms associated with a worsening acid-base alteration, document the status of the alteration, and institute treatment.

Nursing Diagnosis

The nursing diagnosis associated with an acid-base imbalance depends on the cause of the acid-base disturbance. Nursing diagnoses associated with respiratory acidosis reflect a problem with ventilation, and nursing diagnoses associated with respiratory alkalosis reflect the physiological or emotional cause of the imbalance.

Similarly, nursing diagnoses associated with metabolic acidosis or alkalosis reflect the underlying cause of the acid excess or deficit. Frequently metabolic acidosis or alkalosis is a symptom of another disorder.

The nursing diagnoses listed in Table 43-1 are a sample of diagnoses for clients with acid-base disturbances. These nursing diagnoses help to establish a nursing care plan for clients with altered acid-base balance.

Planning

The nursing care plan for clients with acid-base disturbances is based on two goals. First, the care plan treats the underlying cause of the imbalance. For example, if the client has impaired ventilation related to decreased lung expansion, the nurse plans nursing

PROCEDURE 43-1

Arterial Puncture

STEPS	RATIONALE
1. Collect the following equipment and bring it to the bedside:	
a. Heparinized 5 ml syringe	Heparin prevents coagulation of the arterial sample.
b. ⅝-inch 20-gauge needle	This promotes atraumatic cannulization of artery.
c. Crushed ice for arterial blood sample	Ice decreases oxygen metabolism of the arterial blood sample.
d. Local anesthetic	Anesthetic reduces local pain when more than one attempt is necessary and reduces the likelihood of arterial spasm.
e. Topical skin antibacterial scrub, alcohol wipes	These reduce the entry of surface bacteria into the puncture site.
f. Air lock or cap for syringe	This prevents air from entering blood after the sample has been obtained, thus altering the results of the blood gas analysis.
g. 2 × 2 gauze	Gauze allows application of pressure after arterial puncture.
2. Explain the procedure and the client's responsibility to the client.	This prevents hyperventilation owing to anxiety and a resulting temporary change in blood gases.
3. Palpate the radial artery.	The radial artery is selected because it is superficially located, has collateral circulation, and is not adjacent to a large vein.
4. Hyperextend the client's wrist over a rolled towel.	This maintains the radial artery in a superficial position.
5. Cleanse the site with a circular motion with Betadine followed by an alcohol wipe.	This reduces the risk of skin bacteria entering puncture site.
6. Apply local anesthetic. Xylocaine 2% is usually used.	An anesthetic reduces pain and subsequent hyperventilation in some clients. It also decreases the likelihood of arterial spasm.
7. Flush a 5 ml syringe with 0.5 ml of 1:1000 heparin solution and then empty the syringe, leaving heparin in the needle (Metheny, 1983).	Heparin in the needle prevents clotting of the blood sample. Excess heparin in the syringe affects the pH value of the sample blood.
8. Insert the needle at an angle while stabilizing the client's artery with your free hand.	Entering the artery at an angle minimizes the formation of a hematoma at the puncture site.
9. Observe for a pulsating flow of blood into the syringe.	This indicates the puncture of an artery.
10. Withdraw 3 to 5 ml of blood.	This is a sufficient amount for analysis.
11. Remove the needle and syringe from the artery. Cap the needle with cork or the syringe with air lock.	Capping prevents entry of air into syringe. If air enters the syringe, the blood must be discarded to avoid inaccurate blood gas results.
12. Rotate the syringe so blood mixes with heparin.	This prevents clotting of the sample.
13. Submerge the syringe in crushed ice.	Icing reduces the rate of oxygen metabolism of the sampled blood.
14. Label the specimen with client's name, body temperature, and (for clients on oxygen therapy) inspired oxygen concentration.	Normally a 6% change in arterial PaO_2 occurs with each degree of centigrade of body temperature (Metheny, 1983). Measurement of oxygen concentration is important in evaluating the effectiveness of oxygen therapy.
15. Apply pressure to the puncture site by applying 2 × 2 gauze over the site and holding for 5 minutes. Length of time may be increased for clients receiving anticoagulants.	Pressure reduces the risk of hematoma formation and damage to the artery.

therapies to promote or maintain lung expansion (see Chapter 41). If the client has excess metabolic acids related to dehydration, the nurse plans therapies to correct the dehydration (see Chapter 42).

The second goal of the nursing care plan is to restore the hydrogen ion concentration to normal ranges. This is usually achieved once the underlying cause of the imbalance is recognized and treated.

Implementation

Most nursing therapies for clients with acid-base disturbances involve dependent or interdependent nursing functions. Frequently the nurse is responsible for inserting and maintaining an intravenous line (see Chapter 42). With acute acid-base disturbances an intravenous line allows removal of venous blood for serum electrolyte determinations, as well as providing an immediate access route for emergency medications. The nurse should evaluate the patency and functioning of the intravenous line at frequent intervals.

The nurse implements the appropriate nursing measures to promote ventilation and oxygenation (see Chapter 41). This is of particular importance for the client with respiratory acidosis. Stasis of pulmonary secretions and decreased lung expansion worsen the acidotic condition and in some clients can make the difference between life and death.

For clients with respiratory alkalosis resulting from anxiety, the nurse initiates nursing measures to reduce the client's anxiety after first correcting the respiratory alkalosis. To correct the alkalosis the nurse instructs the client to breathe into a paper bag. With this method the client rebreathes exhaled carbon dioxide, thereby providing carbon dioxide that combines with water to form carbonic acid, which increases blood acidity. Once the respiratory alkalosis is corrected, the client's symptoms disappear. At this point the nurse may be able to assist the client in determining the cause of anxiety and methods to control it. Some clients with repeated anxiety attacks need professional counseling from a psychotherapist or psychiatrist, and the nurse should make an appropriate and prompt referral.

The nurse should frequently check the physician's orders for new medications or fluids. Clients with acute acid-base disturbances have continually changing metabolic requirements. The prescribed drugs, such as insulin or sodium bicarbonate, and fluid and electrolyte replacement are to be given promptly. Usually during the acute phase the physician gives both written and oral orders to the nurse. To ensure communication, however, the nurse checks the client's chart hourly for new written orders.

The nurse develops interventions to protect the client from complications. For example, a febrile client needs frequent skin care to prevent skin breakdown. Immobilized clients require frequent position changes and range of motion exercises (see Chapter 30). All the hazards of immobility (see Chapter 31) are potential complications for clients with acid-base imbalances.

Clients with acid-base disturbances usually require repeated arterial blood gas analysis. This procedure provides arterial blood samples for analysis of hydrogen ion concentration.

Arterial Blood Gases

Arterial blood gas determinations require the removal of blood from an artery to determine the client's acid-base status and the adequacy of ventilation and oxygenation. Arterial blood gas samples are drawn from a peripheral artery, such as the radial artery, or from an arterial line. In some agencies nurses are responsible for radial artery punctures. Beginning nursing students do not draw arterial blood gas samples but frequently assist in the sampling process and care for the client after the procedure. Procedure 43-1 presents the steps in arterial puncture.

Evaluation

The evaluation of nursing care delivered to clients with acid-base imbalance is based on two goals of care. First, the underlying condition should be corrected, as with resolution of pneumonia or relief of nausea and vomiting. Second, the arterial blood gas parameters should return to normal ranges or the client's normal baseline levels.

Because severe acid-base imbalances can result in death, it is crucial that the underlying condition be corrected. Otherwise the acid-base imbalance can worsen, creating a vicious circle.

Summary

Acid-base imbalances may result from a number of underlying illnesses. With minor transient imbalances, the body compensates by means of chemical, biological, and physiological regulatory mechanisms. With more severe imbalances, however, medical and nursing interventions are required because acid-base imbalances are life-threatening conditions. Each of the four types of imbalance involves clinical signs and symptoms that the nurse assesses. The nursing process provides a structured approach for nursing care to correct acid-base imbalances and assist the client in maintaining or restoring normal functioning.

KEY CONCEPTS

✓ The individual's acid-base balance depends on the hydrogen ion concentration in the blood.

✓ The body's chemical buffering system responds first to acid-base abnormalities.

✓ Chemical buffers include the carbonic acid–bicarbonate buffering system and protein buffers.

✓ Biological buffering occurs when hydrogen ions are absorbed or released by the cells to compensate for acid-base imbalances.

✓ Physiological buffering involves compensatory responses in the lungs or kidneys.

✓ The buffering response of the lungs occurs immediately.

✓ The buffering response of the kidneys occurs in hours or a few days.

✓ The presence of chronic illnesses increases a client's risk of acid-base imbalance.

✓ Severe acute illness can also result in acid-base disorders.

✓ Clients who are very young or very old are at greater risk for acid-base imbalances.

✓ Fad dieting, anxiety, and alcohol and drug abuse increase a client's risk for acid-base imbalances.

✓ Respiratory acidosis is characterized by increased carbon dioxide concentration, excess carbonic acid, and increased hydrogen ion concentration.

✓ Respiratory acidosis is caused by a primary or secondary failure in ventilation.

✓ Respiratory alkalosis is characterized by decreased carbon dioxide and hydrogen ion concentrations.

✓ Respiratory alkalosis is caused by primary or secondary hyperventilation.

✓ Metabolic acidosis is characterized by a rise in hydrogen ion concentration.

✓ Metabolic acidosis is caused by a primary increase in hydrogen ions or a decrease in bicarbonate.

✓ Metabolic alkalosis is caused by a significant loss of acids or an increased level of bicarbonate.

✓ The goals of therapy for acid-base imbalances are to treat the underlying illness and to restore the client's arterial pH to normal.

REFERENCES

Groër, M.W.: Physiology and pathophysiology of the body fluids, St. Louis, 1981, The C.V. Mosby Co.

Groër, M.W. and Shekleton, M.E.: Basic pathophysiology: a conceptual approach, ed. 2, St. Louis, 1983, The C.V. Mosby Co.

Lee, C.A., Stroot, V.R., and Schaper, C.A.: What to do when acid-base problems hang in the balance, Nursing 75 5:32, 1975.

Luce, J.M., Tyler, M.L., and Pierson, D.J.: Intensive respiratory care, Philadelphia, 1984, W.B. Saunders Co.

Metheny, N.M., and Snively, W.D.: Nurses' handbook of fluid balance, ed. 4, Philadelphia, 1983, J.B. Lippincott Co.

9

Earlier units discuss many elements of nursing care directed toward assisting clients to meet physiological and psychosocial needs. Nursing care related to these needs is appropriate for many clients in most health care settings. Because the nurse also encounters clients with special physiological or psychosocial needs, nursing care for three of the more common types of special needs is addressed in this unit. Clients with sensory impairments may have more difficulty coping with illness or other stresses. Clients with substance abuse problems, including the misuse of alcohol and illegal, prescription, or over-the-counter drugs, face particular health risks as well as psychosocial stresses. Finally, clients experiencing losses related to illness or death, or their own approaching death, may have difficulty adapting through the grieving process. For all three of these special needs, the nurse incorporates special interventions into the nursing care plan to assist the client in maintaining optimal well-being.

Caring for Clients with Special Needs

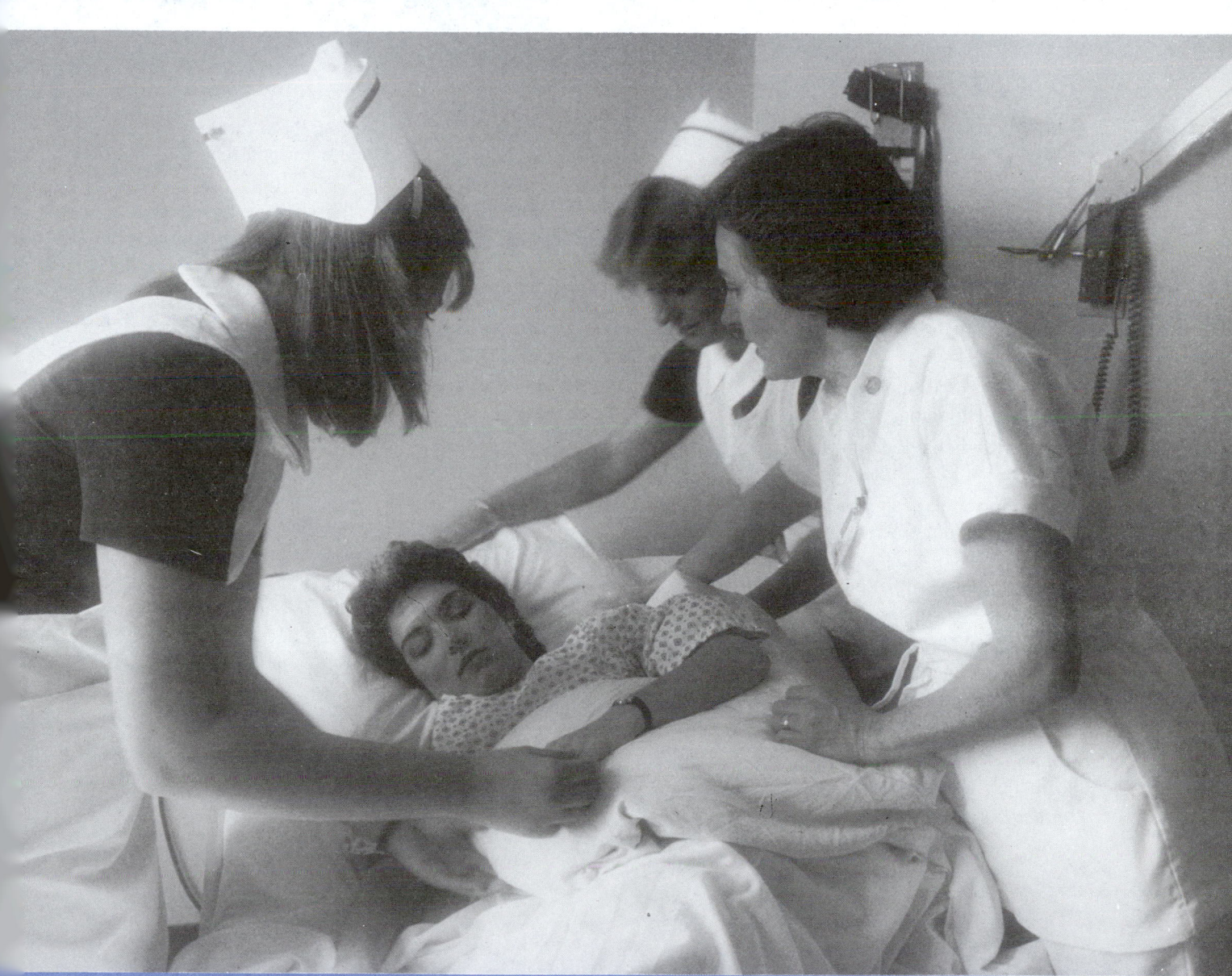

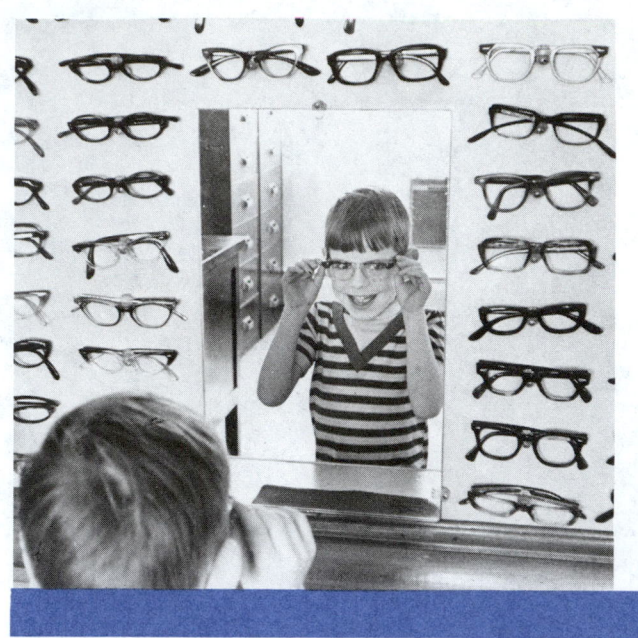

OBJECTIVES

Mastery of content in this chapter will enable the student to:

- Define the terms in the glossary.
- Differentiate among the processes of reception, perception, and reaction to sensory stimuli.
- Discuss common causes of sensory alterations.
- Explain the health problems connected with sensory deficit, sensory deprivation, and sensory overload.
- Discuss common sensory changes that normally occur with aging.
- Describe behaviors that indicate sensory alterations.
- Develop a plan of care for clients with visual, auditory, tactile, speech, and olfactory deficits.
- List interventions for preventing sensory deprivation and controlling sensory overload.
- Describe conditions in the health care agency or the client's home setting that can be adjusted to promote meaningful sensory stimulation.

GLOSSARY

aphasia   Neurological disorder concerning the production and understanding of language.

binocular vision   Vision involving the use of both eyes.

cataract   Abnormal opacity of the lens of the eye causing interference with light reaching the retina.

expressive aphasia   Inability to name common objects or to express simple ideas in words or writing.

gustatory   Pertaining to the sense of taste.

kinesthesia   Perception of position of body parts, weight, and movement.

olfactory   Pertaining to the sense of smell.

ototoxic   Having a harmful effect on the eighth cranial (auditory) nerves or the organs of hearing and balance.

presbyopia   Farsightedness with inability to focus on near objects, resulting from loss of elasticity of the lens; occurs with age.

refractive error   Defect in the ability of the lens of the eye to focus light, such as occurs in nearsightedness and farsightedness.

sensory deficit   Defect in the function of one or more of the senses, resulting in visual, auditory, or olfactory impairments.

sensory deprivation   State in which stimulation to one or more of the senses is lacking, resulting in impaired sensory perception.

sensory overload   State in which stimulation to one or more of the senses is so excessive that the brain disregards or does not meaningfully respond to stimuli.

44 Sensory Alterations

Part of the uniqueness of human beings is the ability to sense a variety of stimuli within the environment, perceive and organize those stimuli, and respond appropriately. Stimulation comes from many sources in and outside of the body, particularly through the senses of sight, hearing, touch (tactile), smell (olfactory), and taste (gustatory). The body also has a kinesthetic sense that enables a person to be aware of the position and movement of body parts without seeing them. The ability to speak is not considered a sense, but it is similar to the senses in that the client unable to talk may lack meaningful stimulation from other human beings. Meaningful stimuli are essential for a person's normal healthy functioning. Stimuli provide a means to learn about the environment and are necessary for normal development of the sensory organs. When a client's sensory function is altered, the ability to relate to and function within the environment changes drastically.

Many clients enter the health care system with preexisting sensory alterations. However, many blind, deaf, or paralyzed clients who have partial or complete loss of a major sensory modality have found alternative ways to function safely within the environment. The nurse should support the client's attempts to adapt to sensory loss and should also control stimuli within the health care environment that may interfere with that adaptation.

A client may also enter the health care setting with normal sensory function. However, a health care setting is often a place of unfamiliar sights, sounds, and smells and minimal contact with family or friends. If a client feels depersonalized and is unable to receive meaningful stimuli, serious sensory alterations can develop.

The nurse's role is to understand and help meet the needs of clients with sensory alterations, as well as to recognize clients most at risk for developing sensory problems. The world can be a frightening place for a client with impaired sensory perception. The nurse should guide the client through the barriers created by sensory alterations and help the client find a meaningful and functional way to live.

Components of Normal Sensation

The nervous system continually receives thousands of bits of information from sensory nerve organs, relays the information through appropriate channels, and integrates the information into a meaningful response. Sensory stimuli reach the sensory organs and can elicit an immediate reaction or present information to the brain to be stored for future use. The nervous system must be intact for sensory stimuli to reach appropriate brain centers and for the individual to perceive the sensation. After interpreting the significance of a given sensation, the person can then react to the stimulus.

Reception, perception, and reaction are the three components of any sensory experience (see Chapter 37). Reception begins with stimulation of a nerve cell called a receptor. For example, the retina of the eye receives light waves, the cochlea of the ear receives sound waves, and the surface of the skin receives sensations from the pressure of tactile stimulation. The body's sensory receptors are usually specifically designed for only one type of stimulus. Only pain receptors are capable of receiving several forms of stimuli, such as pressure, chemicals, or heat. With stimulation of receptors, nerve impulses travel along pathways either to the spinal cord or directly to the brain. For example, light waves stimulate receptors within the retina of the eye, which cause impulses to travel along the optic nerve directly to the occipital lobe of the brain. The movement of a body part stimulates proprioceptors to send impulses along peripheral spinal nerves to the spinal cord. From the spinal cord a second set of nerve fibers, conducting the sensation of position, travel up the cord, cross over at the medulla, and travel to the thalamus. At the thalamus impulses synapse with a third pathway to eventually be sent to the cerebral cortex. Sensory nerve pathways usually cross over to send stimuli to opposite sides of the brain. For example, if a person touches an object with the right hand, the left side of the brain receives the stimulus.

The nerve cells that transmit impulses are very similar in appearance. Impulses travel over all sensory nerves in much the same fashion. The actual perception or awareness of unique sensations thus depends on the region of the cerebral cortex that receives the impulses. Impulses to one region result in a visual image, for example, whereas those to another result in hearing a sound. Specialized brain cells interpret the quality and nature of stimuli. When the person becomes conscious of the sensory stimuli, perception takes place. The person is then a recipient of information about the world.

Perception, however, requires more than just an awareness of stimuli. Perception depends on experience. Multiple stimuli must be organized and integrated to provide meaning. An infant slowly learns to associate meaning with visual images, sounds, and unfamiliar sensations. As a person grows older, a variety of experiences allow the interpretation of numerous sensory stimuli. If sensation is incomplete or if past experience is inadequate for understanding what really is occurring, a person can become confused. The proper perception of time, place, and person is essential for individuals to react appropriately to their environment.

Multiple stimuli constantly bombard the senses. It is impossible to react to each stimulus that enters the nervous system. For example, the professional nurse must concentrate on skills needed to insert an intravenous needle safely and effectively. Auditory stimuli within a client's room such as the television, a noisy suction machine, or the sounds of a stretcher passing by, as well as visual stimuli such as sunlight through the window, a visitor's colorful clothing, or the movement of the client's roommate, could easily distract the nurse from the task at hand. The brain is normally capable of discarding or storing sensory information to prevent sensory bombardment. A person will usually react to stimuli that are most meaningful or significant at the time. After continued reception of the same stimulus, however, a person stops responding and the sensory experience goes unnoticed. For example, a person reading a good novel is not aware of the pressure of resting his body against a pillow. This adaptability phenomenon occurs with most sensory stimuli except for those of pain.

The balance between sensory stimuli entering the brain and those that actually reach the conscious awareness maintains a person's well-being. If an individual attempts to react to every stimulus within the environment or if a variety and quality of stimuli are lacking, sensory alterations will occur.

Types of Sensory Alterations

Three different types of sensory alterations are commonly seen by the nurse: sensory deficits, sensory deprivation, and sensory overload. When a client suffers from more than one sensory alteration, his ability to function and relate effectively within the environment is seriously impaired.

Sensory Deficits

A defect in the normal function of sensory reception and perception is a sensory deficit. A client may no longer be able to receive certain stimuli (for example, the client may be blind or deaf), or stimuli become distorted (for example, the client may have cataracts or be confused). When a deficit develops gradually or when considerable time has passed since the onset of an acute sensory loss, the person learns to rely on unaffected senses. Certain senses may even become more acute to compensate for an alteration. For example, a blind client often develops an acute sense of hearing.

Clients with sensory deficits may change their behaviors in adaptive or maladaptive ways. For example, one client with a hearing impairment may cup his hand around the affected ear or turn the unaffected ear toward a speaker in order to hear better, whereas another client may shun other people to avoid the embarrassment of not being able to understand their speech.

TABLE 44-1

Effects of Sensory Deprivation

Type of Alteration	Associated Symptoms
Cognitive	Reduced capacity to learn, inability to solve problems, poor task performance
Affective	Boredom, restlessness, increased anxiety, emotional lability, increased need for physical stimulation and socialization
Perceptual	Reduced attention span, disorganized visual and motor coordination, temporary loss of color perception, disorientation, confusion of sleeping and waking states

Sensory Deprivation

Sensory stimulation must be of sufficient quality and quantity to maintain a person's awareness. When a person receives an inadequate quality or quantity of stimulation so perception is impaired, sensory deprivation occurs. Three types of sensory deprivation (Ebersole and Hess, 1981) are reduced sensory input (as in clients with sensory deficits), elimination of order or meaning from input (as in clients exposed to a strange, unfamiliar environment), and restriction of the environment that produces monotony and boredom (as in a client confined to bed rest or an isolation room).

The effects of sensory deprivation can be far reaching. Table 44-1 summarizes the cognitive, affective, and perceptual changes a client with deprivation may undergo. The symptoms associated with sensory deprivation can easily confuse nurses or physicians, causing them to believe a client is psychologically ill, senile, suffering from severe electrolyte imbalance, or perhaps under the influence of psychotropic drugs. Therefore the nurse must always remain aware of the client's existing sensory function and the quality of stimuli within the environment.

Sensory Overload

When a person receives multiple sensory stimuli and cannot perceptually disregard or selectively ignore some stimuli, sensory overload occurs. Excessive stimulation of the senses leads to a state in which the brain cannot meaningfully respond to or ignore certain stimuli. Because of the multitude of stimuli lead-

ing to overload, the person no longer perceives the environment in a way that makes sense. Overload thus results in a state similar to that produced by sensory deprivation.

The client who is acutely ill is a good example of one who may fall victim to sensory overload. The constant pain resulting from the disease process, the insertion of needles for blood samples, the nurse's frequent monitoring of vital signs, and the irritation from drainage tubes protruding from the client's body all combine to cause overload. Even if the nurse offers a comforting word or provides a gentle backrub, the client may not benefit because his attention and energy are focused on more stressful stimuli.

Sensory overload differs from deprivation in that the level of stimuli that can cause the condition depends more on individual factors. The point at which stimuli needed for healthy function become enough to tax a person's endurance changes according to the person's level of fatigue, attitude, or emotional and physical well-being. With sensory overload, the person's thoughts begin to race, his attention moves in many directions, and he finds it difficult to remain still. Continued overload can cause the person eventually to develop many of the same symptoms as those associated with sensory deprivation.

Factors Influencing Sensory Function

The sensations a person is capable of receiving or perceiving depend on a number of factors. The nurse's knowledge of these factors influences ways of applying the nursing process to the client's needs.

AGE

An infant possesses all of the special senses at birth; however, the ability to discriminate sensory stimuli is lacking. Nerve pathways have not matured within the cerebral cortex to allow an infant to integrate and process sensory information.

After a person reaches adulthood, sensory acuity declines. By the fourth decade, presbyopia is common. This condition involves a decrease in the eye's ability to focus on near objects for close and detailed work. It also becomes more difficult for persons to adapt their vision in dim light and darkness. By 60 years of age a person needs twice as much light to see objects as was required at the age of 20. Most individuals between the ages of 40 and 50 need glasses for reading and accommodation (adjustment of eyes for near vision) because of degenerative changes in the lens. A cataract, or opacity of the lens, is a common change occurring after the fifth decade of life. Cataracts cause an increased sensitivity to glare. Other visual changes that occur with aging include reductions in the person's field of vision and in lacrimal secretions. An adult over the age of 60 has reduced peripheral visual fields. Thus it is difficult for the person to see fast-moving objects to the side. The reduction in lacrimation causes eyes to take on a lackluster appearance, and a person will experience the sensation of dry, scratchy eyes.

Changes in hearing acuity occur more subtly. By the age of 30, a person may begin to notice deficiencies in hearing acuity, speech intelligibility, discrimination of pitch, and hearing threshold, especially within normal speech frequencies. After the age of 60 it becomes difficult to hear high-pitched and sibilant consonants; for example, "s," "sh," and "ch" are difficult to differentiate. An elderly person is better able to hear low-pitched vowels. Another hearing problem accompanying aging is difficulty in hearing conversation over background noise. Loud music or a paging system in a hospital will mask the conversation an older adult is attempting to hear.

Taste and smell tend to decline together, partly because of their close association. Taste buds atrophy in later years, causing a reduction in taste acuity. Olfactory nerve fibers decrease by the age of 50. Elderly people can still tell the difference between the basic tastes, but it is common to see an older adult use heavy seasoning on foods or add extra sugar to coffee and tea. The elderly also experience a decreased sensitivity to odors (such as a smoldering cigarette) and have difficulty discriminating between them.

Normally a person begins to lose proprioceptive sensation after the age of 60. Without the ability to sense position in space, a person has difficulty with balance, spatial orientation, and coordination. The elderly become accident prone. The reflexive response of bracing oneself from falling and the ability to move around obstacles become slower.

Other sensory changes that accompany aging are reductions in sensitivity to pain, touch, and heat and cold. Conditions that are normally painful, such as appendicitis or a myocardial infarction, may be sensed only as minor discomforts. An inability to perceive pain is obviously dangerous. If an elderly person is unable to perceive extremes in temperature, tissue injury can easily occur during bathing or use of a heating pad. When the individual is confined to bed, the sensation of pressure on bony prominences may go unnoticed, leading to formation of a decubitus ulcer.

MEDICATIONS

Certain types of medications can impair sensory acuity. Antibiotics such as vancomycin, streptomycin, neomycin, and gentamicin can cause permanent damage to the auditory nerve. The antibiotic chloramphenicol has been found to cause irritation of the optic nerve and blindness in some cases.

Narcotic analgesics, sedatives, and antidepressant medications can alter the perception of stimuli. Clients receiving such drugs may become lethargic, drowsy, and less capable of responding to sensory stimuli.

ENVIRONMENT

Sensory stimuli originate from a person's environment. When stimuli from the environment are excessive, infrequent, or nonstimulating, sensory alterations develop.

Clients in an intensive care unit frequently experience numerous sources of stimuli. The number of staff members, the noise of machines, the constant lighting, and the physical discomforts associated with numerous procedures create an environment of sensory overload. Frequently clients within an intensive care unit receive medications that alter the brain's perception of stimuli. Nurses often must interrupt the client's sleep to conduct physical assessments. Also, the customary sights, smells, and sounds of everyday routines are disrupted, and soon the client becomes confused, disoriented, and incapable of decision making. A client who lives alone and who suddenly enters a hospital is at risk for sensory overload because of the significant change in the quantity of sensory stimulation.

Often, however, a client becomes isolated as a result of illness or therapy. When placed under protective asepsis precautions, a client is confined to a room and interacts only with family or staff who are hidden behind gowns, masks, and gloves. Clients immobilized in bed as a result of illness or therapy are also at risk for sensory deprivation. For example, a client may be forced to remain in traction for several weeks or may be restricted to bed because of a debilitating illness. Such a client is unable to experience the normal sensations of rising from bed, sitting up to eat, or having the luxury of taking a refreshing shower.

For certain clients the home living environment provides little meaningful stimulation. The elderly who live alone or are confined to their home or a nursing home are not always able to enjoy the stimulation of socialization with other people. Many nursing homes present drab, unpleasant surroundings, and frequently the care givers are unaware of the residents' sensory problems. This is not to say that all nursing homes ignore the elderly's needs for sensory stimulation. Many agencies consider the elderly's sensory problems and design and construct facilities to provide stimulation.

PREEXISTING ILLNESSES

Various forms of illness can directly or indirectly lead to sensory impairment. Peripheral vascular disease, frequently associated with arteriosclerosis and diabetes mellitus, can cause reduced sensation in the extremities as well as changes in mental function because of impaired blood flow to the extremities and brain. The vascular changes occurring in chronic diabetes can lead to reduced vision or blindness. A cerebrovascular accident or stroke resulting from a clot or hemorrhage in blood vessels within the brain frequently produces loss of speech (aphasia). Also, clients suffering from malignancy of the larynx are often treated by surgical removal of the larynx, which causes a loss of the ability to speak normally. A number of neurological diseases or injuries cause paralysis and loss of sensation in affected body parts.

SMOKING

The chronic use of cigarettes, cigars, or pipes can lead to atrophy of the taste buds. A client can still discriminate between tastes, but perception of flavors is not as acute.

NOISE LEVELS

The constant exposure to high levels of noise predisposes people to hearing loss. Airplane traffic controllers on the ground, construction workers using air-hammers, and industrial workers on a noisy assembly line are examples of people who should wear protective ear covers. Since the advent of loud rock and roll music in the 1950s, band musicians and their audiences are also at risk for hearing loss because of the music's high sound levels.

ENDOTRACHEAL INTUBATION

Clients critically ill as a result of serious respiratory disorders or conditions influencing the body's ability to provide needed oxygen often require an artificial airway (see Chapter 42). However, an endotracheal tube, inserted through the mouth or nose into the trachea, prohibits a client from speaking. This temporary loss of speech can be a frightening experience because the client loses one of the primary ways of relating to the environment. Frequently family members react as though the client were also deaf, speaking loudly in their frustration at being unable to communicate. Without an effective means of communication the client can become highly anxious, which can add to sensory overload.

Assessment

When assessing clients with existing sensory alterations and clients at risk for sensory problems, the nurse considers all of the factors just described. The client's age significantly affects the assessment of the normal sensory level and the extent to which a sensory alteration may be a health problem.

For clients with sensory deficits the nurse must assess the degree to which any impairment influences the client's life-style and ability to relate to the en-

---

TABLE 44-2

Assessing Sensory Function

Sense	Assessment
Vision	Ask the client to read a newspaper, a magazine, or lettering on a menu.
	Measure visual acuity with a Snellen chart.
	Assess pupil size, shape, equality, and reaction to light.
	Assess visual fields.
Hearing	Test the client's ability to hear a watch ticking or a softly spoken word.
	Compare the client's ability to recognize consonants with ability to distinguish vowels.
	Talk to the client while facing him and then while turned away to determine if the client reads lips.
Touch	Check for sensitivity to light touch by using a cotton swab.
	Assess ability to discriminate between sharp and dull stimuli with use of a safety pin.
	Determine if the client can distinguish objects (dime, penny, quarter) in his hand with his eyes closed.
Smell	Have the client close his eyes and identify several nonirritating odors (e.g., coffee or mustard).
Taste	Ask client to sample and distinguish different tastes (lemon, sugar, etc.). (Have the client drink a sip of water and wait 1 minute between each taste.)
Position sense	Ask the client to close his eyes. Grasp the client's finger while supporting the hand and move the finger up, down, and level with the hand. Ask the client to identify the position of the finger.

TABLE 44-3

Behaviors Indicating Sensory Deficits in Children and Adults

Altered Sense	Behaviors in Children	Behaviors in Adults
Vision	Self-stimulation: eye rubbing, body rocking, sniffing or smelling, arm twirling; hitches (uses legs to propel while in sitting position) instead of crawls	Poor coordination; squinting; underreaching or overreaching for objects; uncontrolled eye movements; persistent repositioning of objects
Hearing	Frightened when unfamiliar people approach; no reflex or purposeful response to sounds; failure to be awakened by loud noise; slow or absent development of speech; greater response to movement than to sound; avoidance of social interaction with other children	Blank looks; decreased attention span; lack of reaction to loud noises; increased volume of speech; positioning of head toward sound; smiling and nodding head in approval when someone speaks
Touch	—	Clumsiness; overreaction or underreaction to painful stimulus; failure to respond when touched; avoidance of touch
Taste	—	Change in appetite; excessive use of seasoning and sugar; complaints about taste of food
Smell	—	Failure to react to noxious or strong odor; increase in body odor

vironment. The extent of any sensory problem may be related to the environment in which the client lives, or is restricted to because of illness. Thus, the nurse's assessment must focus on the quality and quantity of stimuli within the client's environment.

Physical Assessment

To identify the presence of sensory deficits the nurse should perform a detailed assessment of the client's vision, hearing, olfaction, sense of taste, and ability to discriminate light touch, temperature, pain, and position (see Chapter 29). Table 44-2 summarizes useful assessment techniques for identifying sensory deficits. As the nurse performs the various measures of care, the client may exhibit certain behaviors indicating specific sensory alterations (Table 44-3).

A neurological assessment of the client's level of consciousness, orientation, and cognitive thought processes helps to reveal symptoms of sensory deprivation or overload. An assessment of neurological functioning can also reveal the client's level of perception. Of course, factors other than sensory deprivation or overload may cause impaired perception, for example, medications, pain, or reduced oxygenation.

Ability to Perform Self-Care

A client with sensory or perceptual alterations is often unable to perform the activities of daily living. The nurse must assess the client's ability to feed, dress, groom, and perform toileting activities. The nurse asks questions to determine the client's abilities: Can the client with altered vision find items on a meal tray? Can the client with diminished touch button a shirt or dress? If the client seems sensorially deprived, does he concern himself with grooming? Does a client's loss of balance prevent him from rising from a toilet seat safely? Any impairment in the ability to perform self-care has implications for the nurse in planning the client's discharge from an acute care setting and in providing resources within the home.

Environment

The nurse should assess the quality and quantity of stimuli within the client's environment. In the home setting of an aged client, the nurse should determine whether potentially meaningful sources of stimuli are present such as pet animals, a record player, television set, or photographs of family members. The nurse observes whether the client's environment is pleasant, characterized by bright colors, good ventilation, clean surroundings, and comfortable furnishings. Drab, dirty, poorly lit surroundings can be conducive to sensory deprivation. On the other hand, if the client's home is noisy because of neighbors, traffic, or other continual environmental noises, sensory overload is a potential problem.

With infants or young children, the nurse should assess the types of toys available. Does the infant's play area or crib have toys of different sizes, shapes, and colors? Is the play area clean, pleasantly lit, and decorated attractively?

When the nurse assesses the hospital or health care environment, it is important to observe the room environment. Is the client in a private or semiprivate room? If semiprivate, is there a roommate who constantly watches television, has frequent visitors, or persistently attempts to converse and prevents the client from resting? Is the client's room located near sources of noise such as the nurses' station, an elevator, or a door leading to stairs? If the client is in protective isolation, does the room include any sources of stimulation such as a window, pictures on the wall, or a television? The client may be confined to a hospital room for several days or even weeks. The presence or absence of meaningful stimuli will have a predictable influence on the client's alertness and ability to participate in care.

A factor to assess within the acute care setting is the level of care the client requires. The nurse should assess the frequency of observations and procedures performed on the client. It may be possible to control the number of procedures in order to minimize stress-producing stimuli. If the client is in pain, has multiple tubes and dressings, or is restricted by casts or traction, excessive stimulation can be a problem.

The nurse also should assess the safety of the environment for clients with sensory deficits. For a client with visual problems, for example, the room should not contain footstools or obstacles on the floor that are easy to stumble over while walking. In the home setting the nurse should look for throw rugs, torn carpets, or unlit stairways that can contribute to accidents.

Family and Significant Others

The amount of contact the client has with supportive family members or significant others can influence the degree of isolation he feels. The nurse should determine whether a client lives alone and whether family, friends, or neighbors frequently visit. The absence of visitors while a client is hospitalized can also have a significant impact on the client's sensory status. The ability to discuss fears or concerns with loved ones is an important coping mechanism for most people. The absence of meaningful conversation can also cause a person to become sensorially deprived.

Communication Methods

Clients with existing sensory deficits often must develop alternative ways of communicating. A deaf or hearing-impaired client may read lips, use sign language, or even communicate with written notes. The visually impaired often learn to read Braille. Clients who have undergone laryngectomies often write notes, use communication boards, speak with mechanical vibrators, or use esophageal speech. The nurse must understand the client's method of communication to interact with the client and promote the client's interaction with others.

The aphasic client may be unable to produce language or to understand it. Expressive aphasia, a motor type of aphasia, is the inability to name common objects or to express simple ideas in words or writing. Sensory or receptive aphasia, on the other hand, is an inability to understand written or spoken language. To determine the nature of the client's communication problem, the nurse should speak slowly in short, simple sentences. Clients can generally respond to simple questions requiring a yes or no answer by a nod or blink of the eye. The manner of the client's response will help to reveal the type of aphasia (Table 44-4).

Clients with endotracheal tubes have a temporary loss of speech. The nurse should observe the client's

---

TABLE 44-4

Communication Characteristics of Persons with Aphasia

Type of Aphasia	Characteristics of Language
Expressive	Slow, nonfluent speech produced with great effort; poor articulation; difficulty in spontaneous speech; poor naming of objects; depression or frustration stemming from knowledge of speech problem; ability to understand written and verbal speech
Receptive	Fluent speech with normal rhythm and articulation but incorrect use of words and sounds; difficulty in repeating words; poor naming of objects; inability to understand written or verbal speech; unawareness of deficit

TABLE 44-5

Examples of Nursing Diagnoses Related to Sensory Alterations

Problem	Causes
Sensory deficit	Related to: Visual alteration Hearing impairment Loss of tactile sense Aphasia
Sensory deprivation	Related to: Isolation for protective asepsis Nonstimulating home environment
Sensory overload	Related to: Pain Intensive care unit syndrome Frequent monitoring by nurse
Self-care deficit	Related to: Visual loss Loss of tactile sense Impaired balance
Actual or potential risk of injury	Related to: Visual loss Reduced hearing Reduced tactile and pain sensation Reduced olfaction
Impaired ability to communicate	Related to: Deafness Aphasia Endotracheal tube insertion

behavior to determine if the client has developed a sign language or system of symbols to communicate needs. Often the client will merely make a noise or shake the side rail of the bed to gain the nurse's attention.

Nursing Diagnosis

Nursing diagnoses of sensory alterations may involve a variety of nursing care problems (Table 44-5). When a client is unable to relate to or perceive the world normally, numerous nursing implications arise. The diagnosis of sensory deficit, deprivation, or overload should include the specific contributing factors. For example, when caring for clients in a health care setting who are experiencing sensory overload, interventions for controlling the pain that is contributing to the overload in one client will be quite different from those to control excess stimulation within an intensive care unit that is causing the problem in another. Problems related to sensory deficits may include risk of injury, self-care deficit, or communication alterations. The nurse can identify related problems by predicting the impact sensory alterations will have on the client's ability to function. Identifying the functional problems (for example, self-care deficit) may be more effective for the development of an individualized care plan than simply diagnosing "sensory deficit." A diagnosis of sensory deficit carries numerous implications for the client's care. The more specific the nurse's diagnosis with respect to factors influencing sensory deficits, the more effective will be the plan of care.

Planning

Because many sensory alterations have the potential for being long-term problems, the nurse's plan of care often must be based on appropriate goals to be achieved within the health care setting and at home. Involvement of family members is important. The family can provide meaningful stimulation to the client, as well as being a source of information for the nurse in understanding the client's needs within the home.

Goals for nursing care of clients with actual or potential sensory alterations include the following:

1. Promoting optimal function of existing senses
2. Controlling the environment to create meaningful sensory stimuli
3. Providing a safe environment
4. Preventing additional sensory loss
5. Promoting optimal effective communication
6. Promoting the client's ability to perform self-care

Implementation

Nursing interventions should focus on helping the client adapt to existing sensory alterations and on preventing conditions that may create sensory disturbances.

Promoting Function of Existing Senses

When clients have sensory deficits, the nurse should use interventions to maintain or stimulate existing function. This requires the nurse to assess remaining function and use techniques to promote continued function.

VISION

CHILDREN. The most common visual problem during childhood is a refractive error such as nearsightedness. The key to the child's care is early detection of visual impairment. The school nurse plays an important role in vision screening of school-age children and adolescents. Parents may need encouragement to pursue eye testing by an ophthalmologist.

ADULTS. With advancing age adults require more light to see objects. The nurse needs to teach the client the importance of increasing illumination and reducing glare. A high-intensity light focused on a newspaper will better enhance the client's ability to read than will increasing the intensity of light in a ceiling lamp. To minimize the effects of glare, clients may benefit from wearing sunglasses outside, especially while driving. In the home a common source of glare is a shiny waxed kitchen floor. This problem may be eliminated by simply washing and not waxing floors.

The aging adult also has reduction in peripheral vision. Therefore the client should be taught to make a habit of looking to the sides to see all objects. This is especially important if the client drives.

When visual ability is reduced, the nurse can offer clients special reading materials with large print.

HEARING

CHILDREN. Chronic middle ear infections are the most common cause of impaired hearing in children. Children with repeated incidents of ear infection should receive auditory testing. Parents must be warned of the risks and should seek medical care whenever the child has symptoms of earache or respiratory infection.

Children should be immunized against childhood diseases capable of causing hearing loss (rubella, mumps, and measles). When infections do develop, it is important that children not receive ototoxic medications.

ADULTS. A hearing loss can be embarrassing, and often clients with partial deficits are unwilling to admit that their hearing is impaired. The nurse must therefore use sensitivity and understanding when encouraging clients to seek evaluation for a hearing aid. Hearing aid companies are usually able to provide information regarding the appropriate aid for a client and the proper care and operation of their products. A client who has a hearing aid must understand how to clean the earpiece and keep the amplifier function-

ing. Mild soap and water are generally safe for cleaning earpieces. Habitually carrying an extra battery is a good idea.

TASTE

The nurse can easily promote the sense of taste by using measures to enhance remaining taste perception. Good oral hygiene keeps the taste buds well hydrated. Allowing secretions or coating of the tongue to build up will reduce taste perception.

Foods should be offered separately. Taste will be more distinctive if the client eats one type of food per mouthful.

Clients also enjoy foods that are well seasoned. However, the nurse should not permit excess use of salt or salt-containing products if the client is on a sodium-restricted diet.

Presenting food with different textures is beneficial. Most clients who can chew and swallow safely do not enjoy pureed foods or soft diets. Breakfast, for example, can consist of crunchy bacon, toasted bread, oatmeal, and a scrambled egg. All of these foods can be eaten easily even without teeth. If a client's perception of taste is improved, food intake and appetite will also improve.

TOUCH

Clients with reduced tactile sensation usually have the impairment only over a limited portion of their bodies. The nurse can stimulate existing function by providing touch therapy.

The nurse must be sure the client is willing to accept touch. A client can easily become anxious when not accustomed to being touched by another person. Hairbrushing and combing, backrubs, and touching on the arms or shoulders are ways of increasing tactile contact. When sensation is reduced, a firm pressure may be necessary when applying touch for the client to feel the nurse's hand. Turning and repositioning can also improve the quality of tactile sensation.

SMELL

If the nurse is assisting the client with eating or setting up a meal tray, identification of foods can help the client imagine the aromas of the food. The nurse should also encourage the client to smell food before eating. Recollection of aromas can often help enhance the sense of smell.

Controlling Environmental Stimulation

When a client's environment presents risks of overstimulation or understimulation of the senses, the nurse should attempt to provide meaningful stimuli or eliminate confusing or irritating stimuli, respec-

Suggestions for Introducing Environmental Stimuli

VISUAL

- Open the drapes to the client's room so outside sights can be seen.
- Raise the head of the bed and draw back any dividing curtains or partitions so the client can see a roommate or movement in the hallway.
- Provide attractive decorations on tables or cabinets, such as fresh flowers, plants, a picture, or greeting cards.
- Encourage family to enrich the client's home environment with clean curtains, familiar objects or keepsakes, and perhaps a fresh coat of paint on bedroom walls.

AUDITORY

- Sit down and speak with the client. Listen to the client's thoughts and experiences. Make the conversation meaningful.
- Turn on a radio with pleasant music of the type the *client* (not the nurse) enjoys. A favorite radio or television program can also be stimulating.

TASTE AND SMELL

- Provide attractive, taste-appealing meals. Be sure tableware and glasses are clean. Foods meant to be served warm should be warm and cold foods cold.
- Provide a variety of textures, aromas, and flavors to enhance the client's appetite.

TOUCH

- The same measures (therapeutic touch) that promote existing sensory function also prove useful in creating meaningful stimuli.

tively. When the client's diagnosis is sensory deprivation, the nurse should introduce meaningful stimuli for all the senses. It is important, however, to select stimuli the client prefers. The nurse should not force stimulation if the client is more concerned with basic functions such as comfort or being able to breathe with ease. The boxed material offers suggestions for increasing environmental stimulation.

REDUCING SENSORY OVERLOAD

When the client's problem is sensory overload, the nurse must control excessive stimuli. The client must have time for rest and freedom from stresses caused by frequent monitoring or repeated tests. Sitting quietly with the client often helps. Involvement in a non-demanding repetitive activity such as combing hair or brushing teeth may produce a feeling of security. When a client experiences stress in the home, meal planning or household chores can be helpful in providing distraction.

Many clients require reorientation to the environment, since sensory overload may distort perception. Name tags on uniforms help clients recognize nursing personnel and other staff. Orientation may also be provided through conversational cues such as, "This morning should be more pleasant," or "Can you believe it's June already?" Addressing the client by name orients him to self. If the client becomes confused about location or place, the nurse can simply remind him that he is in a hospital or at home with family. Often families become frightened by clients' confusion. The nurse can help the family learn not to argue with or contradict the client but to explain calmly where they are, who they are, and the time of day.

The nurse can have significant influence on sources of sensory overload by improving the plan for delivery of care. It may be possible to perform a number of activities, such as changing dressings, emptying urinary drainage bags, and checking vital signs, in one visit. The client becomes exhausted if the nurse enters the room every 10 or 15 minutes. Coordination with laboratory and radiology departments can reduce the amount of time needed for tests and examinations. In the intensive care unit nurses frequently "over-nurse" because of their concern with monitoring the client closely. Anticipating the client's actual needs will help reduce unnecessary stimulation.

In the hospital environment the nurse can try to control extraneous sources of noise. It may be necessary to ask a roommate to reduce the volume of a television set. The nurse may choose to move the client to a quieter room. Nurses themselves should control laughter or conversation so clients with rooms near the nurses' station can gain needed rest and sleep.

Providing a Safe Environment

Clients with existing sensory loss are susceptible to injury and require protective measures. In contrast, clients with normal sensory function but at risk for sensory loss require education about precautions against sensory impairment. The nature of the client's actual or potential sensory loss determines the safety precautions taken.

VISUAL LOSS

The client with recent visual impairment often requires assistance with ambulation. The nurse should stand at the client's nondominant side approximately one step in front of the client (Fig. 44-1). The client

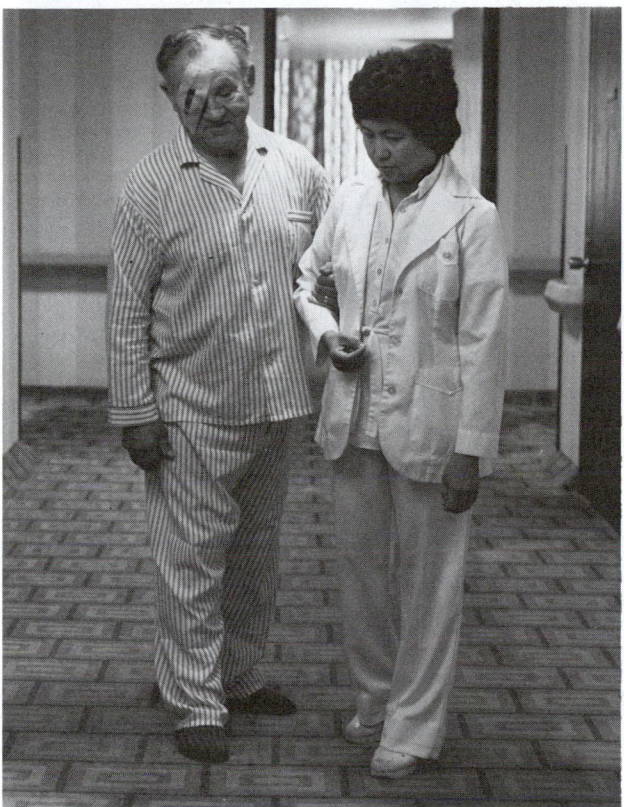

Fig. 44-1 A nurse assists in the ambulation of a client wearing an eye patch.

can use the nondominant hand to grasp the nurse's upper arm. As the nurse and client begin ambulation, the nurse should describe the course of movement, such as, "We are going to make a right turn," or "The hallway is narrow so I will be just in front of you." The client can reach forward with the dominant hand to feel for any barriers or landmarks. The nurse should not allow a client with serious visual impairment to walk in front. Before ambulating a client, the nurse should be sure to remove obstacles such as footstools or chairs.

A client with visual impairment should have necessary objects within safe reach. If the client spends considerable time in bed, a call light should be close by. Toiletry items, Kleenex, or a water pitcher should be placed in front of the client to prevent accidental falls as a result of the client needing to reach over the bedside. Side rails are also important in this regard.

If the client has reduced peripheral vision and difficulty driving in darkness, the nurse should emphasize precautions such as looking to both sides before passing cars or while turning a corner and driving only during the day.

When depth perception and visual acuity are poor, the client has difficulty judging distances. This is a problem even during simple activities such as walking up or down steps. In the home setting it is useful to paint the edges of stairs a bright color. The client is better able to see the stairs and does not stumble.

HEARING LOSS

The client with a hearing loss may be unable to hear sounds of danger. Nurses often rely on clients to report unusual sounds, such as a suction apparatus running improperly or an intravenous pump alarm sounding. However, the client with a hearing loss may not hear such sounds and thus requires more frequent visits by the nurse. The client can also benefit from learning to use the sense of vision to discover sources of danger.

In the home a telephone is a valuable piece of equipment. But if the client cannot hear the phone's ring, family members may be unable to reach the client during emergencies. The phone company can attach a light to the phone that flashes when it rings. Family members should be taught to let the phone ring for a longer period when calling a client with a hearing impairment.

REDUCED OLFACTION

A reduced sensitivity to odors can be dangerous. The client may be unable to detect odors such as leaking gas, a smoldering cigarette or fire, or tainted food. The client should learn to use alternative precautions such as checking ashtrays, placing cigarette butts in water, or observing the color and consistency of leftover foods. Smoke detectors are invaluable for such a client.

REDUCED TACTILE SENSATION

Clients with reduced tactile sensation are at risk for injury when their condition confines them to bed, since they are unable to sense pressure on bony prominences or the need to change position. These clients will need to rely on nurses for timely repositioning and turning.

When a client's ability to sense temperature variations is reduced, the nurse should use extra caution in applying heat and cold therapies (see Chapter 49). The nurse should check the condition of the client's skin frequently to avoid causing burns and tissue injury.

SPEECH ALTERATIONS

A client lacking the ability to speak cannot call out for assistance. Aphasic clients or those with a laryngectomy or endotracheal intubation need an alternative means of communication. In the health care agency a call light should always be close by. For the client at home a small bell at the bedside is helpful.

Communicating with a Deaf or Hearing-Impaired Client

- Get the client's attention. Do not startle him when entering a room. Be sure the client knows you wish to speak.
- Face the client. Be sure your face and lips are illuminated.
- If the client wears glasses, be sure they are clean so he can see your gestures and face.
- Speak slowly and articulate clearly. Use normal tones of voice and inflections of speech.
- Restate with different words when you are not understood.
- Do not shout. Loud sounds are usually of a higher pitch. If it is necessary to raise your voice, speak in lower tones.
- Talk toward the client's best or normal ear.
- Use gestures to enhance the spoken word.

Communicating with an Aphasic Client

- Ask questions the client can answer with a simple yes or no, a nod, or blinking of the eyes.
- Give the client time to understand.
- Talk as though the client does understand.
- Discuss familiar subjects.
- Try not to talk too loud.
- Allow only one person to talk at a time.
- Use visual cues such as pictures, objects, or gestures to accompany words.

Preventing Sensory Loss

Occupation or life-style may place a person at risk for sensory loss. Persons who work around loud noises need to learn of potential dangers to hearing function. Protective ear covers are essential if exposure to loud sound is continuous. Ringing of the ears is an early sign of hearing impairment.

Clients exposed to dangerous chemicals or small flying objects should wear eye goggles for protection. A chemical burn to the cornea or a penetrating eye injury can cause permanent blindness. Children should be discouraged from playing with any kind of sharp object, since it is not uncommon for a child to be blinded accidentally by a playmate.

Promoting Communication

A sensory deficit can cause a person to feel isolated because of inability to communicate with others. The nature of the sensory loss will influence the methods and styles of communication nurses can use with clients. The methods described in the following sections can be taught to the client's family members and significant others.

HEARING IMPAIRMENT

The hearing-impaired client may be able to speak normally. However, if deafness is present, the client's inability to hear his own words may cause serious speech alterations. A child born deaf is not able to speak at all. Clients may use sign language or write

with a pad and pencil. If sign language is difficult for the nurse to learn, use of a pad and pencil is appropriate. The nurse should not rush a client to communicate and should show interest in his ideas and opinions. The box contains suggestions for communication with hearing-impaired clients.

APHASIA

Depending on the type of aphasia, the client's inability to communicate can be frustrating and frightening. The communication a nurse establishes initially should be very basic. The nurse must recognize that aphasia does not mean that the client is intellectually impaired or has a degeneration of personality. The boxed material gives suggestions for communicating with aphasic clients.

The aphasic client often benefits from using a communication board. The board may include pictures reflecting the client's basic needs, such as a toilet, a glass of water, food, or the body in pain. The nurse shows the board to the client and asks the client to point to his needs. Commercially made communication boards are available.

LARYNGECTOMY OR INTUBATION

When a client is not able to speak because of a laryngectomy or intubation, the nurse can provide either a communication board or a pad and pencil for writing. The nurse should position the client comfortably so writing is not difficult. The client should not be rushed, since he may suddenly stop writing or refuse to communicate ideas if he feels pressured.

FAMILY COMMUNICATION WITH CLIENTS

The family can create serious obstacles for clients with communication barriers. Often a family member will try to speak for a client rather than giving the client a chance to express himself. The nurse must explain the importance of allowing clients time to communicate. The nurse should also share with the family the techniques the nurse uses to promote communication.

Promoting Self-Care

The ability to perform self-care is essential for a client's self-esteem. Frequently family members or nurses believe that the sensorially impaired person requires assistance, when in fact the person can help himself. The following are some useful guidelines to assist clients with visual or tactile impairment when they require help with activities of daily living.

FEEDING

A meal tray can be set up as though food on the tray and condiments or drinks around the tray were numbers on the face of a clock. The client can easily orient himself to the items after the nurse explains each item's location. For example, the nurse can say, "Mr. Ray, your potatoes are at 9 o'clock, the meatloaf is at 6 o'clock, and the corn is at 1 o'clock. I placed your coffee on the right side at 3 o'clock. Your ice cream is on the far left at 9 o'clock." With this orientation most visually impaired clients can feed themselves.

DRESSING

If a client's tactile sense is diminished, it may be difficult to grasp objects. Buttons on clothing can be replaced with zippers or Velcro strips. Sweaters or blouses that slip over the head are easy to put on. Pants with elastic waists are also convenient. If a client has partial paralysis in addition to reduced sensation, it is always better to dress the affected side first. For example, if the right arm is paralyzed, the sleeve of a blouse is placed over the right arm first, followed by the left.

GROOMING

When a client is seriously visually impaired, it often becomes a family member's responsibility to select colors and styles of garments. Family members should be encouraged to select the type of clothing the client prefers. Any sensory impairment has a significant influence on a client's body image, and it is important for the client to feel well groomed and attractive. The nurse should offer assistance if needed in brushing, combing, and shampooing of hair.

TOILET

The client with visual problems needs assistance in reaching toilet facilities safely. Toilet paper should be within easy reach. When the nurse leaves the client alone in the bathroom, the call light cord should be close by.

Clients with proprioceptive problems may lose their balance when attempting to use the toilet. The nurse's supervision with ambulation and sitting is essential. The client still can have privacy when using toilet facilities, but the nurse should make frequent checks to prevent falls. Clients should be cautioned against leaning forward, which can cause a loss of balance.

Evaluation

The overall goal of nursing interventions is to provide the client with as normal a sensory environment as possible. The nurse attempts to maintain existing sensory function, in addition to promoting normal sensory reception, perception, and reaction to the environment.

Interventions designed to promote optimal function of existing senses can be evaluated on the basis of the following:
1. The client's ability to read without glare or blurred vision
2. The client's mastery of techniques for checking his peripheral field of vision
3. Parents' understanding of the importance of auditory and visual screening for children
4. The client's maintenance of appetite and adequate food intake
5. The client's ability to relax during touch therapy

Manipulation of the client's environment for the purpose of creating meaningful sensory stimuli is evaluated on the basis of these criteria:
1. Absence of signs or symptoms of sensory deprivation or overload
2. The client's alertness to stimuli and orientation to name, date, and place

The nurse's efforts at promoting a safe environment can be evaluated on these bases:
1. The client's ability to ambulate and climb stairs without fall or an injury
2. The client's understanding of the use of vision to detect sources of danger when hearing or olfaction is impaired
3. Absence of skin breakdown in a client with reduced tactile sensation

The prevention of sensory loss can best be evaluated by judging the client's ability to identify potential risks to visual and auditory function within the home and work setting.

The variety of interventions designed to maintain the client's ability to communicate effectively can be evaluated on the basis of:

1. The hearing-impaired client's ability to comprehend the nurse's messages
2. The hearing-impaired client's willingness to use alternative communication techniques
3. The nurse's and family's identification and meeting of the aphasic client's needs and concerns
4. The willingness of a client with a laryngectomy or intubation to use alternative communication techniques

Summary

The client with sensory alterations often faces a lonely and frightening world. Inability to interact effectively with the environment leads to a loss of security and self-esteem. A healthy balance between incoming sensory stimuli and those to which the person is able to respond is necessary for the person's well-being.

Nurses work with a variety of clients who have actual or potential sensory alterations. Specific physiological changes can create sensory deficits. Exposure to excessive environmental stimulation causes sensory overload. Isolation within an environment devoid of meaningful stimulation causes sensory deprivation. The nature of any sensory change influences the choice of nursing interventions.

The nurse promotes the sensorially deprived client's ability to maintain normal function with existing sensory deficits. Likewise, the nurse attempts to make changes within the environment to provide meaningful stimulation for clients. Sensory changes can affect various aspects of a client's life-style. The nurse uses creative intervention to help clients interact effectively with their world.

KEY CONCEPTS

✓ Sensory reception involves the stimulation of sensory nerve fibers and the transmission of impulses to higher centers within the brain.

✓ Sensory perception involves the organization and integration of sensory information into meaning and conscious awareness.

✓ The brain normally discards or stores sensory information to prevent sensory bombardment.

✓ Since a person learns to rely on unaffected senses after experiencing a sensory loss, the nurse designs interventions to preserve function of these senses.

✓ Sensory deprivation results from an inadequate quality or quantity of sensory stimuli.

✓ Sensory overload differs from sensory deprivation in that the level of stimuli needed to cause overload depends more on the individual.

✓ Aging results in a gradual decline of acuity in all senses.

✓ An intensive care unit places a client at risk for sensory overload.

✓ The isolated confined environment of a client in protective asepsis contributes to sensory deprivation.

✓ The sensorially impaired client exhibits certain behaviors specific to the type of sensory loss.

✓ Within the home a client requires meaningful stimuli to maintain perception and alertness.

✓ The extent of support from family members or significant others can influence the quality of sensory experiences.

KEY CONCEPTS, cont'd

✓ Clients with existing sensory deficits can learn alternative ways to communicate.

✓ Providing optimal illumination of objects and eliminating sources of glare are ways to improve the visual acuity of older adults.

✓ Since clients with hearing loss may be unwilling to admit their deficit because of embarrassment, nursing interventions are required to maintain communication.

✓ Providing oral hygiene and offering foods with a variety of textures and tastes can enhance a client's appetite.

✓ Clients with limited tactile sensation are at risk for skin breakdown because of their inability to sense pressure on bony prominences.

✓ To prevent sensory overload the nurse controls stimuli, orients the client to the environment, and provides care with a minimum of interruptions.

✓ To improve communication with the hearing impaired, the nurse speaks clearly, avoids shouting, and makes sure the client can see facial and lip movements.

✓ Clients with laryngectomy or endotracheal intubation can communicate effectively with communication boards and written messages.

REFERENCE

Ebersole, P., and Hess, P.: Toward healthy aging, St. Louis, 1981, The C.V. Mosby Co.

ADDITIONAL READINGS

Adair, M., and Simonson, J.: Communicative problems in older persons. In Jacobs, B., editor: Working with the impaired elderly, New York, 1976, National Senior Center Foundation.

Aranosian, R.D.: Dealing with the deaf, Emergency Med. 15:29, 1983.

Blanco, K.M.: The aphasic patient, J. Neurosurg. Nurs. 14:34, 1982.

Downs, F.S.: Bedrest and sensory disturbances, Am. J. Nurs. 74:435, 1974.

Kopac, C.A.: Sensory loss in the aged: the role of the nurse and the family, Nurs. Clin. North Am. 18:373, 1983.

Perron, D.M.: Deprived of sound, Am. J. Nurs. 74:1057, 1974.

Whaley, L.F., and Wong, D.L.: Nursing care of infants and children, ed. 2, St. Louis, 1983, The C.V. Mosby Co.

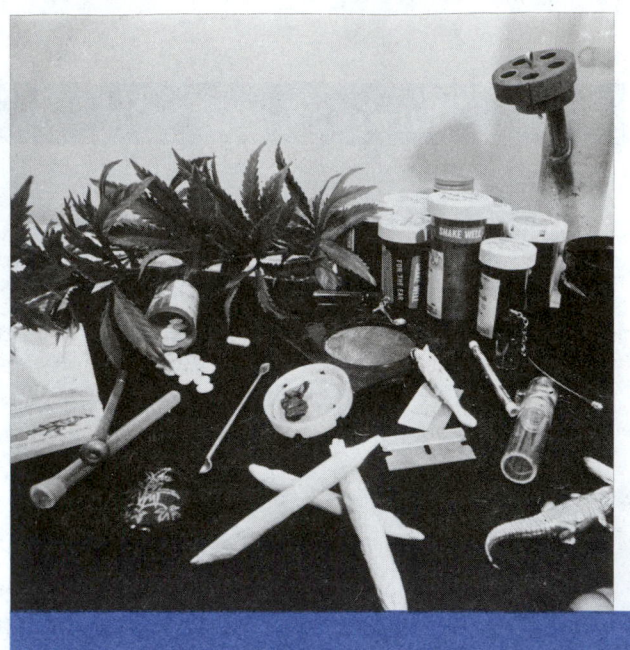

OBJECTIVES

Mastery of the content in this chapter will allow the student to:

- Define the terms in the glossary.
- Discuss the general health risks related to the abuse of any substance.
- Compare and contrast physiological and psychological dependence.
- List nine major groups of drugs and substances and discuss their major effects.
- Describe several psychosocial causative variables in substance abuse.
- Describe the typical course of substance abuse.
- State at least three special groups particularly at risk for substance abuse.
- Describe the nurse's responsibility if a colleague may be abusing a substance.
- Describe special assessment approaches for clients with substance abuse problems.
- List three or more examples of nursing diagnoses related to substance abuse.
- List and discuss five general types of interventions appropriate for substance abusers.
- Describe major characteristics of the evaluation process for nursing care of substance abusers.

GLOSSARY

abuse Indiscriminate chronic or acute use of a drug or other substance such that physiological or psychosocial functioning is impaired.

CNS sympathomimetic Drug, such as cocaine and amphetamines, whose effects mimic the effects of sympathetic nervous system stimulation.

escape mechanism Behavioral response by which a person consciously or unconsciously attempts to avoid a problem or stressor.

fetal alcohol syndrome Fetal abnormalities associated with heavy alcohol consumption by the pregnant woman.

hallucinogens Drugs such as LSD and PCP that cause excitation of the central nervous system, including hallucinations, sensory distortions, and other effects.

inhalants Substances abused by inhalation because of their depressant effects on the central nervous system.

misuse Indiscriminate use of a drug or substance but to a lesser extent than with chronic abuse and dependence.

physiological dependence Condition in which the body is so accustomed to a drug or substance that functioning is impaired without it.

45 Substance Abuse and Dependence

psychological dependence   Chronic emotional or psychological reliance on a drug or substance such that the person feels unable to handle stress without it.

psychotomimetic   Drug or substance whose effects mimic the symptoms of psychosis, such as hallucinations.

sedative-hypnotics   Drugs, such as barbiturates, that depress the central nervous system and produce a sense of euphoria or relaxation.

substance   Any drug, chemical, or biological entity; specifically, any material capable of being self-administered or abused because of its physiological or psychological effects.

withdrawal syndrome   Physiological and psychological responses that occur when a person physiologically dependent on a substance abruptly withdraws from its use.

Substance abuse is a major problem faced by our society and indeed the world. If it were possible to add up all the direct and indirect results of substance abuse, including automobile accidents involving alcohol, violent crime and behaviors involving drugs, and the full range of health problems associated with the chronic abuse of alcohol and other drugs and substances, substance abuse might prove the major health problem in most industrialized countries today, even though the mortality associated with substance abuse is lower than with many illnesses. If the economic and social effects of substance abuse are added in, including the economic costs of health care, job absenteeism, and reduced functioning and effects on the family and other social units, substance abuse can be considered one of the most serious social problems.

A substance is any drug, chemical, or biological entity that can be self-administered. Substance abuse occurs because of the substance's real or perceived effects or benefits. Even substances the general public may consider harmless, such as vitamins, aspirin, and laxatives, can cause health problems if used improperly. The nurse needs to be aware of problems involved in substance abuse because the effects on physiological and psychosocial health have a wide range and can be serious or even life threatening. Nurses need to be knowledgeable about the many variables that may cause substance abuse, the many effects on the person who abuses a substance, and the various health problems involved with substance abuse.

Basic Concepts of Substance Misuse, Abuse, and Dependence

Drugs and other substances can be used, misused, or abused, and the nurse must be able to distinguish among these different behaviors when providing care to clients with actual or potential drug or substance problems. These terms are defined in varying ways in different contexts, but the following meanings are generally accepted by health care professionals. A drug or substance is being *used* if it is appropriately taken only as prescribed or generally recommended for its intended physiological or psychological effects. A drug or substance is being *misused* if it is taken indiscriminately, whether as prescribed or self-administered as an over-the-counter medication, or taken improperly by a client who does not clearly understand the correct uses and dosage. A drug or substance is being *abused* if it is regularly taken indiscriminately in excessive quantities to the extent that the person's physiological, psychological, or social functioning is impaired.

The meanings given these terms are related to societal attitudes and values. The ingestion of alcohol to the point of intoxication may be accepted in some groups as a social use but be viewed as misuse or, if chronic, abuse by other groups. In addition, these behaviors exist on a continuum from cautious and appropriate use at one extreme to self-destructive, violent, chronic abuse at the other. We can generally categorize the more extreme cases as clear use or abuse, but it is often more difficult to discriminate between use and misuse or misuse and abuse. For example, it is impossible to draw a line between how many alcoholic drinks a month are acceptable and how many constitute abuse.

Many variables are involved in whether the use of any drug or substance becomes misuse, including personality factors, cultural background, social context, and the person's motivations, values, attitudes, and related behavioral patterns. Although misuse of a drug or substance may not immediately compromise the individual's functioning, misuse has the potential for becoming abuse and therefore can be viewed as a major risk factor. The concept of the health-illness continuum (see Chapter 2) is useful in assessing the client's health status and risk factors related to abuse patterns if physiological changes have not yet begun to occur.

The nurse may encounter substance abuse in two ways. A person may enter the health care system with a complaint directly or indirectly related to substance abuse, such as a cigarette smoker with a severe chronic respiratory infection, a teenager seen in the emergency room with PCP-induced seizures, or an alcoholic client being treated for liver disease. The nurse may also discover a client's substance abuse while providing care for other conditions, such as learning in a routine nursing history that the client has been using laxatives daily for several months or in a family counseling situation that a father suspects that his son frequently smokes marijuana. Because any type of drug or substance abuse threatens the person's health, the nurse who discovers abuse in either way can provide care directed toward resolving the abuse problem.

Two additional concepts are necessary for understanding substance abuse: physiological and psychological dependence. *Physiological dependence* is a condition in which the body has become so accustomed to the drug or substance that functioning is significantly impaired without it. Physiological dependence is present if a withdrawal syndrome occurs when administration of the drug is abruptly stopped. Use of alcohol, opiates, barbiturates, antianxiety drugs, and other agents can lead to physiological dependence. Closely related is the phenomenon of tolerance, in which higher doses of the drug are required to produce the same effects.

Psychological dependence is an emotional or psychological reliance on a drug or substance, usually because of its psychological effects. The person prefers the drugged state to a nondrugged state and experiences a desire, craving, or compulsion for the drug or substance. Most physiologically dependent persons are also psychologically dependent on the drug, but psychological dependence can occur alone, as with cocaine, amphetamines, marijuana, and even caffeine.

Any person who is physiologically dependent on a drug or substance can be considered to be abusing it because of the actual or potential impairments to functioning related to the chronic use of any drug or substance. Although a person may believe that drugs that do not lead to physiological dependence are safer, as with the teenager who is aware that marijuana is not "addictive" and who believes that he can stop using it whenever he wants, psychological dependence is often at least as powerful a habit. Chronic abuse of these "nonaddictive" drugs can also lead to impaired functioning and physiological damage.

Drugs and Substances

The general public often considers only medically prescribed substances and highly publicized illegal substances to be drugs, but chemically active substances such as caffeine, nicotine, and alcohol and nonprescription substances such as aspirin, laxatives, and antacids are also drugs and are commonly abused. The following sections describe the major classes of drugs and chemical substances, their prevalence in society today, and their major physiological and psychological effects.

Alcohol

Ethyl alcohol, the form of alcohol present in beer, wine, and other liquors, is the most commonly used and abused drug today. About 7% of adults over the age of 18 in the United States, or about 10 million people, are alcoholics or problem drinkers. Alcohol consumption plays a role in over half of all traffic accidents and leads to more than 28,000 traffic-related fatalities a year. The direct effects of alcoholism, including emotional illness and physiological diseases such as gastritis and liver disease, make it the third greatest health problem in the United States. If the indirect effects such as stress-related illnesses and traffic deaths are considered, alcoholism is the major health problem in society today. Alcohol abuse is a similar problem in Canada. Approximately 80% of the 17,000 Canadians responding to a survey taken in 1978 and 1979 said they had drunk alcohol in the preceding 12 months. Alcohol abuse has been increasing among adolescents; an estimated 3.3 million teenagers between 14 and 17 are problem drinkers.

Although commonly considered a stimulant, alcohol is actually a central nervous system depressant that causes pseudostimulant effects as parts of the brain are released from inhibitory control by the cortex. In the gastrointestinal system, alcohol is an irritant that may cause inflammation, bleeding, and malabsorption at any site. Chronic use of alcohol may lead to gastritis, enteritis, liver disease, and alcoholic pancreatitis. In the neurological system, chronic use may result in brain damage, memory loss and blackouts, sleep disturbances, sensory-motor disturbances, and (with large doses) anesthesia. Cardiovascular effects include diminished cardiac output, arrhythmias, and heat loss as a result of vasodilation of peripheral vessels. In the genitourinary system alcohol has a diuretic effect with rising blood levels and an antidiuretic effect as blood levels fall. Chronic use affects hormone levels and thus primary and secondary sex characteristics. Respiratory effects of chronic use include bronchitis, emphysema, and asthma. In the musculoskeletal system, chronic alcohol myopathy may produce muscle weakness and wasting.

Repeated and prolonged use of alcohol in large doses results in physical tolerance and in physical and psychological dependence.

At intoxicating levels the user's desired effect is often a sense of euphoria produced by depression of the central nervous system. The psychological effects of chronic alcohol use include heightened defense mechanisms, such as denial of reality and rationalization, a tendency to manipulate others, depression, suicidal tendencies, loneliness caused by decreased social skills, dependent behaviors, impulsiveness, and a low frustration tolerance.

Narcotics and Related Drugs

Opiates and opiate derivatives, including heroin, morphine, and codeine, are the most commonly abused narcotic drugs. Estimates of the prevalence of heroin use range from 1 to 3 million users in the United States.

Opiate derivatives are generally administered by sniffing (absorption through the mucous membranes) or subcutaneous or intravenous injection. In addition to physical dependence, opiate abuse leads to severely deteriorated functioning and altered behavioral patterns, often including criminal activities to gain the money for drug purchases.

The opiate derivatives are central nervous system depressants that can lead to tolerance and physical and psychological dependence. The therapeutic effect is the reduction of pain. Depressed respiration is a major side effect, and respiratory arrest can occur with overdose. Nausea and vomiting are common. In the digestive system, motility is delayed, secretions are reduced, and intestinal water absorption is increased. Acute overdosage may result in coma and pulmonary edema.

Opiate derivatives are often abused for their expected effects: mood elevation, relief of tension and anxiety, and a feeling of euphoria and tranquility. The user is generally drowsy and content, with a feeling that all biological needs are met. Usually functioning in all areas is severely impaired, leading to physical problems such as dehydration and malnutrition. As with chronic users of alcohol, social functioning is altered, leading to a range of psychosocial problems.

Sedative-Hypnotics

Sedative-hypnotic drugs include barbiturates, such as pentobarbital, phenobarbital, and primidone, and nonbarbiturates, such as ethchlorvynol, glutethimide, and methaqualone. About 1% of the U.S. adult population uses these prescribed drugs on a daily basis, and another 1% uses them less frequently. Up to 3% of high school seniors use these drugs illicitly. It is not uncommon for individuals who take these prescribed drugs for medical reasons to advance gradually to abuse.

Barbiturates produce central nervous system

depression ranging from mild sedation to deep anesthesia. Large doses cause respiratory depression, aspiration pneumonia, hypotension, and reduced gastrointestinal motility. Less common side effects are nausea and skin rashes. Overdose can cause coma, hypoxia, hypothermia, cardiovascular depression or cardiac arrest, and respiratory failure.

Nonbarbiturate sedatives and hypnotics also depress the central nervous system. There is a wide range of additional effects, including headache, ataxia, dizziness, nausea, and vomiting.

Psychological effects include relaxation or sedation, sleepiness, a sense of euphoria that is often followed by depression, and impaired judgment. Chronic users of barbiturates can become both physically and psychologically dependent on these drugs.

Tranquilizers

Tranquilizers include antianxiety and antipsychotic agents such as phenothiazine, benzodiazepine, diazepam, and chlordiazepoxide. Diazepam follows alcohol as the next most commonly abused drug because it is sometimes viewed as harmless and is often freely prescribed. In 1975 diazepam was the most commonly prescribed drug. The risks have since been recognized, and use of the drug has declined considerably. Nonetheless, about 12% of adults use medically prescribed tranquilizers. Both physical and psychological dependence can result from chronic use.

The physical effects of tranquilizers in large doses include hypotension, respiratory depression or coma, ataxia, hypothermia or hyperthermia, tachycardia, and reduced coordination such as slurred speech.

Psychological effects include reduced activity, decreased attentiveness or confusion, emotional bluntness, lethargy, somnolence, and a feeling of tranquility and increased self-confidence.

Central Nervous System Sympathomimetics

Central nervous system sympathomimetics include cocaine and amphetamines, which are pharmacologically related to epinephrine and norepinephrine. Both drugs stimulate the central nervous system. Amphetamines are ingested or injected, and cocaine is sniffed, injected intravenously, or smoked in converted base form. Amphetamines produce physical tolerance. Neither drug leads to physical dependence, but both can result in strong psychological dependence.

Cocaine is an increasingly popular drug. Approximately 10 million people in the United States use it regularly, and about 5 million people use it less frequently.

The physiological effects of amphetamines can include tachycardia, dyspnea, chest pain, and restlessness. Although users report a greater physical and mental energy, this occurs because of more rapid expenditure of energy resources, not with the creation of any new energy. Because the appetite is reduced, malnutrition is common among chronic abusers.

The effects of cocaine are similar to those of amphetamines. Large doses of cocaine can cause nausea, vomiting, muscle spasms, respiratory failure, convulsions, coma, and circulatory collapse.

The psychological effects of amphetamines and cocaine are similar: mood elevation or euphoria, a reduction in fatigue, a sense of greater alertness and increased energy, potential aggressiveness, and hyperactivity. Behaviors may be repetitious and inefficient. Severe depression, often of suicidal proportions, may follow an amphetamine high.

Marijuana

Marijuana and hashish (a powdered form of the plant's resin) are the most common forms of the cannabis drugs and are derived from a species of hemp. The plant is usually dried and smoked but is sometimes ingested. The pharmacological classification of marijuana is not definite, but the drug seems to act as a central nervous system depressant. Almost one third of high school seniors report smoking marijuana at least once a month, and two thirds of people age 18 to 25 have smoked marijuana at least once in their lives.

The physiological effects of marijuana are less dramatic than with most other drugs affecting the central nervous system. Effects include immediate tachycardia, delayed bradycardia, delayed hypotension, and enhanced appetite. The psychological effects have been the subject of many studies and are still being debated. The drug produces a state of relaxation, distorted perceptions of time and space, moments of excitement or hilarity, impaired decision making, and sometimes fear, panic, or paranoia. Hallucinations occur only with very high doses. Long-term use may be associated with apathy, memory problems, and some loss of mental acuity.

Hallucinogens

Hallucinogens include lysergic acid diethylamide (LSD), mescaline, psilocybin, and phencyclidine (PCP). Of all high school seniors, 15% report having used a hallucinogenic drug at least once. These drugs generally do not lead to physical or psychological dependence but are of concern because unpredictable, often violent behavior is associated with their use.

PCP use has become more widespread in recent years, and it is sometimes smoked in a mixture with marijuana. PCP is particularly dangerous because of its unpredictable behavioral effects.

LSD produces relatively mild autonomic nervous system changes such as tachycardia, hypertension, nausea, and vertigo. The physiological effects of PCP include flushing, sweating, diplopia, nystagmus, analgesia, sedation, ataxia, seizures, hypertension, numbness of extremities, impaired motor skills, respiratory depression, and coma.

LSD causes perceptual changes or hallucinations, impaired judgment, and toxic psychosis characterized by panic, paranoia, and unpredictable behavior. The psychological effects of PCP include perceptual distortions, apathy, disorganized thought processes, impaired attention span, hallucinations that can recur unpredictably for days or weeks after use, paranoid behavior, and self-destructive acts.

Inhalants

Inhalants are substances such as volatile hydrocarbons and aerosols that are abused for their central nervous system depressant effect. Inhalants include toluene, xylene, benzene, gasoline, paint thinner, lighter fluid, and airplane glue. Thirteen percent of high school seniors report using an inhalant at least once. Inhalants are frequently used by preteens because of their accessibility and low cost.

The physiological effects of inhalants include bronchial and laryngeal irritation, headache, vertigo, and ataxia. Coma may occur with large doses.

The psychological effects of inhalants include inebriation, exhilaration, dizziness, euphoria, abandonment, and aggressiveness. Depression may follow the initial mood elevation.

Nonprescription Substances

Any drug or substance that alters consciousness or physiological functioning in any way has the capacity to be misused or abused. For example, nicotine in cigarettes causes central nervous system changes and can be abused for these effects. Similarly, coffee and soft drinks containing caffeine can be misused. Society is generally becoming more aware of the effects and risks of these substances. Many over-the-counter products, however, hold the same potential for misuse and abuse when individuals diagnose their own needs and turn habitually to a commercial product they can easily buy and self-administer. The box lists 26 classes of nonprescription medications having active ingredients that make them attractive as drugs of misuse.

Classes of Nonprescription Medications

- Antacids
- Sedatives and sleep aids
- Cold remedies and antitussives
- Mouthwashes
- Antirheumatics
- Vitamins and minerals
- Laxatives
- Sunburn treatments and preventives
- Stimulants
- Antidiarrheals
- Bronchodilators and antiasthmatics
- Ophthalmics
- Miscellaneous internal products
- Antimicrobials
- Analgesics
- Antihistamines and allergy drugs
- Topical analgesics
- Hematinics
- Antiperspirants
- Dentifrices and dental products
- Contraceptive and vaginal products
- Hemorrhoidals
- Dandruff and athlete's foot preparations
- Antiemetics
- Emetics
- Miscellaneous external products

From Ray, O.: *Drugs, society, and human behavior,* ed. 3, St. Louis, 1983, The C.V. Mosby Co.

The physiological effects of all nonprescription medications are too numerous and varied to be described here. Unlike other drugs and substances discussed so far, most of these medications are overused or misused not for their psychological effects but because the user becomes psychologically dependent if he feels the medication is necessary for continued good health, even in cases when continued use is actually having adverse effects. Some medications, such as laxatives, do result in physical dependence (see Chapter 32).

As a general rule, any nonprescription drug can be misused and with chronic or acute overdoses may result in physiological problems, such as the occult gastrointestinal bleeding caused by large doses of aspirin or the toxic effects of large doses of some vitamin supplements. In addition, some medications may mask the symptoms of an underlying illness, preventing the individual from seeking appropriate health care. Although the chronic misuse of most nonprescription medications cannot be assessed on the basis of altered behaviors, the nurse may learn of a client's misuse pattern through the nursing health history and can give the client information to prevent future misuse and dependence.

TABLE 45-1

Classes of Drugs Taken During a 2-Day Period* Among Adults Aged 15 Years and Over According to a Survey Conducted in Canada,† 1978-79

Type of Drug	Percentage‡ Taking Specified Drugs in Each Age Group					
	All Ages	15-19	20-24	25-44	45-64	65 and Over
Pain relievers	16.0	9.1	11.7	16.2	18.7	21.6
Tranquilizers and sleeping pills	5.9	1.1§	1.5	3.8	10.0	14.0
Cough and cold remedies	4.9	4.8	4.8	5.4	4.7	4.2
Other drugs	45.2	28.2	32.8	34.5	57.3	85.8
No drugs taken	50.0	64.6	59.1	55.0	40.9	27.4
TOTAL	17,492	2,333	2,215	6,472	4,453	2,019

From Canada Health Survey: The health of Canadians—report of the Canada Health Survey, Catalogue No. 82-538, Ottawa, 1981, Health and Welfare Canada and Statistics Canada.
*Drug consumption refers to consumption during the last 2 days prior to the survey.
†Data are based on the results of a Canada-wide survey conducted May 1978 to March 1979. A total of 17,492 persons aged 15 years and over were questioned about their use of drugs.
‡Because of multiple responses resulting from individuals taking several of these types of drugs simultaneously, percentages do not add up to 100%.
§Subject to sampling error of 20% to 39% of cell entry.

Drug and Substance Interactions

The potential for dangerous drug interactions is increased among substance abusers. Because of personality and other factors, a person who abuses one substance may be more likely to abuse other substances as well to attain different kinds of psychological effects. Physiological or psychological dependence on a substance also increases the potential for drug interaction. In some cases a person who commonly abuses a drug may become so familiar with its effects that he "forgets" he is on the drug and takes another. Finally, social changes in recent decades have led to a serious problem of drug mixture experimentation in search of new "highs," particularly among adolescents.

Drug interactions are also more likely among frequent users and misusers of prescription and over-the-counter medications. Table 45-1 shows figures for total drug use by class in Canada; the increasing incidence of drug use by age demonstrates the substantial risk for drug interactions. By age 65, for example, over 85% of people are taking some form of drug every day or two.

Substance Abuse and Psychosocial Health

Because of their mind- and behavior-altering effects, most abused substances can also have serious effects on a person's psychosocial well-being and family functioning. To understand the relationship between abuse and the client's psychosocial dimension, and thus provide nursing care for a client with a substance abuse problem, the nurse needs to understand the psychosocial variables that play a causative role in substance abuse, the typical pattern or course of abuse, and the psychosocial effects on the abuser's family and other social interactions.

Causes of Substance Abuse

Physiological and psychological dependence has a major role in the abuser's pattern or continued use, but the reasons for the person's initial misuse of the substance are more varied. Generally two kinds of conscious or unconscious motivations may explain why a person first misuses a substance (Hahn, Barkin, and Oestreich, 1982). The person using mind-altering drugs may be seeking pleasure, euphoria, a new or unusual experience, or self-discovery; he may be motivated by factors such as curiosity, boredom, peer pressure, or media attention. The person may be consciously or unconsciously seeking to solve or avoid a problem or to cope with stress or other problems. This motivation may apply both to a chronic abuser of self-prescribed laxatives and to a businessman who habitually has three martinis at lunch to relieve tension at the office. Many psychologists have examined substance abuse as an escape mechanism by which the person attempts to reduce inner tensions, depression, self-concept problems, or problems in social interaction with a spouse, family, or peers. There is current debate as to the possible existence of a drug-dependent personality, having the characteristics of psychological dependence, fear of failure, and feelings of inadequacy. Some psychologists argue that everyone has the potential to become dependent on *something*.

It is often difficult to sort out the exact role of causative factors for a particular client with a substance abuse problem. The initial reason might be boredom, for example, but as the person becomes more psychologically dependent on the substance, it may become an escape mechanism for attempting to cope with emotional or other problems. Typically the causative factors are multiple by the time the substance abuse problem becomes chronic or comes to the attention of health care professionals.

STRESS FACTORS

Many theories have been put forth to explain substance abuse in terms of biological, psychological, or sociocultural factors. Since no one theory has successfully explained all substance abuse, the nurse should consider stressors in all these dimensions when providing care for clients with substance abuse problems.

Biological factors may include a genetic tendency for substance abuse. Research has uncovered a high incidence of alcoholism in the children of alcoholics (almost half) and a tendency of alcoholism to occur in families with manic-depressive illness.

Psychological factors include a dependent personality type, low self-esteem, an underdeveloped sense of identity in adolescents, the need for peer approval, an unstable family structure, and emotional states such as shame, depression, guilt, and loneliness.

Sociocultural factors include ease of access to substances of abuse, social group acceptance, peer group pressure, social group ambivalence or permissiveness about the value of drugs, parental misuse behaviors, religious values, cultural values related to substance use patterns, and sex role differences.

ATTITUDES TOWARD SUBSTANCE ABUSE

When providing care for a client with a substance abuse problem, to be objective in understanding the problem and to facilitate a therapeutic nurse-client relationship, the nurse should be aware of personal attitudes and values related to use of the substance. The values clarification process is useful in this respect (see Chapter 13). The nurse who adopts a moralistic, judgmental attitude toward drinking might have difficulty understanding how individual factors have contributed to the client's behavior.

The nurse should also assess the client's and family's attitudes toward the abuse problem. A client who views his drinking as a sin, for example, may experience such guilt after drinking that in a vicious circle he continues to drink to escape the guilt, thus causing

more guilt and leading to still more drinking. On the other extreme, a client who is convinced his drinking is outside his control may not be motivated to attempt to comply with a treatment program unless counseling or teaching methods first lead to an acceptance of his role in attempting to resolve the problem. As current media announcements for treatment programs emphasize, to admit one has a problem is to take the first step toward solving it.

Course of Substance Abuse

Many variables are involved in the individual's pattern of substance misuse leading to abuse. There is no one typical course of substance abuse for most people or most substances with a potential for abuse. Nonetheless, there are certain common behavioral patterns of how abuse develops. The nurse familiar with these patterns may more easily assess the current status of a client with an abuse problem or with the risk of an abuse problem developing.

Alcoholism begins with social drinking in which the person is motivated by peer pressure, family drinking habits, and other reasons. There is evidence as well for a hereditary predisposition for alcoholism, suggesting that one person may be biologically more likely to become an alcoholic than another. Studies have shown also that certain personality traits are more common among teenagers who later become alcoholics, including lower academic performance, less value of church and school, and greater need for peer approval. One must be careful to avoid generalizing from such factors, however, because many alcoholics are very different from this stereotype.

In the second stage the person develops a pattern of drinking larger amounts for longer periods of time more frequently, generally resuming a pattern of drinking again if having stopped for a time. The person is becoming physiologically and psychologically dependent on alcohol and has developed tolerance for the drug. Alcoholism may develop acutely or gradually. As psychological dependence increases, the person may use drinking increasingly as a coping mechanism for stress or as an escape mechanism. Drinking may lead to problems at work, in the family, and in other aspects of the person's life. When tolerance becomes established, the person may appear sober and functional even after consumption of large amounts of alcohol, although judgment and other cognitive and psychomotor skills are impaired. Blackouts (temporary amnesia or memory losses) may become common.

One of two general patterns of drinking may emerge: steady drinking or binge drinking. The steady drinker often increases consumption until problems start occurring and the drinker realizes the seriousness of the problem. The person may give up drinking or attempt to give it up for a time and return, or he may continue drinking steadily until a physiological or other problem interrupts the course of steady drinking. Binge drinkers may drink and remain relatively intoxicated for as long as several days, then stop drinking altogether for a varying length of time until the next binge occurs.

With physiological dependence and tolerance, the person suffers the alcohol withdrawal syndrome after stopping or decreasing alcohol consumption. Symptoms may include tremor, anxiety, convulsions, hallucinations, and delirium tremens, depending on the extent of the dependence. Such symptoms often motivate the person to continue drinking.

The later course of alcoholism, which follows the establishment of dependence, varies widely. The person may recognize the problem, seek help, and successfully stop drinking. The person may for a long time be successful enough in alternating periods of drinking and abstinence to prevent job, family, and physiological problems from occurring. Steady drinking may lead to severe depression and suicide as all aspects of the person's life are disrupted. The person may continue drinking until an accident or health problem brings him into the health care system.

The similarity of patterns of other types of substance abuse to the typical patterns of alcoholism depends on many factors, such as physiological and psychological effects, the presence or absence of physiological dependence, and other threats to the person's health. Generally, the stronger the psychological effects of a substance, the more disruptive the abuse problem will be and the more accelerated the course.

Effects on the Family

Because of the many effects of substance abuse on the person's functioning, roles and relationships within the family are often altered, usually with detrimental effects on family functioning. Because nursing care frequently involves the family, the nurse is often in a unique position to observe altered patterns of functioning and to involve the family in nursing interventions. Chapter 22 details nursing perspectives of the family as the client's environment and of the family unit as the client.

The effects of substance abuse on the person's spouse involve all aspects of their relationship and life together. During a nursing history the spouse may mention such matters as sexual maladjustment, thoughts of separation or divorce, quarreling, economic difficulties, feelings of loneliness, confusion, or resentment about increased responsibilities in child rearing and other family roles. All these may be direct or indirect effects of the person's substance abuse, as usual roles and coping mechanisms break down with increasing psychological dependence. The family 20-question questionnaire, developed as an assessment tool for the spouses of alcoholics, reveals the range of concerns often felt by the spouse (see the boxed material). Most of the items in this questionnaire are important with other types of substance abuse as well, particularly with drugs that have severe psychological effects and the potential for psychological dependence.

The effects of substance abuse by either or both parents on their children is often of particular importance to the nurse. The stresses of having an alcoholic parent in the home can have wide-range effects and lead to physical and emotional problems in the early developmental stages. Emotional neglect is the most common problem, and physical neglect may also occur. The child's self-concept may be seriously damaged because most children and adolescents do not understand the complex abuse problem but tend to blame themselves for the parents' emotional neglect. Family conflicts are more likely, and violence often erupts in the presence of children. Children in such families are also at a high risk for child abuse. Sexual child abuse, for example, is often related to alcoholism. Other effects include necessary role changes by the children, a lack of a good role model in the dependent parent, and alterations in the child's relationships with peers. In addition, children of substance abusers, particularly alcoholics, are at greater risk for later becoming substance abusers themselves.

The nurse's overall goal in providing care for the spouse and children of a client with a substance abuse problem is to help family members adjust to role changes, reduce stress, promote a healthful environment, and maintain emotional and psychological health while preventing future problems.

Substance Abuse in Special Groups

Developmental Stages

Because substance abuse involves many physiological and psychosocial effects and causative variables, people in different developmental stages have different susceptibilities and are affected in different ways. For example, a 40-year-old businessman may increase alcohol consumption in response to an awareness that his physical energy is diminishing, or an adolescent may experiment with drugs because of pressures from his peer group. Each developmental stage presents certain kinds of stresses and the potential for matu-

Family 20-Question Questionnaire

Ask yourself these questions about your husband's or your wife's drinking

1. Do you worry about your spouse's drinking?	Yes ▢	No ▢
2. Have you ever been embarrassed by your spouse's drinking?	Yes ▢	No ▢
3. Are holidays more of a nightmare than a celebration because of your spouse's drinking behavior?	Yes ▢	No ▢
4. Are most of your spouse's friends heavy drinkers?	Yes ▢	No ▢
5. Does your spouse often promise to quit drinking without success?	Yes ▢	No ▢
6. Does your spouse's drinking make the atmosphere in the home tense and anxious?	Yes ▢	No ▢
7. Does your spouse deny a drinking problem because your spouse only drinks beer?	Yes ▢	No ▢
8. Do you find it necessary to lie to employer, relatives, or friends in order to hide your spouse's drinking?	Yes ▢	No ▢
9. Has your spouse ever failed to remember what occurred during a drinking period?	Yes ▢	No ▢
10. Does your spouse avoid conversation pertaining to alcohol or problem drinking?	Yes ▢	No ▢
11. Does your spouse justify his or her drinking problem?	Yes ▢	No ▢
12. Does your spouse avoid social situations where alcoholic beverages will not be served?	Yes ▢	No ▢
13. Do you ever feel guilty about your spouse's drinking?	Yes ▢	No ▢
14. Has your spouse ever driven a vehicle while under the influence of alcohol?	Yes ▢	No ▢
15. Are your children afraid of your spouse while he or she is drinking?	Yes ▢	No ▢
16. Are you afraid of physical or verbal abuse when your spouse is drinking?	Yes ▢	No ▢
16. Has another person mentioned your spouse's unusual drinking behavior?	Yes ▢	No ▢
18. Do you fear riding with your spouse when he or she is drinking?	Yes ▢	No ▢
19. Does your spouse have periods of remorse after a drinking occasion and apologize for behavior?	Yes ▢	No ▢
20. Do you notice your spouse is getting drunk on fewer drinks?	Yes ▢	No ▢

If you have answered yes to any two of the questions, there is a definite warning that a drinking problem may exist in your family.

If you have answered yes to any four of the questions, the chances are that a drinking problem does exist in your family.

If you have answered yes to five or more, there very definitely is a drinking problem in your family.

rational crises, and these may influence the individual's behavior related to abuse patterns. In addition, the physiological and psychological effects of substance abuse vary according to the person's developmental stage. Unit 4 discusses the developmental stages in detail and the developmental changes that influence the individual's susceptibilities.

Special attention should be given to the effects of substance abuse in the fetal stage of development. Chapter 24 describes different kinds of teratogens, drugs that cross the placenta into the embryo's or fetus's circulation with a potential effect on normal growth. Many drugs, including prescription and over-the-counter medications and illegal substances, have detrimental effects on fetal development, including low birth weight, high fetal and infant mortality, and congenital abnormalities.

Fetal alcohol syndrome has been recognized only in the last decade, although its effects are wide ranging and can be tragic. Evidence shows that about one third of children of alcoholic mothers will be born with the fetal alcohol syndrome, characterized by growth deficiencies, motor dysfunctions, cranial and cardiac deficiencies, and mental developmental delays or deficiencies. Why some children are affected and others are not is unclear. The teratogenic effects are related to the amount of alcohol consumed and the frequency of consumption, and nurses and pregnant women should understand that alcohol consumption even by nonalcoholics can have adverse effects. Smith (1982) estimates that an average of two drinks a day can affect birth weight and that four to six drinks a day can lead to physical defects and dysfunctions, with the full fetal alcohol syndrome likely at higher levels of consumption.

The fetal effects of cigarette smoking, caused by the increased level of carbon monoxide in the pregnant woman's blood, have also been recognized increasingly in recent years. Cigarette smoking has been shown to be associated with low-birth-weight infants and higher incidences of stillborn infants and neonatal deaths. Researchers continue to investigate a possible relationship between maternal smoking and a higher incidence of infant bronchitis and pneumonia in the first year. In addition, cigarette smoking has been shown to have an additive effect with the effects of alcohol.

Other drugs associated with congenital malformations include antidepressants, narcotics, and tranquilizers. These effects are generally greater when the drug is taken in the first trimester but are not limited to this period. Drug combinations may intensify the effects. For example, smoking more than triples the risk that tranquilizers will cause malformations.

Much more research is needed to investigate all the potential effects and risks of substances likely to be abused. In addition, more information is needed on the long-term neurological and behavioral effects in the child whose mother engaged in substance abuse during pregnancy. If the nursing history for a pregnant woman or a woman likely to become pregnant indicates the use of any drug or substance with potential fetal effects, the nurse should use teaching and counseling techniques to decrease the health risks, research the current literature on teratogenic effects or obtain a consultation, or make an appropriate referral.

Special Groups

Substance abuse occurs in virtually all age groups, socioeconomic levels, and cultural groups, and in individuals with different educational levels, professions, and personality traits. Because substance abuse is often associated with certain psychosocial variables, however, it tends to be more common among individuals in certain groups.

ALCOHOLISM AND NATIVE AMERICANS

Although the stereotype of the "drunken Indian" accepted by many Americans is generally untrue or exaggerated, for some Native Americans (Indians) alcohol abuse is a serious problem. The incidence of alcoholism with physiological dependence is not higher among Native Americans than in the United States as a whole, but it is estimated that over half of the Native American population consistently abuse alcohol. When the indirect effects of alcohol abuse

are included, it becomes the major health and social problem for this group.

The problem of alcohol abuse among Native Americans for the most part originates in a complex set of psychosocial factors in this cultural group, some of which are unique and some of which are shared by other cultural groups. Native Americans who choose to live on reservations often face problems such as unemployment, poor housing, and inadequate health care. Outside the reservation, common problems include social and economic discrimination and rejection, as well as the problems of acculturation (see Chapter 21). Excessive drinking may begin as an attempt to escape emotional problems, stress, anger, anxiety, helplessness, hopelessness, or conditions of deprivation. As discussed in Chapter 21, many of these problems are shared by other ethnic-cultural groups. In some respects many Native Americans drink in the same patterns and for the same reasons as members of the dominant white culture—but these reasons are often greater in scope or number among Native Americans.

ALCOHOLISM AND WOMEN

In today's society alcoholism and alcohol-related problems are increasing among women but remain less common than among men according to most estimates. As a group women with alcohol problems deserve special attention for several reasons. First, because less research has been directed toward causes and effects of alcohol abuse among women, health care professionals often are not well prepared to understand and manage the problems of women alcoholics. Second, because of differences in family, social, and other roles between men and women, the patterns of drinking and the consequences of alcoholism are often different for women. Finally, certain stressors are more common among women, including frustration felt by working women in male-dominated professions, greater or sole responsibility in child rearing, and depression or loneliness often felt by nonworking mothers after children have left home. In the past, most research in this area focused on the alcohol problems of nonworking women over the age of 40. Women alcoholics in this group tend to drink alone in a pattern significantly different from male drinking patterns. Thus their problem is compounded by emotional and social isolation.

More recently research has been directed to drinking patterns among working women, whose alcohol problems are more similar to the traditional problems of alcoholism among men. This change is related to larger societal changes as traditional sex-related social roles break down or become less rigid. Because of the wide variety of abuse patterns among women, as among men, the nurse should assess the individual variables involved and individualize the care plan when providing care for a woman with a substance abuse problem.

SUBSTANCE ABUSE AND HEALTH CARE PROFESSIONALS

The incidence of substance abuse is generally higher among health care professionals than in the population as a whole. The incidence of narcotic dependence, for example, is about 0.3% for the U.S. population but an estimated 1% to 2% for physicians. Up to 18% of physicians are alcoholics, compared with 10% of the general population. The incidence of alcoholism among nurses is similar, with an estimated 40,000 alcoholic nurses in the United States today.

Health care professionals may abuse alcohol or other drugs for the same reasons as other people, but nurses and physicians are confronted with additional and unique stressors. Interacting with clients who have a variety of illnesses, including incurable and fatal diseases, can lead to frustration and emotional exhaustion. More than workers in many other professions, health professionals often work long or irregular hours with few opportunities for relaxation. The complexities of the health care delivery system and an often unwieldy institutional structure may lead to additional frustrations. Furthermore, nurses and physicians have greater access to medications and may believe more than other people in the "magic" of drugs to solve problems. For all these reasons, substance abuse is a serious problem in the health care professions.

The problems associated with abuse are the same for nurses as for other people, but impairment of the nurse's work performance may have more serious consequences because of the many responsibilities of the nurse. For this reason, and because of societal expectations for health care professionals to be "above" this problem, alcoholism or other substance abuse has in the past frequently led to job dismissal or license revocation or suspension. Many nurses therefore attempted to hide the problem rather than seeking therapy. In recent years, with greater awareness of and sensitivity to the abuse problem, institutions and state nursing boards are increasingly seeking to help nurses with abuse problems. Although license revocation still occurs in some cases, more than half the states now have assistance or prevention programs, and the trend is to put substance-dependent nurses on probation while in therapy rather than revoke their licenses.

Nurses have several responsibilities related to the problem of substance abuse among health care professionals. First, nurses need to be aware of the nature of the problem, how it may arise and develop, and the risk factors involved. Nursing educators in the past often neglected or underemphasized the problem, but being well informed about alcoholism and substance abuse is perhaps the major factor in prevention. Second, nurses can take action to minimize personal and job-related stress that may lead to substance abuse (see Chapter 5). Finally, if a nurse observes that another nurse's or physician's job functioning is impaired, possibly as a result of substance abuse, the nurse should take appropriate actions for the situation and institution, often by speaking to the nurse in charge. Impaired functioning may be demonstrated by mistakes in carrying out procedures or poor judgment in clinical decision making. The nurse must not jump to conclusions about a colleague's behavior. Communication with the appropriate supervisor should concern only the colleague's specific job performance, not suspicion or speculation about abuse. The supervisor's action in many cases is a referral to an employee-assistance or off-site therapy program.

Nursing Process for Substance Abuse

Nurses may encounter clients with substance abuse problems in most settings and in a variety of situations; for example, clients who may have an abuse problem may be seen for other reasons, and clients who have acute health problems directly caused by substance abuse may be seen. As with other health care problems, the nursing process provides a means for individualizing health care for the client with an actual or potential substance abuse problem.

Assessment

Because of the variety of physiological and psychological effects of chronic substance abuse and the often subtle factors that create the potential for an abuse problem to develop, the nursing assessment should be thorough and explore the client's health status in all dimensions. The goals of the assessment are to determine if a substance abuse problem exists, to explore causative factors and effects in all areas of the client's life, to assess the psychological, behavioral, and physiological impact of the abused substance, and to assess the extent of physiological or psychological dependence. Assessment includes the observation of the client's behaviors that may indicate substance abuse, the interview and nursing history, and the physical examination.

A person under the influence of a drug generally

TABLE 45-2

Summary of Behaviors Associated with Substance Abuse

Substance	Route*	Physical Dependence	Psychological Dependence	Expected Behaviors	Behaviors Related to Overdose	Withdrawal Syndrome	Special Considerations
Alcohol	Ingestion	Yes	Yes	Euphoria, followed by depression and sometimes hostility; decreased inhibitions; impaired judgment; incoordination; slurred speech	Unconsciousness, coma, respiratory depression, death	Tremors, hallucinosis, seizure disorder, delirium tremens (alcohol withdrawal delirium)	Chronic use leads to serious disruptions in most organ systems; malnutrition and dehydration are common; vitamin deficiency may lead to Wernicke's encephalopathy and alcoholic amnestic syndrome; alcohol-dependent people are susceptible to other dependencies as well
Opiates							
Heroin	Injection, ingestion, inhalation	Yes	Yes	Euphoria, relaxation, relief from pain, lack of concern, detachment from reality, drowsiness, constricted pupils, nausea, constipation, slurred speech, impaired judgment	Unconsciousness, coma, respiratory depression, circulatory depression, respiratory arrest, cardiac arrest, death	Watery eyes, dilated pupils, anxiety, abdominal cramps, piloerection, yawning, diaphoresis, rhinorrhea, achiness, anorexia, insomnia, fever, nausea, vomiting, diarrhea	Chronic use leads to lack of concern about physical well-being, resulting in malnutrition and dehydration; criminal behavior may take place to acquire money for drugs; injection sites may become infected; multiple drug use is common
Morphine	Injection	Yes	Yes				
Meperidine	Ingestion						
Codeine	Ingestion injection	Yes	Yes				
Opium	Smoking, ingestion	Yes	Yes				
Methadone	Ingestion	Yes	Yes	Relieves craving for drugs without causing impaired functioning	Same	Same	
Barbiturates	Ingestion, injection	Yes	Yes	Euphoria, followed by depression and sometimes hostility; decreased inhibitions; impaired judgment; slurred speech; incoordination; drowsiness	Respiratory depression, coma, death	Postural hypotension, tachycardia, fever, insomnia, tremors, agitation, anxiety; rapid withdrawal causes apprehension, weakness, tremors, postural hypotension, anorexia, grand mal seizures	Frequently used alternately with stimulants; combination with alcohol enhances effects and may lead to overdosage; paradoxical responses of hyperactivity may occur in children and the elderly

Drug	Routes of administration	Physical dependence	Psychological dependence	Effects	Overdose	Withdrawal syndrome	Possible consequences
(Amphetamines)	Ingestion, injection	No	Yes	Euphoria, hyperactivity, irritability, hyperalertness, insomnia, anorexia, weight loss, tachycardia, hypertension	Restlessness, tremor, rapid respiration, confusion, assaultiveness, hallucinations, panic	Depression, fatigue	Prolonged use can result in psychotic behavior; a paradoxical depressant reaction occurs in children; frequently used alternately with depressant substances
Cocaine	Inhalation, smoking, injection	No	Yes	Euphoria, elation, agitation, hyperactivity, irritability, grandiosity, pressured speech, tachycardia, hypertension, diaphoresis, anorexia, weight loss, insomnia	Restlessness, tremor, rapid respiration, confusion, assaultiveness, hallucinations, panic	Depression, fatigue, anxiety	Psychotic behavior may occur following large doses; prolonged use by inhalation may result in destruction of the mucous membranes in the nose and deterioration of the nasal septum; use in combination with other substances is dangerous
Hallucinogens (psychedelics)	Ingestion, smoking	No	No	Distorted perception, heightened sense of awareness, grandiosity, hallucinations, illusions, distortions of time and space, depersonalization, mystical experiences, dilated pupils, increased blood pressure, increased salivation	Panic, psychosis	None	A "bad trip" may result in panic, unpredictable behavior, and psychotic behaviors; "flashbacks" may occur for several months after use; self-destructive behavior may occur while under the effect of the drug
Phencyclidine (PCP)	Smoking, ingestion	No	No	Euphoria, perceptual distortion, agitation, violence, delusions, antisocial behavior, elevated blood pressure, increased salivation, diaphoresis, ataxia, nystagmus, decreased pain response	Drowsiness, stupor, coma, grand mal seizures, death	None	Use may lead to psychotic behavior, irrationality, panic
Marijuana	Smoking, ingestion	No	Yes	Relaxation, mild euphoria, loss of inhibition, decreased motivation, red eyes, dry mouth	Psychosis	None	Physiological consequences of use are under investigation
Antianxiety drugs (benzodiazepines)	Ingestion, injection	Yes	Yes	Relaxation, increased self-confidence, relief of anxiety, drowsiness, ataxia, slurred speech, hypotension	Drowsiness, confusion, hypotension, coma, death	Tremors, agitation, anxiety, grand mal seizures, abdominal cramps, vomiting, diaphoresis	Dependence may occur insidiously; users may underreport the actual amount taken because of guilt about multiple prescriptions and abuse

From Stuart, G.W., and Sundeen, S.J.: Principles and practice of psychiatric nursing, ed. 2, St. Louis, 1983, The C.V. Mosby Co.
*Most common listed first.

manifests a set of behaviors as a result of the drug's psychological and physiological effects. Table 45-2 summarizes the expected behaviors associated with substance abuse and typical behaviors during withdrawal. Observing such behaviors in a client, even when the nurse does not otherwise suspect an abuse problem, should prompt further assessment using interview techniques.

Because many clients are defensive or especially sensitive about their substance use patterns and because many tend to deny the problem both to themselves and to the nurse, the nurse should be cautious in the interview and nursing history. Asking the client if he thinks he drinks too much usually requires a greater degree of tact and sensitivity than, for example, asking the client how many hours of sleep he gets each night.

Estes, Smith-DiJulio, and Heinemann (1980) have described four interviewing styles that can direct the interview process productively. With the *empathetic* style, the nurse demonstrates an acceptance and understanding of the client's problem, and the client may respond by speaking more freely about the problem. A *clarifying* style seeks to sort through the client's perception of his problems with specific questions. It is particularly useful if the client is having difficulty focusing his thoughts or if he is denying the extent of the problem. A style based on *giving advice,* although this may seem to move too rapidly to the intervention stage, is occasionally an effective interview approach because many substance abusers tend to look to outside sources for answers. If the client asks frequent questions during the interview process about how he might manage the problem, the nurse can incorporate general teaching principles to satisfy this need while continuing to gather assessment data. A fourth style is *confrontation,* in which the nurse confronts elements in the interview that are impeding effective interaction. The nurse may, for example, directly raise the question of the client's lack of motivation or involvement in the interview. This technique runs the risk of seeming to reject the client but is occasionally effective in breaking through relationship barriers.

During the interview and nursing history the nurse should also listen for any misconceptions the client may have about the substance itself or the nature of substance abuse. Later interventions may need to include teaching to provide accurate information so the client can participate more effectively in care. In addition, the nurse should pay attention to the client's nonverbal behaviors during the interview, which may reveal if the client feels threatened, defensive, or angry.

Many different assessment scales and nursing history formats have been developed to gather assessment data from clients with alcohol or other substance abuse problems. The boxed material is a specialized nursing history format for clients with alcohol problems. It illustrates the range of information to be obtained about major body systems. Of particular importance in the nursing history is the client's psychosocial status. Questions in this area are generally open ended to explore the full extent of the client's problem.

Finally, assessment includes physical examination. The nurse may choose to perform a complete physical assessment (Chapter 29) if appropriate, focusing on body systems at greatest risk for problems caused by the substance, or a more limited examination may be conducted, depending on the abused substance. For example, assessment for an adult who smokes cigarettes would emphasize the cardiovascular and pulmonary systems, whereas for a client who abuses laxatives examination would focus on the gastrointestinal system. When a client is seen with symptoms of substance overdose, the nurse sets priorities for the assessment of vital physiological function. In the case of an overdose of a substance capable of causing central nervous system depression, the nurse must assess for signs of respiratory depression (such as bradypnea and reduced depth of respirations), loss of consciousness, and cardiovascular alterations (such as hypotension and bradycardia). It obviously becomes necessary for the nurse to assess vital signs frequently.

The nurse should also be alert for indirect effects of substance abuse, such as malnutrition related to poor dietary patterns caused by the substance abuse. Laboratory and other diagnostic tests may also be appropriate to complete the data base.

Nursing Diagnosis

The nursing diagnosis for clients with substance abuse problems should include actual and potential physiological problems relevant to nursing practice, as well as psychosocial problems such as stresses, interpersonal conflicts, altered work or family roles, and self-concept deficits. Many nursing diagnoses for these clients are therefore similar to diagnoses discussed in other chapters, such as those on self-concept (Chapter 18), sexuality (Chapter 19), safety (Chapter 35), hygiene (Chapter 36), and nutrition (Chapter 38), except that the causative factor related to the substance is included. Table 45-3 gives examples of nursing diagnoses of problems related to substance abuse.

Nursing History Tool for Use with Clients with Alcohol Problems

Place of interview _____ Date _____

Name of interviewer _____

Client's name _____

Ethnic group _____ Age _____ Sex _____

Birthplace _____ Occupation _____

Last grade attended _____

1. For what reason did you come to this agency?
2. What do you most want help with at the present time?

DRINKING HISTORY

3. How old were you when you started drinking alcohol regularly?
4. How long have you had problems with alcohol?
5. How often do you drink alcoholic beverages?
6. What kinds of alcoholic beverages do you drink?
7. How much of each alcoholic beverage do you drink?
* 8. When did you have your last drink?
* 9. When did you start your last drinking bout?
*10. What have you been drinking during this last drinking episode?
*11. How much alcohol did you consume each day during your last drinking episode?
*12. Has your drinking created problems for you in any of the following areas?
    □ With spouse   □ On the job
    □ With family   □ With children
    □ With friends
13. Have you ever been injured because of drinking? □ Yes □ No
    □ In fights   □ Auto accident
    □ Accidental fall   □ Other _____
14. Have you ever been arrested because of drinking? □ Yes □ No
    On what charge:
    □ DWI   □ Drunk in public
    □ Fights   □ Other (specify) _____
15. Have you ever been in prison or jail because of drinking? □ Yes □ No
16. What previous treatments have you had for alcohol problems?

    DATE   PLACE

    _____   _____

    _____   _____

SYMPTOMS RELATED TO GASTROINTESTINAL SYSTEM

*17. What have you been eating during this most recent drinking bout?
*18. What is your usual eating pattern?
    a. When not drinking:
    b. When drinking:
19. Have you had recent changes in appetite?
20. Have you had any recent weight changes?
21. Are you on a special diet?
22. What fluids do you drink other than alcohol? Kind of fluid and amount per day.
    □ Regular coffee   □ Tea
    □ Water   □ Decaffeinated coffee
    □ Juices   □ Milk
23. Do you have frequent irritation of your mouth and throat?
24. Are you having pain in your stomach?
25. Are you bothered by heartburn or gas?
*26. Are you nauseated?
*27. Are you vomiting or having dry heaves?
*28. Have you ever vomited blood? If yes, when?
*29. Have you ever had stomach ulcers or other stomach problems?
30. How frequently and for what reason do you use aspirin?
31. What medications do you use to relieve stomach pain?
32. Are you having pain in your abdomen?
33. Are you having diarrhea or constipation?
34. Do you have hemorrhoids?
35. Have you had bleeding from your bowels?
36. Have you noted a change in the color of your stool?
    □ Clay colored
    □ Bright red
    □ Black

*Indicates questions providing important information for a quick survey of intoxicated patients.

Continued.

Modified from Estes, N.J., and Heinemann, M.E.: Alcoholism: development, consequences, and interventions, ed. 2, St. Louis, 1982, The C.V. Mosby Co.

Nursing History Tool for Use with Clients with Alcohol Problems, cont'd

37. What problems have you had in the past with your bowels?

38. What medications do you use to relieve abdominal or bowel pains?

39. Have you ever had problems with your pancreas?

*40. Has your skin or the white of your eyes ever turned yellow?

*41. Have you ever had problems with your liver?

*42. Do you have diabetes? If yes, what medication do you take?

SYMPTOMS RELATING TO NEUROLOGICAL SYSTEM

43. Have you noticed any change in the amount of alcohol it takes to get the effect you desire? If yes, describe the change.

*44. What reactions occur when you stop drinking?
- Tremors
- Hear or see things
- DTs
- Other
- Seizures

*45. Have you ever taken Dilantin or any other drug for seizures?

46. Have you ever experienced a period of time you don't remember when drinking?

47. Have you experienced tingling, pain, or numbness in hands or feet?

48. Have you experienced muscle pain in your legs or arms?

*49. Are you experiencing any difficulty in keeping your balance?

*50. Are you experiencing any difficulty with your vision?

51. Do you have problems with your sleep? If yes, describe.

52. How many hours do you usually sleep?
- When sober
- When drinking

53. Do you feel rested after a night's sleep?

54. What do you do when you are unable to sleep?

55. Have you noticed any recent changes in your sex life? If yes, describe.

SYMPTOMS RELATING TO CARDIOVASCULAR AND PULMONARY SYSTEMS

*56. Do you have heart trouble? If yes, describe.

*57. Do you have swelling of the hands and feet?

*58. Do you have shortness of breath?

*59. Do you have chest pain?

*60. Are you taking any medication for heart disease?

61. Have you had pneumonia?

62. Have you ever had tuberculosis? If yes, are you taking any medication for it?

63. Do you have frequent infections (e.g., colds, flu, boils, sores that don't heal quickly)?

64. Do you have a chronic cough? If yes, describe.

65. Have you ever coughed up blood or phlegm?

66. Describe any other lung problems you have had.

67. Do you smoke? If yes, how many packs a day?

PSYCHOSOCIAL STATUS

68. What is your marital status?

69. With whom do you live?

70. Does this person have alcoholism or use alcohol regularly? □ Yes □ No

71. To whom do you feel close?

72. Do your neighbors, relatives, and/or friends use alcohol regularly? □ Yes □ No

73. How many children do you have?

74. How often do you see your children?

75. Describe the place you live.
Type of residence (i.e., house, apartment, room, etc.)
Cooking facilities
Number of stairs
Availability and type of transportation

76. Have you had mental or emotional problems?
- Depression
- Nervousness (anxiety)
- Loneliness
- Suicidal attempt
- Other _____

77. Are you currently involved in a counseling program?

*78. Are you currently taking medication for emotional problems? If yes, describe.

79. Are you actively affiliated with a religious group?

80. What is your current employment status?

81. Do you have some special job skills?

82. If employed, how does this period of treatment affect your employement?

83. If unemployed, what is your current source of income?

84. What hobbies or special interests do you have?

85. How do you spend a typical day at home?

Nursing History Tool for Use with Clients with Alcohol Problems, cont'd

DRUG TAKING OTHER THAN ALCOHOL

*86. What drugs do you take that you haven't mentioned?

Prescribed drugs _____

_____

Over-the-counter drugs _____

_____

Drugs obtained on the street _____

_____

*87. What is your usual manner of taking drugs?
   ☐ As directed
   ☐ Less than directed
   ☐ More than directed

*88. Are you allergic to any drugs?

FINAL QUESTIONS

89. What are your ideas for managing your drinking when you leave this agency?

90. Are there any further comments you would like to make?

91. Are there any questions you would like to ask?

Write a summary of the nursing history interview.

1. Describe your overall impressions of the client (mood, attitude, intelligence, ability to relate, social skills, general physical and emotional health, level of orientation, reliability of information given).

2. List all the problems identified in order of priority.

3. Suggest a plan of action for each problem identified.

Planning and Implementation

In the planning stage, long- and short-term goals are established and priorities are set for the care of the client with a substance abuse problem. Often the long-range goal is to establish a pattern of abstinence from the substance, but because physiological and psychological dependence is not easily broken, short-term goals must be realistic and individualized for the client. The nurse should recognize that psychological dependence may be transferred to a different drug or substance, particularly if the client has chronically abused the substance as a coping mechanism for daily stresses or as an escape mechanism. Goals should include all the client's dimensions. For example, the long-range goals for an alcoholic client might be complete cessation of drinking and restoration of prealcoholic functioning in family and work roles. Short-term goals might include learning stress management techniques, participating in a therapy program in an agency or community setting, establishing a balanced diet to correct nutritional deficits, and interventions for the physiological symptoms of alcohol withdrawal.

Priorities are set for the goals according to individualized client needs. The withdrawal syndrome of some drugs may be physiologically life threatening, or depression or anxiety may potentially lead to life-threatening behaviors. In some cases emotional support to meet the client's safety and security needs may be as critical as interventions directed toward physiological needs. Modification of goals is an ongoing process when providing care.

A wide range of interventions may be needed to address all the client's needs. With any intervention, however, the nurse-client relationship is usually a critical factor in the client's compliance. If a client begins to lose hope of being able to solve the problem or feels that no one cares whether he is successful, he may retreat to his chronic pattern of coping with such feelings by again abusing the substance. A supportive, empathetic relationship can help minimize the stresses of withdrawal and help the client continue to work with a hopeful attitude toward long-term goals.

Interventions for clients with physiological dependence generally include medical interventions, such as treatments for withdrawal, and referrals to specialized therapy programs such as alcohol treatment centers and group therapy programs. The following types of interventions are generally within the domain of nursing practice:

1. Interventions for abusive behaviors
2. Acute care interventions
3. Teaching
4. Counseling
5. Support system building
6. Family interventions
7. Community resources and referrals

Other types of interventions as described in other chapters may also be used, such as stress management techniques (Chapter 5), self-concept interventions (Chapter 18), interventions for altered sexuality (Chapter 19), and nutritional interventions (Chapter 38).

TABLE 45-3

Examples of Nursing Diagnoses Related to Substance Abuse

Problem	Cause
PHYSIOLOGICAL	
Sleep disturbance	Related to chronic amphetamine abuse
Physiological dependence on morphine	Related to chronic use for pleasure
Nutritional deficits	Related to insufficient dietary intake while drinking
Altered bowel motility	Related to chronic use of laxatives
Chronic respiratory infection	Related to cigarette smoking
Muscle weakness and pain	Related to chronic alcohol abuse
Altered gastrointestinal functioning	Related to withdrawal from antianxiety drugs
Risk of physical injury	Related to substance overdose
PSYCHOSOCIAL	
Low self-esteem	Related to guilt feelings for emotionally neglecting children because of drinking habits
Anxiety for fetal health	Related to smoking and alcohol use in first trimester
Decreased motivation and academic performance	Related to psychological dependence on marijuana
Anxiety about work role	Related to absences because of alcohol withdrawal syndrome
Altered family functioning	Related to binge drinking patterns of both parents
Social isolation	Related to physiological dependence on barbiturates
Depression	Related to past inability to stop drinking

INTERVENTIONS FOR ABUSIVE BEHAVIORS

When a client enters a health care facility in an intoxicated or drugged state, the nurse often falls victim to the client's verbal abuse and attempts at manipulation. The client should not be held responsible for his behavior, since the substance's effects often cause paranoia, fear, and anger. The verbal attacks on a nurse may simply be a client's expression of self-hatred related to the substance abuse. The challenge nurses face in such circumstances is to keep themselves and their clients in an emotional balance. Too often nurses react to the client's abuses and become angry and resentful. Eventually the nurse's interventions become ineffective because of an inability to provide care with understanding and compassion.

When a client makes critical remarks about the nurse's personality or appearance, such as height, weight, or other distinguishing characteristic, the nurse should not become upset. The client may needle or insult the nurse in an attempt to arouse the nurse's anger, pity, or fear. If the nurse reacts emotionally, the client's verbal attacks are likely to continue. A neutral response by the nurse discourages the client from continuing such manipulative efforts. If the client makes a sexual advance toward the nurse, it is better for the nurse to ignore it and instead direct the client's attention to the present situation, including the reason why he is in the nursing unit or the type of care he will receive. The nurse must have a high level of self-esteem in such cases to be able to ignore the client's physical, mental, or emotional harassment.

It is important also for the nurse to take time out occasionally from caring for abusive clients. A coffee or lunch break helps relieve developing emotional tension. The nurse must remember that the client's abusiveness is the result of intoxication and illness, not the client's personality.

ACUTE CARE INTERVENTIONS

Acute care interventions, which depend on the client's current health status and on the body systems affected by the substance, often involve medical interventions, physiological supportive measures, and a variety of nursing interventions. Emergency therapies may be required in cases of alcoholic coma caused by acute intoxication, hepatic coma related to liver malfunctioning, or trauma caused by falls or accidents while under a drug's effects. Emergency treatments may include the administration of narcotic antagonists for opiate overdose, safety measures in cases of acute toxic psychosis, treatment for respiratory or cardiac depression, or treatment for withdrawal syndromes. In most cases the specific substance that resulted in the acute condition must first be identified, followed by a physical assessment and appropriate diagnostic tests.

In acute situations, nursing and medical care generally focuses on physiological problems. As the initial crisis passes, interventions continue to address physiological problems but increasingly include interventions for the client's psychosocial needs, as described in the following sections.

TEACHING AND COUNSELING

Often a primary nursing role is to provide information about the potential physiological and psychological effects of substance abuse and the effects of withdrawal for the substance-dependent client. Such information should stress positive aspects rather than attempt to frighten the client into changing abuse habits. Portraying in grisly terms the physiological condition of lung cancer, for example, will likely cause stress for the chronic cigarette smoker that may increase rather than decrease the person's desire to smoke. Instead, the nurse can provide information about the success rate of an available treatment program. Other teaching activities include stress management techniques and self-care activities for hygiene, nutrition, and other areas affected by the substance abuse.

Counseling clients with a substance abuse problem often requires specialized experience and skills related to the particular substance. A referral to a qualified health professional is generally appropriate, although the nurse may continue to provide other kinds of care for the client and may engage in counseling activities concurrently. Counseling often follows a pattern based on the extent of the client's problem. The goals of counseling, for example, may be first to assist the client in recognizing and accepting the problem, then in adapting to stresses and other problems associated with the abuse or withdrawal (the client's family may be counseled in this regard), and finally in adapting to a nondependent life-style following successful withdrawal.

SUPPORT SYSTEMS

Support from family members, friends, and others is often valuable in assisting a person with a substance abuse problem. Such support can be important at any stage, from accepting the problem to learning to live with new coping mechanisms after successful rehabilitation. Helping the client to build a social support system may include family counseling, referral to a self-help group, and other interventions such as those for altered self-concept (see Chapter 18) that can assist the client in adapting positively to interactions with others.

FAMILY INTERVENTIONS

Earlier sections have discussed the potential effects of substance abuse on other family members. Nursing interventions may be required for individual members or for the family as a whole. Family functioning is also affected by the adjustment process of a parent's or spouse's withdrawal or rehabilitation. Because any kind of family health problem may be precipitated or heightened by substance abuse, the nurse assesses and may intervene in substance abuse–related family problems much as with the similar problems in families without substance abuse problems (see Chapter 22). Interventions for family members include teaching and counseling, values clarification about substance abuse, stress management techniques, interventions adapted to the developmental needs of children, development of support systems, and referral to agencies or self-help groups specializing in family programs.

COMMUNITY PROGRAMS

In many communities there are a range of substance withdrawal and other therapy programs to which the nurse can refer the client. Alcoholics Anonymous (AA) is a self-help group that assists alcoholics through mutual support to acknowledge the problem and work toward solving it. Similar support groups are Al-Anon, an organization for spouses and relatives of alcoholics, and Alateen, for children and adolescents who have an alcoholic parent. In addition, many inpatient or outpatient alcoholism clinics offer treatment programs independently or in association with hospitals or community mental health centers. As with alcoholism, specialized drug treatment programs offer counseling, health education, and medical services such as methadone maintenance or withdrawal programs for narcotic abusers. Other types of community resources include employee programs within businesses and industries and programs provided by student health clinics in colleges and other schools.

Substance abuse prevention programs are becoming more prominent in community health settings such as schools and mental health clinics. The primary focus of preventive programs is to provide drug education, strengthen family functioning, improve social conditions, and assist individuals in the areas of interpersonal skills and self-esteem. Such a focus helps minimize or eliminate factors that may lead to the abuse of substances as a coping or escape mechanism. On the individual level the nurse can also initiate preventive interventions, such as educating the client about drugs, promoting effective coping mechanisms, and providing support.

The nurse is responsible for knowing about community programs and other resources to which to refer the client. Equally important, however, is the appropriateness of any particular program for an individual client. With full knowledge of available resources and assessment data concerning the client's total needs, the nurse, client, and family can most effectively explore possibilities to choose the program most appropriate for the client.

Evaluation

Evaluation of nursing care for clients with substance abuse problems is based on goals of care and expected outcomes. The evaluation process, like the setting of goals, must be realistic and avoid unreasonable hopes, such as expecting a psychologically dependent client to achieve abstinence overnight. Often a more important criterion is that the client makes significant progress toward long-term goals. Other evaluation criteria typically include gaining increased self-esteem, learning to use more effective coping mechanisms and internal resources when confronted by stress, and forming behavioral patterns and activities that replace substance-related behaviors.

The client must be involved in evaluation. Even if the nurse evaluates the client's progress as satisfactory, the client may return to former habits if he has unrealistically high personal goals and thus views his progress with frustration. By involving the client and family in evaluation, the nurse can provide further support, reinforcement, and reassurance. Evaluation may also reveal the need for changes in the nursing care plan.

Summary

Substance abuse takes a variety of forms and may be encountered by the nurse in any setting. Because substance abuse affects the client in all dimensions, the nurse should be alert to both actual and potential health problems associated with abuse patterns. Although any person at any age and in any life situation may become physiologically or psychologically dependent on a drug or substance, including nurses and other health professionals, certain groups may be more susceptible to the problem of abuse at certain developmental stages. The client's family may also be affected in a variety of ways, and the nurse should include the family in the total plan of care.

The nurse's choice of the appropriate interventions for the client with a substance abuse problem depends on both the causative variables and the client's individual health status. Because society is increasingly aware of substance abuse as a health problem, it carries less stigma than in the past, and individuals with abuse problems are now more likely to seek help before physiological problems bring them to the attention of health care professionals. With increasing societal recognition of the problem has come a wider variety of support and treatment services, including prevention programs. Substance abuse remains a sensitive area for many clients, however, and the nurse needs to be particularly aware of communication skills and other aspects of the nurse-client relationship when providing care to clients experiencing the wide range of psychosocial stresses commonly associated with substance abuse.

KEY CONCEPTS

✓ Any substance that produces physiological or psychological effects can potentially be misused or abused.

✓ Substance abuse is the indiscriminate, usually chronic abuse of a substance to the extent that the person's physiological and psychosocial functioning is impaired.

✓ The major groups of abused drugs include alcohol, narcotics, sedative-hypnotics, tranquilizers, central nervous system sympathomimetics, hallucinogens, inhalants, and nonprescription substances, each of which produces distinct psychological and physiological effects.

✓ Substance abusers are more likely to experience health problems as a result of drug interactions.

✓ Many psychosocial variables have a causative role in substance abuse, including pleasure-seeking and problem-solving or avoidance behaviors, personality factors, sociocultural factors, and stressors.

✓ No one cause or set of causes affects all or most persons who abuse a substance.

KEY CONCEPTS, cont'd

✓ To facilitate the therapeutic relationship and work toward solving the problems of substance abuse, both the client and the nurse should be aware of their attitudes toward the abused substance and the causes of the abuse.

✓ The course of substance abuse varies but typically progresses from social misuse or experimentation through a gradually increasing pattern of abuse to a state of dependence in which all aspects of the person's life are affected.

✓ Substance abuse affects family functioning, roles, and responsibilities, often with seriously detrimental psychosocial effects on spouse and children.

✓ Causative variables in substance abuse vary among developmental stages, as do the effects of the abuse, and therefore a developmental perspective should be included when the client's abuse problem is assessed.

✓ The fetus is susceptible to the effects of substance abuse by the mother.

✓ Certain patterns of substance abuse are more common in particular groups sharing common stresses.

✓ Nurses and other health professionals are highly susceptible to abuse problems and need to be aware of how such problems can develop and what interventions may be necessary.

✓ The assessment of a client with a substance abuse problem may include a tactfully obtained history, observation of behaviors linked to substance abuse, and a complete psychosocial and physical assessment.

✓ Nursing diagnoses for clients with abuse problems identify needs for physiological support as well as problems involving stress, interpersonal conflicts, altered work or family roles, and self-concept deficits.

✓ Interventions may address the client's needs in all dimensions and may include acute care, teaching and counseling, support systems, family interventions, and the use of community resources.

✓ Evaluation of the care of substance abusers should be based on realistic goals and often focuses on day-to-day progress toward long-term goals rather than on the expectation that the client will immediately overcome the problems associated with abuse.

REFERENCES

Estes, N.J., Smith-DiJulio, K., and Heinemann, M.E., editors: Nursing diagnosis of the alcoholic person, St. Louis, 1980, The C.V. Mosby Co.

Hahn, A.B., Barkin, R.L., and Oestreich, S.J.K.: Pharmacology in nursing, ed. 15, St. Louis, 1982, The C.V. Mosby Co.

Smith, J.W.: Fetal alcohol syndrome: a tragic and preventable disorder. In Estes, N.J., and Heinemann, M.E., editors: Alcoholism: development, consequences, and interventions, ed. 2, St. Louis, 1982, The C.V. Mosby Co.

ADDITIONAL READINGS

Cody, B.: Alcohol and other drug abuse among adolescents, Stat. Bull. Metropol. Life Insur. Co. 65(1):4, 1984.

Dusek, D., and Girdano, D.A.: Drugs: a factual account, Reading, Mass., 1980, Addison-Wesley Publishing Co., Inc.

Estes, N.J., and Heinemann, M.E.: Alcoholism: development, consequences, and interventions, ed. 2, St. Louis, 1982, The C.V. Mosby Co.

Freedman, A.M.: Opiate dependence. In Kaplan, H.I., Freedman, A.M., and Sadock, B.J.: Comprehensive textbook of psychiatry, ed. 3, Baltimore, 1980, The Williams & Wilkins Co.

Greene, M.H., et al.: Evolving patterns of drug abuse, Ann. Intern. Med. 83:402, 1975.

Hughes, R., and Brewin, R.: The tranquilizing of America: pill popping and the American way of life, New York, 1979, Harcourt Brace Jovanovich, Inc.

Isler, C.: The alcoholic nurse: what we try to deny, RN **41**:48, 1978.

Lawrence, F., et al.: Admitting an intoxicated patient, Am. J. Nurs. 84(5):617 1984.

Ray, O.: Drugs, society, and human behavior, ed. 3, St. Louis, 1983, The C.V. Mosby Co.

Yowell, S., and Brose, C.: Working with drug abuse patients in the ER, Am. J. Nurs. 77:82, 1977.

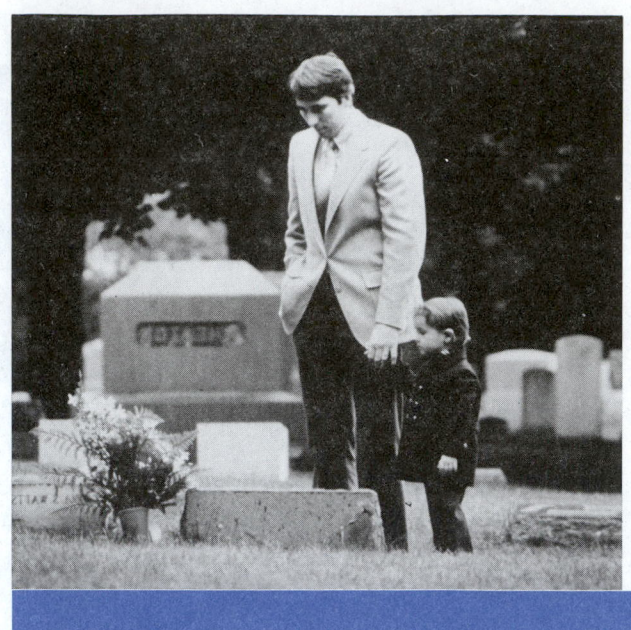

OBJECTIVES

Mastery of the content in this chapter will enable the student to:

- Define the terms in the glossary.
- Identify the nurse's role in assisting clients with problems related to loss, death, and grief.
- Describe and compare the three stages of grieving in Engel's theory and the five stages of Kübler-Ross's theory.
- List and discuss the five basic categories of loss.
- Perform an assessment of the client's grief response and relate it to the stages of the grieving process.
- Identify ways in which the loss reaction is influenced by growth and development, cultural and spiritual beliefs, sex roles, relationships with significant others, and socioeconomic status.
- Describe behavioral patterns useful as assessment criteria for the grieving client.
- Compare and contrast grief after loss, anticipatory grief, and resolved grief.
- Give at least five examples of nursing diagnoses related to grief.
- Implement interventions for grieving clients to provide therapeutic communication, maintain self-esteem, and promote a return to normal activities.
- Describe how the nurse helps meet the special needs of the dying client.
- List and discuss important factors in caring for the body after death.
- Describe criteria to evaluate nursing care for grieving and dying clients.

GLOSSARY

algor mortis Reduction in body temperature after death accompanied by loss of skin elasticity.

anticipatory grief Grief response in which the person begins the grieving process before an actual loss.

grief Form of sorrow involving the person's thoughts, feelings, and behaviors, occurring as a response to an actual or perceived loss.

grief work Adaptation process of mourning a loss, distress, disengagement, reinvestment, and resolution; parallel to the grieving process.

grieving process Sequence of affective, cognitive, and physiological states through which the person responds to and finally accepts an irretrievable loss.

livor mortis Purple discoloration of the skin in dependent body parts after death; results from red blood cell destruction.

maturational loss Loss, usually of an aspect of self, resulting from the normal changes of growth and development.

rigor mortis Stiffening of the body shortly after death because of the contraction of skeletal and smooth muscle.

situational loss Loss of a person, thing, or quality resulting from a change in a life situation, including changes related to illness, body image, environment, and death.

unresolved grief Severe chronic grief reaction in which the person does not complete the resolution stage of the grieving process within a reasonable time.

46 Loss, Death, and the Grieving Process

irth, loss, and death are universal phenomena and individually unique events of the human experience. A person experiences loss in the absence of an object, person, body part or function, or emotion that was formerly present. Losses may be actual or perceived. Actual losses are easily identified, as with the child who loses a favorite toy or whose playmate moves away, or the adult who loses the car keys or a marriage partner through divorce. Perceived losses are less tangible and are easily misunderstood, such as the loss of a person's confidence or the loss of prestige. The more the individual has invested of himself in that which is lost, the greater the feeling of loss. Loss may be maturational or situational or both. The child in learning to walk loses the infantlike body image, the woman experiencing menopause loses the ability to bear children, the man experiencing unemployment loses self-esteem, and the elderly person experiencing visual and hearing changes loses self-reliance.

Death in our culture is difficult for the dying person, as well as for the person's family, friends, and care givers. When a person becomes terminally ill, the people around him are reminded of their own mortality. Feelings of guilt, anger, and fear can cause family members and care givers to withdraw at a time when the dying person is in need of love, reassurance, and support. The style of dying is inherent in a person's style of living, and a person's attitudes about death depend on the systems of beliefs and emotional strengths that person brings to the task of dying.

It is common to hear the phrase "at a loss for words," which expresses the feeling of uncertainty or puzzlement experienced in a situation of loss. The way a person learns to deal with early losses in life affects his adaptation to subsequent losses. An individual brings to the present a repertoire of past behaviors, which intertwine and may help or hinder the process of coping with loss. Life is a series of losses and gains. The child beginning to walk loses dependence yet gains independence with mobility. The adolescent loses his childlike body image yet gains a measure of self-identity. The coping mechanisms a person learns throughout life have much to do with that person's resiliency and adaptability in facing a significant loss.

Grieving Process

A significant loss is one that is perceived by the individual as important to his total well-being. Whether the significant loss is actual or perceived, maturational or situational, it may result in the grieving process. Grief is a form of sorrow involving thoughts, feelings, and behaviors. The grieving person attempts a variety of strategies to cope with grief and sadness. In the past, our society discouraged openness in the grieving processes associated with life events. The unhappy child was told not to cry when his playmate moved away; the awkward adolescent was told not to be embarrassed about his sudden growth spurt; the dying person was told to remain calm and dignified in the face of death. Changes in societal attitudes, beliefs, and values have promoted more open expressions of grief. For example, nurses learn to seek support from peers in expressing their concerns about dealing with clients in a terminal stage of illness. Similarly, family members seek support from care givers to express their anger and fear over loss of a loved one. Grieving can lead to new understanding that can promote growth. Through openness, the encouragement of others, and adequate support systems, the grieving person can learn and grow from experiences of loss.

Loss, Death, Grief, and Nursing

The nurse needs to understand the phenomena of loss, death, and grief. Nursing by its very nature is involved in all of the processes of life from birth to death. The nurse interacts daily with clients and families experiencing loss and grief. At the same time, the nurse is experiencing personal loss as the client-family-nurse relationship ends through transfer, discharge, recovery, or death of the client. The nurse is accustomed to dealing with the biological and physical aspects of a client's care. The nurse may find it easy and nonthreatening to relieve physical symptoms associated with illness and death, but becoming involved in meaningful interpersonal relationships to support a person who is suffering or dying is difficult. The nurse's own feelings, values, and experiences influence the extent to which she can support clients and families during a loss or death. Self-assessment—exploring personal attitudes, feelings, and values—is necessary before the nurse can use a sensitive, therapeutic approach with others. The development of the art of being with the grieving and dying requires an inner strength that arises from the nurse's positive belief in herself. Formulation of a personal philosophy of life will help the nurse function during difficult times. A knowledge of the concepts of loss and the grieving process will enable the nurse to use creative interventions to promote health, prevent illness, and support dying clients.

Concepts and Theories of the Grieving Process

The behaviors and feelings associated with the grieving process occur in individuals suffering such losses as a physical deformity or the death of a close friend, as well as in individuals facing their own death. Both the person undergoing the loss and the significant others in that person's life experience grief. The concept and theories of grief are tools for the nurse who must anticipate the emotional needs of clients and families and plan interventions to help them understand their grief and deal effectively with it. These concepts and theories are not a panacea for dealing

with dying clients. A dying person should not be stereotyped as experiencing a certain phase of grief. All those involved in the care of the dying individual will experience different aspects of the grieving process at different times. The nurse's role is to assess grieving behaviors, recognize how grief is influencing each person's behavior, and provide appropriate empathetic support.

Fairbairn's object relation theory (1963) provides a framework for understanding how individuals become attached to or detached from other persons, places, things, or ideas. The theory of object relations has two major components: object attachment and object detachment. Both components involve the investment of feelings in varying degrees. Object loss is described as an internal state through which the individual determines the significance of the loss and chooses to retain the internal image, displace the internal image with a substitute, or resolve the internal image. Object resolution can be compared to the grieving process in that there is gradual diminishing of attachment to the internal image. The loss is remembered, but with time the emotional investment lessens and new investments occur without substitution. Through the grieving process the individual accepts the loss and its finality and adjusts to the situation.

Groves (1978) defines grief as the sequence of affective, cognitive, and physiological states that directly follows an irretrievable loss. The classic works of Engle (1964) and Kübler-Ross (1969) provide a framework for understanding the dynamics of the grieving process. Each theory proposes that the grieving process has distinct phases or stages (Table 46-1). The term "grief work," applied to the mourning process, involves somatic distress, disengagement, and reinvestment through resolution of the loss. The phase theory of the grieving process is helpful in understanding the concept of grief. Each of the frameworks, which are usually applied to grieving persons, is also applicable to dying persons. Engle's framework is process oriented and incorporates three steps: shock and disbelief, developing awareness, and reorganization and restitution.

In step one the individual denies the reality of the loss and may withdraw from family and friends, sit motionless, or wander aimlessly. It may seem to observers that the full impact has not hit the person. Initial physical reactions may include fainting, diaphoresis, nausea, diarrhea, rapid heart rate, restlessness, insomnia, and fatigue. In stage two, the individual begins to feel the loss acutely and may experience desperation. Suddenly the emotions of anger, guilt, frustration, depression, and emptiness occur. Engle (1964) believes that crying is typical in this

TABLE 46-1

Comparison of Two Approaches for Coping with Grief or Dying

Engle (1964)	Kübler-Ross (1969)
Shock and disbelief	Denial
	Anger
Developing awareness	Bargaining
	Depression
Reorganization and restitution	Acceptance

stage as the individual becomes preoccupied with the loss. Crying seems to involve "both an acknowledgement of the loss and the regression to a more helpless and childlike status" (Engle, 1964). In stage three the inevitability of the loss is acknowledged and there is no longer a need for anger or depression. The loss is clear to the individual, and he begins to reorganize his life. By experiencing the three steps a person moves from a low to a higher level of emotional and intellectual integration and the development of a new self-awareness.

The framework provided by Kübler-Ross (1969) is behavior oriented and includes five stages: denial, anger, bargaining, depression, and acceptance. In the denial stage the individual acts as though nothing has happened and may refuse to believe or understand that a loss has occurred. Statements such as "No, that can't be so," and "It can't be happening to me!" are common. In the anger stage the individual resists the loss and may "act out" to everyone and everything in his environment. In the bargaining stage there is postponement of the reality of the loss. The individual may attempt to make a deal in a subtle or overt way to prevent the loss from occurring. Thoughts such as "I have to hold on until John graduates," or "After Mary's wedding is over, I can face this" are common. Frequently the client seeks the opinions of others during the bargaining stage. A hospitalized client may show model behavior because he is convinced the staff will make him well if he is a "good patient." The depression stage occurs when the loss is realized and the full impact of its significance is apparent. This fourth stage may be accompanied by overwhelming feelings of loneliness and withdrawal from interactions with others. The depression stage provides an opportunity to work through the loss and begin the process of problem solving. In the fifth stage acceptance is reached. Physiological reactions cease and

social interactions resume. Kübler-Ross stresses that acceptance is coming to terms with the situation rather than resignation or hopelessness.

The phases a person experiences during grief or dying may not be concrete or easily identifiable. Grieving is a personal experience for each individual and his family. To be supportive of the client passing through the stages of grief at his own pace requires knowledge and understanding of the dynamics involved in the process. The nurse must be aware of the client's actual grief response rather than anticipate what responses should occur.

Categories of Loss

Personal loss is any significant loss that requires adaptation through the grieving process. Loss occurs when something or someone can no longer be seen, felt, heard, known, or experienced. The type of loss influences the degree of stress the person encounters. For example, it might be assumed that the loss of an object would not generate the same degree of stress

Losses Faced by the Chronically Ill

- Former good health
- Independence
- Sense of control over life
- Privacy
- Modesty
- Body image
- Relationships
- Established roles inside and outside the home
- Social status
- Sense of self-confidence
- Possessions
- Financial security
- Means of productivity and self-fulfillment in a job or at home
- Life-style
- Plans or fantasies for the future
- Fantasy of immortality
- Money
- Familiar daily routine
- Sleep
- Sexual functioning
- Leisure activities

Modified from Lewis, K.: J. Rehabil. **49**:8, 1983.

as the loss of a significant other. However, each individual responds to a given type of loss differently. The death of a family member would be expected to cause more stress than the loss of a pet. But for an elderly woman living alone, the death of a pet that has been a constant companion would likely cause more emotional stress than the death of a cousin the woman had not seen for years. The type of loss is significant to the grieving process, yet the nurse must recognize each person's unique interpretation of a loss.

There are five categories of loss: loss of external objects, loss of a known environment, loss of a significant other, loss of an aspect of self, and loss of life. Nurses may encounter clients who experience more than one type of loss. For the hospitalized chronically ill adult, Lewis (1983) describes numerous potential permanent losses (see boxed material). The losses a client faces threaten his self-concept, self-esteem, and sense of worth. The nurse must recognize the meaning each loss has to a client and the impact on the person's physical and psychological functioning.

Loss of External Objects

Loss of an external object involves any personal possession that is worn out, misplaced, stolen, or ruined by fire or natural disaster such as flood or hurricane. For a child the object may be a toy or a blanket; for an adult it may be a piece of jewelry or an article of clothing. The extent of grieving a person feels for a lost object depends on the object's material value, the sentiment the person attaches to the object, and the object's usefulness.

Loss of a Known Environment

The loss associated with separation from a known environment includes leaving a familiar setting for a short or long period or relocating permanently. Examples of this category of loss include moving to a new neighborhood or city, taking a new job, or hospitalization. Loss through separation from a known environment may occur through maturational or situational circumstances and through injury or illness.

When a person becomes hospitalized for an illness, confinement within an institution isolates him from routine life events. The rules and policies of a hospital create an environment that is often impersonal and demoralizing. The loneliness of an unfamiliar setting threatens a person's self-esteem and makes the process of grieving more difficult.

Loss of a Significant Other

A significant other may be anyone within the individual's constellation of family, friends, and acquaintances. Persons identified as significant others include parents, spouses, children, siblings, teachers, clergy, friends, neighbors, and work associates. In our society entertainment figures and well-known athletes may be significant others for young people. Research shows that many people regard pets as significant others. Loss of significant others occurs as a result of separation, moving, running away, promotion at work, and death.

Loss of an Aspect of Self

The loss of an aspect of self may include the loss of a body part, a physiological function, or a psychological function. Such a loss lessens the individual's well-being. Physical loss includes loss of a body part such as a limb, an eye, hair, teeth, or a breast. Loss of physiological function includes loss of urinary or bowel control, mobility, strength, or sensory function. Loss of psychological function includes loss of memory, humor, self-esteem, self-confidence, power, respect, or love. Illness, injury, or developmental and situational changes result in loss of an aspect of self. A person not only experiences grief over his loss but may experience permanent changes in body image and self-concept (see Chapter 18).

Loss of Life

A person facing death lives until the moment of death, feeling, thinking, and responding to the events and people around him. Frequently a person's concern is not about death itself but about pain and loss of control. Each person responds differently to impending death. For the aged who have lived alone and suffered long terminal illness, death sometimes comes as a relief. Some people perceive death not as a loss but as an entry into an afterlife to be reunited with loved ones in paradise. Others experience fear of dying and displace the emotion to other sources of anxiety such as fear of separation, abandonment, loneliness, or mutilation. The threat of death often causes individuals to become dependent. The helplessness and shame that accompany dependence create a challenge for the nurse whose goal is to meet the dying client's needs.

■ ■ ■ ■ ■

The nurse cannot assume, based on her own values, feelings, or experiences, that she understands the significance any loss has for a client. Many variables affect a person's reaction to loss, including the person's stage of growth and development. The nurse must assess the effect of the loss on the client and family and validate her assessment with them before initiating nursing interventions to assist in the grieving process.

Assessment of the Grieving Client

Assessment of the grieving client begins with exploration of the meaning of the loss through collection of objective and subjective data. By listening, open communication, and alertness to nonverbal cues, the nurse can draw inferences from the client's responses and behavior. These inferences must then be validated with the client to develop a diagnosis and plan effective interventions. The grieving process may be viewed as a sequence of responses and behaviors. An understanding of this sequence is beneficial for planning appropriate nursing interventions.

A major consideration for the nurse in assessing grieving is not how the individual should be reacting but how he is actually reacting. The sequences or stages may occur in order, a stage may be skipped totally, or a stage may recur. Through the assessment process the nurse must consider the many variables affecting the client's reaction to loss and progression through the stages of grief.

Factors Influencing a Loss Reaction
GROWTH AND DEVELOPMENT

A person's stage of growth and development plays a role in the recognition and reaction to loss. The infant is not generally considered able to understand the concepts of loss and death. Loss, separation, and death have little meaning to an infant until he is able to recognize familiar persons, form an attachment to a consistent care giver, usually the mother, and demonstrate anxiety concerning strangers. Once a bond of trust forms between parent and child, even a temporary loss can cause profound anxiety and resistance in the child.

A toddler's cognition is still not sufficiently developed to permit understanding of death. The child's self-centeredness and difficulty in separating fact from fantasy prevent him from comprehending an absence of life. The toddler experiences anxiety over loss of objects, such as a favorite toy, and separation from parents or the familiar setting of his home.

The preschooler has heard the word "death" and perceives it as a kind of sleep or temporary departure. Since the preschooler's concept of time is immature, he does not comprehend the finality of death. A preschooler strongly identifies with the parent of the opposite sex and may wish to take the place of the same-sex parent. This Oedipus or Electra complex eventually resolves, with the child identifying with the role of the same-sex parent. However, if the same-sex parent dies during the child's unresolved psychosexual conflict, the preschooler may feel guilt and shame over the parent's death.

School-age children are very aware of their bodies and will suffer a sense of grief over loss of a body part or function. At this age children are conscious of differences or abnormalities in themselves and others and are strongly affected by such a loss. The school-age child associates misdeeds or bad thoughts with causing death and may feel intense guilt over loss of a significant other. Unlike younger children, however, the school-age child is able to understand logical explanations about death. The child's concept of death is one of destruction. At the age of 6 or 7 years the child associates death with "ghosts" or "evil spirits." By the age of 9 or 10 the child recognizes the universality of death. The child may acquire an unusual fear of the unknown when a death in the family occurs or when the child faces a terminal illness.

For the adolescent physical attributes and strength are essential for a healthy self-concept. The adolescent experiences acute grief when loss of a body part or function occurs. The adolescent fears rejection by peers and views such a loss as interfering with plans for the future. Adolescents have an adult comprehension of the concept of death, yet they are the least likely of any age group to accept the loss of life, particularly their own. The rejection of death is related to the adolescent's developmental task of establishing an identity and purpose in life.

The young adult relates loss to its significance for status, role, and life-style. A loss of job or economic well-being, divorce, or a physical impairment causes considerable grief and threatens the adult's efforts for success in life. A young adult's concept of death is largely a product of religious and cultural beliefs. The death of a young adult is perceived as especially tragic by society, since it represents the loss of a life not yet fully lived.

During middle age a person begins to realize that youthfulness and physical fitness cannot be taken for granted. The middle-aged adult begins to reexamine his life to consider what options are available to gain fulfillment. The person becomes sensitive to the physical changes of aging. Any loss in physical function can create grief. Middle-aged people usually associate actively with friends, since their children are at an age to marry and move away. Loss of significant others creates a significant threat to the middle-aged person's life-style. The career-oriented adult has usually reached a peak professionally or occupationally. Any loss of job or ability to perform a job will cause considerable grief. The middle-aged adult knows that time is at a premium and life is finite. Commonly adults take time to consider what the remainder of life will be like and how death will occur.

The elderly experience anticipatory grief as a result of the physical changes accompanying aging and the fear of losing capabilities for self-care. The loss of independence is perhaps the greatest source of grief in the elderly. In contrast to the stereotypical view, most elderly people are able to meet their own needs and continue socializing with family and significant others. The way an elderly person reacts to death is a reflection of his sense of fulfillment and the contributions made to others. Whether an elderly person can accept death depends on personality traits, feelings of self-worth, and the amount of functional ability retained. The aged often fear the events surrounding death more than death itself and may perceive loneliness, isolation, loss of social role, prolonged illness, and loss of self-determination and dignity as more frightening than death (Gonda, 1971; McGrory, 1978).

CULTURAL AND SPIRITUAL BELIEFS

Values, attitudes, beliefs, and customs are cultural aspects of a person's life-style that influence the reaction to loss, grief, and death. The expression of grief generally emanates from a person's cultural background and family dynamics. Culture influences each person in a different way, and it is essential that the client's uniqueness be considered rather than grouping or stereotyping by cultural or ethnic origins. Expectations of how a person should react and behave in situations of loss are learned throughout life. Chapter 21 explores the overall aspects of culture and ethnicity and stresses the need for self-assessment by the nurse to provide a model for the assessment of clients' values and attitudes and to avoid judgmental or prejudicial reactions. Not only should the nurse be aware of the grieving client's cultural background and how it influences his behavior, but she should also explore his strengths and weaknesses in relation to cultural influences. The nurse should recognize that the grief reaction expressed may not be indicative of the client's true feelings but rather the expression expected by his culture.

Spiritual or religious beliefs include practices, rites, and rituals directed toward loss experiences and the grieving process. Individuals may find solace and meaning in losses through the spiritual dimension. Frequently a grieving person turns to religion for strength and support. The nurse should be alert to the significance of religious practices and rituals, not only for the client but for the family as well. By words and actions the nurse can indicate a sensitivity to the spiritual needs of grieving clients and families. Through openness in responses, the nurse can verify who or what sustains the client and family and plan appropriate interventions. For example, members of the Jewish faith remain at a dying person's bedside to witness death and be assured everything possible was done. If a dying client is Catholic, a priest must perform last rites to ensure the person's resurrection. The nurse must be familiar with the client's and family members' beliefs about rituals surrounding death because the nurse usually has the most contact with a dying client and his family.

For some clients the experience of loss triggers a questioning attitude regarding the meaning of life, personal values, and beliefs. Typically this attitude is demonstrated by the "why me?" response. Internal conflict concerning religious beliefs and practices may occur. The nurse should assess spirituality in her own life and cultivate an awareness of the spiritual dimension for each client and family. Data collection includes clues given by the client about his religious beliefs, which must be validated by the nurse.

SEX ROLES

How an individual reacts to loss is influenced by the social expectations of the male and female roles. In our society it is generally more difficult for men to express grief openly than for women. The nurse must be alert to this and verify with the client feelings and reactions and the personal meaning attached to a loss. Men and women attach different significance to body parts, functions, interpersonal relationships, and objects. The nurse should assess her thoughts and feelings in regard to sex roles and consider these influences as she relates to clients. The nurse should ask herself what her expectations are about how a man or woman should react to a significant loss, and if she expects a woman to cry and a man to be strong and supportive. By being aware of her own values the nurse can be open to the possibilities for each individual, regardless of sex roles and social expectations.

RELATIONSHIPS WITH SIGNIFICANT OTHERS

The relationship one has with a significant other will influence how that person grieves when the significant other dies or suffers a loss. For example, a husband's grief over the death of his wife may be greater than that over the death of a parent because of the impact the wife's death has on the husband's life-style and relationship. When a parent's only child suffers a loss of function of a body part, the grief may be greater than if the child was one of several children. The nurse should assess the quality of relationships between significant others to determine the grief a loss may cause. The nurse determines whether the individuals provide support for one another, if there is a common understanding of each person's needs, and how the client's significant other reacts when the client experiences a loss.

Hampe (1975) conducted a study concerning needs of spouses when attempting to cope with their mate's impending death. The spouse's needs identified include the following:

1. Need to be with the dying person
2. Need to be helpful to the dying person
3. Need for assurance of the spouse's comfort
4. Need to be informed of the spouse's condition
5. Need to be informed of the impending death
6. Need to ventilate emotions
7. Need for comfort and support of family members
8. Need for acceptance, support, and comfort from health professionals

The nurse who is able to anticipate a spouse's or significant other's needs during loss and grief is better equipped to provide emotional support. The nurse must also communicate with physicians to obtain the information sought by spouses or families about their loved one's condition.

SOCIOECONOMIC STATUS

Loss is a universal phenomenon, experienced by all individuals regardless of socioeconomic status. The poor react to loss in the same way as the rich, the middle class in the same way as the poor. Emotional investment is not tied to one's "station in life" but is experienced by everyone. However, assessment of the client's socioeconomic status is essential because it influences the family's ability to utilize resources and available support mechanisms in coping with the loss. The family's financial resources determine their op-

tions in dealing with a loss. In all instances the nurse can identify available options and provide information about resources.

Assessment of Grief Stage

Assessment of the client and family also includes consideration of the stages of grief. By observing behavior the nurse draws inferences regarding the effects of the loss. The nurse carefully assesses the existence of unique individual, family, and situational characteristics such as the relationship of spouses or the events leading to the loss. It may be possible on the basis of careful observations and nurse-client interactions for the nurse to predict the nature of grief resolution.

No two people grieve in exactly the same way. However, grieving patterns have been researched and documented and are observable in persons experiencing significant loss. A person in Engle's shock stage of grief will display significantly different behaviors than a person experiencing the stage of developing awareness (Table 46-2). A client moves back and forth between the stages of grief until final resolution occurs. The ability to recognize behaviors characteristic of grieving will help the nurse formulate nursing diagnoses and identify appropriate means of communicating with and providing support for clients and their families. The box on p. 1312 lists characteristics of dysfunctional grief for an actual or perceived loss.

Assessment of a Dying Person's Grief

The meaning of death varies widely for individuals as a result of numerous variables, including the setting in which death occurs. Most nurses care for dying

TABLE 46-2

Behaviors Common to Stages of Grieving

Stage of Grief	Behaviors
Shock and disbelief	Emotionally denies loss occurred; intellectually can accept loss but does not comprehend implications; withdraws from social interactions; is preoccupied with image of lost object or person; seems to stare or move about aimlessly; has difficulty carrying out normal daily activities; has somatic complaints including shortness of breath, choking, sighing, chills, anorexia, fatigue, faintness
Developing awareness	Begins to realize loss is real; experiences guilt, anger, frustration, depression, frequent episodes of crying
Reorganization and restitution	Accepts loss; desires to renew life and looks to the future; becomes interested in new objects and relationships; seeks pleasurable experiences; is able to talk about loss realistically

Characteristics of People Experiencing Dysfunctional Grief

- Verbal expression of distress at loss
- Denial of loss
- Expression of guilt
- Expression of unresolved issues
- Anger
- Sadness
- Crying
- Difficulty in expressing loss
- Alterations in eating habits
- Alterations in sleep
- Alterations in dream patterns
- Alterations in activity level
- Alterations in libido
- Idealization of the lost object
- Reliving of past experiences
- Interference with life functioning
- Developmental regression
- Labile affect
- Alterations in concentration and pursuit of tasks

clients in a hospital and thus are able to observe client behaviors toward staff members as well as families. It is important for the nurse to know what assessment criteria are appropriate for a dying client, since nursing therapies are very different from those for clients who will live.

The intensity of coping and the rate at which the client and family pass through the stages of grief are influenced by the time period between the client's first awareness that he is going to die and the actual moment of death. In an intensive care unit clients generally either recover or die quickly. The unit often has an aura of death. However, unless a chronic illness has been present, death is sudden and unexpected, and the client and family have little time for expressing grief. In contrast, in units for terminally ill clients the process of dying is usually gradual. Clients have time to go through all the stages of grief and generally can accept death with more grace and dignity.

A client experiences a variety of emotions depending on the stage of dying or grief (Table 46-3). The nurse must recognize that each emotion serves a purpose in helping the client cope with death. The nurse must not identify the client's grief stage on the basis of a single behavior or emotion displayed by the client. However, the client's responses determine the techniques used by the nurse to relate to the client. For example, in the acceptance stage of death the nurse can encourage a client to discuss his feelings about leaving family members behind. This approach

---

TABLE 46-3

Behaviors Representative of Kübler-Ross's Stages of Dying

Stage	Behaviors
Denial	Avoids reality, cannot deal with decisions about treatment; may attempt activities of which he is no longer physically capable; isolates self from sources of accurate information; fails to comply with medical therapy; uses considerable emotional energy to deny truth; may appear artificially happy
Anger	May retaliate against family members, nursing staff, or physicians; becomes demanding and accusing; anger may arouse guilt because client knows he depends on care givers; guilt may foster feelings of anxiety and low self-esteem
Bargaining	Is fearful of losing body functions, experiencing uncontrollable pain, and losing control; is willing to do anything to change prognosis or fate; accepts new forms of therapies
Depression	Recognizes potential loss of loved ones; may withdraw from important relationships to avoid painful feelings; may become quiet and noncommunicative when feeling loss of control; may express feelings of loneliness; does little to maintain his appearance; may become suicidal when unrealistic hopes of a cure fade
Acceptance	Accepts terms of death; begins to make plans for his death, e.g., writes a will, completes financial arrangements for the family, gives up personal possessions; is able to discuss feelings about death; reminisces about the past

Focus Assessment Criteria

SUBJECTIVE DATA
Family

- Previous copying patterns to crisis or loss
- Quality of the relationship of the ill or deceased person to each family member
- Position or role responsibilities of the ill or deceased person
- Sociocultural expectations for bereavement

Individual Family Members

- Previous experiences with loss and grief (as child, adolescent, or adult): Did family talk out their grief? Did they practice any particular religious rituals associated with grieving?
- Present interactions between or among family members
  - Adults
  - Children
    Maturational level
    Understanding of crisis
    Degree of participation
- Knowledge of expected grief reactions
- Relationship of ill or deceased person

Expressions of Emotions

- Ambivalence
- Denial
- Fear
- Concerns
- Anger
- Depression
- Guilt

Report of Physical Complaints

- Gastrointestinal disturbances
  - Indigestion
  - Nausea or vomiting
  - Anorexia
  - Weight gain or loss
  - Constipation or diarrhea
- Insomnia
- Preoccupation with sleep
- Fatigue (decreased or increased activity level)

OBJECTIVE DATA
Normative (simple bereavement)

- Shock
- Disbelief
- Anger
- Crying
- Sorrow
- Withdrawal
- Preoccupation with lost object or person
- Hopelessness

Pathological Pattern (profound; increases in intensity; continuous over 6 months)

- Anger
- Depression
- Isolation
- Denial
- Regression
- Obsession
- Despair
- Worthlessness
- Guilt
- Suicidal thoughts
- Hallucinations
- Delusions
- Phobias

Modified from Carpenito, L.J.: Nursing diagnosis—application to clinical practice, Philadelphia, 1983, J.B. Lippincott Co.

would not be successful if the client were in the anger stage.

Assessment Criteria

When assessing the client's or family members' responses to loss, the nurse will find it helpful to have a framework for collecting data. The focus assessment criteria (see boxed material) uses Engle's process framework as a guideline for assessing a person's grief response. The subjective data collected allow the nurse to determine relationships between the family and client that may affect their response to loss. The criteria focus on individual family members, their experiences with grief, their understanding of loss, and their knowledge of grief reactions. The nurse also ob-

serves the level of communication between the client and family members. Any expressions of anger, guilt, or emotions reflecting the stages of grief can be helpful in identifying the needs of the client and family.

Within the subjective realm of data the nurse also assesses the client and family for symptoms of somatic disturbances. During the initial stage of grief the client may have numerous physical complaints. The criteria can also be useful for the dying client, who may display fatigue or insomnia during the depression stage.

Objective data result from the nurse's observation of actual client and family behaviors. For example, within the criteria for shock, the nurse looks for behaviors such as aimless staring, inability to perform activities of daily living, or a preoccupation with discussing the lost object or person. The level and intensity of the client's behavior indicate the severity of the grief response.

Anticipatory and Unresolved Grief

In assessing the grieving client, two concepts identified by Lindemann (1965) merit the nurse's attention: anticipatory grief and unresolved grief.

ANTICIPATORY GRIEF

The phenomenon of anticipatory grief refers to the process of accomplishing part of the grief work before an actual loss. For example, a hospitalized woman scheduled for a mastectomy may have begun the grieving process from the moment a breast mass was discovered. Before admission she may have worked through the phases of disbelief and anger. When the nurse first meets her, she may be developing awareness of the significance of the loss. Similarly, a family member commonly experiences anticipatory grief before the loss of a loved one. Nurses also feel anticipatory grief while watching their clients experience the stages of dying. Anticipatory grief can be beneficial if it helps a person progress to a healthier emotional state after the loss has occurred. Nursing diagnoses related to anticipatory grieving have been defined based on the following characteristics:

1. Potential loss of significant object
2. Expression of distress at potential loss
3. Denial of potential loss
4. Guilt
5. Anger
6. Sorrow
7. Choked feelings
8. Changes in eating habits
9. Alterations in sleep patterns
10. Alterations in activity level
11. Altered libido
12. Altered communication patterns

The phenomenon of anticipatory grief underlines the importance of not stereotyping clients. A client who enters a health care facility after experiencing a loss may be at any stage of grief.

UNRESOLVED GRIEF

Lindemann (1965) describes unresolved grief as a severe reaction to separation through loss, characterized by unexplained somatic responses, specific medical diseases, and altered relationships with relatives, friends, and others. The nurse must recognize that as a person moves through the grieving process to resolution of a loss, there may be recurring feelings of intense sorrow. For example, individuals often reexperience the pain of grief on the anniversary date of a loss. This response may be anticipated and does not necessarily indicate unresolved grief. Usually grief for a significant loss is resolved within 6 months to 2 years. If resolution does not occur within a reasonable time, grieving may become chronic and be expressed through depressive responses (Werner-Beland, 1980) or through actual somatic illness. The client may have the need to work through the phases of the grief process that were previously unresolved. For example, a daughter who continues to feel guilt over the loss of her mother after 3 years may need assistance to express the anger she felt when her mother died and left her alone.

The nurse attempts to identify patterns indicative of unresolved grief reaction. Carpenito (1983) lists the following characteristics as potential "pathological grieving reactions":

1. Delusion
2. Hallucinations
3. Phobias
4. Obsessions
5. Isolation
6. Conversion hysteria
7. Agitated depression
8. Delay in grief work
9. Suicidal indications
10. Difficulty crying or controlling crying
11. Loss of control of environment leading to hopelessness and helplessness
12. Intense reactions lasting longer than 6 months with few signs of relief
13. Restrictions of pleasure

■ ■ ■ ■ ■

A detailed nursing assessment enables the nurse to establish tentative nursing diagnoses. The nurse makes inferences from the data base and validates them with the client and family to establish mutual goals and a plan of care. Effective planning and appropriate interventions must focus on the meaning of the loss for the client and the family.

The nurse should recognize that not all people experiencing loss grieve. A phenomenon known as absence of grief is evident in the absence of a strong attachment. Without significant attachment, the stage of detachment that begins the grieving process will not occur. The nurse who expects a client and his family to grieve in a prescribed manner might search for evidence of the grieving process when in fact the client and the family have experienced no significant loss.

The nurse must also be aware that some people who do grieve do not express grief outwardly. For example, an individual may memorialize a loss, focusing on memories of the past rather than resolution in the present. This phenomenon often occurs in the elderly, who may show little or no grieving because they are coping with loss through memorializing.

Nursing Diagnosis

Nursing diagnoses are based on the client's and family members' patterns of behavior and responses to loss. A diagnosis of grief reaction indicates that patterns of grieving have been identified and validated. Defining contributing factors helps the nurse develop specific interventions appropriate to the client's needs. For example, the diagnosis "grief reaction related to loss of job" might direct the nurse to refer the client to a resource (such as a social worker) for help with any financial problems. The diagnosis "grief reaction related to loss of body part" will require very different interventions to ensure the client's physical and emotional well-being. Table 46-4 gives examples of nursing diagnoses related to grief.

Grief reaction is a normal response to loss and an adaptive mechanism to overcome the stress of loss. As a result of grieving the client may exhibit other health-related problems. Alterations in sleep patterns or eating habits may become significant enough to warrant the nurse's attention.

TABLE 46-4

Examples of Nursing Diagnoses Related to Grief

Problem	Causes
Grief reaction	Related to: Loss of body part Role loss Loss of significant other Loss of job Fear over impending loss of life
Anticipatory grieving	Related to: Impending diagnostic testing Impending surgery Impending loss of a loved one
Unresolved grieving	Related to: Loss of loved one Loss of body part or function
Alterations in sleep pattern	Related to actual, anticipatory, or unresolved grief
Alterations in eating habits	Related to actual, anticipatory, or unresolved grief

The dying client requires special consideration when nursing diagnoses are formulated. The need to grieve is only one of many problems presented by such a client. A client with a terminal illness that may cause deformity or physical disabilities is likely to undergo alterations in body image or self-concept. Examples of this are a client with leukemia who receives chemotherapeutic drugs that cause loss of hair, or a client with bone cancer who becomes disabled because of chronic pain. As a dying client's condition worsens, the nurse makes diagnoses relevant to basic needs such as alterations in comfort, alterations in elimination, ineffective breathing patterns, or sensory alterations. Because of the nature and severity of terminal illness, physical assessment data are collected frequently and can be used to validate diagnoses.

Planning

Grieving is the natural response to loss. Grieving has a therapeutic value, enabling people to think through their loss, recollect their thoughts, and resume life with new insights and direction. In planning care for clients and family members the nurse's goals include the following:

1. Promoting open communication for the expression of feelings
2. Increasing the client's understanding of the grieving process
3. Maintaining and promoting the client's self-esteem
4. Facilitating the client's return to the routines of life

These goals can also be applied when planning care for a dying client. In addition, the nurse's responsibilities extend to the dying client's physical needs and the unique psychological and social problems associated with dying. Care of a dying client also involves intimate bodily care. Although the nurse's tasks may be similar to those required by a client who will recover from illness (such as bathing, feeding, or turning), the nurse's awareness of the client's approach to death influences her attitude toward the client. The nurse must be tolerant and willing to spend more time with dying clients, to listen to their expressions of grief, and to maintain their quality of living. Additional goals of care for dying clients include the following:

1. Maintaining comfort
2. Maintaining independence
3. Conserving energy
4. Preventing isolation or sensory deprivation
5. Promoting spiritual comfort
6. Supporting the family unit in grief

Implementation

Therapeutic Communication

Nursing care of the grieving client begins with establishing the significance of the loss for the client. This is difficult if the client is unwilling to express feelings or is in a phase of shock or denial. The nurse observes the client's response to the loss and then attempts to identify the client's strengths in dealing with it. To identify client's strengths the nurse uses open-ended questions and reflective statements such as "You appear concerned about your brother's condition" or "When the doctor informed you about the test results, you appeared frightened." The nurse must schedule adequate time with the client and family to promote open communication and must provide a private location for the interview that is conducive to sharing of perceptions. The nurse's words and actions should convey acceptance of all grief reactions. For example, if a client begins to cry, the nurse quietly remains at his side ready to offer comfort, rather than abandoning the client when his needs are the greatest. Acknowledging grief through touching the client and expressing concern evokes the client's trust.

If a client chooses not to share feelings or concerns, the nurse conveys a willingness to be available when needed. Many people are embarrassed about showing their emotions. When the nurse is reassuring and acknowledges the client's beliefs and values, a therapeutic relationship may evolve. Sometimes the client needs to begin resolving the grief before he can discuss the loss.

When considering a client's potential reactions to loss, the nurse is alert to the possibility of expressions of denial, anger, depression, or guilt. An initial denial of the loss when it is felt most acutely and perhaps cannot yet be faced is normal. If the nurse encourages the client to face the reality of the loss before the client is ready, she may become the target of the client's anger or fear once denial is resolved. Since it is difficult not to take anger personally, the nurse may avoid a client who expresses anger or guilt. In an effective relationship the nurse must deal with her personal feelings before encouraging the client's expression of anger. The nurse remains supportive by letting the client and family know that such expressions are normal. For example, the nurse might say, "You are obviously upset, but so are most people in this situation. I just want to let you know I'm available to talk if you'd like." It is helpful to explain to the client's significant others that anger may be a way of controlling the situation in the face of loss.

Most important, the nurse must avoid erecting barriers to communication by denying the client's grief, providing false reassurance, or avoiding discussion of the problem. For example, when a client is expressing anger about his terminal illness, the nurse avoids making statements such as "Don't worry, you'll probably outlive us all" or "Since you're so upset, why don't we discuss something else?"

When a client demonstrates a readiness to move on to the awareness stage, the nurse might explain the recognized grief reactions. Effective listening techniques and communication of concern and understanding also help the client move through the grieving process.

No topic should be avoided that a dying client wishes to discuss. If a client introduces the subject of dying, he is reaching out for support and understanding. The client will be more likely to discuss his impending death with a person who is willing to listen. The client may initially test the nurse by offering a statement that does not explicitly express his true concerns. For example, the client may make an open-ended statement, such as "My doctor talked with me today. . .," hoping the nurse will respond with interest.

If the nurse senses the client's desire to begin a discussion, it is important to let the client discuss *his* concerns. The nurse responds to any questions as honestly and positively as possible without giving false reassurance.

When a client's condition is terminal, the nurse should not encourage expressions of denial. However, the nurse can help the client develop a hopeful attitude while the client is still physically strong. It is easy for the dying client to become depressed because of new or unexpected symptoms, stressors related to treatment, financial concerns, or the temporary unavailability of a physician. If the nursing staff can instill feelings of hope and cheer when the client is still receiving active treatment, the client will be better able to participate in the treatment. The refusal to die or accept the feeling of helplessness serves as a motivator. Clients who remain confident and determined despite severe illness are better able to tolerate side effects of treatment, make fewer emotional demands on staff, serve as models for other clients, and often live longer than predicted. By teaching clients and families the early signs of hopelessness and despair (such as asking few questions about treatment, avoiding discussions of the client's condition, refusing to eat, or ignoring efforts to maintain personal hygiene), the nurse can help the client assume healthier behaviors. The nurse's support shows the client that he has something to live for.

As the grieving client moves to the resolution stage, the nurse can encourage discussion of how the loss has affected his life and his perceptions of the current situation. The nurse may share with the client and the family the signs of resolution, notably the client's desire to establish new roles, relationships, and goals. When the client is ready to loosen ties with the past and begin to look to the future, the nurse should encourage him as he plans for the future and participates in the decision-making process.

The nurse should recognize her own limitations in providing appropriate interventions for a grieving client. When the expertise of other professionals is needed, the nurse explores with the client and family alternatives in selecting appropriate resource persons, community agencies, or groups to enhance grief work. Some groups available in communities are self-help groups, bereavement groups, widow-to-widow groups, and parent groups. Signs of unresolved grief and pathological grieving reactions may require referral to a psychologist, psychiatrist, or counselor.

Maintenance of Self-Esteem

Nursing interventions with the grieving client and family focus on promoting the client's sense of identity, dignity, and self-esteem. The nurse can help by listening, responding quickly and positively to requests, maintaining confidentiality and privacy, and providing comfort and support. The quality and quantity of time spent with the client are important in creating a therapeutic environment for the grieving process. Frequently nurses and other health team members say they have no time to spend with grieving clients and family members. Nurses may become preoccupied with the physical tasks of care. However, the real problem is often the nurse's lack of knowledge and inability to deal with the client's grief. Davitz and Davitz (1980) explored the characteristics of nurses who demonstrate a "highly refined" empathetic response to their clients. These nurses identified the nurse's relationship with the client as the very core of nursing.

Measures that provide comfort and support should be implemented in a caring, nonhurried manner to reinforce the client's feelings of self-worth and dignity and to decrease the fear of rejection, isolation, and the sense of hopelessness. When self-esteem is low, pain and aloneness will have a greater effect on the client. Specific comfort measures for the hospitalized client will depend on the type of physical loss.

Self-esteem and dignity complement each other. Dignity is the person's ability to maintain his concept of himself as a person. The disabilities experienced by the dying client may threaten the client's dignity. Care givers often take control of the client's life. Taking away the client's right to make decisions about his care will foster hopelessness and feelings of de-

spair. The client loses the will to live. To maintain self-esteem the client must believe that his opinions are valuable in decisions that will affect the course of his dying.

The nurse can maintain and promote the dying client's self-esteem by giving attention to the client's appearance. Cleanliness, a lack of body odors, attractive clothing, and personal grooming (shaving or wearing ribbons in the hair) are ways to promote a sense of worth. If the nurse assumes management of the client's body functions, she must show an attitude of respect and helpfulness rather than encourage dependence or feelings of guilt.

Promotion of a Return to Life Activities

As clients enter the acceptance stage of grieving, it is important for the nurse to encourage a return to a normal life-style. If clients and families are able to express grief openly and to progress through the grief process with support and understanding, the resolution of grief is easier. Depending on the nature of a client's loss, many demands may be placed on the client's and family members' resources. Vocational or educational plans, role relationships, financial stability, and general life-style may be disrupted.

The nurse can help by encouraging clients to participate in decisions about relationships and resources for the future. The identification of usual life-style practices helps bring a sense of closure to the loss. For example, if a woman has begun to accept the loss from a mastectomy, the nurse introduces the client to a member of Reach for Recovery who shows the client breast prostheses, talks about clothing and grooming, and discusses ways to resume normal activities.

Special Needs of the Dying
PROMOTION OF COMFORT

The dying client may suffer acute or chronic pain (see Chapter 37). Problems arise when staff members hold misconceptions about the nature and treatment of pain. Often nurses administer narcotic analgesics sparingly, fearing a client will develop a tolerance to or dependence on the drug. However, narcotic addiction should not be an issue for a dying client, and the relief of pain is critically important. The sooner the dying client obtains pain relief, the more energy the client can direct toward maintaining quality in the remainder of his life.

The dying client's physical needs can be numerous. Any source of physical irritation will exacerbate the client's pain and make relief more difficult to achieve. Thorough skin care, including provision of daily baths, massage to pressure areas, exercises to promote circulation, and dry, clean bed linen, will eliminate irritants and minimize pain. Mouth care can be extremely important. Often as the client approaches death the mouth remains open, the tongue becomes edematous and dry, and cracks develop in the lips. As long as the client can swallow, water should be offered. To prevent accidental choking a water-soaked gauze can be placed between the lips. Sucking is one of the body's last instinctive reactions, and thirst is the last craving. When swallowing becomes impossible, a light film of petrolatum jelly applied to the lips and tongue relieves discomfort from drying. The nurse cleans the oral cavity and moistens the mucosa with a soft toothbrush or sponge-tipped applicator to prevent bleeding from sensitive tissues. Since the client's ability to talk provides a link with the world, the mouth should be kept as comfortable, usable, and attractive as possible.

As the client loses the ability to move or turn, maintaining proper alignment becomes an essential comfort measure. Misalignment of extremities or pressure from bony prominences will prevent a client from being able to relax or sleep. The nurse helps the client find the most comfortable position possible. Normally the nurse does not place pillows under a client's knees, since this might impair circulation. For the dying client support with pillows or blankets relieves pressure and strain on the extremities. Frequent repositioning of the client ensures maximum comfort.

MAINTENANCE OF INDEPENDENCE

The dying client gains considerable satisfaction from being able to help himself as long as he has the will and energy to do so. Allowing the client to perform simple tasks such as washing his face, putting on eyeglasses, or feeding himself maintains the client's dignity and sense of worth. When a client becomes physically unable to perform any self-care, the nurse still encourages the client's participation in decision making to give him a sense of control. The nurse must look for any nonverbal cues from the client that suggest unwillingness to participate in care. The nurse should not force the client to participate, particularly if physical limitations make it difficult.

CONSERVATION OF ENERGY

Meeting the physical and emotional stress of a terminal illness requires a great deal of energy. In the exhaustion phase of the general adaptation syndrome (see Chapter 5), continued stress can lead to death. The nurse's role is to conserve the client's energy. An elderly client poses the greatest challenge because of diminished energy reserves.

The nurse must determine what the client is capable of doing without becoming physically and emotionally drained. What are the priorities of care? Should the nurse bathe the client so he can feed himself? Would it be best to feed the client so he can sit in a chair for half an hour? Will the client require considerable energy to talk with family members who are about to visit? Careful planning of nursing care activities throughout the day can make a difference in the client's ability to remain active.

Limiting physical activity is not the only way the nurse can conserve the client's energy. Anxiety consumes energy. Listening, touching the client gently, and staying at the client's side reduce the emotional fears that can exhaust the client.

PREVENTION OF LONELINESS AND ISOLATION

When the nurse caring for the dying person is detached, directing her attention to physical care and avoiding discussion of the client's situation, the client experiences an overwhelming loneliness. It takes time and experience for a nurse to react positively toward dying clients. Nurses are oriented to the cure of clients and may find it difficult to provide the necessary support for those who die. For many health care providers death symbolizes failure. Furthermore, the process of dying may cause a client to be unpleasant. If the client's condition causes offensive odors, incontinence, confusion, or combativeness, nurses may avoid the client. Often the dying person is confined to a private room to avoid exposing other clients to his suffering. The room may be dimly lit with curtains drawn and environmental sounds reduced to a minimum. Without meaningful sensory stimulation the dying person feels abandoned and isolated.

To prevent loneliness and sensory deprivation the nurse intervenes to improve the quality of the client's immediate environment. Dying clients should not be routinely placed in private rooms in out-of-the-way locations. Clients feel a sense of involvement when sharing a room and watching the nurse's activities. The client can then also share conversation and companionship with his roommate and any visitors. When the client dies, however, the nurse should give attention to the client's roommate, since the experience of watching a person die can be frightening.

Providing meaningful environmental stimulation comforts the client. Rooms should be brightly lit and decorated with attractive colors. A pleasant view outside the room window can become an important source of stimulation as the client watches activities outside. Pictures, cherished objects, cards or letters from family members, and live plants and flowers console the client. Familiar objects provide security in an alien environment. A portable radio or television allows the client to keep in touch with the outside world.

Perhaps the most important factor in preventing a client's sense of loneliness is visits by family members or significant others. Visitors should be allowed to remain with dying clients at any time. If the client shares a semiprivate room, however, the nurse should be sure the visitors will not disturb the client's roommate. If several family members visit, it may be necessary to provide a private room. The elderly client becomes particularly lonely at night and may feel more secure if someone stays at the bedside during the night. The nurse should know how to contact family members at any time if the client requests a visit or the client's condition worsens.

It is very important for the dying person to have someone who can share the dying experience with him. Nurses should not feel guilty if they cannot provide this support. The nurse may not have the time, skill, or love for the dying person that is required. However, the nurse must be available to meet the client's bodily needs. Care at this level may require long intervals of time with the client. It is the nurse's responsibility to stay with dying clients when they are needed and to show concern and compassion. The mere presence of the nurse can offer the client a sense of security and freedom from loneliness.

PROMOTION OF SPIRITUAL COMFORT

Providing a client with spiritual comfort means much more than asking a member of the clergy to visit the client. The nurse must support the client in his expression of the philosophy he has chosen for his life. As death approaches, the client will often seek comfort by reviewing and analyzing the values and beliefs that have structured his life and that now influence his perceptions of the meaning of death.

Values clarification (see Chapter 13) may assist the nurse in learning what beliefs are most significant for the client. Many clients do not practice a formal religion, and those who do have diverse interpretations of the meaning of death.

It is important for the nurse to feel comfortable about personal spiritual beliefs and values before attempting to support the client. Attentive listening encourages the client to express feelings, clarify them, and accept his fate. If the nurse feels comfortable in providing spiritual support, it is appropriate to pray silently with the client. When clients look for support from a member of the clergy and do not have their own clergyman, the nurse makes referrals through the hospital's or institution's spiritual counseling office.

SUPPORT FOR THE GRIEVING FAMILY

Family members must be supported through the dying and death of the client and simultaneously be encouraged to provide support to the client. In an institutional setting the family has greater difficulty carrying out supportive activities. The nurse must recognize the value of family members as resources and assist them in working with the dying person.

To use family members as resources the nurse must assess family relationships. Identifying how family roles are being influenced by the client's death is crucial. Family members have their own need to express

---

Suggestions for Involving the Family in the Care of a Dying Client

- Assist in planning a visitation schedule for family members to prevent client and family from becoming fatigued.
- Allow young children to visit a dying parent when the client is able to communicate.
- Be willing to listen to family complaints about the client's care, as well as positive or negative feelings about the client.
- Help family members learn how to interact with the dying person (e.g., using attentive listening, avoiding false reassurances, conducting conversations about normal family activities or problems).
- Allow family members to help with simple care measures such as feeding, bathing, and straightening bed linen. Family members are often more successful than nursing staff in persuading the client to eat.
- When the family becomes fatigued with care activities, relieve them from their duties so they can acquire needed rest and support. Refer them to resources for meals and lodging.
- Support the act of grieving between client and family. Provide privacy when preferred. Do not discourage open expression of grief between family and client.
- Provide information daily with regard to the client's condition. Prepare the family for sudden changes in the client's appearance and behavior.
- Communicate news of impending death when the family is together if possible. Members can provide support for one another. Convey the news in a private area and be willing to stay with the family.
- At the time of death, help the family stay in communication with the dying person through short visits, caring silence, touch, and telling the client of their love for him.
- After death assist the family with decision making, such as selection of a mortician, transportation of family members, and collection of the client's belongings.

their feelings, and they must also deal directly with the client's expressions of anger, denial, and fear. Sometimes the family becomes unwilling to face the client's hostility or aggressive behavior and refuses to care for him at home or visit him in the institution. In contrast, the family may show excessive concern for the client and seek to spend more time with him than the client desires.

The nurse cannot work with dying clients without involving the family. The family is facing the loss of someone they love. The nurse must consistently deal with families and clients by showing kindness, respect, and courtesy. The box on p. 1319 provides guidelines for supporting families in their grief and helping them become supportive of the client.

Care after Death

The nurse may be the best person to care for the client's body after death because she maintained a therapeutic relationship with the client during his life and therefore is more sensitive to the need of caring for the body with dignity and sensitivity. After death the body undergoes numerous physical changes (Table 46-5). The care of the body should occur as soon as possible after death to prevent damage to tissues or disfigurement of body parts.

If the deceased's family asks to view the body, the nurse prepares the room and the body so as to minimize the stress of the experience. The nurse removes all supplies and equipment from countertops or bedside stands. Dirty linen should be disposed of properly and any clutter on the floor should be removed. If there are any unpleasant odors in the room, the nurse uses a spray deodorizer.

The nurse prepares the body by making it look as natural and comfortable as possible. If the body is placed in a supine position with arms at the sides,

palms down, or across the abdomen, the mortician will be better able to prepare the body for internment. The nurse places a small pillow or folded towel under the head to prevent discoloration from blood pooling. If gently held closed for a few seconds the eyelids will usually remain closed. The nurse inserts the client's dentures to maintain the normal facial features. A rolled-up towel placed under the chin will help keep the mouth closed.

The nurse washes any soiled body parts, dresses the body in a clean gown, and covers the body up to the shoulders with clean linen. Most shroud kits contain absorbent pads that are placed under the perineal and rectal area to collect any oozing feces or urine. The nurse removes all jewelry and presents it and any other valuables to the family. In some agencies a single wedding band may be left in place as long as it is taped securely to the finger. After the body is prepared, the family is allowed to enter the room. The nurse should not allow a single family member to enter the room alone. The nurse or another family member should accompany the person to provide emotional support.

After the family views the body, the nurse removes the gown and wraps the body in a large plastic sheet or shroud before delivering it to the morgue. Special tags containing the deceased's name and other identification information are placed on the wrist and toe and on the outside of the shroud. In the morgue the body is placed in a special cooling unit to slow decomposition. Institutions vary as to the methods for transporting the body through the hallways.

Evaluation

The desired outcome criteria suggested by Carpenito (1983) can be used to evaluate nursing care and

---

TABLE 46-5

Physiological Changes after Death

Change	Related Interventions
Stiffening of body (rigor mortis), developing in 2 to 4 hours after death; involves contraction of skeletal and smooth muscle owing to lack of ATP	Position body in normal anatomical alignment. Close eyelids and mouth. Insert dentures in mouth.
Reduction in body temperature (algor mortis) with loss of skin elasticity	Remove tape and dressings gently to avoid tissue breakdown. Avoid pulling on skin or body parts.
Purple discoloration of skin (livor mortis) in dependent areas owing to breakdown of red blood cells	Elevate head to prevent discoloration.

intervention strategies used with the grieving client and family. Broadly stated, these criteria include expression of grief, description of the personal meaning of the loss, participation in decision making for the future, and sharing of grief with significant others. Evaluation occurs throughout the nursing process. The nurse continually collects assessment data and plans daily care based on careful observation of responses and behavior. Although resolution of grief may require 6 months to 2 years, the majority of clients are in the hospital for only a short time. The nurse may become frustrated when, just as she feels she has begun to help the client and family express their grief, the discharge order is written or the client dies. It is helpful to remember that grieving is an individualized process, and resolution of loss does not proceed according to a set schedule.

The following are questions for evaluating change in the client and family's responses and behavior:

1. Is the client or family able to express grief?
2. Is the client or family able to describe the significance of the loss?
3. Is the client able to share his grief with significant others?
4. Has the client participated in plans for the future?
5. Have attitudes toward loss been altered?
6. Is the present life-style different from the past?
7. Is the client or family able to identify strengths and support systems?

The care of the dying client requires that the nurse evaluate whether the client has accepted his fate and whether the nurse was able to sustain the quality of the person's life. The success of the nurse's evaluation will depend on the bond formed with the client. Unless the client has learned to trust the nurse, he will be unlikely to share his true feelings and concerns.

Questions for evaluating the client's acceptance of death include the following:

1. Is the client able to use such terms as "death," "cancer," or "terminal"?
2. Is the client able to discuss the impact of his death on remaining family members?
3. Has the client completed any final tasks or responsibilities such as writing a will or paying off the mortgage?
4. Is the client able to reminisce about days in the past without anger or depression?
5. Is the client able to say good-bye to family members?

Summary

Loss is a universal phenomenon experienced throughout life. Categories of loss include loss of an aspect of self, loss of external objects, loss of a significant other, loss experienced in separation from a known environment, and loss of life. Nurses interact daily with clients and families experiencing loss. Knowledge of the concepts and theories concerning loss, death, and the grieving process provides a framework for assessment, nursing diagnosis, and the planning and implementation of appropriate therapies. Evaluation of the nurse's therapies determines whether grief is successfully resolved or death has been accepted.

The nurse's responses and interactions with the grieving client and family create the climate for openness in expressing grief. The nurse explores the strengths of the client and support systems available to him through listening, being with the client when needed, and conveying respect for the client's values and beliefs. A trust relationship creates a therapeutic environment that enhances grief work and fosters the client's sense of dignity and self-esteem. The nurse who has explored her personal attitudes, beliefs, values, and responses to loss, death, and grief is able to assess her interactions with clients and families. Her understanding promotes growth and paves the way for effective nursing care of the grieving or the dying client and their families.

KEY CONCEPTS

✓ A loss is the absence of an object, person, body part or function, or emotion.

✓ The grieving process involves a set of emotional, cognitive, and behavioral responses to an actual or perceived loss.

✓ Individuals experience different aspects of the grieving process at different times.

✓ The stages of the grieving process vary among theories but progress from distress and shock to resolution and acceptance.

✓ With all five categories of loss, the nurse considers the meaning of the loss to the client rather than attempting to assess the value of the loss itself.

✓ The chronically ill face many different kinds of losses.

✓ Dying may lead to a grief response similar to that with other kinds of losses.

✓ Assessment of the grieving client focuses on how the individual is actually responding rather than how he theoretically should respond.

✓ The individual's loss reaction is influenced by many factors including developmental stage, beliefs, roles, relationships, and socioeconomic status.

✓ Assessment of the grieving client considers behavioral characteristics that suggest the client's stage of grieving.

✓ Assessment of the dying client focuses on grieving stage as a basis for planning care to assist the client in coping.

✓ Nursing diagnoses related to grief allow the nurse to incorporate interventions for coping with loss into the client's holistic care plan.

✓ Therapeutic communication is an important nursing intervention to assist both the grieving and the dying client in coping with loss.

✓ Nursing care of the grieving and dying client should promote the client's sense of identity, dignity, and self-esteem.

✓ Nursing interventions to promote a return to life activities assist the client in resolving grief and accepting the loss.

✓ Nursing interventions for dying clients address the psychosocial and spiritual needs of the client and family, as well as physiological needs.

✓ Nursing care for the client's body after death continues to be based on dignity and sensitivity.

✓ The evaluation of nursing care for the grieving and dying client is ongoing and based on identifiable behavioral changes through the grieving process.

REFERENCES

Carpenito, L.J.: Nursing diagnosis—application to clinical practice, Philadelphia, 1983, J.B. Lippincott Co.

Davitz, L., and Davitz, J.: Nurses' responses to patients' suffering, New York, 1980, Springer Publishing Co.

Engle, G.L.: Grief and grieving, Am. J. Nurs. 64:93, 1964.

Fairbairn, W.: Synopsis of an object-relations theory of the personality, Int. J. Psychoanal. 44:244, 1963.

Gonda, T.A.: Coping with dying and death, Geriatrics 26:71, 1971.

Groves, J.: Differentiating grief, mourning and bereavement, Am. J. Psychiatry 135(7):875, 1978.

Hampe, S.O.: Needs of the grieving spouse in a hospital setting, Nurs. Res. 24:113, 1975.

Kübler-Ross, E.: On death and dying, New York, 1969, Macmillan, Inc.

Lewis, K.: Grief in chronic illness and disability, J. Rehabil. 49:8, 1983.

Lindemann, E.: Symptomatology and management of acute grief. In Parad, H., editor: Crisis intervention, New York, 1965, Family Association of America.

McGrory, A.: A well model approach to care of the dying client, New York, 1978, McGraw-Hill Book Co.

Werner-Beland, J.A.: Grief response of long term illness and disability, Reston, Va., 1980, Reston Publishing Co., Inc.

ADDITIONAL READINGS

Bowlby, J.: Attachment and loss, vols. I and II, New York, 1969 and 1973, Basic Books, Inc.

Castles, M.R., and Murray, R.B.: Dying in an institution: nurse patient perspectives, New York, 1979, Appleton-Century-Crofts.

Ebersole, P., and Hess, P.: Toward healthy aging: human needs and nursing responses, St. Louis, 1981, The C.V. Mosby Co.

Engle, G.L.: Psychological development in health and disease, Philadelphia, 1962, W.B. Saunders Co.

Kim, M.J., McFarland, G.K., and McLane, A.M., editors: Classification of nursing diagnoses, St. Louis, 1984, The C.V. Mosby Co.

Kim, M.J., et al.: Pocket guide to nursing diagnoses, St. Louis, 1984, The C.V. Mosby Co.

Lee, R.: Object loss and counseling the bereaved. In Fruehling, J., editor: Sourcebook on death and dying, Chicago, Ill., 1982, Marquis Professional Publications.

Miles, H.S., and Hays, D.R.: Widowhood, Am. J. Nurs. 75:280, 1975.

Smith, S., and Duell, D.: Nursing skills and evaluation: a nursing process approach, Los Altos, Calif., 1982, National Nursing Review.

10

In hospitals, clinics, and other health care settings, nurses provide care for clients before and after surgical procedures. Special skills are required for the care of these clients, as well as preparatory teaching activities. Because the anticipation of surgery creates emotional stresses for many clients and their families, the nurse also provides care to promote successful coping with these stresses and to help the client adapt to changes after surgery during the recovery and rehabilitation stages. Specific nursing skills are required also to care for the surgical wound, and therefore this unit includes a chapter on wound healing, in which nursing care for other types of wounds is discussed as well.

Caring for the Perioperative Client

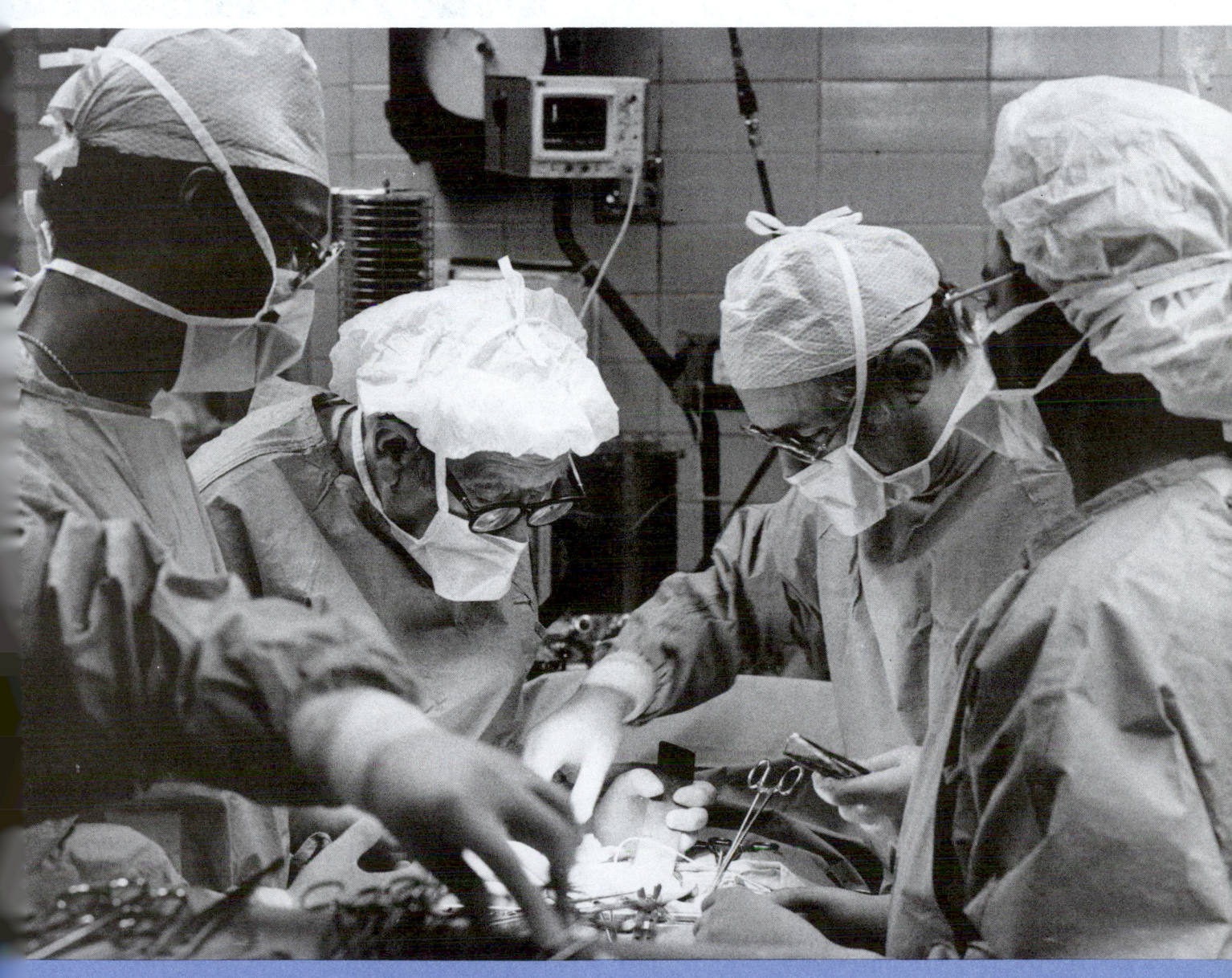

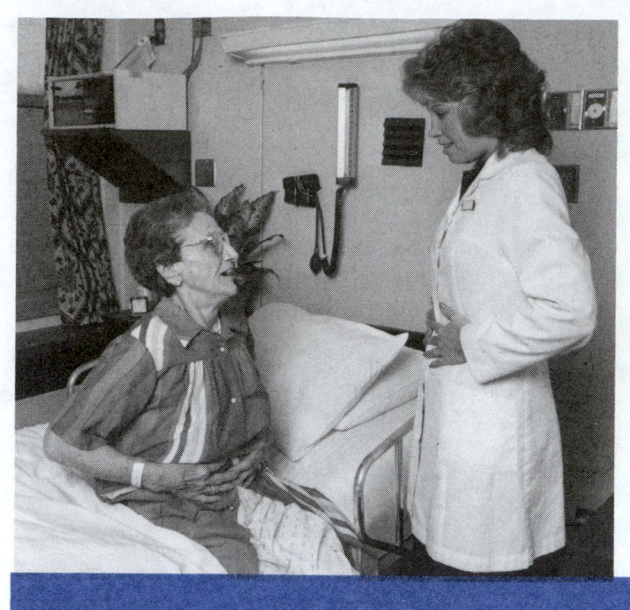

OBJECTIVES

Mastery of content in this chapter will enable the student to:

- Define the terms in the glossary.
- Explain the concept of perioperative nursing care.
- Differentiate between classifications of surgery.
- List factors to include in the preoperative assessment of a surgical client.
- Properly witness a client's informed consent for surgery.
- Demonstrate postoperative exercises: diaphragmatic breathing, coughing, turning, leg exercises.
- Design a preoperative teaching program.
- Prepare a client for surgery on the morning of a scheduled operation.
- Compare and contrast the side effects of general and regional anesthesia.
- Identify factors to include in the postoperative assessment of a client in recovery.
- Describe the rationale for nursing interventions designed to prevent postoperative complications.
- Identify potential sources of a postoperative client's pain.

GLOSSARY

anesthesia Absence of normal sensation, especially sensitivity to pain.

autopsy Postmortem examination performed to confirm or determine the cause of death.

cholecystectomy Surgical removal of the gallbladder.

convalescence Period of recovery after an illness, injury, or surgery.

dehiscence Separation of a wound's edges, revealing underlying tissues.

depilatory Substance that removes hair.

embolus Small amount of air, fat, or other substance that circulates in the blood until becoming lodged in a blood vessel.

evisceration Protrusion of visceral organs through a surgical wound.

excise To remove completely, as in the surgical excision of the appendix.

gangrene Necrosis or death of tissue, usually the result of loss of blood supply.

induction of anesthesia All portions of the anesthetic process that occur before attaining the desired stage of anesthesia, including premedication, intubation, and administration of oxygen.

intraoperative Pertaining to the period of time during a surgical procedure.

47 *Nursing Care of the Surgical Client*

intubation   Passage of a tube into a body opening, for example, endotracheal intubation—passage of an endotracheal tube into the trachea through the mouth or nose.

necrotic   Of or pertaining to the death of tissue in response to disease or injury.

postoperative   Pertaining to the period of time after surgery.

preoperative   Pertaining to the period of time before surgery.

serosanguineous   Thin red drainage composed of serum and blood.

suture   Surgical stitch taken to repair an incision or wound.

vascularization   Process by which body tissue becomes vascular and develops proliferating capillaries.

venous stasis   Disorder in which the normal flow of blood through a vein is slowed or halted.

A client faces a variety of stressors when surgery becomes the therapy of choice. Anticipating surgery leads to fear and anxiety for clients, who tend to associate surgery with pain, possible disfigurement, dependence, and perhaps even loss of life. Family members often fear a disruption in their life-style and experience a sense of powerlessness as the client's surgery approaches. Part of the nurse's role is to provide adequate emotional and physical support to clients and family members so they become better able to cope with the surgical experience.

The trauma a client sustains during an operation creates physical needs requiring close supervision and skilled intervention by the nurse and physician. The nurse learns to anticipate the client's needs on the basis of the person's overall health and the specific type of surgery performed. The client is better able to cooperate and participate in the care plan if the nurse has provided information about events occurring before and after surgery.

Most surgery is performed in hospitals. However, as a result of changes in health care economics, outpatient surgical units are increasingly common. A client enters the unit, undergoes the scheduled surgery, and returns home the same day. Nurses working in a variety of settings—for example, home health care and clinics as well as hospitals—must understand the principles of caring for surgical clients.

Perioperative Nursing Care

In the midnineteenth century surgery evolved as a medical specialty. Surgery became a means for physicians to treat conditions that were difficult or impossible to manage by pure medical means. However, early surgeons had little knowledge of the principles of asepsis, and anesthesia techniques were primitive and unsafe. A surgeon in an early operating room did not wear gloves but used cleansing solution for handwashing. The same surgical instruments were used for different clients. The incidence of infection, gangrene, and hemorrhage was so high that surgeons performed only minor corrective surgery or procedures that were a last resort for a client. Nurses working in the first operating rooms cleaned the rooms and equipment, performed such technical tasks for surgeons as obtaining equipment, and occasionally accompanied the client to the surgical ward to deliver nursing care.

With the advent of antiseptic and later aseptic practices, surgery became a treatment of choice for many conditions. The development of safer anesthetic gases allowed the surgeon to conduct longer operative procedures. The risk of surgical mortality was reduced. Operating room nurses required special training for new responsibilities in caring for surgical clients.

In 1876 Massachusetts General Hospital provided the first operating room education for nurses (Metzger, 1976). This trend continued into the 1900s as nursing schools included operating room experience in each nurse's clinical instruction. Nurses gained valuable experience in actually assisting physicians during surgery by passing instruments and other necessary equipment. The nurses acquired an understanding of the value of strict aseptic technique and observed firsthand the delicate anatomy of body parts. As the number and types of surgical procedures grew, so too did the role of the nurse as a vital member of the surgical team.

In 1956 the Association of Operating Room Nurses (AORN) was formed with the purpose of gaining new knowledge and exploring methods to improve nursing care of surgical clients. The association met many challenges, including the fight to overcome the notion that operating room nurses were only technically skilled practitioners. The organization developed standards of nursing practice in the operating room to establish the need for registered nurses in the operating room. The association also originated the term "perioperative nursing," which defines the role of the operating room nurse during the preoperative, intraoperative, and postoperative phases of a client's surgical experience. The concept of perioperative nursing stresses the importance of providing continuity of care for the client undergoing surgery.

In many hospitals, operating room nurses assess a client's health status preoperatively, identify specific client needs, provide teaching and counseling, attend to the client's needs in the operating room, and then follow the client's postoperative recovery. The nurse's role can thus be quite diversified. However, in many other institutions different nurses care for the surgical client during each phase of the surgical experience. Nurses in general nursing divisions attend to the client's needs before and after surgery, and the operating room nurse practices only in the operating room setting. Involvement of the operating room nurse in each phase of the client's care provides a smooth course for the client's therapy. To avoid an assembly line style of treatment, nurses in general divisions and operating room nurses must establish lines of communication. Whatever system for the delivery of care is used, the nurse's major responsibility is to provide safe, consistent, and effective nursing care during each phase of surgery.

Classification of Surgery

The classification for the types of surgical procedures performed relates to the seriousness, urgency, or purpose of surgery (Table 47-1). A given procedure may fall into more than one classification. For example, the surgical removal of a disfiguring scar is minor in seriousness, elective in urgency, and reconstructive in purpose. Frequently, the classes overlap. A procedure that is urgent is also considered major in seriousness. The same operation may be performed for different reasons on different clients. For example, a gastrectomy may be performed as an emergency procedure to resect a bleeding ulcer or as an urgent procedure to remove a cancerous growth. The classification indicates to the nurse the level of care a client might require.

Preoperative Surgical Phase

Surgical clients enter the health care setting in different stages of health. A client may enter the hospital on a predetermined day feeling relatively healthy and prepared to face impending elective surgery. In contrast, a victim of a motor vehicle accident may face emergency surgery with no time to prepare for the surgical experience. The surgical client must undergo a battery of tests and procedures to confirm or rule out the presence of alterations requiring surgery. The

TABLE 47-1			

Classification for Surgical Procedures

Classification	Type	Description	Example
Seriousness	Major	Involves extensive reconstruction or alteration in body parts; poses great risks to a client's well-being	Coronary artery bypass, colon resection, laryngectomy, mastectomy
	Minor	Involves minimal alteration in body parts; often designed to correct deformities; physical risks minimal compared with major procedures	Cataract extraction, facial plastic surgery, skin graft, tooth extraction, arthrotomy
Urgency	Elective	Performed on the basis of a client's choice; is not essential and may not be necessary for the client's physical health	Bunionectomy, facial plastic surgery, hernia repair, breast reconstruction
	Urgent	Necessary for the client's health; may prevent additional problems from developing, e.g., tissue destruction or impaired organ function; not necessarily an emergency	Excision of cancerous tumor, removal of gallbladder for stones, vascular repair for obstructed artery, e.g., coronary artery bypass
	Emergency	Must be done immediately to save the client's life or preserve function of a body part	Repair of perforated appendix, repair of traumatic amputation, control of internal hemorrhaging
Purpose	Diagnostic	Surgical exploration that allows a physician to confirm a diagnosis; may involve removal of tissue for further diagnostic testing	Exploratory laparotomy (incision into peritoneal cavity to inspect abdominal organs), breast mass biopsy
	Ablative	Excision or removal of a diseased body part	Amputation, appendectomy, cholecystectomy
	Palliative	Designed to relieve or reduce the intensity of disease symptoms; will not produce a cure	Colostomy, debridement of necrotic tissue, resection of nerve roots
	Reconstructive	Restores function or appearance to traumatized or malfunctioning tissues	Internal fixation of fractures, scar revision
	Transplant	Performed to replace malfunctioning organs or structures	Kidney, cornea, or liver transplant, total hip replacement
	Constructive	Restores function lost or reduced as a result of congenital anomalies	Repair of cleft palate, closure of atrial septal defect in the heart

client meets many health care personnel, including surgeons, nurse anesthetists or anesthesiologists, laboratory technicians, therapists, and nurses, all of whom play a role in the client's care and recovery. Family members attempt to provide support through their presence, yet face many of the same stressors as the client.

The nurse's role in the preoperative surgical phase is to assess the client's physical and emotional well-being, recognize the degree of surgical risk, coordinate performance of diagnostic tests, identify nursing diagnoses reflecting the client's and family members'

needs, prepare the client physically and mentally for surgery, and communicate pertinent information to members of the surgical team.

Assessment

The nurse's assessment of the surgical client involves collecting a nursing history, performing a physical examination, reviewing the client's and family members' emotional health, and analyzing risk factors and diagnostic data. The length of the preoperative period will determine how thorough the nurse's

---

TABLE 47-2

Medical Conditions That Increase the Risks of Surgery

Type of Condition	Reason for Risk
Bleeding disorders (thrombocytopenia, leukemia, hemophilia, bone marrow depression following use of chemotherapeutic drugs)	Increases risk of hemorrhaging during and after surgery
Diabetes mellitus	Impairs wound healing and increases risk of infection from altered glucose metabolism and associated circulatory impairment; blood sugar levels may cause CNS malfunction during anesthesia
Heart disease (recent myocardial infarction, arrhythmias, congestive heart failure)	Stress of surgery causing increased demands on myocardium to maintain cardiac output; general anesthetic agents that depress cardiac function
Upper respiratory infection	Increases risk of respiratory complications during anesthesia, e.g., pneumonia and spasm of the laryngeal muscles
Liver disease	Alters metabolism and elimination of drugs administered during surgery; impairs wound healing because of alterations in protein metabolism
Fever	Predisposes client to fluid and electrolyte imbalances; may indicate underlying infection
Chronic respiratory disease (emphysema, bronchitis, asthma)	Reduces client's means to compensate for acid-base alterations (see Chapter 43); anesthetic agents reduce respiratory function, increasing risk for severe hypoventilation

---

assessment will be. If the client enters a hospital only a few hours before surgery, the nurse sets priorities in terms of the client's most significant needs.

NURSING HISTORY

The nurse collects a history similar to that described in Chapter 7. Key elements in the history pertain to the surgical client's needs. If a client is unable to relate all of the necessary information, the nurse may use family members as primary resources.

MEDICAL HISTORY. A review of the client's medical history should include past illnesses and the primary reason for seeking medical care. When the nurse first assesses the client, the reasons for surgery may be unclear or the client may not yet know that surgery will be required. Preexisting illnesses can influence the client's ability to tolerate surgery and reach full recovery. Examples of medical conditions that increase the risk of surgery are listed in Table 47-2.

PREVIOUS SURGERIES. A client's past experience with surgery can significantly influence both physical and psychological responses to a procedure. The type of previous surgery, the level of discomfort experienced, the extent of disability, and the overall level

of care provided are some of the factors the client recalls when faced with another surgical experience. The nurse determines what unpleasant factors the client experienced. It is also helpful to know if any complications developed, such as a wound infection or clotting disorder. This information helps the nurse anticipate the client's needs preoperatively and postoperatively. For example, if the client recalls experiencing great discomfort while turning, the nurse initiates emotional support preoperatively and plans to explain the importance of physical activity postoperatively, demonstrating ways for the client to turn with minimal stress on the surgical wound.

A client's past surgery may also influence the level of physical care required after a surgical procedure. For example, a client who has had a previous thoracotomy for the resection of a lung lobe is at a greater risk for postoperative pulmonary complications than a client with intact normal lungs. Thus knowledge of the client's previous surgical alteration enables the nurse to initiate aggressive pulmonary care.

CLIENTS' AND FAMILY MEMBERS' PERCEPTIONS AND UNDERSTANDING OF SURGERY. A client may be admitted to a surgical nursing division without an understanding of what surgery entails. Often the client must undergo diagnostic procedures before

TABLE 47-3

Drugs with Special Implications for the Surgical Client

Drug Class	Effects during Surgery
Antibiotics	Potentiate action of anesthetic agents; if taken within 2 weeks preoperatively, aminoglycosides (gentamicin, tobramycin, neomycin) may cause mild respiratory depression from depressed neuromuscular transmission
Antiarrhythmics	Have potential for reducing cardiac contractility and impairing conduction during anesthesia
Anticoagulants	Alter normal clotting factors and thus increase risk of hemorrhaging; should be discontinued at least 48 hours preoperatively
Anticonvulsants	Long-term use of certain anticonvulsants—e.g., phenytoin (Dilantin) and phenobarbital—alters metabolism of anesthetic agents
Antihypertensives	Interact with anesthetic agents to cause bradycardia, hypotension, and impaired circulation; inhibit synthesis and storage of norepinephrine in sympathetic nerve endings
Corticosteroids	With prolonged use cause adrenal atrophy, which reduces body's ability to withstand stress; before and during surgery dosages may be temporarily increased
Insulin	Diabetic client's need for insulin preoperatively is reduced since client fasts; postoperatively, stress response and IV administration of glucose solutions can increase dosage requirements
Diuretics	Potentiate electrolyte imbalances postoperatively (particularly potassium)

the surgeon determines the exact type of surgery to perform. Identifying the client's perceptions and expectations allows the nurse to plan teaching and emotional preparation measures for a client. Often clients and family members have misconceptions about surgery because of misleading stories from well-meaning friends. The nurse is confronted with an ethical dilemma when a client is unaware of the real reason for surgery. In this situation the nurse confers with the physician before revealing specific information related to the client's medical diagnosis. When a client is well prepared and knows what to expect, the nurse's role is to reinforce the client's knowledge and maintain consistency in regard to the client's expectations.

MEDICATION HISTORY. If a client regularly uses prescription or over-the-counter medications, the physician may temporarily discontinue the drugs before surgery or adjust the dosages (Table 47-3). Anticoagulants, for example, increase the risk of intraoperative and postoperative hemorrhaging and must be discontinued. Other drugs—for example, antibiotics and anticonvulsants—may create adverse effects during general anesthesia. All prescription medications taken preoperatively are automatically discontinued postoperatively unless a physician reorders the medications.

ALLERGIES. The nurse is particularly alert for a client's allergies to medications that may be given during a phase of the surgical experience. The client receives a special allergy identification band before going to surgery. The nurse also makes sure that the front of the client's chart contains a listing of all allergies.

SMOKING HABITS. The client who smokes is at a greater risk for postoperative pulmonary complications than a nonsmoker. The chronic smoker already has an increased amount and thickness of mucous secretions in the tracheobronchial tree. General anesthetics stimulate production of pulmonary secretions, which are retained as a result of reduction in ciliary activity during anesthesia (see Chapter 41). After surgery the client who smokes has greater difficulty clearing the airways of mucous secretions. Smoke also causes local irritation to the tracheobronchial mucosa, and exposure to general anesthetic agents worsens airway irritation.

ALCOHOL INGESTION. Habitual use of alcohol predisposes the client to adverse reactions to anesthetic agents. The client also experiences a cross-tolerance to anesthetic agents, necessitating higher than normal doses of anesthetics. In addition, the physician may need to increase postoperative dosage requirements of analgesics.

FAMILY SUPPORT. It is important for the nurse to determine the extent of the client's support from family members or friends. Surgery often results in temporary or permanent disability that necessitates added assistance from family members during the client's recovery. The surgical client cannot always immediately assume the same level of physical activity enjoyed before an illness. Often a client returns home with dressings to change or exercises to perform. The family is an important resource in assisting the client with physical limitations and providing the emotional support needed to motivate the client to return to a previous state of health.

OCCUPATION. Surgery may result in physical alterations that hinder or prevent a person from returning to work. For example, back surgery affects a laborer who lifts heavy objects, and eye surgery has an influence on a seamstress. The nurse assesses the client's occupational history to anticipate the effects surgery might have on the client's work performance. This information prepares the nurse to explain any restrictions the client will have before returning to work. Clients are frequently concerned over the time it will take before they are allowed to return to work. When a client is unable to return to a job, the nurse may confer with a social worker to refer the individual to job-training programs or to seek economic assistance for the client.

REVIEW OF EMOTIONAL HEALTH

Surgery poses a psychological crisis for any individual. The client undergoes considerable anxiety in anticipation of what will happen during surgery and whether the procedure will bring an improved level of health. It is often difficult for individuals to face impending surgery calmly because they feel they have little control over their situation.

Family members perceive the client's surgery as a disruption in their life-style. Hospitalization, as well as the recovery period at home, may be lengthy. The family is usually concerned as to whether or not the client will be able to return to a normal productive life. When the client has chronic illness, the family becomes fearful that surgery may result in further disability.

To understand the impact surgery has on a client and family's emotional health, the nurse assesses the client's feelings about surgery and the client's self-concept, coping resources, and body image.

FEELINGS. How does a client really feel about having surgery? The nurse may be able to detect the client's emotions from mannerisms or behaviors. A fearful client often asks numerous questions, seems uneasy when strangers enter the room, or actively seeks the company of friends and relatives.

The nurse should choose a time for discussion after preliminary admitting or diagnostic tests are completed. It should be explained to the client that it is normal to have fears and concerns. The client's ability to share feelings depends on the nurse's willingness to listen, to be supportive, and to take time to clarify any of the client's misconceptions.

If the client describes a feeling of being powerless, the nurse determines what factors have caused this emotion. Perhaps the client's medical diagnosis generates apprehension of increased dependence and loss of physical or mental function. The thought of being "put to sleep" under anesthesia creates concern, since the client has no choice but to trust members of the surgical team while the level of consciousness is impaired. It is also important for many clients to retain the power to make decisions about their treatment. The nurse must assure clients of their right to ask questions and seek information about their condition.

A client may be angry about the need for surgery. A young person may feel it is unfair to have a disorder that typically affects older people. Surgery may occur at a time when it is inconvenient or potentially disruptive to a client's plans. It is common for the client to express anger by verbally attacking the nurse or physician. Being argumentative or overly demanding, refusing to cooperate, and criticizing the nurse's efforts to provide care are manifestations of anger and anxiety.

SELF-CONCEPT. A client with a positive self-concept is more likely to approach the surgical experience in a healthy manner. The nurse can assess a client's self-concept by asking the client to identify personal strengths and weaknesses. The client who is quick to criticize or scorn personal characteristics is likely either to have little self-regard or to be testing the nurse's opinion of his character. A poor self-concept hinders a client's ability to adapt to the stress of surgery and aggravates any feelings of guilt or inadequacy.

COPING RESOURCES. Assessment of a client's feelings and self-concept will help reveal whether the client has the ability to cope with the stress of surgery. It is also valuable to ask the client about past management of anxiety. If the client has had previous surgery, the nurse determines what behaviors helped resolve any tension or nervousness. Perhaps the client talked about the surgery or stayed busy with an activity such as reading. The nurse may instruct the client on relaxation exercises (see Chapter 37), which can be useful in helping control apprehension.

The nurse should inquire if there are family members or friends who can provide support during the surgical experience. The client may want a family member or friend present when the nurse provides instructions or explanations about surgery. Often a family member can become the client's coach, offering valuable support during the postoperative period when the client's participation in care is vital.

BODY IMAGE. The surgical removal of a diseased body part often leaves permanent disfigurement or alteration in body function. Concern over mutilation or loss of a body part compounds a surgical client's fears. The nurse can often detect the significance an attractive physical appearance holds for a client by the client's clothes and grooming.

The nurse determines what body image alterations the client perceives will result from surgery. A young woman is likely to be more threatened by the prospect of a mastectomy than by an appendectomy. A teacher facing a laryngectomy, a musician requiring hand surgery, or an athlete in need of an amputation are persons whose life-styles and body images would be significantly changed by surgery.

Often surgery changes the physical or psychological aspects of a client's sexuality. Sexuality is an important part of a person's identity and body image. The excision of breast tissue, a colostomy (see Chapter 40), a ureterostomy (see Chapter 39), or the removal of the prostate gland are just a few surgical alterations that may permanently affect a person's sexuality. Surgery such as a hernia repair or cataract extraction forces clients to refrain from sexual intercourse until they can return to normal physical activity.

It is important for the nurse to encourage clients to express any concerns surrounding their sexuality. The client who is to face even temporary sexual dysfunction requires the nurse's understanding and support. Any discussions about the client's sexuality should be held in the presence of the client's sexual partner so they can gain a shared understanding of how to cope with limitations in sexual function.

PHYSICAL EXAMINATION

The nurse conducts a partial or complete physical examination depending on the time available and the client's preoperative condition. Chapter 29 describes the techniques used in physical assessment. The assessment focuses on findings related to the client's medical history and on body systems to be affected by the surgery.

GENERAL SURVEY. The nurse observes the client's general appearance. The client's gestures and body movements may reflect energy or weakness caused by illness. The client may appear malnourished. Height and body weight are important indicators of the client's nutritional status.

Preoperative assessment of the client's vital signs provides an important baseline with which to compare alterations that occur during and after surgery. Anxiety and fear commonly cause elevations in heart rate and blood pressure. Anesthetic agents typically depress all vital functions; however, adverse drug reactions may include elevations in heart rate and blood pressure. As the effects of anesthesia diminish after surgery, the nurse closely monitors vital signs and compares findings with preoperative baselines.

Preoperative assessment of vital signs is also important to rule out the presence of fluid and electrolyte abnormalities (see Chapter 42). An elevated heart rate may result from a plasma fluid volume deficit, potassium deficit, or sodium excess. If the pulse is full and bounding, a fluid volume excess may be the cause. Cardiac arrhythmias are commonly caused by electrolyte imbalances.

An elevated temperature preoperatively is a cause for concern. If the client has an underlying infection, the surgeon may choose to postpone surgery until the infection has been treated. An increased body temperature increases the risk of fluid and electrolyte imbalance postoperatively.

HEAD AND NECK. The condition of oral mucous membranes reveals the client's level of hydration. A dehydrated client is at risk for developing serious fluid and electrolyte imbalances during surgery.

Inspection of the soft palate and nasal sinuses can reveal sinus drainage indicative of respiratory or sinus infection. To rule out the possibility of local or systemic infection the nurse palpates for cervical lymph node enlargement.

The nurse inspects the jugular veins for distention. An excess of fluid within the circulatory system or failure of the heart to contract efficiently may lead to jugular vein distention.

INTEGUMENT. The nurse carefully inspects the skin overlying all body parts. Particular attention is paid to bony prominences such as elbows, the sacrum, or scapula. During surgery a client must lie in a fixed position, often for several hours. Thus a client is susceptible to pressure sores (see Chapter 31) if the skin is thin and dry and has poor turgor. The overall condition of the skin also reveals the client's level of hydration.

THORAX AND LUNGS. Assessment of the client's breathing pattern and chest excursion will aid the nurse in determining the client's ventilatory capacity. Clients are encouraged to deep breathe and cough postoperatively (see section on preoperative teaching). A decline in ventilatory function may place the client at risk for respiratory complications.

Auscultation of breath sounds will indicate whether the client has pulmonary congestion or narrowing of the airways. The presence of crackles or rales signifies moisture in the airways, a condition that will be aggravated during surgery. Certain anesthetic agents can cause spasm of laryngeal muscles. If the nurse auscultates wheezing in the airways preoperatively, the client is at risk for further airway narrowing during surgery.

HEART AND VASCULAR SYSTEM. If the client has known cardiac disease, it is essential for the nurse to assess the character of the apical pulse. Postoperatively the nurse compares the rate and rhythm of the pulse with preoperative baselines. Anesthetic agents, alterations in fluid balance, and sympathetic stimulation from the surgical stress response can cause cardiac arrhythmias.

The nurse assesses peripheral pulses preoperatively to determine a client's circulatory status. This is particularly important for the client having vascular surgery or for a client who may have casts or constricting bandages applied to the extremities postoperatively. The postoperative development of a weak or absent pulse in a client who had adequate circulation before surgery is a sign that the client's circulation is impaired.

ABDOMEN. It is important to assess the client's abdomen for size, shape, symmetry, and the presence of distention. If the client undergoes abdominal surgery, the nurse makes frequent postoperative assessments of the abdominal incisional area and compares findings with preoperative data. Alteration in gastrointestinal function postoperatively may be manifest by the development of distention. The nurse should know whether the client is simply obese or the abdomen has become distended following surgery.

Assessment of preoperative bowel sounds is likewise useful as a baseline. The nurse also determines whether the client has regular bowel movements. If the client's surgery requires manipulation of portions of the gastrointestinal tract, normal peristalsis will not return and bowel sounds will be absent or diminished for several days postoperatively.

NEUROLOGICAL STATUS. During the health history and physical assessment the nurse observes the client's level of orientation, alertness, and mood. The nurse notes whether the client answers questions appropriately and is able to recall recent and past events. A client's level of consciousness will change as a result of general anesthesia; however, once the effects of

anesthesia disappear, the client should return to the preoperative level of responsiveness.

If a client is to have spinal anesthesia, preoperative assessment of gross motor function and strength is important. Spinal anesthesia causes temporary paralysis of the lower extremities. If the client enters surgery with weakness or impaired mobility of the lower extremities, the nurse should be aware of this to avoid becoming alarmed when full motor function does not return postoperatively.

RISK FACTORS

Various conditions and factors increase a person's risk in surgery. Knowledge of risk factors enables the nurse to take necessary precautions in planning a client's care.

AGE. Very young and elderly clients are surgical risks as a result of an immature or a declining physiological status. The infant cannot respond physically to the stress of surgery as well as an older child. During surgery nurses and physicians are especially concerned with maintaining an infant's normal body temperature. The infant's shivering reflex is underdeveloped, and often wide temperature variations occur. Anesthesia adds to the risk, since anesthetics can cause vasodilation and heat loss.

During surgery an infant has difficulty maintaining a normal circulatory blood volume. The total blood volume of infants is considerably less than that of older children and adults. Even a small amount of blood loss can be serious in an infant. For this reason the infant is highly susceptible to dehydration. However, if blood or fluids are replaced too quickly in an infant, overhydration may occur. A reduced circulatory volume makes it difficult for the infant to respond to the need for increased oxygen during surgery.

With advancing age a client's physical capacity to adapt to the stress of surgery is hampered because of deterioration in certain body functions. Despite the risk the majority of clients undergoing surgery are elderly. In urology and orthopedic wards the population is largely elderly. Table 47-4 summarizes physiological factors that place elderly clients at risk for surgery.

NUTRITION. Normal tissue repair and the resistance to infection depend on an adequate supply of nutrients. Surgery intensifies the body's need for nutrients. Postoperatively a client requires at least 1500 kcal per day just to maintain energy reserves (Keithley, 1982). A malnourished client is prone to improper wound healing, reduced energy stores, and the development of infection following surgery. If a client undergoes elective surgery, any nutrient imbalances

T A B L E 47 - 4

Physiological Factors That Place an Elderly Client at Risk for Surgery

System	Alterations	Risks	Preoperative Nursing Implications
Cardiovascular	Degenerative change in myocardium and valves	Reduced cardiac reserve	Assessing baseline vital signs
	Rigidity of arterial walls and reduction in sympathetic and parasympathetic innervation to heart	Predisposes client to postoperative hemorrhage and rise in systolic and diastolic blood pressure	
	Increase in calcium and cholesterol deposits within small arteries; arterial walls thickened	Predisposes client to clot formation in lower extremities	Instructing client on techniques for performing leg exercises and proper turning
Pulmonary	Rib cage stiffened and reduced in size	Reduced vital capacity	Instructing client on proper technique for coughing and deep breathing exercises
	Reduced range of movement in diaphragm	Greater residual capacity or volume of air left in lung after normal breath increases, reducing amount of new air brought into lungs with each inspiration	
	Lung tissue stiffened and airspaces enlarged	Reduced blood oxygenation	
Renal	Reduced blood flow to kidneys	Increases danger of shock when blood loss occurs	Determining baseline urinary output for 24 hour period
	Reduced glomerular filtration rate and excretory times	Limits ability to remove drugs or toxic substances	
	Reduced bladder capacity	Voiding frequency increases, and larger amount of urine stays in the bladder after voiding	Instructing client to notify nurse immediately when sensation of bladder fullness develops
		Sensation of need to void may not occur until bladder is filled	Keeping call light and/or bedpan within easy reach
Neurological	Sensory losses: reduced tactile sense, increased pain tolerance	Client less able to respond to early warning signs of surgical complications	Orienting client to surrounding environment
	Decreased reaction time	Becomes confused easily following anesthesia	
Metabolic	Lower basal metabolic rate	Reduces total oxygen consumption	
	Reduced number of red blood cells and hemoglobin levels	Reduces ability to carry adequate oxygen to tissues	Administering necessary blood products preoperatively
	Change in total amounts of body potassium and water volume	Greater risk for fluid or electrolyte imbalance	Monitoring electrolyte levels preoperatively

can be corrected beforehand (see Chapter 38). However, if a malnourished client must undergo emergency surgery, efforts to restore necessary nutrients occur postoperatively.

Obesity is a nutritional disorder that increases a client's surgical risk. The obese client usually has reduced ventilatory and cardiac function and experiences difficulty in resuming normal physical activity after surgery. The obese client is susceptible to poor wound healing and wound infection because of the structure of fatty tissue. Fatty tissue contains a very poor blood supply, which slows the delivery of essential nutrients, antibodies, and enzymes needed for wound healing. It is also often difficult to close the surgical wound of an obese client because of the thick adipose layer.

RADIOTHERAPY. For the client with cancer, surgery may be only one form of treatment. Radiotherapy is often given preoperatively to reduce the size of the cancerous tumor so it can be removed surgically. Radiation has some unavoidable effects on normal tissue, such as excess thinning of skin layers, destruction of collagen, and impaired vascularization of tissue. Ideally the surgeon waits to perform surgery 4 to 6 weeks after the completion of radiation treatments. If this is impossible, the client may face serious wound healing problems postoperatively.

FLUID AND ELECTROLYTE BALANCE. The body responds to surgery as a form of trauma. As a result of the adrenocortical stress response, hormonal reactions cause sodium and water retention and potassium loss within the first 2 to 5 days after surgery. Protein breakdown causes a negative nitrogen balance. The severity of the stress response influences the degree of fluid and electrolyte imbalance. The more extensive the surgery, the more severe the stress. A client who is hypovolemic or who has serious electrolyte alterations preoperatively is at significant risk during and after surgery. For example, an excess or depletion of potassium preoperatively increases the chance of arrhythmias developing during or after surgery. If the client has preexisting renal, gastrointestinal, or cardiovascular abnormalities, the risk of fluid and electrolyte alterations is even greater.

DIAGNOSTIC SCREENING

Before a client undergoes surgery, the surgeon will order an array of diagnostic tests to screen for the presence of preexisting abnormalities. Many clients are able to obtain the tests on an outpatient basis before entering the hospital. However, a client may also enter the hospital several days in advance to complete all testing procedures. If diagnostic tests reveal sufficiently severe problems, the surgeon may choose to cancel surgery until the client's condition stabilizes.

The nurse is responsible for coordinating the completion of tests and for being sure all clients are prepared properly for the diagnostic studies. The nurse also reviews diagnostic results as they become available so as to alert physicians to findings and to plan appropriate therapy.

Routine screening tests include a complete blood count (CBC), serum electrolytes, serum creatinine or blood urea nitrogen (BUN), urinalysis, and a chest x-ray study.

COMPLETE BLOOD COUNT. A CBC is an analysis of a peripheral venous blood specimen that includes measurement of a client's red blood cell count, hemoglobin concentration, and hematocrit (packed red cell volume). The laboratory of each health institution has a standard for normal laboratory values. An abnormal CBC may be indicative of a number of alterations, for example, dietary deficiency and chronic blood loss, placing the client at risk for cardiovascular and pulmonary complications. In such a case the surgeon may choose to administer blood products before surgery.

SERUM ELECTROLYTES. Analysis of serum electrolyte levels also requires the collection of a peripheral venous blood sample. Serum electrolyte tests routinely include measurement of sodium, potassium, chloride, and carbon dioxide content. Because of the potential for fluid and electrolyte imbalances following surgery, the surgeon screens preoperative electrolyte levels to determine if electrolyte replacement is necessary before surgery.

SERUM CREATININE. To assess the client's renal function the physician orders a serum creatinine test. Creatinine is the by-product of muscle metabolism. The body excretes a constant amount through the kidneys, which serves as an excellent measure of the glomerular filtration rate. The creatinine level can be a sensitive indicator of renal failure when the value rises. In the past, many physicians used the serum BUN test to assess renal function. Unlike creatinine, BUN is affected by a variety of conditions unrelated to kidney function, for example, diet, infection, exercise, or fluid intake.

URINALYSIS. Analysis of a urine specimen consists of screening for the presence of urinary infection, renal disease, and diabetes mellitus. The nurse collects a clean voided specimen. Included in a urinalysis is measurement of urine color, pH, and specific gravity. There is also a determination of the presence of protein, glucose, ketones, and blood. Chapter 39 discusses normal values in a urinalysis.

CHEST X-RAY STUDY. A chest film allows the physician to examine the condition of the heart and lungs before surgery. Although the x-ray study does not always detect subtle pathological changes, it can reveal the overall size and shape of the heart, presence of lung lesions and chest wall abnormalities, and position of the diaphragm and aorta. If the physician detects any lung abnormalities, a different type and dosage of sedatives or anesthetic agents may be used. Before sending the female client for x-ray examination, the nurse should be sure she is not pregnant. Exposure of the fetus to radiation may cause injury.

ADDITIONAL SCREENING TESTS. If a client is over the age of 40 or has heart disease, the physician orders an electrocardiogram (ECG). The test involves the painless application of electrodes to the client's chest and extremities. An ECG measures the heart's electrical activity to determine if the heart rate and rhythm and other factors are normal. The procedure takes less than 5 minutes and requires the client simply to lie flat and relax.

Depending on the type of surgery the client will undergo, there are a variety of diagnostic tests for specific anatomical structures and physiological functions. (See Unit 8 for a more detailed discussion of these tests.)

If the client is likely to lose a significant amount of blood during surgery, the physician orders a blood specimen for type and cross-matching. The test enables the laboratory to determine the proper blood type and Rh factor for the client. The surgeon usually designates the number of blood units to have available during the client's surgery.

Diagnosis

The nurse's assessment of the surgical client leads to the formation of nursing diagnoses with implications for care during one or all of the surgical phases. Preoperative nursing diagnoses allow the nurse to take necessary precautions so care provided during the intraoperative and postoperative phases is consistent with the client's needs. For example, if the nurse identifies a problem of altered skin integrity preoperatively, an attempt can be made to position the client on the operating table so that bony prominences are protected. The nurse caring for the client postoperatively will continue to position the client and provide skin care until the client is able to resume normal physical movement and maintain personal hygiene.

Nursing diagnosis also focuses on the potential risks a client may face postoperatively. For example, a client with a preoperative diagnosis of inadequate food intake may be a candidate for poor wound healing after surgery. Thus the client's postoperative nurs-

---

TABLE 47-5

Examples of Nursing Diagnoses That Focus on Potential Risks of Surgery

Diagnosis	Surgical Risk
Knowledge deficit related to physiological and psychological responses to surgery	Client unable to understand implications of surgery; will have difficulty cooperating and participating in plan of care without extensive teaching
Alteration in nutrition	
Related to excessive intake	Obese client at risk for poor wound healing, infection, and pulmonary and cardiovascular problems
Related to deficient intake	Malnourished client more susceptible to infection and poor wound healing
Impaired skin integrity related to radiation exposure	Client prone to skin breakdown and impaired wound healing
Anxiety related to impending surgery	Client's fears or concerns may interfere with ability to participate in care
Ineffective airway clearance	Client who is fatigued or unable to effectively cough and clear secretions at risk for developing further pulmonary congestion postoperatively
Fluid volume deficit	Fluid imbalance will become aggravated postoperatively as a result of surgical stress response

ing care will include efforts to maintain an adequate nutritional intake and to minimize exposure of the surgical wound to infectious agents. Table 47-5 presents some typical nursing diagnoses that pose nursing challenges for reducing a client's risks during surgery.

Communication of the client's diagnoses among care givers is essential throughout the surgical experience. Preoperative diagnoses that direct the care provided to a client before surgery can be found in the client's care plan in the chart or Kardex. Operating room nurses often have checklists and intraoperative care plans on which they record the client's nursing care. The nurse uses preoperative and intraoperative diagnoses as standards for supportive and preventive care after surgery. The nurse in the surgical unit also reassesses the client for any new problems that develop following surgery.

Planning

Although it is essential to include any client in health care planning, this is especially important for the surgical client. Early involvement of the client in developing the surgical plan of care will minimize surgical risks and postoperative complications. For example, nursing research has shown that structured preoperative teaching can reduce the surgical client's hospital stay (Lindeman and VanAernam, 1971).

The plan of care is based on the nursing diagnoses. Therefore the preoperative preparation of the surgical client is an individualized process. However, there are also basic types of preparation each surgical client must undergo. Goals to include in the client's preparation include the following:

1. Promoting the client's and family's understanding of the physiological and psychological responses to surgery
2. Promoting return of normal physiological function postoperatively
3. Maintaining the client's normal fluid and electrolyte balance
4. Minimizing skin contamination by microorganisms
5. Preventing bowel or bladder incontinence intraoperatively
6. Promoting the client's rest and comfort
7. Protecting the client from physical harm

Preoperative Preparation

Nursing interventions during the preoperative surgical phase provide the client with a complete understanding of what surgery involves and prepare the client physically for surgical intervention.

INFORMED CONSENT

A surgeon cannot legally perform surgery until a client understands the need for a procedure, what is involved, the risks, expected results, and alternative treatments. Primary responsibility for informing the client rests with the surgeon. Consent is not informed if the client is confused, unconscious, mentally incompetent, or under the influence of sedatives. All consent forms must be signed before the nurse administers preoperative medications.

The surgeon's explanation to the client should be witnessed by a qualified member of the health care team. The consent form's structure allows the physician to write in information related to the client's surgery. A client's signature on a consent form implies that the client has been thoroughly informed about the procedure. The nurse frequently witnesses signing of the form and examines the document for the correct date, time, and signature, which must be in ink. A client who is illiterate can sign by making a mark as long as it is properly witnessed. As a witness the nurse is able to attest that the client's signature is on the form but not that the client was properly informed. In many institutions a time limit is placed on consent forms, for example, 30 days.

Individuals must personally sign the consent form if they are (1) of legal age (varies among states and Canadian provinces), (2) under legal age but have a valid marriage certificate, (3) designated as an emancipated minor (certain states), and (4) not at present under legal guardianship. In some Canadian provinces a teenager may sign a consent form under certain conditions. If the client is a minor or legally considered to be incompetent and is not included in any of these categories, a parent or legal guardian signs the consent form. A spouse or next of kin signs for an adult who is unconscious or mentally incompetent.

In emergency situations the client may be unable to sign and family members may be unavailable. The surgeon is legally permitted to perform surgery without consent in such a case; however, every effort must be made to obtain permission from a responsible family member by telephone or telegram. A telephone consent must be witnessed by two persons who hear the family member's oral consent. The two witnesses sign the consent with the name of the family member, noting that an oral consent was obtained. The acquisition of informed consent is critical to protect not only the client but also health personnel so the surgical team can practice without fear of legal reprisal.

Once the client's consent form has been completed, the nurse makes sure the form is placed in the client's record. The record goes to the operating room with the client. Chapter 17 discusses in detail the nurse's responsibilities for informed consent.

PREOPERATIVE TEACHING

With some nursing interventions it is difficult to prove that the action positively influences a client's overall health status. However, structured preoperative teaching has proven benefits. Preoperative teaching concerning a client's expected postoperative behaviors, provided in a systematic and structured format with teaching and learning principles, has a positive influence on the client's recovery. Structured preoperative teaching can influence such postoperative factors as the following:

1. *Ventilatory function.* Teaching improves the client's ability to cough and deep breathe effectively.
2. *Physical functional capacity.* Teaching improves the client's ability to ambulate and resume activities of daily living early.
3. *Sense of well-being.* Clients who are prepared for surgery experience less anxiety and report a greater sense of psychological well-being.
4. *Length of hospital stay.* Structured preoperative teaching can reduce the length of stay.

The most effective type of teaching program for surgical clients is planned so all clients receive the same information. Detailed discussion and demonstration of postoperative exercises, including diaphragmatic breathing, effective coughing, turning, and leg exercises, are vital. If the client understands why these exercises are important to postoperative recovery and knows how to perform them correctly, the recovery period will be less complicated.

Including family members in the client's preoperative preparation is highly advantageous. Often it is a family member who serves as the coach for postoperative exercises when the client returns from surgery. If anxious relatives do not understand routine postoperative events, it is likely their anxiety will heighten the client's fears or concerns. Preoperative preparation of family members minimizes their anxiety and misunderstanding.

The nurse should provide the client with information about sensations typically experienced after surgery. A person who faces an event different from anything experienced previously is inadequately prepared to interpret that event. Preparatory information (see Chapter 16) helps clients anticipate what will happen during a procedure and thus helps them form a realistic image of the surgical experience. When events occur as predicted, the client is better able to cope and attend to the experiences. For example, in the operating room the anesthesiologist may apply petrolatum ointment to the client's eyes to prevent corneal damage. Warning the client about the sensation of blurred vision will reduce the client's anxiety on awakening from surgery. Other sensations the nurse may describe include the expected pain at the surgical site, the tightness of dressings, dryness of the mouth, or the sensation of a sore throat resulting from insertion of an endotracheal tube.

It is highly advantageous to begin preoperative teaching well in advance of a client's scheduled surgery. If the nurse is able to teach a client 1 or 2 days before surgery, the client will be better able to attend to learning. Anxiety and fear are significant barriers to learning, and both emotions are heightened as surgery approaches. As is the case with any client education program, the nurse assesses the surgical client's readiness and ability to learn. If the client is capable and receptive to learning, the nurse presents information in a logical sequence beginning with preoperative events and advancing to intraoperative and postoperative routines. Preoperative teaching checklists give nurses useful guidelines for presenting clients with comprehensive instructions.

The Association of Operating Room Nurses (1982) has established criteria by which the client demonstrates understanding of the surgical experience. Extensive preoperative teaching will not only improve the client's understanding but will promote the return of the client's normal physiological function as well. The AORN's recommendations and a discussion of each follow.

1. *The client cites reasons for each of the preoperative instructions provided and exercises explained or practiced.* Given a rationale for the various preoperative and postoperative procedures, the client is better prepared to participate in nursing care. Every preoperative teaching program includes explanation and demonstration of the four postoperative exercises: diaphragmatic breathing, coughing, turning, and leg exercises. These exercises are designed to prevent postoperative complications (Procedure 47-1).

While a client is under general anesthesia, the lungs do not ventilate fully. The cough reflex is suppressed, and mucus accumulates within the airway passages. Postoperatively the client has a reduced lung volume and needs greater effort to breathe.

During surgery the venous blood flow to the legs slows. Stasis of the circulation may lead to formation of thrombi or clots. A clot can break off from the point of origin and travel to the brain, heart, or lungs to cause potentially fatal complications.

Diaphragmatic breathing improves lung expansion and oxygen delivery without excessive energy expenditure. The client learns how to use the diaphragm

PROCEDURE 47-1

Demonstrating the Postoperative Exercise Regimen

STEPS	RATIONALE

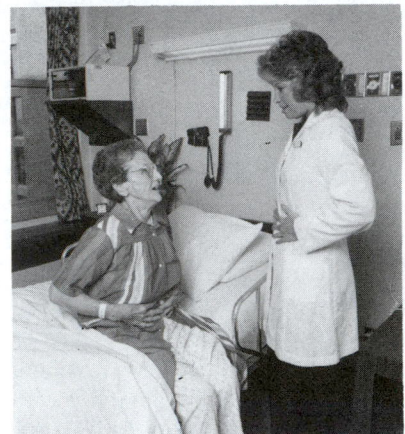

DIAPHRAGMATIC BREATHING

1. Sit or stand upright placing the hands palm down along the lower borders of the anterior rib cage.

An upright position facilitates diaphragmatic excursion. This placement of hands allows the individual to feel movement of the chest and abdomen as the diaphragm descends and lungs expand.

2. Take a slow deep breath, inhaling through the nose.

This discourages panting or hyperventilation. Breathing through the nose warms, humidifies, and filters air.

3. Give attention to the normal downward movement of the diaphragm during inspiration. The abdominal organs descend, and the thorax expands slowly.

The nurse's explanation focuses on normal ventilatory movements so the client can anticipate how diaphragmatic breathing feels.

4. Avoid using chest and shoulders while inhaling.

Use of auxiliary chest and shoulder muscles increases energy expenditure during breathing.

5. After holding the breath to a count of 3, slowly exhale through the mouth.

This allows gradual expulsion of all air.

6. Repeat the exercise three to five times.

This establishes a slow, rhythmical breathing pattern.

7. Have the client practice the exercise.

This reinforces learning.

COUGHING

1. Assume an upright position.

This position facilitates diaphragm movement and enhances expansion of lungs.

2. Take two or three slow diaphragmatic breaths.

This expands the lungs fully to move air behind mucus in airways.

3. Inhale deeply, hold the breath to a count of 3, and cough once, then again.

Two successive coughs help remove mucus more effectively and completely than one forceful cough.

4. Caution the client against merely clearing the throat.

Clearing of the throat does not remove mucus from deep in the airways.

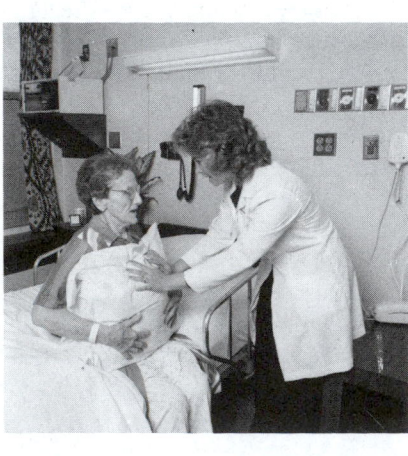

5. If the surgical incision is to be in the chest or abdominal area, place one hand over the incisional area and the other hand on top of the first hand. During inhalation and coughing press gently against the incisional area to splint the incision. (A pillow over the incision is optional.)

A surgical incision results in the cutting of muscles and tissues. Breathing and coughing place strain on a suture line and cause discomfort. Splinting minimizes incisional pulling. The hands provide firm support to the incision.

6. Have the client practice coughing with splinting.

The nurse emphasizes the value of deep coughing with splinting to effectively expectorate mucus with minimal discomfort.

STEPS	RATIONALE

TURNING

NOTE: This is for turning to the left side.

1. Instruct the client to assume a supine position to the right half of the bed. (Side rails are up on both sides of the bed).

   The nurse cannot demonstrate the exercise in the client's bed for obvious reasons of asepsis. Positioning begins toward the right side of the bed so turning to the left will not cause the client to roll toward the bed's edge.

2. Have the client place the left hand over the incisional area for splinting.

   This supports the incisional area to minimize pulling of suture line during turning.

3. Have the client keep the left leg straight and flex the right knee up and over the left leg.

   A straight left leg stabilizes the client's position. The flexed right leg shifts weight for easier turning.

4. Have the client grasp the side rail on the left side of the bed with the right hand. Then the client pulls toward the left and rolls onto the left side.

   Pulling toward the side rail minimizes the effort needed to turn.

LEG EXERCISES

1. Place the client in a flat supine position in bed. Demonstrate leg exercises by putting the client through passive range of motion.

   This provides for normal anatomical position of lower extremities.

   NOTE: If the client's surgery involves one or both extremities, a surgeon's order is required before exercises can be performed postoperatively. Legs unaffected by surgery can be safely exercised unless a client has preexisting alterations.

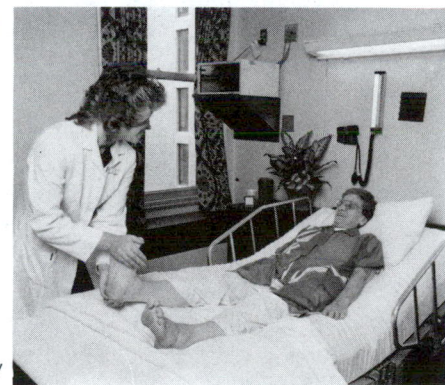

2. Rotate each ankle in a complete 360-degree circle by having the client pretend to draw circles with the big toe

   Leg exercise maintains joint mobility and promotes venous return.

2. Alternate dorsiflexion and plantar flexion of the feet. The client will feel the calf muscles alternately contract and relax.

   This stretches and contracts the gastrocnemius muscles.

3. Have the client alternately flex and extend the knees.

4. Have the client alternately raise each leg straight up from the bed surface, keeping the legs straight.

   This promotes contraction and relaxation of quadriceps muscles.

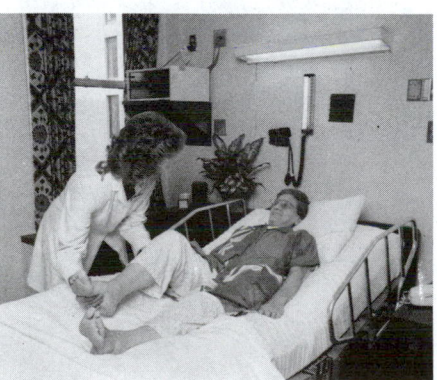

during deep breathing to take slow, deep, and relaxed breaths. Eventually the client's lung volume improves postoperatively. Deep breathing also helps to clear out any anesthetic gases remaining in the airways. To facilitate deep breathing the physician may order an incentive spirometer for the client. This device encourages effective deep breathing through sustained maximal inspiration (see Chapter 41).

Coughing assists in the removal of retained mucus in the airways. A deep productive cough is more beneficial than merely clearing the throat. It is especially important for a client to practice this exercise after surgery. Postoperative incisional pain makes coughing difficult. Unless the client anticipates the pain and understands the importance of coughing, it is unlikely that coughing will be successful. The nurse also teaches the client how to splint an incision to minimize pain during coughing. Nurses direct clients to cough and deep breathe at least every 2 hours while awake.

Leg exercises and turning improve blood flow to the extremities and thus reduce stasis. Contraction of lower leg muscles promotes venous return, making it difficult for clots to form. When a client has learned how to turn and perform leg exercises, the nurse encourages the individual to perform each at least every 2 hours while awake. The client can easily exercise in bed.

After explaining each exercise, the nurse demonstrates it. The client observes the proper position for each exercise and the performance of each step. The nurse then acts as a coach, guiding the client through each exercise. For example, the nurse says whether the client is sitting properly and helps the client place the hands in the proper position during breathing. The nurse then allows the client time (at least 15 minutes) for independent practice. The nurse can attend to other clients' needs before returning to watch the learner demonstrate each exercise independently. The nurse gives the client feedback as to the performance, telling the client what aspect of each exercise is done correctly and what needs improvement.

2. *The client states the time surgery is scheduled.* The client and family should be informed of the approximate time when surgery will begin. If the hospital has a busy operating room schedule, it is best to let the client know the order of surgery—that is, how many procedures are scheduled before the client's. It is unwise to tell the client and family the anticipated length of surgery. Unanticipated delays may occur for many reasons—delays in room cleaning, slow transport of the client, or complications during surgery. If the client fails to return at the time expected by the family, they will be highly anxious. Family members should be told that nurses in the postoperative surgical division will inform them of the client's arrival in the recovery room.

3. *The client states the unit to which he will return after surgery and the location of family during the intraoperative and immediate recovery periods.* The unit to which the client is admitted before surgery may be different from the postoperative unit. It is important for the family to know where the client will be taken after surgery. The nurse also explains where the family can wait and where the surgeon will attempt to find family members when surgery is completed. If the client is to be taken to a special unit, it is helpful before surgery to familiarize both the client and family members with the unit's environment.

4. *The client discusses anticipated monitoring and therapeutic devices or materials likely to be used postoperatively.* The client and family want to know what to expect. For example, nurses routinely monitor vital signs postoperatively to detect complications and the aftereffects of anesthesia. If the client and family understand this before surgery, they will not be apprehensive when nurses make frequent postoperative assessments. The nurse can also explain whether the client is likely to have intravenous lines, dressings, drainage tubes, or other types of equipment. The nurse should take the precaution of neither overpreparing nor underpreparing the client and family. It is difficult for the nurse to predict every type of therapy or equipment the client will require. Each surgeon tends to follow different practices for each type of surgery. Although the nurse becomes familiar with each surgeon's preferences, as well as the surgical procedure itself, it is easy to misinform a client about a therapy that may not be initiated. Contradictions between what the nurse explains and what actually occurs postoperatively can cause great anxiety for the client and family.

5. *The client describes in general terms the surgical procedures and subsequent treatment plan.* After the surgeon has explained the basic purpose of a surgical procedure and what it involves, the client may ask the nurse additional questions to clarify any misunderstandings. The nurse is careful to avoid saying anything that contradicts the surgeon's explanation. One way to avoid problems is to first ask what the client has been told. For example, if the client says, "I know I'm having my gallbladder removed," it is within the nurse's role to explain basically how the procedure is performed. When the client has little or no understanding about the surgery, the nurse first checks with the physician to determine what explanations can be given.

Postoperatively there are certain predictable aspects of the client's treatment plan, for example, dressing changes, respiratory therapy, and level of supportive nursing care to be offered. The nurse can also describe plans for postoperative rehabilitation and drug therapy.

6. *The client describes anticipated steps in post-operative activity resumption.* Two questions clients ask commonly before surgery are "How soon will I be able to get up?" and "When will I be able to eat?" The type of surgery a client undergoes will affect the speed with which normal physical activity and regular eating habits can be resumed. For example, the client with extensive back surgery may not be able to walk as early as the client with a simple hernia repair. Likewise, the client who undergoes abdominal surgery will not be able to eat solid foods as soon as the client who has had a repair of a clotted artery in the leg.

The nurse explains that it is normal for the client to progress gradually in activity and eating. If the client tolerates activity and diet well, activity levels will progress more quickly.

7. *The client verbalizes expectations about pain relief and the measures likely to be taken to alleviate pain.* One of the surgical client's greatest fears is the amount of pain to be experienced postoperatively. The family also has a primary concern for the client's comfort. Pain after surgery is normal. The nurse informs the client and family of therapies available for pain relief, for example, analgesics, positioning, splinting, and relaxation exercises. The client should understand what an "as needed" (p.r.n.) medication for pain really means (see Chapter 32). Often a client is misled into believing pain medication is available on request.

The client should be encouraged to inform the nurses as soon as the pain becomes a constant discomfort. If a client waits until postoperative pain becomes excruciating, an analgesic will not provide relief. The client should also know that it takes time for a medication to act and that rarely will all the discomfort be eliminated.

Often surgical clients avoid taking pain medications for fear of becoming dependent on the drug. Normally this is unlikely, since the drug dosages and the required intervals between "as needed" medications are not sufficient to cause dependence. The nurse should encourage the client to use analgesics as needed. Unless the pain is controlled, it will be difficult for the client to participate in postoperative exercises, ambulation, and self-care activities. Clients initially receive parenteral injections. As they become able to tolerate food, the physician replaces parenteral analgesics with oral dosage forms.

8. *The client expresses feelings regarding surgical intervention and its expected outcomes.* The client may feel like part of an assembly line during the pre-operative surgical phase. Frequent visits by physicians and nurses, diagnostic testing, and the physical preparation for surgery consume a large amount of time and the client has few opportunities to reflect on what is happening. The nurse has an important role in making sure the surgical client does not feel like a "case" or "number." The client and family need time to express any feelings about surgery. The client's level of anxiety will influence how often the nurse should provide time for discussion. While delivering routine care the nurse can offer the client the opportunity to express any concerns. Late in the evening after tests and procedures have been completed is an opportune time for the nurse and client to sit together and discuss the client's feelings at length. The family may wish to discuss their concerns without the client in attendance so that their fears will not frighten the client.

PHYSICAL PREPARATION

The degree of preoperative physical preparation depends on the client's health status, the type of surgery to be performed, and the surgeon's own preferences. A seriously ill client will receive more supportive care in the form of medications, intravenous fluid therapy, and monitoring than the client facing a minor elective procedure. The nurse explains to the client the purpose of all procedures. The nurse's responsibilities include the following.

1. *The nurse maintains normal fluid and electrolyte balance.* The surgical client is vulnerable to fluid and electrolyte imbalances as a result of inadequate preoperative intake or excessive fluid losses intraoperatively. A client is given nothing by mouth (NPO) after midnight before the morning of surgery. After 6 to 8 hours of fasting the client's gastrointestinal tract will be relatively empty, so the risks of vomiting or aspirating emesis during surgery are minimal. General anesthetics typically cause slowing of gastrointestinal peristalsis. The nurse removes all fluids and solid foods from the client's bedside and posts a sign over the bed to alert hospital personnel and family members about fasting restrictions. The nurse can allow the client to rinse the mouth with water or mouthwash and brush the teeth as long as the client does not swallow water. The nurse notifies the surgeon immediately if the client eats or drinks during the fasting period.

During surgery the normal mechanisms for controlling fluid and electrolyte balance, including respiration, digestion, circulation, and elimination, are disturbed. The surgical procedure itself may cause extensive losses of blood and other body fluids. The surgical stress response aggravates any fluid and electrolyte imbalance. The nurse determines if the client

PROCEDURE 47-2

Shaving the Surgical Site

EQUIPMENT:

1. Portable lamp to illuminate site
2. Bath blanket for draping the client
3. Wet shave:
    Razor with extra blade
    Clean basin with warm water
    Gauze sponges
    Basin with liquid antiseptic soap mixed with water
    Waterproof underpad or towels
    Washcloth
    Cotton balls, cotton-tipped applicator, and antiseptic solution (optional)

4. Dry shave:
    Electric clippers
    Scissors
    Towel
    Antiseptic solution (optional)

---

has eaten and drunk sufficient amounts preoperatively before fasting to ensure adequate fluid and nutrition intake. The client's diet should include foods high in protein, with sufficient amounts of carbohydrates, fat, and vitamins. If a client is unable to eat because of gastrointestinal alterations or impairments in consciousness, an intravenous route for fluid replacement is started. The physician relies on serum electrolyte levels to determine the type of intravenous fluids and electrolyte additives to administer. Clients with severe nutritional imbalances may require intravenous supplements that contain concentrated protein and glucose (see Chapter 42).

2. *The nurse minimizes skin contamination by microorganisms.* The skin is a favorite site for microorganisms to grow and multiply. Without proper skin preparation the risk of postoperative wound infection is high.

The evening before surgery the client showers with an antiseptic soap to remove resident and transient bacteria. Depending on the surgical procedure the client may repeat the shower the morning of surgery. The nurse directs the client to pay particular attention to scrubbing the operative site. Often the surgeon will order two or more applications of soap with each shower. If the surgical procedure involves the head, neck, or upper chest area, the client may also be required to shampoo the hair. Cleaning and trimming of fingernails and toenails are necessary when the surgeon desires strict asepsis.

Many surgeons order shaving of the surgical site because body hair harbors large numbers of microorganisms. Thick or coarse hair also interferes with visibility of the surgical site. Although some physicians order a preoperative shave the night before surgery, it is preferable to shave hair immediately before surgery. This often occurs in a special holding area

outside the surgical suite. Hair removal can injure the skin, especially if a razor is used. Minor nicks or cuts in the skin are prime sites for bacterial growth, and the longer the period between the shave and surgery, the greater the potential for bacterial growth.

Shaving is not as routine a procedure as in the past. The wound infection rate for clients shaved before surgery is higher than for clients who were not shaved. The Centers for Disease Control recommends using clippers or a depilatory to remove hair. The nurse should consult agency policy for the preoperative shave procedure. Procedure 47-2 describes the procedure for shaving surgical sites.

3. *The nurse prevents bowel and bladder incontinence.* At one time clients routinely received enemas before surgery because general anesthesia slows gastrointestinal motility. Emptying the client's intestinal tract reduces the chance that constipation will develop postoperatively.

Today a client may not receive a bowel preparation unless surgery involves the gastrointestinal system. Manipulation of portions of the gastrointestinal tract during surgery results in absence of peristalsis for 24 hours and sometimes longer. Enemas and cathartics cleanse the gastrointestinal tract to prevent postoperative constipation, as well as incontinence during surgery. An empty bowel reduces risk of injury to the intestines and prevents contamination of the operative wound should a portion of the bowel be incised or opened. The surgeon's order may read "give enemas until clear." This means the nurse is to administer enemas until the time when the enema return contains no fecal material (see Chapter 40). Too many enemas given over a short period of time, however, can cause serious fluid and electrolyte imbalances. Most agencies recommend a limit to the number of enemas a nurse may administer successively.

PROCEDURE 47-2, cont'd

Shaving the Surgical Site

STEPS	RATIONALE

WET SHAVE

1. Explain the purpose of the shave to the client and the reason for preparation of a large skin surface area.

This minimizes the client's anxiety (the client may fear surgical incision will be as large as shaved site).

2. Refer to the physician's order to determine the portion of body to shave.

Shaving of a wide area around the incision site further reduces risk of contamination by hair.

3. Provide for the client's privacy by closing the room divider and door. Drape the client. Leave only the area to be shaved at one time (4 to 8 inches) exposed.

This promotes comfort and reduces anxiety.

4. Place a towel or waterproof pad under the body part to be shaved.

This prevents soiling of bed linen.

5. Lather the skin with gauze sponges dipped in antiseptic soap.

This softens hair and reduces friction against the skin from the razor.

6. Shave a small area at a time (approximately 4 to 8 inches). With the nondominant hand gently stabilize the skin, and with the razor held in the dominant hand at a 45-degree angle shave in the same direction the hair grows. Use short gentle strokes with the razor.

Shaving a small area minimizes cutting. The direction of shave prevents pulling of hair.

7. Rinse the razor as soap and hair accumulate on the blade. Discard blades as they become dull.

This maintains a clean, sharp razor edge to promote the client's comfort.

8. Rearrange drapes as each portion of the shave is completed.

This maintains the client's comfort.

9. Use washcloth and warm water to wash off remaining hair and soap solution. Discard the waterproof pad or towel.

This reduces skin irritation.

10. Observe for any nicks or cuts in the skin. Report them to the physician.

A break in skin integrity increases the risk of infection.

11. Dispose of equipment according to agency policy.

This prevents spread of infection and reduces the risk of injury from razor blades.

12. Record the area of skin preparation in the client's chart.

DRY SHAVE

1. Follow steps 1 through 3 of the wet shave procedure.

2. Lightly dry the area to be shaved with a towel.

This eliminates moisture, which can interfere with clean cut of clippers.

3. Hold the clippers approximately 1 cm above the skin, and shave in the direction hair grows.

This prevents abrasion of skin and pulling of hair.

4. Rearrange drapes as necessary.

5. Lightly brush off cut hair with a towel.

This removes contaminated hair and promotes the client's comfort.

6. Follow steps 11 and 12 of wet shave procedure.

7. (Optional) When the shaved area is over body crevices, e.g., umbilicus or groin, clean the crevices with cotton-tipped applicators or cotton balls dipped in antiseptic solution. Dry with cotton balls or applicators.

This removes secretions, dirt, and any remaining hair clippings, which harbor microorganisms.

The bladder is not prepared until the morning of surgery. The nurse instructs the client to void just before leaving for the operating room. An empty bladder prevents a client from being incontinent during surgery. This is particularly important during abdominal surgery when it may become necessary for the surgeon to manipulate the bladder. An empty bladder also makes abdominal organs more accessible during surgery. Often the nurse in the operating room will insert a Foley catheter in the client to maintain an empty bladder.

4. *The nurse promotes rest and comfort.* Rest is essential for normal restoration and healing of the body. Anxiety about surgery can easily interfere with the client's ability to relax or sleep. The underlying condition necessitating surgery may be a painful one, further impairing rest.

The nurse should attempt to make the client's environment as comfortable as possible. A loud boisterous roommate, a television program, or talkative family members are some stimuli the nurse may need to control. Frequently, the physician orders a sedative for the night before surgery. Drugs such as pentobarbital (Nembutal) and secobarbital (Seconal) produce a calming effect and relieve the client's apprehension. The nurse should administer the sedative when the client is prepared for sleep and after all tests and procedures have been completed.

DAY OF SURGERY

On the morning before surgery the nurse completes a number of routine procedures before releasing the client for surgery.

1. *The nurse checks medical record contents and completes recording.* Before the client goes to the operating room, the nurse checks the contents of the medical record to be sure all pertinent laboratory and test results are present. The nurse checks all consent forms for accuracy of information. A preoperative checklist (Fig. 47-1) provides the nurse with guidelines for ensuring completion of all nursing interventions. The nurse also checks the nurse's notes to be sure documentation of nursing care is current. This is especially important if the client experienced any unpredicted problems the night before surgery.

2. *The nurse checks vital signs.* The nurse makes a final preoperative assessment of vital signs. The anesthesiologist will use these values as a baseline for comparing the client's intraoperative vital signs. If the client's preoperative vital signs prove to be abnormal, there may be a need to postpone surgery. For example, an elevated temperature increases the client's surgical risk. The nurse notifies the physician of any vital sign abnormalities before sending the client to the operating room.

3. *The nurse provides hygiene.* Basic hygiene measures provide the client with an additional level of comfort before surgery. If the client is unwilling to take a complete bath, a partial bath is refreshing and removes any irritating secretions or drainage from the skin. Since the client cannot wear personal nightwear to the operating room, the nurse provides a clean hospital gown. After being allowed nothing by mouth throughout the night, the client usually has a very dry mouth. The nurse may offer mouthwash and toothpaste, again cautioning the client not to swallow water.

4. *The nurse checks hair and cosmetics.* During surgery under general anesthesia the anesthesiologist positions the client's head in order to introduce an endotracheal tube into the client's airway (see Chapter 41). This procedure may involve manipulation of

---

BEND PEEL TAB - FORM #52-1 REVISED 1/77

BARNES HOSPITAL SURGICAL CHECK LIST

NAME: DATE:

ITEM	YES	NO	NURSE SIGNATURE
I.D. band on			
Face sheet in chart			
Name plate in chart			
Operative Permit signed			
History & Physical in chart			
Patient on proper service			
Operative area prepped and checked			
Blood work in chart and within normal limits			
Urinalysis in chart			
Allergies noted as to whether or not present			
Chest X-ray done if ordered EKG			
V.S. taken & charted			
Jewelry removed or secured to patient			
Dentures, eyeglasses, contact lenses, nail polish, hairpins, or prothesis removed			
Patient in hospital pajamas			
Voided or catheterized			
Has patient been NPO			
Pre-op med given			
TIME_____			

Fig. 47-1 Preoperative checklist.
Courtesy Barnes Hospital, St. Louis.

the client's hair and scalp. To avoid injury the nurse asks the client to remove any hairpins or clips before leaving for surgery. Clients should also remove any hairpieces or wigs. Long hair can be braided to keep it in place. The client will be asked to wear a paper hair net before entering the operating room.

During and after surgery the anesthesiologist and nurses assess skin and mucous membranes to determine the client's level of oxygenation and circulation. The client must remove all makeup (lipstick, powder, blush, nail polish) to expose normal skin and nail coloring.

5. *The nurse checks removal of prosthetics.* It is easy for any type of prosthetic device to become lost or damaged during surgery. The client must remove all prosthetics including partial or complete dentures, artificial limbs, artificial eyes, and contact lenses. Hearing aids, false eyelashes, and eyeglasses must also be removed. If a client has a brace or splint, the nurse checks with the physician to determine if it should remain with the client.

For many clients it is embarrassing to remove dentures or other devices that enhance the client's appearance. Thus the client should be offered privacy as the dentures are removed. Dentures must be placed in special containers for safekeeping to prevent breakage, and the client assessed for any loose teeth. A broken tooth can become dislodged during insertion of an endotracheal tube and obstruct the client's airway.

In many agencies nurses must inventory all prosthetic devices and have them locked away for safekeeping. It is also common practice for nurses to give prosthetics to family members or to keep the devices at the client's bedside.

6. *The nurse prepares the bowel and bladder.* The client may require an enema or cathartic the morning of surgery. If so, it should be given at least an hour before the client is scheduled to leave, allowing time for the client to void without rushing. If the client is unable to void, it should be noted on the preoperative checklist.

7. *The nurse checks antiembolic stockings.* Many physicians prefer clients to wear antiembolic stockings during surgery. The stockings are designed to provide support to the lower extremities and maintain compression of small veins and capillaries. The constant compression forces blood into larger vessels, thus promoting venous return and preventing circulatory stasis. When correctly sized and applied properly, antiembolism stockings can prevent formation of thrombi. Chapter 31 reviews the procedure for sizing and application.

8. *The nurse checks special procedures.* A client's condition may warrant special interventions before leaving for the operating room. The surgeon's orders inform nurses of the need to start intravenous infusions, insert Foley catheters, or administer specific medications preoperatively.

One special procedure involves insertion of a nasogastric tube, a pliable plastic tube, through the client's nasopharynx into the stomach. The tube has a hollow lumen that allows the removal of gastric secretions, as well as the introduction of solutions into the stomach. There are several purposes for nasogastric intubation (Table 47-6). For a surgical client the main purpose is stomach decompression to prevent abdominal distention. Often the physician waits to order nasogastric tube insertion until the client is in the operating room.

The Levin and Salem sump tubes are the most common for stomach decompression. The Levin tube is a single-lumen tube with holes near the tip. The tube may be connected to a drainage bag or intermittent suction device to drain stomach secretions. The Salem sump tube is preferable for stomach decompression.

TABLE 47-6

Purposes of Nasogastric Intubation

Purpose	Description	Type of Tube
Decompression	Removal of secretions and gaseous substances from the gastrointestinal tract; prevention or relief of abdominal distention	Levin, Salem sump, Miller-Abbott
Feeding (gavage)	Instillation of liquid nutritional supplements or feedings into the stomach for clients unable to swallow fluid	Duo, Dobhoff, Levin
Compression	Internal application of pressure by means of an inflated balloon to prevent internal gastrointestinal hemorrhage	Sengstaken-Blakemore
Lavage	Irrigation of stomach in cases of active bleeding, poisoning, or gastric dilation	Levin, Ewald, Salem sump

PROCEDURE 47-3

Inserting a Nasogastric Tube

EQUIPMENT:

1. #14 or #16 French nasogastric tube
2. Water-soluble lubricating jelly
3. Stethoscope
4. Tongue blade
5. Flashlight
6. Asepto bulb syringe or cone tip (30 to 50 cc) syringe
7. 2.5 cm (1-inch) wide hypoallergenic tape
8. Safety pin and rubber band
9. Clamp, drainage bag, or suction machine
10. Bath towel
11. Emesis basin with ice (optional)
12. Glass of water with straw
13. Facial tissues
14. Normal saline (for irrigation only)

STEPS	RATIONALE
TUBE INSERTION	
1. Explain the procedure fully to the client, as well as the purpose of nasogastric decompression.	The procedure is easier to complete with the client's full cooperation.
2. Assemble all equipment at the bedside.	An organized procedure can be performed in a timely fashion, limiting the client's discomfort.
3. If the nasogastric tube is too pliable, place it in emesis basin and cover with ice.	This stiffens the tube for easier insertion.
4. Position the client in high Fowler's position with pillows behind head and shoulders.	This position promotes the client's ability to swallow.
5. Place bath towel over client's chest, and keep facial tissues close to client's reach.	This prevents soiling of the client's gown. Insertion of tube through nasal passages may cause tearing.
6. Stand on the right side of the bed of right-handed client and left side of bed of left-handed client.	This allows easier manipulation of tubing.
7. Instruct the client to relax and breathe normally while occluding one naris. Then repeat the procedure for the other naris. Select the nostril with the greater air flow.	The tube passes more easily through the naris that is more patent.
8. Estimate the distance to insert the tube by placing the tip of tube at client's nose and extending the tube to tip of earlobe and down to xiphoid process of sternum.	The tube should extend from naris to the stomach; distance varies for each client.

9. Curve 10 to 15 cm (4 to 6 inches) of the end of the tube tightly around the index finger, and then release.	Curving of tube tip aids insertion.
10. Lubricate 7.5 to 10 cm (3 to 4 inches) of the end of the tube with the water-soluble lubricating jelly.	This minimizes friction against nasal mucosa (water-soluble lubricant cannot cause aspiration pneumonia if it accidentally enters lungs).
11. Instruct the client to initially extend the neck and insert the tube slowly through naris with curved end pointing downward.	This facilitates initial passage of tube through naris and maintains clear airway for open naris.
12. Continue to pass the tube along the floor of the nasal passage. When resistance is felt, apply gentle downward pressure to advance the tube (do not force past a resistance).	This minimizes discomfort of tube rubbing against upper nasal turbinates. Resistance is created by the posterior nasopharynx.
13. If the tube meets resistance, withdraw it, relubricate, and insert in other naris.	Forcing against resistance can cause trauma to mucosa.
14. Stop tube advancement briefly. Allow the client to relax, and provide tissues. Explain that the next step requires the client to swallow.	This relieves the client's anxiety. Tearing is a natural response to mucosal irritation.

STEPS	RATIONALE
15. With the tube just above the oropharynx, instruct the client to flex head forward and dry swallow or suck in air through a straw. Advance the tube 2.5 to 5 cm (1 to 2 inches) with each swallow. If the client has trouble swallowing and can take fluids, offer a glass of water. Advance the tube with each swallow of water.	Flexed position closes off upper airway to trachea and opens esophagus. Swallowing aids the entrance of tube into the esophagus; swallowing water reduces gagging.
16. If the client begins to cough, gag, or choke, stop tube advancement momentarily. Have the client breathe easily, and offer another sip of water.	Tubing may accidentally enter the larynx to initiate a cough reflex. Gagging can be eased by swallowing water.
17. Withdraw the tube slightly if the client continues coughing.	Tube entering larynx will obstruct airway.
18. If gagging continues, check the back of the pharynx with a tongue blade and flashlight.	Tubing may slide in back of throat.
19. Once the client is at ease, continue to advance the tube the desired distance.	Tip of tube should be within stomach to decompress properly.

CHECKING TUBE PLACEMENT

1. Attach a syringe to the end of nasogastric tube. Place the diaphragm of the stethoscope over the upper left quadrant of the client's abdomen just below the costal margin. Inject 10 to 20 ml of air while auscultating abdomen.	Air entering stomach creates a "whooshing" sound and confirms tube placement. Absence of sound indicates tip of tube is in esophagus.
2. Aspirate gently back on the syringe to obtain gastric contents.	This is another effective test for tube placement. If tip is not in stomach, contents cannot be aspirated.
3. If the tube is not in the stomach, advance another 2.5 to 5 cm (1 to 2 inches), and again check position	Tubing must be in stomach to provide adequate decompression.

ANCHORING TUBE

1. Once the tube is properly inserted, either clamp the end or connect it to a drainage bag or suction machine.	Client going to OR often will have tube clamped. Drainage bag provides for gravity drainage. Intermittent suction is most effective in providing decompression.
2. Tape the tube to the client's nose, avoiding pressure on the naris. Take a 10 cm (4-inch) long piece of tape. Split one end lengthwise 5 cm (2 inches). Place the tab of tape over the bridge of the nose. Wrap the 1.3 cm (½-inch) strips around the tube as it exits the nose.	This prevents tissue necrosis.
3. Fasten the end of the nasogastric tube to the client's gown by looping a rubber band around the tube in a slip knot and pinning the rubber band to the gown. (Allow slack for movement.)	This reduces traction on the naris during movement of the tube.
4. Record insertion procedure. Note type of tube inserted, checking of tube placement, drainage return, and client's tolerance.	Timely recording accurately documents performance of the procedure.

TUBE IRRIGATION

1. Check tube placement.	This prevents accidental entrance of irrigating solution into the lungs.
2. Draw up 30 ml of normal saline into Asepto or GU syringe.	Isotonic solution maintains osmotic pressure and minimizes loss of electrolytes from the stomach.
3. Kink or clamp off tubing proximal to the connection site of drainage or suction apparatus. Disconnect the tubing and lay the end on a towel.	This prevents backflow of secretions and soiling of client's gown and bed linen.

Continued.

PROCEDURE 47-3, cont'd

Inserting a Nasogastric Tube

STEPS	RATIONALE
4. Insert the tip of the irrigating syringe into the end of the nasogastric tube. Release the clamp or kink in the tube. Holding the syringe with the tip toward the floor, inject the saline slowly but evenly. (Do not force solution.)	The position of the syringe prevents introduction of air into the tubing. Air can cause distention, and fluid introduced under pressure can cause trauma.
5. When resistance occurs, check for kinks in tubing. Turn the client onto one side. Repeated resistance should be reported to the physician.	Buildup of secretions will cause distention.
6. After instilling the saline, immediately aspirate or pull back on the syringe to withdraw the fluid. Measure the volume returned.	The stomach should remain empty. Fluid remaining in the stomach is measured as intake.
7. Reconnect nasogastric tube to drainage or suction. (If flow does not return, irrigation may be repeated.)	Reestablish means to collect drainage.

DISCONTINUATION

1. Turn off suction and disconnect nasogastric tube from drainage tube or bag. Remove tape from bridge of nose and remove pin from gown.	Tube should be free of connection when removed.
2. Explain the procedure to the client, reassuring him that removal is less distressing than insertion.	This minimizes the client's anxiety.
3. Hand the client a facial tissue. Instruct the client to take a deep breath and hold.	The airway may be temporarily obstructed during removal of tube.
4. Pull the tube steadily and smoothly as the client is holding his breath. (Do not pull either too slowly or too rapidly.)	This reduces trauma to mucosa and minimizes the client's discomfort.
5. Dispose of tube and drainage equipment.	This prevents transfer of microorganisms.
6. Clean the client's nares and provide mouth care.	This promotes comfort.
7. Record procedure, tube removal, final volume of secretions collected in drainage system, and client's response.	Timely recording accurately documents procedure.

The tube has two lumina: one for removal of gastric contents and one to provide an air vent. A blue "pigtail" is the air vent that connects with the second lumen. When the sump tube's main lumen is connected to suction, the air vent permits free, continuous drainage of secretions. The air vent should never be clamped off or connected to suction.

The procedure for tube insertion (Procedure 47-3) does not require sterile technique. The nurse simply uses adequate clean technique to minimize transfer of organisms from the client's nasal passages or oropharynx. The procedure is an uncomfortable one. The client experiences a burning sensation as the tube passes through the sensitive nasal mucosa. When the tube reaches the back of the pharynx, the client may begin to gag. It is important for the nurse to clarify the purpose of the procedure and to elicit the client's full cooperation. If the client is able to swallow voluntarily, tube passage is easier to achieve. A reluctance or inability of the client to cooperate makes tube insertion difficult.

One of the greatest problems in caring for a client with a nasogastric tube is maintenance of client comfort. The tube provides a constant irritation to the nasal mucosa. The nurse anchors the tubing with tape to the client's nose to prevent excess tube movement. The nurse also pins the end of the tubing to the client's gown to avoid excessive pulling. The nurse must assess the condition of the nares and mucosa daily for signs of inflammation and excoriation. As the tape becomes soiled, the nurse changes it to lessen irritation. Frequent lubrication of the nares also minimizes excoriation. With one naris occluded, the client may breathe through the mouth. Frequent mouth care (at least every 2 hours) helps minimize dehydration of the oral mucosa. Keeping a glass of cool water for rinsing the mouth close to the client's reach is useful, but the client who is to receive nothing by mouth should be cautioned not to swallow the water. The client will frequently complain of a sore throat as a result of the tube rubbing against the pharynx. An ice bag applied externally to the throat sometimes provides relief.

Once the client is intubated, the nurse must maintain patency of the nasogastric tube. If the tip of the tubing rests against the stomach wall or if the tube becomes blocked with thick secretions, it is necessary for the nurse to irrigate the tube regularly. Flushing the tube with normal saline by way of an Asepto or cone-tipped syringe clears any blockage within the tube. Procedure 47-3 outlines the steps for tube irrigation. If a nasogastric tube continues to drain improperly after irrigation, it is necessary for the nurse to reposition the tube by advancing or withdrawing it slightly. Any change in position requires reassessment of tube placement.

The nasogastric tube can actually cause distention unless the nurse manages the client correctly. Presence of the tube in the nose causes many clients to swallow large volumes of air. Channels of gastric secretions also form along the walls of the stomach and bypass the suction holes. The nurse must turn the client regularly to collapse the channels and promote emptying of stomach contents.

9. *The nurse safeguards valuables.* If a client has any valuables, the nurse should either turn them over to family members or secure them for safekeeping. The accidental loss of jewelry or money could lead to legal suits against the hospital. Many hospitals require clients to sign a release to free the institution of responsibility for lost valuables. Valuables can usually be stored and locked in a designated location in the nursing division or in the hospital security department. Often clients are reluctant to remove wedding rings or religious medals. A wedding band can be taped in place; however, if there is a risk that the client will experience swelling of the hand or fingers, the band should be removed. Many hospitals allow clients to pin religious medals to their gowns, although the risk of loss increases.

10. *The nurse administers preoperative medications.* The anesthesiologist or surgeon will order preanesthetic drugs that reduce the client's anxiety, the amount of general anesthesia required, and respiratory tract secretions. Tranquilizers such as chlorpromazine (Thorazine) or diazepam (Valium) reduce

the client's anxiety and relax skeletal muscles. Narcotic analgesics such as meperidine (Demerol) or morphine provide sedation, reduce pain and anxiety, and reduce the amount of anesthetic required during surgery. Drugs such as glycopyrrolate (Robinul) or atropine create anticholinergic effects to inhibit mucous secretions in the oral and respiratory passages and prevent spasm of laryngeal muscles.

Typically the physician orders preoperative medications to be administered when the client leaves for the operating room or at an earlier prescribed time. The nurse provides all nursing care measures before giving the client preoperative medications. Since the drugs cause sedation, the client should not be allowed to leave bed until the surgical orderlies and nurses arrive to transport the client to the operating room. The client should be warned to anticipate drowsiness and dry mouth, although the medications usually do not induce sleep. The bed side rails should be raised and the bed kept in the low position for client safety.

Evaluation of Preoperative Care

Often there is limited time available to evaluate the outcomes of the nurse's preoperative plan of care. The client's surgery may be an emergency, or the performance of various procedures may make it difficult for the nurse to find time for evaluation.

The most essential evaluation to make is that of the effectiveness of preoperative teaching. Interventions designed to improve the client's and family's knowledge and understanding of intraoperative and postoperative events are evaluated on the basis of the client's and family members' ability to identify (1) approximate time of surgery, (2) the unit the client will return to postoperatively, (3) the routine types of postoperative monitoring to be performed by the nurses, (4) the basic purpose of surgery, and (5) the routine types of treatment required postoperatively.

Performance of postoperative exercises is essential for a smooth recovery period. The nurse evaluates success at instructing clients in postoperative exercises on the basis of the client's ability to demonstrate the following exercises and techniques independently and correctly: deep breathing, coughing, splinting, foot and leg exercises, and turning.

The nurse's success at promoting the client's physical and emotional comfort can be evaluated on the basis of the client's falling asleep within half an hour after bedtime, sleeping through the night, and feeling rested the next morning.

It is difficult to measure the influence of the nurse's preoperative preparation on the client's postoperative pain or anxiety. Many factors come into play once the client experiences pain for the first time and observes the various therapies the nurse must perform. When a client appears to be relatively free of anxiety as evidenced by a willingness to cooperate, absence of nonverbal expressions of anxiety, and a minimal number of questions about previously discussed topics, the nurse can only surmise that preparations were effective. Likewise, if the client does not require frequent pain medications and demonstrates an understanding of the pain relief therapies postoperatively, the nurse's interventions were likely successful.

Transport to the Operating Room

Personnel in the operating room notify the nursing division when it is time for the client's surgery. In many hospitals a nursing orderly or transporter brings a stretcher for transporting the client. The transporter checks the client's identification bracelet against the client's chart to be sure the right person is going to surgery. Since the client has already received a preoperative medication, the nurses and transporter will assist the client in transferring from bed to stretcher.

The family gets one last opportunity to visit before the client is transported to the operating room. The nurses then direct the family to the appropriate waiting area. Most waiting areas have telephones, vending machines, and reading material for the family members' convenience.

Once the client leaves the nursing division, the nurse prepares the bed and room for the client's return, if the client will return to the same nursing division. A postoperative bedside unit should include:
1. Sphygmomanometer, stethoscope, and thermometer
2. Emesis basin
3. Clean gown
4. Washcloth, towel, and facial tissues
5. Intravenous pole
6. Suction equipment
7. Oxygen equipment
8. Extra pillows for positioning the client comfortably
9. Bed pads to protect bed linen from drainage

The nurse will be better prepared to care for the client postoperatively if the room is readied well in advance of the client's return. The need for any additional monitoring equipment will depend on the client's postoperative status.

Intraoperative Surgical Phase

Care of the client during surgery requires careful preparation and knowledge of the events that occur during the surgical procedure.

Holding Area

In most hospitals the client enters a small unit or room immediately outside the operating room. In the holding area the nurse explains the steps to be taken in preparing the client for surgery. Nurses in the holding area are part of the operating room staff and wear surgical scrub suits, hats, and footwear in accordance with infection control policies.

In the holding area the nurses or anesthesiologist will insert an intravenous catheter into the client's arm to establish a route for fluid replacement and intravenous medications. A large-bore intravenous catheter is used for easy infusion of all fluids, including blood products.

The nurse will also apply a blood pressure cuff to the client's arm. The cuff will remain in place throughout surgery in order for the anesthesiologist to assess blood pressure readings.

By this time the client begins to feel drowsy. Since the temperature in the holding area and adjacent operating room suites is usually cool, the client should be offered an extra blanket for comfort. The client's stay in the holding area while the staff prepares the operating suite for surgery should be brief.

Admission to the Operating Room

The nurses will transfer the client to the operating room via stretcher. The client is usually still awake and will notice nurses and physicians wearing complete surgical masks and gowns. The staff carefully transfers the client to the operating table, being sure both the stretcher and table are locked in place. Once the client is on the table, the nurse fastens a safety strap around the client to prevent falls.

The operating room nurse goes through a checklist similar to that used by the nurses preoperatively. The nurse makes a final check of the client's identification bracelet and chart. A review of consent forms, medical history, physical assessment findings, and diagnostic test results ensures that all medical record information is complete and available to the surgeon. The nurse examines the client to check that all prosthetic devices and valuables have been removed. Finally, the operating room nurse reviews the client's nursing care plan to establish an intraoperative plan of care that meets the client's continuing needs.

The nurse applies monitoring devices to the client before surgery begins. All clients undergo continuous electrocardiographic monitoring during surgery. Small plastic electrodes are placed on the client's chest and extremities to record the electrical activity of the heart. A monitor in the operating room displays the heart's electrical activity.

Introduction of Anesthesia

Two types of anesthesia are used during surgical procedures: general and regional.

GENERAL ANESTHESIA

Under general anesthesia a client loses all sensation and consciousness. Muscles of the body relax to make the surgeon's job of manipulating and moving body parts easier. The client also experiences amnesia of all events occurring during the actual surgical procedure. Surgery performed under general anesthesia involves major procedures requiring extensive tissue manipulation, for example, resection of organs, exploration for tumors, and reconstruction of organ parts.

An anesthesiologist administers general anesthetics by intravenous and inhalation routes through the four stages of anesthesia:

Stage 1	Begins with client being awake; client gradually becomes drowsy and loses consciousness; state of analgesia begins
Stage 2	Stage of excitement; client's muscles are often tense and almost spasmodic; swallowing and vomiting reflexes remain intact; client may have an irregular breathing pattern
Stage 3	Begins with onset of regular rhythmical breathing; vital functions depressed; client's reflexes are depressed or temporarily lost; surgeon begins operation during this phase
Stage 4	Stage of complete respiratory depression; can be fatal

To move the client quickly to stage 3 of general anesthesia the anesthesiologist usually administers an intravenous dose of a barbiturate. To prevent possible aspiration and other respiratory complications the anesthesiologist introduces an endotracheal tube into the client's airway. Succinylcholine is a paralyzing agent that causes temporary paralysis of vocal cords and respiratory muscles while the client is intubated. With the endotracheal tube in place the anesthesiologist provides artificial ventilation until succinylcholine's effects wear off and the client again breathes spontaneously. From that point anesthetic gases or vapors are usually delivered by inhalation through the endotracheal tube. The client also receives a continuous supply of oxygen. It is common for a client to complain of a sore throat on awakening after surgery. The irritation is a result of trauma caused by the endotracheal tube.

The duration of anesthesia depends on the length of surgery. The client's surgical risks influence how long a surgeon is willing to prolong surgery. The greatest risks from general anesthesia are the side effects of anesthetic agents, including cardiovascular depression or irritability, respiratory depression, and liver and kidney damage.

REGIONAL ANESTHESIA

The induction of regional anesthesia results in loss of sensation in an area of the body. The method of induction influences which portion of the client's sensory pathways is anesthetized. The anesthesiologist administers regional anesthetics by infiltration and local application. (See Chapter 37 for local anesthesia.) In major surgery, such as a hernia repair, vaginal hysterectomy, or vascular repair of leg blood vessels, only infiltrative induction is used.

Infiltration of anesthetic agents may involve any one of three induction methods:

1. *Nerve block.* Local anesthetic is injected into a nerve plexus, blocking the nerve supply to the operative site. The area affected is usually localized.
2. *Spinal anesthesia.* The anesthesiologist performs a lumbar puncture and introduces the local anesthetic into the cerebrospinal fluid in the spinal subarachnoid space. Anesthesia can extend from the tip of the xiphoid process down to the client's feet. Positioning of the client influences the movement of the anesthetic agent up or down the spinal cord. For example, in prostate surgery, the male client sits until the anesthetic block takes full effect.
3. *Epidural anesthesia.* This is a safer procedure than spinal anesthesia, since the anesthetic agent is injected into the epidural space outside the dura mater, and the level of anesthesia is not as great as spinal anesthesia. Since epidural anesthesia provides an effective loss of sensation in the vaginal and perineal areas, it is the anesthetic of choice for obstetrical procedures.

There are risks involved with infiltrative anesthetics, particularly in the case of spinal anesthesia, since the level of anesthesia may rise. The client may experience a sudden fall in blood pressure, which results from extensive vasodilation caused by the anesthetic block to sympathetic vasomotor nerves, pain, and motor fibers. If the level of anesthesia rises, respiratory paralysis may develop, necessitating resuscitation by the anesthesiologist. The client requires careful monitoring during and immediately after surgery.

The client under regional anesthesia is awake throughout the surgical procedure unless the physician orders a tranquilizer that allows the client to sleep. Because the client is responsive and capable of breathing voluntarily, it is not necessary for the anesthesiologist to introduce an endotracheal tube. Operating room personnel often gain a false sense of security because of the client's relative alertness. Nurses must remember that burns and other trauma can occur on the anesthetized part of the body without the client being aware of the injury. It is therefore necessary frequently to observe the position of the client's extremities, as well as the condition of the skin.

Positioning the Client for Surgery

During general anesthesia the nursing personnel and surgeon often do not position the client until the stage of complete relaxation. The choice of position is usually determined by the surgical approach. Ideally the client's position provides good access to the operative site and sustains adequate circulatory and respiratory function; it should not impair neuromuscular structures. The client's comfort and safety must be considered.

It is sometimes difficult for nurses in postoperative divisions to appreciate the discomfort a client may feel after surgery—for example, discomfort of the right arm or side in a client whose left kidney was removed (Fig. 47-2). Normal range of motion is maintained in an alert person by pain and pressure receptors. If a joint is extended too far, pain stimuli provide a warning that muscle and joint strain are too great. In a client who is anesthetized, normal defense mechanisms cannot guard against joint damage, muscle stretch, and strain. The client's muscles are so relaxed that it is relatively easy to place the client in a position

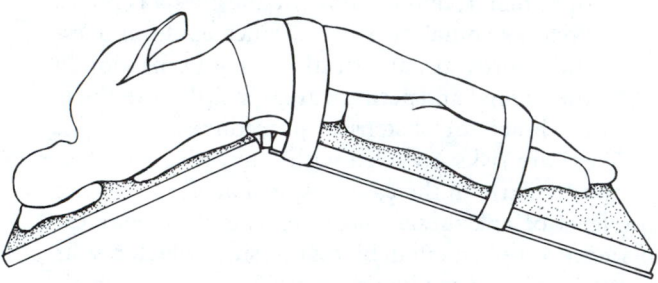

Fig. 47-2 Client's position on operating room table for a nephrectomy.

the individual normally could not assume while awake. The client often remains in a given position for several hours. Although it may be necessary to place a client in an unusual position, the nurse should attempt to maintain correct physiological alignment and protect the client from pressure, abrasion, and other injuries. Special attachments to the operating table allow for proper protection and padding of extremities and bony prominences. Positioning should not impede normal movement of the diaphragm or interfere with circulation to body parts. If restraints are necessary, the nurse uses blankets to prevent trauma to the skin.

Nurse's Role during Surgery

The nurse assumes one of two roles during the surgical procedure: scrub nurse or circulating nurse. The scrub nurse provides the surgeon with appropriate instruments and supplies, which requires strict surgical asepsis (see Chapter 33), as well as familiarity with an extensive array of surgical instruments. Each surgical instrument is designed for a specific purpose during a certain phase or step in surgery. It takes considerable knowledge and skill to anticipate which instrument the surgeon requires and to pass the instrument quickly and smoothly. In addition to assisting the surgeon, the scrub nurse also disposes of soiled gauze sponges and accounts for all sponges, needles, and instruments on the surgical field and in body cavities. Since few schools of nursing provide clinical scrub nurse training, most nurses learn on the job.

The circulating nurse works within the operating room suite as an assistant to the scrub nurse and surgeon. When the client first enters the operating room, the circulator helps in positioning the client and applying necessary equipment and surgical drapes. During surgery the circulator provides the scrub nurse with supplies, disposes of soiled equipment and sponges, and keeps a careful count of instruments, needles, and sponges used. If there is a need to help reposition the client or move the operating room lights, the circulating nurse is available to assist. Like all members of the surgical team the circulator follows surgical aseptic technique. If a break in asepsis occurs, the circulator assists team members with regowning and regloving.

At the end of each surgical procedure the scrub nurse and circulator count the number of used instruments, needles, and gauze sponges. This procedure prevents the accidental loss of such items within the client's surgical wound. It is not difficult for a sponge saturated with blood to be overlooked within a wound. Careful monitoring of all items is essential for the client's safety. The nurse who fails to make accurate counts can be held legally accountable. If a client is injured by a misplaced needle or instrument, the nurse may be judged negligent (see Chapter 17).

Postoperative Surgical Phase

Postoperative care of the client poses a challenge for the nurse because of the complex physiological changes that can occur. To assess the client's postoperative condition the nurse relies on information from the preoperative nursing assessment and on knowledge regarding the type of surgical procedure performed and events occurring intraoperatively. The nurse must be skilled at noticing change. A slight variation in respiratory rhythm, an increase in wound drainage, or an increase in restlessness may indicate development of surgically related complications.

The client's postoperative course involves two phases: the immediate recovery period and the postoperative convalescence, which lasts through discharge from the hospital.

Immediate Postoperative Recovery

Before the arrival of the client in the recovery room (RR), or postanesthesia room (PAR), the recovery room nurse communicates with the surgical team in the operating room to determine the client's general status and the need for special equipment and nursing care. Careful planning allows the nursing staff to consider placement of clients in the recovery room. For example, clients who undergo spinal anesthesia are aware of their surroundings and may benefit from being in a quieter part of the recovery room, away from clients needing frequent monitoring. The client with a serious infection should be isolated from other clients.

When the client enters the recovery room, the nurse and members of the surgical team confer about the client's status. The surgical team's report includes a review of anesthetic agents administered so the recovery room nurse can anticipate the ease with which a client should regain consciousness. A report on intravenous fluids or blood products administered during surgery alerts the nurse to the client's fluid and electrolyte balance. The surgeon often reports any special concerns, for example, if the client is at risk for hemorrhaging or the development of infection. The operating room nurse discusses whether the client experienced any complications during surgery such as excessive blood loss or cardiac irregularities.

After reviewing events occurring in the operating room, the recovery room nurse makes a complete assessment of the client's status. Until stabilized, the client remains in the recovery room.

The recovery room personnel notify the nursing division of the client's arrival. This allows the nursing staff to inform family members of the client's operative course. The nurse usually advises family members to remain in the designated waiting area so they can be found when the surgeon arrives to explain the client's condition.

Problems can arise if the surgeon informs the family preoperatively of the anticipated length of surgery and the client remains in the operating room past this time. Families become highly anxious when they expect the client's surgery to last 2 hours, yet have heard nothing after 3 hours. Nurses in the division can help relieve family members' concerns by explaining the normal types of delays that occur, such as room preparation or delay in the previous surgery. If the client's stay in recovery is extended, the nurses can explain to the family that the client is being held longer for observation. Should the client suffer complications, it is the surgeon's responsibility to explain to family members what actually occurred during surgery.

If the client's surgery was unsuccessful or the surgeon discovered an inoperable condition (for example, a malignant tumor), it becomes the nurse's responsibility to provide support to the family. Directing the family to the location of public telephones, providing a cup of hot coffee, or encouraging verbalization of fears in a private location are a few ways to help the family cope with the waiting period before the client's return. The family's initial shock requires the nurse to be available and serve as a resource for the family.

After the initial assessment on the client's arrival to recovery, the nurse repeats evaluation of vital signs and other key observations pertinent to the individual's condition at least every 15 minutes.

RESPIRATION

Certain anesthetic agents may continue to cause respiratory depression. For this reason the nurse is especially alert for shallow, slow breathing and a weak cough. The nurse assesses respiratory rate, rhythm, depth of ventilation, symmetry of chest wall movement, breath sounds, and color of mucous membranes. If the client's breathing is unusually shallow, placement of the nurse's hand over the client's face or mouth allows the nurse to feel exhaled air.

The client often has an oral or nasal airway (see Chapter 41) inserted to maintain a patent airway until comfortable breathing at a normal rate resumes. As respiratory function returns, the nurse will ask the client to spit out the airway. The client's ability to do so signifies a return of a normal gag reflex.

One of the nurse's greatest concerns is airway obstruction resulting from (1) aspirations of emesis, (2) accumulation of mucous secretions in the pharynx, or (3) swelling or spasm of the larynx. The following measures maintain airway patency:

1. The nurse positions the client on his side with the face down and the neck slightly extended. A small folded towel serves to support the client's head. The neck extension prevents occlusion of the airway at the pharynx. When the face is kept turned downward, the tongue moves forward and mucous secretions flow out of the mouth instead of accumulating in the pharynx. If the nature of the surgery prevents turning the client on one side, the head of the bed is slightly elevated and the client's neck slightly extended, with the head turned to the side. The client should never be positioned with arms over or across the chest. This position reduces maximal chest expansion.

2. The nurse begins coughing and deep breathing exercises as soon as the client is responsive to commands.

3. The nurse suctions artificial airways and the oral cavity for mucous secretions. Care must be taken to avoid continually eliciting the gag reflex, which might cause vomiting. Before the nurse or client removes an airway, the back of the airway should be suctioned so mucus plugs and secretions are not retained.

4. The nurse provides oxygen therapy as ordered.

CIRCULATION

The client is at risk for cardiovascular complications resulting from actual or potential blood loss from the surgical site, side effects of anesthesia, electrolyte imbalances, and depression of normal circulatory regulating mechanisms. Careful assessment of heart rate and rhythm, along with blood pressure, reveals the client's cardiovascular status. The nurse compares preoperative vital signs with postoperative values. The surgeon's postoperative orders may specify when vital sign changes should be reported. For example, a heart rate above 110 per minute or below 60 usually should be reported immediately. However, the nurse must use judgment in reporting vital sign changes. If the client's blood pressure drops progressively after each check or if the heart rate becomes more irregular, the physician should be notified.

The nurse assesses circulatory perfusion by noting the color of nail beds and skin. If the client has had vascular surgery or has casts or constricting devices that may impair circulation, the nurse assesses peripheral pulses distal to the site of surgery. For example, after surgery to the femoral artery, the nurse assesses popliteal and dorsalis pedis pulses. The nurse also compares pulses in the affected extremity with those in the nonaffected extremity.

A common circulatory problem to observe for is hemorrhage. A client's blood loss may occur externally through a drain or incision or internally within the surgical wound. Either type of hemorrhage may manifest itself by the classic signs of fall in blood pressure, elevated heart and respiratory rate, thready pulse, cool, clammy, pale skin, and restlessness. If hemorrhage is external, the nurse will note increased bloody drainage on dressings or through drains. If a dressing becomes saturated, the blood will ooze down the client's sides and collect in a pool under bedclothes. An alert nurse always checks under the client for drainage. When hemorrhage is internal, the operative site becomes swollen and tight. For example, if a client bleeds within the abdomen, the abdomen becomes tight and distended. The first signs of suspected hemorrhaging should be reported to the physician immediately. The nurse will maintain intravenous fluid infusion and monitor vital signs every 15 minutes or more frequently until the client's condition stabilizes.

TEMPERATURE CONTROL

The operating room and recovery room environments are extremely cool. The client's depressed level of body function results in a lowering of metabolism and fall in body temperature. When clients begin to awaken, they complain of feeling cold and uncomfortable.

The nurse measures the client's body temperature and provides specially warmed blankets. Increasing body warmth causes the client's metabolism to rise and circulatory and respiratory functions to improve.

Often clients exhibit postoperative shivering. This may not be a sign of hypothermia but rather a side effect of certain anesthetic agents. Deep breathing and coughing will help expel any retained anesthetic gases. In rare instances the complication malignant hyperpyrexia develops. A life-threatening complication of anesthesia, the condition causes a high fever, tachycardia, metabolic changes, and even convulsions. Without proper treatment it can be fatal.

NEUROLOGICAL FUNCTIONS

The client on arrival in the recovery room is usually asleep or reacting to verbal commands. However, medications, electrolyte and metabolic changes, pain, and emotional factors can influence the client's level of consciousness. The nurse rouses the client by calling his name in a moderate tone of voice. The nurse notes if the client responds appropriately or seems confused and disoriented. If the client remains asleep or unresponsive, the nurse attempts arousal through touch or by gently moving a body part. If a painful stimulus is needed to arouse the client, the nurse should notify the anesthesiologist.

As the effects of anesthesia wear off, the client's reflexes return and muscle strength is regained. The nurse can easily check for pupillary and gag reflexes (see Chapter 29). If a client has had surgery involving a portion of the neurological system, the nurse conducts a more thorough neurological assessment. For example, if the client had low back surgery, the nurse assesses leg movement, sensation, and strength.

Orientation to the recovery room environment is important in maintaining the client's alertness. The nurse explains that surgery is completed and describes all procedures and nursing measures within the recovery area. The client who was properly prepared preoperatively will not be as anxious when the recovery nurses begin their care.

SURGICAL WOUND

Following surgery most surgical wounds are covered with a type of dressing, which protects the wound site and serves to collect any form of drainage. The nurse observes the amount, color, odor, and consistency of drainage on dressings. The nurse estimates the amount of drainage by noting the number of saturated gauze sponges. If drainage appears on the outer surface of a dressing, another way of assessing drainage is by drawing a circle around the outer perimeter of the drainage. If the perimeter expands, drainage is increasing. Chapter 48 describes wound care in detail.

Many physicians prefer to change a client's dressing the first time so they can personally inspect the incisional area. Therefore the recovery room nurse may simply reinforce a dressing if it becomes soiled. Reinforcing means to add an extra layer of gauze on top of the original dressing.

GENITOURINARY FUNCTION

A client may not regain voluntary control over urinary function for 6 to 8 hours after anesthesia. A spinal anesthetic may prevent the client from feeling bladder fullness or distention. The nurse palpates the lower abdomen just above the symphysis pubis for bladder distention. Because a full bladder can be painful and is often the cause of a client's restlessness in recovery, it may become necessary to catheterize a client. If the client has a Foley catheter, there should be a continuous flow of urine of at least 30 ml per hour. The nurse observes the color and odor of urine. Surgery involving portions of the urinary tract normally causes bloody urine for at least 12 to 24 hours, depending on the type of surgery.

GASTROINTESTINAL FUNCTION

Anesthetics slow gastrointestinal motility and cause nausea. Normally during the immediate recovery phase a nurse will hear faint or absent bowel sounds in all four quadrants. Inspection of the abdomen rules out the presence of distention that may be caused by the accumulation of gas. In a client who has had abdominal surgery, distention will develop if internal bleeding occurs.

To minimize nausea the nurse avoids sudden movement of the client. If the client has a nasogastric tube, it is important to keep the tube patent by regular irrigations. Occlusion of nasogastric tubes results in the accumulation of gastric contents within the stomach. Since stomach emptying slows under anesthesia, the accumulated contents cannot escape and nausea and vomiting develop. Normally a client does not receive fluids to drink in the recovery room because of the risk of vomiting.

FLUID AND ELECTROLYTE BALANCE

Because of the surgical client's risk for fluid and electrolyte abnormalities, the nurse assesses the hydration status and monitors cardiac and neurological function for signs of electrolyte alterations (see Chapter 42). The nurse also has an important responsibility for maintaining patency of intravenous infusions. The client's only source of fluid intake immediately after surgery is through intravenous catheters. The nurse inspects a catheter insertion site to be sure it is properly positioned within a vein so fluid flows freely. The physician orders a prescribed rate for each infusion. To ensure the client's receiving an adequate fluid intake the nurse should not allow the infusion of fluids to fall behind. The client may also receive blood products postoperatively depending on the blood loss suffered during surgery.

Accurate recording of intake and output helps to assess the client's renal and circulatory function. The nurse measures all sources of output including urine, gastric drainage, drainage from wounds, and any insensible loss from diaphoresis. Mucus suctioned from the client's airways is not included in output measurements.

COMFORT

As a client awakens from general anesthesia, the sensation of pain becomes prominent. Acute incisional pain causes the client to become restless and may be responsible for changes in vital signs. It is difficult for clients to begin coughing and deep breathing exercises when they experience pain. The client who had spinal anesthesia usually does not experience pain initially, since the incisional area is still anesthetized.

Surgeons routinely order postoperative analgesics by the parenteral route. Nurses in the recovery room often administer only one half or a third of the prescribed dose for fear that a full dose may depress vital signs and the client's level of consciousness. However, a low blood pressure may be caused by a client's acute pain. In such a situation an analgesic may improve vital sign values. Judgment is needed in determining the proper dose of an analgesic. It may be to the client's advantage to withhold analgesics in the recovery room so that a full dose can be administered once the client reaches the postoperative nursing division.

Postoperative Convalescence

Once the client's condition stabilizes in recovery, it is time for the client to return to the postoperative nursing division. Nursing care focuses on returning the client to a functional level of wellness as soon as possible within the limitations created by surgery. The speed of a client's convalescence will depend on the type or extent of surgery, risk factors, incidence of postoperative complications, and the nurse's plan of care.

DISCHARGE FROM THE RECOVERY ROOM

The nurse evaluates a client's readiness for discharge from recovery on the basis of the following criteria: vital sign stability, body temperature control, good ventilatory function, orientation to surroundings, absence of surgical or anesthetic complications, minimal pain and nausea, controlled wound drainage, adequate urine output, and fluid-electrolyte balance. If the client's condition continues to be poor after 2 to 3 hours, the stay in recovery will lengthen or the surgeon may transfer the client to an intensive care unit (ICU) for closer monitoring.

When the client is discharged from recovery, the nurse calls the nursing division to report the client's vital signs, the type of surgery and anesthesia performed, blood loss, level of consciousness, general physical condition, and whether any intravenous lines or drainage tubes are present. The nurse's report helps the nurses in the division to anticipate special client needs and obtain necessary equipment.

A nurse and transporter bring the client to the nursing division on a stretcher. Staff members assist in safely transferring the client to a bed (see Chapter 30). At this time the recovery room nurse shows the division nurse the recovery room record and reviews the client's course in recovery. The recovery room nurse also points out any physician orders that require attention now that the client has returned. Before the recovery nurse leaves, the division nurse takes a complete set of vital signs to compare with recovery room findings. Minor vital sign variations normally occur after transporting the client.

ASSESSMENT

The nurse's assessment includes an initial check of the client's general condition, including vital signs, level of consciousness, condition of dressings and drains, intravenous fluid status, comfort level, and skin integrity.

The same physical measurements and observations performed in the recovery room (such as circulatory and respiratory assessment) are also carried out in the postoperative division. The nurse routinely assesses the client at least every 15 minutes the first hour, every 30 minutes for 1 to 2 hours, every hour for 4 hours, and then every 4 hours. Frequency of assessment depends on the client's condition. A nurse should not assume that further monitoring is unnecessary if the client appears normal during the initial assessment. A client's condition can change rapidly. A wound may begin to hemorrhage, respiratory airway obstruction may still develop, or an intravenous infusion may clot off. A nurse is guilty of neglect when failing to follow the assessment schedule for a postoperative client.

The nurse thoroughly documents the initial assessment and makes successive entries in the nurse's notes. Vital signs, intravenous fluid intake, and urinary output can be entered on flowsheets. The nurse's initial findings serve as a baseline for comparing any postoperative changes the client may undergo.

After the nurse completes the first assessment of the client and has attended to any immediate needs—for example, repositioning the client or regulating an intravenous infusion—the family is allowed to visit. This is a good opportunity for the nurse to explain the purpose of procedures or equipment, such as intravenous lines and drainage tubes. The family will want to know how the client is doing. The nurse explains if vital signs are stable and if the client seems to be awakening without difficulty. The family should know that the client will fall in and out of sleep for most of the remainder of the day from the effects of general anesthesia. The family should also be reminded that frequent assessments of the client's condition are to be expected and that, if the client had spinal anesthesia, loss of sensation and movement in the extremities remains for several hours.

NURSING DIAGNOSES

The nurse determines the status of problems identified from preoperative diagnoses and identifies new diagnoses pertinent to postoperative problems (Table 47-7). Previously defined diagnoses such as alteration in skin integrity may continue to be a postoperative

TABLE 47-7

Examples of Nursing Diagnoses for the Postoperative Client

Problem	Causes
Alteration in comfort	Related to incisional pain
Impaired mobility	Related to: Activity restrictions Pain Altered function of body part
Ineffective breathing pattern	Related to: Pain Altered consciousness
Potential for skin breakdown	Related to: Impaired mobility Wound drainage
Potential for fluid imbalance	Related to: Wound drainage Inadequate fluid intake
Ineffective family member coping	Related to: Inoperable condition Severity of client's illness Appearance of client
Grieving	Related to client's impending death
Altered body image	Related to surgical removal of body part

problem. During the immediate postoperative period the client is less mobile. Wound drainage may collect on bed linen and cause softening or maceration of the skin. The client remains at risk for skin breakdown until able to resume more normal activity.

Many of the nurse's postoperative diagnoses relate to potential problems. For example, the client is at risk for complications of immobilization (see Chapter 31) and impaired wound healing. The nurse plans interventions of a preventive nature so that such problems do not develop. Nursing diagnoses will also pertain to alterations resulting directly from surgery, for example, alteration in comfort, altered body image related to loss of a body part, or alteration in elimination.

The nurse cannot forget the family when identifying nursing diagnoses. The inability of the members to cope with the client's condition or with the knowledge that the client's surgery was unsuccessful requires the nurse's intervention. To be of assistance to the client

during the recovery process the family needs support. Likewise, if the client's condition becomes terminal, the family will require the nurse's help to cope with the grieving process (see Chapter 46).

PLANNING POSTOPERATIVE CARE

At the convalescent phase of the client's recovery the nurse has a wealth of information to plan the client's care. Current physical assessment data coupled with analysis of the preoperative nursing history allows the nurse to plan specific nursing interventions. The surgeon's postoperative orders also offer guidelines for the type of therapy to provide. Typical postoperative orders include:

1. Frequency of vital signs and special assessments, for example, circulation or neurological checks
2. Types of intravenous fluids and rate of infusion
3. Postoperative medications, for example, analgesics and antibiotics
4. Fluids and food allowed by mouth
5. Level of activity the client is allowed to resume such as bed rest or sitting in chair
6. Position the client is to maintain while in bed, for example, supine or not on left side
7. Intake and output
8. Laboratory tests and x-ray studies
9. Special directions, for example, materials for dressing changes, use of incentive spirometers

The nurse considers the effects of the stress of surgery and the resultant limitations it produces when establishing goals of care such as the following:

1. To prevent onset of medical complications
2. To promote rest and comfort
3. To promote client's return to a functional state of health within limitations posed by surgery
4. To maintain the client's self-esteem

POSTOPERATIVE INTERVENTIONS

PREVENTING MEDICAL COMPLICATIONS. The creation of a surgical wound, the effects of prolonged immobilization during surgery and convalescence, and the influence of anesthesia and analgesics are the principal causes for postoperative complications. Failure on the part of the client to become actively involved in the recovery process adds to the risk of complications. Table 47-8 reviews the most common postoperative complications. Respiratory complications result primarily from immobilization and the depressant effects of anesthesia. The client's ventilatory function is reduced during anesthesia. Mucus accumulates in airways, and alveoli collapse from lack of expansion. Resultant pulmonary problems such as atelectasis and pneumonia usually develop early during the client's recovery. With pulmonary embolism the alteration occurs as a result of circulatory changes.

TABLE 47-8

Postoperative Complications

System	Complication	Description	Cause
Respiratory	Atelectasis	Collapse of alveoli with retained mucous secretions; signs and symptoms elevated respiratory rate, dyspnea, fever, crackles auscultated over involved lobes of lungs, productive cough	Inadequate lung expansion; anesthesia, analgesics, and immobilized position prevent full lung expansion; greater risk in clients with upper abdominal surgery who have pain during inspiration and repress deep breathing
	Pneumonia	Inflammation of alveoli caused by infectious process; may involve one or several lobes of lung; development of pneumonia in lower dependent lobes of lung common in immobilized surgical client; signs and symptoms fever, chills, productive cough, chest pain, purulent mucus, dyspnea	Poor lung expansion with retained secretions; common resident bacteria in respiratory tract is *Diplococcus pneumoniae,* which causes most cases of pneumonia
	Hypoxia	Inadequate concentration of oxygen in arterial blood; signs and symptoms restlessness, dyspnea, high blood pressure, tachycardia, diaphoresis, cyanosis	Respirations depressed by anesthetics or analgesics; increased retention of mucus with impaired ventilation because of pain or poor positioning
	Pulmonary embolism	Embolus blocking pulmonary artery and disrupting blood flow to one or more lobes of lung; signs and symptoms dyspnea, sudden chest pain, cyanosis, tachycardia, drop in blood pressure	Same factors that lead to formation of thrombus or embolus; immobilized surgical client with preexisting circulatory or coagulation disorders at high risk
Circulatory	Hemorrhage	Loss of a large amount of blood either externally or internally in short period of time; signs and symptoms same as hypovolemic shock (see below)	Slipping of suture or dislodged clot at incisional site, clients with coagulation disorders at greater risk
	Hypovolemic shock	Inadequate perfusion of tissues and cells from loss of circulatory fluid volume; signs and symptoms hypotension, weak and rapid pulse, cool clammy skin, rapid breathing, restlessness, reduced urine output	In surgical client usually caused by hemorrhage

TABLE 47-8, cont'd

Postoperative Complications

System	Complication	Description	Cause
	Thrombophlebitis	Inflammation of vein often accompanied by clot formation; veins in legs most commonly affected; signs and symptoms swelling and inflammation of involved site, aching or cramping pain; vein feels hard, cord-like, and sensitive to touch; pain in calf when client walks or dorsiflexes foot (Homans' sign)	Venous stasis aggravated by prolonged sitting or immobilization; trauma to vessel wall and hypercoagulability of blood increase risk of vessel inflammation
	Thrombus and embolus	Thrombus is formation of clot attached to interior wall of a vein or artery, which can occlude the vessel lumen; embolus is piece of thrombus that has dislodged and circulates in bloodstream until it lodges in another vessel, commonly the lungs, hearts, or brain	Venous stasis (see thrombophlebitis) and vessel trauma; venous injury common following surgery of legs, abdomen, pelvis, and major vessels; thrombi also form from increased coagulability of blood, e.g., polycythemia and use of birth control pills containing estrogen
Gastrointestinal	Abdominal distention	Retention of air within intestines; signs and symptoms increased abdominal growth and tympanic percussion note over abdominal quadrants; client complains of fullness and "gas pains"	Slowed peristalsis from anesthesia, bowel manipulation, or immobilization
	Constipation	Infrequent passage of stools; should not be a concern immediately postoperatively, especially if client had a preoperative bowel preparation; after client resumes a solid diet, failure to pass a stool within 48 hours is cause for concern	Slowed peristalsis (see causes of distention) and delay in resuming normal diet
	Nausea and vomiting	Symptoms of improper gastric emptying or chemical stimulation of vomiting center; client complains of gagging, feeling full or sick to the stomach	Severe pain, abdominal distention, fear, medications, eating, or drinking before peristalsis returns, initiating gag reflex
Genitourinary	Urinary retention	Involuntary accumulation of urine in the bladder as result of loss of muscle tone; signs and symptoms inability to void, restlessness, bladder distention; common 6-8 hours after surgery	Effects of anesthesia and narcotic analgesics; local manipulation of tissues surrounding bladder and edema interfere with bladder tone; poor positioning of client impairs voiding reflexes

TABLE 47-8, cont'd

Postoperative Complications

System	Complication	Description	Cause
Integumentary	Wound infection	Invasion of deep or superficial wound tissues by pathogenic microorganisms; signs and symptoms skin around incision warm to touch, red, and tender; client may have fever and chills; purulent material may exit from drains or from separated wound edges; appears 3-6 days postoperatively	Poor aseptic technique; dirty wound before surgical exploration
	Wound dehiscence	Separation of wound edges at the suture line; signs and symptoms increased drainage and appearance of underlying tissues, usually occurs 6-8 days after surgery	Malnutrition; preoperative radiation to surgical site; old age; poor circulation to tissues; unusual strain on suture line
	Wound evisceration	Protrusion of internal organs and tissues through incision; usually occurs 6-8 days after surgery	See dehiscence; client with dehiscence at risk for developing evisceration

Clients who smoke or have preexisting lung disease are more prone to complications.

Complications affecting the client's circulatory status may be caused by the surgeon's lack of skill. A slipped suture or an overlooked bleeding vessel can result in hemorrhage at the surgical site. More commonly the development of hemorrhage is caused by underlying coagulation problems or surgical repair of fragile tissues. Circulatory alterations such as thrombus formation and thrombophlebitis commonly result from inactivity and the resultant impairment in normal blood flow. Clients with circulatory alterations because of arteriosclerosis, diabetes, and chronic lung disease require more aggressive care to prevent complications.

Disturbances of the gastrointestinal system result largely from inactivity, effects of anesthesia, and a delay in assuming normal dietary habits. Clients who have abdominal surgery will have slowing of peristalsis longer than clients whose surgery did not involve the gastrointestinal tract.

General anesthetic agents temporarily depress urinary bladder tone. Manipulation of organs and tissues surrounding the bladder may cause spasm of the bladder sphincter. For these reasons the client has difficulty voiding voluntarily, and often the bladder does not empty completely. The retention of urine within the bladder coupled with inactivity and poor fluid intake increases the chances of urinary infection developing (see Chapter 39).

A break in skin integrity immediately places a client at risk for infection. Strict aseptic practices may not be enough to prevent an impairment in wound healing. A poor nutritional status, circulatory alterations, and an alteration in integrity of skin layers will increase susceptibility to complications in wound healing. Prolonged coughing can place stress on a suture line and lead to a break in wound edges (see Chapter 48). The nurse should also be alert with an obese client whose general physical condition is poor.

Maintaining Respiratory Function. In an effort to prevent respiratory complications the nurse begins aggressive pulmonary hygiene measures early. The benefits of thorough preoperative teaching are realized when the client is able to participate actively in the nurse's plan of care. The following measures promote expansion of the lung.

1. The nurse encourages diaphragmatic breathing exercises at least every 2 hours while the client is awake. Maximal inspirations lasting 3 to 5 seconds open up alveoli.

2. The nurse instructs the client on use of an incentive spirometer to promote maximum inspiration.

3. The nurse encourages early ambulation. Walking causes the client to assume an anatomical position that does not restrict chest wall expansion and stimulates an increased respiratory rate.

4. The nurse assists clients who are restricted to bed to turn on their sides every 1 to 2 hours while awake and assume a sitting position when possible. Turning permits expansion of lungs that were previously in a dependent position. Sitting causes lowering of abdominal organs, thus facilitating diaphragmatic movement and lung expansion.

The following measures promote the removal of pulmonary secretions.

1. The nurse encourages coughing exercises every 2 hours while the client is awake and maintains pain control to promote a full productive cough.

2. The nurse provides oral hygiene to facilitate expectoration of mucus. Oral mucosa becomes dry when the client is allowed nothing by mouth or placed on limited fluid intake.

3. The nurse initiates nasotracheal suction for clients who are too weak or unable to cough (see Chapter 41).

Preventing Circulatory Stasis. Measures directed at preventing circulatory complications serve to prevent circulatory stasis. It is again important for the client to begin these activities early. Some clients are at greater risk of venous stasis because of the nature of their surgery, for example, orthopedic surgery necessitating immobilization of extremities and vascular bypass and repair. The following measures promote normal venous return and circulatory blood flow.

1. The nurse encourages clients to perform leg exercises at least every hour while awake. Exercise may be contraindicated in an affected extremity involving vascular repair or realignment of fractured bones and torn cartilage.

2. The nurse applies elastic support stockings as ordered by the physician. The stockings should be removed every 8 hours and left off for 1 hour. It is convenient to remove stockings when the client is bathing, ambulating, or sitting up in a chair.

3. The nurse encourages early ambulation. Most clients are ordered to ambulate the evening of surgery depending on the severity of surgery and the client's condition. The degree of activity allowed progresses as the client's condition improves. For example, the physician may order "up in a chair this evening; ambulate t.i.d. [three times a day] beginning tomorrow." Before ambulation the nurse assesses vital signs. Any abnormalities may contraindicate ambulation. If vital signs are normal, the nurse first assists the client to a sitting position on the side of the bed. If the client complains of dizziness, this is a sign of postural hy-

potension. A recheck of the client's blood pressure will determine if ambulation is safe. The nurse assists with ambulation by standing at the client's side, making sure the client is able to walk with a steady gait. The first few times out of bed the client may be able to walk only a few feet. This will improve each time. The nurse evaluates the client's tolerance to activity by periodically assessing pulse rate during ambulation.

4. The nurse avoids positioning the client in a manner that interrupts blood flow to the extremities. While in bed the client should not have pillows or rolled blankets placed under the knees. Compression of the popliteal vessels can promote thrombus formation. When sitting in a chair, clients should elevate their legs on a footstool. The postoperative client should never be allowed to sit with one leg crossed over the other.

5. The nurse administers anticoagulant medications as ordered. It is common for physicians to order small doses of anticoagulants such as heparin for clients at greatest risk for thrombus formation. Orthopedic clients often receive aspirin for its anticoagulation properties.

6. The nurse promotes adequate fluid intake orally or intravenously. Adequate hydration prevents the concentrated buildup of formed blood elements such as platelets and red blood cells. When a client's plasma volume is low, these elements may gather to form small clots within blood vessels.

Promoting Normal Elimination and Adequate Nutrition. The nurse's interventions for preventing gastrointestinal complications ultimately promote the return of normal elimination and faster resumption of normal nutritional intake. It takes several days for a client who has had surgery on gastrointestinal structures, for example, colon resection, cholecystectomy, or gastrectomy, to be able to resume a normal dietary intake. Normal peristalsis may not return for 2 to 3 days. In contrast, the client whose gastrointestinal tract is unaffected directly by surgery must simply endure the effects of anesthesia before resuming dietary intake. For example, the client who undergoes orthopedic surgery, a mastectomy, or plastic surgery is usually able to begin taking fluids as soon as nausea subsides.

The following measures promote return of normal elimination.

1. The nurse assesses for return of peristalsis. The nurse routinely auscultates the abdomen to detect the return of normal bowel sounds: five to 30 loud gurgles per minute over each quadrant indicates that peristalsis has returned. The presence of high-pitched tinkling sounds accompanied by abdominal distention

suggests the bowel is not functioning properly. The nurse asks if the client is passing flatus. This may be embarrassing for the client, but it is an important sign indicating normal bowel function.

2. The nurse maintains a gradual progression in dietary intake. For the first few hours postoperatively a client receives only intravenous fluids. If the physician orders resumption of a normal diet the first evening postoperatively, the nurse first provides clear liquids such as water, apple juice, or tea after the client's nausea subsides. Overloading a client with large amounts of fluids may lead to distention and vomiting. If the client tolerates liquids without nausea, the diet is advanced as ordered. Clients who have had abdominal surgery are usually allowed nothing by mouth the first 24 to 48 hours. As peristalsis returns, the nurse provides clear liquids, followed by full liquids, a light diet of solid foods, and finally a regular diet.

3. The nurse promotes ambulation and exercise. Physical activity stimulates a return of peristalsis. The client who suffers abdominal distention and "gas pain" will often acquire relief while walking.

4. The nurse maintains an adequate fluid intake. Fluids keep fecal material soft for easy passage during bowel elimination. Fruit juices and warm liquids are especially effective.

5. The nurse administers enemas, rectal suppositories, and rectal tubes as ordered. If constipation or distention develops, the physician will attempt to stimulate peristalsis through the use of cathartics or enemas. A rectal tube promotes passage of flatus.

The following measures maintain an adequate dietary intake.

1. The nurse removes sources of noxious odors. Drainage that has collected on a client's dressing, soiled linen, and drainage-collecting devices may be sources of noxious odors that cause nausea and loss of appetite.

2. The nurse assists the client to a comfortable position during mealtime. The client should sit if possible to minimize pressure on the abdomen and allow for easy access to the food tray.

3. The nurse provides small servings of food. A client will be more willing to face the first meal when servings are not large.

4. The nurse provides frequent oral hygiene. Adequate hydration and cleansing of the oral cavity eliminate dryness and bad tastes in the client's mouth.

5. The nurse provides meals when the client is rested and free from pain. Often a surgical client will lose interest in eating if mealtime has been preceded by exhausting activities such as ambulation, coughing and deep breathing exercises, or extensive dressing changes. When a client is experiencing pain, often the associated nausea causes a loss of appetite.

Promoting Urinary Elimination. The depressant effects of anesthesia and analgesics impair the client's sensation of bladder fullness. If bladder tone is reduced, the client has difficulty starting urination. Clients who undergo surgery of the urinary system frequently have Foley catheters inserted to maintain free urinary flow until voluntary control of urination returns.

The following measures promote normal urinary elimination.

1. The nurse assists clients to assume normal positions during voiding. The male client may need assistance to stand to void. The client will be less embarrassed if a male nurse is available to assist. Bedpans make voiding difficult. A female client will have better results if she is able to use a toilet.

2. The nurse checks the client frequently for the need to void. A surgical client restricted to bed will need assistance in handling and using bedpans or urinals. Often the client acquires a sudden feeling of bladder fullness and urgency to void. In this case the nurse must respond quickly when the client calls for help.

3. The nurse assesses for bladder distention. If a client does not void within 8 hours of surgery, it may be necessary to insert a urinary catheter. A physician's order is needed for a catheter insertion.

4. The nurse monitors intake and output. An accepted level of urine output is at least 30 ml per hour. If the client's urine is dark, concentrated, and low in volume, a physician should be notified. A surgical client can easily become dehydrated as a result of fluid loss from the surgical wound. The nurse will measure intake and output for several days postoperatively until normal fluid intake and urinary output are achieved.

Promoting Wound Healing. A surgical wound undergoes considerable stress during the client's convalescence. The stress of inadequate nutrition, impaired circulation, and metabolic alterations increases the client's risk for delayed healing. A wound may also undergo considerable physical stress. Strain on sutures from coughing, vomiting, distention, and movement of body parts can disrupt the wound layers. The nurse is responsible for protecting the wound and promoting the healing process. A critical time for wound healing is 24 to 72 hours following surgery. If a wound becomes infected, it usually occurs 3 to 6 days after surgery. A clean surgical wound usually does not regain strength against normal stress for 15 to 20 days postoperatively. Nursing measures for care of the surgical wound are detailed in Chapter 48.

PROMOTING REST AND COMFORT. A surgical client's pain increases as the effects of anesthesia wear off. The client becomes more aware of surroundings and more perceptive of any sources of discomfort. The incisional area may be only one source of pain. Irritation from drainage tubes, tight dressings, or casts and the muscular strains caused from positioning on the operating room table are examples of factors that can make the client feel miserable.

Pain can significantly slow a surgical client's recovery. The client becomes reluctant to cough, deep breathe, turn, ambulate, or perform necessary exercises. It is important for the nurse to assess the client's pain thoroughly (see Chapter 37). It should not be assumed that the pain is incisional. When the client calls for a pain medication, the nature and character of the pain should be determined. For example, a nurse may prepare an injection for a client who has a repair of a fractured leg only to learn when entering the room that the client is having chest pain. Chapter 37 discusses the administration of analgesics and non-pharmacological measures for pain relief.

PROMOTING SELF-CONCEPT. The appearance of wounds, bulky dressings, and extruding drains and tubes are just some of the factors that threaten a client's self-concept. The nature of the surgery may create permanent change, such as disfiguring scars and excised body parts, in the client's body image. If surgery leads to impairment in body function, the client's role within the family can change significantly.

Often a nurse becomes so involved with the physical aspects of a surgical client's care that the nurse forgets a person lies in the bed. It is important for the nurse, however, to observe the client for alterations in self-concept. Clients may show a revulsion toward their appearance by refusing to look at an incision, carefully covering dressings with bedclothes, or refusing to get out of bed because of various tubes and devices. The fear of not being able to return to a functional role in the family may even cause the client to avoid participating in the nurse's plan of care.

The family becomes an important part of the nurse's efforts to improve the client's self-concept. The nurse explains to the family what the client's appearance is like and how to avoid nonverbal expressions of revulsion or surprise. The family needs to adopt an accepting attitude toward the client's needs and still encourage the client's independence. If the client's condition is terminal, the family learns how to assist the client through the grieving process so both client and family can reach a stage of acceptance.

The following measures maintain the client's self-concept.

1. The nurse provides privacy during dressing changes or inspection of the wound. The room curtains are kept closed around the bed and the client is draped so only the dressing or incisional area is exposed.

2. The nurse maintains the client's hygiene. Wound drainage and antiseptic solutions from the surgical skin preparation dry on the skin's surface and act as sources of irritation. A complete bath the first day after surgery can make the client feel like a new person. Whenever the client's gown becomes soiled by wound drainage, the nurse offers a clean gown and washcloth. The nurse keeps the client's hair neatly combed and offers frequent oral hygiene, especially for the client who is allowed nothing by mouth.

3. The nurse prevents drainage sets from overflowing. Typically the physician orders contents of drainage sets to be measured every 8 hours for output recording. The client sometimes becomes preoccupied with observing the gradual collection of drainage, and some drainage sets can leak contents if they become too full. The nurse should empty the sets periodically to prevent hampering the client's movement and accidental spills.

4. The nurse maintains a pleasant environment. A client's self-concept is heightened by being in pleasant, comfortable surroundings. Frequently the room of a surgical client becomes cluttered with extra dressings, rolls of tape, and bottles of antiseptic solution. If the client requires frequent dressing changes, the room may take on the appearance of a supply room. The nurse should store or remove all unused supplies and keep the client's bedside orderly and clean.

5. The nurse offers opportunities for clients to discuss feelings about their appearance. If the nurse notices that the client avoids looking at an incision, the client may need to discuss any fears or concerns. A client having surgery for the first time is often more anxious than a client who has had multiple surgeries. Both male and female clients may worry about permanent scarring. A client is more apt to look at an incision several days after surgery when healing is occurring and the client begins to gain more energy and a feeling of well-being. If the client chooses to look at an incision for the first time, the area should be clean. Eventually the client should be able to care for the incision site by applying simple dressings or bathing the affected area.

6. The nurse provides the family with opportunities to discuss ways to promote the client's self-concept.

Encouraging the client's independence can be difficult for a family member who has a strong desire to assist the client in any way. By knowing what a wound or incision looks like, family members can be supportive during dressing changes. The topic or tone of a conversation can also help family members distract clients from dwelling on their fears and concerns. Family members should not avoid discussing the future. However, the nurse must help them know when it is appropriate to discuss future plans with the client. Then the client and family can work together to discuss realistic plans for the client's return home.

Promoting Return to a Functional State of Health.

Throughout the postoperative convalescent period the nurse strives to promote the client's independence and active participation in care. When a surgical client is in pain or suffers from postoperative complications, there is little motive for self-care. The nurse must maintain a balance of providing for clients' needs when they are physically dependent and promoting more involvement by clients when their conditions allow it.

The goals a nurse sets for a client's involvement in care must be realistic. Surgery may limit a client's ability to participate effectively. For example, a nurse will frequently encourage a client to assist with bathing. However, the surgical client may be "tied down" by intravenous lines, a nasogastric tube, wound drainage systems, or a Foley catheter. It is unrealistic for the nurse to involve the client if movement is highly restricted or if participation increases the client's discomfort.

The nurse should keep the client and family informed of progress made toward recovery. Many clients become depressed if they think their recovery is slow. The nurse explains that it normally takes many days to reach a level of maximal recovery. Surgery may also cause permanent physical limitations that will require time for the client to accept and adjust to.

The nurse plans care on a daily basis, keeping in mind the ultimate goals for a client's recovery. For example, if the client is having a joint replacement for an arthritic knee, the nurse begins on the first postoperative day with graded exercises ordered by the physician. The client's physical therapy progresses to maintain existing function and regain function temporarily lost from surgery. From the moment the client enters the hospital, through surgery, and during the postoperative phase, the nurse anticipates the client's return home.

Involvement of family members in the client's plan of care can facilitate the client's recovery. If the client requires additional care at home such as dressing changes, assistance with ambulation, or medication administration, the nurse instructs family members on proper care techniques. If family members are unable to assist the client, the nurse works with the physician in making plans for home care through a visiting nurse agency. The client will be more able to assume a functional state of health when family members understand the limitations a client faces.

Evaluation

The nurse evaluates the effectiveness of care provided the surgical client on the basis of the expected outcomes of nursing interventions.

Efforts to promote respiratory function are evaluated on the following bases:
1. The client's lung sounds becoming clear
2. Normal chest excursion
3. Nonproductive cough
4. Normal color of skin and nail beds

Evaluation of good circulatory function is indicated by the following:
1. Absence of pain in calves
2. Normal peripheral pulses
3. Warm extremities with good capillary filling in the nail beds

The surgical client's elimination status is judged by these criteria:
1. Soft and formed stools
2. Normal bowel sounds
3. Resumption of regular bowel movements

Effort to promote normal nutrition are evaluated on the basis of these criteria:
1. Absence of weight loss
2. Absence of wound complications such as dehiscence

A client has normal genitourinary function postoperatively if these characteristics are present:
1. Voluntary voiding without urgency or difficulty in starting urination
2. Urine output equal to or greater than 30 ml per hour

Evaluation of normal wound healing is indicated by these:
1. The edges of the incision being closed or well approximated
2. An absence of drainage or minimal serous drainage
3. An absence of inflammation or tenderness at the incision

A surgical client will likely have a degree of discomfort or pain even at the time of discharge. However, the pain should not seriously impair function, that is, normal ventilatory movement or ambulation.

If range of joint motion is reduced as a result of surgery, pain should not lead to further reduction in joint movement at the time of discharge.

Whether a client has maintained or regained a sense of self-esteem can be evaluated on the following bases:

1. The client's level of grooming and hygiene
2. The client's willingness to discuss surgery and any related limitations
3. The client's ability to care for the incision

Attainment of a functional level of health is evaluated on the basis of the nature of the client's surgery and the client's physical condition postoperatively. The nurse must understand to what extent physical function will be temporarily or permanently impaired. Evaluative outcomes thus will be based on the optimal level of function the client can achieve.

KEY CONCEPTS

✓ With the evolution of surgical asepsis and the development of modern anesthetic practices, the nurse's role in the operating room expanded.

✓ Perioperative nursing is the professional nursing care afforded the surgical client before, during, and after surgery.

✓ Surgery is classified by level of severity, urgency, and purpose.

✓ In addition to the nature of nursing care provided, previous illnesses and past surgeries influence the client's ability to tolerate surgery.

✓ The duration of the preoperative period may be several days or only a few hours.

✓ All medications taken preoperatively are automatically discontinued postoperatively unless a physician reorders the drugs.

✓ Family members are important in assisting clients with any physical limitations and in providing emotional support during postoperative recovery.

✓ Preoperative assessment of vital signs and physical findings provides an important baseline with which to compare postoperative assessment data.

✓ A client's feelings about surgery can have significant impact on relationships with nursing staff and the client's ability to participate in care.

✓ The surgical removal of a body part may permanently alter a person's body image as well as the individual's sexuality.

✓ Routine diagnostic tests used to screen for preexisting abnormalities preoperatively include a complete blood count (CBC), serum electrolytes, urinalysis, and chest x-ray study.

✓ Nursing diagnoses of the surgical client may pose implications for nursing care during one or all of the phases of surgery.

✓ Primary responsibility for informed consent rests with the client's surgeon.

✓ A consent form cannot be signed after a nurse administers preoperative medications.

✓ Structured preoperative teaching has a positive influence on a client's postoperative recovery.

✓ Basic to preoperative teaching is explanation of all preoperative and postoperative routines, as well as demonstration of postoperative exercises.

✓ Shaving of a surgical site should be done as close as possible to the time of surgery to minimize infection.

KEY CONCEPTS, *cont'd*

✓ A routine preoperative checklist provides a guide for the final preparation of the client before surgery.

✓ Many of the responsibilities of nurses within the operating room focus on protecting the client from potential harm.

✓ Administration of an agent for general anesthesia usually requires intubation of the client with an endotracheal tube.

✓ A major risk with regional infiltrative anesthetics is a sudden drop in the client's blood pressure.

✓ Improper positioning on the operating table may cause the client serious respiratory, circulatory, and neuromuscular complications, as well as postoperative pain.

✓ The nurse's assessment of the postoperative client centers on the body systems most likely to be affected by anesthesia, immobilization, and surgical trauma.

✓ Because a surgical client's condition may change rapidly in recovery, the nurse monitors the client's status every 15 minutes.

✓ The recovery room nurse reports to the nurse on the postoperative division any information pertaining to the client's current physical status and risk for postoperative complications.

✓ Many of the nurse's postoperative interventions serve to prevent more than one type of medical complication.

✓ A surgical client's pain may arise from sources other than the surgical wound.

✓ From the time of admission to the hospital the nurse plans for the surgical client's discharge home.

REFERENCES

American Nurses' Association and Association of Operating Room Nurses: Standards of perioperative nursing care, Kansas City, Mo., 1982, The Associations.

Keithley, J.K.: Wound healing in malnourished patients, J. Am. Assoc. OR Nurs. 35:1094, 1982.

Lindeman, C., and VanAernam, B.: Nursing intervention with the presurgical patient—the effects of structured and unstructured preoperative teaching, Nurs. Res. 20:319, 1971.

Metzger, R.S.: The beginning of OR nursing education, J. Am. Assoc. OR Nurs. 24:73, 1976.

ADDITIONAL READINGS

Breslin, E.F.: Prevention and treatment of pulmonary complications in patients after surgery of the upper abdomen, Heart Lung 10:511, 1981.

Croushore, T.M.: Postoperative assessment: the key to avoiding the most common nursing mistakes, Nursing 79 9:47, 1979.

Fortin, F., and Kirovac, S.: A randomized controlled trial of preoperative patient education, Int. J. Nurs. Stud. 13:11, 1976.

Frogge, M.H.: Promoting wound healing in the irradiated patient, J. Am. Assoc. OR Nurs. 35:1088, 1982.

Gruendemann, B.J., and Meeker, M.H.: Alexander's care of the patient in surgery, ed. 7, St. Louis, 1983, The C.V. Mosby Co.

Horsley, J., and Crane, J.: Structured preoperative teaching, New York, 1981, Grune & Stratton, Inc.

Kneedler, J., and Dodge, G.: Perioperative patient care, Boston, 1983, Blackwell Scientific Publications, Inc.

McHugh, N.G., et al.: Preparatory information: what helps and why, Am. J. Nurs. 82:780, 1982.

Metheny, N.: Preoperative fluid balance assessment, J. Am. Assoc. OR Nurs. 33:51, 1981.

Pagana, K.D., and Pagana, T.J.: Diagnostic testing and nursing implications, St. Louis, 1982, The C.V. Mosby Co.

Volden, C., and Grinde, J.: Taking the trauma out of nasogastric intubation, Nursing 80 10:64, 1980.

Wells, N.: The effect of relaxation on postoperative muscle tension and pain, Nurs. Res. 31:236, 1982.

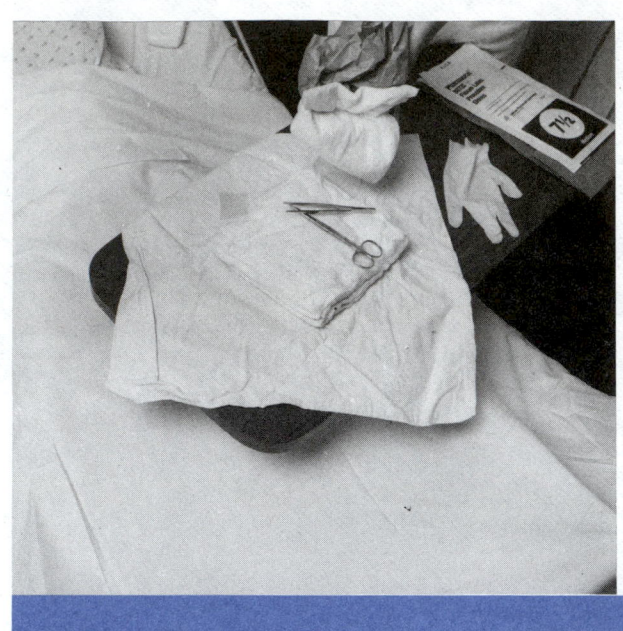

OBJECTIVES

Mastery of content in this chapter will enable the student to:

- Define the terms in the glossary.
- Describe the relationship of normal integumentary function to wound healing.
- Discuss the body's response during each stage of the wound healing process.
- Classify a wound according to the state of skin integrity, severity, cleanliness, and descriptive qualities.
- Differentiate healing by primary and secondary intention.
- Discuss common complications of wound healing.
- Explain the factors that impair or promote normal wound healing.
- Conduct an assessment of a surgical and open wound.
- List and discuss the three purposes of wound first aid.
- Apply a sterile dry dressing using sterile technique.
- Describe the purposes and precautions taken during wound irrigations.
- Discuss the purpose of bandages and binders.
- Apply a warm and a cold compress safely to an injured body part.

GLOSSARY

approximate To come close together, as in the edges of a wound.

binder Bandage made of a large piece of material to fit a specific body part.

compress Soft pad of gauze or cloth used to apply heat, cold, or medications to the surface of a body part.

desquamation Normal process in which the dead cells of the epidermal skin layer slough off.

drainage tube Catheter used for evacuation of air or fluid from a cavity or wound in the body.

ecchymosis Discoloration of skin or bruise caused by leakage of blood into subcutaneous tissues as a result of trauma to underlying vessels.

fibrin Protein product formed from the action of thrombin on fibrinogen in the clotting process.

fistula Abnormal passage from an internal organ to the body surface or between two internal organs.

granulation tissue Soft, pink, fleshy projections of tissue that form during the healing process in a wound not healing by primary intention.

hematoma Collection of blood trapped in the tissues of the skin or an organ.

hemostasis Termination of bleeding by mechanical or chemical means or by the coagulation process of the body.

48 Nursing Care of Wounds

laceration Torn, jagged wound.

primary intention Primary union of the edges of a wound, progressing to complete scar formation without granulation.

secondary intention Wound closure in which the edges are separated, granulation tissue develops to fill the gap, and finally, epithelium grows in over the granulation, producing a larger scar than results with primary intention.

sitz bath Bath in which only the hips or buttocks are immersed in fluid.

The body's integument provides a protective barrier against disease-causing organisms and serves as a sensory organ for pain, temperature, and touch. Any disruption in skin or mucous membrane integrity poses risks to a person's safety and physical well-being. When a person suffers injury to the integument, the body responds in a complex series of steps to achieve wound healing. The nurse's knowledge of normal patterns of wound healing permits easier recognition of alterations in wound repair. The type of wound and the conditions that promote or retard healing influence the nurse's choice of interventions. The nurse's primary responsibilities are to prevent the invasion of microorganisms into wounds and to support the body's defenses in achieving wound repair.

The impact of wounds on a client's self-esteem and body image cannot be ignored. A surgical scar or a traumatic laceration of the skin can leave permanent changes in a person's appearance. The pain associated with a wound adds further demands on the nurse in selecting therapies appropriate for the client's needs. The client's psychological well-being also influences the ability of the client to comply with wound-healing therapies.

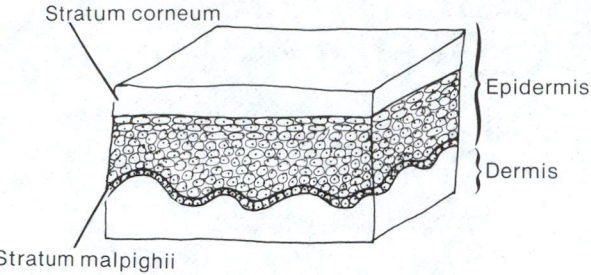

Fig. 48-1 Layers of the integument.

Review of the Normal Integument

In relation to wound healing the integument has two principal layers: the epidermis and the dermis (Fig. 48-1). The epidermis or outer skin layer consists of two layers. The stratum corneum, the thin, outermost layer of the epidermis, consists of flattened, dead cells. The cells originate from the second epidermal layer, the stratum malpighii. Cells in the stratum malpighii divide, proliferate, and migrate toward the epidermal surface. Once the cells reach the stratum corneum they flatten and die. The constant movement of epidermal cells ensures replacement of cells sloughed at the surface during normal desquamation. The thin stratum corneum protects underlying cells and tissues from dehydration and prevents entrance of certain chemical agents. However, the stratum corneum does allow evaporation of water from the skin and permits absorption of certain locally applied medications.

The dermal skin layer differs from the epidermis in that the dermis contains no skin cells. Collagen (a tough fibrous protein), blood vessels, and nerves comprise the dermis. Fibroblasts, which are responsible for collagen formation, are the only distinctive cell type within the dermis.

Understanding the integument's layers helps the nurse promote the process of wound healing. The epidermis functions to resurface wounds and restore the barrier to invading organisms. The dermis responds during wound healing to restore the structural integrity and physical properties of the skin. Even though a wound may close in the upper epidermal layer, the client is at risk for infection, circulatory impairment, and tissue breakdown if the underlying dermis fails to heal.

Wound Classifications

There are numerous ways to classify wounds. Wound classifications focus on the status of skin in-

tegrity, the cause of the wound, the severity of tissue injury, the cleanliness of the wound, or the descriptive qualities of the wound. These classifications overlap. For example, a penetrating knife wound is also an open wound, and a contused wound is a closed wound. Table 48-1 outlines various wound classifications. Wound classifications enable the nurse to understand the potential risks associated with a wound and the implications for wound care. For example, an open wound presents a greater risk of infection than a closed wound. An abrasion will require less extensive dressings than a deep penetrating wound. A surgical incision is generally cleaner than a traumatic wound.

Wound Healing Process

The process of wound healing involves a series of integrated physiological processes. The nature of healing is the same for all wounds with variations depending on the location, severity, and extent of injury. The ability of cells and tissues to regenerate or return to normal structure by cell growth also affects healing. Cells of the liver, renal tubules, and neurons of the central nervous system typically regenerate slowly or not at all.

In general terms, there are two different types of wounds with respect to tissue loss: those with loss and those without. A clean surgical incision is an example of a wound with little tissue loss. The surgical wound heals by *primary intention*. The skin edges approximate, or close together, and the risk of infection developing is lower. In contrast, a wound involving loss of tissue, such as a burn, decubitus ulcer, or severe laceration, heals by *secondary intention*. The wound edges do not approximate. The wound is left open until it becomes filled by scar tissue. It takes longer for a wound to heal by secondary intention, and thus the chance of infection is greater. If scarring from secondary intention is severe, there may be permanent loss of tissue function.

Regardless of the type of wound, the healing process involves an orderly series of physiological responses. When healing occurs by secondary intention, a particular response may take longer or certain cellular responses may be altered.

Healing by Primary Intention

A good example of the normal healing process is the repair of a clean surgical wound. The healing process occurs in three stages as described by Bruno (1979): defensive, reconstructive, and maturative. The *defensive stage* begins immediately at the time of

TABLE 48-1

Wound Classifications

Classification	Type	Description	Causes	Implications for Healing
Status of skin integrity	Open	Wound involving a break in skin or mucous membranes	Trauma by sharp object or blow, e.g., surgical incision, venipuncture, gunshot wound	Break in skin exposes body to invasion by microorganisms; loss of blood and body fluids through wound; reduced function of body part
	Closed	Wound involving no break in skin integrity	Part of body being struck by a blunt object; twisting, straining, or deceleration force against the body, e.g., bone fracture, tear of visceral organ	May predispose person to internal hemorrhage; reduced function of affected body part
Cause	Intentional	Wound resulting from therapy	Surgical incision; introduction of needle into body part	Usually performed under aseptic technique, which minimizes chances of infection; wound edges usually smooth and clean
	Unintentional	Wound that occurs unexpectedly	Traumatic injury, e.g., knife wound, burn	Occurs under unsterile conditions; wound edges often jagged
Severity of injury	Superficial	Wound that involves only epidermal layer of skin	Result of friction applied to skin surface, e.g., abrasion, first- or second-degree burn	Break in skin creates risk of infection; does not involve underlying injury to tisues or organs; blood supply to area intact
	Penetrating	Wound involving break in epidermal skin layer as well as dermis and deeper tissues or organs	Foreign object or instrument entering deep into body tissues; usually unintentional, e.g., gunshot wound, stab wound	High risk of infection, since foreign object is contaminated; may cause internal as well as external hemorrhage; damage to internal organs causes temporary or permanent loss of function
	Perforating	Penetrating wound in which foreign object enters and exits an internal organ	See penetrating wound	High risk of infection; nature of injury depends on organ perforated: lung—compromised oxygenation; major vessel—serious hemorrage; intestine—contamination of abdominal cavity by feces

Continued.

TABLE 48-1, cont'd

Wound Classifications

Classification	Type	Description	Causes	Implications for Healing
Cleanliness	Clean	Wound containing no pathogenic organisms	Surgical wound that does not enter the gastrointestinal tract, respiratory tract, or oropharyngeal cavity	Low risk of infection
	Clean-contaminated	Wound made under aseptic conditions but involving entrance into body cavity that normally harbors microorganisms	Surgical wound entering gastrointestinal or respiratory tract or oropharyngeal cavity	Greater risk of infection than with clean wound
	Contaminated	Wound existing under conditions in which presence of microorganisms is likely	Open, traumatic wounds; surgical wound in which a break in asepsis occurred	Tissues often not healthy and show inflammation; high risk of infection
	Infected	Bacterial organisms present in wound site	Any wound that does not properly heal and grows organisms; old traumatic wound; surgical incision into area infected, e.g., ruptured bowel	Wound presents signs of infection, e.g., inflammation, purulent drainage, skin separation
Descriptive qualities	Laceration	Tearing of tissues with irregular wound edges	Severe traumatic injury, e.g., knife wound, industrial accident involving machinery, tissues cut by broken glass	Wound usually created by a contaminated object; depth of wound determines other complications
	Abrasion	Superficial wound involving scraping or rubbing of skin's surface by friction	Often results from a fall, e.g., skinned knee or elbow; also result of a dermatological procedure for removing scar tissue	Painful owing to exposure of superficial nerves; deeper tissues uninvolved; risk of infection from exposure to contaminated surface
	Contusion	Closed wound caused by a blow to the body by a blunt object; contusion or bruise characterized by swelling, discoloration, and pain	Bleeding in underlying tissues caused by blunt force against body part	More severe if internal organ contused; may cause temporary loss of function of body part; localized bleeding into the tissues may form a hematoma, or collection of blood

injury and lasts 4 to 6 days. Reparative processes work to control bleeding (hemostasis), deliver blood and cells to the injured area (inflammation), and form epithelial cells at the injury site (epithelial cell migration). During hemostasis injured blood vessels constrict and platelets gather to stop bleeding. Clots form a fibrin matrix that later provides a framework for cell repair. A scab consisting of clot and dead tissue provides an external protection against infectious organisms. The inflammatory response increases blood flow to the wound and vascular permeability to plasma, resulting in localized redness and edema. Leukocytes reach the wound within a few hours. The primary acting white blood cell is the neutrophil, which begins to ingest bacteria and small debris. The neutrophils die in a few days and leave behind an enzyme exudate that can either attack bacteria or interfere with tissue repair. In chronic inflammation the dying neutrophils create wound pus. The second important leukocyte is the monocyte, which transforms into macrophages. The macrophages are "garbage cells" that clean a wound of bacteria, dead cells, and debris by phagocytosis. The macrophages also digest and recycle substances such as amino acids and sugars that aid in wound repair.

After the macrophages debride the wound and make it ready for tissue repair, epithelial cells move from the wound margins toward the base of the clot or scab. Epithelial cells continue to gather under the wound space for approximately 48 hours. Eventually a thin layer of epithelial tissue forms over the wound to act as a barrier against infectious organisms and toxic materials.

The stage of *reconstruction* begins before the defensive stage ends. During this period the wound begins to close with new tissue. Reconstruction begins on the third or fourth day following trauma and lasts from 2 to 3 weeks.

First the epithelial cells multiply to fill the wound. Fibroblasts, cells that originate from the wound, function to synthesize collagen, the main component of scar tissue. Fibroblasts require vitamins B and C, oxygen, and amino acids to function properly. The collagen provides strength and structural integrity to a wound. As reconstruction progresses, the risk of wound separation or rupture is less likely. After 15 to 20 days the wound can resist normal stress such as tension or twisting. The degree of stress on a wound influences the amount of scar tissue formed. For example, more scar tissue forms in an extremity wound than in a less mobile area such as the scalp or chest.

The final phase of reconstruction is the differentiation of epithelial cells. The epithelial cells assume the characteristics of previously damaged cells; for example, epidermal cells flatten and intestinal mucosal cells acquire their columnar appearance.

Maturation, the final stage of healing, may take more than a year, depending on the depth and extent of the wound. The collagen scar continues to gain strength for several months. However, a healed wound usually does not have the strength of the tissue it replaces. The collagen fibers undergo remodeling or organization before assuming their normal appearance. Usually scar tissue contains fewer pigmented cells (melanocytes) and has a lighter color than the normal skin color.

Healing by Secondary Intention

When tissue loss in a wound is extensive, the process of healing takes longer. A large open wound typically drains more fluid than a closed wound. Inflammation is often chronic, and tissue defects become filled with fragile granulation tissue rather than collagen. Granulation tissue is a form of connective tissue that has a more abundant blood supply than collagen. Since the wound is larger, the amount of connective tissue scarring is larger.

When epithelial and connective tissue cells are unable to close a wound defect, contraction may occur. Wound contraction involves the movement of the dermis and epidermis on each side across a wound surface. The wound fills in part with normal skin rather than scar tissue. Wound contraction is not the same as a contracture or deformity resulting from muscle shortening and joint fixation. The wound contraction results in thinning of surrounding tissue. The size and shape of the final scar correspond to tension lines in the damaged area. For example, a square wound in the abdomen assumes the shape of a four-point star because of stress along the scar lines.

Complications of Wound Healing

When a wound fails to heal properly, a number of complications may develop.

Hemorrhage

Bleeding from a wound site is normal during and immediately after the initial trauma. Hemostasis occurs within several minutes unless large blood vessels are involved or the client has poor clotting function. Hemorrhage occurring after the period of hemostasis indicates a slipped surgical suture, a dislodged clot, infection, or the erosion of a blood vessel by a foreign object (for example, a drain). Hemorrhage may occur externally or internally. For example, if a surgical suture slips off a blood vessel, bleeding will occur within the tissues and there will be no visible signs of blood unless a surgical drain is present. (The surgeon often inserts a drain into tissues beneath a wound to remove fluid that collects in underlying tissues.) The nurse can detect internal bleeding by looking for distention or swelling of the affected body part or the development of signs of hypovolemic shock (fall in blood pressure, increased thready pulse, increased respirations, restlessness, and diaphoresis). A hematoma is a localized collection of blood underneath the tissues. It will appear as a localized swelling or mass that often takes on a bluish discoloration. A hematoma near a major artery or vein is dangerous because the pressure from the expanding hematoma may obstruct blood flow through the vessel.

External hemorrhaging is more obvious. The nurse observes dressings covering the wound for bloody drainage. If bleeding is extensive, the dressing soon becomes saturated and frequently blood escapes along the sides of the dressing and pools beneath the client. The nurse observes all wounds closely, particularly surgical wounds in which the risk of hemorrhage is great during the first 24 to 48 hours after surgery.

Infection

Wound infection is one of the most common nosocomial (hospital-related) infections. According to the Centers for Disease Control (Simmons, 1983), a wound is infected if purulent material drains from it, even if culture is not taken or has negative results. A sample of drainage from an infected wound may not reveal presence of bacteria in a culture because of poor culture technique or because the client has already received antibiotics. Positive culture findings do not always indicate an infection, since many wounds contain colonies of noninfective resident bacteria. The chances of wound infection are greater when the wound contains dead or necrotic tissue, when there are foreign bodies in or near the wound, and when blood supply and local tissue defenses are reduced. Bacterial wound infection inhibits wound healing by increasing tissue damage and by causing alterations in the healing process.

A contaminated or traumatic wound may show signs of infection early, within 2 to 3 days. A surgical wound infection usually does not develop until the fourth or fifth day. The client will have a fever, tenderness and pain at the wound site, and an elevated white blood cell count. The edges of the wound appear inflamed. Drainage is purulent and has a yellow, green, or brown color depending on the causative organism. For example, the gram-negative bacterium *Pseudomonas aeruginosa,* a common organism in incisional wound infections, causes a greenish discharge.

Dehiscence

When a wound fails to heal properly, the layers of skin and tissue may separate. This most commonly occurs before collagen formation (3 to 11 days after injury). Dehiscence is the partial or total separation of wound layers. Any client with poor wound healing is at risk for dehiscence. However, obese clients have a high risk because of the constant strain placed on their wounds and the poor healing qualities of fatty tissue. Dehiscence most often involves abdominal surgical wounds and occurs after a sudden strain such as coughing, vomiting, or sitting up in bed. Clients often report feeling as though something had given way. When there is an increase in serosanguineous drainage from a wound, the nurse should be alert for dehiscence.

Evisceration

When wound layers separate, evisceration, or the protrusion of visceral organs through a wound opening, may occur. The condition is a medical emergency that necessitates surgical repair. When evisceration occurs, the nurse places sterile towels soaked in sterile saline over the extruding tissues to reduce chances of bacterial invasion and drying. As long as the organs protrude through the wound, blood supply to the tissues is compromised.

Fistulas

A fistula is an abnormal passage between two organs or between an organ and the outside of the body. A surgeon may create a fistula for therapeutic purposes, for example, making an opening between the stomach and the outer abdominal wall to insert a gastrostomy tube for feeding purposes. Most fistulas, however, form as a result of poor wound healing. Trauma, infection, radiation exposure, and disease such as cancer prevent tissue layers from closing properly and allow the fistula tract to form. Fistulas increase the risk of infection, as well as fluid-electrolyte imbalance resulting from fluid loss. Chronic drainage of fluids through a fistula can also predispose a person to skin breakdown.

Factors Influencing Wound Healing

Numerous factors promote or retard wound healing. The nurse's knowledge of conditions influencing wound healing will aid in the selection of appropriate nursing therapies.

Age

The process of aging has direct impact on each of the stages of wound healing. An elderly client has undergone alterations in the defensive, reconstructive, and maturational responses that promote healing. Vascular changes that accompany aging, for example, reduction in number of capillaries and atherosclerosis (plaque formation in blood vessels), impair circulation to the wound site. Aging can also alter synthesis of clotting factors because of a reduction in liver function. The inflammatory response may be slowed or less extensive in nature. The aged client often has nutritional deficiencies that reduce numbers of red blood cells and leukocytes. Therefore there is a reduction in oxygen delivery to a wound and phagocytosis is impaired. Changes in the elderly client's immune system reduce the formation of antibodies and lymphocytes, thus increasing risk of infection.

Because of a slowing in cell growth and differentiation, the reconstructive stage of wound healing does not progress normally in the aged client. If the client's nutritional status is also poor, the components needed to promote collagen formation are lacking.

The maturation stage of wound healing also does not progress normally in an aged client. The older person's connective tissues contain more elastic fibers, and collagen tissue is less pliable. Scar tissue is tauter and firmer, increasing the risk of altered body part function. The long process of wound maturation in an elderly client may be a special challenge to the nurse. The nurse must give special attention to helping the elderly client learn and understand the principles of wound care and healing. Often the aged person requires support persons in the home setting to reinforce compliance with the nurse's therapies.

Nutrition

Malnutrition is a significant factor in impaired wound healing. Tissue repair and resistance to infection depend on a balanced diet, including protein, carbohydrates, lipids, vitamins, and minerals. If the client has undergone significant stress, as in the case of surgery, severe trauma, or a burn injury, the normal nutritional requirements are greater. For example, a well-nourished surgical client without postoperative complications needs at least 1500 kcal per day for dietary maintenance (Keithley, 1982). If a serious infection develops, the nutritional requirements increase 50%.

Obesity

Fatty tissue does not contain an abundant supply of blood vessels. Poor vascularization impairs delivery of nutrients and cellular elements needed for healing. The obese client has a greater risk for wound infection. It is also more difficult for a surgeon to close or suture adipose tissue. If the tissue heals by secondary intention, the chance of dehiscence or evisceration is greater.

Extent of Wound

The deeper the wound and the greater the tissue loss, the greater the risk of impaired wound healing. Healing by secondary intention takes longer, increasing the vulnerability to complications. A superficial wound such as an abrasion or cut of the skin heals more quickly and does not expose the client to chances of serious tissue injury.

Oxygenation

A reduction in oxygen delivered to the tissues inhibits wound repair. Low arterial oxygen tension alters the synthesis of collagen and the formation of epithelial cells. A wound heals more slowly when local circulating blood flow is poor and when the wound surface is not exposed to oxygen. Thus certain wounds, such as a small, closed surgical wound, will likely heal more quickly when exposed to air. In contrast, even though a large open wound may benefit from exposure to air, the risk of infection is too great.

Local blood flow is not the only factor contributing to oxygenation of tissues. The percentage of red blood cells that carry oxygen can also influence healing. Anemia is a condition characterized by a decrease in hemoglobin in the blood, resulting from decreased hemoglobin or red cell production, blood loss, or increased destruction of hemoglobin and red cells. In cases of mild anemia the body responds by improving oxygen delivery to tissues through increased cardiac output and greater release of oxygen to the tissues. However, if anemia is severe enough to cause a reduction in arterial Po_2 in capillaries or extracellular fluid adjacent to the wound, healing may be affected. A hematocrit value below 33% (normal: men 42% to 52%; women 37% to 47%) or a hemoglobin value below 10 g/100 ml (normal: men 14 to 18 g; women 12 to 16 g) can interfere with tissue repair.

Smoking

A smoker has a reduced amount of functional hemoglobin capable of carrying oxygen. Smoking also interferes with the normal cellular mechanisms that promote release of oxygen in the tissues. If the client has undergone surgery and is under the influence of anesthetics or analgesics, the reduction in lung ventilation will add to the smoker's risk of poor tissue oxygenation.

Immunosuppression

Any agent or disease state that reduces a person's immune response adds to the likelihood of poor wound healing. The administration of steroids (anti-inflammatory drugs) reduces the inflammatory response and slows collagen synthesis. Cortisone is one steroid that depresses fibroblast activity and capillary growth and thereby impairs wound closure. The masking of the inflammatory response by steroids also prevents the nurse from being able to detect early signs of inflammation or infection such as redness, swelling, or tenderness.

Chemotherapeutic drugs used in the treatment of various forms of cancer can depress bone marrow function. The resultant decrease in the formation of leukocytes will impair the defensive stage of wound healing and increase the risk of infection. Cancerous diseases involving the bone marrow or lymphatic system, for example, Hodgkin's disease, multiple myeloma, and leukemia, also interfere with leukocyte production and the immune response.

Diabetes

Diabetes mellitus deserves special consideration with respect to wound healing. The diabetic client has a small blood vessel disease that impairs tissue perfusion. The diabetic client with poorly controlled disease also has the problem of poor oxygen delivery, since the hemoglobin has a greater affinity for oxygen and fails to release it to the tissues. Hyperglycemia, the elevation in blood glucose concentration symptomatic of diabetes, alters the ability of leukocytes to perform phagocytosis. The wound will not debride cleanly, adding to the infection risk.

Radiation

Clients with cancerous tumors often receive radiotherapy that shrinks the cancerous mass to make it operable or halt its growth. Postoperative wound healing becomes a problem if surgery is not performed within 4 to 6 weeks of irradiation. Fibrosis and vascular scarring eventually develop in the irradiated skin layers. A delay in surgery will result in the client's wound attempting to heal when tissues are fragile and poorly perfused.

Wound Stress

Continual stress to an abdominal suture line and wound tissues can disrupt wound layers. In a surgical client the three factors that most commonly contribute to wound stress are vomiting, abdominal distention, and respiratory effort. During vomiting, abdominal muscles contract sharply. The sudden unexpected tension on an incision inhibits the formation of endothelial cell and collagen networks. The gradual accumulation of gastrointestinal secretions and swallowed air causes distention of the bowel with stretching of an abdominal wound.

Coughing is essential to a surgical client's well-being but poses a risk to wound healing. Coughing clears secretions that accumulate within the airways. With vigorous coughing the straining of abdominal muscles may tear open an abdominal wound. Splinting abdominal incisions while performing a series of short successive coughs will minimize stress to a wound and still ensure productive coughing.

Wound Assessment

The nurse often assesses wounds under two different conditions: (1) at the time of injury before the initiation of treatment and (2) after therapy when the wound is relatively stable. Each condition requires the nurse to make different observations and to take different actions. The nurse uses the skills of inspection and palpation to assess the condition of a wound. Further information is available through laboratory analysis of wound cultures.

Emergency Setting

The nurse may see wounds in any setting: the clinic, the emergency room, a rural Girl Scout camp, or the nurse's own backyard. The type of wound determines the criteria for inspection. For example, the nurse need not inspect for signs of internal bleeding after an abrasion but should do so in the event of a puncture wound.

When a client's condition is judged to be stable because of the presence of spontaneous breathing, a clear airway, and a strong carotid pulse (see Chapter 41), the nurse inspects the wound for bleeding. An *abrasion* is usually superficial with little bleeding. The wound may appear "weepy" because of the leakage of plasma from damaged capillaries. A *laceration* may bleed more profusely depending on the wound's depth and location. For example, minor scalp lacerations tend to bleed profusely because of the rich blood supply to the scalp. Lacerations greater than 5 cm (2 inches) long or 2.5 cm (1 inch) deep can cause serious bleeding. *Puncture* wounds bleed in relation to the depth and size of the wound; obviously a nail puncture does not cause as much bleeding as a knife wound. The primary dangers of puncture wounds are internal bleeding and infection.

The nurse next inspects the wound for the presence of foreign bodies or contaminant material. Most traumatic wounds are dirty. Soil, broken glass, shreds of cloth, and foreign substances clinging to penetrating objects can become embedded in the wound.

The size of the wound is the next criterion for inspection. A deep laceration will require suturing by a physician. A large open wound may expose bone or tissue that should be protected.

When the client's injury is the result of trauma from a dirty penetrating object, the nurse inquires when the client last received a tetanus toxoid injection. The tetanus bacteria reside in soil and infect wounds containing dead tissue. A tetanus antitoxin injection is necessary if the client has not had one within 5 years.

Stable Setting

When the client's condition is stabilized, for example, after surgery or treatment, the nurse assesses the wound to determine its progress toward healing. If the wound is covered by a dressing and the physician has not ordered the dressing changed, the nurse should avoid direct inspection of the wound unless serious complications are suspected. In such a situation the nurse should inspect only the dressing and any external drains. If the physician prefers to be the one to change the dressing, the physician will assess the wound at least daily. When the nurse removes dressings, special care is necessary to avoid accidentally removing or displacing underlying drains. Since removal of dressings can be painful for a client, it may be helpful to administer an analgesic at least 30 minutes before exposing a wound.

The nurse first inspects the *appearance of a wound*. The nurse notes the approximation of wound edges. A surgical incision should have clean, well-approximated edges. Crusts often form along the wound edges as a result of exudate. A puncture wound is usually a small circular wound with the edges coming together toward the center. If a wound is open, the wound edges will be separated and the nurse inspects the condition of underlying tissue such as adipose and connective tissue. This is also the time to look for complications such as dehiscence and evisceration. The outer edges of a wound normally appear inflamed for the first 2 to 3 days, but this slowly disappears. Within 7 to 10 days a normally healing wound fills with epithelial cells and the edges close. If infection develops, the wound edges become brightly inflamed and swollen.

Skin discoloration usually results from bruising of interstitial tissues or possibly hematoma formation. Blood collecting beneath the skin first takes on a bluish or purple appearance. Gradually, as the clotted blood is broken down, shades of brown and yellow appear.

The nurse also assesses the *character of wound drainage* by noting the amount, color, odor, and consistency. The amount of drainage depends on the location and extent of the wound. For example, drainage is minimal after a simple appendectomy. In contrast, wound drainage is moderate for 1 to 2 days after resection of a portion of the small bowel. If the nurse needs an accurate measurement of the amount of drainage within a dressing, the dressing can be weighed and the result compared with the weight of the same dressing when clean and dry.

The color and consistency of wound drainage vary depending on the constituents. Serous drainage consists of clear, watery plasma. Presence of old blood may cause serous drainage to be slightly brown. Sanguineous or bloody drainage indicates fresh bleeding, which is common in a new wound. Serosanguineous drainage, a combination of plasma and red cells, appears paler and more watery than sanguineous drainage. Purulent drainage is thick, indicating the presence of dead or living organisms and white blood cells. The type of infectious organism influences whether the color of purulent drainage is yellow, green, or brown.

If the drainage has a pungent or strong odor, an infection is likely. Some experienced nurses can detect the type of infectious organism by the drainage odor.

The nurse should objectively record the integrity of a wound and the character of drainage. Phrases such as "appears to be healing well" or "minimal drainage" do not give a clear picture of the wound's condition. The nurse should describe the wound's appearance according to characteristics observed. The nurse describes drainage by the diameter of drainage collected on dressings or the number of dressings containing drainage. Examples of accurate recording include:

Abdominal incision is approximately 5 cm long across RLQ [right lower quadrant]; edges well approximated without inflammation or exudate. 1.2 cm diameter circle of serous drainage on one 4 × 4 gauze.

Wound extends 5-7 cm across inner aspect of right calf, edges separated 1.2 cm. Tissues pink without purulent drainage. Three 4 × 4 gauze pads soaked with serosanguineous drainage.

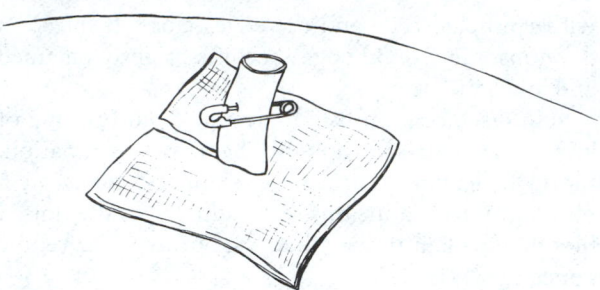

Fig. 48-2 Penrose drain.

The *presence of drains* is another important assessment criterion. There are several types of drains. The physician inserts a drain into or close to a surgical wound if a large amount of drainage is expected and if keeping wound layers closed is especially important. If fluid is allowed to accumulate under the tissues, the inner wound edges may never close.

A drain may lie under a dressing, extend through a dressing, or be connected to a drainage bag or a suction apparatus. The physician often places a pin or clip through the drain to prevent it from slipping farther into a wound (Fig. 48-2). It is usually the physician's responsibility to pull or advance the drain to permit healing deep within the drain site. As drainage decreases, the physician gradually withdraws the drain completely.

The nurse assesses the placement of the drain, the character of drainage, and the condition of any collecting apparatus. First, the nurse observes the security of the drain and its location with respect to the wound. Next the nurse notes the character of drainage. If there is a collecting device, the nurse measures the volume of drainage. Since a drainage system must be patent, the nurse pays particular attention to the flow of drainage through the tubing. A sudden decrease in the amount of drainage may indicate a blocked drain, and the physician should be notified. When a drain is connected to suction, the nurse assesses the system to be sure the correct pressure is being exerted. Evacuator units such as a Hemovac or VacuDrain (Fig. 48-3) exert a constant low pressure as long as the suction bladder or bag is fully compressed. When drains are connected to portable or wall suction units, the physician may order a specific pressure level.

In the case of a surgical wound the nurse inspects the *staples, sutures,* or *wound closures.* A popular form of skin closure is the stainless steel staple. The staple provides more strength than nylon or silk sutures and tends to cause less irritation to the skin. The nurse looks for irritation around staple or suture sites and notes if the closures are intact. The nurse may choose to count sutures when the physician has

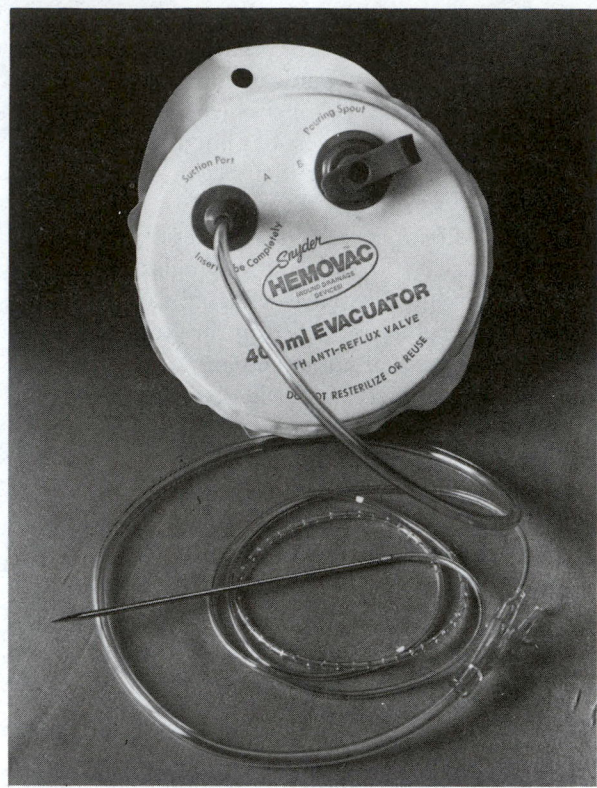

Fig. 48-3 Hemovac wound drainage evacuator.

removed a portion of them. Normally for the first 2 to 3 days postoperatively the skin around sutures or staples is swollen. Eventually the swelling subsides; continued swelling may indicate that the closures are too tight. The skin can be cut by overly tight suture material, leading to wound separation. Excessively tight sutures are a common cause of wound dehiscence. Early suture removal reduces formation of defects along the suture line and minimizes chances of unattractive scar formation. Physicians typically apply Steri-strips, which are thin adhesive strips, across the incision to bring wound edges together after suture removal.

When inspecting a wound the nurse may observe swelling or separation of wound edges. With light *palpation* to wound edges the nurse can detect localized areas of tenderness or collection of drainage. The nurse should don sterile gloves before palpating any wound. The nurse gently applies the fingertips along the wound edges. If pressure causes fluid to be expressed from the wound, the nurse notes the character of the drainage. It may be necessary to collect the drainage for purposes of culturing. The client normally is sensitive to palpation of wound edges; however, extreme tenderness may indicate development of an infection.

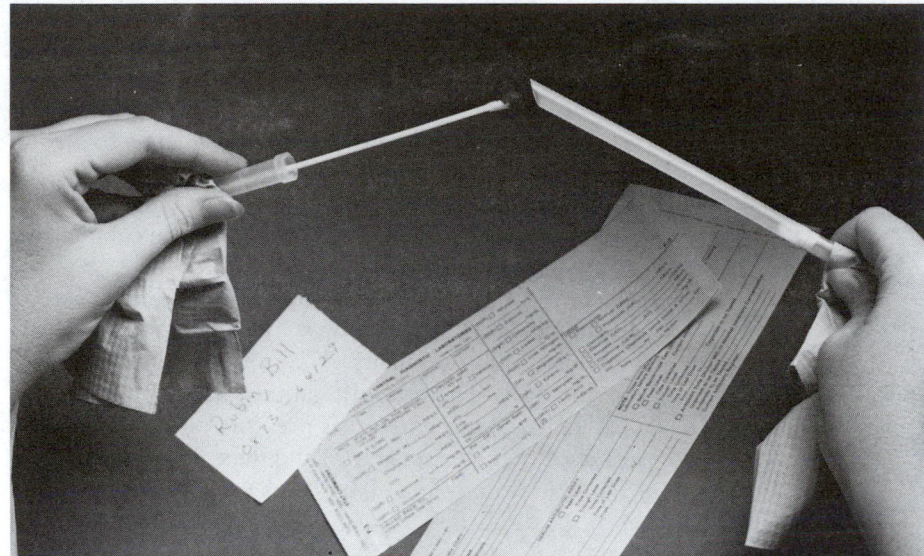

Fig. 48-4 Wound culturette tube.

Pain assessment is an important component of wound assessment, in terms of detecting complications as well as planning for future wound care. If the client experiences serious discomfort while the nurse inspects or palpates the wound, the nurse should look for underlying problems. If the wound is extensive and discomfort seems to be related to dressing removal or application, the nurse plans to administer analgesics before future dressing changes.

Wound Cultures

If the nurse's assessment detects the presence of purulent or suspicious-looking drainage, collecting a specimen for culture may be necessary (see Chapter 33). The nurse should never collect a wound culture sample from old drainage. Resident colonies of bacteria from the skin grow within exudate and may not be the true causative organisms of a wound infection. The nurse cleans a wound first to remove skin flora. Aerobic organisms grow in superficial wounds exposed to the air, and anaerobic organisms tend to grow within body cavities. The nurse uses a different method of specimen collection for each type of organism.

To collect an aerobic specimen the nurse uses a sterile swab from a culturette tube (Fig. 48-4). If wound edges are separated, the nurse slowly and gently inserts the tip of the swab into the wound to collect deeper secretions. After collecting the specimen the nurse returns the swab to the culturette tube, caps the tube, and crushes the inner ampule containing the medium for organism growth. The medium must moisten and coat the swab tip. The nurse then sends the labeled specimen to the lab immediately.

If drainage from a deep body cavity has a foul odor, there is a chance of anaerobic organism growth. The nurse uses a sterile syringe tip to aspirate drainage from the *inner* wound. After collecting the specimen the nurse applies a sterile needle to the syringe, expels any air from the syringe and needle, and places a cork over the needle to prevent entrance of air. In some institutions the nurse may inject the specimen into a special vacuum container with a culture medium.

Nursing Diagnosis

The identification of nursing diagnoses related to wound healing directs the nurse in anticipating the need for supportive or preventive care. If the nurse's assessment reveals that a wound is healing poorly, the diagnosis "impaired wound integrity" focuses on the need to initiate interventions that promote the healing process. When an assessment indicates that a wound is healing normally, the diagnosis "potential for injury" helps define the risks involved when layers of the skin are broken.

The client may be at risk for poor wound healing because of any number of the previously defined factors that impair healing. Thus, even though the client's wound may appear normal, the nurse identifies diagnoses such as "altered nutrition" or "reduced tissue perfusion," which direct nursing care toward support of wound repair.

The nature of a wound can cause problems unrelated to wound healing. Alteration in comfort, impaired mobility, and ineffective breathing pattern are problems that have implications for the client's eventual recovery. For example, a large abdominal inci-

TABLE 48-2

Examples of Nursing Diagnoses Related to Problems of Wound Healing

Problem	Causes
Impairment of skin integrity	Related to: Wound infection Dehiscence Wound drainage Evisceration
Potential for injury	Related to: Open wound Presence of drain Immunosuppression
Alteration in nutrition	Related to inadequate dietary intake
Alteration in comfort	Related to: Incisional wound Wound drainage
Impaired mobility	Related to: Painful incision Constricting bandages
Ineffective breathing pattern	Related to incisional or wound pain

sion can cause sufficient pain to interfere with the client's ability to turn in bed and cough secretions effectively.

Table 48-2 lists examples of nursing diagnoses related to problems of wound healing.

Evaluation

The criteria the nurse uses to evaluate the progress of wound healing are similar to those used in assessment. By recognizing the phases of wound healing, the nurse anticipates the changes that will occur as the wound bed fills and skin edges close. Wound healing is evaluated with each dressing change, after application of heat and cold therapies, after wound irrigations, and after the client experiences any stress to the wound site.

The changes that occur in the appearance of the wound should normally be progressive. The nurse looks for the following:

1. Wound edges gradually approximating or closing together
2. Reduction in inflammation and swelling of skin edges
3. Filling of tissue defects by epithelial cells, which

first appears as exudate and gradually assumes a scablike appearance

4. Gradual reduction in amount of drainage
5. Change in character of drainage progressing from sanguineous or serosanguineous to serous (time required for character of drainage to change influenced by type of wound)
6. Reduction in tenderness or pain along the wound site

It is important for the nurse to evaluate wound healing before applying any topical medications such as antibiotic ointments. The ointment may discolor skin edges or take on the appearance of exudate or drainage. If any exudate is present on the wound, the nurse notes its appearance and then cleans the wound in order to observe all of its characteristics.

Objectives of Wound Care

The same objectives of care apply for all types of wounds, although the priority of objectives depends on whether the client's condition is an emergency or stable one. The methods for meeting each objective depend on the type, extent, and location of the wound. Following is a discussion of the significant objectives of wound care.

Promoting Wound Hemostasis

The control of blood loss is especially important during the time of injury when bleeding may be profuse. The nurse uses basic first aid techniques to control bleeding. Later, as a wound becomes stabilized, the nurse avoids disrupting superficial wound layers. Further trauma to the skin may prompt bleeding. The use of pressure dressings during the first 24 to 48 hours after injury can also help maintain hemostasis.

Preventing Transmission of Infection to the Wound Site

The nurse uses principles of medical and surgical asepsis (see Chapter 33) in wound care. Handwashing reduces organisms residing on the nurse's skin. Techniques for cleansing a wound prevent transfer of organisms from the skin to exposed tissues. The dressing is applied in an environment where transfer of organisms through the air is minimal. The nurse changes dressings before accumulated drainage can become a medium for infection.

Preventing Further Wound Injury

Covering a wound with dressings protects skin and tissues from further accidental trauma. Immobilizing wounds through the use of binders or slings reduces strain on wound edges. Instructing clients on the proper methods for turning, coughing, and ambulating also protects wounds from muscular stress. Techniques for dressing removal prevent the accidental disruption of epithelial cell layers.

Preventing Transmission of Infection from an Infected Wound to the Client or Health Care Personnel

If a wound becomes infected the nurse uses protective aseptic techniques (isolation precautions; see Chapter 33).

Supporting the Process of Wound Healing

Nutritional support is a key measure the nurse uses to promote healing. The application of heat and cold improves circulation to a wound, minimizes inflammation and swelling, and promotes comfort for optimal relaxation of the affected area. Proper positioning of injured body parts also serves to improve circulation. The proper maintenance of drains and suction apparatus ensures that accumulated fluid will be evacuated from underlying tissue layers.

Maintaining Skin Integrity

Draining wounds expose skin surfaces to moisture and irritation. To prevent skin breakdown the nurse changes dressings as they become saturated, minimizes removal of tape from and reapplication to the skin, and keeps the skin clean and dry. The nurse often applies special skin barriers around drainage sites for added skin protection. Disposable pouches can be placed over drains and fistulas to collect drainage.

Promoting a Return to Normal Function

The nurse clarifies and reinforces the physician's instructions regarding activity restrictions. A surgical wound of the abdomen, for example, contraindicates lifting of objects for several weeks. The client also must be encouraged to maintain ambulation and safe exercise to prevent loss of muscle and joint function.

Management of Wounds

In an emergency setting the nurse employs first aid measures for wound care. Under more stable conditions the nurse is able to use a variety of interventions to ensure wound healing.

First Aid for Wounds

When a client suffers a traumatic wound, the nurse may be the only person available to provide first aid. Interventions for stabilizing cardiopulmonary function are described in chapter 41. Wound care focuses on promoting hemostasis, cleansing the wound, and protecting the wound from further injury.

HEMOSTASIS

After assessing the type and extent of the wound the nurse controls bleeding by applying direct pressure on a wound. For lacerations up to 5 cm (2 inches) long and 2.5 cm (1 inch) deep the nurse presses a sterile or clean dressing, such as a washcloth or handkerchief, over the wound. Once bleeding subsides, an adhesive bandage strip or gauze dressing taped over the laceration will allow skin edges to close and a blood clot to form. More extensive lacerations require longer application of pressure. If a dressing becomes saturated with blood, the nurse does not remove it, since bleeding may increase. Instead the nurse adds another layer of dressing and continues to apply pressure. Elevation of the affected part can slow bleeding. The client should be taken to an emergency clinic or hospital so a physician can suture the more serious lacerations.

When the client has a puncture wound, the nurse allows it to bleed. Bleeding helps to remove dirt and other contaminants, such as saliva from a dog bite. If a penetrating object such as a knife blade remains in the client's body, the nurse does not remove it, since this could cause massive, uncontrolled bleeding. The nurse may apply pressure around the object but not on it or on adjacent tissues.

CLEANSING

Cleansing of a wound removes contaminants that might serve as sources of infection. Removing embedded dirt and particles is important; however, if the wound is deep or extensive, vigorous cleaning can increase bleeding.

For abrasions, minor lacerations, and small puncture wounds the nurse first rinses the wound in running water and then cleans it with mild soap and water. An over-the-counter antiseptic can be helpful in initially reducing microorganisms in the wound. However, continued application of antibiotic ointments can foster bacterial growth. When a laceration is bleeding profusely, the nurse should only brush away surface contaminants. In this situation hemostasis becomes a priority until the client can be cared for in a clinic or hospital.

PROTECTION

Regardless of whether the wound has stopped bleeding or continues to bleed, the nurse protects the wound by applying sterile or clean dressings and immobilizing the body part. A light dressing applied over minor wounds prevents entrance of microorganisms. In the case of small abrasions it is acceptable to leave the wound open to air so a scab can form.

The more extensive the wound, the larger the bandage required. In the home setting a clean towel or diaper may be the best dressing. A bulky dressing applied with pressure minimizes movement of underlying tissues and helps immobilize the entire body part. A bandage or cloth wrapped around a penetrating object should immobilize it adequately.

Dressings

The use of dressings requires an understanding of wound healing. A variety of dressing materials are commercially available. Unless a dressing is suited to the characteristics of a wound, the dressing can hinder wound repair.

The choice of dressings and the method of dressing a wound influence the progress of wound healing. The proper dressing should not allow a draining wound to become overly dry with extensive scab formation. When this occurs, the dermis dehydrates and crusts. As a result, a barrier forms against normal epidermal cell growth, leaving a depression or defect in the new epidermal surface. Furthermore, dryness of the wound may increase the client's discomfort. Ideally a dressing leaves a wound slightly moist to promote normal epidermal cell migration. The dressing should also absorb drainage to prevent pooling of exudate that may promote bacterial growth.

For surgical wounds that heal by primary intention, it is common to remove dressings as soon as drainage stops. In contrast, when the nurse dresses an open wound healing by secondary intention, the dressing material becomes a means for mechanically removing exudate and necrotic tissue.

PURPOSES OF DRESSINGS

A dressing may serve several purposes:
1. Protecting a wound from microorganism contamination
2. Aiding hemostasis
3. Promoting healing by absorbing drainage and debriding a wound
4. Supporting or splinting the wound site
5. Hiding the wound from the client

When the body's first line of defense against infection is breached, a dressing helps to reduce exposure to microorganisms. However, when wound drainage is minimal, the healing process forms a fibrin seal. This natural protection can eliminate the need for a dressing, although some risk for infection remains. A dressing is a necessity for extensive wounds.

Pressure dressings promote hemostasis. Applied with elastic bandages, a pressure dressing exerts localized downward pressure over an actual or potential bleeding site. For example, after an arteriogram (injection of a radiopaque dye into an artery), the puncture wound site is usually covered by a pressure dressing to prevent a hematoma from forming. A pressure dressing also eliminates dead space in underlying tissues so wound healing progresses normally. The nurse must check pressure dressings to be sure they do not interfere with circulation to a body part. The nurse assesses skin color, pulses in distal extremities, the client's comfort, and any changes in sensation.

One of the primary functions of a dressing is to absorb drainage. Most surgical dressings have three layers: (1) a contact or primary dressing, (2) an absorbent dressing, and (3) an outer protective layer. The contact dressing covers the incision and part of the adjacent skin. Fibrin, blood products, and debris adhere to the contact dressing's surface. A problem occurs if the wound drainage dries, causing the dressing to stick to the suture line. Early or improper removal of the dressing can cause tearing of the healing epidermal surface. The nurse must either remove the dressing gently and moisten the attached area with sterile normal saline before removal or leave the dressing unchanged for several days. When wounds require debriding, such as infected or necrotic wounds, the contact dressing serves to debride necrotic tissue and debris. Even though the contact dressing may stick to underlying tissue, the mechanical removal of exudate helps clean the wound. Dressings applied to a draining wound require frequent changing to prevent microorganism growth. Bacteria grow readily in the dark, warm, moist environment underneath a dressing.

The absorbent dressing layer serves as a reservoir for additional secretions. The wicking action of gauze dressings pulls excess drainage into the dressing and away from the wound.

The final outer layer of a dressing helps to prevent bacteria and other external contaminants from reaching the wound surface. Usually the outer dressing is made of a thicker dressing material.

A dressing can also support or immobilize a body part. Firmly taped or wrapped dressings minimize movement of the underlying incision and traumatized tissues. For example, the more layers of dressings applied around an extremity, the more difficult it is for a client to flex or extend the body part. Thus less stress occurs along the wound site.

Clients can become highly anxious over the appearance of a wound. The dressing hides what can often be an unpleasant sight. It is not uncommon for clients to look away or appear frightened as the nurse performs a dressing change. It can be helpful for the client to know that the gradual reduction in size and shape of dressings usually indicates progress toward healing.

TYPES OF DRESSINGS

Dressings can be categorized by the types of materials used or whether the dressings are applied wet or dry. Dressings are available in numerous sizes and materials. A dressing should be easy to apply, comfortable for the client, and made of materials that promote wound healing.

Gauze dressings are the most common type. The gauze dressing does not interact with wound tissues and thus causes little wound irritation. Even when physiological solutions such as normal saline or lactated Ringer's are applied to gauze, the dressing remains safe. If substances such as iodine are poured onto gauze, however, the dressing can cause irritation to healthy tissue. Gauze is available in squares of 10 × 10 cm (4 × 4 inches) or 5 × 5 cm (2 × 2 inches), rectangles of 10 × 20 cm (4 × 8 inches), and rolls of various lengths. Certain gauze dressings are more finely woven than others to provide different textures suited to the extent and nature of wound drainage.

The nurse applies gauze either wet or dry. Dry dressings are best for wounds with minimal drainage. Wet dressings are the treatment of choice for wounds requiring debridement. The nurse moistens the contact dressing layer that touches the wound surface. The moistened gauze increases the absorptive ability of the dressing to collect all exudate and wound debris. The second or absorbent dressing layer is a dry dressing. This *wet-to-dry* dressing is very effective in cleansing infected and necrotic wounds.

Gauze dressings that contain a shiny, nonadherent surface on one side are called Telfa gauze. When used as a contact layer, the Telfa gauze does not stick to incisions or wound openings. Drainage passes through the nonadherent surface to the softened gauze above.

Dressings are also available as thin, self-adhesive elastic films (for example, Op-site). The dressing is a synthetic permeable membrane that acts as a temporary second skin. This type of dressing has several advantages: (1) it adheres to undamaged skin to contain exudate and minimize wound contamination, (2) it serves as a barrier to external fluids and bacteria but still allows the wound surface to "breathe," (3) it promotes a moist environment that speeds epithelial cell growth, and (4) it can be removed without damaging underlying tissues. The disadvantage of such a dressing is that it cannot debride an infected or necrotic wound. Op-site is ideal for small, superficial wounds or those that do not require debridement. It is also useful as a dressing over an intravenous catheter site. The transparent film allows the nurse to assess the wound without removing the dressing.

CHANGING DRESSINGS

When a nurse changes a dressing, it is important to know what type of dressing it is, whether there are underlying drains or tubing, and the type of supplies needed for wound care. Performing a dressing change without proper preparation can result in a break in aseptic technique, accidental dislodging of drains, and improper use of dressing materials. The nurse's judgment is important during wound care, particularly if the character of a wound changes. The nurse is able to adjust the type and amount of dressings used if the character or amount of drainage changes or if a wound becomes deeper. Notifying the physician of any changes is essential.

The physician usually assesses the client's wound at least daily and adjusts orders accordingly. The physician's order for dressing changes should indicate the type of dressing, for example, dry or wet-to-dry, the frequency of dressing changes, and whether special solutions or ointments should be applied to the wound. The medical or operating room record usually reveals whether drains are present and from what body cavity they drain. After the initial dressing change the nurse communicates in the nursing Kardex the type of dressing materials and solutions to use, as well as the type and location of drains.

At times the physician may order the nurse to "reinforce dressing p.r.n." This means the nurse is not to remove the dressing but should only add dressings to the existing ones. The order is most common immediately after surgery when the physician does not want accidental disruption of the suture line or loss of hemostasis.

The most important principles to follow during dressing change procedures are those of aseptic technique. Thorough handwashing is necessary before handling sterile supplies. Some institutions recommend use of a face mask for surgical dressing changes. The nurse dons the mask before handwashing and assembling supplies. Sterile gloves allow the nurse to handle supplies and sterile solutions without risk of contamination.

The preparation of the client before a dressing change is an essential responsibility of the nurse. If the client is likely to experience pain, the nurse should time administration of the appropriate analgesic to allow the drug's peak effect to occur during the dressing change. The nurse should also ensure that the client understands the steps of the procedure, for ex-

Changing a Dry Dressing

EQUIPMENT:

1. A sterile dressing set or individual supplies of the following items:
   a. Sterile gloves
   b. Dressing set (scissors and forceps),
   c. Sterile drape (optional)
   d. Gauze dressings and pads
   e. Basin for antiseptic or cleaning solution
   f. Antiseptic ointment (optional)
2. Cleaning solution prescribed by physician

3. Sterile saline or water
4. Clean disposable gloves
5. Tape, ties, or bandage as needed
6. Waterproof bag for disposal
7. Extra gauze dressings and surgipads or ABD pads.
8. Bath blanket
9. Acetone (optional)

STEPS	RATIONALE
1. Explain the procedure to the client by describing steps of wound care.	This relieves the client's anxiety and promotes understanding of the healing process.
2. Assemble all necessary supplies at bedside table (do not yet open supplies).	Preprocedural organization of supplies prevents chances of a break in sterile technique by accidental omission of a needed supply.
3. Take a disposable bag and make a cuff at the top. Place the bag within reach of your work area.	The cuff prevents accidental contamination of the top of the outer bag surface. The nurse should not reach across a sterile field to dispose of a soiled dressing.
4. Close room or cubicle curtains or arrange a partition around the bed. Close any open windows.	This provides client privacy and reduces air currents that may transmit microorganisms.
5. Position the client in a comfortable position and drape the client with a bath blanket to expose only the wound site. Instruct the client not to touch the wound area or sterile supplies.	Sudden movement on the client's part during dressing change can cause contamination of wound or supplies. Draping provides access to the wound and minimizes unnecessary exposure.
6. Wash hands thoroughly (see Chapter 33).	Washing hands removes microorganisms resident on skin surface and reduces transmission of pathogens to exposed tissues.
7. Don clean disposable gloves and remove tape, ties, or bandage.	Gloves prevent transmission of infectious organisms from soiled dressings to the nurse's hands.
8. Remove tape by loosening the end and pulling gently, parallel to the skin and toward the dressing. (If adhesive remains on the skin, it may be removed with acetone.)	Removing tape in this way reduces tension against suture line or wound edges.
9. With the gloved hand or forceps lift the dressings off, keeping the soiled undersurface away from the client's sight. NOTE: If drains are present, remove only a layer at a time.	The appearance of drainage may upset the client emotionally. Cautious removal of dressings prevents accidental withdrawal of the drain.
10. If dressing sticks to the wound, loosen it by applying sterile saline or water.	This prevents disruption of the epidermal surface.

STEPS	*RATIONALE*
11. Observe the character and amount of drainage on dressings.	This provides an estimate of the amount of drainage lost and assessment of the wound's condition.
12. Dispose of soiled dressings in a trash bag, avoiding contamination of the bag's outer surface. Remove disposable gloves by pulling them inside out and dispose of them properly.	These procedures reduce transmission of microorganisms to other persons.
13. Open the sterile dressing tray or individually wrapped sterile supplies (see Chapter 33). Place it on the bedside table or at the client's side on the bed. Dressings, scissors, and forceps remain in the sterile tray or can be placed on open sterile drape used as a sterile field. Open the bottle or packet of antiseptic solution and pour it into a sterile basin or over sterile gauze.	Sterile dressings and supplies remain sterile while on or within a sterile surface. Preparation of all supplies prevents a break in technique during the actual dressing change. 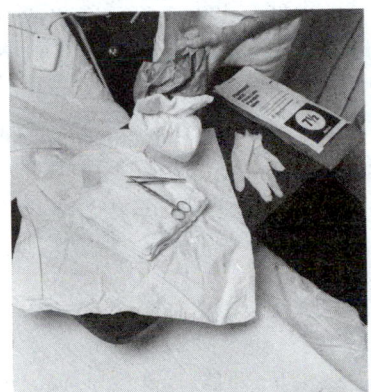
14. If the sterile drape or gauze packages become wet from antiseptic solution, repeat preparation of the supplies.	Fluids move through material by capillary action. Microorganisms travel from an unsterile environment on table top or bed linen through the dressing package to the dressing itself.
15. Don sterile gloves (see Chapter 33).	Gloves allow the nurse to handle sterile dressings, instruments, and solutions without contaminating them with microorganisms. 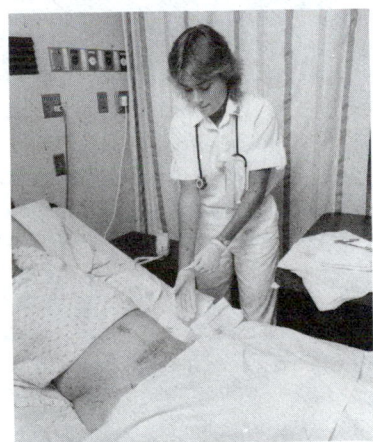
16. Inspect the wound. Note the condition of the wound, drain placement, suture or skin closure integrity, and character of drainage. (Palpate wound, if necessary, with portion of nondominant hand that will not touch sterile supplies.)	Observations determine state of wound healing. (Contact with skin surface or drainage contaminates glove.) 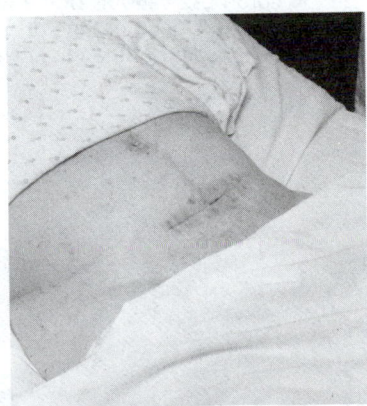

Continued.

Changing a Dry Dressing

STEPS	RATIONALE
17. Cleanse the wound with prescribed antiseptic solution or normal saline. Grasp the gauze moistened in solution with forceps. Use a separate gauze swab for each cleansing stroke. Clean from the least contaminated area to the most contamined. Move in progressive strokes away from the incision line or wound edges.	Use of forceps prevents contamination of gloved fingers. This direction of cleansing prevents introduction of organisms into the wound.
18. Use dry gauze to dry the wound or incision line. Swab in the same manner as described in step 17.	Drying reduces moisture at the wound site that eventually could harbor microorganisms.
19. Apply antiseptic ointment (if ordered), using the same technique as for cleansing. Do not apply over the drainage site.	Application of ointment directly to the dressing or the drainage site can occlude drainage.
20. Apply dry sterile dressings to the incision or wound site.	
a. Apply dressings one at a time.	Applying dressings one at a time prevents application of large bulky dressings that may impair the client's movement and ensures proper coverage of the entire wound.
b. Apply loose woven gauze (4 × 4) or Telfa as a contact layer.	Layering of gauze promotes proper absorption of drainage.
c. If a drain is present, take scissors and cut a gauze 4 × 4 to fit around the drain (see Fig. 48-2).	Dressing around the drain secures its placement and absorbs drainage at the site.
d. Apply a second layer of gauze as an absorbent layer.	
e. Apply a thicker woven surgipad or ABD pad (blue line down middle of pad marks outside surface).	A thick pad protects the wound from the entrance of microorganisms.
21. Apply tape over the dressing or secure with Montgomery ties, bandage, or binder.	This provides support to wound and ensures complete coverage of the wound to minimize exposure to microorganisms.
22. Remove the gloves and dispose of them properly in container.	Proper disposal of gloves reduces transmission of microorganisms
23. Dispose of all supplies and help the client return to a comfortable position.	A clean environment enhances client comfort.
24. Wash hands.	Clean hands reduce microorganism transmission.
25. Record observatioins of the wound, dressing, and drainage. Document the dressing change, includings statement of the client's response.	Accurate, timely documentation notifies personnel of any changes in wound condition and the status of the client.

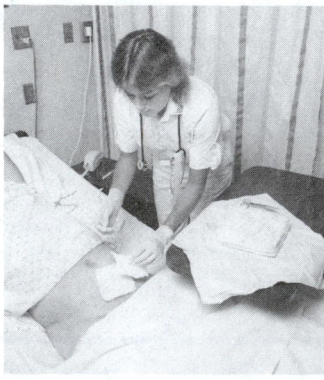 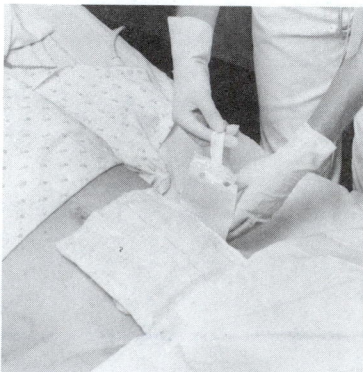 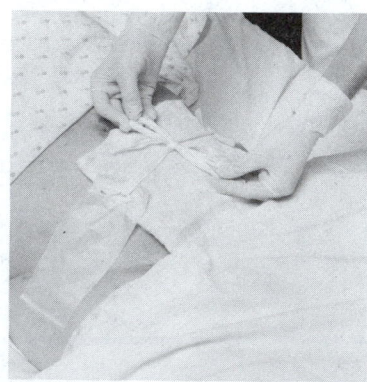

PROCEDURE 48-2

Changing Wet-to-Dry Dressings

EQUIPMENT:
Same as Procedure 48-1 in addition to:
1. Thin fine-mesh gauze
2. Sterile solution prescribed to moisten dressing
3. Waterproof pad

STEPS	RATIONALE
1. Explain the procedure to the client as in Procedure 48-1.	
2. Assemble all equipment and prepare the client as in steps 2 through 6 of Procedure 48-1.	
3. Place a waterproof pad under the client.	A waterproof pad prevents soiling of bed linen.
4. Wash hands thoroughly.	Washing removes microorganisms from the skin's surface.
5. Remove the dressing according to steps 7 through 9 of Procedure 48-1.	
6. If the dressing adheres to underlying tissues, do not moisten it. Gently free the dressing from dried exudate. Warn the client about pulling and possible discomfort.	A wet-to-dry dressing is designed to clean contaminated or infected wounds by debridement of necrotic tissue and exudate.
7. Follow steps 11 and 12 of Procedure 48-1.	
8. Prepare sterile dressing supplies. Pour the prescribed solution into a sterile basin and add fine-mesh gauze.	The contact layer of gauze must be totally moistened to increase the dressing's absorptive abilities.
9. Follow steps 15 through 17 of Procedure 48-1.	
10. Apply moist fine-mesh gauze directly on the wound surface. If the wound is deep, gently pack it by first picking up the end of the gauze with forceps. Gradually feed gauze into the wound so all surfaces of the wound are in contact with moist gauze.	Moist gauze absorbs drainage and adheres to debris. The wound should be backed so gauze is evenly distributed within the wound bed.
11. Apply dry sterile gauze (4 × 4) over the wet gauze.	The dry layer serves as an absorbent layer to pull moisture from the wound surface.
12. Cover with gauze, surgipad, or ABD pad.	The gauze or pad protects the wound from entrance of microorganisms.
13. Secure the dressing and dispose of supplies (see Procedure 48-1).	
14. Assist the client to a comfortable position.	The client's comfort enhances a sense of well-being.
15. Wash hands.	Washing reduces microorganism transmission.
16. Record observations of the wound, dressing, and drainage.	Accurate and timely documentation notifies personnel of any changes in wound condition and status of the client.

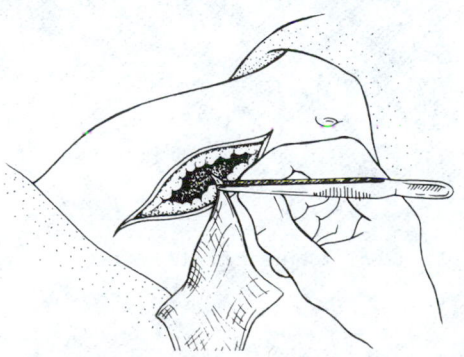
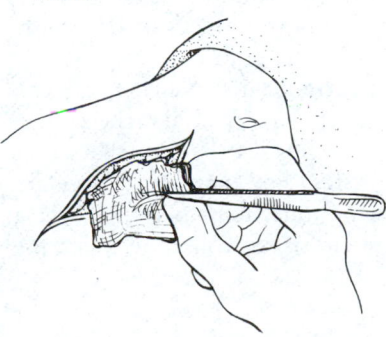

ample, removing tape and dressings, inspecting the wound, using solutions to clean the wound, and reapplying the dressing. The client who knows the purpose of the dressing and the techniques for changing dressings will experience less anxiety. A family member may be asked to observe the procedure if wound care will be needed in the home setting. While changing the dressing the nurse describes normal signs of the healing process, for example, "the wound is clean" or "the incision is closing well." If the client is able to look at the wound, the nurse offers to answer any questions about what the client observes.

Often the physician orders clients to learn how to change dressings so they will be prepared for home care. In this situation the nurse must demonstrate dressing change to the client and family and then provide an opportunity for the client or family member to practice. Usually in this situation wound healing has progressed to the point that risks of complications such as dehiscence or evisceration are minimal. The client should be able to change a dressing independently or with assistance from a family member before discharge.

Procedures 48-1 and 48-2 outline the steps for changing dry and wet-to-dry dressings.

SECURING DRESSINGS

The nurse may use tape, ties, or bandages and cloth binders to secure a dressing over a wound site. It is important for the nurse to assess the wound size, location, presence of drainage, frequency of dressing changes, and client's level of activity. For example, a dressing over a small laceration across the lower arm will require a different type of anchoring than a dressing covering a long incision over the client's hip.

The nurse most often uses strips of tape to secure dressings. Before applying tape the nurse determines if the client has an allergy to tape. Adhesive tape is most likely to cause skin irritation. Skin sensitive to adhesive can become severely inflamed and excoriated and may even slough off after the tape is removed.

A variety of kinds of tapes are available. Nonallergenic paper and plastic tapes minimize skin reactions. The common adhesive tape has the advantage of adhering well to the skin's surface. Elastic adhesive tape is useful in applying pressure bandages because the tape compresses closely around a dressing. Elasticized tape also permits more movement of a body part.

Tape is available in various widths such as 1.2 cm, 2.5 cm, 5 cm, and 7.5 cm (½ inch, 1 inch, 2 inch, and 3 inch). The nurse chooses the size that sufficiently secures the dressing. For example, a large abdominal wound dressing must remain secure over a large area despite frequent stress from movement, the

client's respiratory effort, and possibly abdominal distention. Strips of 7.5 cm (3-inch) adhesive will more likely stabilize such a large dressing so it will not continually slip off. Whenever a nurse applies tape, it is important that the tape adhere to several inches of skin on both sides of the dressing, in addition to being placed across the middle of the dressing. When securing the dressing the nurse presses the tape gently, exerting pressure away from the wound. This way tension occurs in both directions away from the wound, minimizing skin distortion and irritation. Tape is never applied over irritated or broken skin.

To remove tape safely the nurse first loosens the tape ends and then gently pulls the outer end parallel with the skin surface toward the wound. The nurse applies gentle traction to the skin in a direction away from the wound as the tape is loosened and removed. The traction minimizes pulling of the skin. If tape covers areas of hair growth, the client will experience less discomfort if the nurse pulls the tape in the direction of hair growth.

To prevent the need for repeated removal of tape from sensitive skin, Montgomery ties are used for securing dressings (Fig. 48-5). The ties come in pairs,

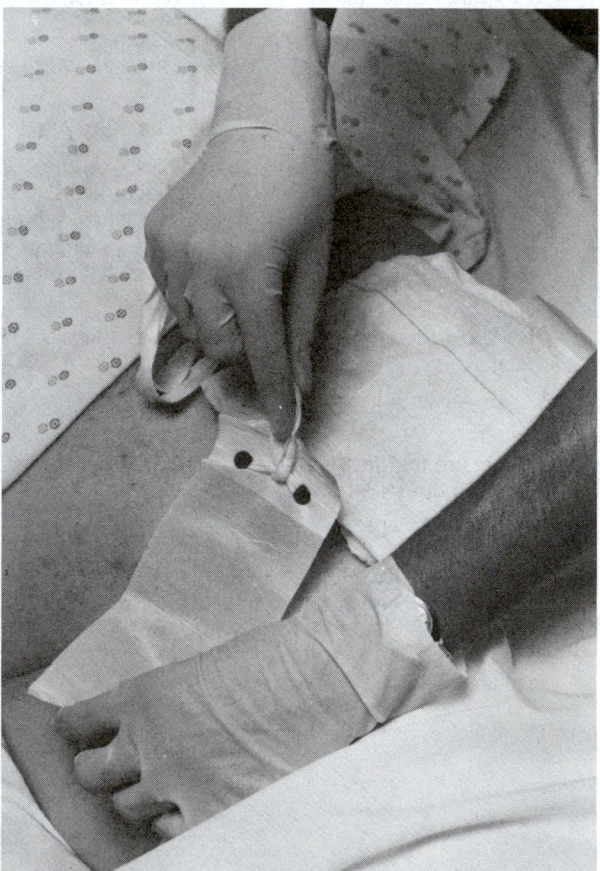

Fig. 48-5 Montgomery tie.

one on each side of a dressing. Each tie consists of a long strip; half contains an adhesive backing to apply to the skin and the other half folds back and contains a cloth tie. The nurse removes a dressing by simply untying the Montgomery ties. When the dressing is reapplied, the ties can be reused. If a dressing is large and bulky, the nurse may use two or more sets of Montgomery ties.

To provide even support to a wound and immobilize a body part the nurse may apply elastic gauze or cloth bandages and binders over a dressing. Bandages are available in rolls of various widths (1.5 to 7.5 cm [½ to 3 inches]) and lengths. The nurse wraps the bandage over the dressing as an added layer of support and protection. Binders support dressings applied over a large area. Binders come in shapes that conform to special body parts. For example, a breast binder looks like a small vest or large bra.

Cleansing Wounds and Drain Sites

If drainage is not absorbed appropriately by a dressing or if an open drain, for example, a Penrose drain (see Fig. 48-2), deposits drainage onto the skin, it may be necessary to cleanse the wound or drain site. Reducing pathogens by removing tissue debris promotes healing. Not all wounds require cleansing; a moderate amount of wound exudate is desirable for optimal growth of epithelial cells. Physicians differ as to their preference for wound cleansing and the solutions to use.

The most important techniques to follow in wound cleansing are good handwashing and use of aseptic techniques. The nurse may apply antiseptics locally to the skin to remove pathogens or may use the technique of irrigation to remove debris.

The most effective antiseptic solutions for wound cleansing are tincture of chlorhexidine (Hibiclens) and the iodophors (such as Betadine). These antiseptics have persistent activity against bacteria if they are not wiped from the skin. Alcohol 70% acts rapidly on bacteria but has no persistent effect since it evaporates. Hydrogen peroxide is useful when cleaning open wounds. The oxidizing property of peroxide exerts an antiseptic action against organic material and debris. Peroxide is less effective on intact skin.

PREOPERATIVE SKIN PREPARATION

The client undergoing surgery has an extensive skin preparation (see Chapter 47) before the procedure. The Centers for Disease Control recommends that preoperative preparation include bathing of the operative site with antiseptics; hair removal, if necessary, should be done with clippers just before the operation (Simmons, 1983). In the operating room

the nurse may be the one to prepare the operative site. First, using sterile technique, the nurse scrubs the skin thoroughly with a detergent solution to remove resident bacteria, soil, and debris. Second, the nurse applies an antiseptic solution over the area to be incised to kill more adherent and deeper-residing bacteria. Often the surgeon places a special transparent sterile drape, which resembles the self-adhesive Opsite, directly over the skin as a final protective barrier before making an incision.

BASIC WOUND CLEANSING

When cleansing surgical or traumatic wounds, the nurse applies antiseptic solutions with sterile gauze or by irrigation. Three principles are important when cleaning an incision or the area surrounding a drain:
1. Cleanse in a direction from the least contaminated area to the most contaminated.
2. Use friction when applying antiseptics locally to the skin.
3. When irrigating, allow the solution to flow from the least contaminated to the most contaminated area.

The wound is considered to be less contaminated than the surrounding skin. The nurse applies the gauze containing antiseptic on the incision or wound site and then cleans away from the wound (Fig. 48-

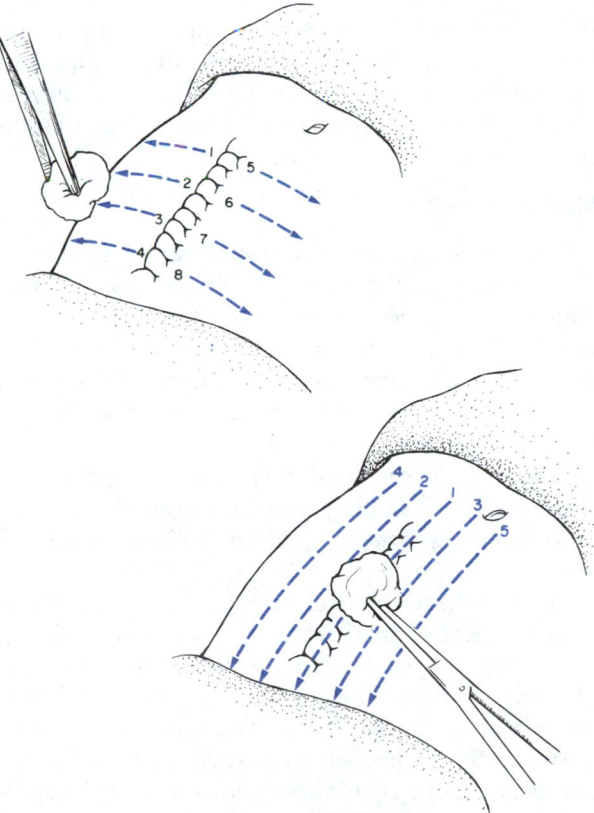

Fig. 48-6 Methods for cleansing wound site.

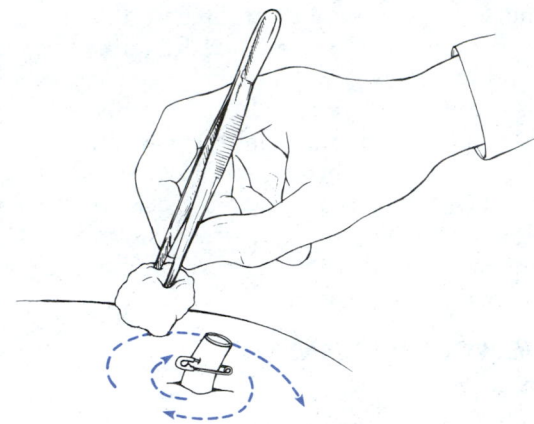

Fig. 48-7 Cleansing of a drain site.

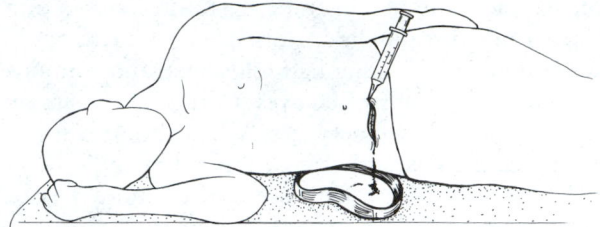

Fig. 48-8 Position of the client for abdominal wound irrigation.

6). The nurse never uses the same piece of gauze to cleanse across an incision or wound twice. A drain site is considered highly contaminated, since the moist drainage harbors microorganisms. If a wound has a dry incisional area and a moist drain site, cleansing moves from the incisional area toward the drain. The nurse uses two separate swabs; one to clean from the top of the incision toward the drain and one to clean from the bottom of the incision toward the drain. To cleanse the area of an isolated drain site (Fig. 48-7) the nurse swabs around the drain, moving in circular rotations outward from a point closest to the drain. In this situation the skin near the site is more contaminated than the site itself. To cleanse circular wounds the nurse uses the same technique as cleansing around a drain.

IRRIGATIONS

Irrigations are a special means of cleansing wounds. The nurse uses an irrigating syringe to flush the area with a constant flow of solution. The gentle washing action of the irrigation cleans a wound of exudate and debris. Irrigations are particularly useful for open deep wounds, when access to all wound surfaces is limited. When a wound involves an inaccessible body part such as the ear canal, irrigations are very useful. Cleansing sensitive body parts, for example, the conjunctival lining of the eye, is more easily accomplished by irrigations.

In addition to wound cleansing, irrigations serve to (1) apply heat to an affected area to promote healing and (2) apply locally acting medications in the form of sterile solutions. The nurse administers the solution prescribed by the physician. The solution is usually sterile water, saline, or an antiseptic solution. Administration of irrigating solutions at body temperature enhances the client's comfort and provides the added benefit of local heat application.

WOUND IRRIGATIONS. Irrigation of an open wound requires sterile technique. The nurse uses a large Asepto or cone-tipped syringe to deliver the solution, since large volumes of solution are often necessary. It is important never to occlude a wound opening with a syringe, since this would result in the introduction of irrigating fluid into a closed space. The pressure of the fluid could cause tissue damage and discomfort to the client. A wound should always be irrigated with the syringe tip over but not in the drainage site. Fluid should flow directly into the wound and not over a contaminated area before entering the wound (Fig. 48-8). Procedure 48-3 lists steps for wound irrigation.

EAR IRRIGATIONS. A client usually requires ear irrigations for cleansing purposes. The external auditory canal may contain excess cerumen or exudate from a lesion or inflamed area. When a lesion or infection is present, the nurse should remember that the skin lining the auditory canal can be very sensitive. The nurse should avoid pulling the auricle excessively or introducing the tip of the irrigating syringe into the canal. The auditory canal should never be occluded with the syringe tip. Introduction of irrigating fluid under pressure could cause rupture of the tympanic membrane. An irrigating solution must be at room temperature. Introduction of hot or cold fluids into the auditory canal causes discomfort, severe dizziness, and occasionally nausea resulting from irritation to the semicircular canals. A small syringe is usually adequate for irrigation, since a large volume of fluid is seldom necessary. Procedure 48-4 describes the technique for ear irrigations.

EYE IRRIGATIONS. Irrigations of the eye are usually not for actual wound care but rather to relieve local inflammation of the conjunctiva, apply antiseptic solution, or flush out exudate or caustic or irritating solutions. Inflammation of the conjunctiva typically causes exudate to collect in the inner canthus, which can be effectively cleaned by irrigation. Usually warm normal saline is used for cleansing purposes. A small

PROCEDURE 48-3

Wound Irrigation

EQUIPMENT:

1. Sterile basin
2. 200 to 500 ml of irrigating solution as ordered (warmed to body temperature 32° to 37° C [90° to 98.6° F])
3. Sterile irrigating syringe (sterile red rubber catheter as an attachment for deep wounds with small openings)
4. Clean basin to receive solution
5. Sterile dressing tray and supplies for dressing change (see Procedures 48-1 and 48-2)
6. Waterproof pad
7. Lubricating jelly and tongue blade (optional)

STEPS	RATIONALE
1. Explain the procedure to the client. Describe the sensations to be felt during the irrigation.	The client's anxiety will be reduced through an awareness of what the procedure involves and the sensations to expect.
2. Assemble supplies at the bedside.	Organization of equipment prevents a break in procedure.
3. Position the client so irrigating solution will flow from the upper end of the wound into a basin held below the wound's lower end.	Fluid flows by gravity. Fluid flows from least to most contaminated area.
4. Place waterproof pad under the client.	A pad prevents soiling of bed linen.
5. Wash hands.	This reduces microorganism transmission.
6. Remove the wound dressing following the steps in Procedure 48-1 and inspect the wound.	This allows assessment of wound healing.
7. Prepare sterile supplies. Open the sterile basin and pour in solution (volume varies depending size of wound and extent of drainage). Open the sterile syringe. Prepare the dressing tray. Don sterile gloves.	Use of sterile equipment prevents introduction of microorganisms into the wound.
8. Place the clean basin against the client's skin below the incision or wound site.	The basin collects contaminated irrigating solution.
9. Draw up the volume of solution into the syringe. While holding the syringe tip just above the top of the wound, irrigate the wound slowly but continuously with enough force to flush away drainage and debris. Avoid sudden spurts or splashing of fluid. Irrigate pockets in the wound.	Irrigation mechanically removes drainage and debris. Debris collects easily in pockets or depressions in the wound bed.
10. Continue irrigating until the solution draining into the basin is clear.	This ensures that all debris has been removed.
11. With sterile dry gauze dry off the wound edges (use the technique for cleansing a wound in Procedures 48-1 and 48-2).	This removes excess moisture that can serve as a medium for microorganism growth or as an irritant to the skin.
12. Apply a sterile dressing.	A sterile dressing prevents infection and promotes wound healing.
13. Assist the client to a comfortable position.	This promotes client comfort.
14. Dispose of equipment and wash hands.	Washing controls transfer of microorganisms.
15. Record the irrigation: volume and type of solution, character of drainage, appearance of wound, and client's response.	Timely recording provides accurate documentation of therapy and progress to wound healing.

PROCEDURE 48-4

Ear Irrigation

EQUIPMENT:

1. Irrigating solution prescribed (volume depends on purpose; 200-500 ml at 37° C [98.6° F])
2. Sterile basin for solution
3. Asepto or small-bulb syringe
4. Curved emesis basin
5. Moisture-proof towel or pad
6. Cotton-tip applicators
7. Bath thermometer
8. Cotton balls

STEPS	RATIONALE
1. Explain the steps of the procedure and warn the client about the sensations that might be experienced.	Understanding of what will occur relieves the client's anxiety.
2. Assist the client to a lying or sitting position with head tilted toward the affected ear. Position the emesis basin under the affected ear. (The client may help hold the basin.)	Irrigating solution will flow from the auditory canal into the basin.
3. Place a towel over the client's shoulder just under the ear and emesis basin.	A towel prevents soiling of the client's gown and bed linen.
4. Inspect the ear canal for any accumulation of cerumen or debris. Remove with cotton applicator and solution.	Removal of drainage prevents reentrance into the canal during irrigation.
5. Check the irrigating solution for proper temperature. Fill the bulb syringe with the appropriate volume.	Irrigating solution at body temperature minimizes the onset of dizziness and discomfort.
6. Straighten the auditory canal for introduction of solution. In infants, pull the auricle or pinna down and back. In adults, pull the auricle or pinna up and back.	Straightening of the canal facilitates the entrance and flow of irrigating solution.
7. With the tip of the syringe just above the canal opening, irrigate gently by creating a steady flow of solution against the roof of the auditory canal.	Occlusion of the canal with the syringe causes pressure against the tympanic membrane during irrigation. The flow of solution drains safely out of the canal while loosening debris.
8. Continue irrigation until all debris has been removed or all solution has been used.	The purpose of irrigation may be to cleanse the canal, to instill antiseptics, or to provide local heat.
9. Assess the client for the onset of dizziness or nausea. Onset of symptoms may require temporary cessation of the procedure.	Irritation of semicircular canals may cause dizziness and nausea.
10. Dry off the external ear and apply a cotton ball to the auditory meatus.	Drying promotes the client's comfort. The cotton ball collects excess drainage.
11. Position the client on the side of the affected ear for 10 minutes.	Remaining solution in the auditory canal will drain out.
12. Remove equipment and wash hands.	This controls transfer of microorganisms.
13. Return to the client to assess the character and amount of drainage and determine the client's level of comfort.	The nurse can identify the client's tolerance of procedure.
14. Record the client's response to irrigation and note the type, temperature, and volume of solution used and the character of the drainage.	Timely recording provides accurate documentation of the client's response to the procedure.
15. Return to the client after 10 minutes to remove the cotton ball and reassess drainage. The client may return to a normal level of activity.	Increase in drainage or onset of pain may indicate injury to the tympanic membrane.

PROCEDURE 48-5

Eye Irrigation

EQUIPMENT:

1. Prescribed irrigating solution; volume varies: 30-180 ml at 37° C (98.6° F) (For chemical flushing: tap water in volume to provide continuous irrigation over 15 minutes)
2. Sterile basin for solution
3. Curved emesis basin
4. Waterproof pad or towel
5. Cotton balls
6. Soft bulb syringe or eye dropper
7. Disposable gloves (optional)

STEPS	RATIONALE
1. Explain the procedure fully to the client. Explain that the client will be allowed to close the eye periodically and that no object will touch the eye.	An understanding of the procedure relieves the client's anxiety and improves the client's ability to cooperate with the procedure.
2. Assist the client to a lying position on the side of the affected eye. Turn the client's head toward the affected eye.	Irrigating solution will flow from the inner to the outer canthus of the eye into the collecting basin.
3. Wash hands.	This reduces the number of microorganisms on the skin's surface.
4. Don disposable gloves (if client's eye is infected).	Gloves prevent exposure of the nurse's hands to pathogens.
5. Place a waterproof pad under the client's face.	A pad prevents soiling of bed linen.
6. With cotton ball moistened in prescribed solution (or normal saline) gently clean the lid margins and eyelashes. Clean from inner to outer canthus.	This minimizes entrance of debris on lids or lashes into the eye during irrigation. The cleaning motion prevents entrance of drainage into the nasolacrimal duct.
7. Place a curved emesis basis just below the client's cheek on the side of the affected eye.	The basin collects irrigating solution.
8. Fill the irrigating syringe or eye dropper. Gently retract the lower conjunctival sac and upper eyelid by applying pressure to the lower bony orbit and bony prominence beneath the eyebrow. Do not apply pressure over the eye.	Retraction minimizes blinking and exposes the upper and lower conjunctival membrane for irrigation. Pressure exerted on internal eye structures can cause permanent injury.
9. Hold the irrigating syringe or dropper approximately 2.5 cm (1 inch) above the inner canthus.	If the dropper or syringe touches the eye, there is risk of injury and the dropper or syringe becomes contaminated.
10. Ask the client to look up and *gently* irrigate by directing solution into the lower conjunctival sac toward the outer canthus. Use force sufficient to remove secretions gently.	Flushing of the conjunctival sac prevents exposure of the sensitive cornea to solution. Fluid flows away from the nasolacrimal duct, minimizing absorption of contaminated solution.
11. Allow the client to close the eye periodically, particularly if burning or excess blinking occurs. Encourage the client's cooperation.	Closure of lids moves secretions from the upper conjunctival sac to the lower sac. It also promotes the client's ability to relax during procedure.
12. Continue irrigation until all solution is used or secretions have been cleaned. (Remember that a 15-minute irrigation is needed to flush chemicals.)	Eye irrigation serves to clean exudate, relieve inflammation, or flush caustic solution.
13. Dry the eyelids and facial area with a sterile cotton ball. The client may return to normal position and activity.	Drying removes excess solution and provides for the client's comfort.
14. Remove equipment and wash hands.	Washing prevents transfer of microorganisms.
15. Record the client's response to irrigation (burning, itching, pain) and note the volume and type of solution used, character of drainage, and appearance of conjunctiva.	Timely recording provides accurate documentation of the client's response to the procedure.

syringe or eye dropper is adequate, since rarely is more than a few hundred millimeters of solution required.

In emergencies when caustic chemicals enter the eye, the nurse must flush the eye continuously for at least 15 minutes with tap water. The continuous flushing prevents burning of the sensitive cornea. After the irrigation the client should be seen immediately by a physician to assess the presence or extent of eye injury.

In the home setting it is difficult for a client to irrigate the eye continuously. A family member can easily learn to perform the procedure. However, if the client has no support person to assist, an eye irrigation can be performed by the client with an eye cup. These cups are made of plastic or glass and are available in most drugstores. The nurse should instruct the client on proper cleansing of the cup between uses and on the need to check for chipped glass. Procedure 48-5 outlines eye irrigation.

Suture Care

In closing a wound the surgeon attempts to bring the wound edges as close together as possible to minimize the formation of scar tissue, which is weaker than normal tissue. Proper wound closure requires layers of tissue to be closely approximated with minimal trauma and tension and with control of bleeding.

Sutures are threads or wires used to sew body tissues together. The client's history of wound healing, the site of surgery, the tissues involved, and the purpose of the sutures determine the suture material to be used. For example, if a client has had repeated surgery for an abdominal hernia, the physician might choose wire sutures to provide greater strength for wound closure. In contrast, a small laceration of the face calls for the use of very fine Dacron (polyester) sutures to minimize scar formation.

Sutures are available in a variety of materials, including silk, steel, cotton, nylon, and Dacron. Sutures come with or without sharp surgical needles attached. Growing in popularity are steel staples, a type of outer skin closure that causes less trauma to tissues than sutures yet provides extra strength. Fewer staples are needed to close a wound effectively.

Sutures are placed within tissue layers in deep wounds and superficially as the final means for wound closure. The deeper sutures are usually an absorbable material that disappears in several days. Sutures are foreign bodies and thus capable of causing local inflammation. The surgeon can minimize tissue injury by using the finest suture possible and the smallest number necessary.

In some settings, such as clinics, community first aid centers, and physician's offices, the nurse removes sutures. The procedure requires a physician's order. Special scissors with curved cutting tips or special staple removers slide under the skin closures for their removal. The physician usually signifies the number of sutures or staples to remove. If the suture line appears to be healing in certain locations better than in others, the physician may choose to have only some of the sutures removed (for example, every other one).

The nurse must have knowledge of the type of suturing method the physician used (Fig. 48-9). With interrupted suturing the surgeon ties each individual suture made in the skin. Continuous suturing, as the name implies, is a series of sutures with only two knots, one at the beginning and one at the end of the suture line. The manner in which the suture crosses and penetrates the skin determines the method for removal. The most important principle in suture removal is *never pull the visible portion of a suture through underlying tissue*. Sutures on the skin's surface harbor microorganisms and debris. The portion of the suture beneath the skin is sterile. Pulling the contaminated portion of the suture through tissues may lead to an infection. The nurse clips suture materials as close to the skin edge on one side as possible and then pulls the suture through from the other side (Fig. 48-10).

Drainage Evacuation

Wounds that produce large amounts of drainage or wounds that will not heal properly if even small amounts of accumulated drainage require drainage evacuation to promote proper healing. A simple drain may serve this purpose, or it may become necessary to apply constant suction to a drainage tube. Drainage evacuators are convenient portable units that connect to tubular drains lying within a wound bed. The evacuator exerts a safe, constant, low-pressure vacuum to remove wound drainage. Drainage collects within the

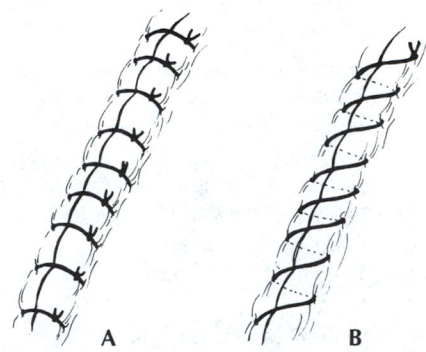

Fig. 48-9 Examples of suturing methods. **A,** Intermittent. **B,** Continuous.

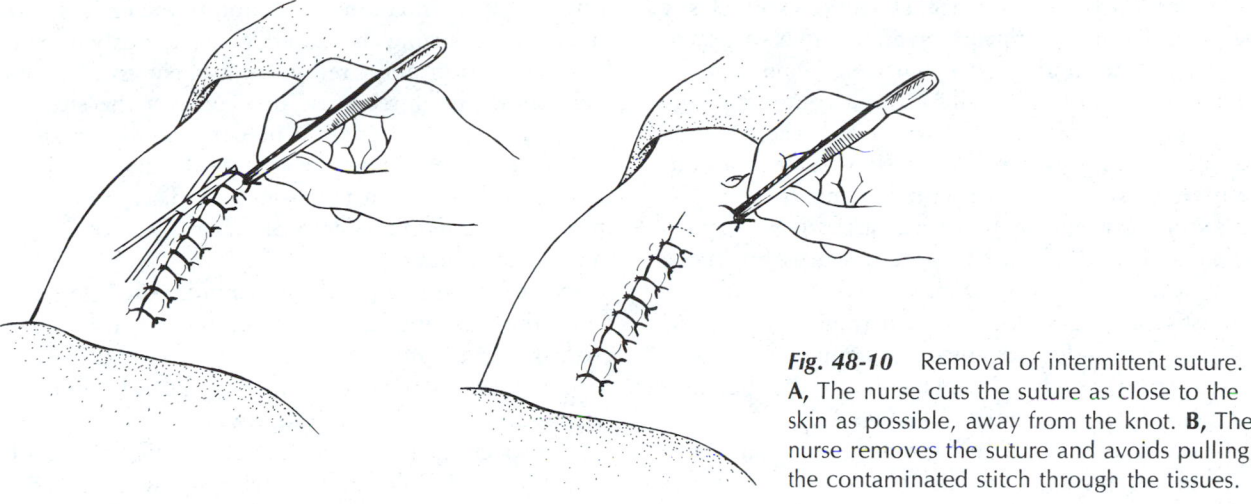

Fig. 48-10 Removal of intermittent suture. **A,** The nurse cuts the suture as close to the skin as possible, away from the knot. **B,** The nurse removes the suture and avoids pulling the contaminated stitch through the tissues.

Fig. 48-11 Setting the suction on a drainage evacuator. **A,** With drainage port open, the lever to the vacuum diaphragm is raised. **B,** The nurse pushes straight down on the lever to lower the diaphragm. Closure of the port prevents escape of air and creates vacuum pressure.

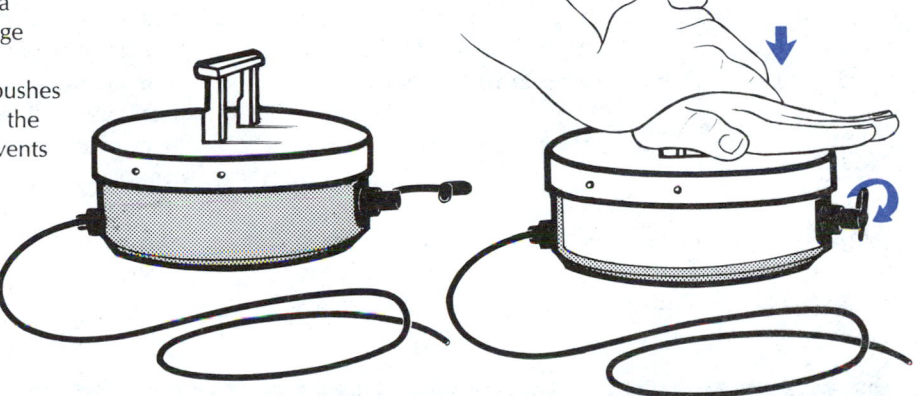

evacuator, maintaining sterility of the system and providing a means for the nurse to measure drainage output.

The nurse's responsibilities include being sure the evacuator is exerting suction, keeping all connection points between the evacuator and tubing intact, and observing for the character and amount of drainage. Fig. 48-11 shows the proper way to exert suction for one type of evacuator unit. When the evacuator fills with drainage, the nurse measures output by emptying the contents into a graduated cylinder. The nurse then immediately resets the evacuator to apply suction. As the volume of drainage decreases, the physician gradually withdraws the drainage tube from the wound bed so deeper tissues can heal. The physician discontinues use of the evacuator once the drain is removed.

Bandages and Binders

A simple gauze dressing is often not enough to immobilize or provide support to a wound. Binders and bandages applied over or around dressings give wounds extra protection and also provide therapeutic benefits for wound healing.

Purposes of binders and bandages include:
1. Creating pressure over a body part, for example, an elastic pressure bandage applied over an arterial puncture site
2. Immobilizing a body part, for example, an elastic bandage applied around a sprained ankle
3. Supporting a wound, for example, an abdominal binder applied over a large abdominal incision and dressing
4. Reducing or preventing edema, for example, a breast binder used to minimize swelling between skin and tissue layers following a mastectomy
5. Securing a splint, for example, a bandage applied around hand splints for correction of deformities
6. Securing dressings, for example, elastic webbing applied around leg dressings following a vein stripping

Bandages are rolls of gauze, elasticized knit, elastic webbing, flannel, or muslin, available in a variety of widths. Gauze bandages are lightweight and have the advantage of molding easily around contours of the body, for example, elbows or knees. The gauze is porous and thus permits circulation of air to an underlying body part to prevent skin maceration. The nurse discards gauze bandages after they become soiled or frayed. Gauze bandages are useful in the home setting because of their low cost.

Elastic bandages also conform well to body parts and have the added advantage of being able to exert pressure over a body part. The common Ace bandage is an example of an elastic bandage.

Flannel and muslin bandages have a thicker weave than gauze and are thus stronger for supporting or applying pressure to body parts. A flannel bandage also insulates to provide body warmth.

Binders are bandages made of large pieces of material to fit a specific body part. Most binders are made of cotton, muslin, or flannel. An arm sling and a breast binder are two examples of binders.

PRINCIPLES FOR APPLYING BANDAGES AND BINDERS

The correct application of bandages and binders involves taking precautions against causing injury to an underlying or nearby body part. For example, applying an elastic bandage too tightly around a client's arm can cause impaired circulation to the fingers and hand. A tight-fitting chest binder can seriously impair lung ventilation and predispose a client to alveolar atelectasis. The nurse must also consider the client's comfort. Failure to apply a binder smoothly results in folds or creases that can irritate the skin. A tight bandage can be a constant source of discomfort and may interfere with a client's ability to sleep or maintain use of a body part.

Before applying a bandage or binder the nurse assesses the skin and underlying body part to be covered. It may also be necessary to protect the area to be bandaged to prevent further injury. The nurse's responsibilities include the following:

1. Inspecting the skin for abrasions, areas of edema, discoloration, or exposed wound edges
2. Covering any exposed wounds or open abrasions with a sterile dressing
3. Assessing the condition of underlying dressings—a soiled dressing should be changed before bandage application
4. Assessing the skin of underlying body parts and parts that will be distal to the bandage for signs of circulatory impairment (coolness, pallor or cyanosis, diminished or absent pulses, swelling, numbness, and tingling) to provide a means for comparing changes in circulation after bandage application

---

TABLE 48-3

Principles for Bandage and Binder Application

Principle	Rationale
Position body part to be bandaged in a comfortable position of normal anatomical alignment.	Bandages cause restriction in movement. Immobilization in a normal functioning position reduces the risks of deformity or injury.
Prevent friction between and against skin surfaces by applying gauze or cotton padding.	Skin surfaces in contact with each other (e.g., between toes, under breasts) can rub against each other to cause abrasion or chafing. Bandages over bony prominences may rub against the skin to cause breakdown.
Apply bandages securely to prevent slippage during client's movement.	Friction between bandage and skin can cause skin breakdown.
When bandaging extremities, apply bandage first at the distal end and progress toward the trunk.	Gradual application of pressure from distal toward proximal portion of extremity promotes venous return and minimizes risk of edema or circulatory impairment.
Apply bandages firmly with equal tension exerted over each turn or layer. Avoid excess overlapping of bandage layers.	This prevents unequal pressure distribution over bandaged body part. Localized pressure causes circulatory impairment.
Position pins, knots, or ties away from the wound or any sensitive skin areas.	Pins and ties used to secure bandages and binders can exert localized pressure and irritation.

Table 48-3 outlines the principles of bandage and binder application. Once a bandage is applied, it is the nurse's responsibility to assess routinely for circulatory or nerve impairment, reduced body function such as decreased ventilation, discomfort, or changes in skin integrity. Any changes should be documented thoroughly in the nurse's notes and reported to the physician immediately. Any bandage the nurse applies can be loosened or readjusted by the nurse as necessary. When the physician has applied a bandage, the nurse should seek an order before loosening or removing the bandage. Loosening a pressure bandage, for example, could cause more damage than leaving the bandage intact. The nurse explains to the client that any bandage or binder will feel relatively firm or tight. The client's initial reaction to bandage application thus may not be as significant as during a period of time after application. The nurse must assess the bandage carefully to be sure it is applied properly and is providing therapeutic benefit. The nurse discards bandages whenever they become soiled and reapplies clean ones. Like a damp dressing, a bandage or binder can harbor microorganisms.

BINDER APPLICATION

Binders are especially designed for the body part to be supported. The most common types of binders are the breast binder, abdominal binders (Scultetus and straight), T binder, and sling.

BREAST BINDER. A breast binder looks like a tight-fitting sleeveless vest. The binder conforms to the shape of the chest wall and is available in different sizes. Breast binders provide support after surgery to the breast and exert pressure when the goal is to reduce lactation in a woman after childbirth.

For an optimal fit the nurse instructs the client to lie supine after placing her arms through the binder's armholes. Safety pins secure the binder in front. The nurse first secures the binder at the nipple line as the client supports the breasts, and then carefully secures the binder above and below the point of initial attachment. The binder should not impair chest expansion. If the client's pulmonary secretions are increased, the nurse must encourage active pulmonary hygiene exercises. It is essential that excess pressure be avoided when clients or family members are learning how to apply a breast binder.

ABDOMINAL BINDERS. A physician frequently uses abdominal binders to support large abdominal incisions that are vulnerable to tension or stress as the client moves or coughs. An abdominal binder is a rectangular piece of cotton or elasticized material that either has many tails attached to the two longer sides

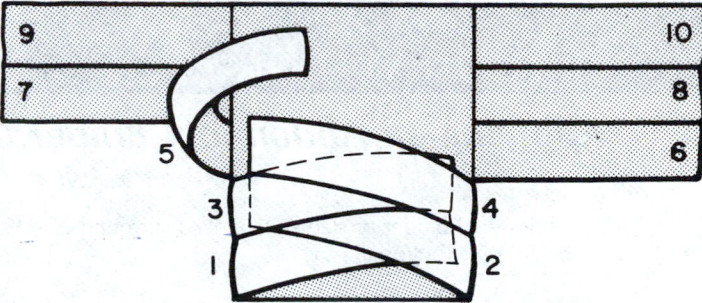

Fig. 48-12 Scultetus binder. Each successive tail overlaps and secures the previous tail.

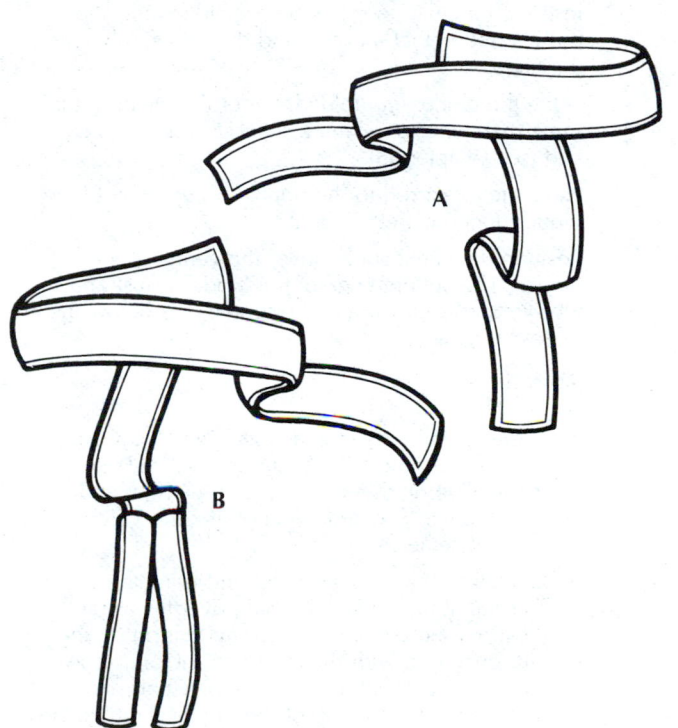

Fig. 48-13 T binders. **A,** Female. **B,** Male.

(Scultetus; Fig. 48-12) or has long extensions on each side to surround the abdomen. The nurse secures an abdominal binder with safety pins, Velcro strips, or metal stays. Procedure 48-6 describes steps for an abdominal binder application.

T BINDERS. As the name implies, the T binder looks like the letter **T** (Fig. 48-13) with either a single or double tail. The single **T** is for female clients and the double **T** fits male clients. The binders secure rectal or perineal dressings.

The belt of the **T** binder fits securely around the client's waist. The tail passes between the client's legs from back to front and attaches to the belt's front. It is important for the nurse to be sure the tail fits

PROCEDURE 48-6

Applying an Abdominal Binder (Straight and Scultetus)

EQUIPMENT:
1. Abdominal binder of size sufficient to surround client's abdomen
2. Safety pins (optional)

STEPS	RATIONALE
1. Explain to the client that the binder serves to support the abdominal incision and provides comfort.	This reduces the client's anxiety.
2. Instruct the client to roll onto one side while supporting abdominal incision and dressing firmly with the hands.	Splinting of the incision during movement reduces pain.
3. Place the binder (fan folded) under the client in the same manner as applying a sheet for an occupied bed (see Chapter 35).	This method will allow the client to roll over the binder to ease positioning and centering.
4. Have the client roll to the opposite side. Unfold the binder underneath the client.	
5. Position the client supine over the center of the binder. The bottom edge of the binder is just above the symphysis pubis, and the top edge is below the costal margins.	Proper positioning of the binder ensures that adequate pressure will be applied over the wound and prevents interference with chest expansion.
6. Close the binder.	A firm, even application of pressure provides optimal wound support and comfort.
a. *Straight.* Pull the left end of the binder toward the center of the client's abdomen. While keeping tension on the left end, pull the right end over the left. Secure by smoothing the Velcro edges together.	
b. *Scultetus.* Take the left hand and bring the bottom tail at the client's left side over toward the center of the abdomen. Keeping tension on the tail, overlap it with the bottom right tail. Repeat the procedure with each successive pair of tails moving toward the top of the binder. Double the ends of the tails back on themselves to prevent bulging or pressure areas. Be sure each pair of tails overlaps the pair below. Secure the top pair of tails with a safety pin for each end.	
7. Assess the client's ability to deep breathe and cough. Readjust as necessary.	The binder should not impair chest expansion or exert increased pressure over the abdomen.
8. Record application in the nurse's notes.	Prompt documentation improves accuracy of the record.

smoothly against the dressings. T binders usually are soiled easily and thus require frequent changing. Special care is needed to prevent irritating the female's urethra and the male's scrotum.

SLINGS. Slings provide support to arms injured from muscular sprains or fractures. The nurse applies the sling in a manner that supports the entire arm and does not exert excess pressure to neck structures. A commercially made sling consists of a long sleeve that fits around the client's elbow and a strap that fits around the neck. In the home setting a large triangular piece of cloth can be used as a sling.

When a sling is being applied the client may sit or lie supine (Fig. 48-14). The nurse instructs the client to bend the affected arm, bringing the forearm straight across the chest. The open sling fits under the client's arm and over the chest, with the base of the

PROCEDURE 48-7

Applying a Spiral Turn Roller Bandage

STEPS	RATIONALE
1. Stand in front of the body part to be bandaged.	This improves access to the body part and ease of handling the bandage.
2. Hold the free end of the bandage in the nondominant hand and place the outer surface against the client's skin. Hold the body of the bandage in the dominant hand.	Holding the body of the bandage with the outer surface against the skin improves the ease of unrolling the remainder of the bandage.
3. With firm, even tension make a circular turn around the distal portion of the body part, anchoring the free end.	Application from the distal end toward the trunk promotes venous return. Anchoring of the bandage end prevents slippage.
4. Pass the body of the bandage from hand to hand while making even spiral turns up the body part. (Each turn overlaps the previous turn by one-half or two-thirds the width of the bandage.)	Gradual, even unwinding of the bandage applies equal pressure to the body part.
5. Once the full roll of bandage is applied, make a final circular turn and secure the terminal end with tape or metal stays.	This prevents slippage. Tape and stays do not place pressure against the client's skin.
6. Assess the circulation and sensation of the distal body part.	Too firm an application can impair blood flow.

triangle under the wrist and the triangle's point at the client's elbow. One end of the sling fits around the back of the client's neck. The nurse brings the other end up over the affected arm while supporting the extremity. The nurse ties the two ends at the side of the neck so the knot does not press against the cervical spine. The loose fold at the elbow can be folded evenly around the elbow and pinned. The lower arm should always be supported at a level above the elbow to prevent the formation of dependent edema.

BANDAGE APPLICATION

The nurse uses rolls of bandage to secure or support dressings over irregularly shaped body parts such as an extremity or an amputated stump. Each roll has an initial or free outer end and a terminal end at the center of the roll. The rolled portion of the bandage is its body. The bandage's outer surface faces the outside of the body of the bandage and is the surface that touches the client's skin or dressing. The inner surface faces the center of the bandage roll. Procedure 48-7 describes the steps for applying a roller bandage using simple spiral turns. The nurse may use a variety of other turns depending on the body part to be bandaged (Table 48-4).

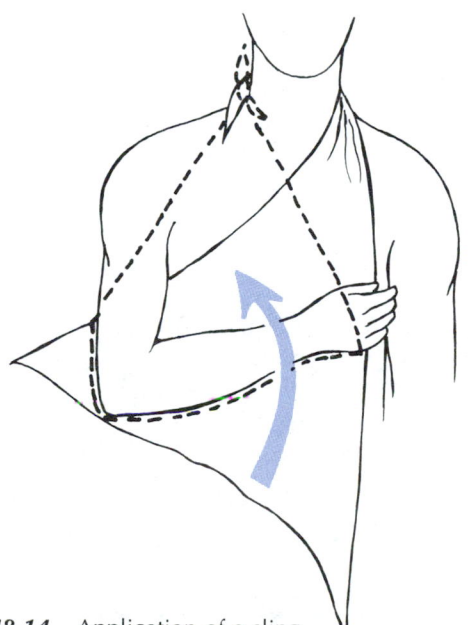

Fig. 48-14 Application of a sling.

Heat and Cold Therapy

The local application of heat and cold to an injured body part can provide therapeutic benefits. To use heat and cold therapies safely, the nurse must understand the manner in which the body normally responds to local temperature variations. Clients with alterations in sensory reception or perception (see

TABLE 48-4

Types of Bandage Turns

Type	Description	Purpose or Use	
Circular	Bandage turn overlapping previous turn completely	Anchors a bandage at the first and final turn; covers a small part (e.g., finger or toe)	
Spiral	Bandage ascending body part with each turn overlapping previous one by ½ or ⅔ width of bandage.	Covers cylindrical body parts such as wrist or upper arm	
Spiral—reverse	Turn requires a twist (reversal) of bandage halfway through each turn	Covers cone-shaped body parts such as the forearm, thigh, or calf; useful with nonstretching bandages such as gauze or flannel	
Figure-eight	Oblique overlapping turns alternately ascending and descending over bandaged part; each turn crossing previous one to form a figure-eight	Covers joints; snug fit provides excellent immobilization	
Recurrent	Bandage first secured with two circular turns around proximal end of body part; half turn made perpendicular up from bandage edge; body of bandage brought over distal end of body part to be covered with each turn folded back over on itself	Covers uneven body parts such as head of amputated limb	

Chapter 44) can easily be injured by heat and cold applications. The nurse assesses the integrity of any body part carefully and determines the client's ability to sense temperature variations before making any applications. The temperature of the device or compress must be within a safe range and all equipment parts must operate efficiently so that the client cannot suffer injury. The nurse is legally responsible for the safe administration of all heat and cold applications.

Bodily Responses to Heat and Cold

Exposure to heat and cold can cause both systemic and local responses. Chapter 28 describes the mechanisms for the control of body temperature. When exposed to excessively warm surroundings, the body normally reacts through heat loss mechanisms such as sweating and vasodilation. If the body becomes exposed to cold temperatures, mechanisms promoting heat conservation (vasoconstriction, piloerection) and heat production (shivering) come into play.

The local response to heat and cold involves stimulation of temperature-sensitive nerve endings within the skin. Stimulation of the nerve endings causes impulses to travel from peripheral afferent nerve fibers to the spinal cord and ascend the cord to the hypothalamus, which becomes aware of local temperature sensations. The reception of impulses at the level of the hypothalamus triggers adaptive responses for the maintenance of normal body temperature. Prolonged local exposure to temperature changes can require systemic adaptive responses. If any alterations occur along temperature sensation pathways, the reception and eventual perception of stimuli will be altered.

The body also possesses a protective reflex response for exposure to extremely hot or cold stimuli. The response is similar to the body's pain response (see Chapter 37). When a person comes in contact with an extremely hot or cold stimulus, impulses travel to the spinal cord, synapse within the cord, and then return by way of a motor nerve to cause withdrawal from the stimulus. The person simultaneously becomes aware of the discomfort. For example, if a person touches a hot iron, the reflex response causes rapid withdrawal of the person's hand.

The body is capable of adapting to wide variations in temperature. Temperature receptors become stimulated when temperatures reach levels above or below that of the skin's surface (34° C [93.2° F]). Ranges of temperature sensation are subjective and vary among individuals. Generally people describe temperatures as very cold, cold, cool, tepid (at body temperature), warm, hot, and very hot. Pain impulses develop when local temperatures reach extremes of 45° C (113° F) or 15° C (59° F). Excessive heat causes an intense burning sensation. Cold produces a numbing sensation before pain is noticeable.

The ability of temperature receptors to adapt quickly to temperature changes creates the major problem in protecting clients from injury resulting from temperature extremes. A person initially feels an extreme change in temperature but within a short time hardly notices the temperature variation. For example, when the hand is placed in a basin of hot

---

TABLE 48-5

Conditions That Increase Risk of Injury from Heat and Cold Application

Condition	Risk Factors
Very young; elderly	Thinner skin layers in children increase risk of burns; elderly have reduced sensitivity to pain
Open wounds, broken skin, stomas	Subcutaneous and visceral tissues more sensitive to temperature variations; also contain no temperature and fewer pain receptors
Areas of edema or scar formation	Reduced sensation to temperature stimuli because of thickening of skin layers from fluid buildup or scar formation
Peripheral vascular disease (e.g., diabetes or arteriosclerosis)	Body's extremities less sensitive to temperature and pain stimuli because of circulatory impairment and local tissue injury; cold application would further compromise blood flow
Confusion or unconsciousness	Reduced perception of sensory or painful stimuli
Spinal cord injury	Alterations in nerve pathways preventing reception of sensory or painful stimuli
Abscessed tooth or appendix	Infection highly localized; application of heat may cause rupture with spread of microorganisms systemically

water, initially an uncomfortable sensation is felt. However, the sensory receptors adapt quickly, and soon the person can keep the hand immersed even though the water temperature has not dropped. The same response occurs with exposure to cold stimuli. This adaptive phenomenon can be dangerous, since a person insensitive to heat and cold extremes can suffer serious tissue injury. The nurse must be familiar with clients most at risk for injuries from heat and cold applications (Table 48-5).

Local Effects of Heat and Cold

Heat and cold stimuli create different physiological responses, including changes in the diameter and permeability of cutaneous (skin) blood vessels, blood flow and viscosity, local metabolism, and muscular contraction. The choice of heat or cold therapy depends on the local physiological responses desired for wound healing. Table 48-6 summarizes the benefits of heat and cold application.

EFFECTS OF HEAT APPLICATION

The initial response to local heat application is vasodilation of skin vessels. As vessels dilate, blood flow increases, causing the skin to become pink and warm. The improved blood flow helps relieve discomfort and edema in congested tissues. Vasodilation also promotes the local inflammatory response. Heat reduces blood viscosity, enabling leukocytes and antibodies to reach injured tissues more quickly. Heat applied to an infected wound causes consolidation of pus, preventing its spread through the body. The increases in circulation and in permeability of capillaries improve the exchange of oxygen, nutrients, and waste products between tissues and blood vessels.

Local heat application also reduces muscle spasm through muscle relaxation. As the muscle relaxes,

---

TABLE 48-6

Therapeutic Effects of Heat and Cold Applications

Therapy	Physiological Response	Therapeutic Benefit	Examples of Conditions Treated
Heat	Vasodilation	Improves blood flow to injured body part; promotes delivery of nutrients and removal of wastes; lessens venous congestion in injured tissues	Inflamed or edematous body part; new surgical wound; infected wound; arthritis, degenerative joint disease; localized joint pain, muscle strains; low back pain; menstrual cramping; hemorrhoidal, perianal, and vaginal inflammation; local abscesses
	Reduced blood viscosity	Improves delivery of leukocytes and antibiotics to wound site	
	Reduced muscle tension	Promotes muscle relaxation and reduces pain from spasm or stiffness	
	Increased tissue metabolism	Increases blood flow; provides local warmth	
	Increased capillary permeability	Promotes movement of waste products and nutrients	
Cold	Vasoconstriction	Reduces blood flow to injured body, preventing edema formation; reduces inflammation	Immediately after direct trauma, e.g., sprains, strains, fractures, muscle spasms; superficial laceration or puncture wound; minor burn; when malignancy is suspected in area of injury or pain; after injections; arthritis, joint trauma
	Local anesthesia	Reduces localized pain	
	Reduced cell metabolism	Reduces oxygen needs of tissues	
	Increased blood viscosity	Promotes blood coagulation at injury site	
	Decreased muscle tension	Relieves pain	

pain dissipates. Local tissue metabolism increases. Blood flow increases, transferring heat either to other body parts or through the skin to the outside.

If heat applications remain in place for 1 hour or more, blood flow is reduced by a reflex vasoconstriction. The response is the body's attempt to control heat loss from the area. The periodic removal and reapplication of local heat will restore vasodilation. Continuous exposure to heat damages epithelial cells, causing redness, localized tenderness, and even blistering of the skin.

EFFECTS OF COLD APPLICATION

Application of cold to the skin surface causes vasoconstriction. The skin becomes pale and cool. With vasoconstriction local blood flow falls, causing a reduction in the vascular response of inflammation. The reduced blood flow also prevents edema formation at an injury site, since less blood reaches the damaged vessels. Vasoconstriction results in increased blood viscosity, promoting blood coagulation and thus controlling hemorrhaging.

Cold lowers local tissue metabolism. Oxygen utilization is reduced and less waste accumulates within tissues. Cold also has an anesthetic effect when applied to the skin. A person may become unaware of superficial pain or sensory stimuli after only a few minutes of cold application.

Prolonged exposure of the skin to cold will result in a reflex vasoconstriction. The cell's inability to receive adequate blood flow and nutrients results in tissue ischemia. The skin initially takes on a reddened appearance, followed by a bluish purple mottling with numbness and a burning type of pain. The skin's tissues can actually freeze from exposure to extreme cold.

Factors Influencing Heat and Cold Tolerance

The body's response to heat and cold therapies depends on a number of factors. The nurse uses knowledge of each factor to ensure the safe administration of therapies. The factors are as follows:

1. *Duration of application.* A person is better able to tolerate temperature extremes when the duration of exposure is short. Continued exposure to safe temperatures eventually results in increased tolerance.
2. *Body part.* Certain areas of the skin are more sensitive to temperature variations. The neck, inner aspect of the wrist and forearm, and perineal regions are sensitive. The foot and the palm of the hand are less sensitive.
3. *Damage to body surface.* Exposed skin layers are more sensitive to temperature variations.

4. *Prior skin temperature.* The body responds best to minor temperature adjustments. If a body part is cool and a hot stimulus touches the skin, the response is greater than if the stimulus were only warm.
5. *Body surface area.* A person has less tolerance to temperature changes when a large area of the body is exposed to heat or cold.
6. *Age and physical condition.* Tolerance to temperature variations changes with age. The very young and elderly are most sensitive to heat and cold. If a client's physical condition reduces the reception or perception of sensory stimuli, the tolerance to temperature extremes is high but the risk of injury is also high.

Assessment

Before applying heat or cold therapies the nurse assesses the client's physical condition for signs of potential intolerance to heat and cold. The nurse first observes the area to be treated. Alterations in skin integrity, such as abrasions, open wounds, edema, bruising, bleeding, or localized areas of inflammation, increase the client's risk of injury. Since the physician commonly orders heat and cold applications to be placed on traumatized areas, the nurse's baseline assessment provides a guide for evaluating skin changes that might occur during therapy.

The nurse's assessment includes identification of conditions that contraindicate heat or cold therapy. If the client has a localized malignant tumor, heat should not be applied over the site because of the risk of increasing cell growth. An active area of bleeding should also not be covered by a warm application, since bleeding will continue. Warm applications are contraindicated when the client has an acute localized inflammation such as appendicitis, since the heat could cause the appendix to rupture. If a client has cardiovascular problems, it is unwise to apply heat to large portions of the body. The massive vasodilation may disrupt blood supply to vital organs.

Cold is contraindicated if the site of injury is already edematous. Cold will further retard circulation to the area and prevent absorption of the interstitial fluid. If the client has impairment in circulation, for example, arteriosclerosis, cold will further reduce blood supply to the affected area. One other contraindication for cold therapy is the presence of shivering. Cold applications may intensify shivering and dangerously increase the client's body temperature. The nurse also assesses the client's response to stimuli. Sensation to light touch, pinprick, and mild temperature variations (see Chapter 29) will reveal the ability of the client to recognize when heat or cold becomes excessive. If a client has peripheral vascular disease, the nurse pays particular attention to the integrity of the extremities. For example, if the physician's order is to apply a cold compress to a lower extremity, the nurse should assess circulation to the leg by observing skin color and palpating skin temperatures, distal pulses, and any edematous areas. If signs of circulatory inadequacy are present, the nurse should question the order.

A client's level of consciousness will influence the ability to perceive heat, cold, or pain. The nurse assesses the client's level of alertness and orientation. If a client is confused or unresponsive, the nurse must make frequent observations of skin integrity once the therapy begins.

The nurse must also assess the condition of all equipment being used. Any electrical equipment should be checked for cracked cords, frayed wires, damaged insulation, or exposed heating components. Equipment containing circulating fluids should not have leaks. The nurse also checks equipment for evenness of temperature distribution. For example, a heating pad's entire surface should be warm. Uneven temperature distribution suggests that the equipment is functioning improperly.

Client Education and Safety

The safety of heat and cold therapy depends in part on the client's understanding of the procedure. Before the application of any therapy the client should understand its purpose, the symptoms of temperature exposure, and the precautions taken to prevent injury. The nurse also provides a safe environment for the therapy. The box provides hints for applying heat and cold therapy.

Implementation

A physician's order is needed before using any form of heat or cold application. The order should include the type of application, the body site to be treated, the frequency of the application, and the duration of each application. If the physician does not designate the duration of therapy, the nurse must use judgment in determining a safe time period for the application. The correct temperature to use for heat and cold applications varies according to agency policy. The nurse should consult the agency's procedure manual.

CHOICE OF MOIST OR DRY

Both heat and cold applications can be administered in dry or moist forms. Dry heat includes use of a heating pad, a hot water bag, a heat lamp, aquathermia (water flow) pads, and commercial hot packs.

Safety Suggestions for Applying Heat or Cold Therapy

- **Do** explain to the client the sensations to be felt during the procedure.
- **Do** instruct the client to report any changes in sensation or any discomfort immediately.
- **Do** provide a timer, clock, or watch so the client can help the nurse time the application.
- **Do** keep the call light within the client's reach.
- **Do** refer to the institution's policy and procedure manual for safe temperatures.
- **Do not** allow the client to adjust temperature settings.
- **Do not** allow the client to move an application or place his hands on the wound site.
- **Do not** place the client in a position that prevents movement away from the temperature source.
- **Do not** leave unattended a client who is unable to sense temperature changes or move from the temperature source.

Examples of moist heat are moist hot compresses, sitz baths and warm baths, and hot soaks. Moist compresses and cold soaks are forms of moist cold therapies. The forms of dry cold applications include ice bags, collars, or packs and aquathermia pads. There are advantages and disadvantages to both dry and moist applications. The type of wound or injury, the location of the body part, and the presence of drainage or inflammation are factors considered in selecting dry or moist applications. Table 48-7 summarizes advantages and disadvantages of both.

MOIST HEAT THERAPIES

HOT MOIST COMPRESSES. For open wounds hot moist compresses are effective in improving circulation, relieving edema, and promoting consolidation of pus and drainage. A compress is a piece of gauze dressing moistened in a prescribed warmed solution. Commercially packaged sterile, premoistened compresses are available in many agencies. The nurse simply applies an infrared lamp to the pack to heat the solution. A pack is a larger cloth or dressing applied to a larger body area.

In the case of open wounds the nurse applies compresses and packs using sterile technique. Compresses applied over an intact skin area, such as a swollen sprained ankle, need not be sterile.

Heat from hot compresses evaporates quickly. To

TABLE 48-7

Choice of Dry or Moist Applications

Type	Advantages	Disadvantages
Moist applications	Moist application reduces drying of skin and softens wound exudate.	Prolonged exposure can cause maceration of the skin.
	Moist compresses conform well to body area being treated.	Moist heat will cool rapidly because of moisture evaporation.
	Moist heat penetrates deeply into tissue layers.	Moist heat creates a greater risk for burns to the skin since moisture conducts heat.
	Warm moist heat does not promote sweating and insensible fluid loss.	
Dry applications	Dry heat has less risk of burns to skin than moist applications.	Dry heat increases body fluid loss through sweating.
	Dry application does not cause skin maceration.	Dry applications do not penetrate deep into tissues.
	Dry heat retains temperature longer, since it is not influenced by evaporation.	Dry heat causes increased drying of skin.

maintain a constant temperature the nurse must either change the compress frequently or apply a warm aquathermic pad, waterproof heating pad, or warm water bottle over the compress. It is important to remember that moisture conducts heat. The temperature setting on any device applied to a moist compress need not be as high as if the device were used for a dry application. If a heating device is unavailable, the nurse uses a layer of plastic wrap or a dry towel to insulate the compress and retain heat.

Moist heat promotes vasodilation and evaporation of heat from the skin's surface. For this reason a client may feel chilly. The nurse controls drafts within the room and keeps the client covered with a blanket or robe. Procedure 48-8 describes the steps for applying a warm compress.

WARM SOAKS. Immersion of a body part in a warmed solution promotes circulation, lessens edema, and increases muscle relaxation. Warm soaks also provide a means to debride wounds and apply medicated solution. Usually the physician orders soaks for a body extremity. If the body part is too large to immerse, a soak can be accomplished by wrapping the part in dressings and saturating them with the warmed solution.

The nurse positions the client comfortably and places waterproof pads under the area to be treated. The nurse uses a sterile or clean container for the solution, which is heated to approximately 40.5° to 43° C (105° to 110° F). The problem is to keep the

solution at a constant temperature. A soak generally lasts 20 minutes, and during that time the solution can cool quickly. After immersing the body part the nurse covers the container and extremity with a towel to reduce heat loss. It is usually necessary to remove the cooled solution and add heated solution after about 10 minutes. The client must remove the extremity from the soak while warmer solution is being added. When medications are used, changing the solution may dilute the drug's concentration. After any soak the nurse dries the body part thoroughly to prevent maceration.

SITZ BATH. The client who has had rectal surgery or an episiotomy during childbirth or who has painful hemorrhoids or vaginal inflammation may benefit from immersing the pelvic area in warmed water. A sitz or hip bath is given in a special tub or chair or in a basin that fits on the toilet seat. The client sits in a sitz bath so that the legs and feet remain out of the water. The basins are disposable and especially useful in the home setting. Resting in a bathtub does not provide the same therapeutic benefit as a sitz bath. Immersing the entire body causes widespread vasodilation and nullifies the effect of local heat application to the pelvic area.

The desired temperature for a sitz bath varies depending on whether the purpose is to promote relaxation or to clean a wound. Agency procedures must be checked for recommended temperatures. The nurse should prevent overexposure of the client by draping

PROCEDURE 48-8

Applying a Hot Moist Compress to an Open Wound

EQUIPMENT:
1. Prescribed solution warmed to proper temperature (approximately 43° to 46° C [110° to 115° F])
2. Sterile gauze dressings
3. Sterile container for solution
4. Commercially prepared compresses (optional)
5. Sterile gloves
6. Petrolatum jelly
7. Sterile cotton swabs
8. Waterproof pad
9. Tape or ties
10. Dry bath towel
11. Aquathermic or heating pad (optional)
12. Disposable gloves
13. Bath thermometer

STEPS	RATIONALE
1. Explain the procedure to the client, including sensations to be felt, e.g., feeling of warmth and wetness. Explain precautions to prevent burning.	The client's understanding of the procedure will improve cooperation and lessen anxiety.
2. Assist the client in assuming a comfortable position in proper body alignment.	The compress remains in place for several minutes up to an hour. Limited mobility in an uncomfortable position causes muscular stress.
3. Place a waterproof pad under the area to be treated.	A waterproof pad prevents soiling of bed linen.
4. Expose the body part to be covered with a compress and drape the client with a bath blanket.	This prevents unnecessary cooling and exposure of the body part.
5. Wash hands.	Washing prevents infection transmission.
6. Assemble equipment. Pour warmed solution in sterile container. (If using a portable heating source, keep the solution warm. Commericially prepared compresses may remain under an infrared lamp until just before use.) Open sterile packages and drop the gauze into the container to become immersed in solution. Turn the electrical heating pad to the correct temperature.	Compresses must retain warmth for therapeutic benefit.
7. Don disposable gloves. Remove the existing dressing covering the wound. Dispose of the gloves and dressings in the proper receptacle.	Proper disposal techniques prevent spread of microorganisms.
8. Assess the condition of the wound and surrounding skin.	This provides a baseline to determine skin changes following compress application.
9. Don sterile gloves.	Sterile touching sterile remains sterile.
10. Apply sterile petrolatum jelly with a cotton swab to the skin surrounding the wound. Do not place jelly in broken areas of skin.	Petrolatum jelly protects the skin from the possible burns and maceration.
11. Pick up one layer of the immersed gauze and wring out any excess water.	Excess moisture macerates the skin and increases the risk of burns and infection.
12. Apply gauze lightly to the open wound. Watch the client's response and ask if the client feels discomfort. In a few seconds lift the edge of the gauze to assess for redness.	Skin is most sensitive to a sudden change in temperature. Redness indicates a burn.
13. If the client tolerates the compress, pack the gauze snugly against the wound. Be sure all wound surfaces are covered by the hot compress.	Packing of the compress prevents rapid cooling from underlying air currents.

STEPS	RATIONALE
14. Wrap the moist compress with a dry bath towel. If necessary, pin or tie in place.	A towel insulates the compress to prevent heat loss.
15. Change the hot compress every 5 minutes.	This prevents cooling, thus maintaining the therapeutic benefit of the compress.
16. (Optional) Apply aquathermic or waterproof heating pad over the towel. Keep it in place for the desired duration of application (approximately 20 to 30 minutes)	This provides a constant temperature to the compress.
17. Ask the client periodically if there is any discomfort or a burning sensation.	Continued exposure to heat can cause burning of skin.
18. Remove the pad, towel, and compress. Assess the wound and the condition of surrounding skin.	Continued exposure to moisture will macerate the skin.
19. Replace the sterile dressing.	Replacing the dressing prevents entrance of microorganisms into the wound site.
20. Dispose of equipment and wash hands.	
21. Record the type of application, solution, temperature of solution, duration of application, and condition of skin before and after procedure.	Accurate documentation provides legal protection for the nurse.

bath blankets around the client's shoulders and thighs and controlling for drafts. To promote comfort the client should be able to sit in the basin or tub with feet flat on the floor. The client should avoid assuming a position that places pressure on the sacrum or the thighs.

Since a large portion of the body becomes exposed to heat, the extensive vasodilation may cause the client to become light-headed and faint. The nurse assesses the client's pulse and facial color and asks if the client feels light-headed or nauseated. A pale facial color and rapid pulse may signal a fainting episode.

A sitz bath usually lasts 20 minutes. As in the case of warm soaks, it may become necessary to add hot water during the procedure. A disposable basin contains a special attachment that resembles an enema bag and allows the gradual introduction of warmer water.

PARAFFIN BATHS. A paraffin bath consists of a mixture of heated paraffin wax and mineral oil (1 part oil to 5 parts paraffin). Clients with painful arthritis or other joint discomforts of the hands and feet benefit most from the baths. In many institutions only physical therapists administer the applications.

Clients often heat paraffin baths at home in double boilers (53.3° to 54.4° C [128° to 130° F]). After heating, the paraffin cools to form a white film on the surface. It is then safe for the client to immerse the foot or hand. The client holds the fingers or toes still while slowly dipping the extremity in and out of the bath. Should the client move, cracks in the paraffin may form, allowing additional hot paraffin to seep in and increase the risk of burns. After approximately six to 10 repetitions a paraffin glove forms over the extremity. The nurse or client then wraps the extremity in a dry towel for approximately 20 minutes. After the time elapses, the client can simply peel the paraffin off like a glove or sock. The same paraffin can be remelted and used three or four times a day.

An advantage of paraffin baths is the lubricating effect of the mineral oil. The nurse cautions a client never to use paraffin baths on skin rashes or open wounds.

DRY HEAT THERAPIES

AQUATHERMIA (WATER FLOW) PADS. A popular device in health care institutions is the aquathermia (water flow) pad (Fig. 48-15). The device is useful for treating muscle sprains and areas of mild inflammation or edema. The aquathermia unit consists of a waterproof plastic or rubber pad connected by two hoses to an electrical control unit that has a heating element and motor. Distilled water circulates through

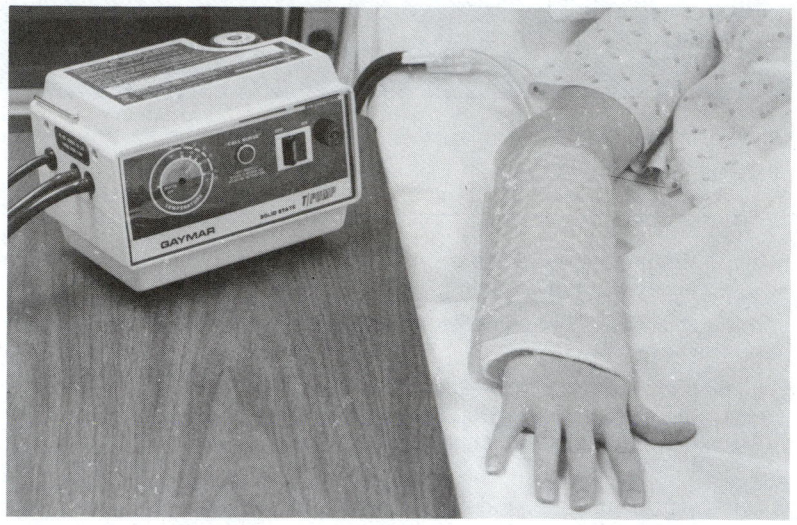

Fig. 48-15   Aquathermia pad.

hollowed channels within the pad to the control unit where water is heated or cooled (depending on temperature setting). The units are safer than the conventional heating pad. However, the nurse should still check for any equipment malfunctions. The temperature setting is fixed by inserting a plastic key into the temperature regulator. In many institutions the central supply room sets the regulators to the recommended temperature (40.5° to 43° C [110° to 115° F]). If the distilled water in the unit runs low, the nurse simply adds water to the reservoir at the top of the control unit. Plain tap water is never added, since it might leave mineral deposits in the unit.

To avoid burning the client's skin the nurse does not place the pad directly on it. A thin towel or pillow case fits easily over the heating pad. Tape, ties, or a gauze roll holds the pad in place. Pins are never used because they might cause a leak. The nurse checks the client's skin frequently for signs of burning. An application should last only 20 to 30 minutes. The nurse does not allow a client to lie on a pad. Pressure against a mattress prevents normal heat dissipation. If the pad is to be applied to a region of the back, the client should lie prone or on one side.

HEAT LAMP. An advantage of a heat lamp over other forms of heat therapy is that nothing touches the client's skin surface. This is valuable in clients with sensitive or painful skin conditions or wounds.

A heat lamp works best for applying heat to small areas such as a decubitus ulcer or venous stasis ulcer. The heat lamp is used primarily to increase circulation to a wound. The lamps come with infrared and regular household 40- to 50-watt light bulbs. Both lamps expose only superficial layers of the skin to heat.

The nurse's primary concerns include providing the client with privacy, protecting the exposed skin, and

positioning the lamp a safe distance away to avoid causing burns. After explaining the procedure to the client the nurse closes the room door and cubicle curtains. It is often necessary to expose large areas of the body. The nurse drapes as much of the area not to be exposed as possible. The nurse never uses the bed sheets to form a tent over the lamp, since this produces a fire hazard. Next the nurse inspects the skin for scars or stomas. These areas should be covered because they are insensitive to heat and the chest may burn without feeling the heat. The nurse also wipes off any moisture on the skin that can conduct heat. The distance between the heat lamp bulb and the exposed body surface depends on the bulb wattage and the client's tolerance. A 60-watt bulb should be placed at least 50 cm (24 inches) away. A larger watt bulb should be approximately 75 cm (30 inches) away. The nurse checks the client's skin at 5-minute intervals throughout the duration of the procedure (approximately 20 minutes). The client is instructed not to touch the lamp's surface, since it generates considerable heat.

HEAT CRADLE. A heat cradle is a long, metal, half-circle frame that fits over a large body part such as a leg or the lower trunk. A series of small (25-watt) light bulbs emits heat over a broad area to promote circulation. The nurse may place bed sheets over the frame to prevent exposure of the client's body and to prevent cooling from air currents. The sheets should not come in contact with the light bulb.

The nurse follows the same precautions for protecting the client's skin as with heat lamps. Because of the light bulbs' low temperatures it is safe to keep the cradle on for up to an hour. The bulbs should be at least 40 to 45 cm (16 to 18 inches) away from the client's skin.

HOT WATER BOTTLES. In the home or health care institution the hot water bottle has always been an economical means of applying heat to an injured body part. However, institutions are using water bottles less often because of the danger of leakage. Nurses must give clients and family members the following instructions on the safe use of water bottles:

1. First check the bottle for leaks. Fill it with hot tap water, secure the cap, and turn the bottle upside down. There should be no leaks.
2. Fill the bag with warm tap water at a temperature of 40.5° to 46° C (105° to 115° F).
3. Fill the bag only two-thirds full, expel any air at the top, and secure the cap. The bag is then easier to mold over a body part.
4. Wipe off any moisture on the outside of the bag.
5. Never apply a water bottle directly to the skin surface. Cover it with a towel or pillow case.
6. Keep the bottle in place for 20 to 30 minutes.

ELECTRIC HEATING PADS. Another conventional form of heat therapy is the heating pad. The pad consists of an electric coil enclosed within a waterproof covering. A cotton or flannel cloth covers the outer pad. The pad is connected to an electric cord that has a temperature-regulating unit for a high, medium, or low setting. Nurses should advise clients to avoid using the high setting.

The same precautions for application of an aquathermia pad apply to a conventional heating pad. It is safe to apply the flannel or cotton covering against the client's skin. The client should never lie directly on a pad. A safety pin inserted through a pad can result in an electrical shock.

MOIST COLD THERAPIES

COLD MOIST COMPRESSES. The procedure for applying cold moist compresses is the same as that for warm compresses. Cold compresses should be at a temperature of 15° C (59° F). The nurse checks the compresses frequently to avoid warming. Cold compresses are effective for areas of inflammation and swelling. They may be clean or sterile. The nurse observes for adverse reactions such as burning or numbness, mottling of the skin, redness, extreme paleness, or a bluish skin discoloration. Application of cold compresses lasts for 20 minutes.

COLD SOAKS. The procedure for preparing cold soaks and immersing a body part is the same as for warm soaks. The temperature for a cold soak is 15° C (59° F). The nurse takes precautions to protect the client from chilling. During the 20-minute application it may be necessary to remove solution that has warmed and add cooler solution.

DRY COLD THERAPIES

ICE BAG OR COLLAR. For a client who has a muscle sprain, localized hemorrhage, or hematoma or has undergone dental surgery, an ice bag is ideal to prevent edema formation, control bleeding, and anesthetize the body part. Ice bags come in various sizes and shapes to fit different body parts. A bag is made of rubber and has a cap and flannel cloth cover. Proper use of the bag requires the following:

1. Filling the bag with water, securing the cap, inverting the bag to check for leaks, and pouring out the water
2. Filling the bag two-thirds full with small pieces of crushed ice, which enables the bag to mold easily over a body part
3. Releasing any air from the bag by squeezing its sides before securing the cap (since excess air interferes with conduction of cold)
4. Wiping the bag dry of excess moisture
5. Applying a flannel cover, towel, or pillow case over the bag
6. Applying the bag to the injury site for 30 minutes; the bag can be reapplied in an hour

COLD PACKS. Commercially prepared ice packs come in various sizes and shapes. When the pack is squeezed or kneaded, an alcohol-based solution is released inside to create the cold temperature. The bags cannot be frozen for reuse. The soft outer coverings can usually be safely applied directly to the skin surface.

Nutritional Support

Despite the nurse's efforts with wound care, wound healing will not occur if the client is malnourished. Malnutrition lowers the client's capacity to fight wound infection and the complications of healing. During tissue repair the body uses more protein, carbohydrates, fats, minerals, water, and oxygen than during normal tissue metabolism. Each nutritional element plays a vital role in the steps of wound healing. The delivery of nutritional substances to tissues depends on a healthy circulatory system. In malnourished clients the supply of the nutritional elements needed for wound repair is insufficient. Malnutrition also causes alterations in blood vessel integrity. For example, with protein deficiency (hypoalbuminemia), edema forms in interstitial spaces, impairing nutrient exchange. The malnourished client thus has few resources for wound repair.

The nurse works closely with dietitians to provide the client with a well-balanced diet. Client education becomes an important means of ensuring that the client understands the importance of good dietary habits. For clients weakened or debilitated by their illness, supportive nutritional therapies in the form of supplemental tube feedings (see Chapter 38) or parenteral nutrition (see Chapter 42) become necessary.

The postoperative client who is malnourished and unable to eat presents a significant challenge. The surgical client who is well nourished and has no complications requires at least 1500 kcal per day for nutritional maintenance. A typical postoperative client receives only 3 liters of parenteral fluids (5% dextrose in water) a day, which contains only a total of 500 kcal. The well-nourished client with no complications is able to resume eating soon enough that few problems arise. However, if the client is malnourished from the beginning or if an infection develops that increases energy requirements by as much as 50%, nutritional support becomes a serious problem.

Enteral Feedings

The client with impaired gastrointestinal function will require enteral feedings (nutrients introduced directly into the gastrointestinal tract). A nasogastric tube (see Chapter 48), gastrostomy tube (tube introduced through the abdomen into the stomach), or jejunostomy tube (tube introduced through the abdomen into the jejunum) provides a route for enteral feeding. The dietitian selects the type of feeding that meets the client's nutritional needs and promotes normal digestion.

Parenteral Nutrition

If a client is unable to tolerate enteral feedings, the physician may order parenteral nutrition. Clients with high energy demands receive intravenously administered solutions with high carbohydrate, protein, and electrolyte content. Large intravenous catheters introduced into a client's subclavian vein provide the safest route for the highly concentrated intravenous solutions. The large diameter of the subclavian vein minimizes the risk of vein inflammation (phlebitis) and breakdown of circulating red blood cells (hemolysis). Chapter 42 describes the nursing implications for safe monitoring of parenteral nutrition.

Summary

The nurse administers various forms of therapy to clients with surgical or traumatic wounds. The type of wound healing determines the types of dressing used, their method of application, the manner of caring for drains and sutures, and the observations to make for monitoring wound repair. Clients most at risk for impaired wound healing require close observation and may benefit from the use of bandages and binders to support and protect wounds.

Principles the nurse follows to promote wound healing include use of aseptic technique, protection of the wound from further injury, and promotion of the stages of healing. These principles are employed in the application of hot and cold therapies. In addition, the nurse uses knowledge of the effects of heat and cold to recognize wounds that will benefit from heat or cold applications.

The successful healing of any wound depends on provision of a balanced diet. The client's energy and nutritional requirements are increased as a result of tissue injury. The nurse works in collaboration with the dietitian to find a diet that is palatable and includes the nutrients needed by the client.

KEY CONCEPTS

- ✓ In normal wound healing the epidermal skin layer resurfaces wounds while the dermis restores the structural integrity and physical properties of the skin.
- ✓ A clean surgical incision with little tissue loss heals by primary intention.
- ✓ Healing by primary intention proceeds through three stages: defensive, reconstruction, and maturation.
- ✓ When there is extensive tissue loss, a wound heals by secondary intention.
- ✓ Hemorrhaging most often occurs during the defensive stage of wound healing.
- ✓ The chances of wound infection are greater when the wound contains dead or necrotic tissue, when foreign bodies lie on or near the wound, and when blood supply and tissue defenses are reduced.

KEY CONCEPTS, *cont'd*

✓ Any factor that lowers a client's immune response impairs wound healing.

✓ Physical stress from vomiting, coughing, or sudden muscular contraction can cause separation of wound edges.

✓ A wound assessment requires a description of the appearance of the wound, character of drainage, presence of drains and wound closures, and presence of pain.

✓ Wound drains remove secretions within tissue layers to promote wound closure.

✓ The nurse never collects a wound culture from old drainage.

✓ Principles of wound first aid include control of bleeding, wound cleansing, and wound protection.

✓ The layers of a dry dressing protect the wound edges, absorb drainage, and prevent entrance of bacteria.

✓ The wet-to-dry dressing mechanically removes dead tissue and wound exudate to cleanse the wound.

✓ When cleaning wounds or drain sites, an important principle is to clean from the least to most contaminated area, away from wound edges.

✓ The type of suture securing a wound influences the method of suture removal.

✓ A bandage or binder should be applied in a manner that does not impair the client's circulation or irritate the skin.

✓ The safe use of heat and cold therapy requires an assessment of the client's sensory function, identification of risk factors, and understanding of the physiological effects of heat and cold.

✓ An acute sprain, fracture, or bruise responds best to cold applications.

✓ Warm applications are effective for improving circulation to wound sites and promoting muscle relaxation.

✓ The choice of moist or dry applications depends on the type of wound, location of body part, and presence of drainage or inflammation.

REFERENCES

Bruno, P.: The nature of wound healing: implications for nursing practice, Nurs. Clin. North Am. **14**:667, 1979.

Keithley, J.K.: Wound healing in malnourished patients, AORN J. **35**:1094, 1982.

Simmons, B.P.: CDC guidelines for prevention of surgical wound infections, Am. J. Infect. Control **11**:133, 1983.

ADDITIONAL READING

Alterescu, V.: Toward a physiologic approach to the topical treatment of opened wounds, J. Enterostomal Ther. **10**:101, 1983.

Brubacher, L.L.: To heal a draining wound, RN **45**:30, 1982.

Bruno, P., and Craven, R.F.: Age challenges to wound healing, J. Gerontol. Nurs. **8**:686, 1982.

Croushore, T.M.: Postoperative assessment: the key to avoiding the most common nursing mistakes, Nursing 79 **9**:47, 1979.

Flynn, M.E., and Rovee, D.T.: Wound healing mechanisms, Am. J. Nurs. **82**:1544, 1982.

Greenburg, A.G., et al.: Wound dehiscence, pathophysiology and prevention, Arch. Surg. **114**:143, 1979.

Hotter, A.N.: Physiologic aspects and clinical implications of wound healing, Heart Lung **11**:522, 1982.

Marchiondo, K.: The very fine art of collecting culture specimens, Nursing 79 **9**:34, 1979.

Pollack, S.: Wound healing: a review. I. The biology of wound healing, J. Enterostomal Ther. **8**:16, 1981.

Pollack, S.: Wound healing: a review. II. Environmental factors affecting wound healing, J. Enterostomal Ther. **9**:14, 1982.

Pollack, S.: Wound healing: a review. III. Nutritional factors affecting wound healing, J. Enterostomal Ther. **9**:28, 1982.

Schumann, D.: Preoperative measures to promote wound healing, Nurs. Clin. North Am. **14**:683, 1979.

Wright, N.E.: Abdominal wounds: breakdown and dehiscence, J. Enterostomal Ther. **10**:143, 1983.

11

Contemporary nursing, as a profession, involves more than the day-to-day provision of care to individual clients. Because most nurses work with other nurses and health care professionals, leadership skills are often needed to ensure the successful cooperation and direction of the group to provide health care of the highest quality. Nursing, like other professions related to the sciences, is engaged in research to gain new knowledge about client care, and nurses need to be aware of the principles of research in order to incorporate new knowledge into nursing practice. The chapters in this unit address these additional dimensions of the profession in its dynamic relationship with the world around us.

Contemporary Nursing: Dimensions and Dynamics

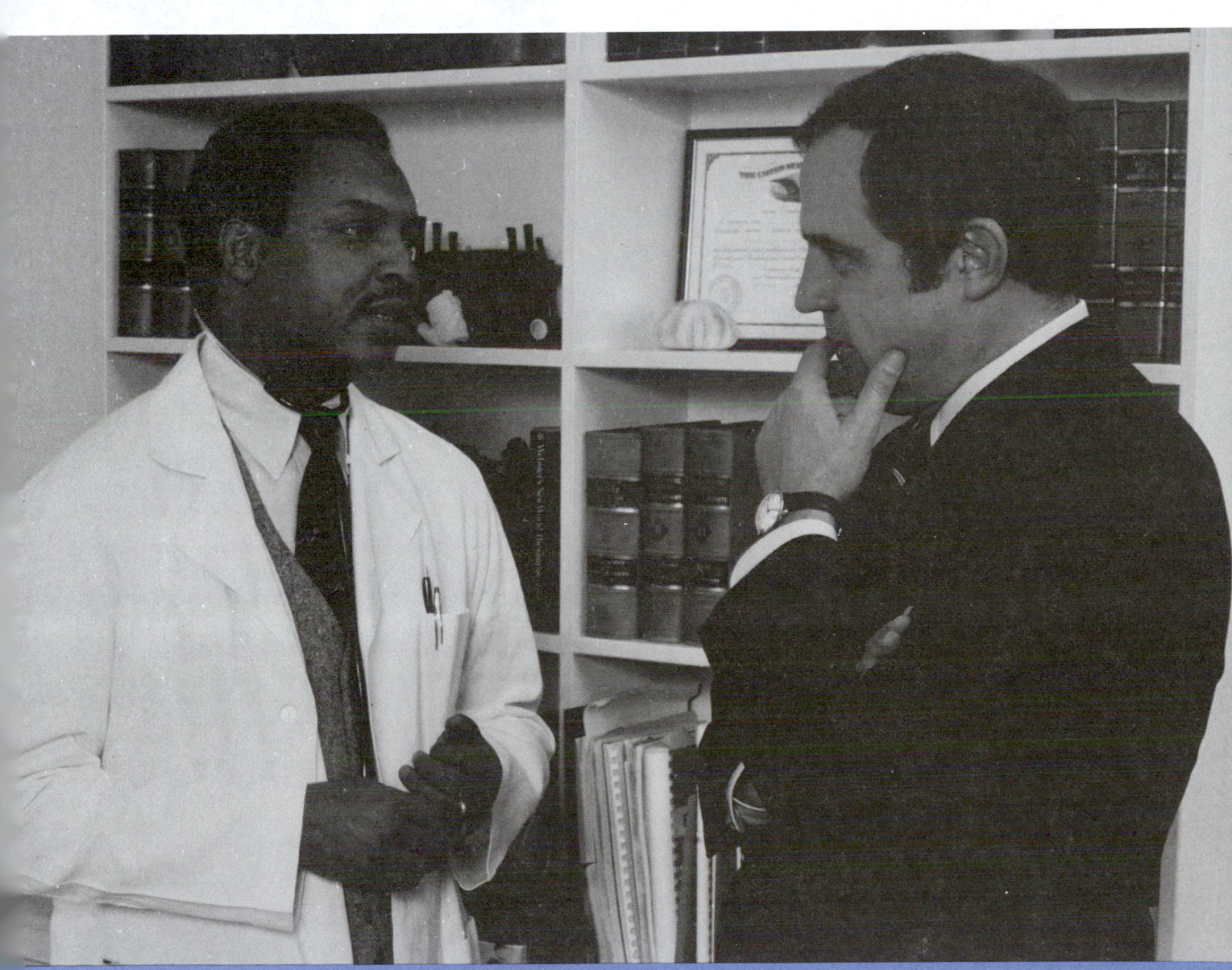

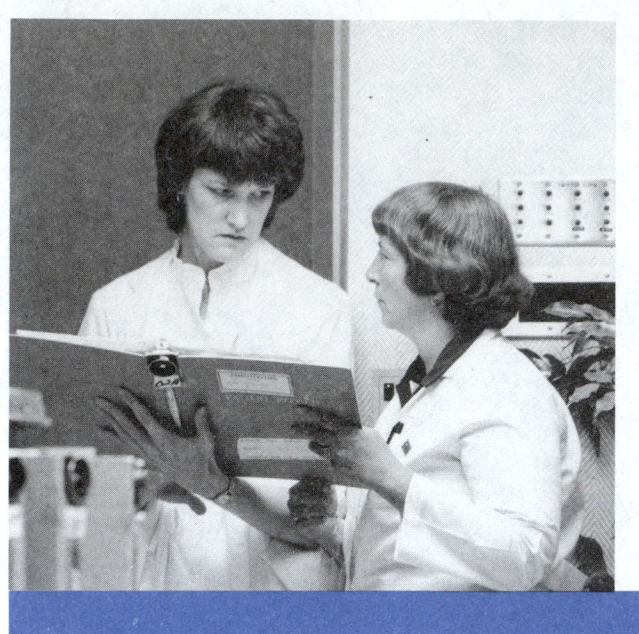

OBJECTIVES

Mastery of the content in this chapter will allow the student to:

- Define the terms in the glossary.
- Differentiate between leadership and management.
- Compare and contrast the scientific management theory and the human relations movement in their perspectives for improving productivity.
- Identify the primary principles of situational leadership theories.
- Describe and give examples of the four classic leadership styles: authoritarian, democratic, laissez-faire, and situational.
- Explain why leadership is important for nursing.
- List and give examples of the four primary types of leadership skills student nurses can begin to develop.

GLOSSARY

authoritarian style Leadership style in which the leader retains all authority and responsibility and is concerned primarily with tasks and goal achievement.

democratic style People-centered leadership style in which the group participates openly in decision making for group goals.

human relations movement Leadership theory that emphasizes the role of interpersonal relationships and human needs for improving productivity in the workplace.

laissez-faire style Leadership style in which the leader denies responsibility, abdicates authority, and allows the group to direct themselves.

leader Person with the ability to influence the behavior of others toward the accomplishment of common goals; not necessarily a manager.

leadership style Specific means by which a leader influences a group to accomplish goals.

manager Person with an official organizational position to guide and direct the work of subordinate employees; not necessarily a leader.

scientific management theory Leadership theory that emphasizes technology and task analysis, rather than human factors, as a means of improving productivity.

situational theory Leadership theory in which the manager chooses a leadership style to match the particular situation.

trait development theory Leadership theory that analyzes successful leadership in terms of the leader's personal qualities, including intelligence, energy level, aggressiveness, and friendliness.

49 | *Nursing Leadership and Management*

Successful organizations have one major characteristic that sets them apart from unsuccessful organizations: effective and dynamic leadership. In hospitals and other health care facilities, certain nursing units have a reputation for delivering superior nursing care. These units generally have head nurses who are recognized leaders within their institutions and who motivate the nursing staff to maintain higher standards of nursing care. Effective nursing leaders such as these head nurses are generally successful because of their early commitment to developing leadership skills.

Drucker (1954), a well-known authority on management, identifies a need for effective leaders in many areas of modern society. Effective leaders are the most basic and scarcest resource in any business, as well as in government and religious, educational, and health care institutions. According to other authorities in this area, there is not only a shortage of leaders who can get the job done effectively but also a scarcity of people willing to assume significant leadership roles in our society (Hersey and Blanchard, 1977). Leadership is needed in nursing as in other areas.

Leadership skills are usually developed by individuals early in their careers. To meet the need for more effective leaders in nursing, therefore, it is important for nursing students to understand leadership concepts, to begin to develop leadership skills early in their careers, and to commit themselves to exercising leadership skills in their everyday nursing activities.

Definition of Leadership

Leadership is the ability to influence others toward the accomplishment of a goal. The leader possesses skills required for directing, controlling, predicting, and changing the actions of others. Leadership is generally needed whenever a group of people is acting toward a common goal, and thus leadership occurs in all areas of life: in the family, in the school dormitory, in the classroom, and in a nursing division. Not all effective leaders have the same capabilities or leadership style. What effective leaders do have in common, however, is the ability to lead others on an ongoing basis, day after day, year after year, in a wide variety of situations and circumstances.

Understanding what constitutes leadership and what skills, abilities, and traits are necessary to be a good leader is important for the nursing student, just as leaders are important for the nursing profession. This understanding provides a basis for the learning and development of leadership skills.

Leadership and Management Theories

Leadership has been an area of study since the turn of the century, when psychological testing became popular and provided tools for objective research. A number of theories about the qualities of leadership have been developed. The review of these theories in the following sections can help the student nurse better understand what is involved in leadership.

Early leadership studies concentrated on the traits and qualities of leaders. Trait development theorists generally believed that the leader was born with certain qualities that determined his leadership ability and success. These qualities were considered to include intelligence, aggressiveness, high energy level, and friendliness. The trait theorists believed that these leadership traits were applicable in all situations. Effective leaders were studied to identify the traits they had in common. Many attempts were made to put this theory into practice. From a group of job applicants, for example, only those possessing the identified traits were considered potential leaders and were selected for positions requiring leadership. Leadership training was provided only for those who possessed the desired leadership traits. This method of selecting and developing leaders, however, was not particularly effective.

As more research has been conducted in the area of leadership, the theory that a leader possesses certain traits has been proved to be incorrect. Research into necessary leadership traits showed few consistent findings. The list of traits grew to over 100 traits that were considered essential to successful leadership. Gradually it became clear that very few successful leaders could possess all these traits identified as essential for the successful leader. In a review of this research, Jennings (1961) concluded, "Fifty years of study have failed to produce one personality trait or set of qualities that can be used to discriminate leaders and non-leaders."

Scientific Management Theory

Another approach to the study of leadership was developed by Taylor in the early 1900s. Taylor's scientific management theory emphasized technology as the basis for increasing the productivity of employees. Taylor's theory has been interpreted to mean that people are instruments or machines that are manipulated by their leaders. This approach suggested that management should be divorced from human affairs and emotions and that employees should adjust to management, not management to the workers.

The scientific management movement introduced time and motion studies to analyze tasks, based on the belief that improving the performance of tasks would improve every aspect of the organization. Attempts were made to satisfy the needs of employees through various incentives. If this approach had been applied to nursing, for example, a nurse might have received a cash bonus for shortening a client's period of hospitalization. This approach has proved ineffective and simplistic because it ignores complex human needs and encourages shortcuts and short-term goals at the expense of long-term goals. Therefore it is not practiced in nursing.

In the scientific management theory the leader's function was to set up and enforce performance criteria through close supervision. The leader provided direction in an authoritarian manner, focusing on the needs of the organization rather than the needs of the employees or customers.

Human Relations Movement

Mayo and his associates in the 1920s and 1930s argued that managers attempting to improve productivity must be concerned with human affairs rather than solely with technological methods. The human relations theorists believed that the real power centers within an organization were the interpersonal relationships established within the work environment. They suggested that organizations be developed around human relationships, including those between leaders and employees, and consider human feelings and attitudes.

The role of the leader, according to this approach, was to ensure that employees cooperated to attain their goals while also encouraging the employees' personal growth and development. The leader was to focus more on the workers' needs than the needs of the organization. In this respect the human relations movement was in direct opposition to the scientific management movement.

Michigan Leadership Studies

University of Michigan researchers studied leadership to identify clusters of characteristics related to the leader's effectiveness. According to their studies the two primary kinds of leaders are those who are employee oriented and those who are production oriented. Production-oriented leaders are more concerned about the technical aspects of the job, whereas employee-oriented leaders stress the importance of the employees' needs.

Theory X and Theory Y

McGregor described two kinds of management theories, which he called theory X and theory Y. Managers who believe in theory X assume that people inherently dislike work and will avoid it whenever possible. The manager therefore must force employees to work, control and direct them continually, and threaten them with punishment if they are to work toward the accomplishment of organizational goals. Theory X assumes that human beings prefer to be directed, have little ambition, reject responsibility, and are most concerned about job security. McGregor believed that managers who used the theory X approach would never be able to reach high levels of production because only employees' low-level needs were satisfied.

Theory Y, in contrast, assumes that employees can enjoy physical and mental work just as they enjoy play and rest. Employees are capable of self-motivation and job satisfaction if they are happy in the organization and committed to its goals. Most human beings want responsibility, and if employees have responsibility rather than being controlled authoritatively, many organizational problems can be solved through group interaction. Theory Y managers believe that the organization is more successful when employees are self-directed and exercise self-control in their work. For this to occur, the employee must share the organization's goals and feel a commitment to the organization. McGregor suggests that theory Y organizations will satisfy higher human needs, resulting in greater employee responsibility and, in turn, higher productivity.

Ohio State Leadership Studies

The Bureau of Business Research at Ohio State University conducted studies in the 1940s to identify various dimensions of leadership behaviors. Leadership behaviors were described in terms of two dimensions: structure and consideration. Consideration behaviors reflect friendship, mutual trust, respect, and warmth between the leader and employee. Structure behaviors are those that clearly define the structured organizational relationship between the leader and employees.

Researchers collected data on the behaviors of leaders through a specially designed questionnaire. The results of the research indicated that structure and consideration behaviors are separate and distinct dimensions, each on a continuum that ranges from low to high. Any leader may have any combination of characteristics in these two dimensions. A high level in one dimension does not necessarily mean a low level in the other. Thus there are four general types of leaders, with many variations in specific characteristics:

1. High consideration, high structure
2. High consideration, low structure
3. Low consideration, high structure
4. Low consideration, low structure

Fig. 49-1 describes the characteristics of these four types of leaders. This study is particularly important because it represents the first multidimensional approach to leadership behavior.

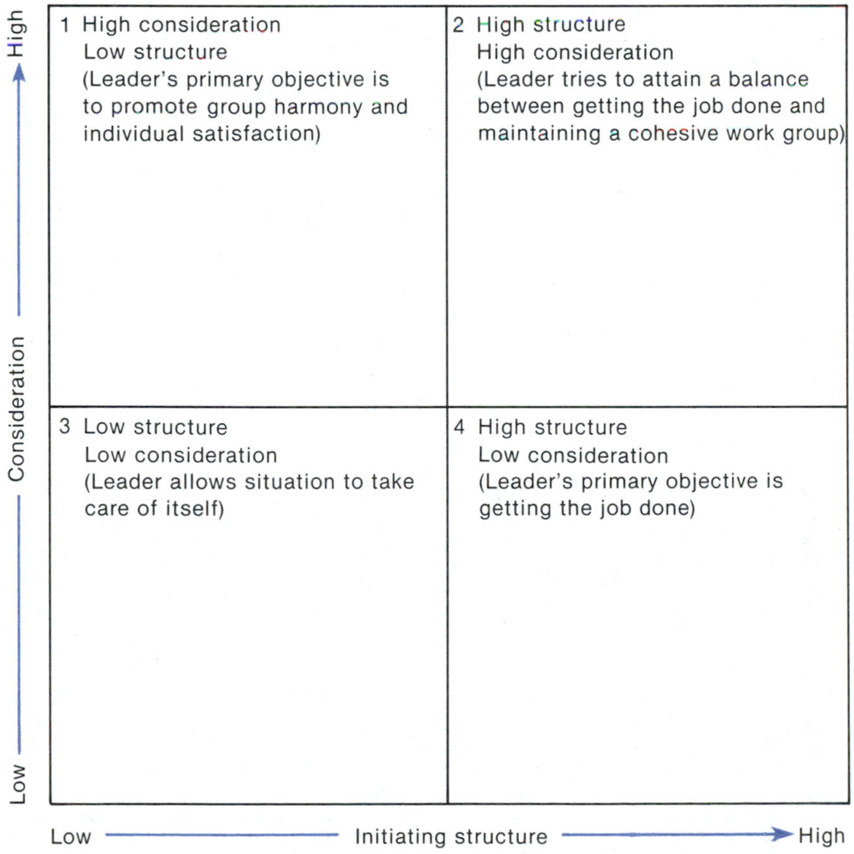

Fig. 49-1 Ohio State leadership quadrants.

These types of leadership behaviors involve different approaches to the manager-employee relationship. For example, a head nurse who believes the staff's scheduling requests are more important than the needs of the nursing unit would rate high in consideration and low in structure. A head nurse who considers only the needs of the nursing unit and not the needs of the staff would rate low in consideration and high in structure. The first head nurse may achieve a more harmonious working relationship with staff nurses, but the second head nurse may be more effective in ensuring that short-staffing does not occur. Neither is necessarily a better leader because effective leadership also depends on many other factors and skills.

Managerial Grid

The managerial grid theory of Blake and Mouton focuses on management purposes and organizational improvement. Organizations are seen to have three universal characteristics: organizational purposes, employees, and a power structure or hierarchy. The power structure involves the supervision of employees by leaders. Management styles in this approach involve two concerns: task accomplishment and the development of human relationships. As in the Ohio State Study, these two concerns exist on continuums, here represented with a grid (Fig. 49-2). The position of a manager on this grid is determined by the extent of his concern for employees and for organizational goals. There are four extreme types of leadership styles:

1. Impoverished
2. Country club
3. Task
4. Team

The ultimate management style in this theory is the team management style. The team manager is both committed to the organization and concerned for the employees. The team manager makes decisions through employee involvement, participation, and exchange of ideas. Team managers are even tempered, maintain a sense of humor, are dependable in difficult situations, and are willing to change their ideas.

Situational Theories

In recent years human relations theorists have influenced how managers deal with the needs, feelings,

Fig. 49-2 Managerial grid leadership styles.

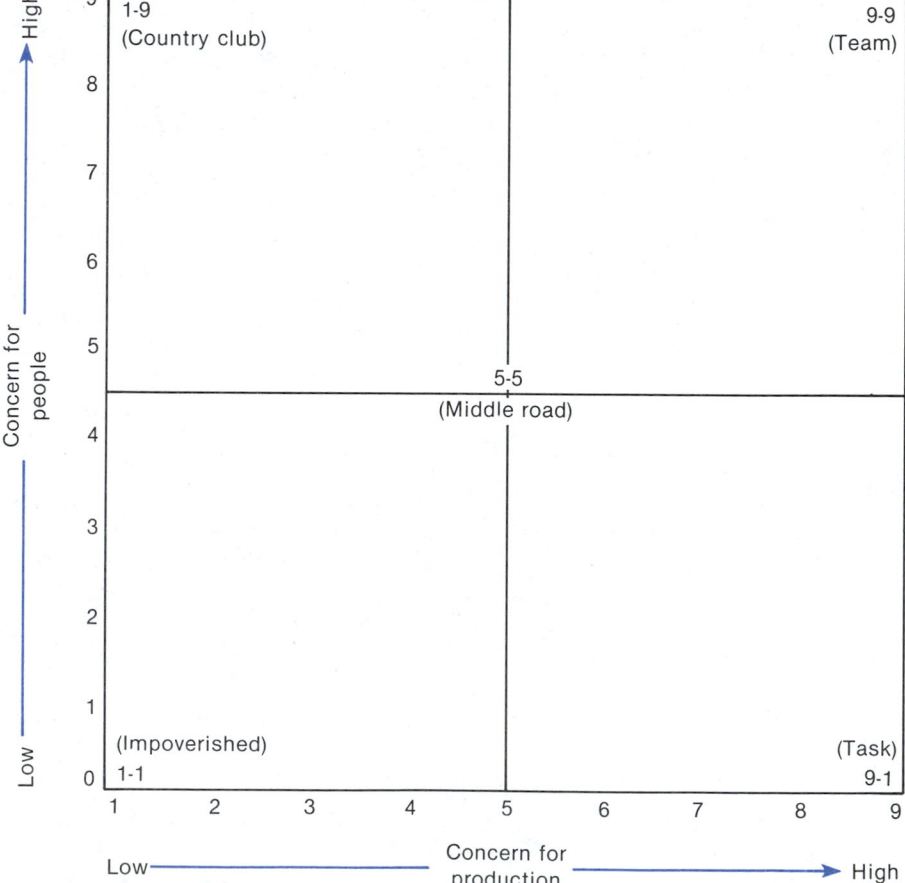

and general working conditions of employees. Because of this humanistic approach to management, a problem has arisen for the modern manager, who must maintain a balance between managing in a "democratic" manner and exercising the necessary control and authority to complete the specified tasks or goals.

Management style can thus be described on a continuum that ranges from highly autocratic leadership to a democratic process in which the group makes decisions within prescribed limits (Tannenbaum and Schmidt, 1958). The leader chooses a style on this continuum that reflects what is practical and desirable for the situation. According to situational theory, the manager's traits, employee factors, and situational factors must be considered in this choice. Managerial factors include confidence in employees, leadership philosophy, values, and feelings of security in any given situation. Employee factors include the need for independence, readiness to accept responsibility, understanding of the organizational goals, and previous knowledge and experience to manage the problem. Situational factors are important in the manager's choice of leadership style. One key factor is the extent of employee's understanding of organizational values within the situation. Other situational factors include the effectiveness of the working group, the problems under consideration, time limitations, and available resources.

Managers are concerned about their responsibilities and the effectiveness and productivity of the employees they supervise. They are also concerned about the motivation and needs of employees. Several theorists have analyzed this double concern in leadership with a situational approach.

Redden (1970) developed an approach to managerial effectiveness based on the Ohio State studies. In this approach no one style of leadership is seen as always effective. Effectiveness depends, instead, on the leader's qualities and skills. Three managerial skills are necessary for effective leadership: situational sensitivity, style flexibility, and situational management. Situational sensitivity is the manager's ability to read and diagnose a working situation. Style flexibility is the leader's ability to choose from a variety of management styles the most appropriate style for a given situation; this does not involve avoiding pressure or simply keeping employees happy but rather maintaining efficiency, even in a stressful situation, by balancing the needs of employees and the organization. Situational management is the process of working to change from an unfavorable situation to a more favorable one.

Another situational management theorist, Likert (1961, 1967), addresses human factors while recog-

nizing the impact of situational variables. This approach suggests that managers who are helpful and oriented to employees achieve higher productivity and greater effectiveness within the organization. Management style is based on supportive relationships, group decision making, group methods of supervision, and high performance goals. Each employee views the institution as supportive and interested in developing the employee's personal worth and importance. The organization is arranged in working groups rather than the usual structure in which one manager supervises many employees working individually.

Working groups overlap within the organizational structure to promote communication. Important decisions are made by the group. The group's goals include high productivity, high quality, and low costs. The manager is accountable for the group's decisions, productivity, and results.

Likert's System 4 Management theory is effective only if each person within the organization belongs to one or more effectively functioning work groups characterized by strong group loyalty, effective skills, and high performance goals. Situational factors are important and can affect the group decision-making process. If the group is unable to reach a united decision, the leader must make the decision. If the leader disagrees with the group's decision, he may try to persuade the group to act in another direction. If the leader follows the group's decision, he is responsible for the outcome. The leader must also make decisions when time or other factors restrict the use of the group decision-making process.

The situational approach of Fiedler (1967) emphasizes fitting the job to the style of the leader rather than the leader changing styles according to the situation. The two major styles of leadership are the task-oriented and employee-oriented styles. According to this theory, every leader has a certain predominant style, and effective management should not attempt to change a leader's style but should choose a leader with the style most appropriate to the situation. Three major situational variables affect what type of leader is most appropriate in a particular situation: the acceptance and personal feelings of the group for the leader, the structured or unstructured nature of the task, and the need for authority to accomplish the group's task. The personal relationship between the leader and group is the most important factor in the group's interaction and effectiveness. The second variable, the nature of the task, is important because some situations involve highly regimented tasks, whereas others require more creativity and personal or group initiative. Finally, in some situations groups require directive leadership to accomplish the job, while in others the group requires more permissive leadership.

Fiedler describes eight possible combinations of these situational variables. In a difficult situation in which the tasks must be accomplished by group effort, for example, the autocratic, task-oriented manager produces the most favorable results. In less difficult or less structured situations, the nondirective, permissive leader is more successful. Based on studies showing that leaders are generally unaware of their own leadership styles, Fiedler concludes that the most effective approach is to teach leaders how to identify their styles and to diagnose the working situation in order to match the leader to the situation. This has been applied successfully in various organizations.

Hersey and Blanchard's situational leadership theory (1977), originally called the life cycle theory of leadership, is concerned with the extent of structure and socioemotional support from the leader necessary according to the maturity of employees. As the leader and group develop a working relationship based on mutual trust and respect, the process encourages mature and effective followers. The effective leader must be flexible in using more than one style of leadership. Leadership depends on three key skills: technical skills required to perform definite tasks, human skills required to work with and through other people, and conceptual skills necessary to understand the leader's responsibility within the organization and the organization's overall goals and structures.

The leader uses task behaviors to organize the group and task, establish goals, and direct employees. The leader uses relationship behavior to establish and maintain personal relationships with followers, to open channels of communication, and to provide emotional support for employees. The effective leader combines these two types of behaviors in ways most appropriate for a specific situation. Four basic types of leadership styles are derived from these combinations:

1. *High task/low relationship.* By one-way communication the leader defines the roles of the followers and tells them what, how, when, and where to do various tasks.
2. *High task/high responsibility.* The leader provides most of the direction to employees but also attempts through two-way communication and socioemotional support to motivate employees to accept decisions that have been made.
3. *High relationship/low task.* Employees participate in decision making through two-way communication. The leader only guides the employees, who have the ability and knowledge to do the task.
4. *Low relationship/low task.* The leader allows employees to make their own decisions with only general supervision. In this case the employees are mature in terms of both the task and the ability to accept responsibility.

Leadership style therefore depends on the maturity of the employee group in relation to specific work situations. An employee may be mature and capable of accepting responsibility in one situation but immature and requiring directive management in another. The concept of maturity applies to both individuals and groups. In addition, maturity depends on both job maturity (technical skill and ability to do the task) and psychological maturity (feeling of self-confidence needed to complete the task). The leader's responsibility is to diagnose the situation, determine the maturity of employees, and select the appropriate leadership style. As the maturity of the followers increases, the leader should gradually move from a task style into a relationship style. The reverse is true in situations where the individual or group demonstrates immaturity. As followers develop higher maturity levels, the leader should be able to reduce both task and relationship behaviors. Employees who achieve a high level of maturity in their performance can provide their own direction and achieve on their own the necessary psychological satisfaction.

Leadership and Management Style

A leader is not necessarily a manager, nor is a manager necessarily a leader. A manager is a person whose official position within an organization is to guide and direct the work of others. The manager has been given authority and responsibility by the organization to enforce decisions and policies. A manager may or may not have leadership abilities. Examples of management positions in nursing are head nurses and charge nurses for specific shifts. In contrast, a leader must possess the ability to direct the actions of others. The leader may or may not hold an official management position within the organization. There are two types of leaders. The formal leader is appointed by the organization and therefore is a manager. The informal leader does not have an official appointment within the organization but nonetheless influences the behaviors of others. If that influence is lost, the person is no longer a leader. In the following discussion on leadership styles, the term "leader" refers to a formal leader who is a manager, but many of the general qualities of leadership styles are true of informal leaders as well.

Leadership style is an important factor influencing

the extent to which a leader is effective. Style in general involves the ways in which something is said or done, including particular behaviors associated with an individual. Leadership style specifically refers to how the leader uses his influence on the group to accomplish goals. Leadership styles, like other behaviors, can be learned, regulated, and developed. Research indicates that no one leadership style is effective in all situations but that each has unique strengths for different situations. The three classical styles of leadership are the authoritarian, democratic, and laissez-faire.

Authoritarian Style

The authoritarian leader retains all authority and responsibility and is concerned primarily with tasks and goal accomplishment. This type of leader assigns people to clearly defined tasks and establishes one-way communication patterns with the group. The authoritarian leader is firm, insistent, self-assured, and dominating. Such a leader stresses prompt, orderly, and predictable performance from employees or followers. The leader displays little trust or confidence in employees, and generally employees are fearful of this type of manager. The authoritarian leader tends to stifle individual initiative and creativity.

The authoritarian leader may also be benevolent and value employees both as people and for their capabilities. This kind of authoritarian leader issues orders but allows employees to comment on them. Employees are permitted some flexibility to carry out their tasks within specific limits and procedures. A benevolent authoritarian leader may give orders, praise employees, demand their loyalty, and make followers feel they are participating in the decision process even though they continue to do as the leader directs. The benevolent authoritarian leader generally has a condescending attitude toward employees, who therefore tend to be cautious when dealing with the leader.

Authoritarian leaders have always been present in nursing. The authoritarian nurse leader manages by giving orders and expecting staff members to accept them without question. The authoritarian manager stresses adherence to hospital policies and procedures. Staff members are expected to conform in nursing practice to the example and direction of the manager (Douglass, 1980).

The authoritarian style of leadership is appropriate in some situations. Some nursing staff members function more productively under the direction of authoritarian leaders because this leadership style meets their needs for security and job satisfaction. In situations when immediate action is required and there is no time for a group decision-making process, the authoritarian leader is able to take action quickly. Authoritarian leaders excel in times of crisis and in situations of disorder; they often can remain calm while others falter. Authoritarian leaders have the reputation for being able to get difficult assignments completed.

Democratic Style

The democratic leadership style is a people-centered approach. The democratic leader allows greater individual participation in the decision-making process. The manager delegates authority but retains ultimate responsibility. The democratic leader maintains active two-way communication that is open, friendly, and trusting with employees.

This style of management enhances employees' personal commitment to the organization through group participation. The manager encourages goal setting by the group. The democratic manager has a sense of responsibility for the good of the group and for individual achievements. The democratic manager uses performance standards to assist the group in knowing job responsibilities rather than to control employees.

In nursing practice, democratic nurse managers have introduced a variety of mechanisms to promote staff involvement in the management of the nursing unit. Some examples are staff involvement in the development of the time schedule, group problem solving through quality control circles, and mutual goal setting during performance appraisals.

Laissez-Faire Style

The last classical leadership style is called laissez-faire. Laissez-faire leadership is also referred to as the free-run style or as permissive leadership. This type of leader denies responsibility and abdicates authority to the group. The laissez-faire manager may simply tell group members to work things out themselves and do the best they can. Communication between the manager and employees is open and lacks control and direction.

The laissez-faire manager wants everyone to feel good, including himself. This management style allows the group to drift aimlessly because the leader provides no direction. The principal management functions, such as decision making, planning, structuring, and controlling organization goals, are carried out by the group.

This style is not generally useful in the health care

system because organization and control are necessary for day-to-day operation. Laissez-faire leadership may be beneficial for employees involved in research projects, however, because self-direction assists in the creative process (Douglass, 1980). This style is probably most beneficial to a staff of highly motivated professionals who have shown the capacity for independent work.

■ ■ ■ ■ ■

There is no one best leadership style. The effectiveness of each of the three classical leadership styles depends on the situation. As the situation changes, the effective manager adapts by changing leadership behaviors. Hersey (1967) concludes about differences in leadership styles, "The more managers adapt their style of leader behaviors to meet the particular situations and the needs of their followers, the more effective they will tend to be in reaching personal and organizational goals."

Situational Leadership

Situational leadership theory best describes the necessary skills for effective leadership in nursing. The effective nurse manager is able to use different leadership styles and skills depending on the specific situation and the maturity of employees. Employees who have limited technical skills or who are unwilling or unable to take responsibility require an authoritarian leader style. With employees who are more skilled or more willing to take responsibility, a democratic management style in which employees participate in decision making can be effective. With the laissez-faire style the leader can allow employees to make decisions, if employees have the skills to handle tasks and are psychologically mature. The nurse manager must diagnose the particular nursing situation to determine which leadership style is most appropriate for which employees to accomplish what specific tasks.

The following example demonstrates how situational leadership styles can be applied. After a hospital institutes a new client classification system, the head nurse uses authority leadership behaviors to tell staff nurses how to use a new classification form. The head nurse cannot use democratic behaviors at this point because the decision to use the new approach has already been made. If some staff members are less mature and resist using the new system, the head nurse uses more authoritarian methods to ensure that they carry out this task. As the nursing staff become more familiar with this new task, the head nurse allows increasing staff participation in working out the details of the new system. With a democratic leadership style the head nurse encourages the group decision-making process to resolve problems within the system. Finally, when this new client classification system is so familiar to all nursing staff that all staff members have demonstrated they have the knowledge and ability to continue using the system without direction from the head nurse, the head nurse can use the laissez-faire style to allow staff nurses to continue with the new system on their own. If problems occur, the head nurse returns to an authoritarian or democratic style as needed to resolve the problem. It is important to note that these shifts in leadership style apply only to the situation of the new client classification system. At the same time the head nurse is using a democratic style to make decisions in this area, she may be using an authoritarian style in another

Primary Leadership Skills for Nurses

SKILLS OF PERSONAL BEHAVIOR

The effective leader:
- Is sensitive to feelings of the group
- Identifies self with the needs of the group
- Listens attentively
- Does not ridicule or criticize another's suggestions
- Helps others feel important and needed
- Does not argue

SKILLS OF COMMUNICATION

The effective leader:
- Makes sure everyone understand what is needed and the reason why
- Establishes positive communication with the group as a routine part of the job
- Recognizes that everyone's contributions are important

SKILLS OF ORGANIZATION

The effective leader helps the group:
- Develop long-range and short-range objectives
- Break big problems into small ones
- Share responsibilities and opportunities
- Plan, act, follow-up, and evaluate
- Be attentive to details

SKILLS OF SELF-EXAMINATION

The effective leader:
- Is aware of personal motivations
- Is aware of group members' level of hostility so that appropriate countermeasures are taken
- Helps the group be aware of their attitudes and values

area, such as ensuring the incorporation of a new standard of care into the nursing practice of staff nurses.

Leadership Skills for Student Nurses

Nursing continues to need new effective leaders in all practice areas. Leadership is most important when changes are occurring in health care, such as the current changes being implemented in financing of the health care system. Changes are coming about in both Medicare and private health care insurance programs (see Chapter 3). For this and other reasons, it is imperative that student nurses begin early to prepare for future leadership and management roles. The box lists skills in four areas that are important for effective leadership and that the student nurse can begin to develop. These skills can be applied by leaders using any leadership style in any situation.

Summary

As the nursing profession and health care agencies become increasingly specialized and complex, the need for effective leadership in nursing is even more important than in the past. Many nursing roles and responsibilities involve group activities, and for a group to function optimally, the leader must be able to motivate and influence the behavior of others. Successful leadership, whether in nursing, business, or other areas of group effort, depends on an effective leadership style. For this reason many theorists have analyzed the components of leadership that result in success. Although these theories do not agree entirely about the components of successful leadership, it is clear that the leader must remain flexible and adapt the leadership style to the particular group situation and goals.

In any situation the nurse in a leadership role needs certain skills, including skills related to personal behavior, communication skills, organization skills, and the skills of self-examination. These are all skills the nursing student can begin to develop while learning other nursing skills. By developing these skills early in their careers, individual nurses will be better prepared to meet the needs for leadership in professional groups, health care agencies, and practice settings.

KEY CONCEPTS

✓ Leadership is the ability to influence the behaviors of others toward the accomplishment of a goal.

✓ Studies of leadership have demonstrated that the effective leader is concerned with both the needs of employees and the needs of the organization.

✓ No single set of personality traits is true of all effective leaders.

✓ Situational leadership theory proposes that the leader should adapt the style of leadership to the needs of the situation.

✓ A leader may or may not have an official appointment within the organization.

✓ A manager has authority and responsibility to enforce decisions and policies of the organization but is not necessarily an effective leader.

✓ The three classical leadership styles are the authoritarian, the democratic, and the laissez-faire.

✓ There is no one best leadership style because effective leaders alter their behaviors to fit the situation.

✓ Leadership style is important in all nursing practice areas just as in other types of organizations.

✓ Leadership skills the nurse can begin to develop while still a student include those of personal behaviors, communication, organization, and self-examination.

REFERENCES

Douglass, L.M.: The effective nurse, St. Louis, 1980, The C.V. Mosby Co.

Drucker, P.F.: The practice of management, New York, 1954, Harper & Row, Publishers, Inc.

Fiedler, F.: A theory of leadership effectiveness, New York, 1967, McGraw-Hill Book Co.

Hersey, P.: Management concepts and behavior: programmed instruction for managers, Little Rock, Ark., 1967, Mancin Publishing Co.

Hersey, P., and Blanchard, K.H.: Management of organizational behavior: utilizing human resources, ed. 3, Englewood Cliffs, N.J., 1977, Prentice-Hall, Inc.

Jennings, E.E.: The anatomy of leadership, Management Personnel Quarterly 1(1):1, 1961.

Likert, R.: New patterns of management, New York, 1961, McGraw-Hill Book Co.

Likert, R.: The human organization, New York, 1967, McGraw-Hill Book Co.

Redden, W.: Managerial effectiveness, New York, 1970, McGraw-Hill Book Co.

Tannenbaum, R., and Schmidt, W.: How to choose a leadership pattern, Harvard Business Review **36**:95, 1958.

ADDITIONAL READINGS

Blake, R.R., and Mouton, J.S.: The new managerial grid, Houston, 1964, Gulf Publishing Co.

Fiedler, F.: Engineer the job to fit the manager, Harvard Business Review **43**:115, 1965.

Fiedler, F.: Responses to Sergiovanni, Educational Leadership **36**:394, 1979.

Grammatteo, M., and Grammatteo, D.: Forces on leadership, Reston, Va., 1981, The National Association of Secondary School Principals.

McMurry, R.: The case for the benevolent autocrat, Harvard Business Review **36**:82, 1958.

Stagdill, R.M., and Coons, A.E., editors: Leader behaviors: its description and measurement, Research Monogr. 88, Columbus, 1957, Bureau of Business Research, The Ohio State University.

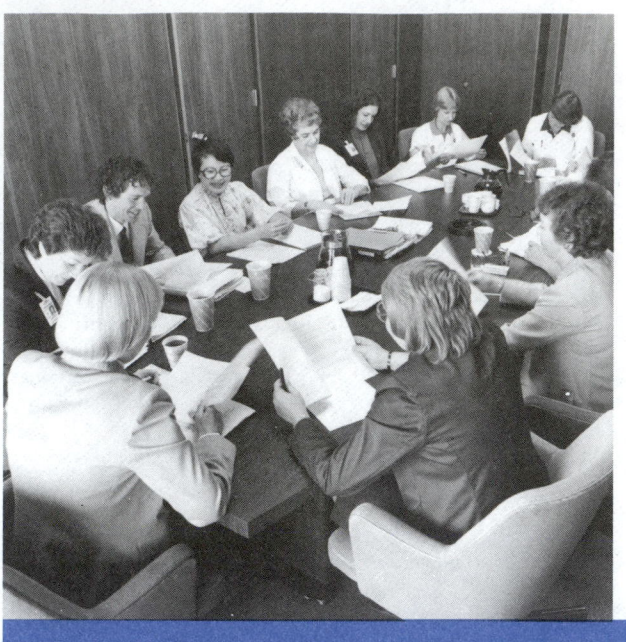

OBJECTIVES

Mastery of content in this chapter will enable the student to:

- Define the terms in the glossary.
- List and compare various ways for acquiring knowledge.
- List the characteristics of scientific investigation.
- Compare methods for developing new knowledge in nursing.
- Define scientific and nursing research.
- Compare the research process to nursing process.
- List ANA priorities for nursing research.
- Explain the rights of human research subjects.
- Explain the rights of others who assist in the conduct of human research studies.
- Describe a typical research report.
- Discuss methods of locating research reports in nursing and related areas.
- Explain how to organize information from a research report.
- List the characteristics of a clinical nursing problem that can be researched.
- List the criteria for using research findings in nursing practice.

GLOSSARY

bias   Prejudice or mental inclination to collect or interpret data according to a person's opinions or beliefs.

citation   Reference notation to the source of an idea or quotation.

comparison group   Group of subjects in a study who are equivalent to the subjects in the experimental group but do not receive the treatment or intervention the study is examining; also known as a control group.

concept   Abstract idea summarized in a word or phrase.

control   To regulate or limit error or distortion of information.

empirical data   Information that has been collected through the human senses and can be verified through research.

experiment   Research study designed to examine a cause-and-effect relationship.

generalization   Application of findings from a research study in a broader situation.

phenomena   Data that can be observed in reality.

primary source   Research report written by an investigator in an original study.

proposition   Statement that defines or explains a relationship between two or more concepts.

random selection   Method of choosing subjects for a research study in which all members of a particular group are equally likely to be included.

research process   Systematic collection and analysis of data to obtain new knowledge, add to existing knowledge, or find solutions to problems.

sample   Portion of a larger group of subjects.

secondary source   Report that interprets research data written by someone not involved in the original research.

statistics   Mathematical science concerned with measuring, classifying, and analyzing objective information.

subjects   People or events selected for a study in order to examine a particular variable or condition.

theory   General statement about relationships among concepts or facts, based on existing information.

50 Research in Nursing Care

For the past two decades many nursing leaders and organizations have made considerable efforts to increase nurses' awareness of the importance of conducting nursing studies and using research as a foundation for nursing practice. In 1974 the American Nurses' Association (ANA) House of Delegates passed a resolution calling for more nursing research to focus on clinical problems that nurses face in professional practice. Until the 1970s nursing studies tended to focus on the roles and characteristics of nurses rather than on problems in delivering professional care to patients (Gortner, 1980). In 1976 the ANA recommended that nursing research be included in baccalaureate, master's degree, and continuing education nursing programs, and in 1981 the ANA published specific recommendations for studying research at the different nursing education levels. The Institute of Medicine's study of nursing (1983) recommended that the federal government increase funds for scientific research in nursing and that steps be taken to establish a national organization that would place nursing research "in the mainstream of scientific investigation." In 1983 the U.S. Congress considered legislation to establish a National Institute of Nursing. The ANA Cabinet on Nursing Research (1983) supported this plan because it seemed to be a realistic, viable way for increasing and stabilizing the funds available for nursing research.

Nursing research is important even for nursing students studying the fundamentals of the profession. The subjects discussed in this chapter should help the student (1) gain an appreciation of the importance of research in furthering the status of nursing as a science, and (2) develop basic skills for understanding and using nursing research to gain knowledge and practice skills.

Scientific Research in Nursing

Acquiring Knowledge

Human beings can acquire knowledge in many ways. A person continually takes in and processes numerous pieces of information to understand experiences. The scientific researcher also seeks to explain or understand reality, but the scientist's process of acquiring knowledge is systematic and logical. This process, referred to as the scientific method, is the foundation of research. Scientific research is the most reliable and objective of all human methods of gaining knowledge.

One way of knowing is through tradition. One generation passes knowledge on to the next. For example, children often learn about traditional holidays such as Christmas and Passover through traditional or customary family practices. In nursing there are certain traditional methods of practice, such as the change-of-shift report and other daily hospital work practices, which are passed from one practitioner to the next. Tradition is an efficient way of knowing, but it can also limit the ability to seek new ways of doing things. If tradition becomes so ingrained that a person does not question the custom, the person may overlook other ways that would be more appropriate or efficient.

Knowledge is also acquired by seeking information from people who are experts in a particular field. Experts are often asked to solve problems or answer questions. For example, at income tax time an accountant's help is sought to fill out tax forms. Similarly, nursing students often seek the advice of instructors and practicing nurses in assessing and caring for clients. Authority, like tradition, is not infallible, although it is commonly treated as absolute truth.

A third way of knowing is by learning through experience. Without this process, a person would have to relearn a procedure every time it was performed. Practice leads to the development of routines that help build skills. For example, a student nurse taking a client's blood pressure for the first time may feel awkward and unsure of hearing the sounds, but with practice the student's technique and confidence improve. While experience is an important way of knowing, it has limitations. A person may continue to do something simply because it was learned that way and may overlook improved or other ways of doing the same thing. If experience prevents the learning of a legitimate improvement, it is being used inappropriately.

Learning by trial and error is yet another way of gaining knowledge. Making mistakes or repeatedly trying various ways of accomplishing something will result in a better way of solving the problems. This method of learning is practical, but it is unsystematic and often a haphazard way of acquiring knowledge. In nursing, because clients' health status depends on nursing actions, trial and error is not an appropriate way of acquiring new knowledge.

The scientific method is the most advanced, objective means of acquiring knowledge. The scientific method is characterized by systematic, orderly procedures that, while not infallible, seek to limit the possibility for error and minimize the likelihood that any bias or opinion by the researcher might influence the results of research and thus the knowledge gained. Polit and Hungler (1983) described the characteristics of scientific investigation as follows:

1. The steps of planning and conducting an investigation are undertaken in a systematic, orderly fashion.
2. Scientists attempt to control exterior factors that can influence a relationship between phenomena they are studying. For example, if a scientist were studying the relationship between diet and heart disease, other characteristics such as stress would have to be eliminated as contributing factors to this disease.
3. Evidence that is part of reality (empirical data) is gathered directly or indirectly through use of the human senses and is the basis for discovering new knowledge.
4. The goal is to understand phenomena in such a way that the knowledge gained can be applied generally, not just to isolated cases or circumstances.
5. Scientists strive to conduct investigations that contribute to testing or developing theories, thereby advancing the knowledge that can be applied toward increasing understanding of people, places, or life events.

Nursing and the Scientific Method

Compared with other ways of acquiring knowledge, the scientific method is more orderly and objective in its approach. Nurses are now increasingly using this approach to develop knowledge. In the past, much of the information used in nursing practice was borrowed from other fields such as biology, physiology, psychology, and sociology. Often this information has been applied in nursing without testing or comparing various ways for caring for clients. For example, nurses use several different methods to help clients sleep. Interventions such as giving a client a backrub, making sure the bed is clean and comfortable, preparing the environment by dimming the lights, and talking to a client who is worried or anxious are frequently used nursing measures, and in general these are logical, common-sense approaches. However, when these measures are considered in greater depth, questions may arise about their applications for different clients in different situations. Will all these approaches work with all clients at all times? If not, why not? Which ones are more effective and why? In what order should a nurse try these various nursing interventions to promote sleep? How can the nurse know which interventions are appropriate for certain clients? What are the sleep problems clients with a particular health care problem tend to experience? These are some of the questions that can be raised about sleeping difficulties and the nursing measures that might be appropriate to promote sleep. Through research these questions could be studied in greater depth. At the present time nurses generally rely on personal experience with helping patients sleep or what nursing experts say should work. If an intervention works for most clients, the nurse may be satisfied with this success without questioning if there might be a better way. If the intervention is not successful, the nurse might resort to trial and error by trying different approaches or a different sequence of accepted measures to promote sleep. Even if an intervention discovered with this approach is effective for one or more clients, however, the questions raised above about applications for other clients in other settings still remain.

Definitions of Scientific and Nursing Research

According to Kerlinger (1973), "scientific research is systematic, controlled, empirical and critical investigation of hypothetical propositions about the presumed relations among natural phenomena." When scientists use systematic, controlled methods for studying events or problems, they can have greater confidence that what has been observed is accurate rather than influenced by opinion or belief. For a study to be empirical, the evidence collected must come from objective findings. Other researchers should be able to examine the evidence and see the same phenomena as the original investigator. To guide the design of a research study, scientists make a hypothetical proposition about they expect to see before conducting the study. Finally, scientists generally study how characteristics or events are related to one another. A relationship may mean that an attribute changes as another changes, but this does not necessarily mean that a change in one attribute causes a change in the other. For example, as people get older they tend to lose their hair and their skin becomes wrinkled. Hair loss and skin wrinkles are related to each other as part of the aging process, but this does not necessarily mean that either factor causes the other to occur. Both these changes are associated with the aging process, but what causes aging is not known. Scientists can and do study how attributes or events cause other things to happen, as well as other kinds of relationships. Yet when reading research studies, it is important to avoid inappropriately interpreting results in terms of cause and effect, because there is a difference between cause-and-effect relationships and other kinds of relationships. Researchers often study how changes in attributes are related to each other without being able to determine why or how these changes take place.

The Commission on Nursing Research of the ANA (1981) has defined nursing research as follows:

Nursing research develops knowledge about health and the promotion of health over the full lifespan, care of persons with health problems and disabilities, and nursing actions to enhance the ability of individuals to respond effectively to actual or potential health problems.

Biomedical research is concerned mainly with discovering what causes disease and how it should be treated. In contrast, nursing research is directed toward helping well people improve their health status and stay healthy, as well as assisting clients who are sick or disabled by an illness. Nursing also focuses on the full range of human responses rather than only the biological or physical ones. For example, the effect(s) of preoperative teaching on postoperative recovery is an area of nursing that has been studied extensively. Some studies (Schmidt and Wooldridge, 1973; Wolfer and Davis, 1970) have examined the emotional reaction of clients to a surgical experience, such as postoperative anxiety and fear, as well as physiological responses such as the return to usual oral intake and urinary retention. Teaching clients what they can expect on the day of surgery and in the immediate postoperative period is now an accepted nursing measure that is widely implemented in nursing practice. Such teaching often includes, for example, information about how often their vital signs will be monitored after surgery and the deep breathing and coughing techniques they will be asked to perform. This information is provided to relieve clients' fear and anxiety and to help them recover from surgery.

Since nurses are interested in acquiring knowledge about a wide range of human needs and responses to health problems, nursing research uses various methods to study clinical problems. The hallmark of scientific research is the experiment. In a true experimental study the conditions under which a measure is investigated are tightly controlled. Usually the study includes a comparison or control group that does not receive the nursing measure being investigated. The results for this group are compared with those of a study or experimental group that does receive some form of treatment or intervention. The subjects selected for the comparison and experimental groups are chosen at random from among those eligible for the study. Designing an experiment to study physical causes of disease is less difficult than designing an investigation that also includes psychological or social aspects of health. For example, to study the relationship between postoperative anxiety and preoperative teaching, the researcher can control one psychological factor by using only subjects having surgery for the first time. However, the researcher cannot control other experiences the clients may have had, such as hearing a friend's "horror" stories about surgery or reading about surgical experiences in the newspapers. These psychological factors that cannot be controlled may influence the subject client's level of anxiety.

Nursing studies use various methods for investigating clinical problems, some of which may be similar to the experimental approach. Other methods may be similar to those used in the social sciences such as anthropology and sociology. The actual problem being investigated is one of the factors that determine which method is appropriate. To the extent that the particular problem allows, a study strives to follow the criteria of scientific investigation described earlier.

Nursing Research and the Nursing Process

The research process (Seaman and Verhonick, 1982) consists of phases or steps that can be compared to and contrasted with those of the nursing process. Both are problem-solving processes used by nurses in practice (Table 50-1). The two processes are very different, however, because the nursing process is used to determine health needs and structure nursing care for individual clients. The nursing process is employed as a basis for gaining and using information about clients to help them restore, maintain, or promote their health. Depending on the nursing diagnosis, knowledge from a variety of disciplines may be used in the nursing process to help clients solve particular health problems.

In contrast, the research process is used to gain knowledge that can be used in other similar situations. Nurses may want to gain knowledge about why a particular event happens or the best way to provide care for a group of clients with a certain health problem. The research process is used to gain knowledge that can be applied to a whole group or class of clients.

In the assessment step the nurse caring for a client with sleeping difficulties would determine what factors are present that might interfere with the client's ability to sleep. Is the client concerned about his health status? Is the client experiencing pain? Is the environment noisy? Is the bed messy or uncomfortable? After assessing these aspects the nurse determines a nursing diagnosis, plans interventions, implements these interventions, and evaluates the subjective and objective evidence that indicates whether or not the patient is now able to sleep.

In contrast, a researcher studying sleeping difficulties is interested in gaining new information that can be applied to more than one client. For example, a nurse notices that many clients seem to have a difficult time sleeping the night before a particular diagnostic procedure. Based on work with these clients, the nurse determines that most of them express concerns about what the test may discover. In this situation the nurse might design a research study in which some of the clients receive the usual nursing care and others receive a different approach that is based on relieving clients' anxiety about the procedure. After collecting information about the effects of the usual care for one group and the new approach for the other, the nurse researcher compares the results to determine if the clients who received the new care had less difficulty sleeping than those who received the normal nursing care. If the clients receiving the new care slept better, the nurse has acquired new knowledge about how *generally* to help clients sleep better who are undergoing the diagnostic procedure.

TABLE 50-1

Comparison of Phases in the Nursing Process and the Research Process

Phases in Nursing Process	Phases in Research Process*
Assessment	Identify the research problem
	Formulate a summary of the proposed research
	Define concepts and variables to be studied
Diagnosis	State hypotheses about expected observations
Planning	Determine ethical implications of the proposed study
	Review the literature for theory and other related studies
	Identify assumptions and limitations
	Describe the research design and methods
	Plan for communicating findings
Intervention	Collect data from subjects
Evaluation	Analyze and interpret data
	Communicate findings in written and other forms

*Data from Seaman, C.H., and Verhonick, P.J.: Research methods for undergraduate students in nursing, ed. 2, Norwalk, Conn., 1982, Appleton-Century-Crofts.

Nurse Researchers

In 1981 the ANA published the following list of priorities for nursing research:

1. Promoting health, well-being, and competency for personal care among all age groups
2. Preventing health problems throughout the life span that have the potential to reduce productivity and satisfaction
3. Decreasing the negative impact of health problems on coping abilities, productivity, and life satisfaction of individuals and families
4. Ensuring that the care needs of particularly vulnerable groups are met through appropriate strategies
5. Designing and developing health care systems that are cost effective in meeting the nursing needs of the population

6. Promoting health, well-being, and competency for personal health in all age groups

These priorities demonstrate to nurses, other health care professionals, and the general public what the profession sees as important areas in which nurses need further knowledge to improve the services they provide. These priorities can be used by researchers to develop research projects, by funding agencies to set priorities for funding research, and by student nurses to help determine whether to participate in a research project when asked to do so.

Nurses conduct research in a variety of settings. Both student nurses and practitioners may be asked to participate in research that investigates the effectiveness of nursing care. This type of research is commonly called quality assurance. Data are collected to determine what impact nurses are having on achievement of client care objectives in a particular clinical setting. Because the results of such research are usually applicable only in one institution, this is not scientific research as discussed earlier. However, such research is important to the institution because the nursing department can use it to demonstrate the contributions made by nurses to patient care.

Clinical nursing research should be undertaken by nurses who are trained to conduct scientific investigations. Generally nurse researchers hold master's and doctoral degrees. A student nurse who is asked to participate in a nursing study as a subject or by collecting data is entitled to receive information about the qualifications of the person who is conducting the study. The researcher's educational background and biographical sketch give some information about the person's qualifications for conducting research. Usually an experienced researcher is more qualified to undertake a complex, long-term project than a beginning researcher. Nurses who are new to research may, however, make an important contribution by conducting less complex studies investigating important nursing problems (Seaman and Verhonick, 1982).

Ethical Issues in Research

Rights of Human Subjects

In order to refine existing knowledge and develop new knowledge, clinical research is sometimes directed toward trying new procedures whose outcome is doubtful or unknown (American Nurses' Association, 1975). This kind of research may contrast with the purpose of nursing practice, which is to meet specific clients' needs. In such cases the researcher is responsible for structuring the investigation in such a way that harm to the subjects is avoided or minimized. Although it is not always possible to anticipate all potential undesirable effects, researchers are obligated to inform everyone involved about the potential risks. Other basic human rights must also be observed when people are involved as subjects in a study. These principles, as set forth by the Canadian Nurses' Association (CNA), are outlined on p. 1434.

Informed consent means that research subjects are (1) given full and complete information about the purpose of the study, procedures, how data will be collected, potential harm and benefits, and alternative methods of treatment; (2) capable of fully understanding the research and the implications of participation; and (3) assured of free choice in giving their consent, including the right to withdraw from the study at any time. Procedures for obtaining informed consent must be outlined in the study protocol.

Confidentiality means that the privacy of subjects will be respected. Anonymity is often used to ensure privacy, and if anonymity is promised, it must be respected.

In addition, the researcher planning to conduct a study must possess the knowledge and skills necessary to undertake the research. Current ANA and CNA guidelines state that qualified nurse researchers have a right to engage in research and a right of access to resources needed to conduct studies.

In the United States any agency that receives federal funds must have an institutional review board (Armiger, 1977). This group reviews all studies being conducted in the institution to ensure that the ethical principles described above are being observed. Not all research undertaken in clinical areas involves experimentation with human subjects. Research that does not use a new treatment with subjects may involve minimal or no risk to clients. Nonetheless, a major responsibility of the institutional board is to determine the risk status of all research projects.

Rights of Other Research Participants

Student nurses and practicing nurses may be asked to participate in research as data collectors or may be involved in the care of clients participating in a study. All participants have the right to be fully informed about the study, its procedures, including informed consent and risk factors, and any physical or emotional injury that clients could experience as a result of their participation. Often the physical risks are more obvious than those of an emotional nature. Depending on the problem area being studied, clients may be asked to give information that is highly personal and intrusive. Because participating in this type of research can lead to anxiety or stress for some

Canadian Nurses' Association Ethics of Nursing Research

THE SUBJECT

Respect for the value of human life, for the worth and dignity of human beings, and their rights to knowledge, privacy, and self-determination must underlie research practices in nursing as in other health disciplines. The legitimacy of involving human subjects in nursing research must be assessed within the context of these values. The right of the subject to informed consent, confidentiality, positive risk value, and competence of the investigator must be assured.

Free and Informed Consent

When individuals are involved as subjects of research, the researcher must obtain free and informed consent. Informed consent implies that every effort be made to have the subject understand the purpose and nature of the research and the use or usages to which the findings will be put, in such a way that he can appreciate the implications of participation or non-participation. He must also be informed that if any significant change in purpose, nature, or use of findings is contemplated, he will also be informed and have the right to consent or refuse to participate further.

Free consent means that the relationship between the researcher and the subject, and persons or institutions involved in his care will not place him under any obligation to agree or take part in the project against his own personal inclinations. It also means that his refusal to take part, or his withdrawal after having once consented, should not lead to any repercussions or recriminations. Free consent implies informing the subject that he has the right to withdraw at any point during the research.

If the nature of the research is such that fully informing subjects before the study would invalidate results, then this fact must be stated to the subject, together with whatever explanations can be given. There must be provision for appropriate explanation to the subject on completion of the study.

If the subject for any reason is unable to appreciate the implications of participation, informed consent must be obtained from the legal guardian or an impartial committee acting on behalf of the subject. If the research should impinge on the privacy or other rights of any third party, such as the spouse of the subject, this person's consent must also be obtained.

Confidentiality

Subjects must be assured that confidentiality will be respected. Where anonymity is promised, it must be provided. Hidden coding to enable the researcher to identify individuals must not be resorted to. Every effort must be made to ensure that individuals and institutions cannot be identified.

Injury, Risk, and Priorities

Research subjects must be assured protection against physical, mental or emotional injury. Should the research involve risk of injury, such risks must be weighed against the good to be achieved. Should the risk outweigh the positive value of the research, the project must not be pursued.

Where there is conflict between the rights of the subject and the needs of the researcher for freedom of inquiry, the conflict must be resolved with priority given to the concerns and rights of the subject.

THE RESEARCHER

In order to maintain high ethical standards, the nurse researcher must possess knowledge and skills compatible with the demands of the investigation to be undertaken. The researcher has responsibility to acknowledge personal limitations and to correct misrepresentations made by others. The researcher is obligated to develop the design and procedures appropriate to the study.

The researcher is accountable in varying ways to those participating in the investigation. The purpose of the research must be honestly represented, and any uses to which the findings may be put, made known to persons or institutions involved. In order to justify the investigation, the researcher must ensure that the purposes and anticipated outcomes are compatible with the financial investment and the people and resources used.

In order to ensure the integrity of the investigation, the researcher must present the project for review to a group of professional peers. With certain studies, ongoing reviews by a peer group may be mandatory.

THE SETTING

The milieu in which an investigation is to be conducted, must be assessed in terms of the potential for a nurse researcher to conduct a study that is consistent with these guidelines. While the board and/or administrators of an institution or agency may require approval by its research committee of a nursing study as well as of any other proposal, any such approval body should include nursing representation. There should be ongoing provisions for coping with setting-related ethical problems during the course of the investigation.

Nurse researchers ought to be the principal investigators in the study of nursing problems and must be collaborators with other researchers in the study of interprofessional problems of health care. This interprofessional involvement indicates that a common code of ethics for health research should be developed to facilitate research in nursing and its related professions.

From Canadian Nurses' Association: Can. Nurse **68**:23, 1972.

clients, the researcher should prepare all participants, including nurses who are delivering care, for this possibility and assist them in coping with the effects. Participants also have the right to see review forms from the institutional review board certifying that the study has been approved. Any student, nurse, or other participant has the right to refuse to carry out any research procedures if concerned about ethical aspects of the study.

Besides dealing with the harmful effects of a research project, nurses may be faced with other ethical dilemmas (Brink and Wood, 1983). For instance, some clients may feel they have to participate in an investigation to please the health care professionals on whom they depend for care. They may feel that they will receive inferior care if they refuse to participate. Research ethics require that clients not be made to feel that they are obliged to participate in a study. The ultimate decision rests with the client. Withholding proper care from clients who refuse to participate is unethical.

Another ethical dilemma in research involves withholding a new intervention from clients who might benefit from its use. In an experiment investigating a new intervention, for example, the experimental group may receive the new intervention while the comparison group receives the usual care. In such cases comparison group clients are deprived of a new treatment that could be beneficial to them. One way of managing this dilemma is to offer the new nursing care to the comparison group after data necessary to the experimental study have been collected.

Using Research in Nursing Practice

Identifying Research Studies

When reading nursing literature, the practicing or student nurse must be able to differentiate a research report or article from other types of writing. This may not be as simple as it seems; even if the title has the word research in it, the article does not necessarily report the results of a research study. The nurse can determine whether an article reports a research study only by examining its contents.

Sometimes, however, an article's title can give a clue to its contents. Phrases such as "a study of" or "comparison of" suggest that it may be a research report. The abstract and the introductory paragraphs of an article can also indicate whether the article is based on research. The abstract is a short summary of the purpose of a study, the subjects included in the research, how the study was conducted, and the results obtained in the investigation. An abstract is often

very brief and does not contain all the essential information from the article. The first few paragraphs of the article should provide further clues about whether it describes a research study. Phrases such as "the purpose of this study was" and "this research was carried out to determine" are indications that the article is a research report. If the article describes only the author's *experience* with a particular aspect of nursing care, it probably is not a research article.

A typical research report (1) includes an introductory section that presents the purpose, a summary of literature used to formulate the study, and the hypotheses that were tested; (2) describes the methods used to conduct the study, including the sample (what or who was studied), and to collect data, including the device or instrument used to measure empirical information; (3) describes the results obtained in the study, including statistical tests used to analyze data; and (4) presents the author's interpretation of the results, including conclusions and implications that can be drawn from the study. If the report is written by one of the researchers in the study, it is a primary source. Any other article about the study is considered a secondary source, in which the author was not directly involved in conducting the study but collected the information from a primary or another secondary source. Most nursing textbooks are secondary sources of information. Authors of these texts incorporate knowledge and information gathered from nursing and related literature, including research written by original investigators.

The fact that a report is a primary source does not guarantee that it is accurate. Accuracy depends on the ability of researchers to be scientific, impersonal, and impartial in conducting studies. However, a primary source does report firsthand knowledge, whereas secondary sources may include another person's interpretation of the original work.

Finding Research Studies

Students and practicing nurses often need to find research articles on subjects in which they are interested. In the health care field a number of resources are useful when searching the literature for research articles.

To find primary research sources related to a particular subject, the first source is the journals where original research reports are usually published. The most efficient way to locate research articles is to consult an index of journal articles. The *Cumulative Index to Nursing and Allied Health Literature*, published bimonthly, contains listings from approximately 250 English language nursing and allied health journals. The *International Nursing Index*, published four times a year, contains listings from over 200 nursing journals from around the world. *Index Medicus,* an international index that is published monthly, includes listings from approximately 2200 biomedical journals, including about 60 nursing journals. The *Hospital Literature Index,* published quarterly, contains listings from journals dealing with planning and providing health care programs and services. These indexes are generally found in reference sections of medical and nursing libraries. Information about which indexes are available in a particular library is available from the reference librarian.

Using these indexes can save time in finding articles. Each index uses a list of key words that form subject headings and subheadings under which article listings are grouped or organized. An author listing is also available, making it possible to find articles published during a certain time period by a particular person. Articles on a particular subject are found by first checking the subject headings to see if the key term listed in the index matches the subject. The key term listing may also lead to other subject groupings in the index that contain articles similar in meaning to the original subject. Using an index may at first seem time consuming, but in the long run it saves time, since the alternative is paging through journals trying to find articles pertinent to the subject.

Many nursing and medical libraries provide computerized searches for articles. MEDLINE, for example, is a system available in many libraries for locating research materials. Information in this system is retrieved from *Index Medicus* and the *International Nursing Index.* A list of articles and abstracts is transmitted over telephone lines within hours of being requested. Computer searches generally involve a user's fee. Reference librarians generally have information about this type of resource.

The major nursing journals that publish research studies include *Nursing Research, Research in Nursing and Health,* and *Western Journal of Research in Nursing.* Although not all articles published in these journals are research reports, most issues are devoted to primary reports of nursing studies. Other nursing journals also publish original reports of research studies. For instance, *Heart & Lung,* a specialty journal published under the auspices of the American Association of Critical-Care Nurses, often includes research reports. As mentioned previously, it is important to determine whether an article is a research report.

Secondary literature sources such as books can be helpful in finding primary research sources. Nursing students seeking research articles often overlook reference lists or bibliographies at the end of textbook chapters. To document the scientific basis for their writing, authors frequently cite primary sources as references, and these references are a valuable resource for nursing students who want more information.

Another secondary resource that is helpful in finding primary nursing research articles is the *Annual Review of Nursing Research.* Each volume is devoted to certain topics; for example, the 1983 edition (Werley and Fitzpatrick, 1983) contains a chapter on death and dying written by Jean Quint Benoliel, a prominent nurse researcher in this area. A review can be helpful in determining the current status of research on a topic and can direct the reader toward other primary research sources. Research reviews are relatively new in nursing.

Organizing Information from a Research Study

Articles listed in a bibliography or reference section are called citations. A citation provides the author's name and information about where *ideas* or *quotations* were originally published. Writers are ethically obligated to give credit to others whose thoughts are used, even if the original author's exact words are not quoted.

There are many ways to list a citation. One format widely used in nursing literature is the style recommended by the American Psychological Association (1983). This format has the advantage of avoiding footnotes; all citations are arranged alphabetically at the end of the report. Schools of nursing use various formats, however, and nursing students should determine which citation format is currently being used in their own school. Listing citations according to the recommended guidelines prevents the problem of incomplete citations.

A book citation includes author name(s), date of publication, title, edition if appropriate, place of publication, and publisher. Journal citations include author name(s), date of publication, title of article, name of the journal in which the article appeared, volume number, and the exact page numbers of the article. The page number should also be noted with direct quotations from either a book or journal article. The order of this information in the citation, the punctuation used, and the use of underlining and quotation marks depend on the particular format.

The use of index cards for recording information helps in maintaining consistency and accuracy in record keeping. One card is used for notations about each article. Besides the complete citation, other categories of information should be noted for future use of the research study as a foundation for nursing practice. These categories include (1)*when* the study was

Sample Bibliography Card

WHEN

Walike, B.C. & Walike, J.W. (1977). Relative lactose intolerance: A clinical study of tube-fed patients. *Journal of American Medical Association, 238*, 948-951.

WHAT Lactose intolerance of tube-fed patients.

HOW Consistency, frequency and composition of stools; body weight; selected blood studies including electrolyte levels, protein, glucose, cholesterol, total bilirubin, and BUN; 24-hour urine studies; glucose tolerance test; lactose tolerance test; symptoms of gastrointestinal distress.

WHO 20 white patients between the ages of 46 and 74 receiving both lactose and lactose-free nasogastric tube feedings after head or neck surgery for cancer; 4 patients were dropped from the study due to complications unrelated to tube feeding.

WHERE Inpatient hospital clinical research unit (14 patients) in Seattle, WA; location of 6 patients not stated.

RESULTS Significant differences in stool frequency and consistency were found for patients on tube feeding diets that contained lactose (milk sugar) when compared to how these same patients tolerated lactose-free diets. Nine patients also experienced at least one other symptom of gastrointestinal distress. Lactose intolerance is relative and should be viewed in relation to both increased amount and ability of the intestines to breakdown milk sugar.

"The results indicate that lactose should be reduced or eliminated from tube-feeding diets to improve patient tolerance and comfort and to reduce diarrhea." (p. 948)

---

conducted; (2) *what* problem area was studied; (3) *how* information and data were collected; (4) the subjects *who* were included in the study; (5) *where* the study was conducted, including type of setting and geographical region; and (6) a brief summary of the *results,* including major findings and conclusions of the study. Any direct quotation from the report should be noted on the index card with quotation marks and the exact page number on which the quotation appears. For a sample bibliography card, see the box.

The date of publication gives an approximation of the time when the study was conducted. Sometimes researchers define the exact time period in the article, because a considerable time, as long as 2 years, may pass between the time a study was completed and the time of publication. Noting when a study was conducted allows tracing the development of knowledge in a particular area.

In nursing, many kinds of clinical problems can be studied. Knowing exactly *what* was studied involves information about the various topics that have been investigated by nurse researchers. Studies undertaken in a particular problem area can then be evaluated.

There are often many ways to investigate a particular research problem. Knowing *how* researchers studied a question helps in the evaluation of how thoroughly aspects of the problem have been investigated.

A major purpose of scientific research is to increase knowledge about general classes of people or events. Knowing *who* the subjects were in a research study gives information about to whom the conclusions may be applied. When similar results are obtained with different groups of clients, nurses can be more confident in applying the conclusions to other groups of clients.

Nursing care is provided for clients in varying circumstances. Knowing *where* the research was undertaken can influence whether the results might apply in a different setting or region. This information is particularly relevant for research involving psychosocial aspects of nursing care. Different regions of the country have unique traditions and customs. Nursing interventions that are appropriate for people with certain specific attitudes and beliefs may not be relevant in regions or settings where clients differ substantially in attitudes and beliefs.

A summary of the results concerns what has or has not been demonstrated in a particular problem area. When the findings and conclusions reached are similar in a number of research studies, the conclusions are considered more significant than in the case of an isolated research project. The effects of preoperative teaching on the postoperative recovery of clients is an example of a problem area in which the collective evidence provides a reasonable scientific foundation for nursing practice.

■ ■ ■ ■ ■

This section on identifying, finding, and organizing information from research studies is intended as an introduction. Many books and journal articles published in nursing and related disciplines provide more detailed information about reading and evaluating research studies. Learning to find and read nursing research studies is not a simple task, but nursing research is based on principles of logic, and with a thoughtful approach the nursing student can learn to understand and evaluate nursing research studies.

Identifying Clinical Nursing Problems

Diers (1979) defines a clinical nursing problem as "a difference between two states of affairs, a discrepancy between the way things are and the way they ought to be, or between what one knows and what one needs to know to eliminate the problem." The question raised in this definition is that, given the current nursing interventions recommended for a group of clients, how might the suggested care be improved so the results are better for the clients? Given the present knowledge about how to provide nursing care, what additional information would be needed to plan new interventions for clients with a particular health care problem?

Experience can make it possible to identify a researchable clinical nursing problem. A nurse does not need to have completed years of clinical practice to identify a nursing problem; sometimes a person who is relatively new in a situation can more easily see how things could be improved than others with longer experience who take present conditions for granted. The nurse also needs to consider whether the problem frequently occurs in a particular client group, whether it can be consistently and accurately measured, and whether there is a possible solution that might change how nursing care is delivered (Fuller, 1982).

Sometimes nursing students or practicing nurses think their ideas about nursing problems for study are not worthwhile unless they are certain in advance that the proposed clinical study would make a radical change in client care. Research efforts also may have to refine ideas about a clinical problem before the investigator can test alternative nursing interventions. The researcher may have to spend time devising correct ways for measuring the results before the actual experiment can be undertaken. All these factors may discourage a nurse from undertaking a nursing re-

search project. On the other hand, they can be viewed as stimulating challenges because much information has yet to be scientifically tested for its relevance to nursing practice.

The series of studies by Dr. Barbara Walike Hansen and associates to investigate tube feeding problems illustrates how research can progress from the phase of clinical problem refinement to the testing of new nursing measures. An early study (Walike et al., 1974) documented the need for further research into tube feeding procedures and how clients are affected by this method of meeting nutritional needs. As a result of this early work, a variety of factors associated with clients' responses to tube feedings were identified, including (1) tube location for proper formula administration; (2) temperature, volume, and rate of formula administration; (3) the attitudes and adjustments of clients toward tube feeding procedures; and (4) the nutritional contents and gastrointestinal responses of clients to tube feeding. The researchers then performed further research into these various aspects of caring for people who receive tube feedings.

Determining the proper insertion length for a nasogastric tube so it is located properly in the stomach is a topic frequently covered in nursing texts. Hanson (1979, 1980) described an improved method for determining the proper length of insertion. The new measurement method, as compared with the traditional ear–to–nose–to–xiphoid process technique, increased the likelihood that the tube would be properly located in the body or fundus of the stomach from 72% to 91% (Hanson, 1979).

The temperature, volume, and rate of administration of tube-feeding formula are regulated and monitored by nurses. The effects of cold, room, and warm (body) temperature feedings on gastrointestinal function have been reported by Kugawa-Busby and Associates (1980). In this study, normal volunteer subjects tolerated room-temperature feedings as well as they tolerated warmed formula. Some subjects experienced cramping and diarrhea 6 to 9 hours after receiving cold feedings. No differences were reported in gastric motility based on the three formula temperatures. The volume and rate of administering feedings to normal volunteer subjects were found to be related to subjective symptoms of gastrointestinal distress (Heitkemper et al., 1981). The recommended rate for tube feeding in this study was less than 60 ml per minute for the usual volume feeding of 250 ml. When larger volumes (up to 750 ml per feeding) were needed to meet nutritional needs, subjects were able to tolerate this amount when administered at a rate of 30 ml per minute. Six of the 14 subjects experienced nausea or abdominal discomfort with the initial (first) feeding; tolerance improved with subsequent formula administrations.

Two additional studies investigated the distressful objective and subjective symptoms experienced by tube-fed clients. The first study (Padilla et al., 1979) described the psychosensory irritations and deprivations commonly experienced by 30 clients. Sensory irritations included dry mouth, sore throat, and thirst. Deprivation of taste when chewing and swallowing food were reported by these clients as being distressful. A follow-up study (Padilla et al., 1981) explored the effects on reducing client distress of four different ways of providing clients with information about tube feeding procedures. The teaching intervention most effective for subjects in this study was one that provided sensory information about the procedure, as well as information about coping behaviors to increase comfort during and after feeding tube insertion. This latter study also examined the relationship between clients' perception of control and level of distress. Clients who perceived that they had control over their environment and behavior did not express less distress than clients who perceived that they had no control over the situation.

Results of an additional study (Walike and Walike, 1977) dealing with the effects of lactose (milk sugar) on stool frequency and consistency are shown in the box on p. 1437. As a result of this research, commercially prepared tube-feeding formulas that do not contain lactose are now available. One problem in this study was the difficulty experienced by Dr. Hansen (Hansen, 1984) in finding a reliable and uniform way to measure stool consistency. The investigators found that the nurses used "very creative and imaginative descriptions" to describe the characteristics of stool, and these descriptions differed among the nurses who participated in data collection. A stool consistency rating form (Fig. 50-1) was developed to group nurses' descriptions into nine categories. The actual water content of stools in each category was analyzed to confirm these categories objectively. At the time of the study, only one rating form for stool consistency of infant meconium existed in the research literature. The experience of these investigators in having to develop a reliable, valid way for measuring a human phenomenon is common among nursing researchers. Much of nursing practice deals with identifying and describing human responses to health care problems that have not been sufficiently defined and classified to permit general agreement among nurses about observations.

These articles represent a sample of the research that has been conducted by the Tube Feeding Consortium Group. Through collaborative efforts (Bergstrom et al., 1984), the group studied a large number

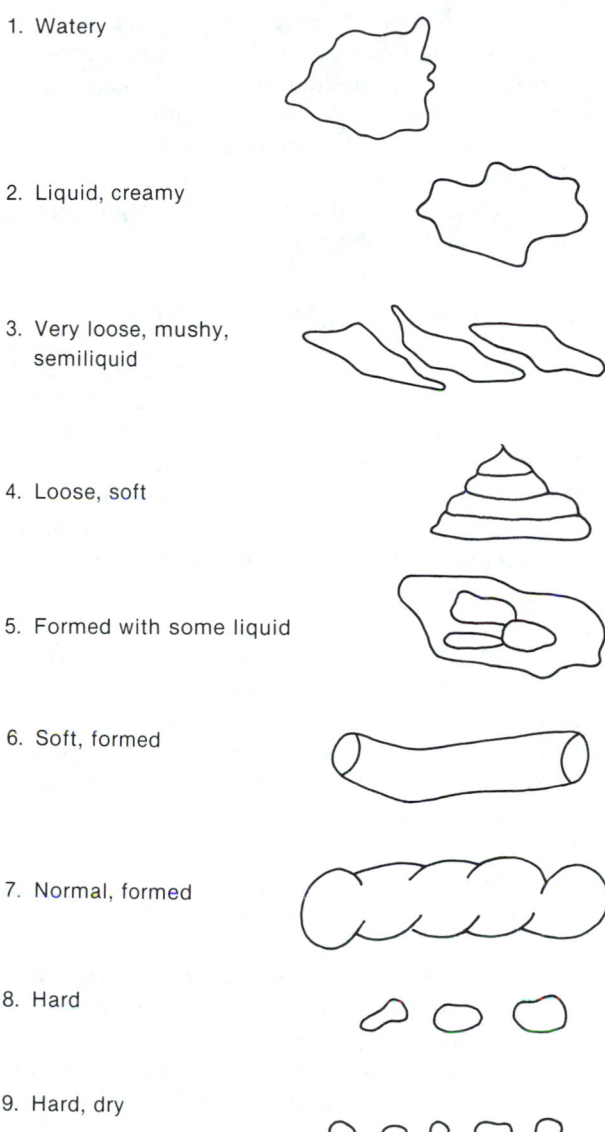

1. Watery

2. Liquid, creamy

3. Very loose, mushy, semiliquid

4. Loose, soft

5. Formed with some liquid

6. Soft, formed

7. Normal, formed

8. Hard

9. Hard, dry

Fig. 50-1   Stool consistency diagram.

Modified from Horsley, J.A., Crane, J., and Haller, K.B.: Reducing diarrhea in tube-fed patients, CURN project, New York, 1981, Grune & Stratton, Inc.

of subjects in various locations to improve the generalizability of findings. The clinical nursing problems addressed in these various studies involve aspects of care with which nurses must deal in everyday practice. Client safety might be improved, for example, if the new method for determining length of inserting a feeding tube were widely used in professional nursing practice. The problem of diarrhea of clients receiving tube feedings can be eliminated by changing the contents of the tube-feeding formula. In the past, this has been a significant nursing problem, especially with clients who are bedridden or have a decreased level of consciousness. The scientific foundation on which decisions about the nursing care of tube-fed patients can be based has been strengthened by the work of the Tube Feeding Consortium Group. It is interesting that these studies originated in questions about procedures and clients' responses to a common nursing measure. The results of these studies did not lead to the invention of a completely new nursing intervention, but there has been a substantial improvement in nursing care for tube-fed patients.

Using Findings in Nursing Practice

To use research findings in clinical practice, the nurse must be aware of what problems have been studied. Therefore nurses should read journals in nursing and related fields that contain research reports, as well as textbooks and other sources.

Not all research related to clinical nursing problems can or should be applied in practice. The nurse must judge the scientific worth of a study before considering its use in nursing practice. This chapter can provide only a foundation for judging the worth of a research study. Other aspects that should be considered are as follows (Stetler and Marram, 1976):

1. How much substantiating evidence is provided by other scientific studies that have obtained similar results
2. Whether the subjects and environment in the study are similar to the patients for whom the nurse provides care in the particular practice setting
3. The theoretical basis for present nursing care and the effectiveness of current theory in solving clinical nursing problems
4. The feasibility of applying findings, including ethical and legal limitations, institutional policy, changes in the organization of nursing services that might be required, and potential costs in time, money, and equipment

As these considerations suggest, nurses should not change from accepted to unproven ways of providing client care without careful deliberation and consultation with their colleagues. Experimenting with new nursing measures is inappropriate, especially if there may be an increased risk to the health of clients.

Some people estimate that the half-life of knowledge in the health care field is about 5 years. This means that about half of what a nurse learns today may be out of date in 5 years. By developing the skills necessary to read and understand nursing research studies, nurses can remain current throughout their professional nursing careers.

Summary

Research is an essential part of the nursing profession because it is an advanced, objective method of gaining new knowledge about human needs and physiological and psychosocial responses to illness, treatments and therapies, and other health-related factors. The nursing research process, a problem-solving method, involves a number of phases from the identification of the problem to be researched, through the development and testing or hypotheses, to the analysis, interpretation, and communication of findings. To gain new knowledge in a variety of nursing areas, nurses conduct clinical research in many different settings, involving many kinds of research subjects whose rights the nurse must carefully protect.

Nurses not directly involved in conducting research also gain from nursing research findings relevant to their study and practice. Nurses therefore must develop skills for finding and identifying research studies and for organizing information from research for clinical application. Successful use of research findings in nursing practice depends on the skills of judging the scientific worth of a study, determining the similarity of the practice setting and clients to those in the study, and considering practical issues such as ethical implications, institutional policies, and implementation costs. These skills are important for all nurses because of continually evolving nursing knowledge about skills used in all practice settings.

KEY CONCEPTS

✓ People acquire knowledge through tradition, from authorities in a particular field, through experience, by trial and error, and through application of the scientific method.

✓ The scientific method is the most objective method of gaining new knowledge.

✓ A scientific investigation is an orderly, planned, and controlled way of studying reality that can be applied to general situations and contributes to the testing of theories about people, places, or life events.

✓ Nursing research is conducted to study the physical or psychosocial responses of people of all ages in both health and illness.

✓ An experimental research study controls undesirable factors that could influence the results, includes both a comparison and an experimental treatment group of subjects, and uses a random means for selecting study subjects.

✓ The nursing process is a systematic method for providing nursing care for specific clients.

✓ The research process is a systematic means for gaining knowledge about how to provide care for a group of people with a particular health care problem.

✓ Participation of human subjects in research studies requires the researcher to obtain informed consent of study subjects, to maintain the confidentiality of subjects, and to protect subjects from undue risk or injury.

✓ The researcher conducting a study is required to inform everyone assisting in the study, as by collecting information, about the purposes of the study and to prepare them for any untoward effects the subjects could experience.

✓ Research reports are most commonly found in specialized journals.

✓ A number of indexes are available in the health care field for finding research journal articles.

✓ When summarizing data reported in a particular research study, the nurse should note when, how, where, and by whom the investigation was conducted, who was studied, and what was studied.

✓ A researchable clinical nursing problem is one that is not satisfactorily resolved by present nursing interventions, that occurs frequently in a particular client group, that can be consistently and accurately measured, and that has a possible solution within the realm of nursing practice.

✓ To determine whether research findings can be used as a basis for nursing practice, the nurse should consider the scientific worth of the study, the substantiating evidence provided in other studies, the similarity of the research setting to the nurse's own clinical practice setting, the status of current nursing theory, and factors affecting the feasibility of application.

REFERENCES

American Nurses' Association: Human rights guidelines for nurses in clinical and other research, Kansas City, Mo., 1975, The Association.

American Psychological Association: Publication manual of the American Psychological Association, ed. 3, Washington, D.C., 1983, The Association.

Armiger, B.: Ethics of nursing research: profile, principles, perspective, Nurs. Res. 26:330, 1977.

Bergstrom, N., et al.: Collaborative nursing research: anatomy of a successful consortium, Nurs. Res. 33:20, 1984.

Brink, P.J., and Wood, M.J.: Basic steps in planning nursing research: from question to proposal, ed. 2, North Scituate, Mass., 1983, Duxbury Press.

Cabinet on Nursing Research, American Nurses' Association: Establishment of a National Institute of Nursing: statement of rationale (Mimeographed), Kansas City, Mo., 1983, The Association.

Commission on Nursing Research, American Nurses' Association: Guidelines for the investigative function of nurses, Kansas City, Mo., 1981, The Association.

Diers, D.: Research in nursing practice, Philadelphia, 1979, J.B. Lippincott Co.

Fuller, E.D.: Selecting a clinical nursing problem, Image 14:60, 1982.

Gortner, S.R.: Nursing research: out of the past and into the future, Nurs. Res. 29:204, 1980.

Hansen, B.W.: Personal communication, February 14, 1984.

Hanson, R.L.: Predictive criteria for length of nasogastric tube insertion for tube feeding, J. Parenter. Enter. Nutr. 3:160, 1979.

Hanson, R.L.: New approach to measuring adult nasogastric tubes for insertion, Am. J. Nurs. 80:1334, 1980.

Heitkemper, M.E., et al.: Rate and volume of intermittent enteral feeding, J. Parenter. Enter. Nutr. 5:125, 1981.

Institute of Medicine, Division of Health Care Services: Nursing and nursing education: public policies and private actions, Washington, D.C., 1983, National Academic Press.

Kagawa-Busby, K.S., et al.: Effects of diet temperature on tolerance of enteral feedings, Nurs. Res. 29:276, 1980.

Kerlinger, F.N.: Foundations of behavioral research, ed. 2, New York, 1973, Holt, Rinehart & Winston.

Padilla, G.V., et al.: Subjective distresses of nasogastric tube feeding, J. Parenter. Enter. Nutr. 3:53, 1979.

Padilla, G.V., et al.: Distress reduction and the effects of preparatory teaching films and patient control, Res. Nurs. Health 4:375, 1981.

Polit, D.V., and Hungler, B.P.: Nursing research: principles and practice, ed. 2, Philadelphia, 1983, J.B. Lippincott Co.

Schmidt, F.E., and Wooldridge, P.J.: Psychological preparation of surgical patients, Nurs. Res. 22:108, 1973.

Seaman, C.H., and Verhonick, P.J.: Research methods for undergraduate students in nursing, ed. 2, Norwalk, Conn., 1982, Appleton-Century-Crofts.

Stetler, C.B., and Marram, G.: Evaluating research findings for applicability in practice, Nurs. Outlook 24:559, 1976.

Walike, B.C., and Walike, J.W.: Relative lactose intolerance: a clinical study of tube-fed patients, J.A.M.A. 238:948, 1977.

Walike, B.C., et al.: Patient problems related to tube feeding. In Batey, M.V., editor: Communicating nursing research, vol. 7, Boulder, Colo., 1974, Western Interstate Commission for Higher Education.

Werley, H.H., and Fitzpatrick, J.: Annual review of nursing research, vol. 1, New York, 1983, Springer Publishing Co.

Wolfer, J.A., and Davis, C.E.: Assessment of surgical patients' preoperative emotional condition and postoperative welfare, 19:402, 1970.

ADDITIONAL READINGS

Binger, J.L., and Jensen, L.M.: Lippincott's guide to nursing literature: a handbook for students, writers, and researchers, Philadelphia, 1980, J.B. Lippincott Co.

Commission on Nursing Research, American Nurses' Association: Research priorities for the 1980's, generating a scientific basis for nursing practice, Kansas City, Mo., 1981, The Association.

Fox, D.A.: Fundamentals of research in nursing, Norwalk, Conn., 1983, Appleton-Century-Crofts.

Horsley, J.A., Crane, J., and Haller, K.B.: Reducing diarrhea in tube-fed patients, CURN project, New York, 1981, Grune & Stratton, Inc.

Trussell, P., Brandt, A., and Knapp, S.: Using nursing research: discovery, analysis and interpretation, Wakefield, Mass., 1981, Nursing Resources.

Appendixes

Professional Nursing Organizations in the United States and Canada

NURSING ASSOCIATIONS IN THE UNITED STATES

National Organizations

Alpha Tau Delta National Fraternity
for Professional Nurses
489 Serento Circle
Thousand Oaks, California 91360

American Association of Colleges of
Nursing
Suite 430
11 DuPont Circle
Washington, D.C. 20036

American Hospital Association
Division of Nursing
840 N. Lake Shore Drive
Chicago, Illinois 60611

American Indian/Alaska Native
Nurses Association, Inc.
P.O. Box 1588
Norman, Oklahoma 73070

American Nurses' Association
2420 Pershing Road
Kansas City, Missouri 64108

Committee on Nursing of the
Catholic Hospital Association
1438 S. Grand Boulevard
St. Louis, Missouri 63104

Gay Nurses' Alliance
P.O. Box 115
Brownsville, Texas 78520

Lutheran Hospital Association of
America
Room 607 W
840 N. Lake Shore Drive
Chicago, Illinois 60611

National Black Nurses Association,
Inc.
425 Ohio Building
175 S. Main Street
Akron, Ohio 44308

National Center for Nursing Ethics
P.O. Box 2237
Cincinnati, Ohio 45201

National League for Nursing
10 Columbus Circle
New York, New York 10019

National Male Nurses' Association
2308 State Street
Saginaw, Michigan 48602

National Nurses for Life
1998 Menold
Allison Park, Pennsylvania 15101

National Student Nurses' Association,
Inc.
10 Columbus Circle
New York, New York 10019

Nurses Christian Fellowship
233 Langdon Street
Madison, Wisconsin 53703

Nurses Educational Funds
10 Columbus Circle
New York, New York 10019

Sigma Theta Tau
National Honor Society of Nursing
1100 West Michigan Street
Indianapolis, Indiana 46202

Specialty Associations

American Association for Respiratory
Therapy
1720 Regal Row
Dallas, Texas 75235

American Association of Critical Care
Nurses
P.O. Box C-19528
Irvine, California 92664

American Association of Nephrology
Nurses and Technicians
Suite 219
505 N. Tustin
Santa Ana, California 92705

American Association of
Neurosurgical Nurses
Suite 1519
625 North Michigan Avenue
Chicago, Illinois 60611

American Association of Nurse
Anesthetists
Suite 929
111 East Wacker Drive
Chicago, Illinois 60601

American Association of
Occupational Health Nurses, Inc.
575 Lexington Avenue
New York, New York 10022

American Board of Urologic Allied
Health Professionals
Suite 256
2222 N.W. Lovejoy
Portland, Oregon 97210

American Burn Association
c/o Dr. Charles E. Hartford
Burn Treatment Center
Crozier-Chester Medical Center
15th and Upland Avenue
Chester, Pennsylvania 19013

American College of Nurse
Mid-Wives
Suite 1120
1522 K Street N.W.
Washington, D.C. 20005

American Geriatric Society
Room 1470
10 Columbus Circle
New York, New York 10019

Association for Practitioners in
Infection Control
c/o Katherine R. Holl
557 N. Pinecrest
Wichita, Kansas 67208

Association of Operating Room
Nurses
10170 E. Mississippi Avenue
Denver, Colorado 80231

Association of Pediatric Oncology
Nurses
c/o Lorraine Bivalec
Pacific Medical Center
P.O. Box 7999
San Francisco, California 94120

Association of Rehabilitation Nurses
2506 Gross Point Road
Evanston, Illinois 60201

Emergency Department Nurses'
Association
Suite 1729
666 N. Lake Shore Drive
Chicago, Illinois 60611

International Association for
Enterostomal Therapy
1701 Lake Avenue
Glenview, Illinois 60025

National Association of Orthopaedic
Nurses
Scottish Rite Hospital
1001 Johnson Ferry Road, N.E.
Atlanta, Georgia 30342

National Association of Pediatric
Nurse Associates and Practitioners
North Woodbury Road, Box 56
Pitman, New Jersey 08071

Nurses Association of the American
College of Obstetricians and
Gynecologists
Suite 2700
1 East Wacker Drive
Chicago, Illinois 60601

Oncology Nursing Society
c/o Donna Liberto
P.O. Box 33
Oakmont, Pennsylvania 15129

CANADIAN ASSOCIATIONS

Canadian Association of Enterostomal
Therapy
Royal Jubilee Hospital
Victoria, British Columbia V8R 1J8

Canadian Association of Neurological
and Neurosurgical Nurses
296 Palace Road
Kingston, Ontario
K7L 4T3

Canadian Association of Practical and
Nursing Assistants
R.R. No. 4
St. Stephen, New Brunswick
E3L 2Y2

Canadian Association of University
Schools of Nursing
1200-151 Slater
Ottawa, Ontario
K1P 5N1

Canadian Council of Cardiovascular
Nurses
1200-1 Nicholas Street
Ottawa, Ontario
K1N 7B7

Canadian Hospital Infection Control
Association
McMaster University
Medical Centre
1200 Main Street W.
Hamilton, Ontario
L8S 4J9

Canadian Nurses' Association
50 The Driveway
Ottawa, Ontario
K2P 1E2

Canadian Nurses Foundation
50 The Driveway
Ottawa, Ontario
K2P 1E2

Canadian Nurses Respiratory Society
Nurses Section
Canadian Lung Association
908-75 Albert Street
Ottawa, Ontario
K1P 5E7

Canadian Orthopedic Nurses
Association
43 Wellesley Street E.
Toronto, Ontario
M4Y 1H1

Canadian University Nursing Students
1468 Summer Street
Halifax, Nova Scotia
B3H 3A3

National Conference of Operating
Room Nurses
c/o Operating Room
St. Boniface General Hospital
Winnipeg, Manitoba
R2H 2A6

Nursing Sisters Association of Canada
8500 Francis Road
Richmond, British Columbia
V6Y 1A6

Psychiatric Nurses Association of
Canada
1854 Portage Avenue
Winnipeg, Manitoba
R3J 0G9

Registered Nurses of Canadian Indian
Ancestry
500-275 Portage Avenue
Winnipeg, Manitoba
R3B 2B3

APPENDIX B
Normal Reference Laboratory Values

Blood, Plasma, or Serum Values

Determination	Reference Range	
	Conventional	SI
Acetoacetate plus acetone	0.3-2.0 mg/100 ml	3-20 mg/l
Aldolase	1.3-8.2 mU/ml	12-75 nmol · s^{-1}/l
Alpha amino nitrogen	3.0-5.5 mg/100 ml	2.1-3.9 mmol/l
Ammonia	80-110 µg/100 ml	47-65 µmol/l
Ascorbic acid	0.4-1.5 mg/100 ml	23-85 µmol/l
Barbiturate	0	0 µmol/l
	Coma level: phenobarbital, approximately 10 mg/100 ml; most other drugs, 1-3 mg/100 ml	
Bilirubin (van den Bergh test)	One minute: 0.4 mg/100 ml	Up to 7 µmol/l
	Direct: 0.4 mg/100 ml	Up to 17 µmol/l
	Total: 1.0 mg/100 ml	
	Indirect is total minus direct	
Blood volume	8.5-9.0% of body weight in kg	80-85 ml/kg
Bromide	0	0 mmol/l
	Toxic level: 17 mEq/l	
Bromsulfalein (BSP)	Less than 5% retention 45 min after 5 mg/kg IV	<0.051
Calcium	8.5-10.5 mg/100 ml (slightly higher in children)	2.1-2.6 mmol/l
Carbon dioxide content	24-30 mEq/l	24-30 mmol/l
	20-26 mEq/l in infants (as HCO_3^-)	
Carbon monoxide	Symptoms with over 20% saturation	0(1)
Carotenoids	0.8-4.0 µg/ml	1.5-7.4 µmol/l
Ceruloplasmin	27-37 mg/100 ml	1.8-2.5 µmol/l
Chloride	100-106 mEq/l	100-106 mmol/l
Cholinesterase (pseudocholinesterase)	0.5 pH U or more/h	0.5 or more arb. unit
	0.7 pH U or more/h for packed cells	
Copper	Total: 100-200 µg/100 ml	16-31 µmol/l
Creatine phosphokinase (CPK)	Female 5-35 mU/ml	0.08-0.58 µmol · s^{-1}/l
	Male 5-55 mU/ml	
Creatinine	0.6-1.5 mg/100 ml	60-130 µmol/l
Ethanol	0.3-0.4%, marked intoxication; 0.4-0.5%, alcoholic stupor; 0.5% or over, alcoholic coma	65-87 mmol/l 87-109 mmol/l >109 mmol/l
Glucose	Fasting: 70-110 mg/100 ml	3.9-5.6 mmol/l
Iron	50-150 µg/100 ml (higher in males)	9.0-26.9 µmol/l
Iron-binding capacity	250-410 µg/100 ml	44.8-73.4 µmol/l
Lactic acid	0.6-1.8 mEq/l	0.6-1.8 mmol/l
Lactic dehydrogenase	60-120 U/ml	1.00-2.00 µmol · s^{-1}/l
Lead	50 µg/100 ml or less	Up to 2.4 µmol/l
Lipase	2 U/ml or less	Up to 2 arb. unit
Lipids		
Cholesterol	120-220 mg/100 ml	3.10-5.69 mmol/l
Cholesterol esters	60-75% of cholesterol	

Modified from Kaye, D.A., and Rose, L.F.: Fundamentals of internal medicine, St. Louis, 1983, The C.V. Mosby Co. Adapted by permission from the New England Journal of Medicine, Vol. 302, pages 37-48, 1980.
Abbreviations used: SI, Système international d'Unités (The SI for the Health Professions. World Health Organization, Office of Publications, Geneva, Switzerland, 1977); d, 24 hours; P, plasma; S, serum; B, blood; U, urine; l, liter; h, hour; and s, second.

Blood, Plasma, or Serum Values, cont'd

Determination	Reference Range	
	Conventional	SI
Phospholipids	9-16 mg/100 ml as lipid phosphorus	2.9-5.2 mmol/l
Total fatty acids	190-420 mg/100 ml	1.9-4.2 g/l
Total lipids	450-1000 mg/100 ml	4.5-10.0 g/l
Triglycerides	40-150 mg/100 ml	0.4-1.5 g/l
Lithium	Toxic level 2 mEq/l	2 mmol/l
Magnesium	1.5-2.0 mEq/l	0.8-1.3 mmol/l
5'Nucleotidase	0.3-3.2 Bodansky U	30-290 nmol · s^{-1}/l
Osmolality	285-295 mOsm/kg water	285-295 mmol/kg
Oxygen saturation (arterial)	96-100%	0.96-1.00 l
P$_{CO_2}$	35-43 mm Hg	4.7-6.0 kPa
pH	7.35-7.45	Same
P$_{O_2}$	75-100 mm Hg (dependent on age) while breathing room air	
	Above 500 mm Hg while on 100% O_2	10.0-13.3 kPa
Phenylalanine	0-2 mg/100 ml	0-120 μmol/l
Phenytoin (Dilantin)	Therapeutic level, 5-20 μg/ml	19.8-79.5 μmol/l
Phosphorus (inorganic)	3.0-4.5 mg/100 ml (infants in 1st yr up to 6.0 mg/100 ml)	1.0-1.5 mmol/l
Potassium	3.5-5.0 mEq/l	3.5-5.0 mmol/l
Primidone (Mysoline)	Therapeutic level 4-12 μg/ml	18-55 μmol/l
Protein: Total	6.0-8.4 g/100 ml	60-84 g/l
Albumin	3.5-5.0 g/100 ml	35-50 g/l
Globulin	2.3-3.5 g/100 ml	23-35 g/l
Electrophoresis	% of total protein	Of total protein
Albumin	52-68	0.52-0.68
Globulin:		
Alpha$_1$	4.2-7.2	0.042-0.072
Alpha$_2$	6.8-12	0.068-0.12
Beta	9.3-15	0.093-0.15
Gamma	13-23	0.13-0.23
Pyruvic acid	0-0.11 mEq/l	0-0.11 mmol/l
Quinidine	Therapeutic: 1.5-3 μg/ml	4.6-9.2 μmol/l
	Toxic: 5-6 μg/ml	15.4-18.5 μmol/l
Salicylate:	0	
Therapeutic	20-25 mg/100 ml; 25-30 mg/100 ml to age 10 yr 3 h post dose	1.4-1.8 mmol/l 1.8-2.2 mmol/l
Toxic	Over 30 mg/100 ml	Over 2.2 mmol/l
	Over 20 mg/100 ml after age 60	Over 1.4 mmol/l
Sodium	135-145 mEq/l	135-145 mmol/l
Sulfate	0.5-1.5 mg/100 ml	0.05-1.2 mmol/l
Sulfonamide	0 mg/100 ml	0 mmol/l
	Therapeutic: 5-15 mg/100 ml	
Transaminase (SGOT) (aspartate amino-transferase)	10-40 U/ml	0.08-0.32 μmol · s^{-1}/l
Urea nitrogen (BUN)	8-25 mg/100 ml	2.9-8.9 mmol/l
Uric acid	3.0-7.0 mg/100 ml	0.18-0.42 mmol/l
Vitamin A	0.15-0.6 μg/ml	0.5-2.1 μmol/l
Vitamin A tolerance test	Rise to twice fasting level in 3 to 5 h	

Urine Values

Determination	Reference Range	
	Conventional	**SI**
Acetone plus acetoacetate (quantitative)	0	0 mg/l
Alpha amino nitrogen	64-199 mg/d; not over 1.5% of total nitrogen	4.6-14.2 mmol/d
Amylase	24-76 U/ml	24-76 arb. unit
Calcium	150 mg/d or less	3.8 or less mmol/d
Catecholamines	Epinephrine: under 20 μg/d	<55 nmol/d
	Norepinephrine: under 100 μg/d	<590 nmol/d
Copper	0-100 μg/d	0-1.6 μmol/d
Coproporphyrin	50-250 μg/d	80-380 nmol/d
	Children under 80 lb 0-75 μg/d	0-115 nmol/d
Creatine	Under 100 mg/d or less than 6% of creatinine. In pregnancy: up to 12%. In children under 1 yr: may equal creatinine. In older children: up to 30% of creatinine	<0.75 mmol/d
Cystine or cysteine	0	0
Follicle-stimulating hormone:		
Follicular phase	5-20 IU/d	Same
Midcycle	15-60 IU/d	
Luteal phase	5-15 IU/d	
Menopausal	50-100 IU/d	
Men	5-25 IU/d	
Hemoglobin and myoglobin	0	
5-Hydroxyindole acetic acid	2-9 mg/d (women lower than men)	10-45 μmol/d
Lead	0.08 μg/ml or 120 μg or less/d	0.39 μmol/l or less
Phenolsulfonphthalein (PSP)	At least 25% excreted by 15 min; 40% by 30 min; 60% by 120 min	0.25 l
Phosphorus (inorganic)	Varies with intake; average 1 g/d	32 mmol/d
Porphobilinogen	0	0
Protein:		
Quantitative	<150 mg/d	<0.15 g/d
Steroids		

Steroids

	Age (yr)	Male (mg)	Female (mg)	Male (μmol/d)	Female (μmol/d)
17-Ketosteroids (per day)	10	1-4	1-4	3-14	3-14
	20	6-21	4-16	21-73	14-56
	30	8-26	4-14	28-90	14-49
	50	5-18	3-9	17-62	10-31
	70	2-10	1-7	7-35	3-24

Determination	Conventional	SI
17-Hydroxysteroids	3-8 mg/d (women lower than men)	8-22 μmol/d as hydrocortisone
Sugar:		
Quantitative glucose	0	0 mmol/l
Identification of reducing substances		
Fructose	0	0 mmol/l
Pentose	0	0 mmol/l
Titratable acidity	24-40 mEq/d	20-40 mmol/d
Urobilinogen	Up to 1.0 Ehrlich U	To 1.0 arb. unit
Uroporphyrin	0	0 nmol/d
Vanillylmandelic acid (VMA)	Up to 9 mg/d	Up to 45 μmol/d

Special Endocrine Tests

Determination	Reference Range Conventional	SI
STEROID HORMONES		
Aldosterone	Excretion: 5-19 µg/d	14-53 nmol/d
Fasting, at rest, 210 mEq sodium diet	Supine: 48 ± 29 pg/ml	180 ± 64 pmol/l
	Upright: (2 h) 65 ± 23 pg/ml	
Fasting, at rest, 110 mEq sodium diet	Supine: 107 ± 45 pg/ml	279 ± 125 pmol/l
	Upright: (2 h) 239 ± 123 pg/ml	663 ± 341 pmol/l
Fasting, at rest, 10 mEq sodium diet	Supine: 175 ± 75 pg/ml	485 ± 208 pmol/l
	Upright: (2 h) 532 ± 228 pg/ml	1476 ± 632 pmol/l
Cortisol		
Fasting	8 AM: 5-25 µg/100 ml	0.14-0.69 µmol/l
At rest	8 PM: Below 10 µg/100 ml	0-0.28 µmol/l
20 U ACTH	4 h ACTH test: 30-45 µg/100 ml	0.83-1.24 µmol/l
Dexamethasone at midnight	Overnight suppression test: Below 5 µg/100 ml	<0.14 nmol/l
	Excretion: 20-70 µg/d	
		55-193 nmol/d
11-Deoxycortisol	Responsive; over 7.5 µg/100 ml (after metyrapone)	>0.22 µmol/l
Testosterone	Adult male: 300-1100 ng/100 ml	10.4-38.1 nmol/l
	Adolescent male: over 100 ng/100 ml	>3.5 nmol/l
	Female: 25-90 ng/100 ml	0.87-3.12 nmol/l
Unbound testosterone	Adult male: 3.06-24.0 ng/100 ml	106-832 pmol/l
	Adult female: 0.09-1.28 ng/100 ml	3.1-44.4 pmol/l
POLYPEPTIDE HORMONES		
Adrenocorticotropin (ACTH)	15-70 pg/ml	3.3-15.4 pmol/l
Calcitonin	Undetectable in normals	0
	>100 pg/ml in medullary carcinoma	>29.3 pmol/l
Growth hormone		
Fasting, at rest	Below 5 ng/ml	<233 pmol/l
After exercise	Child: Over 10 ng/ml	>465 pmol/l
	Male: Below 5 ng/ml	<233 pmol/l
	Female: Up to 30 ng/ml	0-1395 pmol/l
After glucose	Male: Below 5 ng/ml	<233 pmol/l
	Female: Below 10 ng/ml	0-465 pmol/l
Insulin		
Fasting	6-26 µU/ml	43-187 pmol/l
During hypoglycemia	Below 20 µU/ml	<144 pmol/l
After glucose	Up to 150 µU/ml	0-1078 pmol/l
Leuteinizing hormone	Male: 6-18 mU/ml	6-18 u/l
Pre- or postovulatory	Female: 5-22 mU/ml	5-22 u/l
Midcycle peak	30-250 mU/ml	30-250 u/l
Parathyroid hormone	<10 µl equiv/ml	<10 ml equiv/l
Prolactin	2-15 ng/ml	0.08-6.0 nmol/l
Renin activity		
Normal diet	Supine: 1.1 ± 0.8 ng/ml/h	0.9 ± 0.6 (nmol/l)h
	Upright: 1.9 ± 1.7 ng/ml/h	1.5 ± 1.3 (nmol/l)h
Low-sodium diet	Supine: 2.7 ± 1.8 ng/ml/h	2.1 ± 1.4 (nmol/l)h
	Upright: 6.6 ± 2.5 ng/ml/h	5.1 ± 1.9 (nmol/l)h
Low-sodium diet	Diuretics: 10.0 ± 3.7 ng/ml/h	7.7 ± 2.9 (nmol/l)h

Determination	Reference Range Conventional	SI
THYROID HORMONES		
Thyroid-stimulating hormone (TSH)	0.5-3.5 µU/ml	0.5-3.5 mU/l
Thyroxine-binding globulin capacity	15-25 µg T_4/100 ml	193-322 nmol/l
Total triiodothyronine by radioimmunoassay (T_3)	70-190 ng/100 ml	1.08-2.92 nmol/l
Total thyroxine by RIA (T_4)	4-12 µg/100 ml	52-154 nmol/l
T_3 resin uptake	25-35%	0.25-0.35
Free thyroxine index (FT_4I)	1-4 ng/100 ml	12.8-51.2 pmol/l

Cerebrospinal Fluid Values

Determination	Reference Range Conventional	SI	Determination	Reference Range Conventional	SI
Bilirubin	0	0 µmol/l	Glucose	50-75 mg/100 ml	2.8-4.2 mmol/l
Chloride	120-130 mEq/l (20 mEq/l higher than serum)			(30-50% less than blood)	
			Pressure (initial)	70-180 mm of water	70-80 arb. units
Albumin	Mean: 29.5 mg/100 ml	0.295 g/l	Protein:		
	±2 SD: 11-48 mg/100 ml	±2 SD: 0.11-0.48	Lumbar	15-45 mg/100 ml	0.15-0.45 g/l
IgG	Mean: 4.3 mg/100 ml	0.043 g/l	Cisternal	15-25 mg/100 ml	0.15-0.25 g/l
	±2 SD: 0-8.6 mg/100 ml	±2 SD: 0-0.086	Ventricular	5-15 mg/100 ml	0.05-0.15 g/l

Hematologic Values

Determination	Reference Range Conventional	SI
Coagulation factors:		
Factor I (fibrinogen)	0.15-0.35 g/100 ml	4.0-10.0 μmol/l
Factor II (prothrombin)	60-140%	0.60-1.40
Factor V (accelerator globulin)	60-140%	0.60-1.40
Factor VII-X (proconvertin-Stuart)	70-130%	0.70-1.30
Factor X (Stuart factor)	70-130%	0.70-1.30
Factor VIII (antihemophilic globulin)	50-200%	0.50-2.0
Factor IX (plasma thromboplastic cofactor)	60-140%	0.60-1.40
Factor XI (plasma thromboplastic antecedent)	60-140%	0.60-1.40
Factor XII (Hageman factor)	60-140%	0.60-1.40
Coagulation screening tests:		
Bleeding time (Simplate)	3-9 min	180-540 s
Prothrombin time	Less than 2-s deviation from control	Less than 2-s deviation from control
Partial thromboplastin time (activated)	25-37 s	25-37 s
Whole-blood clot lysis	No clot lysis in 24 h	0/d
Fibrinolytic studies:		
Euglobin lysis	No lysis in 2 h	0 (in 2 h)
Fibrinogen split products	Negative reaction at greater than 1:4 dilution	0 (at >1:4 dilution)
Thrombin time	Control ± 5 s	Control ± 5 s
"Complete" blood count:		
Hematocrit	Male: 45-52%	Male: 0.42-0.52
	Female: 37-48%	Female: 0.37-0.48
Hemoglobin	Male: 13-18 g/100 ml	Male 8.1-11.2 mmol/l
	Female: 12-16 g/100 ml	Female: 7.4-9.9 mmol/l
Leukocyte count	4300-10,800/mm^3	4.3-10.8 × 10^9/l
Erythrocyte count	4.2-5.9 million/mm^3	4.2-5.9 × 10^{12}/l
Mean corpuscular volume (MCV)	80-94 μm^3	80-94 fl
Mean corpuscular hemoglobin (MCH)	27-32 pg	1.7-2.0 fmol
Mean corpuscular hemoglobin concentration (MCHC)	32-36%	19-22.8 mmol/l
Erythrocyte sedimentation rate (Westergren method)	Male: 1-13 mm/h	Male: 1-13 mm/h
	Female: 1-20 mm/h	Female: 1-20 mm/h
Erythrocyte enzymes:		
Glucose-6-phosphate dehydrogenase	5-15 U/gHb	5-15 U/g
Pyruvate kinase	13-17 U/gHb	13-17 U/g
Ferritin (serum)		
Iron deficiency	0-20 ng/ml	0-20 μg/l
Iron excess	Greater than 400 ng/l	>400 μg/l
Folic acid		
Normal	Greater than 1.9 ng/ml	>4.3 mmol/l
Borderline	1.0-1.9 ng/ml	2.3-4.3 mmol/l
Haptoglobin	100-300 mg/100 ml	1.0-3.0 g/l
Hemoglobin studies:		
Electrophoresis for A$_2$ hemoglobin	1.5-3.5%	0.015-0.035
Hemoglobin F (fetal hemoglobin)	Less than 2%	<0.02
Hemoglobin, met- and sulf-	0	0
Serum hemoglobin	2-3 mg/100 ml	1.2-1.9 μmol/l
Thermolabile hemoglobin	0	0

Determination	Reference Range	
	Conventional	SI
L.E. (lupus erythematosus) preparation:		
Heparin as anticoagulant	0	0
Defibrinated blood	0	0
Leukocyte alkaline phosphatase:		
Quantitative method	15-40 mg of phosphorus liberated/h/ 10^{10} cells	15-40 mg/h
Qualitative method	Males: 33-188 U	33-188 U
	Females (off contraceptive pill): 30-160 U	30-160 U
Muramidase	Serum, 3-7 µg/ml	3-7 mg/l
	Urine, 0-2 µg/ml	0-2 mg/l
Osmotic fragility of erythrocytes	Increased if hemolysis occurs in over 0.5% NaCl; decreased if hemolysis is incomplete in 0.3% of NaCl	
Peroxide hemolysis	Less than 10%	<0.10
Platelet count	150,000-350,000/mm^3	150-350 × 10^9/l
Platelet function tests:		
Clot retraction	50-100%/2 h	0.50-1.00/2 h
Platelet aggregation	Full response to ADP, epinephrine, and collagen	1.0
Platelet factor 3	33-57 s	33-57 s
Reticulocyte count	0.5-1.5% red cells	0.005-0.015
Vitamin B$_{12}$	90-280 pg/ml (borderline: 70-90)	66-207 pmol/l (borderline: 52-66)

Miscellaneous Values

Determination	Reference Range Conventional	SI
Autoantibodies in serum		
Thyroid colloid and microsomal antigens	Absent	
Stomach parietal cells	Absent	
Smooth muscle	Absent	
Kidney mitochondria	Absent	
Rabbit renal collecting ducts	Absent	
Cytoplasm of ova, theca cells, testicular interstitial cells	Absent	
Skeletal muscle	Absent	
Adrenal gland	Absent	
Carcinoembryonic antigen (CEA) in blood	0-2.5 ng/ml, 97% healthy nonsmokers	0-2.5 µg/l, 97% healthy nonsmokers
Cryoprecipitable proteins in blood	0	0 arb. unit
Digitoxin in serum	17 ± 6 ng/ml	22 ± 7.8 nmol/l
Digoxin in serum		
0.25 mg/d	1.2 ± 0.4 ng/ml	1.54 ± 0.5 nmol/l
0.5 mg/d	1.5 ± 0.4 ng/ml	1.92 ± 0.5 nmol/l
Duodenal drainage:		
pH	5.5-7.5	5.5-7.5
Amylase	Over 1200 U/total sample	>1.2 arb. unit
Trypsin	Values from 35 to 160% "normal"	0.35-1.60
Viscosity	3 min or less	180 s or less
Gastric analysis	Basal:	
	Females 2.0 ± 1.8 mEq/h	0.6 ± 0.5
	Males 3.0 ± 2.0 mEq/h	0.8 ± 0.6 µmol/s
	Maximal: (after histalog or gastrin)	
	Females 16 ± 5 mEq/h	4.4 ± 1.4 µmol/s
	Males 23 ± 5 mEq/h	6.4 ± 1.4 µmol/s
Gastrin-I in blood	0-200 pg/ml	0-95 pmol/l
Immunologic tests		
Alpha-feto-globulin	Abnormal if present	
Alpha 1-antitrypsin	200-400 mg/100 ml	2.0-4.0 g/l
Antinuclear antibodies	Positive if detected with serum diluted 1:10	
Anti-DNA antibodies	Less than 15 units/ml	
Complement, total hemolytic	150-250 U/ml	
C3	Range 55-120 mg/100 ml	0.55-1.2 g/l
C4	Range 20-50 mg/100 ml	0.2-0.5 g/l
Immunoglobulins in blood:		
IgG	1140 mg/100 ml	11.4 g/l
	Range 540-1663	5.5-16.6 g/l
IgA	214 mg/100 ml	2.14 g/l
	Range 66-344	0.66-3.44 g/l
IgM	168 mg/100 ml	1.68 g/l
	Range 39-290	0.39-2.9 g/l
Viscosity	1.4-1.8 expressed as relative viscosity of serum compared to water	
Iontophoresis	Children: 0-40 mEq sodium/l	0-40 mmol/l
	Adults: 0-60 mEq sodium/l	0-60 mmol/l
Propranolol (includes bioactive 4-OH metabolite) in serum 4h after last dose	100-300 ng/ml	386-1158 nmol/l

Determination	Reference Range	
	Conventional	**SI**
Stool fat	Less than 5 g in 24 h or less than 4% of measured fat intake in 3-d period	<5 g/d
Stool nitrogen	Less than 2 g/d or 10% of urinary nitrogen	<2 g/d
Synovial fluid:		
Glucose	Not less than 20 mg/100 ml lower than simultaneously drawn blood sugar	See blood glucose mmol/l
Mucin	Type 1 or 2 Grades as: Type 1-tight clump Type 2-soft clump Type 3-soft clump that breaks up Type 4-cloudy, no clump	1-2 arb. unit
D-Xylose absorption	5-8 g/5 h in urine 40 mg/100 ml in blood 2 h after ingestion of 25 g of D-xylose	33-53 mmol 2.7 mmol/l

Index